STOELTING'S

Pharmacology and Physiology in Anesthetic Practice

FIFTH EDITION

STOELTING'S

Pharmacology and Physiology in Anesthetic Practice

FIFTH EDITION

Pamela Flood, MD, MA

Professor of Anesthesiology, Perioperative and Pain Medicine
Stanford University
Palo Alto, California

James P. Rathmell, MD

Executive Vice Chair and Chief, Division of Pain Medicine
Department of Anesthesia, Critical Care and Pain Medicine
Massachusetts General Hospital
Henry Knowles Beecher Professor of Anaesthesia, Harvard Medical School
Boston, Massachusetts

Steven Shafer, MD

Professor of Anesthesiology, Perioperative and Pain Medicine
Stanford University
Palo Alto, California

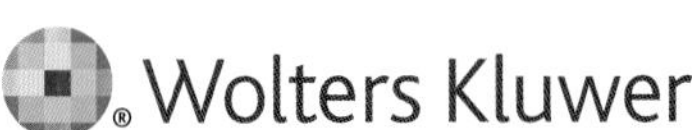

Philadelphia • Baltimore • New York • London
Buenos Aires • Hong Kong • Sydney • Tokyo

Acquisitions Editor: Brian Brown
Product Development Editor: Nicole Dernoski
Editorial Assistant: Lindsay Burgess
Senior Production Project Manager: Alicia Jackson
Design Coordinator: Stephen Druding
Illustration Coordinator: Jennifer Clements
Manufacturing Coordinator: Beth Welsh
Marketing Manager: Daniel Dressler
Prepress Vendor: Absolute Service, Inc.

Fifth Edition

9 8 7 6 5 4

Printed in China

Library of Congress Cataloging-in-Publication Data

Shafer, Steven L., author.
Stoelting's pharmacology and physiology in anesthetic practice / Steven Shafer, James P. Rathmell, Pamela Flood. — Fifth edition.
p. ; cm.
Pharmacology and physiology in anesthetic practice
Preceded by: Pharmacology & physiology in anesthetic practice / Robert K. Stoelting, Simon C. Hillier. 4th ed. c2006.
Includes bibliographical references and indexes.
ISBN 978-1-60547-550-9 (hardback)
I. Rathmell, James P., author. II. Flood, Pamela, 1963- , author. III. Title. IV. Title: Pharmacology and physiology in anesthetic practice.
[DNLM: 1. Anesthetics—pharmacology. 2. Physiological Phenomena. QV 81]
RD82.2
615.7'81—dc23

2014039745

LWW.com

CCS0119

CONTRIBUTORS

Nicholas Anast, MD
Cardiovascular Anesthesia Fellow
Stanford University
Palo Alto, California

Bihua Bie, MD, PhD
Postdoctoral Research Fellow
Anesthesiology Institute
Cleveland Clinic
Cleveland, Ohio

Mark Burbridge, MD
Clinical Instructor
Stanford University
Palo Alto, California

Kenneth Cummings III, MD, MS
Assistant Professor of Anesthesiology
Anesthesiology Institute
Cleveland Clinic
Cleveland, Ohio

Hesham Elsharkawy, MD, MSc
Assistant Professor of Anesthesiology
Cleveland Clinic Lerner College of Medicine
Staff
Department of Outcomes Research
Anesthesiology Institute
Cleveland Clinic
Cleveland, Ohio

Pamela Flood, MD, MA
Professor of Anesthesiology, Perioperative and Pain Medicine
Stanford University
Palo Alto, California

Sumeet Goswami, MD, MPH
Associate Professor of Anesthesiology
Columbia University Medical Center
New York, New York

David A. Grossblatt, MD
Postdoctoral Residency Fellow
Mayo Clinic
Phoenix, Arizona

Jonathan Hastie, MD
Assistant Professor of Anesthesiology
Department of Anesthesiology
Columbia University Medical Center
New York, New York

Maya Jalbout Hastie, MD
Assistant Professor of Anesthesiology
Department of Anesthesiology
Columbia University Medical Center
New York, New York

Bessie Kachulis, MD
Assistant Professor of Anesthesiology
Department of Anesthesiology
Columbia University Medical Center
New York, New York

Mihir M. Kamdar, MD
Instructor, Harvard Medical School
Associate Director, Palliative Care Service
Massachusetts General Hospital
Boston, Massachusetts

Joseph Kwok, MD
Clinical Instructor
Department of Anesthesiology and Pain Medicine
Stanford University School of Medicine
Stanford, California

Barrett Larson, MD
Resident in Anesthesiology
Department of Anesthesiology, Perioperative, and Pain Medicine
Stanford University School of Medicine
Stanford, California

Jerrold H. Levy, MD
Professor of Anesthesiology
Associate Professor of Surgery
Codirector
Cardiothoracic Intensive Care Unit
Duke University School of Medicine
Durham, North Carolina

Sansan S. Lo, MD
Assistant Professor of Anesthesiology
Division of Cardiothoracic Anesthesia
Columbia University
New York, New York

Kamal Maheshwari, MD
Staff Anesthesiologist
Regional Anesthesia and Acute Pain Management
Department of Outcomes Research
Cleveland Clinic
Cleveland, Ohio

Jillian A. Maloney, MD
Department of Anesthesiology
Mayo Clinic
Phoenix, Arizona

Steven Miller, MD
Assistant Professor
Department of Anesthesiology
Columbia University Medical Center
New York-Presbyterian Hospital
New York, New York

Vivek K. Moitra, MD
Associate Professor of Anesthesiology
Department of Anesthesiology
Division of Critical Care
Columbia University Medical Center
New York, New York

Teresa A. Mulaikal, MD
Assistant Professor of Anesthesiology
Columbia University Medical Center
Divisions of Cardiothoracic and Critical Care Medicine,
Department of Anesthesiology
Columbia University Medical Center
New York, New York

Michael J. Murray, MD, PhD
Consultant
Department of Anesthesiology
Mayo Clinic
Phoenix, Arizona
Professor of Anesthesiology
Mayo Medical School
Scottsdale, Arizona

Mohamed A. Naguib, MD, MSc, FFARCSI
Professor of Anesthesiology
Cleveland Clinic Lerner College of Medicine
Faculty
Department of General Anesthesiology
Cleveland Clinic
Cleveland, Ohio

Carter Peatross, MD
Cardiovascular and Thoracic Anesthesiology Fellow
Mayo Clinic
Rochester, Minnesota

James Ramsay, MD
Professor of Anesthesiology
Department of Anesthesia and Perioperative Care
University of California
San Francisco, California

James P. Rathmell, MD
Executive Vice Chair and Chief, Division of Pain Medicine
Department of Anesthesia, Critical Care and Pain Medicine
Massachusetts General Hospital
Henry Knowles Beecher Professor of Anaesthesia,
Harvard Medical School
Boston, Massachusetts

Carl E. Rosow, MD, PhD
Professor
Department of Anesthesia, Critical Care and Pain Medicine
Massachusetts General Hospital
Boston, Massachusetts

Steven Shafer, MD
Professor of Anesthesiology, Perioperative and Pain Medicine
Stanford University
Palo Alto, California

Jack S. Shanewise, MD, FASE
Professor of Anesthesiology
Columbia University Medical Center
New York, New York

Peter Slinger, MD, FRCPC
Professor of Anesthesiology
University of Toronto
Toronto, Canada

Sarah C. Smith, MD
Assistant Professor of Anesthesiology
Division of Cardiothoracic Anesthesiology
Department of Anesthesiology
Columbia University Medical Center
New York, New York

Jessica Spellman, MD
Assistant Professor of Anesthesiology
Department of Anesthesiology
Division of Adult Cardiothoracic Anesthesiology
Columbia University Medical Center
New York, New York

Robert K. Stoelting, MD
Emeritus Professor
Department of Anesthesia
Indiana University School of Medicine
Indianapolis, Indiana

Hui Yang, MD, PhD
Anesthesiology Institute
Cleveland Clinic
Cleveland, Ohio

FOREWORD

My journey with *Pharmacology and Physiology in Anesthetic Practice* began in the early 1980s with what seemed an impossible dream, a single-author anesthesia textbook devoted to the *daily application of principles of pharmacology and physiology in the care of patients*. Many yellow tablets later (my computer skills were in their infancy), an understanding family, residents and faculty in the Department of Anesthesia at Indiana University School of Medicine, and the unwavering support and encouragement of a special friend and publisher, the first edition of *Pharmacology and Physiology in Anesthetic Practice* appeared in the fall of 1986.

The acceptance of the textbook by students, trainees, and practitioners over the years has been incredibly rewarding to me personally and served as the stimulus to create revisions for the next three editions with Simon C. Hillier, MB, ChB joining me as a coeditor for the fourth edition that appeared in 2006.

It is clearly time for a new edition and a new approach if *Pharmacology and Physiology in Anesthetic Practice* is going to continue to meet its original goal of *providing an in-depth but concise and current presentation of those aspects of pharmacology and physiology that are relevant either directly or indirectly to the perioperative anesthetic management of patients*.

In this regard, I could not be more pleased and honored that Drs. James P. Rathmell, Steven Shafer, and Pamela Flood agreed to act as coeditors of a multiauthored fifth edition. Their unique expertise and access to recognized authorities in the wide and expanding areas of pharmacology and physiology that impact the perioperative care of patients is clearly evident in this fifth edition.

On behalf of myself and all our past (and future) readers, I thank the new coeditors and their authors for keeping *Stoelting's Pharmacology and Physiology in Anesthetic Practice* current with the times and fulfilling the dream I had more than 30 years ago.

Robert K. Stoelting, MD

PREFACE TO THE FIFTH EDITION

Robert Stoelting is among the best writers in our specialty. His signature textbook, *Pharmacology and Physiology in Anesthetic Practice*, resonated with residents and young faculty, including us, because it was exceptionally well written. Dr. Stoelting's clear prose succinctly covered the drugs we were using in our daily practice. His explanations of physiology were intuitive and sensible. Every chapter in the earlier editions spoke with the same voice, reflecting the many years he invested in a single-authored textbook. Even though Dr. Hillier joined him as coauthor of the fourth edition, the text always resonated as a single voice.

When first approached about revising the textbook, we turned down the project. It seemed impossible to reproduce the clarity of Dr. Stoelting's work. However, the option for the publisher was to transform *Pharmacology and Physiology in Anesthetic Practice* into a conventional multiauthored textbook. That felt like sacrilege, reducing one of the revered texts in our specialty to a "me too" multiauthored textbook. We agreed to take on the task.

It took a half decade longer than expected. Too much had changed in the 30 years since Dr. Stoelting produced his initial textbook to simply revise the chapters. The textbook required a complete reorganization. Every chapter was nearly completely rewritten.

The job was too much for one person or even three. We chose a hybrid model, in which a small number of authors oversaw major blocks. The final editing was done by two editors, Flood and Rathmell, to approximate the single voice that distinguished the first four editions.

We have to acknowledge the efforts of our publishers Brian Brown and Nicole Dernoski, who never gave up on us during the 7 years it took to produce this textbook. The final book reflects their dedication to Dr. Stoelting's textbook. They knew he had created a gem. They were determined to keep it polished.

We are proud to bring the fifth edition of Dr. Stoelting's textbook to anesthesiology residents, clinicians, and investigators. The name has been changed, forever, to reflect where this started. It is now *Stoelting's Pharmacology and Physiology in Anesthetic Practice*. Making no pretense of reproducing the elegant writing of Dr. Stoelting's original textbook, we have tried to capture the current state-of-the-art in anesthetic pharmacology and physiology.

Is everything in this book correct? No. The authors of each chapter have imperfect understanding; knowledge changes and mistakes happen. Wikipedia brilliantly addresses this by allowing readers who catch errors to fix them. We can't implement the Wikipedia approach in a textbook, but we can come close by inviting you, the reader compulsive enough to read the Preface, to bring any errors, corrections, or suggestions to our attention. The e-mail address is StoeltingSuggestions@gmail.com. We invite our readers to become "peer reviewers," pointing out errors, out-of-date references, drugs no longer used, or missing content relevant to pharmacology and physiology in anesthesia practice. In this manner, readers will become collaborators for all future editions.

This fifth edition is our tribute to the profound contribution to education and clinical practice made by Dr. Stoelting with his now eponymous textbook.

Pamela Flood, MD
James P. Rathmell, MD
Steven Shafer, MD

CONTENTS

CHAPTER 1

Basic Principles of Physiology

Pamela Flood • Steven Shafer

This chapter will review the basic principles of the composition of the body and the structure of cells. Although very basic, these principles are essential for everything that follows.

Body Composition

Water is the most abundant single constituent of the body and is the medium in which all metabolic reactions occur. Water accounts for about 60% of the weight in an adult man and about 50% of the body weight in an adult woman (Fig. 1-1)[1]; the difference is due to increased body fat in women. In a neonate, total body water may represent 70% of body weight. Total body water is less in obese individuals, reflecting the decreased water content of adipose tissue. Advanced age is also associated with increased fat content and decreased total body water (Table 1-1).

Body fluids can be divided into intracellular and extracellular fluid, depending on their location relative to the cell membrane (see Fig. 1-1).[1] Approximately two-thirds of the total body fluid in an adult are contained inside the estimated 100 trillion cells of the body. The fluid in these cells, despite individual differences in constituents, is collectively designated ***intracellular fluid***. The one-third of fluid outside the cells is referred to as ***extracellular fluid***. Extracellular fluid is divided into interstitial fluid and plasma (intravascular fluid) by the capillary membrane (see Fig. 1-1).[1]

Interstitial fluid is present in the spaces between cells. An estimated 99% of this fluid is held in the gel structure of the interstitial space. Plasma is the noncellular portion of blood. The average plasma volume is 3 L, a little over half of the blood volume of 5 L. Plasma is in dynamic equilibrium with the interstitial fluid through pores in the capillaries; the interstitial fluid serving as a reservoir from which water and electrolytes can be mobilized into the circulation. Loss of plasma volume from the intravascular space is minimized by colloid osmotic pressure exerted by the plasma proteins.

Other extracellular fluid that may be considered as part of the interstitial fluid includes cerebrospinal fluid, gastrointestinal fluid (because it is mostly resorbed), and fluid in potential spaces (pleural space, pericardial space, peritoneal cavity, synovial cavities). Excess amounts of fluid in the interstitial space manifest as peripheral edema.

The normal daily intake of water (drink and internal product of food metabolism) by an adult averages 2.5 L, of which about 1.5 L is excreted as urine, 100 mL is lost in sweat, and 100 mL is present in feces. All gases that are inhaled become saturated with water vapor (47 mm Hg at 37°C). This water vapor is subsequently exhaled, accounting for an average daily water loss through the lungs of 300 to 400 mL. The water content of inhaled gases decreases with decreases in ambient air temperature such that more endogenous water is required to achieve a saturated water vapor pressure at body temperature. As a result, insensible water loss from the lungs is greatest in cold environments and least in warm temperatures. The remaining 400 mL is lost by diffusion through the skin. This is insensible water loss, not perceived as sweat. Insensible water loss is limited by the mostly impermeable layer of the skin (cornified squamous epithelium). When the cornified layer is removed or interrupted, as after burn injury, the loss of water through the skin is greatly increased.

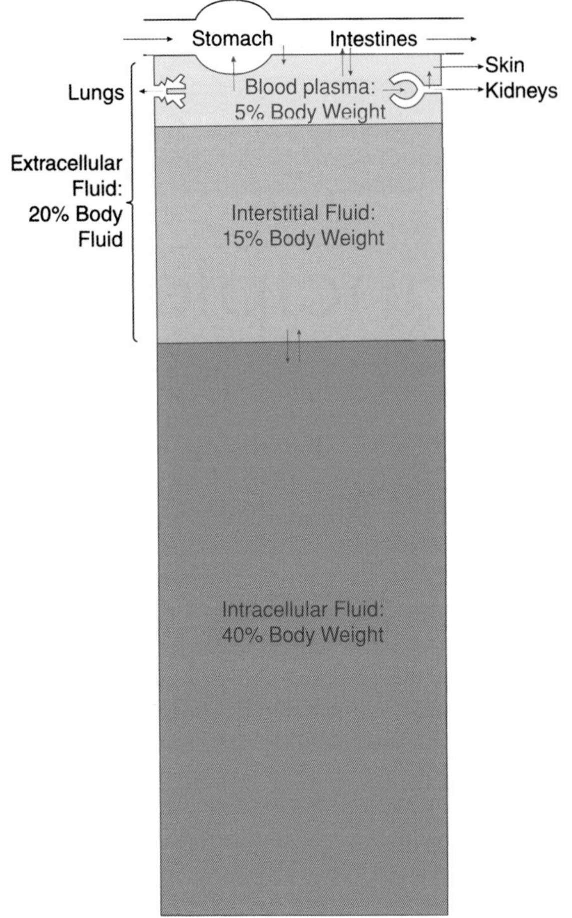

FIGURE 1-1 Body fluid compartments and the percentage of body weight represented by each compartment. The location relative to the capillary membrane divides extracellular fluid into plasma or interstitial fluid. *Arrows* represent fluid movement between compartments. (From Gamble JL. *Chemical Anatomy, Physiology, and Pathology of Extracellular Fluid.* 6th ed. Boston, MA: Harvard University Press; 1954, with permission.)

Blood Volume

Blood contains extracellular fluid, the plasma, and intracellular fluid, mostly held in erythrocytes. The body has multiple systems to maintain intravascular fluid volume, including renin-angiotensin system, and arginine vasopressin (antidiuretic hormone) that increase fluid reabsorption in the kidney and evoke changes in the renal tubules that lead to restoration of intravascular fluid volume (see Chapter 17).

The average blood volume of an adult is 5 L, comprising about 3 L of plasma and 2 L of erythrocytes. These volumes vary with age, weight, and gender. For example, in nonobese individuals, the blood volume varies in direct proportion to the body weight, averaging 70 mL/kg for lean men and women. The greater the ratio of fat to body weight, however, the less is the blood volume in milliliter per kilogram because adipose tissue has a decreased vascular supply. The hematocrit or packed cell volume is approximately the erythrocyte fraction of blood volume. The normal hematocrit is about 45% for men and postmenopausal women and about 38% for menstruating women, with a range of approximately ± 5%.

Table 1-1

Total Body Water by Age and Gender

	Total Body Water	
Age (yrs)	Men (%)	Women (%)
18–40	61	51
40–60	55	47
>60	52	46

Constituents of Body Fluid Compartments

The constituents of plasma, interstitial fluid, and intracellular fluid are identical, but the quantity of each substance varies among the compartments (Fig. 1-2).[2] The most striking differences are the low protein content in interstitial fluid compared with intracellular fluid and plasma and the fact that sodium and chloride ions are largely extracellular, whereas most of the potassium ions (approximately 90%) are intracellular. This unequal distribution of ions results in establishment of a potential (voltage) difference across cell membranes.

The constituents of extracellular fluid are carefully regulated by the kidneys so that cells are bathed in a fluid containing the proper concentrations of electrolytes and nutrients. The normal amount of sodium and potassium in the body is about 58 mEq/kg and 45mEq/kg, respectively (note that normal serum level of sodium is 137 to 142 mEq/L and potassium is 3.5 to 5.5 mEq/L, reflecting the intracellular and extracellular predominance of each electrolyte). Trauma is associated with progressive loss of potassium through the kidneys due in large part to the increased secretion of vasopressin and in variable part (depending on the type of surgery) to the role of nasogastric suctioning and direct potassium loss. For example, a patient undergoing surgery excretes about 100 mEq of potassium in the first 48 hours postoperatively and, after this period, about 25 mEq daily. Plasma potassium concentrations are not good indicators of total body potassium content because most potassium is intracellular. There is a correlation, however, between the potassium and hydrogen ion content of plasma; the two are increasing and decreasing together.

Osmosis

Osmosis is the movement of water (solvent molecules) across a semipermeable membrane from a compartment in which the nondiffusible solute (ion) concentration is

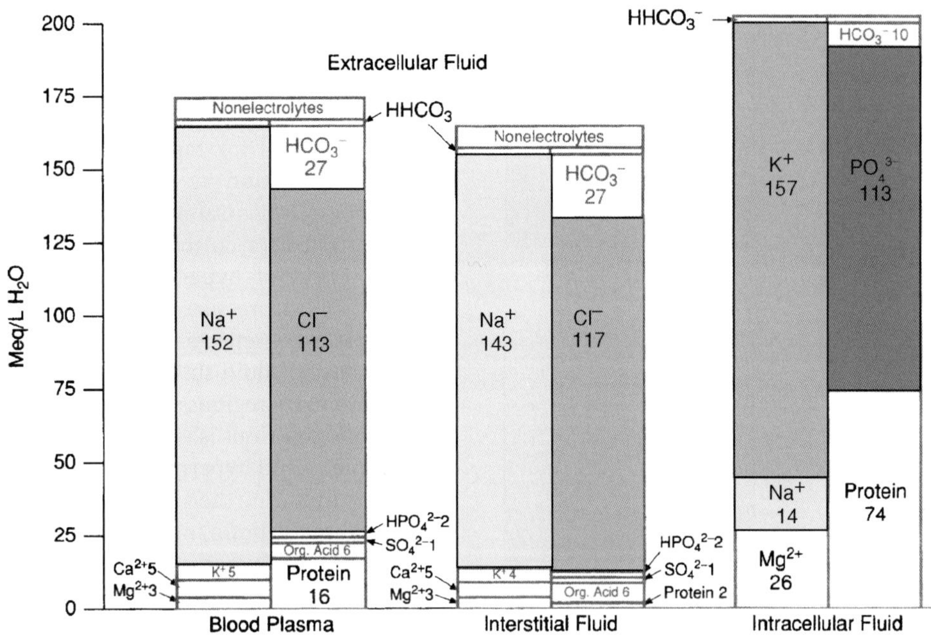

FIGURE 1-2 Electrolyte composition of body fluid compartments. (From Leaf A, Newburgh LH. *Significance of the Body Fluids in Chemical Medicine.* 2nd ed. Springfield, IL: Thomas; 1955, with permission.)

lower to a compartment in which the solute concentration is higher (Fig. 1-3).[3] The lipid bilayer that surrounds all cells is freely permeable to water but is impermeable to ions. As a result, water rapidly moves across the cell membrane to establish osmotic equilibration, which happens almost instantly.

Cells control their size by controlling intracellular osmotic pressure. The maintenance of a normal cell volume and pressure depends on sodium–potassium adenosine triphosphatase (ATPase) (sodium–potassium exchange pump), which maintains the intracellular–extracellular ionic balance by removing three sodium ions from the cell for every two potassium ions brought into the cell. The

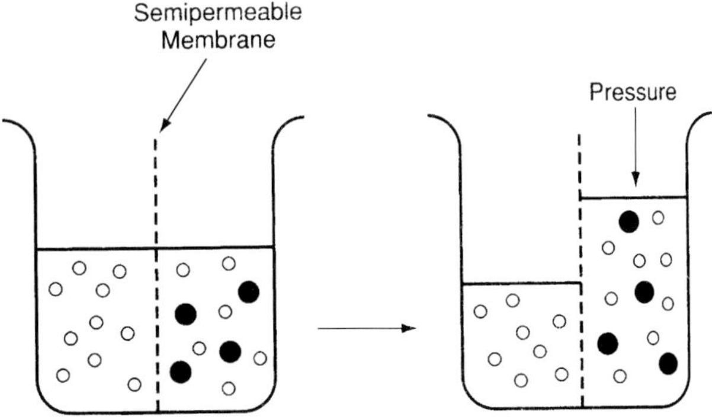

FIGURE 1-3 Diagrammatic representation of osmosis depicting water molecules *(open circles)* and solute molecules *(solid circles)* separated by a semipermeable membrane. Water molecules move across the semipermeable membrane to the area of higher concentration of solute molecules. Osmotic pressure is the pressure that would have to be applied to prevent continued movement of water molecules. (From Ganong WF. *Review of Medical Physiology.* 21st ed. New York, NY: Lange Medical Books/McGraw-Hill; 2003.)

sodium–potassium pump also maintains the transmembrane electrical potential and the sodium and potassium concentration gradients that power many cellular processes, including neural conduction.

The osmotic pressure exerted by nondiffusible particles in a solution is determined by the number of particles in the solution (degree of ionization) and not the type of particles (molecular weight) (see Fig. 1-3).[3] Thus a 1-mol solution of glucose or albumin and 0.5-mol solution of sodium chloride exert the same osmotic pressure, because the sodium chloride exists as independent sodium and chloride ions, each having a concentration of 0.5 mol. Osmole is the unit used to express osmotic pressure in solutes, but the denominator for osmolality is kilogram of *water*. ***Osmolarity*** is the correct terminology when osmole concentrations are expressed in liters of body fluid (e.g., plasma) rather than kilogram of water (***osmolality***). Because it is much easier to express body fluids in liters of fluid rather than kilograms of free water, almost all physiology calculations are based on osmolarity. Plasma osmolarity is important in evaluating dehydration, overhydration, and electrolyte abnormalities.

Normal plasma has an osmolarity of about 290 mOsm/L. All but about 20 mOsm of the 290 mOsm in each liter of plasma are contributed by sodium ions and their accompanying anions, principally chloride and bicarbonate. Proteins normally contribute <1 mOsm/L. The major nonelectrolytes of plasma are glucose and urea, and these substances can contribute significantly to plasma osmolarity when hyperglycemia or uremia is present, as suggested by the standard calculation of plasma osmolarity:

$$\text{Plasma osmolarity} = 2\,(\text{Na}^+) + 0.055\,(\text{glucose}) + 0.36\,(\text{blood urea nitrogen}).$$

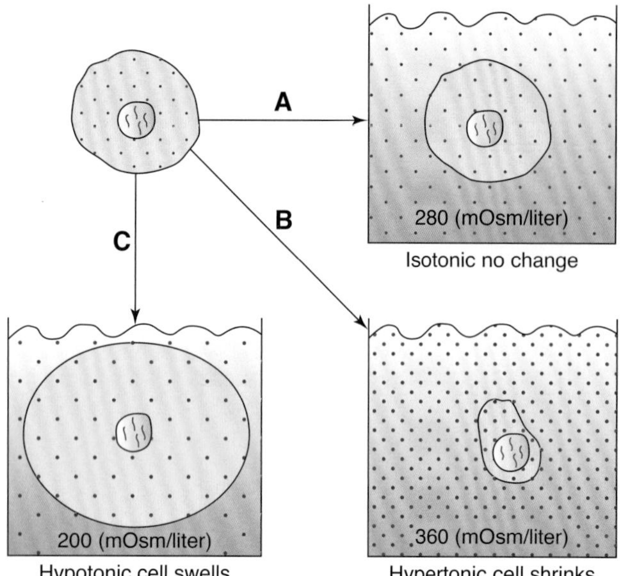

FIGURE 1-4 Effects of isotonic *(A)*, hypertonic *(B)*, and hypotonic *(C)* solutions on cell volume. (Modified from Guyton AC, Hall JE. *Textbook of Medical Physiology.* 10th ed. Philadelphia, PA: W.B. Saunders; 2000.)

Tonicity of Fluids

Packed erythrocytes must be suspended in ***isotonic*** solutions to avoid damaging the cells (e.g., Fig. 1-4).[4] A 0.9% solution of sodium chloride is isotonic and remains so because there is no net movement of the osmotically active particles in the solution into cells, and the particles are not metabolized. A solution of 5% glucose in water is initially isotonic when infused, but glucose is metabolized, so the net effect is that of infusing a hypotonic solution. Lactated Ringer solution plus 5% glucose is initially hypertonic (about 560 mOsm/L), but as glucose is metabolized, the solution becomes less hypertonic.

Fluid Management

The goal of fluid management is to maintain normovolemia and thus hemodynamic stability. Crystalloids consist of water; electrolytes; and, occasionally, glucose that freely distribute along a concentration gradient between the two extracellular spaces. After 20 to 30 minutes, an estimated 75% to 80% of an isotonic saline or a lactate-containing solution will have distributed outside the confines of the circulation, thus limiting the efficacy of these solutions in treating hypovolemia. Indeed, the ability of crystalloids to restore perfusion in the microcirculation is doubtful.[5]

Hypotonic intravenous fluids equilibrate with extracellular fluid, causing it to become hypotonic with respect to intracellular fluid. When this occurs, osmosis rapidly increases intracellular water, causing cellular swelling. Increased intracellular fluid volume is particularly undesirable in patients with intracranial mass lesions or increased intracranial pressure. Protection from excessive fluid accumulation in the interstitium (extravascular lung water) is mediated by lymphatic flow, which can increase as much as 10-fold.

Hypertonic saline solutions (7.5% sodium chloride) have been useful for rapid intravascular fluid repletion during resuscitation as during hemorrhagic and septic shock. Hypertonic saline solutions compare favorably with mannitol for lowering intracranial pressure.[6] The primary effect of hypertonic saline solutions (increase systemic blood pressure and decrease intracranial pressure) most likely reflects increased intravascular fluid volume because of fluid shifts and movement of water away from uninjured regions of the brain. The use of hypertonic saline solutions is viewed as short-term treatment as hypertonicity and hypernatremia are likely with sustained administration. Furthermore, patients with hypotension due to traumatic brain injury who received prehospital resuscitation with hypertonic saline solutions have similar neurologic outcomes to those treated with conventional fluids when assessed 6 months after the initial injury.[7]

Dehydration

Loss of water by gastrointestinal or renal routes or by diaphoresis (excessive sweating) is associated with an initial deficit in extracellular fluid volume. At the same instant, intracellular water passes to the extracellular fluid compartment by osmosis, thus keeping the osmolarity in both compartments equal despite decreased absolute volume (dehydration) of both compartments. The ratio of extracellular fluid to intracellular fluid is greater in infants than adults, but the absolute volume of extracellular fluid is obviously less, explaining why dehydration develops more rapidly and is often more severe in the very young. Clinical signs of dehydration are likely when about 5% to 10% (severe dehydration) of total body fluids have been lost in a brief period of time. Physiologic mechanisms can usually compensate for acute loss of 15% to 25% of the intravascular fluid volume, whereas a greater loss places the patient at risk for hemodynamic decompensation.

Cell Structure and Function

The basic living unit of the body is the cell. It is estimated that the entire body consists of 100 trillion or more cells, of which (amazingly) about 25 trillion are red blood cells.[4] Each organ is a mass of cells held together by intracellular supporting structures. A common characteristic of all cells is dependence on oxygen to combine with nutrients (carbohydrates, lipids, proteins) to release energy necessary for cellular function. Almost every cell is within 25 to 50 μm of a capillary, assuring prompt diffusion of oxygen to cells. All cells exist in nearly the same composition of extracellular fluid (***milieu interieur*** or interior milieu, the extracellular fluid environment), and the organs of the body (lungs, kidneys, gastrointestinal tract) function to

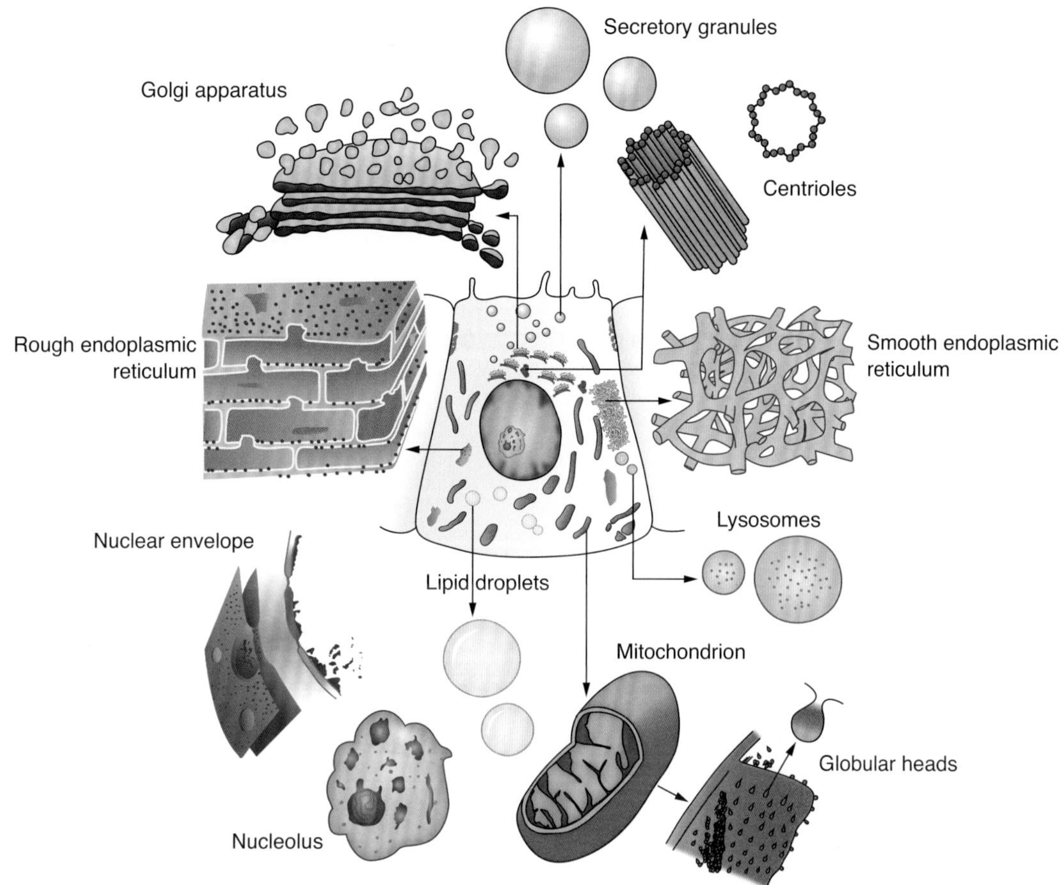

FIGURE 1-5 Schematic diagram of a hypothetical cell *(center)* and its organelles.

maintain a constant composition (homeostasis) of extracellular fluid.

Cell Anatomy

The principal components of cells include the nucleus (except for mature red blood cells), and the cytoplasm, which contains structures known as ***organelles*** (Fig. 1-5).[8] The nucleus is separated from the cytoplasm by a nuclear membrane, and the cytoplasm is separated from surrounding fluids by a cell (plasma) membrane. The membranes around the cell, the nucleus, and organelles are lipid bilayers.

Cell Membrane

Each cell is surrounded by a lipid bilayer that acts as a permeability barrier, allowing the cell to maintain a cytoplasmic composition different from the extracellular fluid. Proteins and phospholipids are the most abundant constituents of cell membranes (Table 1-2). The lipid bilayer is interspersed with large globular proteins (Fig. 1-6).[9] The lipid bilayer of cell membranes is readily permeable to water, both through passive diffusion and through aquaporins, specialized proteins in the membrane that function as water channels (described in the following text). Lipid bilayers are nearly impermeable to water-soluble substances, such as ions and glucose. Conversely, fat-soluble substances (e.g., steroids) and gases readily cross cell membranes.

There are several types of proteins in the cell membrane (see Table 1-2). In addition to structural proteins

Table 1-2

Cell Membrane Composition

Phospholipids
- Lecithins (phosphatidylcholines)
- Sphingomyelins
- Amino phospholipids (phosphatidylethanolamine)

Proteins
- Structural proteins (microtubules)
- Transport proteins (sodium–potassium ATPase)
- Ion channels
- Receptors
- Enzymes (adenylate cyclase)

ATPase, adenosine triphosphatase.

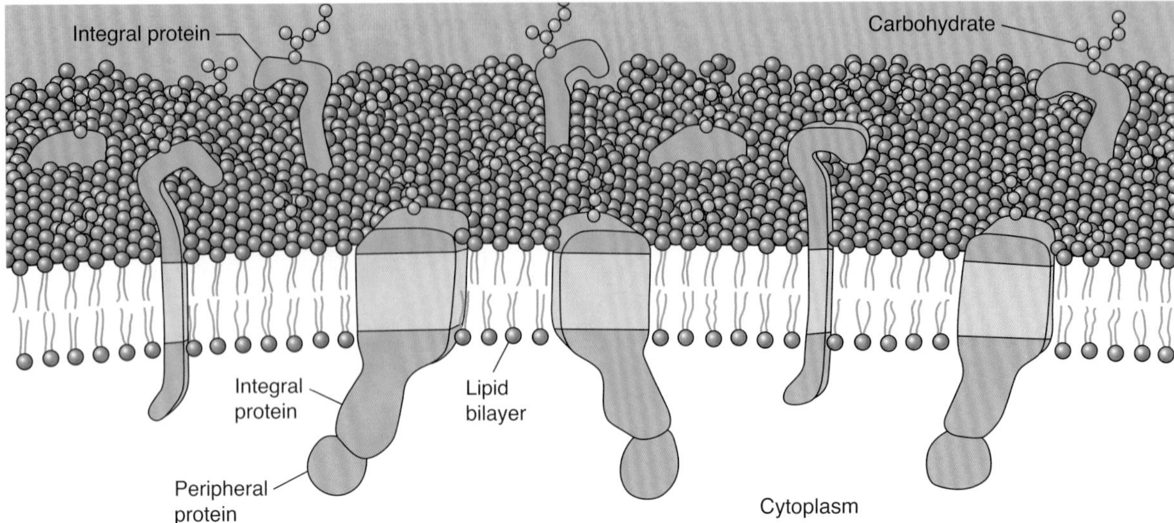

FIGURE 1-6 The cell membrane is a two molecule–thick lipid bilayer containing protein molecules that extend through the bilayer.

(microtubules), there are transport proteins (sodium–potassium adenosine ATPase) that function as pumps, actively transporting ions across cell membranes. Other proteins function as passive channels for ions that can be opened or closed by changes in the conformation of the protein. There are proteins that function as receptors to bind ligands (hormones or neurotransmitters), thus initiating physiologic changes inside cells. Another group of proteins functions as enzymes (adenylate cyclase) catalyzing reactions at the surface of cell membranes. The protein structure of cell membranes, especially the enzyme content, varies from cell to cell.

Transfer of Molecules through Cell Membranes

Diffusion

Oxygen, carbon dioxide, and nitrogen move through cell membranes by simple diffusion through the lipid bilayer. Because of the slowness of diffusion over macroscopic distances, organisms have developed circulatory systems to deliver nutrients within reasonable diffusion ranges of cells (Table 1-3). Water is also able to diffuse through cells, although not as freely as gases. Lipids generally diffuse readily through the lipid bilayer. However, cell membranes are virtually impermeable to ions and charged water-soluble molecules, especially those with molecular weights of greater than 200 daltons.

Poorly lipid-soluble substances, such as glucose and amino acids, may pass through lipid bilayers by facilitated diffusion. For example, glucose combines with a carrier to form a complex that is lipid soluble. This lipid-soluble complex can diffuse to the interior of the cell membrane where glucose is released into the cytoplasm, and the carrier moves back to the exterior of the cell membrane, where it becomes available to transport more glucose from the extracellular fluid (Fig. 1-7).[4] As such, the carrier renders glucose soluble in cell membranes that otherwise would prevent its passage. Insulin greatly speeds facilitated diffusion of glucose and some amino acids across cell membranes.

Table 1-3

Predicted Relationship between Diffusion Distance and Time

Diffusion Distance (mm)	Time Required for Diffusion
0.001	0.5 ms
0.01	50 ms
0.1	5 s
1	498 s
10	14 h

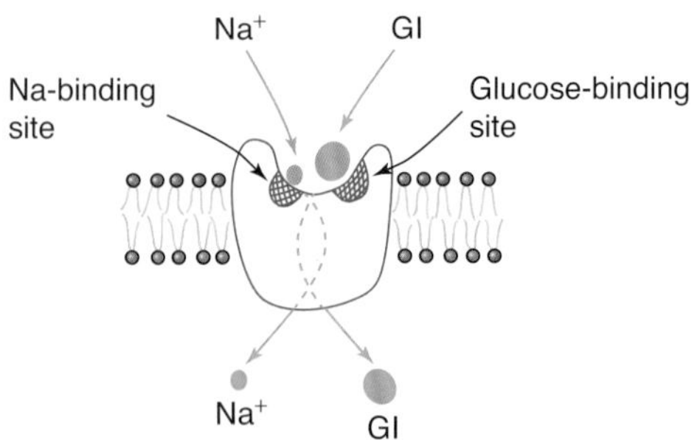

FIGURE 1-7 Glucose (Gl) can combine with a sodium cotransport carrier system at the outside surface of the cell membrane to facilitate diffusion (carrier-mediated diffusion) of Gl across the cell membrane. At the inside surface of the cell membrane, Gl is released to the interior of the cell and the carrier again becomes available for reuse.

Endocytosis and Exocytosis

Endocytosis and exocytosis transfer molecules such as nutrients across cell membranes without the molecule actually passing through the cell membrane. The uptake of particulate matter (bacteria, damaged cells) by cells is termed phagocytosis, whereas uptake of materials in solution in the extracellular fluid is termed pinocytosis (Fig. 1-8).[10] The process of phagocytosis is initiated when antibodies attach to damaged tissue and foreign substances (opsonization), facilitating binding to specialized proteins on the cell surface and endocytosis. Fusion of phagocytic or pinocytic vesicles with lysosomes allows intracellular digestion of materials to proceed. Neurotransmitters are ejected from cells by exocytosis, a process that requires calcium ions and resembles endocytosis in reverse.

Sodium–Potassium Adenosine Triphosphatase

As mentioned previously, sodium–potassium ATPase, also known as the sodium–potassium pump, is an ATP-dependent sodium and potassium transporter on the cell membrane that ejects three sodium ions from the cell in exchange for the import of two potassium ions (Fig. 1-9).[4] This action maintains oncotic equilibration across the cell membrane, reducing the number of intracellular ions to balance the large number of protein and other intracellular constituents. It also is responsible for the transmembrane electrical potential, creating a net positive charge on the outside of the cell from the excess of positive sodium ions outside compared to number of positive potassium ions inside of the cell. Lastly, it creates the sodium gradients responsible for propagation of the action potential and the potassium gradient that rapidly restores the resting membrane potential after conduction of an action potential. In the brain, the sodium–potassium pump accounts for nearly 50% of energy consumption.[11]

Other ion transporters include hydrogen–potassium ATPases in the gastric mucosa and renal tubules, the transporter that exchanges protons for potassium ions. Calcium ATPases are responsible for maintaining very low cytoplasmic concentrations of calcium either by ejecting calcium from the cell (plasma membrane calcium ATPase) or sequestering calcium in the endoplasmic reticulum via the sarcoplasmic/endoplasmic reticulum calcium ATPase (SERCA ATPase).[12]

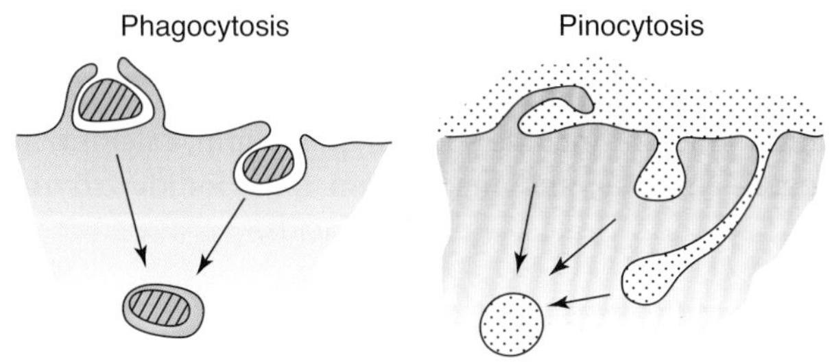

FIGURE 1-8 Schematic depiction of phagocytosis (ingestion of solid particles) and pinocytosis (ingestion of dissolved particles).

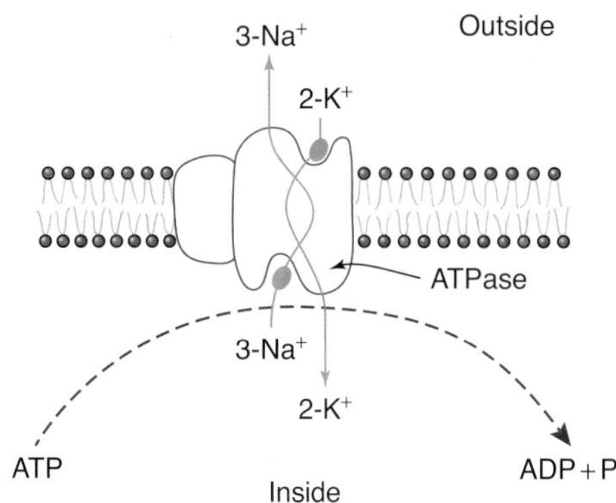

FIGURE 1-9 Sodium–potassium adenosine triphosphatase is an enzyme present in all cells that catalyzes the conversion of adenosine triphosphate (ATP) to adenosine diphosphate (ADP). The resulting energy is used by the active transport carrier system (sodium–potassium pump) that is responsible for the outward movement of three sodium ions across the cell membrane for every two potassium ions that pass inward. (From Guyton AC, Hall JE. *Textbook of Medical Physiology*. 10th ed. Philadelphia, PA: Saunders; 2000, with permission.)

Ion Channels

Ion channels are transmembrane proteins that generate electrical signals in the brain, nerves, heart, and skeletal muscles (Fig. 1-10).[13] Ion channels use the energy stored in the chemical and electrical gradients created by sodium–potassium ATPase to rapidly initiate changes in transmembrane potential, causing conduction of an action potential.

Because of their charge, most ions are relatively insoluble in cell membranes such that their passage across these membranes is thought to occur through protein channels. These channels are likely to be intermolecular spaces in proteins that extend through the entire cell membrane. Some channels are highly specific with respect to ions allowed to pass (sodium, potassium), whereas other channels allow all ions below a certain size to pass (Table 1-4). Tetrodotoxin is a specific blocker of sodium ion channels as a result of binding to the extracellular side of the channel, whereas tetraethylammonium blocks potassium ion channels by attaching to the inside surface of the membrane.

Genes encoding the protein ion channels may be defective, leading to diseases such as cystic fibrosis (chloride channel defects), long Q-T interval syndrome (mutant potassium or, less commonly, sodium channels), hereditary nephrolithiasis (chloride channel), hereditary myopathies including myotonia congenital (chloride channel), and malignant hyperthermia (calcium channel defects).[13] Many drugs target ion channels, including common intravenous anesthetics and, perhaps, inhalational anesthetics. Ion channels are discussed in detail in Chapter 3.

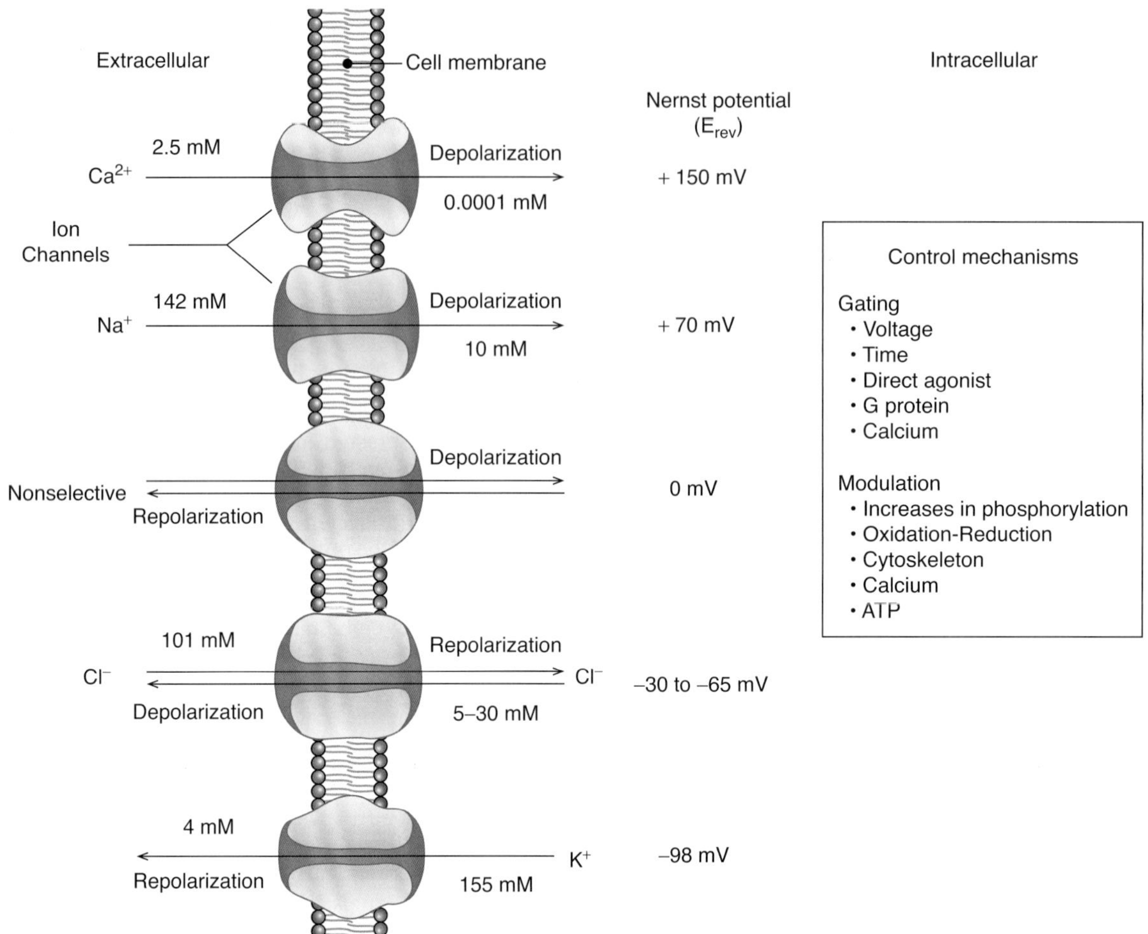

FIGURE 1-10 The five major types of protein ion channels are calcium, sodium, nonselective, chloride, and potassium. Flow of ions through these channels (calcium and sodium into cells and potassium outward) determines the transmembrane potential of cells. (Modified from Ackerman MJ, Clapham DE. Ion channels—basic science and clinical disease. *N Engl J Med.* 1997;336:1575–1586, with permission.)

Protein-Mediated Transport

Protein-mediated transport is responsible for movement of specific substrates across cell membranes. P glycoprotein is responsible for the movement of many drugs across the cell membrane, notably including the transport of morphine out of the central nervous system (CNS), slowing the rate of rise of morphine in the CNS. Virtually all transport of molecules against concentration gradients requires proteins, which use energy provided by ATP to pump the molecule against the concentration gradient.

Active transport via proteins requires energy that is most often provided by hydrolysis of ATP. Indeed, carrier molecules are enzymes known as ATPases that catalyze the hydrolysis of ATP. The most important of the ATPases is sodium–potassium ATPase, which is also known as the sodium–potassium pump. Substances that are actively transported through cell membranes against a concentration gradient include sodium, potassium, calcium, hydrogen, chloride, and magnesium ions; iodide (thyroid gland); carbohydrates; and amino acids.

Sodium Ion Cotransport

Despite the widespread presence of sodium–potassium ATPase, the active transport of sodium ions in some tissues is coupled to the transport of other substances. For example, a carrier system present in the gastrointestinal tract and renal tubules will transport sodium ions only in

Table 1-4

Diameters of Ions, Molecules, and Channels

	Diameter (nm)[a]
Channel (average)	0.80
Water	0.30
Sodium (hydrated)	0.51
Potassium (hydrated)	0.40
Chloride (hydrated)	0.39
Glucose	0.86

[a]1 nm = 10 Å.

combination with a glucose molecule. As such, glucose is returned to the circulation, thus preventing its excretion. Sodium ion cotransport of amino acids is an active transport mechanism that supplements facilitated diffusion of amino acids into cells. Epithelial cells lining the gastrointestinal tract and renal tubules are able to reabsorb amino acids into the circulation by this mechanism, thus preventing their excretion.

Other substances, including insulin, steroids, and growth hormone, influence amino acid transport by the sodium ion cotransport mechanism. For example, estradiol facilitates transport of amino acids into the musculature of the uterus, which promotes development of this organ.

Aquaporins

Aquaporins are protein channels that permit the free flux of water across cell membranes.[14] In the absence of aquaporins, diffusion of water might not be sufficiently rapid for some physiologic processes. Genetic defects in aquaporins are responsible for several clinical diseases, including some cases of congenital cataracts[15] and nephrogenic diabetes insipidus.[16]

Nucleus

The nucleus is primarily made up of the 46 chromosomes, except the nucleus of the egg cell, which contains 23. Each chromosome consists of a molecule of DNA covered with proteins. The nucleus is surrounded by a membrane that separates its contents from the cytoplasm, through which substances, including RNA, pass from the nucleus to the cytoplasm.

The nucleolus is a non–membrane-bound structure within the nucleus responsible for the synthesis of ribosomes. Centrioles are present in the cytoplasm near the nucleus and are concerned with the movement of chromosomes during cell division.

Structure and Function of DNA and RNA

DNA consists of two complementary nucleotide chains composed of adenine, guanine, thymine, and cytosine (Fig. 1-11).[17] The genetic message is determined by the sequence of nucleotides. DNA is transcribed to RNA, which transfers the genetic message to the site of protein synthesis (ribosomes) in cytoplasm. Cell reproduction (mitosis) is determined by the DNA genetic system. The human genome has now been 99% sequenced and is composed of just 20,000 to 25,000 genes.[18] The protein encoding genes account for only 1% to 2% of our DNA, the rest being regulatory sequences, non–protein-encoding RNA sequences, introns, and a considerable amount of DNA termed "junk" because it has no known function. Our genome differs from that of chimpanzees by just 1%.[19]

Genes are regulated by specific regulatory proteins and RNA molecules. Regulatory proteins are the target of many hormones, such as steroids, and drugs (antineoplastic drugs).

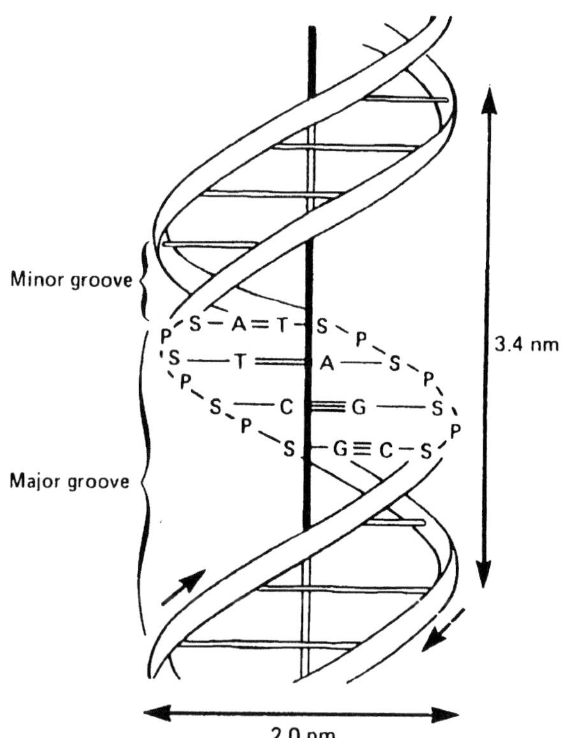

FIGURE 1-11 Double helical structure of DNA with adenine (A) bonding to thymine (T) and cytosine (C) to guanine (G). (From Murray RK, Granner DK, Mayes PA, et al. *Harper's Biochemistry*. 21st ed. Norwalk, CT: Appleton & Lange; 1988, with permission.)

Cytoplasm

The cytoplasm consists of water; electrolytes; and proteins including enzymes, lipids, and carbohydrates. About 70% to 80% of the cell volume is water. Cellular chemicals are dissolved in the water, and these substances can diffuse to all parts of the cell in this fluid medium. Proteins are, next to water, the most abundant substance in most cells, accounting for 10% to 20% of the cell mass.

The cytoplasm contains numerous organelles with specific roles in cellular function.

Mitochondria

Mitochondria are the power-generating units of cells containing both the enzymes and substrates of the tricarboxylic acid cycle (Krebs cycle) and the electron transport chain. As a result, oxidative phosphorylation and synthesis of adenosine triphosphate (ATP) are localized to mitochondria. ATP leaves the mitochondria and diffuses throughout the cell, providing energy for cellular functions. Mitochondria consist of two lipid bilayers, the outer bilayer in contact with the cytoplasm, and the inner layer that houses most of the biochemical machinery and the mitochondrial DNA. The space between these two membranes functions as a reservoir for protons created during electron transport. It is the movement of these protons back to the matrix, through the inner membrane, that drives most of the conversion of ADP to ATP, the primary form of intercellular energy, by ATP synthase.[20]

Increased need for ATP in the cell leads to an increase in the number of mitochondria. A number of diseases are known to be based on aberrant mitochondrial function.[21] The common element of mitochondrial diseases is aberrant cellular energetics. There are approximately 1,500 proteins responsible for mitochondrial function. Of these, only 13 are encoded by mitochondrial DNA, the balance being encoded by nuclear DNA. Thus, the vast majority of mitochondrial diseases follow standard models of genetic inheritance.

Endoplasmic Reticulum

The endoplasmic reticulum is a complex lipid bilayer that wraps and folds, creating tubules and vesicles in the cytoplasm. Ribosomes, composed mainly of RNA, attach to the outer portions of many parts of the endoplasmic reticulum membranes, serving as the sites for protein synthesis (hormones, hemoglobin). The portion of the membrane containing these ribosomes is known as the ***rough endoplasmic reticulum***. The part of the membrane that lacks ribosomes is the ***smooth endoplasmic reticulum***. This smooth portion of the endoplasmic reticulum membrane functions in the synthesis of lipids, metabolism of carbohydrates, and other enzymatic processes. The sarcoplasmic reticulum is found in muscle cells, where it serves as a reservoir for calcium.

Lysosomes

Lysosomes are lipid membrane–enclosed globules scattered throughout the cytoplasm, providing an intracellular digestive system. Lysosomes are filled with digestive (hydrolytic) enzymes. When cells are damaged or die, these digestive enzymes cause autolysis of the remnants. Bactericidal substances in the lysosome kill phagocytized bacteria before they can cause cellular damage. These bactericidal substances include (a) lysozyme, which dissolves the cell membranes of bacteria; (b) lysoferrin, which binds iron and other metals that are essential for bacterial growth; (c) acid that has a pH of <4; and (d) hydrogen peroxide, which can disrupt some bacterial metabolic systems.

Lysosomal storage diseases are genetic disorders caused by inherited genetic defect in lysosomal function, resulting in accumulation of incompletely degraded macromolecules. There are about 50 known lysosomal storage diseases, including Tay-Sachs, Gaucher, Fabry, and Niemann-Pick disease.[22]

Golgi Apparatus

The Golgi apparatus is a collection of membrane-enclosed sacs that are responsible for storing proteins and lipids as well as performing postsynthetic modifications including glycosylation and phosphorylation. Proteins synthesized in the rough endoplasmic reticulum are transported to the Golgi apparatus, where they are stored in highly concentrated packets (secretory vesicles) for subsequent release into the cell's cytoplasm, or transport to the surface for extracellular release via exocytosis. Exocytotic vesicles continuously release their contents, whereas secretory vesicles store the packaged material until a triggering signal is received. Neurotransmitter release is a highly relevant (to anesthesia) example of regulated secretion. The Golgi apparatus is also responsible for creating lysosomes.

References

1. Gamble JL. *Chemical Anatomy, Physiology, and Pathology of Extracellular Fluid*. 6th ed. Boston, MA: Harvard University Press; 1954.
2. Leaf A, Newburgh LH. *Significance of the Body Fluids in Chemical Medicine*. 2nd ed. Springfield, IL: Charles C Thomas; 1955.
3. Ganong WF. *Review of Medical Physiology*. 21st ed. New York, NY: Lange Medical Books/McGraw-Hill; 2003.
4. Guyton AC, Hall JE. *Textbook of Medical Physiology*. 10th ed. Philadelphia, PA: W.B. Saunders; 2000.
5. Funk W, Baldinger V. Microcirculatory perfusion during volume therapy. A comparative study using crystalloid or colloid in awake animals. *Anesthesiology*. 1995;82:975–982.
6. Qureshi AI, Suarez JI. Use of hypertonic saline solutions in treatment of cerebral edema and intracranial hypertension. *Crit Care Med*. 2000;28:3301–3313.
7. Cooper DJ, Myles PS, McDermott FT, et al. Prehospital hypertonic saline resuscitation of patients with hypotension and severe traumatic brain injury. A randomized controlled trial. *JAMA*. 2004;291:1350–1357.
8. Junqueira LC, Carneiro J, Kelley RO. *Basic Histology*. 7th ed. Norwalk, CT: Appleton & Lange; 1992.
9. Lodish HF, Rothman JE. The assembly of cell membranes. *Sci Am*. 1979;240:48–63.
10. Berne RM, Levy MN, Koeppen BM, et al. *Physiology*. 5th ed. St. Louis, MO: Mosby; 2004.
11. Kety SS. The general metabolism of the brain in vivo. In: Richter D, ed. *Metabolism of the Nervous System*. London, United Kingdom: Pergamon; 1957:221–237.
12. Uhlén P, Fritz N. Biochemistry of calcium oscillations. *Biochem Biophys Res Commun*. 2010;396:28–32.
13. Ackerman MJ, Clapham DE. Ion channels—basic science and clinical disease. *N Engl J Med*. 1997;336:1575–1586.
14. Agre P, King LS, Yasui M, et al. Aquaporin water channels—from atomic structure to clinical medicine. *J Physiol*. 2002;542:3–16.
15. Kozono D, Yasui M, King LS, et al. Aquaporin water channels: atomic structure and molecular dynamics meet clinical medicine. *J Clin Invest*. 2002;109:1395–1399.
16. Bichet DG. Nephrogenic diabetes insipidus. *Adv Chronic Kidney Dis*. 2006;13:96–104.
17. Murray RK, Granner DK, Mayes PA, et al. *Harper's Biochemistry*. 21st ed. Norwalk, CT: Appleton & Lange; 1988.
18. International Human Genome Sequencing Consortium. Finishing the euchromatic sequence of the human genome. *Nature*. 2004; 431:931–945.
19. Chimpanzee Sequencing and Analysis Consortium. Initial sequence of the chimpanzee genome and comparison with the human genome. *Nature*. 2005;437:69–87.
20. Walker JE, Cozens AL, Dyer MR, et al. Structure and genes of ATP synthase. *Biochem Soc Trans*. 1987;15:104–106.
21. Scharfe C, Lu HH, Neuenburg JK, et al. Mapping gene associations in human mitochondria using clinical disease phenotypes. *PLoS Comput Biol*. 2009;5:e1000374.
22. Parkinson-Lawrence EJ, Shandala T, Prodoehl M, et al. Lysosomal storage disease: revealing lysosomal function and physiology. *Physiology*. 2010;25:102–115.

CHAPTER 2

Basic Principles of Pharmacology

Pamela Flood • Steven Shafer

This chapter combines Dr. Stoelting's elegant description of pharmacology with a mathematical approach first presented by Dr. Shafer[1] in 1997, and most recently in *Miller's Anesthesia* textbook.[2,3] The combination of approaches sets a foundation for the pharmacology presented in the subsequent chapters. It also explains the fundamental principles of drug behavior and drug interaction that govern our daily practice of anesthesia.

Receptor Theory

A drug that activates a receptor by binding to that receptor is called an ***agonist***. Most agonists bind through a combination of ionic, hydrogen, and van der Waals interactions (the sum of the attractive or repulsive forces between molecules), making them reversible. Rarely, an agonist will bind covalently to the receptor, rendering the interaction irreversible. Receptors are often envisioned as proteins that are either unbound or are bound to the agonist ligand. When the receptor is bound to the agonist ligand, the effect of the drug is produced. When the receptor is not bound, there is no effect. The receptor state is seen as binary: It is either unbound, resulting in one conformation, or it is bound, resulting in another conformation. Agonists are often portrayed as simply activating a receptor (Fig. 2-1). In this view, the magnitude of the drug effect reflects the total number of receptors that are bound. In this simplistic view, the "most" drug effect occurs when every receptor is bound.

This simple view helps to understand the action of an antagonist (Fig. 2-2). An ***antagonist*** is a drug that binds to the receptor without activating the receptor. Antagonists typically bind with ionic, hydrogen, and van der Waals interactions, rendering them reversible. Antagonists block the action of agonists simply by getting in the way of the agonist, preventing the agonist from binding to the receptor and producing the drug effect. ***Competitive antagonism*** is present when increasing concentrations of the antagonist progressively inhibit the response to the agonist. This causes a rightward displacement of the agonist dose-response (or concentration-response) relationship. ***Noncompetitive antagonism*** is present when, after administration of an antagonist, even high concentrations of agonist cannot completely overcome the antagonism. In this instance, either the agonist is bound irreversibly (and probably covalently) to the receptor site, or it binds to a different site on the molecule and the interaction is allosteric (based on a change in shape and thereby the activity of the receptor). Noncompetitive antagonism causes both a rightward shift of the dose-response relationship as well as a decreased maximum efficacy of the concentration versus response.

Although this simple view of activated and inactivated receptors explains agonists and antagonists, it has a more difficult time with ***partial agonists*** and ***inverse agonists*** (Fig. 2-3). A partial agonist is a drug that binds to a receptor (usually at the agonist site) where it activates the receptor but not as much as a full agonist. Even at supramaximal doses, a partial agonist cannot cause the full drug effect. Partial agonists may also have antagonist activity in which case they are also called ***agonist-antagonists***. When a partial agonist is administered with a full agonist, it decreases the effect of the full agonist. For example, butorphanol acts as a partial agonist at the μ opioid receptor. Given alone, butorphanol is a modestly efficacious analgesic. Given along with fentanyl, it will partly reverse the fentanyl analgesia, and in individuals using opioids chronically, may precipitate withdrawal. Inverse agonists bind at the same site as the agonist (and likely compete with it), but they produce the opposite effect of the agonist. Inverse agonists "turn off" the constitutive activity of the receptor. The simple view of receptors as bound or unbound does not explain partial agonists or inverse agonists.

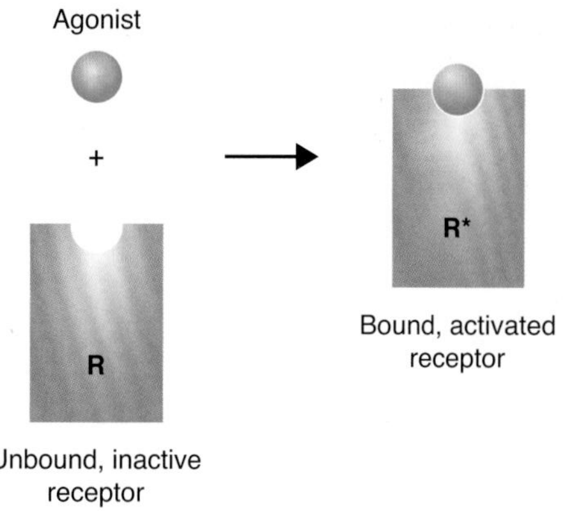

FIGURE 2-1 The interaction of a receptor with an agonist may be portrayed as a binary bound versus unbound receptor. The unbound receptor is portrayed as inactive. When the receptor is bound to the agonist ligand, it becomes the activated, *R**, and mediates the drug effect. This view is too simplistic, but it permits understanding of basic agonist behavior.

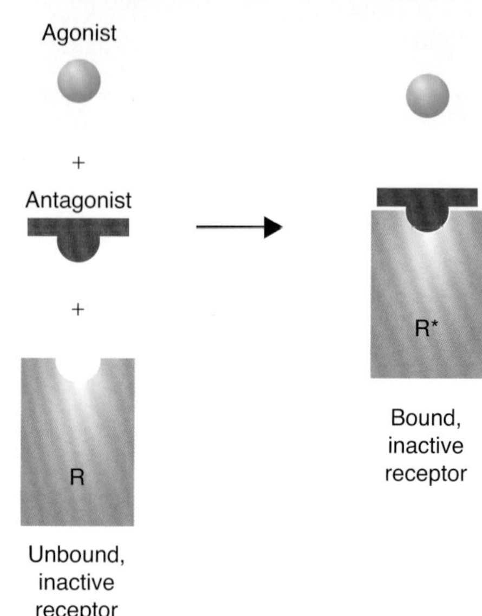

FIGURE 2-2 The simple view of receptor activation also explains the action of antagonist. In this case, the antagonist *(red)* binds to the receptor, but the binding does not cause activation. However, the binding of the antagonist blocks the agonist from binding, and thus blocks agonist drug effect. If the binding is reversible, this is competitive antagonism. If it is not reversible, then it is noncompetitive antagonism.

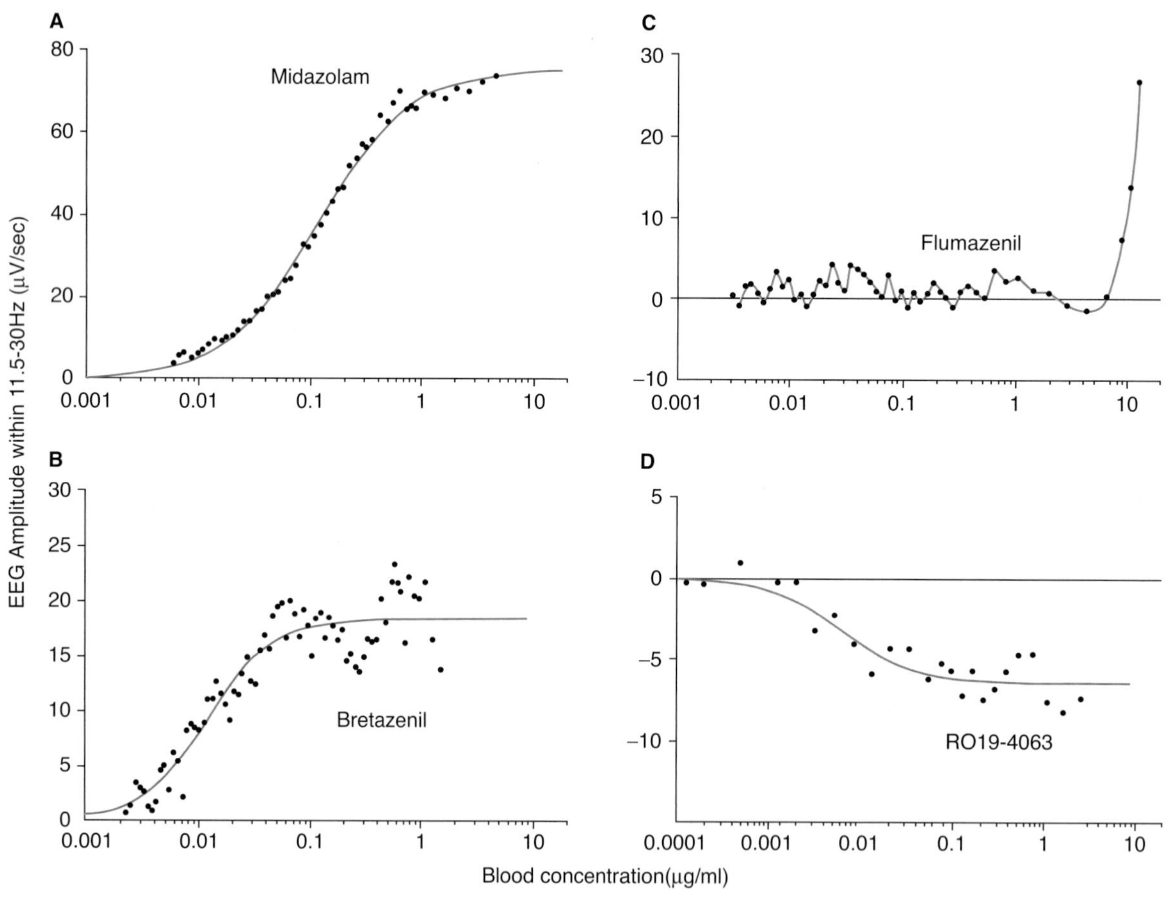

FIGURE 2-3 The concentration versus EEG response relationship for four benzodiazepine ligands: midazolam (full agonist), bretazenil (partial agonist), flumazenil (competitive antagonist), and RO 19-4063 (inverse agonist). (From Shafer S. Principles of pharmacokinetics and pharmacodynamics. In: Longnecker DE, Tinker JH, Morgan GE, eds. *Principles and Practice of Anesthesiology.* 2nd ed. St. Louis, MO: Mosby-Year Book; 1997:1159, based on Mandema JW, Kuck MT, Danhof M. In vivo modeling of the pharmacodynamic interaction between benzodiazepines which differ in intrinsic efficacy. *J Pharmacol Exp Ther.* 1992;261[1]:56–61.)

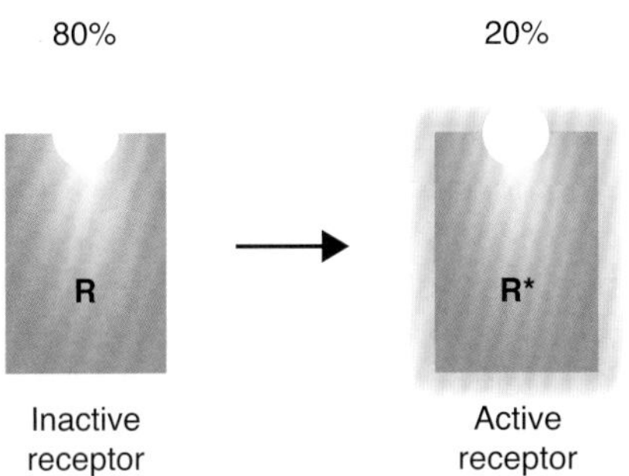

FIGURE 2-4 Receptors have multiple states, and they switch spontaneously between them. In this case, the receptor has just two states. It spends 80% of the time in the inactive state and 20% of the time in the active state in the absence of any ligand.

It turns out that receptors have many natural conformations, and they naturally fluctuate between these different conformations (Fig. 2-4). Some of the conformations are associated with the pharmacologic effect, and some are not. In the example shown, the receptor only has two states: an inactive state and an active state that produces the same effect as if an agonist were bound to the receptor, although at a reduced level because the receptor only spends 20% of its time in this activated state.

In this view, ligands do not cause the receptor shape to change. That happens spontaneously. However, ligands change the ratio of active to inactive states by (thermodynamically) favoring one of the states. Figure 2-5 shows the receptor as seen in Figure 2-4 in the presence of an agonist, a partial agonist, an antagonist, and an inverse agonist. Presence of the full agonist causes the conformation of the active state to be strongly favored, causing the receptors to be in this state nearly 100% of the time. The partial agonist is not as effective in stabilizing the receptor in the active state, so the bound receptor only spends 50% of its time in this state. The antagonist does not favor either state; it just gets in the way of binding (as before; see Fig. 2-2). The inverse agonist favors the inactive state, reversing the baseline receptor activity.

Using this information, we can now interpret the action of several ligands for the benzodiazepine receptor (see Fig. 2-3). The actions include full agonism (midazolam), partial agonism (bretazenil), competitive antagonism (flumazenil), and inverse agonism (RO 19-4063). This range of actions can be explained by considering receptor states. Assume that the γ-aminobutyric acid (GABA) receptor has several conformations, one of which is particularly sensitive to endogenous GABA. Typically, there are some GABA receptors in this more sensitive conformation. As a full agonist, midazolam causes nearly all of the GABA receptors to be in the confirmation with increased sensitivity to GABA. Bretazenil does the same thing but not as well. Even when every benzodiazepine receptor is occupied by bretazenil, fewer GABA receptors are in the more sensitive confirmation. Bretazenil simply does not favor

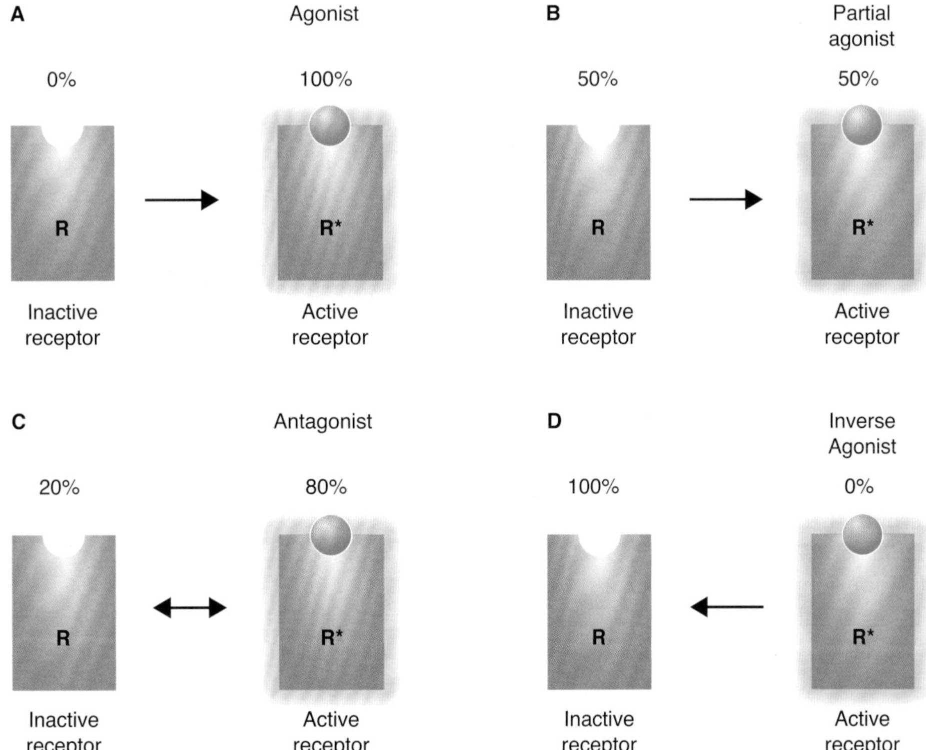

FIGURE 2-5 The action of agonists **(A)**, partial agonists **(B)**, antagonists **(C)**, and inverse agonists **(D)** can be interpreted as changing the balance between the active and inactive forms of the receptor. In this case, in the absence of agonist, the receptor is in the activated state 20% of the time. This percentage changes based on nature of the ligand bound to the receptor.

that conformation as well as midazolam. When flumazenil is in the binding pocket, it does not change the relative probabilities of the receptor being in any conformation. Flumazenil just gets in the way of other drugs that would otherwise bind to the pocket. RO 19-4063 actually decreases the number of GABA receptors in the more sensitive conformation. Usually, some of them are in this more sensitive conformation, but that number is decreased by the inverse agonist RO 19-4063 (which was never developed as a drug because endogenous benzodiazepines, although anticipated, have not been described). The notion of the drugs having multiple conformations, and drugs acting through favoring particular conformations, helps to understand the action of agonists, partial agonists, antagonists, and inverse agonists.

Receptor Action

The number for receptors in cell membranes is dynamic and increases (upregulates) or decreases (downregulates) in response to specific stimuli. For example, a patient with pheochromocytoma has an excess of circulating catecholamines. In response, there is a decrease in the numbers of β-adrenergic receptors in cell membranes in an attempt to maintain homeostasis. Likewise, prolonged treatment of asthma with a β agonist may result in tachyphylaxis (decreased response to the same dose of β agonist, also called ***tolerance***) because of the decrease in β adrenergic receptors. Conversely, lower motor neuron injury causes an increase in the number of nicotinic acetylcholine receptors in the neuromuscular junction, leading to an exaggerated response to succinylcholine. Changing receptor numbers is one of many mechanisms that contribute to variability in response to drugs.

Receptor Types

Receptors for drug action can be classified by location. Many of the receptors thought to be the most critical for anesthetic interaction are located in the lipid bilayer of cell membranes. For example, opioids, intravenous sedative hypnotics, benzodiazepines, β blockers, catecholamines, and muscle relaxants (most of which are actually antagonists) all interact with membrane-bound receptors. Other receptors are intracellular proteins. Drugs such as caffeine, insulin, steroids, theophylline, and milrinone interact with intracellular proteins. Circulating proteins can also be drug targets; for example, the many drugs that affect components of the coagulation cascade.

There are also drugs that do not interact with proteins at all. Stomach antacids such as sodium citrate simply work by changing gastric pH. Chelating drugs work by binding divalent cations. Iodine kills bacteria by osmotic pressure (intracellular desiccation), and intravenous sodium bicarbonate changes plasma pH. The mechanism of action of these drugs does not involve receptors per se, and hence these drugs will not be further considered in this section.

Proteins function in the body as small machines, catalyzing enzymatic reactions and acting as ion channels among other functions. When a drug binds to a receptor, it changes the activity of the machine, typically by enhancing its activity (e.g., propofol increases the sensitivity of the GABA-A receptor to GABA, the endogenous ligand), decreasing its activity (ketamine decreases the activity of the *N*-methyl-D-aspartate [NMDA] receptor), or triggering a chain reaction (opioid binding to the μ opioid receptor activates an inhibitory G protein that decreases adenylyl cyclase activity). The protein's response to binding of the drug is responsible for the drug effect.

Pharmacokinetics

Pharmacokinetics is the quantitative study of the absorption, distribution, metabolism, and excretion of injected and inhaled drugs and their metabolites. Thus, pharmacokinetics describes what the body does to a drug. Pharmacodynamics is the quantitative study of the body's response to a drug. Thus, pharmacodynamics describes what the drug does to the body. This section will introduce the basic principles of pharmacokinetics. The next section discusses the basic principles of pharmacodynamics.

Pharmacokinetics determines the concentration of a drug in the plasma or at the site of drug effect. Pharmacokinetic variability is a significant component of patient-to-patient variability in drug response and may result from genetic modifications in metabolism; interactions with other drugs; or disease in the liver, kidneys, or other organs of metabolism.[4]

The basic principles of pharmacokinetics are absorption, metabolism, distribution, and elimination. These processes are fundamental to all drugs. They can be described in basic physiologic terms or using mathematical models. Each serves a purpose. Physiology can be used to predict how changes in organ function will affect the disposition of drugs. Mathematical models can be used to calculate the concentration of drug in the blood or tissue following any arbitrary dose, at any arbitrary time. We will initially tackle the physiologic principles that govern distribution, metabolism, elimination, and absorption, in that order. We will then turn to the mathematical models.

Distribution

When drugs are administered, they mix with body tissues and are immediately diluted from the concentrated injectate in the syringe to the more dilute concentration measured in the plasma or tissue. This initial distribution (within 1 minute) after bolus injection is considered mixing within the "central compartment" (Fig. 2-6). The

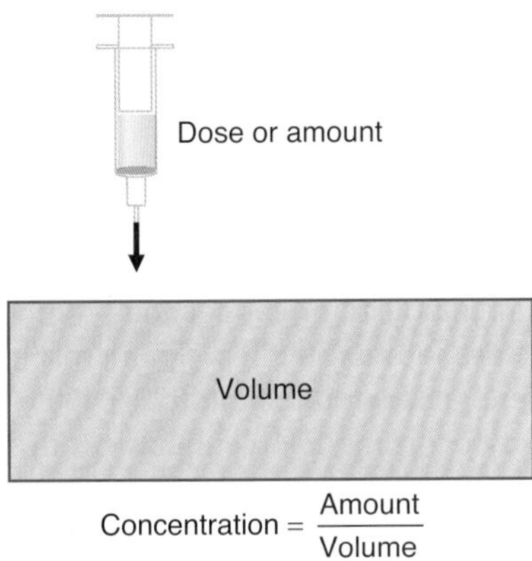

FIGURE 2-6 The central volume is the volume that intravenously injected drug initially mixes into. (From Shafer S, Flood P, Schwinn D. Basic principles of pharmacology. In: Miller RD, Eriksson LI, Fleisher LA, et al, eds. *Miller's Anesthesia*. Vol 1. 7th ed. Philadelphia, PA: Churchill Livingstone; 2010:479–514, with permission.)

central compartment is physically composed of those elements of the body that dilute the drug within the first minute after injection: the venous blood volume of the arm, the volume of the great vessels, the heart, the lung, and the upper aorta, and whatever uptake of drug occurs in the first passage through the lungs. Many of these volumes are fixed, but drugs that are highly fat soluble may be avidly taken up in the first passage through the lung, reducing the concentration measured in the arterial blood and increasing the apparent size of the central compartment. For example, first-pass pulmonary uptake of the initial dose of lidocaine, propranolol, meperidine, fentanyl, sufentanil, and alfentanil exceeds 65% of the dose.[5]

The body is a complex space, and mixing is an ongoing process. Almost by definition, the central compartment is the mixing with a small portion of the blood volume and the lung tissue. Several minutes later, the drug will fully mix with the entire blood volume. However, it may take hours or even days for the drug to fully mix with all bodily tissues because some tissues have very low perfusion.

In the process of mixing, molecules are drawn to other molecules, some with specific binding sites. A drug that is polar will be drawn to water, where the polar water molecules find a low energy state by associating with the charged aspects of the molecule. A drug that is nonpolar has a higher affinity for fat, where van der Waals binding provides numerous weak binding sites. Many anesthetic drugs are highly fat soluble and poorly soluble in water. High fat solubility means that the molecule will have a large volume of distribution because it will be preferentially taken up by fat, diluting the concentration in the plasma. The extreme example of this is propofol, which is almost inseparable from fat. The capacity of body fat to hold propofol is so vast that in some studies the total volume of distribution of propofol has been reported as exceeding 5,000 L. Of course, nobody has a total volume of 5,000 L. It is important to understand that those 5,000 L refer to imaginary aqueous liters or the amount of plasma that would be required to dissolve the initial dose of propofol. Because propofol is so fat soluble, a large amount of propofol is dissolved in the body's fatty tissues and the concentration measured in the plasma will be low.

Following bolus injection, the drug primarily goes to the tissues that receive the bulk of arterial blood flow: the brain, heart, kidneys, and liver. These tissues are often called ***the vessel rich group***. The rapid blood flow ensures that the concentration in these highly perfused tissues rises rapidly to equilibrate with arterial blood. However, for highly fat soluble drugs, the capacity of the fat to hold the drug greatly exceeds the capacity of highly perfused tissues. Initially, the fat compartment is almost invisible because the blood supply to fat is quite limited. However, with time, the fat gradually absorbs more and more drug, sequestering it away from the highly perfused tissues. This redistribution of drug from the highly perfused tissue to the fat accounts for a substantial part of the offset of drug effect following a bolus of an intravenous anesthetic or fat-soluble opioid (e.g., fentanyl). Muscles play an intermediate role in this process, having (at rest) blood flow that is intermediate between highly perfused tissues and fat.

Protein Binding

Most drugs are bound to some extent to plasma proteins, primarily albumin, α_1-acid glycoprotein, and lipoproteins.[6] Most acidic drugs bind to albumin, whereas basic drugs bind to α_1-acid glycoprotein. Protein binding effects both the distribution of drugs (because only the free or unbound fraction can readily cross cell membranes) and the apparent potency of drugs, again because it is the free fraction that determines the concentration of bound drug on the receptor.

The extent of protein binding parallels the lipid solubility of the drug. This is because drugs that are hydrophobic are more likely to bind to proteins in the plasma and to lipids in the fat. For intravenous anesthetic drugs, which tend to be quite potent, the number of available protein binding sites in the plasma vastly exceeds the number of sites actually bound. As a result, the fraction bound is not dependent on the concentration of the anesthetic and only dependent on the protein concentration.

Binding of drugs to plasma albumin is nonselective, and drugs with similar physicochemical characteristics may compete with each other and with endogenous substances for the same protein binding sites. For example, sulfonamides can displace unconjugated bilirubin from binding sites on albumin, leading to the risk of bilirubin encephalopathy in the neonate.

Age, hepatic disease, renal failure, and pregnancy can all result in decreased plasma protein concentration. Alterations in protein binding are important only for drugs that are highly protein bound (e.g., >90%). For such drugs, the free fraction changes as an inverse proportion with a change in protein concentration. If the free fraction is 2% in the normal state, then in a patient with 50% decrease in plasma proteins, the free fraction will increase to 4%, a 100% increase.

Theoretically, an increase in free fraction of a drug may increase the pharmacologic effect of the drug, but in practice, it is far from certain that there will be any change in pharmacologic effect at all. The reason is that it is the unbound fraction that equilibrates throughout the body, including with the receptor. Plasma proteins only account for a small portion of the total binding sites for drug in the body. Because the free drug ***concentration*** in the plasma and tissues represents partitioning with all binding sites, not just the plasma binding sites, the actual free drug concentration that drives drug on and off receptors may change fairly little with changes in plasma protein concentration.

Metabolism

Metabolism converts pharmacologically active, lipid-soluble drugs into water-soluble and usually pharmacologically inactive metabolites. However, this is not always the case. For example, diazepam and propranolol may be metabolized to active compounds. Morphine-6-glucuronide, a metabolite of morphine, is a more potent opioid than morphine itself. In some instances, an inactive parent compound (prodrug) metabolized to an active drug. This is the case with codeine, which is an exceedingly weak opioid. Codeine is metabolized to morphine, which is responsible for the analgesic effects of codeine.

Pathways of Metabolism

The four basic pathways of metabolism are (a) oxidation, (b) reduction, (c) hydrolysis, and (d) conjugation. Traditionally, metabolism has been divided into phase I and phase II reactions. Phase I reactions include oxidation, reduction, and hydrolysis, which increase the drug's polarity and prepare it for phase II reactions. Phase II reactions are conjugation reactions that covalently link the drug or metabolites with a highly polar molecule (carbohydrate or an amino acid) that renders the conjugate more water soluble for subsequent excretion. Hepatic microsomal enzymes are responsible for the metabolism of most drugs. Other sites of drug metabolism include the plasma (Hofmann elimination, ester hydrolysis), lungs, kidneys, and gastrointestinal tract and placenta (tissue esterases).

Hepatic microsomal enzymes, which participate in the metabolism of many drugs, are located principally in hepatic smooth endoplasmic reticulum. These microsomal enzymes are also present in the kidneys, gastrointestinal tract, and adrenal cortex. Microsomes are vesicle-like artifacts re-formed from pieces of the endoplasmic reticulum when cells are homogenized; microsomal enzymes are those enzymes that are concentrated in these vesicle-like artifacts.

Phase I Enzymes

Enzymes responsible for phase I reactions include cytochrome P450 enzymes, non–cytochrome P450 enzymes, and flavin-containing monooxygenase enzymes. The cytochrome P450 enzyme (CYP) system is a large family of membrane-bound proteins containing a heme cofactor that catalyze the metabolism of endogenous compounds. P450 enzymes are predominantly hepatic microsomal enzymes although there are also mitochondrial P450 enzymes. The designation cytochrome P450 emphasizes this substance's absorption peak at 450 nm when it is combined with carbon monoxide. The cytochrome P450 system is also known as the mixed function oxidase system because it involves both oxidation and reduction steps; the most common reaction catalyzed by cytochrome P450 is the monooxygenase reaction, for example, insertion of one atom of oxygen into an organic substrate while the other oxygen atom is reduced to water. Cytochrome P450 functions as the terminal oxidase in the electron transport chain.

Individual cytochrome P450 enzymes have evolved from a common protein.[7] Cytochrome P450 enzymes, often called ***CYPs***, that share more than 40% sequence homology are grouped in a family designated by a number (e.g., "CYP2"), those that share more than 55% homology are grouped in a subfamily designated by a letter (e.g., "CYP2A"), and individual CYP enzymes are identified by a third number (e.g., "CYP2A6"). Ten isoforms of cytochrome P450 are responsible for the oxidative metabolism of most drugs. The preponderance of CYP activity for anesthetic drugs is generated by CYP3A4, which is the most abundantly expressed P450 isoform, comprising 20% to 60% of total P450 activity. P450 3A4 metabolizes more than one-half of all currently available drugs, including opioids (alfentanil, sufentanil, fentanyl), benzodiazepines, local anesthetics (lidocaine, ropivacaine), immunosuppressants (cyclosporine), and antihistamines (terfenadine).

Drugs can alter the activity of these enzymes through induction and inhibition. Induction occurs through increased expression of the enzymes. For example, phenobarbital induces microsomal enzymes and thus can render drugs less effective through increased metabolism. Conversely, other drugs directly inhibit enzymes, increasing the exposure to their substrates. Famously, grapefruit juice (not exactly a drug) inhibits CYP 3A4, possibly increasing the concentration of anesthetics and other drugs.

Oxidation

Cytochrome P450 enzymes are crucial for oxidation reactions. These enzymes require an electron donor in the form of reduced nicotinamide adenine dinucleotide (NAD) and molecular oxygen for their activity. The molecule of oxygen is split, with one atom of oxygen oxidizing each molecule of drug and the other oxygen atom being incorporated into a molecule of water. Examples of oxidative metabolism of drugs catalyzed by cytochrome P450 enzymes include hydroxylation, deamination, desulfuration, dealkylation, and dehalogenation. Demethylation of morphine to normorphine is an example of oxidative dealkylation. Dehalogenation involves oxidation of a carbon-hydrogen bond to form an intermediate metabolite that is unstable and spontaneously loses a halogen atom. Halogenated volatile anesthetics are susceptible to dehalogenation, leading to release of bromide, chloride, and fluoride ions. Aliphatic oxidation is oxidation of a side chain. For example, oxidation of the side chain of thiopental converts the highly lipid-soluble parent drug to the more water-soluble carboxylic acid derivative. Thiopental also undergoes desulfuration to pentobarbital by an oxidative step.

Epoxide intermediates in the oxidative metabolism of drugs are capable of covalent binding with macromolecules and may be responsible for some drug-induced organ toxicity, such as hepatic dysfunction. Normally, these highly reactive intermediates have such a transient existence that they exert no biologic action. When enzyme induction occurs, however, large amounts of reactive intermediates may be produced, leading to organ damage. This is especially likely to occur if the antioxidant glutathione, which is in limited supply in the liver, is depleted by the reactive intermediates.

Reduction

Cytochrome P450 enzymes are also essential for reduction reactions. Under conditions of low oxygen partial pressures, cytochrome P450 enzymes transfer electrons directly to a substrate such as halothane rather than to oxygen. This electron gain imparted to the substrate occurs only when insufficient amounts of oxygen are present to compete for electrons.

Conjugation

Conjugation with glucuronic acid involves cytochrome P450 enzymes. Glucuronic acid is synthesized from glucose and added to lipid-soluble drugs to render them water soluble. The resulting water-soluble glucuronide conjugates are then excreted in bile and urine. In premature infants, reduced microsomal enzyme activity interferes with conjugation, leading to neonatal hyperbilirubinemia and the risk of bilirubin encephalopathy. The reduced conjugation ability of the neonate increases the effect and potential toxicity of drugs that are normally inactivated by conjugation with glucuronic acid.

Hydrolysis

Enzymes responsible for hydrolysis of drugs, usually at an ester bond, do not involve the cytochrome P450 enzyme system. Hydrolysis often occurs outside of the liver. For example, remifentanil, succinylcholine, esmolol, and the ester local anesthetics are cleared in the plasma and tissues via ester hydrolysis.

Phase II Enzymes

Phase II enzymes include glucuronosyltrasferases, glutathione-S-transferases, N-acetyl-transferases, and sulfotransferases. Uridine diphosphate glucuronosyltransferase catalyzes the covalent addition of glucuronic acid to a variety of endogenous and exogenous compounds, rendering them more water soluble. Glucuronidation is an important metabolic pathway for several drugs used during anesthesia, including propofol, morphine (yielding morphine-3-glucuronide and the pharmacologically active morphine-6-glucuronide), and midazolam (yielding the pharmacologically active 1-hydroxymidazolam). Glutathione-S-transferase (GST) enzymes are primarily a defensive system for detoxification and protection against oxidative stress. N-acetylation catalyzed by *N*-acetyltransferase (NAT) is a common phase II reaction for metabolism of heterocyclic aromatic amines (particularly serotonin) and arylamines, including the inactivation of isoniazid.

Hepatic Clearance

The rate of metabolism for most anesthetic drugs is proportional to drug concentration, rending the clearance of the drug constant (i.e., independent of dose). This is a fundamental assumption for anesthetic pharmacokinetics. Exploring this assumption will provide insight into what clearance actually is and how it relates to the metabolism of drugs.

Although the metabolic capacity of the body is large, it is not possible that metabolism is *always* proportional to drug concentration because the liver does not have infinite metabolic capacity. At some rate of drug flow into the liver, the organ will be metabolizing drug as fast as the metabolic enzymes in the organ allow. At this point, metabolism can no longer be proportional to concentration because the metabolic capacity of the organ has been exceeded.

Understanding metabolism starts with a simple mass balance: the rate at which drug flows *out* of the liver must be the rate at which drug flows *into* the liver, minus the rate at which the liver metabolizes drug. The rate at which drug flows into the liver is liver blood flow, Q, times the concentration of drug flowing in, C_{inflow}. The rate at which drug flows out of the liver is liver blood flow, Q, times the concentration of drug flowing out, $C_{outflow}$. The rate of hepatic metabolism by the liver, R, is the difference between the drug concentration flowing into the liver and the drug concentration flowing out of the liver, times the rate of liver blood flow:

$$\text{Rate of drug metabolism} = R = Q(C_{inflow} - C_{outflow})$$

Equation 2-1

This relationship is illustrated in Figure 2-7.

Metabolism can be saturated because the liver does not have infinite metabolic capacity. A common equation used for this saturation processes is:

$$\text{Response} = \frac{C}{C_{50} + C}$$

Equation 2-2

"Response" in **Equation 2-2** varies from 0 to 1, depending on the value of *C*. In this context, Response is the

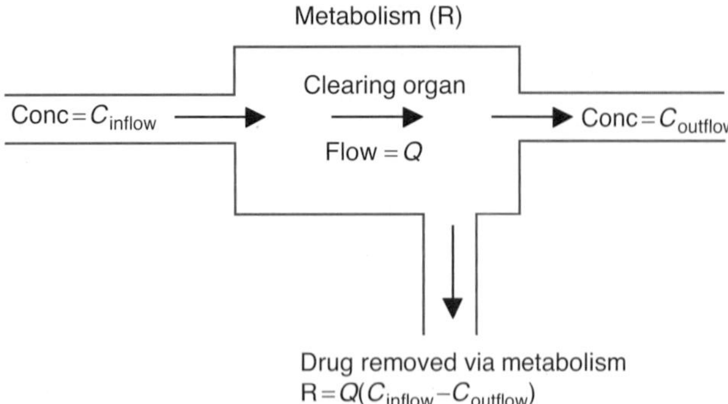

FIGURE 2-7 The relationship between drug rate of metabolism can be computed as the rate of liver blood flow times the difference between the inflowing and outflowing drug concentrations. This is a common approach to analyzing metabolism or tissue uptake across an organ in mass-balance pharmacokinetic studies. (From Shafer S, Flood P, Schwinn D. Basic principles of pharmacology. In: Miller RD, Eriksson LI, Fleisher LA, et al, eds. *Miller's Anesthesia.* Vol 1. 7th ed. Philadelphia, PA: Churchill Livingstone; 2010: 479–514, with permission.)

fraction of maximal metabolic rate. Response = 0 means no metabolism, and Response = 1 means metabolism at the maximal possible rate. C refers to whatever is driving the response. In this chapter, C means drug concentration. When C is 0, the response is 0. If C is greater than 0 but much less than C_{50}, the denominator is approximately C_{50} and the response is nearly proportional to C: Response $\approx \frac{C}{C_{50}}$. If we increase C even further to exactly C_{50}, then the response is $\frac{C_{50}}{C_{50} + C_{50}}$, which is simply 0.5. That is where the name "C_{50}" comes from: it is the concentration associated with 50% response. As C becomes much greater than C_{50}, the equation approaches $\frac{C}{C}$, which is 1. The shape of this relationship is shown in Figure 2-8. The relationship is nearly linear at low concentrations, but at high concentrations, the response saturates at 1.

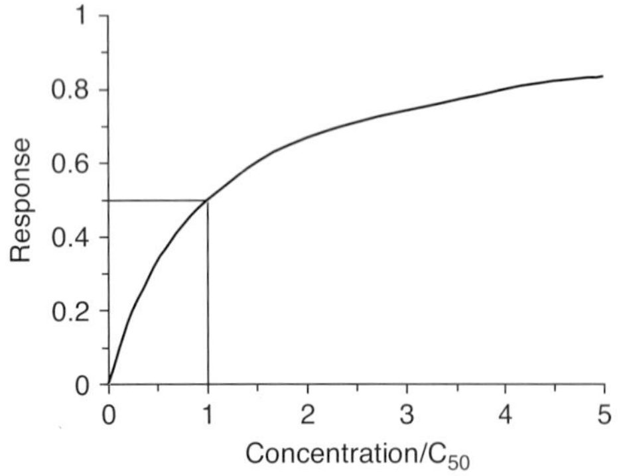

FIGURE 2-8 The shape of the saturation equation. (From Shafer S, Flood P, Schwinn D. Basic principles of pharmacology. In: Miller RD, Eriksson LI, Fleisher LA, et al, eds. *Miller's Anesthesia.* Vol 1. 7th ed. Philadelphia, PA: Churchill Livingstone; 2010:479–514, with permission.)

To understand hepatic clearance, we must understand the relationship between hepatic metabolism and drug concentration. But what concentration determines the rate of metabolism: the concentration flowing into the liver, the average concentration within the liver, or the concentration flowing out of the liver? All have been used, but the most common views the rate of metabolism as a function of the concentration flowing *out* of the liver, $C_{outflow}$.

We can expand our equation of metabolism to include the observation that the rate of metabolism, R, approaches saturation at the maximum metabolic rate, Vm, as a function of $C_{outflow}$:

$$\text{Rate of drug metabolism} = R = Q\,(C_{inflow} - C_{outflow}) = Vm\frac{C_{outflow}}{Km + C_{outflow}} \quad \text{Equation 2-3}$$

The saturation equation appears at the end of the aforementioned equation. Vm is the maximum possible metabolic rate. The saturation part of this equation, $\frac{C_{outflow}}{Km + C_{outflow}}$, determines fraction of the maximum metabolic rate. Km, the "Michaelis constant," is the outflow concentration at which the metabolic rate is 50% of the maximum rate (Vm). This relationship is shown in Figure 2-9. The x-axis is the outflow concentration, $C_{outflow}$, as a fraction Km. The y-axis is the rate of drug metabolism as a fraction of Vm. By normalizing the x- and y-axis in

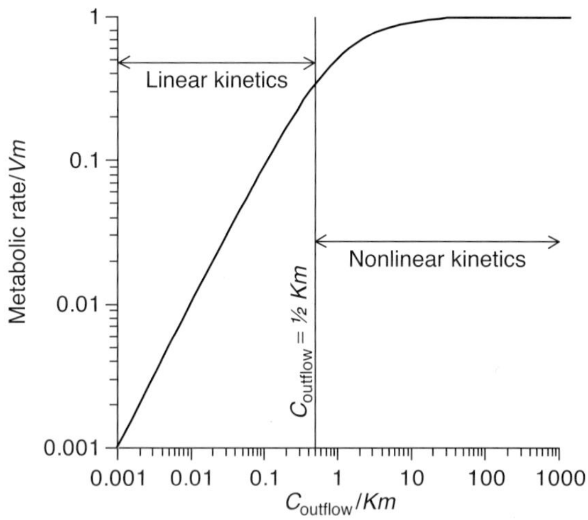

FIGURE 2-9 The relationship between concentration, here shown as a fraction of the Michaelis constant (Km), and drug metabolism, here shown as a fraction of the maximum rate (Vm). Metabolism increases proportionally with concentration as long as the outflow concentration is less than half Km, which corresponds to a metabolic rate that is roughly one-third of the maximal rate. Metabolism is proportional to concentration, meaning that clearance is constant, for typical doses of all intravenous drugs used in anesthesia. (From Shafer S, Flood P, Schwinn D. Basic principles of pharmacology. In: Miller RD, Eriksson LI, Fleisher LA, et al, eds. *Miller's Anesthesia.* Vol 1. 7th ed. Philadelphia, PA: Churchill Livingstone; 2010:479–514, with permission.)

this manner, the relationship shown in Figure 2-9 is true for all values of Vm and Km. As long as the outflow concentration is less than one-half of Km (true for almost all anesthetic drugs), there is a nearly proportional change in metabolic rate with a proportional change in outflow concentration. Another interpretation is that metabolism will be proportional to concentration as long as the metabolic rate is less than one-third of the maximum metabolic capacity.

So far, we have talked about the rate of metabolism and not about hepatic clearance. If the liver could completely extract the drug from the afferent flow, then clearance would equal liver blood flow, Q. However, the liver cannot remove every last drug molecule. There is always some drug in the effluent plasma. The fraction of inflowing drug extracted by the liver is $\frac{C_{inflow} - C_{outflow}}{C_{inflow}}$. This is called the ***extraction ratio***. Clearance is the amount of blood completely cleared of drug per unit time. We can calculate clearance as the liver blood flow times the extraction ratio

$$\text{Clearance} = Q \times ER = Q\left(\frac{C_{inflow} - C_{outflow}}{C_{inflow}}\right)$$

Equation 2-4

With this basic understanding of clearance, let us divide each part of Equation 2-3 by C_{inflow}:

$$\frac{\text{Rate of drug metabolism}}{C_{inflow}} = \frac{R}{C_{inflow}} =$$

$$Q\left(\frac{C_{inflow} - C_{outflow}}{C_{inflow}}\right) = \frac{C_{outflow}}{C_{inflow}}\left(\frac{Vm}{Km + C_{outflow}}\right)$$

Equation 2-5

The third term is clearance as defined in Equation 2-4: Q times the extraction ratio. Thus, each term in Equation 2-4 must be clearance. Let us consider them in order.

The first term tells us that Clearance $= \frac{\text{Rate of drug metabolism}}{C_{inflow}}$. This indicates that clearance is a proportionality constant that relates inflowing (e.g., arterial) concentration to the rate of metabolism. If we want to maintain a given steady-state arterial drug concentration, we must infuse drug at the same rate that it is being metabolized. With this understanding, we can rearrange the equation to say: Infusion rate = metabolic rate = Clearance $\times C_{inflow}$. Thus, the infusion rate to maintain a given concentration is the clearance times the desired concentration.

The third and fourth terms,

$$\text{Clearance} = Q\left(\frac{C_{inflow} - C_{outflow}}{C_{inflow}}\right)$$

and

$$\text{Clearance} = \frac{C_{outflow}}{C_{inflow}}\left(\frac{Vm}{Km + C_{outflow}}\right)$$

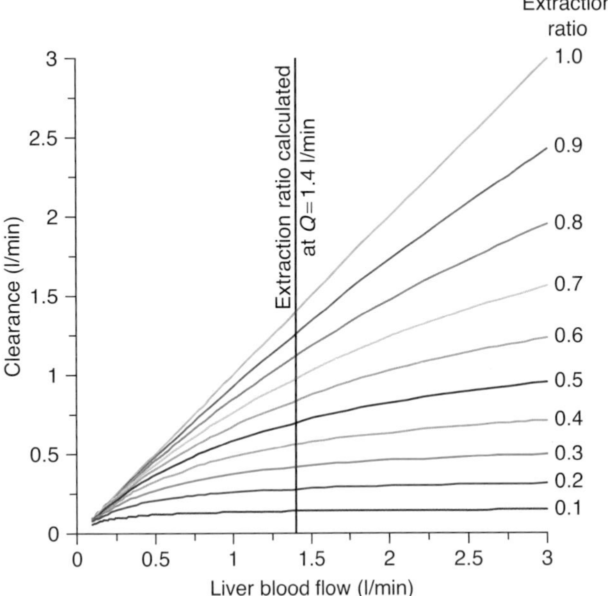

FIGURE 2-10 The relationship between liver blood flow (Q), clearance, and extraction ratio. For drugs with a high extraction ratio, clearance is nearly identical to liver blood flow. For drugs with a low extraction ratio, changes in liver blood flow have almost no effect on clearance. (From Shafer S, Flood P, Schwinn D. Basic principles of pharmacology. In: Miller RD, Eriksson LI, Fleisher LA, et al, eds. *Miller's Anesthesia*. Vol 1. 7th ed. Philadelphia, PA: Churchill Livingstone; 2010:479–514, with permission.)

are more interesting if taken together. Remembering that $\frac{C_{inflow} - C_{outflow}}{C_{inflow}}$ is the extraction ratio, these equations relate clearance to liver blood flow and the extraction ratio, as shown in Figure 2-10.[8] For drugs with an extraction ratio of nearly 1 (e.g., propofol), a change in liver blood flow produces a nearly proportional change in clearance. For drugs with a low extraction ratio (e.g., alfentanil), clearance is nearly independent of the rate of liver blood flow. This makes intuitive sense. If nearly 100% of the drug is extracted by the liver, then the liver has tremendous metabolic capacity for the drug. In this case, flow of drug to the liver is what limits the metabolic rate. Metabolism is "flow limited." The reduction in liver blood flow that accompanies anesthesia can be expected to reduce clearance. However, moderate changes in hepatic metabolic function per se will have little impact on clearance because hepatic metabolic capacity is overwhelmingly in excess of demand.

Conversely, for drugs with an extraction ratio considerably less than 1, clearance is limited by the capacity of the liver to take up and metabolize the drug. Metabolism is "capacity limited." Clearance will change in response to any change in the capacity of the liver to metabolize such drugs, such as might be caused by liver disease or enzymatic induction. However, changes in liver blood flow, as might be caused by the anesthetic state itself, usually have

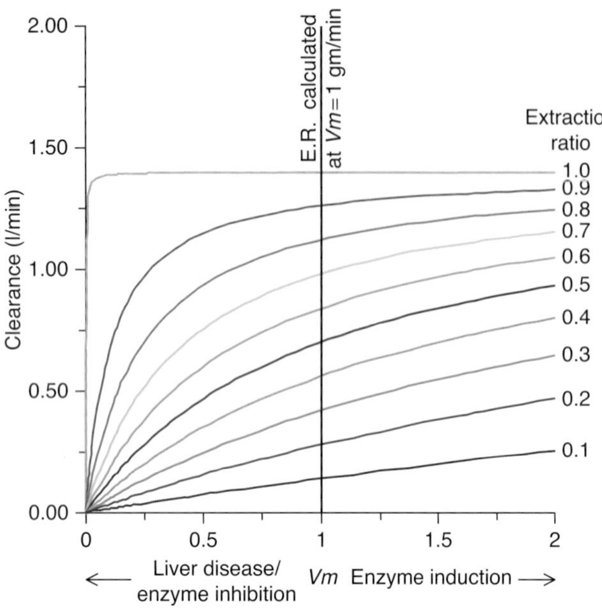

FIGURE 2-11 Changes in maximum metabolic velocity (*Vm*) have little effect on drugs with a high extraction ratio but cause a nearly proportional decrease in clearance for drugs with a low extraction ratio. (From Shafer S, Flood P, Schwinn D. Basic principles of pharmacology. In: Miller RD, Eriksson LI, Fleisher LA, et al, eds. *Miller's Anesthesia.* Vol 1. 7th ed. Philadelphia, PA: Churchill Livingstone; 2010: 479–514, with permission.)

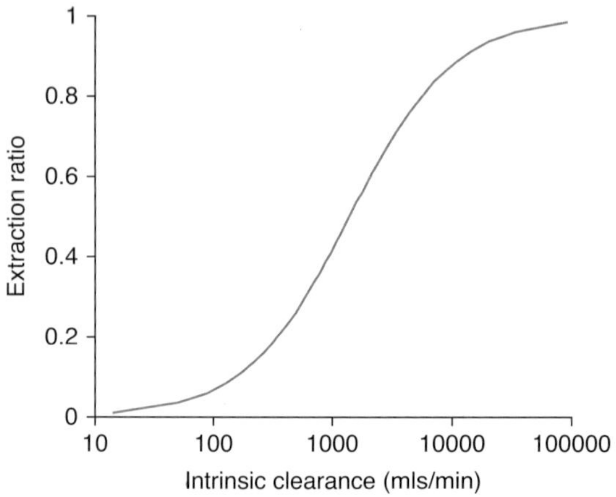

FIGURE 2-12 The extraction ratio as a function of the intrinsic calculated for a liver blood flow of 1,400 mL/min. (From Shafer S, Flood P, Schwinn D. Basic principles of pharmacology. In: Miller RD, Eriksson LI, Fleisher LA, et al, eds. *Miller's Anesthesia.* Vol 1. 7th ed. Philadelphia, PA: Churchill Livingstone; 2010:479–514, with permission.)

little influence on the clearance because the liver only handles a fraction of the drug it sees. This relationship can be seen in Figure 2-11.

We can also put the third and fourth terms of the clearance equation together to show how extraction ratio governs the response of clearance to changes in metabolic capacity (*Vm*). Figure 2-11 shows the clearance for drugs with an extraction ratio ranging from 0.1 to 1, based on a liver blood flow of 1.4 L per minute. The extraction ratios were calculated for a $Vm = 1$. Changes in *Vm*, as might be caused by liver disease (reduced *Vm*) or enzymatic induction (increased *Vm*) have little effect on drugs with a high extraction ratio. However, drugs with a low extraction ratio have a nearly linear change in clearance with a change in intrinsic metabolic capacity (*Vm*).

Vm and *Km* are usually not known and condensed into a single term, $\frac{Vm}{Km}$. This term summarizes the hepatic metabolic capacity and is called ***intrinsic clearance***. Because clearance $= \frac{C_{outflow}}{C_{inflow}}\left(\frac{Vm}{Km + C_{outflow}}\right)$, consider what happens if hepatic blood flow increases to infinity (this is a thought experiment). At super high hepatic blood flow, $C_{outflow}$ becomes indistinguishable from C_{inflow} because the finite hepatic capacity only metabolizes an infinitesimal fraction of the drug flowing through the liver. As a result, clearance becomes $\frac{Vm}{Km + C_{outflow}}$. We can solve for this in the "linear range" by finding clearance when $C_{inflow} = 0$, $\frac{Vm}{Km}$. This is the intrinsic clearance, Cl_{int}. It can be demonstrated algebraically from the definition of Cl_{int} that in the linear range, Cl_{int} is directly related to the extraction ratio: $\frac{Cl_{\text{int}}}{Q + Cl_{\text{int}}}$. Combining this with Equation 2-5 yields the relationship between hepatic clearance and Cl_{int}:

$$\text{Hepatic Clearance} = \frac{Q\,Cl_{\text{int}}}{Q + Cl_{int}} \qquad \text{Equation 2-6}$$

The relationship between intrinsic clearance and extraction ratio is shown in Figure 2-12, calculated at a hepatic blood flow of 1,400 mL/min. In general, true hepatic clearance and extraction ratio are more useful concepts for anesthetic drugs than the intrinsic clearance. However, intrinsic clearance is introduced here because it is occasionally used in pharmacokinetic analyses of drugs used during anesthesia.

So far, we have focused on linear pharmacokinetics, that is, the pharmacokinetics of drugs whose metabolic rate at clinical doses is less than *Vm*/3. The clearance of such drugs is generally expressed as a constant (e.g., propofol clearance = 1.6 L per minute). Some drugs, such as phenytoin, exhibit saturable pharmacokinetics (i.e., have such low *Vm* that typical doses exceed the linear portion of Figure 2-9). The clearance of drugs with saturable metabolism is a function of drug concentration, rather than a constant.

Renal Clearance

Renal excretion of drugs involves (a) glomerular filtration, (b) active tubular secretion, and (c) passive tubular reabsorption. The amount of drug that enters the renal tubular lumen depends on the fraction of drug bound to protein and the glomerular filtration rate (GFR). Renal tubular secretion involves active transport processes, which may be selective for certain drugs and metabolites, including protein-bound compounds. Reabsorption from renal tubules removes drug that has entered tubules by glomerular filtration and tubular secretion. This reabsorption is most prominent for lipid-soluble drugs that can easily cross cell membranes of renal tubular epithelial cells to enter pericapillary fluid. Indeed, a highly lipid-soluble drug, such as thiopental, is almost completely reabsorbed such that little or no unchanged drug is excreted in the urine. Conversely, production of less lipid-soluble metabolites limits renal tubule reabsorption and facilitates excretion in the urine.

The rate of reabsorption from renal tubules is influenced by factors such as pH and rate of renal tubular urine flow. Passive reabsorption of weak bases and acids is altered by urine pH, which influences the fraction of drug that exists in the ionized form. For example, weak acids are excreted more rapidly in alkaline urine. This occurs because alkalinization of the urine results in more ionized drug that cannot easily cross renal tubular epithelial cells, resulting in less passive reabsorption.

Renal blood flow is inversely correlated with age, as is creatinine clearance, which is closely related to GFR because creatinine is water soluble and not resorbed in the tubules. Creatinine clearance can be predicted from age and weight according to the equation of Cockroft and Gault[9]:

Men:

$$\text{Creatinine Clearance (ml/min)} = \frac{[140 - \text{age(years)}] \times \text{weight(kgs)}}{72 \times \text{serum creatinine (mg\%)}} \quad \text{Equation 2-7}$$

Women:

85% of the aforementioned equation.

Equation 2-7 shows that age is an independent predictor of creatinine clearance. Elderly patients with normal serum creatinine have about half the GFR than younger patients. This can be seen graphically in Figure 2-13.

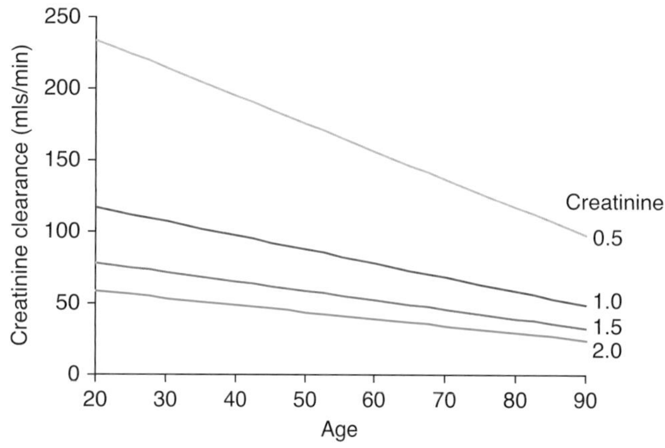

FIGURE 2-13 Creatinine clearance as a function of age and serum creatinine based on the equation of Cockroft and Gault. (From Cockcroft DW, Gault MH. Prediction of creatinine clearance from serum creatinine. *Nephron*. 1976;16:31–41, with permission.)

Absorption

Classically, pharmacokinetics is taught as "absorption, distribution, metabolism, and elimination." Because most anesthetic drugs are administered intravenously and inhaled anesthetic pharmacokinetics are discussed elsewhere, this order has been changed in this textbook to put absorption at the end of the list. Absorption is simply not particularly relevant for most anesthetic drugs.

Ionization

Most drugs are weak acids or bases that are present in solutions in ionized and nonionized form. The nonionized molecule is usually lipid soluble and can diffuse across cell membranes including the blood–brain barrier, renal tubular epithelium, gastrointestinal epithelium, placenta, and hepatocytes (Table 2-1). As a result, it is usually the nonionized form of the drug that is pharmacologically active, undergoes reabsorption across renal tubules, is absorbed from the gastrointestinal tract, and is susceptible to hepatic metabolism. Conversely, the ionized fraction is poorly lipid soluble and cannot penetrate lipid cell membranes easily (see Table 2-1). A high degree of ionization thus impairs absorption of drug from the gastrointestinal tract, limits access to drug-metabolizing enzymes in the hepatocytes, and facilitates excretion of unchanged drug, as reabsorption across the renal tubular epithelium is unlikely.

Determinants of Degree of Ionization

The degree of drug ionization is a function of its dissociation constant (pK) and the pH of the surrounding fluid. When the pK and the pH are identical, 50% of the drug exists in both the ionized and nonionized form. Small changes in pH can result in large changes in the extent of ionization, especially if the pH and pK values are similar. Acidic

Table 2-1

Characteristics of Nonionized and Ionized Drug Molecules

	Nonionized	Ionized
Pharmacologic effect	Active	Inactive
Solubility	Lipids	Water
Cross lipid barriers (gastrointestinal tract, blood–brain barrier, placenta)	Yes	No
Renal excretion	No	Yes
Hepatic metabolism	Yes	No

drugs, such as barbiturates, tend to be highly ionized at an alkaline pH, whereas basic drugs, such as opioids and local anesthetics, are highly ionized at an acid pH. Acidic drugs are usually supplied in a basic solution to make them more soluble in water and basic drugs are usually supplied in an acidic solution for the same reason, unless the pH affects drug stability, as is the case for most ester local anesthetics.

Ion Trapping

Because it is the nonionized drug that equilibrates across lipid membranes, a concentration difference of total drug can develop on two sides of a membrane that separates fluids with different pHs,[10] because the ionized concentrations will reflect the local equilibration between ionized and nonionized forms based on the pH. This is an important consideration because one fraction of the drug may be more pharmacologically active than the other fraction.

Systemic administration of a weak base, such as an opioid, can result in accumulation of ionized drug (ion trapping) in the acid environment of the stomach. A similar phenomenon occurs in the transfer of basic drugs, such as local anesthetics, across the placenta from mother to fetus because the fetal pH is lower than maternal pH. The lipid-soluble nonionized fraction of local anesthetic crosses the placenta and is converted to the poorly lipid-soluble ionized fraction in the more acidic environment of the fetus. The ionized fraction in the fetus cannot easily cross the placenta to the maternal circulation and thus is effectively trapped in the fetus. At the same time, conversion of the nonionized to ionized fraction maintains a gradient for continued passage of local anesthetic into the fetus. The resulting accumulation of local anesthetic in the fetus is accentuated by the acidosis that accompanies fetal distress. The kidneys are the most important organs for the elimination of unchanged drugs or their metabolites. Water-soluble compounds are excreted more efficiently by the kidneys than are compounds with high lipid solubility. This emphasizes the important role of metabolism in converting lipid-soluble drugs to water-soluble metabolites. Drug elimination by the kidneys is correlated with endogenous creatinine clearance or serum creatinine concentration. The magnitude of change in these indices provides an estimate of the necessary change adjustment in drug dosage. Although age and many diseases are associated with a decrease in creatinine clearance and requirement for decreased dosing, pregnancy is associated with an increase in creatinine clearance and higher dose requirements for some drugs.

Route of Administration and Systemic Absorption of Drugs

The choice of route of administration for a drug should be determined by factors that influence the systemic absorption of drugs. The systemic absorption rate of a drug determines the magnitude of the drug effect and duration of action. Changes in the systemic absorption rate may necessitate an adjustment in the dose or time interval between repeated drug doses.

Systemic absorption, regardless of the route of drug administration, depends on the drug's solubility. Local conditions at the site of absorption alter solubility, particularly in the gastrointestinal tract. Blood flow to the site of absorption is also important in the rapidity of absorption. For example, increased blood flow evoked by rubbing or applying heat at the subcutaneous or intramuscular injection site enhances systemic absorption, whereas decreased blood flow due to vasoconstriction impedes drug absorption. Finally, the area of the absorbing surface available for drug absorption is an important determinant of drug entry into the circulation.

Oral Administration

Oral administration of a drug is often the most convenient and economic route of administration. Disadvantages of the oral route include (a) emesis caused by irritation of the gastrointestinal mucosa by the drug, (b) destruction of the drug by digestive enzymes or acidic gastric fluid, and (c) irregularities in absorption in the presence of food or other drugs. Furthermore, drugs may be metabolized by enzymes or bacteria in the gastrointestinal tract before systemic absorption can occur.

With oral administration, the onset of drug effect is largely determined by the rate and extent of absorption from the gastrointestinal tract. The principal site of drug absorption after oral administration is the small intestine due to the large surface area of this portion of the gastrointestinal tract. Changes in the pH of gastrointestinal fluid that favor the presence of a drug in its nonionized (lipid-soluble) fraction thus favor systemic absorption. Drugs that exist as weak acids (such as aspirin) become highly ionized in the alkaline environment of the small intestine, but absorption is still great because of the large surface area. Furthermore, absorption also occurs in the stomach, where the fluid is acidic.

First-Pass Hepatic Effect

Drugs absorbed from the gastrointestinal tract enter the portal venous blood and thus pass through the liver before entering the systemic circulation for delivery to tissue receptors. This is known as the ***first-pass hepatic effect***. For drugs that undergo extensive hepatic extraction and metabolism (propranolol, lidocaine), it is the reason for large differences in the pharmacologic effect between oral and intravenous doses.

Oral Transmucosal Administration

The sublingual or buccal route of administration permits a rapid onset of drug effect because this blood bypasses the liver and thus prevents the first-pass hepatic effect on the initial plasma concentration of drug. Venous drainage from the sublingual area is into the superior vena cava. Evidence of the value of bypassing the first-pass hepatic effect is the efficacy of sublingual nitroglycerin. Conversely, oral administration of nitroglycerin is ineffective because extensive first-pass hepatic metabolism prevents establishment of a therapeutic plasma concentration. Buccal administration is an alternative to sublingual placement of a drug; it is better tolerated and less likely to stimulate salivation. The nasal mucosa also provides an effective absorption surface for certain drugs.

Transdermal Administration

Transdermal administration of drugs provides sustained therapeutic plasma concentrations of the drug and decreases the likelihood of loss of therapeutic efficacy due to peaks and valleys associated with conventional intermittent drug injections. This route of administration is devoid of the complexity of continuous infusion techniques, and the low incidence of side effects (because of the small doses used) contributes to high patient compliance. Characteristics of drugs that favor predictable transdermal absorption include (a) combined water and lipid solubility, (b) molecular weight of $<1,000$, (c) pH 5 to 9 in a saturated aqueous solution, (d) absence of histamine-releasing effects, and (e) daily dose requirements of <10 mg. Scopolamine, fentanyl, clonidine, estrogen, progesterone, and nitroglycerin are drugs available in transdermal delivery systems. Unfortunately, sustained plasma concentrations provided by transdermal absorption of scopolamine and nitroglycerin may result in tolerance and loss of therapeutic effect.

It is likely that transdermal absorption of drugs initially occurs along sweat ducts and hair follicles that function as diffusion shunts. The rate-limiting step in transdermal absorption of drugs is diffusion across the stratum corneum of the epidermis. Differences in the thickness and chemistry of the stratum corneum are reflected in the skin's permeability. For example, skin may be 10 to 20 μm thick on the back and abdomen compared with 400 to 600 μm on the palmar surfaces of the hands. Likewise, skin permeation studies have shown substantial regional differences for systemic absorption of scopolamine. The postauricular zone, because of its thin epidermal layer and somewhat higher temperature, is the only area that is sufficiently permeable for predictable and sustained absorption of scopolamine. The stratum corneum sloughs and regenerates at a rate that makes 7 days of adhesion the duration limit for one application of a transdermal system. Contact dermatitis at the site of transdermal patch applications occurs in a significant number of patients.

Rectal Administration

Drugs administered into the proximal rectum are absorbed into the superior hemorrhoidal veins and subsequently transported via the portal venous system to the liver (first-pass hepatic effect), where they are exposed to metabolism before entering the systemic circulation. On the other hand, drugs absorbed from a low rectal administration site reach the systemic circulation without first passing through the liver. These factors, in large part, explain the unpredictable responses that follow rectal administration of drugs. Furthermore, drugs may cause irritation of the rectal mucosa.

Pharmacokinetic Models

In the following section, several common, useful pharmacokinetic models are derived. Although it is not necessary for every clinician to be able to derive these models, a consideration of where they come from takes them out of the "black box" and allows consideration of their representative parts.

Zero- and First-Order Processes

The consumption of oxygen and production of carbon dioxide are processes that happen at a constant rate. These are called ***zero-order processes***. The rate of change (dx/dt) for a zero-order process is $\frac{dx}{dt} = k$. This says the rate of change is constant. If x represents an amount of drug and t represents time, then the units of k are amount/time. If we want to know the value of x at time t, $x(t)$, we can compute it as the integral of this equation from time 0 to time t, $x(t) = x_0 + k \cdot t$, where x_0 is the value of x at time 0. This is the equation of a straight line with a slope of k and an intercept of x_0.

Many processes occur at a rate proportional to the amount. For example, the interest payment on a loan is proportional to the outstanding balance. The rate at which water drains from a bathtub is proportional to amount (height) of water in the tub. These are examples of first-order processes. The rate of change in a first-order process is only slightly more complex than for a zero-order process, $\frac{dx}{dt} = k \cdot x$. In this equation, x has units of amount already, so the units of k are 1/time. The value of x at time t, $x(t)$, can be computed as the integral from time 0 to time t, $x(t) = x_0\, e^{kt}$, where x_0 is the value of x at time 0. If $k > 0$, $x(t)$ increases exponentially to infinity. If $k < 0$, $x(t)$ decreases exponentially to 0. In pharmacokinetics, k is negative because concentrations decrease over time. For clarity, the minus sign is usually explicit, so k is expressed as a positive number. Thus, the identical equation for pharmacokinetics, with the minus sign explicitly written, is

$$x(t) = x_0\, e^{-kt} \qquad \text{Equation 2-8}$$

Figure 2-14A shows the exponential relationship between x and time. x continuously decreases over time. Taking the natural logarithm of both sides of $x(t) = x_0\, e^{-kt}$ gives:

$$\begin{aligned} \ln\left[x(t)\right] &= \ln\left(x_0 \cdot e^{-kt}\right) \\ &= \ln\left(x_0\right) + \ln\left(e^{-kt}\right) \\ &= \ln\left(x_0\right) - k \cdot t \end{aligned} \qquad \text{Equation 2-9}$$

This is the equation of a straight line, as shown in Figure 2-14B, where the vertical axis is $\ln\left[x(t)\right]$, the

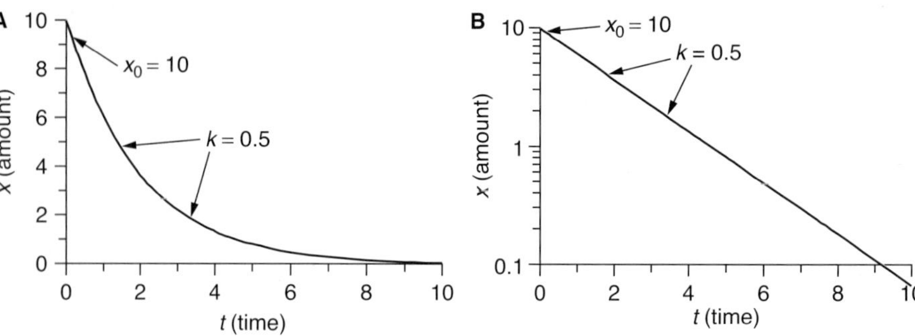

FIGURE 2-14 Exponential decay curve, as given by $x(t) = x_0e^{-kt}$, plotted on standard axis **(A)** and a logarithmic axis **(B)**.

horizontal axis is t, the intercept is $\ln(x_0)$, and the slope of the line is $-k$. How long will it take for x to go from some value, x_1, to half that value, $x_{1/2}$? Because k is the slope of a straight line relating $\ln(x)$ to time, it follows that

$$k = \frac{\Delta \ln(x)}{\Delta t} = \frac{\ln(x_1) - \ln\left(\frac{x_1}{2}\right)}{t½} = \frac{n\left[\frac{x_1}{\left(\frac{x_1}{2}\right)}\right]}{t½}$$

$$= \frac{\ln(2)}{t½} \approx \frac{0.693}{t½} \qquad \text{Equation 2-10}$$

where $t½$ is the "half-life," the time required for a 50% decrease in x. The natural log of 2 is close enough to 0.693 for the authors' purposes that "$\approx$" is replaced with "$=$" for readability. Thus, the relationship of the slope (or "rate constant"), k, to half-life, $t½$ is $k = \frac{0.693}{t½}$. If we measure the time it takes for x to fall by 50%, $t½$, then we know the rate constant, k. Conversely, if we know k, the rate constant, we can easily calculate the time it will take for x to fall by 50% as

$$t½ = \frac{0.693}{k} \qquad \text{Equation 2-11}$$

Physiologic Pharmacokinetic Models

It is possible to analyze volumes and clearances for each organ in the body and construct models of pharmacokinetics by assembling the organ models into physiologically and anatomically accurate models of the entire animal. Figure 2-15 shows such a model for thiopental in rats.[11] However, models that work with individual tissues are mathematically cumbersome and do not offer a better prediction of plasma drug concentration than models that lump the tissues into a few compartments. If the goal is to determine how to give drugs in order to obtain therapeutic plasma drug concentrations, then all that is needed is to mathematically relate dose to plasma concentration. For this purpose, "compartmental" models are usually adequate.

Compartmental Pharmacokinetic Models

Compartmental models are built on the same basic concepts as physiologic models. The "one-compartment model" (Fig. 2-16A) contains a single volume and a single clearance, as though we were buckets of fluid. For anesthetic drugs, we resemble several buckets connected by pipes. These are usually modeled using two- or three-compartment models, Figure 2-16B,C. The volume to the left in the two-compartment model and in the center of the three-compartment model is the central volume where drug is injected. The other volumes are peripheral volumes of distribution. The sum of the all volumes is the volume of distribution at steady state, Vd_{ss}. The clearance leaving the central compartment for the outside is the "systemic" clearance, in that it clears drug from the entire system. The clearances between the central compartment and the peripheral compartments are the "intercompartmental" clearances. Although the concept of compartments yields useful mathematics for planning dosing, when experimental animals were flash frozen at different times following administration of anesthetic drugs, and characterized using physiologic models, compartments identified in simple compartment model could not be anatomically identified.[12] Other than clearance, none of the parameters of compartment models readily translates into any anatomic structure or physiologic process.

One-Compartment Model

Bolus Pharmacokinetics

Returning to the one-compartment bucket, call the amount of drug poured into the bucket x_0 (x at time 0). The initial concentration is x_0/V, where V is the volume of fluid in the bucket. Remembering that the definition of concentration is dose (or amount) per volume, we can rearrange this to calculate the dose required to achieve a specific target concentration, C_T (target concentration), based on V, the volume in the bucket: Dose $= C_T \times V$.

Let us assume that the fluid is being circulated through a clearing organ at a constant rate, which we will call ***clearance***, *Cl*. What is the rate, dx/dt, that drug, x, is leaving the bucket? Because concentration is x/V and Cl is the rate that the fluid in the bucket is through the clearing organ, then the rate at which the drug is leaving must be $x/V \times Cl$, which is the concentration times the flow rate. This rate is a first-order process if, and only if, it equals a constant, k, times the amount of drug, x, in the bucket. It does because we can arrange the equation as $x \times Cl/V$. Because Cl and V are both constants,

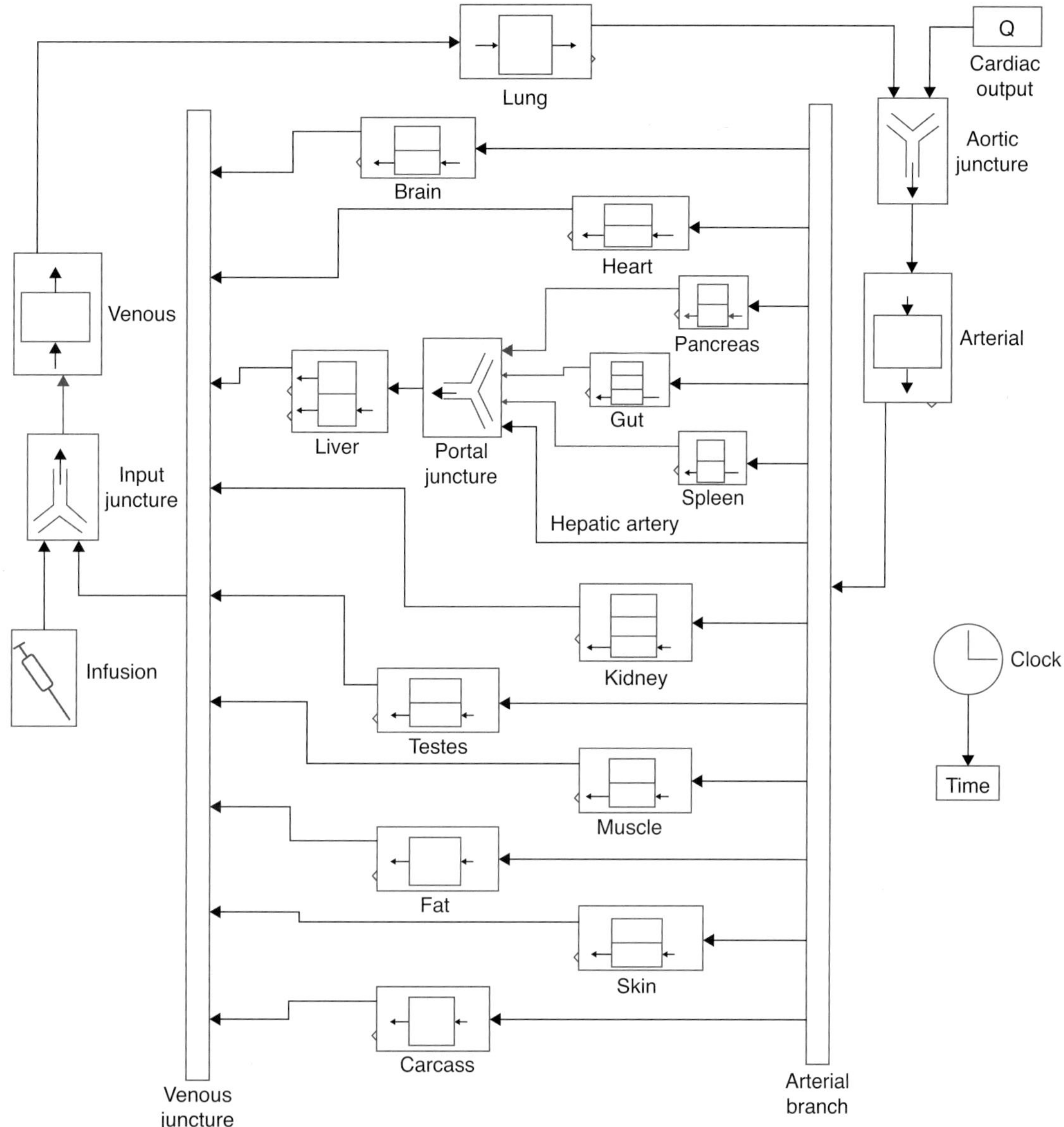

FIGURE 2-15 Physiologic model for thiopental in rats. The pharmacokinetics of distribution into each organ has been individually determined. The components of the model are linked by zero-order (flow) and first-order (diffusion) processes. (From Ebling WF, Wada DR, Stanski DR. From piecewise to full physiologic pharmacokinetic modeling: applied to thiopental disposition in the rat. *J Pharmacokinetic Biopharm.* 1994;22:259–292, with permission.)

we can define k as Cl/V. Therefore, the rate is $x \times k$, which defines a first-order process. This can be rearranged to yields the fundamental identity of linear pharmacokinetics:

$$Cl \text{ (clearance)} = k \text{ (rate constant)} \times V \text{ (volume of distribution)}$$

What does this identity tell us about the relationship between half-life, volume, and clearance? Rearranging the aforementioned equation as $k = \frac{Cl}{V}$ and remembering that $t½ = \frac{0.693}{k}$, we can conclude that half-life is proportional to volume and inversely proportional to clearance.

$$t½ = 0.693 \frac{V}{Cl} \qquad \text{Equation 2-12}$$

Consider two alternative models, one with a large volume and a small clearance, Figure 2-17A, and one with a small volume and a large clearance, Figure 2-17B. It is (hopefully) intuitively obvious that following bolus injection, concentrations will fall more quickly (shorter half-life) with the larger clearance, as predicted by Equation 2-12.

Because this is a first-order process, let us calculate the concentration of drug that remains in the bucket as drug is being cleared following bolus injection. Using the equation that describes first-order processes, $x(t) = x_0 e^{-kt}$, $x(t)$ is the amount of drug at time t, x_0 is the amount of drug right after bolus injection, and k is the rate constant (Cl/V). If we divide both sides by V, and remember that x/V is the definition of concentration, we get the equation

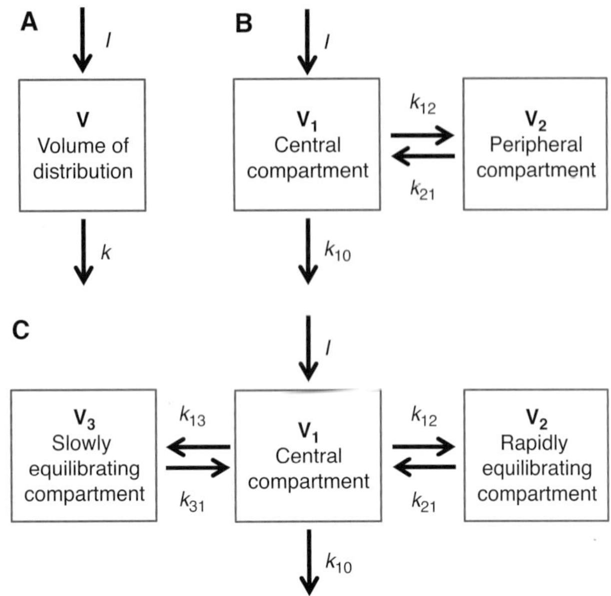

FIGURE 2-16 Standard one- **(A)**, two- **(B)**, and three-compartment **(C)** mammillary pharmacokinetic models. *I* represents any input into the system (e.g., bolus or infusion). The volumes are represented by *V* and the rate constants by *k*. The subscripts on rate constants indicate the direction of flow, noted as $k_{\text{from to}}$.

that relates concentration following an intravenous bolus to time and initial concentration:

$$C(t) = C_0\, e^{-kt} \qquad \text{Equation 2-13}$$

This equation defines the "concentration over time" curve for a one-compartment model and has the log linear shape seen in Figure 2-14B.

In a typical experiment, we start with the concentrations, as seen in Figure 2-14, and calculate clearance in one of two ways. First, we can calculate *V* by rearranging the definition of concentration, V = dose/initial concentration = $dose/C_0$. If you know the dose and you measure C_0 in the experiment, you can calculate *V*. If you then fit the log (*C*) line versus time line to a straight line, you can directly measure the slope, $-k$. You can then calculate clearance as $k \cdot V$.

A more general solution is to consider the integral of the concentration over time curve, $C(t) = C_0\, e^{-kt}$, known in pharmacokinetics as the area under the curve, or AUC:

$$\begin{aligned} AUC &= \int_0^\infty C_0 e^{-kt} dt \\ &= \int_0^\infty \frac{x_0}{V}\left(e^{-\frac{Cl}{V}t}\right) dt \text{ (substituting for } C_0 \text{ and } k) \\ &= \frac{x_0}{V} \times \frac{V}{Cl} \text{ (evaluating the above integral)} \\ &= \frac{x_0}{Cl} \end{aligned} \qquad \text{Equation 2-14}$$

We can rearrange the right side and the last term on the left side to solve for clearance, *Cl*:

$$Cl = \frac{x_0}{AUC} \qquad \text{Equation 2-15}$$

Because x_0 is the dose of drug, clearance equals the dose divided by the AUC. This fundamental property of *linear* pharmacokinetic models applies to one-compartment models, multicompartment models, and to any type of intravenous drug dosing (provided the *total* dose

FIGURE 2-17 The relationship between volume and clearance and half-life can be envisioned by considering two settings: a big volume and a small clearance **(A)** and a small volume with a big clearance **(B)**. Drug will be eliminated faster in the latter case.

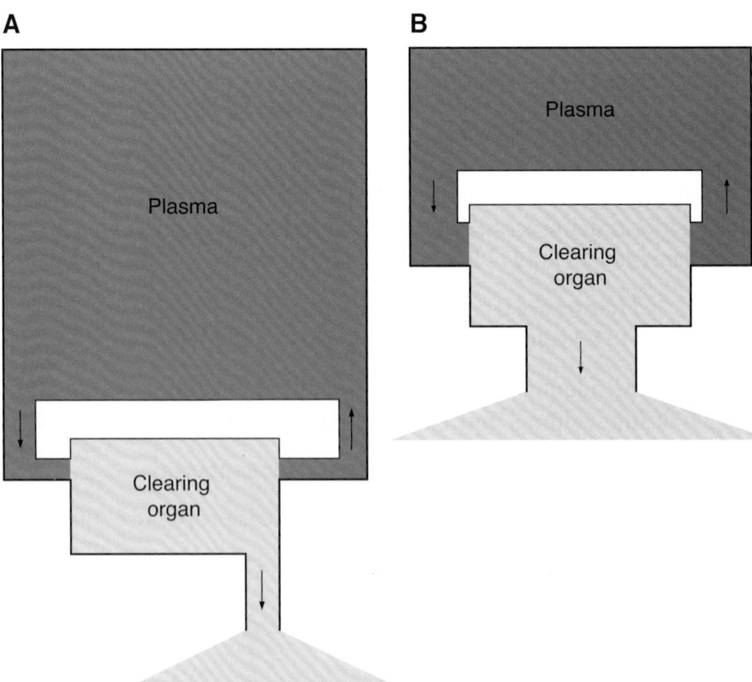

administered systemically is used as the numerator). It directly follows that AUC is proportional to dose for linear models (i.e., models where Cl is constant).

Infusion Pharmacokinetics

If you give an infusion at a rate of I (for Input), the plasma concentration will rise as long as the rate of drug going in the body, I, exceeds the rate at which drug leaves the body, $C \cdot Cl$, where C is the drug concentration. Once, $I = C \cdot Cl$, drug is going in and coming out at the same rate, and the body is at steady state. We can calculate the concentration at steady state by observing that the rate of drug going in must equal the rate of drug coming out. We have determined that that rate of drug metabolism at steady state is themetabolic rate $= C_{ss} \cdot Cl$, where C_{ss} is the arterial concentration at steady state. Because by definition at steady state the infusion rate equals the metabolic rate, the infusion rate, I, at steady state must be $I = C_{ss} \cdot Cl$. Solving this for the concentration at steady state, C_{ss} gives $C_{ss} = \frac{I}{Cl}$. Thus, the steady-state concentration during an infusion is the rate of drug input divided by the clearance. It follows that if we want to calculate the infusion rate that will achieve a given target concentration, C_T, at steady state, then the infusion rate must be $C_T \cdot Cl$.

$C_\infty = \frac{I}{Cl}$ is similar in form to the equation describing the concentration following a bolus injection: $C_0 = \frac{x_0}{V}$. Thus, volume is a scalar relating bolus to initial concentration, and clearance is a scalar relating infusion rate to steady-state concentration. It follows that the initial concentration following a bolus is independent of the clearance, and the steady-state concentration during a continuous infusion is independent of the volume.

During an infusion, the rate of change in the amount of drug, x, is rate of inflow, I, minus the rate of outflow, $k \cdot x$, which is represented as $\frac{dx}{dt} = I - kx$. We can calculate x at any time t as the integral from time 0 to time t. Assuming that we are starting with no drug in the body (i.e., $x_0 = 0$) the result is $x(t) = \frac{I}{k}\left(1 - e^{-kt}\right)$. If we divide both sides by volume, V, and remember that $Cl = k \cdot V$, we can solve this equation for concentration: $C(t) = \frac{I}{Cl}\left(1 - e^{-kt}\right)$. This is the equation for concentration during an infusion in a one-compartment model.

As $t \to \infty$, $e^{-kt} \to 0$, the equation $x(t) = \frac{I}{k}\left(1 - e^{-kt}\right)$ reduces to $x_{ss} = \frac{I}{k}$. During an infusion, the amount in the body approaches x_{ss} (steady state) asymptotically, only reaching it at infinity. However, we can calculate how long does it take to get to half of the steady-state amount, $\frac{x_{ss}}{2}$. If $x_{ss} = \frac{I}{k}$, then $\frac{x_{ss}}{2} = \frac{I}{2k}$. Because $\frac{I}{2k}$ is the amount of drug when we are halfway to steady state, we can substitute that for the amount of drug in our formula $x(t) = \frac{I}{k}\left(1 - e^{-kt}\right)$, giving us $\frac{I}{2k} = \frac{I}{k}\left(1 - e^{-kt}\right)$, and solve that for t. The solution is $t\tfrac{1}{2} = \frac{\ln(2)}{k}$. This is the time to rise to half steady state. Recall that $t\tfrac{1}{2}$, the half time to decrease to 0, following a bolus injection was $\frac{\ln(2)}{k}$. We again have a parallel between boluses and infusions. Following a bolus, it takes 1 half-life to reduce the concentrations by half, and during an infusion, it takes 1 half-life to increase the concentration halfway to steady state. Similarly, it takes 2 half-lives to reach 75%, 3 half-lives to reach 87.5%, and 5 half-lives to reach 97% of the steady-state concentration. By 4 to 5 half-lives, we typically consider the patient to be at steady state, although the concentrations only asymptotically approach the steady-state value.

Absorption Pharmacokinetics

When drugs are given intravenously, every molecule reaches the systemic circulation. When drugs are given by a different route, such as orally, transdermally, or intramuscularly, the drug must first reach the systemic circulation. Oral drugs may be only partly absorbed. What is absorbed then has to get past the liver ("first-pass hepatic metabolism") before reaching the systemic circulation. Transdermally applied drugs may be rubbed off, removed with soap or alcohol, or be sloughed off with the stratum corneum without being absorbed. The dose of drug that eventually reaches the systemic circulation with alternative routes of drug delivery is the administered dose times f, the fraction "bioavailable."

Alternative routes of drug delivery are often modeled by assuming the drug is absorbed from a reservoir or depot, usually modeled as an additional compartment with a monoexponential rate of transfer to the systemic circulation, $A(t) = f \cdot D_{oral} \cdot k_a \cdot e^{-k_a t}$, where $A(t)$ is the absorption rate at time t, f is the fraction bioavailable, D_{oral} is the dose taken orally (or intramuscularly, applied to the skin, etc). k_a is the absorption rate constant. Because the integral of $k_a\, e^{-k_a t}$ is 1, the total amount of drug absorbed is $f \cdot D_{oral}$. To compute the concentrations over time, we first reduce the problem to differential equations and integrate. The differential equation for the amount, x, with oral absorption into a one-compartment disposition model is:

$$\frac{dx}{dt} = \text{inflow} - \text{outflow} = A(t) - k \cdot x = f \cdot D_{oral} \cdot k_a \cdot e^{-k_a t} - k \cdot x \quad \text{Equation 2-16}$$

This is simply the rate of absorption at time t, $A(t)$, minus the rate of exit, $k \cdot x$. The amount of drug, x, in the compartment at time t is the integral of this from 0 to time t:

$$x(t) = \frac{D_{oral} f\, k_a}{k - k_a}\left(e^{-k_a t} - e^{-kt}\right) \quad \text{Equation 2-17}$$

This equation describes the amount of drug in the systemic circulation following first-order absorption from a depot, such as the stomach, an intramuscular injection, the skin, or even an epidural dose. To describe the concentrations, rather than amounts of drug, it is necessary to divide both sides by V, the volume of distribution.

Multicompartment Models

The previous section used one-compartment model to introduce concepts of rate constants and half-lives and relate them to the physiologic concepts of volume and clearance. Unfortunately, none of the drugs used in anesthesia can be accurately characterized by one-compartment models because anesthetic drugs distribute extensively into peripheral tissues. To describe the pharmacokinetics of intravenous anesthetics, we must extend the one-compartment model to account for this distribution.

The plasma concentrations over time following an intravenous bolus resemble the curve in Figure 2-18. In contrast to Figure 2-14, Figure 2-18 is not a straight line even though it is plotted on a log y-axis. This curve has the characteristics common to most drugs when given by intravenous bolus. First, the concentrations continuously decrease over time. Second, the rate of decline is initially steep but becomes less steep over time until we get to a portion that is "log-linear."

Many anesthetic drugs appear to have three distinct phases, as suggested by Figure 2-18. There is a "rapid distribution" phase (*red* in Fig. 2-18) that begins immediately after bolus injection. Very rapid movement of the drug from the plasma to the rapidly equilibrating tissues characterizes this phase. Often, there is a second "slow distribution" phase (*blue* in Fig. 2-18) that is characterized by movement of drug into more slowly equilibrating tissues and return of drug to the plasma from the most rapidly equilibrating tissues. The terminal phase (*green* in Fig. 2-18) is a straight line when plotted on a semilogarithmic graph. The distinguishing characteristic of the terminal elimination phase is that the plasma concentration is lower than the tissue concentrations, and the relative proportion of drug in the plasma and peripheral volumes of distribution remains constant. During this "terminal phase," drug returns from the rapid and slow distribution volumes to the plasma and is permanently removed from the plasma by metabolism or excretion.

The presence of three distinct phases following bolus injection is a defining characteristic of a mammillary model with three compartments (a mammillary model consists of a central compartment with peripheral compartments connecting to it. There are no interconnections among other compartments). It is possible to develop "hydraulic" models, as shown in Figure 2-19, for intravenous drugs.[13] In this model, there are three tanks, corresponding (from left to right) with the slowly equilibrating peripheral compartment, the central compartment (the plasma, into which drug is injected), and the rapidly equilibrating peripheral compartment. The horizontal pipes represent intercompartmental clearance or (for the pipe draining onto the page) metabolic clearance. The volumes of each tank correspond with the volumes of the compartments for fentanyl. The cross-sectional areas of the pipes correlate with fentanyl systemic and intercompartmental clearances. The height of water in each tank corresponds to drug concentration.

We can follow the processes that decrease drug concentration over time following bolus injection. Initially, drug flows from the central compartment to both peripheral compartments and is eliminated via the drain pipe through metabolic clearance. Because there are three places for drug to go, the central compartment concentration decreases very rapidly. At the transition between

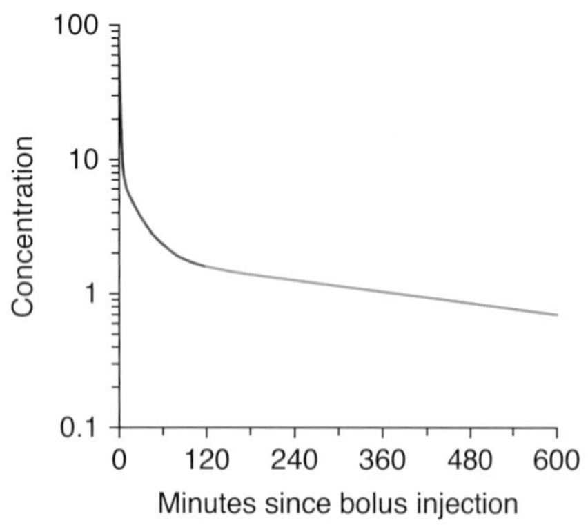

FIGURE 2-18 Typical time course of plasma concentration following bolus injection of an intravenous drug, with a rapid phase *(red)*, an intermediate phase *(blue)*, and a slow log-linear phase *(green)*. The simulation was performed with the pharmacokinetics of fentanyl. (From Scott JC, Stanski DR. Decreased fentanyl and alfentanil dose requirements with age. A simultaneous pharmacokinetic and pharmacodynamics evaluation. *J Pharmacol Exp Ther.* 1987;240: 159–166, with permission.)

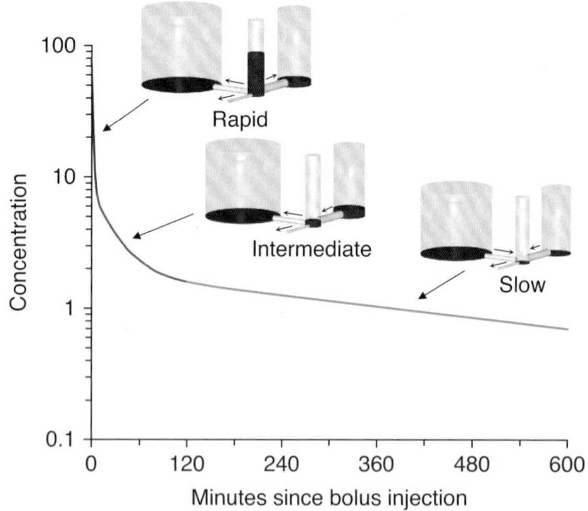

FIGURE 2-19 Hydraulic equivalent of the model in Figure 2-18. (Adapted from Youngs EJ, Shafer SL. Basic pharmacokinetic and pharmacodynamic principles. In: White PF, ed. *Textbook of Intravenous Anesthesia.* Baltimore, MD: Lippincott Williams & Wilkins; 1997:10, with permission.)

the red and the blue lines, there is a change in the role of the most rapidly equilibrating compartment. At this transition, the central compartment concentration falls below the concentration in the rapidly equilibrating compartment, and the direction of flow between them is reversed. After this transition *(blue line)*, drug in the plasma only has two places to go: the slowly equilibrating compartment or out the drain pipe. These processes are partly offset by the return of drug to the plasma from the rapidly equilibrating compartment, which slows the decrease in plasma concentration. Once the concentration in the central compartment falls below both the rapidly and slowly equilibrating compartments *(green line)*, then the only method of decreasing the plasma concentration is clearance out the drain pipe. Drug accumulated in the rapidly and slowly equilibrating compartments acts as an enormous drag on the system, and the little drain pipe now is working against the entire body store of drug.

Curves that continuously decrease over time, with a continuously increasing slope (i.e., curves that look like Figs. 2-18 and 2-19), can be described by a sum of negative exponentials, as shown in Figure 2-20, which shows how three single exponential curves are added together to get a sum of exponentials that describes the plasma concentrations over time after bolus injection:

$$C(t) = Ae^{-\alpha t} + Be^{-\beta t} + Ce^{-\gamma t} \qquad \text{Equation 2-18}$$

where t is the time since the bolus; $C(t)$ is the drug concentration following a bolus dose; and A, α, B, β, C, and γ are parameters of a pharmacokinetic model. A, B, and C are called ***coefficients***, whereas α, β, and γ are called ***exponents***. Following a bolus injection, all six of the parameters (A, α, B, β, C, and γ) will be greater than 0.

The main reason that polyexponential equations are used is that they work. These equations describe reasonably accurately the plasma concentrations observed after bolus injection, except for the misspecification in the first few minutes mentioned previously.

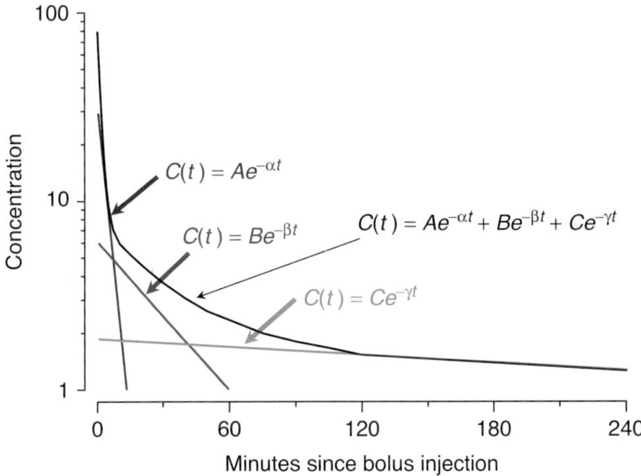

FIGURE 2-20 The polyexponential equation that describes the decline in plasma concentration for most intravenous anesthetics, is the algebraic sum of the exponential terms that represent rapid phase shown in *red*, intermediate phase shown in *blue* and slow phase shown in *green*.

Polyexponential equations permit us to use the one-compartment ideas just developed, with some generalization of the concepts. $C(t) = Ae^{-\alpha t} + Be^{-\beta t} + Ce^{-\gamma t}$ says that the concentrations over time are the algebraic sum of three separate functions, $Ae^{-\alpha t}$, $Be^{-\beta t}$, and $Ce^{-\gamma t}$. Typically, $\alpha > \beta > \gamma$ by about 1 order of magnitude. At time 0 ($t = 0$), Equation 2-18 reduces to $C_0 = A + B + C$. In other words, the sum of the coefficients A, B, and C equals the concentration immediately following a bolus. It thus follows that $A + B + C =$ bolus amount / V_1.

Constructing pharmacokinetic models represents a trade-off between accurately describing the data, having confidence in the results, and mathematical tractability. Adding exponents to the model usually provides a better description of the observed concentrations. However, adding more exponents terms usually decreases our confidence in how well we know each coefficient and exponential, and *greatly* increases the mathematical burden of the models. This is why most pharmacokinetic models are limited to two or three exponents.

Polyexponential models can be mathematically transformed from the admittedly unintuitive exponential form $C(t) = Ae^{-\alpha t} + Be^{-\beta t} + Ce^{-\gamma t}$ to a more easily visualized compartmental form, as shown in Equation 2-16. Micro-rate constants, expressed as k_{ij}, define the rate of drug transfer from compartment i to compartment j. Compartment 0 is the compartment outside the model, so k_{10} is the micro-rate constant for irreversible removal of drug from the central compartment (analogous to k for a one-compartment model). The intercompartmental micro-rate constants (k_{12}, k_{21}, etc.) describe the movement of drug between the central and peripheral compartments. Each peripheral compartment has at two micro-rate constants, one for drug entry and one for drug exit. The micro-rate constants for the two- and three-compartment models can be seen in Figure 2-16. The differential equations describing the rate of change for the amount of drugs in compartments 1, 2, and 3 follow directly from the micro-rate constants. For the two-compartment model, the differential equations for each compartment are:

$$\frac{dx_1}{dt} = I + x_2k_{21} - x_1k_{10} - x_1k_{12}$$

$$\frac{dx_2}{dt} = x_1k_{12} - x_2k_{21} \qquad \text{Equation 2-19}$$

where I is the rate of drug input. For the three-compartment model, the differential equations for each compartment are:

$$\frac{dx_1}{dt} = I + x_3k_{31} + x_2k_{21} - x_1k_{10} - x_1k_{12} - x_1k_{13}$$

$$\frac{dx_2}{dt} = x_1k_{12} - x_2k_{21}$$

$$\frac{dx_3}{dt} = x_1k_{13} - x_3k_{31} \qquad \text{Equation 2-20}$$

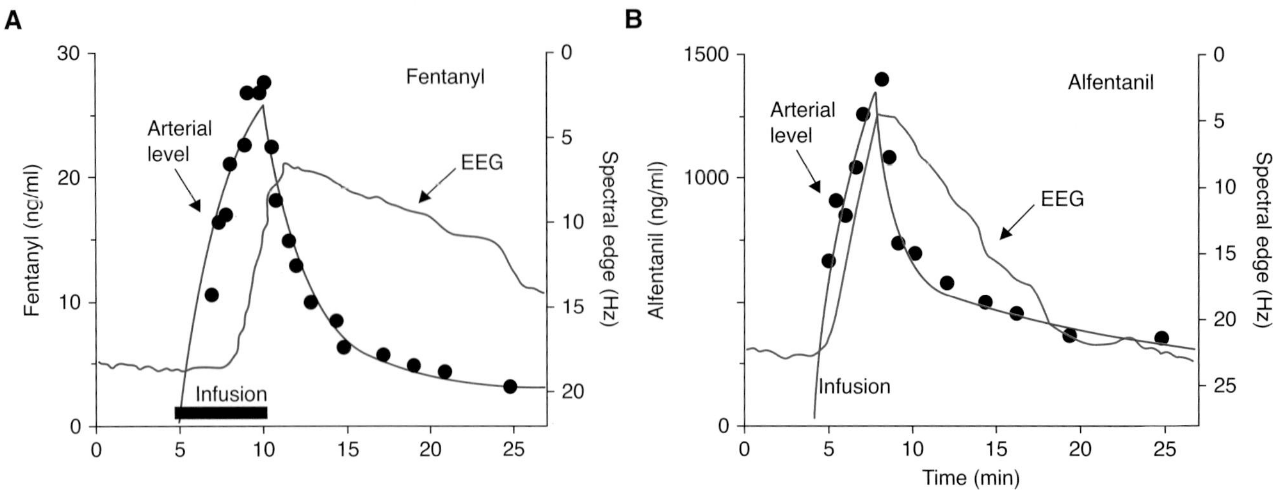

FIGURE 2-21 Fentanyl and alfentanil arterial concentrations *(circles)* and electroencephalographic (EEG) response *(irregular line)* to an intravenous infusion. Alfentanil shows a less time lag between the rise and fall of arterial concentration and the rise and fall of EEG response than fentanyl because it equilibrates with the brain more quickly. (Modified from Scott JC, Ponganis KV, Stanski DR. EEG quantitation of narcotic effect: the comparative pharmacodynamics of fentanyl and alfentanil. *Anesthesiology.* 1985;62:234–241, with permission.)

For the one-compartment model, *k* was both the rate constant and the exponent. For multicompartment models, the relationships are more complex. The interconversion between the micro-rate constants and the exponents becomes exceedingly complex as more exponents are added, because every exponent is a function of every micro-rate constant and vice versa. Individuals interested in such interconversions can find them in the Excel spreadsheet "convert.xls," which can be downloaded from *http://anesthesia.stanford.edu/pkpd*. This is useful because publications on pharmacokinetics may use one or another system and it is difficult to compare without converting the exponents to micro-rate constants.

The Time Course of Drug Effect

The plasma is not the site of drug effect for anesthetic drugs. There is a time lag between plasma drug concentration and effect site drug concentration. Consider the different rate of onset for fentanyl and alfentanil. Figure 2-21 is from work by Stanski and colleagues.[14,15] The black bar in Figure 2-21A shows the duration of a fentanyl infusion.[14] Rapid arterial samples document the rise in fentanyl concentration. The time course of EEG effect (spectral edge) lags 2 to 3 minutes behind the rapid rise in arterial concentration. This lag is called ***hysteresis***. The plasma concentration peaks at the moment the infusion is turned off. Following the peak plasma concentration (and the Disney logo that appears at peak plasma concentration), the plasma fentanyl concentration rapidly decreases. However, the offset of fentanyl drug effect lags well behind the decrease in plasma concentration. Figure 2-21B shows the same study design in a patient receiving alfentanil. Because of alfentanil's rapid blood–brain equilibration, there is less hysteresis (delay) with alfentanil than with fentanyl.

The relationship between the plasma and the site of drug effect is modeled with an "effect site" model, as shown in Figure 2-22. The site of drug effect is connected to the plasma by a first-order process. The equation that relates effect site concentration to plasma concentration is:

$$\frac{dCe}{dt} = k_{e0} \cdot Cp - k_{e0} \cdot Ce \qquad \text{Equation 2-21}$$

where *Ce* is the effect site concentration and *Cp* is the plasma drug concentration. k_{e0} is the rate constant for elimination of drug from the effect site. It is most easily understood in terms of its reciprocal, $0.693/k_{e0}$, the half-time for equilibration between the plasma and the site of drug effect.

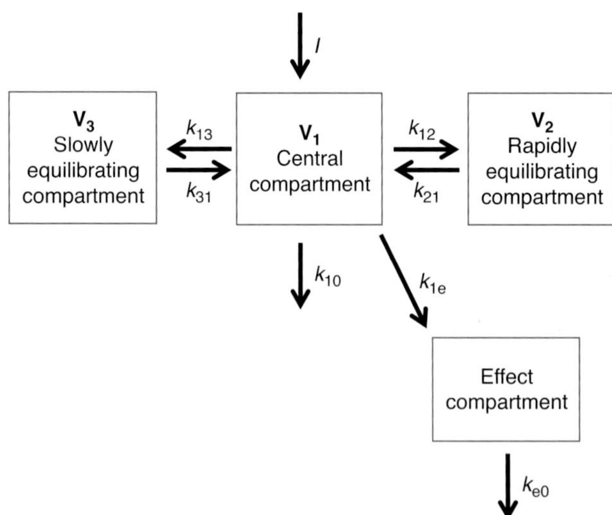

FIGURE 2-22 The three-compartment model from Figure 2-16 with an added effect site to account for the equilibration delay between the plasma concentration and the observed drug effect. The effect site has a negligible volume. As a result, the only parameter that affects the delay is k_{e0}.

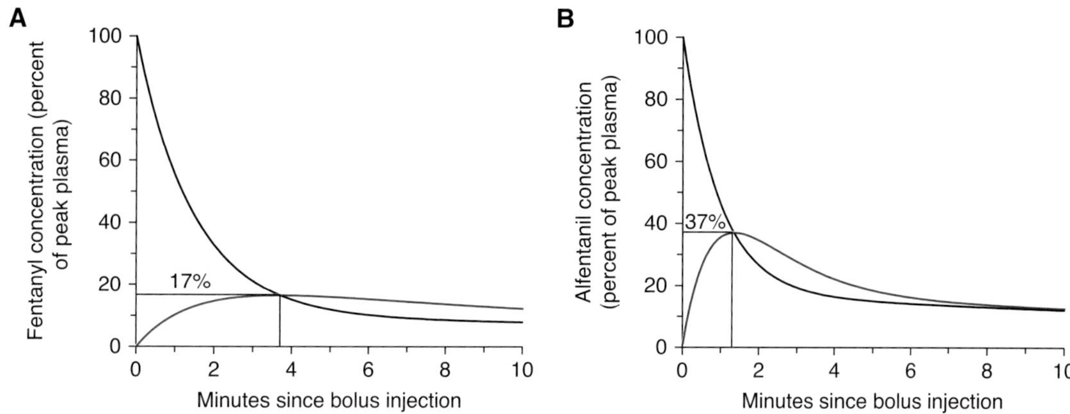

FIGURE 2-23 Plasma *(black line)* and effect site *(red line)* concentrations following a bolus dose of fentanyl **(A)** or alfentanil **(B)**. (Adapted from Shafer SL, Varvel JR. Pharmacokinetics, pharmacodynamics, and rational opioid selection. *Anesthesiology*. 1991;74:53–63, with permission.)

Figure 2-23 shows the plasma and effect site concentrations predicted by the model (see Fig. 2-22) for fentanyl and alfentanil. The plasma concentrations *(black lines)* are not very different. However, the effect site concentrations *(red lines)* show that alfentanil equilibrates more quickly. There are two consequences. First, the peak effect is sooner (obviously). Second, the rapid equilibration of alfentanil allows the brain to "see" the initial high plasma concentrations, producing a relatively greater rise in effect site concentrations than observed with fentanyl. This permits alfentanil to deliver relatively more "bang" for a bolus.

The constant k_{e0} has a large influence on the rate of rise of drug effect, the rate of offset of drug effect, the time to peak effect,[16] and the dose that is required to produce the desired drug effect.

Dose Calculations

Bolus Dosing

We noted previously that we can rearrange the definition of concentration to find the amount of drug required to produce any desired target concentration for a known volume, amount = $C_T \times$ volume. Many introductory pharmacokinetic texts suggest using this formula to calculate the loading bolus required to achieve a given concentration. The problem with applying this concept to the anesthetic drugs is that there are several volumes: V_1 (central compartment), V_2 and V_3 (the peripheral compartments), and Vd_{ss}, the sum of the individual volumes. V_1 is usually much smaller than Vd_{ss}, and so it is tempting to say that the loading dose should be something between $C_T \times V_1$ and $C_T \times Vd_{ss}$.

That proves to be a useless suggestion. Consider the initial dose of fentanyl. The C_{50} for fentanyl to attenuate hemodynamic response to intubation (when combined with an intravenous hypnotic) is approximately 2 ng/mL. The V_1 and Vd_{ss} for fentanyl are 13 L and 360 L, respectively. The dose of fentanyl thus ranges from a low of 26 μg (based on the V_1 of 13 L) to a high 720 μg (based on the Vd_{ss} of 360 L). A fentanyl bolus of 26 μg achieves the desired concentration in the plasma for an initial instant (Fig. 2-24). Unfortunately, the plasma levels almost instantly decrease below the desired target, and the effect site levels are never close to the desired target. A fentanyl bolus of 720 μg, not surprisingly, produces an enormous overshoot in the plasma levels that persists for hours. It is absurd to use equations to calculate the fentanyl dose if the resulting recommendation is "pick a dose between 26 and 720 μg."

Conventional approaches to calculate a bolus dose are designed to produce a specific plasma concentration. This makes little sense because the plasma is not the site of drug effect. By knowing the k_{e0} (the rate constant for elimination of drug from the effect site) of an intravenous anesthetic, we can design a dosing regimen that yields the desired concentration *at the site of drug effect*. If we do not want to overdose the patient, we should select the bolus that produces the desired peak concentration in the effect site.

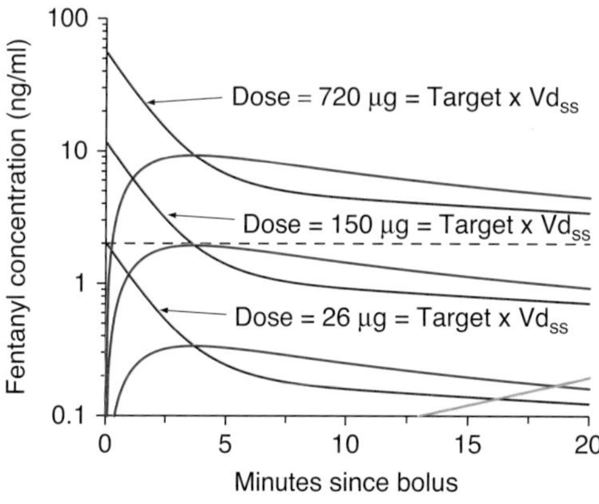

FIGURE 2-24 The volume of the central compartment of fentanyl is 13 L. The volume of distribution at steady state is 360 L. For a target concentration of 2 μg/L *(dotted line)*, the dose calculated on V_1, 26 μg, results in a substantial undershoot. The dose calculated using Vd_{ss}, 720 μg, produces a profound overshoot. Only a dose based on $Vd_{peak\ effect}$, 150 μg, produces the desired concentration in the effect site. The *black lines* show plasma concentration over time. *Red lines* show effect site concentration over time.

The decline in plasma concentration after the bolus, up to the time of peak effect, can be thought of as a dilution of the bolus into a larger volume than the volume of the central compartment. One interesting characteristic of the equilibration between the plasma and the effect site is that at the time of peak effect, the plasma and the effect site concentrations are the same (if they were not the same, then it would not be the peak because there would be a gradient driving drug in or out of the effect site). This introduces the concept of Vd_{pe}, the apparent volume of distribution at the time of peak effect. The size of this volume can be readily calculated from the observation that the plasma and effect site concentrations are the same at the time of peak effect:

$$Vd_{pe} = \frac{\text{bolus amount}}{C_{pe}} \qquad \text{Equation 2-22}$$

where C_{pe} is the plasma concentration at the time of peak effect. We can arrange this equation to calculate the dose that provides the desired peak effect site concentration: bolus dose $= C_T \times Vd_{pe}$. For example, the Vd_{pe} for fentanyl is 75 L. Producing a peak fentanyl effect site concentration of 2 ng/mL requires 150 μg for the typical patient, which produces a peak effect in 3.6 minutes. This is a much more reasonable dosing guideline than the previous recommendation of picking a dose between 26 and 760 μg. Table 2-2 lists V_1 and Vd_{pe} for fentanyl, alfentanil, sufentanil, remifentanil, propofol, thiopental, and midazolam. Table 2-3 lists the time to peak effect and the t ½ k_{e0} (half-life at the site of drug effect) of the commonly used intravenous anesthetics. Of course, individuals may differ from the typical patient. The individual characteristics that drive the differences may be known (age, weight, renal or hepatic dysfunction) in which case they can be built into the pharmacokinetic model if they are found to be significant. On the other hand, they may be unknown, in which case pharmacodynamic monitoring is required to fine tune dosing.

Table 2-2

Volume of Distribution at the Time of Peak Effect.

Drug	V_1 (L)	Vd_{pe} (L)
Fentanyl	12.7	75
Alfentanil	2.19	5.9
Sufentanil	17.8	89
Remifentanil	5.0	17
Propofol	6.7	37
Thiopental	5.6	14.6
Midazolam	3.4	31

V_1, volume of the central compartment; Vd_{pe}, apparent volume of distribution at the time of peak effect.

From Glass PSA, Shafer S, Reves JG. Intravenous drug delivery systems. In: Miller RD, Eriksson LI, Fleisher LA, et al., eds. *Miller's Anesthesia*. Vol 1. 7th ed. Philadelphia, PA: Churchill Livingstone; 2010:825–858.

Table 2-3

The Time to Peak Effect and t ½ k_{e0} following a Bolus Dose

Drug	Time to Peak Drug Effect (min)	t ½ k_{e0} (min)[a]
Fentanyl	3.6	4.7
Alfentanil	1.4	0.9
Sufentanil	5.6	3.0
Remifentanil	1.6	1.3
Propofol	2.2	2.4
Thiopental	1.6	1.5
Midazolam	2.8	4.0
Etomidate	2.0	1.5

[a] t ½ $k_{e0} = 0.693/k_{e0}$, the effect site half-life, where k_{e0} is the rate constant for elimination of drug from the site of drug effect and t ½ k_{e0} is the time required for the concentration at the site of drug effect to fall to half of its value.

From Glass PSA, Shafer S, Reves JG. Intravenous drug delivery systems. In: Miller RD, Eriksson LI, Fleisher LA, et al., eds. *Miller's Anesthesia*. Vol 1. 7th ed. Philadelphia, PA: Churchill Livingstone; 2010:825–858.

Maintenance Infusion Rate

As explained previously, to maintain a given target concentration, C_T, drug must be delivered at the same rate that drug is exiting the body. Thus, the maintenance infusion rate at steady state is maintenance infusion rate $= C_T \times Cl_S$. However, this equation only applies after peripheral tissues have fully equilibrated with the plasma, which may require many hours. At all other times, this maintenance infusion rate underestimates the infusion rate to maintain a target concentration.

In some situations, this simple rate calculation may be acceptable. For example, if an infusion at this rate is used after a bolus based on Vd_{pe} (apparent volume of distribution at time of peak effect), and the drug has a long delay between the bolus and peak effect, then much of the distribution of drug into the tissues may have occurred by the time of peak effect site concentration. In this case, the maintenance infusion rate calculated as clearance times target concentration may be satisfactory because Vd_{pe} is sufficiently higher than V_1 to account for the distribution of drug into peripheral tissues. Unfortunately, most drugs used in anesthesia have sufficiently rapid plasma-effect site equilibration that Vd_{pe} does not adequately encompass the distribution process, making this approach unsuitable.

The mathematically and clinically sound approach accounts for tissue distribution. Initially, the infusion rate is higher than the simple calculation because it is necessary to replace the drug that gets taken up by peripheral tissues. However, the net flow of drug into peripheral tissues

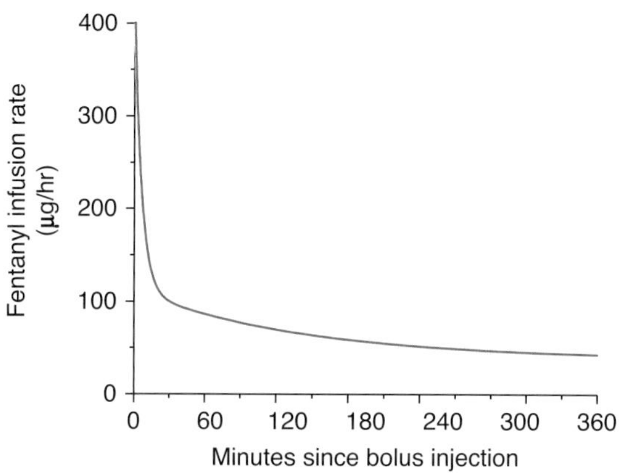

FIGURE 2-25 Fentanyl infusion rate to maintain a plasma concentration of 1 μg/hr. The rate starts off quite high because fentanyl is avidly taken up by body fat. The necessary infusion rate decreases as the fat equilibrates with the plasma.

decreases over time. Therefore, the infusion rate required to maintain any desired concentration must also decrease over time. Following bolus injection, the equation to maintain the desired concentration is:

$$\text{Maintenance infusion rate} = C_T \times V_1 \times (k_{10} + k_{12}e^{-k_{21}t} + k_{13}e^{-k_{31}t})$$

Equation 2-23

This equation indicates that a high infusion rate is initially required to maintain C_T. Over time, the infusion rate gradually decreases (Fig. 2-25). At equilibrium ($t = \infty$), the infusion rate decreases to $C_T\ V_1\ k_{10}$, which is the same as $C_T \times Cl$. Nobody wants to mentally solve such an equation during administration of an anesthetic. Fortunately, there are simple techniques that can be used in place of solving such a complex expression.

Figure 2-26 is a nomogram in which the Equation 2-14 has been solved, showing the infusion rates over time necessary to maintain any desired concentration of fentanyl, alfentanil, sufentanil, and propofol. This nomogram is complex, and not even the authors use it. The point in including it is to show how infusion rates must be turned down over time as drug accumulates. The *y*-axis represents the target concentration, C_T. The suggested target initial concentrations (shown in *red*) are based on the work of Vuyk and colleagues,[17] and appropriately scaled for fentanyl and sufentanil. The *x*-axis is the time since the beginning of the anesthetic. The intersections of the target concentration line and the diagonal lines indicates the infusion rate appropriate at each point in time. For example, to maintain a fentanyl concentration of 1.0 ng/mL, the appropriate rates are 3.0 μg/kg/hour at 15 minutes, 2.4 μg/kg/hour at 30 minutes, 1.8 μg/kg/hour at 60 minutes, 2.1 μg/kg/hour at 120 minutes, and 0.9 μg/kg/hour at 180 minutes.

Another approach to determine infusion rates for maintenance of anesthesia to a desired target concentration is through the use of a specialized slide rule.[18] Figure 2-27 illustrates such a slide rule for propofol. As described by Bruhn et al.,[18] "The bolus dose required to reach a given target plasma concentration is the product of the (weight-related) distribution volume and required concentration. Similarly, the infusion rate at a particular time point is the product of target concentration, body weight, and a correction factor that depends on the time elapsed from the start of the initial infusion. This factor can be determined for each time point using a PK simulation program."

The best approach is through the use of target-controlled drug delivery. With target-controlled drug delivery, the user simply sets the desired plasma or effect site concentration. Based on the drug's pharmacokinetics and the mathematical relationship between patient covariates (e.g., weight, age, gender) and individual pharmacokinetic parameters, the computer calculates the dose of drug necessary to rapidly achieve and then maintain any desired concentration. Most critically, it can raise and lower concentrations in a controlled fashion, a calculation that cannot be captured in any simple nomogram. Such computerized controlled drug delivery systems are now widely available.

Context Sensitive Half-time

Special significance is often ascribed to the smallest exponent, which determines the slope of the final log-linear portion of the curve. When the medical literature refers to the half-life of a drug, unless otherwise stated, the half-life is based on the terminal half-life (i.e., 0.693/smallest exponent). However, the terminal half-life for drugs with more than 1 exponential term is nearly impossible to interpret. The terminal half-life sets an upper limit on the time required for the concentrations to decrease by 50% after drug administration. Usually, the time for a 50% decrease will be much faster than that upper limit. A more useful concept is the "context-sensitive half-time," shown in Figure 2-28,[19] which is the time for the plasma concentration to decrease by 50% from an infusion that maintains a constant concentration. The "context" is the duration of the infusion. The context-sensitive half-time increases with longer infusion durations, because it takes longer for the concentrations to fall if drug has accumulated in peripheral tissues.

The context-sensitive half-time is based on the time for a 50% decrease, which was chosen both to provide an analogy to half-life, and because, very roughly, a 50% reduction in drug concentration appears necessary for recovery after administration of most intravenous hypnotics at the termination of surgery. Of course, decreases other than 50% may be clinically relevant. Additionally, the context-sensitive half-time does not consider plasma-effect site disequilibrium and thus may be misleading for drugs with very slow plasma-effect site equilibration. A related but more clinically relevant representation is the

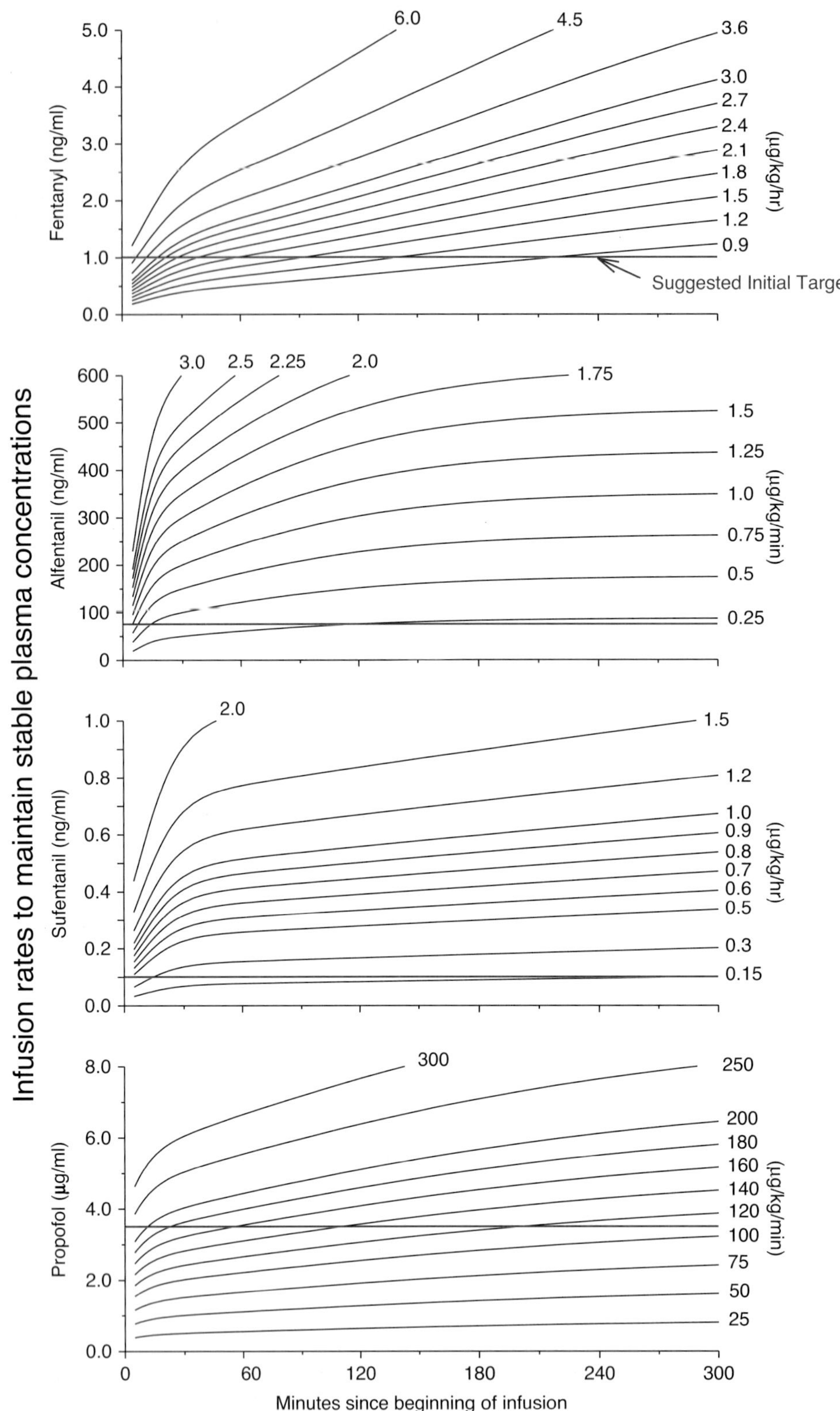

FIGURE 2-26 Dosing nomogram, showing the infusion rates (numbers on the perimeter) required to maintain stable concentrations of fentanyl (1.0 µg/mL), alfentanil (75 µg/mL), sufentanil (0.1 µg/mL), and propofol (3.5 ng/mL).

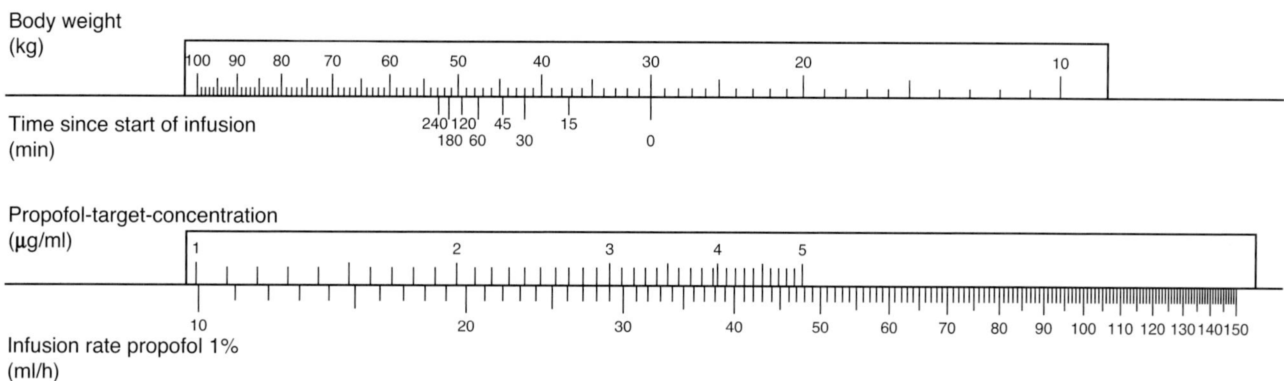

FIGURE 2-27 Propofol slide ruler to calculate maintenance infusion rate, based on the patient's weight and the time since the start of the infusion, as proposed by Bruhn and colleagues (Adapted from Bruhn J, Bouillon TW, Ropcke H, et al. A manual slide rule for target-controlled infusion of propofol: development and evaluation. *Anesth Analg.* 2003;96:142–147.). To make use of the calculator, make a photocopy and cut in to top (body weight), middle (time since start of infusion/propofol target concentration), and bottom (infusion rate propofol 1%) sections—calculation requires sliding the middle piece in relationship to the top and bottom segments, which are fixed.

context-sensitive effect site decrement time, as shown in Figure 2-29. For example, the upper black line in Figure 2-29 is the context-sensitive 20% effect site decrement time for fentanyl, that is, the time required for fentanyl effect site concentrations to fall by 20%, based on the duration of a fentanyl infusion. Context-sensitive half-time and effect site decrement times are more useful than elimination half-time in characterizing the clinical responses to drugs.[20]

Pharmacodynamics

Pharmacodynamics is the study of the intrinsic sensitivity or responsiveness of the body to a drug and the mechanisms by which these effects occur. Thus, pharmacodynamics may be viewed as what the drug does to the body. Structure–activity relationships link the actions of drugs to their chemical structure and facilitate the design of drugs with more desirable pharmacologic properties. The intrinsic sensitivity is determined by measuring plasma concentrations of a drug required to evoke specific pharmacologic responses. The intrinsic sensitivity to drugs varies among patients and within patients over time with aging. As a result, at similar plasma concentrations of a drug, some patients show a therapeutic response, others show no response, and in others, toxicity develops.

The basic principles of receptor theory were covered in the first section of this chapter. This section focuses on methods of evaluating clinical drug effects such as dose-response curves, efficacy, potency, the median effective dose (ED_{50}), the median lethal dose (LD_{50}), and the therapeutic index.

Concentration versus Response Relationships

The most fundamental relationship in pharmacology is the concentration (or dose) versus response curve, shown in Figure 2-30. This is the time-independent relationship between exposure to the drug (x-axis) and the measured effect (y-axis). The exposure can be the concentration, the dose, the area under the concentration versus time curve, or any other measure of drug exposure that is clinically

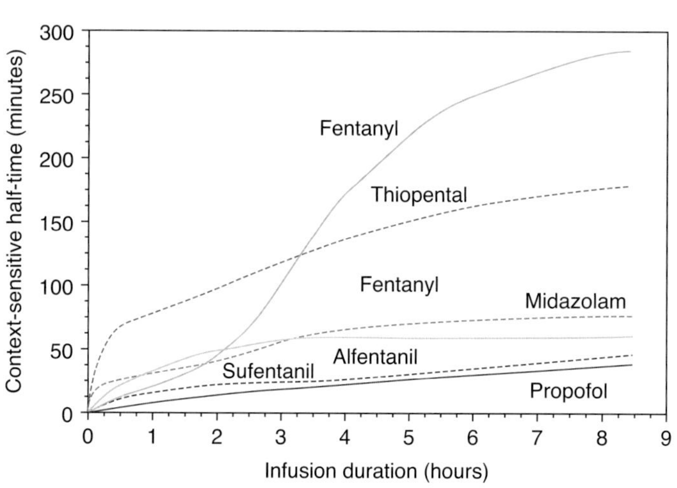

FIGURE 2-28 Context-sensitive half-times as a function of the duration of intravenous drug infusion for each fentanyl, alfentanil, sufentanil, propofol, midazolam, and thiopental. (From Hughes MA, Glass PSA, Jacobs JR. Context-sensitive half-time in multicompartment pharmacokinetic models for intravenous anesthetic drugs. *Anesthesiology.* 1992;76:334–341, with permission.)

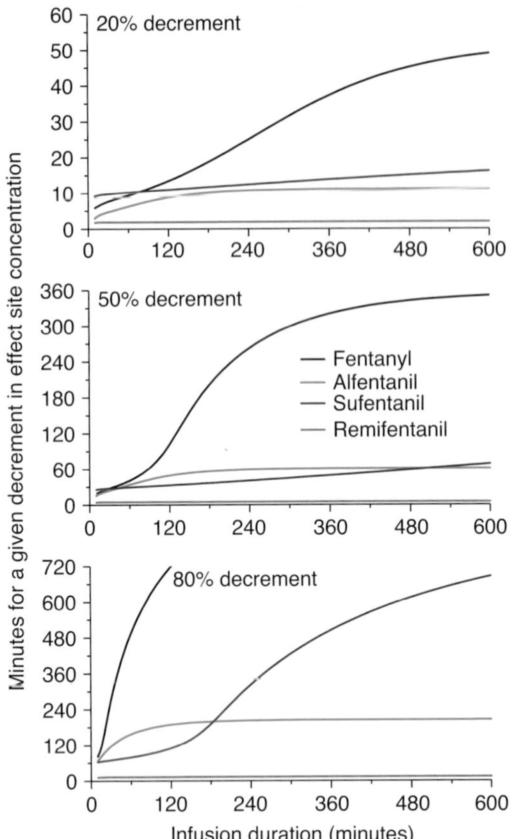

FIGURE 2-29 Effect site decrement times. The 20%, 50%, and 80% decrement times for fentanyl *(black)*, alfentanil *(green)*, sufentanil *(red)*, and remifentanil *(blue)*. When there is substantial plasma-effect site disequilibrium, the effect site decrement time will provide a better estimate of the time required for recover than the context-sensitive half-time. (Adapted from Youngs EJ, Shafer SL. Pharmacokinetic parameters relevant to recovery from opioids. *Anesthesiology*. 1994;81:833–842, with permission.)

meaningful. The measured effect can be an absolute response (e.g., twitch height), a normalized response (e.g., percentage of twitch depression), a population response (e.g., fraction of subjects moving at incision), or any physiologic response (chloride current). The standard

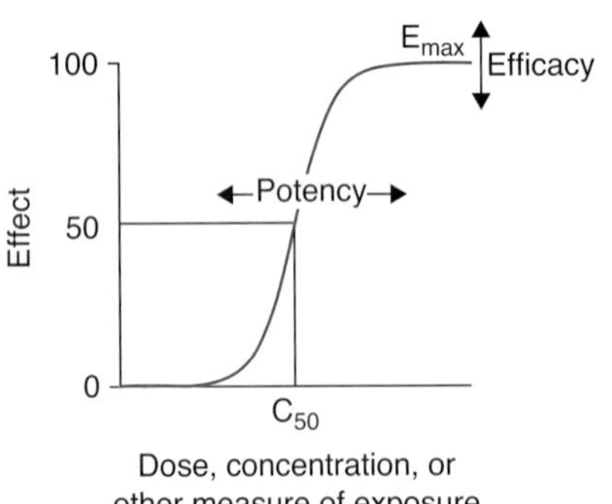

FIGURE 2-30 Drug exposure (dose, concentration, etc.) versus drug effect relationship. Potency refers to the position of the curve along the *x*-axis. Efficacy refers to the position of the maximum effect on the *y*-axis.

equation for this relationship is the "Hill" equation, sometimes called the ***sigmoid-E_{max} relationship***:

$$Effect = E_0 + (E_{\max} - E_0)\frac{C^{\gamma}}{C_{50}{}^{\gamma} + C^{\gamma}} \qquad \text{Equation 2-24}$$

In this equation, E_0 is the baseline effect in the absence of drug, and $E_{\max}$ is the maximum possible drug effect. C is typically concentration or dose, although other measures of drug exposure (e.g., dose, peak concentration, area under the concentration vs. time curve) can be used. C_{50} is the concentration associated with 50% of peak drug effect and is a measure of drug potency. The term $\frac{C^{\gamma}}{C_{50}{}^{\gamma} + C^{\gamma}}$ is a modification of the saturation equation $\frac{C}{C_{50} + C}$ presented in the prior section. Previously, it did not have an exponent. However, when used in pharmacodynamic models, the exponent γ, also called the ***Hill coefficient***, appears. The exponent relates to the "sigmoidicity" and steepness of the curve. If γ is less than 1 and the curve is plotted on a standard x-axis, then the curve appears hyperbolic (see Fig. 2-8). If γ is greater than 1, then the curve appears sigmoidal, as in Figure 2-30. If the x-axis is plotted on a log scale, then the curve will always appear sigmoidal regardless of the value of γ.

Potency and Efficacy

There are two problems with the term ***potency***. Clinicians often use potency to refer to the relative dose of two drugs, such as the relative potency of fentanyl and morphine. The problem with this definition is that when drugs have very different time courses, the relative potency varies depending on the time of the measurement. Fentanyl reaches peak effect 3.5 minutes after injection. Morphine reaches peak effect 90 minutes after injection. As a result, the "relative potency" 3.5 minutes after injection indicates that fentanyl is far more potent than morphine. However, when morphine has reached its peak effect 90 minutes after injection, the effect of the fentanyl has almost entirely dissipated. Measured 90 minutes after injection, morphine is more potent. From therapeutic perspective, potency is often defined in terms of relative doses.

However, from a pharmacologic perspective, potency is more logically described in terms of the concentration versus response relationship. As shown in Figure 2-31, a drug with a left-shifted concentration versus response curve (i.e., lower C_{50}) is considered more potent, whereas a drug with a right-shifted dose versus response curve is less potent. To be precise, potency should be defined in terms of a specific drug effect (e.g., 50% of maximal effect of a full agonist). This is particularly important if the two drugs have differing Hill coefficients or efficacies ($E_{\max}$).

Efficacy is a measure of the intrinsic ability of a drug to produce a given physiologic or clinical effect (see Fig. 2-30). Consider the example of benzodiazepines given

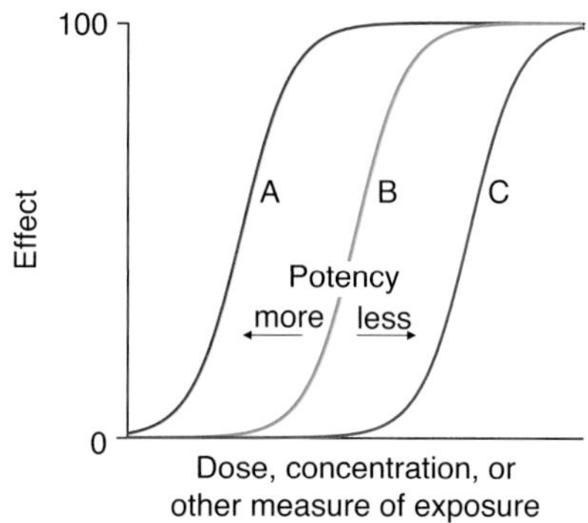

FIGURE 2-31 Dose versus response relationship for three drugs with potency. Drug A is the most potent, and drug C is the least potent.

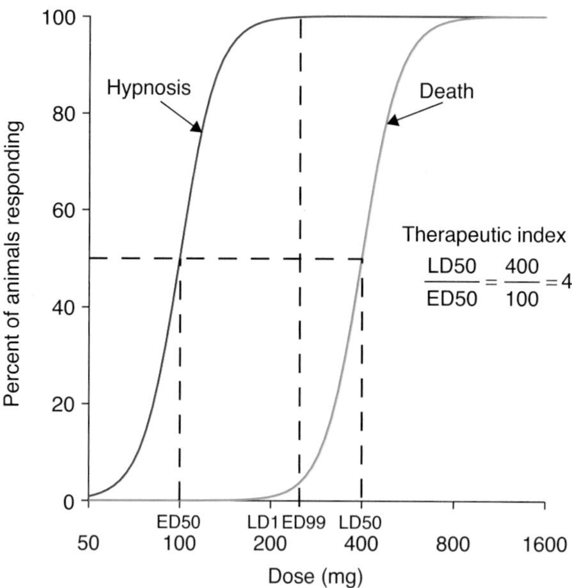

FIGURE 2-33 Analysis to determine the LD_{50}, the LD_{99}, and the therapeutic index of a drug.

earlier (see Fig. 2-3). Intrinsic efficacy ranged from full effect for midazolam to partial effect for bretazenil, to no effect for flumazenil. The difference between a full agonist, a partial agonist, and an antagonist represents differences in efficacy. Efficacy refers to the position of the concentration versus response curve in the *y*-axis, whereas potency refers to relative drug concentration for a particular response on the *y*-axis.

Two drugs may have the same C_{50}, but different efficacies. Because C_{50} is defined relative to the maximum drug effect, the drug with lower efficacy demonstrates less effect at C_{50} (Fig. 2-32) and is therefore less potent. This introduces the second problem with the term potency. One can only compare potencies by comparing C_{50} values if the maximum effect and the Hill coefficient are identical for both drugs. If not, then potency must be described in terms of a specific drug effect (a specific point on the *y*-axis of the dose vs. response curve).

Effective Dose and Lethal Dose

The ED_{50} is the dose of a drug required to produce a specific desired effect in 50% of individuals receiving the drug. The LD_{50} is the dose of a drug required to produce death in 50% of patients (or, more often, animals) receiving the drug. The therapeutic index is the ratio between the LD_{50} and the ED_{50} (LD_{50}/ED_{50}). The larger the therapeutic index of a drug, the safer the drug is for clinical administration. The relationship among ED_{50}, LD_{50}, and therapeutic index is shown in Figure 2-33. The classic calculation of LD_{50} is not clinically very helpful in anesthesia where we expect 100% of patients to fall asleep and nobody to die. A more effective ratio is the LD_1/ED_{99} ratio. That ratio shows a far smaller margin of safety and actually is reversed in Figure 2-33, meaning that there is appreciable risk of death, even at subtherapeutic doses in some individuals. Anesthetic drugs have uniquely low therapeutic ratio, and thus require enormous vigilance for their safe use.

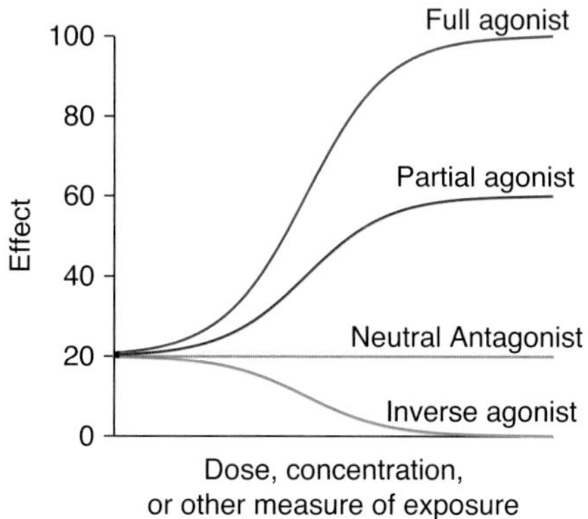

FIGURE 2-32 Concentration versus response curves for drugs with differing efficacies. Although the C_{50} of each curve is the same, the partial agonist is less potent than the full agonist because of the decreased efficacy.

Drug Interactions

Actions at Different Receptors

Opioids potently reduce the minimum alveolar concentration (MAC) of inhaled anesthetics required to suppress movement to noxious stimulation (Fig. 2-34).[21,22] Initially, the interaction is profound, with approximately 50% reduction in MAC at a plasma fentanyl concentration of 1.5 ng/mL. However, after the initial reduction in MAC, there is fairly limited benefit from additional fentanyl. The clinical pearl is that a modest amount of opioid dramatically reduces the concentrations of inhalational anesthetic required to prevent movement. The second pearl is that even with huge doses of opioids, some hypnotic component must be added to the anesthetic to prevent movement.

Similar work has been done for propofol. Vuyk and colleagues[17] characterized the interaction of propofol with

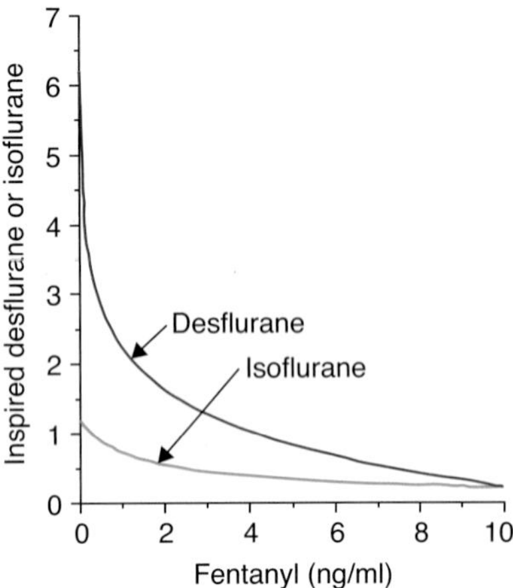

FIGURE 2-34 Interaction between fentanyl and isoflurane or desflurane on the minimum alveolar concentration required to suppress movement to noxious stimulation. (Adapted from Sebel PS, Glass PS, Fletcher JE, et al. Reduction of the MAC of desflurane with fentanyl. *Anesthesiology.* 1992;76:52–59; McEwan AI, Smith C, Dyar O, et al. Isoflurane minimum alveolar concentration reduction by fentanyl. *Anesthesiology.* 1993;78:864–869.)

alfentanil. As shown in Figure 2-35, the interaction is markedly synergistic, with modest amounts of alfentanil greatly decreasing the amount of propofol associated with 50% chance of response to intubation or surgical incision. Vuyk and colleagues[17] also documented a similar interaction of propofol and alfentanil on return of consciousness.

Hendrickx and colleagues[23] have recently surveyed the interaction of anesthetic drugs that affect nociception, analgesia, and hypnosis (Fig. 2-36). They examined two endpoints: "hypnosis," defined as loss of consciousness in humans and loss of righting reflex in animals, and "immobility," defined as the loss of movement response to noxious stimulation in a nonparalyzed subject. As shown in

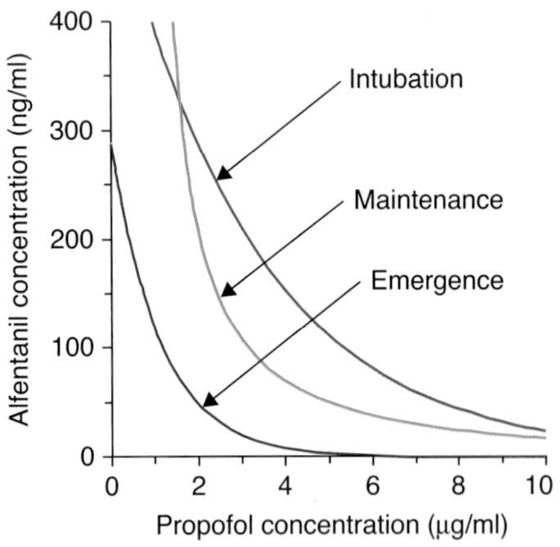

FIGURE 2-35 Interaction of propofol with alfentanil on the concentration required to suppress response to intubation, maintain nonresponsiveness during surgery, and then awaken from anesthesia. (Adapted from Vuyk J, Lim T, Engbers FH, et al. The pharmacodynamics interaction of propofol and alfentanil during lower abdominal surgery in women. *Anesthesiology.* 1995;83:8–22, with permission.)

Figure 2-36, the interaction between pairs of intravenous drugs and intravenous drugs and inhaled anesthetics is typically synergistic. An exception is the combination of the NMDA antagonists, ketamine and nitrous oxide, which demonstrate synergy, additivity, or infra-additivity in different models that have been studied. By contrast, the inhaled anesthetics are strictly additive in their interactions with other inhaled anesthetics, potentially suggesting a common mechanism of action.

Classic interaction studies, such as those described earlier, examine the concentrations associated with a particular response (such as a 50% chance of moving) for two drugs, evaluated separately and in combination. However, a more general view is that any combination of two drugs is associated with a response. This is best viewed as a "response surface" in which the *x*-axis and *y*-axis of the surface are concentrations (or doses) of drugs A and B, and the Z axis is the response to the particular combination. Minto et al.[24] have proposed a mathematical framework for response surfaces for a variety of interaction surfaces of interest to anesthesiologists. Figure 2-37 shows six examples of possible response surfaces, depending on the nature of the interaction.

Stereochemistry

Stereochemistry is the study of how molecules are structured in three dimensions.[25,26] ***Chirality*** is a unique subset of stereochemistry, and the term ***chiral*** is used to designate a molecule that has a center (or centers) of three-dimensional asymmetry. This kind of molecular configuration is almost always a function of the unique, tetrahedral bonding characteristics of the carbon atom.

Chirality is the structural basis of ***enantiomerism***. Enantiomers (substances of opposite shape) are a pair of molecules existing in two forms that are mirror images of one another (right and left hand) but cannot be superimposed. In every other aspect, enantiomers are chemically identical. A pair of enantiomers is distinguished by the direction in which, when dissolved in solution, they rotate polarized light either clockwise (dextrorotatory, d [+]) or counterclockwise (levorotatory, l [−]). These observed signs of rotation, d(+) and l(−), are often confused with the designations D and L used in protein and carbohydrate chemistry. The characteristic of rotation of polarized light is the origin of the term ***optical isomers***. When the two enantiomers are present in equal proportions (50:50), they are referred to as a ***racemic mixture***. A racemic mixture does not rotate polarized light because the optical activity of each enantiomer is canceled by the other. The most applicable and unambiguous convention for designating isomers is the *sinister (S)* and *rectus (R)* classification that specifies the absolute configuration in the name of the compound.[26] Molecular interactions that are the mechanistic foundation of pharmacokinetics and

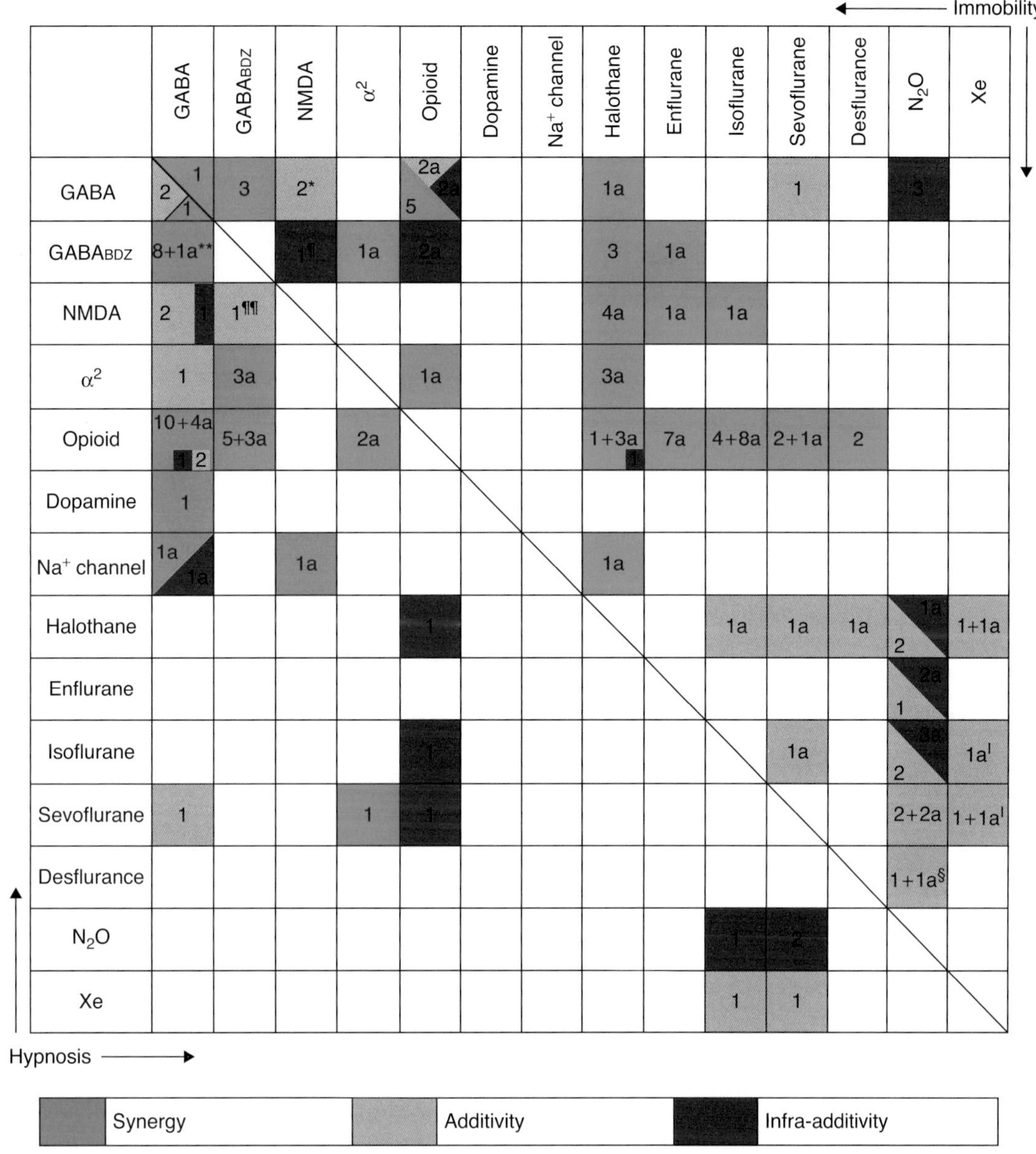

FIGURE 2-36 Survey of interactions between hypnotics and analgesics by Hendrickx et al. (From Hendrickx JF, Eger EI II, Sonner JM, et al. Is synergy the rule? A review of anesthetic interactions producing hypnosis and immobility. *Anesth Analg.* 2008;107:494–550, with permission.)

pharmacodynamics are stereoselective (relative difference between enantiomers) or stereospecific (absolute difference between enantiomers).[26] The "lock and key" hypothesis of enzyme-substrate activity emphasizes that biologic systems are inherently stereospecific. The pharmacologic extension of this concept is that drugs can be expected to interact with other biologic components in a geometrically specific way.[25] Pharmacologically, not all enantiomers are created equal. Drug-specific, drug-enzyme, and drug-protein binding interactions are virtually always three-dimensionally exacting. Enantiomers can exhibit differences in absorption, distribution, clearance, potency, and toxicity (drug interactions). Enantiomers can even antagonize the effects of one another.

The administration of a racemic drug mixture may in fact represent pharmacologically two different drugs with distinct pharmacokinetic and pharmacodynamic properties. The two enantiomers of the racemic mixture may have different rates of absorption, metabolism, and excretion as well as different affinities for receptor binding sites. Although only one enantiomer is therapeutically active, it is possible that the other enantiomer contributes to side effects. The therapeutically inactive isomer in a racemic mixture should be regarded as an impurity.[27] A cogent theoretical argument is that studies on racemic mixtures may be scientifically flawed if the enantiomers have different pharmacokinetics or pharmacodynamics.[25] An estimated one-third of drugs in clinical use are administered

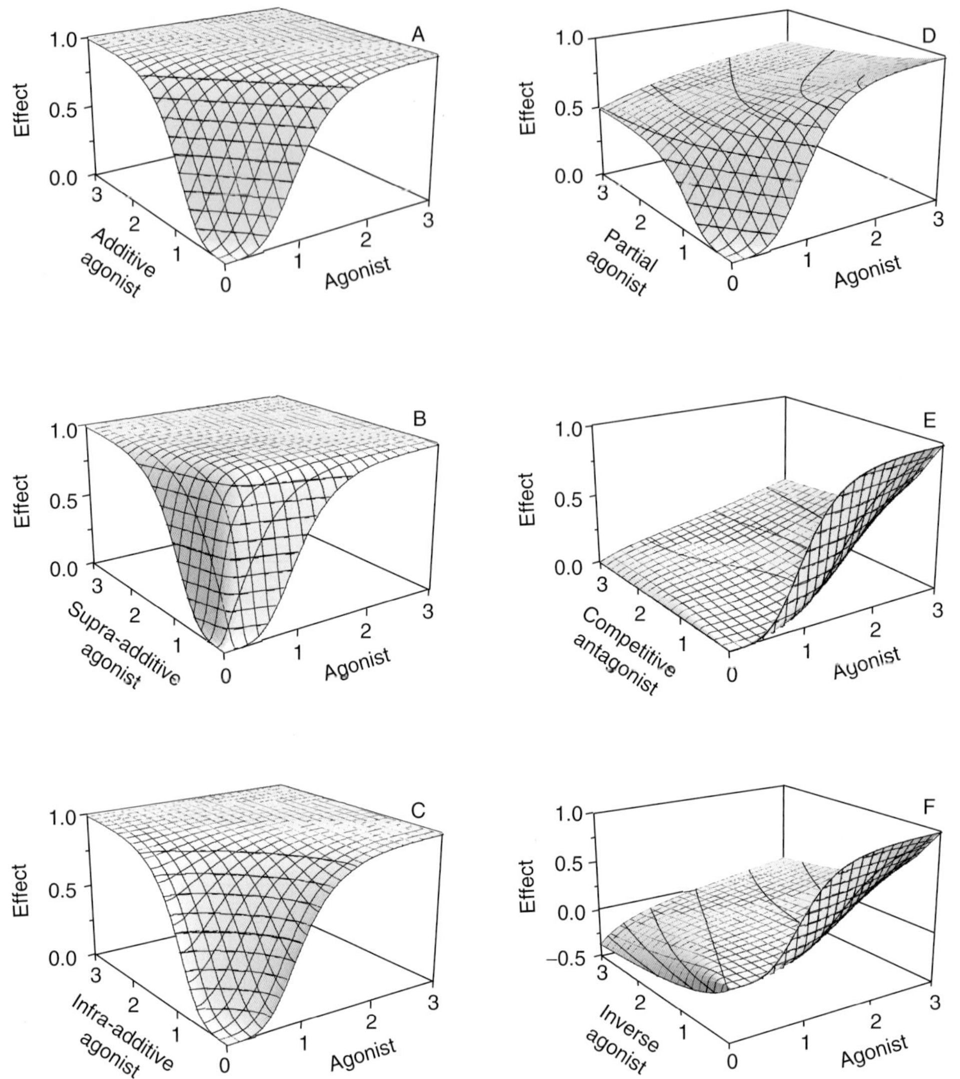

FIGURE 2-37 Interaction surfaces, showing simple additivity **(A)**, synergy **(B)**, and infra-additivity **(C)**. More complex relationships exist between agonists and partial agonists **(D)**, agonists and competitive antagonists **(E)**, and agonists and inverse agonists **(F)**. (From Minto CF, Schnider TW, Short TG, et al. Response surface model for anesthetic drug interactions. *Anesthesiology*. 2000;92:1603–1616, with permission.)

as racemic mixtures, but their use is likely to decrease in the future although the clinical advantages of single enantiomers must be balanced against the increased costs of drugs.[26] Enantiomer-specific drug studies are likely to become more common in the future. Regulatory agencies and pharmaceutical companies are increasingly aware of the importance of identification of the therapeutic enantiomer in pharmacology and are likely to avoid the scientific ambiguities associated with the development of racemic drugs.[25,28] Progress in chemical engineering technology has greatly simplified the separation and the preparation of individual enantiomers.

Clinical Aspects of Chirality

More than one-third of all synthetic drugs are chiral, although most of them are utilized clinically as racemic mixtures.[26,29] In addition to thiopental, methohexital and ketamine are administered as racemic mixtures. The majority of inhaled anesthetics are chiral with the notable exception of sevoflurane. Most evidence suggests that enantiomer-selective effects for volatile anesthetics are relatively weak in contrast to much stronger evidence for specific drug-receptor interactions for intravenous anesthetics.[29] Local anesthetics, including mepivacaine, prilocaine, and bupivacaine, have a center of molecular asymmetry. The S (+) enantiomer of ketamine is more potent than the R (−) form and is also less likely to produce emergence delirium. Similarly, in addition to pharmacokinetic differences, the cardiac toxicity of bupivacaine is thought to be predominantly due to the *R*-bupivacaine isomer. Ropivacaine is the S-enantiomer of a bupivacaine homolog, which has decreased cardiac toxicity. Likewise, the S-enantiomer of bupivacaine, levobupivacaine is associated with less cardiac toxicity than bupivacaine. Cisatracurium is an isomer of atracurium that lacks histamine-releasing potential. Drugs used in anesthesia that occur naturally reflect the importance of stereochemistry, with morphine (actually *l*-morphine) and *d*-tubocurarine being examples. Because these drugs are synthesized by nature's stereospecific enzymatic machinery, they exist in a single form before they are extracted and purified.[25]

Individual Variability

The response to many drugs varies greatly among patients.[30] After administration of identical doses, some patients may have clinically significant adverse effects, whereas others may exhibit no therapeutic response. Some of this diversity of response can be ascribed to differences in the rate of drug metabolism, particularly by the cytochrome P450 family of enzymes. The incorporation of pharmacogenetics into clinical medicine may become useful in predicting patient responses to drugs.

Variability of individual responses to a drug often reflects differences in pharmacokinetics and/or pharmacodynamics among patients (Table 2-4).[4] This may even account for differences in pharmacologic effects of drugs in the same patient at different times. Accurate dosing is difficult to achieve in the presence of interindividual variability and it is not unusual to find a twofold or more variation in plasma concentrations achieved in different individuals using the same dosing scheme. This is true for inhaled as well as injected drugs. Furthermore, there may be a fivefold range in the plasma concentrations of a drug required to achieve the same pharmacologic effect in different individuals, and this range may be even greater if tolerance has developed in some individuals.

The relative importance of the numerous factors that contribute to variations in individual responses to drugs depends, in part, on the drug itself and its usual route of excretion. Drugs excreted primarily unchanged by the kidneys tend to exhibit smaller differences in pharmacokinetics than do drugs that are metabolized. The most important determinant of metabolic rate is genetic. Changes in metabolic rate have little impact on drugs with a high extraction ratio as the efficiency of extraction is so great that hepatic blood flow is a more rate-limiting factor than metabolism. Conversely, the systemic clearance of low-extraction drugs is highly susceptible to small changes in the rate of metabolism. For example, the systemic clearance of alfentanil is exquisitely sensitive to CYP induction and inhibition, whereas clearance of high-extraction opioids such as fentanyl and sufentanil is minimally influenced.[31] Interindividual variability in the response to the prodrug codeine is determined by activity of CYP2D6-mediated *O*-demethylation to morphine and morphine-6-glucuronide. CYP2D6-deficient individuals have diminished or absent morphine formation following administration of codeine, whereas individuals with CYP2D6 gene amplification experience exaggerated opioid effects following administration of codeine ("codeine intoxication").[32] Quinidine inhibits CYP2D6 and markedly diminishes codeine metabolism the active metabolite, morphine. The dynamic state of receptor concentrations, as influenced by diseases and other drugs, also influences the variation in drug responses observed among patients. Finally, inhaled anesthetics, by altering circulatory, hepatic, and renal function, may influence the pharmacokinetics of injected drugs.

In clinical practice, the impact of interpatient variability may be masked by the administration of high doses of a drug. For example, the administration of 2 to 3 $\times$ ED_{95} of a nondepolarizing neuromuscular blocking drug is common practice for achieving a skeletal muscle paralysis in all patients. Inter-patient variability, however, is manifest if the level of neuromuscular blockade and duration of action is monitored. Furthermore, it is common practice in anesthesia to administer drugs in proportion to body weight although pharmacokinetic and pharmacodynamic principles may not support this practice. In attempts to minimize interindividual variability, computerized infusion systems (target-controlled infusion systems) have been developed to deliver intravenous drugs (alfentanil, remifentanil, etomidate, propofol) to achieve a desired (target) concentration (reviewed in reference 3).

Table 2-4

Events Responsible for Variations in Drug Responses between Individuals

- Pharmacokinetics
  - Bioavailability
  - Renal function
  - Hepatic function
  - Cardiac function
  - Patient age
- Pharmacodynamics
  - Enzyme activity
  - Genetic differences
  - Drug interactions

Elderly Patients

In elderly patients, variations in drug response most likely reflect (a) decreased cardiac output, (b) increased fat content, (c) decreased protein binding, and (d) decreased renal function. Decreased cardiac output decreases hepatic blood flow and, thus, delivery of drug to the liver for metabolism. This decreased delivery, combined with the possibility of decreased hepatic enzyme activity, may prolong the duration of action of drugs such as lidocaine and fentanyl.[33] An enlarged fat compartment may increase the *Vd* and lead to the accumulation of lipid-soluble drugs such as diazepam and thiopental.[34] Increased total body fat content and decreased plasma protein binding of drugs accounts for the increased *Vd* that accompanies aging. A parallel decrease in total body water accompanies increased fat stores. The net effect of these changes is an increased vulnerability of elderly patients to cumulative drug effects. Effects of age on PK and PD are discussed in detail in Chapter 46.

Enzyme Activity

Alterations in enzyme activity as reflected by enzyme induction may be responsible for variations in drug responses among individuals. For example, cigarette smoke contains polycyclic hydrocarbons that induce mixed-function hepatic oxidases, leading to increased dose requirements for drugs such as theophylline and tricyclic antidepressants. Acute alcohol ingestion can inhibit metabolism of drugs. Conversely, chronic alcohol use (>200 g per day) induces microsomal enzymes that metabolize drugs. Because of enzyme induction, this accelerated metabolism may manifest as tolerance to drugs such as barbiturates.

Genetic Disorders

Variations in drug responses among individuals are due, in part, to genetic differences that may also affect receptor sensitivity. Genetic variations in metabolic pathways (rapid vs. slow acetylators) may have important clinical implications for drugs such as isoniazid and hydralazine. ***Pharmacogenetics*** describes genetically determined disease states that are initially revealed by altered responses to specific drugs. Examples of diseases that are unmasked by drugs include (a) atypical cholinesterase enzyme revealed by prolonged neuromuscular blockade after administration of succinylcholine or mivacurium; (b) malignant hyperthermia triggered by succinylcholine or volatile anesthetics; (c) glucose-6-phosphate dehydrogenase deficiency, in which certain drugs cause hemolysis; and (d) intermittent porphyria, in which barbiturates may evoke an acute attack.

Drug Interactions

A drug interaction occurs when a drug alters the intensity of pharmacologic effects of another drug given concurrently. Drug interactions may reflect alterations in pharmacokinetics (increased metabolism of neuromuscular blocking drugs in patients receiving anticonvulsants chronically) or pharmacodynamics (decrease in volatile anesthetic requirements produced by opioids). The net result of a drug interaction may be enhanced or diminished effects of one or both drugs, leading to desired or undesired effects. A physicochemical drug interaction occurs when two incompatible drugs are mixed in the same solution (precipitate of the conjugate salt of a weak acid and weak base when pancuronium and thiopental are mixed together in the same intravenous tubing). The potential for drug interactions in the perioperative period is great, considering the large number of drugs from different chemical classes that are likely to be part of anesthesia management. For example, a typical "balanced anesthetic" may include benzodiazepines, sedative-hypnotics, opioids, neuromuscular blocking drugs, anticholinergics, anticholinesterases, sympathomimetics, sympathetic nervous system blocking drugs, and antibiotics.

An example of a beneficial drug interaction is the concurrent administration of propranolol with hydralazine to prevent compensatory increases in heart rate that would offset the blood pressure–lowering effects of hydralazine. Interactions between drugs are frequently used to counter the effects of agonist drugs, as reflected by the use of naloxone to antagonize opioids. Adverse drug interactions typically manifest as impaired therapeutic efficacy and/or enhanced toxicity. In this regard, one drug may interact with another to (a) impair absorption, (b) compete with the same plasma protein-binding sites, (c) alter metabolism by enzyme induction or inhibition, or (d) change the rate of renal excretion.

References

1. Shafer S. Principles of pharmacokinetics and pharmacodynamics. In: Longnecker DE, Tinker JH, Morgan GE, eds. *Principles and Practice of Anesthesiology*. 2nd ed. St. Louis, MO: Mosby-Year Book; 1997:1159.
2. Shafer S, Flood P, Schwinn D. Basic principles of pharmacology. In: Miller RD, Eriksson LI, Fleisher LA, et al, eds. *Miller's Anesthesia*. Vol 1. 7th ed. Philadelphia, PA: Churchill Livingstone; 2010: 479–514.
3. Glass PSA, Shafer S, Reves JG. Intravenous drug delivery systems. In: Miller RD, Eriksson LI, Fleisher LA, et al, eds. *Miller's Anesthesia*. Vol 1. 7th ed. Philadelphia, PA: Churchill Livingstone; 2010: 825–858.
4. Wood M. Variability of human drug response. *Anesthesiology*. 1989;71:631–634.
5. Boer F, Bovill JG, Burm AGL, et al. Effect of ventilation on first-pass pulmonary retention of alfentanil and sufentanil in patients undergoing coronary artery surgery. *Br J Anaesth*. 1994;73: 458–463.
6. Wood M. Plasma drug binding: implications for anesthesiologists. *Anesth Analg*. 1986;65:786–804.
7. Nelson DR. Cytochrome P450 and the individuality of species. *Arch Biochem Biophys*. 1999;369:1–10.
8. Wilkinson GR, Shand DG. Commentary: a physiological approach to hepatic drug clearance. *Clin Pharmacol Ther*. 1975;18:377–390.
9. Cockcroft DW, Gault MH. Prediction of creatinine clearance from serum creatinine. *Nephron*. 1976;16:31–41.
10. Hug CC. Pharmacokinetics of drugs administered intravenously. *Anesth Analg*. 1978;57:704–723.
11. Ebling WF, Wada DR, Stanski DR. From piecewise to full physiologic pharmacokinetic modeling: applied to thiopental disposition in the rat. *J Pharmacokinet Biopharm*. 1994;22:259–292.
12. Wada DR, Björkman S, Ebling WF, et al. Computer simulation of the effects of alterations in blood flows and body composition on

thiopental pharmacokinetics in humans. *Anesthesiology*. 1997;87: 884–899.

13. Youngs EJ, Shafer SL. Basic pharmacokinetic and pharmacodynamic principles. In: White PF, ed. *Textbook of Intravenous Anesthesia*. Baltimore, MD: Lippincott Williams & Wilkins; 1997:10.
14. Scott JC, Ponganis KV, Stanski DR. EEG quantitation of narcotic effect: the comparative pharmacodynamics of fentanyl and alfentanil. *Anesthesiology*. 1985;62:234–241.
15. Scott JC, Stanski DR. Decreased fentanyl and alfentanil dose requirements with age. A simultaneous pharmacokinetic and pharmacodynamic evaluation. *J Pharmacol Exp Ther*. 1987;240:159–166.
16. Minto CF, Schnider TW, Gregg KM, et al. Using the time of maximum effect site concentration to combine pharmacokinetics and pharmacodynamics. *Anesthesiology*. 2003;99:324–333.
17. Vuyk J, Lim T, Engbers FH, et al. The pharmacodynamic interaction of propofol and alfentanil during lower abdominal surgery in women. *Anesthesiology*. 1995;83:8–22.
18. Bruhn J, Bouillon TW, Ropcke H, et al. A manual slide rule for target-controlled infusion of propofol: development and evaluation. *Anesth Analg*. 2003;96:142–147.
19. Hughes MA, Glass PSA, Jacobs JR. Context-sensitive half-time in multicompartment pharmacokinetic models for intravenous anesthetic drugs. *Anesthesiology*. 1992;76:334–341.
20. Fisher DM. (Almost) everything you learned about pharmacokinetics was (somewhat) wrong! *Anesth Analg*. 1996;83:901–903.
21. Sebel PS, Glass PS, Fletcher JE, et al. Reduction of the MAC of desflurane with fentanyl. *Anesthesiology*. 1992;76:52–59.
22. McEwan AI, Smith C, Dyar O, et al. Isoflurane minimum alveolar concentration reduction by fentanyl. *Anesthesiology*. 1993;78: 864–869.
23. Hendrickx JF, Eger EI II, Sonner JM, et al. Is synergy the rule? A review of anesthetic interactions producing hypnosis and immobility. *Anesth Analg*. 2008;107:494–506.
24. Minto CF, Schnider TW, Short TG, et al. Response surface model for anesthetic drug interactions. *Anesthesiology*. 2000;92:1603–1616.
25. Egan TD. Stereochemistry and anesthetic pharmacology: joining hands with the medicinal chemists. *Anesth Analg*. 1996;83:447–450.
26. Nau C, Strichartz GR. Drug chirality in anesthesia. *Anesthesiology*. 2002;97:497–502.
27. Ariens EJ. Stereochemistry, a basis for sophisticated nonsense in pharmacokinetics and clinical pharmacology. *Eur J Clin Pharmacol*. 1984;26:663–668.
28. Nation RL. Chirality in new drug development. Clinical pharmacokinetic considerations. *Clin Pharmacokinet*. 1994;27:249–255.
29. Burke D, Henderson DJ. Chirality: a blueprint for the future. *Br J Anaesth*. 2002;88:563–576.
30. Caraco Y. Genes and the response to drugs. *N Engl J Med*. 2004; 351:2867–2869.
31. Kharasch ED, Russell M, Mautz D, et al. The role of cytochrome P450 3A4 in alfentanil clearance: implications for interindividual variability in disposition and perioperative drug interactions. *Anesthesiology*. 1997;87:36–50.
32. Gasche Y, Daali Y, Fathi M, et al. Codeine intoxication associated with ultrarapid CYP2D6 metabolism. *N Engl J Med*. 2004;351: 2827–2831.
33. Bentley JB, Borel JD, Nad RE, et al. Age and fentanyl pharmacokinetics. *Anesth Analg*. 1982;61:968–971.
34. Jung D, Mayersohn M, Perrie D, et al. Thiopental disposition as a function of age in female patients undergoing surgery. *Anesthesiology*. 1982;56:263–268.

CHAPTER 3

Neurophysiology

Pamela Flood • Steven Shafer

The most amazing aspect of the daily miracle of anesthesia is turning off consciousness to permit surgery to proceed and then fully restoring consciousness in a controlled manner. We still do not fully understand how this miracle occurs. A full understanding of consciousness, and the biology that underlies it, is probably decades in the future, if it is tractable at all.[1] However, recent advances in neurophysiology are providing insight into how drugs interact with receptors throughout the nervous system to mediate anesthesia and analgesia.

How Nerves Work

Neurons

Neurons are the basic elements of all rapid signal processing within the body. A neuron consists of a cell body, also called the ***soma***; dendrites; and the nerve fiber, also called the ***axon*** (Fig. 3-1). Dendrites are highly specialized extensions of the cell body. The axon of one neuron commonly terminates (synapses) near the cell body or dendrites of another neuron. The axon connects to a neighboring cell with a ***presynaptic terminal***. The ***synaptic cleft*** separates the presynaptic terminal and the cell body or dendrites of the next neuron in the signaling cascade (Fig. 3-2). Transmission of impulses between responsive neurons at a synapse is mediated by the release of a chemical mediator (neurotransmitter), such as ***glutamate*** or ***γ-aminobutyric acid*** (GABA) from the presynaptic terminal. The membrane of the postsynaptic neurons contains receptors that bind neurotransmitters released from presynaptic nerve terminals, transducing the signal.

The impulse travels along the nerve membrane as an ***action potential***. This is entirely mediated by the receptors within the membrane. Indeed, removal of the axoplasm from the nerve fiber does not alter conduction of impulses. Nerve fibers derive their nutrition from the cell body. Interruption of a nerve fiber causes the peripheral portion to degenerate (Wallerian degeneration). The axon of a peripheral neuron is able to regenerate, as does the myelin sheath. Regeneration is the exception in most of the brain and spinal cord. Extensive research is underway to better understand the conditions that are required for central neuron regeneration to improve recovery from central neuronal injury.

Classification of Afferent Nerve Fibers

Nerve fibers are called ***afferent*** if they transmit impulses from peripheral receptors to the central nervous system (CNS) and efferent if they transmit impulses from the CNS to the periphery. Afferent nerve fibers are classified as A, B, and C on the basis of fiber diameter and velocity of conduction of nerve impulses (Table 3-1). Conduction speed increases with nerve diameter, because the larger diameter nerves have decreased longitudinal resistance to ion flux.[2] The largest, and hence fastest, nerves are designated type A. Type A fibers are subdivided into α, β, γ, and δ. Type A-α_1 fibers innervate muscle spindles and A-α_{1b} innervate the Golgi tendon organ. Both A-α afferents are important to muscle reflexes and control of muscle tone.

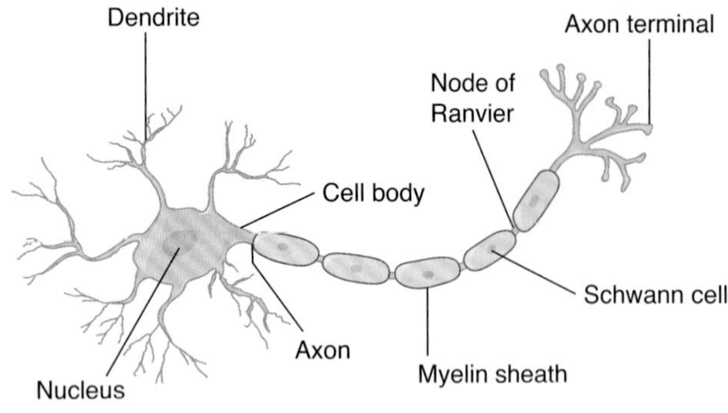

FIGURE 3-1 Anatomy of a neuron.

All cutaneous mechanoreceptors (Meissner's corpuscles, hair receptors, Pacinian corpuscles) transmit signals in type A-β fibers. Touch and fast pain are transmitted by lightly myelinated type A-δ fibers with free nerve endings. Type C fibers transmit slow pain, pruritus, and temperature sensation.

Myelin that surrounds type A and B nerve fibers acts as an insulator that prevents flow of ions across nerve membranes. Type C fibers are unmyelinated. The myelin sheath is interrupted approximately every 1 to 2 mm by the nodes of Ranvier (see Fig. 3-1).[3] Ions can flow freely between nerve fibers and extracellular fluid at the nodes of Ranvier. Action potentials are conducted from node to node by the myelinated nerve rather than continuously along the entire fiber as occurs in unmyelinated nerve fibers. This successive excitation of nodes of Ranvier by an action potential that jumps between successive nodes is termed ***saltatory conduction*** (Fig. 3-3).[3] Saltatory conduction allows for a 10-fold increase in the velocity of nerve transmission.[2] It also conserves the membrane potential because only the membrane at the node of Ranvier depolarizes, resulting in less ion transfer than would otherwise occur. Furthermore, because depolarization is limited to the nodes of Ranvier, little energy is needed for to reestablish the transmembrane sodium and potassium ion concentration gradients necessary for signal transmission. The energy savings is more than a hundred fold. As brilliantly understated by Hartline and Colman,[2] "For a nervous system such as ours, which already accounts for 20% of the body's resting metabolic energy budget, this is not an inconsequential advantage." If myelin did not exist, you would not be reading about it.

Evaluation of Peripheral Nerve Function

Peripheral nerves may be injured by ischemia of the intraneural vasa nervorum, as might be caused by excessive stretch of the nerve or external compression. Nerve conduction studies are useful in the localization and assessment of peripheral nerve dysfunction. Focal demyelination of nerve fibers causes slowing of conduction and decreased amplitudes of compound muscle and sensory action potentials. The presence of denervation potentials in skeletal muscle indicates axonal or anterior horn cell damage. Changes in motor unit potentials also arise from reinnervation of skeletal muscle fibers by surviving axons. Signs of denervation on the electromyogram after acute nerve injury require 18 to 21 days to develop.[4] Electromyographic testing is helpful in determining the etiology of neurologic dysfunction that may occur after surgery.

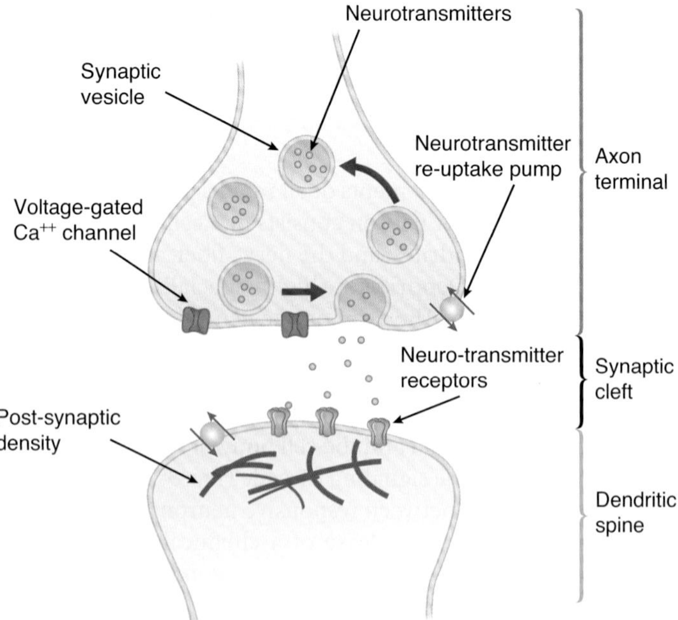

FIGURE 3-2 Basic structure of the synapse. The signal arrives at the axon terminal, where it causes the release of neurotransmitters into the synapse. These cross the synaptic cleft, where they may or may not result in a propagation of the signal. Many synapses simply render the postsynaptic cell excited or inhibited without actually triggering an action potential.

Table 3-1

Classification of Peripheral Nerve Fibers

	Myelinated	Fiber Diameter (mm)	Conduction Velocity (m/s)	Function	Sensitivity to Local Anesthetic (Subarachnoid, Procaine, %)
A-α	Yes	12–20	70–120	Innervation of skeletal muscles Proprioception	1
A-β	Yes	5–12	30–70	Touch Pressure	1
A-γ	Yes	3–6	15–30	Skeletal muscle tone	1
A-δ	Yes	2–5	12–30	Fast pain Touch Temperature	0.5
B	Yes	3	3–15	Preganglionic autonomic fibers	0.25
C	No	0.4–1.2	0.5–2.0	Slow pain Touch Temperature Postganglionic sympathetic fibers	0.5

The Action Potential

Electrical potentials exist across nearly all cell membranes, reflecting principally the difference in transmembrane concentrations of sodium and potassium ions. This unequal distribution of ions is created and maintained by the membrane-bound enzyme sodium-potassium ATPase, sometimes called the ***sodium-potassium pump***. The sodium-potassium pump transfers three sodium ions out of the cell in exchange for two potassium ions brought into the cell. This causes a net transfer of positive charges out of the cell. The resulting voltage difference across the cell membrane is called the ***resting membrane potential***. The cytoplasm is electrically negative (typically −60 to −80 mV) relative to the extracellular fluid (Fig. 3-4).[5]

When channels open to specific ions, the ions generally flow in the direction of their concentration gradients. An action potential is the rapid change in transmembrane potential due to the opening of sodium channels (***depolarization***) and rapid influx of sodium ions down the concentration gradient, reversing the net negative charge within the cell. The membrane resting potential is restored by the closing of the sodium channels and the opening of potassium channels (***repolarization***) after the action potential has passed. The outward flux of potassium ions down their concentration gradient restores the net negative charge within the cell. This is discussed in greater detail under the "Ion Channels" section.

Propagation of Action Potentials

Propagation of action potentials along the entire length of a nerve axon is the basis of rapid signal transmission along nerve cells. The size and shape of the action potential varies among excitable tissues (see Fig. 3-4).[5]

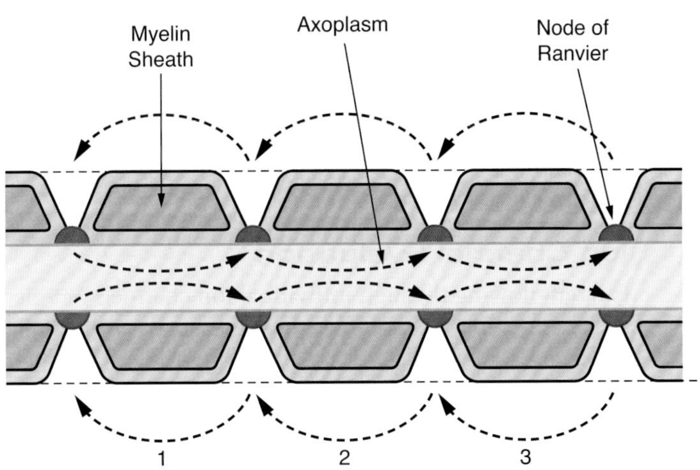

FIGURE 3-3 Saltatory conduction is transmission of nerve impulses that jump between successive nodes of Ranvier of myelinated nerves.

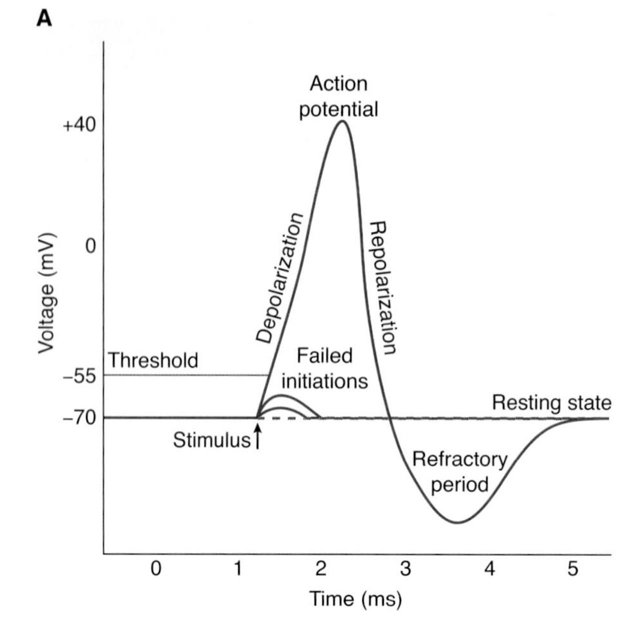

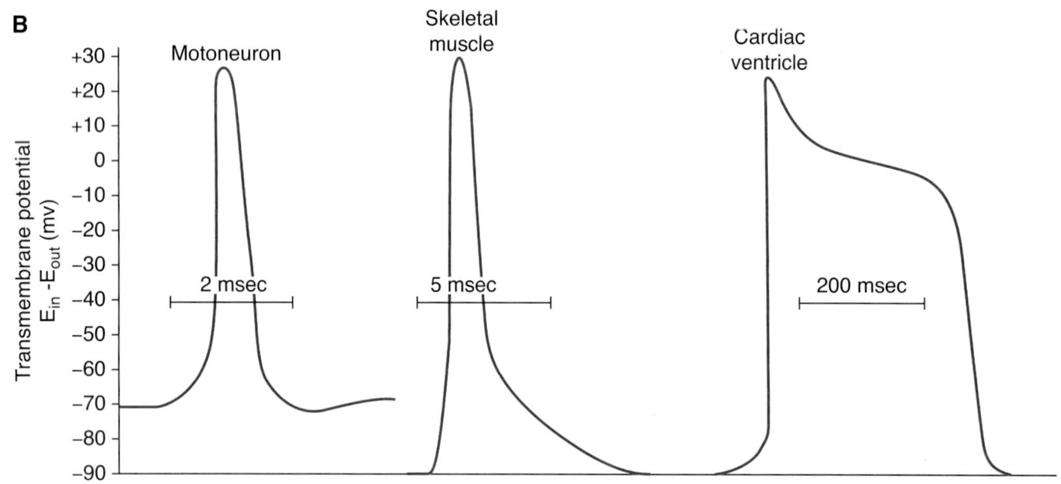

FIGURE 3-4 **A:** The elements of the action potential. **B:** The transmembrane potential and duration of the action potential varies with the tissue site. (From Berne RM, Levy MN, Koeppen B, et al. *Physiology.* 5th ed. St. Louis, MO: Mosby; 2004, with permission.)

Action potentials are conducted along nerve or muscle fibers by local current flow that produces depolarization of adjacent areas of the cell membrane (Fig. 3-5). These propagated action potentials travel in both directions along the entire extent of the fiber. The transmission of the depolarization process along nerve or muscle fibers is called a ***nerve*** or ***muscle impulse***. The entire action potential usually occurs in less than 1 millisecond.

During much of the action potential, the cell membrane is completely refractory to further stimulation. This is termed the ***absolute refractory period*** and is due to the presence of a large fraction of inactivated sodium ion channels. During the last portion of the action potential, a stronger than normal stimulus can evoke a second action potential. This "relative refractory period" reflects the need to activate a critical number of sodium ion channels to trigger an action potential.

The action potential is dynamic, which is difficult to illustrate with a static textbook image. We encourage the motivated reader to search for the text "action potential animation" on the Internet. There are many high-quality animations of the action potential that dynamically display how it propagates.

Ion Channel Evaluation

Current flowing through individual ion channels or voltage changes in a membrane can be measured with patch-clamping, a method used in electrophysiology.[6] In patch clamping, an electrode is connected with a cell (or piece of membrane) with a tight seal. This electrode is able to control either the voltage or the current so that the other

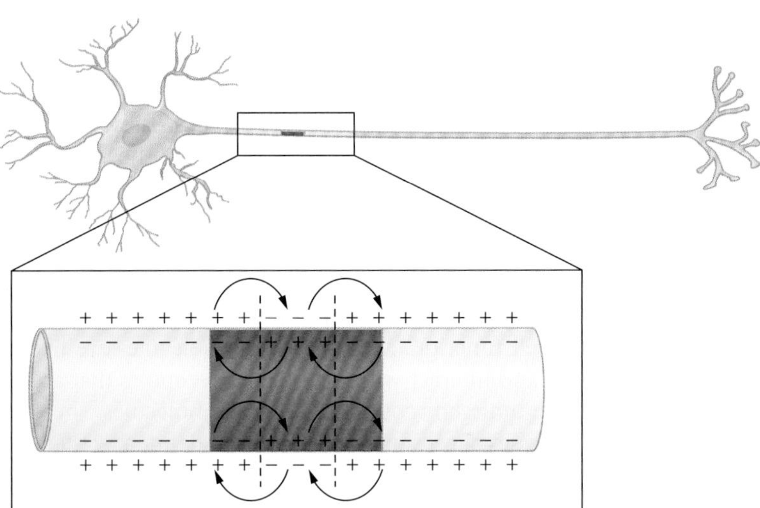

FIGURE 3-5 Depolarization spreads in both directions along cell membranes, resulting in propagation of an action potential.

can be measured. Currents carried through different types of channels can be isolated by the use of specific inhibitors. For example, tetraethylammonium blocks many types of potassium ion channels, whereas tetrodotoxin blocks many types of sodium ion channels. Channels that are not normally expressed in a cell can be added through heterologous expression. With these methods, the impact of specific naturally occurring or synthetic channel elements on function can be evaluated. Using DNA manipulation, entire genes that code for channels/receptors can be *knocked out*. Specific amino acids in the receptor proteins can be altered by manipulating the DNA encoding the receptor, resulting in a *knocked in* receptor with specific amino acid substitutions. Enormous strides have been made in understanding the mechanism of action of anesthetic drugs using these genetic methods and assessments of electrophysiology and animal behavior studies.[7]

Abnormal Action Potentials

A deficiency of calcium ions in the extracellular fluid (hypocalcemia) prevents the sodium channels from closing between action potentials. The resulting continuous leak of sodium contributes to sustained depolarization or repetitive firing of cell membranes (tetany). Conversely, high calcium ion concentrations decrease cell membrane permeability to sodium and thus decrease excitability of nerve membranes. Low potassium ion concentrations in extracellular fluid increase the negativity of the resting membrane potential, resulting in hyperpolarization and decreased cell membrane excitability. Skeletal muscle weakness that accompanies hypokalemia presumably reflects hyperpolarization of skeletal muscle membranes. Local anesthetics decrease permeability of nerve cell membranes to sodium ions, preventing achievement of a threshold potential that is necessary for generation of an action potential. Blockage of cardiac sodium ion channels by local anesthetics may result in altered conduction of cardiac impulses and decreases in myocardial contractility.

Neurotransmitters and Receptors

Neurotransmitters are chemical mediators that are released into the synaptic cleft in response to the arrival of an action potential at the nerve ending. Neurotransmitter release is voltage dependent and requires the influx of calcium ions into the presynaptic terminals (see Fig. 3-2). Synaptic vesicles of the cell body and dendrites of neurons are the sites of continuous synthesis and storage of neurotransmitters. These vesicles may contain and release more than one neurotransmitter. Neurotransmitters may be excitatory or inhibitory, depending on the ion selectivity of the protein receptor. A postsynaptic receptor may be excited or inhibited, reflecting the existence of both types of receptors in the same postsynaptic neuron. Furthermore, the same neurotransmitter may be inhibitory at one site and excitatory at another. This is particularly applicable to G protein–coupled receptors as the associated G protein determines the polarity of the response. Some neurotransmitters function as neuromodulators or coagonists in that they influence the sensitivity of receptors to other neurotransmitters. For example, glycine is an important coagonist at the *N*-methyl-d-aspartate (NMDA) receptor.

Volatile anesthetics produce a broad spectrum of actions, as reflected by their ability to modify both inhibitory and excitatory neurotransmission at presynaptic and postsynaptic loci within the CNS. The precise mechanism of these effects remains uncertain. It is likely that volatile anesthetics interact with multiple neurotransmitter systems by a variety of mechanisms.[8] In general, volatile anesthetics inhibit excitatory receptors (NMDA and nicotinic acetylcholine receptors) and potentiate the action of inhibitory receptors ($GABA_A$ and glycine). To quote Ted Eger, "How do they know?" Inhaled anesthetics may depress excitable tissues at all levels of the nervous system by interacting with neuronal membranes,[9] resulting in a decreased release of neurotransmitters and transmission

Table 3-2

Chemicals that Act at Synapses as Neurotransmitters

Glutamate
Acetylcholine
Norepinephrine
Glycine
Endorphins
Serotonin
Histamine
Oxytocin
Cholecystokinin
Gastrin
γ-Aminobutyric acid
Dopamine
Epinephrine
Substance P
Vasopressin
Prolactin
Vasoactive intestinal peptide
Glucagon

of impulses at synapses as well as a general depression of excitatory postsynaptic responsiveness.

The list of chemical mediators functioning as excitatory or inhibitory neurotransmitters continues to increase (Table 3-2). Glutamate is the major excitatory neurotransmitter in the CNS, whereas GABA is the major inhibitory neurotransmitter.[8] Acetylcholine, dopamine, histamine, and norepinephrine are widely distributed and play important roles in sleep pathways that are impacted upon by general anesthetics. Neuromodulators coexist in presynaptic terminals with neurotransmitters but do not themselves cause substantive voltage or conductance changes in postsynaptic cell membranes. They can, however, amplify, prolong, decrease, or shorten the postsynaptic response to selected neurotransmitters.

Receptors can be classified by their cellular localization. Receptors on the cell membrane act as signal transducers by binding the extracellular signal molecule and converting this information into an intracellular signal that alters target cell function. Most signaling molecules are hydrophobic and interact with cell surface receptors that are directly or indirectly coupled to effector molecules. There are three classes of cell surface receptors as defined by their signal transduction mechanisms: guanine nucleotide-binding protein ("G protein") coupled receptors, ligand-gated ion channels, and enzyme-linked transmembrane receptors.

G protein–coupled receptors in the plasma membrane are coupled to specific intracellular G proteins (Fig. 3-6). The binding of the receptor to the ligand activates the G protein, which then activates or inhibits an enzyme, ion channel, or other target. G protein–coupled receptors constitute the largest family of cell surface receptors. A number of different isoforms of G protein subunits (α, β, γ) are present and mediate stimulation or inhibition of functionally diverse effector enzymes and ion channels. Most hormones and many neurotransmitters interact with G protein–coupled cell-surface receptors to produce the cellular response.[10–12] The resulting response is often a change in transmembrane voltage and thus neuronal excitability. There is great diversity in the number of G protein–coupled receptors for the same ligand as reflected by multiple receptors for catecholamines and opioids.[13]

Ligand-gated ion channels are channels in the plasma membrane that respond directly to extracellular ligands,

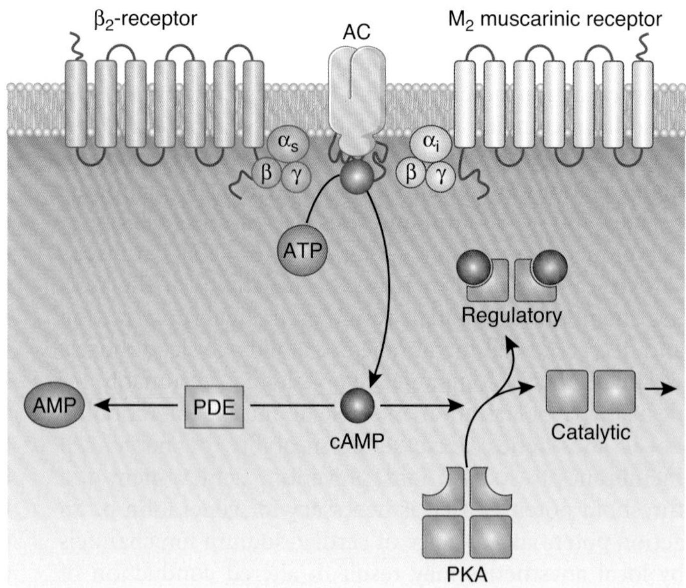

FIGURE 3-6 Schematic presentation showing G protein–coupled receptors; the β_2 adrenergic receptor, which upregulates adenylyl cyclase; and the M_2 muscarinic receptor, which downregulates adenylyl cyclase (AC). The effects of these G protein–coupled receptors are then mediated through the intercellular concentration of cyclic adenosine monophosphate (cAMP). ATP, adenosine triphosphate; AMP, adenosine monophosphate; PDE, phosphodiesterase; PKA, protein kinase A.

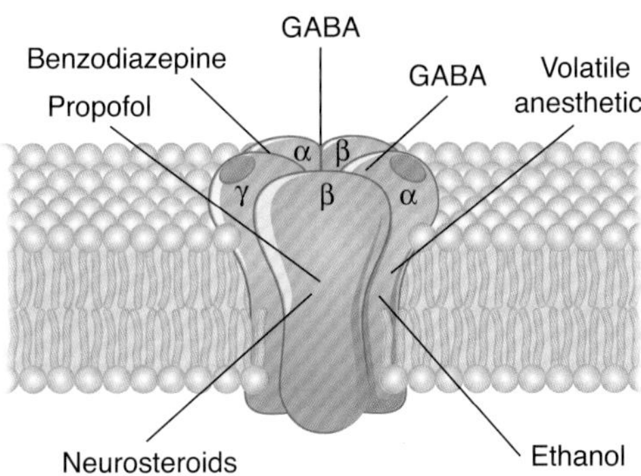

FIGURE 3-7 Schematic illustration of the $GABA_A$ ligand-gated ion channel. The ligand binds to the external binding domain, modulating the conductance of ions through the central pore. The receptor is a pentamer of two α subunits, two β subunits, and one γ subunit. The binding sites show where several sedatives are known to act. These sedatives increase the flux of chloride through the channel, leading to hyperpolarization of the cell.

rather than require coupling through G proteins (Fig. 3-7). They are one of three classes of ion channels, the other two being ***voltage-gated ion channels*** that respond to transmembrane voltage flux, and ***"other" gated ion channels*** that are gated by a huge variety of mechanisms. Rapid synaptic transmission is entirely accomplished through voltage-gated ion channels, which propagate action potentials, and ligand-gated ion channels, which transmit the signal across the synapse.

Enzyme-linked transmembrane receptors are not involved in neuronal signaling per se, as they have relatively slow effects on cells. Most enzyme-linked transmembrane receptors are tyrosine kinases that phosphorylate an intracellular second messenger when the extracellular ligand binds to the receptor (Fig. 3-8). The insulin receptor,[14] the atrial natriuretic peptide receptor, and the receptors for many growth factors (nerve growth factor, epidermal growth factor, fibroblast growth factor, and vascular endothelial growth factor) are all examples of tyrosine kinase–linked transmembrane receptors.

There are also ***intracellular receptors***. For example, steroid receptors and thyroid hormone receptors act in the nucleus where they directly regulate the transcription of specific genes, whereas phosphodiesterase inhibitors (e.g., caffeine, milrinone, and sildenafil) act in the cytosol by inhibiting the activity of phosphodiesterase, increasing the cytosolic concentration of cyclic adenosine monophosphate (cAMP). These receptors are also not involved in neuronal signaling per se, because the cellular response is quite slow.

G Protein–Coupled Receptors

G protein–coupled receptors consist of three separate components: a receptor protein, three G proteins (α, β, and γ), and an effector mechanism (see Fig. 3-6). The recognition site faces the exterior of the cell membrane to facilitate access of water-soluble endogenous ligands and exogenous drugs, whereas the catalytic site faces the interior of the cell. There are at least 16 G_α, 5 G_β, and 11 G_γ proteins,[15] providing G protein–coupled receptors that mediate an enormous variety of cellular effects.

The G protein–coupled receptor consists of a single protein with seven transmembrane spanning domains (Fig. 3-9). Binding of an extracellular ligand to the G protein–coupled receptor triggers a conformational change of the protein. That change causes activation of the G_α protein coupled to the interior portion of the receptor. The activation occurs by exchanging a guanine diphosphate (GDP) moiety that is bound to the protein for a guanine triphosphate (GTP) moiety. The activated G_α protein is liberated, where it interacts as a "second messenger" with other proteins in the cell.[11] When the G_α protein finds its target, the GTP is hydrolyzed to GDP, and the energy liberated by that hydrolysis powers the effect of the G_α protein on the target protein.

G_α proteins can either be stimulatory, promoting a specific enzymatic reaction within the cell, or inhibitory, depressing a specific enzymatic reaction. For example, β-adrenergic receptors couple with stimulatory $G_{\alpha s}$ proteins and increase the activity of adenylyl cyclase (also called ***adenylate cyclase***). Opioid receptors associate with inhibitory $G_{\alpha i}$ proteins that decrease the activity of adenylyl cyclase. By regulating the level of activity of adenylyl cyclase, the β-adrenergic and opioid receptors modulate the internal level of cAMP, which functions as an intercellular second messenger (see Fig. 3-6).

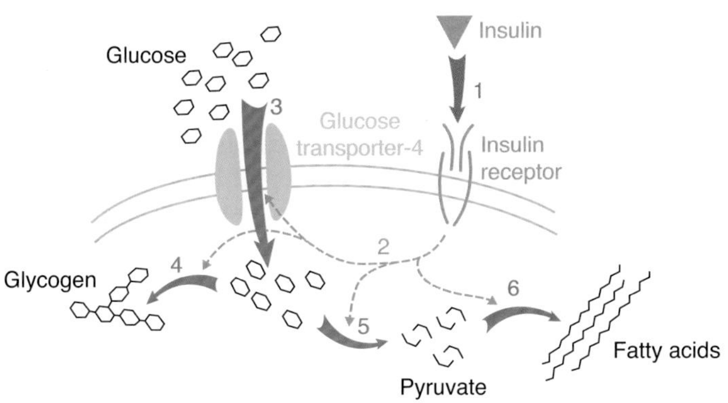

FIGURE 3-8 The insulin receptor is a transmembrane tyrosine kinase receptor that binds extracellular insulin, resulting in phosphorylation of intracellular proteins and increased expression of glucose transporter proteins on the cell membrane.

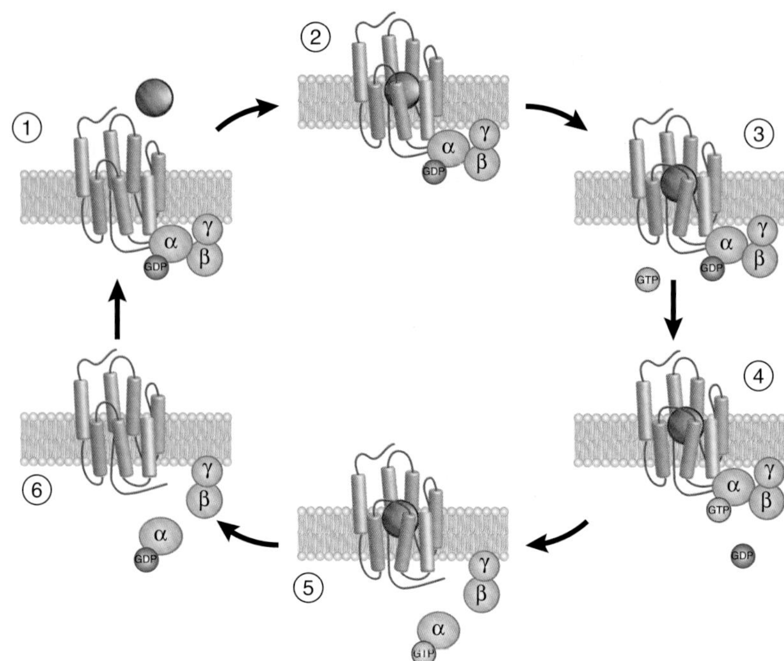

FIGURE 3-9 Activation of G protein following coupling of a ligand *(brown oval)* to the seven transmembrane domain G protein–coupled receptor *(blue)*. The G protein–coupled receptor awaits the binding of the ligand, with the G_α protein bound to GDP *(1)*. The ligand binds to the G protein–coupled receptor *(2)*. The bound G protein–coupled receptor undergoes a conformational change *(3)*. The conformational change allows the G protein–coupled receptor to substitute GTP for GDP on the G_α protein *(4)*. The GTP-bound G_α protein diffuses away from the complex, functioning as a second messenger *(5)*. The GTP-bound G_α protein, having delivered its message, returns bound to GDP *(6)*. In the meantime, the ligand has diffused away from the G protein–coupled receptor. The GDP-bound G_α protein is again bound to the G protein receptor, awaiting the next ligand *(1)*.

Just as $G_{\alpha s}$ and $G_{\alpha i}$ modulate adenylyl cyclase, other types of G_a proteins modulate other specific cellular targets. In some cases, the message is transmitted via $G_{\beta\gamma}$ rather than G_α, as described below for G protein regulation of potassium channels.

Many hormones and drugs act through G protein–coupled receptors, including catecholamines, opioids, anticholinergics, and antihistamines. In contrast to the immediate cellular responses associated with ion channels, signals that use G protein–coupled receptors are involved in functions that operate with time courses of seconds to minutes. Some ion channels are also gated by G proteins. These are discussed below with the ion channels.

Dopamine

Dopamine represents more than 50% of the CNS content of catecholamines, with high concentrations in the basal ganglia. Dopamine can be either inhibitory or excitatory, depending on the specific dopaminergic receptor that it activates. Dopamine is important to the reward centers of the brain and plays a key role in addiction and tolerance to anesthetic and analgesic drugs.

Norepinephrine

Norepinephrine is present in large amounts in the reticular activating system and the hypothalamus, where it plays a key role in natural sleep and analgesia. Neurons responding to norepinephrine send excitatory (through α_1) and inhibitory (through α_2) signals to widespread areas of the brain, including the cerebral cortex. The sedative action of dexmedetomidine is mediated by activation of α_2 adrenergic receptors in the locus ceruleus that inhibit firing of the ventral lateral preoptic nucleus of the hypothalamus (VLPO), an endogenous sleep pathway.[16] Descending noradrenergic fibers that project to the dorsal horn of the spinal cord play an important tonic inhibitory role in pain transmission. These pathways are augmented by epidural clonidine for postoperative and intrapartum analgesia.

Substance P

Substance P is an excitatory neurotransmitter coreleased by terminals of pain fibers that synapse in the substantia gelatinosa of the spinal cord. Substance P activates the neurokinin-1 G protein–coupled receptor.

Endorphins

Endorphins are endogenous opioid peptide agonists that are secreted by nerve terminals in the pituitary, thalamus, hypothalamus, brainstem, and spinal cord. Endorphins act through the μ opioid receptor, the same receptor responsible for the effects of administered opioids. Endorphins are secreted after exercise and during pain and anxiety. Endorphins facilitate dopamine release and activate inhibitory pain pathways.

Serotonin

Serotonin (5-HT) is present in high concentrations in the brain, where it acts on both ligand-gated ion channels and G protein–coupled receptors. Serotonin receptors are located in the chemoreceptor trigger zone, where they are inhibited by ondansetron, granisetron, and other common antiemetic drugs

Histamine

Histamine is present in high concentrations in the hypothalamus and the reticular activating system. Histaminergic neurons present in the tuberomammillary nucleus of the hypothalamus are active during the wake cycle. The sleep promoting properties of antihistamine drugs that cross the blood–brain barrier are due to inhibition of H_1 G protein–coupled receptors.

Ion Channels

As pointed out earlier, the normal resting membrane potential is −60 to −80 mV, with the interior of the cell negative relative to the extracellular fluid. The lipid bilayer is mostly impermeable to ions, which must pass in and out of the cell through ion-specific channels. If the flux of ions makes the inside of the cell more negative ("hyperpolarized"), then it is harder for the cell to initiate an action potential. If the flux of ions makes the inside of the cell less negative ("depolarized"), then it is easier for the cell to initiate an action potential.

When ion channels open, ions usually flow in the direction favored by their concentration gradient. Extracellular concentrations of sodium, calcium, and chloride greatly exceed intracellular concentrations, and thus these ions flow into cells when the appropriate ion channel opens. Intracellular concentrations of potassium greatly exceed extracellular concentrations, and thus potassium follows out of cells whenever a potassium channel is opened. The inwardly rectifying potassium channel is an exception in that potassium flows into the cell, opposite the concentration gradient, in response to the electrical gradient.

When sodium flows into a cell, it makes the interior less negative. Sodium channels are thus depolarizing. When potassium flows out of a cell, it makes the interior more negative. Therefore, potassium channels are hyperpolarizing. Sodium channels open to conduct action potentials, after which potassium channels open to restore the resting negative potential and terminate the action potential.

When chloride flows into a cell, the interior becomes more negative, or hyperpolarized. Because it is harder for a hyperpolarized cell to initiate an action potential, chloride channels are "inhibitory," at least after birth. When calcium flows into a cell, the interior becomes less negative, or "depolarized." Because it is easier for a depolarized cell to initiate an action potential, calcium channels are "excitatory." Calcium can also act as a second messenger within the cell.

When cell membranes are depolarized (the outside becomes less negative relative to the inside) or the appropriate ligand is present, these ion channels undergo conformational changes, the ion channel opens, and ions pass through. About 10^4 to 10^5 ions flow per millisecond per channel and thousands of channels may open during a single action potential.

As mentioned previously, there are three basic types of ion channels: (a) ligand-gated ion channels (ionotropic receptors), (b) voltage-sensitive ion channels, and (c) ion channels that respond to other types of gating.

Ligand-Gated Ion Channels

Ligand-gated ion channels (ionotropic receptors) are complexes of protein subunits that act as switchable portals for ions. Ligand-gated ion channels are involved principally with fast synaptic transmission between excitable cells. Binding of signaling molecules to these receptors causes an immediate conformational change in the ion channels, opening (usually) or closing (rarely) the channel to alter the ion permeability of the plasma membranes and therefore the membrane potential. Ligand-gated ion channels are activated by ligands for which they are named. Nicotinic acetylcholine receptors (nAChRs), serotonin receptors (5-HT_3), γ-aminobutyric acid receptors ($GABA_A$) (see Fig. 3-7), and glycine receptors are opened in the presence of acetylcholine, serotonin, GABA, and glycine, respectively. Sometimes the agonist for which the channel is named is not the native agonist. For example, NMDA and α-amino-3-hydroxyl-5-methyl-4-isoxazole-propionate (AMPA) receptors are opened selectively by NMDA and AMPA, but the native agonist for both receptors is glutamate.

Excitatory Ligand-Gated Ion Channels

Excitatory ligand-gated ion channels cause the inside of the cell to become less negative, typically by facilitating the influx of cations into the cell.

Acetylcholine

Acetylcholine is an excitatory neurotransmitter that activates muscarinic and nicotinic receptors in the CNS. Nicotinic acetylcholine receptors are nonspecific cation channels, permitting sodium and in some cases calcium to flow into cells, and potassium to flow out of cells. Because the flow of sodium and calcium is driven both by concentration and electrical gradients, the channel produces a net positive inward flux of cations and is therefore depolarizing (the interior becomes less negative). Nicotinic acetylcholine receptors in the brain are most commonly in a presynaptic location where they act as a "gain control mechanism" to enhance the release of other neurotransmitters. Acetylcholine-releasing neurons play an important role in native sleep pathways where acetylcholine mediates arousal. Although all volatile anesthetics are highly potent inhibitors of the nicotinic acetylcholine receptors that mediate this response,[17] direct nicotinic inhibition is not likely responsible for the hypnotic actions of volatile anesthetics. Nicotinic acetylcholine receptors are largely antagonized at volatile anesthetic concentrations; 1/10 of that induce immobility and thus at concentrations associated with a fully awake patient.[18,19] Injection of nicotine into the central medial thalamus reversed the hypnotic effect of continued sevoflurane.[20] However, in this case, nicotine was acting as an arousing stimulus. Microinfusion of the broad-spectrum nicotinic antagonist mecamylamine did not add to the hypnotic potential of sevoflurane by reducing the dose necessary for hypnosis.

The excitatory effect on the CNS mediated through nicotinic ion channels contrasts with the inhibitory effects that are mediated by the G protein–coupled muscarinic acetylcholine receptors in the peripheral parasympathetic nervous system.

Nicotinic acetylcholine receptors are also responsible for activating muscle contraction. Nondepolarizing muscle relaxants work by blocking the acetylcholine binding site. Because these channels cause depolarization, they are excitatory.

Glutamate

Glutamate is the major excitatory amino acid neurotransmitter in the CNS. Glutamate receptors are nonselective cation channels, permitting sodium and some calcium to flow into cells, and potassium to flow out of cells. Because nonspecific cation channels primarily favor net inward flux of cations down the electrical gradient, glutamate receptors are depolarizing and excitatory. Glutamate-responsive receptors are distributed widely in the CNS. Glutamate plays a key role in learning, and memory, central pain transduction, and pathologic processes such as excitotoxic neuronal injury following CNS trauma or ischemia.

Glutamate is synthesized by the deamination of glutamine via the tricarboxylic acid cycle. Glutamate is released into the synaptic cleft in response to depolarization of the presynaptic nerve terminal. The release of glutamate from presynaptic terminals is a calcium ion-dependent process regulated by multiple types of calcium channels. In common with many other central neurotransmitter systems, the actions of glutamate within the synaptic cleft are terminated by high-affinity sodium-dependent reuptake of glutamate.

The two main subgroups of glutamate receptors are ***inotropic*** and ***metabotropic*** receptors.[8] Ionotropic glutamate receptors (NMDA, AMPA, and kainate receptors) are ligand-gated ion channels. Glutamate receptors that respond to NMDA are associated with neuropathic pain and opioid tolerance and are blocked by ketamine. NMDA receptors are highly calcium permeable. Glutamate receptors that respond to AMPA and kainate are involved with fast synaptic transmission and synaptic plasticity, including long-term potentiation.

Metabotropic glutamate receptors are transmembrane receptors that are linked to G proteins that modulate intracellular second messengers such as inositol phosphates and cyclic nucleotides.

Serotonin

The serotonin (5-HT) receptor is also excitatory, permitting passage of sodium, potassium, and calcium cations as described for the nicotinic acetylcholine receptor.

Inhibitory Ligand-Gated Ion Channels

Inhibitory ligand-gated ion channels cause the inside of the cell to become less negative, typically by facilitating the flux of chloride into the cell. Potassium channels that facilitate the efflux of potassium ions are also inhibitory.

γ-Aminobutyric Acid

GABA is the major inhibitory neurotransmitter in the brain. When two molecules of GABA bind to the GABA receptor, the chloride channel in the center of the receptor opens and chloride ions enter the cell following their concentration gradient (see Fig. 3-7).[11] The negatively charged chloride ion hyperpolarizes the interior of the cell, rendering GABA receptors inhibitory shortly after birth. It is estimated that as many as one-third of the synapses in the brain are GABAergic. The chloride channel is formed from the α and β subunits, with or without γ and δ subunits.

In the developing brain neurons have higher concentrations of chloride then the extracellular fluid. As a result, opening of the GABA chloride channel initiates a flux of negatively charged chloride ions out of the cell, depolarizing the cell. Later in development, the potassium/chloride cotransporter appears. This transporter decreases intracellular chloride in exchange for extracellular potassium, creating a concentration gradient for chloride that favors inward flux.[21] The change in chloride concentration gradient renders the GABA receptor hyperpolarizing and hence inhibitory.

GABA receptors are the target of propofol, etomidate, and thiopental, which can directly open the channel at high concentration, or at lower concentration increase sensitivity to exogenous GABA. Benzodiazepines also work through GABA receptors but increase the sensitivity of the receptor to exogenous GABA only rather than directly opening the ion channel. There is increasing evidence that extrasynaptic GABA receptors are important in volatile anesthetic-induced behavioral responses.

Glycine

Glycine is the principal inhibitory neurotransmitter in the spinal cord, acting through the glycine receptor to increase chloride ion conductance into the cell, causing hyperpolarization. Glycine receptors are also present in the brain. These channels are involved in many neurologic processes and are modulated by a variety of anesthetic drugs but are not known to be responsible for any specific anesthetic induced behavior.

Strychnine and tetanus toxin result in seizures because they antagonize the effects of glycine on postsynaptic inhibition. Visual disturbances after transurethral resection of the prostate in which glycine is the irrigating solution may reflect the role of this substance as an inhibitory neurotransmitter in the retina.[22] Amplitude and latency of visual evoked potentials are altered by infusions of glycine.[23]

Voltage-Gated Ion Channels

Voltage-gated ion channels are complexes of protein subunits that act as switchable portals sensitive to membrane potential through which ions can pass through the cell membrane. They are "voltage-sensitive" because they open and close in response to changes in voltage across cell membranes. Charged portions of the molecule physically move in response to voltage changes to energetically favor the open or closed state of the channel. For example, the sodium channel opens in response to a sudden depolarization, propagating the action potential in nerves. Voltage-gated ion channels are present in neurons, skeletal muscles, and endocrine cells. They are often named based on the ion that passes through the channel (e.g., sodium, chloride, potassium, and calcium channels).

The voltage-gated sodium channel is of particular interest to anesthesiologists, because it is the site of local anesthetic action. Local anesthetics block neural conduction by blocking passage of sodium through the voltage-gated sodium channel.

The human *ether-a-go-go* related gene (hERG) potassium channel is a voltage-gated inwardly rectifying potassium channel, mostly famous for its association with prolonged QT syndrome. The hERG potassium channel is sensitive to many drugs and is responsible for sudden death from drugs that predispose the patient to *torsades de point*. Inhibition of the hERG potassium channel is also responsible for the U.S. Food and Drug Administration (FDA) black box warning on droperidol.

G Protein–Gated Ion Channels

Some ion channels are directly gated by G proteins (Fig. 3-10). G protein–gated potassium channels are the most well studied of the G protein–regulated ion channels.[24] The first identified G protein–regulated ion channel was the cardiac potassium channel, which is directly regulated by the M_2 muscarinic acetylcholine G protein–coupled receptor.[25] This is one of many inward rectifying potassium channels that share the unusual property of permitting influx of potassium ions into the cell following the electrical gradient, rather than the more typical outward flux of potassium following the ionic concentration gradient. G protein regulated inwardly, rectifying potassium channels, commonly referred to as ***GIRKs***, are regulated by $G_{\beta\gamma}$ rather than G_α. In addition to acetylcholine, A_1 adenosine, α_2 adrenergic, D_2 dopamine, opioid, serotonin, and $GABA_B$ receptors are coupled directly to GIRKs.[24,26]

Other Gated Ion Channels

Other types of ion channel gating include gating by other ions (e.g., hydrogen, calcium), second messengers (e.g., cAMP, cyclic guanosine monophosphate [cGMP]), and tissue injury (acid, stretch, temperature, cytokines).

Receptor Concentration

Receptors in cell membranes are not static components of cells. Excess circulating concentrations of ligand often results in a decrease in the density of the target receptors in cell membranes. For example, the excessive circulating norepinephrine in patients with pheochromocytoma leads to downregulation of β-adrenergic receptors. Desensitization of receptor responsiveness is the waning of a physiologic response over time despite (and, caused by) the presence of a constant stimulus.[12] Drug-induced antagonism of receptors often results in an increased density of receptors in cell membranes (upregulation). Abrupt discontinuation of the antagonist can result in an exaggerated response to the endogenous agonist. This is one reason that most cardiovascular medicines should be continued throughout the perioperative period.

Receptor Diseases

Numerous diseases are associated with receptor dysfunction. For example, failure of parathyroid hormone and arginine vasopressin to produce increases in cAMP

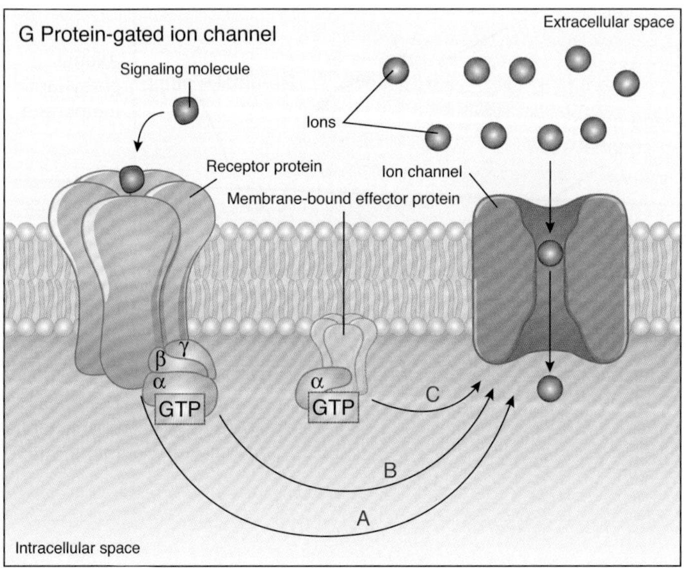

FIGURE 3-10 G protein–gated ion channel. When the signaling molecule binds to the G protein–coupled receptor, the G proteins either directly activate the ion channel (*line B* for activation by G_α; *line C* for activation by $G_{\beta\gamma}$) or activate an intermediary membrane-bound effector protein, which in turn activates the ion channel (*line A*).

in target organs manifests as pseudohypoparathyroidism and nephrogenic diabetes insipidus, respectively. Grave's disease and myasthenia gravis reflect development of antibodies against thyroid-stimulating hormone and nicotinic acetylcholine receptors, respectively.

The Synapse

Structure

The synapse functions as a diode that transmits an action potential from the presynaptic membrane to the postsynaptic membrane across the synaptic cleft (Fig. 3-11). The presynaptic membrane contains the vesicles of neurotransmitter and the reuptake pump that returns the neurotransmitter to the presynaptic axoplasm following neurotransmitter release. It also contains the voltage-gated calcium channel. Synaptic transmission starts when an afferent action potential arrives at the voltage-gated calcium channel.

The depolarization permits the influx of calcium ions through the voltage-gated calcium channel. Calcium ions bind to specialized proteins called the ***release apparatus*** on axonal and vesicular membranes. Calcium triggers the fusion of the vesicle to the cell membrane and the release of the neurotransmitter into the synaptic cleft through exocytosis, resulting in the extrusion of the contents of the synaptic vesicles. Calcium in the extracellular fluid is essential to the release of neurotransmitters in response to an action potential. The effect of calcium is antagonized by magnesium.

The neurotransmitter in the cleft binds to receptors in the postsynaptic membrane. This binding initiates an efferent action potential in the dendrite of the efferent nerve, which is then propagated. Immediately behind the postsynaptic membrane is the postsynaptic density. The postsynaptic density contains a variety of receptors and structural proteins responsible for maintaining synapse homeostasis.

There are several common misconceptions conveyed by the usual representation of the synapse. First, Figure 3-11 suggests that the synapse consists of two distinct plug-shaped entities that are joined together to form a synapse. Often, the presynaptic neuron may be no more than a slight widening of the axon, the "synaptic varicosity" or "bouton," because of the presence of the vesicles containing the neurotransmitter. Second, the synapse often appears as a wide gap, as in Figure 3-11. However, the synapse is extremely narrow, on the order of just 20 nm, as shown in Figure 3-12. When the vesicle releases its content into the synapse, the concentration of neurotransmitter is extraordinarily high for a very brief period of time. Lastly, both dendrites and axons have extensive arborizations. The interconnection of hundreds of arborizations across tens of billions of brain cells creates circuits of unimaginable complexity.

Synaptic Modulation

The resting transmembrane potential of neurons in the CNS is about −70 mV, less than the −90 mV in large peripheral nerve fibers and skeletal muscles. The resting transmembrane potential is important for controlling the responsiveness of neurons and is impacted on by extrasynaptic receptors as well as the sodium-potassium ATP exchanger. Postsynaptic inhibitory and excitatory potentials modulated by synaptic and nonsynaptic signaling pathways sum to determine the likelihood of depolarization in response to an incoming stimulus.

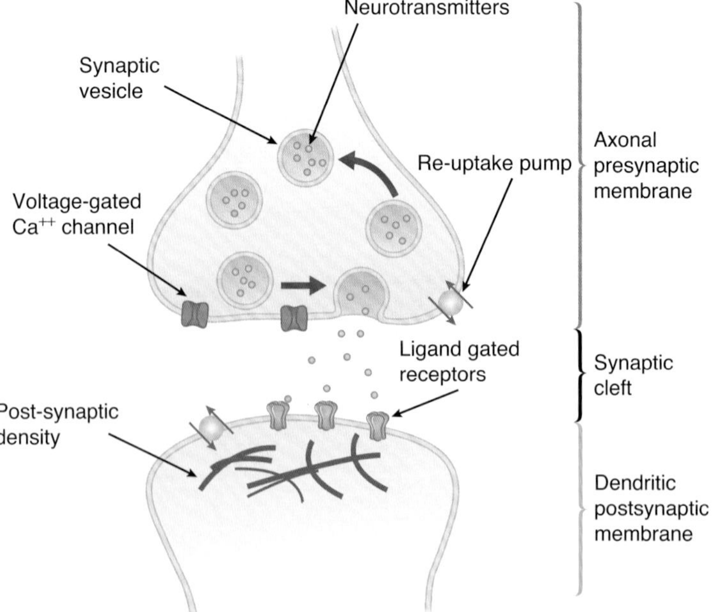

FIGURE 3-11 Structure of the synapse. Axons typically have many synapses, not just the single synapse implied by the conventional typical rendition below. The presynaptic membrane encloses the synaptic vesicles that contain the neurotransmitters, the reuptake pump that removes the neurotransmitter following synaptic transmission, and the voltage-gated calcium channel that responds to the incoming action potential. The ligand-gated receptors in the postsynaptic membrane trigger an efferent action potential. The postsynaptic density contains multiple proteins and receptors and appears responsible for organizing the structure of the receptors on the synapse.

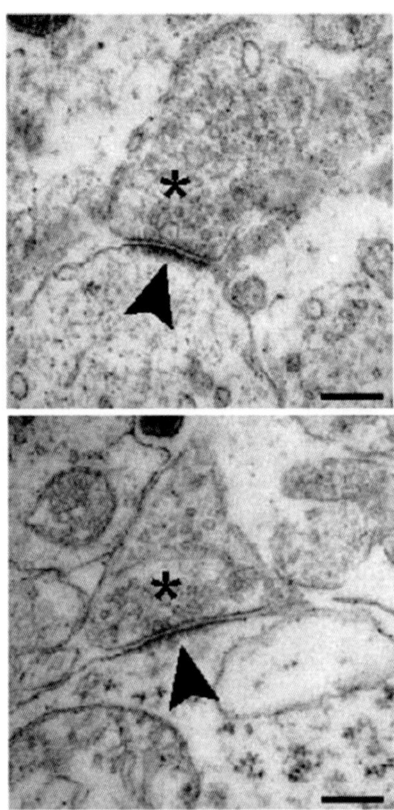

FIGURE 3-12 Presynaptic vesicles are marked with an *asterisk* in this figure, and the postsynaptic density is marked with an *arrow*. The extremely narrow gap between them is the synapse. (From Heupel K, Sargsyan V, Plomp JJ, et al. Loss of transforming growth factor-beta 2 leads to impairment of central synapse function. *Neural Dev.* 2008;3:25, used with permission as an Open Access article distributed under the terms of the Creative Commons Attribution License.)

Synaptic Delay

Synaptic delay is the 0.3 to 0.5 millisecond necessary for the transmission of an impulse from the synaptic varicosity to the postsynaptic neuron.[27] This synaptic delay reflects the time for release of the neurotransmitter from the synaptic varicosity, diffusion of the neurotransmitter to the postsynaptic receptor, and the subsequent change in permeability of the postsynaptic membrane to various ions.

Synaptic Fatigue

Synaptic fatigue is a decrease in the number of discharges by the postsynaptic membrane when excitatory synapses are repetitively and rapidly stimulated. For example, synaptic fatigue decreases excessive excitability of the brain as may accompany a seizure, thus acting as a protective mechanism against excessive neuronal activity. The mechanism of synaptic fatigue is presumed to be exhaustion of the stores of neurotransmitter in the synaptic vesicles. Synaptic fatigue is unmasked at the neuromuscular junction in myasthenia gravis when the enormous reserve for neuromuscular transmission is limited by either pre- or postsynaptic autoimmune damage.

Posttetanic Facilitation

Posttetanic facilitation is increased responsiveness of the postsynaptic neuron to stimulation after a rest period that was preceded by repetitive stimulation of an excitatory synapse. This phenomenon reflects increased release of neurotransmitters due to enhanced local concentrations of intracellular calcium. Posttetanic facilitation may be a mechanism for short-term memory and sensory neuron wind-up.

Factors that Influence Neuron Responsiveness

Neurons are highly sensitive to changes in the pH of the surrounding interstitial fluids. For example, alkalosis enhances neuron excitability. Voluntary hyperventilation can evoke a seizure in a susceptible individual. Conversely, acidosis depresses neuron excitability, with a decrease in arterial pH to 7.0, potentially causing coma. Hypoxia can cause total refractoriness in neurons within 3 to 5 seconds as reflected by the almost immediate onset of unconsciousness following cessation of cerebral blood flow. This response is in part protective because the metabolic activity of inactive neurons is an order of magnitude less than that of active neurons.

Central Nervous System

The brain, brainstem, and spinal cord constitute the CNS. The brain is a complex collection of neural networks that regulate their own and each other's activity. Activity within the CNS reflects a balance between excitatory and inhibitory influences, a homeostasis that is normally maintained within relatively narrow limits. Anatomic divisions of the brain reflect the distribution of brain functions (Fig. 3-13).

The two cerebral hemispheres constitute the cerebral cortex, where sensory, motor, and associational information is processed. The limbic system lies beneath the cerebral cortex and integrates the emotional state with motor and visceral activities. The thalamus lies in the center of the brain beneath the cerebral cortex and basal ganglia and above the hypothalamus. The neurons of the thalamus are arranged in nuclei that act as relays between the incoming sensory pathways and the cerebral cortex, hypothalamus, and basal ganglia. The hypothalamus is the principal integrating region for the autonomic nervous system and regulates other functions, including systemic blood pressure, body temperature, water balance, secretions of the pituitary gland, emotions, and sleep.

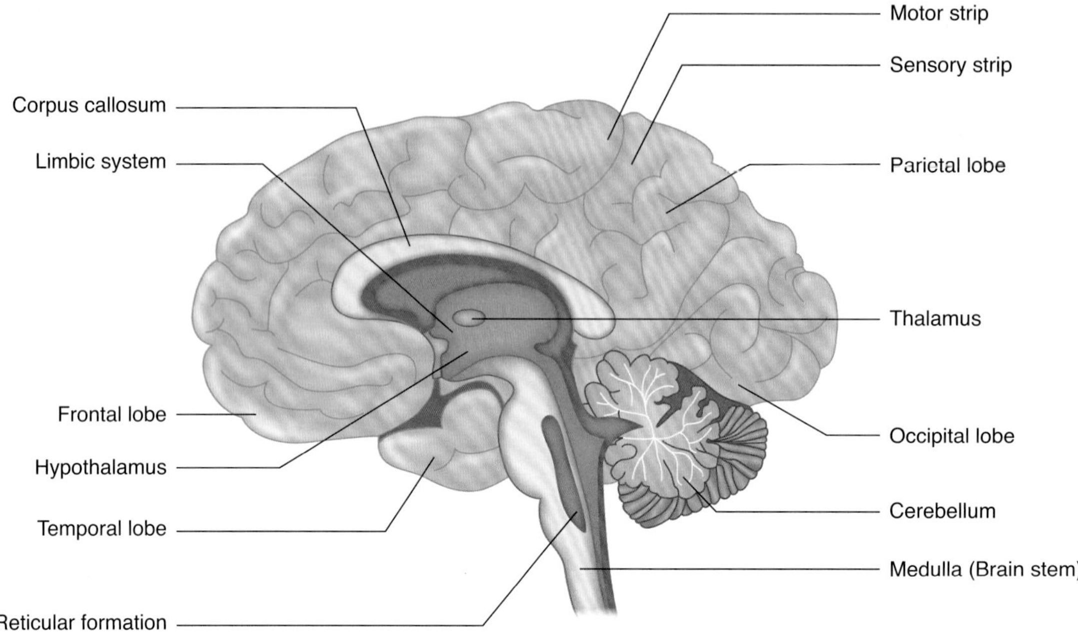

FIGURE 3-13 Brain anatomy.

The brainstem connects the cerebral cortex to the spinal cord and contains most of the nuclei of the cranial nerves and the reticular activating system. The reticular activating system is essential for regulation of sleep and wakefulness. The cerebellum arises from the posterior pons and is responsible for coordination of movement, maintenance of body posture, and certain types of motor memory.

The spinal cord extends from the medulla oblongata to the lower lumbar vertebrae. Ascending and descending tracts are located within the white matter of the spinal cord, whereas intersegmental connections and synaptic contacts are concentrated in the gray matter. Sensory information flows into the dorsal portion (posterior) of the gray matter, and motor outflow exits from the ventral (anterior) portion. Preganglionic neurons of the autonomic nervous system are found in the intermediolateral portions of the gray matter.

Cerebral Hemispheres

The two cerebral hemispheres, known as the ***cerebral cortex***, constitute the largest division of the human brain. Regions of the cerebral cortex are classified as ***sensory***, ***motor***, ***visual***, ***auditory***, and ***olfactory***, depending on the type of information that is processed. ***Frontal***, ***temporal***, ***parietal***, and ***occipital*** designate anatomic positions of the cerebral cortex (Fig. 3-14). For each area of the cerebral cortex, there is a corresponding and connecting area to the thalamus such that stimulation of a small portion of the thalamus activates the corresponding and much larger portion of the cerebral cortex. Indeed, the cerebral cortex is actually an evolutionary outgrowth of the lower regions of the nervous system, especially the thalamus. The functional part of the cerebral cortex is composed mainly of a 2- to 5-mm layer of neurons covering the surface of all the convolutions. It is estimated that the cerebral cortex contains 50 to 100 billion neurons.

Anatomy of the Cerebral Cortex

The sensorimotor cortex is the area of the cerebral cortex responsible for receiving sensation from sensory areas of the body and for controlling body movement (see Fig. 3-14).[3] The premotor cortex is important for controlling the functions of the motor cortex. The motor cortex lies anterior to the central sulcus. Its posterior portion

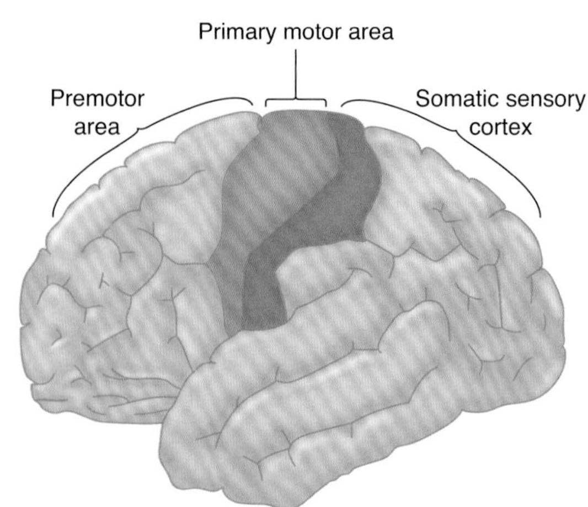

FIGURE 3-14 The sensorimotor cortex consists of the motor cortex, pyramidal (Betz) cells, and somatic sensory cortex.

is characterized by the presence of large, pyramid-shaped (pyramidal or Betz) cells.

Topographic Areas

The area of the cerebral cortex to which the peripheral sensory signals are projected from the thalamus is designated the ***somesthetic cortex*** (see Fig. 3-14).[3] Each side of the cerebral cortex receives sensory information exclusively from the opposite side of the body. The size of these areas is directly proportional to the number of specialized sensory receptors in each respective area of the body. For example, a large number of specialized nerve endings are present in the lips and the thumbs, whereas only a few are present in the skin of the trunk.

The motor cortex is organized into topographic areas corresponding to different regions of the skeletal muscles. The spatial organization is similar to that of the sensory cortex. In general, the size of the area in the motor cortex is proportional to the preciseness of the skeletal muscle movement required. As such, the digits, lips, tongue, and vocal cords have large representations in humans. The various topographic areas in the motor cortex were originally determined by electrical stimulation of the brain during local anesthesia and observation of the evoked skeletal muscle response. Such stimulation can be used intraoperatively to identify the location of the motor cortex and thus avoid damage to this area. The motor cortex is commonly damaged by loss of blood supply as occurs during a stroke.

Corpus Callosum

The two hemispheres of the cerebral cortex, with the exception of the anterior portions of the temporal lobes, are connected by fibers in the corpus callosum. The anterior portions of the temporal lobes, including the amygdala, are connected by fibers that pass through the anterior commissure. The corpus callosum and anterior commissure make information processed or stored in one hemisphere available to the other hemisphere.

Dominant versus Nondominant Hemisphere

Language function and interpretation is typically localized in the dominant cerebral hemisphere, whereas spatiotemporal relationships (ability to recognize faces) is localized in the nondominant hemisphere. The left hemisphere is dominant in 90% of right-handed individuals and 70% of left-handed individuals. Destruction of the dominant cerebral hemisphere in adults results in loss of nearly all intellectual function.

The historical failure to document an important role of prefrontal lobes in intellectual function (frontal lobotomy) is surprising because the principal difference between the brains of humans and monkeys is the prominence of human prefrontal areas. It seems that the function of the prefrontal areas in humans is to provide additional cortical area in which thought processing can occur. Furthermore, selection of behavior patterns for different situations may be an important role of the prefrontal areas that transmit signals to the limbic areas of the brain. Persons without prefrontal lobes may react precipitously in response to incoming signals or manifest undue anger at slight provocations. Ability to maintain a sustained level of concentration is lost in the absence of the prefrontal lobes.

Memory

The cerebral cortex, especially the temporal lobes, serves as a storage site for information that is often characterized as memory.[28] The mechanisms for short-term and long-term memory are not completely understood but are thought to be encoded through selective synaptic strengthening in response to experience.

Short-Term Memory

The favored explanation for short-term memory is posttetanic potentiation. For example, tetanic stimulation of a synapse for a few seconds causes increased excitability of the synapse that lasts for seconds to hours. This change in excitability of the synapse is mediated by increased local intracellular calcium concentrations that facilitate transmitter release and act as a second messenger to activate genetic programs that result in structural synaptic stabilization.

Long-Term Memory

Long-term memory depends on stable synaptic changes that are induced by experience. The stability of this system is evidenced by total inactivation of the brain by hypothermia or anesthesia without detectable significant loss of long-term memory. Long-term memory is thought to rely on long-term synaptic potentiation mediated by structural changes. Long-term potentiation is the enhanced synaptic transmission observed after repeatedly stimulating a presynaptic neuron. The mechanism often involves increased expression of NMDA receptors and voltage-gated calcium channels in the postsynaptic neuron.[29] Thus, protein transcription and synaptic remodeling are an essential component of long-term memory. The hippocampus and amygdala are critically involved in creating new long-term memories. However, long-term memories are not actually stored in the hippocampus and amygdala. Sleep is known to play an important role in the formation of long-term memory.[30] However, the actual mechanism by which long-term memories are stored remains a fascinating unsolved puzzle.

Everyone knows from personal experience that repetition is essential to forming long-term memory. There is an old joke about a man asking a fellow pedestrian in New York, "How do you get to Carnegie Hall?" The pedestrian replies, "Practice, practice, practice." It has been repeatedly demonstrated in animal studies as well that repetition is key to forming long-term memories. Long-term potentiation is the synaptic consequence of repeated stimulation, which is one reason that long-term potentiation is thought to be the fundamental building block of long-term memory.

We also know that memories are transferred from short-term memory to long-term memory. Because the creation of long-term memory requires anatomic changes in the synapse, this transfer requires time. This suggests, and studies confirm, that if the brain is not given adequate time to make this transfer, there will be no transfer from short-term memory to long-term memory. This has direct applicability to the practice of anesthesia. During the provision of general anesthesia, we are vigilant for signs of inadequate anesthesia and intraoperative awareness (discussed further at the end of this section). If a patient has conscious perception of the surgery, this will initially be part of the patient's short-term memory. Rapid deepening of the anesthesia, for example by administering a bolus of propofol in response to patient movement, will prevent transfer of the recall from short-term memory to the long-term memory, and the patient will be amnestic. Conversely, if the patient is paralyzed and is awake for many minutes without the anesthesiologist being aware of the situation, then there has been adequate time for transfer of the short-term memory to long-term memory.

Because the neural substrate of memory is not well understood, memory is often discussed from a psychological point of view. Memories typically involve multiple senses (sight, hearing, touch), emotions (fear, satisfaction, pleasure, anger), and cognitive assessment ("I remember thinking that. . ."). These are thought to be held together in a facilitated circuit that has been called a ***memory engram*** or ***memory trace.*** Initially the circuit is facilitated through posttetanic potentiation in short-term memory. If memory is to persist, this is replaced with long-term potentiation. The pieces of the engram are consolidated through hypothalamic circuitry. The memory engram is reinforced with every subsequent recall of the memory. An important feature of the process of consolidation is that long-term memory is encoded into different categories. New memories are not stored randomly in the brain but seem to be associated with previously encoded and similar information. This permits scanning of memory to retrieve desired information at a later date. We also know that memory scanning is often a subconscious process. This is confirmed by the daily experience of struggling to recall a fact or event, only to have the memory suddenly jump into our consciousness hours later.

Postoperative Cognitive Dysfunction

Postoperative cognitive dysfunction (impaired memory) persisting after 3 months has been described in 10% of elderly patients receiving general anesthesia without known arterial hypoxemia or systemic hypotension.[31] Inhaled anesthetics are known to alter the proteins involved in the formation of Alzheimer's disease.[32] It is unclear whether the postoperative cognitive dysfunction is caused by anesthetic injury to the aged brain, as might be caused by increasing the polymerization of β amyloid, or is caused by the combined effects of surgical trauma, inflammation, social interruption, anesthesia, and other unidentified causes.

Awareness and Recall during Anesthesia

Awareness, defined as conscious memory of events during anesthesia, has been a recurrent problem particularly since the introduction of neuromuscular-blocking drugs.[33] Neuromuscular blocking drugs permit inadequate anesthesia to be administered without obvious patient withdrawal from the noxious stimulus. The use of neuromuscular blockade is a risk factor for awareness under general anesthesia, particularly awareness that is associated with memories of pain and complicated by posttraumatic stress disorder.[34]

Memory may be considered to be conscious (explicit) or unconscious (implicit). Conscious memory includes spontaneous recall and recognition memory. Unconscious memory is manifest by altered performance or behavior due to experiences that are not consciously remembered. By definition, general anesthesia abolishes conscious memory, but the extent to which it also abolishes unconscious memory is controversial. Behavioral disturbances manifest as night terrors in children after anesthesia may be an expression of implicit memory in the dream state.

The incidence of awareness with recall (conscious memory) following general anesthesia has been estimated at between 1 and 5 in 1,000 general anesthetics, depending on the risk group.[35–37] Although the incidence of conscious recall of intraoperative events is rare and the development of posttraumatic stress disorder is even more uncommon, the fact that approximately 20 million general anesthetics are administered annually in the United States would correspond to 26,000 cases of awareness (0.13% of approximately 20 million) each year. The incidence of awareness in patients undergoing cesarean section was 0.4% and for cardiac surgery was 1.14% to 1.50% .[38,39] A higher incidence of awareness has been described for major trauma cases (11% to 43%) where the concentration of anesthetic administered is limited by hemodynamic instability.[40] Many cases of conscious awareness during surgery can be attributed to intentionally or unintentionally low concentrations of administered anesthetic.

Subanesthetic doses of inhaled anesthetics have powerful inhibitory effects on short-term memory, and the decrease in the transfer of information from the periphery to the cerebral cortex associated with general anesthesia prevents the recall of intraoperative events.[8]

Isoflurane (and presumably other volatile anesthetics) and nitrous oxide suppress memory in a dose-dependent manner, and isoflurane is more potent than equivalent

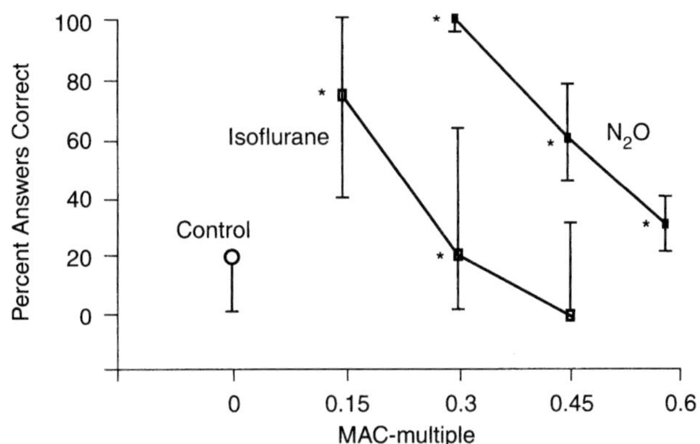

FIGURE 3-15 Percentage of correct answers for each anesthetic at increasing anesthetic concentrations. (From Dwyer R, Bennett HL, Eger EI, et al. Effects of isoflurane and nitrous oxide in subanesthetic concentrations on memory and responsiveness in volunteers. *Anesthesiology*. 1992;77: 888–898, with permission.)

concentrations of nitrous oxide (Fig. 3-15).[41] For example, conscious memory was prevented by 0.45 minimum alveolar concentration to prevent movement (MAC) isoflurane or 0.6 MAC nitrous oxide. Isoflurane concentrations of ≥0.6 MAC prevent conscious recall and unconscious learning of factual information and behavioral suggestions.[42]

Recognizing Awareness

Monitoring patients during general anesthesia for the presence of awareness is challenging. Despite a variety of monitoring methods, awareness may be difficult to recognize in real time. Indicators of awareness (heart rate, blood pressure, and skeletal muscle movement) are often masked by anesthetic and adjuvant drugs (β-adrenergic blockers and/or neuromuscular-blocking drugs). Several different monitors, based on analysis of electroencephalogram (EEG) and somatosensory evoked potential patterns, have been introduced in hopes of addressing this issue.

Brainstem

Homeostatic life-sustaining processes are controlled subconsciously in the brainstem. Examples of subconscious activities of the body regulated by the brainstem include control of systemic blood pressure and breathing in the medulla. The thalamus serves as a relay station for most afferent impulses before they are transmitted to the cerebral cortex. The hypothalamus receives fibers from the thalamus and is also closely modulated by the cerebral cortex.

Limbic System and Hypothalamus

Behavior associated with emotions is primarily a function of structures known as the ***limbic system*** (hippocampus, basal ganglia) located in the basal regions of the brain. The hypothalamus functions in many of the same roles as the limbic system and is considered by some to be part of the limbic system rather than a separate structure. In addition, the hypothalamus controls many internal conditions of the body, such as core temperature, thirst, and appetite. The great Oxford neurophysiologist Sir Charles Sherrington called the ***hypothalamus*** the ***head ganglion*** of the autonomic nervous system. The suprachiasmatic nucleus of the hypothalamus helps to maintain the body clock by secreting melatonin and other mediators according to the circadian rhythm. This nucleus sits just above the optic chiasm and receives inputs from the optic nerve that serve to entrain the circadian rhythm to environmental light. At high doses, melatonin and its analogs have properties similar to a general anesthetic.[43]

Basal Ganglia

The basal ganglia include the caudate nucleus, putamen, globus pallidus, substantia nigra, and subthalamic nucleus. Many of the impulses from basal ganglia are inhibitory mediated by dopamine and GABA. The balance between agonist and antagonist skeletal muscle contractions is an important role of the basal ganglia. A general effect of diffuse excitation of the basal ganglia is inhibition of skeletal muscles, reflecting transmission of inhibitory signals from the basal ganglia to both the motor cortex and the lower brainstem. Therefore, whenever destruction of the basal ganglia occurs, there is associated skeletal muscle rigidity. For example, damage to the caudate and putamen nuclei that normally secrete GABA results in choreiform random and continuous uncontrolled movements. Destruction of the substantia nigra and loss of dopaminergic neurons results in a predominance of the excitatory neurotransmitter acetylcholine, manifesting as the skeletal muscle rigidity of Parkinson's disease. As such, dopamine precursors or anticholinergic drugs are used in the treatment of Parkinson's disease in an attempt to restore the balance between excitatory and inhibitory impulses traveling from the basal ganglia.

Reticular Activating System

The reticular activating system is a polysynaptic pathway that is intimately concerned with electrical activity of the cerebral cortex. Neurons of the reticular activating system are both excitatory and inhibitory. The reticular activating system determines the overall level of CNS activity, including nuclei important in determining wakefulness and sleep. Selective activation of certain areas of the cerebral cortex by the reticular activating system is crucial for the direction of the attention of certain aspects of mental activity. It is likely that many injected and inhaled anesthetics exert their sedative effects through interaction with the brainstem and midbrain nuclei that mediate arousal and sleep.[44] This is not to say that general anesthesia is equivalent to sleep. Although the EEG response to many anesthetics resembles deep slow-wave sleep, a key difference is that afferent stimulation does not cause arousal.

Slow-Wave Sleep

Most of the sleep that occurs each night is slow-wave sleep. The EEG is characterized by the presence of high-voltage δ waves occurring at a frequency of <4 cycles per second. Presumably, decreased activity of the reticular activating system that accompanies sleep permits an unmasking of this inherent rhythm in the cerebral cortex. Slow-wave sleep is restful and devoid of dreams. During slow-wave sleep, sympathetic nervous system activity decreases, parasympathetic nervous system activity increases, and skeletal muscle tone is greatly decreased. As a result, there is a 10% to 30% decrease in systemic blood pressure, heart rate, breathing frequency, and basal metabolic rate.

Desynchronized Sleep

Periods of desynchronized sleep typically occur for 5 to 20 minutes during each 90 minutes of sleep. These periods tend to be shortest when the person is extremely tired. This form of sleep is characterized by active dreaming, irregular heart rate and breathing, and a desynchronized pattern of low-voltage β waves on the EEG similar to those that occur during wakefulness. This brain wave pattern emphasizes that desynchronized sleep is associated with an active cerebral cortex, but this activity does not permit persons to be aware of their surroundings and thus be awake. Despite the inhibition of skeletal muscle activity, the eyes are an exception, exhibiting rapid movements. For this reason, desynchronized sleep is also referred to as ***paradoxical sleep*** or ***rapid eye movement (REM) sleep***.

Cerebellum

The cerebellum operates subconsciously to monitor and elicit corrective responses in motor activity caused by stimulation of other parts of the brain and spinal cord. Rapid repetitive skeletal muscle activities, such as typing, playing musical instruments, and running, require intact function of the cerebellum. Loss of function of the cerebellum causes incoordination of fine skeletal muscle activities even though paralysis of the skeletal muscles does not occur. The cerebellum is also important in the maintenance of equilibrium and postural adjustments of the body. For example, sensory signals are transmitted to the cerebellum from receptors in muscle spindles, Golgi tendon organs, and receptors in skin joints. These spinocerebellar pathways can transmit impulses at velocities exceeding 100 m per second, which is the most rapid conduction of any pathway in the CNS. This extremely rapid conduction is important for instantaneous appraisal by the cerebellum of changes that take place in the positional status of the body.

Dysfunction of the Cerebellum

In the absence of cerebellar function, a person cannot predict prospectively how far movements will go. This results in overshoot of the intended mark (past pointing). This overshoot is known as ***dysmetria***, and the resulting incoordinate movements are called ***ataxia***. Dysarthria is present when rapid and orderly succession of skeletal muscle movements of the larynx, mouth, and chest do not occur. Failure of the cerebellum to dampen skeletal muscle movements results in intention tremor when a person performs a voluntary act. Cerebellar nystagmus is associated with loss of equilibrium, presumably because of dysfunction of the pathways that pass through the cerebellum from the semicircular canals. In the presence of cerebellar disease, a person is unable to activate antagonist skeletal muscles that prevent a certain portion of the body from moving unexpectedly in an unwanted direction. For example, a person's arm that was previously contracted but restrained by another person will move back rapidly when it is released rather than automatically remain in place.

Spinal Cord

The spinal cord extends from the medulla oblongata to the lower border of the first and, occasionally, the second lumbar vertebra. Below the spinal cord, the vertebral canal is filled by the roots of the lumbar and sacral nerves, which are collectively known as the ***cauda equina***. The spinal cord is composed of gray and white matter, spinal nerves, and covering membranes.

Gray Matter

The gray matter of the spinal cord functions as the initial processor of incoming sensory signals from peripheral somatic receptors and as a relay station to send these signals to the brain.

In addition, this area of the spinal cord is the site for final processing of motor signals that are being transmitted downward from the brain to skeletal muscles. Anatomically, the gray matter of the spinal cord is divided into anterior, lateral, and dorsal horns consisting of nine separate laminae that are H-shaped when viewed in cross-section (Fig. 3-16). The anterior horn is the location of α and γ motor neurons that give rise to nerve fibers that leave the spinal cord via the anterior (ventral) nerve roots and innervate skeletal muscles. Cells of Renshaw are intermediary neurons in the anterior horn, providing nerve fibers that synapse in the gray matter with anterior motor neurons. These cells inhibit the action of anterior motor neurons to limit excessive activity. Cells of the preganglionic neurons of the sympathetic nervous system are located lateral to the thoracolumbar portions of the spinal cord. Cells of the intermediate neurons located in the portion of the dorsal horns of the spinal cord known as the ***substantia gelatinosa*** (laminae II to III) transmit afferent tactile, temperature, and pain impulses to the spinothalamic tract. The dorsal horn serves as a gate where impulses in sensory nerve fibers are translated into impulses in

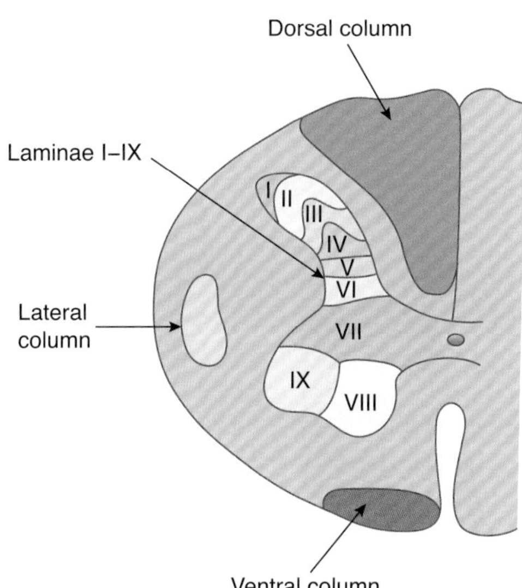

FIGURE 3-16 Schematic diagram of a cross-section of the spinal cord depicting anatomic laminae I to IX of the spinal cord gray matter and the ascending dorsal, lateral, and ventral sensory columns of the spinal cord white matter.

ascending tracts. There is evidence for a form of memory in the dorsal horn of the spinal cord that is evoked by intense stimulation. Resulting increases in intracellular calcium set into motion long-lasting changes that are associated with central sensitization and result in increased sensitivity to subsequent inoffensive stimuli.

White Matter

The white matter of the spinal cord is formed by the axons that make up their respective ascending and descending tracts. This area of the spinal cord is divided into dorsal, lateral, and ventral columns (see Fig. 3-16). The dorsal column of the spinal cord is composed of spinothalamic tracts that transmit touch and pain impulses to the brain.

Pyramidal and Extrapyramidal Tracts

A major pathway for transmission of motor signals from the cerebral cortex to the anterior motor neurons of the spinal cord is through the pyramidal (corticospinal) tracts (Fig. 3-17).[3] All pyramidal tract fibers pass downward through the brainstem and then cross to the opposite side to form the pyramids of the medulla. After crossing the midline at the level of the medulla, these fibers descend in the lateral corticospinal tracts of the spinal cord and terminate on motor neurons in the dorsal horn of the spinal cord. A few fibers do not cross to the opposite side of the medulla but rather descend in the ventral corticospinal tracts. In addition to these pyramidal fibers, a large number of collateral fibers pass from the motor cortex into the basal ganglia, forming the extrapyramidal tracts. Extrapyramidal tracts are all those tracts beside the pyramidal tracts that transmit motor impulses from the cerebral cortex to the spinal cord.

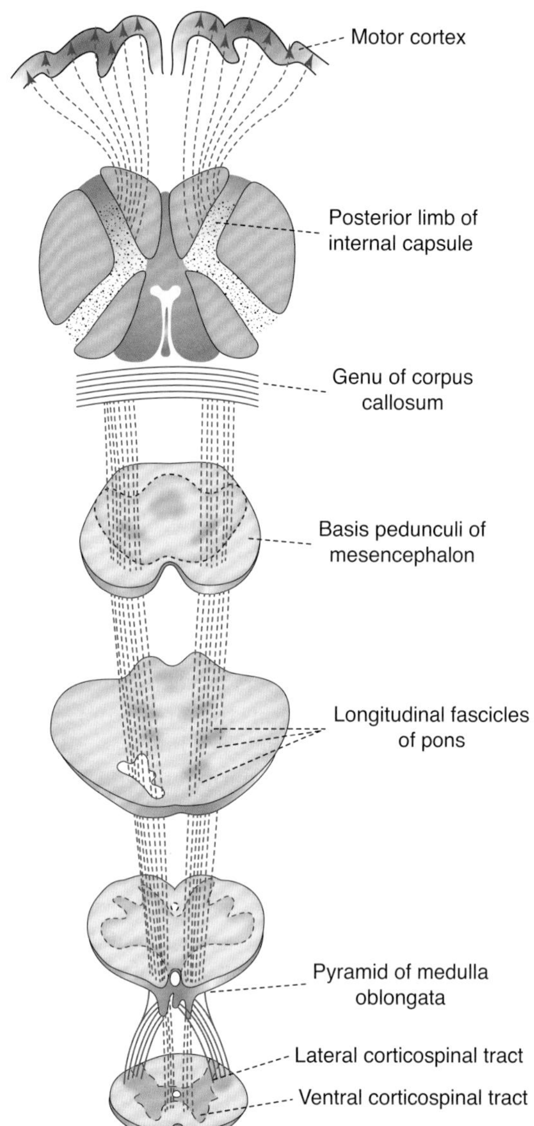

FIGURE 3-17 The pyramidal tracts are major pathways for transmission of motor signals from the cerebral cortex to the spinal cord.

The pyramidal and extrapyramidal tracts have opposing effects on the tone of skeletal muscles. For example, the pyramidal tracts cause continuous facilitation and therefore a tendency to produce increases in skeletal muscle tone. Conversely, the extrapyramidal tracts transmit inhibitory signals through the basal ganglia with resultant inhibition of skeletal muscle tone. Selective or predominant damage to one of these tracts manifests as spasticity or flaccidity.

Babinski Sign

A positive Babinski sign is characterized by upward extension of the first toe and outward fanning of the other toes in response to a firm tactile stimulus applied to the dorsum of the foot. A normal response to the same tactile stimulus is downward motion of all the toes. A positive

Babinski sign reflects damage to the pyramidal tracts. Damage to the extrapyramidal tracts does not cause a positive Babinski sign.

Thalamocortical System

The thalamocortical system serves as the pathway for passage of nearly all afferent impulses from the cerebellum; basal ganglia; and visual, auditory, taste, and pain receptors as they pass through the thalamus on the way to the cerebral cortex. Signals from olfactory receptors are the only peripheral sensory signals that do not pass through the thalamus. Overall, the thalamocortical system controls the activity level of the cerebral cortex.

Spinal Nerve

A pair of spinal nerves arises from each of 31 segments of the spinal cord. Spinal nerves are made up of fibers of the ventral (anterior) and dorsal (posterior) roots. Efferent motor fibers travel in the anterior roots that originate from axons in the anterior and lateral horns of the spinal cord gray matter. Sensory fibers travel in the dorsal nerve roots that originate from axons that arise from cell bodies in the spinal cord ganglia. These cell bodies send branches to the spinal cord and to the periphery. The anterior and dorsal nerve roots each leave the spinal cord through an individual intervertebral foramen enclosed in a common dural sheath that extends just past the spinal cord ganglia where the spinal nerve originates.

Each spinal nerve innervates a segmental area of skin designated a ***dermatome*** and an area of skeletal muscle known as a ***myotome***. A dermatome map is useful in determining the level of spinal cord injury or level of sensory anesthesia produced by a neuraxial anesthetic (Fig. 3-18).[3] Despite common depictions of dermatomes as having distinct borders, there is extensive overlap between segments. For example, three consecutive dorsal nerve roots need to be interrupted to produce complete denervation of a dermatome. The scrotum has considerable sensory overlap, with innervation coming from T1 (variable) and L1–L2 and S2–S4 despite common depictions on dermatome charts as being limited to sacral innervation.[45] Segmental innervation of myotomes is even less well defined than that of dermatomes, emphasizing that skeletal muscle groups receive innervation from several anterior nerve roots.

Sensory signals from the periphery are transmitted through spinal nerves into each segment of the spinal cord, resulting in automatic motor responses that occur instantly (muscle stretch reflex, withdrawal reflex) in response to sensory signals. Spinal cord reflexes are important in emptying the bladder and rectum. Segmental temperature reflexes allow localized cutaneous vasodilation or vasoconstriction in response to changes in skin temperature. The function of the spinal cord component of the CNS and spinal cord reflexes is particularly apparent in patients with transection of the spinal cord.

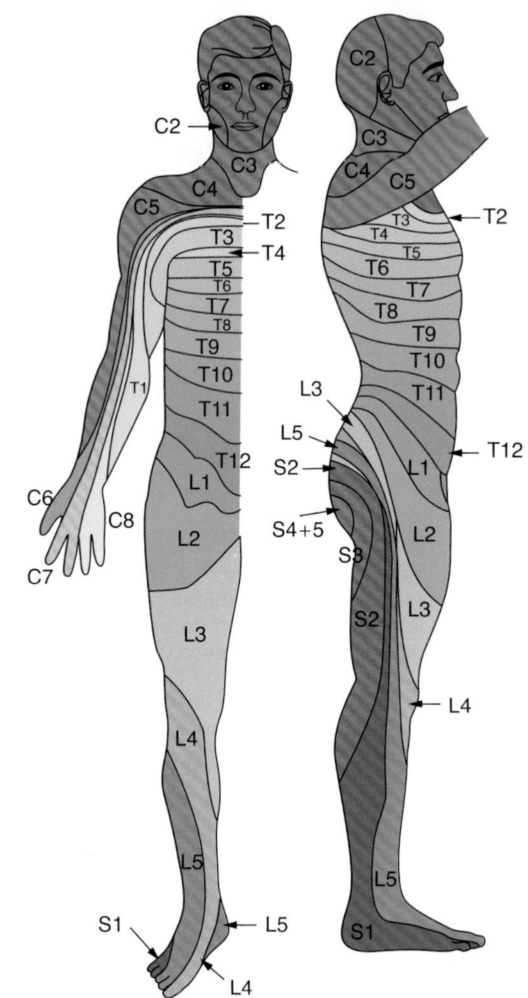

FIGURE 3-18 Dermatome map that may be used to evaluate the level of sensory anesthesia produced by regional anesthesia.

Covering Membranes

The spinal cord is enveloped by membranes (dura, arachnoid, pia) that are direct continuations of the corresponding membranes surrounding the brain. The dura consists of an inner and an outer layer. The outer periosteal layer in the cranial cavity is the periosteum of the skull, whereas this layer in the spine is the periosteal lining of the spinal cord. The epidural space is located between the inner and outer layers of the dura. The fact that the inner layer of the dura adheres to the margin of the foramen magnum and blends with the periosteal layer means that the epidural space does not extend beyond this point. As a result, drugs such as local anesthetics or opioids cannot travel cephalad in the epidural space beyond the foramen magnum. However, there is extensive equilibration between epidural and subarachnoid drug concentrations. Because of this equilibration hydrophilic opioids such as morphine given to the lumbar epidural space may cause delayed respiratory depression in patients at risk. The inner layer of the dura extends as a dural cuff that blends with the perineurium of spinal nerves. The cerebral arachnoid extends as the spinal arachnoid, ending at the second sacral vertebra. The pia is in close contact with the spinal cord.

CT scans demonstrate the occasional presence of a connective tissue band (dorsomedian connective tissue band or plica mediana dorsalis) that divides the epidural space at the dorsal midline.[46] This band binds the dura mater and the ligamentum flavum at the midline, making it difficult to feel loss of resistance during attempted midline identification of the epidural space. The band may also explain the occasional occurrence of unilateral analgesia after injection of local anesthetic solutions into the epidural space.[47] In some patients, there is a failure of midline fusion of the dura. This is particularly common in at higher thoracic levels.[48]

Autonomic Reflexes

Segmental autonomic reflexes occur in the spinal cord and include changes in vascular tone, diaphoresis, and evacuation of the bladder and colon. Simultaneous excitation of all the segmental reflexes is the mass reflex (denervation hypersensitivity or autonomic hyperreflexia). The mass reflex typically occurs in the presence of spinal cord transection when a painful stimulus is applied to the skin below the level of the spinal cord transection, or following distension of a hollow viscus, such as the bladder or gastrointestinal tract. The principal manifestation of the mass reflex is systemic hypertension due to intense peripheral vasoconstriction, reflecting an inability of vasodilating inhibitory impulses from the CNS to pass beyond the site of spinal cord transection. Carotid sinus baroreceptor-mediated reflex bradycardia accompanies the systemic hypertension associated with the mass reflex.

Spinal Shock

Spinal shock is a manifestation of the abrupt loss of spinal cord reflexes that immediately follows transection of the spinal cord. It emphasizes the dependence of spinal cord reflexes on continual tonic discharges from higher centers. The immediate manifestations of spinal shock are hypotension due to loss of vasoconstrictor tone and absence of all skeletal muscle reflexes. Within a few days to weeks, spinal cord neurons gradually regain their intrinsic excitability. Sacral reflexes for control of bladder and colon evacuation are completely suppressed for the first few weeks after spinal cord transection, but these spinal cord reflexes also eventually return, although their conscious control does not.

Imaging of the Nervous System

Until the introduction of computed tomography (CT), imaging studies of the brain included skull radiography, cerebral angiography, and pneumoencephalography.[49] These techniques allowed only examination of the skull, the cerebral blood vessels, and the fluid-containing spaces of the brain. CT and magnetic resonance imaging (MRI) provide high-resolution images of brain tissue and clear discrimination between gray and white matter. Positron emission tomography (PET) and single photon emission computed tomography (SPECT) permit imaging of both structure and functional characteristics (blood flow, metabolism, and concentrations of neurochemicals and receptors) of the brain.

Comparative studies indicate that MRI is superior to CT in evaluating most cerebral parenchymal lesions because of better spacial discrimination.[49] CT is used in patients who cannot undergo MRI because of the presence of artificial cardiac pacemakers, mechanical heart valves, or magnetizable intracranial metal clips. CT is also useful in visualizing intracranial blood that may be present in patients with subdural hematomas or cerebral hemorrhage.

Cerebral Blood Flow

Cerebral blood flow averages 50 mL/100 g per minute of brain tissue. For an adult, this is equivalent to 750 mL per minute, or about 15% of the resting cardiac output, delivered to an organ that represents only about 2% of the body's mass. The gray matter of the brain has a higher cerebral blood flow (80 mL/100 g per minute) than the white matter (20 mL/100 g per minute). As in most other tissues of the body, cerebral blood flow parallels cerebral metabolic requirements for oxygen (3 to 5 mL/100 g per minute). $Paco_2$ and Pao_2 influence cerebral blood flow, whereas sympathetic and parasympathetic nerves play little or no role in the regulation of cerebral blood flow (Fig. 3-19). Changes in the $Paco_2$ between about 20 and 80 mm Hg produce corresponding changes in cerebral blood flow. For example, in this range, a 1-mm Hg increase in the $Paco_2$ evokes a 1 to 2 mL/100 g per minute increase in cerebral blood flow (Table 3-3).[50]

Carbon dioxide increases cerebral blood flow by combining with water in body fluids to form carbonic acid, with

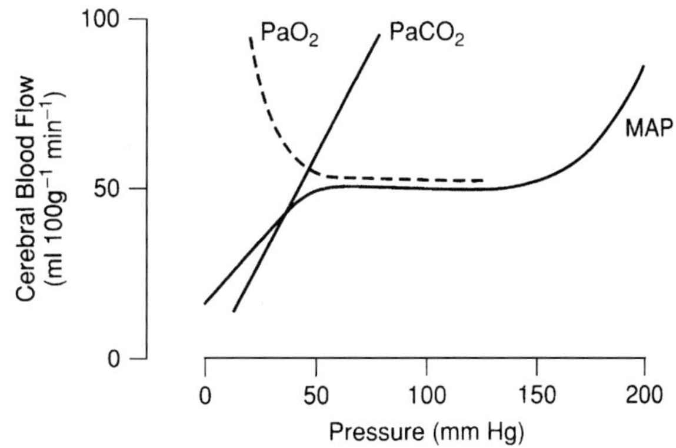

FIGURE 3-19 Cerebral blood flow is influenced by Pao_2, $Paco_2$, and mean arterial pressure (MAP).

Table 3-3

Carbon Dioxide and Cerebral Physiology

Cerebral blood flow (CBF)
- Changes 1–2 mL/100 g per minute for each 1 mm Hg change in $Paco_2$ between 20 and 80 mm Hg
- Slope of the response depends on normocapnic CBF
- CBF returns to baseline over several hours during sustained alterations in $Paco_2$ (reflects correction of brain extracellular fluid pH)
- Response to hypocapnia not altered by aging if CBF is maintained
- Response to changes in $Paco_2$ not altered by untreated hypertension
- Hypothermia decreases normocapnic CBF and the response of CBF to changes in $Paco_2$

Cerebral blood volume (CBV)
- Changes 0.05 mL/100 g for each 1 mm Hg change in $Paco_2$
- Returns to baseline during sustained alterations in $Paco_2$

Cerebral autoregulation
- Modest hypercapnia impairs and marked hypercapnia abolishes
- Hypotension below the lower limit of autoregulation abolishes hypocapnic cerebral vasoconstriction

Carbon dioxide response and anesthetics
- Maintained during inhaled and intravenous anesthetics
- Relative response to hypocapnia depends on normocapnic CBF (anesthetics that increase CBF enhance the reduction of CBF by hypocapnia)

Carbon dioxide response in presence of disease or injury
- Hypercapnic response intact with hypertension
- Hypocapnia response present with brain injury (subarachnoid hemorrhage) but may be attenuated if vasospasm is present

subsequent dissociation to form hydrogen ions. Hydrogen ions produce vasodilation of cerebral vessels that is proportional to the increase in hydrogen ion concentration.

Any other acid that increases hydrogen ion concentration, such as lactic acid, also increases cerebral blood flow. Increased cerebral blood flow in response to increases in $Paco_2$ serves to carry away excess hydrogen ions that would otherwise greatly depress neuronal activity.

Unlike the continuous response of cerebral blood flow to changes in $Paco_2$, the response to Pao_2 is a threshold phenomenon (see Fig. 3-19). If the $Paco_2$ is maintained, cerebral blood flow begins to increase when the Pao_2 decreases below 50 mm Hg or the cerebral venous Po_2 decreases from its normal value of 35 mm Hg to about 30 mm Hg.

Autoregulation

Cerebral blood flow is closely autoregulated between a mean arterial pressure of about 60 and 140 mm Hg (see Fig. 3-19). As a result, changes in systemic blood pressure within this range will not significantly alter cerebral blood flow. Chronic systemic hypertension shifts the autoregulation curve to the right such that decreases in cerebral blood flow may occur at a mean arterial pressure of >60 mm Hg. Autoregulation of cerebral blood flow is attenuated or abolished by hypercapnia, arterial hypoxemia, and volatile anesthetics. Furthermore, autoregulation is often abolished in the area surrounding an acute cerebral infarction. For example, reactivity of blood vessels in areas surrounding cerebral infarcts and tumors is abolished. These blood vessels are maximally vasodilated, presumably reflecting accumulation of acidic metabolic products. As a result, cerebral blood flow to this area is already maximal (luxury perfusion), and changes in $Paco_2$ have no effect on its local blood flow. If $Paco_2$ should increase, however, it is theoretically possible that resulting vasodilation in normal blood vessels would shunt blood flow away from the diseased area (intracerebral steal syndrome). Conversely, a decrease in $Paco_2$ that constricts normal cerebral vessels could divert blood flow to diseased areas ("Robin Hood" phenomenon). Increases in mean arterial pressure above the limits of autoregulation can cause leakage of intravascular fluid through capillary membranes, resulting in cerebral edema. Because the brain is enclosed in a solid vault, the accumulation of edema fluid increases intracranial pressure and compresses blood vessels, decreasing cerebral blood flow and leading to destruction of brain tissue.

Measurement of Cerebral Blood Flow

Cerebral blood flow can be measured by injecting a radioactive substance, usually xenon, into the carotid artery and measuring the rate of decay of the radioactivity in each tissue segment using scintillation detectors. Using this technique, it can be demonstrated that cerebral blood flow changes within seconds in response to changes in local neuronal activity. For example, clasping the hand can be shown to cause an immediate increase in blood flow in the motor cortex of the opposite cerebral hemisphere. Reading increases blood flow in the occipital cortex and the language areas of the temporal cortex. This measuring procedure can be used to localize the origin of epilepsy because blood flow increases acutely at the site of origin of the seizure.

Electroencephalogram

The EEG is a recording of the brain waves that result from the summed electrical activity in the brain. The intensity of the electrical activity recorded from the surface of the scalp ranges from 0 to 300 μV, and the frequency may

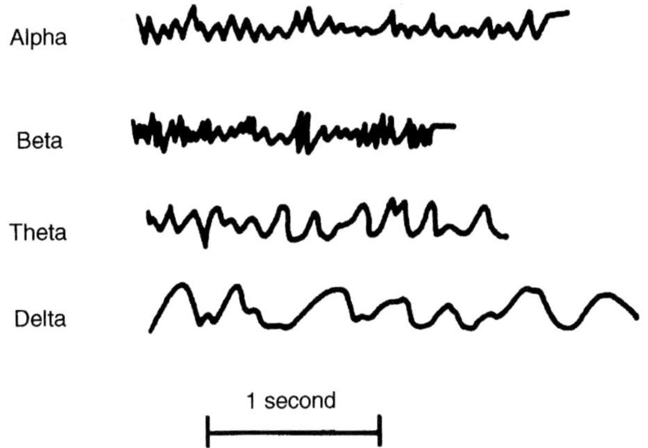

FIGURE 3-20 The electroencephalogram consists of α, β, θ, and δ waves.

exceed 50 cycles per second. The character of the waves greatly depends on the level of activity of the cerebral cortex and the degree of wakefulness. There is a direct relationship between the degree of cerebral activity and the frequency of brain waves. Furthermore, during periods of increased mental activity, brain waves become asynchronous rather than synchronous, so the voltage decreases despite greater cortical activity.

Classification of Brain Waves

Brain waves are classified as α, β, θ, and δ waves depending on their frequency and amplitude (Fig. 3-20). The classic EEG is a plot of voltage against time, usually recorded by 16 channels on paper moving at 30 mm per second. One page of recording is 10 seconds of data.

α Waves

α waves occur at a frequency of 8 to 12 Hz and a voltage of about 50 μV. These waves are typical of an awake, resting state of cerebration with the eyes closed. During sleep, α waves disappear. Because α waves do not occur when the cerebral cortex is not connected to the thalamus, it is assumed these waves result from spontaneous activity in the thalamocortical system.

β Waves

β waves occur at a frequency of 13 to 30 Hz and a voltage usually of <50 μV. These high-frequency and low-voltage asynchronous waves replace α waves in the presence of increased mental activity or visual stimulation.

θ Waves

θ waves occur at a frequency of 4 to 7 Hz. These waves occur in healthy children during sleep and also during general anesthesia.

δ Waves

δ waves include all the brain waves with a frequency of less than 4 Hz. These waves occur (a) in deep sleep, (b) during general anesthesia, and (c) in the presence of organic brain disease. δ waves occur even when the connections of the cerebral cortex to the reticular activating system are severed, indicating these waves originate in the cerebral cortex independently of lower brain structures.

Clinical Uses

The EEG is useful in diagnosing different types of epilepsy and for determining the focus in the brain causing seizures. Brain tumors, which compress surrounding neurons and cause abnormal electrical activity, may be localized using the EEG. Monitoring of the EEG during carotid endarterectomy, cardiopulmonary bypass, or controlled hypotension may provide an early warning of inadequate cerebral blood flow. In this regard, the EEG may be influenced by anesthetic drugs, depth of anesthesia, and hyperventilation of the patient's lungs. Several different monitors of EEG activity that use different algorithms designed to process EEG recordings and decompose them into a number that may be predictive of anesthetic depth.

Brain Wave Monitors

Numerous quantitative EEG processing techniques have been developed to monitor brain depression during anesthesia, including Bispectral Index, Narcotrend, SEDLine, and Entropy monitors. These are discussed in hundreds of manuscripts and review articles. Only two will be presented here.

Bispectral Index

The Bispectral Index (BIS) is a variable derived from the EEG that is a quantifiable measure of the sedative and hypnotic effects of anesthetic drugs on the CNS.[51] BIS is a processed EEG descriptor that predicts depth of anesthesia. Bispectral analysis is based on the correlation of the phase between different frequency components of the EEG in which the EEG signal is converted into its component sine waves using Fourier transformation. Electromyographic activity is specifically filtered with modern BIS algorithm but can still result in artifact. A set of bispectral features is calculated by analyzing the phase relations between the component waves. These bispectral features are combined with other EEG features into a single measurement, the BIS, expressed as a dimensionless numerical index from 0 to 100. Decreasing numerical values correlate with sedation and predict the response of patients to surgical stimulation (values of <60 are associated with a low probability of recall and a high probability of unresponsiveness during surgery) (Fig. 3-21).[52,53] Titrating desflurane and sevoflurane using the BIS monitor to maintain a numerical value of 60 results in decreased use of drug and faster awakening.[54] Likewise, titration of propofol to maintain a numerical value of 45 to 60 and then permitting an increase to 60 to 75 during the last 15 minutes of the operation results in decreased propofol use and more rapid recovery.[55] In this regard, BIS monitoring may serve as a useful intraoperative monitor for guiding drug administration, particularly for intravenous hypnotics (e.g., propofol).

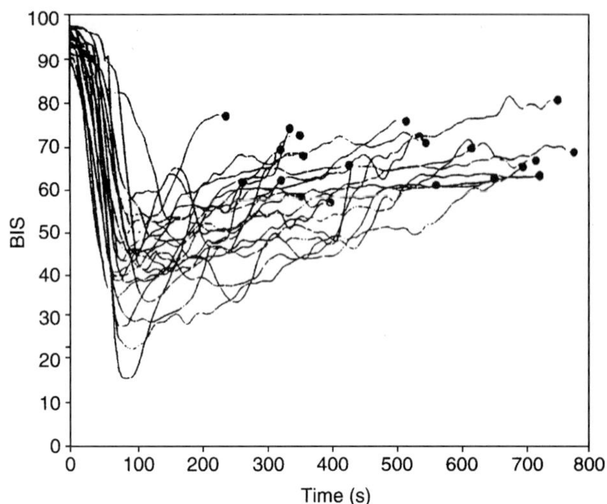

FIGURE 3-21 Plot of bispectral index (BIS) against time from induction of anesthesia to recovery of consciousness after administration of propofol. (From Flaishon R, Windsor A, Sigl J, et al. Recovery of consciousness after thiopental or propofol. Bispectral index and the isolated forearm technique. *Anesthesiology.* 1997;86:613–619, with permission.)

Based on published studies, the FDA determined that use of BIS monitoring to guide anesthetic administration may be associated with a reduction of the incidence of awareness with recall in adults during general anesthesia and sedation.[36,56,57] However, these findings have been challenged by a recent study that found that the BIS monitor performed similarly to rigorous monitoring of end-tidal inhaled anesthetic concentration[37,58] in preventing awareness. It may be that monitors of processed EEG are pharmacodynamic monitors of the complex interplay between the concentration of anesthetic agents and surgical stimulation, and thus the use of monitoring may be a function of the anesthetic technique, the drugs used, and the availability of methodology to easily the concentration in the patient.

Spectral Entropy

Spectral entropy (SE) represents an alternative concept to bispectral analysis for quantifying the EEG. SE and response entropy (RE) are computed over specific frequency ranges of the EEG. RE includes electromyographic activity. SE, RE, and BIS reveal similar information about the level of sedation.[59] BIS and SE measurement are similar during propofol anesthesia. However, they are not interchangeable. For example, SE measurements are lower than BIS measurements during anesthesia with xenon.[60]

Epilepsy

Epilepsy is characterized by excessive activity of either a part or all of the CNS. Grand mal epilepsy is characterized by intense neuronal discharges in multiple areas of the cerebral and reticular activating system. These impulses are transmitted to the spinal cord, resulting in alternating skeletal muscle contractions known as ***tonic-clonic seizures***. Profound autonomic activity often results in defecation and urination. The grand mal seizure lasts from a few seconds to several minutes and is followed by generalized depression of the entire CNS (the postictal state). The EEG during a grand mal seizure reveals high-voltage, synchronous brain wave discharges over the entire cerebral cortex. Synaptic fatigue is a likely mechanism that contributes to spontaneous cessation of a grand mal seizure and postictal depression.

Status epilepticus is present when grand mal seizure activity is sustained. Judicious doses of an intravenous sedative hypnotics can stop seizures and permit resumption of effective breathing. In the rare instance in which conventional drug therapy is ineffective, volatile anesthetics such as isoflurane may be administered in an attempt to stop status epilepticus.[61] When volatile anesthetics are administered for this purpose, it is likely that systemic blood pressure will need to be supported with intravenous administration of fluids and/or sympathomimetics. If the underlying cause of the seizure has not been addressed then the seizure is likely to recur when the volatile anesthetic is discontinued.

Evoked Potentials

Evoked potentials are the electrophysiologic responses of the CNS to sensory, motor, auditory, or visual stimulation. The waveforms resulting from sensory stimulation reflect transmission of impulses through specific sensory pathways. Poststimulus latency is the time in milliseconds from application of the stimulus to a peak in the recorded waveform. The amplitude and latency of evoked potentials may be influenced by a number of events, especially volatile anesthetics. Evoked potentials are used to monitor (a) spinal cord function during operations near or on the spinal cord, and (b) auditory nerve and brainstem function, as during operations on pituitary tumors or other lesions that impinge on the optic nerves or optic chiasm. The modes of sensory stimulation used to produce evoked potentials in the operating room are somatosensory, auditory, and visual.

Somatosensory Evoked Potentials

Somatosensory evoked potentials are produced by application of a low-voltage electrical current that stimulates a peripheral nerve such as the median nerve at the wrist or the posterior tibial nerve at the ankle. The resulting evoked potentials reflect the integrity of sensory neural pathways from the peripheral nerve to the somatosensory cortex. Somatosensory stimulation follows the dorsal column pathways of proprioception and vibration. These pathways are supplied by the posterior spinal artery, leaving the motor pathway, which is supplied by the anterior spinal artery, unmonitored. Indeed, postoperative paraplegia has been described in patients despite the preservation of somatosensory evoked potentials intraoperatively.[62] Inhaled anesthetics, especially volatile anesthetics, produce dose-dependent depression of

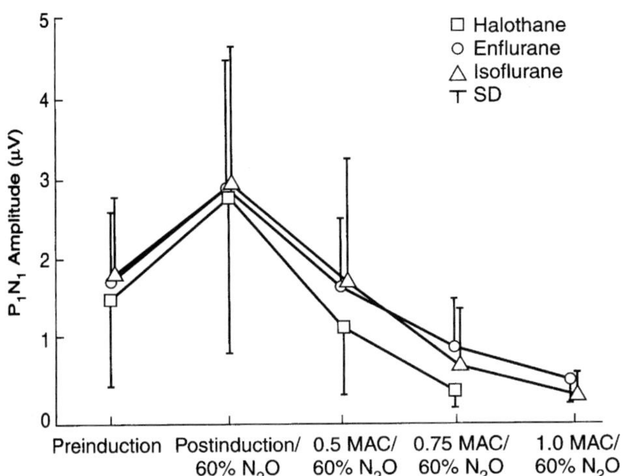

FIGURE 3-22 Peak-to-peak amplitudes (and latencies—not shown) decrease significantly with increasing MAC levels. (From Pathak KS, Ammadio M, Kalamchi A, et al. Effects of halothane, enflurane, and isoflurane on somatosensory evoked potentials during nitrous oxide anesthesia. *Anesthesiology*. 1987;66:753–757, with permission.)

somatosensory evoked potentials (see Chapter 4). Although less so than volatile anesthetics, morphine and fentanyl also produce depressant effects on somatosensory evoked potentials, with a low-dose continuous infusion of the opioid producing less depression than intermittent injections (Fig. 3-22).[63] Ketamine and etomidate may increase the amplitude of somatosensory evoked potentials (see Chapter 5). Acute hyperventilation of the patient's lungs to produce a $Paco_2$ near 20 mm Hg does not significantly alter the amplitude or latencies of somatosensory evoked potentials.[64]

Motor Evoked Potentials

The use of motor evoked potentials remains limited, as their recording requires direct (epidural) or indirect (transosseous) stimulation of the brain or spinal cord.[65] These evoked potentials reflect the integrity of motor neural pathways from the motor cortex to the muscle. Motor evoked potentials are extremely sensitive to depression by anesthetics. Furthermore, it is not possible to monitor motor evoked potentials in the presence of significant drug-induced neuromuscular blockade. During scoliosis surgery or other operations that place spinal cord motor function at risk, the use of motor evoked potentials obviates the need for an intraoperative wake-up test. In many instances, it is useful to monitor both motor and sensory evoked potentials to fully evaluate the functional integrity of both motor and sensory pathways. As an alternative to motor evoked potentials, transcranial motor stimulation may be used to monitor spinal cord function during spinal surgery. Total intravenous anesthesia with propofol and an opioid with judicious infusion of neuromuscular blocker is a useful technique when monitoring of somatosensory and motor evoked potentials is desired.

Auditory Evoked Potentials

Auditory evoked potentials arise from brainstem auditory pathways. Volatile anesthetics produce dose-dependent depression of auditory evoked potentials. Auditory evoked potentials may provide an objective electrophysiologic alternative to the clinical assessment of sedation.[66]

Visual Evoked Potentials

Visual evoked potentials are produced by flashes from light-emitting diodes that are mounted on goggles placed over the patient's closed eyes. Visual evoked potentials may be useful to monitor the visual pathways during transphenoidal or anterior fossa neurosurgical procedures. Volatile anesthetics produce dose-dependent depression of visual evoked potentials, especially above concentrations equivalent to about 0.8 MAC.[67]

Cerebrospinal Fluid

Cerebrospinal fluid (CSF) is present in the (a) ventricles of the brain, (b) cisterns around the brain, and (c) subarachnoid space around the brain and spinal cord (Fig. 3-23). The total volume of CSF is about 150 mL and the specific gravity is 1.002 to 1.009. A major function of CSF is to cushion the brain in the cranial cavity. A blow to the head moves the entire brain simultaneously, causing no one portion of the brain to be selectively contorted by the blow. When a blow to the head is particularly severe, it usually does not damage the brain on the ipsilateral side, but instead damage manifests on the opposite side. This phenomenon is known as ***contrecoup*** and reflects the creation of a vacuum between the brain and skull opposite the blow caused by sudden movement of the brain at this site away from the skull. When the skull is no longer being accelerated by the blow, the vacuum suddenly collapses and the brain strikes the interior of the skull.

Formation

The choroid plexuses (cauliflower-like growths of blood vessels covered by a thin layer of epithelial cells) in the four cerebral ventricles are the major site of formation of CSF, which continually exudes from the surface of the choroid plexus at a rate of about 30 mL per hour. In comparison with other extracellular fluids, the concentration of sodium and chloride in CSF is 7% greater and the concentration of glucose and potassium is 30% and 40% less, respectively. This difference in composition from other extracellular fluids emphasizes that CSF is a choroid secretion and not a simple filtrate from the capillaries. The pH of CSF is closely regulated and maintained at 7.32. Changes in $Paco_2$, but not arterial pH, promptly alter CSF pH, reflecting the ability of carbon dioxide, but not hydrogen ions, to cross the blood–brain barrier easily. As a result, acute respiratory acidosis or alkalosis produces corresponding changes in CSF pH. Active transport of bicarbonate ions eventually returns CSF pH to 7.32, despite the persistence of alterations in arterial pH.

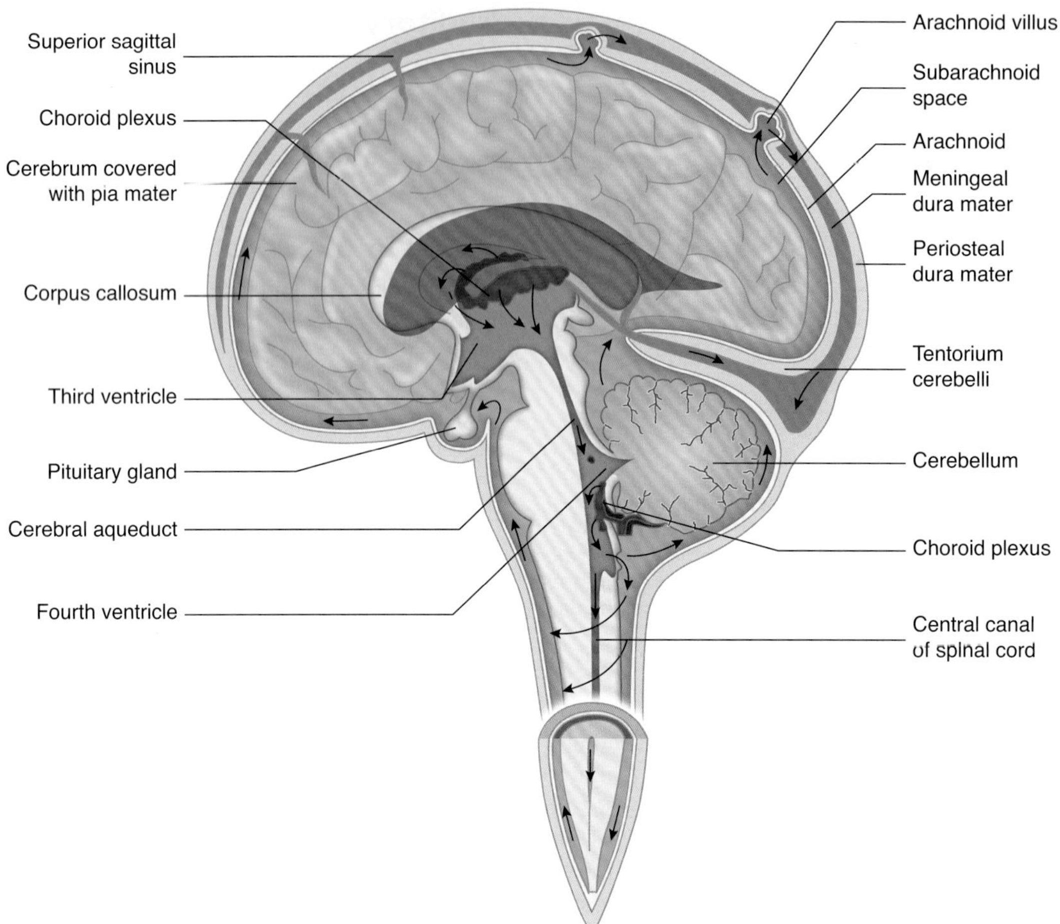

FIGURE 3-23 Cerebral spinal fluid fluxes in and out of the ventricles with the cardiac cycle.

Reabsorption

Almost all the CSF formed each day is reabsorbed into the venous circulation through special structures known as ***arachnoid villi*** or ***granulations***. These villi project the subarachnoid spaces into the venous sinuses of the brain and occasionally into veins of the spinal cord. Arachnoid villi are actually trabeculae that protrude through venous walls, resulting in highly permeable areas that permit relatively free flow of CSF into the circulation. The magnitude of reabsorption depends on the pressure gradient between the CSF and the venous circulation.

Circulation

CSF formed in the lateral cerebral ventricles passes into the third ventricle through the foramen of Monro (see Fig. 3-23), where it mixes with CSF formed there. From there, it passes along the aqueduct of Sylvius into the fourth cerebral ventricle, where still more CSF is formed. The CSF then passes into the cisterna magna through the lateral foramen of Luschka and via a middle foramen of Magendie. From this point, CSF flows through the subarachnoid spaces upward toward the cerebrum, where most of the arachnoid villi are located.

Hydrocephalus

Obstruction to free circulation of CSF in the neonate results in hydrocephalus. For example, blockage of the aqueduct of Sylvius results in expansion of the lateral and third cerebral ventricles and compression of the brain (see Fig. 3-23). This type of obstruction producing a noncommunicating type of hydrocephalus is treated by surgical creation of an artificial pathway for flow of CSF between the cerebral ventricular system and the subarachnoid space.

Intracranial Pressure

Normal intracranial pressure (ICP) is $<$15 mm Hg. This pressure is regulated by the rate of CSF formation and resistance to CSF reabsorption through arachnoid villi as determined by venous pressure. In addition, increases in cerebral blood flow, as during inhalation of volatile anesthetics, can cause the ICP to increase because of the concomitant increase in cerebral blood flow and cerebral blood volume. Systemic blood pressure does not alter ICP within the range of normal autoregulation. Phasic variations in systemic blood pressure, however, are transmitted as variations in ICP.

Papilledema

Anatomically, the dura of the brain extends as a sheath around the optic nerve and then connects with the sclera of the eye. Increases in ICP are transmitted to the optic nerve sheath. Increased pressure in the optic sheath impedes blood flow in the retinal veins, leading to increases in the retinal capillary pressure and retinal edema. The tissues of the optic disc are more distensible than the rest of the retina, so the disc becomes edematous and swells into the cavity of the eye. This swelling of the optic disc is termed ***papilledema***.

Blood–Brain Barrier

The blood–brain barrier reflects the impermeability of capillaries in the CNS, including the choroid plexuses, to circulating substances such as electrolytes and exogenous drugs or toxins. As a result, the neural and glial cells in the CNS live in a tightly controlled milieu that varies little in the healthy individual. The blood–brain barrier is maintained by the tight junction between endothelial cells of brain capillaries. Envelopment of brain capillaries by glial cells further decreases their permeability. The blood–brain barrier is less developed in the neonate and tends to break down in areas of the brain that are irradiated, infected, or compromised by neoplasm. The blood–brain barrier is also relatively permeable in the area around the posterior pituitary and the chemoreceptor trigger zone. The blood–brain barrier is characterized by active transport mediated by p-glycoprotein transporters (p-GP). These proteins are of the ATP binding cassette (ABC) family. Active transport of morphine out of the CNS by a p-GP is responsible for the >90-minute delay between morphine bolus and peak morphine drug effect.

Vision

The eye is optically equivalent to a photographic camera in that it contains a lens system, a variable aperture system (pupil), and light-sensitive surface (retina) (Fig. 3-24).[68] The lens system of the eye focuses an image on the retina. Relaxation and contraction of the ciliary muscles are responsible for altering the tension of ligaments attached to the lens, causing its refractive power to change. One diopter is equivalent to the ability of a lens to converge parallel light rays to a focal point 1 meter beyond the lens (59 diopters equals the total refractive power of the eye). Stimulation of parasympathetic nervous system fibers to the ciliary muscle causes this muscle to relax, which in turn relaxes the ligaments of the lens and increases its refractive power. This increased refractive power allows the eye to focus on objects that are nearby. Interference with this process of accommodation may be noted by patients in the postoperative period who have received an anticholinergic drug in the preoperative medication or as part of the pharmacologic reversal of nondepolarizing neuromuscular blockade. The principal function of the pupil is to increase or decrease the amount of light that enters the eye. For example, the pupil may vary from 1.5 to 8.0 mm in diameter, permitting a 30-fold variation in the amount of light that enters the eye.

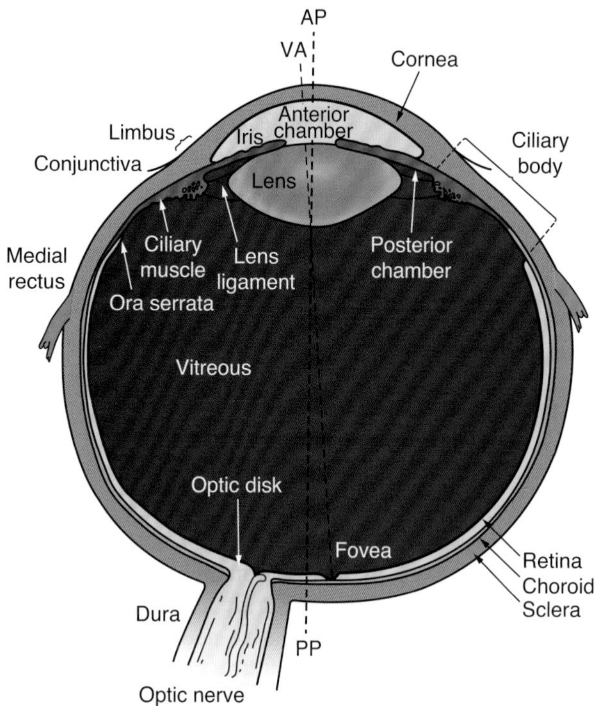

FIGURE 3-24 Schematic diagram of the eye. AP, anterior pole; PP, posterior pole; VA, visual axis.

The lens loses its elastic nature with aging because of progressive denaturation of the len's proteins. As a result, the ability to accommodate is almost totally absent by 45 to 50 years of age. This lack of ability to accommodate is known as ***presbyopia***.

Progressive denaturation of the proteins in the lens leads to the formation of a cataract. In later stages, calcium is often deposited in the coagulated proteins, thus further increasing the opacity. If the cataract impairs vision, the lens can be replaced by an artificial convex lens that compensates for the loss of refractive power created by removal of the lens.

Intraocular Fluid

Intraocular fluid consists of aqueous humor, which lies in front and at the sides of the lens, and vitreous humor, which lies between the lens and retina. Aqueous humor is freely flowing fluid that is continuously formed (2 to 3 mL per minute) and reabsorbed. This fluid is secreted by ciliary processes of the ciliary body in a manner similar to formation of CSF by the choroid plexus. After flowing into the anterior chamber, aqueous humor enters the canal of Schlemm, a thin vein that extends circumferentially around the eye. Vitreous humor is a gelatinous mass into which substances can diffuse slowly, but there is little flow of fluid.

Intraocular Pressure

Intraocular pressure is normally 15 to 25 mm Hg. This pressure is measured clinically by tonometry, in which the amount of displacement of the tonometer is calibrated in terms of intraocular pressure. It is believed that intraocular pressure is regulated primarily by resistance to outflow of aqueous humor from the anterior chamber into the canal of Schlemm. Glaucoma is associated with increased intraocular pressure sufficient to compress retinal artery inflow to the eye, leading to ischemic pain and eventually blindness. When medical control of glaucoma fails, it may be necessary to surgically create an artificial outflow tract for aqueous humor.

Retina

The retina is the light-sensitive portion of the eye containing the cones, which are responsible for color vision, and the rods, which are mainly responsible for vision in the dark. When the cones and rods are stimulated, impulses are transmitted through successive neurons in the retina and optic nerve before reaching the cerebral cortex. The presence of melanin in the pigment layer of the retina prevents reflection of light throughout the globe. Without this pigment, light rays would be reflected in all directions within the globe, causing visual acuity to be impaired. Indeed, albinos, who lack melanin, have greatly decreased visual acuity.

The nutrient blood supply for the retina is largely derived from the central retinal artery, which accompanies the optic nerve. This independent retinal blood supply prevents rapid degeneration of the retina should it become detached from the pigment epithelium and allows time for surgical correction of a detached retina. The main arterial supply to the globe and orbital contents is from the ophthalmic artery, which is a branch of the internal carotid artery.[69]

Ischemic Optic Neuropathy

Ischemic optic neuropathy (ION) results from infarction of the optic nerve and is the most frequently reported cause of vision loss following general anesthesia.[70] ION is classified as ***anterior ION*** (nonarteritic or arteritic) and ***posterior ION***. Nonarteritic anterior ION occurs more often in patients with congenitally small optic discs. It is presumed that the small cross-sectional area of the optic disc results in little room for expansion of optic nerve fibers in response to ischemia-induced edema.

Posterior ION has been reported after diverse surgical procedures (prolonged spinal fusion surgery, cardiac operations requiring cardiopulmonary bypass, radical neck surgery) and its etiology appears to be multifactorial—including intraoperative anemia and hypotension combined with at least one other factor (e.g., congenital absence of the central retinal artery, increased venous pressure owing to venous obstruction, large amounts of fluid administration, prolonged head-down position, administration of vasopressors).[70–73] Prone positioning increases IOP during anesthesia and could contribute to decreases in ocular perfusion pressure (Fig. 3-25).[74] Despite the multifactorial etiology of ION, some cases do not have any of the speculated associated factors (anemia, hypotension), except perhaps for a large amount of intravenous fluids.[75]

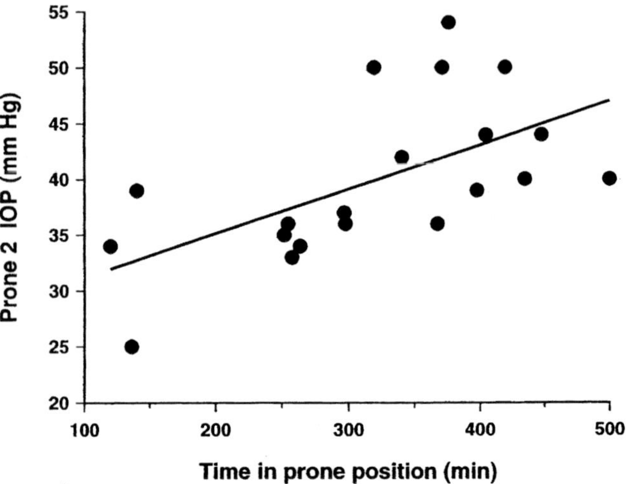

FIGURE 3-25 Intraocular pressure (IOP) at the conclusion of prone positioning (prone 2) is correlated with the total time spent in the prone position (minutes). (From Cheng MA, Todorov A, Tempelhoff R, et al. The effect of prone positioning on intraocular pressure in anesthetized patients. *Anesthesiology*. 2001;95:1351 1355, with permission.)

Other Causes of Postoperative Blindness

Cortical blindness, retinal occlusion, and ophthalmic venous obstruction need to be excluded when postoperative blindness occurs and ION is a consideration. Cortical blindness is characterized by loss of visual sensation with retention of pupillary reaction to light and normal funduscopic examination results. CT or MRI abnormalities in the parietal or occipital lobe confirm the diagnosis. A rare cause of cortical blindness is cyclosporine-induced neurotoxicity that is usually reversible.[71] Central retinal artery occlusion presents as painless, monocular blindness. Ophthalmoscopic examination of the eyes with retinal artery occlusion shows a pale edematous retina, a cherry-red spot at the fovea, and platelet-fibrin or cholesterol emboli in the narrowed retinal arteries. Obstruction of venous drainage from the eye may occur intraoperatively when patient positioning results in external pressure on the eyes.

Photochemicals

The light-sensitive photochemical continuously synthesized in rods is rhodopsin. Cones contain photochemicals that resemble rhodopsin. Vitamin A is an important precursor of photochemicals, which explains the occurrence of night blindness when this vitamin becomes deficient. Photochemicals in rods and cones decompose on exposure to light and in the process stimulate fibers in the optic nerve. Decomposition of rhodopsin decreases conductance of the membranes of rods for sodium ions. The resulting hyperpolarization in rods is opposite to the effect that occurs in almost all other sensory receptors. The intensity of the hyperpolarization signal is proportional to the logarithm of light energy, in contrast to the more linear response of most other receptors. This logarithmic response is important to vision because it allows the eyes to detect contrasts on the image even when light intensities vary several thousand fold.

If a person is in bright light for a prolonged period, large proportions of photochemicals in the rods and cones are depleted, resulting in decreased sensitivity of the eye to light (light adaptation). Conversely, during total darkness, the sensitivity of the retina is increased, reflecting conversion of photochemicals to rhodopsin (dark adaptation). The eye can also adapt to changes in light intensity by changing the size of the pupillary opening up to 30-fold.

Visual Pathway

Impulses from the retina pass backward through the optic nerve (Fig. 3-26).[68] The macula is a small area in the center of the retina that is composed mainly of cones to permit detailed vision. The fovea is the central portion of the macula and is the site of the clearest vision. At the optic chiasm, all the fibers from the nasal halves of the retina cross to the opposite side to join fibers from the opposite temporal retina to form the optic tracts. Fibers of the optic tract synapse in the lateral geniculate body before passing into the visual (occipital) area of the cerebral cortex. Specific points of the retina connect with specific points of the visual cortex, which results in the detection of lines, borders, and colors.

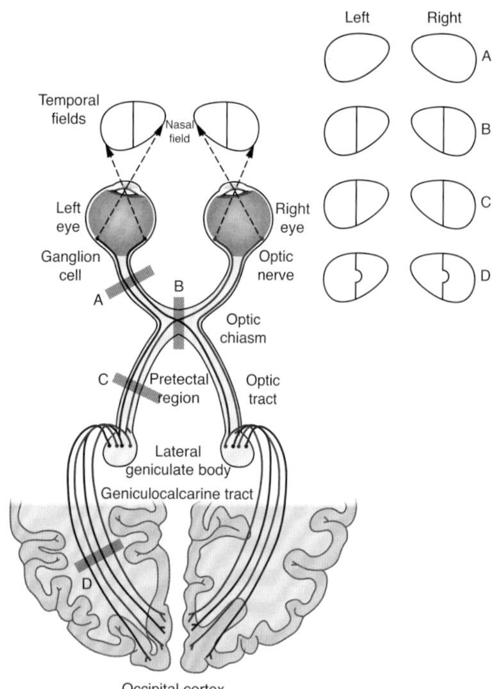

FIGURE 3-26 Visual impulses from the retina pass to the optic chiasm, where fibers from the nasal halves of the retina cross to the opposite side to join temporal fibers and form the optic tract. These fibers synapse in the lateral geniculate body before passing to the visual (occipital) area of the cerebral cortex. Visual field defects reflect lesions at various sites *(A–D)* in the nerve pathways.

Field of Vision

The field of vision is the area seen by the eye at a given instant. The area seen to the nasal side is called the ***nasal field of vision***, and the area seen to the lateral side is called the ***temporal field of vision*** (see Fig. 3-26).[68] An important use of visual fields is localization of lesions in the visual neural pathway. For example, anterior pituitary tumors may compress the optic chiasm, causing blindness in both temporal fields of vision (called ***bitemporal hemianopia***). Thrombosis of the posterior cerebral artery is a cause of infarction of the visual cortex.

Muscular Control of Eye Movements

The cerebral control system for directing the eyes toward the object to be viewed is as important as the cerebral system for interpretation of the visual signals. Movements of the eyes are controlled by three pairs of skeletal muscles designated as the (a) medial and lateral recti, (b) superior and inferior recti, and (c) superior and inferior obliques. The medial and lateral recti contract reciprocally to move the eyes from side to side; the superior and inferior recti move the eyes upward or downward; and rotation of the globe is accomplished by the superior and inferior obliques. Each of the three sets of eye muscles is reciprocally innervated by cranial nerves III, IV, and VI so that one muscle of the pair contracts while the other relaxes.

Simultaneous movement of both eyes in the same directions is called ***conjugate movement of the eyes***. Occasionally, abnormalities occur in the control system for eye movements that cause continuous nystagmus. Nystagmus is likely to occur when one of the vestibular apparatuses is damaged or when deep nuclei in the cerebellum are damaged or under the influence of ketamine anesthesia.

Innervation of the Eye

The eyes are innervated by the sympathetic and parasympathetic nervous system. The preganglionic fibers of the parasympathetic nervous system arise in the Edinger-Westphal nucleus of cranial nerve III and then pass to the ciliary ganglion, which gives rise to nerve fibers that innervate the ciliary muscle and sphincter of the iris. Sympathetic nervous system fibers innervate the radial fibers of the iris as well as several extraocular structures. Stimulation of the parasympathetic nervous system fibers to the eye excites the ciliary sphincter, causing miosis. Conversely, stimulation of sympathetic nervous system fibers to the eye excites the radial fibers of the iris and causes mydriasis. Volatile anesthetics cause midrange pupillary dilation, whereas opioids cause papillary constriction. Monitoring of papillary diameter provides some indication of the residual opioid activity on anesthetic emergence.

Horner Syndrome

Interruption of the superior cervical chain of the sympathetic nervous system innervation to the eye results in miosis, ptosis, and vasodilation with absence of sweating on the ipsilateral side of the body, commonly referred to as ***Horner's syndrome***. Miosis occurs because of interruption of sympathetic nervous system innervation to the radial fibers of the iris. Ptosis reflects the normal innervation of the superior palpebral muscle by the sympathetic nervous system. Horner's syndrome often occurs following stellate ganglion block and is occasionally a complication of interscalene block of the brachial plexus.

Hearing

Receptors for hearing and equilibrium are housed in the inner ear (Fig. 3-27).[68] The external ear focuses sound waves on the ear drum, which oscillates in contact with the bones of the middle ear. The sound is amplified at the oval window, where the vibrations are transmitted to the hair cells of the cochlea in the inner ear. The anatomic arrangement of the hair cells results in their responding to different frequencies, performing a mechanical Fourier transformation of the incoming sound waves. The electrical current generated from activation of a hair cell travels from the auditory nerve to the inferior colliculus and auditory cortex.

The Eustachian tube connects the middle ear with the posterior tonsillar pillars and allows pressures on both sides of the tympanic membrane to be equalized during chewing or swallowing. Nitrous oxide may increase middle ear pressure and has been associated with rupture of the tympanic membrane when inflammation or scarring of the Eustachian tube opening into the nasopharynx prevents spontaneous decompression of the middle ear.[76]

Deafness

Nerve deafness is due to an abnormality of the cochlear or auditory nerve. Certain drugs such as streptomycin, gentamicin, kanamycin, and chloramphenicol may damage the organ of Corti, causing nerve deafness. Conduction deafness is caused by injury to the mechanisms that conduct sound waves from the tympanic membrane to the oval window. Conduction deafness is often caused by fibrosis of the structures in the middle ear after repeated infections in the middle ear by the hereditary disease known as ***osteosclerosis***.

Perioperative Hearing Impairment

Perioperative hearing impairment is often subclinical and may go unnoticed unless audiometry is performed.[77] Hearing loss (incidence may be as high as 50%) after dural puncture in the low-frequency range is most likely due to CSF leak and should resolve completely within days. Hearing loss following general anesthesia for surgery not requiring cardiopulmonary bypass does not appear to have a uniform prognosis, likely reflecting the myriad of etiologies (e.g., CSF leak after ear, nose, and throat [ENT] and

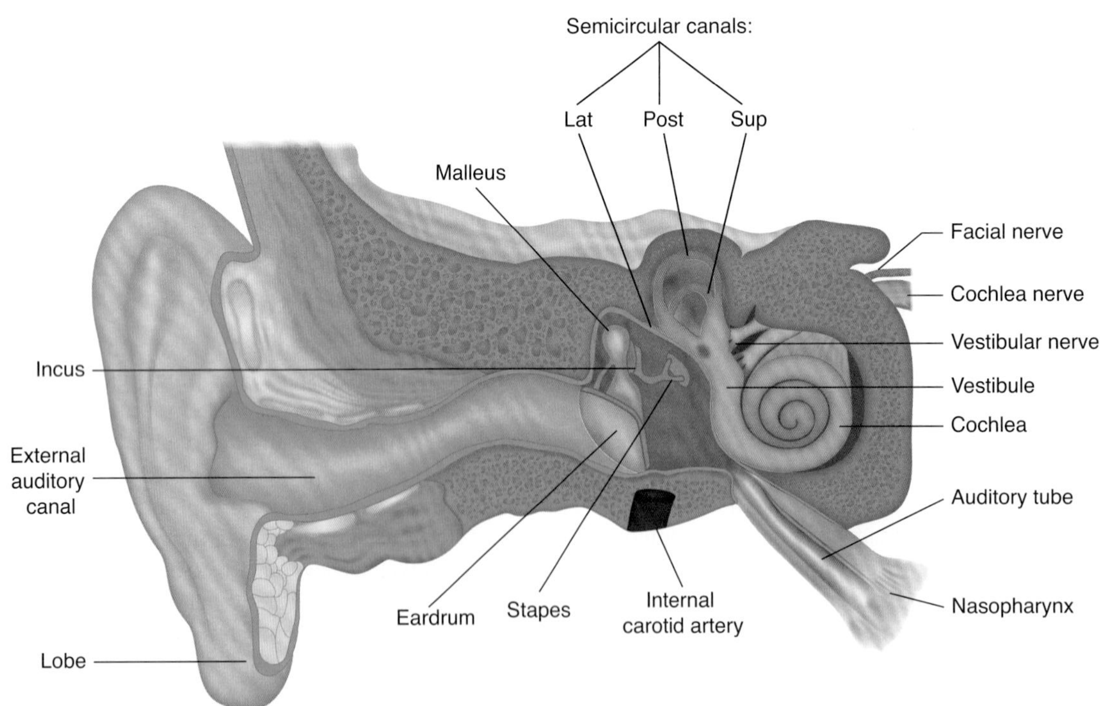

FIGURE 3-27 Schematic diagram of the outer and inner ear. Lat, lateral; Post, posterior; Sup, superior.

neurosurgery, barotrauma from nitrous oxide, embolism during cardiac surgery, or preexisting vasculopathy). Recovery in hearing appears to be independent of treatment. Unilateral hearing loss following cardiopulmonary bypass is often permanent and probably due to embolism and subsequent ischemic injury to areas of the organ of Corti.

Equilibrium

The semicircular canals (the utricle and saccule of the inner ear) are important for maintaining equilibrium (see Fig. 3-27).[68] The utricle and saccule contain cilia that transmit nerve impulses to the brain necessary for maintaining orientation of the head in space. Endolymph present in the semicircular canals flows with changes in head position, causing signals to be transmitted via the vestibular nerve nuclei and the cerebellum.

Taste

Taste is mainly a function of taste buds located principally in the papillae of the tongue. Sweet, sour, salty, and bitter are the four primary sensations of taste. Sour taste is caused by acids. Sour taste intensity is approximately proportional to the logarithm of the hydrogen ion concentration (i.e., pH). Sweet and salt are pleasurable tastes, of course. Bitter tastes are generally unpleasant. The bitter taste of alkaloids causes the individual to reject these substances. This may be protective as many plant toxins are alkaloids.

Adaptation to taste sensations is almost complete in 1 to 5 minutes of continuous stimulation. Individuals with upper respiratory tract infections complain of loss of taste sensation when, in fact, taste bud function is normal, emphasizing that most of what is considered taste is actually smell. Taste preference is presumed to be a CNS phenomenon but may be influenced by common polymorphisms in the many genes for taste receptors.

Smell

Olfactory receptors are located high in the nasal cavity. Each olfactory receptor is located on a single cilium. Olfactory receptors are coupled to G proteins. G protein activation increases activity of adenylyl cyclase, increasing the concentration of cAMP. A substance must be volatile and lipid soluble to stimulate olfactory cells. The importance of upward air movement in smell acuity is the reason sniffing improves the sense of smell, whereas holding one's breath prevents the sensation of unpleasant odors. Olfactory receptors adapt extremely rapidly, such that smell sensation may become extinct in about 60 seconds. Compared with lower animals, the sense of smell in humans is almost rudimentary. Humans have over 1,000 genes for odorant receptors but only about 40% of those are functional. Nevertheless, the threshold for smell is low as reflected by the detection of trace concentrations of methyl mercaptan that is mixed with odorless natural gas to alert one to a gas leak.

Nausea and Vomiting

Nausea is the conscious recognition of excitation of an area in the medulla that is associated with the vomiting (emetic) center (Fig. 3-28).[78] Impulses are transmitted by afferent fibers of the parasympathetic and sympathetic nervous system to the vomiting center. Motor impulses transmitted via cranial nerves V, VII, IX, X, and XII to the gastrointestinal tract and through the spinal nerves to the diaphragm and abdominal muscles are required to cause the mechanical act of vomiting.

The medullary vomiting center is located close to the fourth cerebral ventricle and receives afferents from the (a) chemoreceptor trigger zone, (b) cerebral cortex, (c) labyrinthovestibular center, and (d) neurovegetative system. Impulses from these afferents lead to nausea and vomiting. The chemoreceptor trigger zone includes receptors for serotonin, dopamine, histamine, and opioids. Stimulation of the chemoreceptor trigger zone located on the floor of the fourth cerebral ventricle initiates vomiting independent of the vomiting center. The chemoreceptor trigger zone is not protected by the blood–brain barrier

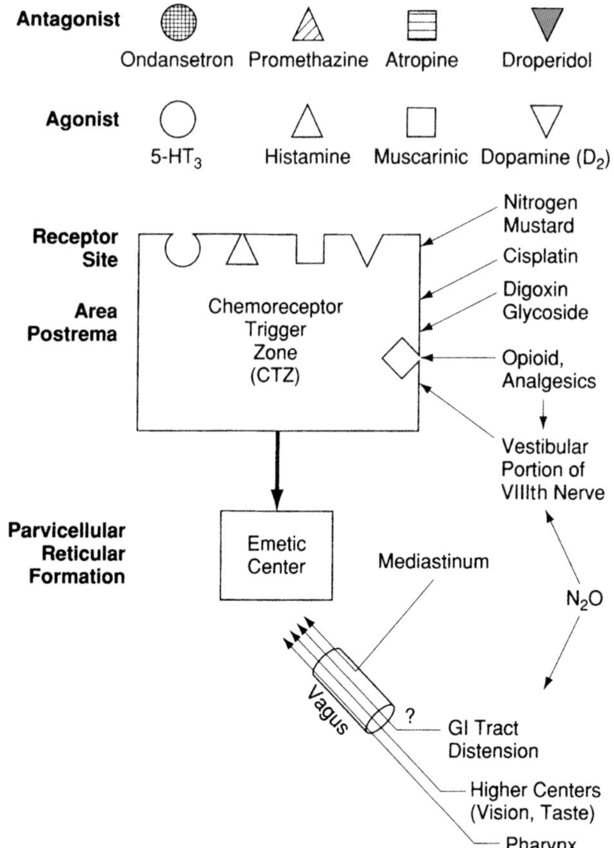

FIGURE 3-28 The chemoreceptor trigger zone and emetic center respond to a variety of stimuli resulting in nausea and vomiting. 5-HT_3, 5-hydroxytryptamine; GI, gastrointestinal. (From Watcha MR, White PF. Postoperative nausea and vomiting. Its etiology, treatment, and prevention. *Anesthesiology.* 1992;77:162–184, with permission.)

and thus this zone can be activated by chemical stimuli received through the systemic circulation as well as the CSF. The cerebral cortex stimulates vomiting through as a response to certain smells and physiologic stresses. Motion can stimulate equilibrium receptors in the inner ear, which may also stimulate the medullary vomiting center. The neurovegetative system is sensitive principally to gastrointestinal stimulation. Blocking of impulses from the chemoreceptor trigger zone does not prevent vomiting due to irritative stimuli (ipecac) arising in the gastrointestinal tract.

Peripheral Nervous System

The peripheral nervous system is composed of the sensory and motor nerves that connect the CNS to the tissues and organs (Fig. 3-29). These nerves are familiar to anesthesiologists as the targets for regional anesthetic techniques, and the anatomy is well reviewed in many atlases of regional anesthesia.

Pathways for Peripheral Sensory Impulses

The peripheral nerves extend from the dendrite in the periphery to the dorsal root ganglion, where the cell body is located, and from there to the spinal cord by way of the dorsal root (Fig. 3-30). By definition, dendrites conduct impulses toward the cell body, whereas axons conduct impulses away from the cell body. Thus, the portion of the nerve from the cell body to the peripheral receptor is a dendrite, whereas the relatively shorter connection from the dorsal root ganglion to the spinal cord is the axon. However, structurally, the dendrite and the axon are indistinguishable, and the nerve behaves like one long axon, giving rise to the term ***pseudounipolar neuron*** that occasionally is used to describe peripheral nerves.

After entering the spinal cord, peripheral sensory neurons synapse in the dorsal horn and give rise to long, ascending fiber tracts that transmit sensory information to the brain. These sensory signals are transmitted to the brain by the dorsal-lemniscal system, which includes dorsal column pathways and spinocervical tracts, and by anterolateral spinothalamic tracts (Figs. 3-31 and 3-32).[3] Impulses in the dorsal column pathways cross in the spinal cord to the opposite side before passing upward to the thalamus. Synapses in the thalamus are received by neurons that project into the somatic sensory area of the cerebral cortex. Nerve fibers of the anterolateral spinothalamic system cross in the anterior commissure to the opposite side of the spinal cord, where they turn upward toward the brain as the ventral and lateral spinothalamic tracts. Sensory signals from the anterolateral spinothalamic system are relayed from the thalamus to the somatic sensory area of the cerebral cortex. All sensory information that enters the cerebral cortex, with the exception of the olfactory system, passes through the thalamus.

Pathways for Peripheral Motor Responses

Sensory information is integrated at all levels of the nervous system and causes appropriate motor responses, beginning in the spinal cord with relatively simple reflex responses. Motor responses originating in the brainstem are more complex, whereas the most complicated and precise motor responses originate from the cerebral cortex.

Anterior motor neurons in the anterior horns of the spinal cord gray matter give rise to A-α fibers that leave the spinal cord by way of anterior nerve roots and innervate skeletal muscles. Skeletal muscles and tendons contain muscle spindles and Golgi tendon organs that operate at a subconscious level to relay information to the spinal cord and brain relative to changes in length and tension of skeletal muscle fibers. The stretch reflex is a reflex contraction of the skeletal muscle whenever stretch of the opposite balanced muscle results in stimulation of the muscle spindle. Tapping the patellar tendon elicits a knee jerk, which is a stretch reflex of the quadriceps femoris muscle. The ankle jerk is due to reflex contraction of the gastrocnemius muscle. Transmission of large numbers of facilitatory impulses from upper regions of the CNS to the spinal cord results in exaggerated stretch reflex responses. For example, lesions in the contralateral motor areas of the cerebral cortex, as caused by a cerebral vascular accident or brain tumor, cause greatly enhanced stretch reflexes. Clonus occurs when evoked muscle jerks oscillate. This phenomenon typically occurs when the stretch reflex is sensitized by facilitatory impulses from the brain, resulting in exaggerated facilitation of the spinal cord. When associated with recovery from general anesthesia, clonus as initiated by abrupt dorsiflexion of the foot can be eliminated by flexing the knees and keeping them in a flexed position.[79]

Transection of the brainstem at the level of the pons (isolates the spinal cord from the rest of the brain) results in spasticity known as ***decerebrate rigidity***. Decerebrate rigidity reflects diffuse facilitation of stretch reflexes.

The motor system is often divided into upper and lower motor neurons. Lower motor neurons originate in the spinal cord and directly innervate skeletal muscles. A lower motor neuron lesion is associated with flaccid paralysis, atrophy of skeletal muscles, and absence of stretch reflex responses. Spastic paralysis with accentuated stretch reflexes is due to destruction of upper motor neurons in the brain. Upper motor neurons originate in the cerebral cortex or brainstem and traverse down the anterior and lateral corticospinal paths until they connect with the lower motor neuron in the ventral horn of the spinal cord.

Withdrawal flexor reflexes are a lower motor neuron reflex, typically elicited by a painful stimulus. Associated

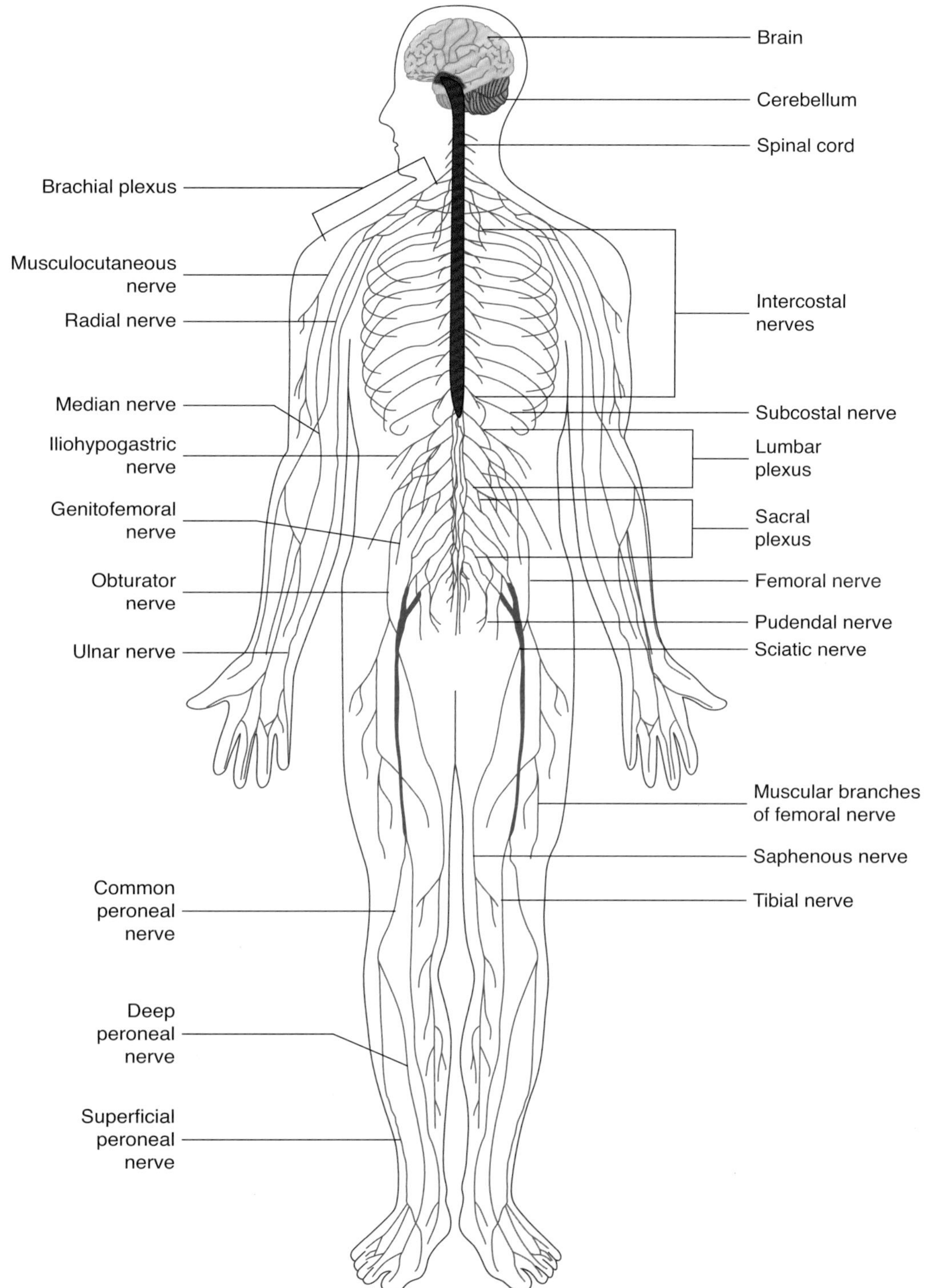

FIGURE 3-29 The peripheral nervous system connects the body tissues to the spinal cord and central nervous system.

with withdrawal of the stimulated limb is extension of the opposite limb (cross-extensor reflex) that occurs 0.2 to 0.5 second later and serves to push the body away from the object causing the painful stimulus. The delayed onset of the cross-extensor reflex is due to the time necessary for the signal to pass through the additional neurons to reach the opposite side of the spinal cord.

Autonomic Nervous System

The autonomic nervous system controls the visceral functions of the body. In addition, the autonomic nervous system modulates systemic blood pressure, gastrointestinal motility and secretion, urinary bladder emptying, sweating, and body temperature maintenance. Activation of the

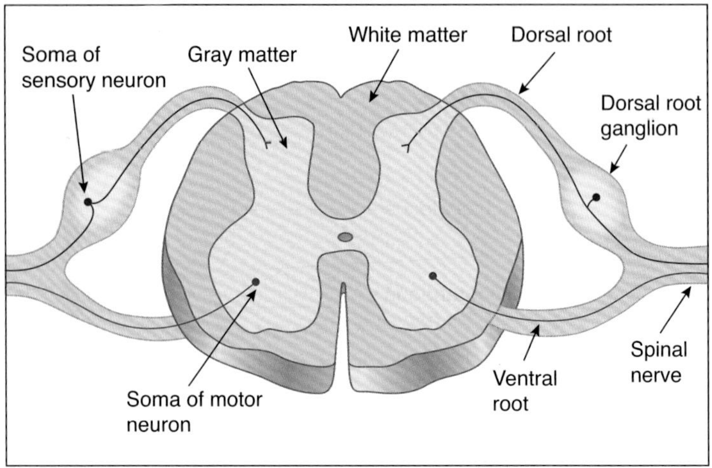

FIGURE 3-30 Cross section of the spinal cord, showing the dorsal (posterior) and ventral (anterior) roots. The cell body of peripheral sensory nerves is in the dorsal root ganglion. The cell body of motor nerves is in the anterior horn.

autonomic nervous system occurs principally via centers located in the hypothalamus, brainstem, and spinal cord. The ANS is divided into the sympathetic, parasympathetic, and enteric nervous systems.

The sympathetic and the parasympathetic nervous systems usually function as physiologic antagonists such that the compiled action on any organ represents a balance of the influence of each component (Table 3-4). The sympathetic nervous system functions as an amplification response, whereas the parasympathetic nervous system evokes discrete and narrowly targeted responses.

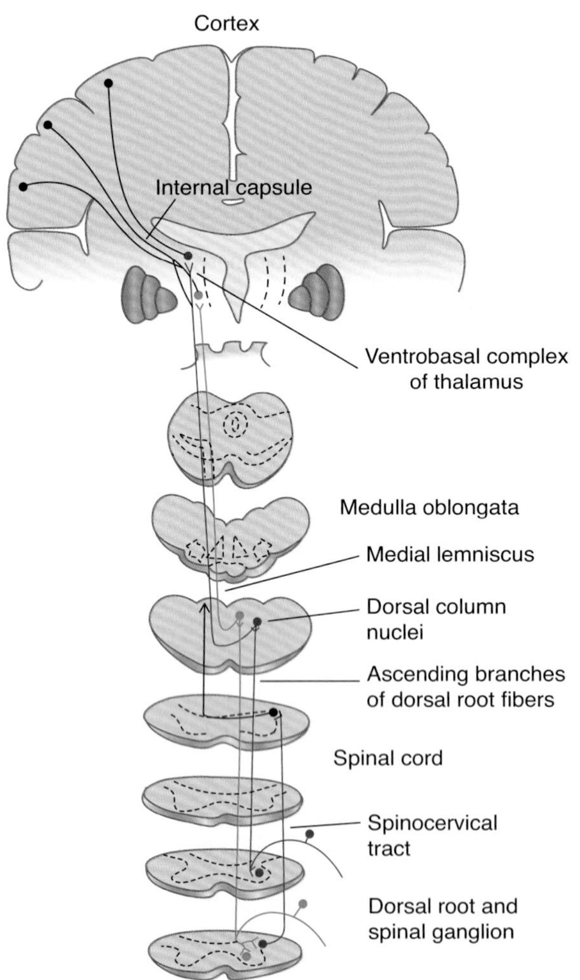

FIGURE 3-31 Sensory signals are transmitted to the brain by the dorsal column pathways and spinocervical tracts of the dorsal-lemniscal system.

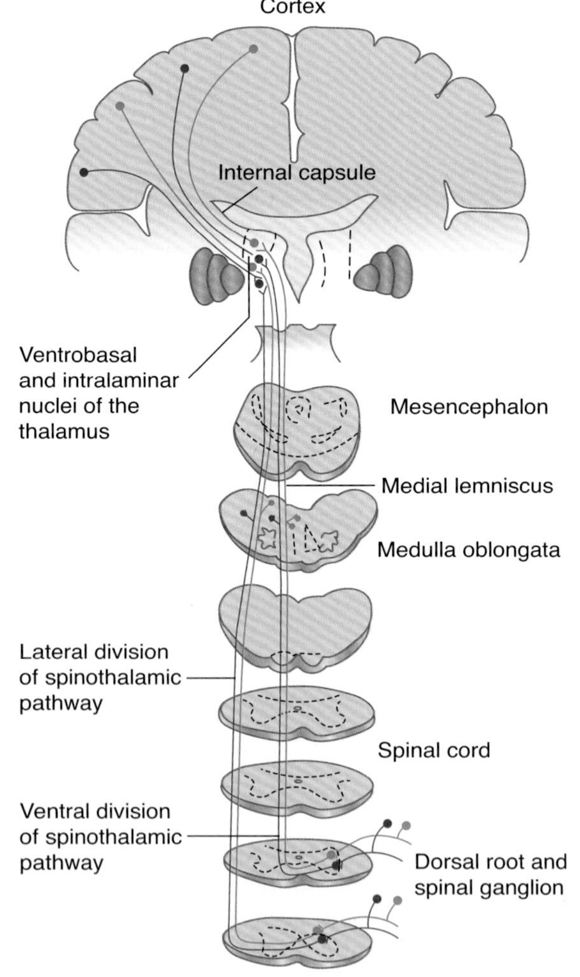

FIGURE 3-32 The anterolateral spinothalamic system fibers cross in the anterior commissure of the spinal cord before ascending to the brain. The fibers of this system transmit signals via ventral and lateral spinothalamic tracts.

Table 3-4

Responses Evoked by Autonomic Nervous System Stimulation

	Sympathetic Nervous System Stimulation	Parasympathetic Nervous System Stimulation
Heart		
Sinoatrial node	Increase heart rate	Decrease heart rate
Atrioventricular node	Increase conduction velocity	Decrease conduction velocity
His-Purkinje system	Increase automaticity, conduction velocity	Minimal effect
Ventricles	Increase contractility, conduction velocity Automaticity	Minimal effects, slight decrease in contractility (?)
Bronchial smooth muscle	Relaxation	Contraction
Gastrointestinal tract		
Motility	Decrease	Increase
Secretion	Decrease	Increase
Sphincters	Contraction	Relaxation
Gallbladder	Relaxation	Contraction
Urinary bladder		
Smooth muscle	Relaxation	Contraction
Sphincter	Contraction	Relaxation
Uterus	Contraction	Variable
Ureter	Contraction	Relaxation
Eye		
Radial muscle	Mydriasis	
Sphincter muscle		Miosis
Ciliary muscle	Relaxation for far vision	Contraction for near vision
Liver	Glycogenolysis Gluconeogenesis	Glycogen synthesis
Pancreatic β cell secretion	Decrease	
Salivary gland secretion	Increase	Marked increase
Sweat glands	Increase[a]	Increase
Apocrine glands	Increase	
Arterioles		
Coronary	Constriction (α) Relaxation (β)	Relaxation (?)
Skin and mucosa	Constriction	Relaxation
Skeletal muscle	Constriction (α) Relaxation (β)	Relaxation
Pulmonary	Constriction	Relaxation

[a]Postganglionic sympathetic fibers to sweat glands are cholinergic.

The enteric nervous system is arranged nontopographically and its neurons and cells are located in the walls of the gastrointestinal tract. Although the gastrointestinal tract is influenced by sympathetic and parasympathetic nervous system activity, it is the enteric nervous system through the myenteric and submucous plexi that regulates digestive activity even in the presence of spinal cord transection.

An understanding of the anatomy and physiology of the autonomic nervous system is required for predicting the pharmacologic effects of drugs that act on either the sympathetic or parasympathetic nervous systems (Table 3-5).

Anatomy of the Sympathetic Nervous System

Nerves of the sympathetic nervous system arise from the thoracolumbar (T1 to L2) segments of the spinal cord (Fig. 3-33).[3] These nerve fibers pass to the paravertebral sympathetic chains located lateral to the spinal cord. From the paravertebral chain, nerve fibers pass to tissues and organs innervated by the sympathetic nervous system.

Each nerve of the sympathetic nervous system consists of a preganglionic neuron and a postganglionic neuron (Fig. 3-34). Cell bodies of preganglionic neurons are

Table 3-5

Mechanism of Action of Drugs that Act on the Autonomic Nervous System

Mechanism	Site	Drug
Inhibition of neurotransmitter synthesis	Central SNS	α-Methyldopa
False neurotransmitter	Central SNS	α-Methyldopa
Inhibition of uptake of neurotransmitter	Central noradrenergic synapses	Tricyclic antidepressants, cocaine
Displacement of neurotransmitter from storage sites	Central SNS	Amphetamine
	PNS	Carbachol
Prevention of neurotransmitter release	SNS	Bretylium
	PNS	Botulinum toxin
Mimic action of neurotransmitter at receptor	SNS	
	α_1	Phenylephrine, methoxamine
	α_2	Clonidine dexmedetomidine
	β_1	Dobutamine
	β_2	Terbutaline, albuterol
Inhibition of action of neurotransmitter on post-synaptic receptor	SNS	
	α_1	Prazosin
	α_2	Yohimbine
	α_1 and α_2	Phentolamine
	β_1	Metoprolol, esmolol
	β_1 and β_2	Propranolol
	PNS	
	M_1	Pirenzepine
	M_1, M_2	Atropine
	N_1	Hexamethonium
	N_2	*d*-Tubocurarine
Inhibition of metabolism of neurotransmitter	SNS	Monoamine oxidase inhibitors
	PNS	Neostigmine, pyridostigmine, edrophonium

PNS, parasympathetic nervous system; SNS, sympathetic nervous system; N_1, ganglionic nicotinic aceylcholine receptors; N_2, muscle nicotinic receptors. Note to editor, these abbreviations are not standard.

located in the intermediolateral horn of the spinal cord. Fibers from these preganglionic cell bodies leave the spinal cord with anterior (ventral) nerve roots and pass via white rami into 1 of 22 pairs of ganglia composing the paravertebral sympathetic chain. Axons of preganglionic neurons are mostly myelinated, slow-conducting type B fibers (see Table 3-1). In the ganglia of the paravertebral sympathetic chain, the preganglionic fibers can synapse with cell bodies of postganglionic neurons or pass cephalad or caudad to synapse with postganglionic neurons (mostly unmyelinated type C fibers) in other paravertebral ganglia. Postganglionic neurons then exit from paravertebral ganglia to travel to various peripheral organs. Other postganglionic neurons return to spinal nerves by way of gray rami and subsequently travel with these nerves to influence vascular smooth muscle tone and the activity of piloerector muscles and sweat glands.

Fibers of the sympathetic nervous system are not necessarily distributed to the same part of the body as the spinal nerve fibers from the same segments. For example, fibers from T1 usually ascend in the paravertebral sympathetic chain into the head, T2 into the neck, T3–T6 into the chest, T7–T11 into the abdomen, and T12 and L1–L2 into the legs. The distribution of these sympathetic nervous system fibers to each organ is determined in part by the position in the embryo from which the organ originates. In this regard, the heart receives many sympathetic nervous system fibers from the neck portion of the paravertebral sympathetic chain because the heart originates in the neck of the embryo. Abdominal organs receive their sympathetic nervous system innervation from the lower thoracic segments, reflecting the origin of the gastrointestinal tract from this area.

Anatomy of the Parasympathetic Nervous System

Nerves of the parasympathetic nervous system leave the CNS through cranial nerves III, V, VII, IX, and X (vagus) and from the sacral portions of the spinal cord (Fig. 3-35).[3] About 75% of all parasympathetic nervous system fibers are in the vagus nerves passing to the thoracic and

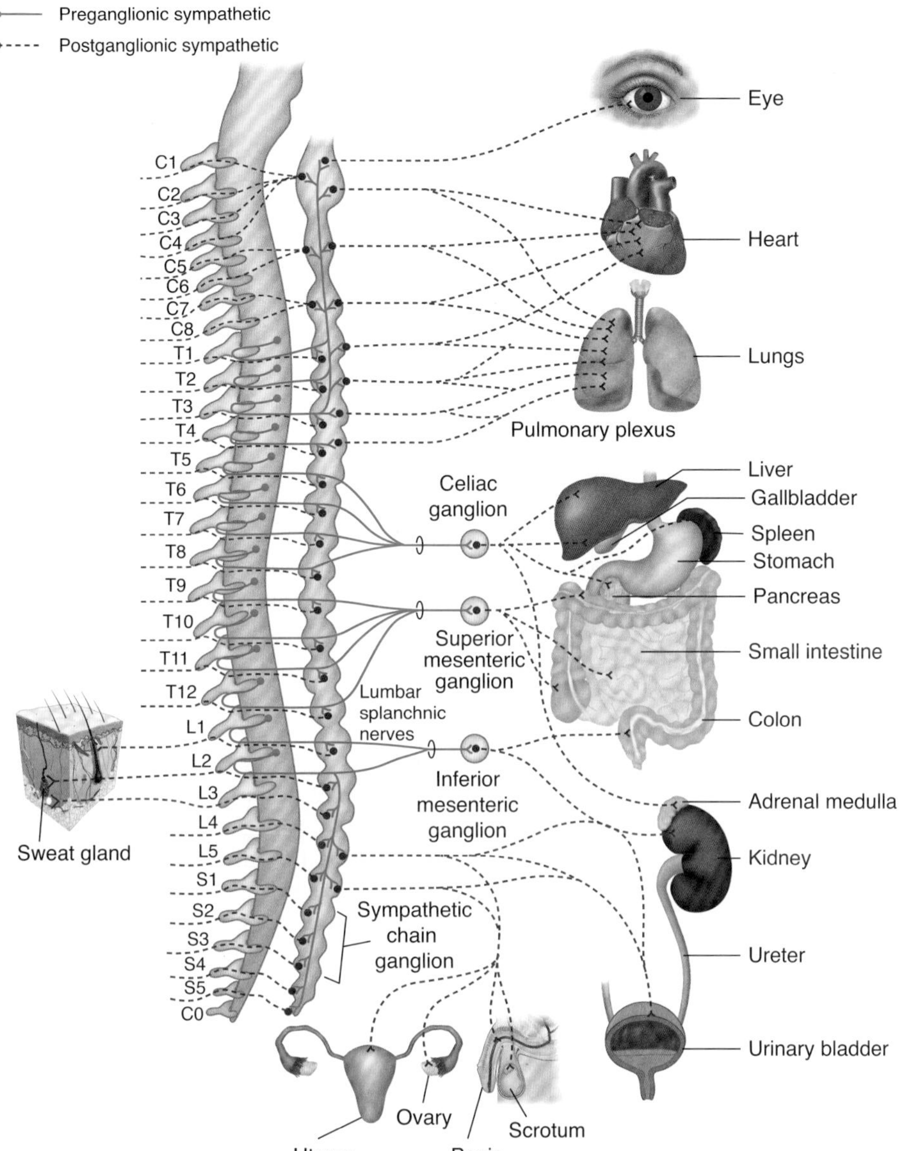

FIGURE 3-33 Anatomy of the sympathetic nervous system. Dashed lines represent postganglionic fibers in gray rami leading to spinal nerves for subsequent distribution to blood vessels and sweat glands.

abdominal regions of the body. As such, the vagus nerves supply parasympathetic innervation to the heart, lungs, esophagus, stomach, small intestine, liver, gallbladder, pancreas, and upper portions of the uterus. Fibers of the parasympathetic nervous system in cranial nerve III pass to the eye. The lacrimal, nasal, and submaxillary glands receive parasympathetic nervous system fibers via cranial nerve VII, whereas the parotid gland receives parasympathetic nervous system innervation via cranial nerve IX.

The sacral part of the parasympathetic nervous system consists of the second and third sacral nerves, and, occasionally, the first and fourth sacral nerves. Sacral nerves form the sacral plexus on each side of the spinal cord. These nerves distribute fibers to the distal colon, rectum, bladder, and lower portions of the uterus. In addition, parasympathetic nervous system fibers to the external genitalia transmit impulses that elicit various sexual responses.

In contrast to the sympathetic nervous system, preganglionic fibers of the parasympathetic nervous system pass uninterrupted to ganglia near or in the innervated organ (see Fig. 3-35).[3] Postganglionic neurons of the parasympathetic nervous system are short because of the location of the corresponding ganglia. This situation contrasts with the sympathetic nervous system, in which postganglionic neurons are relatively long, reflecting their origin in the ganglia of the paravertebral sympathetic chain, which is often distant from the innervated organ. Furthermore, unlike the amplified and diffuse discharges characteristic of sympathetic nervous system responses, activation of the parasympathetic nervous system is tonic and discrete. The vasodilatory effects of acetylcholine depend on the integrity of the vascular endothelium because activation of muscarinic receptors on the endothelium results in the release of nitric oxide.[80]

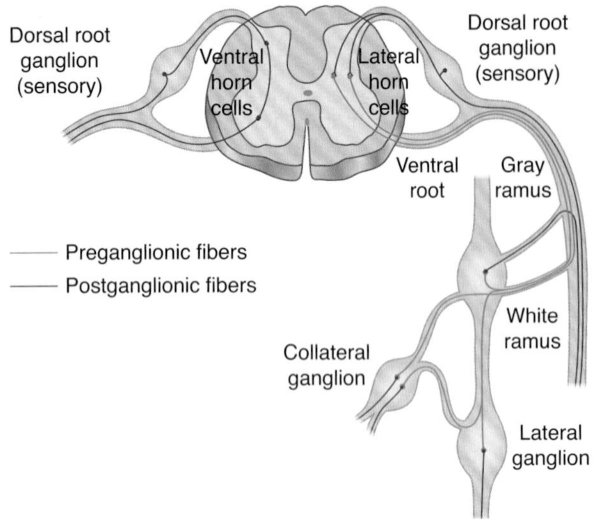

FIGURE 3-34 Anatomy of a sympathetic nervous system nerve. Preganglionic fibers pass through the white ramus to a paravertebral ganglia, where they may synapse, course up the sympathetic chain to synapse at another level, or exit the chain without synapsing to pass to an outlying collateral ganglion.

Physiology of the Autonomic Nervous System

Postganglionic fibers of the sympathetic nervous system secrete norepinephrine as the neurotransmitter (Fig. 3-36). These norepinephrine-secreting neurons are classified as ***adrenergic fibers***. Postganglionic fibers of the parasympathetic nervous system secrete acetylcholine as the neurotransmitter (see Fig. 3-36). These acetylcholine-secreting neurons are classified as ***cholinergic fibers***. In addition, innervation of sweat glands and some blood vessels is by postganglionic sympathetic nervous system fibers that release acetylcholine as the neurotransmitter. All preganglionic neurons of the sympathetic and parasympathetic nervous system release acetylcholine as the neurotransmitter and are thus classified as *cholinergic fibers*. For this reason, acetylcholine release at preganglionic fibers activates both sympathetic and parasympathetic postganglionic neurons.

Norepinephrine as a Neurotransmitter

Synthesis

Synthesis of norepinephrine involves a series of enzyme-controlled steps that begin in the cytoplasm of postganglionic sympathetic nerve endings (varicosities) and are completed in the synaptic vesicles (Fig. 3-37). For example, the initial enzyme-mediated steps leading to the formation of dopamine take place in the cytoplasm. Dopamine then enters the synaptic vesicle, where it is converted to norepinephrine by dopamine β-hydroxylase. It is likely that the enzymes that participate in the synthesis of norepinephrine are produced in postganglionic sympathetic nerve endings. These enzymes are not highly specific, and other endogenous substances, as well as certain drugs, may be acted on by the same enzyme. For example, dopa-decarboxylase can convert the antihypertensive drug α-methyldopa to α-methyldopamine, which is subsequently converted by dopamine β-hydroxylase to the weakly active (false) neurotransmitter α-methylnorepinephrine that decreases the activation of central α1-adrenergic synapses and results in the reduction of blood pressure.

Storage and Release

Norepinephrine is stored in synaptic vesicles for subsequent release in response to an action potential.[81] Adrenergic fibers can sustain output of norepinephrine during prolonged periods of stimulation. Tachyphylaxis in response to repeated administration of ephedrine and other indirect-acting sympathomimetics may reflect depletion of the norepinephrine stored in sympathetic nerve endings.

Termination of Action

Termination of the action of norepinephrine is by (a) uptake (reuptake) back into postganglionic sympathetic nerve endings, (b) dilution by diffusion from receptors, and (c) metabolism by the enzymes monoamine oxidase (MAO) and catechol-*O*-methyltransferase (COMT). Norepinephrine released in response to an action potential exerts its effects at receptors for only a brief period, reflecting the efficiency of these termination mechanisms.

Reuptake

Uptake of previously released norepinephrine back into postganglionic sympathetic nerve endings is probably the most important mechanism for terminating the action of this neurotransmitter on receptors. As much as 80% of released norepinephrine undergoes reuptake. Reuptake provides a source for reuse of norepinephrine in addition to synthesis.

It is likely that two active transport systems are involved in reuptake of norepinephrine, with one system responsible for uptake into the cytoplasm of the varicosity and a second system for passage of norepinephrine into the synaptic vesicle for storage and reuse. The active transport system for norepinephrine uptake can concentrate the neurotransmitter 10,000-fold in postganglionic sympathetic nerve endings. Magnesium and adenosine triphosphate are essential for function of the transport system necessary for the transfer of norepinephrine from the cytoplasm into the synaptic vesicle. The transport system for uptake of norepinephrine into cytoplasm is blocked by numerous drugs, including cocaine and tricyclic antidepressants.

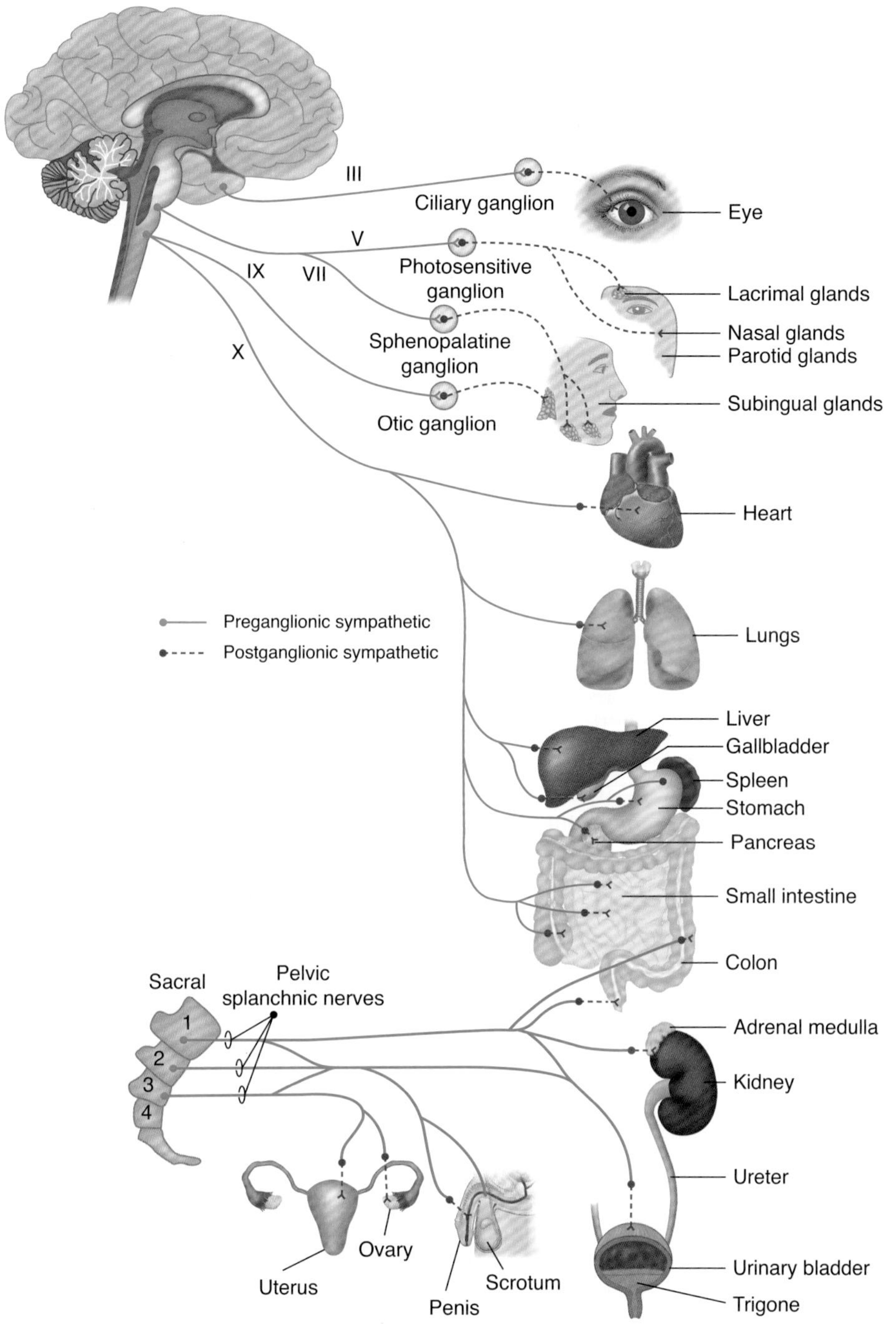

FIGURE 3-35 Anatomy of the parasympathetic nervous system.

Metabolism

Metabolism of norepinephrine is of relatively minor significance in terminating the actions of endogenously released norepinephrine. The exception may be at some blood vessels, where enzymatic breakdown and diffusion account for the termination of action of norepinephrine. Norepinephrine that undergoes uptake is vulnerable to metabolism in the cytoplasm of the varicosity by MAO. Any neurotransmitter that escapes reuptake is vulnerable to metabolism by COMT, principally in the liver. Inhibitors of MAO cause an increase in tissue levels of norepinephrine and may be accompanied by a variety of pharmacologic effects. Conversely, no striking pharmacologic change accompanies inhibition of COMT.

The primary urinary metabolite resulting from metabolism of norepinephrine by MAO or COMT is 3-methoxy-4-hydroxymandelic acid. This metabolite is also referred to as ***vanillylmandelic acid (VMA)***. Normally, the 24-hour urinary excretion of 3-methoxy-4-hydroxymandelic acid is 2 to 4 mg, representing primarily norepinephrine that is

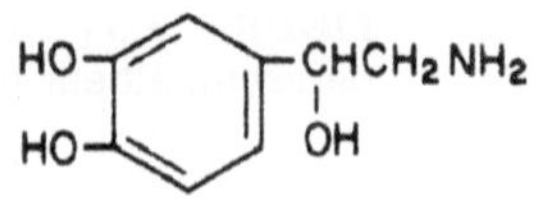

HO–C₆H₃(HO)–CHCH₂NH₂ (OH)

Norepinephrine

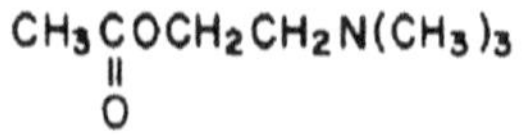

$CH_3COCH_2CH_2N(CH_3)_3$ (C=O)

Acetylcholine

FIGURE 3-36 Neurotransmitters of the autonomic nervous system.

deaminated by MAO in the cytoplasm of the varicosity of the postganglionic sympathetic nerve endings. Elevated levels of urinary VMA suggest pheochromocytoma.

Acetylcholine as a Neurotransmitter

Synthesis

Acetylcholine is synthesized in the cytoplasm of varicosities of the preganglionic and postganglionic parasympathetic nerve endings. The enzyme choline acetyltransferase is responsible for catalyzing the combination of choline with acetyl coenzyme A to form acetylcholine. Choline enters parasympathetic nerve endings from the extracellular fluid through an active transport system. Acetyl coenzyme A is synthesized in mitochondria present in high concentrations in parasympathetic nerve endings.

Tyrosine (HO–ring–CH_2CHNH_2, $COOH$)
↓ hydroxylase
DOPA (HO, HO–ring–CH_2CHNH_2, $COOH$)
↓ decarboxylase
Dopamine (HO, HO–ring–$CH_2CH_2NH_2$)
↓ dopamine beta-hydroxylase
Norepinephrine (HO, HO–ring–$CHCH_2NH_2$, OH)
↓ phenylethanolamine N-methyltransferase
Epinephrine (HO, HO–ring–$CHCH_2NH$, OH, CH_3)

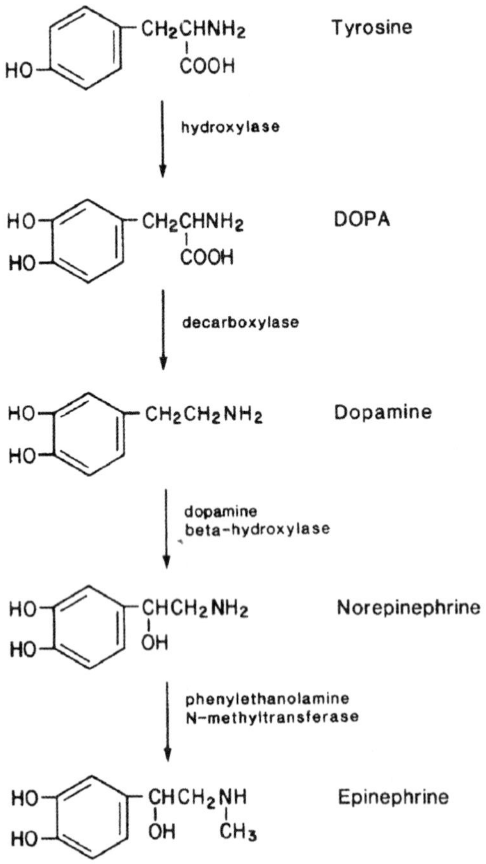

FIGURE 3-37 Steps in the enzymatic synthesis of endogenous catecholamines and neurotransmitters.

Storage and Release

Acetylcholine is stored in synaptic vesicles for release in response to an action potential. Arrival of an action potential at a parasympathetic nerve ending results in the release of 100 or more vesicles of acetylcholine. It is estimated that a single nerve ending contains >300,000 presynaptic vesicles of acetylcholine.

Metabolism

Acetylcholine has a brief effect at receptors (<1 millisecond) because of its rapid hydrolysis by acetylcholinesterase to choline and acetate. Choline is transported back into parasympathetic nerve endings, where it is used for synthesis of new acetylcholine. Plasma cholinesterase is an enzyme found in low concentrations around acetylcholine receptors, being present in the highest amounts in plasma. The physiologic significance of plasma cholinesterase is unknown, as it is too slow to be physiologically important in the metabolism of acetylcholine. Absence of plasma cholinesterase produces no detectable clinical signs or symptoms until a drug such as succinylcholine or mivacurium is administered.

Interactions of Neurotransmitters with Receptors

Norepinephrine and acetylcholine, acting as neurotransmitters, interact with receptors (protein macromolecules) in lipid cell membranes (Table 3-6). This receptor-neurotransmitter interaction most often activates or inhibits effector enzymes, such as adenylate cyclase, or alters flux of sodium and potassium ions across cell membranes via protein ion channels. The net effect of these changes is transduction of external stimuli into intracellular signals.

Norepinephrine Receptors

The pharmacologic effects of catecholamines led to the original concept of α- and β-adrenergic receptors.[82] Subdivision of these receptors into α_1, α_2, β_1 (cardiac), and β_2 (noncardiac) allows an understanding of drugs that act as either agonists or antagonists at these sites (see Table 3-5). Genetic cloning has borne out the original pharmacologic distinctions. However, there are splice variants of each gene that create receptors with different pharmacologic properties. The α_2 receptors are also present on platelets, where they mediate platelet aggregation. In the CNS, stimulation of postsynaptic α_2 receptors by drugs such as clonidine or dexmedetomidine results in enhanced potassium ion conductance and membrane hyperpolarization

Table 3-6

Classification and Characterization of Adrenergic and Cholinergic Receptors

Classification	Molecular Pharmacology	Signal Transduction	Effectors
Adrenergic receptors			
α_1	α_{1A1D}	G_{q11}	Activates phospholipase C
	α_{1B}	G_{q11}	Activates phospholipase C
	α_{1C}	G_{q11}	Activates phospholipase C
α_2	α_{2A}	G_i and G_o	Inhibits adenylate cyclase, calcium and potassium ion channels
	α_{2B}	G_i and G_o	Inhibits adenylate cyclase, calcium and potassium ion channels
	α_{2C}	G_i and G_o	Inhibits adenylate cyclase, calcium and potassium ion channels
β_1	β_1'	G_s	Stimulates adenylate cyclase and calcium ion channels
β_2	β_2'	G_s	Stimulates adenylate cyclase and calcium ion channels
β_3	β_3'	G_s	Stimulates adenylate cyclase and calcium ion channels
Cholinergic receptors			
Nicotinic	Autonomic ganglia Neuromuscular junction Central nervous system	Ion channels	
Muscarinic	M_1	G_q	Phospholipase activation
	M_3	G_q	Phospholipase activation
	M_5	G_q	Phospholipase activation
	M_2	G_1 and G_o	Inhibits adenylate cyclase
	M_4	G_1 and G_o	Inhibits adenylate cyclase

manifesting as decreased anesthetic requirements and analgesia.

Dopamine receptors were originally pharmacologically subdivided as dopamine$_1$ and dopamine$_2$. However, molecular cloning has allowed for the identification of five dopamine receptor genes. However, it is still possible to classify the dopamine receptors into D1 such as DRD1 and DRD5 and D2 such as DRD2, DRD3, and DRD4. Dopamine receptors play important roles on smooth muscle and in the kidney as well as in the CNS where they are targets of many neuropsychiatric drugs and the unwitting target of many drugs of abuse. Activation of dopamine$_1$ receptors is responsible for vasodilation of the splanchnic and renal circulations. D4 receptors are present in the human heart where there stimulation with dopamine results in an increase in contractility and intrinsic heart rate. α_2 adrenergic and dopamine$_2$ receptors function as a negative feedback loop such that their activation inhibits subsequent release of neurotransmitter (Table 3-7).

Signal Transduction

Adrenergic and dopaminergic receptors are G protein–coupled receptors. The bound receptor activates the G protein, typically resulting in activation of protein kinases and phosphorylation of target proteins. Catecholamines activate β_1-adrenergic receptors resulting in dramatic increases in intracellular cAMP through activation of G_s. Increased intracellular cAMP initiates a series of intracellular events, including cascading protein phosphorylation reactions and stimulation of the sodium-potassium pump, which results in the metabolic and pharmacologic effects typical of epinephrine and other catecholamines. In contrast to β receptors, α_1-adrenergic receptors are linked to G_q receptors which when activated increase phospholipase 3, increasing inositol trisphosphate (IP3) and liberating the release of intracellular calcium stores. The α_2-adrenergic and dopamine 2 receptors are linked to the G_i protein, activation of which decreases adenylate cyclase.

Adrenergic Receptor Concentrations

Concentrations of β-adrenergic receptors in the postsynaptic membrane adjust dynamically to the concentration of norepinephrine in the synaptic cleft and plasma. Desensitization reflects the rapid waning of responses to hormones and neurotransmitters despite continuous exposure to adrenergic agonists.[83] Downregulation is different from the rapid appearance of desensitization occurring only hours after exposure to agonists. During downregulation, receptors are destroyed and new receptors must be synthesized before a return to baseline is possible.

Table 3-7

Responses Evoked by Selective Stimulation of Adrenergic Receptors

α_1 (postsynaptic) receptors
- Vasoconstriction
- Mydriasis
- Relaxation of gastrointestinal tract
- Contraction of gastrointestinal sphincters
- Contraction of bladder sphincter

α_2 (presynaptic) receptors
- Inhibition of norepinephrine release

α_2 (postsynaptic) receptors
- Platelet aggregation
- Hyperpolarization of cells in the central nervous system

β_1 (postsynaptic) receptors
- Increased conduction velocity
- Increased automaticity
- Increased contractility

β_2 (postsynaptic) receptors
- Vasodilation
- Bronchodilation
- Gastrointestinal relaxation
- Uterine relaxation
- Bladder relaxation
- Glycogenolysis
- Lipolysis

Dopamine_1 (postsynaptic) receptors
- Vasodilation

Dopamine_2 (presynaptic) receptors
- Inhibition of norepinephrine release

Similarly, in the presence of long-term blockade, β_1 receptor numbers increase. Drug-induced alteration in adrenergic receptor number is consistent with rebound tachycardia and myocardial ischemia that may accompany sudden discontinuation of chronic β-adrenergic receptor blockers.

Chronic congestive heart failure (CHF) results in depletion of catecholamines in the myocardium and compensatory increases in plasma concentrations of norepinephrine to maintain systemic vascular resistance and perfusion pressure. Accompanying decreases in the concentrations of β_1 receptors in the heart are likely responsible for the failure of β agonists to effectively treat CHF.[84] Long-term treatment with pharmacologic doses of β-adrenergic agonists is also associated with myocardial toxicity, whereas paradoxically treating chronic CHF with judicious doses of β blockers is efficacious by upregulating β_1-adrenergic receptors.

Acetylcholine Receptors

Cholinergic receptors are classified as ***nicotinic*** and ***muscarinic***. The links between stimulus and response are different in nicotinic and muscarinic receptors (see Table 3-6). Nicotinic receptors are ligand-gated receptors, whereas muscarinic receptors are G protein linked.

Nicotinic Receptors

Acetylcholine can affect nicotinic receptors at either the neuromuscular junction, at autonomic ganglia and in the CNS. Nicotinic receptors belong to the superfamily of ligand-gated ion channels that includes GABA_A, 5-HT_3, and glycine receptors. Muscle-type nicotinic receptors are membrane proteins (two α subunits, β, ε, and δ) that form nonselective ion channels.[85] In human muscle, the γ subunit is replaced by the ε subunit within the first 2 weeks of life. This change in structure converts the receptor from one with low conductance and long duration of opening to a receptor with high conductance and brief duration of opening. In the setting of immobilization and burns, the fetal-type receptor is upregulated and expressed outside the neuromuscular junction, resulting in excessive potassium release in response to succinylcholine.

Nicotinic acetylcholine receptors in nerves are composed of 2 to 5 α subunits with or without 3 β subunits. Ten α and 3 β subunits have been cloned. The nicotinic acetylcholine receptors that act as the preganglionic receptor in the sympathetic nervous system are primarily composed of α_3 and β_4 subunits. The nicotinic receptors in the brain are mostly presynaptic where they act as a gain control on the release of glutamate, GABA, dopamine, norepinephrine, and serotonin. They are highly expressed in and around the cholinergic nuclei that mediate arousal. The α_4 β_2 combination is also highly expressed in the reward centers leading to the high addictive potential of nicotine. Activation of α_4 β_2 and α_7-type nicotinic receptors has analgesic effects in animals and humans and nicotinic ligands may serve as analgesic adjuvants.

Muscarinic Receptors

In contrast to ligand-gated nicotinic receptors, muscarinic receptors belong to the superfamily of G protein–coupled receptors and are more homologous to adrenergic receptors than to nicotinic receptors. Five muscarinic receptors have been identified. All muscarinic subtypes are expressed in the CNS but M_4 and M_5 seem to be restricted there. M_1 receptors are important in autonomic ganglia and for salivary and stomach secretion. M_2 is expressed in the heart where its activation slows heart rate and nodal activity and decreases atrial contractility. M_3 receptors are involved in smooth muscle contraction and eye accommodation. Their activation induces emesis and their antagonism with scopolamine has antiemetic properties. Atropine is a broad-spectrum muscarinic agonist.

Signal Transduction

Muscarinic receptors exhibit different signal transduction mechanisms. Odd-numbered muscarinic receptors (M_1,

M_3, and M_5) link to G_q and work predominantly through hydrolysis of phosphoinositide and release of intracellular calcium, whereas even-numbered receptors (M_2 and M_4) work primarily through G_i proteins to regulate adenylate cyclase.[86]

Residual Autonomic Nervous System Tone

The sympathetic and parasympathetic nervous systems are continually active, and this basal rate of activity is referred to as ***sympathetic*** or ***parasympathetic tone***. The value of this tone is that it permits alterations in sympathetic or parasympathetic nervous system activity to mediate a fine increase or decrease in responses at innervated organs. For example, sympathetic nervous system tone normally keeps blood vessels about 50% constricted. As a result, increased or decreased sympathetic nervous system activity produces corresponding changes in systemic vascular resistance. If sympathetic tone did not exist, the sympathetic nervous system could only cause vasoconstriction.

In addition to continual direct sympathetic nervous system stimulation, a portion of overall sympathetic tone reflects basal secretion of norepinephrine and epinephrine by the adrenal medulla. The normal resting rate of secretion of norepinephrine is about 0.05 μg/kg per minute and epinephrine is about 0.2 μg/kg per minute. These secretion rates are nearly sufficient to maintain systemic blood pressure in a normal range even if all direct sympathetic nervous system innervation to the cardiovascular system is removed.

Determination of Autonomic Nervous System Function

Autonomic dysfunction associated with aging and diabetes mellitus may increase operative risk and can be associated with increased morbidity and mortality.[87] Diagnosis of autonomic neuropathy in patients with diabetes mellitus is facilitated by tests of cardiovascular function (Table 3-8). Tests involving variability in heart rate measure activity of the sympathetic and parasympathetic nervous systems and precede changes in the measures of blood pressure. In addition to clinical tests of autonomic function, sensitive techniques for measuring plasma catecholamines are available. Interpretation of these data is

Table 3-8

Clinical Assessment of Autonomic Nervous System Function

Clinical Observation	Method of Measurement	Normal Value
Parasympathetic nervous system		
Heart rate response to Valsalva	Patient blows into a mouthpiece maintaining a pressure of 40 mm Hg for 15 s.	
	The Valsalva ratio is the ratio of the longest R-R interval on the electrocardiogram immediately after release to the shortest R-R interval during the maneuver.	Ratio >1.21
Heart rate response to standing	Heart rate is measured as the patient changes from the supine to standing position (increase maximal around 15th beat after standing and slowing maximal around 30th beat).	
	The response to standing is expressed as the "30:15" ratio and is the ratio of the longest R-R interval (around 30th beat) to the shortest R-R interval (around 15th beat).	Ratio >1.04
Heart response to deep breathing	Patient takes six deep breaths in 1 min.	
	The maximum and minimum heart rates during each cycle are measured and the mean of the differences (maximum heart rate–minimum heart rate) during three successive breathing cycles is taken as the maximum–minimum heart rate.	Mean difference >15 beats/minute
Sympathetic nervous system		
Blood pressure response to standing	The patient changes from the supine to standing position and the standing systolic blood pressure is subtracted from the supine systolic blood pressure.	Difference <10 mm Hg
Blood pressure response to sustained handgrip	The patient maintains a handgrip of 30% of maximum squeeze for up to 5 min.	Difference >16 mm Hg
	The blood pressure is measured every minute and the initial diastolic blood pressure is subtracted from the diastolic blood pressure just prior to release.	

confounded by other influences. Plasma epinephrine concentrations (normally 100 to 400 pg/mL) reflect adrenal release but vary greatly with psychological and physical stress. Plasma norepinephrine concentrations (normally 100 to 400 pg/mL) reflect both sympathetic nervous system and adrenal activity. Unlike plasma epinephrine levels, plasma norepinephrine concentrations reflect spillover from neuroeffector junctions, which may represent 10% to 20% of total release and vary among various organ systems.

Aging and Autonomic Nervous System Dysfunction

Common clinical manifestations of autonomic nervous system dysfunction in elderly patients are orthostatic hypotension, postprandial hypotension, hypothermia, and heat stroke. These responses reflect limited ability of elderly patients to adapt to stresses with vasoconstriction and vasodilation as mediated by the autonomic nervous system. Decreased autonomic nervous system function in elderly patients is due to fewer prejunctional terminals as plasma epinephrine concentrations and the numbers of β-adrenergic receptors are unchanged with aging. Plasma norepinephrine concentrations increase with age, suggesting a primary physiologic deficit in reuptake mechanisms.[88]

Clinically, there is attenuation of physiologic responses to β-adrenergic stimulation in the elderly. Exogenous β-adrenergic agonists have less profound effects on heart rate.[89] This decreased response to adrenergic stimulation seems to reflect decreased affinity (number of receptors unchanged) of β receptors for the neurotransmitter and decreases in coupling of stimulatory G proteins and adenylate cyclase units.

Diabetic Autonomic Neuropathy

Diabetic autonomic neuropathy is present in 20% to 40% of insulin-dependent diabetic patients. Common manifestations of diabetic autonomic neuropathy include impotence, diarrhea, postural hypotension, sweating abnormalities, and gastroparesis. When impotence or diarrhea is the sole manifestations of autonomic neuropathy, there is little impact on survival. Conversely, 5-year mortality rates may exceed 50% when postural hypotension or gastroparesis is present. Anesthetic risk is increased in diabetic patients with autonomic neuropathy associated with gastroparesis (aspiration hazard), postural hypotension (hemodynamic instability), and is a marker for vasculopathy in other organs including the heart.[90]

Chronic Sympathetic Nervous System Stimulation

Chronic sympathetic nervous system stimulation may increase morbidity and mortality. Pheochromocytoma is characterized by explosive release of catecholamines. Even physiologic responses and surgical stress that lead to sustained autonomic nervous system hyperactivity can result in metabolic and endocrine responses. Interventions that attenuate stress responses during the entire perioperative period (continuous epidural infusions of local anesthetics, perioperative administration of β-adrenergic blocking drugs, α_2 agonists) may decrease perioperative morbidity and mortality.[91–93] Inhaled anesthetics and adjuvants that block the stress response may also be beneficial in long-term outcomes following surgery.[94]

Acute Denervation

Acute removal of sympathetic nervous system tone, as produced by a regional anesthetic or spinal cord transection, results in immediate maximal vasodilation of blood vessels (spinal shock). In the anesthetic setting, this is transient and can be treated with fluid or α vasoconstrictors. In the chronic setting, over several days, intrinsic tone of vascular smooth muscle increases, usually restoring almost normal vasoconstriction.

Denervation Hypersensitivity

Denervation hypersensitivity is the increased responsiveness (decreased threshold) of the innervated organ to norepinephrine or epinephrine that develops during the first week or so after acute interruption of autonomic nervous system innervation. The presumed mechanism for denervation hypersensitivity is the proliferation of receptors (upregulation) on postsynaptic membranes that occurs when norepinephrine or acetylcholine is no longer released at synapses. As a result, more receptor sites become available to produce an exaggerated response when circulating neurotransmitter does become available.

Adrenal Medulla

The adrenal medulla is innervated by preganglionic fibers that bypass the sympathetic chain. As a result, these fibers pass directly from the spinal cord to the adrenal medulla. Cells of the adrenal medulla are derived embryologically from neural tissue and are analogous to postganglionic sympathetic neurons. Stimulation of the sympathetic nervous system causes release of epinephrine (80%) and norepinephrine from the adrenal medulla. As such, epinephrine and norepinephrine, released by the adrenal medulla into the blood, function as hormones and not as neurotransmitters.

Synthesis

In the adrenal medulla, most of the synthesized norepinephrine is converted to epinephrine by the action of phenylethanolamine-*N*-methyltransferase (see Fig. 3-37). Activity of this enzyme is enhanced by cortisol, which is carried by the intraadrenal portal vascular system directly to the adrenal medulla. For this reason, any stress that releases glucocorticoids also results in increased synthesis and release of epinephrine.

Release

The triggering event in the release of epinephrine and norepinephrine from the adrenal medulla is the liberation of acetylcholine by preganglionic cholinergic fibers. Acetylcholine acts on α_3 and β_4 subunit containing nicotinic receptors, resulting in a change in permeability (localized depolarization) that permits entry of sodium, potassium, and calcium ions through extracellular nicotinic acetylcholine channels. Calcium ions result in extrusion, by exocytosis, of synaptic vesicles containing epinephrine.

Norepinephrine and epinephrine released from the adrenal medulla evoke responses similar to direct stimulation of the sympathetic nervous system. The difference, however, is that effects are greatly prolonged (10 to 30 seconds) compared with the brief duration of action on receptors that is produced by norepinephrine released as a neurotransmitter from postganglionic sympathetic nerve endings. The prolonged effect of circulating epinephrine and norepinephrine released by the adrenal medulla reflects the time necessary for metabolism of these substances by COMT and MAO.

Circulating norepinephrine from the adrenal medulla causes vasoconstriction of blood vessels, inhibition of the gastrointestinal tract, increased cardiac activity, and dilation of the pupils (see Table 3-4). The effects of circulating epinephrine differ from those of norepinephrine in that the cardiac and metabolic effects of epinephrine are greater, whereas relaxation of blood vessels in skeletal muscles reflects a predominance of β over α effects at low concentrations of epinephrine. Circulating norepinephrine and epinephrine released by the adrenal medulla and acting as hormones can substitute for sympathetic nervous system innervation of an organ. Another important role of the adrenal medulla is the ability of circulating norepinephrine and epinephrine to stimulate areas of the body that are not directly innervated by the sympathetic nervous system. For example, the metabolic rate of all cells can be influenced by hormones released from the adrenal medulla, even though these cells are not directly innervated by the sympathetic nervous system.

Thermoregulation

Body temperature is determined by the relationship between heat production and heat dissipation. Heat is continually being produced in the body as a product of metabolism. As heat is produced, it is also continuously being lost to the environment. Mammals are homeotherms. Both heat generation and heat loss are adjusted in order to regulate body temperature within narrow limits. Normal core body temperatures range from about 36°C to 37.5°C and undergo circadian fluctuations, being lowest in the morning and highest in the evening. This is consistent with a 10% to 15% decrease in basal metabolic rate during physiologic sleep, presumably reflecting decreased activity of skeletal muscles and the sympathetic nervous system. An estimated 55% of the energy in nutrients is converted to heat during the formation of adenosine triphosphate. The average daily caloric requirement for basal function is approximately 2,000 calories.

Heat Loss

The important mechanisms of heat loss from the body include radiation, conduction, convection, and evaporation. Their relative contributions vary, and depend upon the environmental circumstances.[95] The skin is the most important route for heat dissipation, whereas the lungs account for only about 10% of heat loss. Under typical circumstances, most heat (about 60%) is lost by radiation. A warm object emits energy in the form of radiation, predominantly in the infrared range, independent of ambient air temperature. The unclothed human is an excellent source of radiant heat. Significant radiant losses can occur from the unclothed patient in the operating room. In infant incubators, radiant heat losses occur from the exposed infant. Radiant heat loss is countered by heating the surrounding surfaces, so that radiant heat loss is offset by the absorption of radiant heat from nearby surfaces. Radiant heat loss is also countered by blankets, which absorb and then return radiant heat. The extreme example is the "space blanket" which directly reflects infrared radiation back toward the patient.

Conduction of heat from the body occurs by direct contact with a cooler object; for example, between the patient and cold air or an adjacent mattress. The area of the conducting surfaces, the temperature difference, and the heat capacity affect conductive heat transfer. Conductive loss to still air is limited because a stationary layer of air next to the skin acts as a good insulator. Air has a very low heat capacity and warms quickly, thus promptly eliminating the temperature gradient. In humans, piloerection reduces heat loss by trapping a layer of air next to the skin.

Although pure conduction accounts for <5% of heat loss, conductive heat loss to air is greatly facilitated by air movement and is termed ***convection*** or ***facilitated conduction***. Thus, a fan is comfortable on a hot summer day because it facilitates heat loss. The rate of convective loss depends on both the air temperature and its velocity (the "wind-chill" phenomenon). Convection accounts for approximately 15% to 30% of heat loss in the operating room, but increases significantly in high wind-chill environments such as a laminar flow unit. However, significant convective heat loss occurs even in a draft-free environment because warmed air rises to be replaced by denser cold air, thus maintaining cutaneous airflow.

Evaporative heat losses are important because significant energy is required to vaporize water. Evaporation from the skin accounts for about 20% of total heat loss. The magnitude of evaporative loss depends on environmental humidity, exposed skin surface area, presence of diaphoresis, wound and bowel exposure, and application of fluid to the skin (prep solutions). Evaporation is the only mechanisms by which the body can eliminate excess heat when the temperature of the surroundings is higher than that of the skin. Diaphoresis occurs in response to stimulation of the preoptic area of the hypothalamus. A normal individual has a maximal sweat production of about 700 mL per hour. With continued exposure to a warm environment, sweat production may increase to 1,500 mL per hour. Evaporation of this amount of sweat can remove heat from the body at a rate of >10 times the normal basal rate of heat production. Evaporation accounts for two-thirds of the heat loss from the respiratory tract. Evaporative heat and fluid loss is an important consideration during surgery in which large segments of moist bowel are exposed for evaporation.

Reductions in core temperature also follow infusions of cold intravenous fluids and blood products.

Regulation of Body Temperature

Body temperature is regulated by feedback mechanisms predominantly mediated by the preoptic nucleus of the anterior hypothalamus,[96] which integrates afferent input from thermoreceptors in the skin, deep tissues, and spinal cord. Afferent thermoregulatory input is modulated in the brainstem and spinal cord before arrival in the hypothalamus. Heat-sensitive neurons in the preoptic nucleus receive additional thermal input from extrahypothalamic areas of the brain. Reflex responses to cold (vasoconstriction, piloerection, shivering, and nonshivering thermogenesis) originate in the posterior hypothalamus. Reflex responses to heat (vasodilation, sweating) originate in the anterior hypothalamus.

The hypothalamic thermostat detects body temperature changes and initiates autonomic, somatic, and endocrine thermoresponses when the various set points are reached. However, in the awake individual, behavioral responses (putting on a jacket) usually occur before the core temperature reaches the set points. If the behavioral response to hypothermia fails or is abolished by anesthesia, the hypothalamic thermostat stimulates vasoconstriction at 36.5°C and shivering at 36.2°C. As a result, the rate of heat transfer to the skin is decreased, heat product rises from shivering, and body temperature increases.

There is a narrow range of normal core temperature, 36.7°C to 37.1°C, within which thermoregulatory responses are not triggered. General anesthesia abolishes much of the ability to regulate temperature through drug-induced vasodilation and muscle relaxation. Maintenance of body temperature at a value close to the optimum for enzyme activity assures a constant rate of metabolism, optimal enzyme function, nervous system conduction, and skeletal muscle contraction. Even modest hypothermia (<36°C) reduces the drug metabolism, delaying emergence from anesthesia. Hyperthermia is even less well tolerated, as protein denaturation begins at about 42°C.

Nonshivering Thermogenesis

Nonshivering thermogenesis (alternatively called ***chemical thermogenesis***) is an increase in the rate of cellular metabolism in brown adipose tissue evoked by sympathetic nervous system stimulation or by circulating catecholamines. In adults, who have almost no brown fat, it is rare that chemical thermogenesis increases the rate of heat production by >15%. In infants, however, chemical thermogenesis in brown fat located in the interscapular space and around the great vessels in the thorax and abdomen can increase the rate of heat production by as much as 200%. In contrast to other fat depots, brown fat contains large numbers of mitochondria and has extensive sympathetic innervation. Within these mitochondria, the generation of adenosine triphosphate is uncoupled as oxidative phosphorylation is short-circuited to generate heat. This process is dependent on an uncoupling protein (UCP 1). Lipolysis and heat generation in brown fat is mediated via β-adrenergic receptors.

Shivering

Skeletal muscle activity is a major source of heat. Shivering increases body heat production in response to decreased core temperature. The posterior hypothalamic area responsible for the response to hypothermia controls reflex shivering. Shivering occurs due to both increased motor traffic via anterior motor neurons and to upregulation of the muscle stretch reflex. However, shivering is inefficient and induces significant metabolic demand. Awake patients find shivering intensely unpleasant.

Causes of Increased Body Temperature

A variety of disorders can increase body temperature. Those disorders resulting from thermoregulatory failure (excessive metabolic production of heat, excessive environmental heat, and impaired heat dissipation) are properly characterized as ***hyperthermia***, whereas those resulting from intact homeostatic responses are categorized as ***fever*** (Table 3-9).[96]

In hyperthermic states, the hypothalamic set point is normal but peripheral mechanisms are unable to maintain body temperature that matches the set point. In contrast, fever occurs when the hypothalamic set point is increased by the action of circulating pyrogenic cytokines, causing intact peripheral mechanisms to conserve and generate heat until the body temperature increases to the elevated set point. Despite their physiologic differences, hyperthermia and fever cannot be differentiated clinically based on the height of the temperature or its pattern. However, the clinical management of hyperthermia and fever are very different. The treatment of hyperthermia should be directed at promoting heat dissipation and terminating excessive heat production (e.g., administration of dantrolene for malignant hyperthermia), whereas the treatment of fever should be directed at identification and eradication of pyrogens and lowering the thermoregulatory set point

Table 3-9

Causes of Hyperthermia

- Disorders associated with excessive heat production
  - Malignant hyperthermia
  - Neuroleptic malignant syndrome
  - Thyrotoxicosis
  - Delirium tremens
  - Pheochromocytoma
  - Salicylate intoxication
  - Drug abuse (cocaine, amphetamine, MDMA)
  - Status epilepticus
  - Exertional hyperthermia
- Disorders associated with decreased heat loss
  - Autonomic nervous system dysfunction
  - Anticholinergics
  - Drug abuse (cocaine)
  - Dehydration
  - Occlusive dressings
  - Heat stroke
- Disorders associated with dysfunction of the hypothalamus
  - Trauma
  - Tumors
  - Idiopathic hypothalamic dysfunction
  - Cerebrovascular accidents
  - Encephalitis
  - Neuroleptic malignant syndrome

with antipyretic drugs such as aspirin, acetaminophen, and cyclooxygenase inhibitors.

Fever

Pyrogens are bacterial and viral toxins that indirectly cause the set point of the hypothalamic thermostat to increase. Bacterial pyrogens stimulate host inflammatory cells (mononuclear phagocytes) to generate endogenous pyrogens, including interleukins, prostaglandins, and tumor necrosis factor. Viruses do not release pyrogens directly, but stimulate infected cells to release interferons α and β that act as endogenous pyrogens. All known endogenous pyrogens are polypeptides and are therefore unlikely to cross the blood–brain barrier. However, endogenous pyrogens have actions in the organum vasculosum of the lamina terminalis (OVLT), which is a structure adjacent to the lateral ventricles that lies outside the blood–brain barrier. It is likely that endogenous pyrogens acting in the OVLT evoke the release of prostaglandins in the CNS, leading to stimulation of the preoptic nucleus and generation of the febrile response.[68]

Chills

Sudden resetting of the hypothalamic thermostat to a higher level because of tissue destruction, pyrogens, or dehydration, results in a lag between blood temperature and the new hypothalamic set point. During this period, the person experiences chills and feels cold even though body temperature may be increased. The skin is cold because of cutaneous vasoconstriction. Chills continue until the body temperature increases to the new set point of the hypothalamic thermostat. As long as the process causing the hypothalamic thermostat to be set at a higher level is present, the body's core temperature will remain increased above normal. Sudden removal of the factor that is causing the body temperature to remain increased is accompanied by intense diaphoresis and feeling of warmth because of generalized cutaneous vasodilation.

Cutaneous Blood Flow

Cutaneous blood flow is a major determinant of heat loss. The cutaneous circulation is among the most variable in the body, reflecting its primary role in regulation of body temperature in response to alterations in the rate of metabolism and the temperature of the external surroundings. The skin's metabolic needs are so low that the typical cutaneous blood flow is about 10 times higher than needed to supply nutritive needs of the skin.

Cutaneous blood flow is largely regulated by the sympathetic nervous system. Vascular structures concerned with heat loss from skin consist of subcutaneous venous plexuses that can hold large quantities of blood. The cutaneous circulation of the fingers, palms, toes, and earlobes has richly innervated arteriovenous anastomoses that facilitate significant heat loss. In an adult, typical total cutaneous blood flow is about 400 mL per minute. This flow can decrease to as little as 50 mL per minute in severe cold and may increase to as much as 2,800 mL per minute in extreme heat. Patients with borderline cardiac function may become symptomatic in hot environments as the heart attempts to supply increased blood flow to the skin. During acute hemorrhage, the sympathetic nervous system can produce sufficient cutaneous vasoconstriction to transfer large amounts of blood into the central circulation. As such, the cutaneous veins act as an important blood reservoir that can supply 5% to 10% of the blood volume in times of need. Acute hemorrhage may be less well tolerated in a warm environment because the hypothalamic vasodilator response may override the vasoconstrictor response to hypovolemia. Inhaled anesthetics increase cutaneous blood flow, perhaps by inhibiting the temperature-regulating center of the hypothalamus.[97]

Skin Color

Skin color in light-skinned individuals with little melanin expression is principally due to the color of blood in the cutaneous capillaries and veins. The skin has a pinkish hue when arterial blood is flowing rapidly through these tissues. Conversely, when the skin is cold and blood is flowing slowly, the removal of oxygen for nutritive purposes gives the skin the bluish hue (cyanosis) of deoxygenated blood. Severe vasoconstriction of the skin forces most of this blood into the central circulation, and skin takes on the whitish hue (pallor) of underlying connective tissue, which is composed primarily of collagen fibers.

Perioperative Temperature Changes

The thermoregulatory system contains three key elements: afferent input, central processing, and the efferent response. General anesthesia affects all three elements and regional anesthesia affects both the afferent and efferent components. Thus, anesthesia and surgery in a cool environment makes perioperative hypothermia a likely occurrence (Table 3-10).[98,99] General and regional anesthesia increase the interthreshold range to 4.0°C, approximately 20 times the normal range. Typically, the threshold for sweating and vasodilation is increased about 1°C, and the threshold for vasoconstriction and shivering is decreased about 3°C. As a result, anesthetized patients are relatively poikilothermic, with body temperatures determined by the environment. Anesthetics inhibit thermoregulation in a dose-dependent manner and inhibit vasoconstriction and shivering about three times as much as they restrict sweating (Fig. 3-38).[100]

Alfentanil and propofol similarly lower the threshold for vasoconstriction and sweating. Volatile anesthetics such as isoflurane and desflurane decrease the threshold temperatures for cold responses in a nonlinear fashion. Nonshivering thermogenesis does not occur during general anesthesia in adults or infants.

Table 3-10

Events that Contribute to Decreases in Body Temperature during Surgery

Resetting of the hypothalamic thermostat
Ambient temperature <21°C
Administration of unwarmed intravenous fluids
Drug-induced vasodilation
Basal metabolic rate decreased
Attenuated shivering response
Core compartment exposed to ambient temperature
Heat required to humidify inhaled dry gases

Sequence of Temperature Changes during Anesthesia

In the awake individual, body heat is unevenly distributed. Tonic thermoregulatory vasoconstriction maintains a temperature gradient between the core and periphery of 2°C to 4°C. The core compartment, which is insulated from the environment by the peripheral compartment, consists of the major viscera and includes the head, chest, abdomen, and pelvis. Under general anesthesia, tonic vasoconstriction is attenuated and heat contained in the core compartment will move to the periphery, thus allowing the core temperature to decrease toward the anesthetic-induced lowered threshold for vasoconstriction. This core

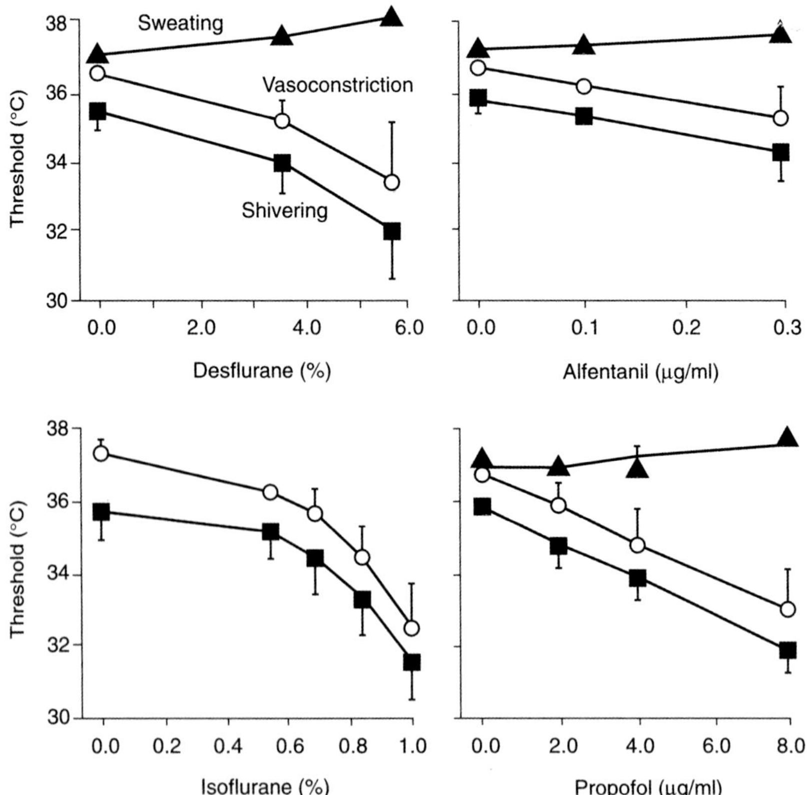

FIGURE 3-38 Changes in the thermoregulatory threshold for sweating, vasoconstriction, and shivering in the presence of increasing concentrations of inhaled or injected anesthetics. (From Sessler DI. Mild perioperative hypothermia. *N Engl J Med.* 1997;336:1630–1637, with permission.)

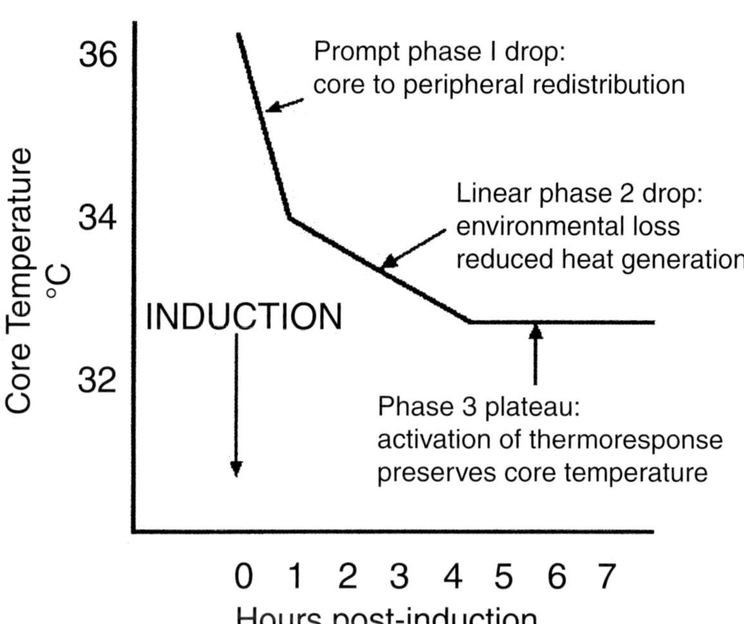

FIGURE 3-39 Graphic representation of the typical triphasic core temperature pattern that occurs after induction of anesthesia. Note that the phase 3 plateau may not occur, particularly during regional anesthesia or during combined regional and general anesthesia. Although core temperature is preserved during the phase 3 plateau, heat will continue to be lost to the environment from the peripheral compartment.

to peripheral heat redistribution is responsible for the 1°C to 5°C decrease in core temperature that occurs during the first hour of general anesthesia (Fig. 3-39). For this reason, protection from heat loss early in a surgical procedure is important to reduce the temperature gradient from the environment to the peripheral compartment as significant heat energy has been shunted to the periphery.

After the first hour of general anesthesia, the core temperature usually decreases at a slower rate. This decrease is nearly linear and occurs because continuing heat loss to the environment exceeds the metabolic production of heat. After 3 to 5 hours of anesthesia, the core temperature often stops decreasing (see Fig. 3-39). This thermal plateau may reflect a steady state in which heat loss equals heat production. This type of thermal steady state is especially likely in patients who are well insulated or effectively warmed. However, if a patient becomes sufficiently hypothermic, activation of thermoregulatory vasoconstriction will occur, decreasing cutaneous heat loss and retaining heat in the core compartment. Intraoperative vasoconstriction thus reestablishes the normal core-to-periphery temperature gradient by preventing the loss of centrally generated metabolic heat to peripheral tissues. Although vasoconstriction may effectively maintain the core temperature plateau, mean body temperature and the total heat content of the body continue to decrease as continued loss of heat occurs from the peripheral compartment to the environment. Because reflex vasoconstriction is usually effective in maintaining core temperature, the intraoperative core temperature rarely decreases the additional 1°C necessary to trigger shivering during general anesthesia.[99]

Although regional anesthesia is thought to have minimal effect upon the central processing and integration of the thermoregulatory response, afferent cold input from the lower body may be overridden by a sense of warmth from cutaneous vasodilation. Decreases in core temperature of a similar or greater magnitude to those experienced during general anesthesia may occur during spinal or epidural techniques despite the sensation of warmth. The initial redistributive temperature drop may be less precipitous during regional anesthesia because vasodilation is restricted to the blocked area. However, because reflex vasoconstriction is abolished below the level of the block, the plateau phase seen during general anesthesia may not occur during regional anesthesia (see Fig. 3-39). Indeed, core temperature may decrease sufficiently during regional anesthesia to trigger the shivering response. However, the ability of reflex shivering to generate heat is markedly attenuated because it is restricted to the unblocked upper body. The risk of significant core hypothermia during regional anesthesia strongly supports the routine use of temperature monitoring. Combined general and regional anesthetic techniques predispose the patient to a greater degree of heat loss than either technique used alone.

Beneficial Effects of Perioperative Hypothermia

Oxygen consumption is decreased by approximately 5% to 7% per degree Celsius of cooling. Thus even moderate decreases in core temperature of 1°C to 3°C below normal provide substantial protection against cerebral ischemia and arterial hypoxemia. Indeed, induced hypothermia to 28°C, as used during cardiopulmonary bypass, will reduce cerebral metabolic rate by 50%. Mild hypothermia (33°C to 36°C) may be recommended during operations likely to be associated with cerebral ischemia such as carotid endarterectomy, aneurysm clipping, and cardiac surgery.

Operations involving aortic cross-clamping can jeopardize spinal cord perfusion and may also benefit from the increased margin of safety afforded by mild hypothermia. Mild hypothermia also slows the triggering of malignant hyperthermia.[101] Outside the operating room, there has been renewed interest in mild hypothermia during the resuscitation of survivors of cardiac arrest, stroke, traumatic brain injury, acute myocardial infarction, and birth injury,[102,103] although recent large trials suggest that the hypothermia is less protective than thought.[104,105] The main benefit of mild hypothermia accrues from a reduction in metabolic demand. Typical approaches to achieve mild hypothermia often include surface cooling. However, surface cooling may induce shivering, which will delay core cooling.

Adverse Consequences of Perioperative Hypothermia

Perioperative hypothermia may predispose to several significant complications (Table 3-11). These include postoperative shivering (significantly increasing metabolic rate and cardiac work) and impaired coagulation (impaired platelet function, decreased activation of the coagulation cascade). Indeed, hypothermia-induced coagulopathy is associated with increased transfusion requirements. A 1°C decrease in temperature is associated with a 5% reduction in anesthetic requirements (MAC) and an increase in volatile anesthetic blood/gas solubility. Drug metabolism is decreased by hypothermia, particularly that of nondepolarizing neuromuscular-blocking drugs. These factors all conspire to delay emergence from anesthesia and delay recovery room discharge. Hypothermia also impairs wound healing and is associated with decreased resistance to surgical wound infection.[100] The underlying mechanism is thought to be hypothermia-induced vasoconstriction, which decreases wound perfusion and local tissue oxygen partial pressure. Perioperative hypothermia is also associated with delayed hospital discharge and an increased catabolic state. Shivering occurs in approximately 40% of unwarmed patients who are recovering from general anesthesia and is associated with substantial sympathetic nervous system activation and discomfort from the sensation of cold. Core hypothermia equal to a 1.5°C decrease triples the incidence of ventricular tachycardia and morbid cardiac events.[106]

Perioperative Temperature Measurement

The significant adverse physiologic effects of changes in body temperature are a compelling reason to monitor body temperature during anesthesia. Unless hypothermia is specifically indicated, as for protection against tissue ischemia, it is recommended that intraoperative core temperature be maintained at ≥36°C.[100] Measuring the temperature of the lower 25% of the esophagus (about 24 cm beyond the corniculate cartilages or site of the loudest heart sounds heard through an esophageal stethoscope) gives a reliable approximation of blood and cerebral temperature. Readings elsewhere in the esophagus are more likely to be influenced by the temperature of inhaled gases. A nasopharyngeal temperature probe positioned behind the soft palate gives a less reliable measure of cerebral temperature than a correctly positioned esophageal probe. Leakage of gases around the tracheal tube may also influence nasopharyngeal temperature measurements. Heat-producing bacteria in the gastrointestinal tract, cold blood returning from the lower limbs, and insulation of the probe by feces, can all influence rectal temperature. Bladder temperature is also subject to a prolonged response time, particularly if urine flow is <270 mL per hour.[107] Tympanic membrane and aural canal temperatures provide a rapidly responsive and accurate estimate of hypothalamic temperature and correlate well with esophageal temperature. Potential damage to the tympanic membrane has limited the acceptance of tympanic membrane probes. However, infrared thermometers allow atraumatic measurement of tympanic temperature. However, the accuracy of individual infrared thermometers is dependent on instrumental design and positioning. Thermistors in pulmonary artery catheters provide the best continuous estimate of body temperature but are invasive. Skin temperature gives no information other than the temperature of that area of the skin.

Table 3-11

Immediate Adverse Consequences of Perioperative Hypothermia

Adverse Outcome	Mechanism
Increased operative blood loss	Coagulopathy and platelet dysfunction
Increased morbid cardiac events	Increased myocardial work load
Dysrhythmias and myocardial ischemia	Increased sympathetic activity
Wound infection	Sympathetic mediated cutaneous vasoconstriction
Delayed wound healing	Decreased drug metabolism and increased volatile agent solubility, decreased MAC
Delayed anesthetic emergence	
Delayed recovery room discharge	Postanesthetic shivering, delayed recovery

Prevention of Perioperative Hypothermia

Passive or active airway heating and humidification contribute little to perioperative thermal management in adults because <10% of metabolic heat is lost via ventilation.[100] Each liter of intravenous fluid at ambient temperature that is infused into adult patients, or each unit of blood at 4°C decreases the mean core body temperature about 0.25°C. In this regard, the administration of unwarmed fluids can markedly decrease body temperature. Warming fluids to near 37°C is useful for preventing hypothermia, especially if large volumes of fluid are being infused.

The skin is the predominant source of heat loss during anesthesia and surgery, although evaporation from large surgical incisions may also be important. A high ambient temperature maintains normothermia in anesthetized patients, but temperatures of >25°C are uncomfortable for operating room personnel.

Covering the skin with surgical drapes or blankets can decrease cutaneous heat loss. A single layer of insulator decreases heat loss by approximately 30%, but additional layers do not proportionately increase the benefit.[108] For this reason, active warming is needed to prevent intraoperative hypothermia. Forced-air warming is probably the most effective method available, although any method or combination of methods that maintains core body temperature near 36°C is acceptable (Fig. 3-40).[100] Circulating warm water mattresses are generally ineffective because cutaneous blood flow to the back is limited in the supine position. Patients undergoing minor operations in a warm environment may not require active warming, whereas forced-air warming, alone or combined with fluid warming, is helpful for maintaining normal intraoperative core temperature in most other instances.

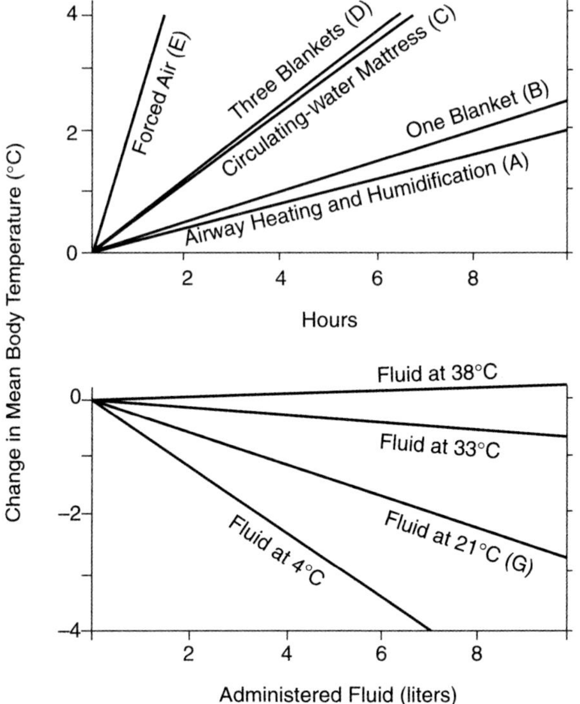

FIGURE 3-40 The effects of different warming techniques on mean body temperature plotted according to the elapsed hours of treatment *(top)* and changes in mean body temperature according to the volume of fluid administered *(bottom)*. (From Sessler DI. Mild perioperative hypothermia. *N Engl J Med.* 1997;336:1630–1637, with permission.)

References

1. Alkire MT, Hudetz AG, Tononi G. Consciousness and anesthesia. *Science.* 2008;322:876–880.
2. Hartline DK, Colman DR. Rapid conduction and the evolution of giant axons and myelinated fibers. *Curr Biol.* 2007;17:R29–R35.
3. Guyton AC, Hall JE. *Textbook of Medical Physiology.* 10th ed. Philadelphia, PA: Saunders; 2000.
4. Perreault L, Drolet P, Farny J. Ulnar nerve palsy at the elbow after general anaesthesia. *Can J Anaesth.* 1992;39:499–503.
5. Berne RM, Levy MN, Koeppen BM, et al. *Physiology.* 5th ed. St. Louis, MO: Mosby; 2004.
6. Ackerman MJ, Clapham DE. Ion channels-basic science and clinical disease. *N Engl J Med.* 1997;336:1575–1586.
7. Zecharia AY, Nelson LE, Gent TC, et al. The involvement of hypothalamic sleep pathways in general anesthesia: testing the hypothesis using the GABAA receptor beta3N265M knock-in mouse. *J Neurosci.* 2009;29:2177–2187.
8. Hudspith MJ. Glutamate: a role in normal brain function, anaesthesia, analgesia and CNS injury. *Br J Anaesth.* 1997;78:731–747.
9. Sonner JM. A hypothesis on the origin and evolution of the response to inhaled anesthetics. *Anesth Analg.* 2008;107:849–854.
10. Gelman AC. G proteins: transducers of receptor-generated signals. *Annu Rev Biochem.* 1987;56:615–649.
11. Maze M. Transmembrane signaling and the Holy Grail of anesthesia. *Anesthesiology.* 1990;72:959–961.
12. Schwinn DA. Adrenoceptors as models for G protein-coupled receptors: structure, function, and regulation. *Br J Anaesth.* 1993;71:77–85.
13. Doyle GA, Sheng XR, Lin SS, et al. Identification of five mouse mu-opioid receptor (MOR) gene (Oprm1) splice variants containing a newly identified alternatively spliced exon. *Gene.* 2007;395:98–107.
14. Ward CW, Lawrence MC. Ligand-induced activation of the insulin receptor: a multi-step process involving structural changes in both the ligand and the receptor. *Bioessays.* 2009;31:422–434.
15. Bourne HR. How receptors talk to trimeric G proteins. *Curr Opin Cell Biol.* 1997;9:134–142.
16. Nelson LE, Lu J, Guo T, et al. The alpha2-adrenoceptor agonist dexmedetomidine converges on an endogenous sleep-promoting pathway to exert its sedative effects. *Anesthesiology.* 2003;98:428–436.
17. Flood P, Ramirez-Latorre J, Role L. alpha 4 beta 2 Neuronal nicotinic acetylcholine receptors in the central nervous system are potently inhibited by both isoflurane and propofol: alpha 7 Type nAChRs are unaffected. *Anesthesiology.* 1997;86:859–865.
18. Violet JM, Downie DL, Nakisa RC, et al. Differential sensitivities of mammalian neuronal and muscle nicotinic acetylcholine receptors to general anesthetics. *Anesthesiology.* 1997;86:866–874.
19. Evers AS, Steinbach JH. Supersensitive sites in the central nervous system. Anesthetics block brain nicotinic receptors. *Anesthesiology.* 1997;86:760–762.
20. Alkire MT, McReynolds JR, Hahn EL, et al. Thalamic microinjection of nicotine reverses sevoflurane-induced loss of righting reflex in the rat. *Anesthesiology.* 2007;107:264–272.
21. Rivera C, Voipio J, Payne JA, et al. TheK+/Cl− co-transporter KCC2 renders GABA hyperpolarizing during neuronal maturation. *Nature.* 1999;397:251–255.
22. Ovassapian A, Joshi CW, Brunner EA. Visual disturbances: an unusual symptom of transurethral prostatic resection reaction. *Anesthesiology.* 1982;57:332–334.

23. Wang JML, Creel DJ, Wong KC. Transurethral resection of the prostate: serum glycine levels and ocular evoked potentials. *Anesthesiology.* 1989;70:36–41.
24. Yamada M, Inanobe A, Kurachi Y. G protein regulation of potassium ion channels. *Pharmacol Rev.* 1998;50:723–760.
25. Pfaffinger PJ, Martin JM, Hunter DD, et al. GTP-binding proteins couple cardiac muscarinic receptors to a K channel. *Nature.* 1985;317:536–538.
26. Kubo Y, Adelman JP, Clapham DE, et al. International Union of Pharmacology. LIV. Nomenclature and molecular relationships of inwardly rectifying potassium channels. *Pharmacol Rev.* 2005;57:509–526.
27. Brooks CM, Eccles JC. Electrical investigation of the monosynaptic pathway through the spinal cord. *J Neurophysiol.* 1947;10: 251–273.
28. Budson AE, Price BH. Memory dysfunction. *N Engl J Med.* 2005; 352:692–699.
29. Blundon JA, Zakharenko SS. Dissecting the components of long-term potentiation. *Neuroscientist.* 2008;14:598–608.
30. Born J. Slow-wave sleep and the consolidation of long-term memory. *World J Biol Psychiatry.* 2010;11(suppl 1):16–21.
31. Moller JT, Cluitmans P, Rasmussen LS, et al. Long-term postoperative cognitive dysfunction in the elderly. *Lancet.* 1998;351: 857–861.
32. Carnini A, Lear JD, Eckenhoff RG. Inhaled anesthetic modulation of amyloid beta(1-40) assembly and growth. *Curr Alzheimer Res.* 2007;4:233–241.
33. Ghoneim MM. Awareness during anesthesia. *Anesthesiology.* 2000;92:597–602.
34. Sandin RH, Enlund G, Samuelsson P, et al. Awareness during anaesthesia: a prospective case study. *Lancet.* 2000;355:707–711.
35. Sebel PS, Bowdle TA, Ghoneim MM, et al. The incidence of awareness during anesthesia: a multicenter United States study. *Anesth Analg.* 2004;99:833–839.
36. Myles PS, Leslie K, McNeil J, et al. Bispectral index monitoring to prevent awareness during anaesthesia: the B-Aware randomized controlled trial. *Lancet.* 2004;363:1757–1763.
37. Avidan MS, Zhang L, Burnside BA, et al. Anesthesia awareness and the bispectral index. *N Engl J Med.* 2008;358(11):1097–1108.
38. Lyons G, MacDonald R. Awareness during cesarean section. *Anaesthesia.* 1991;46:62–64.
39. Ranta S, Jussila J, Hynyen M. Recall of awareness during cardiac anaesthesia: influence of feedback information to the anaesthesiologist. *Acta Anaesthesiol Scand.* 1996;40:554–560.
40. Bogetz MS, Katz JA. Recall of surgery for major trauma. *Anesthesiology.* 1984;61:6–9.
41. Dwyer R, Bennett HL, Eger EI II, et al. Effects of isoflurane and nitrous oxide in subanesthetic concentrations on memory and responsiveness in volunteers. *Anesthesiology.* 1992;77:888–898.
42. Dwyer R, Bennett HL, Eger EI II, et al. Isoflurane anesthesia prevents unconscious learning. *Anesth Analg.* 1992;75:107–112.
43. Naguib M, Schmid PG III, Baker MT. The electroencephalographic effects of IV anesthetic doses of melatonin: comparative studies with thiopental and propofol. *Anesth Analg.* 2003;97: 238–243.
44. Franks NP. General anaesthesia: from molecular targets to neuronal pathways of sleep and arousal. *Nat Rev Neurosci.* 2008;9: 370–386.
45. Sprung J, Wilt S, Bourke D, et al. Is it time to correct the dermatome chart of the anterior scrotal region? *Anesthesiology.* 1993;79: 381–383.
46. Savolaine ER, Pandya JB, Greenblatt SH, et al. Anatomy of the human lumbar epidural space. New insights using CT-epidurography. *Anesthesiology.* 1988;68:217–220.
47. Gallart L, Blanco D, Samso E, et al. Clinical and radiologic evidence of the epidural plica medina dorsalis. *Anesth Analg.* 1990;71: 698–701.
48. Lirk J, Colvin B, Steger B, et al. Incidence of lower thoracic ligamentum flavum midline gaps. *Br J Anaesth.* 2005;94:852–855.
49. Gilman S. Advances in neurology. *N Engl J Med.* 1992;326: 1608–1616.
50. Brian JE. Carbon dioxide and the cerebral circulation. *Anesthesiology.* 1998;88:1365–1386.
51. Sigl J, Chamoun N. An introduction to bispectral analysis for the electroencephalogram. *J Clin Monit.* 1994;10:392–404.
52. Flaishon R, Windsor A, Sigl J, et al. Recovery of consciousness after thiopental or propofol. Bispectral index and the isolated forearm technique. *Anesthesiology.* 1997;86:613–619.
53. Kearse LA, Manberg P, Chamoun N, et al. Bispectral analysis of the electroencephalogram correlates with patient movement to skin incision during propofol/nitrous oxide anesthesia. *Anesthesiology.* 1994;81:1365–1370.
54. Song D, Joshi G, White PF. Titration of volatile anesthetics using bispectral index facilitates recovery after ambulatory anesthesia. *Anesthesiology.* 1997;87:842–848.
55. Gan TJ, Glass PS, Windsor A, et al. Bispectral index monitoring allows faster recovery from propofol, alfentanil, and nitrous oxide anesthesia. *Anesthesiology.* 1997;87:808–815.
56. Ekman A, Lindholm M-L, Lennmarken C, et al. Reduction in the incidence of awareness using BIS monitoring. *Acta Anaesthesiol Scand.* 2004;48:20–26.
57. Lennmarken C, Sandin R. Neuromonitoring for awareness during surgery. *Lancet.* 2004;363:1747–1748.
58. Orser BA. Depth-of-anesthesia monitor and the frequency of intraoperative awareness. *N Engl J Med.* 2008;358:1189–1191.
59. Schmidt GN, Bischoff P, Standl T, et al. Comparative evaluation of the Datex-Ohmeda S/5 entropy module and the Bispectral Index® monitor during propofol-remifentanil anesthesia. *Anesthesiology.* 2004;101:1283–1290.
60. Höcker J, Raitschew B, Meybohm P, et al. Differences between bispectral index and spectral entropy during xenon anaesthesia: a comparison with propofol anaesthesia. *Anaesthesia.* 2010;65: 595–600.
61. Kofke WA, Young RSK, Davis P, et al. Isoflurane for refractory status epilepticus: a clinical series. *Anesthesiology.* 1989;71:653–659.
62. Ginsburg HH, Shetter AG, Raudzens PA. Postoperative paraplegia with preserved intraoperative somatosensory evoked potentials. *J Neurosurg.* 1985;63:296–299.
63. Pathak KS, Ammadio M, Kalamchi A, et al. Effects of halothane, enflurane, and isoflurane on somatosensory evoked potentials during nitrous oxide anesthesia. *Anesthesiology.* 1987;66: 753–757.
64. Schubert A, Drummond JC. The effect of acute hypocapnia on human median nerve somatosensory evoked responses. *Anesth Analg.* 1986;65:240–244.
65. Adams DC, Emerson RG, Heyer EJ, et al. Monitoring of intraoperative motor-evoked potentials under condition of controlled neuromuscular blockade. *Anesth Analg.* 1993;77:913–918.
66. Haenggi M, Ypparila H, Takala J, et al. Measuring depth of sedation with auditory evoked potentials during controlled infusion of propofol and remifentanil in health volunteers. *Anesth Analg.* 2004;99:1728–1736.
67. Chi OZ, Field C. Effects of isoflurane on visual evoked potentials in humans. *Anesthesiology.* 1986;65:328–330.
68. Ganong WF. *Review of Medical Physiology.* 21st ed. New York, NY: Lange Medical Books/McGraw-Hill; 2003.
69. Johnson RW. Anatomy for ophthalmic anaesthesia. *Br J Anaesth.* 1995;75:80–87.
70. Williams EL, Hart WM, Tempelhoff R. Postoperative ischemic optic neuropathy. *Anesth Analg.* 1995;80:1018–1029.
71. Janicki PK, Pai R, Wrights JK, et al. Ischemic optic neuropathy after liver transplantation. *Anesthesiology.* 2001;94:361–363.
72. Myers MA, Hamilton SR, Bogosian AJ, et al. Visual loss as a complication of spine surgery. *Spine.* 1997;22:1325–1329.

73. Roth S, Barach P. Postoperative visual loss: still no answers—yet. *Anesthesiology*. 2001;95:575–577.
74. Cheng MA, Todorov A, Tempelhoff R, et al. The effect of prone positioning on intraocular pressure in anesthetized patients. *Anesthesiology*. 2001;95:1351–1355.
75. Lee LA, Lam AM. Unilateral blindness after prone lumbar spine surgery. *Anesthesiology*. 2001;95:793–795.
76. Owens WD, Gustave F, Schlaroff A. Tympanic membrane rupture with nitrous oxide anesthesia. *Anesth Analg*. 1978;57:283–286.
77. Sprung J, Bourke DL, Contreras MG, et al. Perioperative hearing impairment. *Anesthesiology*. 2003;98:241–257.
78. Watcha MR, White PF. Postoperative nausea and vomiting. Its etiology, treatment, and prevention. *Anesthesiology*. 1992;77:162–184.
79. Azzam FJ. A simple and effective method for stopping post-anesthesia clonus. *Anesthesiology*. 1987;66:98.
80. Johns RA. EDRF/nitric oxide. the endogenous nitrovasodilator and a new cellular messenger. *Anesthesiology*. 1991;75:927–933.
81. Sudhof TC. The synaptic vesicle cycle revisited. *Neuron*. 2000;28:317–323.
82. Ahlquist RP. A study of adrenotropic receptors. *Am J Physiol*. 1948;53:586–606.
83. Insel PA. Adrenergic receptors—evolving concepts and clinical implications. *N Engl J Med*. 1996;334:580–589.
84. Lefkowitz RJ, Rockman HA, Koch WJ. Catecholamines, cardiac beta-adrenergic receptors, and heart failure. *Circulation*. 2000;101:1634–1640.
85. Martyn JA, White DA, Gronert GA, et al. Up-and-down regulation of skeletal muscle acetylcholine receptors. Effects on neuromuscular blockers. *Anesthesiology*. 1992;76:822–830.
86. Hosey MM. Diversity of structure, signaling and regulation within the family of muscarinic cholinergic receptors. *FASEB J*. 1992;6:845–851.
87. Charlson ME, MacKenzie CR, Gold JP. Preoperative autonomic function abnormalities in patients with diabetes mellitus and patients with hypertension. *J Am Coll Surg*. 1994;179:1–6.
88. Veith RC, Featherstone JA, Linares OA, et al. Age differences in plasma norepinephrine kinetics in humans. *J Gerontol*. 1986;41:319–325.
89. Lakatta ED. Deficient neuroendocrine regulation of the cardiovascular system with advancing age in healthy humans. *Circulation*. 1993;87:631–637.
90. Burgos LG, Ebert TJ, Asiddao C, et al. Increased intraoperative cardiovascular morbidity in diabetics with autonomic neuropathy. *Anesthesiology*. 1989;70:591–599.
91. Mangano DT, Layug EL, Wallace A, et al. Effect of atenolol on mortality and cardiovascular morbidity after noncardiac surgery. *N Engl J Med*. 1996;335:1713–1719.
92. Kehlet H. Manipulation of the metabolic response in clinical practice. *World J Surg*. 2000;24:690–698.
93. Wallace AW, Galindez D, Salahieh A, et al. Effect of clonidine on cardiovascular morbidity and mortality after noncardiac surgery. *Anesthesiology*. 2004;101:284–293.
94. Ebert TJ, Perez F, Uhrich TD, et al. Desflurane-mediated sympathetic activation occurs in humans despite preventing hypotension and baroreceptor unloading. *Anesthesiology*. 1998;88:1227–1235.
95. Buggy DJ, Crossley AWA. Thermoregulation, mild perioperative hypothermia, and post-anaesthetic shivering. *Br J Anaesth*. 2000;84:615–628.
96. Simon HB. Hyperthermia, fever and fever of undetermined origin. In: Rubenstein E, Federman D, eds. *ACP Medicine*. New York, NY: WebMD, Inc; 2003.
97. Heistad DD, Abboud FM. Factors that influence blood flow in skeletal muscle and skin. *Anesthesiology*. 1974;41:139–156.
98. Giesbrecht GG. Human thermoregulatory inhibition by regional anesthesia. *Anesthesiology*. 1994;81:277–281.
99. Sessler DI. Perioperative heat balance. *Anesthesiology*. 2000;92:578–599.
100. Sessler DI. Mild perioperative hypothermia. *N Engl J Med*. 1997;336:1630–1637.
101. Iaizzo PA, Kehler CH, Carr RJ, et al. Prior hypothermia attenuates malignant hyperthermia in susceptible swine. *Anesth Analg*. 1996;82:803–809.
102. Zviman MM, Roguin A, Jacobs A, et al. A new method for inducing hypothermia during cardiac arrest. *Crit Care Med*. 2004;32:S369–S373.
103. Gunn AJ, Thoresen M. Hypothermic neuroprotection. *NeuroRx*. 2006;3:154–169.
104. Todd MM, Hindman BJ, Clarke WR, et al. Intraoperative Hypothermia for Aneurysm Surgery Trial (IHAST) Investigators. Mild intraoperative hypothermia during surgery for intracranial aneurysm. *N Engl J Med*. 2005;352:135–145.
105. Hindman BJ, Bayman EO, Pfisterer WK, et al. IHAST Investigators. No association between intraoperative hypothermia or supplemental protective drug and neurologic outcomes in patients undergoing temporary clipping during cerebral aneurysm surgery: findings from the Intraoperative Hypothermia for Aneurysm Surgery Trial. *Anesthesiology*. 2010;112:86–101.
106. Frank SM, Fleisher LA, Breslow MJ, et al. Perioperative maintenance of normothermia reduces the incidence of morbid cardiac events: a randomized clinical trial. *JAMA*. 1997;277:1127–1134.
107. Imrie MM, Hall GM. Body temperature and anaesthesia. *Br J Anaesth*. 1990;64:346–354.
108. Sessler DI, Schroeder M. Heat loss in humans covered with cotton hospital blankets. *Anesth Analg*. 1993;77:73–77.

CHAPTER 4

Inhaled Anesthetics

Pamela Flood • Steven Shafer

History

The discovery of the anesthetic properties of nitrous oxide, diethyl ether, and chloroform in the 1840s was followed by a hiatus of about 80 years before other inhaled anesthetics were introduced (Fig. 4-1).[1] In 1950, all inhaled anesthetics, with the exception of nitrous oxide, were flammable or potentially toxic to the liver. Recognition that replacing a hydrogen atom with a fluorine atom decreased flammability led to the introduction, in 1951, of the first halogenated hydrocarbon anesthetic, fluroxene. Fluroxene was used clinically for several years before its voluntary withdrawal from the market due to its potential flammability and increasing evidence that this drug could cause organ toxicity.[2]

Halothane was synthesized in 1951 and introduced for clinical use in 1956. However, the tendency for alkane derivatives such as halothane to enhance the arrhythmogenic effects of epinephrine led to the search for new inhaled anesthetics derived from ethers. Methoxyflurane, a methyl ethyl ether, was the first such derivative. Methoxyflurane was introduced into clinical practice in 1960. Although methoxyflurane did not enhance the arrhythmogenic effects of epinephrine, its high solubility in blood and lipids resulted in a prolonged induction and slow recovery from anesthesia. More importantly, methoxyflurane caused hepatic toxicity. Extensive hepatic metabolism increased plasma concentrations of fluoride, which caused nephrotoxicity, especially with prolonged exposures to the anesthetic. Methoxyflurane has analgesic properties at concentrations far below those that induce anesthesia. Although its use was abandoned in the United States and Canada in the 1970s, it continues to be used in Australia for brief painful procedures and emergency transport.[3] Enflurane, the next methyl ethyl ether derivative, was introduced for clinical use in 1973. This anesthetic, in contrast to halothane, does not enhance the arrhythmogenic effects of epinephrine or cause hepatotoxicity. Nevertheless, side effects were present, including metabolism to inorganic fluoride and stimulation of the central nervous system (CNS), lowering the seizure threshold. In search of a drug with fewer side effects, isoflurane, a structural isomer of enflurane, was introduced in 1981. This drug was resistant to metabolism, making organ toxicity unlikely after its administration.

Inhaled Anesthetics for the Present and Future

The search for even more pharmacologically "perfect" inhaled anesthetics did not end with the introduction and widespread use of isoflurane. The exclusion of all halogens except fluorine results in nonflammable liquids that are poorly lipid soluble and extremely resistant to metabolism. Desflurane, a totally fluorinated methyl ethyl ether, was introduced in 1992 and was followed in 1994 by the totally fluorinated methyl isopropyl ether, sevoflurane.[4,5] The low solubility of these volatile anesthetics in blood facilitated rapid induction of anesthesia, precise control of end-tidal anesthetic concentrations during maintenance of anesthesia, and prompt recovery at the end of anesthesia independent of the duration of administration. The development, introduction, and rapid clinical acceptance of desflurane and sevoflurane reflects market forces (ambulatory surgery and the desire for rapid awakening possible with poorly soluble but potent anesthetics) more than an improved pharmacologic profile on various organ systems as compared with isoflurane. The challenge to the anesthesiologist is to exploit the pharmacokinetic advantages of these drugs while minimizing the risks (airway irritation, sympathetic nervous system stimulation, carbon monoxide production from interaction with carbon dioxide absorbent and complex vaporizer technology with desflurane, and compound A production from sevoflurane) and the increased expense associated with the manufacture and increased cost of administration of desflurane and sevoflurane.

Cost Considerations

Cost is an important consideration in the adoption of new drugs, including inhaled anesthetics. Factors that may

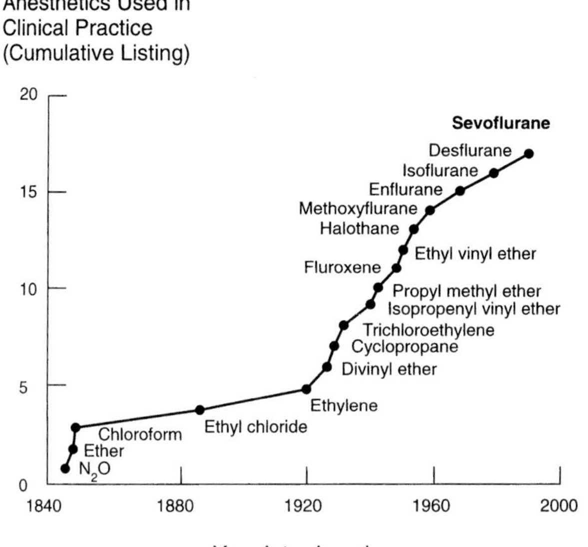

FIGURE 4-1 Inhaled anesthetics introduced into clinical practice beginning with the successful use of nitrous oxide in 1844 for dental anesthesia followed by recognition of the anesthetic properties of ether in 1846 and of chloroform in 1847. Modern anesthetics, beginning with halothane, differ from prior anesthetics in being fluorinated and nonflammable. (Modified from Eger EI. *Desflurane [Suprane]: A Compendium and Reference*. Nutley, NJ: Anaquest, 1993:1–119, with permission.)

influence the cost of a new inhaled anesthetics include (a) price (cost per milliliter of liquid); (b) inherent characteristics of the anesthetic, such as its vapor pressure (milliliter of vapor available per milliliter of liquid), potency, and solubility; and (c) fresh gas flow rate selected for delivery of the anesthetic.[6] The costs of new inhaled anesthetics can be decreased by using low fresh gas flow rates. Less soluble anesthetics are more suitable for use with low gas flow rates because their poor solubility permits better control of the delivered concentration. Furthermore, there is less depletion of these anesthetics from the inspired gases so that fewer molecules need to be added to the returning rebreathed gases. This conservation offsets the decreased potency of a drug such as desflurane compared with isoflurane. For example, desflurane is one-fifth as potent as isoflurane, yet the amount of desflurane that must be delivered to sustain minimal alveolar concentration (MAC) is only slightly more than threefold the amount of isoflurane. Similarly, although MAC of sevoflurane is 74% greater than isoflurane, the amount of sevoflurane that must be delivered to sustain MAC is only 30% greater.

Current Clinically Useful Inhaled Anesthetics

Commonly administered inhaled anesthetics include the inorganic gas nitrous oxide and the volatile liquids isoflurane, desflurane, and sevoflurane (Table 4-1) (Fig. 4-2).[4,5] Halothane and enflurane are administered infrequently but are included in the discussion of the comparative pharmacology of volatile anesthetics since halothane in particular has been studied extensively.[4,5]

Volatile liquids are administered as vapors after their vaporization in devices known as ***vaporizers***. Diethyl ether and chloroform are still available, but mostly used only in veterinary medicine. Xenon is an inert gas with anesthetic properties, but its clinical use is hindered by its high cost.[7]

Nitrous Oxide

Nitrous oxide is a low-molecular-weight, odorless to sweet-smelling nonflammable gas of low potency and poor blood solubility (blood:gas partition coefficient 0.46) that is most commonly administered in combination with opioids or volatile anesthetics to produce general anesthesia. Although nitrous oxide is nonflammable, it will support combustion.[8] Its poor blood solubility permits rapid achievement of an alveolar and brain partial pressure of the drug (Fig. 4-3). The analgesic effects of nitrous oxide are prominent but short lived, dissipating after about 20 minutes of use while sedative effects persist.[9] Nitrous

Table 4-1

Physical and Chemical Properties of Inhaled Anesthetics

	Nitrous Oxide	Halothane	Enflurane	Isoflurane	Desflurane	Sevoflurane
Molecular weight	44	197	184	184	168	200
Boiling point (°C)		50.2	56.5	48.5	22.8	58.5
Vapor pressure (mm Hg; 20°C)	Gas	244	172	240	669	170
Odor	Sweet	Organic	Ethereal	Ethereal	Ethereal	Ethereal
Preservative necessary	No	Yes	No	No	No	No
Stability in soda lime (40°C)	Yes	No	Yes	Yes	Yes	No
Blood:gas partition coefficient	0.46	2.54	1.90	1.46	0.42	0.69
MAC (37°C, 30–55 years old, P_B 760 mm Hg) (%)	104	0.75	1.63	1.17	6.6	1.80

```
                                F  Cl     F
                                |  |      |
                              F-C--C--O--C-H
                                |  |      |
        N≡N=O                   F  H      F
     Nitrous oxide               Isoflurane

    F  F      F                 CF3       F
    |  |      |                   \       |
  F-C--C--O--C-H                H-C--O--C-H
    |  |      |                   /       |
    F  H      F                 CF3       F
     Desflurane                  Sevoflurane
```

FIGURE 4-2 Inhaled anesthetics.

oxide causes minimal skeletal muscle relaxation. The speculated role of nitrous oxide in postoperative nausea and vomiting is controversial. Although much studied, the results of double-blind randomized trials have varied. A recent meta-analysis that included 30 published studies suggests that avoidance of nitrous oxide is associated with a lower risk of postoperative nausea and vomiting (RR = 0.80 [0.71–0.90]).[10] Nitrous oxide has no effect on tissue Po_2 measurements but does cause a small increase in the P_{50} (about 1.6 mm Hg).[11] The benefits of nitrous oxide must be balanced against its possible adverse effects

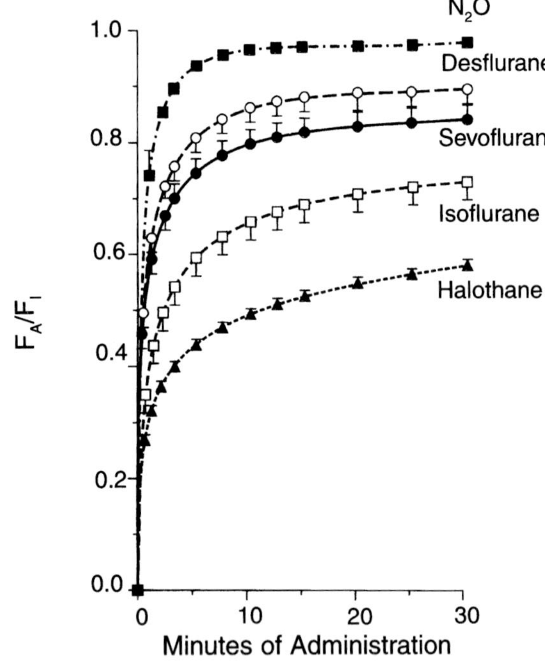

FIGURE 4-3 The pharmacokinetics of inhaled anesthetics during the induction of anesthesia is defined as the ratio of the end-tidal anesthetic concentration (F_A) to the inspired anesthetic concentration (F_I). Consistent with their relative blood:gas partition coefficients, the F_A/F_I of poorly soluble anesthetics (nitrous oxide, desflurane, sevoflurane) increases more rapidly than that of anesthetics with greater solubility in blood. A decrease in the rate of change in the F_A/F_I after 5 to 15 minutes (three time constants) reflects decreased tissue uptake of the anesthetic as the vessel-rich group tissues become saturated. (Data are mean ± SD.) (From Yasuda N, Lockhart SH, Eger EI, et al. Comparison of kinetics of sevoflurane and isoflurane in humans. *Anesth Analg.* 1991;72:316–324, with permission.)

related to the high-volume absorption of nitrous oxide in gas-containing spaces, potential increase in the risk of postoperative nausea and vomiting, and its ability to inactivate vitamin B_{12}.

Halothane

Halothane is a halogenated alkane derivative that exists as a clear, nonflammable liquid at room temperature. The vapor of this liquid has a sweet, nonpungent odor. An intermediate solubility in blood, combined with a high potency, permits intermediate onset and recovery from anesthesia using halothane alone or in combination with nitrous oxide or injected drugs such as opioids.

Halothane was developed on the basis of predictions that its halogenated structure would provide nonflammability, intermediate blood solubility, anesthetic potency, and molecular stability. Specifically, carbon-fluorine decreases flammability, and the trifluorocarbon contributes to molecular stability. The presence of a carbon-chlorine and carbon-bromine bond plus the retention of a hydrogen atom ensures anesthetic potency. Despite its chemical stability, halothane is susceptible to decomposition to hydrochloric acid, hydrobromic acid, chloride, bromide, and phosgene. For this reason, halothane is stored in amber-colored bottles, and thymol is added as a preservative to prevent spontaneous oxidative decomposition. Thymol that remains in vaporizers after vaporization of halothane can cause vaporizer turnstiles or temperature-compensating devices to malfunction.

Enflurane

Enflurane is a halogenated methyl ethyl ether that exists as a clear, nonflammable volatile liquid at room temperature and has a pungent, ethereal odor. Its intermediate solubility in blood combined with a high potency permits intermediate onset and recovery from anesthesia, using enflurane alone or in combination with nitrous oxide or injected drugs such as opioids. Enflurane decreases the threshold for seizures. Enflurane is oxidized in the liver to produce inorganic fluoride ions that can be nephrotoxic. It is primarily used for procedures in which a low threshold for seizure generation is desirable, such as electroconvulsive therapy.

Isoflurane

Isoflurane is a halogenated methyl ethyl ether that exists as a clear, nonflammable liquid at room temperature and has a pungent, ethereal odor. Its intermediate solubility in blood combined with a high potency permits intermediate onset and recovery from anesthesia using isoflurane alone or in combination with nitrous oxide or injected drugs such as opioids.

Although isoflurane is an isomer of enflurane, their manufacturing processes are not similar. The compounds used at the start of manufacturing are different, with 2,2,2-trifluoroethanol the starting compound for isoflurane and chlorotrifluoroethylene for enflurane. The subsequent purification of isoflurane by distillation is complex and expensive. Isoflurane is characterized by extreme physical stability, undergoing no detectable deterioration during 5 years of storage or on exposure to carbon dioxide absorbents or sunlight. The stability of isoflurane obviates the need to add preservatives such as thymol to the commercial preparation.

Desflurane

Desflurane is a fluorinated methyl ethyl ether that differs from isoflurane only by substitution of a fluorine atom for the chlorine atom found on the alpha-ethyl component of isoflurane. Fluorination rather than chlorination increases vapor pressure (decreases intermolecular attraction), enhances molecular stability, and decreases potency. Indeed, the vapor pressure of desflurane exceeds that of isoflurane by a factor of three such that desflurane would boil at normal operating room temperatures. A new vaporizer technology addressed this property, producing a regulated concentration by converting desflurane to a gas (heated and pressurized vaporizer that requires electrical power), which is then blended with diluent fresh gas flow. The only evidence of metabolism of desflurane is the presence of measurable concentrations of serum and urinary trifluoroacetate that are one-fifth to one-tenth those produced by the metabolism of isoflurane. The potency of desflurane as reflected by MAC is about fivefold less than isoflurane.

Unlike halothane and sevoflurane, desflurane is pungent, making it unlikely that inhalation induction of anesthesia would be feasible or pleasant for the patient. Indeed, the pungency of desflurane produces airway irritation and an appreciable incidence of salivation, breath-holding, coughing, or laryngospasm when >6% inspired desflurane is administered to an awake patient.[4] Carbon monoxide results from degradation of desflurane by the strong base present in desiccated carbon dioxide absorbents. Desflurane produces the highest carbon monoxide concentrations, followed by enflurane and isoflurane, whereas amounts produced from halothane and sevoflurane are trivial.

Solubility characteristics (blood:gas partition coefficient 0.45) and potency (MAC 6.6%) permit rapid achievement of an alveolar partial pressure necessary for anesthesia followed by prompt awakening when desflurane is discontinued. It is this lower blood-gas solubility and more precise control over the delivery of anesthesia and more rapid recovery from anesthesia that distinguish desflurane (and sevoflurane) from earlier volatile anesthetics.

Sevoflurane

Sevoflurane is a fluorinated methyl isopropyl ether. The vapor pressure of sevoflurane resembles that of halothane and isoflurane, permitting delivery of this anesthetic via a conventional unheated vaporizer. The solubility of sevoflurane (blood:gas partition coefficient 0.69) resembles that of desflurane, ensuring prompt induction of anesthesia and recovery after discontinuation of the anesthetic. Compared with isoflurane, recovery from sevoflurane anesthesia is 3 to 4 minutes faster and the difference is magnified in longer duration surgical procedures (>3 hours) (Fig. 4-4).[12] Sevoflurane is nonpungent, has minimal odor, produces bronchodilation similar in degree to isoflurane, and causes the least degree of airway irritation among the currently available volatile anesthetics. For these reasons, sevoflurane, like halothane, is acceptable for inhalation induction of anesthesia.

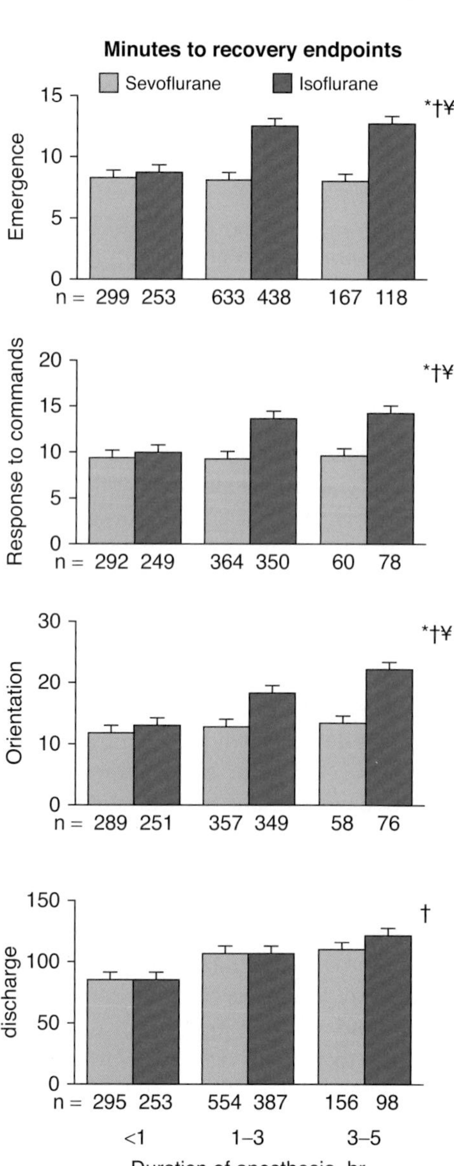

FIGURE 4-4 Analysis of variance results showing times to emergence, responses to commands, orientation, and discharge from the postanesthesia care unit (PACU) with differing durations of anesthesia. Mean ± SEM. n, Number of patients studied; *, significant difference between sevoflurane and isoflurane; †, significant difference with increasing duration of anesthesia; ¥, significant interaction between anesthetic and duration of anesthesia. (From Ebert TJ, Robinson BJ, Uhrich TD, et al. Recovery from sevoflurane anesthesia: a comparison to isoflurane and propofol anesthesia. *Anesthesiology.* 1998;89:1524–1531, with permission.)

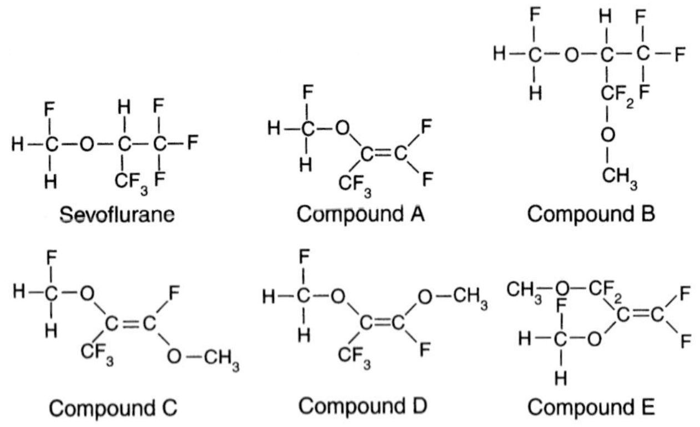

Sevoflurane Compound A Compound B

Compound C Compound D Compound E

FIGURE 4-5 Degradation products of sevoflurane on exposure to soda lime. The formation of these degradation products is increased under experimental conditions in which the soda lime is heated to ≥65°C.

Sevoflurane may be 100-fold more vulnerable to metabolism than desflurane, with an estimated 3% to 5% of the dose undergoing biodegradation. The resulting metabolites include inorganic fluoride (plasma concentrations exceed those that occur after enflurane) and hexafluoroisopropanol. The chemical structure of sevoflurane is such that it cannot undergo metabolism to an acyl halide. Sevoflurane metabolism does not result in the formation of trifluoroacetylated liver proteins and therefore cannot stimulate the formation of antitrifluoroacetylated protein antibodies. In this regard, sevoflurane differs from halothane, enflurane, isoflurane, and desflurane, all of which are metabolized to reactive acyl halide intermediates with the potential to produce hepatotoxicity as well as cross-sensitivity between drugs.[13] Sevoflurane is the least likely volatile anesthetic to form carbon monoxide on exposure to carbon dioxide absorbents. In contrast to other volatile anesthetics, sevoflurane breaks down in the presence of the strong bases present in carbon dioxide absorbents to form compounds that are toxic in animals (Fig. 4-5).[5] The principal degradation product is fluoromethyl-2, 2-difluoro-1-(trifluoromethyl) vinyl-ether (compound A). Compound A is a dose-dependent nephrotoxin in rats, causing renal proximal tubular injury. Although this finding is a concern, the levels of these compounds (principally compound A) that occur during administration of sevoflurane to patients are far below speculated toxic levels, even when total gas flows are 1 L per minute.[13,14]

Xenon

Xenon is an inert gas with many of the characteristics considered important for an ideal inhaled anesthetic.[7] MAC is 63% to 71% in humans, suggesting that this gas is more potent than nitrous oxide (MAC 104%).[15] MAC_{awake} for xenon is 33%.[16] Unlike MAC for other volatile anesthetics, there is evidence that xenon MAC is gender-dependent, being less in females.[17] Xenon is nonexplosive, nonpungent, odorless, and chemically inert as reflected by absence of metabolism and low toxicity. Unlike other inhaled anesthetics, it is not harmful to the environment because it is prepared by fractional distillation of the atmospheric air. To date, its high cost has hindered its acceptance in anesthesia practice. This disadvantage may be offset to some degree by using low fresh gas flow rates and development of a xenon-recycling system. Nevertheless, even if cost considerations can be negated, acceptance of xenon as a replacement for current inhaled anesthetics (that also share many of the same advantages of xenon) will be based more on evidence that morbidity and mortality is less when this drug is administered during anesthesia.[7]

Xenon has a blood:gas partition coefficient of 0.115, which is lower than that of other clinically useful anesthetics and even lower than that of nitrous oxide (0.46), sevoflurane (0.69), and desflurane (0.42). Like nitrous oxide, xenon anesthesia results in gas exchange conditions that favor air bubble expansion, which could worsen neurologic injury from venous air embolism.[18] Diffusion of xenon into highly compliant bowel occurs but is less compared with nitrous oxide (Fig. 4-6).[19] It is possible this minimal effect on bowel may be different when xenon diffuses into less compliant cavities as represented by pneumothorax, pneumoperitoneum, and pneumopericardium. Xenon does not trigger malignant hyperthermia in susceptible swine.[20] Emergence from xenon anesthesia, regardless of the duration of anesthesia, is two to three times faster than that from equal-MAC nitrous oxide plus isoflurane or sevoflurane.[21] Xenon is a potent hypnotic and analgesic, resulting in suppression of hemodynamic and catecholamine responses to surgical stimulation. Unlike other inhaled and injected anesthetics, xenon does not produce hemodynamic depression

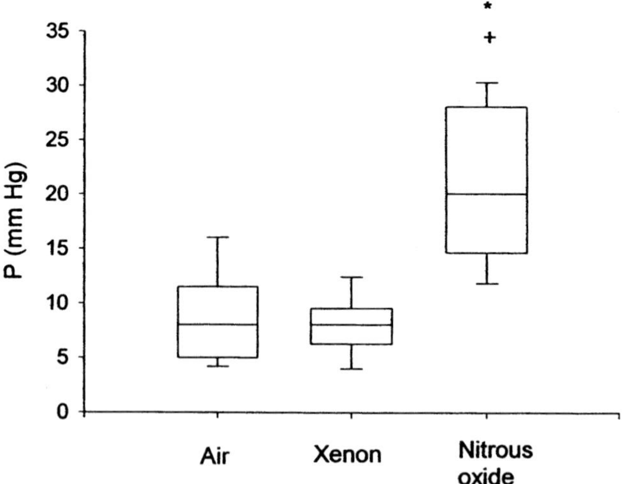

FIGURE 4-6 Pressures in obstructed bowel segments after 4 hours of air or anesthesia administration. After 4 hours of anesthesia, intraluminal pressures were significantly higher in the presence of nitrous oxide. +, Nitrous oxide compared to control; *, nitrous oxide compared to xenon. (From Reinelt H, Schirmer U, Marx T, et al. Diffusion of xenon and nitrous oxide into the blood. *Anesthesiology.* 2001;94:475-7, with permission.)

in healthy adults. Neuromuscular blocking effects of rocuronium are not different when given during propofol versus xenon anesthesia.[22] A risk of recall would seem to be present but has not been observed in small numbers of patients. Like ketamine, xenon exerts antagonist effects at *N*-methyl-D-aspartate (NMDA) subtypes of glutamate receptors, which have been shown to have both neuroprotective and neurotoxic properties. Xenon is unique among known NMDA antagonists in exhibiting neuroprotection without coexisting psychotomimetic behavioral changes.[23] The reason why ketamine and nitrous oxide, but not xenon, produce neurotoxicity may reflect actions on dopaminergic pathways that do not occur in the presence of xenon.

Pharmacokinetics of Inhaled Anesthetics

The pharmacokinetics of inhaled anesthetics describes their (a) absorption (uptake) from alveoli into pulmonary capillary blood, (b) distribution in the body, (c) metabolism, and (d) elimination, principally via the lungs. The pharmacokinetics of volatile anesthetics may be influenced by aging, reflecting decreases in lean body mass and increases in body fat.[24] The volume of distribution (Vd) of the central compartment (plasma volume) is smaller, whereas the apparent Vd (steady state) for these drugs in the elderly is larger, especially for those anesthetics most soluble in fat. In addition, impaired pulmonary gas exchange may decrease anesthetic clearance with age. Furthermore, reduced cardiac output in the elderly decreases tissue perfusion, increases time constants, and may be associated with an altered regional distribution of anesthetics. Opposite effects on the pharmacokinetics of inhaled anesthetics might be expected in the very young.

A series of partial pressure gradients beginning at the anesthetic machine serve to propel the inhaled anesthetic across various barriers (alveoli, capillaries, cell membranes) to their sites of action in the CNS. The principal objective of inhalation anesthesia is to achieve a constant and optimal brain partial pressure of the inhaled anesthetic.

The brain and all other tissues equilibrate with the partial pressures of inhaled anesthetics delivered to them by arterial blood (Pa). Likewise, arterial blood equilibrates with the alveolar partial pressures (PA) of anesthetics. This emphasizes that the PA of inhaled anesthetics mirrors the brain partial pressure (P_{BRAIN}) at steady state. This is the reason that PA is used as an index of (a) depth of anesthesia, (b) recovery from anesthesia, and (c) anesthetic equal potency (MAC). It is important to recognize that equilibration between the two phases means the same partial pressure exists in both phases. Equilibration does not mean equality of concentrations in two biophases. Understanding those factors that determine the PA and thus the P_{BRAIN} permits control of the doses of inhaled anesthetics delivered to the brain so as to maintain a constant and optimal depth of anesthesia. This relationship is applicable because volatile anesthetics are only minimally metabolized and as such are excreted from the lung. The availability of an "online" readout of end-tidal partial pressure, which at equilibrium matches brain partial pressure, makes volatile anesthetic dosing easier than intravenous anesthetic dosing.

Determinants of Alveolar Partial Pressure

The PA and ultimately the P_{BRAIN} of inhaled anesthetics are determined by input (delivery) into alveoli minus uptake (loss) of the drug from alveoli into arterial blood (Table 4-2). Input of anesthetics into alveoli depends on the (a) inhaled partial pressure (PI), (b) alveolar ventilation, and (c) characteristics of the anesthetic breathing (delivery) system. Uptake of inhaled anesthetics from alveoli into the pulmonary capillary blood depends on (a) solubility of the anesthetic in body tissues, (b) cardiac output, and (c) alveolar-to-venous partial pressure differences (A-vD).

Inhaled Partial Pressure

A high PI delivered from the anesthetic machine is required during initial administration of the anesthetic. A high initial input offsets the impact of uptake, accelerating induction of anesthesia as reflected by the rate of rise in the PA and thus the P_{BRAIN}. With time, as uptake into the blood decreases, the PI should be decreased to match the decreased anesthetic uptake and therefore maintain a constant and optimal P_{BRAIN}. If the PI is maintained constant

Table 4-2

Factors Determining Partial Pressure Gradients Necessary for Establishment of Anesthesia

Transfer of inhaled anesthetic from anesthetic machine to alveoli (anesthetic input)
Inspired partial pressure
Alveolar ventilation
Characteristics of anesthetic breathing system
Functional residual capacity
Transfer of inhaled anesthetic from alveoli to arterial blood (anesthetic loss)
Blood:gas partition coefficient
Cardiac output
Alveolar-to-venous partial pressure difference
Transfer of inhaled anesthetic from arterial blood to brain (anesthetic loss)
Brain:blood partition coefficient
Cerebral blood flow
Arterial-to-venous partial pressure difference

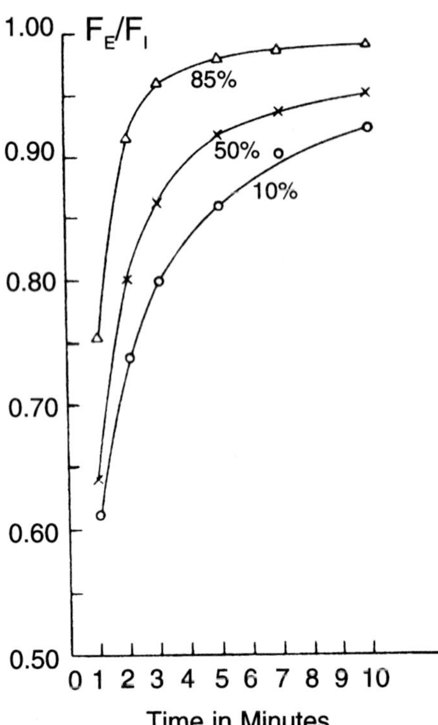

FIGURE 4-7 The impact of the inhaled concentration of an anesthetic on the rate at which the alveolar concentration increases toward the inspired (F_E/F_I) is known as the *concentration effect.* (From Eger EI. Effect of inspired anesthetic concentration on the rate of rise of alveolar concentration. *Anesthesiology.* 1963;24:153–157, with permission.)

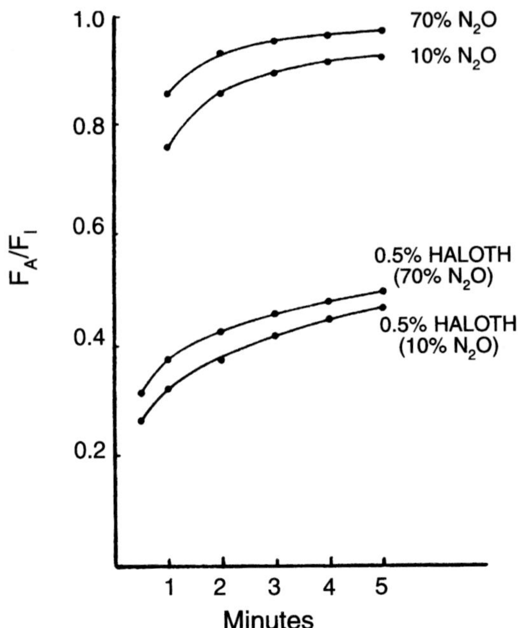

FIGURE 4-8 The second-gas effect is the accelerated increase in the alveolar concentration of a second gas, halothane (HALOTH), toward the inspired (F_A/F_I) in the presence of a high inhaled concentration of the first gas (N_2O). (From Epstein RM, Rackow H, Salanitre E, et al. Influence of the concentration effect on the uptake of anesthetic mixtures: the second gas effect. *Anesthesiology.* 1964;25:364–371, with permission.)

with time, the PA and P_{BRAIN} will increase progressively as uptake diminishes.

Concentration Effect

The impact of PI on the rate of rise of the PA of an inhaled anesthetic is known as the ***concentration effect*** (Fig. 4-7).[25] The concentration effect states that the higher the PI, the more rapidly the PA approaches the PI. The higher PI provides anesthetic molecule input to offset uptake and thus speeds the rate at which the PA increases.

The concentration effect results from (a) a concentrating effect and (b) an augmentation of tracheal inflow.[26] The concentrating effect reflects concentration of the inhaled anesthetic in a smaller lung volume due to uptake of all gases in the lung. At the same time, anesthetic input via tracheal inflow is increased to fill the space (void) produced by uptake of gases.

Second-Gas Effect

The second-gas effect reflects the ability of high-volume uptake of one gas (first gas) to accelerate the rate of increase of the PA of a concurrently administered "companion" gas (second gas) (Fig. 4-8).[27] For example, the initial large-volume uptake of nitrous oxide accelerates the uptake of companion (second) gases such as oxygen and volatile anesthetics. This increased uptake of the second gas reflects increased tracheal inflow of all the inhaled gases (first and second gases) and higher concentration of the second gas or gases in a smaller lung volume (concentrating effect) due to the high-volume uptake of the first gas (Fig. 4-9).[26] Conceptually, the loss of lung volume may be compensated for by decreased expired ventilation as well as increased inspired ventilation (increased tracheal inflow). The implication that extra gas is routinely drawn into the lungs to compensate for loss of lung volume is misleading if compensatory changes include decreased expired ventilation and/or a decrease in lung volume.[28]

Alveolar Ventilation

Increased alveolar ventilation, like PI, promotes input of anesthetics to offset uptake. The net effect is a more rapid

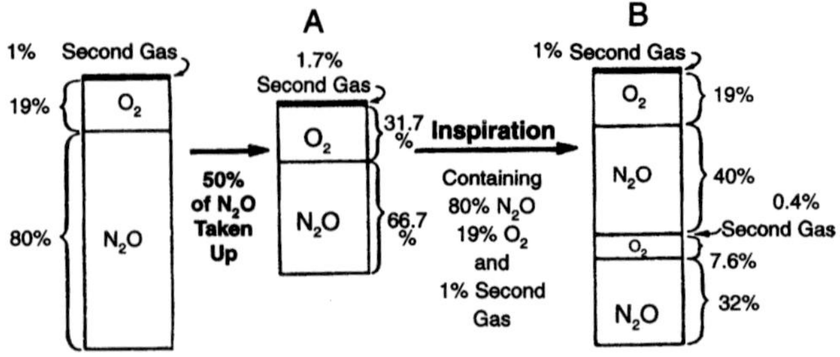

FIGURE 4-9 The second-gas effect results from a concentrating effect **(A)** and an augmentation of tracheal inflow **(B)**. (From Stoelting RK, Eger EI. An additional explanation for the second gas effect: a concentrating effect. *Anesthesiology.* 1969;30:273–277, with permission.)

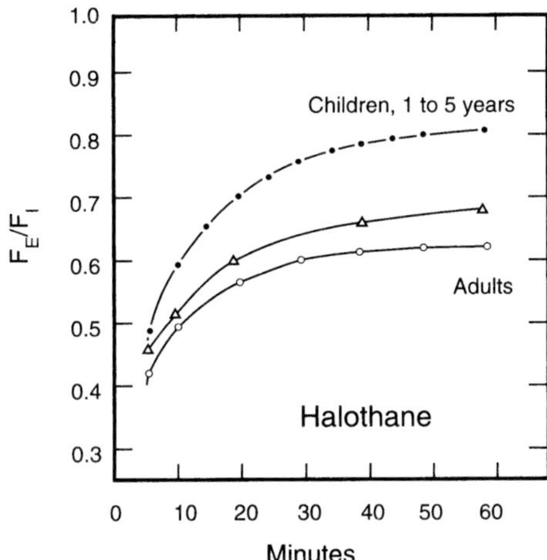

FIGURE 4-10 The rate at which the alveolar concentration (F_E) increases toward the inspired (F_I) for halothane (HALO 0.5%) in children 1 to 5 years of age is more rapid than in adults. (From Salanitre E, Rackow H. The pulmonary exchange of nitrous oxide and halothane in infants and children. *Anesthesiology*. 1969;30:388–392, with permission.)

rate of increase in the PA toward the PI and thus induction of anesthesia. In addition to the increased input, the decreased $Paco_2$ produced by hyperventilation of the lungs decreases cerebral blood flow. Conceivably, the impact of increased input on the rate of rise of the PA would be offset by decreased delivery of anesthetic to the brain. Decreased alveolar ventilation decreases input and thus slows the establishment of a PA and P_{BRAIN} necessary for the induction of anesthesia. The greater the alveolar ventilation to functional residual capacity (FRC) ratio, the more rapid is the rate of increase in the PA. In neonates, this ratio is approximately 5:1 compared with only 1.5:1 in adults, reflecting the greater metabolic rate in neonates compared with adults. As a result, the rate of increase of PA toward the PI and thus the induction of anesthesia is more rapid in neonates than in adults (Fig. 4-10).[29]

Spontaneous versus Mechanical Ventilation

Inhaled anesthetics influence their own uptake by virtue of dose-dependent depressant effects on alveolar ventilation. This, in effect, is a negative feedback protective mechanism that prevents establishment of an excessive depth of anesthesia (delivery of anesthesia is decreased when ventilation is decreased) when a high PI is administered during spontaneous breathing (Fig. 4-11).[30] As anesthetic input decreases in parallel with decreased ventilation, anesthetic present in tissues is redistributed from tissues in which it is present in high concentrations (brain) to other tissues in which it is present in low concentrations (skeletal muscles). When the concentration (partial pressure) in the brain decreases to a certain threshold, ventilation increases and delivery of the anesthetic to the lungs increases. This protective mechanism against development of an excessive depth of anesthesia (anesthetic overdose) is lost when mechanical ventilation of the lungs replaces spontaneous breathing.

Impact of Solubility

The impact of changes in alveolar ventilation on the rate of increase in the PA toward the PI depends on the solubility of the anesthetic in blood. For example, changes in alveolar ventilation influence the rate of increase of the

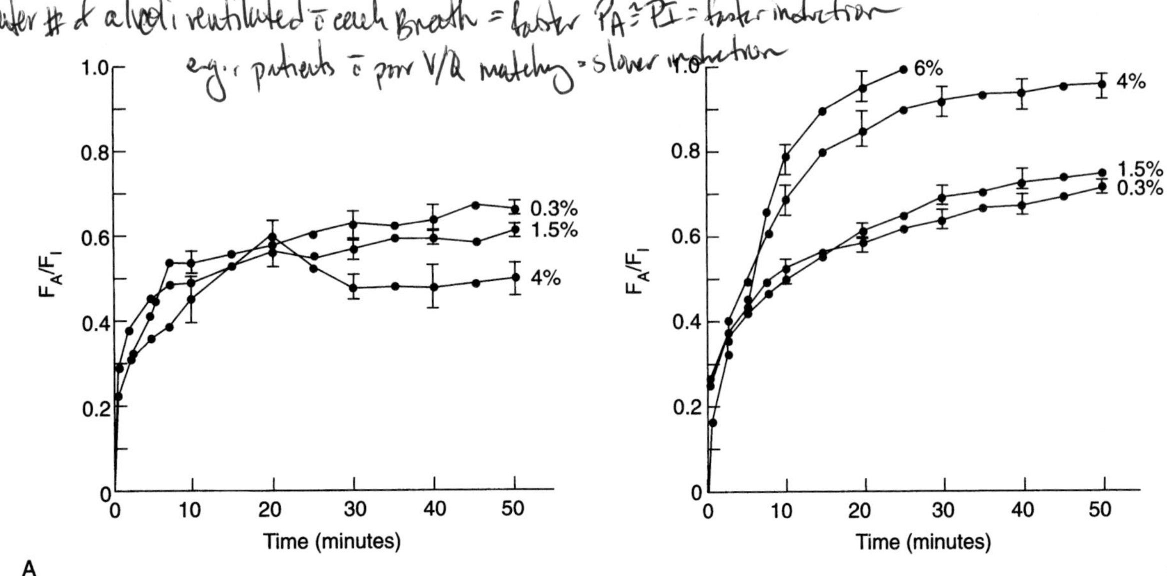

FIGURE 4-11 Effect of the mode of ventilation on the rate of increase of the alveolar concentration (F_A) of halothane toward the inspired concentration (F_I) as determined in an animal model. Negative feedback inhibition of spontaneous ventilation **(A)** limits the F_A/F_I to 0.6 for all the inspired concentrations of halothane. The positive feedback effect of controlled ventilation **(B)** results in ratios of the F_A/F_I that approach 1.0 and excessive depressant effects of halothane on the cardiovascular system at the higher inspired concentrations of the anesthetic. (Data are mean ± SD.) (From Gibbons RT, Steffey EP, Eger EI. The effect of spontaneous versus controlled ventilation on the rate of rise in the alveolar halothane concentration in dogs. *Anesth Analg*. 1977;56:32–37, with permission.)

PA of a soluble anesthetic (halothane, isoflurane) more than a poorly soluble anesthetic (nitrous oxide, desflurane, sevoflurane). Indeed, the rate of increase in the PA of nitrous oxide is rapid regardless of the alveolar ventilation. This occurs because uptake of nitrous oxide is limited because of its poor solubility in blood. Conversely, uptake of a more blood-soluble anesthetic is larger, and increasing alveolar ventilation will accelerate the rate at which the PA of the soluble anesthetic approaches the PI. This emphasizes that changing from spontaneous breathing to mechanical (controlled) ventilation of the lungs, which also is likely to be associated with increased alveolar ventilation, will probably increase the depth of anesthesia (PA) produced by a more blood-soluble anesthetic.

Anesthetic Breathing System

Characteristics of the anesthetic breathing system that influence the rate of increase of the PA are the (a) volume of the external breathing system, (b) solubility of the inhaled anesthetics in the rubber or plastic components of the breathing system, and (c) gas inflow from the anesthetic machine. The volume of the anesthetic breathing system acts as a buffer to slow achievement of the PA. High gas inflow rates (5 to 10 L per minute) from the anesthetic machine negate this buffer effect. Solubility of inhaled anesthetics in the components of the anesthetic breathing system initially slows the rate at which the PA increases. At the conclusion of the administration of an anesthetic, however, reversal of the partial pressure gradient in the anesthetic breathing system results in elution of the anesthetic, which slows the rate at which the PA decreases.

Solubility

The solubility of the inhaled anesthetics in blood and tissues is denoted by the partition coefficient (Table 4-3).[1,31] A partition coefficient is a distribution ratio describing how the inhaled anesthetic distributes itself between two phases at equilibrium (partial pressures equal in both phases). For example, a blood:gas partition coefficient of 0.5 means that the concentration of inhaled anesthetic in the blood is half that present in the alveolar gases when the partial pressures of the anesthetic in these two phases is identical. Similarly, a brain:blood partition coefficient of 2 indicates a concentration of anesthetic in the brain is twice that in the blood when the partial pressures of anesthetic are identical at both sites.

Partition coefficients may be thought of as reflecting the relative capacity of each phase to accept anesthetic. Partition coefficients are temperature dependent such that the solubility of a gas in a liquid is decreased when the temperature of the liquid increases.

Blood:Gas Partition Coefficients

The rate of increase of the PA toward the PI (maintained constant by mechanical ventilation of the lungs) is inversely related to the solubility of the anesthetic in blood (see Fig. 4-3).[32,33] Based on their blood:gas partition coefficients, inhaled anesthetics are categorized traditionally as soluble, intermediately soluble, and poorly soluble (see Table 4-3).[1,31] Blood can be considered a pharmacologically inactive reservoir, the size of which is determined by the solubility of the anesthetic in blood. When the blood:gas partition coefficient is high, a large amount of anesthetic must be dissolved in the blood before the Pa equilibrates

Table 4-3

Comparative Solubilities of Inhaled Anesthetics

	Blood:Gas Partition Coefficient	Brain:Blood Partition Coefficient	Muscle:Blood Partition Coefficient	Fat:Blood Partition Coefficient	Oil:Gas Partition Coefficient
Soluble					
Methoxyflurane	12	2	1.3	48.8	970
Intermediately soluble					
Halothane	2.54	1.9	3.4	51.1	224
Enflurane	1.90	1.5	1.7	36.2	98
Isoflurane	1.46	1.6	2.9	44.9	98
Poorly soluble					
Nitrous oxide	0.46	1.1	1.2	2.3	1.4
Desflurane	0.42	1.3	2.0	27.2	18.7
Sevoflurane	0.69	1.7	3.1	47.5	55
Xenon	0.115				

Data from Eger EI. *Desflurane (Suprane): A Compendium and Reference*. Nutley, NJ: Anaquest; 1993:1–119; Yasuda N, Targ AC, Eger EI. Solubility of I-653, sevoflurane, isoflurane, and halothane in human tissues. *Anesth Analg*. 1989;69:370–373.

with the PA. For example, the high blood solubility of methoxyflurane slows the rate at which the PA and Pa increase relative to the PI, and the induction of anesthesia is slow. The impact of high blood solubility on the rate of increase of the Pa can be offset to some extent by increasing the PI above that required for maintenance of anesthesia. This is termed the ***overpressure*** technique and may be used to speed the induction of anesthesia, recognizing that sustained delivery of a high PI will result in an anesthetic overdose.

When blood solubility is low, minimal amounts of inhaled anesthetic must be dissolved before equilibration is achieved; therefore, the rate of increase of PA and Pa, and thus onset-of-drug effects such as the induction of anesthesia, are rapid. For example, the inhalation of a constant PI of nitrous oxide, desflurane, or sevoflurane for about 10 minutes results in a PA that is ≥80% of the PI (see Fig. 4-3).[32,33] Use of an overpressure technique with sevoflurane is more readily accepted by patients because this anesthetic is less pungent than desflurane. Indeed, one or more vital capacity breaths of high concentrations of sevoflurane (7% with 66% nitrous oxide) may result in loss of the eyelash reflex.[34]

Associated with the rapid increase in the Pa of nitrous oxide is the absorption of several liters (up to 10 L during the first 10 to 15 minutes) of this gas, reflecting its common administration at inhaled concentrations of 60% to 70%. This high-volume absorption of nitrous oxide is responsible for several unique effects of nitrous oxide when it is administered in the presence of volatile anesthetics or air-containing cavities (see the sections "Concentration Effect," "Second-Gas Effect," and "Nitrous Oxide Transfer to Closed Gas Spaces").

Percutaneous loss of inhaled anesthetics occurs but is too small to influence the rate of increase in the PA.[35] With the possible exception of methoxyflurane, the magnitude of metabolism of inhaled anesthetics is too small to influence the rate of increase of the PA. This lack of effect reflects the large excess of anesthetic molecules administered and the saturation, by anesthetic concentrations of inhaled drugs, of enzymes responsible for anesthetic metabolism.[36]

Blood:gas partition coefficients are altered by individual variations in water, lipid, and protein content and by the hematocrit of whole blood.[37,38] For example, blood:gas partition coefficients are about 20% less in blood with a hematocrit of 21% compared with blood with a hematocrit of 43%. Presumably, this decreased solubility reflects the decrease in lipid-dissolving sites normally provided by erythrocytes. Conceivably, decreased solubility of volatile anesthetics in anemic blood would manifest as an increased rate of increase in the PA and a more rapid induction of anesthesia. Ingestion of a fatty meal alters the composition of blood, resulting in an approximately 20% increase in the solubility of volatile anesthetics in blood.[39]

The solubility of inhaled anesthetics in blood varies with age (Fig. 4-12).[40] The blood solubilities of halothane,

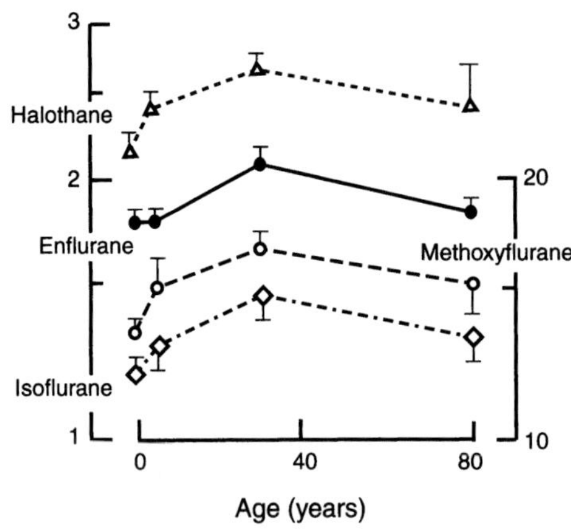

FIGURE 4-12 Blood:gas partition coefficients are 18% less in neonates compared with adults. (Mean ± SD.) (From Lerman J, Gregory GA, Willis MM, et al. Age and solubility of volatile anesthetics in blood. *Anesthesiology*. 1984;61:139–143, with permission.)

enflurane, methoxyflurane, and isoflurane are about 18% less in neonates and the elderly compared to young adults. In contrast, the solubility of the less soluble anesthetic sevoflurane (presumably also true for desflurane) is not different in neonates and adults.[41]

Tissue:Blood Partition Coefficients

Tissue:blood partition coefficients determine uptake of anesthetic into tissues and the time necessary for equilibration of tissues with the Pa. This time for equilibration can be estimated by calculating a time constant (amount of inhaled anesthetic that can be dissolved in the tissue divided by tissue blood flow) for each tissue. One time constant on an exponential curve represents 63% equilibration. Three time constants are equivalent to 95% equilibration. For volatile anesthetics, equilibration between the Pa and P_{BRAIN} depends on the anesthetic's blood solubility and requires 5 to 15 minutes (three time constants). Fat has an enormous capacity to hold anesthetic, and this characteristic, combined with low blood flow to this tissue, prolongs the time required to narrow anesthetic partial pressure differences between arterial blood and fat. For example, equilibration of fat with isoflurane (three time constants) based on this drug's fat:blood partition coefficient and an assumed fat blood flow of 2 to 3 mL per minute per 100 g fat is estimated to be 25 to 46 hours. Fasting before elective operations results in transport of fat to the liver, which could increase anesthetic uptake by this organ and modestly slow the rate of increase in the PA of a volatile anesthetic during induction of anesthesia.[42]

Oil:Gas Partition Coefficients

Oil:gas partition coefficients parallel anesthetic requirements. For example, an estimated MAC can be calculated as 150 divided by the oil:gas partition coefficient. The constant, 150, is the average value of the product of oil:gas solubility and MAC for several inhaled anesthetics with widely divergent lipid solubilities. Using this constant, the calculated MAC for a theoretical anesthetic with an oil:gas partition coefficient of 100 would be 1.5%.

Nitrous Oxide Transfer to Closed Gas Spaces

The blood:gas partition coefficient of nitrous oxide (0.46) is about 34 times greater than that of nitrogen (0.014). This differential solubility means that nitrous oxide can leave the blood to enter an air-filled cavity 34 times more rapidly than nitrogen can leave the cavity to enter blood. As a result of this preferential transfer of nitrous oxide, the volume or pressure of an air-filled cavity increases. Passage of nitrous oxide into an air-filled cavity surrounded by a compliant wall (intestinal gas, pneumothorax, pulmonary blebs, air bubbles) causes the gas space to expand (Fig. 4-13).[43] Conversely, passage of nitrous oxide into an air-filled cavity surrounded by a noncompliant wall (middle ear, cerebral ventricles, supratentorial space) causes an increase in intracavitary pressure.

The magnitude of volume or pressure increase is influenced by (a) partial pressure of nitrous oxide, (b) blood flow to the air-filled cavity, and (c) duration of nitrous oxide administration. In an animal model, the inhalation of 75% nitrous oxide doubles the volume of a pneumothorax in 10 minutes (see Fig. 4-7).[43] The finding emphasizes the high blood flow to this area. Likewise, air bubbles (emboli) expand rapidly when exposed to nitrous oxide (Fig. 4-14).[44] Nevertheless, in neurosurgical patients operated on in the sitting position, 50% nitrous oxide has no measurable effect on the incidence or severity of venous air embolism if its administration is discontinued immediately upon Doppler detection of venous air embolism.[45] In contrast to the rapid expansion of a pneumothorax, the increase in bowel gas volume produced by nitrous oxide is slow but can result in an increase in distention and postoperative pain after a 3-hour surgery.

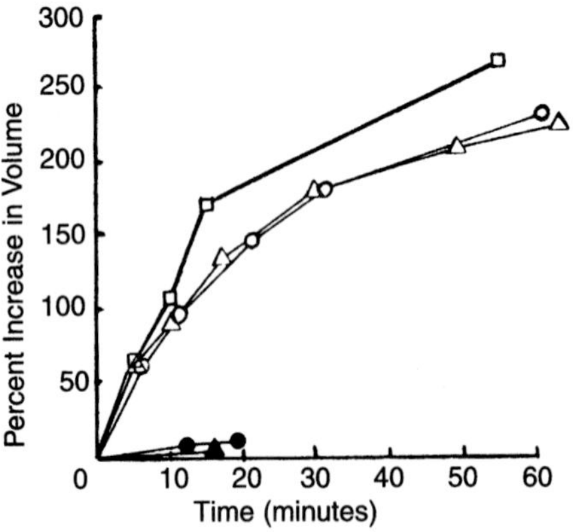

FIGURE 4-13 Inhalation of 75% nitrous oxide rapidly increases the volume of a pneumothorax *(open symbols)*. Inhalation of oxygen *(solid symbols)* does not alter the volume of the pneumothorax. (From Eger EI, Saidman LJ. Hazards of nitrous oxide anesthesia in bowel obstruction and pneumothorax. *Anesthesiology*. 1965;26:61–66, with permission.)

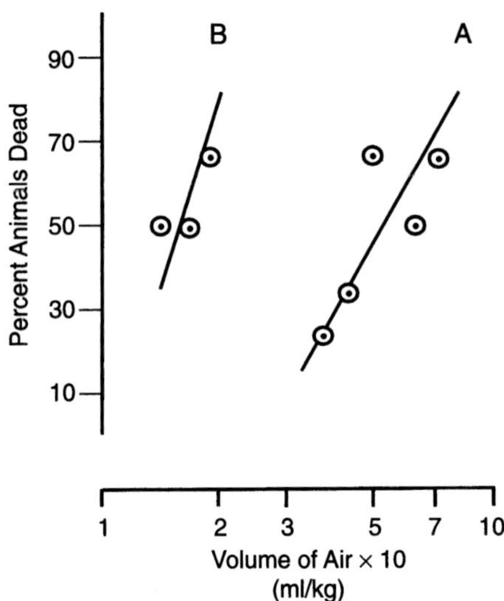

FIGURE 4-14 Nitrous oxide rapidly expands air bubbles as reflected by the volume of injected air necessary to produce 50% mortality in animals breathing nitrous oxide (0.16 mL/kg) **(A)** compared with animals breathing oxygen (0.55 mL/kg) **(B)**. (From Munson ES, Merrick HC. Effect of nitrous oxide on venous air embolism. *Anesthesiology*. 1966;27:783–787, with permission.)

The middle ear is an air-filled cavity that vents passively via the Eustachian tube when pressure reaches 20 to 30 cm H_2O. Nitrous oxide diffuses into the middle ear more rapidly than nitrogen leaves, and middle ear pressures may increase if Eustachian tube patency is compromised by inflammation or edema. Indeed, tympanic membrane rupture has been attributed to this mechanism after administration of nitrous oxide. Negative middle ear pressures may develop after discontinuation of nitrous oxide, leading to serous otitis. Nausea and vomiting that may follow general anesthesia may be due to multiple mechanisms, but the role of altered middle ear pressures as a result of nitrous oxide is a consideration.

Intraocular gas bubbles as used for internal retinal tamponade (retinal detachment, macular hole repair, complicated vitrectomy) may persist in the eye for up to 10 weeks following ocular surgery. Administration of nitrous oxide for periods as brief as 1 hour during this time period may result in rapid increases in the volume of intraocular gas within the rigid closed eye that is sufficient to compress the retinal artery with resulting visual loss.[46]

Cardiopulmonary Bypass

Cardiopulmonary bypass produces changes in blood-gas solubility that depend on the constituents of the priming solution and temperature.[47] Nevertheless, the overall effect of hypothermic cardiopulmonary bypass and a crystalloid prime on blood-gas solubility is only 2%. Volatile anesthetics initiated during cardiopulmonary bypass take longer to equilibrate, whereas the same drugs already present when cardiopulmonary bypass is initiated are diluted, potentially decreasing the depth of anesthesia.

Cardiac Output

Cardiac output (pulmonary blood flow) influences uptake and therefore PA by carrying away either more or less anesthetic from the alveoli. An increased cardiac output results in more rapid uptake, so the rate of increase in the PA and thus the induction of anesthesia are slowed. A decreased cardiac output speeds the rate of increase of the PA, because there is less uptake to oppose input.

The effect of cardiac output on the rate of increase in the PA may seem paradoxical. For example, the uptake of more drugs by an increased cardiac output should speed the rate of increase of partial pressures in tissues and thus narrow the A-vD for anesthetics. Indeed, an increase in cardiac output does hasten equilibration of tissue anesthetic partial pressures with the Pa. Nevertheless, the Pa is lower than it would be if cardiac output were normal. Conceptually, a change in cardiac output is analogous to the effect of a change in solubility. For example, doubling cardiac output increases the capacity of blood to hold anesthetic, just as solubility increases the capacity of the same volume of blood.

As with alveolar ventilation, changes in cardiac output most influence the rate of increase of the PA of a soluble anesthetic. Conversely, the rate of increase of the PA of a poorly soluble anesthetic, such as nitrous oxide, is rapid regardless of physiologic deviations of the cardiac output around its normal value. As a result, changes in cardiac output exert little influence on the rate of increase of the PA of nitrous oxide. In contrast, doubling the cardiac output will greatly increase the uptake of soluble anesthetic from alveoli, slowing the rate of increase of the PA. Conversely, a low cardiac output, as with shock, could produce an unexpectedly high PA of a soluble anesthetic.

Volatile anesthetics that depress cardiac output can exert a positive feedback response that contrasts with the negative (protective) feedback response on spontaneous breathing exerted by these drugs. For example, decreases in cardiac output due to an excessive dose of volatile anesthetic results in an increase in the PA, which further increases anesthetic depth and thus cardiac depression. The administration of a volatile anesthetic that depresses cardiac output, plus controlled ventilation of the lungs, results in a situation characterized by unopposed input of anesthetic via alveolar ventilation combined with decreased uptake because of decreased cardiac output. The net effect of this combination of events can be an unexpected, abrupt increase in the PA and an excessive depth of anesthesia.

Distribution of cardiac output will influence the rate of increase of the PA of an anesthetic. For example, increases in cardiac output are not necessarily accompanied by proportional increases in blood flow to all tissues. Preferential perfusion of vessel-rich group tissues when the cardiac output increases results in a more rapid increase in the PA of anesthetic than would occur if the increased cardiac output was distributed equally to all tissues. Indeed, infants have a relatively greater perfusion of vessel-rich group tissues than do adults and, consequently, show a faster rate of increase of the PA toward the PI (see Fig. 4-10).[29]

Impact of a Shunt

In the absence of an intracardiac or intrapulmonary right-to-left shunt, it is valid to assume that the PA and Pa of inhaled anesthetics are essentially identical. When a right-to-left shunt is present, the diluting effect of the shunted blood on the partial pressure of anesthetic in blood coming from ventilated alveoli results in a decrease in the Pa and a slowing in the induction of anesthesia. Monitoring the end-tidal concentration of anesthetic or carbon dioxide reveals a gradient between the PA and Pa in which the PA underestimates the Pa. A similar mechanism is responsible for the decrease in PaO_2 and the gradient between the PA and Pa in the presence of a right-to-left shunt.

The relative impact of a right-to-left shunt on the rate of increase in the Pa depends on the solubility of the anesthetic. For example, a right-to-left shunt slows the rate of increase of the Pa of a poorly soluble anesthetic more than that of a soluble anesthetic.[48] This occurs because uptake of a soluble anesthetic offsets dilutional effects of shunted blood on the Pa. Uptake of a poorly soluble drug is minimal, and dilutional effects on the Pa are relatively unopposed. This impact of solubility in the presence of a right-to-left shunt is opposite to that observed with changes in cardiac output and alveolar ventilation. All factors considered, it seems unlikely that a right-to-left shunt alone will alter the speed of induction of anesthesia significantly.

Left-to-right tissue shunts (arteriovenous fistulas, volatile anesthetic–induced increases in cutaneous blood flow) result in delivery to the lungs of blood containing a higher partial pressure of anesthetic than that present in blood that has passed through tissues. As a result, left-to-right shunts offset the dilutional effects of a right-to-left shunt on the Pa. Indeed, the effect of a left-to-right shunt on the rate of increase in the Pa is detectable only if there is a concomitant presence of a right-to-left shunt. Likewise, the effect of a right-to-left shunt on the rate of increase in the PA is maximal in the absence of a left-to-right shunt.

Alveolar-to-Venous Partial Pressure Differences

The A-vD reflects tissue uptake of the inhaled anesthetic. Tissue uptake affects uptake at the lung by controlling the rate of increase of the mixed venous partial pressure of anesthetic. Factors that determine the fraction of anesthetic removed from blood traversing a tissue parallel those factors that determine uptake at the lungs (tissue solubility, tissue blood flow, and arterial-to-tissue partial pressure differences).

Table 4-4

Body Tissue Composition

	Body Mass (% of 70-kg Adult)	Blood Flow (% of Cardiac Output)
Vessel-rich group	10	75
Muscle group	50	19
Fat group	20	6
Vessel-poor group	20	<1

Highly perfused tissues (brain, heart, kidneys) in the adult account for <10% of body mass but receive 75% of the cardiac output (Table 4-4). As a result of the small mass and high blood flow, these tissues, known as ***vessel-rich group tissues***, equilibrate rapidly with the Pa. Indeed, after about three time constants, approximately 75% of the returning venous blood is at the same partial pressure as the PA. For this reason, uptake of a volatile anesthetic is decreased greatly after three time constants (5 to 15 minutes, depending on the blood solubility of the inhaled anesthetic), as reflected by a narrowing of the inspired-to-alveolar partial pressure difference. Continued uptake of anesthetic after saturation of vessel-rich group tissues reflects principally the entrance of anesthetic into skeletal muscles and fat. Skeletal muscles and fat represent about 70% of the body mass but receive only about 25% of the cardiac output (see Table 4-4). As a result of the large tissue mass, sustained tissue uptake of the inhaled anesthetic continues and the effluent venous blood is at a lower partial pressure than the PA. For this reason, the A-vD difference for anesthetic is maintained and uptake from the lungs continues, even after several hours of continuous administration of inhaled anesthetics.

The time for equilibration of vessel-rich group tissues is more rapid for neonates and infants than for adults. This difference reflects the greater cardiac output to vessel-rich group tissues in the very young as well as decreased solubility of anesthetics in the tissues of neonates. Furthermore, skeletal muscle bulk comprises a small fraction of body weight in neonates and infants.

Recovery from Anesthesia

Recovery from anesthesia is depicted by the rate of decrease in the P_{BRAIN} as reflected by the PA (Fig. 4-15).[32,33] The rate of washout of anesthetic from the brain should be rapid because inhaled anesthetics are not highly soluble in brain and the brain receives a large fraction of the cardiac output. Although similarities exist between the rate of induction and recovery, as reflected by changes in the PA of the inhaled anesthetic, there are important differences between the two events. In contrast to induction of anesthesia, which may be accelerated by the concentration effect, it is not possible to speed the decrease in PA by this mechanism (you cannot administer less than zero). Furthermore, at the conclusion of every anesthetic, the concentration of the inhaled anesthetic in tissues depends highly on the solubility of the inhaled drug and the duration of its administration. This contrasts with tissue concentrations of zero at the initiation of induction of anesthesia. The failure of certain tissues to reach equilibrium with the PA of the inhaled anesthetic during maintenance of anesthesia means that the rate of decrease of the PA during recovery from anesthesia will be more rapid than the rate of increase of the PA during induction of anesthesia (see Figs. 4-3 and 4-15).[32,33] Indeed, even after a prolonged anesthetic, skeletal muscles probably, and fat almost certainly, will not have equilibrated with the PA of the inhaled anesthetic. Thus, when the PI of an anesthetic is abruptly decreased to zero at the conclusion of an anesthetic, these tissues initially cannot contribute to the transfer of drug back to blood for delivery to the liver for metabolism or to the lungs for exhalation. As long as gradients exist between the Pa and tissues, the tissues will continue to take up anesthetic. Thus, during recovery from anesthesia, the continued passage of anesthetic from blood to tissues, such as fat, acts to speed the rate of decrease in the PA of that anesthetic. Continued tissue uptake of anesthetic will depend on the solubility of the inhaled anesthetic and the duration of anesthesia, with the impact being most

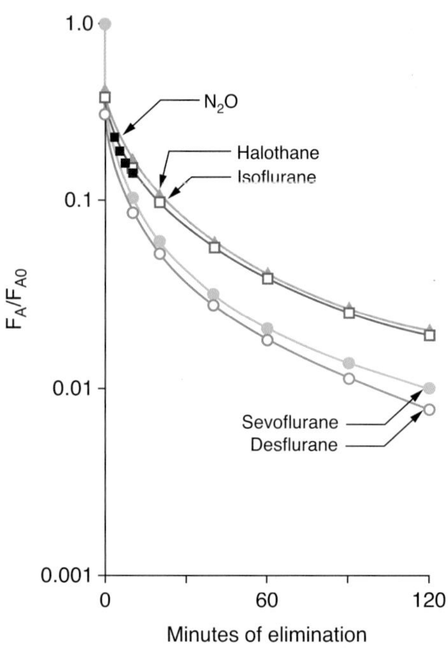

FIGURE 4-15 Elimination of inhaled anesthetics is defined as the ratio of the end-tidal anesthetic concentration (F_A) to the F_A immediately before the beginning of elimination (F_{AO}). The rate of decrease (awakening from anesthesia) in the F_A/F_{AO} is most rapid with the anesthetics that are least soluble in blood (nitrous oxide, desflurane, sevoflurane). (From Yasuda N, Lockhart SH, Eger EI, et al. Comparison of kinetics of sevoflurane and isoflurane in humans. *Anesth Analg.* 1991;72:316–324, with permission.)

important with soluble anesthetics.[49] For example, time to recovery is prolonged in proportion to the duration of anesthesia for soluble anesthetics (halothane and isoflurane), whereas the impact of duration of administration on time to recovery is minimal with poorly soluble anesthetics (sevoflurane and desflurane) (Fig. 4-16).[1]

Anesthetic that has been absorbed into the components of the anesthetic breathing system will pass from the components back into the gases of the breathing circuit at the conclusion of anesthesia and retard the rate of decrease in the PA of the anesthetic. Likewise, exhaled gases of the patient contain anesthetic that will be rebreathed unless fresh gas flow rates are increased (at least 5 L per minute of oxygen) at the conclusion of anesthesia.

In contrast to the rate of increase of the PA during induction of anesthesia, the rate of decrease in the PA during recovery from anesthesia is not entirely consistent with what might be predicted from the inhaled anesthetic's blood:gas partition coefficient (Fig. 4-17).[50,51] For example, the PA for halothane decreases more rapidly than that for isoflurane and enflurane despite the greater blood solubility of halothane. Similarly, the PA of methoxyflurane decreases below that of enflurane even though methoxyflurane is about six times more soluble in blood than is enflurane. The more rapid decrease in the PA for halothane and methoxyflurane is, in large part, due to the metabolism of these drugs in the liver[50,51] (see Chapter 2). This suggests that metabolism can significantly influence the rate of recovery from halothane and methoxyflurane anesthesia. In contrast, the rate of induction of anesthesia is not influenced by the magnitude of metabolism even for drugs such as halothane and methoxyflurane.

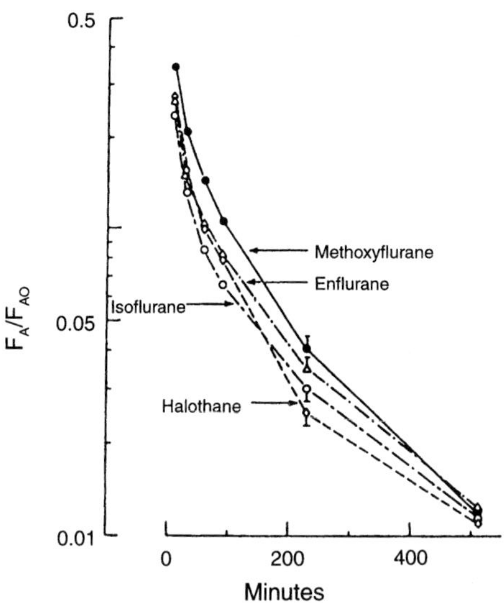

FIGURE 4-17 The decrease in the alveolar concentration is expressed as the ratio of the alveolar partial pressure at a given time (F_A) to the alveolar concentration present immediately before discontinuation of the administration of the anesthetic (F_{AO}). Unlike induction of anesthesia, the rate of decrease in anesthetic concentrations during recovery from anesthesia does not precisely follow predictions based on blood:gas partition coefficients of halothane and methoxyflurane due to the influence of metabolism of these drugs. (From Carpenter RL, Eger EI, Johnson BH, et al. Pharmacokinetics of inhaled anesthetics in humans: measurements during and after the simultaneous administration of enflurane, halothane, isoflurane, methoxyflurane, and nitrous oxide. *Anesth Analg.* 1986;65:575–582, with permission.)

Context-Sensitive Half-Time

The pharmacokinetics of the elimination of inhaled anesthetics depends on the length of administration and the blood-gas solubility of the inhaled anesthetic. As with injected anesthetics, it is possible to use computer simulations to determine context-sensitive half-times for volatile anesthetics. In this regard, the time needed for a 50% decrease in anesthetic concentration of enflurane, isoflurane, desflurane, and sevoflurane is <5 minutes and does not increase significantly with increasing duration of anesthesia.[52] Presumably, this is a reflection of the initial phase of elimination, which is primarily a function of alveolar ventilation. Determination of other decrement times (80% and 90%) reveals differences between various inhaled anesthetics. For example, the 80% decrement times of desflurane and sevoflurane are <8 minutes and do not increase significantly with the duration of anesthesia, whereas 80% decrement times for enflurane and isoflurane increase significantly after about 60 minutes, reaching plateaus of approximately 30 to 35 minutes. The 90% decrement time of desflurane increases slightly from 5 minutes after 30 minutes of anesthesia to 14 minutes after 6 hours of anesthesia, which is significantly less than sevoflurane (65 minutes), isoflurane (86 minutes), and enflurane (100 minutes) after 6 hours of administration. Based on the simulated context-sensitive half-times and assuming that MAC-awake is 0.5 MAC, there would be little difference in recovery time among these volatile anesthetics when a pure inhalation anesthetic technique is

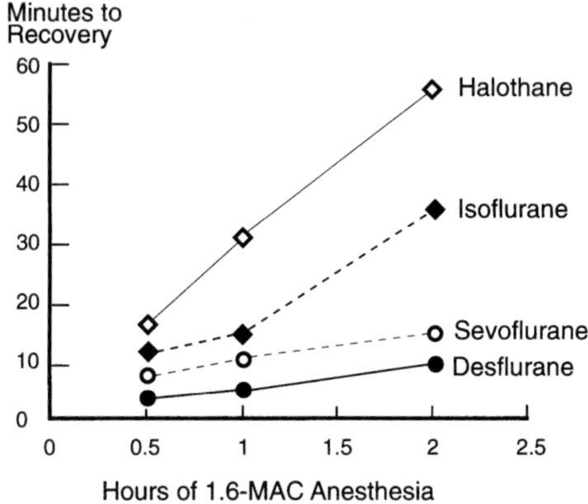

FIGURE 4-16 An increase in the duration of anesthesia during a constant dose of anesthetic (1.6 MAC) is associated with increases in the time to recovery (motor coordination in an animal model), with the greatest increases occurring with the most blood-soluble anesthetics. (From Eger EI. *Desflurane [Suprane]: A Compendium and Reference.* Nutley, NJ: Anaquest, 1993:1–119, with permission.)

used. The major differences in the rates at which desflurane, sevoflurane, isoflurane, and enflurane are eliminated occur in the final 20% of the elimination process.

Diffusion Hypoxia

Diffusion hypoxia occurs when inhalation of nitrous oxide is discontinued abruptly, leading to a reversal of partial pressure gradients such that nitrous oxide leaves the blood to enter alveoli.[53] This initial high-volume outpouring of nitrous oxide from the blood into the alveoli can so dilute the PAO_2 that the PaO_2 decreases. In addition to dilution of the PAO_2 by nitrous oxide, there is also dilution of the $PACO_2$, which decreases the stimulus to breathe.[54] This decreased stimulus to breathe exaggerates the impact on PaO_2 of the outpouring of nitrous oxide into the alveoli. Outpouring of nitrous oxide into alveoli is greatest during the first 1 to 5 minutes after its discontinuation at the conclusion of anesthesia. Thus, it is common practice to fill the lungs with oxygen at the end of anesthesia to ensure that arterial hypoxemia will not occur as a result of dilution of the PAO_2 by nitrous oxide.

Pharmacodynamics of Inhaled Anesthetics

Minimal Alveolar Concentration

MAC of an inhaled anesthetic is defined as that concentration at 1 atmosphere that prevents skeletal muscle movement in response to a supramaximal painful stimulus (surgical skin incision) in 50% of patients.[55] MAC is an anesthetic 50% effective dose (ED_{50}). Immobility produced by inhaled anesthetics as measured by MAC is mediated principally by effects of these drugs on the spinal cord and only a minor component of immobility results from cerebral effects.[56] For example, in animals, MAC for isoflurane is 1.2% when delivered to the intact animal but delivery of inhaled anesthetic only to the brain results in isoflurane MAC increasing to nearly 3%.[57] Further evidence that MAC reflects effects of the inhaled anesthetics at the spinal cord is the observation that decerebration does not change MAC (Fig. 4-18).[58]

MAC is among the most useful concepts in anesthetic pharmacology as it establishes a common measure of potency (partial pressure at steady state) for inhaled anesthetics. This concept is used to provide uniformity in dosages of inhaled anesthetics, to establish relative amounts of inhaled anesthetics to reach specific endpoints (MAC_{awake}), and to guide the search for mechanisms responsible for mechanisms of anesthetic action.[59] A unique feature of MAC is its consistency varying only 10% to 15% among individuals. This small degree of pharmacodynamic variability for inhaled anesthetics is unique in pharmacology. The use of equally potent doses (comparable MAC concentrations) of inhaled anesthetics is mandatory for comparing effects of these drugs not only at the

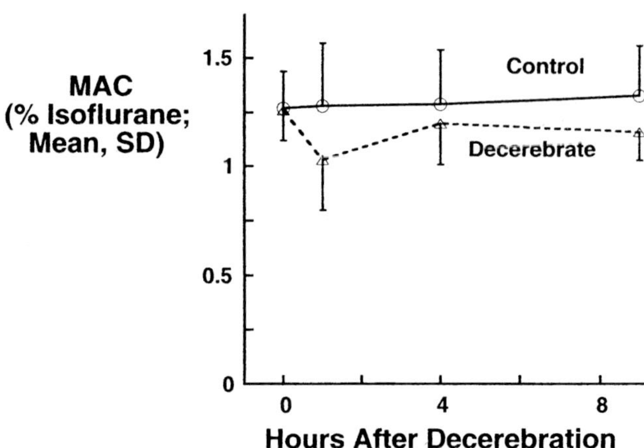

FIGURE 4-18 Decerebration does not change the minimum alveolar anesthetic concentration of isoflurane in rats confirming that the effects of volatile anesthetics on the spinal cord determine MAC. (From Rampil IJ, Mason P, Singh H. Anesthetic potency [MAC] is independent of forebrain structures in the rat. *Anesthesiology*. 1993;78:707–712, with permission.)

spinal cord but also at all other organs (Table 4-5). For example, similar MAC concentrations of inhaled anesthetics produce equivalent depression of the spinal cord, whereas effects on cardiopulmonary parameters may be different for each drug (see Chapter 2). This emphasizes that MAC represents only one point on the dose-response curve of effects produced by inhaled anesthetics and that these dose-response curves are not parallel. It is remarkable though that MAC_{awake}, the concentration of anesthetic that prevents consciousness in 50% of persons, is reliably about half of MAC and that MAC_{memory}, the concentration of anesthetic that is associated with amnesia in 50% of patients, is significantly less than MAC_{awake}. If this were not the case, an ED_{50} would not be satisfactory endpoint for clinical anesthesia! A surgeon may tolerate 50% of his or her patients moving but having 50% of patients have awareness under anesthesia would clearly not be acceptable.

Table 4-5

Comparative Minimum Alveolar Concentration of Inhaled Anesthetics

	MAC (%, 30 to 55 Years Old at 37°C, PB 760 mm Hg)
Nitrous oxide[a]	104
Halothane	0.75
Enflurane	1.63
Isoflurane	1.17
Desflurane	6.6
Sevoflurane	1.80
Xenon	63–71

[a] Determined in a hyperbaric chamber in males 21 to 55 years old.
MAC, minimum alveolar concentration

Factors that Alter Minimal Alveolar Concentration

Inhalation anesthetic requirements are remarkably uniform in humans, mainly being affected by age and body temperature. MAC allows a quantitative analysis of the effect, if any, of various physiologic and pharmacologic factors on anesthetic requirements (Table 4-6).[60,61] For example, increasing age results in a progressive decrease in MAC of about 6% per decade that is similar for all inhaled anesthetics (Figs. 4-19 and 4-20).[62,63] MAC is decreased nearly 30% during pregnancy and in the early

Table 4-6

Impact of Physiologic and Pharmacologic Factors on Minimum Alveolar Concentration

Increases in MAC
- Hyperthermia
- Excess pheomelanin production (red hair)
- Drug-induced increases in central nervous system catecholamine levels
- Cyclosporine
- Hypernatremia

Decreases in MAC
- Hypothermia
- Increasing age
- Preoperative medication
- Drug-induced decreases in central nervous system catecholamine levels
- α-2 agonists
- Acute alcohol ingestion
- Pregnancy
- Postpartum (returns to normal in 24–72 hours)
- Lithium
- Lidocaine
- Neuraxial opioids (?)
- Ketanserin
- Pao_2 <38 mm Hg
- Mean blood pressure <40 mm Hg
- Cardiopulmonary bypass
- Hyponatremia

No change in MAC
- Anesthetic metabolism
- Chronic alcohol abuse
- Gender
- Duration of anesthesia (?)
- $Paco_2$ 15–95 mm Hg
- Pao_2 >38 mm Hg
- Blood pressure >40 mm Hg
- Hyperkalemia or hypokalemia
- Thyroid gland dysfunction

MAC, minimum alveolar concentration.

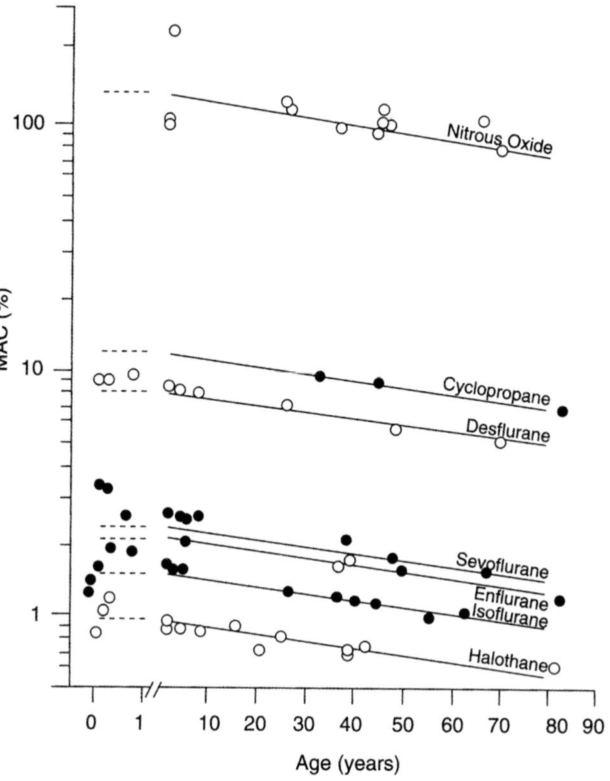

FIGURE 4-19 Effect of age on minimum alveolar concentration (MAC). (From Mapleson WW. Effect of age on MAC in humans: a meta-analysis. *Br J Anaesth.* 1996;76:179–185, with permission.)

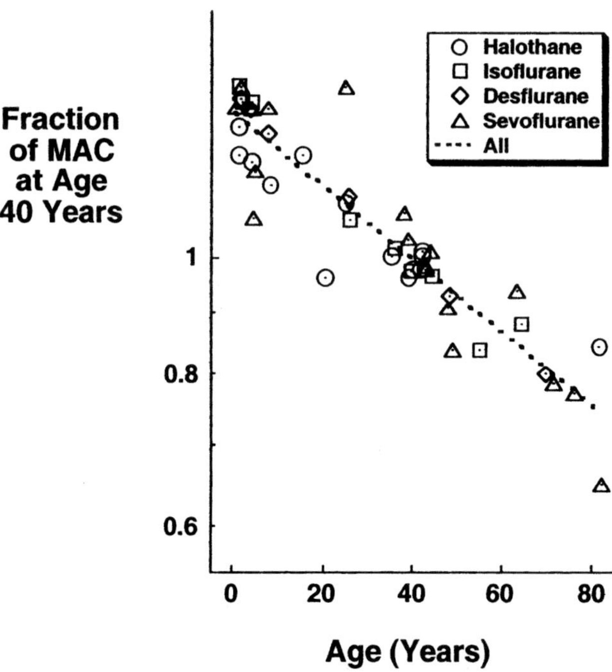

FIGURE 4-20 Minimum alveolar anesthetic concentration (MAC) (as a fraction of MAC at 40 years of age) with increasing age. (From Eger EI. Age, minimum alveolar anesthetic concentration, and minimum alveolar anesthetic concentration-awake. *Anesth Analg.* 2001;93:947–953, with permission.)

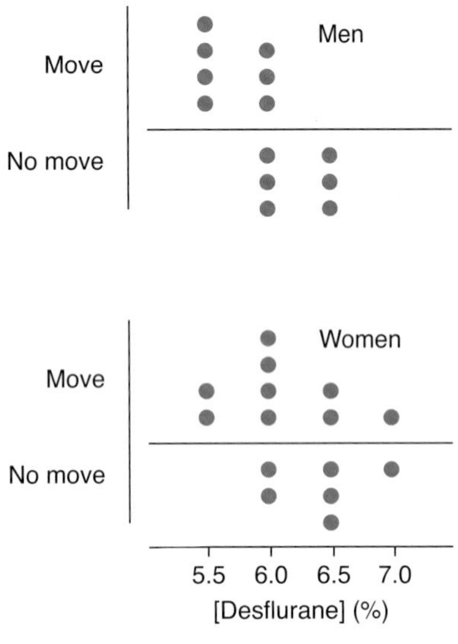

FIGURE 4-21 End-tidal concentrations of desflurane were tested for "Move" or "No move" in men and women. MAC for desflurane in men was 6.0% to 0.3% and in women it was 6.2% to 0.4%. P = 0.31 (mean − SD). (From Wadhwa A, Durrani J, Sengupta P, et al. Women have the same desflurane minimum alveolar concentration as men: a prospective study. *Anesthesiology*. 2003;99:1062–1065, with permission.)

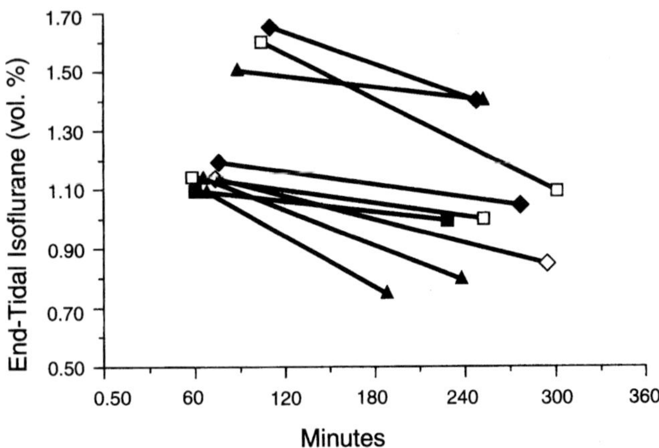

FIGURE 4-23 Preoperative (60 minutes) and postoperative (180 to 300 minutes) individual minimum alveolar concentration (MAC) determinations using continuous electrical stimulation (MAC tetanus). Each line represents an individual patient. (From Petersen-Felix S, Zbinden AM, Fischer M, et al. Isoflurane minimum alveolar concentration decreases during anesthesia and surgery. *Anesthesiology*. 1993;79: 959–965, with permission.)

postpartum period, returning to normal values in 12 to 72 hours.[64,65] Nevertheless, gender does not influence MAC (Fig. 4-21).[66,67] MAC is increased in women with natural red hair, presumably reflecting mutations of the melanocortin-1 receptor gene and increased pheomelanin concentrations (Fig. 4-22).[68] Although most reports describe MAC as independent of the duration of anesthesia, there is evidence that MAC for isoflurane decreases during the administration of anesthesia and the performance of surgery (Fig. 4-23).[69] The effect of cardiopulmonary bypass on MAC is uncertain, with some studies showing a decrease, whereas others fail to demonstrate any change.[47] Despite prolongation of sleeping times in animals, cyclosporine increases rather than decreases isoflurane MAC.[70] MAC is defined by the response to a surgical incision, which is considered to be a supramaximal stimulus. MAC values may vary with the type of stimulus; tetanic stimulation and trapezius squeeze are considered noninvasive stimulation patterns that are relatively equivalent to surgical skin incision, although in contrast to skin incision, these events can be repeated (Fig. 4-24).[71] Tracheal intubation requires the highest MAC to prevent skeletal muscle responses and may represent a true supramaximal stimulation (see Fig. 4-24).[71]

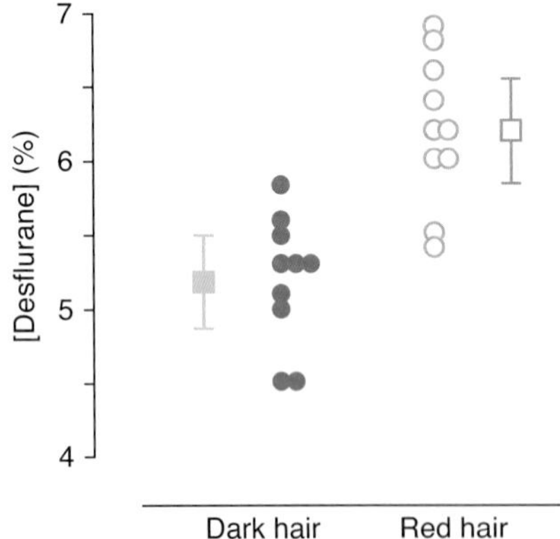

FIGURE 4-22 Anesthetic requirements for individual participants *(circles)* with group means *(squares)*. The desflurane requirement in redheads (6.2%) was significantly greater than in dark-haired women (5.2%) (From Liem ER, Lin C-M, Suleman M-I, et al. Anesthetic requirement is increased in redheads. *Anesthesiology*. 2004;101:279–283, with permission.)

MAC values for inhaled anesthetics are additive.[72] For example, 0.5 MAC of nitrous oxide plus 0.5 MAC isoflurane has the same effect at the brain as does a 1 MAC concentration of either anesthetic alone. The strict additivity of the interactions among inhaled anesthetics implies either a common site of action or that anesthetic action occurs with only a small fraction of the binding sites occupied.[73]

Opioids synergistically decrease anesthetic requirements for volatile anesthetics. For example, 25 minutes after the administration of fentanyl, 3 μg/kg or 6 μg/kg IV, MAC for desflurane is decreased 48% and 68%, respectively.[74] Similar decreases in isoflurane MAC are also produced by these doses of fentanyl.[75]

Dose-response curves for inhaled anesthetics, although not parallel, are all steep. This is emphasized by the fact that a 1 MAC dose prevents skeletal muscle movement in response to a painful stimulus in 50% of patients, whereas a modest increase to about 1.3 MAC prevents movement in at least 95% of patients.

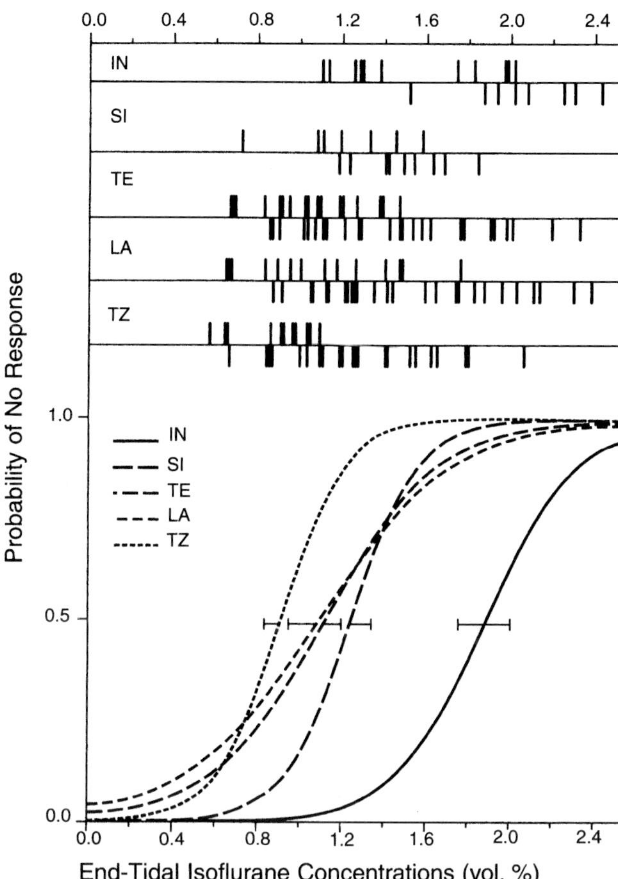

FIGURE 4-24 Responses (movement *[horizontal line above]*) or no movement *(horizontal line below)* to preoperative stimulation represented by tracheal intubation (IN), skin incision (SI), response to a continuous (tetanus) electrical stimulation (TE), direct laryngoscopy (LA), and trapezius muscle squeeze (TZ). The probability of response versus end-tidal isoflurane concentration is plotted. (From Zbinden AM, Maggiorini M, Peterson-Felix S, et al. Anesthetic depth defined using multiple noxious stimuli during isoflurane/oxygen anesthesia. I. Motor reactions. *Anesthesiology.* 1994; 80:253–260, with permission.)

Mechanisms of Anesthetic Action

Meyer-Overton Theory (Critical Volume Hypothesis)

Correlation between the lipid solubility of inhaled anesthetics (oil:gas partition coefficient) and anesthetic potency has historically been presumed to be evidence that inhaled anesthetics act by disrupting the structure or dynamic properties of the lipid portions of nerve membranes. For example, when a sufficient number of molecules dissolve (critical concentration) in crucial hydrophobic sites such as lipid cell membranes, there is distortion of channels necessary for ion flux and the subsequent development of action potentials needed for synaptic transmission. Likewise, changes in the lipid matrix produced by dissolved anesthetic molecules could alter the function of proteins in cell membranes, thus decreasing sodium conductance. Evidence supporting distortion of sodium channels by dissolved anesthetic molecules is the observation that high pressures (40 to 100 atm) partially antagonize the action of inhaled anesthetics (pressure reversal), presumably by returning (compressing) lipid membranes and their sodium channels to their "awake" contour.[76]

The most compelling evidence against the Meyer-Overton theory of anesthesia is the fact that effects of inhaled anesthetics on the fluidity of lipid bilayers is implausibly small and can generally be mimicked by temperature changes of 1°C.[77] Furthermore, not all lipid-soluble drugs are anesthetics, and, in fact, some are convulsants. For example, the observation that, among *n*-alcohols, dodecanol is anesthetic and decanol is not (for *n*-alkanes the cutoff is after octane) suggests that anesthetic binding to protein pockets or clefts and not lipid membranes is important in the mechanism of anesthesia. Based on these negative observations, lipid theories have been refined to postulate that specialized domains in membranes (boundary membranes surrounding proteins) are not only particularly sensitive to anesthetics but also are critical to membrane function. Indeed, either binding to proteins or dissolving in lipids can account for the Meyer-Overton correlation.

Stereoselectivity

The effects of inhaled anesthetics on ion channels responsible for neuronal action are readily demonstrated (Fig. 4-25).[77] The most definitive evidence that general anesthetics act by binding directly to proteins and not a lipid bilayer comes from observations of stereoselectivity.[78] Inhalation anesthetics exist as isomers, and isoflurane has been shown to act stereoselectively on neuronal channels, with the levoisomer being more potent than the

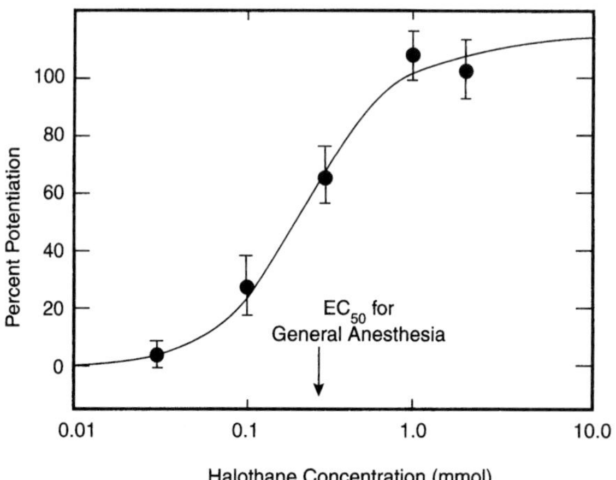

FIGURE 4-25 Clinically relevant concentrations of halothane (0.23 mmol is near the EC_{50} for anesthesia) potentiate responses to low levels of γ-aminobutyric acid in dissociated rat brain neurons. (From Franks NP, Lieb WR. Molecular and cellular mechanisms of general anesthesia. *Nature.* 1994;367:607–614, with permission.)

dextroisomer in enhancing potassium conductance in neurons[79] and in with respect to the loss of righting reflex in animals.[80] The relevance to anesthetic mechanisms of the differing effects of enantiomers of volatile anesthetics on in vitro nerve conduction would be supported by parallel changes in MAC in the intact animal. Indeed, in rats, MAC for the levoisomer of isoflurane was 60% more potent than the dextroisomer.[81] In contrast, others have not found a significant difference in the effects of the enantiomers of isoflurane and desflurane on anesthetic effects in animals.[82] Receptor specificity is also suggested by conversion of an anesthetic to a nonanesthetic by increasing the molecular volume, despite corresponding increases in lipid solubility. Nevertheless, there is evidence that molecular shape (bulkiness) and size provide limited insight into the structure of the anesthetic site of action.[83]

Potential Mediators of Anesthetic Action

Ionotropic and Metabotropic Receptors

Neurotransmitters signal through two families of receptors designated as ionotropic and metabotropic. Ionotropic receptors are also known as ***ligand-gated ion channels*** because the neurotransmitter binds directly to ion channel proteins and this interaction causes opening (gating) of the ion channels allowing transmission of specific ions resulting in changes in membrane potential. Ionotropic receptors are often composed of several subunits. Indeed the γ-aminobuteric acid receptor type A ($GABA_A$) and nicotinic acetylcholine receptors are constructed from large families of evolutionarily related subunits that come together to make pleiomorphic receptors. In contrast, metabotropic receptors are usually monomeric receptors consisting of seven transmembrane segments. Binding of neurotransmitters (acetylcholine) to metabotropic receptors causes activation of guanosine triphosphate binding proteins (G proteins) associated with the receptors, and these G proteins act as second messengers to activate other signaling molecules such as protein kinases, or potassium or calcium channels.[56]

Inhaled anesthetics do not seem to stimulate the release of endogenous opioids and do not suppress ventilatory responses to surgical stimulation at concentrations that suppress movement. The fact that small doses of opioids decrease MAC reflects their ability to provide an effect (analgesia) that is not present with inhaled anesthetics alone.

Inhibitory Ligand-Gated and Voltage-Gated Channels (Glycine and $GABA_A$ Receptors)

Glycine receptors are major mediators of inhibitory neurotransmission in the spinal cord and may mediate part of the immobility produced by inhaled anesthetics.[84] Their spinal localization and potentiation by volatile anesthetics at clinical concentrations is consistent with their being a target for mediating immobility as defined by MAC. Intravenous and intrathecal administration of strychnine, a glycine receptor antagonist increases MAC. An argument in favor of a role for glycine receptor potentiation in mediating MAC is the fact that strychnine only reverses the effect of ketamine (which does not affect glycinergic currents) to a threshold while it affects dose dependent reversal of volatile anesthetic effect.

Although β3-subunit containing $GABA_A$ receptors mediate hypnosis and part of the immobility produced by injected anesthetics (propofol, etomidate),[85] there is evidence that $GABA_A$ receptors do not mediate immobility produced by inhaled anesthetics. In this regard, although $GABA_A$ receptors are potentiated at MAC concentrations of all clinically used volatile anesthetics, their enhancement of $GABA_A$ receptor activation minimally influences MAC.[86]

Glutamate (NMDA, AMPA, and Kainate Receptors)

Inhaled anesthetics decrease excitatory neurotransmission in the CNS. Glutamate is the principal excitatory neurotransmitter in the mammalian CNS. Glutamate receptors include G protein–coupled receptors and the ligand-gated receptors (NMDA, AMPA, and kainate). NMDA receptors may mediate some important behavioral effects of inhaled anesthetics. Volatile anesthetics separate into two different classes in terms of their efficacy for NMDA blockade. At 1 MAC concentration, different volatile anesthetics inhibit NMDA receptors by between 12% and 74% with those anesthetics having cation-π interactions having the greatest NMDA blockade.[87]

Two-Pore Potassium Channels

Two-pore potassium channels are intrinsic membrane receptor/ion channels that normally act to maintain the cell's resting potential and responds to internal stimuli such as a change in pH. Several members of this family have been recently found to be sensitive to volatile anesthetics at clinically used concentrations. TREK and TASK channel activity is potentiated by volatile anesthetics in an agent-specific manner.[88] TASK-3 receptors are an anesthetic sensitive receptor that play a role in maintaining theta oscillations in the EEG that are associated with anesthesia and natural deep sleep.[89]

Voltage-Gated Sodium Channels

Despite the historical notion that inhaled anesthetics do not block axonal conduction and thus voltage-dependent sodium channels, it is now clear that there are many subtypes of sodium channels. Although sodium channels that mediate axonal conduction are not significantly effected at MAC concentrations of volatile anesthetics, those that modulate the release of neurotransmitter may be more sensitive to anesthetics. There is evidence that by interacting with specific subtypes of sodium channel that are expressed at the presynaptic junction, these drugs can inhibit the release of neurotransmitters, particularly glutamate.[90] Indeed, intravenous administration of lidocaine, which is a nonspecific sodium channel blocker, decreases MAC.

Hyperpolarization-Activated Cyclic Nucleotide–Gated Channels

Hyperpolarization-activated cyclic nucleotide–gated (HCN) channels are voltage-gated ion channels that are expressed throughout the body but are particularly important in regulating rhythmogenicity in heart and brain. There is some suggestion that halothane may affect HCN channels in motor neurons to induce anesthetic immobility.[91]

Mechanism of Immobility

MAC is based on the characteristic ability of inhaled drugs to produce immobility by virtue of actions of these drugs principally on the spinal cord rather than on higher centers.[56] The observation that immobility during noxious stimulation does not correlate with electroencephalographic activity reflects the fact that cortical electrical activity does not control motor responses to noxious stimulation. Effects of inhaled anesthetics on the spinal cord leading to immobility are diverse. In this regard, inhaled anesthetics depress excitatory AMPA and NMDA receptor-mediated currents by actions independent of inhibitory $GABA_A$ and glycine receptor-mediated currents. Actions on two-pore potassium channels may also be important in producing immobility. Conversely, cholinergic receptors do not seem to exert a significant role in anesthetic-induced immobility at the spinal cord level.[92] Likewise, although opioids and stimulation of α_2 adrenergic receptors (clonidine) decrease MAC, it is unlikely that immobility produced by inhaled anesthetics is due to activation of these receptors.[66] Inhaled anesthetics do not act via opioid receptors. Overall, no inhaled anesthetic action on a single group of receptors yet described can explain immobility, and immobility as a result of concurrent actions on many receptors is unlikely.[56,93]

Mechanism of Anesthesia-Induced Unconsciousness

A comprehensive explanation of the mechanism by which volatile anesthetics cause loss of consciousness (suppression of awareness) is not known.[94] Hypnosis is typically studied in animal models as loss of righting reflex. In human studies, it can be measured as loss of response to command and in the presence of neuromuscular blockers the spared arm technique uses a tourniquet to block muscle relaxant access to an arm, which is then used to indicate consciousness. Subtle differences in the clinical effects of inhaled anesthetics may be attributed to distinct actions on a number of critical molecular targets. There is evidence that loss of consciousness (hypnosis), amnesia, and the response to skin incision (immobility as defined by MAC) are not a single continuum of increasing anesthetic depth but rather separate phenomena.[95,96] Combining these two observations, it has been proposed that general anesthesia is a process requiring a state of unconsciousness of the brain (produced by volatile or injected anesthetics) plus immobility in response to a noxious stimulus (surgical skin incision) that is mediated by the action of volatile anesthetics on the spinal cord administered at concentrations equivalent to MAC for that drug.

It has been proposed that clinical anesthesia is a hierarchical process in which afferent sensory impulses are diminished by some drugs (opioids, regional anesthesia, ketamine) while the central activating systems are depressed by another mechanism and sometimes other drugs (benzodiazepines, barbiturates, propofol, etomidate, ketamine and volatile anesthetics) and motor reflexes are depressed by yet another mechanism (volatile anesthetics, propofol, etomidate, barbiturates). As defined by MAC, only agents which depress motor reflexes in addition to the other actions can be properly considered general anesthetics but many agents are able to provide one or the other behavioral outcome and can be used as part of a general anesthetic regimen. Volatile anesthetics have been called ***total anesthetics*** because they can be used as a single agent to provide general anesthesia. It was long assumed that they decreased pain transmission, but after more thorough consideration, it appears that volatile anesthetics have a biphasic dose response for nociceptive influences such that they are increased at very low volatile anesthetic concentrations (about 10% MAC) and they diminish thereafter.[97]

Presynaptic inhibition of neurotransmitter release may explain how certain inhaled anesthetics can inhibit synaptic transmission. Inhibition of neurotransmitter release by inhaled anesthetics appears to be mediated by inhibition of neurosecretion rather than by inhibition of transmitter synthesis or storage. The mechanism by which anesthetics act to inhibit neurotransmitter release might reflect actions at ion channels that regulate the probability of neurotransmitter release or could act on the machinery of release itself. As mentioned earlier, halogenated volatile anesthetics inhibit some types of sodium channels in native neurons and in heterologous expression systems.[98] Although sodium channels can presynaptically modulate the release of both glutamate and GABA, their effect on the release of glutamate is greater than on the release of GABA.[99]

Comparative Pharmacology of Gaseous Anesthetic Drugs

Inhaled anesthetics evoke different pharmacologic effects at comparable percentages of MAC concentrations, emphasizing that dose-response curves for these drugs are not necessarily parallel. Measurements obtained from normothermic volunteers exposed to equal potent concentrations of inhaled anesthetics during controlled

Table 4-7

Variables that Influence Pharmacologic Effects of Inhaled Anesthetics

Anesthetic concentration
Rate of increase in anesthetic concentration
Spontaneous versus controlled ventilation
Variations from normocapnia
Surgical stimulation
Patient age
Coexisting disease
Concomitant drug therapy
Intravascular fluid volume
Preoperative medication
Injected drugs to induce and/or maintain anesthesia or skeletal muscle relaxation
Alterations in body temperature

ventilation of the lungs to maintain normocapnia have provided the basis of comparison for pharmacologic effects of these drugs on various organ systems.[100] In this regard, it is important to recognize that surgically stimulated patients who have other confounding variables may respond differently than healthy volunteers (Table 4-7).

Desflurane and sevoflurane provide one specific advantage over other currently available potent inhaled anesthetics.[4] Their lower blood and tissue solubility permit more precise control over the induction of anesthesia and a more rapid recovery when the drug is discontinued. Most of the other properties of these new volatile anesthetics resemble their predecessors, especially at concentrations of ≤1 MAC.

Central Nervous System Effects

Mental impairment is not detectable in volunteers breathing 1,600 ppm (0.16%) nitrous oxide or 16 ppm (0.0016%) halothane.[101] It is therefore unlikely that impairment of mental function in the personnel who work in the operating room using modern anesthetic scavenging techniques can result from inhaling trace concentrations of anesthetics. Reaction times do not increase significantly until 10% to 20% nitrous oxide is inhaled.[102]

Cerebral metabolic oxygen requirements are decreased in parallel with drug-induced decreases in cerebral activity. Drug-induced increases in cerebral blood flow may increase intracranial pressure (ICP) in patients with space-occupying lesions. The effects of desflurane and sevoflurane on the CNS do not differentiate these inhaled anesthetics from the older inhaled drugs.

Electroencephalogram

Volatile anesthetics in concentrations of <0.4 MAC similarly increase the frequency and voltage on the electroencephalogram (EEG). This enhancement is representative of the "excitement stage" of anesthesia. At about 0.4 MAC, there is an abrupt shift of high-voltage activity from posterior to anterior portions of the brain.[103] Cerebral metabolic oxygen requirements also begin to decrease abruptly at about 0.4 MAC. It is likely that these changes reflect a transition from wakefulness to unconsciousness. Furthermore, amnesia probably occurs at this dose of volatile anesthetic. As the dose of volatile anesthetic approaches 1 MAC, the frequency on the EEG decreases and maximum voltage occurs. During administration of isoflurane, burst suppression appears on the EEG at about 1.5 MAC, and at 2 MAC, electrical silence predominates.[104] Electrical silence does not occur with enflurane, and only unacceptably high concentrations of halothane (>3.5 MAC) produce this effect. The effects of nitrous oxide on the EEG are similar to those produced by volatile anesthetics. Slower frequency and higher voltage develop on the EEG as the dose of nitrous oxide is increased or when nitrous oxide is added to a volatile anesthetic to provide a greater total MAC concentration.

Desflurane and sevoflurane cause dose-related changes in the EEG similar to those that occur with isoflurane.[4] With desflurane, the EEG progresses from an initial increase in frequency and lowering of voltage at low anesthetic concentrations to increased voltage at anesthetizing concentrations. Higher concentrations of desflurane produce decreasing voltage and increasing periods of electrical silence with an isoelectric EEG at 1.5 to 2.0 MAC. The addition of nitrous oxide to a given level of anesthesia with desflurane causes little or no change in the EEG.

Seizure Activity

Enflurane can produce fast frequency and high voltage on the EEG that often progresses to spike wave activity that is indistinguishable from changes that accompany a seizure. This EEG activity may be accompanied by tonic-clonic twitching of skeletal muscles in the face and extremities. The likelihood of enflurane-induced seizure activity is increased when the concentration of enflurane is >2 MAC or when hyperventilation of the lungs decreases the $Pa{CO_2}$ to <30 mm Hg. Repetitive auditory stimuli can also initiate seizure activity during the administration of enflurane. There is no evidence of anaerobic metabolism in the brain during seizure activity produced by enflurane. Furthermore, in an animal model, enflurane does not enhance preexisting seizure foci, with the possible exception being certain types of myoclonic epilepsy and photosensitive epilepsy.[105]

Isoflurane does not evoke seizure activity on the EEG, even in the presence of deep levels of anesthesia, hypocapnia, or repetitive auditory stimulation. Indeed, isoflurane possesses anticonvulsant properties; it is able to suppress seizure activity produced by flurothyl.[106] An undocumented speculation is that the greater MAC value for enflurane compared with its isomer, isoflurane, reflects the need for a higher concentration to suppress the stimulating effects of enflurane in the CNS.

Desflurane and sevoflurane, like isoflurane, do not produce evidence of convulsive activity on the EEG either at deep levels of anesthesia or in the presence of hypocapnia or auditory stimulation. Nevertheless, there are reports of pediatric patients with epilepsy and otherwise healthy adults who developed EEG evidence of seizure activity during sevoflurane anesthesia.[107,108] Sevoflurane can suppress convulsive activity induced with lidocaine.

The administration of nitrous oxide may increase motor activity with clonus and opisthotonus even in clinically used concentrations.[109] When nitrous oxide is administered in high concentrations in a hyperbaric chamber, abdominal muscle rigidity, catatonic movements of extremities, and periods of skeletal muscle activity may alternate with periods of skeletal muscle relaxation, clonus, and opisthotonus.[110] Although very rare, tonic-clonic seizure activity has been described after administration of nitrous oxide to an otherwise healthy child.[111] Animals suspended by their tails may experience seizures in the first 15 to 90 minutes after discontinuation of nitrous oxide but not of volatile anesthetics.[112] It is possible that these withdrawal seizures reflect acute nitrous oxide dependence. In patients, delirium or excitement during recovery from anesthesia that included nitrous oxide could reflect this phenomenon.

Evoked Potentials

Volatile anesthetics cause dose-related decreases in the amplitude and increases in the latency of the cortical component of median nerve somatosensory evoked potentials, visual evoked potentials, and auditory evoked potentials.[113,114] Decreases in amplitude are more marked than increases in latencies. In the presence of 60% nitrous oxide, waveforms adequate for monitoring cortical somatosensory evoked potentials are present during administration of 0.50 to 0.75 MAC halothane and 0.5 to 1.0 MAC enflurane and isoflurane.[115] Peri-MAC concentrations of desflurane (0.5 to 1.5 MAC) increasingly depress somatosensory evoked potentials in patients.[4] Even nitrous oxide alone may decrease the amplitude of cortical somatosensory evoked potentials.

Mental Function and Awareness

By definition, inhaled anesthetics cause loss of response to verbal command at MAC-awake concentrations. Subtle effects on mental function (learning) may occur at lower anesthetic concentrations (0.2 MAC).[116] Gaseous anesthetics may not be equally effective in preventing awareness. For example, 0.4 MAC isoflurane prevents recall and responses to commands, whereas nitrous oxide requires greater than 0.5 to 0.6 MAC to produce similar effects. Surgical stimulation may increase the anesthetic requirement to prevent awareness.

Cerebral Blood Flow

Volatile anesthetics produce dose-dependent increases in cerebral blood flow (CBF). The magnitude of this

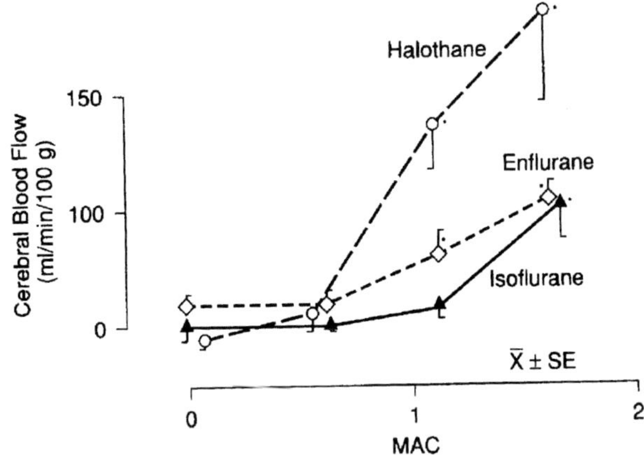

FIGURE 4-26 Cerebral blood flow measured in the presence of normocapnia and in the absence of surgical stimulation. (*P <.05.) (From Eger EI. *Isoflurane [Forane]: A Compendium and Reference.* 2nd ed. Madison, WI: Ohio Medical Products; 1985:1–110, with permission; Eger EI. Pharmacology of isoflurane. *Br J Anaesth.* 1984;56:71S–99S, with permission.)

increase is dependent on the balance between the drug's intrinsic vasodilatory actions and vasoconstriction secondary to flow-metabolism coupling. Volatile anesthetics administered during normocapnia in concentrations of >0.6 MAC produce cerebral vasodilation, decreased cerebral vascular resistance, and resulting dose-dependent increases in CBF (Fig. 4-26).[100] This drug-induced increase in CBF occurs despite concomitant decreases in cerebral metabolic requirements. Sevoflurane has an intrinsic dose-dependent cerebral vasodilatory effect but this effect is less than that of isoflurane.[117] Desflurane and isoflurane are similar in terms of increases in CBF and the preservation of reactivity to carbon dioxide (Fig. 4-27).[118] Nitrous oxide also increases CBF, but its restriction to concentrations of <1 MAC limits the magnitude of this change. In fact, nitrous oxide may be a more potent cerebral vasodilator than an equipotent dose of isoflurane alone in humans.[119]

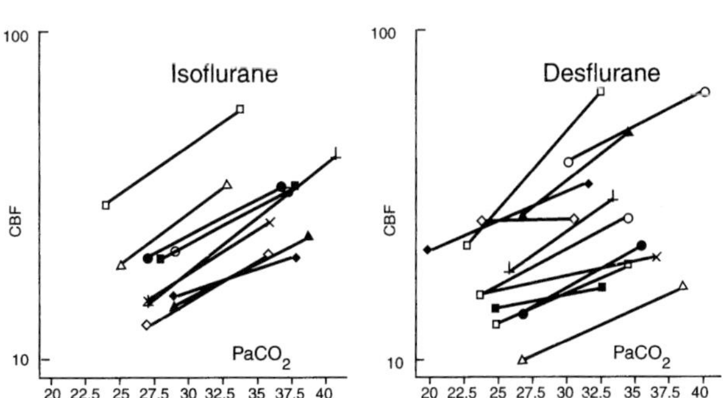

FIGURE 4-27 Individual cerebral blood flow (CBF) measurements (mL/100 g/min) plotted against $PaCO_2$ (mm Hg) in patients receiving 1.25 MAC isoflurane or desflurane. (From Ornstein E, Young WL, Fleischer LH, et al. Desflurane and isoflurane have similar effects on cerebral blood flow in patients with intracranial mass lesions. *Anesthesiology.* 1993;79:498–502, with permission.)

Anesthetic-induced increases in CBF occur within minutes of initiating administration of the inhaled drug and whether blood pressure is unchanged or decreased, emphasizing the cerebral vasodilating effects of these drugs. Animals exposed to halothane demonstrate a time-dependent return to baseline from the previously increased CBF beginning after about 30 minutes and reaching predrug levels after about 150 minutes.[120] This normalization of CBF reflects a concomitant increase in cerebral vascular resistance that is not altered by α- or β-adrenergic blockade and is not the result of changes in the pH of the cerebrospinal fluid.[121]

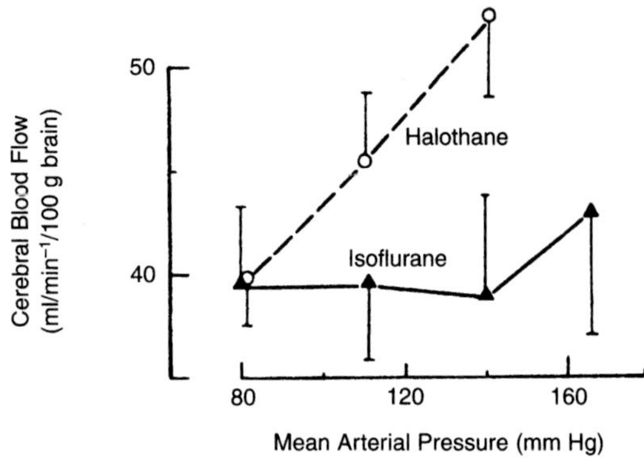

FIGURE 4-29 Autoregulation of cerebral blood flow (mean ± SE) as measured in animals. (From Eger EI. Pharmacology of isoflurane. *Br J Anaesth.* 1984;56:71S–99S, with permission.)

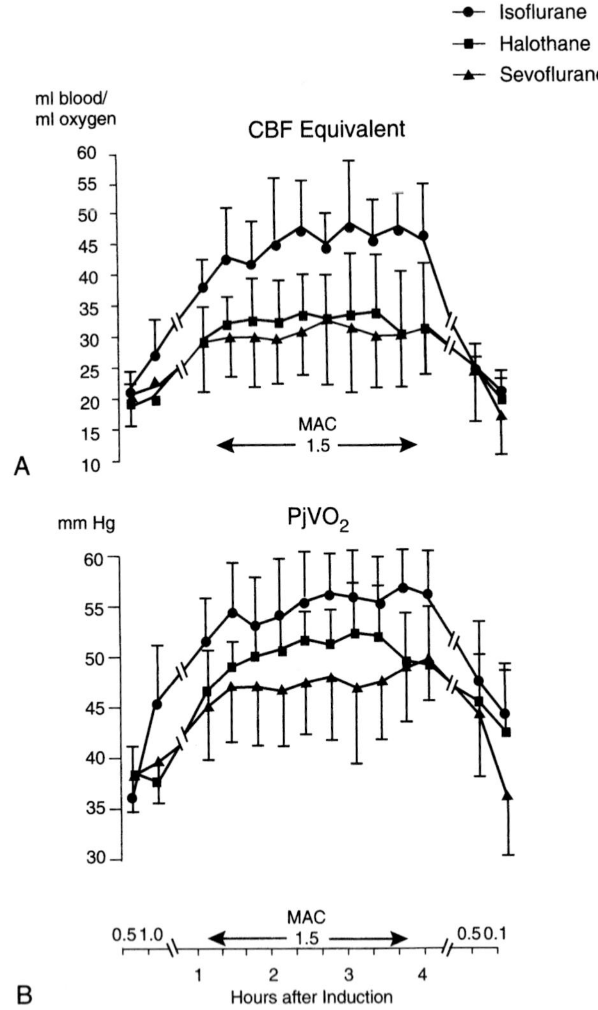

FIGURE 4-28 **A:** When compared at 1.5 MAC, the average increase in cerebral blood flow (CBF) in the patients receiving isoflurane is greater than in those receiving halothane or sevoflurane. **B:** Likewise, the average value of the internal jugular venous oxygen tension ($PjVO_2$) is higher in patients receiving isoflurane. The increased CBF present at 1.5 MAC was sustained over time. (From Kuroda Y, Murakami M, Tsuruta J, et al. Preservation of the ratio of cerebral blood flow/metabolic rate for oxygen during prolonged anesthesia with isoflurane, sevoflurane, and halothane in humans. *Anesthesiology.* 1996;84:555–561, with permission.)

Unlike the decay in CBF with time observed in animals, CBF remains increased relative to cerebral metabolic oxygen requirements for as long as 4 hours during administration of halothane, isoflurane, or sevoflurane to patients during surgery (see Fig. 4-26).[122] Furthermore, in these patients, isoflurane possesses greater capability to maintain global CBF relative to cerebral metabolic oxygen requirements than does halothane or sevoflurane (Fig. 4-28).[122] An unchanging EEG during this period suggests that CBF is increased over time without decay rather than a parallel change in CBF and cerebral metabolic oxygen requirements.

In animals, autoregulation of CBF in response to changes in systemic blood pressure is retained during administration of 1 MAC isoflurane but not halothane (Fig. 4-29).[100,123] Indeed, increases in systemic blood pressure produce smaller increases in brain protrusion during administration of isoflurane and enflurane compared with halothane.[123] It is speculated that loss of autoregulation during administration of halothane is responsible for the greater brain swelling seen in animals anesthetized with this drug. Inhaled anesthetics including desflurane and sevoflurane do not alter autoregulation of CBF as reflected by the responsiveness of the cerebral circulation to changes in $Paco_2$.[118,124,125] For example, cerebrovascular carbon dioxide reactivity is described as intact during administration of 1 MAC desflurane.[126] Nevertheless, others describe impairment of autoregulation by desflurane with 1.5 MAC nearly abolishing autoregulation.[127]

Cerebral Metabolic Oxygen Requirements

Inhaled anesthetics produce dose-dependent decreases in cerebral metabolic oxygen requirements that are greater during the administration of isoflurane than with an equivalent MAC concentration of halothane.[128] When the EEG becomes isoelectric, an additional increase in the concentration of the volatile anesthetics does not produce further decreases in cerebral metabolic oxygen requirements. The greater decrease in cerebral metabolic oxygen requirements produced by isoflurane may explain why CBF is not predictably increased by this anesthetic at concentrations lower than 1 MAC. For example, decreased cerebral metabolism means less carbon dioxide is produced, which thus opposes any increase in CBF. It is conceivable that isoflurane could evoke unexpected increases in CBF if administered to a patient in whom cerebral metabolic oxygen requirements were already decreased by drugs. Desflurane and sevoflurane decrease cerebral metabolic oxygen requirements similar to isoflurane.

Cerebral Protection

In animals experiencing temporary focal ischemia, there is no difference in neurologic outcome when cerebral function is suppressed by isoflurane or thiopental if systemic blood pressure is maintained.[129] In humans undergoing carotid endarterectomy, the CBF at which ischemic changes appear on the EEG is lower during administration of isoflurane than during enflurane or halothane (Fig. 4-30).[130] Although neurologic outcome is not different based on the volatile anesthetic administered, these data suggest that relative to enflurane and halothane, isoflurane may offer a degree of cerebral protection (blunts necrotic processes resulting from cerebral ischemia) from transient incomplete regional cerebral ischemia during carotid endarterectomy.[131] Unchanged CBF and decreased cerebral metabolic oxygen requirements during isoflurane-induced controlled hypotension for clipping of cerebral aneurysms indicates that global cerebral oxygen supply-demand balance is favorably altered in patients anesthetized with this anesthetic.[132]

Intracranial Pressure

Inhaled anesthetics produce increases in ICP that parallel increases in CBF produced by these drugs. Patients with space-occupying intracranial lesions are most vulnerable to these drug-induced increases in ICP. In hypocapnic humans with intracranial masses, desflurane concentrations of <0.8 MAC do not increase ICP, whereas 1.1 MAC increases ICP by 7 mm Hg.[133] Hyperventilation of the lungs to decrease the Pa_{CO_2} to about 30 mm Hg opposes the tendency for inhaled anesthetics to increase ICP.[134] With enflurane, it must be remembered that hyperventilation of the lungs increases the risk of seizure activity, which could lead to increased cerebral metabolic oxygen requirements and carbon dioxide production. These enflurane-induced changes will tend to increase CBF, which could further increase ICP. The ability of nitrous oxide to increase ICP is probably less than that of volatile anesthetics, reflecting the restriction of the dose of this drug to <1 MAC.

Cerebrospinal Fluid Production

Enflurane increases both the rate of production and the resistance to reabsorption of cerebrospinal fluid (CSF), which may contribute to sustained increases in ICP associated with administration of this drug.[135] Conversely, isoflurane does not alter production of CSF and, at the same time, decreases resistance to reabsorption.[136] These observations are consistent with minimal increases in ICP observed during the administration of isoflurane. Increases in ICP associated with administration of nitrous oxide presumably reflect increases in CBF, because enhanced production of CSF does not occur in the presence of this inhaled anesthetic.[137]

Circulatory Effects

Inhaled anesthetics produce dose-dependent and drug-specific circulatory effects. The circulatory effects of desflurane and sevoflurane parallel many of the characteristics

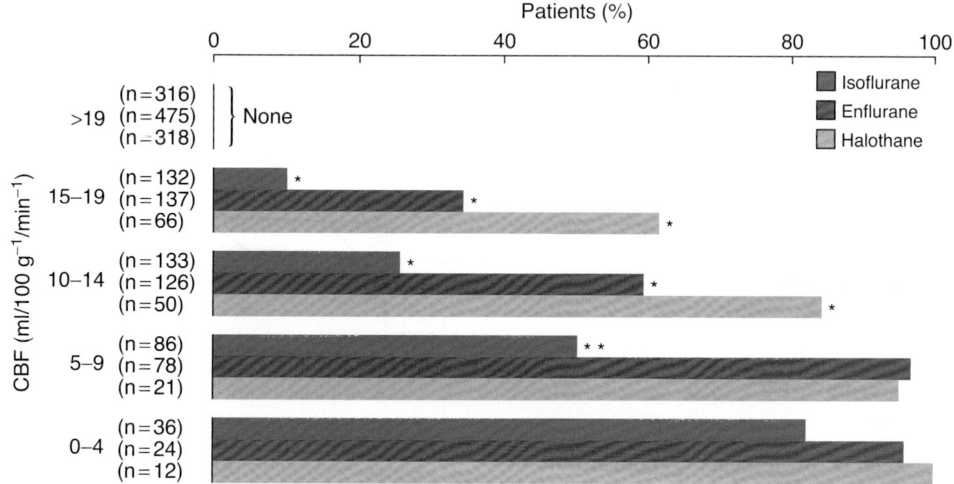

FIGURE 4-30 The number of patients (%) manifesting signs of cerebral ischemia on the electroencephalogram during administration of different volatile anesthetics and various ranges of cerebral blood flow (CBF). *, Significantly different from each other; **, significantly different from the other two. (From Michenfelder JD, Sundt TM, Fode N, et al. Isoflurane when compared to enflurane and halothane decreases the frequency of cerebral ischemia during carotid endarterectomy. *Anesthesiology.* 1987;67:336–340, with permission.)

of older inhaled anesthetics with desflurane most closely resembling isoflurane, whereas sevoflurane has characteristics of both isoflurane and halothane.[4,138]

Drug-induced circulatory effects manifest as changes in systemic blood pressure, heart rate, cardiac output, stroke volume, right atrial pressure, systemic vascular resistance, cardiac rhythm, and coronary blood flow. Circulatory effects of inhaled anesthetics may be different in the presence of (a) controlled ventilation of the lungs compared with spontaneous breathing, (b) preexisting cardiac disease, or (c) drugs that act directly or indirectly on the heart. The mechanisms of circulatory effects are diverse but often reflect the effects of inhaled anesthetics on (a) myocardial contractility, (b) peripheral vascular smooth muscle tone, and (c) autonomic nervous system activity (see the section "Mechanisms of Circulatory Effects").

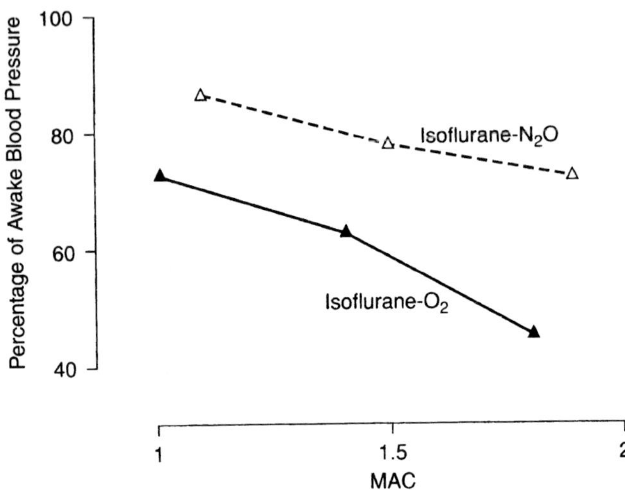

FIGURE 4-32 The substitution of nitrous oxide for a portion of isoflurane produces less decrease in blood pressure than the same dose of volatile anesthetic alone. (From Eger EI. *Isoflurane (Forane): A Compendium and Reference.* 2nd ed. Madison, WI: Ohio Medical Products; 1985:1–110, with permission.)

Mean Arterial Pressure

Halothane, isoflurane, desflurane, and sevoflurane produce similar and dose-dependent decreases in mean arterial pressure when administered to healthy human volunteers (Fig. 4-31).[139] The magnitude of decrease in mean arterial pressure in volunteers is greater than that which occurs in the presence of surgical stimulation. Likewise, artificially increased preoperative levels of systemic blood pressure, as may accompany apprehension, may be followed by decreases in blood pressure that exceed the true pharmacologic effect of the volatile anesthetic. In contrast with volatile anesthetics, nitrous oxide produces either no change or modest increases in systemic blood pressure.[100,140] Substitution of nitrous oxide for a portion of the volatile anesthetic decreases the magnitude of blood pressure decrease produced by the same MAC concentration of the volatile anesthetic alone (Fig. 4-32).[100] The decrease in blood pressure produced by halothane is, in part or in whole, a consequence of decreases in myocardial contractility and cardiac output, whereas with isoflurane, desflurane, and sevoflurane, the decrease in systemic blood pressure results principally from a decrease in systemic vascular resistance (see the section "Mechanism of Anesthesia-Induced Unconsciousness").

Heart Rate

Isoflurane, desflurane, and sevoflurane, but not halothane, increase heart rate when administered to healthy human volunteers (Fig. 4-33).[139] Sevoflurane increases heart rate only at concentrations of >1.5 MAC, whereas isoflurane and desflurane tend to increase heart rate at lower concentrations. Heart rate effects seen in patients undergoing surgery may be quite different than those documented

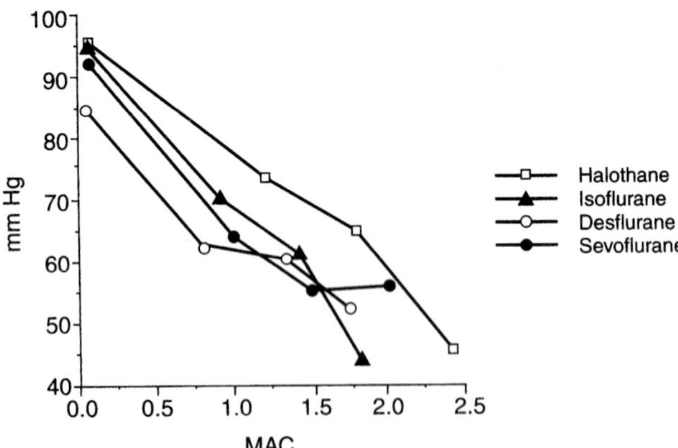

FIGURE 4-31 The effects of increasing concentrations (MAC) of halothane, isoflurane, desflurane, and sevoflurane on mean arterial pressure (mm Hg) when administered to healthy volunteers. (From Cahalan MK. *Hemodynamic Effects of Inhaled Anesthetics [Review Courses].* Cleveland, OH: International Anesthesia Research Society; 1996:14–18, with permission.)

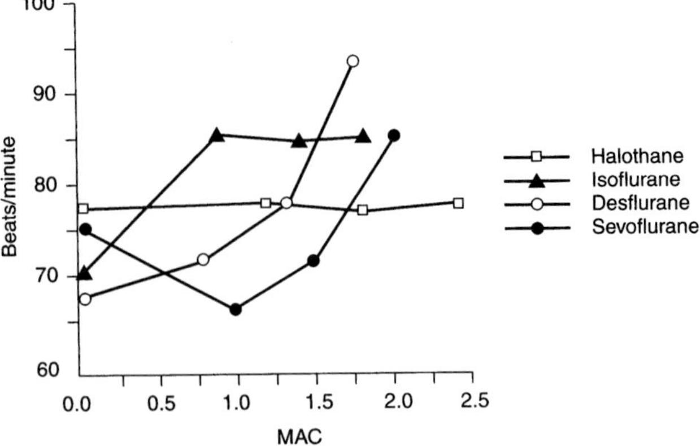

FIGURE 4-33 The effects of increasing concentrations (MAC) of halothane, isoflurane, desflurane, and sevoflurane on heart rate (beats/minute) when administered to healthy volunteers. (From Cahalan MK. *Hemodynamic Effects of Inhaled Anesthetics [Review Courses].* Cleveland, OH: International Anesthesia Research Society; 1996:14–18, with permission.)

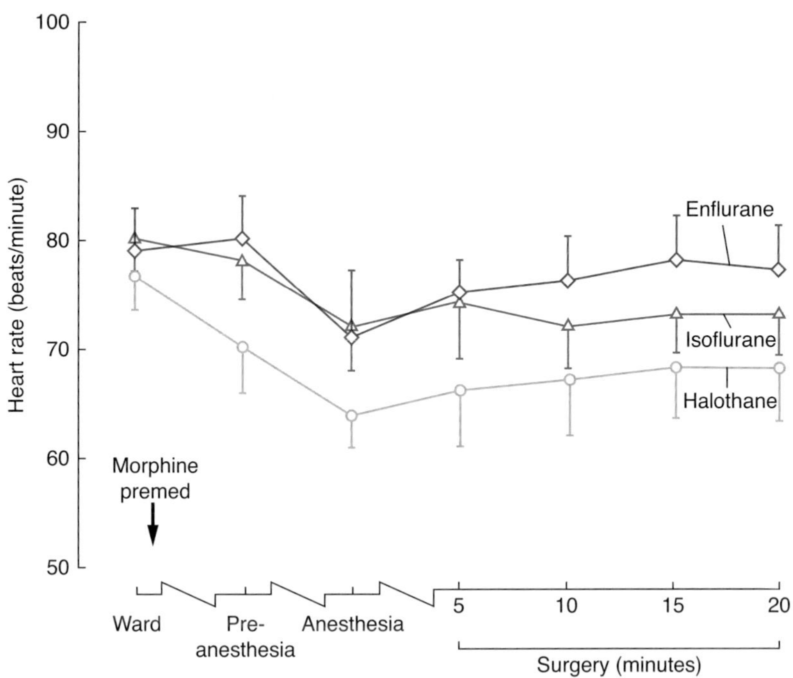

FIGURE 4-34 Morphine premedication is not associated with increases in heart rate (mean ± SE) during administration of volatile anesthetics with or without surgical stimulation. (From Cahalan MK, Lurz FW, Eger EI, et al. Narcotics decrease heart rate during inhalational anesthesia. *Anesth Analg*. 1987;66:166–170, with permission.)

in volunteers because so many confounding variables influence heart rate. For example, a small dose of opioid (morphine in the preoperative medication or fentanyl intravenously immediately before induction of anesthesia) can prevent the heart rate increase associated with isoflurane and presumably the other volatile anesthetics (Fig. 4-34).[141] Increased sympathetic nervous system activity, as accompanies apprehension, may artificially increase heart rate and the magnitude of the true pharmacologic effect of the volatile anesthetic. Similarly, excessive parasympathetic nervous system activity may result in unexpected increases in heart rate when anesthesia is established.

The common observation of an unchanged heart rate despite a decrease in blood pressure during the administration of halothane may reflect depression of the carotid sinus (baroreceptor-reflex response) by halothane, as well as drug-induced decreases in the rate of sinus node depolarization. Junctional rhythm and associated decreases in systemic blood pressure most likely reflect suppression of sinus node activity by halothane. Halothane also decreases the speed of conduction of cardiac impulses through the atrioventricular node and His-Purkinje system. At 0.5 MAC, desflurane produces decreases in systemic blood pressure similar to those caused by isoflurane but does not evoke an increased heart rate as does isoflurane. This difference is not explained by disparate effects of these anesthetics on the baroreceptor-reflex response.[142] In neonates, administration of isoflurane is associated with attenuation of the carotid sinus reflex response, as reflected by drug-induced decreases in blood pressure that are not accompanied by increases in heart rate.[143] Heart rate responses during administration of isoflurane also seem to be blunted in elderly patients, whereas isoflurane-induced increases in heart rate are more likely to occur in younger patients and may be accentuated by the presence of other drugs (atropine, pancuronium) that exert vagolytic effects. Nitrous oxide also depresses the carotid sinus, but quantitating this effect is difficult because of its limited potency and its frequent simultaneous administration with other injected or inhaled drugs.

Cardiac Output and Stroke Volume

Halothane, but not isoflurane, desflurane, and sevoflurane, produces dose-dependent decreases in cardiac output when administered to healthy human volunteers (Fig. 4-35).[139] Sevoflurane did decrease cardiac output at 1 and 1.5 MAC, but at 2 MAC cardiac output had recovered to nearly awake values. Sevoflurane causes a

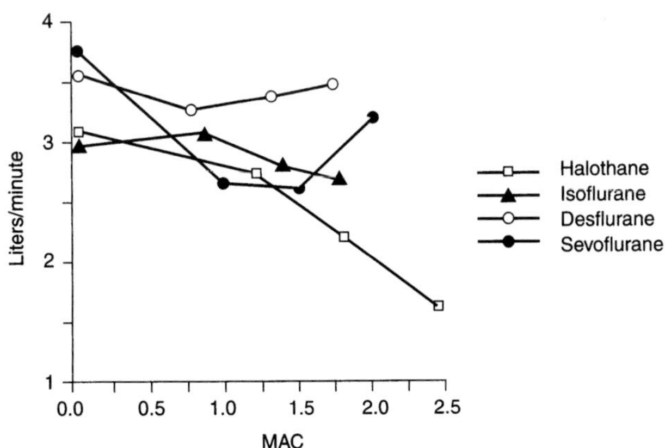

FIGURE 4-35 The effects of increasing concentrations (MAC) of halothane, isoflurane, desflurane, and sevoflurane on cardiac index (Liters per minute) when administered to healthy volunteers. (From Cahalan MK. *Hemodynamic Effects of Inhaled Anesthetics [Review Courses]*. Cleveland, OH: International Anesthesia Research Society; 1996:14–18, with permission.)

smaller decrease in cardiac output than does halothane when administered to infants.[144] Due to different effects on heart rate (halothane causes no change and heart rate increases in the presence of the other volatile anesthetics), the calculated left ventricular stroke volume was similarly decreased 15% to 30% for all the volatile anesthetics. In patients, the increase in heart rate may tend to offset drug-induced decreases in cardiac output. Cardiac output is modestly increased by nitrous oxide, possibly reflecting the mild sympathomimetic effects of this drug.

In addition to better maintenance of heart rate, isoflurane's minimal depressant effects on cardiac output could reflect activation of homeostatic mechanisms that obscure direct cardiac depressant effects. Indeed, volatile anesthetics, including isoflurane, produce similar dose-dependent depression of myocardial contractility when studied in vitro using isolated papillary muscle preparations. The vasodilating effects of the ether-derivative volatile anesthetics make the direct myocardial depression produced by these drugs less apparent than that of halothane. Indeed, excessive concentrations of these drugs administered to patients can produce cardiovascular collapse. In vitro depression of myocardial contractility produced by nitrous oxide is about one-half that produced by comparable concentrations of volatile anesthetics. Direct myocardial depressant effects in vivo are most likely offset by mild sympathomimetic effects of nitrous oxide.

Another possible explanation for the lesser impact of isoflurane on myocardial contractility may be its greater anesthetic potency relative to that of halothane.[100] For example, the multiple of MAC times the oil:gas partition coefficient for halothane is 168 and 105 for isoflurane. The implication is that isoflurane may more readily depress the brain and thus, at a given MAC value, appear to spare the heart. Indeed, in animals, the lesser myocardial depression associated with the administration of isoflurane manifests as a greater margin of safety between the dose that produces anesthesia and that which produces cardiovascular collapse.[145]

Right Atrial Pressure

Halothane, isoflurane, and desflurane, but not sevoflurane, increase right atrial pressure (central venous pressure) when administered to healthy human volunteers (Fig. 4-36).[139] These differences are not predictable based on the many other similarities between sevoflurane, desflurane, and isoflurane. The peripheral vasodilating effects of volatile anesthetics would tend to minimize the effects of direct myocardial depression on right atrial pressure produced by these drugs. Increased right atrial pressure during administration of nitrous oxide most likely reflects increased pulmonary vascular resistance due to the sympathomimetic effects of this drug.[146]

Systemic Vascular Resistance

Isoflurane, desflurane, and sevoflurane, but not halothane, decrease systemic vascular resistance when administered to healthy human volunteers (Fig. 4-37).[139] Thus, although these four volatile anesthetics decrease systemic blood pressure comparably, only halothane does so principally by decreasing cardiac output. For example, the absence of changes in systemic vascular resistance during administration of halothane emphasizes that decreases in systemic blood pressure produced by this drug parallel decreases in myocardial contractility. The other volatile anesthetics decrease blood pressure principally by decreasing systemic vascular resistance. Nitrous oxide does not change systemic vascular resistance.

Decreases in systemic vascular resistance during administration of isoflurane principally reflect substantial (up to fourfold) increases in skeletal muscle blood flow.[147] Cutaneous blood flow is also increased by isoflurane. The implications of these alterations in blood flow may include (a) excess (wasted) perfusion relative to oxygen needs, (b) loss of body heat due to increased cutaneous

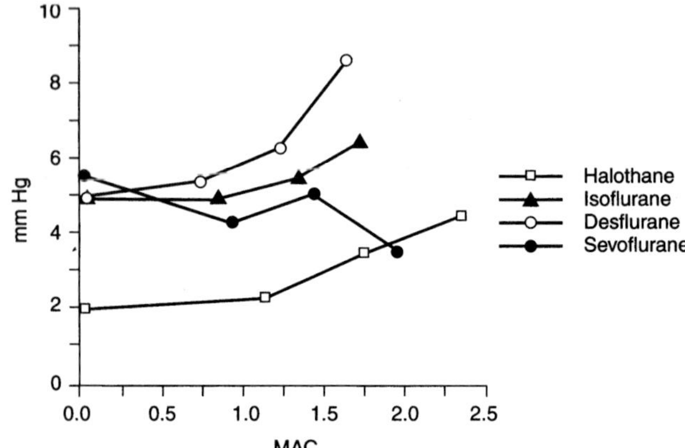

FIGURE 4-36 The effects of increasing concentrations (MAC) of halothane, isoflurane, desflurane, and sevoflurane on central venous pressure (mm Hg) when administered to healthy volunteers. (From Cahalan MK. *Hemodynamic Effects of Inhaled Anesthetics [Review Courses]*. Cleveland, OH: International Anesthesia Research Society; 1996:14–18, with permission.)

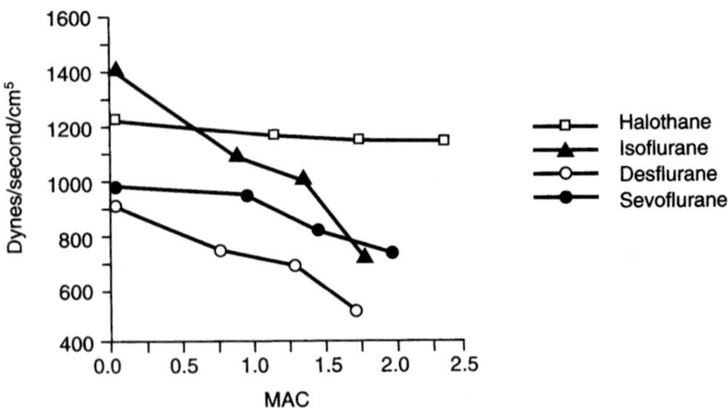

FIGURE 4-37 The effects of increasing concentrations (MAC) of halothane, isoflurane, desflurane, and sevoflurane on systemic vascular resistance (dynes/second/cm^5) when administered to healthy volunteers. [From Cahalan MK. *Hemodynamic Effects of Inhaled Anesthetics [Review Courses]*. Cleveland, OH: International Anesthesia Research Society; 1996:14–18, with permission.)

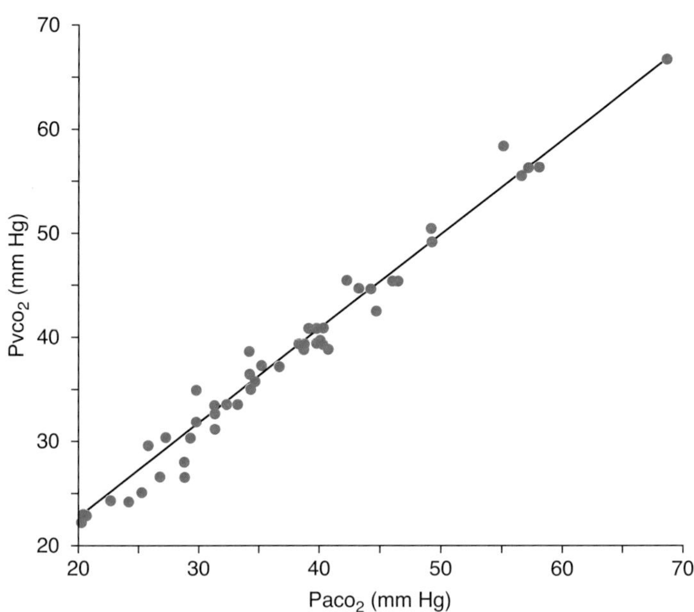

FIGURE 4-38 There is a linear relationship between $Pvco_2$ measured in "arterialized" peripheral venous blood and the $Paco_2$. (From Williamson DC, Munson ES. Correlation of peripheral venous and arterial blood gas values during general anesthesia. *Anesth Analg.* 1982;61: 950–952, with permission.)

blood flow, and (c) enhanced delivery of drugs, such as muscle relaxants, to the neuromuscular junction.

Failure of systemic vascular resistance to decrease during administration of halothane does not mean that this drug lacks vasodilating effects on some organs. Clearly, halothane is a potent cerebral vasodilator and cutaneous vasodilation is prominent. These vasodilating effects of halothane, however, are offset by absent changes or vasoconstriction in other vascular beds such that the overall effect is unchanged calculated systemic vascular resistance.

The increase in cutaneous blood flow produced by all volatile anesthetics arterializes peripheral venous blood, providing an alternative to sampling arterial blood for evaluation of pH and $Paco_2$ (Fig. 4-38).[148] These drug-induced increases in cutaneous blood flow most likely reflect a central inhibitory action of these anesthetics on temperature-regulating mechanisms. In contrast to volatile anesthetics, nitrous oxide may produce constriction of cutaneous blood vessels.[149]

Pulmonary Vascular Resistance

Volatile anesthetics appear to exert little or no predictable effect on pulmonary vascular smooth muscle. Conversely, nitrous oxide may produce increases in pulmonary vascular resistance that is exaggerated in patients with preexisting pulmonary hypertension.[150,151] The neonate with or without preexisting pulmonary hypertension may also be uniquely vulnerable to the pulmonary vascular vasoconstricting effects of nitrous oxide.[152] In patients with congenital heart disease, these increases in pulmonary vascular resistance may increase the magnitude of right-to-left intracardiac shunting of blood and further jeopardize arterial oxygenation.

Duration of Administration

Administration of a volatile anesthetic for 5 hours or longer is accompanied by recovery from the cardiovascular depressant effects of these drugs. For example, compared with measurements at 1 hour, the same MAC concentration after 5 hours is associated with a return of cardiac output toward predrug levels (Figs. 4-39 and 4-40).[153,154] After 5 hours, heart rate is also increased, but systemic blood pressure is unchanged, as the increase in cardiac output is offset by decreases in systemic vascular resistance.

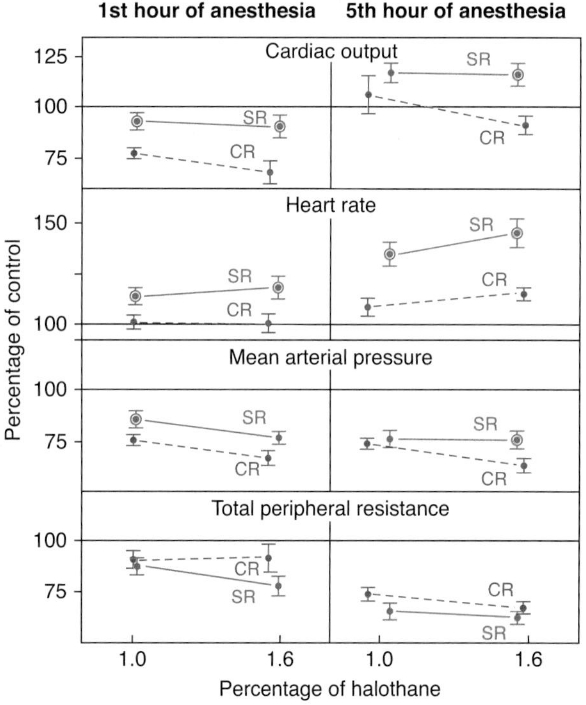

FIGURE 4-39 Comparison of circulatory effects of halothane during spontaneous breathing (SR) and controlled ventilation of the lungs (CR) after 1 and 5 hours of administration of halothane. (From Bahlman SH, Eger EI, Halsey MJ, et al. The cardiovascular effects of halothane in man during spontaneous ventilation. *Anesthesiology.* 1972;36:494–502, with permission.)

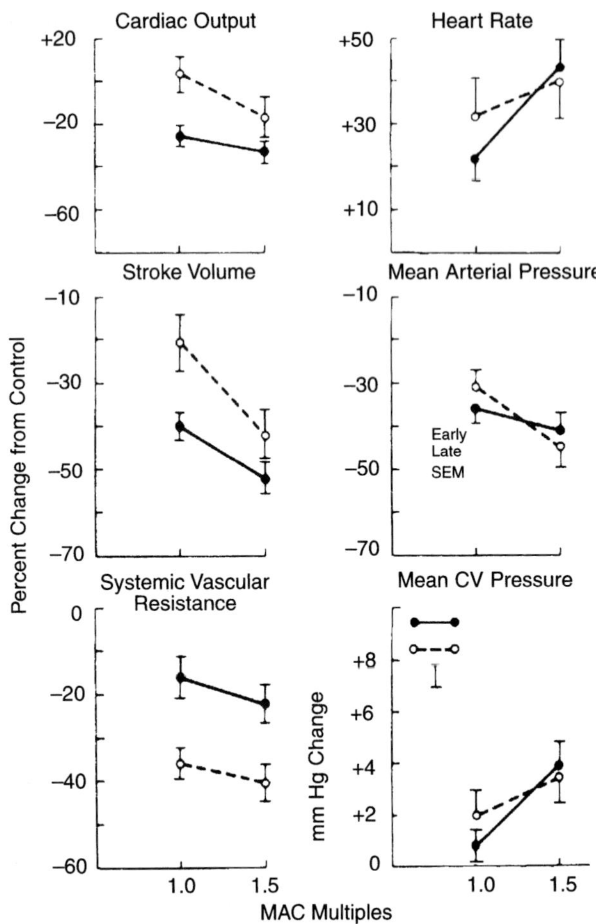

FIGURE 4-40 Comparison of circulatory effects of enflurane after 1 hour *(solid line)* and 6 hours *(broken line)* of administration during controlled ventilation of the lungs to maintain normocapnia. CV, cardiovascular. (From Calverley RK, Smith NT, Prys-Roberts C, et al. Cardiovascular effects of enflurane anesthesia during controlled ventilation in man. *Anesth Analg.* 1978;57:619–628, with permission.)

Evidence of recovery with time is most apparent during administration of halothane and is minimal during inhalation of isoflurane. Minimal evidence of recovery during administration of isoflurane (and presumably desflurane and sevoflurane) is predictable, because this drug does not substantially alter cardiac output even at 1 hour.

The return of cardiac output toward predrug levels with time, in association with increases in heart rate and peripheral vasodilation, resembles a β-adrenergic agonist response. Indeed, pretreatment with propranolol prevents evidence of recovery with time from the circulatory effects of volatile anesthetics.[155]

Cardiac Dysrhythmias

The ability of volatile anesthetics to decrease the dose of epinephrine necessary to evoke ventricular cardiac dysrhythmias is greatest with the alkane derivative halothane and minimal to nonexistent with the ether derivatives isoflurane, desflurane, and sevoflurane (Figs. 4-41 to 4-43).[156–158] In contrast to adults, children tolerate larger

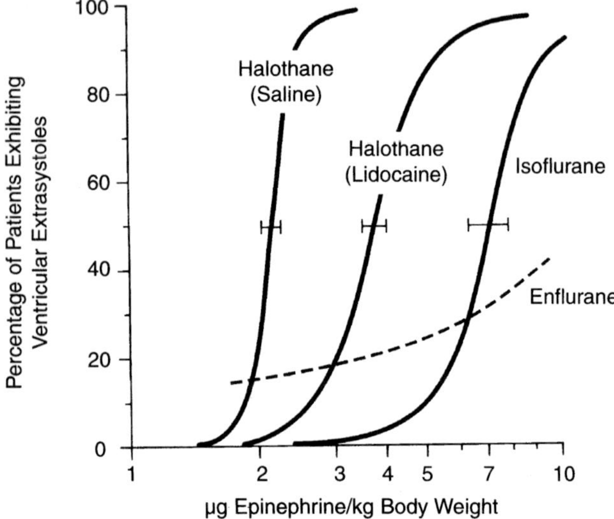

FIGURE 4-41 Percentage of patients developing ventricular cardiac dysrhythmias (three or more premature ventricular contractions [PVCs]) with increasing doses of submucosal epinephrine injected during administration of 1.25 MAC of halothane, isoflurane, or enflurane. (From Johnston PR, Eger EI, Wilson C. A comparative interaction of epinephrine with enflurane, isoflurane, and halothane in man. *Anesth Analg.* 1976;55:709–712, with permission.)

doses of subcutaneous epinephrine (7.8 to 10.0 μg/kg) injected with or without lidocaine during halothane anesthesia.[159,160] Mechanical stimulation associated with injection of epinephrine for repair of cleft palate has been associated with cardiac dysrhythmias.[160]

Inclusion of lidocaine 0.5% in the epinephrine solution that is injected submucosally nearly doubles the dose of epinephrine necessary to provoke ventricular cardiac dysrhythmias (see Fig. 4-41).[156] A similar response occurs

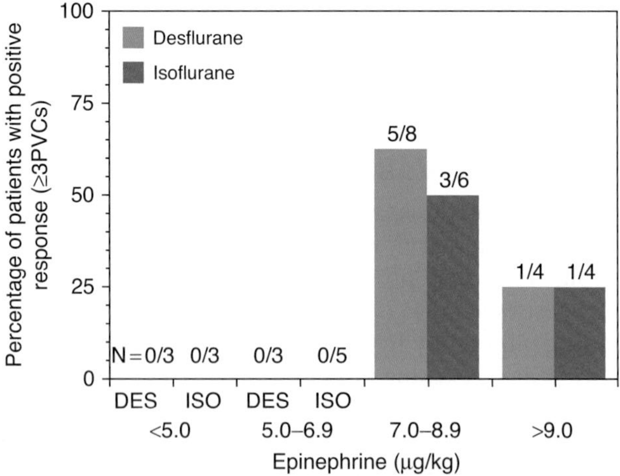

FIGURE 4-42 Responses to submucosally injected epinephrine in patients receiving desflurane (DES) or isoflurane (ISO) anesthesia. PVCs, premature ventricular contractions. (From Moore MA, Weiskopf RB, Eger EI, et al. Arrhythmogenic doses of epinephrine are similar during desflurane or isoflurane anesthesia in humans. *Anesthesiology.* 1993;79:943–947, with permission.)

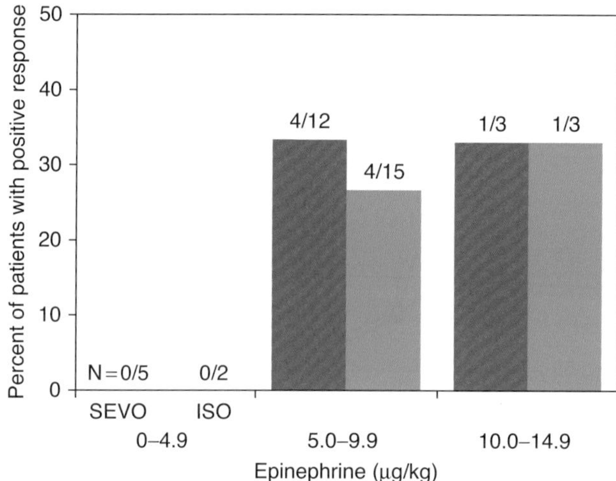

FIGURE 4-43 Responses to submucosally injected epinephrine in patients receiving sevoflurane (SEVO) or isoflurane (ISO) anesthesia. (From Navarro R, Weiskopf RB, Moore MA, et al. Humans anesthetized with sevoflurane or isoflurane have similar arrhythmic response to epinephrine. *Anesthesiology*. 1994;80:545–549, with permission.)

when lidocaine is combined with epinephrine injected submucosally during administration of enflurane.[161] Despite the apparent protective effect of lidocaine, the systemic concentrations of the local anesthetic are <1 μg/mL after its subcutaneous injection with epinephrine.[162]

In animals, enhancement of the arrhythmogenic potential of epinephrine is independent of the dose of halothane between alveolar concentrations of 0.5% and 2%.[163] If true in patients, it is likely that cardiac dysrhythmias due to epinephrine will persist until the halothane concentration decreases to <0.5%. For this reason, therapeutic interventions other than decreasing the inhaled concentration of halothane may be required to treat cardiac dysrhythmias promptly due to epinephrine.

The explanation for the difference between volatile anesthetics and the arrhythmogenic potential of epinephrine may reflect the effects of these drugs on the transmission rate of cardiac impulses through the heart's conduction system. Nevertheless, halothane and isoflurane both slow the rate of sinoatrial node discharge and prolong His-Purkinje and ventricular conduction times.[164]

QTc Interval

Halothane, enflurane, and isoflurane prolong the QTc interval on the ECG in healthy patients.[165] Nevertheless, similar changes may not occur in patients with idiopathic long QTc interval syndrome suggesting that generalizations from healthy patients to patients with long QTc interval syndrome may not be valid. Likewise, thiopental prolongs the QTc interval in healthy patients but has no effect in patients with long QTc syndrome. Conversely, there is a report of a patient with long QTc syndrome of prolongation of the QT interval in response to the administration of sevoflurane.[166] Furthermore, in healthy patients, administration of sevoflurane, but not propofol, results in prolongation of the QTc interval on the ECG.[167]

Accessory Pathway Conduction

Isoflurane increases the refractoriness of accessory pathways and the atrioventricular conduction system thus interfering with interpretation of postablative studies used to determine successful ablation. In contrast, sevoflurane has no effect on the atrioventricular or accessory pathways and is considered an acceptable anesthetic drug for patients undergoing ablative procedures.[168]

Spontaneous Breathing

Circulatory effects produced by volatile anesthetics during spontaneous breathing are different from those observed during normocapnia and controlled ventilation of the lungs. This difference reflects the impact of sympathetic nervous system stimulation due to accumulation of carbon dioxide (respiratory acidosis) and improved venous return during spontaneous breathing. In addition, carbon dioxide may have direct relaxing effects on peripheral vascular smooth muscle. Indeed, systemic blood pressure, and heart rate are increased and systemic vascular resistance is decreased compared with measurements during administration of volatile anesthetics in the presence of controlled ventilation of the lungs to maintain normocapnia (see Figs. 4-39 and 4-40).[153,169,170]

Coronary Blood Flow

Volatile anesthetics induce coronary vasodilation by preferentially acting on vessels with diameters from 20 μm to 50 μm, whereas adenosine, in addition, has a pronounced impact on the small precapillary arterioles.[171] It has been suggested that isoflurane as well as other coronary vasodilators (adenosine, dipyridamole, nitroprusside) that preferentially dilate the small coronary resistance coronary vessels would be capable of redistributing blood from ischemic to nonischemic areas, producing the phenomenon known as ***coronary steal syndrome***. Nevertheless, this phenomenon is not clinically significant and volatile anesthetics, including isoflurane, are cardioprotective (see the section "Cardiac Protection [Anesthetic Preconditioning]").

Neurocirculatory Responses

The solubility characteristics of desflurane make this volatile anesthetic a good choice to treat abrupt increases in systemic blood pressure and/or heart rate as may occur in response to sudden changes in the intensity of surgical stimulation. Nevertheless, abrupt increases in the alveolar concentrations of isoflurane and desflurane from 0.55 MAC (0.71% isoflurane and 4% desflurane) to 1.66 MAC (2.12% isoflurane and 12% desflurane) increase sympathetic nervous system and renin-angiotensin activity and cause transient increases in mean arterial pressure

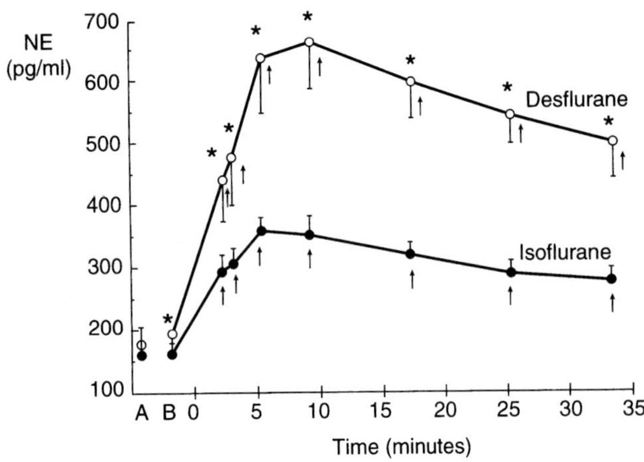

FIGURE 4-44 Plasma norepinephrine (NE) concentrations increased from awake levels *(A)* and those present during administration of 0.55 MAC desflurane or isoflurane *(B)* when the anesthetic concentrations were abruptly increased to 1.66 MAC *(0)*. The increase was greater in the presence of desflurane than isoflurane (*P <.05). Data are mean ± SE. (From Weiskopf RB, Moore MA, Eger EI, et al. Rapid increase in desflurane concentration is associated with greater transient cardiovascular stimulation than with rapid increases in isoflurane concentration in humans. *Anesthesiology*. 1994;80:1035–1045, with permission.)

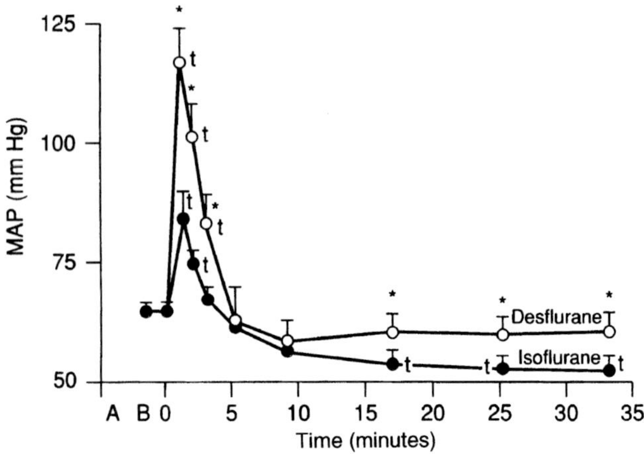

FIGURE 4-45 An abrupt and sustained increase in the concentration of desflurane from 0.55 MAC to 1.66 MAC *(0)* resulted in a substantial but transient increase in mean arterial pressure (MAP). A similar increase in isoflurane MAC produced an increase in MAP that was substantially less than that observed in patients receiving desflurane. Within 5 minutes after increasing the anesthetic concentration, the MAP had decreased below awake **(A)** and 0.55 MAC values **(B)** reflecting the greater depth of anesthesia present at this time. (t, P <.05 compared with the value at 0.55 MAC of the same anesthetic; *P <.05 compared with isoflurane at the same time point.) (From Weiskopf RB, Moore MA, Eger EI, et al. Rapid increase in desflurane concentration is associated with greater transient cardiovascular stimulation than with rapid increases in isoflurane concentration in humans. *Anesthesiology*. 1994;80:1035–1045, with permission.)

and heart rate (Figs. 4-44 to 4-46).[172] Desflurane causes significantly greater increases than isoflurane. The magnitude of the response to a rapid increase from 4% to 8% desflurane was similar to that produced by a rapid increase from 4% to 12%, suggesting that the stimulus provided by 8% desflurane produced a maximum response. Small (1%) increases in the desflurane concentration also transiently increase systemic blood pressure and heart rate, but the magnitude is less than those same changes that occur with an increase from 4% to 12%.[173] Sites mediating sympathetic nervous system activation in response to desflurane are present in the upper airway (larynx and above) and in the lungs.[174] These sites may respond to direct irritation. The increase in basal levels of sympathetic nervous system activity that accompany increasing inhaled concentrations of desflurane does not reflect the effects of drug-induced hypotension or alterations in baroreceptor activity.

In contrast to desflurane and isoflurane, neurocirculatory responses do not accompany abrupt increases in the delivered concentration of sevoflurane (Fig. 4-47).[175]

Fentanyl (1.5 to 4.5 μg/kg IV administered 5 minutes before the abrupt increase in desflurane concentration), esmolol (0.75 mg/kg IV 1.5 minutes before), and clonidine (4.3 μg/kg orally 90 minutes before) blunt the transient cardiovascular responses to rapid increases in desflurane concentration.[176] Fentanyl may be the most clinically useful of these drugs because it blunts the increase in heart rate and blood pressure, has minimal cardiovascular depressant effects, and imposes little postanesthetic sedation. Alfentanil, 10 μg/kg IV, in conjunction with the induction

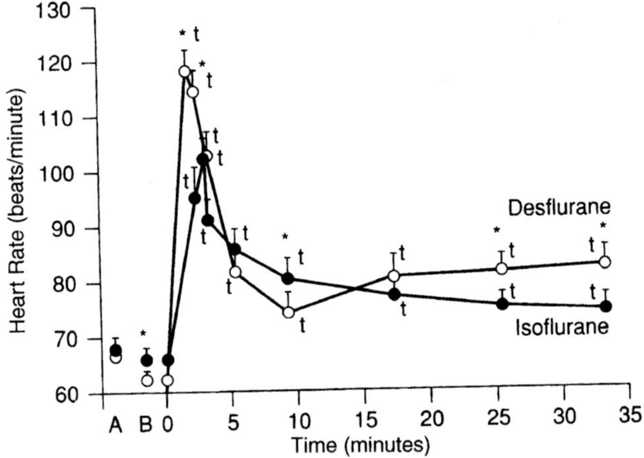

FIGURE 4-46 An abrupt and sustained increase in the concentration of desflurane from 0.55 MAC to 1.66 MAC *(0)* resulted in a substantial but transient increase in heart rate. A similar increase in isoflurane MAC produced an increase in heart rate that was substantially less than that observed in patients receiving desflurane. Within 5 minutes after increasing the anesthetic concentration, the heart rate remained above awake **(A)** and baseline values at 0.55 MAC **(B)**, reflecting the greater depth of anesthesia present at this time. (t, P <.05 compared with the value at 0.55 MAC of the same anesthetic; *P <.05 compared with isoflurane at the same time point.) (From Weiskopf RB, Moore MA, Eger EI, et al. Rapid increase in desflurane concentration is associated with greater transient cardiovascular stimulation than with rapid increases in isoflurane concentration in humans. *Anesthesiology*. 1994;80:1035–1045, with permission.)

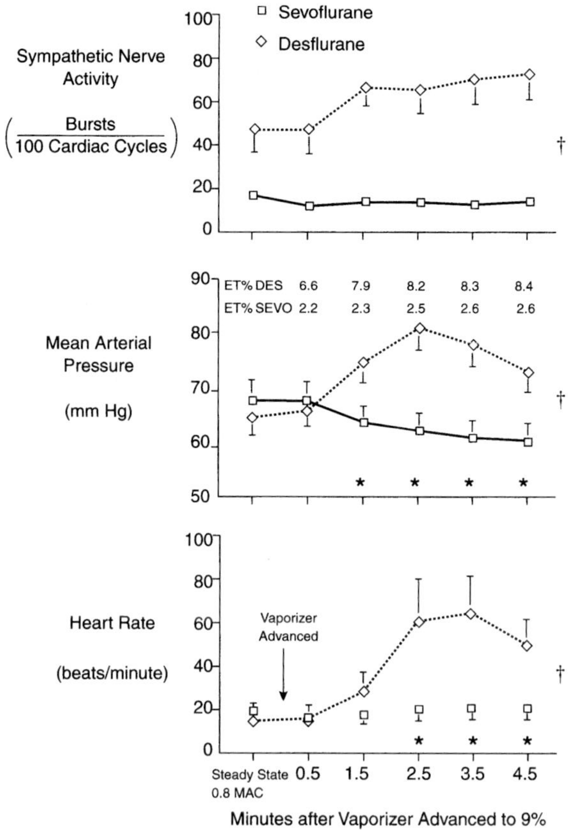

FIGURE 4-47 A rapid increase in the inspired concentration of sevoflurane (SEVO) from 0.8 MAC to 3% did not alter sympathetic nerve activity, mean arterial pressure, or heart rate. Conversely, a rapid increase in the inspired concentration of desflurane (DES) from 0.8 MAC to 9% significantly increased sympathetic nerve activity, mean arterial pressure, and heart rate. (Mean ± SE; *P <.05; ET, end-tidal.) (From Ebert TJ, Muzi M, Lopatka CW. Neurocirculatory responses to sevoflurane in humans: a comparison to desflurane. *Anesthesiology.* 1995;83:88–95, with permission.)

of anesthesia, also blunts the hemodynamic responses to an abrupt increase in the delivered concentration of desflurane; however, the increase in plasma norepinephrine concentrations that accompany the abrupt increase in desflurane concentration are not predictably prevented by the prior administration of opioids.[177]

Preexisting Diseases and Drug Therapy

Preexisting cardiac disease may influence the significance of circulatory effects produced by inhaled anesthetics. For example, volatile anesthetics decrease myocardial contractility of normal and failing cardiac muscle by similar amounts, but the significance is greater in diseased cardiac muscle because contractility is decreased even before administration of depressant anesthetics. Neurocirculatory responses evoked by abrupt increases in the concentration of desflurane may be undesirable in patients with coronary artery disease. In patients with coronary artery disease, administration of 40% nitrous oxide produces evidence of myocardial depression that does not occur in patients without heart disease.[178] Valvular heart disease may influence the significance of anesthetic-induced circulatory effects. For example, peripheral vasodilation produced by isoflurane (presumably also desflurane and sevoflurane) is undesirable in patients with aortic stenosis but may be beneficial by providing afterload reduction in those with mitral or aortic regurgitation. Arterial hypoxemia may enhance the cardiac depressant effects of volatile anesthetics. Conversely, anemia does not alter anesthetic-induced circulatory effects compared with measurements from normal animals.

Prior drug therapy that alters sympathetic nervous system activity (antihypertensives, β-adrenergic antagonists) may influence the magnitude of circulatory effects produced by volatile anesthetics. Calcium entry blockers decrease myocardial contractility and thus render the heart more vulnerable to direct depressant effects of inhaled anesthetics.

Mechanisms of Circulatory Effects

There is no known single mechanism that explains the cardiovascular depressant effects of volatile anesthetics, just as there is none for the neurobehavioral effects. Proposed mechanisms include (a) direct myocardial depression, (b) inhibition of CNS sympathetic activity, (c) peripheral autonomic ganglion blockade, (d) attenuated carotid sinus reflex activity, (e) decreased formation of cyclic adenosine monophosphate, (f) decreased release of catecholamines, and (g) decreased influx of calcium ions through slow channels. Indeed, negative inotropic, vasodilating, and depressant effects on the sinoatrial node produced by volatile anesthetics are similar to the effects produced by calcium entry blockers.[179] However, voltage-gated calcium channels are only inhibited to a small extent by inhalational anesthetics.[180] Plasma catecholamine concentrations typically do not increase during administration of volatile anesthetics except during the initiation of desflurane anesthesia and isoflurane anesthesia to some extent, which is evidence that these drugs do not activate and may even decrease activity of the central and peripheral sympathetic nervous systems.

Isoflurane may be unique among the volatile anesthetics in possessing mild β-adrenergic agonist properties. This effect is consistent with the maintenance of cardiac output, increased heart rate, and decreased systemic vascular resistance that may accompany administration of isoflurane.[147] A β agonist effect of isoflurane, however, is not supported by animal data that fail to demonstrate a difference between volatile anesthetics with or without β-adrenergic blockade.[181] The increase in blood pressure that is associated with rapid increases in desflurane concentration is accompanied by a significant increase in plasma epinephrine suggesting enhanced release from the adrenal gland.[176]

Nitrous oxide administered alone or added to unchanging concentrations of volatile anesthetics produces signs of mild sympathomimetic stimulation characterized by (a) increases in the plasma concentrations of catecholamines, (b) mydriasis, (c) increases in body temperature, (d) diaphoresis, (e) increases in right atrial pressure, and (f) evidence of vasoconstriction in the systemic and pulmonary circulations. It is presumed that this mild sympathomimetic effect masks any direct depressant effects of nitrous oxide on the heart. Nitrous oxide-induced increases in sympathetic nervous system activity may reflect activation of brain nuclei that regulate β-adrenergic outflow from the CNS.[182] Sympathetic nervous system stimulation may also result because nitrous oxide can inhibit uptake of norepinephrine by the lungs, making more neurotransmitter available to receptors.[183] Interestingly, nitrous oxide shares its sympathomimetic aspect with another NMDA blocking anesthetic, ketamine.

In contrast to sympathomimetic effects observed with the administration of nitrous oxide alone or added to volatile anesthetics, the inhalation of nitrous oxide in the presence of opioids results in evidence of profound circulatory depression, characterized by decreases in systemic blood pressure and cardiac output and increases in left ventricular end-diastolic pressure and systemic vascular resistance.[184,185] It is possible that opioids inhibit the centrally mediated sympathomimetic effects of nitrous oxide, thus unmasking its direct depressant effects on the heart.

Cardiac Protection (Anesthetic Preconditioning)

Brief episodes of myocardial ischemia occurring before a subsequent longer period of myocardial ischemia providing protection against myocardial dysfunction and necrosis is termed ischemic preconditioning (IPC).[186] The preconditioning protection seems to be mediated by release of adenosine, which binds to adenosine receptors and increases protein kinase C activity. The resulting phosphorylation of adenosine triphosphate (ATP) sensitive mitochondrial potassium channels (K_{ATP}) results in these channels being less sensitive to inhibition by ATP. These channels are important in regulating vascular smooth muscle tone by causing hyperpolarization and relaxation when oxygen delivery results in decreased ATP production. When K_{ATP} channel activity is increased, there is a decrease in the voltage gradient and decrease in calcium ion accumulation, the cardiac action potential shortens, accompanied by a mild negative inotropic action and remarkable protection against subsequent sustained ischemic or hypoxic insult. Opening of K_{ATP} channels is critical for the beneficial cardioprotective effects of IPC. Brief exposure to a volatile anesthetic (isoflurane, sevoflurane, desflurane) can activate K_{ATP} channels resulting in cardioprotection (anesthetic preconditioning) against subsequent prolonged ischemia and myocardial reperfusion injury that is identical to IPC.[187–191] Concentrations of isoflurane as low as 0.25 MAC are sufficient to precondition myocardium against ischemic injury, although higher doses may provide even greater cardiac protection.[192] Combined administration of isoflurane and morphine enhances protection against myocardial infarction to a greater extent than either drug alone.[193]

Reperfusion injury is defined as cellular injury that is caused by reperfusion itself and not the preceding ischemia. Manifestations of reversible reperfusion injury include cardiac dysrhythmias, contractile dysfunction ("stunning"), and microvascular injury.[194] In addition to myocardium, a similar effect induced by volatile anesthetics on vascular endothelium may result in protection from ischemia in other tissues. If anesthetic preconditioning is to be of clinical value, it will most likely be because it affords additional time before occurrence of dysfunction and/or infarction that will allow either spontaneous reperfusion or application of therapies such as angioplasty to relieve a coronary occlusion.[195] The preconditioning effects of volatile anesthetics may be beneficial in patients who are susceptible to myocardial infarction during and following surgery. Indeed, patients receiving sevoflurane for cardiac surgery (off-bypass or cardiopulmonary bypass) had less myocardial injury (lower release of troponin I) during the first 24 postoperative hours than patients receiving propofol (Figs. 4-48 and 4-49).[196,197] In patients undergoing coronary artery surgery with cardiopulmonary bypass, the cardioprotective effects of sevoflurane were clinically more apparent when this volatile anesthetic was administered throughout the operation compared with administration during only a part of the anesthetic (see Fig. 4-49).[198] Cardiac output was improved in patients receiving sevoflurane but not propofol suggesting better maintenance of myocardial function.

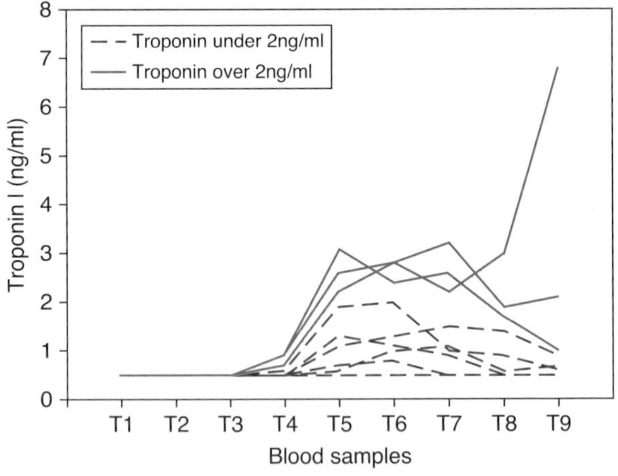

FIGURE 4-48 Cardiac troponin I concentrations in sevoflurane-anesthetized patients during and after anesthesia. Samples were obtained before induction of anesthesia (T1), before ischemia (T2), 15 minutes after reperfusion (T3), at arrival in the postanesthesia care unit (T4), and 3 (T5), 6 (T6), 12 (T7), 18 (T8), and 24 hours (T9) after arrival. (From Conzen PF, Fischer S, Detter C, et al. Sevoflurane provides greater protection of the myocardium than propofol in patients undergoing off-pump coronary artery bypass surgery. *Anesthesiology*. 2003;99:826–833, with permission.)

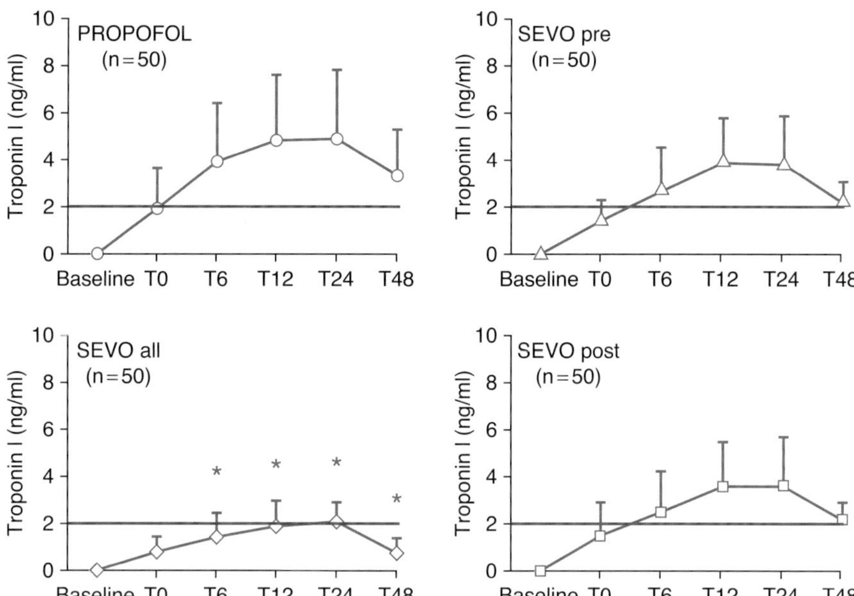

FIGURE 4-49 Cardiac troponin I concentrations in four patient groups before surgery (baseline), at arrival in the intensive care unit (T0), and after 6 (T6), 12 (T12), 24 (T24), and 48 (T48) hours. Mean ± SD. A transient increase in troponin I concentrations was observed in all groups. The increase in the SEVO (sevoflurane) group was significantly less than in the propofol group. (From DeHert, Van der Linden PJ, Cromheecke S, et al. Cardioprotective properties of sevoflurane in patients undergoing coronary surgery with cardiopulmonary bypass are related to its modalities of its administration. *Anesthesiology*. 2004;101:299–310, with permission.)

IPC is a fundamental endogenous protective mechanism against tissue injury (best characterized in the heart but also present in other tissues) ubiquitous to all species in which it has been studied. An early phase of IPC persists for 1 to 2 hours before disappearing and then reoccurring 24 hours. This second or late window of preconditioning may last for as long as 3 days.

Ventilation Effects

Inhaled anesthetics produce dose-dependent and drug-specific effects on the (a) pattern of breathing, (b) ventilatory response to carbon dioxide, (c) ventilatory response to arterial hypoxemia, and (d) airway resistance. The Pa_{O_2} predictably declines during administration of inhaled anesthetics in the absence of supplemental oxygen. Drug-induced inhibition of hypoxic pulmonary vasoconstriction as a mechanism for this decrease in oxygenation has not been confirmed during one-lung ventilation in patients breathing halothane or isoflurane. Changes in intraoperative Pa_{O_2} and the incidence of postoperative pulmonary complications are not different in patients anesthetized with halothane, enflurane, or isoflurane.[199]

Pattern of Breathing

Inhaled anesthetics, except for isoflurane, produce dose-dependent increases in the frequency of breathing.[200] Isoflurane increases the frequency of breathing similarly to other inhaled anesthetics up to a dose of 1 MAC. At a concentration of >1 MAC, however, isoflurane does not produce a further increase in the frequency of breathing. Nitrous oxide increases the frequency of breathing more than other inhaled anesthetics at concentrations of >1 MAC. The effect of inhaled anesthetics on the frequency of breathing presumably reflects CNS stimulation. Volatile anesthetics stimulate central respiratory chemoreceptor neurons likely through activation of THIK-1 receptors, a two-pore potassium channel that is responsible for a background potassium current.[201] Activation of pulmonary stretch receptors by inhaled anesthetics has not been demonstrated. The exception may be nitrous oxide, which, at anesthetic concentrations of >1 MAC, may also stimulate pulmonary stretch receptors.

Tidal volume is decreased in association with anesthetic-induced increases in the frequency of breathing. The net effect of these changes is a rapid and shallow pattern of breathing during general anesthesia. The increase in frequency of breathing is insufficient to offset decreases in tidal volume, leading to decreases in minute ventilation and increases in Pa_{CO_2}. There is evidence in patients that isoflurane produces a greater decrease in minute ventilation than does halothane (Fig. 4-50).[202] The pattern of breathing during general anesthesia is also characterized as regular and rhythmic in contrast to the awake pattern of intermittent deep breaths separated by varying intervals.

Ventilatory Response to Carbon Dioxide

Volatile anesthetics produce dose-dependent depression of ventilation characterized by decreases in the ventilatory response to carbon dioxide and increases in the Pa_{CO_2} (Fig. 4-51).[1] Desflurane and sevoflurane depress ventilation, producing profound decreases in ventilation leading to apnea between 1.5 and 2.0 MAC. Both of these volatile anesthetics increase Pa_{CO_2} and decrease the ventilatory response to carbon dioxide. Depression of ventilation produced by anesthetic concentrations up to 1.24 MAC desflurane are similar to the depression produced by isoflurane.[203]

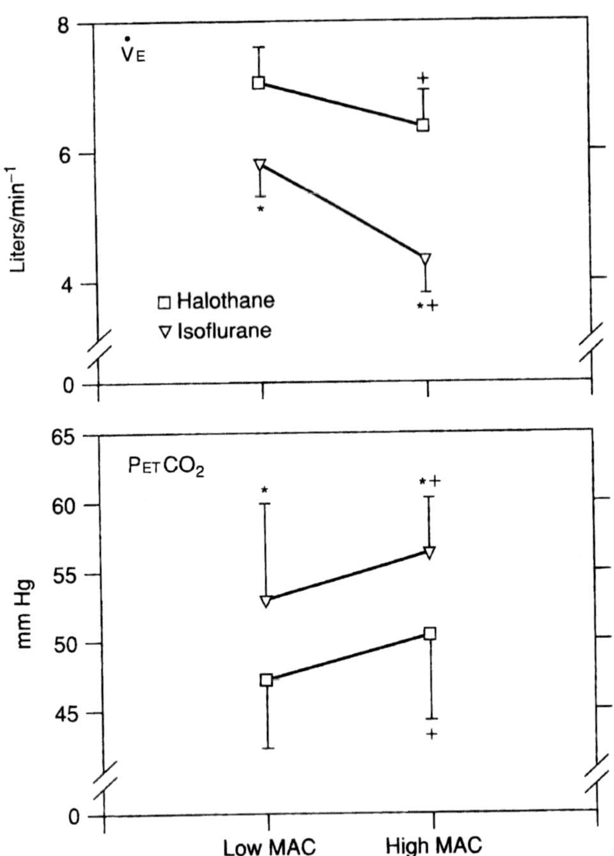

FIGURE 4-50 Minute ventilation ($\dot{V}_E$) and end-tidal carbon dioxide concentration ($P_{ET}CO_2$), as measured in volunteers breathing halothane or isoflurane in oxygen spontaneously at 1.2 (low) and 2.0 (high) MAC. (*P <.05 compared with halothane; +, P <.05 compared with low MAC.) (From Canet J, Sanchis J, Zegri A, et al. Effects of halothane and isoflurane on ventilation and occlusion pressure. *Anesthesiology.* 1994;81: 563–571, with permission.)

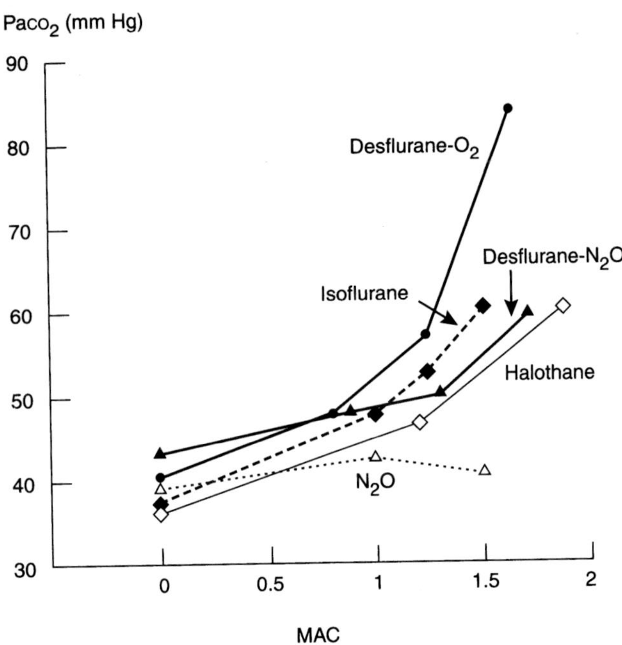

FIGURE 4-51 Inhaled anesthetics produce drug-specific and dose-dependent increases in $Paco_2$. (From Eger EI. *Desflurane [Suprane]: A Compendium and Reference.* Nutley, NJ: Anaquest; 1993:1–119, with permission.)

The presence of chronic obstructive pulmonary disease (COPD) may accentuate the magnitude of increase in $Paco_2$ produced by volatile anesthetics.[204] Nitrous oxide does not increase the $Paco_2$, suggesting that substitution of this anesthetic for a portion of the volatile anesthetic would result in less depression of ventilation. Indeed, nitrous oxide combined with a volatile anesthetic produces less depression of ventilation and increase in $Paco_2$ than does the same MAC concentration of the volatile drug alone.[205] This ventilatory depressant–sparing effect of nitrous oxide is detectable with all volatile anesthetics (see Fig. 4-49).[1]

Despite the apparent benign effect of nitrous oxide on ventilation, the slope of the carbon dioxide response curve is decreased similarly and shifted to the right by anesthetic concentrations of all inhaled anesthetics (Fig. 4-52).[1] Subanesthetic concentrations (0.1 MAC) of inhaled anesthetics, however, do not alter the ventilatory response to carbon dioxide. In addition to nitrous oxide, painful stimulation (surgical skin incision) and duration of drug administration influence the magnitude of increase in $Paco_2$ produced by volatile anesthetics.

Surgical Stimulation

Surgical stimulation increases minute ventilation by about 40% because of increases in tidal volume and frequency of breathing. The $Paco_2$, however, decreases only about 10% (4 to 6 mm Hg) despite the larger increase in minute

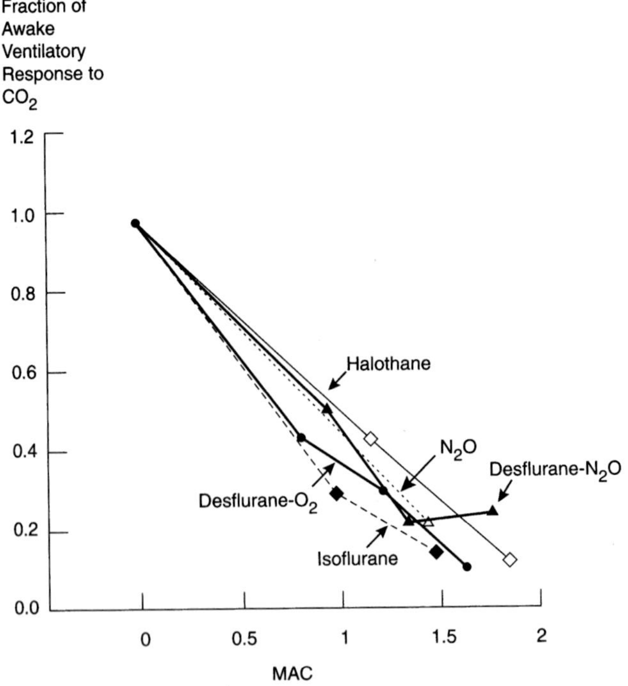

FIGURE 4-52 All inhaled anesthetics produce similar dose-dependent decreases in the ventilatory response to carbon dioxide. (From Eger EI. *Desflurane [Suprane]: A Compendium and Reference.* Nutley, NJ: Anaquest; 1993: 1–119, with permission.)

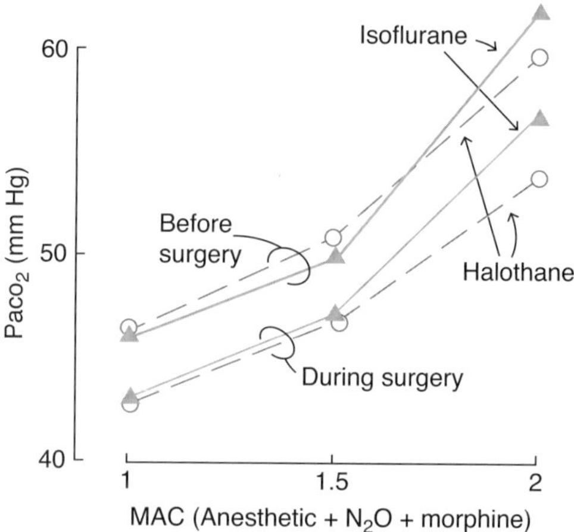

FIGURE 4-53 Impact of surgical stimulation on the resting $Paco_2$ (mm Hg) during administration of isoflurane or halothane. (From Eger EI. *Isoflurane [Forane]: A Compendium and Reference*. 2nd ed. Madison, WI: Ohio Medical Products; 1985:1–110, with permission.)

ventilation (Fig. 4-53).[100] The reason for this discrepancy is speculated to be an increased production of carbon dioxide resulting from activation of the sympathetic nervous system in response to painful surgical stimulation. Increased production of carbon dioxide is presumed to offset the impact of increased minute ventilation on $Paco_2$.

Duration of Administration

After about 5 hours of administration, the increase in $Paco_2$ produced by spontaneous breathing of a volatile anesthetic is less than that present during administration of the same concentration for 1 hour (Table 4-8).[169] Likewise, the slope and position of the carbon dioxide response curve returns toward normal after about 5 hours of administration of the volatile anesthetics.[205] The reason for this apparent recovery from the ventilatory depressant effects of volatile anesthetics with time is not known.

Table 4-8

Evidence for Recovery from the Ventilatory Depressant Effects of Volatile Anesthetics

	Arterial Pco_2	
	1 Hour of Administration	5 Hours of Administration
Enflurane	(mm Hg)	(mm Hg)
1 MAC	61	46
2 MAC	Apnea	67

Data from Calverley RK, Smith NT, Jones CW, et al. Ventilatory and cardiovascular effects of enflurane anesthesia during controlled ventilation in man. *Anesth Analg*. 1978;57:610–618.

Mechanism of Depression

Anesthetic-induced depression of ventilation as reflected by increases in the $Paco_2$ most likely reflects the direct depressant effects of these drugs on the medullary ventilatory center. An additional mechanism may be the ability of halothane and possibly other inhaled anesthetics to selectively interfere with intercostal muscle function, contributing to loss of chest wall stabilization during spontaneous breathing.[206] This loss of chest wall stabilization could interfere with expansion of the chest in response to chemical stimulation of ventilation as normally produced by increases in the $Paco_2$ or arterial hypoxemia. Furthermore, this loss of chest wall stabilization means the descent of the diaphragm tends to cause the chest to collapse inward during inspiration, contributing to decreases in lung volumes, particularly the FRC. It is thus likely that halothane-induced depression of ventilation reflects both central and peripheral effects of the drug. The ventilatory depression associated with sevoflurane may result from a combination of central depression of medullary inspiratory neurons and depression of diaphragmatic function and contractility.[207]

Management of Ventilatory Depression

The predictable ventilatory depressant effects of volatile anesthetics are most often managed by institution of mechanical (controlled) ventilation of the patient's lungs. In this regard, the inherent ventilatory depressant effects of volatile anesthetics facilitate the initiation of controlled ventilation.[208]

Ventilatory Response to Hypoxemia

All inhaled anesthetics, including nitrous oxide, profoundly depress the ventilatory response to hypoxemia that is normally mediated by the carotid bodies. For example, 0.1 MAC produces 50% to 70% depression, and 1.1 MAC produces 100% depression of this response.[209,210] This contrasts with the absence of significant depression of the ventilatory response to carbon dioxide during administration of 0.1 MAC of volatile anesthetics. Inhaled anesthetics also attenuate the usual synergistic effect of arterial hypoxemia and hypercapnia on stimulation of ventilation. Sevoflurane-induced decreases in hypoxic responses are not different in men and women which contrasts with morphine which produces greater depression of the ventilatory response to hypoxia in women.[211] Sevoflurane is useful during thoracic surgery as it is a potent bronchodilator, its low blood-gas solubility permits rapid adjustment of the depth of anesthesia, and effects on hypoxic pulmonary vasoconstriction are small.[212]

Airway Resistance and Irritability

Risk factors for developing bronchospasm during anesthesia include young age (<10 years), perioperative respiratory infection, endotracheal intubation, and the presence of COPD.[213] Nevertheless, isoflurane and

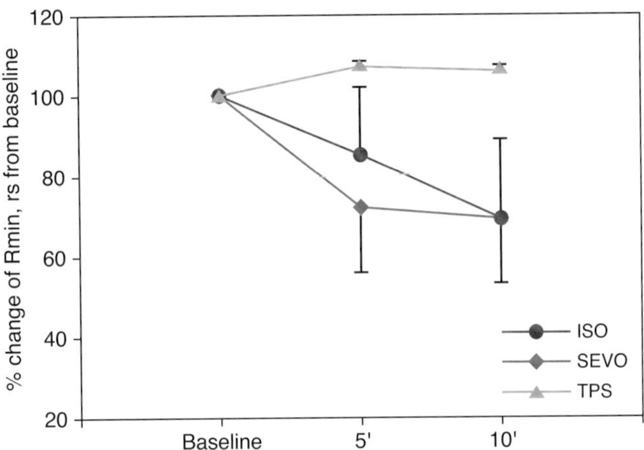

FIGURE 4-54 The percentage change (mean ± SD) in respiratory system resistance (Rmin, rs) after 5 and 10 minutes of maintenance of anesthesia with thiopental (TPS), 1.1 MAC isoflurane (ISO) or 1.1 MAC sevoflurane (SEVO) administered to patients with chronic obstructive pulmonary disease. (From Volta CA, Alvisi V, Petrini S, et al. The effect of volatile anesthetics on respiratory system resistance in patients with chronic obstructive pulmonary disease. *Anesth Analg*. 2005;100:348–353, with permission.)

sevoflurane produce bronchodilation in patients with COPD (Fig. 4-54).[214] Sevoflurane causes moderate bronchodilation that is not observed in patients receiving desflurane or thiopental (Fig. 4-55).[215] Bronchoconstriction produced by desflurane is most likely to occur in patients who smoke (Fig. 4-56).[215] Administration of fentanyl 1 μg/kg IV or morphine 100 μg/kg IV prior to inhalation induction with desflurane and nitrous oxide significantly decreases airway irritability associated with desflurane.[216] After tracheal intubation in patients without asthma, sevoflurane decreases airway resistance as much or more than isoflurane (Fig. 4-57).[217] Sevoflurane and desflurane have been administered without evidence of bronchospasm to patients with bronchial asthma.[4]

The assessment of the cough response to tracheal stimulation by endotracheal tube cuff inflation is a reliable and clinically meaningful measure of upper airway reactivity. At 1 MAC, sevoflurane is superior to desflurane for suppressing moderate and severe responses to this stimulus (Fig. 4-58).[218] However, the irritant effects of desflurane are thought to be as a result of stimulation of TRPA1 receptors in the airways.[219] Administration of desflurane, 1.8% to 5.4%, does not produce secretions, coughing, or breath-holding in human volunteers.[1]

Despite the typical lack of irritant effects of sevoflurane on the airways, there is evidence that exposure of sevoflurane to desiccated carbon dioxide absorbents, especially those containing potassium hydroxide, may result in production of toxic gases and subsequent inhalation of these products causing airway irritation and impaired gas exchange.[220,221] This airway irritation may be caused by formaldehyde which is generated in isomolar concentrations with methanol. Compound A is not an airway irritant.

In the absence of bronchoconstriction, the bronchodilating effects of volatile anesthetics are difficult to demonstrate, because normal bronchomotor tone is low and only minimal additional relaxation is possible. Like other inhaled anesthetics, nitrous oxide decreases FRC; this may be exaggerated by nitrous oxide–induced skeletal muscle rigidity.

Hepatic Effects

Hepatic Blood Flow

In patients receiving 1.5% end-tidal isoflurane, total hepatic blood flow and hepatic artery blood flow was maintained while portal vein blood flow was increased confirming that isoflurane was a vasodilator of the hepatic circulation providing beneficial effects on hepatic oxygen delivery.[222] In contrast, halothane acts as a vasoconstrictor on the hepatic circulation. In another report, patients receiving 1 MAC isoflurane plus nitrous oxide demonstrated increases in hepatic blood flow and increased hepatic venous oxygen saturation, whereas hepatic blood flow did not change in patients receiving 1 MAC halothane plus nitrous oxide.[223] Selective hepatic artery vasoconstriction has been reported in otherwise healthy patients during the administration of halothane.[224] Hepatic blood flow during administration of desflurane and sevoflurane is maintained similar to isoflurane (Fig. 4-59).[4,225] Maintenance of hepatic oxygen delivery relative to demand during exposure to anesthetics is uniquely important in view of the evidence that hepatocyte hypoxia is a significant mechanism in the multifactorial etiology of postoperative hepatic dysfunction.

FIGURE 4-55 Changes in respiratory system resistance as a percentage of the thiopental baseline recorded after tracheal intubation but before the addition of sevoflurane or desflurane to the inhaled gases or beginning the infusion of thiopental. Airway resistance responses to sevoflurane were significantly different from desflurane and thiopental. *P <.05 (From Goff MJ, Arain SR, Ficke DJ, et al. Absence of bronchodilation during desflurane anesthesia. *Anesthesiology*. 2000; 93:404–408, with permission.)

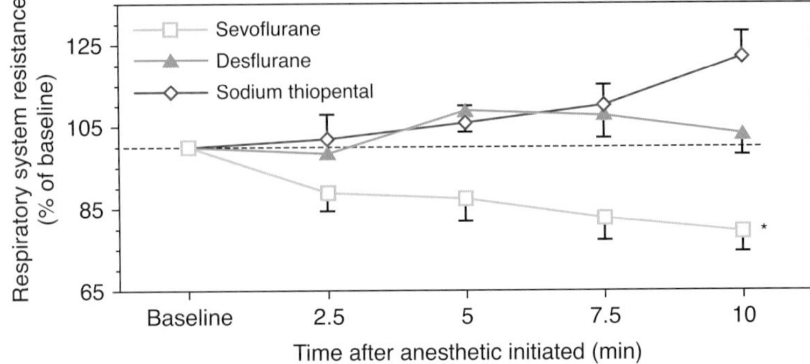

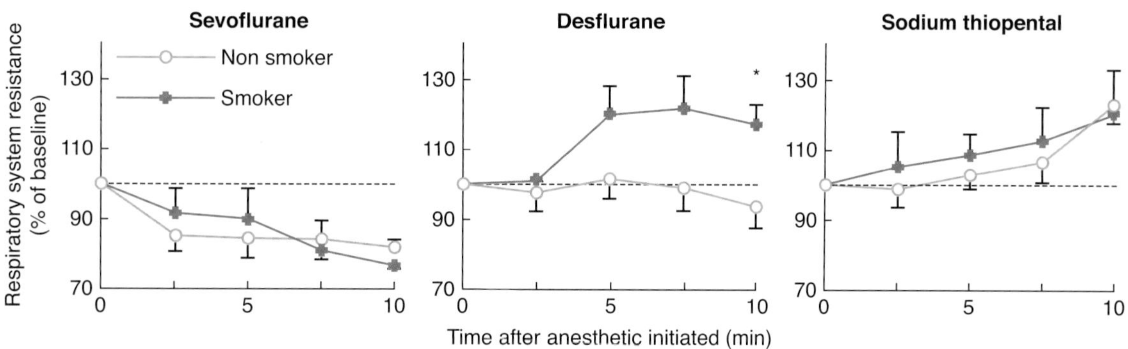

FIGURE 4-56 Respiratory system resistance during the 10 minutes after thiopental (baseline) based on current smoking status. Administration of desflurane to patients who were smokers was associated with significant bronchoconstriction compared with nonsmokers receiving desflurane. *P <.05 (From Goff MJ, Arain SR, Ficke DJ, et al. Absence of bronchodilation during desflurane anesthesia. *Anesthesiology*. 2000;93:404–408, with permission.)

Drug Clearance

Volatile anesthetics may interfere with clearance of drugs from the plasma as a result of decreases in hepatic blood flow or inhibition of drug-metabolizing enzymes. Intrinsic clearance by hepatic metabolism of drugs such as propranolol is decreased by 54% to 68% by inhaled anesthetics.[226] In the overall hepatic clearance of drugs, decreases in hepatic blood flow seem less important than anesthetic-induced inhibition of hepatic drug-metabolizing enzymes.[227]

Liver Function Tests

Transient increases in the plasma alanine aminotransferase activity follow administration of enflurane and desflurane, but not isoflurane administration, to human volunteers (Fig. 4-60).[1,225] Transient increases in plasma concentrations of alpha glutathione transferase (sensitive indicator of hepatocellular injury) follow administration of isoflurane or desflurane for surgical anesthesia.[228] In the presence of surgical stimulation, bromsulphalein retention and increases in liver enzymes follow transiently the administration of even isoflurane, suggesting that changes in hepatic blood flow evoked by painful stimulation can adversely alter hepatic function independent of the volatile anesthetic.

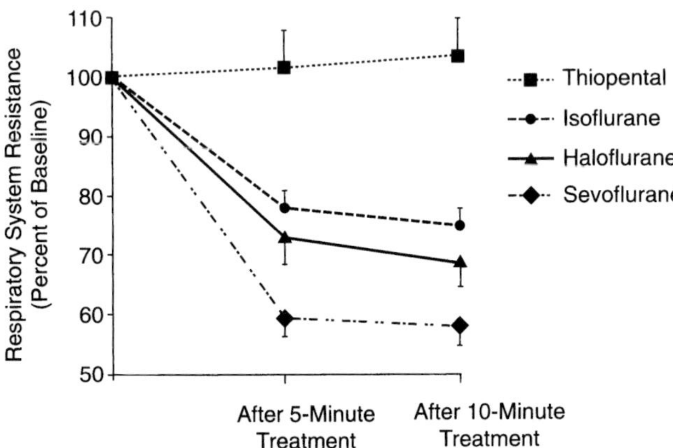

FIGURE 4-57 Respiratory system resistance decreased in the presence of 1.1 MAC isoflurane, halothane, or sevoflurane, whereas no change occurred in patients receiving thiopental 0.25 mg/kg/minute plus 50% nitrous oxide. (From Rooke GA, Choi JH, Bishop MJ. The effect of isoflurane, halothane, sevoflurane, and thiopental/nitrous oxide on respiratory system resistance after tracheal intubation. *Anesthesiology*. 1997;86:1294–1299, with permission.)

Hepatotoxicity

Postoperative liver dysfunction has been associated with most volatile anesthetics, with halothane receiving the most attention.[229] Injected and inhaled anesthetics studied in the hypoxic rat model that includes enzyme induction may produce centrilobular necrosis, but the incidence is greatest with halothane (Fig. 4-61).[230] It is likely that inadequate hepatocyte oxygenation (oxygen supply relative to oxygen demand) is the principal mechanism responsible for hepatic dysfunction that follows anesthesia and surgery. Any anesthetic that decreases alveolar ventilation and/or decreases hepatic blood flow could interfere with adequate hepatocyte oxygenation. Enzyme induction increases oxygen demand and could make patients vulnerable to decreased hepatic oxygen supply due to anesthetic-induced ventilatory or circulatory events that decrease hepatic oxygen delivery. Preexisting liver disease, such as hepatic cirrhosis, may be associated with marginal hepatocyte oxygenation, which would be further jeopardized by the depressant effects of anesthetics on hepatic blood flow and/or arterial oxygenation. Indeed, liver transaminase enzymes are increased more in cirrhotic than noncirrhotic animals exposed to halothane (Fig. 4-62).[231] Hypothermia, which decreases hepatic oxygen demand, may protect the liver from drug-induced events that decrease hepatic oxygen delivery.

Halothane

Halothane produces two types of hepatotoxicity in susceptible patients. An estimated 20% of adult patients

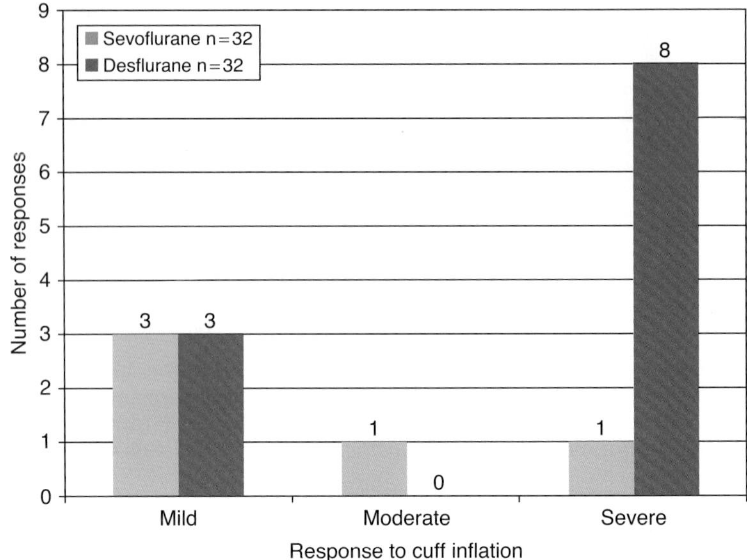

FIGURE 4-58 Responses to tracheal tube cuff inflation during 1 MAC anesthesia with sevoflurane or desflurane. (From Klock PA, Czeslick EG, Klafta JM, et al. The effect of sevoflurane and desflurane on upper airway reactivity. *Anesthesiology.* 2001;94: 963–967, with permission.)

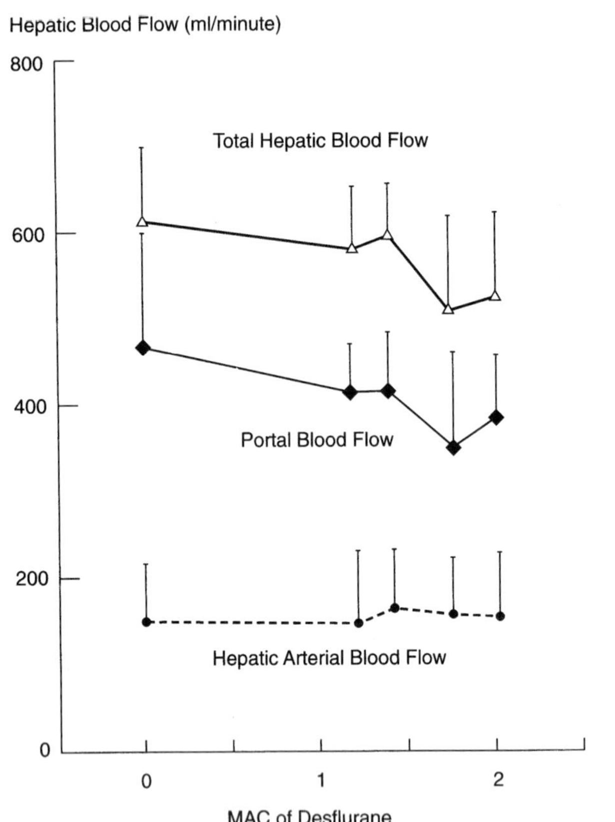

FIGURE 4-59 Administration of desflurane to dogs does not significantly alter hepatic perfusion. (Mean ± SD.) (Modified from Eger EI. *Desflurane [Suprane]: A Compendium and Reference.* Nutley, NJ: Anaquest; 1993:1–119, with permission.)

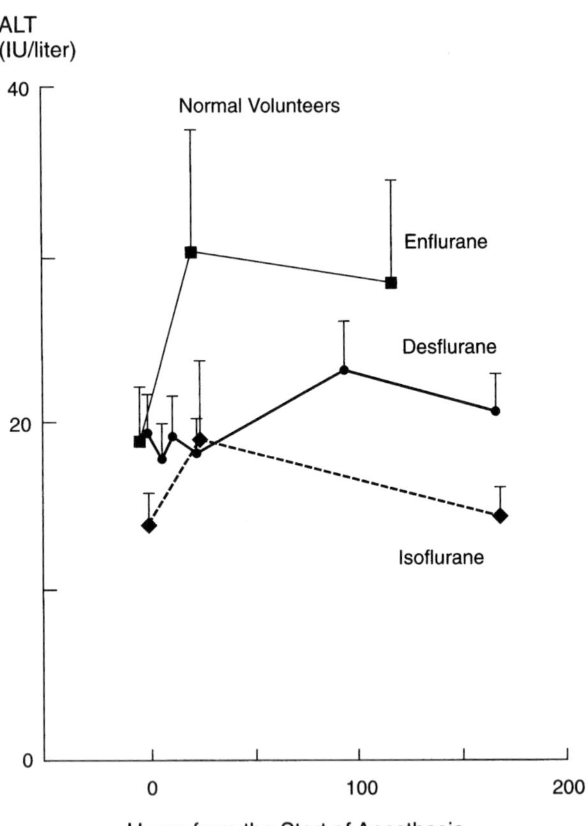

FIGURE 4-60 Plasma alanine aminotransferase (ALT) levels do not change significantly when enflurane, desflurane, or isoflurane are administered to healthy volunteers. (Mean ± SE.) (Modified from Eger EI. *Desflurane [Suprane]: A Compendium and Reference.* Nutley, NJ: Anaquest; 1993:1–119, with permission.)

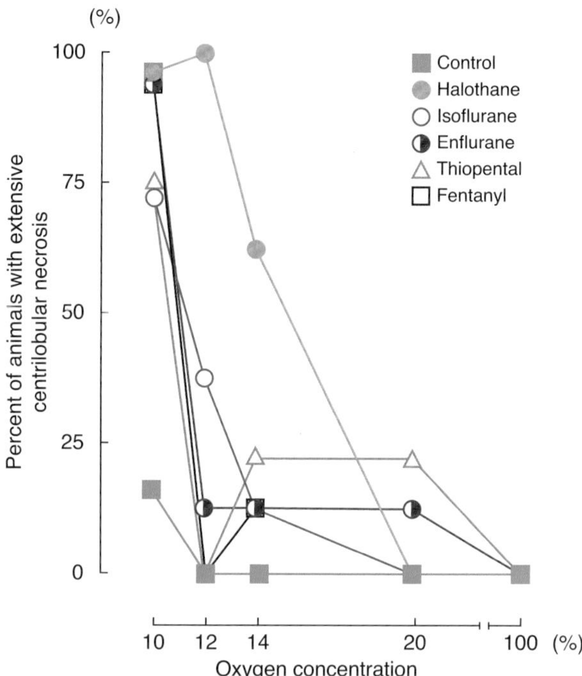

FIGURE 4-61 Hepatic damage may occur in the rat model after administration of inhaled or injected drugs when the inhaled oxygen concentration is 10%. Conversely, hepatic damage occurs after administration of halothane, but not enflurane or isoflurane, when the inhaled concentration of oxygen is 12% or 14%. (From Shingu K, Eger EI, Johnson BH, et al. Effect of oxygen concentration, hyperthermia, and choice of vendor on anesthetic-induced hepatic injury in rats. *Anesth Analg.* 1983;62:146–150, with permission.)

receiving halothane develop a mild, self-limited postoperative hepatotoxicity that is characterized by nausea, lethargy, fever, and minor increases in plasma concentrations of liver transaminase enzymes.[232] The other and rarer type of hepatotoxicity (halothane hepatitis) is estimated to occur in 1 in 10,000 to 1 in 30,000 adult patients receiving halothane and may lead to massive hepatic necrosis and death.[233] Children seem to be less susceptible to this type of hepatotoxicity than adults.[234,235] It is likely that the more common self-limited form of hepatic dysfunction following halothane is a nonspecific drug effect due to changes in hepatic blood flow that impair hepatic oxygenation. Conversely, the rarer, life-threatening form of hepatic dysfunction characterized as halothane hepatitis is most likely an immune-mediated hepatotoxicity.[229]

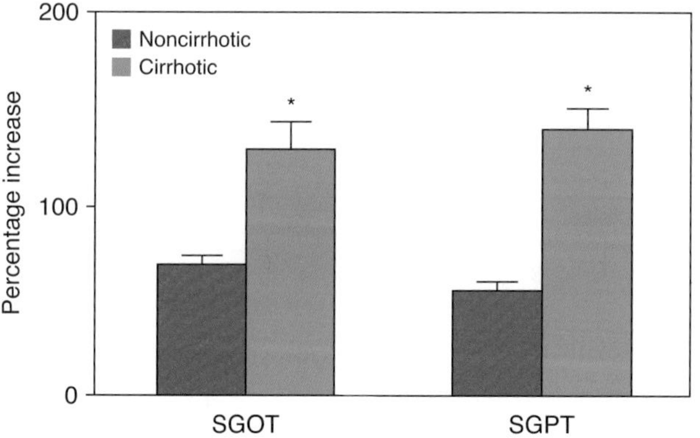

FIGURE 4-62 Increases (mean ± SE) in liver transaminase enzymes after administration of 1.05% halothane for 3 hours to noncirrhotic or cirrhotic rats. (From Baden JM, Serra M, Fujinaga ME, et al. Halothane metabolism in cirrhotic rats. *Anesthesiology.* 1987;67:660–664, with permission.)

Halothane Hepatitis

Clinical manifestations of halothane hepatitis that suggest an immune-mediated response include eosinophilia, fever, rash, arthralgia, and prior exposure to halothane. Risk factors commonly associated with halothane hepatitis include female gender, middle age, obesity, and multiple exposures to halothane. The predominant histologic feature is acute hepatitis. The most compelling evidence for an immune-mediated mechanism is the presence of circulatory immunoglobulin G antibodies in at least 70% of those patients with the diagnosis of halothane hepatitis.[229] These antibodies are directed against liver microsomal proteins on the surface of hepatocytes that have been covalently modified by the reactive oxidative trifluoroacetyl halide metabolite of halothane to form neoantigens (Fig. 4-63).[236] This acetylation of liver proteins in effect changes these proteins from self to nonself (neoantigens), resulting in the formation of antibodies against this new protein. It is presumed that the subsequent antigen–antibody interaction is responsible for the liver injury characterized as halothane hepatitis. The possibility of a genetic susceptibility factor is suggested by case reports of halothane hepatitis in closely related relatives.[237,238] Indeed, metabolism of halothane appears to be under genetic influence in humans.[239]

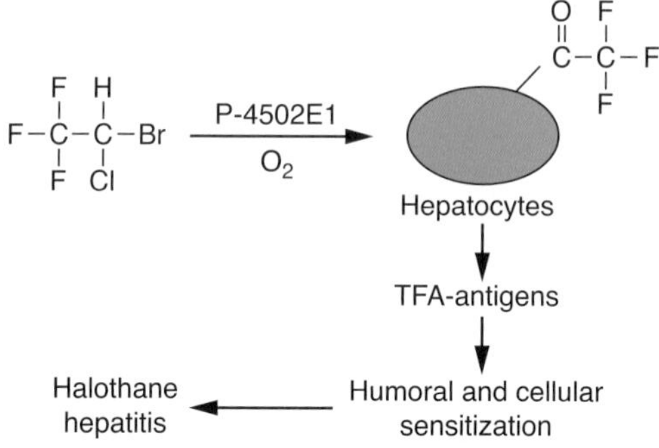

FIGURE 4-63 Halothane is metabolized to a trifluoroacetylated (TFA) adduct that binds to liver proteins. In susceptible patients, this adduct (altered protein) is seen as nonself (neoantigen), generating an immune response (production of antibodies). Subsequent exposure to halothane may result in hepatotoxicity. A similar process may occur in genetically susceptible individuals after anesthetic exposure to other fluorinated volatile anesthetics (enflurane, isoflurane, desflurane) that also generate a TFA adduct. (From Njoku D, Laster MJ, Gong DH, et al. Biotransformation of halothane, enflurane, isoflurane, and desflurane to trifluoroacetylated liver proteins: association between protein acylation and hepatic injury. *Anesth Analg.* 1997;84:173–178, with permission.)

Several observations suggest that reductive metabolism is not the primary mechanism in the development of halothane hepatitis. For example, neither enflurane nor isoflurane undergoes reductive metabolism, yet these drugs both produce centrilobular necrosis in the hypoxic rat model. Furthermore, metabolites produced by reductive metabolism of halothane do not themselves produce hepatotoxicity. Finally, fasting does not alter metabolism but enhances hepatotoxicity by volatile anesthetics.

Enflurane, Isoflurane, and Desflurane

The mild, self-limited postoperative hepatic dysfunction that is associated with all the volatile anesthetics most likely reflect anesthetic-induced alterations in hepatic oxygen delivery relative to demand that results in inadequate hepatocyte oxygenation. More disturbing, however, is the realization that enflurane, isoflurane, and desflurane are oxidatively metabolized by liver cytochrome P450 enzymes to form acetylated liver protein adducts by mechanisms similar to that of halothane (Fig. 4-64).[236,240,241] As a result, acetylated liver proteins capable of evoking an antibody response could occur after exposure to halothane, enflurane, isoflurane, or desflurane. Indeed, trifluoroacetyl-modified proteins have been described in a patient with hepatitis associated with isoflurane.[242] This raises the possibility that enflurane, isoflurane, and desflurane could produce hepatotoxicity by a mechanism similar to that of halothane but at a lower incidence because the degree of anesthetic metabolism appears to be directly related to the potential for hepatic injury. Considering the magnitude of metabolism of these volatile anesthetics, it is predictable that the incidence of anesthetic-induced hepatitis would be greatest with halothane, intermediate with enflurane, and rare with isoflurane.[243–245] Desflurane is metabolized even less than isoflurane, and from the standpoint of immune-mediated hepatotoxicity, desflurane should be very safe because it would have the lowest level of adduct formation. Nevertheless, even very small amounts of adduct may be able

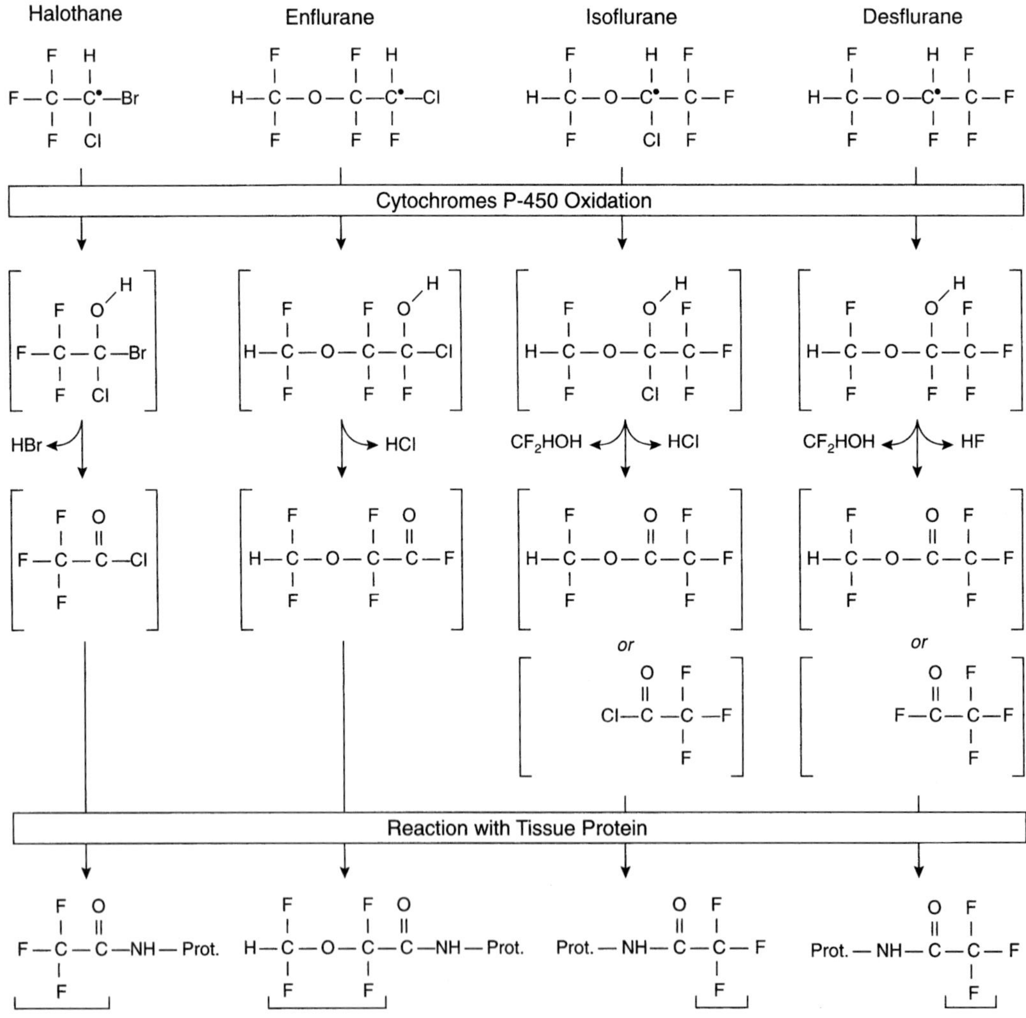

FIGURE 4-64 Pathways for the oxidative metabolism of fluorinated volatile anesthetics by cytochrome P450 enzymes to form acetylated protein adducts. In genetically susceptible individuals, the resulting trifluoroacetylates are thought to produce an immune response manifesting clinically as drug-induced hepatitis. (From Martin JL, Plevak DJ, Flannery KD, et al. Hepatotoxicity after desflurane anesthesia. *Anesthesiology.* 1995;83:1125–1129, with permission.)

to precipitate massive hepatotoxicity, particularly if the patient was previously sensitized against trifluoroacetyl proteins. Indeed, hepatotoxicity after desflurane anesthesia has been described in a patient who may have been previously sensitized by exposure to halothane 18 years and 12 years previously.[241] Fulminant hepatic failure accompanied by high plasma concentrations of CYP2A6 autoantibodies has been observed in a patient 22 years following exposure to enflurane.[246] Similarly, halothane may be able to sensitize patients against protein adducts formed by other fluorinated volatile anesthetics.[240,247]

The risk of fulminant hepatic failure after exposure to enflurane, isoflurane, or desflurane after previous exposure to halothane is probably less than the overall risk associated with anesthesia.[229]

Environmental exposure of operating room personnel to trace concentrations of volatile anesthetics could stimulate antibody production. Indeed, measurement of plasma autoantibody concentrations demonstrated increased levels in pediatric anesthesiologists (especially females) compared with general anesthesiologists and controls.[248] It is presumed that pediatric anesthesiologists experience greater occupational exposure to trace concentrations of volatile anesthetics due to the frequent use of nonrebreathing anesthesia delivery systems and use of uncuffed endotracheal tubes. Despite these higher antibody levels, pediatric anesthesiologists did not have increased liver transaminase enzymes compared with general anesthesiologists, suggesting these antibodies may be insufficient to cause appreciable damage to normal hepatic cells.[249,250]

Sevoflurane

The chemical structure of sevoflurane, unlike that of other fluorinated volatile anesthetics, dictates that it cannot undergo metabolism to an acetyl halide (Fig. 4-65).[251,252] Sevoflurane metabolism does not result in the formation

```
 CF3     H                CF3          O
  |      |                 |           ||      F⁻
H—C—O—C—F   ——→    H—C—O—H   +   C—F→+
  |      |                 |           |       CO2
 CF3     H                CF3          F

Sevoflurane       Hexafluoroisopropanol
                          |
                   UDPGA  |
                          ↓
                         CF3
                          |
                    H—C—O—Glucuronide
                          |
                         CF3

                Hexafluoroisopropanol
                     Glucuronide
```

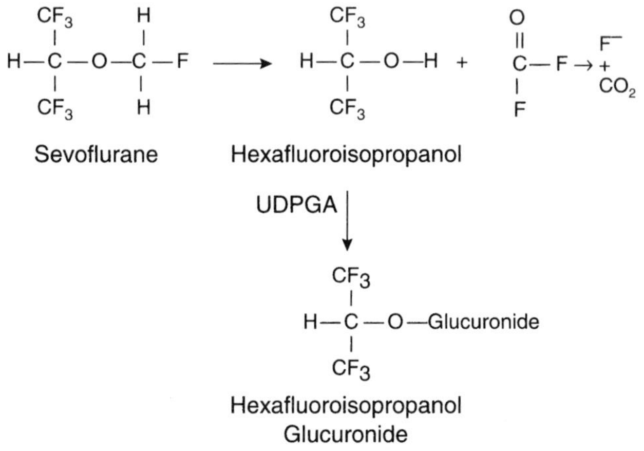

FIGURE 4-65 Proposed pathway for oxidative metabolism of sevoflurane. (UDPGA, uridine diphosphate glucuronic acid.) (From Frink EJ, Ghantous H, Malan TP, et al. Plasma inorganic fluoride with sevoflurane anesthesia: correlation with indices of hepatic and renal function. *Anesth Analg.* 1992;74:231–235, with permission.)

of trifluoroacetylated liver proteins and therefore cannot stimulate the formation of antitrifluoroacetylated protein antibodies. In this regard, sevoflurane differs from halothane, enflurane, and desflurane, all of which are metabolized to reactive acetyl halide metabolites. Therefore, unlike all the other fluorinated volatile anesthetics, sevoflurane would not be expected to produce immune-mediated hepatotoxicity or to cause cross-sensitivity in patients previously exposed to halothane. Rare reported cases of sevoflurane hepatotoxicity are without explanation or proven cause and effect.[4,253,254]

Compound A, a product of sevoflurane interaction with carbon dioxide absorbents, is hepatotoxic in animals, but the concentration present in the anesthesia breathing circuit is far below the toxic level in animals. Nevertheless, small increases in the plasma alanine aminotransferase have been observed in volunteers receiving sevoflurane for prolonged periods of time during which the compound A concentration averaged 41 ppm. Similar changes in the plasma transaminase concentrations did not occur in volunteers receiving desflurane, suggesting that mild transient hepatic injury was limited to the sevoflurane-treated individuals.[255] Conversely, others have not observed differences in liver function enzyme changes in patients receiving sevoflurane compared with isoflurane.[256]

Renal Effects

Volatile anesthetics produce similar dose-related decreases in renal blood flow, glomerular filtration rate, and urine output. These changes are not a result of the release of arginine vasopressin hormone but rather most likely reflect the effects of volatile anesthetics on systemic blood pressure and cardiac output. Preoperative hydration attenuates or abolishes many of the changes in renal function associated with volatile anesthetics. Renal function after kidney transplantation is not uniquely influenced by the volatile anesthetic administered.[257] Volatile anesthetics appear to induce a protective activity on the kidney similar to that of the heart via spingosine kinase and spingosine-1-phosphate generation.[258]

Fluoride-Induced Nephrotoxicity

Fluoride-induced nephrotoxicity (polyuria, hypernatremia, hyperosmolarity, increased plasma creatinine, inability to concentrate urine) was first recognized in patients after the administration of methoxyflurane, which undergoes extensive metabolism (70% of the absorbed dose) to inorganic fluoride, which acts as a renal toxin. In these patients, no renal effects were observed when peak plasma fluoride was <40 μmol/L, subclinical toxicity was accompanied by peak plasma fluoride concentrations of 50 to 80 μmol/L, and clinical toxicity occurred when peak plasma fluoride concentrations were >80 μmol/L. The methoxyflurane nephrotoxicity theory has been extended to other fluorinated volatile anesthetics despite the absence of data to support this extrapolation. Furthermore, a plasma fluoride concentration of 50 μmol/L has been adopted as an indicator that renal toxicity may occur from other volatile anesthetics. Nevertheless, all volatile anesthetics introduced since methoxyflurane undergo significantly less metabolism, and their decreased solubility compared with methoxyflurane means that substantial amounts of the anesthetic are exhaled and thus not available for hepatic metabolism to fluoride. The absence of renal toxicity despite peak plasma fluoride concentrations exceeding 50 μmol/L after administration of enflurane or sevoflurane suggests that this peak value alone cannot be accepted as an indicator for fluoride-induced nephrotoxicity after administration of these volatile anesthetics. Reversible depression of urine concentrating ability observed in healthy volunteers following prolonged enflurane administration (8 hours) may reflect alkaline degradation products of enflurane that are conjugated to thiol compounds, forming S-conjugates.[259] Enzyme induction, obesity, and preexisting renal dysfunction appear to be risk factors for enflurane nephrotoxicity.

Sevoflurane

Sevoflurane is metabolized to inorganic fluoride, and peak plasma fluoride concentrations consistently exceed those peak levels that occur after a comparable dose of enflurane (Fig. 4-66).[260–263] Despite higher peak plasma fluoride concentrations compared with enflurane, prolonged sevoflurane anesthesia does not impair renal concentrating function as evaluated with desmopressin testing 1 and 5 days postanesthesia in healthy volunteers (Fig. 4-67).[260,262] In the same report, two patients receiving enflurane developed transient impairment of renal concentrating ability despite lower peak plasma fluoride concentrations than the patients receiving sevoflurane.[262] In another report, there were no significant differences between urine concentrating abilities after enflurane (6 MAC hours) or sevoflurane (9 MAC hours).[263]

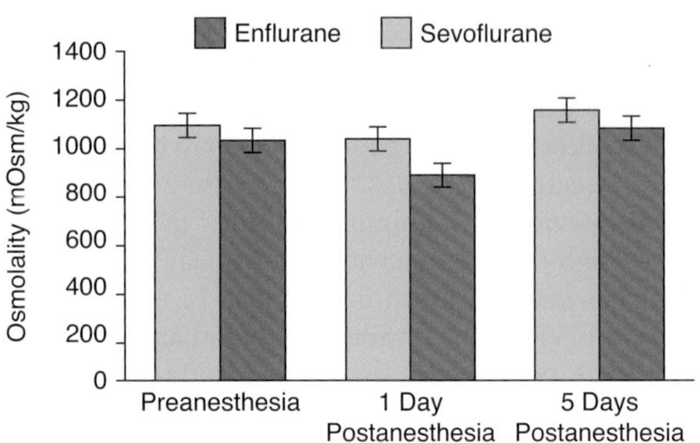

FIGURE 4-67 Maximal urinary osmolalities (mean ± SE) in adult male volunteers after administration of desmopressin before and after prolonged administration (>9 MAC hours) of enflurane or sevoflurane. (From Frink EJ, Malan TP, Isner RJ, et al. Renal concentrating function with prolonged sevoflurane or enflurane anesthesia in volunteers. *Anesthesiology.* 1994;80:1019–1025, with permission.)

Despite reports failing to show renal impairment after the administration of sevoflurane, there are observations of transient impairment of renal concentrating ability and increased urinary excretion of β-*N*-acetylglucosaminidase (NAG) in patients exposed to sevoflurane and developing peak plasma inorganic fluoride concentrations >50 μmol/L (Figs. 4-68 and 4-69).[264] Urinary excretion of NAG is considered an indicator of acute proximal renal tubular injury. Despite these changes, the blood urea nitrogen and plasma creatinine did not change, and the authors concluded that clinically significant renal damage did not accompany administration of sevoflurane to patients with no preexisting renal disease. Concern that

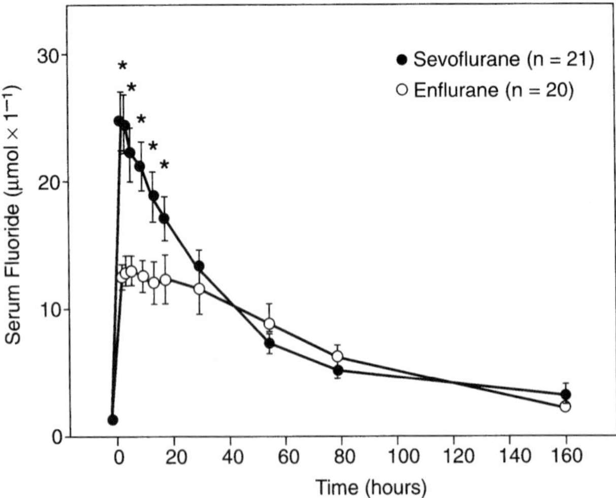

FIGURE 4-66 Plasma fluoride concentrations during and after sevoflurane or enflurane anesthesia. (Mean ± SE.) (From Conzen PF, Nuscheler M, Melotte A, et al. Renal function and serum fluoride concentrations in patients with stable renal insufficiency after anesthesia with sevoflurane or enflurane. *Anesth Analg.* 1995;81:569–575, with permission.)

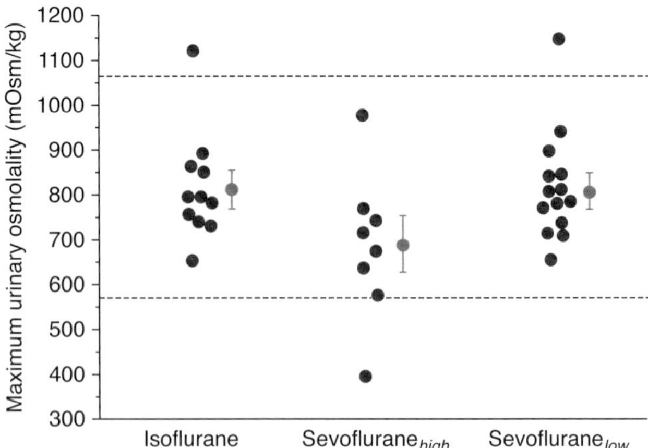

FIGURE 4-68 Maximum urinary osmolality in response to vasopressin 16.5 hours after cessation of anesthesia was not significantly different between the three anesthesia groups. $Sevoflurane_{high}$ included only patients with a peak plasma inorganic fluoride concentration >50 μmol/L. *Solid circles* and *bars* represent mean ± SE. (From Higuchi H, Sumikura H, Sumita S, et al. Renal function in patients with high serum fluoride concentrations after prolonged sevoflurane anesthesia. *Anesthesiology.* 1995;83:449–458, with permission.)

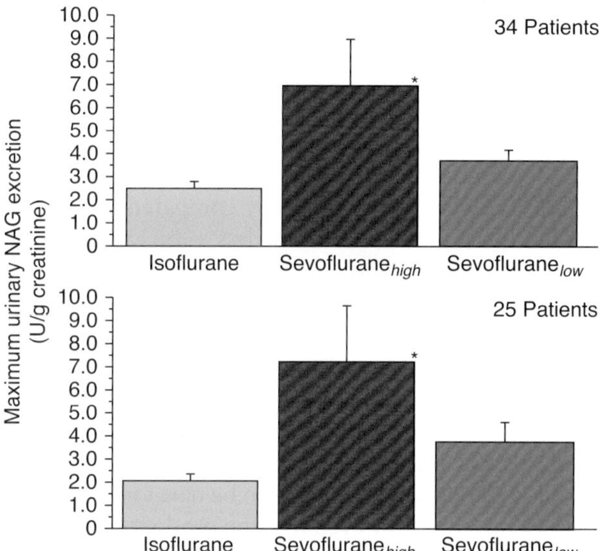

FIGURE 4-69 Urinary excretion of the renal enzyme β-N-acetylglucosaminidase (NAG) was significantly greater (*P <.05) in the sevoflurane-high patients (peak plasma inorganic fluoride concentration >50 μm/L) compared with the other anesthesia groups. (From Higuchi H, Sumikura H, Sumita S, et al. Renal function in patients with high serum fluoride concentrations after prolonged sevoflurane anesthesia. *Anesthesiology*. 1995;83:449–458, with permission.)

administration of sevoflurane to patients with preexisting renal disease could accentuate renal dysfunction was not confirmed when this volatile anesthetic was administered to patients with chronic renal disease as reflected by increased plasma creatinine concentrations.[260,265] Likewise, administration of desflurane or isoflurane did not aggravate renal impairment in patients with preexisting chronic renal insufficiency (Fig. 4-70).[266]

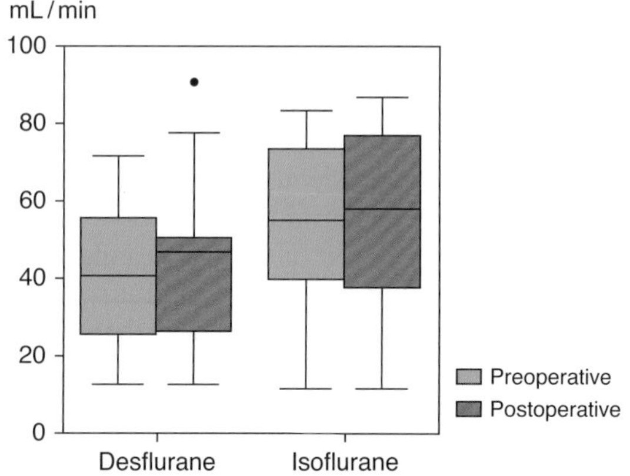

FIGURE 4-70 Preoperative and postoperative creatinine clearance values (mL/min). *Thick lines* represent median values, the *box boundaries* represent 25th to 75th percentiles, and the *bar lines* represent the 10th to 90th percentiles. The single outlier beyond the 90th percentile is shown as an individual data point (*). There were no differences between desflurane and isoflurane. (From Litz RJ, Hubler M, Lorenz W, et al. Renal responses to desflurane and isoflurane in patients with renal insufficiency. *Anesthesiology*. 2002;97:1133–1136, with permission.)

It has been postulated that intrarenal production of inorganic fluoride may be a more important factor for nephrotoxicity than hepatic metabolism that causes increased plasma fluoride concentrations.[251,267] This would explain why patients with increased plasma concentrations of fluoride after administration of sevoflurane occasionally experience less renal dysfunction than patients receiving enflurane and manifesting lower plasma fluoride concentrations (see Figs. 4-66 and 4-67).[260,262,268] Presumably, inhaled anesthetics such as methoxyflurane and enflurane undergo greater intrarenal metabolism to fluoride than sevoflurane whereas sevoflurane undergoes greater hepatic metabolism, thus accounting for the higher plasma concentrations of fluoride.

Vinyl Halide Nephrotoxicity

Carbon dioxide absorbents containing potassium and sodium hydroxide react with sevoflurane and eliminate hydrogen fluoride from its isopropyl moiety to form breakdown products (see Fig. 4-5).[5,269] The degradation product produced in greatest amounts is fluoromethyl-2,2-difluro-1-(trifluoromethyl) vinyl ether (compound A). Compound A is a dose-dependent nephrotoxin in rats causing proximal renal tubular injury at concentrations of 50 to 100 ppm.[270] The concentration of compound A fatal to 50% of rats after a 3-hour exposure is about 400 ppm.[271] In patients, the mean maximum concentration of compound A in the anesthesia breathing circuit averages 19.7, 8.1, and 2.1 ppm during fresh gas flows of 1, 3, and 6 L per minute, respectively (Fig. 4-71).[272,273] During closed-circuit anesthesia with sevoflurane administered to patients undergoing operations lasting longer than 5 hours, the average concentration of compound A in the anesthesia circuit was <20 ppm and no evidence of renal dysfunction occurred based on measurements of blood urea nitrogen and plasma creatinine concentrations (Fig. 4-72).[14] Higher concentrations of compound A

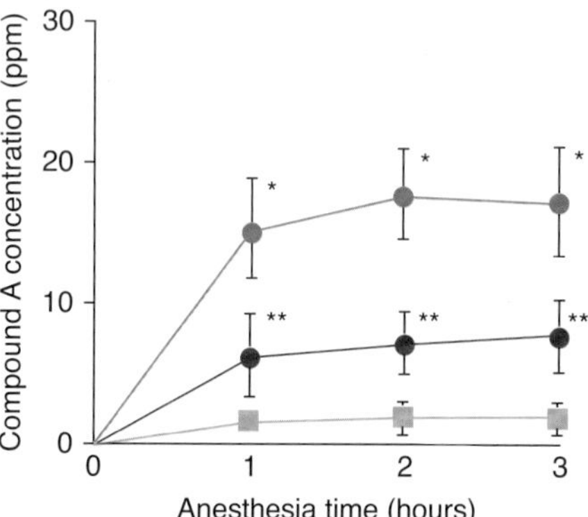

FIGURE 4-71 Inhaled compound A concentrations during administration of sevoflurane at fresh gas flow rates of 1 L per minute *(blue circles)*, 3 L per minute *(red circles)*, and 6 L per minute *(squares)*. (*P <.05 versus 3 L per minute; **P <.05 versus 6 L per minute.) (From Bito H, Ikeda K. Effect of total flow rate on the concentration of degradation products generated by reaction between sevoflurane and soda lime. *Br J Anaesth*. 1995;74:667–669, with permission.)

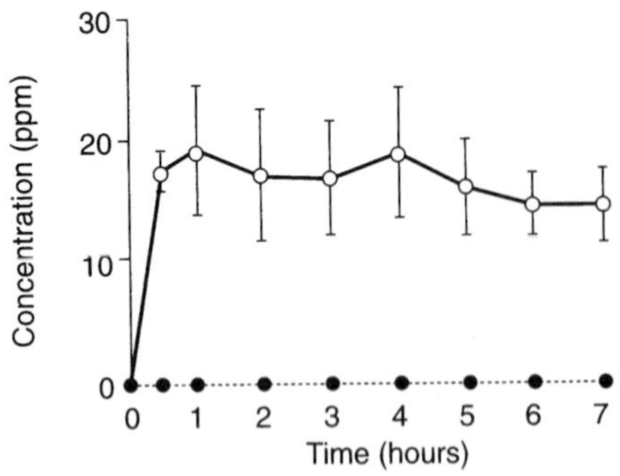

FIGURE 4-72 Inhaled compound A concentrations *(open circles)* and compound B concentrations *(solid circles)* during closed-circuit sevoflurane anesthesia. (Mean ± SD.) (From Bito H, Ikeda K. Closed-circuit anesthesia with sevoflurane in humans: effects on renal and hepatic function and concentrations of breakdown products with soda lime in the circuit. *Anesthesiology*. 1994;80:71–76, with permission.)

occurred in the presence of Baralyme (no longer clinically available) probably as a result of higher absorbent temperatures compared with soda lime.[5,82] Similarly, carbon dioxide production increases the absorbent temperature and thus the production of compound A. Probenecid is a selective inhibitor of organic anion transport and pretreatment with this drug prevents compound A–induced renal injury in rats and may provide similar protection in humans.[274]

The rationale for utilizing at least a 2 L per minute fresh gas flow rate when administering sevoflurane is intended to minimize the concentration of compound A that may accumulate in the anesthesia breathing circuit. To assess the adequacy of this recommendation, the nephrotoxicity of 2, 4, or 8 hours of anesthesia with 1.25 MAC sevoflurane has been compared with a similar exposure to desflurane.[255,275] Compound A concentrations ranged from 40 to 42 ppm during the three different durations of sevoflurane administration. In patients receiving 1.25 MAC sevoflurane for 8 hours or 4 hours, there was transient evidence of injury to the glomeruli (albuminuria), proximal renal tubules (glucosuria and increased urinary excretion of glutathione-S-transferase), and distal renal tubules (increased urinary excretion of glutathione-S-transferase) that was greater in the 8-hour group. Urine-concentrating ability and plasma creatinine were not altered despite these findings in the patients receiving sevoflurane. Desflurane administered at 1.25 MAC for 2, 4, or 8 hours or sevoflurane exposure for 2 hours did not produce any evidence of renal injury. Conversely, comparisons of the renal effects of sevoflurane and isoflurane using fresh gas flows of 1 L per minute or less demonstrated no difference between these drugs based on measurement of indices of renal function.[276,277] In children, sevoflurane anesthesia lasting 4 hours using total fresh gas flows of 2 L per minute produced concentrations of compound A of <15 ppm, and there was no evidence of renal dysfunction.[278]

The amount of compound A produced under clinical conditions has consistently been far below those concentrations associated with nephrotoxicity in animals.[5] A proposed mechanism for nephrotoxicity is metabolism of compound A via the beta-lyase pathway to a reactive thiol. Because humans have less than one-tenth of the enzymatic activity for this pathway compared to rats, it is possible that humans should be less vulnerable to injury by this mechanism. Nevertheless, there are data indicating that humans are not less vulnerable to injury from compound A compared with rats.[255]

Halothane, like sevoflurane, is degraded by carbon dioxide absorbents to unsaturated volatile compounds that are nephrotoxic to rats. Based on the long history of halothane use without evidence of nephrotoxicity, it has been suggested the same may also be true for sevoflurane. There is evidence, however, that the product of halothane breakdown ($CF_2 = CBrCl$) from exposure to carbon dioxide absorbents is less nephrotoxic than compound A.[279] For this reason, the clinical absence of halothane nephrotoxicity does not necessarily indicate a similar absence for sevoflurane.

Skeletal Muscle Effects

Neuromuscular Junction

Volatile anesthetics inhibit muscle type nicotinic receptors incompletely at MAC concentrations.[280] Ether derivative fluorinated volatile anesthetics produce skeletal muscle relaxation that is about twofold greater than that associated with a comparable dose of halothane. Nitrous oxide does not relax skeletal muscles, and in doses of >1 MAC (delivered in a hyperbaric chamber) it may produce skeletal muscle rigidity.[140] This effect of nitrous oxide is consistent with enhancement of skeletal muscle rigidity produced by opioids when low concentrations of nitrous oxide are administered. The ability of skeletal muscles to sustain contractions in response to continuous stimulation is impaired in the presence of increasing concentrations of ether derivative volatile anesthetics but not in the presence of halothane or nitrous oxide (Fig. 4-73).[1]

Volatile anesthetics produce dose-dependent enhancement of the effects of neuromuscular-blocking drugs, with the effects of enflurane, isoflurane, desflurane, and sevoflurane being similar and greater than halothane. In vitro, isoflurane and halothane produce similar potentiation of the effects of neuromuscular-blocking drugs.[281] Nitrous oxide does not significantly potentiate the in vivo effects of neuromuscular-blocking drugs.

Malignant Hyperthermia

All volatile anesthetics including desflurane and sevoflurane can trigger malignant hyperthermia in genetically susceptible patients even in the absence of concomitant administration of succinylcholine.[282–284] In one report, malignant hyperthermia did not manifest until 3 hours

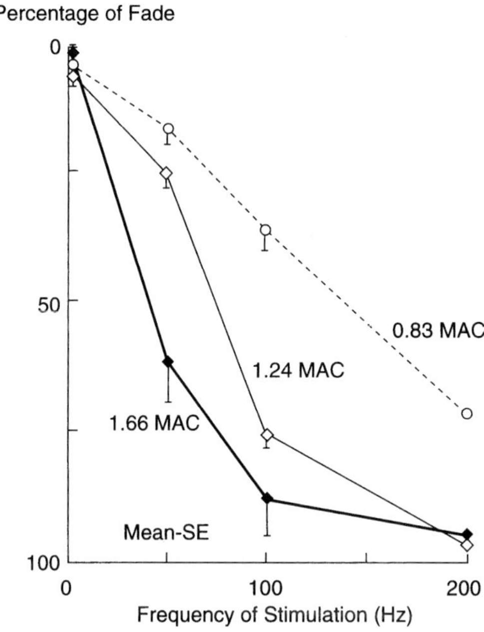

FIGURE 4-73 Increases in fade with tetanic stimulation accompany increasing doses of desflurane or increasing frequency of stimulation. [From Eger EI. *Desflurane [Suprane]: A Compendium and Reference.* Nutley, NJ: Anaquest; 1993: 1–119, with permission.)

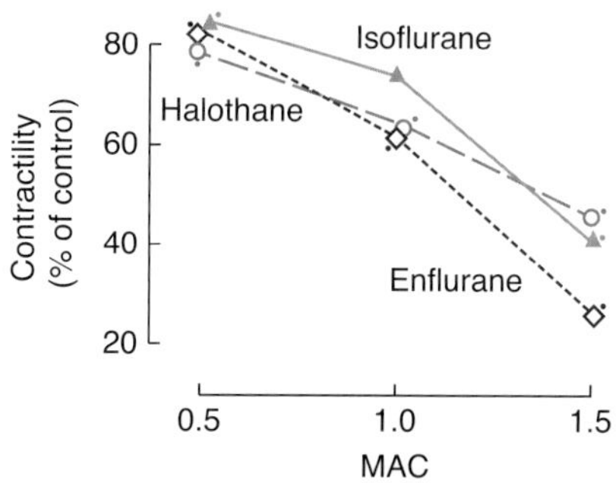

FIGURE 4-74 Impact of volatile anesthetics on contractility of uterine smooth muscle strips studied in vitro. (*P >.05.) (From Eger EI. *Isoflurane [Forane]: A Compendium and Reference.* Madison, WI: Ohio Medical Products; 1985:1–110, with permission.)

following uneventful desflurane anesthesia.[285] Among the volatile anesthetics, however, halothane is the most potent trigger. Nitrous oxide compared with volatile anesthetics is a weak trigger for malignant hyperthermia. For example, augmentation of caffeine-induced contractures of frog sartorius muscle by nitrous oxide is 1.3 times, whereas that for isoflurane is 3 times, enflurane 4 times, and halothane 11 times.[286] Xenon can be given safely to a patient with a history of malignant hyperthermia, although current anesthesia machines need longer flushing times than earlier simpler machines and manufacturer's instructions should be followed.[287]

Obstetric Effects

Volatile anesthetics produce similar and dose-dependent decreases in uterine smooth muscle contractility and blood flow (Fig. 4-74).[100,288,289] These changes are modest at 0.5 MAC (analgesic concentrations) and become substantial at concentrations of >1 MAC. Nitrous oxide does not alter uterine contractility in doses used to provide analgesia during vaginal delivery. As such, nitrous oxide is particularly useful in obstetrical anesthesia to reduce the need to volatile anesthetic that promotes uterine atony while avoiding opioids and benzodiazepines that may cause prolonged depression of the newborn.

In some settings, anesthetic-induced uterine relaxation may be desirable to facilitate removal of retained placenta; nitroglycerine can also be used for this purpose. Conversely, uterine relaxation produced by volatile anesthetics may contribute to blood loss due to uterine atony. Indeed, blood loss during therapeutic abortion is greater in patients anesthetized with a volatile anesthetic compared with that in patients receiving nitrous oxide–barbiturate–opioid anesthesia.[290,291] Propofol inhibits uterine contractility only slightly at anesthetic concentrations.[292]

In animals, evidence of fetal distress does not accompany anesthetic-induced decreases in maternal uterine blood flow as long as the anesthetic concentration is <1.5 MAC.[293] Furthermore, volatile anesthetics at about 0.5 MAC concentrations combined with 50% nitrous oxide ensure amnesia during cesarean section and do not produce detectable effects in the neonate.[294] Inhaled anesthetics rapidly cross the placenta to enter the fetus, but these drugs are likewise rapidly exhaled by the newborn infant. Nitrous oxide–induced analgesia for vaginal delivery develops more rapidly than with most volatile anesthetics (desflurane and sevoflurane may be exceptions), but, after about 10 minutes, all inhaled drugs provide comparable analgesia. Despite the popularity of nitrous oxide for intrapartum analgesia, in animal models, nitrous oxide–induced analgesia dissipates rapidly while only sedative properties remain.[295] It is not known over what period of time the analgesic properties recover.

Resistance to Infection

Many normal functions of the immune system are depressed after patient exposure to the combination of anesthesia and surgery.[296] It would seem that many of the immune changes seen in surgical patients are primarily the result of surgical trauma and the subsequent endocrine (catecholamines and corticosteroids) and inflammatory responses (cytokines and chemokines) rather than the result of the anesthetic exposure itself. However, inhaled anesthetics, particularly nitrous oxide, produce dose-dependent inhibition of polymorphonuclear leukocytes and their subsequent migration (chemotaxis) for phagocytosis, which is necessary for the inflammatory response to infection. Nevertheless, decreased resistance to bacterial infection due to inhaled anesthetics seems unlikely, considering the duration of administration and dose of these drugs. Furthermore, when leukocytes reach the site of infection, their ability to phagocytize bacteria appears to be normal.

Inhaled anesthetics do not have bacteriostatic effects at clinically used concentrations. Conversely, the liquid form of volatile anesthetics may be bactericidal.[297] All volatile anesthetics (doses as low as 0.2 MAC) produce dose-dependent inhibition of measles virus replication and decrease mortality in mice receiving intranasal influenza virus.[298] This inhibition may reflect anesthetic-induced decreases in DNA synthesis.

Genetic Effects

The Ames test, which identifies chemicals that act as mutagens and carcinogens, is negative for enflurane, isoflurane, desflurane, sevoflurane, and nitrous oxide, and their known metabolites.[13,231,299] Compound A, which is formed from sevoflurane degradation by carbon dioxide absorbents, might be expected to be an alkylating agent (and thus a mutagen), but tests of this product do not reveal mutagenicity.[270] Halothane also results in a negative Ames test, but some of its potential metabolites may be positive.[300] In animals, nitrous oxide administered during vulnerable periods of gestation may result in adverse reproductive effects manifesting as an increased incidence of fetal resorptions (abortions).[301,302] Conversely, administration of volatile anesthetics during these vulnerable periods does not increase the incidence of fetal resorptions.[303] Learning may be impaired in newborn animals exposed in utero to inhaled anesthetics.[304,305] Early exposure to common anesthetic agents causes widespread neurodegeneration in the developing rat brain and persistent learning deficits.[306] The widespread neuronal degeneration that results is thought to be a natural programmed response to synaptic silencing. Prolonged anesthesia with ketamine in neonatal monkeys (more than 9 hours) results in neuronal degeneration in the frontal cortex.[307] Whether normal exposures of young children to anesthesia for typical time periods could have neurodevelopmental effects is not known but is being actively studied.

Studies of the risk of spontaneous abortion in operating room personnel that were conducted before modern scavenging procedures have suggested an increase in risk. A more recent meta-analysis that considered the relative value of comparison groups has placed the relative risk of anesthetic exposure at 1.9.[308] The increased incidence of spontaneous abortions in operating room personnel in older studies may reflect a teratogenic effect from chronic exposure to trace concentrations of inhaled anesthetics, especially nitrous oxide.[302] Nitrous oxide irreversibly oxidizes the cobalt atom of vitamin B_{12} such that the activity of vitamin B_{12}–dependent enzymes (methionine synthetase and thymidylate synthetase) is decreased. In patients undergoing laparotomy with general anesthesia including 70% nitrous oxide, the half-time for inactivation of methionine synthetase is about 46 minutes (Fig. 4-75).[309] Volatile anesthetics do not alter activity of vitamin B_{12}–dependent enzymes.

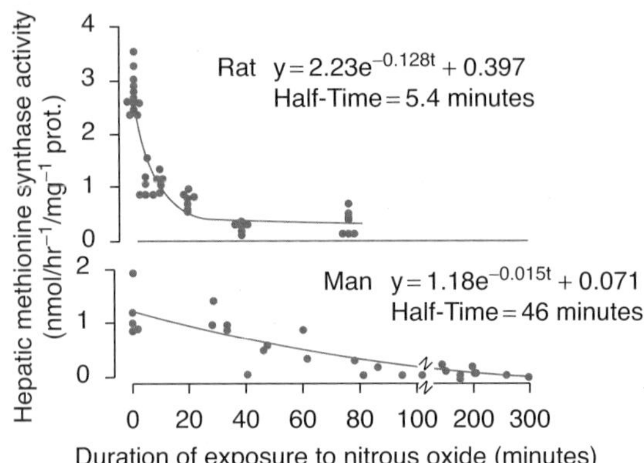

FIGURE 4-75 Time course of inactivation of hepatic methionine synthase (synthetase) activity during administration of 50% nitrous oxide to rats or 70% nitrous oxide to humans. (From Nunn JF, Weinbran HK, Royston D, et al. Rate of inactivation of human and rodent hepatic methionine synthase by nitrous oxide. *Anesthesiology*. 1988;68:213–216, with permission.)

Methionine synthetase converts homocysteine to methionine, which is necessary for the formation of myelin. Thymidylate synthetase is important for DNA synthesis. Interference with myelin formation and DNA synthesis could have significant effects on the rapidly growing fetus, manifesting as spontaneous abortions or congenital anomalies. Inhibition of these enzymes could also manifest as depression of bone marrow function and neurologic disturbances. The speculated but undocumented role of trace concentrations of nitrous oxide in the production of spontaneous abortions has led to the use of scavenging systems designed to remove waste anesthetic gases, including nitrous oxide, from the ambient air of the operating room. Health care workers exposed to nitrous oxide have lower levels of vitamin B_{12} in proportion to their exposure.[310]

Bone Marrow Function

Interference with DNA synthesis is responsible for the megaloblastic changes and agranulocytosis that may follow prolonged administration of nitrous oxide. Megaloblastic changes in bone marrow are consistently found in patients who have been exposed to anesthetic concentrations of nitrous oxide for 24 hours.[311] Exposure to nitrous oxide lasting 4 days or longer results in agranulocytosis. These bone marrow effects occur as a result of nitrous

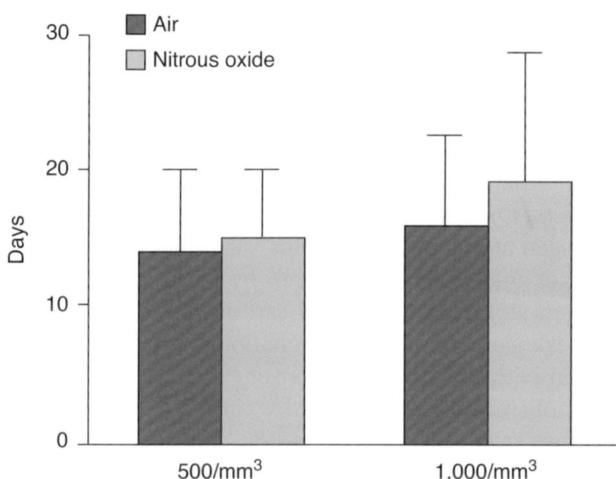

FIGURE 4-76 Nitrous oxide administered during bone marrow harvest did not alter the subsequent number of days needed for cultures to grow 500 to 1,000 cells/mm^3. (Mean ± SD.) (From Lederhaas G, Brock-Utne JG, Negrin RS, et al. Is nitrous oxide safe for bone marrow harvest? *Anesth Analg.* 1995;80:770–772, with permission.)

oxide–induced interference with activity of vitamin B_{12}–dependent enzymes, which are necessary for synthesis of DNA and the subsequent formation of erythrocytes (see the section "Genetic Effects"). Despite these potential adverse effects on bone marrow function, the administration of nitrous oxide to patients undergoing bone marrow transplantation does not influence bone marrow viability (Fig. 4-76).[312]

It is presumed that a healthy surgical patient could receive nitrous oxide for 24 hours without harm. Because the inhibition of methionine synthetase is rapid and its recovery is slow, it is to be expected that repeated exposures at intervals of $<$3 days may result in a cumulative effect. This relationship may be further complicated by other factors influencing levels of methionine synthetase and tetrahydrofolate (necessary for the transmethylation reaction) that might be important in critically ill patients receiving nitrous oxide. Nevertheless, the contradiction between the serious biochemical effects of nitrous oxide and the apparent absence of adverse clinical effects in routine use of this inhaled anesthetic makes it difficult to draw firm conclusions.

Peripheral Neuropathy

Animals exposed to 15% nitrous oxide for up to 15 days develop ataxia and exhibit evidence of spinal cord and peripheral nerve degeneration. Humans who chronically inhale nitrous oxide for nonmedical purposes may develop a neuropathy characterized by sensorimotor polyneuropathy that is often combined with signs of posterior lateral spinal cord degeneration resembling pernicious anemia.[313] The speculated mechanism of this neuropathy is the ability of nitrous oxide to oxidize irreversibly the cobalt atom of vitamin B_{12} such that activity of vitamin B_{12}–dependent enzymes is decreased (see the section "Genetic Effects").

Total Body Oxygen Requirements

Total body oxygen requirements are decreased by similar amounts by different volatile anesthetics. The oxygen requirements of the heart decrease more than those of other organs, reflecting drug-induced decreases in cardiac work associated with decreases in systemic blood pressure and myocardial contractility. Therefore, decreased oxygen requirements would protect tissues from ischemia that might result from decreased oxygen delivery due to drug-induced decreases in perfusion pressure. Decreases in total body oxygen requirements probably reflect metabolic depressant effects as well as decreased functional needs in the presence of anesthetic-produced depression of organ function.

Metabolism

The metabolism of inhaled anesthetics is very small but is important for two reasons. First, intermediary metabolites, end-metabolites, or breakdown products from exposure to carbon dioxide absorbents may be toxic to the kidneys, liver, or reproductive organs. Second, the degree of metabolism may influence the rate of decrease in the alveolar partial pressure at the conclusion of the anesthetic for the most highly metabolized drugs such halothane and methoxyflurane. Conversely, the rate of increase in the alveolar partial pressure during induction of anesthesia is unlikely to be influenced by metabolism because inhaled anesthetics are administered in great excess to the amount metabolized. Metabolism of modern drugs does not significantly affect either onset of offset of drug concentration.

Assessment of the magnitude of metabolism of inhaled anesthetics is by (a) measurement of metabolites or (b) comparison of the total amount of anesthetic recovered in the exhaled gases with the amount taken up during administration (mass balance). The advantages of the mass balance technique are that knowledge of metabolite pharmacokinetics and identification and collection of metabolites are not necessary. Indeed, recovery of metabolites may be incomplete, leading to an underestimation of the magnitude of metabolism. A disadvantage of the mass balance approach is that loss of anesthetic through the surgical skin incision, across the intact skin, in urine, and in feces may prevent complete recovery, and these losses would be construed as due to metabolism. Nevertheless, the error introduced by these losses is likely to be insignificant, with the occasional exception of large and highly perfused wound surfaces.

Table 4-9

Metabolism of Volatile Anesthetics as Assessed by Metabolite Recovery versus Mass Balance Studies

	Magnitude of Metabolism	
Anesthetic	Metabolite Recovery (%)	Mass Balance (%)
Nitrous oxide	0.004	
Halothane	15–20	46.1
Enflurane	3	8.5
Isoflurane	0.2	0[a]
Desflurane	0.02	
Sevoflurane	5	

[a] Metabolism of isoflurane assumed to be 0 for this calculation.

Data adapted from Carpenter RL, Eger EI, Johnson BH, et al. The extent of metabolism of inhaled anesthetics in humans. *Anesthesiology*. 1986;65: 201–205.

Comparison of metabolite recovery and mass balance studies results in greatly different estimates of the magnitude of metabolism of volatile anesthetics (Table 4-9).[50,51] For example, mass balance estimates of the magnitude of metabolism are 1.5 to 3 times greater than estimates determined by the recovery of metabolites. This is not surprising because recovery of metabolites will underestimate the magnitude of metabolism unless all metabolites are recovered. Based on mass balance studies, it is concluded that alveolar ventilation is principally responsible for the elimination of enflurane and isoflurane (presumably also desflurane and sevoflurane), metabolism plays an increasing role for elimination of halothane, and that metabolism was the most important mechanism for the elimination of methoxyflurane.[50,51]

Determinants of Metabolism

The magnitude of metabolism of inhaled anesthetics is determined by the (a) chemical structure, (b) hepatic enzyme activity, (c) blood concentration of the anesthetic, and (d) genetic factors.

Chemical Structure

The ether bond and carbon-halogen bond are the sites in the anesthetic molecule most susceptible to oxidative metabolism. Oxidation of the ether bond is less likely when hydrogen atoms on the carbons surrounding the oxygen atom of this bond are replaced by halogen atoms. Two halogen atoms on a terminal carbon represent the optimal arrangement for dehalogenation, whereas a terminal carbon with fluorine atoms is very resistant to oxidative metabolism. The bond energy for carbon-fluorine is twice that for carbon-bromine or carbon-chlorine. The absence of ester bonds in inhaled anesthetics negates any role of metabolism by hydrolysis.

Hepatic Enzyme Activity

The activity of hepatic cytochrome P450 enzymes responsible for metabolism of volatile anesthetics may be increased by a variety of drugs, including the anesthetics themselves. Phenobarbital, phenytoin, and isoniazid may increase defluorination of volatile anesthetics, especially enflurane. There is evidence in patients that brief (1 hour) exposures during surgical stimulation increase hepatic microsomal enzyme activity independently of the anesthetic drug (halothane or isoflurane) or technique (spinal) used.[314] Conversely, surgery lasting >4 hours can lead to depressed microsomal enzyme activity.

For unknown reasons, obesity predictably increases defluorination of halothane, enflurane, and isoflurane.[315] Peak plasma fluoride concentrations after administration of sevoflurane are higher in obese compared with nonobese patients (Fig. 4-77).[316] Conversely, another report describes no difference in peak plasma fluoride concentrations based on body weight.[317]

Blood Concentration

The fraction of anesthetic that is metabolized on passing through the liver is influenced by the blood concentration of the anesthetic (Fig. 4-78).[36,318] For example, a 1 MAC

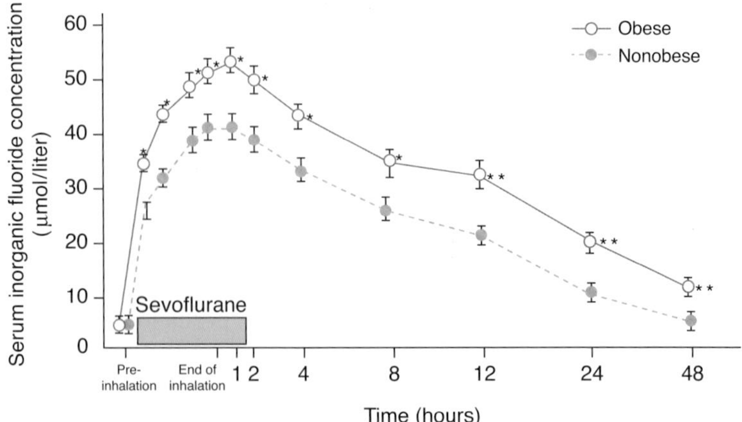

FIGURE 4-77 Plasma inorganic fluoride concentrations during and after sevoflurane administration are higher in obese compared with nonobese patients. (*P <.01 obese vs. nonobese. **P <.001 obese versus nonobese.) (From Higuchi H, Satoh T, Arimura S, et al. Serum inorganic fluoride levels in mildly obese patients during and after sevoflurane anesthesia. *Anesth Analg*. 1993;77:1018–1021, with permission.)

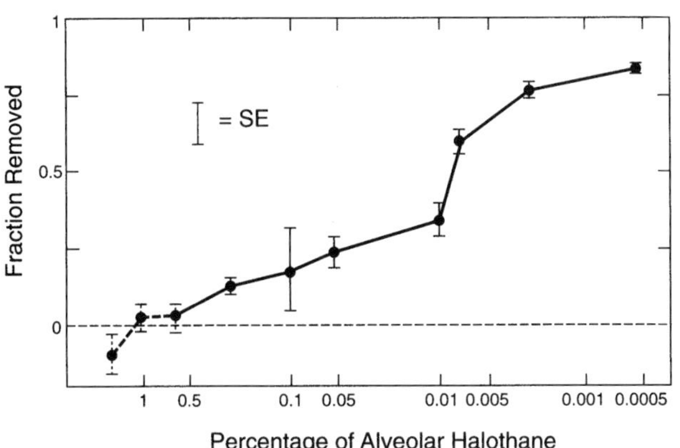

FIGURE 4-78 Fraction of halothane removed during passage through the liver at progressively decreasing alveolar concentrations. (From Sawyer DC, Eger EI, Bahlam SH, et al. Concentration dependence of hepatic halothane metabolism. *Anesthesiology*. 1971;34:230–235, with permission.)

concentration saturates hepatic enzymes and decreases the fraction of anesthetic that is removed (metabolized) during a single passage through the liver. Conversely, subanesthetic concentrations (≤0.1 MAC) undergo extensive metabolism on passage through the liver. Disease states such as cirrhosis of the liver or congestive heart failure could theoretically alter metabolism by decreasing hepatic blood flow and drug delivery or by decreasing the amount of viable liver and thus enzyme activity. Inhaled anesthetics that are less soluble in blood and tissues (nitrous oxide, enflurane, isoflurane, desflurane, sevoflurane) tend to be exhaled rapidly via the lungs at the conclusion of an anesthetic. As a result, less drug is available to pass through the liver continually at low blood concentrations conducive to metabolism. This is reflected in the magnitude of metabolism of these drugs (see Table 4-9).[50,51] Halothane and methoxyflurane are more soluble in blood and lipids and thus likely to be stored in tissues that act as a reservoir to maintain subanesthetic concentrations conducive to metabolism for prolonged periods of time after discontinuation of their administration.

Genetic Factors

Overall, genetic factors appear to be the most important determinant of drug-metabolizing enzyme activity. In this regard, humans are active metabolizers of drugs compared with lower animal species such as the rat.

Metabolism of Specific Inhaled Anesthetics

Nitrous Oxide

An estimated 0.004% of an absorbed dose of nitrous oxide undergoes reductive metabolism to nitrogen in the gastrointestinal tract.[319,320] Anaerobic bacteria, such as *Pseudomonas*, are responsible for this reductive metabolism. Reductive products of some nitrogen compounds include free radicals that could produce toxic effects on cells. The potential toxic role of these metabolites, however, remains undocumented. Oxygen concentrations of >10% in the gastrointestinal tract and antibiotics inhibit metabolism of nitrous oxide by anaerobic bacteria. There is no evidence that nitrous oxide undergoes oxidative metabolism in the liver.[321]

Halothane

An estimated 15% to 20% of absorbed halothane undergoes metabolism (see Table 4-9).[239] Halothane is uniquely metabolized because it undergoes oxidation by cytochrome P450 enzymes when ample oxygen is present but reductive metabolism when hepatocyte Po_2 decreases.

Oxidative Metabolism

The principal oxidative metabolites of halothane resulting from metabolism by cytochrome P450 enzymes are trifluoroacetic acid, chloride, and bromide. In genetically susceptible patients, a reactive trifluoroacetyl halide oxidative metabolite of halothane may interact with (acetylate) hepatic microsomal proteins on the surfaces of hepatocytes (neoantigens) to stimulate the formation of antibodies against this new foreign protein (see Fig. 4-64).[241] These autoantibodies can cause severe necrotic liver failure in rare cases.

The energy bond for carbon-fluorine is strong, accounting for the absence of detectable amounts of inorganic fluoride as an oxidative metabolite of halothane. It is estimated that the plasma concentration of bromide increases 0.5 mEq/L for every MAC hour of halothane administration (Fig. 4-79).[322] Because signs of bromide toxicity, such as somnolence and confusion, do not occur until plasma concentrations of bromide are >6 mEq/L, the likelihood of symptoms from metabolism of halothane to bromide seems remote. Nevertheless, prolonged halothane anesthesia may more likely be associated with

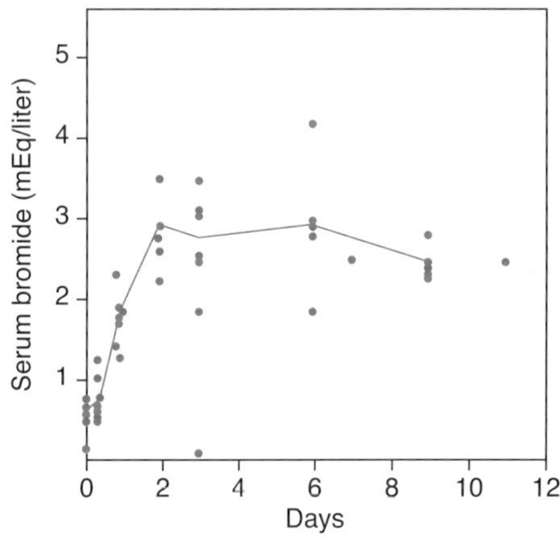

FIGURE 4-79 Serum bromide concentrations in volunteers after prolonged (about 7 hours) exposure to halothane. (From Johnstone RE, Kennell EM, Behar MG, et al. Increased serum bromide concentration after halothane anesthesia in man. *Anesthesiology*. 1975;42:598–601, with permission.)

intellectual impairment than a similar dose of an anesthetic that is not metabolized to bromide.

Reductive Metabolism

Reductive metabolism, which, among the volatile anesthetics, has been documented to occur only during metabolism of halothane, is most likely to occur in the presence of hepatocyte hypoxia and enzyme induction. Reductive metabolites of halothane include fluoride and volatile products, some of which result from the reaction of halothane with carbon dioxide absorbents. In the past, reductive metabolites were considered to be potentially hepatotoxic. Nevertheless, data do not support a role for reductive metabolism in the initiation of halothane hepatitis (see the section "Halothane Hepatitis"). Increased plasma fluoride concentrations reflect reductive metabolism of halothane in obese patients and children with cyanotic congenital heart disease (Fig. 4-80).[323,324] The level of plasma fluoride (<10 μm/L) is far below the level likely to produce even subclinical nephrotoxicity (50 μmol/L), and changes in liver transaminase enzymes as evidence of hepatotoxicity due to reductive metabolism are not seen in these patients.

Enflurane

An estimated 3% of absorbed enflurane undergoes oxidative metabolism by cytochrome P450 enzymes to form inorganic fluoride and organic fluoride compounds (see Table 4-9).[325] Like halothane, enflurane also undergoes cytochrome P450–mediated oxidative metabolism to adducts, which may cause the formation of neoantigens in susceptible patients (see Fig. 4-64)[241] (see the section "Hepatic Effects"). Fluoride results from dehalogenation of the terminal carbon atom. Oxidation of the ether bond and release of additional fluoride does not occur, reflecting the chemical stability imparted to this bond by the surrounding halogens. As with isoflurane, the methyl portion of the molecule seems to be resistant to oxidation, and reductive metabolism does not occur. Minimal metabolism of enflurane reflects its chemical stability and low solubility in tissues such that the drug is exhaled unchanged rather than repeatedly passing through the liver at low plasma concentrations conducive to metabolism.

Enzyme induction with phenobarbital or phenytoin increases the liberation of fluoride from enflurane in vitro but not in vivo.[326] This observation is most likely due to low tissue solubility of enflurane such that, in vivo, the availability of substrate (enflurane) becomes the rate-limiting factor, whereas in vitro, the substrate concentration is controlled and the effect of enzyme induction manifests as increased metabolism of enflurane to inorganic fluoride.[327] For these reasons, it seems unlikely that the nephrotoxic potential of enflurane would be increased by enzyme induction. An exception may be patients who are being treated with isoniazid, because this drug can increase defluorination of enflurane in genetically determined patients who are rapid acetylators.

Isoflurane

An estimated 0.2% of absorbed isoflurane undergoes oxidative metabolism by cytochrome P450 enzymes (see Table 4-9).[328] Metabolism begins with oxidation of the carbon-halogen link of the alpha carbon atom, leading to an unstable compound that subsequently decomposes to difluoromethanol and trifluoroacetic acid (Fig. 4-81).[1] Trifluoroacetic acid is the principal organic fluoride metabolite of isoflurane. Like halothane, isoflurane also undergoes cytochrome P450–mediated oxidative metabolism to adducts, which may cause formation of neoantigens in susceptible patients (see Fig. 4-64)[241] (see the section "Hepatic Effects"). Reductive metabolism of isoflurane does not occur.

Minimal metabolism of isoflurane reflects the drug's chemical stability and low solubility in tissues such that the drug is exhaled unchanged rather than repeatedly passing

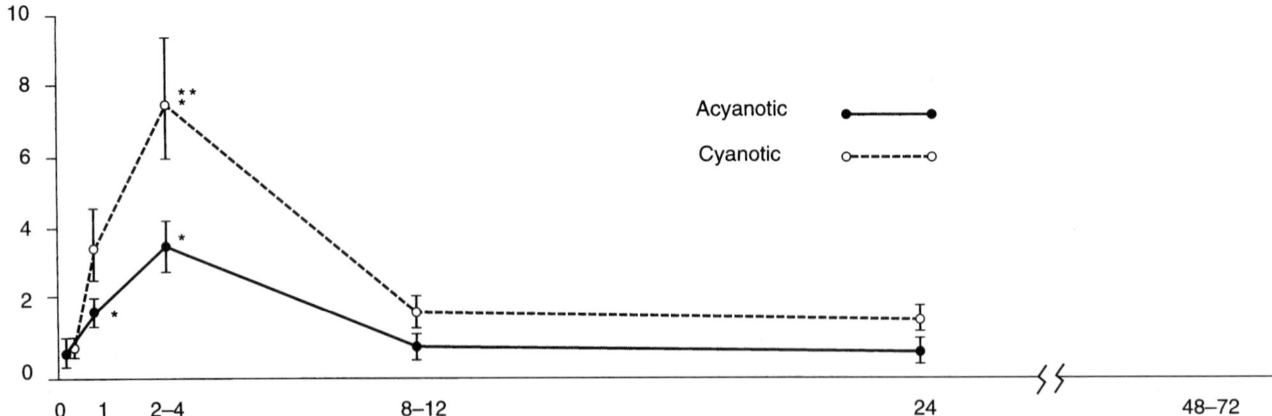

FIGURE 4-80 Plasma concentrations of fluoride are higher after administration of halothane in cyanotic patients than in acyanotic patients. (*P <.05 within groups compared to prehalothane level; **P <.05 between groups.) (Modified from Moore RA, McNicholas KW, Gallagher JD, et al. Halothane metabolism in acyanotic and cyanotic patients undergoing open heart surgery. *Anesth Analg.* 1986;65:1257–1262, with permission.)

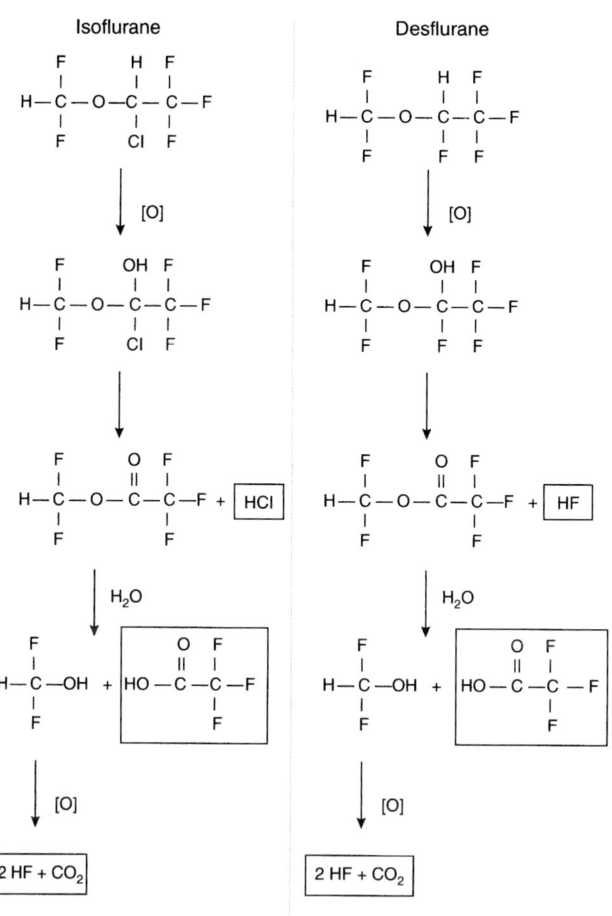

FIGURE 4-81 The proposed metabolic pathways for isoflurane and desflurane are similar. (From Eger EI. *Desflurane [Suprane]: A Compendium and Reference.* Nutley, NJ: Anaquest; 1993:1–119, with permission.)

through the liver at low plasma concentrations conducive to metabolism. The chemical stability of isoflurane is ensured by the trifluorocarbon molecule and the presence of halogen atoms on three sides of the ether bond.

Minimal changes in plasma concentrations of fluoride (peak <5 μm/L) resulting from metabolism of isoflurane plus the absence of other toxic metabolites render nephrotoxicity or hepatotoxicity after administration unlikely. Enzyme induction with phenobarbital or phenytoin increases the liberation of fluoride from isoflurane in vivo.[326] Even in the presence of enzyme induction, however, the metabolism of isoflurane and resulting plasma concentrations of fluoride remain much less than with enflurane. Likewise, isoniazid, which dramatically increases metabolism of enflurane in susceptible patients, fails to significantly alter metabolism of isoflurane.

Desflurane

An estimated 0.02% of absorbed desflurane undergoes oxidative metabolism by cytochrome P450 enzymes (see Table 4-9).[329] The metabolic pathways for desflurane likely parallel those for isoflurane although the greater strength of the carbon-fluorine bond renders desflurane less vulnerable to metabolism than its chlorinated analog, isoflurane (see Fig. 4-81).[1] Metabolism begins with the insertion of an active oxygen atom between the alpha ethyl carbon of desflurane and its hydrogen. The resulting unstable molecule degrades ultimately to inorganic fluoride, trifluoroacetic acid, carbon dioxide, and water. The only evidence of metabolism of desflurane is the presence of measurable concentrations of urinary trifluoroacetic acid equal to about one-fifth to one-tenth that produced by metabolism of isoflurane.[329] Neither plasma fluoride concentrations nor urinary organic fluoride excretion increase significantly after even prolonged administration of desflurane (7.4 MAC hours) to humans.[329] Enzyme induction with phenobarbital or ethanol does not influence the magnitude of metabolism of desflurane in animals.[330] Kinetic studies in humans indicate that all the desflurane absorbed during its administration can be recovered during elimination, emphasizing both the molecular stability of this compound as well as its poor blood and tissue solubility.[32,33] Despite its minimal overall metabolism, desflurane also undergoes cytochrome P450–mediated oxidative metabolism to adducts, which may cause formation of neoantigens in susceptible patients (see Fig. 4-64)[241] (see the section "Hepatic Effects").

Carbon Monoxide Toxicity

Carbon monoxide formation reflects the degradation of volatile anesthetics that contain a CHF_2 moiety (desflurane, enflurane, and isoflurane) by the strong bases present in desiccated carbon dioxide absorbents.[331] Indeed, increases in intraoperative carboxyhemoglobin concentrations have been attributed to this degradation. Factors that influence the magnitude of carbon monoxide production from volatile anesthetics include (a) dryness of the carbon dioxide absorbent with hydration preventing formation, (b) high temperatures of the carbon dioxide absorbent as during low fresh gas flows and/or increased metabolic production of carbon dioxide, (c) prolonged high fresh gas flows that cause desiccation (dryness) of the carbon dioxide absorbent, and (d) type of carbon dioxide absorbent.[332–335] Desflurane produces the highest carbon monoxide concentration (package insert for desflurane describes this risk) followed by enflurane and isoflurane. A carboxyhemoglobin concentration of 36% has been described in a patient receiving desflurane.[336]

Halothane and sevoflurane do not possess a vinyl group and thus carbon monoxide production on exposure to carbon dioxide absorbents has been considered unlikely. Nevertheless, carbon monoxide formation is a risk of sevoflurane administration in the presence of desiccated carbon dioxide absorbent especially when an exothermic reaction between the volatile anesthetic and desiccated absorbent occurs (see the section "Carbon Dioxide Absorber Fires").[337] In the presence of carbon dioxide absorbent temperatures >70°C, hexafluoroisopropanol, an intermediate of sevoflurane metabolism, degrades to carbon monoxide to a small degree. Nevertheless, completely desiccated carbon dioxide absorbent and high patient minute ventilation could result in significant carbon monoxide exposure.[221] As such, it is not possible to completely avoid hazards of carbon monoxide by using sevoflurane. It is concluded that the potential for carbon monoxide formation is a property of all modern volatile anesthetics contacting dry carbon dioxide absorbents that contain potassium hydroxide and/or sodium hydroxide.[337,338] Patients with low hemoglobin quantities (anemia, pediatric patients) are at greater risk for high carboxyhemoglobin concentrations in response to exposure to carbon monoxide.[339] Precautions to ensure carbon dioxide absorbents that contain strong bases have not become desiccated is important for preventing the formation of carbon monoxide during administration of volatile anesthetics. Current Environmental Protection Agency limits for carbon monoxide exposure are 35 ppm for 1 hour.

Intraoperative Diagnosis

Intraoperative detection of carbon monoxide is difficult because pulse oximetry cannot differentiate between carboxyhemoglobin and oxyhemoglobin. Moderately decreased pulse oximetry readings despite adequate arterial partial pressures of oxygen (especially during the first case of the day, "Monday morning phenomena") should suggest the possibility of carbon monoxide exposure and the need to measure carboxyhemoglobin.[339] Furthermore, there is no routinely available means to reliably identify the presence of carbon monoxide in the breathing circuit nor to detect when carbon dioxide absorbent has become desiccated (absorbent color change does not occur in response to desiccation or carbon monoxide formation). In addition to decreased pulse oximeter readings, an erroneous gas analyzer reading (indicates mixed gas readings or enflurane when desflurane is being administered) has been described as an early indirect warning of carbon monoxide formation.[221,336] This erroneous gas analyzer reading was attributed to trifluoromethane, which is produced along with carbon monoxide by degradation of isoflurane, enflurane, and desflurane, but not sevoflurane. Trifluoromethane has an infrared absorption profile similar to enflurane resulting in the gas analyzer indicating administration of this volatile anesthetic when the vaporizer is known to contain desflurane or isoflurane. An erroneous gas analyzer reading as an early warning of carbon monoxide exposure does not occur during administration of sevoflurane.[221] Delayed neurophysiologic sequelae due to carbon monoxide poisoning (cognitive defects, personality changes, gait disturbances) may occur as late as 3 to 21 days after anesthesia. Intraoperative hemolysis has the potential to result in carbon monoxide exposure, which can mimic carbon monoxide production from degradation of volatile anesthetics.[340]

Endogenous Carbon Monoxide

Endogenous carbon monoxide production reflects heme catabolism. The rate-limiting enzyme in formation of carbon monoxide from heme is heme oxygenase-1. This enzyme is induced by its substrate (heme) and by various oxidative stresses. Heme oxygenase-1 is thought to confer protection against oxidative tissue injuries. Conversion of the heme moiety of hemeproteins (hemoglobin, myoglobin, cytochrome P450) to biliverdin (a green bile pigment) results in liberation of carbon monoxide. This endogenous carbon monoxide diffuses from cells into the circulation to form carboxyhemoglobin and is also transported to the lungs where it is exhaled. Independent of volatile anesthetics and carbon dioxide absorbents, the exhaled carbon monoxide and carboxyhemoglobin concentrations are increased on the day following surgery.[341] This suggests that oxidative stress associated with anesthesia and surgery may induce heme oxygenase-1, which catalyzes heme to produce carbon monoxide.

Sevoflurane

An estimated 5% of absorbed sevoflurane undergoes oxidative metabolism by cytochrome P450 enzymes to form organic and inorganic fluoride metabolites (see Table 4-9 and Fig. 4-64).[252] In addition, sevoflurane is degraded by desiccated carbon dioxide absorbents containing strong bases to potentially toxic compounds (see the section "Vinyl Halide Nephrotoxicity").[5] Unlike all the other fluorinated volatile anesthetics, sevoflurane does not undergo metabolism to acetyl halide that could result in formation of trifluoatated liver proteins. As a result, sevoflurane cannot stimulate the formation of antitrifluoroacetylated protein antibodies leading to hepatotoxicity by this mechanism[13] (see the section "Hepatic Effects").

Cytochrome P450–mediated sevoflurane oxidation at the fluoromethoxy carbon produces a transient intermediate that decomposes to inorganic fluoride and the organic fluoride metabolite hexafluoroisopropanol. Hexafluoroisopropanol undergoes conjugation with glucuronic acid and this conjugate is excreted in the urine. There is no evidence that hexafluoroisopropanol is toxic.

Peak plasma fluoride concentrations are higher after administration of sevoflurane than after comparable doses of enflurane.[260,262] Nevertheless, the duration of exposure of renal tubules to fluoride that results from sevoflurane metabolism is limited because of the rapid pulmonary elimination of this poorly blood-soluble anesthetic. Furthermore, hepatic production of fluoride from sevoflurane may be less of a nephrotoxic risk than is intrarenal production of fluoride from enflurane.[267]

Sevoflurane is absorbed and degraded by desiccated carbon dioxide absorbents, especially when the temperature of the absorbent is increased (see Fig. 4-5).[5] Among these compounds, only compound A (and to a lesser extent compound B) is produced under conditions likely to be encountered clinically. The type of carbon dioxide absorbent may influence the magnitude of compound A production.[82] Compound A is nephrotoxic and hepatotoxic in animals (see the sections "Hepatic Effects" and "Renal Effects"). Nevertheless, the amount of compound A produced under clinically relevant circumstances has always been substantially lower than that which produces toxicity in animals.[5]

Carbon Dioxide Absorber Fires

Sevoflurane reacts chemically with desiccated carbon dioxide absorbents (especially Baralyme®, which is no longer clinically available) to produce carbon monoxide and flammable organic compounds, including methanol and formaldehyde. The reaction produces heat and heat increases the reaction speed so the rate of sevoflurane breakdown can accelerate rapidly. Sevoflurane may be so extensively consumed that maintaining anesthesia is difficult. At high temperatures, flammable metabolites can spontaneously combust (formaldehyde gas). A peak absorbent canister temperature of 120° to 140°C is generally reached 10 to 50 minutes after the start of the reaction followed by a rapid decrease in the canister temperature. In nonhuman trials utilizing anesthesia machines the carbon dioxide absorbent temperatures increased rapidly to greater than 300°C and parts of the absorbent canister melted.[221]

In the presence of desiccated carbon dioxide absorbent, temperature increases are greater with sevoflurane than with other volatile anesthetics, and at absorbent temperatures >70°C, there is increased likelihood of degradation of sevoflurane to flammable products and carbon monoxide (Figs. 4-82 and 4-83)[221,337,342] For example, temperatures of desiccated soda lime exposed to 1.5 MAC isoflurane and desflurane peaked at about 100°C and then decreased progressively, whereas temperatures in desiccated carbon dioxide absorbents exposed to 1.5 MAC increased progressively to nearly 200°C and spontaneous combustion in the anesthesia circuit occurred in some instances (see Fig. 4-83).[342] Spontaneous combustion and even explosions involving the carbon dioxide absorber and anesthesia breathing circuit have been described clinically and are most often (perhaps always) associated with Baralyme® carbon dioxide absorbent (no longer clinically available); anesthesia machine use factors that contribute to desiccation of the absorbent (flow of dry gases through the absorber during a weekend, "Monday morning phenomena") and administration of sevoflurane.[221,343–346] Apparently, under certain conditions, exothermic chemical reactions between sevoflurane and desiccated carbon dioxide absorbent creates high temperatures with production of flammable gases (formaldehyde, methanol) and autoignition of plastics and gases in the absorber. The critical observation regarding fires and production of carbon monoxide is that desiccated carbon dioxide absorbents

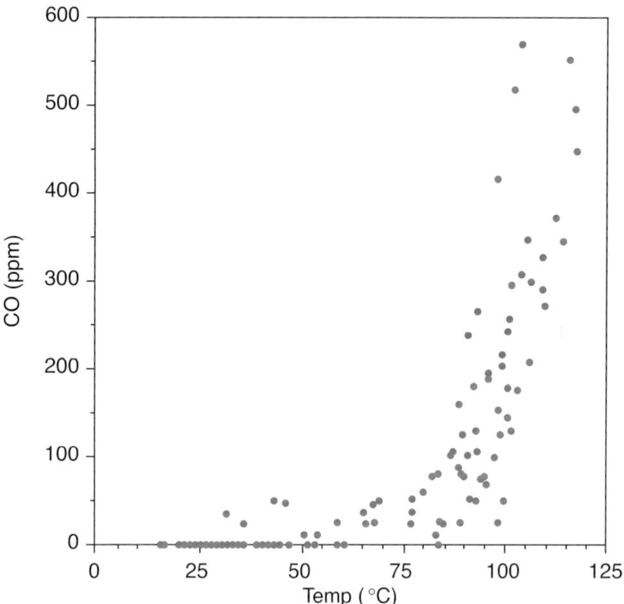

FIGURE 4-82 Carbon monoxide (CO) concentrations in parts per million (ppm) are plotted against absorbent temperatures measured in the center of the canister. Most clinically relevant CO concentrations do not occur until the absorbent temperature exceeds 70°C. (From Holak E, Mei DA, Dunning MB, et al. Carbon monoxide production from sevoflurane breakdown: Modeling of exposures under clinical conditions. *Anesth Analg.* 2003;96:757–764, with permission.)

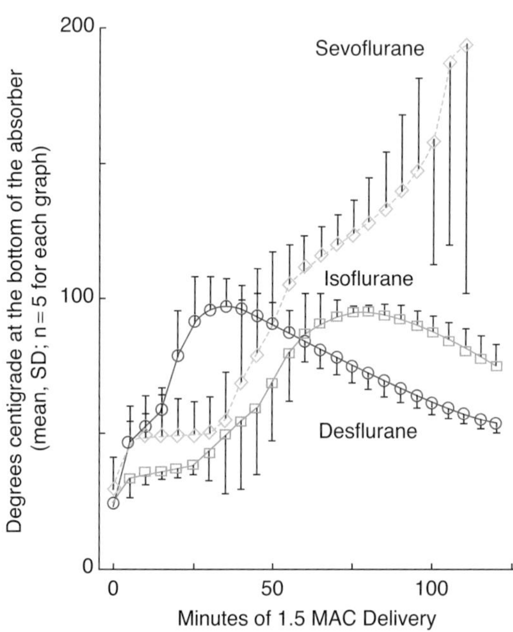

FIGURE 4-83 Temperatures recorded from the bottom of the desiccated carbon dioxide absorbent canister peaked at about 100C¼ when exposed to 1.5 MAC desflurane and isoflurane and then decreased. Temperatures in the desiccated carbon dioxide absorbent canister increased progressively to over 200C¼ when exposed to 1.5 MAC sevoflurane and spontaneous flames occurred in some of the anesthesia circuits. (From Lester M, Roth P, Eger, EI. Fires from the interaction of anesthetics with desiccated absorbent. *Anesth Analg.* 2004;99:769–774, with permission.)

containing strong bases allow these reactions to occur. Clinically, delayed increases or unexpected sudden decreases in inspired sevoflurane concentrations relative to the vaporizer setting may reflect excessive heating of the carbon dioxide absorber canister. Pulmonary injury has been observed following an exothermic reaction between sevoflurane and the carbon dioxide absorbent.[347] Furthermore, formaldehyde alone as a byproduct of sevoflurane breakdown may cause pulmonary injury.

These dangerous chemical reactions can be avoided by utilizing carbon dioxide absorbents devoid of strong bases.[345] Nevertheless, the ability of absorbents lacking strong bases to adequately absorb carbon dioxide in all situations is unclear.[348] Water also inhibits these chemical reactions but may evaporate particularly with prolonged flows through the absorbent when the breathing circuit is not connected to a patient. Strong bases are included in absorbents to enhance carbon dioxide absorption.

References

1. Eger EI. *Desflurane (Suprane): A Compendium and Reference.* Nutley, NJ: Anaquest; 1993.
2. Johnston RR, Cromwell TH, Eger EI, et al. The toxicity of fluroxene in animals and man. *Anesthesiology.* 1973;38:313–319.
3. Buntine P, Thom O, Babl F, et al. Prehospital analgesia in adults using inhaled methoxyflurane. *Emerg Med Australas.* 2007;19:509–514.
4. Eger EI II, Liu J, Koblin DD, et al. Molecular properties of the "ideal" inhaled anesthetic: studies of fluorinated methanes, ethanes, propanes, and butanes. *Anesth Analg.* 1994;79(2):245–251.
5. Smith I, Nathanson M, White PF. Sevoflurane—a long awaited volatile anesthetic. *Br J Anaesth.* 1996;76:435–445.
6. Weiskopf RB, Eger EI. Comparing the costs of inhaled anesthetics. *Anesthesiology.* 1993;79:1413–1418.
7. Goto T, Nakata Y, Morita S. Will xenon be a stranger or a friend? The cost, benefit, and future of xenon anesthesia. *Anesthesiology.* 2003;98:1–2.
8. Neuman GG, Sidebotham G, Negoianu E, et al. Laparoscopy explosive hazards with nitrous oxide. *Anesthesiology.* 1993;78:875–879.
9. Guo TZ, Poree L, Golden W, et al. Antinociceptive response to nitrous oxide is mediated by supraspinal opiate and spinal β2 adrenergic receptors in the rat. *Anesthesiology.* 1996;85:846–852.
10. Fernández-Guisasola J, Gómez-Arnau JI, Cabrera Y, et al. Association between nitrous oxide and the incidence of postoperative nausea and vomiting in adults: a systematic review and meta-analysis. *Anaesthesia.* 2010;65:379–387.
11. Kambam JR, Holaday DA. Effect of nitrous oxide on the oxyhemoglobin dissociation curve and PO2 measurements. *Anesthesiology.* 1987;66:208–209.
12. Ebert TJ, Robinson BJ, Uhrich TD, et al. Recovery from sevoflurane anesthesia: a comparison to isoflurane and propofol anesthesia. *Anesthesiology.* 1998;89:1524–1531.
13. Kharasch ED. Biotransformation of sevoflurane. *Anesth Analg.* 1995;81:S27–S38.
14. Bito H, Ikeda K. Closed-circuit anesthesia with sevoflurane in humans: effects of renal and hepatic function and concentrations of breakdown products with soda lime in the circuit. *Anesthesiology.* 1994;80:71–76.
15. Nakata Y, Goto T, Ishiguro Y, et al. Minimum alveolar concentration (MAC) of xenon with sevoflurane in humans. *Anesthesiology.* 2001;94:611–614.
16. Goto T, Nakata Y, Ishiguro Y, et al. Minimum alveolar concentration-awake of xenon alone and in combination with isoflurane or sevoflurane. *Anesthesiology.* 2000;93:1188–1193.
17. Goto T, Nakata Y, Morita S. The minimum alveolar concentration of xenon in the elderly is sex-dependent. *Anesthesiology.* 2002;97:1129–1132.
18. Maria NS, Eckmann DM. Model predictions of gas embolism growth and reabsorption during xenon anesthesia. *Anesthesiology.* 2003;99:638–645.
19. Reinelt H, Schirmer U, Marx T, et al. Diffusion of xenon and nitrous oxide into the blood. *Anesthesiology.* 2001;94:475–477.
20. Froeba G, Marx T, Pazhur J, et al. Xenon does not trigger malignant hyperthermia in susceptible swine. *Anesthesiology.* 1999;91:1047–1052.
21. Rossaint R, Reyle-Hahn M, Esch JS, et al. Multicenter randomized comparison of the efficacy and safety of xenon and isoflurane in patients undergoing elective surgery. *Anesthesiology.* 2003;98:6–13.
22. Kunitz O, Baumert J-H, Hecker K, et al. Xenon does not prolong neuromuscular block of rocuronium. *Anesth Analg.* 2004;99:1398–1401.
23. Ma D, Wilhelm S, Maze M, et al. Neuroprotective and neurotoxic properties of the "inert" gas, xenon. *Br J Anaesth.* 2002;89:739–746.
24. Strum DP, Eger EI, Unadkat JD, et al. Age affects the pharmacokinetics of inhaled anesthetics in humans. *Anesth Analg.* 1991;73:310–318.
25. Eger EI. Effect of inspired anesthetic concentration on the rate of rise of alveolar concentration. *Anesthesiology.* 1963;24:153–157.
26. Stoelting RK, Eger EI. An additional explanation for the second gas effect: a concentrating effect. *Anesthesiology.* 1969;30:273–277.
27. Epstein RM, Rackow H, Salanitre E, et al. Influence of the concentration effect on the uptake of anesthetic mixtures: the second gas effect. *Anesthesiology.* 1964;25:364–371.
28. Korman B, Mapleson WW. Concentration and second gas effects: can the accepted explanation be improved? *Br J Anaesth.* 1997;78:618–625.
29. Salanitre E, Rackow H. The pulmonary exchange of nitrous oxide and halothane in infants and children. *Anesthesiology.* 1969;30:388–394.
30. Gibbons RT, Steffey EP, Eger EI. The effect of spontaneous versus controlled ventilation on the rate of rise in the alveolar halothane concentration in dogs. *Anesth Analg.* 1977;56:32–37.
31. Yasuda N, Targ AC, Eger EI. Solubility of I-653, sevoflurane, isoflurane, and halothane in human tissues. *Anesth Analg.* 1989;69:370–373.
32. Yasuda N, Lockhart SH, Eger EI, et al. Comparison of kinetics of sevoflurane and isoflurane in humans. *Anesth Analg.* 1991;72:316–324.
33. Yasuda N, Lockhart SH, Eger EI, et al. Kinetics of desflurane, isoflurane, and halothane in humans. *Anesthesiology.* 1991;74:489–498.
34. Meretoja OA, Taivainen T, Raiha L, et al. Sevoflurane-nitrous oxide or halothane-nitrous oxide for pediatric bronchoscopy and gastroscopy. *Br J Anaesth.* 1996;76:767–770.
35. Stoelting RK, Eger EI. Percutaneous loss of nitrous oxide, cyclopropane, ether and halothane in man. *Anesthesiology.* 1969;30:278–283.
36. Sawyer DC, Eger EI, Bahlman SH, et al. Concentration dependence of hepatic halothane metabolism. *Anesthesiology.* 1971;34:230–235.
37. Laasberg HL, Hedley-White J. Halothane solubility in blood and solutions of plasma proteins: effects of temperature, protein composition and hemoglobin concentration. *Anesthesiology.* 1970;32:351–356.
38. Ellis DE, Stoelting RK. Individual variations in fluroxene, halothane and methoxyflurane blood-gas partition coefficients, and the effect of anemia. *Anesthesiology.* 1975;42:748–750.
39. Munson ES, Eger EI, Tham MK, et al. Increase in anesthetic uptake, excretion and blood solubility in man after eating. *Anesth Analg.* 1978;57:224–231.

40. Lerman J, Gregory GA, Willis MM, et al. Age and solubility of volatile anesthetics in blood. *Anesthesiology*. 1984;61:139–143.
41. Malviya S, Lerman J. The blood/gas solubilities of sevoflurane, isoflurane, halothane, and serum constituent concentrations in neonates and adults. *Anesthesiology*. 1990;72:79–83.
42. Fassoulaki A, Eger EI. Starvation increases the solubility of volatile anesthetics in rat liver. *Br J Anaesth*. 1986;58:327–329.
43. Eger EI, Saidman LJ. Hazards of nitrous oxide anesthesia in bowel obstruction and pneumothorax. *Anesthesiology*. 1965;26:61–66.
44. Munson ES, Merrick HC. Effect of nitrous oxide on venous air embolism. *Anesthesiology*. 1966;27:783–787.
45. LoSasso TJ, Muzzi DA, Dietz NM, et al. Fifty percent nitrous oxide does not increase the risk of venous air embolism in neurosurgical patients operated upon in the sitting position. *Anesthesiology*. 1992;77:21–30.
46. Vote BJ, Hart RH, Worsley DR, et al. Visual loss after use of nitrous oxide gas with general anesthetic in patients with intraocular gas still persistent up to 30 days after vitrectomy. *Anesthesiology*. 2002;97:1305–1308.
47. Gedney JA, Ghosh S. Pharmacokinetics of analgesics, sedatives and anaesthetic agents during cardiopulmonary bypass. *Br J Anaesth*. 1995;75:344–351.
48. Stoelting RK, Longnecker DE. Effect of right-to-left shunt on rate of increase in arterial anesthetic concentration. *Anesthesiology*. 1972;36:352–356.
49. Stoelting RK, Eger EI. The effects of ventilation and anesthetic solubility on recovery from anesthesia: an in vivo and analog analysis before and after equilibration. *Anesthesiology*. 1969;30:290–296.
50. Carpenter RL, Eger EI, Johnson BH, et al. Pharmacokinetics of inhaled anesthetics in humans: measurements during and after the simultaneous administration of enflurane, halothane, isoflurane, methoxyflurane, and nitrous oxide. *Anesth Analg*. 1986;65:575–582.
51. Carpenter RL, Eger EI, Johnson BH, et al. The extent of metabolism of inhaled anesthetics in humans. *Anesthesiology*. 1986;65:201–205.
52. Bailey JM. Context-sensitive half-times and other decrement times of inhaled anesthetics. *Anesth Analg*. 1997;85:681–686.
53. Fink BR. Diffusion anoxia. *Anesthesiology*. 1955;16:511–519.
54. Sheffer L, Steffenson JL, Birch AA. Nitrous oxide-induced diffusion hypoxia in patients breathing spontaneously. *Anesthesiology*. 1972;37:436–439.
55. Merkel G, Eger EI. A comparative study of halothane and halopropane anesthesia: including method for determining equipotency. *Anesthesiology*. 1963;24:346–357.
56. Sonner JM, Antognini JF, Dutton RC, et al. Inhaled anesthetics and immobility: mechanisms, mysteries, and minimum alveolar anesthetic concentration. *Anesth Analg*. 2003;97:718–740.
57. Antognini JF, Schwartz K. Exaggerated anesthetic requirements in the preferentially anesthetized brain. *Anesthesiology*. 1993;79:1244–1299.
58. Rampil IJ, Mason P, Singh H. Anesthetic potency (MAC) is independent of forebrain structures in the rat. *Anesthesiology*. 1993;78:707–712.
59. Sani O, Shafer SL. MAC attack? *Anesthesiology*. 2003;99:1249–1250.
60. Hall RI, Sullivan JA. Does cardiopulmonary bypass alter enflurane requirements for anesthesia? *Anesthesiology*. 1990;73:249–255.
61. Quasha AL, Eger EI, Tinker JH. Determination and application of MAC. *Anesthesiology*. 1980;53:315–334.
62. Eger EI, Fisher DM, Dilger JP, et al. Relevant concentrations of inhaled anesthetics for in vitro studies of anesthetic mechanisms. *Anesthesiology*. 2001;94:915–921.
63. Mapleson WW. Effect of age on MAC in humans: a meta-analysis. *Br J Anaesth*. 1996;76:179–185.
64. Chan MTV, Gin T. Postpartum changes in the minimum alveolar concentration of isoflurane. *Anesthesiology*. 1995;82:1360–1363.
65. Zhou HH, Norman P, DeLima LGR, et al. The minimum alveolar concentration of isoflurane in patients undergoing bilateral tubal ligation in the postpartum period. *Anesthesiology*. 1995;82:1364–1368.
66. Eger EI, Laster MJ, Gregory GA, et al. Women appear to have the same alveolar concentration as men: a retrospective study. *Anesthesiology*. 2003;99:1059–1061.
67. Wadhwa A, Durrani J, Sengupta P, et al. Women have the same desflurane minimum alveolar concentration as men: a prospective study. *Anesthesiology*. 2003;99:1062–1065.
68. Liem EB, Lin C-M, Suleman M-I, et al. Anesthetic requirement is increased in redheads. *Anesthesiology*. 2004;101:279–283.
69. Petersen-Felix S, Zbinden AM, Fischer M, et al. Isoflurane minimum alveolar concentration decreases during anesthesia and surgery. *Anesthesiology*. 1993;79:959–965.
70. Niemann CU, Stabernack C, Serkova, et al. Cyclosporine can increase isoflurane MAC. *Anesth Analg*. 2002;95:930–934.
71. Zbinden AM, Maggiorini M, Peterson-Felix S, et al. Anesthetic depth defined using multiple noxious stimuli during isoflurane/oxygen anesthesia. I. Motor reactions. *Anesthesiology*. 1994;80:253–260.
72. Eger EI, Tang M, Liao M, et al. Inhaled anesthetics do not combine to produce synergistic effects regarding minimum alveolar anesthetic concentration in rats. *Anesth Analg*. 2008;107:479–485.
73. Shafer SL, Hendrickx JF, Flood P, et al. Additivity versus synergy: a theoretical analysis of implications for anesthetic mechanisms. *Anesth Analg*. 2008;107:507–524.
74. Sebel PS, Glass PSA, Fletcher JE, et al. Reduction of the MAC of desflurane with fentanyl. *Anesthesiology*. 1992;76:52–59.
75. Manyam SC, Gupta DK, Johnson KB, et al. Opioid-volatile anesthetic synergy: a response surface model with remifentanil and sevoflurane as prototypes. *Anesthesiology*. 2006;105:267–278.
76. Halsey MJ, Smith B. Pressure reversal of narcosis produced by anesthetics, narcotics and tranquilizers. *Nature*. 1975;257:811–813.
77. Franks NP, Lieb WR. Molecular and cellular mechanisms of general anaesthesia. *Nature*. 1994;367:607–614.
78. Lynch C, Pancrazio JJ. Snails, spiders, and stereospecificity—is there a role for calcium channels in anesthetic mechanisms? *Anesthesiology*. 1994;81:1–5.
79. Franks NP, Lieb WR. Stereospecific effects of inhalational general anesthetic optical isomers on nerve ion channels. *Science*. 1991;254:427–430.
80. Dickinson R, White I, Lieb WR, et al. Stereoselective loss of righting reflex in rats by isoflurane. *Anesthesiology*. 2000;93:837–845.
81. Lysko GS, Robinson JL, Casto R, et al. The stereospecific effects of isoflurane isomers in vivo. *Eur J Pharmacol*. 1994;263:25–29.
82. Eger EI, Ionescu P, Laster MJ, et al. Baralyme dehydration increases and soda lime dehydration decreases the concentration of compound A resulting from sevoflurane degradation in a standard anesthetic circuit. *Anesth Analg*. 1997;85:892–898.
83. Fang Z, Sonner J, Laster MJ, et al. Anesthetic and convulsant properties of aromatic compounds and cycloalkanes: implications for mechanisms of narcosis. *Anesth Analg*. 1996;83:1097–1104.
84. Zhang Y, Laster MJ, Hara K, et al. Glycine receptors mediate part of the immobility produced by inhaled anesthetics. *Anesth Analg*. 2003;96:97–101.
85. Jurd R, Arras M, Lambert S, et al. General anesthetic actions in vivo strongly attenuated by a point mutation in the GABA(A) receptor beta3 subunit. *FASEB J*. 2003;17:250–252.
86. Zhang Y, Sonner JM, Eger EI, et al. Gamma-aminobutyric acidA receptors do not mediate the immobility produced by isoflurane. *Anesth Analg*. 2004;95:85–90.
87. Solt K, Eger EI II, Raines DE. Differential modulation of human N-methyl-D-aspartate receptors by structurally diverse general anesthetics. *Anesth Analg*. 2006;102:1407–1411.
88. Franks NP. Molecular targets underlying general anaesthesia. *Br J Pharmacol*. 2006;147(suppl 1):S72–S81.
89. Pang DS, Robledo CJ, Carr DR, et al. An unexpected role for TASK-3 potassium channels in network oscillations with implications for

sleep mechanisms and anesthetic action. *Proc Natl Acad Sci U S A.* 2009;106:17546–17551.
90. Shiraishi M, Harris RA. Effects of alcohols and anesthetics on recombinant voltage-gated Na+ channels. *J Pharmacol Exp Ther.* 2004;309:987–994.
91. Sirois JE, Lynch C III, Bayliss DA. Convergent and reciprocal modulation of a leak K+ current and I(h) by an inhalational anaesthetic and neurotransmitters in rat brainstem motoneurones. *J Physiol.* 2002;541:717–729.
92. Flood P, Sonner JM, Gong D, et al. Heteromeric nicotinic inhibition by isoflurane does not mediate MAC or loss of righting reflex. *Anesthesiology.* 2002;97:902–905.
93. Eger EI. Age, minimum alveolar anesthetic concentration, and minimum alveolar anesthetic concentration-awake. *Anesth Analg.* 2001;93:947–953.
94. John ER, Prichep LS. The anesthetic cascade. A theory of how anesthesia suppresses consciousness. *Anesthesiology.* 2005;102: 447–471.
95. Glass PSA. Anesthetic drug interactions: an insight into general anesthesia-its mechanisms and dosing strategies. *Anesthesiology.* 1998;88:5–6.
96. Mashour GA. Consciousness unbound. Toward a paradigm of general anesthesia. *Anesthesiology.* 2004;100:428–433.
97. Zhang Y, Eger EI II, Dutton RC, et al. Inhaled anesthetics have hyperalgesic effects at 0.1 minimum alveolar anesthetic concentration. *Anesth Analg.* 2000;91:462–466.
98. Hemmings HC Jr. Sodium channels and the synaptic mechanisms of inhaled anaesthetics. *Br J Anaesth.* 2009;103:61–69.
99. Larsen M, Langmoen IA. The effect of volatile anaesthetics on synaptic release and uptake of glutamate. *Toxicol Lett.* 1998;100–101: 59–64.
100. Eger EI. *Isoflurane (Forane): A Compendium and Reference.* 2nd ed. Madison, WI: Ohio Medical Products; 1985.
101. Frankhuizen JL, Vlek CAJ, Burm AGL, et al. Failure to replicate negative effects of trace anesthetics on mental performance. *Br J Anaesth.* 1978;50:229–234.
102. Garfield JM, Garfield FB, Sampson J. Effects of nitrous oxide on decision strategy and sustained attention. *Psycopharmacologia.* 1975;42:5–10.
103. Tinker JH, Sharbrough FW, Michenfelder JD. Anterior shift of the dominant EEG rhythm during anesthesia in the JAVA monkey: correlation with anesthetic potency. *Anesthesiology.* 1977;46:252–259.
104. Eger EI, Stevens WC, Cromwell TH. The electroencephalogram in man anesthetized with Forane. *Anesthesiology.* 1971;35:504–508.
105. Oshima E, Urabe N, Shingu K, et al. Anticonvulsant actions of enflurane on epilepsy models in cats. *Anesthesiology.* 1985;63:29–40.
106. Koblin DD, Eger EI, Johnson BH, et al. Are convulsant gases also anesthetics? *Anesthesiology.* 1980;53:S47.
107. Kaisti KK, Jaaskelainen SK, Rinne JO, et al. Epileptiform discharges during 2 MAC sevoflurane anesthesia in two healthy volunteers. *Anesthesiology.* 1999;91(6):1952–1955.
108. Komatsu H, Taie S, Endo S, et al. Electrical seizures during sevoflurane anesthesia in two pediatric patients with epilepsy. *Anesthesiology.* 1994;81:1535–1537.
109. Henderson JM, Spence DG, Komocar LM, et al. Administration of nitrous oxide to pediatric patients provides analgesia for venous cannulation. *Anesthesiology.* 1990;72:269–271.
110. Russell GB, Snider MT, Richard RB, et al. Hyperbaric nitrous oxide as a sole anesthetic agent in humans. *Anesth Analg.* 1990;70: 289–295.
111. Lannes M, Desparmet JF, Zifkin BG. Generalized seizures associated with nitrous oxide in an infant. *Anesthesiology.* 1997;87: 705–708.
112. Smith RA, Winter PM, Smith M, et al. Convulsion in mice after anesthesia. *Anesthesiology.* 1979;50:501–504.
113. Boisseau N, Madany M, Staccini P, et al. Comparison of the effects of sevoflurane and propofol on cortical somatosensory evoked potentials. *Br J Anaesth.* 2002;88:785–789.
114. Iohom G, Collins I, Murphy D, et al. Postoperative changes in visual evoked potentials and cognitive function tests following sevoflurane anaesthesia. *Br J Anaesth.* 2001;87:855–859.
115. Pathak KS, Ammadio M, Kalamchi A, et al. Effects of halothane, enflurane, and isoflurane on somatosensory evoked potentials during nitrous oxide anesthesia. *Anesthesiology.* 1987;66:753–757.
116. Ghoneim MM, Block RI. Learning and memory during general anesthesia. An update. *Anesthesiology.* 1997;87:387–395.
117. Matta BF, Heath KJ, Tipping K, et al. Direct cerebral vasodilatory effects of sevoflurane and isoflurane. *Anesthesiology.* 1999;91: 677–680.
118. Ornstein E, Young WL, Fleischer LH, et al. Desflurane and isoflurane have similar effects on cerebral blood flow in patients with intracranial mass lesions. *Anesthesiology.* 1993;79:498–502.
119. Lam AM, Mayberg TS, Eng CC, et al. Nitrous oxide-isoflurane anesthesia causes more cerebral vasodilation than an equipotent dose of isoflurane in humans. *Anesth Analg.* 1994;78:462–468.
120. Albrecht RF, Miletich DJ, Madala LR. Normalization of cerebral blood flow during prolonged anesthesia. *Anesthesiology.* 1983;58: 26–31.
121. Warner DS, Boarini DJ, Kassell NE. Cerebrovascular adaptation to prolonged halothane anesthesia is not related to cerebrovascular fluid pH. *Anesthesiology.* 1985;63:243–248.
122. Kuroda Y, Murakami M, Tsuruta J, et al. Preservation of the ratio of cerebral blood flow/metabolic rate for oxygen during prolonged anesthesia with isoflurane, sevoflurane, and halothane in humans. *Anesthesiology.* 1996;84:555–561.
123. Drummond JC, Todd MM, Shapiro HM. CO2 responsiveness of the cerebral circulation during isoflurane anesthesia and N2O sedation in cats. *Anesthesiology.* 1982;57:A333.
124. Cho S, Fujigake T, Uchiyama Y, et al. Effects of sevoflurane with and without nitrous oxide on human cerebral circulation. *Anesthesiology.* 1996;85:755–760.
125. Kitaguchi K, Ohsumi H, Juro M, et al. Effects of sevoflurane on cerebral circulation and metabolism in patients with ischemic cerebrovascular disease. *Anesthesiology.* 1993;79:704–709.
126. Mielck F, Stephan H, Buhre W, et al. Effects of 1 MAC desflurane on cerebral metabolism, blood flow and carbon dioxide reactivity in humans. *Br J Anaesth.* 1998;81:155–160.
127. Bedforth NM, Girling KJ, Skinner HJ, et al. Effects of desflurane on cerebral regulation. *Br J Anaesth.* 2001;87:193–197.
128. Todd MM, Drummond JC. A comparison of the cerebrovascular and metabolic effects of halothane and isoflurane in the cat. *Anesthesiology.* 1984;60:276–282.
129. Milde LN, Milde JH, Lanier WL, et al. Comparison of the effects of isoflurane and thiopental on neurologic outcome and neuropathology after temporary focal cerebral ischemia in primates. *Anesthesiology.* 1988;69:905–913.
130. Michenfelder JD, Sundt TM, Fode N, et al. Isoflurane when compared to enflurane and halothane decreases the frequency of cerebral ischemia during carotid endarterectomy. *Anesthesiology.* 1987;67:336–340.
131. Warner DS. Isoflurane neuroprotection. A passing fantasy, again? *Anesthesiology.* 2000;92:1126–1128.
132. Newman B, Gelb AW, Lam AM. The effect of isoflurane induced hypotension on cerebral blood flow and cerebral metabolic rate for oxygen in humans. *Anesthesiology.* 1986;64:307–310.
133. Muzzi D, Losasso T, Dietz N, et al. The effect of desflurane and isoflurane on cerebrospinal fluid pressure in humans with supratentorial mass lesions. *Anesthesiology.* 1992;76:720–724.
134. Adams RW, Cucchiari RF, Gronert GA, et al. Isoflurane and cerebrospinal fluid pressure in neurosurgical patients. *Anesthesiology.* 1981;54:97–99.
135. Artru AA. Effects of halothane, enflurane, isoflurane and fentanyl on resistance to reabsorption of cerebrospinal fluid. *Anesth Analg.* 1984;63:180.
136. Artru AA. Isoflurane does not increase the rate of CSF production in the dog. *Anesthesiology.* 1984;60:193–197.

137. Artru AA. Anesthetics produce prolonged alterations of CSF dynamics. *Anesthesiology*. 1982;57:A356.
138. Malan TP, DiNardo JA, Isner RJ, et al. Cardiovascular effects of sevoflurane compared with those of isoflurane in volunteers. *Anesthesiology*. 1995;83:918–928.
139. Cahalan MK. *Hemodynamic Effects of Inhaled Anesthetics [Review Courses]*. Cleveland, OH: International Anesthesia Research Society; 1996.
140. Hornbein TF, Eger EI II, Winter PM, et al. The minimum alveolar concentration of nitrous oxide in man. *Anesth Analg*. 1982;61(7): 553–556.
141. Cahalan MK, Lurz FW, Eger EI, et al. Narcotics decrease heart rate during inhalational anesthesia. *Anesth Analg*. 1987;66: 166–170.
142. Muzi M, Ebert TJ. A comparison of baroreflex sensitivity during isoflurane and desflurane anesthesia in humans. *Anesthesiology*. 1995;82:919–925.
143. Murat I, Lapeyre G, Saint-Maurice C. Isoflurane attenuates baroreflex control of heart rate in human neonates. *Anesthesiology*. 1989;70:395–400.
144. Wodey E, Pladys P, Copin C, et al. Comparative hemodynamic depression of sevoflurane versus halothane in infants: an echocardiographic study. *Anesthesiology*. 1997;87:795–800.
145. Wolfson B, Hetrick WD, Lake CL, et al. Anesthetic indices: further data. *Anesthesiology*. 1978;48:187–190.
146. Smith NT, Eger EI II, Stoelting RK, et al. The cardiovascular and sympathomimetic responses to the addition of nitrous oxide to halothane in man. *Anesthesiology*. 1970;32(5):410–421.
147. Stevens WC, Cromwell TH, Halsey MJ, et al. The cardiovascular effects of a new inhalation anesthetic, Forane, in human volunteers at constant arterial carbon dioxide tension. *Anesthesiology*. 1971;35:8–16.
148. Williamson DC, Munson ES. Correlation of peripheral venous and arterial blood gas values during general anesthesia. *Anesth Analg*. 1982;61:950–952.
149. Smith NT, Calverley RK, Prys-Roberts C, et al. Impact of nitrous oxide on the circulation during enflurane anesthesia in man. *Anesthesiology*. 1978;48:345–349.
150. Hilgenberg JC, McCammon RL, Stoelting RK. Pulmonary and systemic vascular responses to nitrous oxide in patients with mitral stenosis and pulmonary hypertension. *Anesth Analg*. 1980;59: 323–326.
151. Schulte-Sasse U, Hesse W, Tarnow J. Pulmonary vascular responses to nitrous oxide in patients with normal and high pulmonary vascular resistance. *Anesthesiology*. 1982;57:9–13.
152. Eisele JH, Milstein JM, Goetzman BW. Pulmonary vascular responses to nitrous oxide in newborn lambs. *Anesth Analg*. 1986;65: 62–64.
153. Bahlman SH, Eger EI, Halsey MJ, et al. The cardiovascular effects of halothane in man during spontaneous ventilation. *Anesthesiology*. 1972;36:494–502.
154. Calverley RK, Smith NT, Prys-Roberts C, et al. Cardiovascular effects of enflurane anesthesia during controlled ventilation in man. *Anesth Analg*. 1978;57:619–628.
155. Price HL, Skovsted P, Pauca AW, et al. Evidence for a receptor activation produced by halothane in normal man. *Anesthesiology*. 1970;32:389–395.
156. Johnston RR, Eger ET, Wilson C. A comparative interaction of epinephrine with enflurane, isoflurane and halothane in man. *Anesth Analg*. 1976;55:709–712.
157. Moore MA, Weiskopf RB, Eger EI, et al. Arrhythmogenic doses of epinephrine are similar during desflurane or isoflurane anesthesia in humans. *Anesthesiology*. 1993;79:943–947.
158. Navarro R, Weiskopf RB, Moore MA, et al. Humans anesthetized with sevoflurane or isoflurane have similar arrhythmic response to epinephrine. *Anesthesiology*. 1994;80:545–549.
159. Karl HW, Swedlow DB, Lee KW, et al. Epinephrine-halothane interactions in children. *Anesthesiology*. 1983;58:142–145.
160. Ueda W, Hirakawa M, Mae O. Appraisal of epinephrine administration to patients under halothane anesthesia for closure of cleft palate. *Anesthesiology*. 1983;58:574–576.
161. Horrigan RW, Eger EI, Wilson EI, et al. Epinephrine-induced arrhythmias during enflurane anesthesia in man: a non-linear dose response relationship and dose-dependent protection from lidocaine. *Anesth Analg*. 1978;57:547–550.
162. Stoelting RK. Plasma lidocaine concentrations following subcutaneous or submucosal epinephrine-lidocaine injection. *Anesth Analg*. 1978;57:724–726.
163. Metz S, Maze M. Halothane concentration does not alter the threshold for epinephrine-induced arrhythmias in dogs. *Anesthesiology*. 1985;62:470–474.
164. Atlee JL, Bosnjak ZJ. Mechanisms for cardiac dysrhythmias during anesthesia. *Anesthesiology*. 1990;72:347–374.
165. Schmeling WT, Warltier DC, McDonald DJ, et al. Prolongation of the QT interval by enflurane, isoflurane, and halothane in humans. *Anesth Analg*. 1991;72:137–144.
166. Gallagher JD, Weindling SN, Anderson G, et al. Effects of sevoflurane on QT interval in a patient with congenital long QT syndrome. *Anesthesiology*. 1998;89:1569–1573.
167. Kleinsasser A, Kuenszberg E, Loeckinger A, et al. Sevoflurane, but not propofol, significantly prolongs the Q-T interval. *Anesth Analg*. 2000;90:25–27.
168. Sharpe MD, Cuillerier DJ, Lee JK, et al. Sevoflurane has no effect on sinoatrial node function or on normal atrioventricular and accessory pathway conduction in Wolff-Parkinson-White syndrome during alfentanil/midazolam anesthesia. *Anesthesiology*. 1999;90:60–65.
169. Calverley RK, Smith NT, Jones CW, et al. Ventilatory and cardiovascular effects of enflurane anesthesia during spontaneous ventilation in man. *Anesth Analg*. 1978;57:610–618.
170. Cromwell TH, Stevens WC, Eger EI, et al. The cardiovascular effects of compound 469 (Forane) during spontaneous ventilation and CO2 challenge in man. *Anesthesiology*. 1971;35:17–25.
171. Conzen PF, Habazettl, Vollmar B, et al. Coronary microcirculation during halothane, enflurane, isoflurane, and adenosine in dogs. *Anesthesiology*. 1992;76:261–270.
172. Weiskopf RB, Moore MA, Eger EI, et al. Rapid increase in desflurane concentration is associated with greater transient cardiovascular stimulation than with rapid increases in isoflurane concentration in humans. *Anesthesiology*. 1994;80:1035–1045.
173. Moore MA, Weiskopf RB, Eger EI, et al. Rapid 1% increases of end-tidal desflurane concentration to greater than 5% transiently increase heart rate and blood pressure in humans. *Anesthesiology*. 1994;81:94–98.
174. Muzi M, Ebert TJ, Hope WG, et al. Site(s) mediating sympathetic activation with desflurane. *Anesthesiology*. 1996;85:737–747.
175. Ebert TJ, Muzi M, Lopatka CW. Neurocirculatory responses to sevoflurane in humans: a comparison to desflurane. *Anesthesiology*. 1995;83:88–95.
176. Weiskopf RB, Eger EI II, Noorani M, et al. Fentanyl, esmolol, and clonidine blunt the transient cardiovascular stimulation induced by desflurane in humans. *Anesthesiology*. 1994;81:1350–1355.
177. Yonker-Sell AE, Muzi M, Hope WG, et al. Alfentanil modifies the neurocirculatory responses to desflurane. *Anesth Analg*. 1996;82: 162–166.
178. Eisele JH, Smith NT. Cardiovascular effects of 40 percent nitrous oxide in man. *Anesth Analg*. 1972;51:956–963.
179. Lynch C, Vogel S, Sperelakis N. Halothane depression of myocardial slow action potentials. *Anesthesiology*. 1981;55:360–368.
180. Hüneke R, Jüngling E, Skasa M, et al. Effects of the anesthetic gases xenon, halothane, and isoflurane on calcium and potassium currents in human atrial cardiomyocytes. *Anesthesiology*. 2001;95:999–1006.
181. Philbin DM, Lowenstein E. Lack of beta-adrenergic activity of isoflurane in the dog: a comparison of circulatory effects of halothane and isoflurane after propranolol administration. *Br J Anaesth*. 1976;48:1165–1170.

182. Fukunaga AF, Epstein RM. Sympathetic excitation during nitrous-oxide-halothane anesthesia in the cat. *Anesthesiology.* 1973;39:23–36.
183. Naito H, Gillis CN. Effects of halothane and nitrous oxide on removal of norepinephrine from the pulmonary circulation. *Anesthesiology.* 1973;39:575–580.
184. Lappas DG, Buckey MJ, Laver MB, et al. Left ventricular performance and pulmonary circulation following addition of nitrous oxide to morphine during coronary artery surgery. *Anesthesiology.* 1975;43:61–69.
185. Stoelting RK, Gibbs PS. Hemodynamic effects of morphine and morphine-nitrous oxide in valvular heart disease and coronary artery disease. *Anesthesiology.* 1973;38:45–52.
186. Lynch C. Anesthetic preconditioning: not just for the heart? *Anesthesiology.* 1999;91:606–608.
187. Hanouz J-L, Yvon A, Massetti M, et al. Mechanisms of desflurane-induced preconditioning in isolated human right atria in vitro. *Anesthesiology.* 2002;97:33–41.
188. Tanaka K, Ludwig LM, Kersten JR, et al. Mechanisms of cardioprotection by volatile anesthetics. *Anesthesiology.* 2004;100: 707–721.
189. Warltier DC, Kersten JR, Pagel PS, et al. Anesthetic preconditioning: serendipity and science. *Anesthesiology.* 2002;97:1–3.
190. Yvon A, Hanouz J-C, Haelewyn B, et al. Mechanisms of sevoflurane-induced myocardial preconditioning in isolated human right atria in vitro. *Anesthesiology.* 2003;99:27–33.
191. Zaugg M, Lucchinetti E, Spahn DR, et al. Volatile anesthetics mimic cardiac preconditioning by priming the activation of mitochondrial KATP channels via multiple signaling pathways. *Anesthesiology.* 2002;97:4–14.
192. Kehl F, Krolikowski JG, Mravoic B, et al. Is isoflurane-induced preconditioning dose related? *Anesthesiology.* 2002;96:675–680.
193. Ludwig LM, Patel HH, Gross GJ, et al. Morphine enhances pharmacological preconditioning by isoflurane. *Anesthesiology.* 2003;98:705–711.
194. Ross S, Foex P. Protective effects of anaesthetics in reversible and irreversible ischaemia-reperfusion injury. *Br J Anaesth.* 1999;82: 622–632.
195. Kevin LE, Katz P, Camara AKS, et al. Anesthetic preconditioning: effects of latency to ischemic injury in isolated hearts. *Anesthesiology.* 2003;99:385–391.
196. Conzen PF, Fischer S, Detter C, et al. Sevoflurane provides greater protection of the myocardium than propofol in patients undergoing off-pump coronary artery bypass surgery. *Anesthesiology.* 2003;99:826–833.
197. DeHert, SG, ten Broecke PW, Mertens E, et al. Sevoflurane but not propofol preserves myocardial function in coronary surgery patients. *Anesthesiology.* 2002;97:42–49.
198. DeHert, Van der Linden PJ, Cromheecke S, et al. Cardioprotective properties of sevoflurane in patients undergoing coronary surgery with cardiopulmonary bypass are related to its modalities of its administration. *Anesthesiology.* 2004;101:299–310.
199. Gold MI, Schwam SJ, Goldberg M. Chronic obstructive pulmonary disease and respiratory complications. *Anesth Analg.* 1983;62: 975–981.
200. Eger EI. *Nitrous Oxide.* New York, NY: Elsevier Science; 1985.
201. Lazarenko RM, Fortuna MG, Shi Y, et al. Anesthetic activation of central respiratory chemoreceptor neurons involves inhibition of a THIK-1-like background K(+) current. *J Neurosci.* 2010;30(27): 9324–9334.
202. Canet J, Sanchis J, Zegri A, et al. Effects of halothane and sevoflurane on ventilation and occlusion pressure. *Anesthesiology.* 1994;81:563–571.
203. Lockhart SH, Rampil IJ, Yasuda N, et al. Depression of ventilation by desflurane in humans. *Anesthesiology.* 1991;74:484–488.
204. Pietak S, Weenig CS, Hickey RF, et al. Anesthetic effects of ventilation in patients with chronic obstructive pulmonary disease. *Anesthesiology.* 1975;42:160–166.
205. Lam AM, Clement JL, Chung DC, et al. Respiratory effects of nitrous oxide during enflurane anesthesia in humans. *Anesthesiology.* 1982;56:298–303.
206. Tusiewicz K, Bryan AC, Froese AB. Contributions of chaining rib cage-diaphragm interactions to the ventilatory depression of halothane anesthesia. *Anesthesiology.* 1977;47:327–337.
207. Ide T, Kochi T, Isono S, et al. Effect of sevoflurane on diaphragmatic contractility in dogs. *Anesth Analg.* 1992;74:739–764.
208. Ravin MB, Olsen MB. Apneic thresholds in anesthetized subjects with chronic obstructive pulmonary disease. *Anesthesiology.* 1972;37:450–454.
209. Knill RL, Clement JL. Variable effects of anaesthetics on the ventilatory response to hypoxemia in man. *Can Anaesth Soc J.* 1982;29:93–99.
210. Nagyova B, Dorrington KL, Poulin MJ, et al. Influence of 0.2 minimum alveolar concentration of enflurane on the ventilatory response to sustained hypoxia in humans. *Br J Anaesth.* 1997;78: 707–713.
211. Sarton E, van der Wal M, Nieuwenhuijs D, et al. Sevoflurane-induced reduction of hypoxic drive is sex-independent. *Anesthesiology.* 1999;90:1288–1293.
212. Beck DH, Doepfmer UR, Sinemus C, et al. Effects of sevoflurane and propofol on pulmonary shunt fraction during one-lung ventilation for thoracic surgery. *Br J Anaesth.* 2001;86:38–43.
213. Olsson GL. Bronchospasm during anesthesia. A computer-aided incidence study of 136,929 patients. *Acta Anaesthesiol Scand.* 1987;31(3):244–252.
214. Volta CA, Alvisi V, Petrini S, et al. The effect of volatile anesthetics on respiratory system resistance in patients with chronic obstructive pulmonary disease. *Anesth Analg.* 2005;100:348–353.
215. Goff MJ, Arain SR, Ficke DJ, et al. Absence of bronchodilation during desflurane anesthesia. *Anesthesiology.* 2000;93:404–408.
216. Kong CF, Chew STH, Ip-Yam PC. Intravenous opioids reduce airway irritation during induction of anaesthesia with desflurane in adults. *Anesthesiology.* 1999;91:A431.
217. Rooke GA, Choi JH, Bishop MJ. The effect of isoflurane, halothane, sevoflurane, and thiopental/nitrous oxide on respiratory system resistance after tracheal intubation. *Anesthesiology.* 1997;86: 1294–1299.
218. Klock PA, Czeslick EG, Klafta JM, et al. The effect of sevoflurane and desflurane on upper airway reactivity. *Anesthesiology.* 2001;94:963–967.
219. Eilers H, Cattaruzza F, Nassini R, et al. Pungent general anesthetics activate transient receptor potential-A1 to produce hyperalgesia and neurogenic bronchoconstriction. *Anesthesiology.* 2010;112: 1452–1463.
220. Funk W, Gruber M, Wild K, et al. Dry soda lime markedly degrades sevoflurane during simulated inhalation induction. *Br J Anaesth.* 1999;82:193–198.
221. Holak E, Mei DA, Dunning MB, et al. Carbon monoxide production from sevoflurane breakdown: Modeling of exposures under clinical conditions. *Anesth Analg.* 2003;96:757–764.
222. Gatecel C, Losser M-R, Didier P. The postoperative effects of halothane versus isoflurane on hepatic artery and portal vein blood flow in humans. *Anesth Analg.* 2003;96:740–745.
223. Goldfarb G, Debaene B, Ang ET, et al. Hepatic blood flow in humans during isoflurane N2O and halothane N2O anesthesia. *Anesth Analg.* 1990;71:349–353.
224. Benumof JL, Bookstein JJ, Saidman LJ, et al. Diminished hepatic arterial flow during halothane administration. *Anesthesiology.* 1976;45:545–551.
225. Frink EJ, Ghantous H, Malan TP, et al. Plasma inorganic fluoride with sevoflurane anesthesia: correlation with indices of hepatic and renal function. *Anesth Analg.* 1992;74:231–235.
226. Whelan E, Wood AJJ, Koshakji R, et al. Halothane inhibition of propranolol metabolism is stereoselective. *Anesthesiology.* 1989;71: 561–564.

227. Reilly CS, Wood AJJ, Koshaji RP, et al. The effect of halothane on drug disposition in intrinsic drug metabolizing capacity and hepatic blood flow. *Anesthesiology*. 1985;63:70–76.
228. Tiainen P, Lindgren L, Rosenberg PH. Changes in hepatocellular integrity during and after desflurane or isoflurane anaesthesia in patients undergoing breast surgery. *Br J Anaesth*. 1998;80:87–89.
229. Elliott RH, Strunin L. Hepatotoxicity of volatile anesthetics. *Br J Anaesth*. 1993;70:339–348.
230. Shingu K, Eger EI, Johnson BH, et al. Effect of oxygen concentration, hyperthermia, and choice of vendor on anesthetic induced hepatic injury rats. *Anesth Analg*. 1983;62:146–150.
231. Baden JM, Serra M, Fujinaga M, et al. Halothane metabolism in cirrhotic rats. *Anesthesiology*. 1987;67:660–664.
232. Wright R, Eade OE, Chilsom M, et al. Controlled prospective study of the effect of liver function on multiple exposure to halothane. *Lancet*. 1975;1:817–820.
233. Moult PJ, Sherlock S. Halothane-related hepatitis. A clinical study of twenty-six cases. *Q J Med*. 1975;44:99–114.
234. Kenna JG, Neuberger J, Mieli-Vergani G, et al. Halothane hepatitis in children. *Br Med J (Clin Res Ed)*. 1987;294:1209–1211.
235. Warner LO, Beach TJ, Garvin JP, et al. Halothane and children: the first quarter century. *Anesth Analg*. 1984;63:838–840.
236. Njoku D, Laster MJ, Gong DH, et al. Biotransformation of halothane, enflurane, isoflurane, and desflurane to trifluoroacetylated liver proteins: association between protein acylation and hepatic injury. *Anesth Analg*. 1997;84:173–178.
237. Farrell G, Prendergast D, Murray M. Halothane hepatitis. Detection of a constitutional susceptibility factor. *N Engl J Med*. 1985;313: 1310–1314.
238. Gourlay GK, Adams JF, Cousins MJ, et al. Genetic differences in reductive metabolism and hepatotoxicity of halothane in three rat strains. *Anesthesiology*. 1981;55:96–103.
239. Cascorbi HF, Blake DA, Helrich M. Differences in the biotransformation of halothane in man. *Anesthesiology*. 1970;32(2):119–123.
240. Christ DD, Kenna JG, Kammerer W, et al. Enflurane metabolism produces covalently bound live adducts recognized by antibodies from patients with halothane hepatitis. *Anesthesiology*. 1988;69: 833–838.
241. Martin JL, Plevak DJ, Flannery KD, et al. Hepatotoxicity after desflurane anesthesia. *Anesthesiology*. 1995;83:1125–1129.
242. Njoku DB, Shrestha S, Soloway R, et al. Subcellular localization of trifluoroacetylated liver proteins in association with hepatitis following isoflurane. *Anesthesiology*. 2002;96:757–761.
243. Brunt EM, White H, Marsh JW, et al. Fulminant hepatic failure after repeated exposure to isoflurane anesthesia: a case report. *Hepatology*. 1991;13:1017–1021.
244. Eger EI, Smuckler EA, Ferrell LD, et al. Is enflurane hepatotoxic? *Anesth Analg*. 1986;65:21–30.
245. Stoelting RK, Blitt CD, Cohen PJ, et al. Hepatic dysfunction after isoflurane anesthesia. *Anesth Analg*. 1987;66:147–154.
246. Martin JL, Keegan MT, Vasdev GMS, et al. Fatal hepatitis associated with isoflurane exposure and CYP2A6 autoantibodies. *Anesthesiology*. 2001;95:551–553.
247. Sigurdsson J, Hreidarson AB, Thjodleifsson B. Enflurane hepatitis: a report of a case with a previous history of halothane hepatitis. *Acta Anaesthesiol Scand*. 1985;29:495–496.
248. Njoku DB, Greenberg RS, Bourdi M, et al. Autoantibodies associated with volatile anesthetic hepatitis found in the sera of a large cohort of pediatric anesthesiologists. *Anesth Analg*. 2002;94:243–249.
249. Eger EI, Zhang Y, Laster M, et al. Acetylcholine receptors does not mediate the immobilization produced by inhaled anesthetics. *Anesth Analg*. 2002;94:1500–1504.
250. Eger EI. Good news, bad news. *Anesth Analg*. 2002;94:239–240.
251. Kharasch ED, Hankins DC, Thummel KE. Human kidney methoxyflurane and sevoflurane metabolism: intrarenal fluoride productions as a possible mechanism of methoxyflurane nephrotoxicity. *Anesthesiology*. 1995;82:689–699.
252. Kharasch ED, Karol MD, Lanni C, et al. Clinical sevoflurane metabolism and disposition. I. Sevoflurane and metabolite pharmacokinetics. *Anesthesiology*. 1995;82:1369–1378.
253. Reich A, Everding AS, Bulla M, et al. Hepatitis after sevoflurane exposure in an infant suffering from primary hyperoxaluria type 1. *Anesth Analg*. 2004;99:370–372.
254. Singhal S, Gray T, Guzman G, et al. Sevoflurane hepatotoxicity: a case report of sevoflurane hepatic necrosis and review of the literature. *Am J Ther*. 2010;17:219–222.
255. Eger EI, Gong D, Koblin DD, et al. Dose-related biochemical markers on renal injury after sevoflurane versus desflurane anesthesia in volunteers. *Anesth Analg*. 1997;85:1154–1163.
256. Kharasch ED. Thorning D, Garton K, et al. Role of renal cysteine conjugate beta-lyase in the mechanism of compound A nephrotoxicity in rats. *Anesthesiology*. 1997;86(1):160–171.
257. Cronnelly R, Salvatierra O, Feduska NJ. Renal allograft function following halothane, enflurane, or isoflurane anesthesia. *Anesth Analg*. 1984;63:202.
258. Kim M, Kim M, Park SW, et al. Isoflurane protects human kidney proximal tubule cells against necrosis via sphingosine kinase and sphingosine-1-phosphate generation. *Am J Nephrol*. 2010;31:353–362.
259. Orhan H, Vermeulen NPE, Sahin G, et al. Characterization of thioether compounds formed from alkaline degradation products of enflurane. *Anesthesiology*. 2001;95:165–175.
260. Conzen PF, Nuscheler M, Melotte A, et al. Renal function and serum fluoride concentrations in patients with stable renal insufficiency after anesthesia with sevoflurane or enflurane. *Anesth Analg*. 1995;81:569–575.
261. Frink EJ, Morgan S, Coetzee A, et al. The effect of sevoflurane, halothane, enflurane, and isoflurane on hepatic blood flow and oxygenation in chronically instrumented greyhound dogs. *Anesthesiology*. 1992;76:85–92.
262. Frink EJ, Malan TP, Isner RJ, et al. Renal concentrating function with prolonged sevoflurane or enflurane anesthesia in volunteers. *Anesthesiology*. 1994;80:1019–1025.
263. Munday IT, Stoddart PA, Jones RM, et al. Serum fluoride concentration and urine osmolality after enflurane and sevoflurane anesthesia in male volunteers. *Anesth Analg*. 1995;81:353–359.
264. Higuchi H, Sumikura H, Sumita S, et al. Renal function in patients with high serum fluoride concentrations after prolonged sevoflurane anesthesia. *Anesthesiology*. 1995;83:449–458.
265. Mazze RI, Jamison R. Renal effects of sevoflurane. *Anesthesiology*. 1995;83(3):443–445.
266. Litz RJ, Hubler M, Lorenz W, et al. Renal responses to desflurane and isoflurane in patients with renal insufficiency. *Anesthesiology*. 2002;97:1133–1136.
267. Brown BR. Sibboleths and jigsaw puzzles: the fluoride nephrotoxicity enigma. *Anesthesiology*. 1995;82:607–608.
268. Mazze RI, Calverley RK, Smith NT. Inorganic fluoride nephrotoxicity: prolonged enflurane and halothane anesthesia in volunteers. *Anesthesiology*. 1977;46:265–271.
269. Yamakage M, Yamada S, Chen X, et al. Carbon dioxide absorbents containing potassium hydroxide produce much larger concentrations of compound A from sevoflurane in clinical practice. *Anesth Analg*. 2000;91:220–224.
270. Morio M, Fujii K, Satoh N, et al. Reaction of sevoflurane and its degradation products with soda lime: toxicity of the byproducts. *Anesthesiology*. 1992;77:1155–1164.
271. Gonsowski CT, Laster MJ, Eger EI, et al. Toxicity of compound A in rats: effect of a 3-hour administration. *Anesthesiology*. 1994;80: 556–565.
272. Bito H, Ikeda K. Effect of total flow rate on the concentration of degradation products generated by reaction between sevoflurane and soda lime. *Br J Anaesth*. 1995;74:667–669.
273. Bito H, Ikeuchi Y, Ikeda K. Area under the compound A concentration curve (compound A AUC) analysis. *Anesthesiology*. 1997;87(3): 715–716.

274. Higuchi H, Wada H, Usua Y, et al. Effects of probenecid on renal function in surgical patients anesthetized with low-flow sevoflurane. *Anesthesiology.* 2001;94:21–31.
275. Eger EI, Koblin DD, Bowland T, et al. Nephrotoxicity of sevoflurane versus desflurane anesthesia in volunteers. *Anesth Analg.* 1997;84:160–168.
276. Conzen PF, Kaharasch ED, Czerner SFA, et al. Low-flow sevoflurane compared with low-flow isoflurane anesthesia in patients with stable renal insufficiency. *Anesthesiology.* 2002;97: 578–584.
277. Kharasch ED, Frink EJ, Artru A, et al. Long-duration low-flow sevoflurane and isoflurane effects on postoperative renal and hepatic function. *Anesth Analg.* 2001;93:1511–1520.
278. Frink EJ, Green WB, Brown EA, et al. Compound A concentrations during sevoflurane anesthesia in children. *Anesthesiology.* 1996;84:566–571.
279. Eger EI, Ionescu P, Laster MJ, et al. Quantitative differences in the production and toxicity of CF2 = BrCl versus Ch2F-O-C(= CF2) (CF3) (Compound A): the safety of halothane does not indicate the safety of sevoflurane. *Anesth Analg.* 1997;85:1164–1170.
280. Paul M, Fokt RM, Kindler CH, et al. Characterization of the interactions between volatile anesthetics and neuromuscular blockers at the muscle nicotinic acetylcholine receptor. *Anesth Analg.* 2002;95:362–367.
281. Vitez TS, Miller RD, Eger EI, et al. Comparison in vitro of isoflurane and halothane potentiation of d-tubocurarine and succinylcholine neuromuscular blockades. *Anesthesiology.* 1974;41:53–56.
282. Papadimos TJ, Almasri M, Padgett JC, et al. A suspected case of delayed onset malignant hyperthermia with desflurane anesthesia. *Anesth Analg.* 2004;98:548–549.
283. Ducart A, Adnet P, Renaud B, et al. Malignant hyperthermia during sevoflurane administration. *Anesth Analg.* 1995;80:609–611.
284. Ochiai R, Toyoda Y, Nishio I, et al. Possible association of malignant hyperthermia with sevoflurane anesthesia. *Anesth Analg.* 1992;74:616–618.
285. Hoenemann CW, Halene-Holtgraeve TB, Booke M, et al. Delayed onset of malignant hyperthermia in desflurane anesthesia. *Anesth Analg.* 2003;96:165–167.
286. Reed SB, Strobel GE. An in vitro model of malignant hyperthermia: differential effects of inhalation anesthetics on caffeine-induced muscle contractures. *Anesthesiology.* 1978;48:254–259.
287. Wappler F. Anesthesia for patients with a history of malignant hyperthermia. *Curr Opin Anaesthesiol.* 2010;23:417–422.
288. Munson ES, Embro WJ. Enflurane, isoflurane and halothane and isolated human uterine muscle. *Anesthesiology.* 1977;46:11–14.
289. Palahniuk RJ, Shnider SM. Maternal and fetal cardiovascular and acid-base changes during halothane and isoflurane anesthesia in the pregnant ewe. *Anesthesiology.* 1974;41:462–472.
290. Cullen BF, Margolis AJ, Eger EI II. The effects of anesthesia and pulmonary ventilation on blood loss during elective therapeutic abortion. *Anesthesiology.* 1970;32(2):108–113.
291. Dolan WM, Eger EI II, Margolis AJ. Forane increases bleeding in therapeutic suction abortion. *Anesthesiology.* 1972;36(1):96–97.
292. Thind AS, Turner RJ. In vitro effects of propofol on gravid human myometrium. *Anaesth Intensive Care.* 2008;36:802–806.
293. Biehl DR, Yarnell R, Wade JG, et al. The uptake of isoflurane by the fetal lamb in utera: effect on regional blood flow. *Can Anaesth Soc J.* 1983;30:581–586.
294. Warren TM, Datta S, Ostheimer GW, et al. Comparison of the maternal and neonatal effects of halothane, enflurane and isoflurane for cesarean delivery. *Anesth Analg.* 1983;62:516–520.
295. Fang F, Guo TZ, Davies MF, et al. Opiate receptors in the periaqueductal gray mediate analgesic effect of nitrous oxide in rats. *Eur J Pharmacol.* 1997;336:137–141.
296. Stevenson GW, Hall SC, Rudnick S, et al. The effect of anesthetic agents on the human immune response. *Anesthesiology.* 1990;72: 542–552.
297. Johnson BH, Eger EI. Bactericidal effects of anesthetics. *Anesth Analg.* 1979;58:136–138.
298. Knight PR, Bedows E, Nahrwold ML, et al. Alterations in influenza virus pulmonary pathology induced by diethyl ether, halothane, enflurane and pentobarbital in mice. *Anesthesiology.* 1983;58:209–215.
299. Baden J, Kelley M, Mazze R. Mutagenicity of experimental inhalational anesthetic agents: sevoflurane, synthane, diozychlorane, and dioxyflurane. *Anesthesiology.* 1982;56:462–463.
300. Sachder K, Cohen EN, Simmou VF. Genotoxic and mutagenic assays of halothane metabolites in Bacillus subtilis and Salmonella typbimurium. *Anesthesiology.* 1980;53:31–39.
301. Bussard DA, Stoelting RK, Peterson C, et al. Fetal changes in hamsters anesthetized with nitrous oxide and halothane. *Anesthesiology.* 1974;41:275–278.
302. Lane GA, Nahrwold ML, Tait AR. Anesthetics as teratogens: nitrous oxide is fetotoxic, xenon is not. *Science.* 1980;210:899–901.
303. Mazze RI, Fujinaga M, Rice SA, et al. Reproductive and teratogenic effects of nitrous oxide, halothane, isoflurane and enflurane in Sprague-Dawley rats. *Anesthesiology.* 1986;64:339–344.
304. Chalon J, Ramanathan S, Turndorf H. Exposure to isoflurane affects learning function of murine progeny. *Anesthesiology.* 1982;57:A360.
305. Mazze RI, Wilson AI, Rice SA, et al. Effects of isoflurane on reproduction and fetal development in mice. *Anesth Analg.* 1984;63:249.
306. Jevtovic-Todorovic V, Hartman RE, Izumi Y, et al. Early exposure to common anesthetic agents causes widespread neurodegeneration in the developing rat brain and persistent learning deficits. *J Neurosci.* 2003;23:876–882.
307. Zou X, Patterson TA, Divine RL, et al. Prolonged exposure to ketamine increases neurodegeneration in the developing monkey brain. *Int J Dev Neurosci.* 2009;27:727–731.
308. Boivin JF. Risk of spontaneous abortion in women occupationally exposed to anaesthetic gases: a meta-analysis. *Occup Environ Med.* 1997;54:541–548.
309. Nunn JF, Weinbran HK, Royston D, et al. Rate of inactivation of human and rodent hepatic methionine synthase by nitrous oxide. *Anesthesiology.* 1988;68:213–216.
310. Krajewski W, Kucharska M, Pilacik B, et al. Impaired vitamin B12 metabolic status in healthcare workers occupationally exposed to nitrous oxide. *Br J Anaesth.* 2007;99:812–818.
311. Nunn JF. Clinical aspects of the interaction between nitrous oxide and vitamin B12. *Br J Anaesth.* 1987;59:3–13.
312. Lederhaas G, Brock-Utne JG, Negrin RS, et al. Is nitrous oxide safe for bone marrow harvest? *Anesth Analg.* 1995;80:770–772.
313. Layzer RB, Fishman RA, Schafer JA. Neuropathy following use of nitrous oxide. *Neurology.* 1978;28:504–506.
314. Loft S, Boel J, Kyst A, et al. Increased hepatic microsomal enzyme activity after surgery under halothane or spinal anesthesia. *Anesthesiology.* 1985;62:11–16.
315. Strube PJ, Hulands GH, Halsey MJ. Serum fluoride levels in morbidly obese patients: enflurane compared with isoflurane anaesthesia. *Anaesthesia.* 1987;42:685–689.
316. Higuchi H, Satoh T, Arimura S, et al. Serum inorganic fluoride levels in mildly obese patients during and after sevoflurane anesthesia. *Anesth Analg.* 1993;77:1018–1021.
317. Frink EJ, Malan TP, Brown EA, et al. Plasma inorganic fluoride levels with sevoflurane anesthesia in morbidly obese and nonobese patients. *Anesth Analg.* 1993;76:1133–1137.
318. White AE, Stevens WC, Eger EI, et al. Enflurane and methoxyflurane metabolism at anesthetic and subanesthetic concentrations. *Anesth Analg.* 1979;58:221–224.
319. Hong K, Trudell JR, O'Neil JR, et al. Metabolism of nitrous oxide by human and rat intestinal contents. *Anesthesiology.* 1980;52: 16–19.
320. Carpenter RL, Eger EI Johnson BH, Unadkat JD, Sheiner LB. The extent of metabolism of inhaled anesthetics in humans. *Anesthesiology.* 1986.65:201–205.

321. Hong K, Trudell JR, O'Neil JR, et al. Biotransformation of nitrous oxide. *Anesthesiology*. 1980;53:354–355.
322. Johnstone RE, Kennell EM, Behar MG, et al. Increased serum bromide concentration after halothane anesthesia in man. *Anesthesiology*. 1975;42:598–601.
323. Moore RA, McNicholas KW, Gallagher JD, et al. Halothane metabolism in acyanotic and cyanotic patients undergoing open heart surgery. *Anesth Analg*. 1986;65:1257–1262.
324. Nawaf K, Stoelting RK. SGOT values following evidence of reductive biotransformation of halothane in man. *Anesthesiology*. 1979;51:185–186.
325. Chase RE, Holaday DA, Fiserova-Bergerova V, et al. The biotransformation of Ethrane in man. *Anesthesiology*. 1971;35:262–267.
326. Mazze RI, Woodruff RE, Heerdt ME. Isoniazid-induced enflurane defluorination in humans. *Anesthesiology*. 1982;57:5–8.
327. Greenstein LR, Hitt BA, Mazze RI. Metabolism in vitro of enflurane, isoflurane, and methoxyflurane. *Anesthesiology*. 1975;42:420–424.
328. Holaday DA, Fiserova-Bergerova V, Latto IP, et al. Resistance of isoflurane to biotransformation in man. *Anesthesiology*. 1975;43:325–332.
329. Sutton TS, Koblin DD, Gruenke LD, et al. Fluoride metabolites after prolonged exposure of volunteers and patients to desflurane. *Anesth Analg*. 1991;73:180–185.
330. Koblin DD, Eger EI, Johnson BH, et al. I-653 resists degradation in rats. *Anesth Analg*. 1988;67:534–538.
331. Baum J, Sachs G, Driesch CVD, et al. Carbon monoxide generation in carbon dioxide absorbents. *Anesth Analg*. 1995;81:144–146.
332. Fang ZX, Eger EI, Laster MJ, et al. Carbon monoxide production from degradation of desflurane, enflurane, isoflurane, halothane, and sevoflurane by soda lime and Baralyme. *Anesth Analg*. 1995;80:1187–1193.
333. Baxter PJ, Kharasch ED. Rehydration of desiccated Baralyme prevents carbon monoxide formation from desflurane in an anesthesia machine. *Anesthesiology*. 1997;86:1061–1065.
334. Baxter PJ, Garton K, Kaharasch ED. Mechanistic aspects of carbon monoxide formation from volatile anesthetics. *Anesthesiology*. 1998;89:929–941.
335. Keijzer C, Perez RS, de Lange JJ. Carbon monoxide production from desflurane and six types of carbon dioxide absorbents in a patient model. *Acta Anaesthesiol Scand*. 2005;49:815–818.
336. Berry PD, Sessler DI, Larson MD. Severe carbon monoxide poisoning during desflurane anesthesia. *Anesthesiology*. 1999;90:613–616.
337. Wissing H, Kuhn K, Warnken U, et al. Carbon monoxide production from desflurane, enflurane, halothane, and sevoflurane with dry soda lime. *Anesthesiology*. 2001;95:1205–1212.
338. Versichelen LFM, Bouche M-P LA, Rolly G, et al. Only carbon dioxide absorbents free of both NaOH and KOH do not generate compound A during in vitro closed-system sevoflurane: evaluation of five absorbents. *Anesthesiology*. 2001;95:750–755.
339. Woehlck HJ, Mei D, Duning MB, et al. Mathematical modeling of carbon monoxide exposures from anesthetics from anesthetic breakdown. Effect of subject size, hematocrit, fraction of inspired oxygen, and quantity of carbon monoxide. *Anesthesiology*. 2001;94:457–460.
340. Wohlfeil ER, Woehlck HJ, Gottschall, et al. Increased carboxyhemoglobin from hemolysis mistaken as intraoperative desflurane breakdown. *Anesth Analg*. 2001;92:1609–1610.
341. Hayashi M, Takahashi T, Morimatsu H, et al. Increased carbon monoxide concentration in exhaled air after surgery and anesthesia. *Anesth Analg*. 2004;99:444–448.
342. Lester M, Roth P, Eger EI. Fires from the interaction of anesthetics with desiccated absorbent. *Anesth Analg*. 2004;99:769–774.
343. Castro BA, Freedman LA, Craig WL, et al. Explosion within an anesthesia machine: Baralyme®, high fresh gas flows and sevoflurance concentration. *Anesthesiology*. 2004;101:537–539.
344. Hazard Report. Anesthesia carbon dioxide absorber fires. *Health Devices*. 2003;32:436–440.
345. Woehlck HJ. Sleeping with uncertainty: anesthetics and desiccated absorbent. *Anesthesiology*. 2004;101:276–278.
346. Wu J, Previte JP, Adler E, et al. Spontaneous ignition, explosion, and fire with sevoflurane and barium hydroxide lime. *Anesthesiology*. 2004;101:534–537.
347. Fatheree RS, Leighton BL. Acute respiratory distress syndrome after an exothermic Baralyme®-sevoflurane reaction. *Anesthesiology*. 2004;101:531–533.
348. Higuchi H, Adachi Y Arimura S, et al. The carbon dioxide absorption capacity of Amsorb is half that of soda lime. *Anesth Analg*. 2001;93:2212–2225.

CHAPTER 5

Intravenous Sedatives and Hypnotics

Updated by: James P. Rathmell • Carl E. Rosow

Overview

No other class of pharmacologic agents is more central to the practice of anesthesiology than the intravenous sedatives and hypnotics. It is this group of agents that we rely upon to provide everything through the spectrum from anxiolysis to light and deep sedation then on to general anesthesia. The term ***sedative*** refers to a drug that induces a state of calm or sleep. The term ***hypnotic*** refers to a drug that induces hypnosis or sleep. There is significant overlap in the two terms as well as with the related term ***anxiolytic***, which refers to any agent that reduces anxiety as nearly all such substances have sedation as a side effect. For practical purposes, we generally combine the terms and refer to all of these drugs as ***sedative-hypnotics***, drugs that reversibly depress the activity of the central nervous system. Depending on the specific agent, the dose, and the rate of administration, the many sedative-hypnotics can be used to allay anxiety with minimal sedation, produce varying degrees of sedation, or rapidly induce the state of drug-induced unconsciousness we call ***general anesthesia***. We will review the pharmacology of these important agents in this chapter.

γ-Aminobutyric Acid Agonists

Propofol

Propofol is a substituted isopropylphenol (2,6-diisopropylphenol) that is administered intravenously as 1% solution in an aqueous solution of 10% soybean oil, 2.25% glycerol, and 1.2% purified egg phosphatide.[1-3] This drug is chemically distinct from all other drugs that act as intravenous (IV) sedative-hypnotics. Administration of propofol, 1.5 to 2.5 mg/kg IV (equivalent to thiopental, 4 to 5 mg/kg IV, or methohexital, 1.5 mg/kg IV) as a rapid IV injection (<15 seconds), produces unconsciousness within about 30 seconds. Awakening is more rapid and complete than that after induction of anesthesia with all other drugs used for rapid IV induction of anesthesia. The more rapid return of consciousness with minimal residual central nervous system (CNS) effects is one of the most important advantages of propofol compared with alternative drugs administered for the same purpose.

Commercial Preparations

Propofol is an insoluble drug that requires a lipid vehicle for emulsification. Current formulations of propofol use a soybean oil as the oil phase and egg lecithin as the emulsifying agent that is composed of long chain triglycerides.[4] This formulation supports bacterial growth and causes increased plasma triglyceride concentrations when prolonged IV infusions are used. Diprivan and generic propofol differ with respect to the preservatives used and the pH of the formulation. Diprivan uses the preservative disodium edetate (0.005%) with sodium hydroxide to adjust the pH to 7 to 8.5. A generic formulation of propofol incorporates sodium metabisulfite (0.25 mg/mL) as the preservative and has a lower pH (4.5 to 6.4). Propofol, unlike thiopental, etomidate, and ketamine, is not a chiral compound.

The mixing of propofol with any other drug is not recommended although lidocaine has been frequently added to propofol in attempts to prevent pain with IV injection. However, mixing of lidocaine with propofol may result in coalescence of oil droplets, which may pose the risk of pulmonary embolism.[5]

A low-lipid emulsion of propofol (Ampofol) contains 5% soybean oil and 0.6% egg lecithin but does not require a preservative or microbial growth retardant.[6] This formulation is equipotent to Diprivan but is associated with a higher incidence of pain on injection.

An alternative to emulsion formulations of propofol and associated side effects (pain on injection, risk of infection, hypertriglyceridemia, pulmonary embolism) is creation of a prodrug (Aquavan) by adding groups to the parent compound that increase its water solubility (phosphate monoesters, hemisuccinates). Propofol is liberated after hydrolysis by endothelial cell surface alkaline phosphatases. In this regard, injection of the water-soluble propofol phosphate prodrug results in propofol and dose-dependent sedative effects.[7,8] However, although the absence of lipid emulsion obviates pain on injection, the release of a small amount of formaldehyde byproduct causes an unpleasant dysesthesia or burning sensation often in the genital area. Compared with propofol, this prodrug has a slower onset, larger volume of distribution, and higher potency.[9]

Another nonlipid formulation of propofol uses cyclodextrins as a solubilizing agent.[10] Cyclodextrins are ring sugar molecules that form guest (propofol)–host complexes migrating between the hydrophilic center of the cyclodextrin molecule and the water-soluble phase. This allows propofol, which is poorly soluble in water, to be presented in an injectable form. After injection, propofol migrates out of the cyclodextrin into the blood. This preparation is in clinical trials and has not been released for general human use.

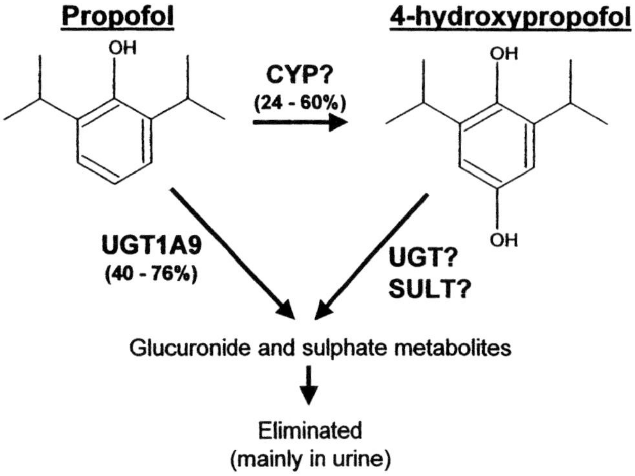

FIGURE 5-1 Major metabolic pathways for propofol. (From Court MH, Duan SX, Hesse LM, et al. Cytochrome P-450 2B6 is responsible for interindividual variability of propofol hydroxylation by human liver microsomes. *Anesthesiology*. 2001;94:110–119, with permission.)

Mechanism of Action

Propofol is a relatively selective modulator of γ-aminobutyric acid ($GABA_A$) receptors although it also has activity at glycine receptors. Propofol is presumed to exert its sedative-hypnotic effects through a $GABA_A$ receptor interaction.[11] GABA is the principal inhibitory neurotransmitter in the brain. When $GABA_A$ receptors are activated, transmembrane chloride conductance increases, resulting in hyperpolarization of the postsynaptic cell membrane and functional inhibition of the postsynaptic neuron. The interaction of propofol (also etomidate and barbiturates) with specific components of $GABA_A$ receptors appears to decrease the rate of dissociation of the inhibitory neurotransmitter, GABA from the receptor, thereby increasing the duration of the GABA-activated opening of the chloride channel with resulting hyperpolarization of cell membranes.

In contrast to volatile anesthetics, spinal motor neuron excitability, as measured by H reflexes, is not altered by propofol, suggesting that immobility during propofol anesthesia is not caused by drug-induced spinal cord depression.[12]

Pharmacokinetics

Clearance of propofol from the plasma exceeds hepatic blood flow, emphasizing that tissue uptake (possibly into the lungs), as well as hepatic oxidative metabolism by cytochrome P450, is important in removal of this drug from the plasma (Fig. 5-1) (Table 5-1).[13] Hepatic metabolism is rapid and extensive, resulting in inactive, water-soluble sulfate and glucuronic acid metabolites that are excreted by the kidneys.[14] Propofol may also undergo ring hydroxylation by cytochrome P450 to form 4-hydroxypropofol which is then glucuronidated or sulfated. Although the glucuronide and sulfate conjugates of propofol appear to be pharmacologically inactive, 4-hydroxypropofol has about one-third the hypnotic activity of propofol. Less than 0.3% of a dose is excreted unchanged in urine. The elimination half-time is 0.5 to 1.5 hours, but more important, the context-sensitive half-time for propofol infusions lasting up to 8 hours is less than 40 minutes.[15] The context-sensitive half-time of propofol is only minimally influenced by the duration of the infusion at times relevant for surgery because of slow return of the drug from tissue storage sites to the circulation. When the infusion is discontinued, this influx from tissues is not sufficient to retard the decrease in plasma concentrations of the drug. However, when used as a sedative for prolonged intensive care unit (ICU) care, the context-sensitive half-time is highly relevant and should be considered. Propofol, like

Table 5-1

Comparative Characteristics of Common Induction Drugs

	Elimination Half-Time (h)	Volume of Distribution (L/kg)	Clearance (mL/kg/min)	Systemic Blood Pressure	Heart Rate
Propofol	0.5–1.5	3.5–4.5	30–60	Decreased	Decreased
Etomidate	2–5	2.2–4.5	10–20	No change to decreased	No change
Ketamine	2–3	2.5–3.5	16–18	Increased	Increased

thiopental and alfentanil, has a short effect-site equilibration time such that effects on the brain occur promptly after IV administration.

The fact that total body clearance of propofol exceeds hepatic blood flow is consistent with extrahepatic clearance (pulmonary uptake and first-pass elimination, renal excretion) of propofol.[14,16] Pulmonary uptake of propofol is significant and influences the initial availability of propofol. Although propofol can be transformed in the lungs to 2,6-diisopropyl-1,4-quiniol, most of the drug that undergoes pulmonary uptake during the first pass is released back into the circulation.[17,18] Glucuronidation is the major metabolic pathway for propofol and uridine 5′-diphospho-glucuronosyltransferase isoforms are expressed in the kidneys and brain.

Despite the rapid clearance of propofol by metabolism, there is no evidence of impaired elimination in patients with cirrhosis of the liver. Plasma concentrations of propofol at the time of awakening are similar in alcoholic and normal patients.[19] Extrahepatic elimination of propofol occurs during the anhepatic phase of orthotopic liver transplantation. Renal dysfunction does not influence the clearance of propofol despite the observation that nearly three-fourths of propofol metabolites are eliminated in urine in the first 24 hours.[20] Patients older than 60 years of age exhibit a decreased rate of plasma clearance of propofol compared with younger adults. The rapid clearance of propofol confirms this drug can be administered as a continuous infusion during surgery without an excessive cumulative effect. Propofol readily crosses the placenta but is rapidly cleared from the neonatal circulation.[21] The effect of instituting cardiopulmonary bypass on the plasma propofol concentration is unpredictable, with some studies reporting a decrease, whereas other observations fail to document any change.[22]

Clinical Uses

Propofol has become the induction drug of choice for many forms of anesthesia, especially when rapid and complete awakening is considered desirable.[3] Continuous IV infusion of propofol, with or without other anesthetic drugs, has become a commonly used method for producing IV "conscious" sedation or as part of a balanced or total IV anesthetic.[1,3] Administration of propofol as a continuous infusion may be used for sedation of patients in the ICU.[2] In this regard, a 2% solution may be useful to decrease the volume of lipid emulsion administered with long-term sedation. In countries outside the United States, a computer controlled infusion pump is available to allow the clinician to select the propofol target concentration and the computer calculates the infusion rates that are necessary to achieve this target concentration based on the pharmacokinetics of propofol.[23]

Induction of Anesthesia

The induction dose of propofol in healthy adults is 1.5 to 2.5 mg/kg IV, with blood levels of 2 to 6 μg/mL producing unconsciousness depending on associated medications and the patient's age. As with barbiturates, children require higher induction doses of propofol on a milligram per kilogram basis, presumably reflecting a larger central distribution volume and higher clearance rate. Elderly patients require a lower induction dose (25% to 50% decrease) as a result of a smaller central distribution volume and decreased clearance rate and increased pharmacodynamic activity.[3] Awakening typically occurs at plasma propofol concentrations of 1.0 to 1.5 μg/mL. The complete awakening without residual CNS effects that is characteristic of propofol is the principal reason this drug has replaced thiopental for induction of anesthesia in many clinical situations. Thiopental is not currently available for use in the United States.

Intravenous Sedation

The short context-sensitive half-time of propofol, combined with the short effect-site equilibration time, make this a readily titratable drug for production of IV sedation.[1] The prompt recovery without residual sedation and low incidence of nausea and vomiting make propofol particularly well suited to ambulatory conscious sedation techniques. The typical conscious sedation dose of 25 to 100 μg/kg/minute IV produces minimal analgesic but marked amnestic effects.[3,24] In selected patients, midazolam or an opioid may be added to propofol for continuous IV sedation. A sense of well-being may accompany recovery from conscious sedation with propofol. When compared with anesthesia based on isoflurane, patients anesthetized with propofol reported less early postoperative pain.[25] A conventional patient-controlled analgesia delivery system set to deliver 0.7 mg/kg doses of propofol with a 3-minute lockout period has been used as an alternative to continuous IV sedation techniques. Propofol has emerged as the agent of choice for sedation for brief gastrointestinal endoscopy procedures. So reliable are the pharmacologic properties of propofol that extensive design and testing have gone in to creation of a computer-assisted personalized sedation for upper endoscopy and colonoscopy, called SEDASYS. A comparative, multicenter randomized study concluded that this system could provide endoscopist/nurse teams a safe and effective means to administer propofol to effect minimal to moderate sedation during routine colonoscopy and esophagogastroduodenoscopy without the need for a trained anesthesia provider.[26] The SEDASYS system received approval from the United States Food and Drug Administration in 2014 and is expected to be introduced in 2014.

Propofol has been administered as a sedative during mechanical ventilation in the ICU in a variety of patient populations including postoperative patients (cardiac surgery, neurosurgery) and patients with head injury.[2] Propofol also provides control of stress responses and has anticonvulsant and amnestic properties. After cardiac surgery, propofol sedation appears to modulate postoperative hemodynamic responses by decreasing the incidence and severity of tachycardia and hypertension.[27] Increasing metabolic acidosis, lipemic plasma, bradycardia, and progressive myocardial failure has been described, particularly in children who were sedated with propofol during management of acute respiratory failure in the ICU.[28]

Maintenance of Anesthesia

The typical dose of propofol for maintenance of anesthesia is 100 to 300 μg/kg/minute, doses that are often lowered by combination with a short acting opioid.[3] General anesthesia that includes propofol is typically associated with minimal postoperative nausea and vomiting, and awakening is prompt, with minimal residual sedative effects.

Nonhypnotic Therapeutic Applications

In addition to its clinical application as an IV induction drug, propofol has been shown to have beneficial effects that were not anticipated when the drug was initially introduced in 1989.[29]

Antiemetic Effects

The incidence of postoperative nausea and vomiting is decreased when propofol is administered, regardless of the anesthetic technique.[29] Subhypnotic doses of propofol (10 to 15 mg IV) may be used in the postanesthesia care unit to treat nausea and vomiting, particularly if it is not of vagal origin. In the postoperative period, the advantage of propofol is its rapid onset of action and the absence of serious side effects. Propofol is generally efficacious in treating postoperative nausea and vomiting at plasma concentrations that do not produce significant sedation. Simulations indicate that antiemetic plasma concentrations of propofol are achieved by a single IV dose of 10 mg followed by 10 μg/kg/minute.[30] Propofol in subhypnotic doses is effective against chemotherapy-induced nausea and vomiting. When administered to induce and maintain anesthesia, it is almost as effective as ondansetron in preventing postoperative nausea and vomiting.[31]

Propofol has a profile of CNS depression that differs from other anesthetic drugs. In contrast to thiopental, for example, propofol uniformly depresses CNS structures, including subcortical centers. Most drugs of known antiemetic efficacy exert this effect via subcortical structures, and it is possible that propofol modulates subcortical pathways to inhibit nausea and vomiting or produces a direct depressant effect on the vomiting center. Nevertheless, the mechanisms mediating the antiemetic effects of propofol remain unknown. An antiemetic effect of propofol based on inhibition of dopaminergic activity is unlikely given that subhypnotic doses of propofol fail to increase plasma prolactin concentrations. A rapid and distinct increase in plasma prolactin concentrations is characteristic of drugs that block the dopaminergic system.[32] Subhypnotic doses of propofol that are effective as an antiemetic do not inhibit gastric emptying and propofol is not considered a prokinetic drug.[33]

Antipruritic Effects

Propofol, 10 mg IV, is effective in the treatment of pruritus associated with neuraxial opioids or cholestasis.[34] The mechanism of the antipruritic effect may be related to the drug's ability to depress spinal cord activity. In this regard, there is evidence that intrathecal opioids produce pruritus by segmental excitation within the spinal cord.

Anticonvulsant Activity

Propofol possesses antiepileptic properties, presumably reflecting GABA-mediated presynaptic and postsynaptic inhibition of chloride ion channels. In this regard, propofol in doses of greater than 1 mg/kg IV decreases seizure duration 35% to 45% in patients undergoing electroconvulsive therapy.[35]

Attenuation of Bronchoconstriction

Compared with thiopental, propofol decreases the prevalence of wheezing after induction of anesthesia and tracheal intubation in healthy and asthmatic patients (Fig. 5-2).[36] However, a newer formulation of propofol uses metabisulfite as a preservative. Metabisulfite may cause bronchoconstriction in asthmatic patients. In an animal model, propofol without metabisulfite attenuated vagal nerve stimulation–induced bronchoconstriction, whereas propofol with metabisulfite did not attenuate vagally or methacholine-induced bronchoconstriction and metabisulfite alone caused increases in airway responsiveness.[37] Following tracheal intubation, in patients with a history of smoking, airway resistance was increased more following the administration of propofol containing metabisulfite than ethylenediaminetetraacetic acid (EDTA).[38]

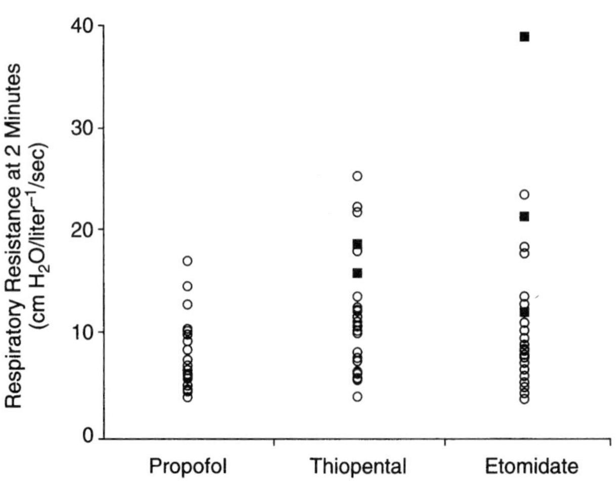

FIGURE 5-2 Respiratory resistance after tracheal intubation is less after induction of anesthesia with propofol than after induction of anesthesia with thiopental or etomidate. The solid squares represent four patients in whom audible wheezing was present. (From Eames WO, Rooke GA, Sai-Chuen R, et al. Comparison of the effects of etomidate, propofol, and thiopental on respiratory resistance after tracheal intubation. *Anesthesiology*. 1996;84:1307–1311, with permission.)

Therefore, the preservative used for propofol can have effects on its ability to attenuate bronchoconstriction. Nevertheless, propofol-induced bronchoconstriction has been described in patients with allergy histories. The formulation of propofol administered to these patients was Diprivan containing soybean oil, glycerin, yolk lecithin, and sodium edetate.[39]

Analgesia

Propofol does not relieve acute nociceptive pain. However in animal models, low-dose propofol equivalent to antiemetic concentrations earlier was highly effective in relieving nociceptive responses to neuropathic pain.[40]

Effects on Organ Systems

Central Nervous System

Propofol decreases cerebral metabolic rate for oxygen ($CMRO_2$), cerebral blood flow, and intracranial pressure (ICP).[41,42] Administration of propofol to produce hypnosis in patients with intracranial space-occupying lesions does not increase ICP.[43] However, large dose propofol may decrease systemic blood pressure sufficiently to decrease cerebral perfusion pressure. Cerebrovascular autoregulation in response to changes in systemic blood pressure and reactivity of the cerebral blood flow to changes in $Paco_2$ are not affected by propofol. Cerebral blood flow velocity changes in parallel with changes in $Paco_2$ in the presence of propofol and midazolam (Fig. 5-3).[44] Propofol produces cortical electroencephalographic (EEG) changes that are similar to those of thiopental, including the ability of high doses to produce burst suppression.[45] Cortical somatosensory evoked potentials as used for monitoring spinal cord function are not significantly modified in the presence of propofol alone but the addition of nitrous oxide or a volatile anesthetic results in decreased amplitude.[46] Propofol does not interfere with the adequacy of electrocorticographic recordings during awake craniotomy performed for the management of refractory epilepsy, provided administration is discontinued at least 15 minutes before recording.[47] At equal levels of sedation, propofol produces the same degree of memory impairment as midazolam, whereas thiopental has less memory effect and fentanyl has none.[24]

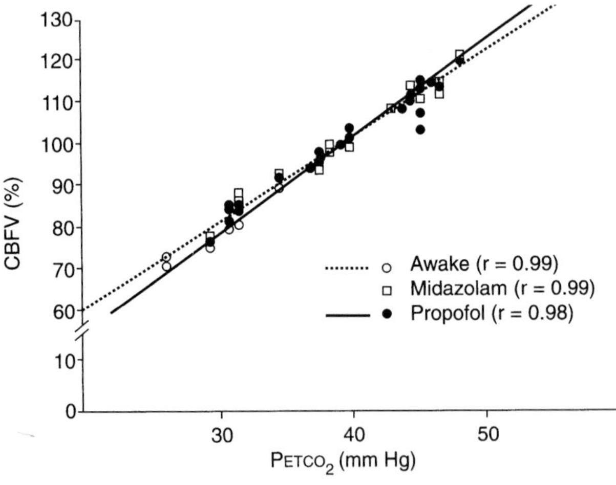

FIGURE 5-3 Changes in the end-tidal Pco_2 ($PETCO_2$) produce corresponding changes in the cerebral blood flow velocity (CBFV) during infusion of propofol or midazolam. (From Strebel S, Kaufmann M, Guardiola PM, et al. Cerebral vasomotor responsiveness to carbon dioxide is preserved during propofol and midazolam anesthesia in humans. *Anesth Analg*. 1994;78:884–888, with permission.)

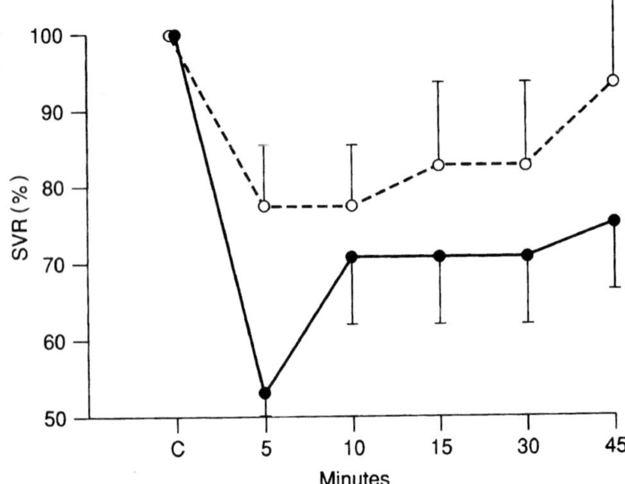

FIGURE 5-4 Comparative changes (expressed in % changes [mean ± SD]) from control values (C) in systemic vascular resistance (SVR) in the 45 minutes after the administration of thiopental, 5 mg/kg IV (*open circles*), or propofol, 2.5 mg/kg IV (*solid circles*). (From Rouby JJ, Andreev A, Leger P, et al. Peripheral vascular effects of thiopental and propofol in humans with artificial hearts. *Anesthesiology*. 1991;75:32–42, with permission.)

Development of tolerance to drugs that depress the CNS is a common finding, occurring with repeated exposure to opioids, sedative-hypnotic drugs, ketamine, and nitrous oxide. However, tolerance to propofol does not develop in children undergoing repeated exposure to the drug during radiation therapy.[48]

Cardiovascular System

Propofol produces decreases in systemic blood pressure, which are greater than those evoked by comparable doses of thiopental (Fig. 5-4).[49] These decreases in blood pressure are often accompanied by corresponding changes in cardiac output and systemic vascular resistance. The relaxation of vascular smooth muscle produced by propofol is primarily due to inhibition of sympathetic vasoconstrictor nerve activity.[50] A negative inotropic effect of propofol may result from a decrease in intracellular calcium availability secondary to inhibition of trans-sarcolemmal calcium influx. Stimulation produced by direct laryngoscopy and intubation of the trachea reverses the blood pressure effects of propofol. Propofol also effectively blunts the hypertensive response to placement of a laryngeal mask airway. The impact of propofol on desflurane-mediated sympathetic nervous system activation is unclear. In one report, propofol 2 mg/kg IV blunted the increase in epinephrine concentration, which accompanied a sudden increase in the delivered desflurane concentration but did not attenuate the transient cardiovascular response.[51] Conversely, in another report, induction of anesthesia with propofol, but not etomidate, blunted the sympathetic nervous system activation and systemic hypertension associated with the introduction of rapidly increasing inhaled concentrations of desflurane.[52] The blood pressure effects of propofol may be exaggerated in hypovolemic patients, elderly patients, and patients with compromised left ventricular function. Adequate hydration before rapid IV administration of propofol is recommended to minimize the blood pressure reduction.

Addition of nitrous oxide does not alter the cardiovascular effects of propofol. The pressor response to ephedrine is augmented by propofol (Fig. 5-5).[53]

Despite decreases in systemic blood pressure, heart rate typically remains unchanged. Baroreceptor reflex control of heart rate may be depressed by propofol.[54] Bradycardia and asystole have been observed after induction of anesthesia with propofol, resulting in the occasional recommendation that anticholinergic drugs be administered when vagal stimulation is likely to occur in association with administration of propofol (see the section "Bradycardia-Related Death"). Propofol may decrease sympathetic nervous system activity to a greater extent than parasympathetic nervous system activity, resulting in a predominance of parasympathetic activity.[1] Propofol does not alter sinoatrial or atrioventricular node function in normal patients or in patients with Wolff-Parkinson-White syndrome, thus making it an acceptable drug to administer during ablative procedures.[55,56] Nevertheless, there is a case report of a patient with Wolff-Parkinson-White syndrome in whom δ waves on the electrocardiogram disappeared during infusion of propofol.[57] Unlike sevoflurane, propofol does not prolong the QTc interval on the electrocardiogram.[58]

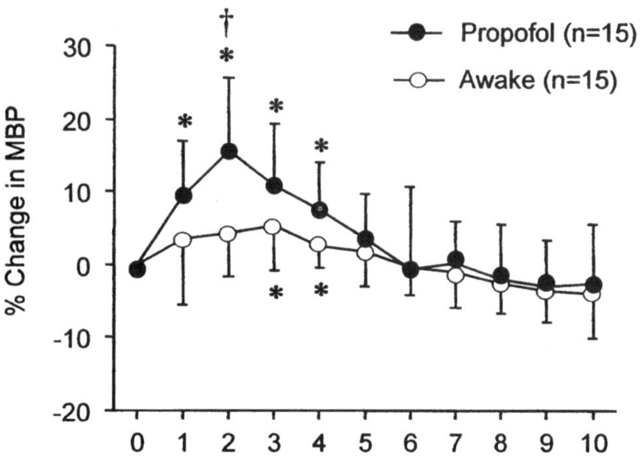

FIGURE 5-5 Mean blood pressure (MBI) increased more following administration of ephedrine (0.1 mg/kg IV) to patients during propofol anesthesia than when awake. (From Kanaya N, Satoh H, Seki S, et al. Propofol anesthesia enhances the pressor response to intravenous ephedrine. *Anesth Analg.* 2002;94:1207–1213, with permission.)

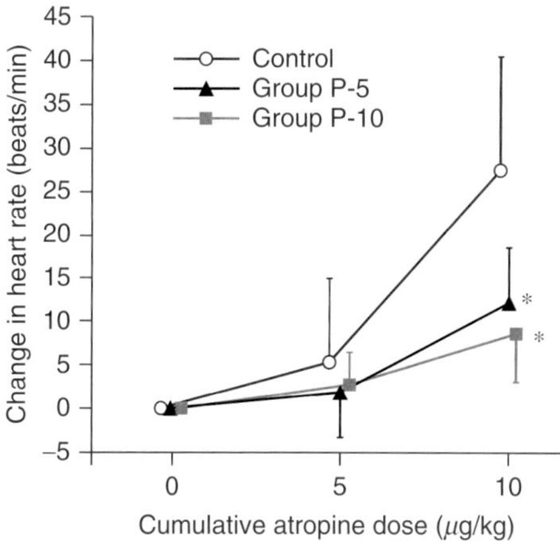

FIGURE 5-6 Heart rate responses to cumulative IV atropine doses in patients receiving no propofol, patients receiving 5 mg/kg/hour IV (group P-5), and patients receiving 10 mg/kg/hour IV (group P-10). Mean ≠ SD. *$P < .05$ compared with the control group. (From Horiguchi T, Nishikawa T. Heart rate response to intravenous atropine during propofol anesthesia. *Anesth Analg.* 2002;95:389–392, with permission.)

Bradycardia-Related Death

Profound bradycardia and asystole after administration of propofol have been described in healthy adult patients, despite prophylactic anticholinergics.[59–62] The risk of bradycardia-related death during propofol anesthesia has been estimated to be 1.4 in 100,000. Propofol anesthesia, compared with other anesthetics, increases the incidence of the oculocardiac reflex in pediatric strabismus surgery, despite prior administration of anticholinergics.[63]

Heart rate responses to IV administration of atropine are attenuated in patients receiving propofol compared with awake patients (Fig. 5-6).[64] This decreased responsiveness to atropine cannot be effectively overcome by larger doses of atropine suggesting that propofol may induce suppression of sympathetic nervous system activity. Treatment of propofol-induced bradycardia may require treatment with a direct β agonist such as epinephrine.

Lungs

Propofol produces dose-dependent depression of ventilation, with apnea occurring in 25% to 35% of patients after induction of anesthesia with propofol.[65] Opioids enhance this ventilatory depression. Painful surgical stimulation is likely to counteract the ventilatory depressant effects of propofol. A maintenance infusion of propofol decreases tidal volume and frequency of breathing. The ventilatory response to arterial hypoxemia are also decreased by propofol due to an effect at the central chemoreceptors.[66] Likewise, propofol at sedative doses significantly decreases the slope and causes a downward shift of the ventilatory response curve to hypoxia.[67] Hypoxic pulmonary vasoconstriction seems to remain intact in patients receiving propofol.

Hepatic and Renal Function

Propofol does not normally affect hepatic or renal function as reflected by measurements of liver transaminase enzymes or creatinine concentrations. Prolonged infusions of propofol have been associated with hepatocellular injury accompanied by lactic acidosis, bradydysrhythmias, and rhabdomyolysis as part of the propofol infusion syndrome described in the following texts. In rare instances, presumed propofol-induced hepatocellular injury following uneventful anesthesia and surgery has been described.[68] Prolonged infusions of propofol may also result in excretion of green urine, reflecting the presence of phenols in the urine. This discoloration does not alter renal function. Urinary uric acid excretion is increased after administration of propofol and may manifest as cloudy urine when the uric acid crystallizes in the urine under conditions of low pH and temperature.[20] This cloudy urine is not considered to be detrimental or indicative of adverse renal effects of propofol.

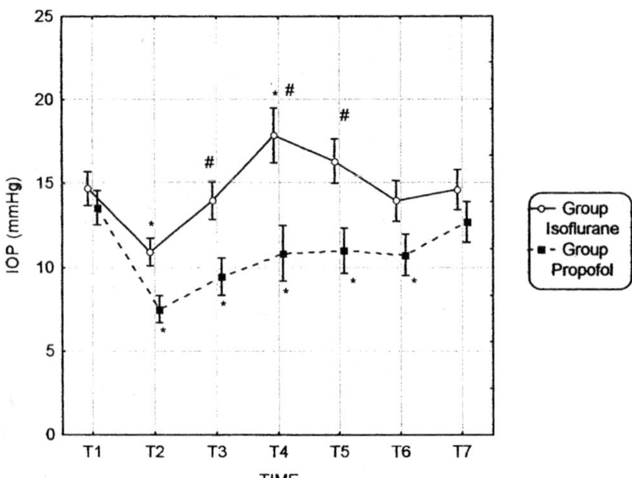

FIGURE 5-7 Changes in intraocular pressure (IOP) in patients receiving isoflurane or propofol. Measurements were made before induction of anesthesia (T1), after induction of anesthesia (T2), after pneumoperitoneum (T3), after head-down position (T4), after return to neutral supine position (T5), after evacuation of pneumoperitoneum (T6), and in the postanesthesia care unit (T7). *, Significant difference compared with T1; #, significant difference between the isoflurane and propofol groups. (From Mowafi HA, Al-Ghamdi A, Rushood A. Intraocular pressure changes during laparoscopy in patients anesthetized with propofol total intravenous anesthesia versus isoflurane inhaled anesthesia. *Anesth Analg.* 2003;97:471–474, with permission.)

Intraocular Pressure

Laparoscopic surgery is associated with increased intraocular pressure and some consider laparoscopic surgery with the head down position a risk in the presence of preexisting ocular hypertension. In this regard, propofol is associated with significant decreases in intraocular pressure that occur immediately after induction of anesthesia and are sustained during tracheal intubation.[1] Total IV anesthesia with propofol for laparoscopic surgery was associated with lower intraocular pressures than in patients undergoing similar surgery with isoflurane anesthesia (Fig. 5-7).[69]

Coagulation

Propofol does not alter tests of coagulation or platelet function. This is reassuring because the emulsion in which propofol is dispensed resembles intralipid, which has been associated with alterations in blood coagulation. However, propofol inhibits platelet aggregation that is induced by proinflammatory lipid mediators including thromboxane A_2 and platelet-activating factor.[70]

Other Side Effects

Side effects of propofol may reflect the parent drug or actions attributed to the oil-in-water emulsion formulation. For example, some of the side effects of propofol (bradycardia, risk of infection, pain on injection, hypertriglyceridemia with prolonged administration, potential for pulmonary embolism) are believed to be due in large part to the lipid emulsion formulation.[7,8,71]

Allergic Reactions

Allergenic components of propofol include the phenyl nucleus and diisopropyl side chain.[72] Patients who develop evidence of anaphylaxis on first exposure to propofol may have been previously sensitized to the diisopropyl radical, which is present in many dermatologic preparations. Likewise, the phenol nucleus is common to many drugs. Indeed, anaphylaxis to propofol during the first exposure to this drug has been observed, especially in patients with a history of other drug allergies, often to neuromuscular blocking drugs.[73] Propofol-induced bronchoconstriction has been described in patients with allergy histories.[39] The formulation of propofol administered to these patients was Diprivan containing soybean oil, glycerin, yolk lecithin, and sodium edetate.

Lactic Acidosis

Lactic acidosis ("propofol infusion syndrome") has been described in pediatric and adult patients receiving prolonged high-dose infusions of propofol (>75 μg/kg/ minute) for longer than 24 hours.[74,75] Severe, refractory, and fatal bradycardia in children in the ICU has been observed with long-term propofol sedation.[76,77] Even short-term infusions of propofol (Diprivan) for surgical anesthesia have been associated with development of metabolic acidosis.[78,79]

Unexpected tachycardia occurring during propofol anesthesia should prompt laboratory evaluation for possible metabolic (lactic) acidosis. Measurement of arterial blood gases and serum lactate concentrations is recommended. Documentation of an increased ion gap is useful but will take time and delay treatment, which includes prompt discontinuation of propofol administration.[80] Metabolic acidosis in its early stages is reversible with discontinuation of propofol administration although cardiogenic shock requiring assistance with extracorporeal membrane oxygenation has been described in a patient receiving a prolonged propofol infusion (Diprivan) for a craniotomy.[81]

The mechanism for sporadic propofol-induced metabolic acidosis is unclear but may reflect poisoning (cytopathic hypoxia) of the electron transport chain and impaired oxidation of long chain fatty acids by propofol or a propofol metabolite in uniquely susceptible patients.[82] Indeed, this propofol infusion syndrome mimics the mitochondrial myopathies, in which there are specific defects in the mitochondrial respiratory chain associated with specific mitochondrial DNA abnormalities, resulting in abnormal lipid metabolism in cardiac and skeletal muscles. These individuals, who are probably genetically susceptible, remain asymptomatic until a triggering event (sepsis, malnutrition) intervenes.

The differential diagnosis when propofol-induced lactic acidosis is suspected includes hyperchloremic metabolic acidosis associated with large volume infusions of 0.9% saline and metabolic acidosis associated with excessive generation of organic acids, such as lactate and ketones (diabetic acidosis, release of a tourniquet). Measurement of the anion gap and individual measurements of anions and organic acids will differentiate hyperchloremic metabolic acidosis from lactic acidosis.

Proconvulsant Activity

The majority of reported propofol-induced "seizures" during induction of anesthesia or emergence from anesthesia reflect spontaneous excitatory movements of subcortical origin.[29] These responses are not thought to be due to cortical epileptic activity. Prolonged myoclonus associated with meningismus has been associated with propofol administration.[83] The incidence of excitatory movements and associated ECG changes are low after the administration of propofol.[84] Propofol resembles thiopental in that it does not produce seizure activity on the EEG when administered to patients with epilepsy, including those undergoing cortical resection.[45] There appears to be no reason to avoid propofol for sedation, induction, and maintenance of anesthesia in patients with known seizures.[10]

Abuse Potential

Intense dreaming activity, amorous behavior, and hallucinations have been reported during recovery from low-dose infusions of propofol.[29] Addiction to virtually all opioids and hypnotics, including propofol, has been described.[85,86] The death of music pop star Michael Jackson in 2009 from an overdose of propofol he was receiving inappropriately as a sleep aid has recently brought the dangers of propofol misuse to public attention.[87]

Bacterial Growth

Propofol strongly supports the growth of *Escherichia coli* and *Pseudomonas aeruginosa*, whereas the solvent (Intralipid) appears to be bactericidal for these same organisms and bacteriostatic for *Candida albicans*.[88] Clusters of postoperative surgical infections manifesting as temperature elevations have been attributed to extrinsic contamination of propofol.[89,90] For this reason, it is recommended that (a) an aseptic technique be used in handling propofol as reflected by disinfecting the ampule neck surface or vial rubber stopper with 70% isopropyl alcohol; (b) the contents of the ampule containing propofol should be withdrawn into a sterile syringe immediately after opening and administered promptly; and (c) the contents of an opened ampule must be discarded if they are not used within 6 hours. In the ICU, the tubing and any unused portion of propofol must be discarded after 12 hours. Despite these concerns, there is evidence that when propofol is aseptically drawn into an uncapped syringe, it will remain sterile at room temperature for several days.[91] Given the cost of propofol, some have questioned the logic of discarding unused drug at the end of an anesthetic or 6 hours, whichever occurs sooner.[3]

Antioxidant Properties

Propofol has potent antioxidant properties that resemble those of the endogenous antioxidant vitamin E.[92,93] Like vitamin E, propofol contains a phenolic hydroxyl group that scavenges free radicals and inhibits lipid peroxidation. A neuroprotective effect of propofol may be at least partially related to the antioxidant potential of propofol's phenol ring structure. For example, propofol reacts with lipid peroxyl radicals and thus inhibits lipid peroxidation by forming relatively stable propofol phenoxyl radicals. In addition, propofol also scavenges peroxynitrite, which is one of the most potent reactive metabolites for the initiation of lipid peroxidation. Because peroxynitrite is a potent bactericidal agent, it is likely that the peroxynitrite-scavenging activity of propofol contributes to this anesthetic's known ability to suppress phagocytosis.[94] Conversely, propofol might be beneficial in disease states, such as acute lung injury, in which peroxynitrite formation is thought to play an important role.[95]

Reintroduction of molecular oxygen into previously ischemic tissues (removal of an aortic cross-clamp) can further damage partially injured cells (reperfusion injury). Oxygen leads to the formation of free oxygen radicals, which react with polyunsaturated fatty acids of cell membranes resulting in disruption of cell membranes. Myocardial cell injury can cause postischemic dysfunction, myocardial stunning, and reperfusion cardiac dysrhythmias. Propofol strongly attenuates lipid peroxidation during coronary artery bypass graft surgery.[96]

Pain on Injection

Pain on injection is the most commonly reported adverse event associated with propofol administration to awake patients. This unpleasant side effect of propofol occurs in fewer than 10% of patients when the drug is injected into a large vein rather than a dorsum vein on the hand. Preceding the propofol with 1% lidocaine, using the same injection site, or by prior administration of a potent short-acting opioid decreases the incidence of discomfort experienced by the patient. The incidence of thrombosis or phlebitis is usually less than 1%. Changing the composition of the carrier fat emulsion for propofol to long and medium chain triglycerides decreases the incidence of pain on injection.[71]

Accidental intraarterial injection of propofol has been described as producing severe pain but no vascular compromise.[97] In an animal model, propofol-exposed arteries showed no changes in the vascular smooth muscle, and the endothelium was not damaged.[98]

Airway Protection

Inhaled and injected anesthetic drugs alter pharyngeal function with the associated risk of impaired upper airway protection and pulmonary aspiration. Subhypnotic concentrations of propofol, isoflurane, and sevoflurane decrease pharyngeal contraction force.[99]

Miscellaneous Effects

Propofol does not trigger malignant hyperthermia and has been administered to patients with hereditary coproporphyria without incident.[100–102] Secretion of cortisol is not influenced by propofol, even when administered for prolonged periods in the ICU. Temporary abolition of tremors in patients with Parkinson's disease may occur after the administration of propofol.[103] For this reason, propofol may not be ideally suited for patients undergoing stereotactic neurosurgery during which the symptom is required to identify the correct anatomic location.

Etomidate

Etomidate is a carboxylated imidazole–containing compound that is chemically unrelated to any other drug used for the IV induction of anesthesia.[104] The imidazole nucleus renders etomidate, like midazolam, water soluble at an acidic pH and lipid soluble at physiologic pH.

Commercial Preparation

The original formulation of etomidate included 35% propylene glycol (pH 6.9) contributing to a high incidence of pain during IV injection and occasional venous irritation. This has been changed to a fat emulsion, which has virtually abolished pain on injection and venous irritation, whereas the incidence of myoclonus remains unchanged. An oral formulation of etomidate for transmucosal delivery has been shown to produce dose-dependent sedation.[105] Administration through the oral mucosa results in direct systemic absorption while bypassing hepatic metabolism. As a result, higher blood concentrations are achieved more rapidly compared with drug that is swallowed.

Mechanism of Action

Etomidate is unique among injected and inhaled anesthetics in being administered as a single isomer.[104] The anesthetic effect of etomidate resides predominantly in the R(+) isomer, which is approximately five times as potent as the S(−) isomer. In contrast to barbiturates, etomidate appears to be relatively selective as a modulator of $GABA_A$ receptors. Stereoselectivity of etomidate supports the concept that $GABA_A$ receptors are the site of action of etomidate. Etomidate exerts its effects on $GABA_A$ receptors by binding directly to a specific site or sites on the protein and enhancing the affinity of the inhibitory neurotransmitter (GABA) for these receptors.[106] Antagonism of steroid-induced psychosis by etomidate is consistent with enhancement of GABA receptor function by this anesthetic drug.[107] Etomidate is not known to modulate other ligand-gated ion channels in the brain at clinically relevant concentrations.

Pharmacokinetics

The volume of distribution (V_d) of etomidate is large, suggesting considerable tissue uptake (see Table 5-1). Distribution of etomidate throughout body water is favored by its moderate lipid solubility and existence as a weak base (pK 4.2, pH 8.2, 99% unionized at physiologic pH). Etomidate penetrates the brain rapidly, reaching peak levels within 1 minute after IV injection. About 76% of etomidate is bound to albumin independently of the plasma concentration of the drug. Decreases in plasma albumin concentrations, however, result in dramatic increases in the unbound pharmacologically active fraction of etomidate in the plasma. Prompt awakening after a single dose of etomidate principally reflects the redistribution of the drug from brain to inactive tissue sites. Rapid metabolism is also likely to contribute to prompt recovery.

Metabolism

Etomidate is rapidly metabolized by hydrolysis of the ethyl ester side chain to its carboxylic acid ester, resulting in a water-soluble, pharmacologically inactive compound. Hepatic microsomal enzymes and plasma esterases are responsible for this hydrolysis. Hydrolysis is nearly complete, as evidenced by recovery of less than 3% of an administered dose of etomidate as unchanged drug in urine. About 85% of a single IV dose of etomidate can be accounted for as the carboxylic acid ester metabolite in urine, whereas another 10% to 13% is present as this metabolite in the bile. Overall, the clearance of etomidate is about five times that for thiopental; this is reflected as a shorter elimination half-time of 2 to 5 hours. Likewise, the context-sensitive half-time of etomidate is less likely to be increased by continuous infusion as compared with thiopental.

Cardiopulmonary Bypass

Institution of hypothermic cardiopulmonary bypass causes an initial decrease of about 34% in the plasma etomidate concentration that then returns to within 11% of the prebypass value only to be followed by a further decrease with rewarming.[22] The return of the plasma concentration toward prebypass levels is attributed to decreased metabolism, and the subsequent decrease on rewarming is attributed to increased metabolism. In addition, hepatic blood flow changes during cardiopulmonary bypass may alter metabolism, as etomidate is a high–hepatic extraction drug.

Clinical Uses

Etomidate may be viewed as an alternative to propofol or barbiturates for the IV induction of anesthesia, especially in the presence of an unstable cardiovascular system. After a standard induction dose of 0.2 to 0.4 mg/kg IV, the onset of unconsciousness occurs within one arm-to-brain circulation time. Involuntary myoclonic movements are common during the induction period as a result of alteration in the balance of inhibitory and excitatory influences on the thalamocortical tract. The frequency of this myoclonic-like activity can be attenuated by prior administration of an opioid. Awakening after a single IV dose of etomidate is more rapid than after barbiturates, and there is little or no evidence of a hangover or cumulative drug effect. Recovery of psychomotor function after administration of etomidate is intermediate between that of methohexital and thiopental. The duration of action is prolonged by increasing the dose of etomidate or administering the drug as a continuous infusion. As with barbiturates, analgesia is not produced by etomidate. For this reason, administration of an opioid before induction of anesthesia with etomidate may be useful to blunt the hemodynamic responses evoked by direct laryngoscopy and tracheal intubation. Etomidate, 0.15 to 0.3 mg/kg IV, has minimal effects on the duration of electrically induced seizures and thus may serve as an alternative to drugs that decrease the duration of seizures (propofol, thiopental) in patients undergoing electroconvulsive therapy.[35]

The principal limiting factor in the clinical use of etomidate for induction of anesthesia is the ability of this drug to transiently depress adrenocortical function (see the section "Adrenocortical Suppression"). It is widely viewed that postoperative nausea and vomiting is increased in patients receiving etomidate for induction of anesthesia.[108] Nevertheless, comparison of etomidate with propofol did not document an increased incidence of nausea and vomiting in the first 24 hours after surgery in patients receiving etomidate.[109]

Side Effects

Central Nervous System

Etomidate is a potent direct cerebral vasoconstrictor that decreases cerebral blood flow and $CMRO_2$ 35% to 45%.[110] As a result, previously increased ICP is lowered by etomidate. These effects of etomidate are similar to those changes produced by comparable doses of thiopental. Suppression of adrenocortical function limits the clinical usefulness for long-term treatment of intracranial hypertension (see the section "Adrenocortical Suppression").

Etomidate produces a pattern on the EEG that is similar to thiopental. However, the frequency of excitatory spikes on the EEG is greater with etomidate than with thiopental or methohexital, suggesting caution in administration of etomidate to patients with a history of seizures.[84] Like methohexital, etomidate may activate seizure foci, manifesting as fast activity on the EEG.[111] For this reason, etomidate should also be used with caution in patients with focal epilepsy. Conversely, this characteristic has been observed to facilitate localization of seizure foci in patients undergoing cortical resection of epileptogenic tissue. Despite the EEG effects: etomidate also possesses anticonvulsant properties and has been used to terminate status epilepticus. Etomidate has been observed to augment the amplitude of somatosensory evoked potentials, making monitoring of these responses more reliable.[112]

Cardiovascular System

Cardiovascular stability is characteristic of induction of anesthesia with 0.3 mg/kg IV of etomidate. After this dose of etomidate, there are minimal changes in heart rate, stroke volume, or cardiac output, whereas mean arterial blood pressure may decrease up to 15% because of decreases in systemic vascular resistance. The decrease in systemic blood pressure in parallel with changes in systemic vascular resistance suggests that administration of etomidate to acutely hypovolemic patients could result in sudden hypotension. When an induction dose of etomidate is 0.45 mg/kg IV, significant decreases in systemic blood pressure and cardiac output may occur.[113] The cardiovascular effects of etomidate and thiopental are similar when continuously infused in patients with severe valvular heart disease.[114]

Effects of etomidate on myocardial contractility are important to consider, as this drug has been proposed for induction of anesthesia in patients with little or no cardiac reserve. It is difficult to document anesthetic-induced negative inotropic effects in vivo because of concurrent changes in preload, afterload, sympathetic nervous system activity, and baroreceptor reflex activity. Therefore, direct effects of anesthetics on intrinsic myocardial contractility may be more accurately assessed in vitro. In this regard,

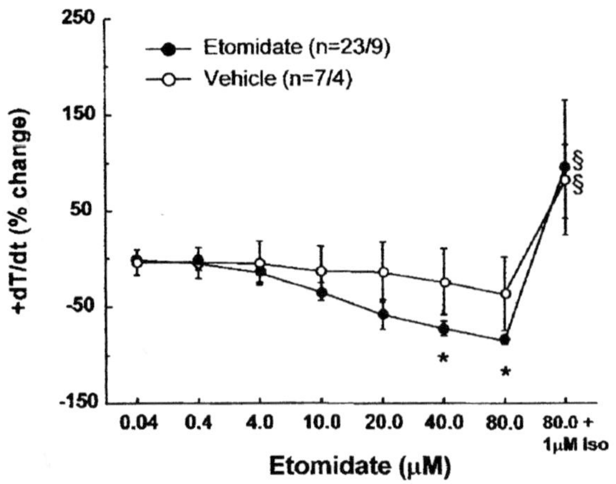

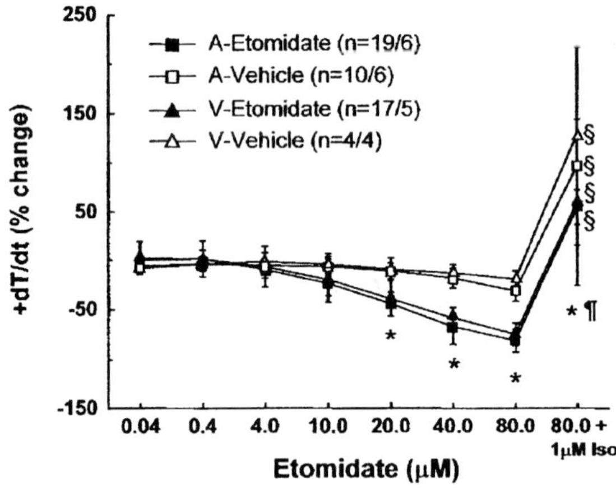

FIGURE 5-8 Effects of etomidate on maximal rate of contraction (+dT/dt) in nonfailing atrial muscle **(A)** and in failing atrial and ventricular muscle **(B)**. Mean ≠ SD. *$P < .05$ versus vehicle. (From Sprung J, Ogletree-Hughes ML, Moravec CS. The effects of etomidate on the contractility of failing and nonfailing human heart muscle. *Anesth Analg*. 2000;91:68–75, with permission.)

etomidate causes dose-dependent decreases in developed tension in isolated cardiac muscle obtained from patients undergoing coronary artery bypass graft operations or cardiac transplantation (Fig. 5-8).[115] This depression was reversible with β-adrenergic stimulation. Nevertheless, concentrations required to produce these negative inotropic effects are in excess of those achieved during clinical use. Etomidate may differ from most other IV anesthetics in that depressive effects on myocardial contractility are minimal at concentrations needed for the production of anesthesia. Hepatic and renal function tests are not altered by etomidate. Intraocular pressure is decreased by etomidate to a similar degree as thiopental. Etomidate does not result in detrimental effects when accidentally injected into an artery.

Ventilation

The depressant effects of etomidate on ventilation seem to be less than those of barbiturates, although apnea may occasionally accompany a rapid IV injection of the drug.[116] In the majority of patients, etomidate-induced decreases in tidal volume are offset by compensatory increases in the frequency of breathing. These effects on ventilation are transient, lasting only 3 to 5 minutes. Etomidate may stimulate ventilation independently of the medullar centers that normally respond to carbon dioxide. For this reason, etomidate may be useful when maintenance of spontaneous ventilation is desirable. Depression of ventilation may be more frequent and more intense when etomidate is combined with inhaled anesthetics or opioids during continuous infusion techniques.

Pain on Injection

Pain on injection and venous irritation has been virtually eliminated with use of etomidate in a lipid emulsion vehicle rather than propylene glycol.

Myoclonus

Most IV anesthetics can cause excitatory effects that manifest as spontaneous movements, such as myoclonus, dystonia, and tremor. These spontaneous movements, particularly myoclonus, occur in 50% to 80% of patients receiving etomidate in the absence of premedication.[84] In one report, 87% of patients receiving etomidate developed excitatory effects, 69% of which were myoclonic. Multiple spikes appeared on the EEG of 22% of these patients.[84] In this same report, the frequency of excitatory effects was 17% after thiopental, 13% after methohexital, and 6% after propofol, and none of the patients treated with other drugs developed myoclonus with spike activity on the EEG.[84] Inclusion of atropine in the preoperative medication can suppress spike activity on the EEG, and prior administration of fentanyl (1 to 2 μg/kg, IV) or a benzodiazepine can decrease the incidence of myoclonus associated with administration of etomidate. Furthermore, the incidence and intensity of myoclonus following the administration of etomidate are dose-related, and so they can be suppressed by pretreatment with a small dose of etomidate (0.03 to 0.075 mg/kg IV) before administration of the induction dose.[117]

The mechanism of etomidate-induced myoclonus appears to be disinhibition of subcortical structures that normally suppress extrapyramidal motor activity. In many patients, excitatory movements are coincident with the early slow phase of the EEG, which corresponds to the beginning of deep anesthesia.[84] It is possible that myoclonus could occur on awakening if the extrapyramidal system emerged more quickly than the cortex that inhibits it.[118] The fact that etomidate-induced myoclonic activity may be associated with seizure activity on the EEG suggests caution in the use of this drug for the induction of anesthesia in patients with a history of seizure activity.[84] Conversely, others have not documented seizure-like activity on the EEG in association with etomidate-induced myoclonus.[117]

Adrenocortical Suppression

Etomidate causes adrenocortical suppression by producing a dose-dependent inhibition of the conversion of cholesterol to cortisol (Fig. 5-9).[119,120] The specific enzyme inhibited by etomidate is 11 β-hydroxylase as evidenced by the accumulation of 11-deoxycorticosterone.[121] This enzyme inhibition lasts more than 8 hours after an induction dose of etomidate. Conceivably, patients experiencing sepsis or hemorrhage and who might require an intact cortisol response would be at a disadvantage should etomidate be administered.[122] Conversely, suppression of adrenocortical function could be considered desirable from the standpoint of "stress-free" anesthesia. In at least one report, it was not possible to demonstrate a difference in the plasma concentrations of cortisol, corticosterone, or adrenocorticotropic hormone in patients receiving a single dose of etomidate or thiopental, even though the response to administration of ACTH was likely suppressed.[123] In a retrospective study of more than 3,000 cardiac surgical patients who received etomidate for induction of anesthesia, there was no evidence to suggest that etomidate exposure was associated with severe hypotension, longer mechanical ventilation hours, longer length of hospital stay, or in-hospital mortality.[124] In stark contrast, another large scale retrospective study demonstrated that anesthetic induction with etomidate, rather than propofol, was associated with increased 30-day mortality and cardiovascular morbidity after noncardiac surgery.[125] The clinical benefit of minimizing cardiac suppression should be carefully weighed against the potential for worsened long-term outcomes when using etomidate in high-risk patients. There have recently been reports of investigational etomidate analogs that do not affect cortisol synthesis. Two of them are currently undergoing human trials.[126]

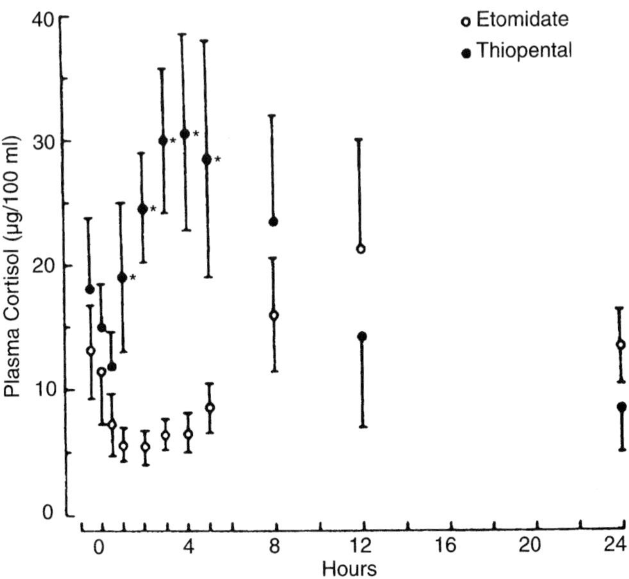

FIGURE 5-9 Etomidate, but not thiopental, is associated with decreases in the plasma concentrations of cortisol. **P* <.05 compared with thiopental; mean ± SD. (From Fragen RJ, Shanks CA, Molteni A, et al. Effects of etomidate on hormonal responses to surgical stress. *Anesthesiology.* 1984; 61:652–656, with permission.)

Allergic Reactions

The incidence of allergic reactions following the administration of etomidate is very low, and the drug does not release histamine from tissue mast cells.[127] When reactions have occurred, it is difficult to separate the role of etomidate from other concomitantly administered drugs (neuromuscular blocking drugs) that are more likely to evoke histamine release than etomidate.

Benzodiazepines

Benzodiazepines are a group of drugs that exert, to slightly varying degrees, five principal pharmacologic effects: anxiolysis, sedation and hypnosis, anticonvulsant actions, spinal cord–mediated skeletal muscle relaxation, and anterograde amnesia (acquisition or encoding of new information).[128] Anxiolysis is most clearly demonstrated in patients with chronic anxiety states, but it may not be as obvious in otherwise normal surgical patients. The amnestic potency of benzodiazepines is greater than their sedative effects, so amnesia can last longer than sedation, or it can occur without much sedation at all. Stored information (retrograde amnesia) is not altered by benzodiazepines.[129] Benzodiazepines do not produce adequate skeletal muscle relaxation for surgical procedures nor does their use influence the required dose of neuromuscular blocking drugs. The frequency of anxiety and insomnia in clinical practice combined with the efficacy of benzodiazepines has led to widespread use of these drugs. For example, it is estimated that 4% of the population uses "sleeping pills" sometime during a given year, and 0.4% of the population uses hypnotics for more than a year.[130] Although benzodiazepines are effective for the treatment of acute insomnia, their use for management of chronic insomnia is decreasing. Compared with barbiturates, benzodiazepines have less tendency to produce tolerance or abuse, a greater margin of safety, and they elicit fewer and less serious drug interactions. Unlike barbiturates, benzodiazepines do not induce hepatic microsomal enzymes. Benzodiazepines are intrinsically far less addicting than opioids, cocaine, amphetamines, or barbiturates.

Midazolam is the most commonly used benzodiazepine in the perioperative period. The context-sensitive half times for diazepam and lorazepam are prolonged, so they are much less satisfactory for this purpose. Midazolam is the only benzodiazepine likely to be used for prolonged administration when a relatively rapid recovery is desired. The longer context-sensitive half time of lorazepam may make this drug an attractive choice for sedation of patients in critical care environments, but it cannot be used easily for a protocol involving intermittent wake-up. Unlike other drugs administered IV to produce CNS effects, benzodiazepines, as a class of drugs, are unique in the availability of a specific pharmacologic antagonist, *flumazenil.*

Structurally, benzodiazepines are similar and many of them share active metabolites.

Mechanism of Action

Benzodiazepines appear to produce all their pharmacologic effects by facilitating the actions of GABA at the $GABA_A$ chloride ionophore.[131] Benzodiazepines do not activate $GABA_A$ receptors directly but bind to a specific site then act allosterically to enhance the affinity of the receptors for GABA (Fig. 5-10).[132] This causes a greater frequency of channel openings, resulting in increased chloride conductance and hyperpolarization of the postsynaptic cell membrane. The postsynaptic neurons are thus rendered more resistant to excitation. This resistance to excitation is presumed to be the mechanism by which benzodiazepines produce anxiolysis, sedation, anterograde amnesia, alcohol potentiation, and anticonvulsant and skeletal muscle relaxant effects.

Benzodiazepines interact with a site located between the α and γ subunits of the $GABA_A$ receptor. The γ subunit is required for benzodiazepine binding. The α_1- and α_5-containing $GABA_A$ receptors are important for sedation, whereas anxiolytic activity is due to interaction with α_2 and α_5 subunit–containing receptors.[133,134] The α_1-containing $GABA_A$ receptors are the most abundant

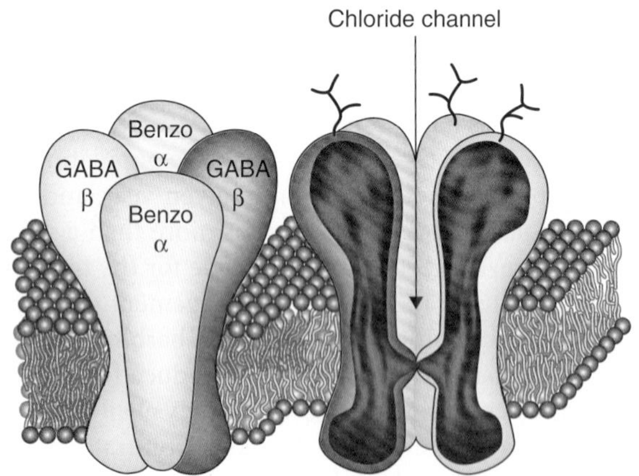

FIGURE 5-10 Model of the γ-aminobutyric acid (GABA) receptor forming a chloride channel. Benzodiazepines (benzo) attach selectively to α subunits and are presumed to facilitate the action of the inhibitory neurotransmitter GABA on α subunits. (From Mohler H, Richards JG. The benzodiazepine receptor: a pharmacologic control element of brain function. *Eur J Anesthesiol Suppl.* 1988;2:15–24, with permission.)

receptor subtypes accounting for approximately 60% of $GABA_A$ receptors in the brain. α_2 Subunits have more restricted expression, principally in the hippocampus and amygdala. The α_5-containing $GABA_A$ receptors are principally extrasynaptic and are responsible for modulation of the resting membrane potential. This anatomic distribution of receptors is consistent with the minimal effects of these drugs outside the CNS (e.g., minimal circulatory effects). In the future, it may be possible to design benzodiazepines that selectively activate specific $GABA_A$ receptor types to produce anxiolysis without sedation.

The $GABA_A$ receptor is a large macromolecule that contains physically separate binding sites (principally α, β, and γ subunits) not only for GABA and the benzodiazepines but also barbiturates, etomidate, propofol, neurosteroids, and alcohol. Acting on a single receptor at different binding sites, the benzodiazepines, barbiturates, and alcohol can produce synergistic effects to increase $GABA_A$ receptor–mediated inhibition in the CNS. This property explains the pharmacologic synergy of these substances and, likewise, the risks of combined overdose, which can produce life-threatening CNS depression. This synergy is also the basis for pharmacologic cross-tolerance between these different classes of drugs and is consistent with the clinical use of benzodiazepines as the first-choice drugs for detoxication from alcohol. Conversely, benzodiazepines are partial agonists and have a low maximal effect on GABA potentiation. The low toxicity of the benzodiazepines and their corresponding clinical safety is attributed to this limitation of their effect on GABAergic neurotransmission.

Differences in the onset and duration of action among commonly administered benzodiazepines reflect differences in potency (receptor binding affinity), lipid solubility (ability to cross the blood–brain barrier and redistribute to peripheral tissues), and pharmacokinetics (uptake, distribution, metabolism, and elimination). All benzodiazepines are highly lipid soluble and are highly bound to plasma proteins, especially albumin. Hypoalbuminemia owing to hepatic cirrhosis or chronic renal failure may increase the unbound fraction of benzodiazepines, resulting in enhanced clinical effects. Following oral administration, benzodiazepines are well absorbed from the gastrointestinal tract and after IV injection, they rapidly enter the CNS and other highly perfused organs.

Nucleoside Transporter Systems

Benzodiazepines decrease adenosine degradation by inhibiting the nucleoside transporter, which is the principal mechanism whereby the effect of adenosine is terminated through reuptake into cells.[135] Adenosine is an important regulator of cardiac function (reduces cardiac oxygen demand by slowing heart rate and increases oxygen delivery by causing coronary vasodilation) and its physiologic effects convey cardioprotection during myocardial ischemia.

Electroencephalogram

The effects of benzodiazepines on the EEG resemble those of barbiturates in that α activity is decreased and low-voltage rapid β activity is increased. This shift from α to β activity occurs more in the frontal and rolandic areas with benzodiazepines, which, unlike the barbiturates, do not cause posterior spread. Midazolam, in contrast to barbiturates and propofol, is unable to produce an isoelectric EEG.

Side Effects

Fatigue and drowsiness are the most common side effects in patients treated chronically with benzodiazepines. Sedation that could impair performance usually subsides within 2 weeks in patients chronically treated with long acting benzodiazepines like lorazepam and diazepam. Patients should be instructed to ingest benzodiazepines before meals and in the absence of antacids because meals and antacids may decrease absorption from the gastrointestinal tract. Chronic administration of benzodiazepines does not adversely affect systemic blood pressure, heart rate, or cardiac rhythm. Although effects on ventilation seem to be absent, it may be prudent to avoid these drugs in patients with chronic lung disease characterized by hypoxemia, since they interact strongly to increase the ventilatory depressant effects of other drugs like opioids (see Drug Interactions). Decreased motor coordination and impairment of cognitive function are also more likely when benzodiazepines are used in combination with other CNS depressant drugs. Acute administration of benzodiazepines often produces transient anterograde amnesia, especially if there is concomitant ingestion of alcohol. There have been reports of profound amnesia in travelers who have ingested triazolam combined with alcohol to facilitate sleep on long airline flights.[136]

Drug Interactions

Benzodiazepines exert synergistic sedative effects with other CNS depressants including alcohol, inhaled and injected anesthetics, opioids, and α_2 agonists. MAC for volatile anesthetics is decreased only modestly by most clinically relevant doses of benzodiazepines, but there is one study suggesting that the analgesic actions opioids may actually be reduced.[137] Another study appeared to support this by finding that antagonism of benzodiazepine effects with flumazenil could enhance the analgesic effects of opioids.[138]

Hypothalamic-Pituitary-Adrenal Axis

Benzodiazepine-induced suppression of the hypothalamic-pituitary-adrenal axis is supported by evidence of suppression of cortisol levels in treated patients.[139] In animals, alprazolam produces dose-dependent inhibition of adrenocorticotrophic hormone and cortisol secretion.[140] Alprazolam's effect may be greater than that of other benzodiazepines and may contribute to its purported efficacy in the treatment of major depression.

Dependence

Even therapeutic doses of benzodiazepines may produce physical dependence as evidenced by the onset of physiological and psychological symptoms after the dosage is decreased or the drug is discontinued. Symptoms of dependence may occur after more than 6 months' use of commonly prescribed low-potency benzodiazepines. It is misleading to consider dependence as evidence of addiction in the absence of inappropriate drug-seeking behaviors. Withdrawal symptoms (irritability, insomnia, tremulousness) have a time of onset that reflects the elimination half-time of the drug being discontinued. These may appear within 1 to 2 days for shorter acting drugs and 2 to 5 days for longer acting drugs. Withdrawal may account for the irritability sometimes experienced in the morning when short acting triazolam is taken for sleep.

Aging

Aging and liver disease affect glucuronidation less than oxidative metabolic pathways. Lorazepam and the two active metabolites of diazepam, oxazepam, and temazepam, are further metabolized only by glucuronidation, and no additional active metabolites are formed. The latter two benzodiazepines are dependably short acting and may be preferable in elderly patients. Elderly patients have increased sensitivity to benzodiazepines based on both pharmacodynamic and pharmacokinetic factors. Administration of long acting benzodiazepines may lead to gait instability, falls and fractures in the elderly, and this can be a cause of increased mortality. Long-term benzodiazepine administration may accelerate cognitive decline in elderly patients. Benzodiazepine withdrawal symptoms in the elderly include confusion. Postoperative confusion is more common in elderly long-term benzodiazepine users (daily use for >1 year) than in short-term users or nonusers of benzodiazepines.[141]

Platelet Aggregation

Benzodiazepines may inhibit platelet-activating factor–induced aggregation resulting in drug-induced inhibition of platelet aggregation. Midazolam-induced inhibition of platelet aggregation may reflect conformational changes in platelet membranes.[142] Although benzodiazepines significantly inhibit platelet aggregation in vitro, they do not appear to affect the risk of hemorrhagic complications in patients with severe, chemotherapy-induced thrombocytopenia[143]; the clinical significance of benzodiazepine-induced inhibition of platelet aggregation in the surgical arena is unclear.

Midazolam

Midazolam is a water-soluble benzodiazepine with an imidazole ring in its structure that accounts for stability in aqueous solutions and rapid metabolism.[144] This benzodiazepine has replaced diazepam for use in preoperative medication and conscious sedation. As with other benzodiazepines, the amnestic effects of midazolam are more potent than its sedative effects. Thus, patients may be awake following administration of midazolam but remain amnestic for events and conversations (postoperative instructions) for several hours.

Commercial Preparation

The pK of midazolam is 6.15, which permits the preparation of salts that are water soluble. The parenteral solution of midazolam used clinically is buffered to an acidic pH of 3.5. Midazolam is unlike other benzodiazepines because it has a substituted imidazole ring. The nitrogen in this ring has a pKa of 6.2, that is protonated (and the drug is therefore water-soluble) in the acidic preparation supplied in the vial. At physiological pH in the bloodstream, 90% of midazolam is unprotonated and lipid soluble.

It should be mentioned that midazolam's water solubility has been attributed incorrectly to the opening of the ring in the benzodiazepine nucleus at acidic pH. In fact, this phenomenon occurs with all benzodiazepines under acidic conditions. At a pH of 3.5 this can account for fewer than 10% of the molecules of midazolam, so it can be responsible for only a small fraction of its water solubility. The water solubility of midazolam obviates the need for a solubilizing preparation, such as propylene glycol required for other benzodiazepines that can produce venoirritation or interfere with absorption after intramuscular (IM) injection. Indeed, midazolam causes minimal to no discomfort during or after IV or IM injection. Midazolam is compatible with lactated Ringer solution and can be mixed with the acidic salts of other drugs, including opioids and anticholinergics.

Pharmacokinetics

Midazolam undergoes rapid absorption from the gastrointestinal tract and prompt passage across the blood–brain barrier. Despite this prompt passage into the brain, midazolam is considered to have a slow effect-site equilibration time ($T_{½}ke0 = 5.6$ minutes) compared with other drugs such as propofol and thiopental. In this regard, IV doses of midazolam should be sufficiently spaced to permit the peak clinical effect to be appreciated before a repeat dose is considered. Only about 50% of an orally administered dose of midazolam reaches the systemic circulation, reflecting a substantial first-pass hepatic effect. As for most benzodiazepines, midazolam is extensively bound to plasma proteins; this binding is independent of the plasma concentration of midazolam (Table 5-2).[144,145] The short duration of a single dose of midazolam is, like diazepam, due to its lipid solubility, which leads to rapid redistribution from the brain to inactive tissue sites. For this reason, the duration of a single dose of midazolam or diazepam is similar. After multiple doses or during continuous infusion, the rate of hepatic clearance becomes an important factor.

The elimination half-time of midazolam is 1.9 hours, which is much shorter than that of diazepam (see Table 5-2).[144] The elimination half-time may be doubled in elderly patients, reflecting age-related decreases in hepatic blood flow and possibly enzyme activity. The volume of distribution (V_d) of midazolam and diazepam are similar, probably reflecting their similar lipid solubility and high degree of protein binding. Elderly and morbidly obese patients have an increased V_d of midazolam resulting from enhanced distribution of the drug into peripheral adipose tissues. The hepatic clearance of midazolam is much more rapid than that of diazepam, as reflected by its context-sensitive half time. As a result, the CNS effects of midazolam are expected to be shorter than those of diazepam, and the difference should be greater as the number of doses is increased.

The institution of cardiopulmonary bypass is associated with a decrease in the plasma concentration of midazolam and an increase on termination of cardiopulmonary bypass.[22] These changes are attributed to redistribution of priming fluid into body tissues. In addition, benzodiazepines are extensively bound to protein, and changes in protein concentrations and pH that accompany institution and termination of cardiopulmonary bypass may have significant effects on the unbound and pharmacologically active fractions of these drugs. The elimination half-time of midazolam is prolonged after cardiopulmonary bypass.

Table 5-2

Comparative Pharmacology of Benzodiazepines

	Equivalent Dose (mg)	Volume of Distribution (L/kg)	Protein Binding (%)	Clearance (mL/kg/min)	Elimination Half-Time (h)
Midazolam	0.15–0.3	1.0–1.5	96–98	6–11	1–4
Diazepam	0.3–0.5	1.0–1.5	96–98	0.2–0.5	21–37
Lorazepam	0.05	0.8–1.3	96–98	0.7–1.0	1–20

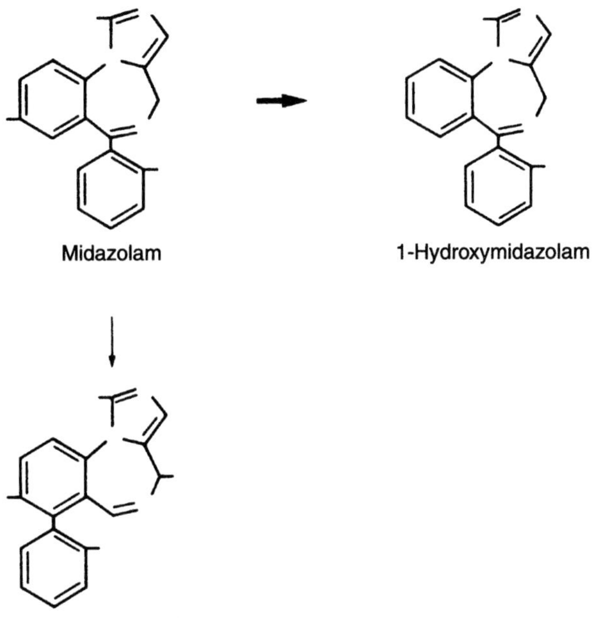

Midazolam

1-Hydroxymidazolam

4-Hydroxymidazolam

FIGURE 5-11 The principal metabolite of midazolam is 1-hydroxymidazolam. A lesser amount of midazolam is metabolized to 4-hydroxymidazolam. (From Reves JG, Fragen RJ, Vinik HR, et al. Midazolam: pharmacology and uses. *Anesthesiology*. 1985;62:310–324, with permission.)

Metabolism

Midazolam is rapidly metabolized by hepatic and small intestine cytochrome P450 (CYP3A4) enzymes to active and inactive metabolites (Fig. 5-11).[144] The principal metabolite of midazolam, 1-hydroxymidazolam, has approximately half the activity of the parent compound.[146] This active metabolite is rapidly conjugated to 1-hydroxymidazolam glucuronide and is subsequently cleared by the kidneys. This glucuronide metabolite has substantial pharmacologic activity when present in high concentrations, as may occur in critically ill patients with renal insufficiency who are receiving continuous IV infusions of midazolam over prolonged periods of time. In these patients, the glucuronide metabolite may have synergistic sedative effects with the parent compound.[147] The other pharmacologically active metabolite of midazolam, 4-hydroxymidazolam, is not present in detectable concentrations in the plasma following IV administration of midazolam.

Metabolism of midazolam is slowed in the presence of drugs (cimetidine, erythromycin, calcium channel blockers, antifungal drugs) that inhibit cytochrome P450 enzymes resulting in unexpected CNS depression.[148] Cytochrome P450 3A enzymes also influence the metabolism of fentanyl. In this regard, the hepatic clearance of midazolam is inhibited by fentanyl as administered during general anesthesia.[149] Overall, the hepatic clearance rate of midazolam is 5 times greater than that of lorazepam and 10 times greater than that of diazepam.

Renal Clearance

The elimination half-time, V_d, and clearance of midazolam are not altered by renal failure.[150] This is consistent with the extensive hepatic metabolism of midazolam.

Effects on Organ Systems

Central Nervous System

Midazolam, like other benzodiazepines, produces decreases in $CMRO_2$ and cerebral blood flow analogous to barbiturates and propofol. Midazolam causes dose-related changes in regional cerebral blood flow in brain regions associated with the normal functioning of arousal, attention, and memory.[151] Cerebral vasomotor responsiveness to carbon dioxide is preserved during midazolam anesthesia.[44] Patients with decreased intracranial compliance show little or no change in ICP when given midazolam doses of 0.15 to 0.27 mg/kg IV. Thus, midazolam is an acceptable alternative to barbiturates for induction of anesthesia in patients with intracranial pathology. There is some evidence, however, that patients with severe head trauma but ICP of less than 18 mm Hg may experience an undesirable increase in ICP when midazolam (0.15 mg/kg IV) is administered rapidly (Fig. 5-12).[152] Similar to thiopental, induction of anesthesia with midazolam does not prevent increases in ICP associated with direct laryngoscopy for tracheal intubation.[153] Although midazolam may improve neurologic outcome after incomplete ischemia, benzodiazepines have not been shown to possess neuroprotective activity in humans. Midazolam is a potent anticonvulsant effective in the treatment of status epilepticus. Prolonged sedation of infants in critical care units (4 to 11 days) with midazolam and fentanyl has been associated with encephalopathy on withdrawal of the benzodiazepine.[154] Paradoxical excitement occurs in less than 1% of all patients receiving midazolam and is effectively treated with a specific benzodiazepine antagonist, flumazenil.[155]

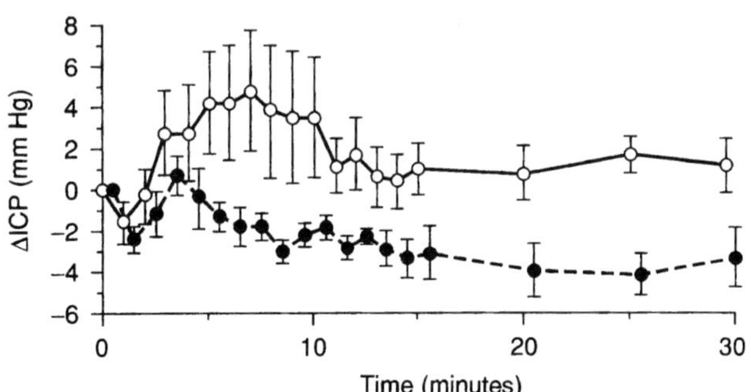

FIGURE 5-12 Administration of midazolam, 0.15 mg/kg IV, to patients with severe head injury (Glasgow coma score ≤6) was associated with an increase in ICP when the control ICP was less than 18 mm Hg (*open circles*) but not when the control ICP was ≥18 mm Hg or greater (*closed circles*). (From Papazian L, Albanese J, Thirion X, et al. Effect of bolus doses of midazolam on intracranial pressure and cerebral perfusion pressure in patients with severe head injury. *Br J Anaesth.* 1993;71:267–271, with permission.)

Ventilation

Midazolam produces dose-dependent decreases in ventilation by decreasing hypoxic drive with 0.15 mg/kg IV producing effects similar to diazepam, 0.3 mg/kg IV.[156] Patients with chronic obstructive pulmonary disease experience even greater midazolam-induced depression of ventilation.[157] Transient apnea may occur after rapid injection of large doses of midazolam (>0.15 mg/kg IV), especially in the presence of preoperative medication that includes an opioid.[158] In one study of healthy volunteers, midazolam 0.05 mg/kg IV produced no ventilatory depressant effects, but adding fentanyl 2 μg/kg IV resulted in apnea in many of the volunteers.[159] Another study found that midazolam 0.05 or 0.075 mg/kg IV depressed resting ventilation in healthy volunteers, whereas spinal anesthesia (mean sensory level T6) stimulated resting ventilation. The combination had a modest synergistic effect for depressing resting ventilation.[160] Benzodiazepines also depress the swallowing reflex and decrease upper airway activity.

Cardiovascular System

Midazolam, 0.2 mg/kg IV, for induction of anesthesia produces a greater decrease in systemic blood pressure and increase in heart rate than does diazepam, 0.5 mg/kg IV.[161] These midazolam-induced hemodynamic changes are similar to the changes produced by thiopental, 3 to 4 mg/kg IV.[162] Cardiac output is not altered by midazolam, suggesting that blood pressure changes are due to decreases in systemic vascular resistance. For this reason, benzodiazepines may be beneficial in improving cardiac output in the presence of congestive heart failure. In the presence of hypovolemia, administration of midazolam results in enhanced blood pressure–lowering effects similar to those produced by other IV induction drugs.[163] Midazolam does not prevent blood pressure and heart rate responses evoked by intubation of the trachea. In fact, this mechanical stimulus may offset the blood pressure–lowering effects of large doses of midazolam administered IV. The effects of midazolam on systemic blood pressure are directly related to the plasma concentration of the benzodiazepine. However, a maximal plasma concentration appears to exist above which little further change in systemic blood pressure occurs.

Clinical Uses

Preoperative Medication

Midazolam is the most commonly used oral preoperative medication for children. Oral midazolam syrup (2 mg/mL) is effective for producing sedation and anxiolysis at a dose of 0.25 mg/kg with minimal effects on ventilation and oxygen saturation even when administered at doses as large as 1 mg/kg (maximum, 20 mg).[164] Midazolam, 0.5 mg/kg administered orally 30 minutes before induction of anesthesia, provides reliable sedation and anxiolysis in children without producing delayed awakening (Fig. 5-13).[165] Although it is recommended that oral midazolam be administered at least 20 minutes before surgery, there is evidence that significant anterograde amnesia is present when 0.5 mg/kg orally is administered 10 minutes before surgery.[166] Midazolam crosses the placenta but the fetal to maternal ratio is significantly less than that for other benzodiazepines.

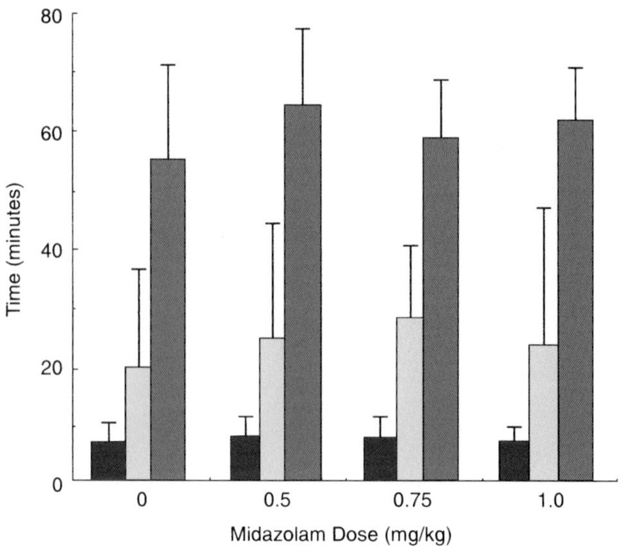

FIGURE 5-13 Increasing doses of oral midazolam premedication administered 30 minutes before the induction of anesthesia did not produce different effects on the interval from the end of surgery until transported to the postanesthesia care unit (*solid bars*), interval from arrival in the postanesthesia care unit until spontaneous eye opening (*light gray bars*), and time in the postanesthesia care unit (*dark gray bars*). (From McMillan CO, Spahr-Schopfer IA, Sikich N, et al. Premedication of children with oral midazolam. *Can J Anaesth.* 1992;39:545–550, with permission.)

Intravenous Sedation

Midazolam in doses of 1.0 to 2.5 mg IV (onset within 30 to 60 seconds, half-time to peak effect 5.6 minutes, duration of sedation 15 to 80 minutes) is effective for sedation during regional anesthesia as well as for brief therapeutic procedures. The effect-site equilibrium time for midazolam must be considered in recognizing the likely time of peak clinical effect and the need for supplemental doses of midazolam.

The most significant side effect of midazolam when used for sedation is depression of ventilation caused by a decrease in the hypoxic drive, particularly in concert with other anesthetic drugs. Midazolam-induced depression of ventilation is exaggerated (synergistic effects) in the presence of opioids and other CNS depressant drugs.[138] Patients with chronic obstructive pulmonary disease may also manifest exaggerated depression of ventilation following administration of benzodiazepines to produce sedation. It is important to appreciate that increasing age greatly increases pharmacodynamic variability and is associated with generally increased sensitivity to the hypnotic effects of midazolam.[167]

Induction of Anesthesia

Although seldom used for this purpose currently, anesthesia can be induced by administration of midazolam, 0.1 to 0.2 mg/kg IV, over 30 to 60 seconds. Nevertheless, thiopental usually produces induction of anesthesia 50% to 100% faster than midazolam (Fig. 5-14).[168] Onset of unconsciousness (synergistic interaction) is facilitated when a small dose of opioid (fentanyl, 50 to 100 μg IV or its equivalent) precedes the injection of midazolam by 1 to 3 minutes. The dose of midazolam required for the IV induction of anesthesia is also less when preoperative medication includes a CNS depressant drug. In healthy patients receiving small doses of benzodiazepines, the cardiovascular depression associated with these drugs is minimal. When significant cardiovascular responses occur, it is most likely a reflection of benzodiazepine-induced peripheral vasodilation. As with depression of ventilation, cardiovascular changes produced by benzodiazepines may be exaggerated in the presence of other CNS depressant drugs such as propofol and thiopental.

Maintenance of Anesthesia

Midazolam may be administered to supplement opioids, propofol, and/or inhaled anesthetics during maintenance of anesthesia. The context-sensitive half-time for midazolam increases modestly with an increasing duration of administration of a continuous infusion of this benzodiazepine.[15] Anesthetic requirements for volatile anesthetics are decreased in a dose-dependent manner by midazolam. Awakening after general anesthesia that includes induction of anesthesia with midazolam is 1.0 to 2.5 times longer than that observed when thiopental is used for the IV induction of anesthesia.[169] Gradual awakening in patients who receive midazolam is rarely associated with nausea, vomiting, or emergence excitement.

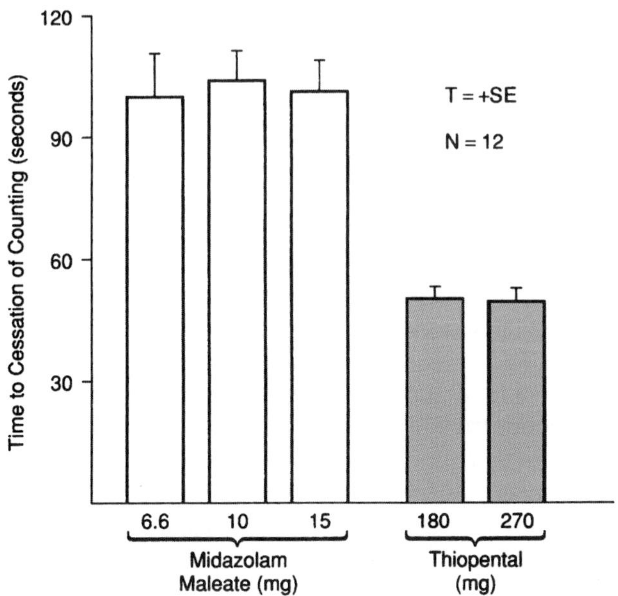

FIGURE 5-14 Induction of anesthesia as depicted by time to cessation of counting occurs in about 110 seconds after the intravenous administration of midazolam compared with about 50 seconds after injection of thiopental. (From Sarnquist FH, Mathers WD, Brock-Utne J, et al. A bioassay of water-soluble benzodiazepine against sodium thiopental. *Anesthesiology*. 1980;52:149–153, with permission.)

Postoperative Sedation

Long-term IV administration of midazolam (loading dose 0.5 to 4 mg IV and maintenance dose 1 to 7 mg per hour IV) to produce sedation in intubated patients resulted loading of peripheral tissues with midazolam and clearance from the systemic circulation becomes less dependent on redistribution into peripheral tissues and more dependent on hepatic metabolism.[170] In addition, pharmacologically active metabolites may accumulate with prolonged IV administration of the parent drug. Under these conditions, plasma concentrations of midazolam decrease more slowly (emergence delayed) after discontinuation of the IV infusion compared with single IV injections. Emergence time is also a function of the plasma concentrations of midazolam at the time the IV infusion is discontinued. Patients maintained at higher plasma concentrations of midazolam take longer to awaken than patients maintained at lower plasma concentrations for comparable periods of time. The concomitant administration of analgesic doses of opioids greatly decreases the needed dose of midazolam and results in a more rapid recovery from sedation following discontinuation of the IV infusion of midazolam.[170] Emergence time from midazolam infusion is increased in elderly patients, obese patients, and in the presence of severe liver disease.

Paradoxical Vocal Cord Motion

Paradoxical vocal cord motion is a cause of nonorganic upper airway obstruction and stridor that may manifest postoperatively. Midazolam 0.5 to 1 mg IV may be an effective treatment for paradoxical vocal cord motion.[171]

Diazepam

Diazepam is a highly lipid-soluble benzodiazepine with a more prolonged duration of action compared with midazolam. Because of the beneficial aspects of midazolam pharmacology, parenteral diazepam is seldom used as part of current anesthetic regimens.

Commercial Preparation

Diazepam is dissolved in organic solvents (propylene glycol, sodium benzoate) because it is insoluble in water. The solution is viscid, with a pH of 6.6 to 6.9. Dilution with water or saline causes cloudiness but does not alter the potency of the drug. Injection by either the IM or IV route may be painful. Diazepam is also available in a unique soybean formulation for IV injection. This formulation is associated with a lower incidence of pain on injection and thrombophlebitis.

Pharmacokinetics

Diazepam is rapidly absorbed from the gastrointestinal tract after oral administration, reaching peak concentrations in about 1 hour in adults but as quickly as 15 to 30 minutes in children. There is rapid uptake of diazepam into the brain, followed by redistribution to inactive tissue sites, especially fat, as this benzodiazepine is highly lipid soluble. The V_d of diazepam is large, reflecting extensive tissue uptake of this lipid-soluble drug (see Table 5-2). Women, with a greater body fat content, are likely to have a larger V_d for diazepam than men. Diazepam rapidly crosses the placenta, achieving fetal concentrations equal to and sometimes greater than those present in the maternal circulation.[172] The duration of action of benzodiazepines is not linked to receptor events but rather is determined by redistribution, then rate of metabolism and elimination.

Protein Binding

Highly lipid-soluble diazepam is extensively bound, primarily to albumin (see Table 5-2). Cirrhosis of the liver or renal insufficiency with associated decreases in plasma concentrations of albumin, may manifest as an increased fraction of unbound diazepam and an increased incidence of drug-related side effects.[173] The high degree of protein binding and the wide distribution to extra-vascular tissues limits the efficacy of hemodialysis in the treatment of diazepam overdose.

Metabolism

Diazepam is principally metabolized by hepatic microsomal enzymes using an oxidative pathway of *N*-demethylation. The two principal metabolites of diazepam are desmethyldiazepam (nordazepam) and oxazepam, with a lesser amount metabolized to temazepam (Fig. 5-15). Desmethyldiazepam is metabolized more slowly than oxazepam and is only slightly less potent than diazepam. Therefore, it is likely that this metabolite contributes to the return of drowsiness that manifests 6 to 8 hours after administration of diazepam, as well as to sustained effects usually attributed to the parent drug. Alternatively, enterothepatic recirculation of diazepam may contribute to recurrence of sedation.[174] Ultimately, desmethyldiazepam is excreted in urine in the form of oxidized and glucuronide conjugated metabolites. Unchanged, diazepam is not appreciably excreted in urine. Benzodiazepines do not produce enzyme induction.

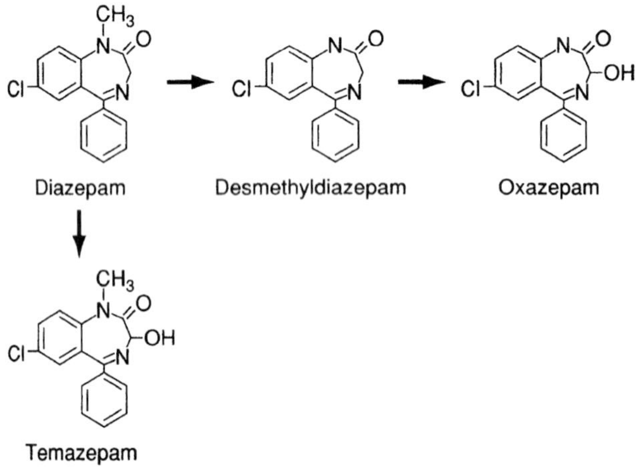

Diazepam → Desmethyldiazepam → Oxazepam

Diazepam → Temazepam

FIGURE 5-15 The principal metabolites of diazepam are desmethyldiazepam and oxazepam. A lesser amount of diazepam is metabolized to temazepam.

Elimination Half-Time

The elimination half time of diazepam is prolonged, averaging over 40 hours in healthy volunteers (see Table 5-2). Cirrhosis of the liver is accompanied by up to fivefold increases in the elimination half-time of diazepam.[175] Likewise, the elimination half-time of diazepam increases progressively with increasing age, which contributes to the increased sensitivity of these patients to the drug's sedative effects.[175] Prolongation of the elimination half time of diazepam in the presence of cirrhosis of the liver is partly due to decreased protein binding of the drug, leading to an increased V_d. In addition, hepatic clearance of diazepam is likely to be decreased, reflecting decreased hepatic blood flow characteristic of cirrhosis of the liver. Compared with lorazepam, diazepam has a longer elimination half-time but shorter duration of action because it dissociates more rapidly than lorazepam from $GABA_A$ receptors, permitting more rapid redistribution to inactive tissue sites.

Desmethyldiazepam, the principal metabolite of diazepam, has an elimination half-time of 48 to 96 hours. As such, the elimination half-time of the metabolite may exceed that of the parent drug. Plasma concentrations of diazepam often decline more rapidly than plasma concentrations of desmethyldiazepam. This pharmacologically active metabolite can accumulate in plasma and tissues during chronic use of diazepam. Prolonged somnolence associated with high doses of diazepam is likely to be caused by sequestration of the parent drug and its active metabolite, desmethyldiazepam, in tissues, presumably fat, for subsequent release back into the circulation. A week or more is often required for elimination of these compounds from plasma after discontinuation of chronic diazepam therapy.

Effects on Organ Systems

Diazepam, like other benzodiazepines, produces minimal effects on ventilation and the systemic circulation. Hepatic and renal functions are not altered appreciably. Diazepam does not increase the incidence of nausea and vomiting. There is no change in the circulating plasma concentrations of stress-responding hormones (catecholamines, arginine vasopressin, cortisol).

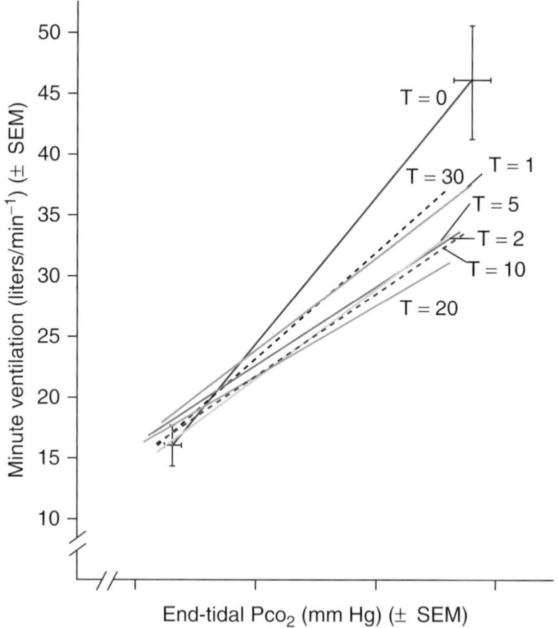

FIGURE 5-16 The slope of the line depicting the ventilatory response to carbon dioxide is decreased (T = minutes) following administration of diazepam, 0.4 mg/kg IV. (From Gross JB, Smith L, Smith TC. Time course of ventilatory response to carbon dioxide after intravenous diazepam. *Anesthesiology.* 1982;57:18–21, with permission.)

Ventilation

Diazepam, in sedative doses, produces minimally depressant effects on ventilation, with detectable increases in $Paco_2$ not occurring until 0.2 mg/kg IV is administered. This slight increase in $Paco_2$ is due primarily to a decrease in tidal volume. Nevertheless, rarely, small doses of diazepam (<10 mg IV) have produced apnea.[176] Combination of diazepam with other CNS depressants (opioids, alcohol) or administration of this drug to patients with chronic obstructive airway disease may result in exaggerated or prolonged depression of ventilation.

The slope of the line depicting the ventilatory response to carbon dioxide is decreased nearly 50% within 3 minutes after the administration of diazepam, 0.4 mg/kg IV (Fig. 5-16).[177] This depression of the slope persists for about 25 minutes and parallels the level of consciousness. Despite the decrease in slope, the carbon dioxide response curve is not shifted to the right as observed with depression of ventilation produced by opioids. These depressant effects on ventilation seem to be a CNS effect because the mechanics of respiratory muscles are unchanged.

Cardiovascular System

Diazepam administered in doses of 0.5 to 1 mg/kg IV for induction of anesthesia typically produces minimal decreases in systemic blood pressure, cardiac output, and systemic vascular resistance that are similar in magnitude to those observed during natural sleep (10% to 20% decreases) (Table 5-3).[178] Because of its relative hemodynamic stability, high-dose diazepam was once used for cardiac surgery. There is a transient depression of baroreceptor-mediated heart rate responses that is less than the depression evoked by volatile anesthetics but that could, in hypovolemic patients, interfere with optimal compensatory changes.[179] In patients with increased left ventricular end diastolic pressure, a small dose of diazepam significantly decreases this pressure. Diazepam appears to have no direct action on the sympathetic nervous system, and it does not cause orthostatic hypotension.

The incidence and magnitude of systemic blood pressure decreases produced by diazepam seem to be less than those associated with barbiturates administered IV for the induction of anesthesia.[180] Nevertheless, occasionally, a patient may unpredictably experience hypotension with even small doses of diazepam.[181] The addition of nitrous oxide after induction of anesthesia with diazepam is not associated with adverse cardiac changes (see Table 5-3).[178] Therefore, nitrous oxide can be administered in the presence of diazepam to ensure absence of patient awareness during surgery. This contrasts with direct myocardial

Table 5-3

Cardiovascular Effects of Diazepam (0.5 mg/kg IV) and Diazepam-Nitrous Oxide

	Awake	Diazepam	Diazepam-Nitrous Oxide
Systolic blood pressure (mm Hg)	144	125[a]	121[a]
Diastolic blood pressure (mm Hg)	81	74	75
Mean arterial pressure (mm Hg)	102	91[a]	91[a]
Heart rate (beats/min)	66	68	65
Pulmonary artery pressure (mm Hg)	18.4	16.3	17.2
Pulmonary artery occlusion pressure (mm Hg)	11.5	10.6	11.9
Cardiac output (L/min)	5.3	5.1	4.8[a]
Systemic vascular resistance (dynes/s/cm^{-5})	1,391	1,344	1,377

*P <.05 compared with the awake value.

From McCammon RL, Hilgenberg JC, Stoelting RK. Hemodynamic effects of diazepam-nitrous oxide in patients with coronary artery disease. *Anesth Analg.* 1980;59:438–441.

depression and decreases in systemic blood pressure that occur when nitrous oxide is administered in the presence of opioids. Likewise, prior administration of diazepam, 0.125 to 0.5 mg/kg IV, followed by injection of a high dose of fentanyl (50 μg/kg IV), is associated with decreases in systemic vascular resistance and systemic blood pressure that do not accompany administration of the opioid alone.

Skeletal Muscle

Skeletal muscle relaxant effects reflect actions of diazepam on spinal internuncial neurons and not actions at the neuromuscular junction.[182] Presumably, diazepam diminishes the tonic facilitatory influence on spinal γ neurons, and, thus, skeletal muscle tone is decreased. Tolerance occurs to the skeletal muscle relaxant effects of benzodiazepines.

Overdose

CNS intoxication can be expected at diazepam plasma concentrations of greater than 1,000 ng/mL. Despite massive overdoses of diazepam, serious sequelae (coma) are unlikely to occur if cardiac and pulmonary functions are supported and other drugs such as alcohol are not present.

Clinical Uses

Diazepam remains a popular oral drug for preoperative medication of adults and continues to be an appropriate choice for management of delirium tremens. Production of skeletal muscle relaxation by diazepam is often used in the management of lumbar disc disease and may be of value in the rare patient who develops tetany. Midazolam has largely replaced diazepam for IV sedation and the preoperative medication of children.

Anticonvulsant Activity

The prior administration of diazepam, 0.25 mg/kg IV, to animals protects against the development of seizures due to local anesthetic toxicity (Fig. 5-17).[183] Diazepam, 0.1 mg/kg IV, is effective in abolishing seizure activity produced by lidocaine, delirium tremens, and status epilepticus.

The efficacy of diazepam as an anticonvulsant reflects its ability to facilitate the actions of the inhibitory neurotransmitter, GABA. In contrast to barbiturates, which inhibit seizures by relatively nonselective action on GABA receptors, diazepam and other benzodiazepines are selective for GABA ionophores containing α-1, α-2, and α-5 subunits. They decrease the frequency of chloride channel opening while barbiturates increase the duration of opening. Benzodiazepines are lower efficacy agonists, and compared to barbiturates, they are capable of much less CNS depression, particularly the hippocampus. If diazepam is administered to terminate seizures, a longer acting antiepileptic drug such as fosphenytoin is also administered.

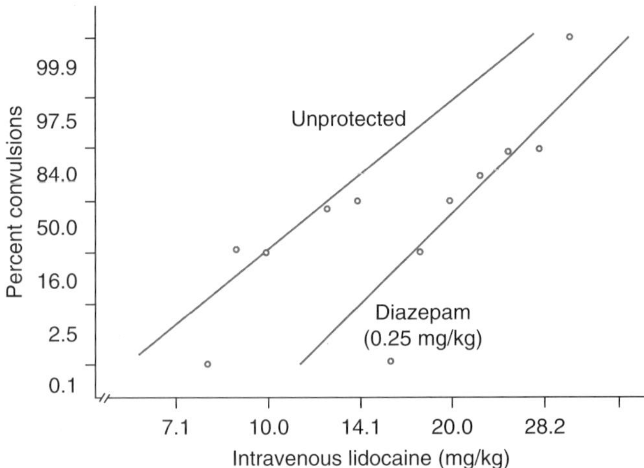

FIGURE 5-17 Prior administration of diazepam, 0.25 mg/kg IV, increases the intravenous dose of lidocaine required to produce seizures compared with untreated (unprotected) animals. (From De Jong RH, Heavner JE. Diazepam prevents and aborts lidocaine convulsions in monkeys. *Anesthesiology*. 1974;49:226–230, with permission.)

Lorazepam

Lorazepam resembles oxazepam, differing only in the presence of an extra chloride atom on the ortho position of the 5-phenyl moiety. Lorazepam is a more potent sedative and amnesic than midazolam and diazepam, whereas its effects on ventilation, the cardiovascular system, and skeletal muscles resemble those of other benzodiazepines.

Pharmacokinetics

Lorazepam is conjugated with glucuronic acid in the liver to form pharmacologically inactive metabolites that are excreted by the kidneys. This contrasts with formation of pharmacologically active metabolites after the administration of midazolam and diazepam. The elimination half time average is 14 hours, with urinary excretion of lorazepam glucuronide accounting for greater than 80% of the injected dose (see Table 5-2). Compared with midazolam, lorazepam has a much slower metabolic clearance. This may be explained by the slower hepatic glucuronidation of lorazepam compared with more rapid oxidative hydroxylation of midazolam. Because formation of glucuronide metabolites of lorazepam is not entirely dependent on hepatic microsomal enzymes, the metabolism of lorazepam is less likely than that of diazepam to be influenced by alterations in hepatic function, increasing age, or drugs that inhibit P450 enzymes such as cimetidine. Indeed, the elimination half-time of lorazepam is not prolonged in elderly patients or in those treated with cimetidine. Lorazepam has a slower onset of action than midazolam or diazepam because of its lower lipid solubility and slower entrance into the CNS.

Clinical Uses

Lorazepam undergoes reliable absorption after oral and IM injection, which contrasts with diazepam. After oral administration, maximal plasma concentrations of lorazepam occur in 2 to 4 hours and persist at therapeutic levels for up to 24 to 48 hours. The recommended oral dose of lorazepam for preoperative medication is 50 μg/kg, not to exceed 4 mg.[184] With this dose, maximal anterograde amnesia lasting up to 6 hours occurs, and sedation is not excessive. Larger oral doses produce additional sedation without increasing amnesia.

Although the plasma pharmacokinetics suggest that lorazepam should have a rapid onset and an intermediate duration of action, the effect of a single IV dose is slower in onset and longer in duration than a comparable dose of diazepam. This is due, in part, to the lower lipid solubility of lorazepam and its slower passage into and out of the CNS. After 1-4 mg IV, the effect starts within 1 to 2 minutes, but the peak effect does not occur for 20 to 30 minutes, and the duration of sedative effects ranges from 6 to 10 hours.[185] Infusions of lorazepam to produce postoperative sedation result in significant delays in emergence from sedation compared with midazolam.[170] Obesity prolongs the sedative effects of lorazepam reflecting the larger volume of distribution and longer elimination half-time.

A slow onset limits the usefulness of lorazepam for (a) IV induction of anesthesia, (b) IV sedation during regional anesthesia, or (c) use as an anticonvulsant. Like diazepam, lorazepam is effective in limiting the incidence of emergence reactions after administration of ketamine. Although it is insoluble in water and thus requires use of solvents such as polyethylene glycol or propylene glycol, lorazepam is alleged to be less painful on injection and to produce less venous thrombosis than diazepam.

Lorazepam may be used as an economic alternative to midazolam for postoperative sedation of intubated patients. The risk of delayed emergence from sedation is increased when lorazepam is used for postoperative sedation and amnestic effects may last for several days. Delayed emergence from sedation may delay weaning from mechanical ventilation.

Oxazepam

Oxazepam, a pharmacologically active metabolite of diazepam, is commercially available (see Fig. 5-15). Its duration of action is slightly shorter than that of diazepam because oxazepam is converted to pharmacologically inactive metabolites by conjugation with glucuronic acid. The elimination half-time is 5 to 15 hours. Like lorazepam, the duration of action of oxazepam is unlikely to be influenced by hepatic dysfunction or administration of cimetidine.

Oral absorption of oxazepam is relatively slow. As a result, this drug may not be useful for the treatment of insomnia characterized by difficulty falling asleep. Conversely, oxazepam may be used for treatment of insomnia characterized by nightly awakenings or shortened total sleep time.

Alprazolam

Alprazolam has significant anxiety-reducing effects in patients with primary anxiety and panic attacks. Based on these effects, alprazolam may be an alternative to midazolam for preoperative medication.[186] Inhibition of adrenocorticotrophic hormone and cortisol secretion may be more prominent with alprazolam than with other benzodiazepines.

Clonazepam

Clonazepam is a highly lipid-soluble benzodiazepine that is well absorbed after oral administration. Clonazepam is metabolized to inactive conjugated and unconjugated metabolites that appear in the urine. The elimination half-time is 24 to 48 hours. Clonazepam is particularly effective in the control and prevention of seizures, especially myoclonic and infantile spasms.

Flurazepam

Flurazepam is chemically and pharmacologically similar to other benzodiazepines but is used exclusively to treat insomnia. After administration of 15 to 30 mg orally to adults, a hypnotic effect occurs in 15 to 25 minutes and lasts 7 to 8 hours. The period of rapid eye movement sleep is decreased by this drug. The principal metabolite of flurazepam is desalkylflurazepam. This metabolite is pharmacologically active and has a prolonged elimination half-time that may manifest as daytime sedation (hangover). Furthermore, repeated doses of flurazepam may result in accumulation of this metabolite, producing cumulative sedation.

Temazepam

Temazepam is an orally active benzodiazepine administered exclusively for the treatment of insomnia. Oral absorption is complete, but peak plasma concentrations do not reliably occur until about 2.5 hours after its administration. Metabolism in the liver results in weakly active to inactive metabolites that are conjugated with glucuronic acid. The elimination half-time is about 15 hours. Temazepam, 15 to 30 mg orally, does not alter the proportion of rapid eye movement sleep to total sleep in adults. Despite the relatively long elimination half-time, temazepam, as used to treat insomnia, is unlikely to be accompanied by residual drowsiness the following morning. Tolerance or signs of withdrawal do not occur, even after nightly administration for 30 consecutive days.

Triazolam

Triazolam is an orally absorbed benzodiazepine with a rapid onset and short duration that is effective in the treatment of insomnia characterized by difficulty falling asleep. Peak plasma concentrations after oral administration of 0.25 to 0.50 mg to adults occur in about 1 hour. The elimination half-time is 1.7 hours, rendering triazolam one of the shortest acting benzodiazepines. The two principal metabolites of triazolam have little if any hypnotic activity, and their elimination half-time is less than 4 hours. For these reasons, residual daytime effects or cumulative sedation effects with repeated doses of triazolam seem less likely than with other benzodiazepines.

Triazolam does not change the proportion of rapid eye movement to total sleep time. Rebound insomnia, however, may occur when this drug is discontinued. Marked anterograde amnesia has developed when this drug has been self-administered in attempts to facilitate sleep when traveling through several time zones.[136] In otherwise healthy elderly patients, triazolam causes a greater degree of sedation or psychomotor impairment than in young persons.[187] These effects are due to decreased clearance and higher plasma concentrations rather than from an increased sensitivity to the drug. For these reasons, it is recommended that the dose of triazolam be decreased 50% in elderly persons.

Flumazenil

Flumazenil, a 1,4-imidazobenzodiazepine derivative, is a selective benzodiazepine antagonist with a high affinity for benzodiazepine receptors, where it exerts minimal agonist activity.[188,189] As a competitive antagonist, flumazenil prevents or reverses, in a dose-dependent manner, all the agonist effects of benzodiazepines. Flumazenil effectively antagonizes only the benzodiazepine component of ventilatory depression that is present during combined administration of a benzodiazepine and opioid.[138] Metabolism of flumazenil is by hepatic microsomal enzymes to inactive metabolites.

Dose and Administration

The dose of flumazenil should be titrated individually to obtain the desired level of consciousness. The recommended initial dose is 0.2 mg IV (8 to 15 μg/kg IV), which typically reverses the CNS effects of benzodiazepine agonists within about 2 minutes. If required, further doses of 0.1 mg IV (to a total of 1 mg IV) may be administered at 60-second intervals. Generally, total doses of 0.3 to 0.6 mg IV have been adequate to decrease the degree of sedation to the required extent in patients sedated or anesthetized with benzodiazepines, whereas total doses of 0.5 to 1.0 mg IV are usually sufficient to completely abolish the effect of a therapeutic dose of a benzodiazepine. In patients who are unconscious due to an overdose with an unknown drug or drugs, failure to respond to IV doses of flumazenil of more than 5 mg probably indicates the involvement of intoxicants other than benzodiazepines or the presence of functional organic disorders. The duration of action of flumazenil is 30 to 60 minutes, and supplemental doses of the antagonist may be needed to maintain the desired level of consciousness. An alternative to repeated doses of flumazenil to maintain wakefulness is a continuous low-dose infusion of flumazenil, 0.1 to 0.4 mg per hour.[188] The administration of flumazenil to patients being treated with antiepileptic drugs for control of seizure activity is not recommended as it could precipitate acute withdrawal seizures.[190]

Side Effects

Flumazenil-induced antagonism of excess benzodiazepine agonist effects is not followed by acute anxiety, hypertension, tachycardia, or neuroendocrine evidence of a stress response in postoperative patients.[191,192] Reversal of benzodiazepine agonist effects with flumazenil is not associated with alterations in left ventricular systolic function or coronary hemodynamics in patients with coronary artery disease.[193] The weak intrinsic agonist activity of flumazenil most likely attenuates evidence of abrupt reversal of agonist effects. Flumazenil does not alter anesthetic requirements (MAC) for volatile anesthetics, suggesting that these drugs do not exert any of their depressant effects on the CNS at benzodiazepine receptors.[194] Flumazenil, administered at about 10 times the clinically recommended dose, has no agonist effects on resting ventilation or psychomotor performance in normal individuals.[195]

Short-Acting Nonbenzodiazepine Benzodiazepines

Benzodiazepine refers to a specific chemical structure consisting of a benzene ring and a diazepine ring, hence the name benzodiazepine. Unfortunately, the name has also come to refer to a pharmacologic class of drugs with a shared clinical activity and a shared molecular binding site on the $GABA_A$ receptor at the interface between the α and γ subunits, the benzodiazepine site. Eventually, drugs were found that bound to the same receptor, and exhibited the same pharmacology, but did not consist of a benzene ring bound to a diazepine ring. These drugs were given the cumbersome but vaguely amusing name: nonbenzodiazepine benzodiazepine. The agents that have been approved are zaleplon (Sonata), zolpidem (Ambien), and more recently, eszopiclone (Lunesta).

Zaleplon, zolpidem, and eszopiclone exert activity at the GABA receptor complex.[196] These drugs seem to have more selectivity for certain subunits of GABA receptors, resulting in a clinical profile for treatment of sleeping disorders that is more efficacious with fewer side effects than occur with conventional benzodiazepines. Their use has steadily risen during the past decade, with 3% of Americans now reporting use of one or more of these agents during the prior month.[197] Due to variations in binding to GABA receptor subunits, these drugs show differences in their effect on sleep stages. Zaleplon (10 mg orally) has a rapid elimination so there are few residual side effects after taking a single dose at bedtime. It may be particularly useful for patients with delayed onset of sleep. By comparison, zolpidem (10 mg orally) has a delayed elimination, prolonging drug effect. This may result in residual sedation and side effects but may be used for sustained treatment of insomnia with less waking during the night. All of these agents are somewhat effective for insomnia, but their ability to produce sustained improvement in sleep is uncertain.[198]

Barbiturates

The introduction of thiopental in 1934 revolutionized the practice of anesthesia. This rapid-acting barbiturate made it possible to induce general anesthesia in seconds, avoiding a slow, often unpleasant, more dangerous induction with diethyl ether. The current edition of this text marks a turning point in anesthetic pharmacology: Thiopental and other barbiturate sedative-hypnotics were imported from manufacturers overseas, but these companies have now ceased exporting barbiturates to the United States in order to protest their use as a part of the lethal injection "cocktail" for capital punishment.[199] We will still include a discussion of barbiturate pharmacology in this chapter, and this is done for several reasons: First, it is conceivable that shipments of these drugs may resume. Second, some anesthesiologists who practice outside of the United States use these drugs. Most importantly, the pharmacokinetics and pharmacodynamics of barbiturates are the prototypes and comparators for almost all of our clinically used IV anesthetics. To understand the literature on drugs like propofol, etomidate, and midazolam, it is critical to know the properties of barbiturates to which they were often compared, as these were the gold standard during their development.

Barbiturates' Use in Anesthesia

The clinically used barbiturates are derived from barbituric acid. The substitutions on this molecule determine the physicochemical properties, pharmacokinetics, and the relative potency to produce various effects. Oxybarbiturates (pentobarbital, secobarbital) have oxygen at the second position. Replacement of the oxygen with a sulfur atom results in the corresponding thiobarbiturates (thiopental, thiamylal), which are much more lipid soluble and have greater hypnotic potency. A phenyl group at the fifth position (phenobarbital) increases the anticonvulsant, but not hypnotic, potency. On the other hand, a methyl group on the nitrogen (as with methohexital) increases hypnotic potency but lowers the seizure threshold and causes myoclonus during induction.

Mechanism of Action

Barbiturates are one of the earliest examples of CNS depressants that act in part by potentiating $GABA_A$ channel activity. At clinically used concentrations, they also act on glutamate, adenosine, and neuronal nicotinic acetylcholine receptors. Studies in knock-in mice have shown that $GABA_A$ receptors containing β_3 subunits are responsible for the immobilizing activity of pentobarbital and partly responsible for the hypnotic activity.[200] The interaction of barbiturates (as well as propofol and etomidate acting at different sites) functions allosterically to increase the affinity of GABA for its binding site, thereby increasing the duration of the $GABA_A$-activated opening of chloride channels (see Fig. 5-10). Barbiturates can also mimic the action of GABA by directly activating $GABA_A$ receptors at higher doses.

Pharmacokinetics

Thiopental causes rapid onset and rapid awakening after a single IV dose due to rapid uptake then rapid redistribution out of the brain into inactive tissues (Fig. 5-18).[201] As previously discussed, this is the basis for the short action of most other highly lipophilic drugs. Ultimately, elimination from the body depends almost entirely on metabolism because less than 1% of thiopental is recovered unchanged in urine.[202] The time required for the plasma concentration of thiopental to decrease 50% after discontinuation of a prolonged infusion (context-sensitive half-time) is lengthy. The drug is sequestered in fat and skeletal muscle then it reenters the circulation and prevents the plasma concentration from dropping rapidly.[15]

Thiobarbiturates are metabolized in hepatocytes and, to a small extent, in extrahepatic sites such as the kidneys and possibly the CNS. Metabolites (particularly hydroxythiopental and the 5-carboxylic acid) are usually inactive and are always more water soluble than the parent compound, which facilitates renal excretion. A small amount of thiopental is metabolized to the active, long-acting oxybarbiturate, pentobarbital. Ultimately, metabolism of thiopental is almost complete (99%). Hepatic clearance of thiopental is characterized by a low hepatic extraction

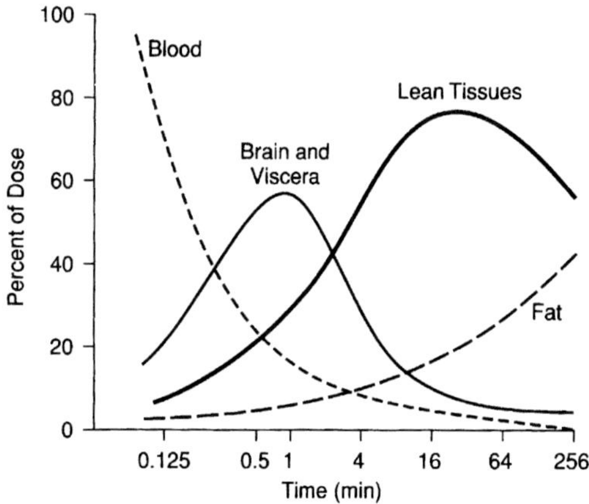

FIGURE 5-18 After a rapid intravenous injection, the percentage of thiopental remaining in the blood rapidly decreases as drug moves from the blood to tissues. Time to achievement of peak levels is a direct function of tissue capacity for barbiturate relative to blood flow. Initially, most thiopental is taken up by the vessel-rich group tissues because of their high blood flow. Subsequently, drug is redistributed to skeletal muscles and, to a lesser extent, to fat. The rate of metabolism equals the early rate of removal by fat, and the sum of these two events is similar to uptake of drug by skeletal muscles. (From Saidman LJ. Uptake, distribution, and elimination of barbiturates. In: Eger EI, ed. *Anesthetic Uptake and Action*. Baltimore, MD: Lippincott Williams & Wilkins; 1974, with permission.)

ratio and capacity-dependent elimination. This means factors affecting hepatic enzyme activity should change clearance. However, the reserve capacity of the liver to oxidize barbiturates is huge, so hepatic dysfunction must be extreme before a prolonged duration of action occurs.

In pediatric patients, the elimination half-time of thiopental is shorter than in adults.[203] This is due to more rapid hepatic clearance of thiopental by pediatric patients. Therefore, recovery after large or repeated doses of thiopental may be more rapid for infants and children than for adults. Protein binding and V_d of thiopental are not different in pediatric and adult patients. Elimination half-time is prolonged during pregnancy because of the increased protein binding of thiopental.

Pharmacodynamics and Clinical Applications

Premedication

Oral and injectable barbiturates have been replaced by benzodiazepines for preanesthetic medication. Drowsiness may last for only a short time after a sedative-hypnotic dose of a barbiturate is administered orally, but residual CNS effects characterized as "hangover" may persist. The rapid onset of action of barbiturates renders these drugs useful for treatment of grand mal seizures, but, again, benzodiazepines are probably superior, providing a more specific site of action in the CNS. Rectal administration of barbiturates, especially methohexital, 20 to 30 mg/kg, has been used to induce anesthesia in uncooperative or young patients.[204] Loss of consciousness after rectal administration of methohexital correlates with a plasma concentration greater than 2 μg/mL.[205]

Induction of Anesthesia

The relative potency of barbiturates used for IV induction of anesthesia assumes that thiopental is 1, thiamylal is 1.1, and methohexital is 2.5. At a blood pH of 7.4, methohexital is 76% nonionized compared with 61% for thiopental, which is consistent with the greater potency of methohexital. These drugs produce minimal to no direct effects on skeletal, cardiac, or smooth muscles. Induction dose requirements for thiopental vary with patient age, weight, and most importantly with cardiac output. The dose of thiopental required to induce anesthesia decreases with age, reflecting a slower passage of barbiturate from the central compartment to peripheral compartments (Fig. 5-19).[206,207] The dose of thiopental needed to produce anesthesia in early pregnancy (7 to 13 weeks' gestation) is decreased about 18% compared with that for nonpregnant females (Fig. 5-20).[208] Thiopental requirements, for unknown reasons, seem to be increased in children for more than 1 year after thermal injury.[209] Despite a contrary clinical impression, thiopental dose requirements (with EEG suppression as the endpoint) are not different between nonalcoholics and alcoholics with abstinence of 9 to 17 days and 30 days (Fig. 5-21).[210]

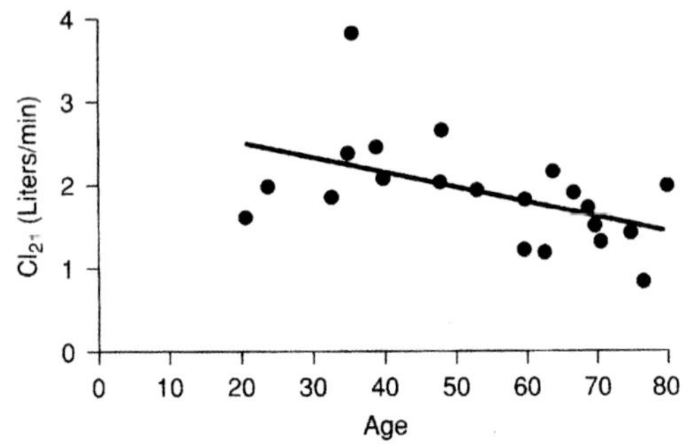

FIGURE 5-19 The rate of intercompartmental clearance of thiopental from the central compartment to the peripheral compartment slows with increasing age. (From Avram JJ, Krejcie TC, Henthorn TK. The relationship of age to the pharmacokinetics to early drug distribution: the concurrent disposition of thiopental and indocyanine green. *Anesthesiology.* 1990;72:403–411, with permission.)

Methohexital is the only barbiturate with pharmacodynamic effects sufficiently different from thiopental and thiamylal to offer an alternative for IV induction. One advantage of methohexital is its effect to lower the seizure threshold. Methohexital, but not thiopental, is effective in inducing seizure activity in patients with psychomotor epilepsy undergoing temporal lobe resection of seizure-producing areas.[211,212] The decreased anticonvulsant effect of methohexital is useful during electroconvulsive therapy because the therapeutic effect is related to the duration of the seizure. The principal disadvantage of methohexital is the incidence of excitatory phenomena, such as involuntary skeletal muscle movements (myoclonus) and other signs of excitatory activity including hiccoughs. These phenomena are dose dependent and may be decreased by pretreatment with opioids.

Occasionally, IV administration of a barbiturate is used as a supplement to inhaled anesthetics or as the sole anesthetic for brief and usually pain-free procedures such

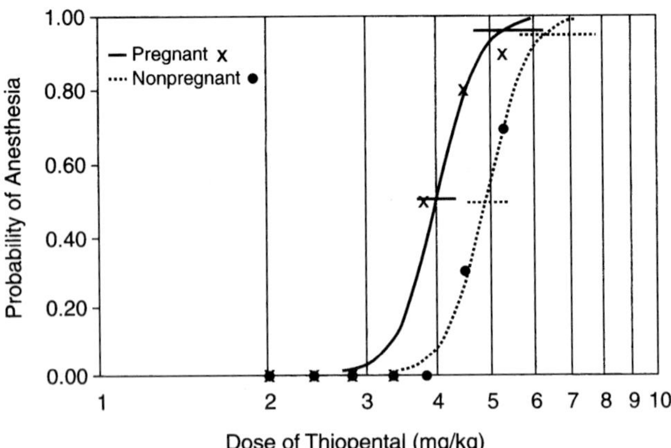

FIGURE 5-20 Dose-response curves for anesthesia in pregnant and nonpregnant females demonstrate a decreased dose requirement during 7 to 13 weeks of gestation. (From Gin T, Mainland P, Chan MT, et al. Decreased thiopental requirements in early pregnancy. *Anesthesiology.* 1997;86:73–78, with permission.)

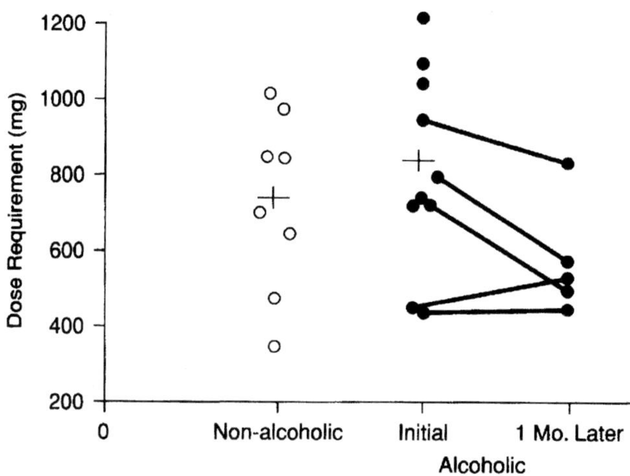

FIGURE 5-21 Thiopental doses needed to achieve burst suppression with 3 seconds of an isoelectric electroencephalogram are similar in nonalcoholic and alcoholic patients with abstinence of 9 to 17 days (initial) and 30 days (1 month later). (From Swerdlow BN, Holley FO, Maitre PO, et al. Chronic alcohol intake does not change thiopental anesthetic requirements, pharmacokinetics, or pharmacodynamics. *Anesthesiology*. 1990;72:455–461, with permission.)

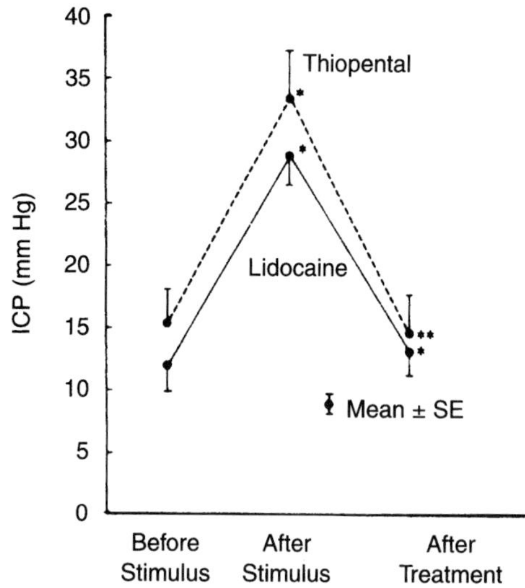

FIGURE 5-22 The administration of thiopental, 3 mg/kg IV, is as effective as lidocaine, 1.5 mg/kg IV, in decreasing intracranial pressure (ICP) after surgical stimulation in patients with brain tumors. *$P < .025$ versus preceding value; **$P < .02$ versus preceding value. (From Bedford RF, Persing JA, Poberskin L, et al. Lidocaine or thiopental for rapid control of intracranial hypertension. *Anesth Analg*. 1980;59:435–437, with permission.)

as cardioversion or electroconvulsive therapy. When high doses of methohexital are administered in a continuous infusion for neuroanesthesia, postoperative seizures occur in about one-third of patients.[213] Thiopental infusion is seldom a satisfactory choice for maintenance of anesthesia because of its long context-sensitive half-time and prolonged recovery period.[15]

Even before the removal of barbiturates from the U.S. market, propofol had replaced them for induction of anesthesia in most cases. The time to awaken from a single induction dose of propofol was not that different, but it produced less nausea and generally patients met recovery milestones (voiding, walking) more rapidly, especially in those where rapid awakening is considered desirable.

Treatment of Increased Intracranial Pressure and Ischemic Injury

Barbiturates can be administered to decrease refractory ICP that remains increased despite other measures. Barbiturates decrease ICP by decreasing cerebral blood volume through drug-induced cerebral vasoconstriction and an associated decrease in cerebral blood flow. The decrease in cerebral blood flow and increase in the perfusion-to-metabolism ratio made thiopental a useful drug for induction of anesthesia in patients with increased ICP (Fig. 5-22).[214] The drug can be titrated to a level that produces EEG burst suppression, and an isoelectric EEG occurs with maximal (~55%) barbiturate-induced depression of $CMRO_2$. However, this therapy produces significant hypotension, and improved outcome after head trauma has not been demonstrated in patients treated with barbiturates, despite the ability of these drugs to decrease and control ICP.[215]

Barbiturate therapy has also been used to improve brain survival after global cerebral ischemia due to cardiac arrest, but the efficacy for this indication remains unproven.[216] There are data suggesting that neuropsychiatric complications after cardiopulmonary bypass (presumably due to embolism) clear more rapidly in patients treated prospectively with thiopental to maintain an isoelectric EEG.[217] There is insufficient evidence, however, to support routine use of this therapy.

In contrast to global cerebral ischemia, animal studies consistently show improved outcome with barbiturate therapy of incomplete (focal) cerebral ischemia that permits drug-induced metabolic suppression.[218] In this regard, barbiturate-induced decreases in $CMRO_2$ exceed decreases in cerebral blood flow, which may provide protection to poorly perfused areas of the brain. The routine use of barbiturates during cardiac surgery or after stroke is not recommended because moderate degrees of hypothermia (33°C to 34°C) appear to provide superior neuroprotection without prolonging the recovery phase.

Side Effects

Side effects, especially on the cardiovascular system, inevitably accompany the clinical use of barbiturates. In normovolemic subjects, thiopental, 5 mg/kg IV, produces a transient 10- to 20-mm Hg decrease in blood pressure that is offset by a compensatory 15 to 20 beats per minute increase in heart rate (Fig. 5-23).[219] The mild and transient decrease in systemic blood pressure that accompanies induction of anesthesia with barbiturates is principally due to peripheral vasodilation, reflecting depression of the medullary vasomotor center and decreased sympathetic

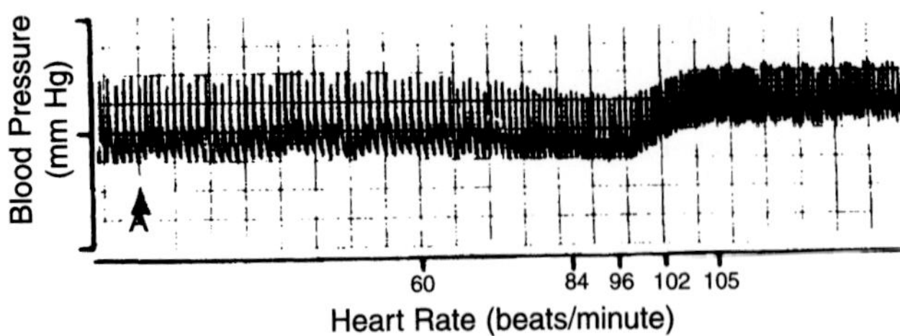

FIGURE 5-23 In normovolemic patients, the rapid administration of thiopental, 5 mg/kg IV (A), is followed by a modest decrease in blood pressure, which is subsequently offset by a compensatory increase in heart rate. (From Filner BF, Karliner JS. Alterations of normal left ventricular performance by general anesthesia. *Anesthesiology.* 1976;45: 610–620, with permission.)

nervous system outflow from the CNS. This dose of thiopental produces minimal to no evidence of direct myocardial depression.

Ventilation

Barbiturates also produce dose-dependent depression of medullary and pontine ventilatory centers. Thiopental decreases the sensitivity of the medullary ventilatory center to stimulation of carbon dioxide, and apnea is especially likely in the presence of other depressant drugs. Resumption of spontaneous ventilation after a single IV induction dose of barbiturate is characterized by a slow frequency of breathing and decreased tidal volume. Laryngeal reflexes and the cough reflex are not depressed until large doses of barbiturates have been administered.

Somatosensory Evoked Responses

Thiopental produces dose-dependent changes in median nerve somatosensory evoked responses and brainstem auditory evoked responses. However, some response is always obtainable,[220] so thiopental is an acceptable drug to administer when the ability to monitor somatosensory evoked potentials is desirable.

Other Effects

Enzyme Induction

Barbiturates, especially phenobarbital, stimulate an increase in liver microsomal protein content (enzyme induction) after 2 to 7 days of sustained drug administration. Altered drug responses and drug interactions may reflect barbiturate-induced enzyme induction, resulting in accelerated metabolism of (a) other drugs, such as oral anticoagulants, phenytoin, and tricyclic antidepressants; or (b) endogenous substances, including corticosteroids, bile salts, and vitamin K. The production of heme is accelerated, and this may exacerbate acute intermittent porphyria in susceptible patients.

Intraarterial Injection

Inadvertent intraarterial injection of thiopental usually results in immediate, intense vasoconstriction and excruciating pain that radiates along the distribution of the artery. Vasoconstriction may obscure distal arterial pulses, and blanching of the extremity is followed by cyanosis. Gangrene and permanent nerve damage may occur.

Treatment of accidental intraarterial injection of a barbiturate includes immediate attempts to dilute the drug, prevention of arterial spasm by injecting vasodilators such as lidocaine or papaverine, and general measures to sustain adequate blood flow.

Allergic Reactions

Allergic reactions in association with IV administration of barbiturates for induction of anesthesia most likely represent anaphylaxis (antigen–antibody interaction). Nevertheless, thiopental can also produce signs of an allergic reaction in the absence of prior exposure, suggesting an anaphylactoid response.[221] Although true anaphylaxis can occur, some of these reactions appear to be anaphylactoid responses due to direct release of histamine from tissue mast cells.[221–223] The incidence of allergic reactions to thiopental is estimated to be 1 per 30,000 patients.[224] The majority of reported cases are in patients with a history of chronic atopy who often have received thiopental previously without adverse responses.

Non–γ-Aminobutyric Acid Sedatives and Hypnotics

Ketamine

Ketamine is a phencyclidine derivative that produces "dissociative anesthesia," which is characterized by evidence on the EEG of dissociation between the thalamocortical and limbic systems.[225,226] Dissociative anesthesia resembles a cataleptic state in which the eyes remain open with a slow nystagmic gaze. The patient is noncommunicative, although wakefulness may appear to be present. Varying degrees of hypertonus and purposeful skeletal muscle movements often occur independently of surgical stimulation. The patient is amnesic, and analgesia is intense. Ketamine has advantages over propofol and etomidate in not requiring a lipid emulsion vehicle for dissolution and in producing profound analgesia at subanesthetic doses. However, the frequency of emergence delirium limits the clinical usefulness of ketamine as a sole agent. Ketamine is a drug with significant abuse potential, emphasizing the need to take appropriate precautions against unauthorized nonmedical use.

Structure–Activity Relationships

Ketamine is a water-soluble molecule that structurally resembles phencyclidine. The presence of an asymmetric carbon atom results in the existence of two optical isomers of ketamine.[225] The left-handed optical isomer of ketamine is designated S(+)-ketamine and the right-handed optical isomer is designated R(−)-ketamine. The racemic form of ketamine has been the most frequently used preparation although S(+)-ketamine is clinically available. When studied separately, S(+)-ketamine produces (a) more intense analgesia, (b) more rapid metabolism and thus recovery, (c) less salivation, and (d) a lower incidence of emergence reactions than R(−)-ketamine.[227,228] For example, the analgesic potency of S(+)-ketamine is approximately twice that of racemic ketamine and four times greater than R(−)-ketamine. Ketamine isomer induces less fatigue and cognitive impairment than equianalgesic small-dose racemic ketamine.[229] Both isomers of ketamine appear to inhibit uptake of catecholamines back into postganglionic sympathetic nerve endings (cocaine-like effect). The fact that individual optical isomers of ketamine differ in their pharmacologic properties suggests that this drug interacts with specific receptors to induce these behaviors. The preservative used for ketamine is benzethonium chloride.

Mechanism of Action

The mechanism of action of ketamine-induced analgesia and dissociative anesthesia is unknown. Ketamine is known to interact with multiple CNS receptors but clear association between receptor interaction and specific behavior has not been established. Ketamine binds noncompetitively to the phencyclidine recognition site on *N*-methyl-D-aspartate (NMDA) receptors. In addition, ketamine exerts effects at other sites including opioid receptors, monoaminergic receptors, muscarinic receptors, and voltage-sensitive sodium and L-type calcium channels and neuronal nicotinic acetylcholine receptors.[230–232] Unlike propofol and etomidate, ketamine has only weak actions at $GABA_A$ receptors. Inflammatory mediators produced locally by compression of nerve roots can activate neutrophils that then adhere to blood vessels and impair blood flow. Ketamine suppresses neutrophil production of inflammatory mediators and improves blood flow.[233] Direct inhibition of cytokines in blood by ketamine may contribute to the analgesic effects of this drug.

N-Methyl-D-Aspartate Receptor Antagonism

NMDA receptors (members of the glutamate receptors family) are ligand-gated ion channels that are unique in that channel activation requires binding of the excitatory neurotransmitter, glutamate with glycine as an obligatory coagonist (Fig. 5-24).[225] Ketamine inhibits activation of NMDA receptors by glutamate and decreases presynaptic release of glutamate. The interaction with phencyclidine binding sites appears to be stereoselective, with the S(+) isomer of ketamine having the greatest affinity.

Opioid Receptors

Ketamine has been reported to directly interact with μ, δ, and κ opioid receptors.[234] In contrast, other studies have suggested ketamine may be an antagonist at μ receptors and an agonist at κ receptors. Ketamine also weakly interacts with σ receptors.

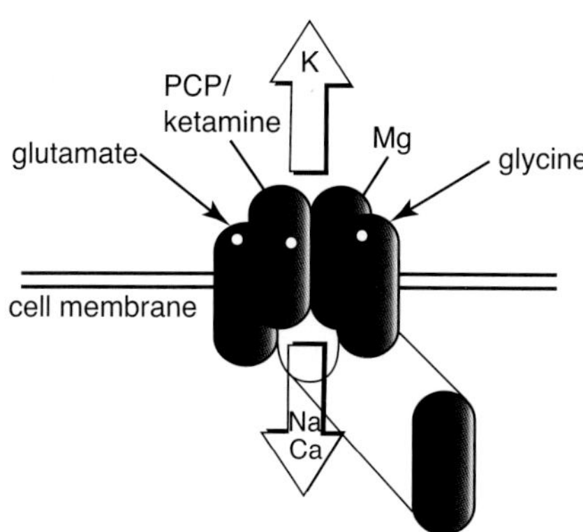

FIGURE 5-24 Schematic diagram of the *N*-methyl-D-aspartate (NMDA) glutamate receptor channel complex. The receptor consists of five subunits surrounding a central ion channel that is permeable to calcium, potassium, and sodium. Binding sites for the agonist glutamate and the obligatory coagonist glycine are indicated. NMDA receptors are ligand-gated ion channels that are activated by the excitatory neurotransmitter glutamate. Glutamate is the most abundant neurotransmitter in the central nervous system. One of the subunits has been removed to show the interior of the ion channel and binding sites for magnesium and ketamine, which produce noncompetitive NMDA receptor blockade. (From Kohrs R, Durieux ME. Ketamine: teaching an old drug new tricks. *Anesth Analg.* 1998;87;1186–1193, with permission.)

Monoaminergic Receptors

The antinociceptive action of ketamine may involve activation of descending inhibitory monoaminergic pain pathways.

Muscarinic Receptors

Ketamine anesthesia is partially antagonized by anticholinesterase drugs. The fact that ketamine produces anticholinergic symptoms (emergence delirium, bronchodilation, sympathomimetic action) suggests that an antagonist effect of ketamine at muscarinic receptors is more likely than an agonist effect.

Sodium Channels

Consistent with its mild local anesthetic–like properties, ketamine interacts with voltage-gated sodium channels, sharing a binding site with local anesthetics.[231]

Neuronal Nicotinic Acetylcholine Receptors

Ketamine interacts with both heteromeric and homomeric α_7 nicotinic acetylcholine receptors.[232] In α_7-type nicotinic receptors, a single subunit has been identified as a binding site in the extracellular loop between transmembrane segments 2 and 3.[235] Nicotinic inhibition by ketamine does not appear to affect sedation or immobility but may play a role in its analgesic effects.[236]

Pharmacokinetics

The pharmacokinetics of ketamine are similar to thiopental in rapid onset of action, relatively short duration of action, and high lipid solubility (see Table 5-1). Ketamine has a pKa of 7.5 at physiologic pH. Peak plasma concentrations of ketamine occur within 1 minute after IV administration and within 5 minutes after IM injection. Ketamine is not significantly bound to plasma proteins and leaves the blood rapidly to be distributed into tissues. Initially, ketamine is distributed to highly perfused tissues such as the brain, where the peak concentration may be four or five times that present in plasma. The extreme lipid solubility of ketamine (5 to 10 times that of thiopental) ensures its rapid transfer across the blood–brain barrier. Furthermore, ketamine-induced increases in cerebral blood flow could facilitate delivery of drug and thus enhance rapid achievement of high brain concentrations. Subsequently, ketamine is redistributed from the brain and other highly perfused tissues to less well-perfused tissues, the release of which results in late psychodynamic effects after emergence. Ketamine has a high hepatic clearance rate (1 L per minute) and a large V_d (3 L/kg), resulting in an elimination half-time of 2 to 3 hours. The high hepatic extraction ratio suggests that alterations in hepatic blood flow could influence ketamine's clearance rate.

Metabolism

Ketamine is metabolized extensively by hepatic microsomal enzymes. An important pathway of metabolism is demethylation of ketamine by cytochrome P450 enzymes to form norketamine (Fig. 5-25).[237] In animals, norketamine is one-fifth to one-third as potent as ketamine. This active metabolite may contribute to prolonged effects of ketamine (analgesia), especially with repeated doses or a continuous IV infusion. Norketamine is eventually hydroxylated and then conjugated to form more water-soluble and inactive glucuronide metabolites that are excreted by the kidneys. After IV administration, less than 4% of a dose of ketamine can be recovered from urine as unchanged drug. Fecal excretion accounts for less than 5% of an injected dose of ketamine. Chronic administration of ketamine stimulates the activity of enzymes responsible for its metabolism. Accelerated metabolism of ketamine as a result of enzyme induction could explain, in part, the observation of tolerance to the analgesic effects of ketamine that occurs in patients receiving repeated doses of this drug. Indeed, tolerance may occur in burn patients receiving more than two short-interval exposures to ketamine.[238] Development of tolerance is also consistent with reports of ketamine dependence.[237]

Clinical Uses

Ketamine is a unique drug evoking intense analgesia at subanesthetic doses and producing prompt induction of anesthesia when administered IV at higher doses. Inclusion of an antisialagogue in the preoperative medication is often recommended to decrease the likelihood of coughing and laryngospasm due to ketamine-induced salivary secretions. Glycopyrrolate may be preferable, as atropine or scopolamine can easily cross the blood–brain barrier and could theoretically increase the incidence of emergence delirium (see the section "Emergence Delirium").

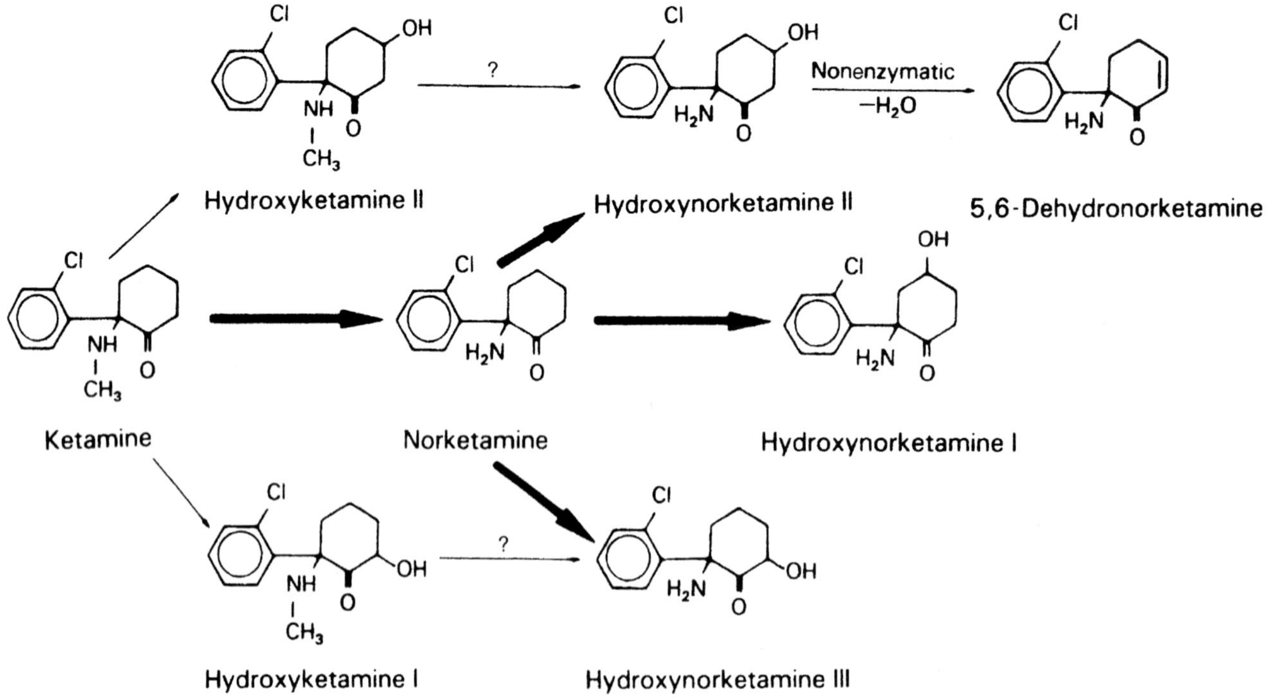

FIGURE 5-25 Metabolism of ketamine. (From White PF, Way WL, Trevor AJ. Ketamine: its pharmacology and therapeutic uses. *Anesthesiology*. 1982;56:119–136, with permission.)

Analgesia

Intense analgesia can be achieved with subanesthetic doses of ketamine, 0.2 to 0.5 mg/kg IV.[239] Plasma concentrations of ketamine that produce analgesia are lower after oral than IM administration, presumably reflecting a higher norketamine concentration due to hepatic first-pass metabolism that occurs after oral administration. Analgesia is thought to be greater for somatic than for visceral pain. The analgesic effects of ketamine are likely due to its activity in the thalamic and limbic systems, which are responsible for the interpretation of painful signals. Small doses of ketamine are also useful adjuvants to opioid analgesia.[240]

Spinal cord sensitization is responsible for pain associated with touching or moving an injured body part that would normally not be painful. Central to the development of spinal cord sensitization is activation of NMDA receptors, which are located in the spinal cord dorsal horn. NMDA receptors are excitatory amino acid receptors that are important in pain processing and the modulation of pain.[241] Excitatory amino acids, particularly glutamate, acting at NMDA receptors play an important role in spinal nociceptive pathways. Inhibition of spinal NMDA receptors by drugs such as ketamine, magnesium, and dextromethorphan is useful in the management of postoperative pain including decreases in analgesic consumption. Analgesia can be produced during labor without associated depression of the neonate.[242,243] Neonatal neurobehavioral scores of infants born by vaginal delivery with ketamine analgesia are lower than those for infants born with epidural anesthesia but higher than the scores in infants delivered with thiopental–nitrous oxide anesthesia.[244] Postoperative sedation and analgesia after pediatric cardiac surgery can be produced by continuous infusions of ketamine, 1 to 2 mg/kg/hour. Ketamine is useful as an analgesic adjuvant in patients with preexisting chronic pain syndromes who require surgery.

Neuraxial Analgesia

The efficacy of extradural ketamine is controversial. Although ketamine has been reported to interact with opioid receptors, the affinity for spinal opioid receptors may be 10,000-fold weaker than that of morphine.[245] It seems likely that extradural effects of ketamine (30 mg) are due to both spinal and systemic effects and possibly interaction with local anesthetic binding sites on voltage-gated sodium ion channels. Overall, the epidural effects of ketamine are relatively small but in combination with other epidural analgesics (opioids, local anesthetics), an additive or synergistic effect may occur.[246] Intrathecal administration of ketamine (5 to 50 mg in 3 mL of saline) produces variable and brief analgesia, unless the ketamine is also combined with epinephrine to slow systemic absorption. The neuraxial use of ketamine to produce analgesia appears to be of limited value and is not an approved indication.[230]

Induction of Anesthesia

Induction of anesthesia is produced by administration of ketamine, 1 to 2 mg/kg IV or 4 to 8 mg/kg IM. Injection of ketamine IV does not produce pain or venous irritation. The need for large IV doses reflects a significant first-pass hepatic effect for ketamine. Consciousness is lost in 30 to 60 seconds after IV administration and in 2 to 4 minutes after IM injection. Unconsciousness is associated with maintenance of normal or only slightly depressed pharyngeal and laryngeal reflexes. Return of consciousness usually occurs in 10 to 20 minutes after an injected induction dose of ketamine, but return to full orientation may require an additional 60 to 90 minutes. Emergence times are even longer after repeated IV injections or a continuous infusion of ketamine. Amnesia persists for about 60 to 90 minutes after recovery of consciousness, but ketamine does not produce retrograde amnesia.

Because of its rapid onset of action, ketamine has been used as an IM induction drug in children and difficult-to-manage mentally challenged patients regardless of age. Due to its intense analgesic activity, ketamine has been used extensively for burn dressing changes, débridements, and skin grafting procedures. The excellent analgesia and ability to maintain spontaneous ventilation in an airway that might otherwise be altered by burn scar contractures are important advantages of ketamine in these patients. Tolerance may develop, however, in burn patients receiving repeated, short-interval anesthesia with ketamine.[238]

Induction of anesthesia in acutely hypovolemic patients is often accomplished with ketamine, taking advantage of the drug's cardiovascular-stimulating effects. In this regard, it is important to recognize that ketamine, like all injected anesthetics, may become a myocardial depressant if endogenous catecholamine stores are depleted and sympathetic nervous system compensatory responses are impaired.[247]

The administration of ketamine to patients with coronary artery disease is complicated by increased myocardial oxygen requirements that may accompany this drug's sympathomimetic effects on the heart. Furthermore, the absence of cardioprotective effects (preconditioning) associated with racemic ketamine is a consideration when this drug is administered to patients with known coronary artery disease (see the section on preconditioning). Nevertheless, induction of anesthesia with administration of diazepam, 0.5 mg/kg IV, and ketamine, 0.5 mg/kg IV, followed by a continuous infusion of ketamine, 15 to 30 μg/kg/minute IV, has been used for anesthesia in patients with coronary artery disease historically.[237] The combination of subanesthetic doses of ketamine with propofol for production of total IV anesthesia has been reported to produce more stable hemodynamics than propofol and fentanyl while avoiding the undesirable emergence reactions that may accompany administration of higher doses of ketamine.[248]

The beneficial effects of ketamine on airway resistance due to drug-induced bronchodilation make this a potentially useful drug for rapid IV induction of anesthesia in patients with asthma.[249]

Ketamine should be used cautiously or avoided in patients with systemic or pulmonary hypertension or increased ICP, although this recommendation may deserve reevaluation based on more recent data (see the sections "Central Nervous System" and "Cardiovascular System"). Nystagmus associated with administration of ketamine may be undesirable in operations or examinations of the eye performed under anesthesia.

Ketamine has been administered safely to patients with malignant hyperthermia and does not trigger the syndrome in susceptible swine.[250] Extensive experience with ketamine for pediatric cardiac catheterization has shown the drug to be useful, but its possible cardiac-stimulating effects must be considered in the interpretation of catheterization data.

Reversal of Opioid Tolerance

Sub anesthetic doses of ketamine have been shown to prevent or reverse morphine-induced tolerance in animals, although this has not been consistently effective in man.[251] Although the mechanism of opioid tolerance is unknown, it is believed to involve, in part, the production of hyperalgesia by an interaction between NMDA receptors, the nitric oxide pathway, and μ-opioid receptors. Administration of sub anesthetic doses of ketamine (0.3 mg/kg/hr) improves analgesia and may reduce the likelihood of opioid tolerance.

Improvement of Psychiatric Disorders

NMDA receptors for glutamate are thought to be involved in the pathophysiology of mental depression and the mechanism of action of antidepressants. Ketamine in small doses improved the postoperative depressive state in patients with mental depression.[252] Intermittent treatment with low-dose ketamine also results in long-term suppression of obsessions and compulsions in patients with obsessive compulsive disorder.[253]

Restless Leg Syndrome

A single case report describes symptomatic improvement in two patients with restless leg syndrome treated with oral ketamine.[254] It is possible that ketamine inhibits neuroinflammation in the spinal cord or higher centers. Within the spinal cord, restless leg syndrome may reflect NMDA receptor activation and production of inflammatory mediators that impair spinal cord blood flow.

Side Effects

Ketamine is unique among injected anesthetics in its ability to stimulate the cardiovascular system and produce emergence delirium.[226] Although generally considered contraindicated in patients with increased ICP, it must be recognized that many of the early studies of ketamine's effects on ICP were conducted on spontaneously breathing subjects.[226]

Central Nervous System

Ketamine is traditionally considered to increase cerebral blood flow and $CMRO_2$, although there is also evidence suggesting that this may not be a valid generalization.[226]

Intracranial Pressure

Ketamine is reported to be a potent cerebral vasodilator capable of increasing cerebral blood flow by 60% in the presence of normocapnia.[255] As a result, patients with intracranial pathology are commonly considered vulnerable to sustained increases in ICP after administration of ketamine. Nevertheless, in mechanically ventilated animals with increased ICP, there was no further increase in ICP after administration of ketamine, 0.5 to 2.0 mg/kg IV.[256] Furthermore, anterior fontanelle pressure, an indirect monitor of ICP, decreases in mechanically ventilated preterm neonates after administration of ketamine, 2 mg/kg IV.[257] In patients requiring craniotomy for brain tumor or cerebral aneurysm resection, administration of ketamine, 1 mg/kg IV, did not increase middle cerebral artery blood flow velocity, and ICP decreased modestly (Fig. 5-26).[258] In patients with traumatic brain injury, the administration of ketamine, 1.5, 3.0, and 5.0 mg/kg IV, during mechanical ventilation of the lungs resulted in significant decreases in ICP regardless of the dose of ketamine.[259] These results in patients suggest that ketamine can be administered to patients with mildly increased ICP if administered with mild hyperventilation without adversely altering cerebral hemodynamics. Prior administration of thiopental, diazepam, or midazolam has been shown to blunt ketamine-induced increases in cerebral blood flow.

Neuroprotective Effects

Activation of NMDA receptors has been implicated in cerebral ischemic damage.[230] The antagonist effect of

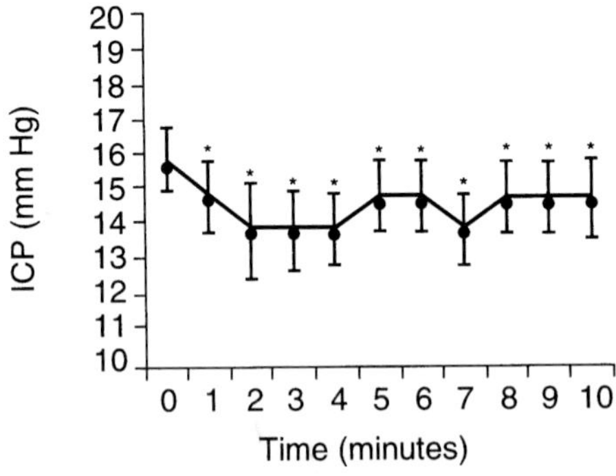

FIGURE 5-26 In patients with a brain tumor or cerebral aneurysm, the administration of ketamine, 1 mg/kg IV, during mechanical ventilation of the lungs with nitrous oxide and isoflurane was associated with a modest decrease in intracranial pressure (ICP). This decrease in ICP was accompanied by a corresponding decrease in cerebral artery blood flow velocity. (From Mayberg TS, Lam AM, Matta BF, et al. Ketamine does not increase cerebral blood flow velocity or intracranial pressure during isoflurane/nitrous oxide anesthesia in patients undergoing craniotomy. *Anesth Analg.* 1995;81:84–89, with permission.)

Table 5-4

Circulatory Effects of Ketamine

	Control	Ketamine (2 mg/kg IV)	Percent Change
Heart rate (beats/min)	74	98	+33
Mean arterial pressure (mm Hg)	93	119	+28
Stroke volume index (mL/m^2)	43	44	
Systemic vascular resistance (units)	16.2	15.9	
Right atrial pressure (mm Hg)	7.0	8.9	
Left ventricular end diastolic pressure (mm Hg)	13.0	13.1	
Pulmonary artery pressure (mm Hg)	17.0	24.5	+44
Minute work index (kg/min/m^2)	5.4	8.9	+40
Tension-time index (mm Hg/s)	2,700	4,600	+68

ketamine on NMDA receptors suggests a possible neuroprotective role for this drug although this remains an unproved hypothesis. Indeed, S(+) ketamine offers no greater neuroprotection than remifentanil.[260]

Electroencephalogram

Ketamine's effects on the EEG are characterized by abolition of alpha rhythm and dominance of θ activity. Onset of δ activity coincides with loss of consciousness. At high doses, ketamine produces a burst suppression pattern. Ketamine-induced excitatory activity occurs in both the thalamus and limbic systems without evidence of subsequent spread of seizure activity to cortical areas.[261] As such, ketamine would be unlikely to precipitate generalized convulsions in patients with seizure disorders. Indeed, ketamine does not alter the seizure threshold in epileptic patients.[262] Although myoclonic- and seizure-like activity may occur in normal patients, EEG evidence of cortical epileptic activity is absent and ketamine is considered to possess anticonvulsant activity.[263]

Somatosensory Evoked Potentials

Ketamine increases the cortical amplitude of somatosensory evoked potentials.[264] This ketamine-induced increase in amplitude is attenuated by nitrous oxide. Auditory and visual evoked responses are decreased by ketamine.

Cardiovascular System

Ketamine produces cardiovascular effects that resemble sympathetic nervous system stimulation. Indeed, a direct negative cardiac inotropic effect is usually overshadowed by central sympathetic stimulation.

Hemodynamic Effects

Systemic and pulmonary arterial blood pressure, heart rate, cardiac output, cardiac work, and myocardial oxygen requirements are increased after IV administration of ketamine (Table 5-4).[265] The increase in systolic blood pressure in adults receiving clinical doses of ketamine is 20 to 40 mm Hg, with a slightly smaller increase in diastolic blood pressure. Typically, systemic blood pressure increases progressively during the first 3 to 5 minutes after IV injection of ketamine and then decreases to predrug levels over the next 10 to 20 minutes. The cardiovascular-stimulating effects on the systemic and pulmonary circulations are blunted or prevented by prior administration of benzodiazepines or concomitant administration of inhaled anesthetics, including nitrous oxide.[226,266] Likewise, ketamine administered to mildly sedated infants fails to produce hemodynamic changes in either the systemic or pulmonary circulation.[267]

Critically ill patients occasionally respond to ketamine with unexpected decreases in systemic blood pressure and cardiac output, which reflect depletion of endogenous catecholamine stores and exhaustion of sympathetic nervous system compensatory mechanisms, leading to an unmasking of ketamine's direct myocardial depressant effects.[247,268] Conversely, ketamine has been shown to decrease the need for inotropic support in septic patients, perhaps reflecting an inhibition of catecholamine reuptake.[269,270]

In shocked animals, ketamine is associated with an increased survival rate compared with animals anesthetized with halothane.[271] Blood pressure may be better maintained in hemorrhaged animals anesthetized with ketamine. However, ketamine administration is associated with greater increases in arterial lactate concentrations than occur in animals with lower systemic blood pressures anesthetized with a volatile anesthetic.[272] This suggests inadequate tissue perfusion despite maintenance of systemic blood pressure by ketamine. Presumably, ketamine-induced vasoconstriction maintains systemic blood pressure at the expense of tissue perfusion.

Cardiac Rhythm

The effect of ketamine on cardiac rhythm is inconclusive. There is evidence that ketamine enhances the dysrhythmogenicity of epinephrine.[273] Conversely, ketamine may abolish epinephrine-induced cardiac dysrhythmias.

Mechanisms of Cardiovascular Effects

The mechanisms for ketamine-induced cardiovascular effects are complex. Direct stimulation of the CNS leading to increased sympathetic nervous system outflow seems to be the most important mechanism for cardiovascular stimulation.[274] Evidence for this mechanism is the ability of inhaled anesthetics, ganglionic blockade, β blockade, cervical epidural anesthesia, and spinal cord transection to prevent ketamine-induced increases in systemic blood pressure and heart rate.[275,276] Furthermore, increases in plasma concentrations of epinephrine and norepinephrine occur as early as 2 minutes after IV administration of ketamine and return to control levels 15 minutes later.[277] In vitro, ketamine produces direct myocardial depression, emphasizing the importance of an intact sympathetic nervous system for the cardiac-stimulating effects of this drug.[278] The role of ketamine-induced inhibition of norepinephrine uptake (reuptake) into postganglionic sympathetic nerve endings and associated increases of plasma catecholamine concentrations on the drug's cardiac-stimulating effects are not known.[273]

Ventilation and Airway

Ketamine does not produce significant depression of ventilation. The ventilatory response to carbon dioxide is maintained during ketamine anesthesia and the $Pa{CO_2}$ is unlikely to increase more than 3 mm Hg.[279] Breathing frequency typically decreases for 2 to 3 minutes after administration of ketamine. Apnea, however, can occur if the drug is administered rapidly IV or an opioid is included in the preoperative medication.

Upper airway skeletal muscle tone is well maintained, and upper airway reflexes remain relatively intact after administration of ketamine.[280] Despite continued presence of upper airway reflexes, ketamine anesthesia does not negate the need for protection of the lungs against aspiration by placement of a cuffed tube in the patient's trachea. Salivary and tracheobronchial mucous gland secretions are increased by IM or IV administration of ketamine, leading to the frequent recommendation that an antisialagogue be included in the preoperative medication when use of this drug is anticipated.

Bronchomotor Tone

Ketamine has bronchodilatory activity and is as effective as halothane or enflurane in preventing experimentally induced bronchospasm in dogs.[249] Ketamine has been used in subanesthetic doses to treat bronchospasm in the operating room and ICU. Successful treatment of status asthmaticus with ketamine has been reported.[281] In the presence of active bronchospasm, ketamine may be recommended as the IV induction drug of choice. The mechanism by which ketamine produces airway relaxation is unclear, although several mechanisms have been suggested, including increased circulating catecholamine concentrations, inhibition of catecholamine uptake, voltage-sensitive calcium channel block, and inhibition of postsynaptic nicotinic or muscarinic receptors.[230]

Hepatic or Renal Function

Ketamine does not significantly alter laboratory tests that reflect hepatic or renal function.

Allergic Reactions

Ketamine does not evoke the release of histamine and rarely, if ever, causes allergic reactions.[282]

Platelet Aggregation

Ketamine inhibits platelet aggregation possibly by suppressed formation of inositol 1,4,5-triphosphate and subsequent inhibition of cytosolic free calcium concentrations.[283] Drug-induced effects on platelet aggregation are a consideration in patients with known bleeding disorders undergoing surgery.

Emergence Delirium (Psychedelic Effects)

Emergence from ketamine anesthesia in the postoperative period may be associated with visual, auditory, proprioceptive, and confusional illusions, which may progress to delirium. Cortical blindness may be transiently present. Dreams and hallucinations can occur up to 24 hours after administration of ketamine. The dreams frequently have a morbid content and are often experienced in vivid color. Dreams and hallucinations usually disappear within a few hours.

Mechanisms

Emergence delirium probably occurs secondary to ketamine-induced depression of the inferior colliculus and medial geniculate nucleus, leading to misinterpretation of auditory and visual stimuli.[237] Furthermore, the loss of skin and musculoskeletal sensations results in decreased ability to perceive gravity, thereby producing a sensation of bodily detachment or floating in space. Opioids that act as κ agonists produce similar psychedelic effects suggesting a potential role for ketamine interaction with κ receptors.

Incidence

The observed incidence of emergence delirium after ketamine ranges from 5% to 30% and is partially dose dependent.[237] Factors associated with an increased incidence of emergence delirium include (a) age older than 15 years, (b) female gender, (c) doses of ketamine of greater than 2 mg/kg IV, and (d) a history of personality problems or frequent dreaming.[237] In healthy volunteers, the incidence of psychedelic effects is related to the plasma concentration of ketamine (Fig. 5-27).[284] It is possible that the incidence of dreaming is similar in children, but this age group is less able to communicate the dream's occurrence. Indeed, there are reports of recurrent hallucinations in children as well as in adults receiving ketamine.[285,286] Nevertheless, psychological changes in children after anesthesia with ketamine or inhaled drugs are not different.[287]

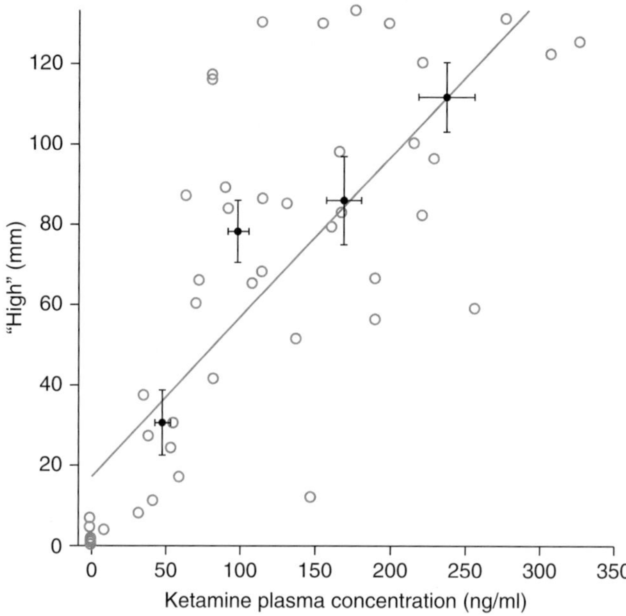

FIGURE 5-27 Visual analog scores for those patients experiencing ketamine-induced psychedelic effects ("high") versus venous plasma concentrations of ketamine. (From Bowdle TA, Radant AD, Cowley DS, et al. Psychedelic effects of ketamine in healthy volunteers: relationship to steady-state plasma concentrations. *Anesthesiology*. 1998;88:82–88, with permission.)

Likewise, no significant long-term personality differences are present in adults receiving ketamine compared with thiopental.[288]

Emergence delirium occurs less frequently when ketamine is used repeatedly. For example, it is rare for emergence delirium to occur after three or more anesthetics with ketamine. Finally, inhaled anesthetics can also produce auditory, visual, proprioceptive, and confusional illusions, but the incidence of such phenomena, especially unpleasant experiences, is indeed greater after anesthesia that includes administration of ketamine.

Prevention

A variety of drugs used in preoperative medication or as adjuvants during maintenance of anesthesia have been evaluated in attempts to prevent emergence delirium after administration of ketamine. Benzodiazepines have proved the most effective in prevention of this phenomenon, with midazolam being more effective than diazepam.[289,290] A common approach is to administer the benzodiazepine IV about 5 minutes before induction of anesthesia with ketamine. Inclusion of thiopental or inhaled anesthetics may decrease the incidence of emergence delirium attributed to ketamine. Conversely, the inclusion of atropine in the preoperative medication may increase the incidence of emergence delirium.[291]

Despite contrary opinions, there is no evidence that permitting patients to awaken from ketamine anesthesia in quiet areas alters the incidence of emergence delirium.[292] Prospective discussion with the patient of the common side effects of ketamine (dreams, floating sensations, blurred vision) is likely to decrease the incidence of emergence delirium and reduce concern if it occurs, as much as any other approach.[237]

Drug Interactions

The importance of an intact and normally functioning CNS in determining the cardiovascular effects of ketamine is emphasized by hemodynamic depression rather than stimulation that occurs when ketamine is administered in the presence of inhaled anesthetics. For example, depression by inhaled anesthetics of sympathetic nervous system outflow from the CNS prevents the typical increases in systemic blood pressure and heart rate that occur when ketamine is administered alone.[275] Ketamine administered in the presence of volatile anesthetics may result in hypotension.[293] Presumably, volatile anesthetics depress sympathetic nervous system outflow from the CNS, thus unmasking the direct cardiac depressant effects of ketamine. Diazepam, 0.3 to 0.5 mg/kg IV, or an equivalent dose of midazolam, is also effective in preventing the cardiac-stimulating effects of ketamine. In the presence of verapamil, the blood pressure–elevating effects of ketamine may be attenuated, whereas drug-induced increases in heart rate are enhanced.[294] β Blockade reduces ketamine-induced increase in heart rate and blood pressure.

Ketamine-induced enhancement of nondepolarizing neuromuscular blocking drugs may reflect interference by ketamine with calcium ion binding or its transport.[295] Alternatively, ketamine may decrease sensitivity of postjunctional membranes to neuromuscular blocking drugs. The duration of apnea after administration of succinylcholine is prolonged, possibly reflecting inhibition of plasma cholinesterase activity by ketamine.

Pharmacologic activation of adenosine triphosphate–regulated potassium (KATP) channels mimics ischemic preconditioning and decreases infarct size or improves functional recovery of ischemic-reperfused viable (stunned) myocardium. Conversely, pharmacologic blockade of (KATP) channels can antagonize the cardioprotective effects of ischemic preconditioning. In an animal model, ketamine blocked the cardioprotective effects of ischemic preconditioning and this effect was due to the R(−) isomer.[296] Conversely, S(+)-ketamine does not block the cardioprotective effects of preconditioning or alter myocardial infarct size (Fig. 5-28).[297] In patients at risk for myocardial infarction during the perioperative period, drugs known to block preconditioning should be used with caution, whereas drugs known to elicit early and late preconditioning (opioids, volatile anesthetics) may be beneficial.

Dextromethorphan

Dextromethorphan (D-isomer of the opioid agonist, levomethorphan) is a low-affinity NMDA antagonist that

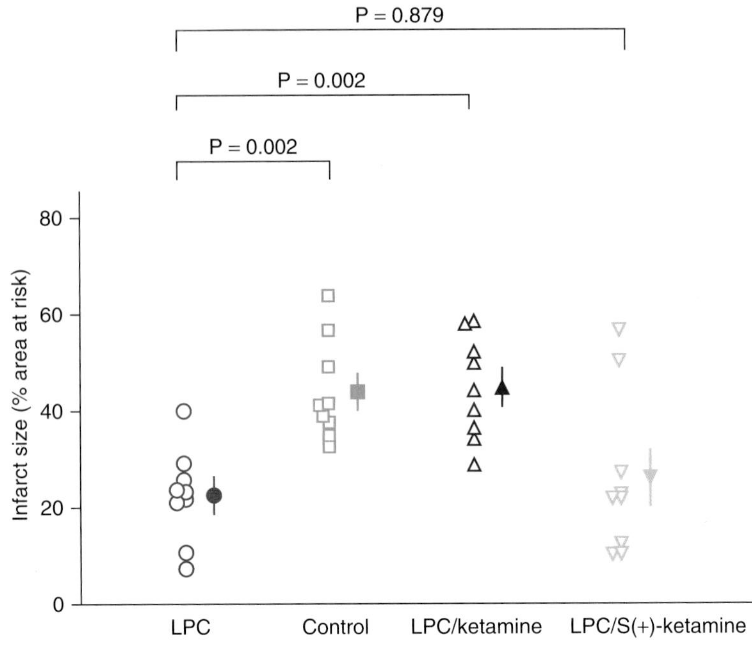

FIGURE 5-28 Infarct size as a percentage of the area at risk in late preconditioning (LPC). Groups are control, LPC, LPC/ketamine, and LPC/S(+)-ketamine. Solid symbols represent mean ≠ SEM. (From Mullenheim J, Rulands R, Wietschorke T, et al. Late preconditioning is blocked by racemic ketamine, but not by S(+)-ketamine. *Anesth Analg.* 2001;93:265–270, with permission.)

is a common ingredient in over-the-counter cough suppressants. It also has activity at multiple other ligands including neuronal nicotinic receptors. It is equal in potency to codeine as an antitussive but lacks analgesic or physical dependence properties. Unlike codeine, this drug rarely produces sedation or gastrointestinal disturbances. Its psychoactive effects lead to a significant abuse potential. Signs and symptoms of intentional excessive intake of dextromethorphan include systemic hypertension, tachycardia, somnolence, agitation, slurred speech, ataxia, diaphoresis, skeletal muscle rigidity, seizures, coma, and decreased core body temperature. Hepatotoxicity may be a consideration when dextromethorphan with acetaminophen is ingested in excessive amounts.

Dexmedetomidine

Dexmedetomidine is a potent α_2 adrenergic agonist that is shorter acting than clonidine and much more selective for α_2 vs. α_1 receptors (dexmedetomidine = 1620:1; clonidine = 220:1).[298,299] One of the highest densities of $\alpha_2$receptors is located in the pontine locus ceruleus, an important nucleus mediating sympathetic nervous system function, vigilance, memory, analgesia, and arousal. The sedative effects produced by dexmedetomidine are largely due to inhibition of this nucleus.[300] Dexmedetomidine is the dextro isomer and pharmacologically active component of medetomidine, which has been used for many years in veterinary practice for its hypnotic, sedative, and analgesic properties. Atipamezole is a specific and selective investigational α_2 receptor antagonist that rapidly and effectively reverses the sedative and cardiovascular effects of IV dexmedetomidine.[301]

The quality of sedation produced by α_2 agonists differs from sedation produced by drugs (midazolam, propofol) that act on GABA.[302] For example, dexmedetomidine, acting on α_2 receptors, produces sedation by decreasing sympathetic nervous system activity and the level of arousal. The result is a calm patient who can be easily aroused to full consciousness. Amnesia is not assured. Drugs that activate GABA receptors produce a clouding of consciousness and can cause paradoxical agitation as well as tolerance and dependence.

Pharmacokinetics

The elimination half-time of dexmedetomidine is 2 to 3 hours compared with 6 to 10 hours for clonidine. Dexmedetomidine is highly protein bound (>90%) and undergoes extensive hepatic metabolism. The resulting methyl and glucuronide conjugates are excreted by the kidneys. Dexmedetomidine has weak inhibiting effects on cytochrome P450 enzyme systems that might manifest as increased plasma concentrations of opioids as administered during anesthesia.[303]

Clinical Uses

As with clonidine, pretreatment with dexmedetomidine attenuates hemodynamic responses to tracheal intubation, decreases plasma catecholamine concentrations during anesthesia, decreases perioperative requirements for inhaled anesthetics and opioids, and increases the likelihood of hypotension.[304,305] Dexmedetomidine decreases MAC for volatile anesthetics in animals by greater than 90% compared with a plateau effect between 25% to 40% for clonidine (Fig. 5-29).[306] In patients, isoflurane MAC was decreased 35% and 48% by dexmedetomidine plasma

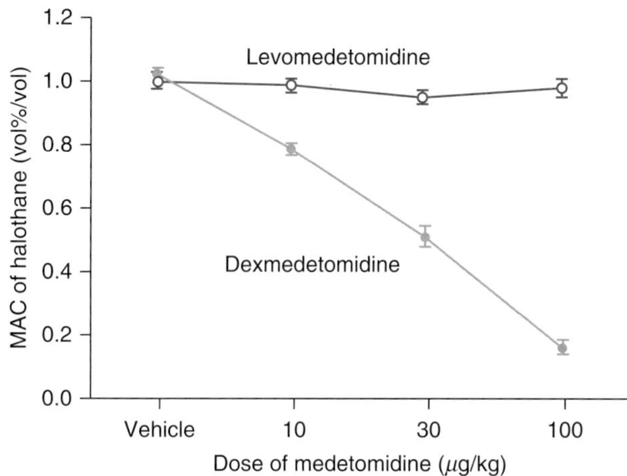

FIGURE 5-29 Dexmedetomidine produces dose-dependent decreases in halothane MAC in rats. Levomedetomidine did not produce any changes in MAC. Data are mean ± SEM. (From Segal IS, Vickery RG, Walton JK, et al. Dexmedetomidine diminishes halothane anesthetic requirements in rats through a postsynaptic alpha-2 adrenergic receptor. *Anesthesiology*. 1988;69:818–823, with permission.)

concentrations of 0.3 ng/mL and 0.6 ng/mL, respectively.[307] Despite marked dose-dependent analgesia and sedation produced by this drug, there is only mild depression of ventilation. Dexmedetomidine in high doses (loading dose of 1 μg/kg IV followed by 5 to 10 μg/kg/hour IV) produces total IV anesthesia without associated depression of ventilation.[308] The preservation of breathing provides a potential anesthetic technique for patients with a difficult upper airway. As with clonidine, dexmedetomidine has been reported to be effective in attenuating the cardiostimulatory and postanesthetic delirium effects of ketamine.[309] Addition of 0.5 μg/kg dexmedetomidine to lidocaine being administered to produce IV regional anesthesia improves the quality of anesthesia and postoperative analgesia without causing side effects.[310] Dexmedetomidine markedly increases the range of temperatures not triggering thermoregulatory defenses. For this reason, dexmedetomidine, like clonidine, is likely to promote perioperative hypothermia and also prove to be an effective treatment for nonthermally induced shivering.[311] Severe bradycardia may follow the administration of dexmedetomidine and cardiac arrest has been reported in a patient receiving a dexmedetomidine infusion as a supplement to general anesthesia.[312]

Postoperative Sedation

Dexmedetomidine (0.2 to 0.7 μg/kg/hour IV) is useful for sedation of postoperative critical care patients in an ICU environment, particularly when mechanical ventilation via a tracheal tube is necessary. In comparison with remifentanil, dexmedetomidine infusions do not result in clinically significant depression of ventilation and sedation exhibits some similarity with natural sleep.[313] Following tracheal extubation, dexmedetomidine-sedated patients breathe spontaneously and appear calm and relaxed.[314] Both clonidine and dexmedetomidine are useful in the ICU to prevent drug withdrawal symptoms following long-term sedation with benzodiazepines. Because of its sympatholytic and vagomimetic actions, dexmedetomidine may be accompanied by systemic hypotension and bradycardia. The ability to specifically antagonize the sedative effects of dexmedetomidine with atipamezole may be useful.[301]

Scopolamine

Scopolamine is a naturally occurring anticholinergic alkaloid derived from the belladonna (deadly nightshade) plant. Scopolamine, also known as ***hyoscine***, is a lipid-soluble tertiary amine that readily crosses the blood–brain barrier, where it binds muscarinic cholinergic receptors.[315] Although chiral, the naturally occurring and biologically active enantiomer is l-scopolamine.

Following IV administration, scopolamine undergoes a biphasic elimination, with an elimination half-life of approximately 4.5 hours.[316] Scopolamine has a volume of distribution of approximately 100 L, hepatic clearance of 1 L per minute, and a renal clearance of just 70 mL per minute. Only 6% of an IV dose appears as unchanged drug in the urine. It is almost never given orally, as the bioavailability is unpredictable, ranging from 10% to 50%.[316]

Clinical Uses

Sedation

As shown in Table 5-5, compared to atropine and glycopyrrolate, the other commonly used anticholinergics, scopolamine is notable for more specificity for the central effects rather than peripheral effects. Scopolamine is the only anticholinergic drug used primarily for sedation. Scopolamine is approximately 100 times more potent than atropine in decreasing the activity of the reticular activating system. Scopolamine, in addition to depressing the cerebral cortex, also affects other areas of the brain, causing amnesia. Typical doses of scopolamine (0.3 to 0.5 mg IM or IV) usually cause sedation, whereas similar doses of atropine produce minimal CNS effects. Scopolamine also greatly enhances the sedative effects of concomitantly administered drugs, especially opioids and benzodiazepines. Indeed, the combination of IM morphine and scopolamine was once a very popular form of preoperative sedation, following introduction of morphine–scopolamine (1.2 mg) combinations for anesthesia in 1900.[317]

Occasionally, CNS effects of anticholinergic drugs, especially scopolamine, cause symptoms ranging from restlessness to somnolence. These symptoms are more likely to occur in elderly patients and should be considered as a possible explanation for delayed awakening from anesthesia or agitation in the early postoperative period.

Table 5-5

Comparative Effects of Anticholinergic Drugs

	Sedation	Antisialagogue	Increase Heart Rate	Relax Smooth Muscle
Atropine	+	+	+ + +	+ +
Scopolamine	+ + +	+ + +	+	+
Glycopyrrolate	0	+ +	+ +	+ +

	Mydriasis, Cycloplegia	Prevent Motion-Induced Nausea	Decrease Gastric Hydrogen Ion Secretion	Alter Fetal Heart Rate
Atropine	+	+	+	0
Scopolamine	+ + +	+ + +	+	?
Glycopyrrolate	0	0	+	0

0, none; +, mild; + +, moderate; + + +, marked.

Inhaled anesthetics can potentiate the effects of anticholinergic drugs on the CNS, leading to an increased incidence of postoperative restlessness or somnolence. Physostigmine is effective in reversing restlessness or somnolence due to CNS effects of tertiary amine anticholinergic drugs. The typical dose of physostigmine for reversal of scopolamine sedation is 2 mg IV. Scopolamine has recently become a drug of abuse.

Antisialagogue Effect

Scopolamine is approximately three times more potent as an antisialagogue than atropine. For this reason, scopolamine is often selected when both an antisialagogue effect and sedation are desired results of preoperative medication. In equivalent antisialagogue doses, scopolamine, 0.3 to 0.5 mg IM, is less likely than atropine, 0.4 to 0.6 mg IM, to produce heart rate changes.

Antiemetic Effect

Scopolamine is commonly administered as a transdermal patch to prevent postoperative nausea and vomiting.

Side Effects

Mydriasis and Cycloplegia

Patients with glaucoma and parturients require special considerations in using anticholinergic drugs for preoperative medication. For example, the mydriatic effects of scopolamine are greater than those of atropine. This suggests that caution should be used in the administration of scopolamine to patients with glaucoma, since mydriasis can block the normal drainage of aqueous humor.[318]

Circular muscles of the iris that constrict the pupil are innervated by cholinergic fibers from the third cranial nerve, whereas fibers from the same nerve cause contraction of the ciliary muscles, allowing the lens to become more convex. Anticholinergic drugs placed topically on the cornea block the action of acetylcholine at both these sites, resulting in mydriasis and cycloplegia (inability to focus for near vision). Mydriasis produced by an anti-cholinergic drug can be completely offset by topical placement on the cornea of a muscarinic agonist such as pilocarpine.

Central Anticholinergic Syndrome

Scopolamine and, to a lesser extent, atropine can enter the CNS and produce symptoms characterized as the central anticholinergic syndrome. Symptoms range from restlessness and hallucinations to somnolence and unconsciousness. Presumably, these responses reflect blockade of muscarinic cholinergic receptors and competitive inhibition of the effects of acetylcholine in the CNS. Physostigmine, a lipid-soluble tertiary amine anticholinesterase drug administered in doses of 15 to 60 μg/kg IV, is a specific treatment for the central anticholinergic syndrome. Treatment may need to be repeated every 1 to 2 hours.

Overdose

Deliberate or accidental overdose with an anticholinergic drug produces a rapid onset of symptoms characteristic of muscarinic cholinergic receptor blockade. The mouth becomes dry, swallowing and talking is difficult, vision is blurred, photophobia is present, and tachycardia is prominent. The skin is dry and flushed, and a rash may appear especially over the face, neck, and upper chest (blush area). Even therapeutic doses of anticholinergic drugs sometimes may selectively dilate cutaneous vessels in the blush area. Body temperature is likely to be increased by anticholinergic drugs, especially when the environmental temperature is also increased. This increase in body temperature largely reflects inhibition of sweating by anticholinergic drugs, emphasizing that innervation of sweat glands is by sympathetic nervous system nerves that release acetylcholine as the neurotransmitter. Small children are particularly vulnerable to drug-induced increases in body temperature, with "atropine fever" occurring occasionally in this age group after administration of even a therapeutic dose of anticholinergic drug. Minute ventilation may be slightly increased due to CNS stimulation and the impact of an increased physiologic dead space due to bronchodilation. Arterial blood gases are usually unchanged. Skeletal muscle weakness and orthostatic hypotension, when present, reflect nicotinic cholinergic receptor blockade. Fatal events due to an overdose of an anticholinergic drug include seizures, coma, and medullary ventilatory center paralysis.

Small children and infants seem particularly vulnerable to developing life-threatening symptoms after an overdose with an anticholinergic drug. Physostigmine, administered in doses of 15 to 60 μg/kg IV, is the specific treatment for reversal of symptoms. Because physostigmine is metabolized rapidly, repeated doses of this anticholinesterase drug may be necessary to prevent the recurrence of symptoms.

References

1. Bryson HM, Fulton BR, Faulds D. Propofol: an update of its use in anaesthesia and conscious sedation. *Drugs.* 1995;50:513–559.
2. Fulton B, Sorkin EM. Propofol: an overview of its pharmacology and a review of its clinical efficacy in intensive care sedation. *Drugs.* 1995;50:636–657.
3. Smith I, White PF, Nathanson M, et al. Propofol: an update on its clinical use. *Anesthesiology.* 1994;81:1005–1043.
4. Ward DS, Norton JR, Guivarc'h PH, et al. Pharmacodynamics and pharmacokinetics of propofol in a medium-chain triglyceride emulsion. *Anesthesiology.* 2002;97:1401–1408.
5. Masaki Y, Tanaka M, Nishikawa T. Physicochemical compatibility of propofol-lidocaine mixture. *Anesth Analg.* 2003;97:1646–1651.
6. Song D, Hamza MA, White PF, et al. Comparison of a lower-lipid propofol emulsion with the standard emulsion for sedation during monitored anesthesia care. *Anesthesiology.* 2004;100:1072–1075.
7. Banaszczyk M, Carlo AT, Millan V, et al. Propofol phosphate, a water-soluble propofol prodrug: in vivo evaluation. *Anesth Analg.* 2002;95:1285–1292.
8. Fechner J, Ihmsen H, Hatterscheid D, et al. Pharmacokinetics and clinical pharmacodynamics of the new propofol prodrug GPI 15715 in volunteers. *Anesthesiology.* 2003;99:303–313.
9. Fechner J, Ihmsen H, Hatterscheid D, et al. Comparative pharmacokinetics and pharmacodynamics of the new propofol prodrug GPI 15715 and propofol emulsion. *Anesthesiology.* 2004;101:626–639.
10. Sneyd JR. Propofol and epilepsy. *Br J Anaesth.* 1999;82:168–169.
11. Yamakura T, Bertaccini E, Trudell JR, et al. Anesthetics and ion channels: molecular models and sites of action. *Annu Rev Pharmacol Toxicol.* 2001;41:23–51.
12. Kerz T, Hennes HJ, Feve A, et al. Effects of propofol on H-reflex in humans. *Anesthesiology.* 2001;94:32–37.
13. Court MH, Duan SX, Hesse LM, et al. Cytochrome P-450 2B6 is responsible for interindividual variability of propofol hydroxylation by human liver microsomes. *Anesthesiology.* 2001;94:110–119.
14. Takizawa D, Hiraoka H, Gota F, et al. Human kidneys play an important role in the elimination of propofol. *Anesthesiology.* 2005;102:327–330.
15. Hughes MA, Glass PSA, Jacobs JR. Context-sensitive half-time in multicompartment pharmacokinetic models for intravenous anesthetic drugs. *Anesthesiology.* 1992;76:334–341.
16. Kuipers JA, Boer F, Olieman W, et al. First-pass lung uptake and pulmonary clearance of propofol: assessment with a recirculatory indocyanine green pharmacokinetic model. *Anesthesiology.* 1999; 91:1780–1787.
17. Dawidowicz AL, Fornal E, Mardarowicz M, et al. The role of human lungs in the biotransformation of propofol. *Anesthesiology.* 2000;93:992–997.
18. He YL, Ueyama H, Tashiro C, et al. Pulmonary disposition of propofol in surgical patients. *Anesthesiology.* 2000;93:986–991.
19. Servin FS, Bourgeois B, Gomeni R, et al. Pharmacokinetics of propofol administered by target controlled infusion to alcoholic patients. *Anesthesiology.* 2003;99:576–585.
20. Masuda A, Asahi T, Sakamaki M, et al. Uric acid excretion increases during propofol anesthesia. *Anesth Analg.* 1997;85:144–148.
21. Dailland P, Cockshott ID, Lirzin JD, et al. Intravenous propofol during cesarean section: placental transfer, concentrations in breast milk, and neonatal effects. A preliminary study. *Anesthesiology.* 1989;71:827–834.
22. Gedney JA, Ghosh S. Pharmacokinetics of analgesics, sedatives and anaesthetic agents during cardiopulmonary bypass. *Br J Anaesth.* 1995;75:344–351.
23. Short TG, Lim TA, Tam YH. Prospective evaluation of pharmacokinetic model-controlled infusion of propofol in adult patients. *Br J Anaesth.* 1996;76:313–315.
24. Veselis RA, Reinsel RA, Feshchenko VA, et al. The comparative amnestic effects of midazolam, propofol, thiopental, and fentanyl at equisedative concentrations. *Anesthesiology.* 1997;87:749–764.
25. Cheng SS, Yeh J, Flood P. Anesthesia matters: patients anesthetized with propofol have less postoperative pain than those anesthetized with isoflurane. *Anesth Analg.* 2008;106:264–269.
26. Pambianco DJ, Vargo JJ, Pruitt RE, et al. Computer-assisted personalized sedation for upper endoscopy and colonoscopy: a comparative, multicenter randomized study. *Gastrointest Endosc.* 2011; 73:765–772.
27. Wahr JA, Plunkett JJ, Ramsay JG, et al. Cardiovascular responses during sedation after coronary revascularization: incidence of myocardial ischemia and hemodynamic episodes with propofol versus midazolam. *Anesthesiology.* 1996;84:1350–1360.
28. Parke TJ, Steven JE, Rice ASC, et al. Metabolic acidosis and fatal myocardial failure after propofol infusion in children: five case reports. *BMJ.* 1992;305:613–616.
29. Borgeat A, Wilder-Smith OHG, Suter PM. The nonhypnotic therapeutic applications of propofol. *Anesthesiology.* 1994;80:642–656.
30. Gan TJ, Glass PSA, Howell ST, et al. Determination of plasma concentrations of propofol associated with 50% reduction in postoperative nausea. *Anesthesiology.* 1997;87:779–784.
31. Apfel CC, Korttila K, Abdalla, M, et al. A factorial trial of six interventions for the prevention of postoperative nausea and vomiting. *N Engl J Med.* 2004;350:2441–2451.
32. Borgeat A. Subhypnotic doses of propofol do not possess antidopaminergic properties. *Anesth Analg.* 1997;84:196–198.
33. Chassard D, Lansiaux S, Duflo F, et al. Effects of subhypnotic doses of propofol on gastric emptying in volunteers. *Anesthesiology.* 2002;97:96–101.
34. Borgeat A, Wilder-Smith OHG, Saiah M, et al. Subhypnotic doses of propofol relieve pruritus induced by epidural and intrathecal morphine. *Anesthesiology.* 1992;76:510–512.
35. Avramov MN, Husain MM, White PF. The comparative effects of methohexital, propofol, and etomidate for electroconvulsive therapy. *Anesth Analg.* 1995;81:596–602.
36. Eames WO, Rooke GA, Sai-Chuen R, et al. Comparison of the effects of etomidate, propofol, and thiopental on respiratory resistance after tracheal intubation. *Anesthesiology.* 1996;84: 1307–1311.
37. Brown RH, Greenberg RS, Wagner EM. Efficacy of propofol to prevent bronchoconstriction: effects of preservative. *Anesthesiology.* 2001;94:851–855.

38. Rieschke P, LaFleur BJ, Janicki PK. Effects of EDTA- and sulfite-containing formulations of propofol on respiratory system resistance after tracheal intubation in smokers. *Anesthesiology*. 2003;98: 323–328.
39. Nishiyama T, Hanaoka K. Propofol-induced bronchoconstriction: two case reports. *Anesth Analg*. 2001;93:645–646.
40. Tibbs GR, Rowley TJ, Sanford RL, et al. HCN1 channels as targets for anesthetic and nonanesthetic propofol analogs in the amelioration of mechanical and thermal hyperalgesia in a mouse model of neuropathic pain. *J Pharmacol Exp Ther*. 2013;345:363–373.
41. Kaisti KK, Langsjo JW, Aalto S, et al. Effects of sevoflurane, propofol, and adjunct nitrous oxide on regional cerebral blood flow, oxygen consumption, and blood volume in humans. *Anesthesiology*. 2003;99:603–613.
42. Pinaud M, Leausque JN, Chetanneau A, et al. Effects of propofol on cerebral hemodynamics and metabolism in patients with brain trauma. *Anesthesiology*. 1990;73:404–409.
43. Girard F, Moumdjian R, Boudreault D, et al. The effect of propofol sedation on the intracranial pressure of patients with space-occupying lesion. *Anesth Analg*. 2004;99:573–577.
44. Strebel S, Kaufmann M, Guardiola PM, et al. Cerebral vasomotor responsiveness to carbon dioxide is preserved during propofol and midazolam anesthesia in humans. *Anesth Analg*. 1994;78:884–888.
45. Hewitt PB, Chu DKL, Polkey CE, et al. Effect of propofol on the electrocorticogram in epileptic patients undergoing cortical resection. *Br J Anaesth*. 1999;82:199–202.
46. Boisseau N, Madany M, Staccini P, et al. Comparison of the effects of sevoflurane and propofol on cortical somatosensory evoked potentials. *Br J Anaesth*. 2002;88:785–789.
47. Herrick IA, Craen RA, Gelb AW, et al. Propofol sedation during awake craniotomy for seizures: electrocorticographic and epileptogenic effects. *Anesth Analg*. 1997;84:1280–1284.
48. Keidan I, Perel A, Shabtai EL, et al. Children undergoing repeated exposures for radiation therapy do not develop tolerance to propofol. *Anesthesiology*. 2004;100:251–254.
49. Rouby JJ, Andreev A, Leger P, et al. Peripheral vascular effects of thiopental and propofol in humans with artificial hearts. *Anesthesiology*. 1991;75:32–42.
50. Robinson BJ, Ebert TJ, O'Brien TJ, et al. Mechanisms whereby propofol mediates peripheral vasodilation in humans. Sympatho-inhibition or direct vascular relaxation? *Anesthesiology*. 1997;86:64–72.
51. Daniel M, Eger IE, Weiskopf RB, et al. Propofol fails to attenuate the cardiovascular response to rapid increases in desflurane concentration. *Anesthesiology*. 1996;84:75–80.
52. Lopatka CW, Muzi M, Eberft JT. Propofol, but not etomidate, reduces desflurane-mediated sympathetic activation in humans. *Can J Anesth*. 1999;46:342–347.
53. Kanaya N, Satoh H, Seki S, et al. Propofol anesthesia enhances the pressor response to intravenous ephedrine. *Anesth Analg*. 2002;94(5):1207–1211.
54. Deutschman CS, Harris AP, Fleisher LA. Changes in heart rate variability under propofol anesthesia: a possible explanation for propofol-induced bradycardia. *Anesth Analg*. 1994;79:373–377.
55. Lavoie J, Walsh EP, Burrows FA, et al. Effects of propofol or isoflurane anesthesia on cardiac conduction in children undergoing radiofrequency catheter ablation for tachydysrhythmias. *Anesthesiology*. 1995;82:884–887.
56. Sharpe MD, Dobkowski WB, Murkin JM, et al. Propofol has no direct effect on sinoatrial node function or on normal atrioventricular and accessory pathway conduction in Wolff-Parkinson-White syndrome during alfentanil/midazolam anesthesia. *Anesthesiology*. 1995;82:888–895.
57. Skei S, Ichimiya T, Hideaki T, et al. A case of normalization of Wolff-Parkinson-White syndrome conduction during propofol anesthesia. *Anesthesiology*. 1999;90:1779–1781.
58. Kleinsasser A, Kuenszberg E, Loeckinger A, et al. Sevoflurane, but not propofol, significantly prolongs the Q-T interval. *Anesth Analg*. 2000;90:25–27.
59. Egan TD, Brock UJG. Asystole after anesthesia induction with a fentanyl, propofol, and succinylcholine sequence. *Anesth Analg*. 1991;73:818–820.
60. Freysz M, Timourt Q, Betrix L, et al. Propofol and bradycardia. *Can J Anaesth*. 1991;28:137–138.
61. James MFM, Reyneke CJ, Whiffler K. Heart block following propofol: a case report. *Br J Anaesth*. 1989;62:213–215.
62. Tramer MR, Moore RA, McQuay HJ. Propofol and bradycardia: causation, frequency and severity. *Br J Anaesth*. 1997;78:642–651.
63. Tramer M, Moore A, McQuay H. Prevention of vomiting after paediatric strabismus surgery: a systematic review using the numbers-needed-to-treat method. *Br J Anaesth*. 1995;75:556–561.
64. Horiguchi T, Nishikawa T. Heart rate response to intravenous atropine during propofol anesthesia. *Anesth Analg*. 2002;95:389–392.
65. Bouillon T, Bruhn J, Radu-Radulescu L, et al. Mixed-effects modeling of the intrinsic ventilatory depressant potency of propofol in the non-steady state. *Anesthesiology*. 2004;100:240–250.
66. Nieuwenhuijs D, Sarton E, Teppema LJ, et al. Respirator sites of action of propofol: Absence of depression of peripheral chemoreflex loop by low-dose propofol. *Anesthesiology*. 2001;95:889–895.
67. Blouin RT, Seifert HA, Babenco HD, et al. Propofol decreases the hypoxic ventilatory response during conscious sedation and isohypercapnia. *Anesthesiology*. 1993;79:1177–1182.
68. Anand K, Ramsay MA, Crippin JS. Hepatocellular injury following the administration of propofol. *Anesthesiology*. 2001;95:1523–1524.
69. Mowafi HA, Al-Ghamdi A, Rushood A. Intraocular pressure changes during laparoscopy in patients anesthetized with propofol total intravenous anesthesia versus isoflurane inhaled anesthesia. *Anesth Analg*. 2003;97:471–474.
70. Fourcade O, Simon MF, Litt L, et al. Propofol inhibits human platelet aggregation induced by proinflammatory lipid mediators. *Anesth Analg*. 2004;99:393–398.
71. Doenicke AW, Roizen MF, Rau J, et al. Pharmacokinetics and pharmacodynamics of propofol in a new solvent. *Anesth Analg*. 1997;85:1399–1403.
72. de Leon-Casasola, Weiss A, Lema MJ. Anaphylaxis due to propofol. *Anesthesiology*. 1992;77:384–386.
73. Laxenaire MC, Mata-Bremejo E, Moneret-Vautrin DA, et al. Life-threatening anaphylactoid reactions to propofol (Diprivan). *Anesthesiology*. 1992;77:275–280.
74. Badr AE, Mychaskiw GH, Eichhorn JH. Metabolic acidosis associated with a new formulation of propofol. *Anesthesiology*. 2001;94:536–538.
75. Cremer OL, Moons KG, Bouman EA, et al. Long-term propofol infusion and cardiac failure in adult head-injured patients. *Lancet*. 2001;357(9250):117–118.
76. Bray RJ. Fatal myocardial failure associated with a propofol infusion in a child. *Anaesthesia*. 1995;50:94.
77. Dearlove O, Dobson A. Does propofol cause death in children? *Anaesthesia*. 1995;50:916.
78. Burow BK, Johnson ME, Packer DL. Metabolic acidosis associated with propofol in the absence of other causative factors. *Anesthesiology*. 2004;101:239–241.
79. Salengros J-C, Velghe-Lenelle CE, Bollens R, et al. Lactic acidosis during propofol-remifentanil anesthesia in an adult. *Anesthesiology*. 2004;101:241–243.
80. Funston JS, Prough DS. Two reports of propofol anesthesia associated with metabolic acidosis in adults. *Anesthesiology*. 2004;101:6–8.
81. Culp KE, Augoustides JG, Ochroch AE, et al. Clinical management of cardiogenic shock associated with prolonged propofol infusion. *Anesth Analg*. 2004;99:221–226.
82. Wolf A, Weir P, Setage P, et al. Impaired fatty acid oxidation in propofol infusion syndrome. *Lancet*. 2001;357:606–607.
83. Hughes NJ, Lyons JB. Prolonged myoclonus and meningismus following propofol. *Can J Anaesth*. 1995;42:744–746.
84. Reddy RV, Moorthy SS, Dierdorf SF, et al. Excitatory effects and electroencephalographic correlation of etomidate, thiopental, methohexital, and propofol. *Anesth Analg*. 1993;77:1008–1011.

85. Follette JW, Farley WJ. Anesthesiologist addicted to propofol. *Anesthesiology.* 1992;77:817–818.
86. Earley PH, Finver T. Addiction to propofol: a study of 22 treatment cases. *J Addict Med.* 2013;7:169–176.
87. Monroe T, Hamza H, Stocks G, et al. The misuse and abuse of propofol. *Subst Use Misuse.* 2011;46:1199–1205.
88. Crowther J, Hrazdil J, Jolly DT, et al. Growth of microorganisms in propofol, thiopental, and a 1:1 mixture of propofol and thiopental. *Anesth Analg.* 1996;82:475–478.
89. Kuehnert MJ, Webb RM, Jochimsen EM, et al. Staphylococcus aureus bloodstream infections among patients undergoing electroconvulsive therapy traced to breaks in infection control and possible extrinsic contamination by propofol. *Anesth Analg.* 1997;85:420–425.
90. Nichols RL, Smith JW. Bacterial contamination of an anesthetic agent. *N Engl J Med.* 1995;333:184–185.
91. Warwick JP, Bladke D. Drawing up propofol [letter]. *Anaesthesia.* 1994;49:172.
92. Daskalopoulos R, Korcok J, Farhangkhgoee P, et al. Propofol protection of sodium-hydrogen activity sustains glutamate uptake during oxidative stress. *Anesth Analg.* 2001;93:1199–1204.
93. Peters CE, Korcok J, Gelb AW, et al. Anesthetic concentrations of propofol protect against oxidative stress in primary astrocyte cultures: comparison with hypothermia. *Anesthesiology.* 2001;94: 313–321.
94. Krumholz W, Endrass J, Hempelmann G. Propofol inhibits phagocytosis and killing of Staphylococcus aureus and Escherichia coli by polymorphonuclear leukocytes in vitro. *Can J Anaesth.* 1994;41:446–449.
95. Kooy NW, Royall JA, Ye YZ, et al. Evidence for in vivo peroxynitrite production in human acute lung injury. *Am J Respir Crit Care Med.* 1995;151:1250–1254.
96. Sayin MM, Ozatamer O, Tasoz R, et al. Propofol attenuates myocardial lipid peroxidation during coronary artery bypass grafting surgery *Br J Anaesth.* 2002;89:242–246.
97. Holley HS, Cuthrell L. Intraarterial injection of propofol. *Anesthesiology.* 1990;73:183–184.
98. MacPherson RD, Rasiah RL, McLeod LJ. Intraarterial propofol is not directly toxic to vascular endothelium. *Anesthesiology.* 1992;76:967–971.
99. Sundman E, Witt HR, Sandin R, et al. Pharyngeal function and airway protection during subhypnotic concentrations of propofol, isoflurane, and sevoflurane: volunteers examined by pharyngeal videoradiography and simultaneous manometry. *Anesthesiology.* 2001;95:1125–1132.
100. Kasraie N, Cousins TB. Propofol and the patient with hereditary coproporphyria. *Anesth Analg.* 1993;77:862–863.
101. Raff M, Harrison GG. The screening of propofol in MHS swine. *Anesth Analg.* 1989;68:750–751.
102. Sebel PS, Lowdon JD. Propofol: a new intravenous anesthetic. *Anesthesiology.* 1989;71:260–277.
103. Krauss JK, Akeyson EW, Giam P, et al. Propofol-induced dyskinesias in Parkinson's disease. *Anesth Analg.* 1996;83:420–422.
104. Tomlin SL, Jenkins A, Lieb WR, et al. Stereoselective effects of etomidate optical isomers on gamma-aminobutyric acid type A receptors and animals. *Anesthesiology.* 1998;88(3):708–717.
105. Streisand JB, Jaarsma RL, Jay MA, et al. Oral transmucosal etomidate in volunteers. *Anesthesiology.* 1998;88:89–95.
106. Tomlin SL, Jenkins A, Lieb WR, et al. Stereoselective effects of etomidate optical isomers on gamma-aminobutyric acid type A receptors and animals. *Anesthesiology.* 1998;88:708–717.
107. Iibeigi MS, Davidson ML, Yarmush JM. An unexpected arousal effect of etomidate in a patient on high-dose steroids. *Anesthesiology.* 1998;89:1587–1589.
108. Holdcroft A, Morgan M, Whitwam JG, et al. Effect of dose and premedication on induction complications with etomidate. *Br J Anaesth.* 1976;48(3):199–205.
109. St Pierre M, Dunkel M, Rutherford A, et al. Does etomidate increase postoperative nausea? A double-blind controlled comparison of etomidate in lipid emulsion with propofol for balanced anaesthesia. *Eur J Anaesthesiol.* 2000;17:634–641.
110. Milde LN, Milde JH, Michenfelder JD. Cerebral functional, metabolic, and hemodynamic effects of etomidate in dogs. *Anesthesiology.* 1985;63:371–377.
111. Ebrahim ZY, DeBoer GE, Luders H, et al. Effect of etomidate on the electroencephalogram of patients with epilepsy. *Anesth Analg.* 1986;65:1004–1006.
112. Sloan TB, Ronai AK, Toleikis R, et al. Improvement of intraoperative somatosensory evoked potentials by etomidate. *Anesth Analg.* 1988;67:582–585.
113. Craido A, Maseda J, Navarro E, et al. Induction of anaesthesia with etomidate: haemodynamic study of 36 patients. *Br J Anaesth.* 1980;52:803–809.
114. Karliczek GF, Brenken U, Schokkenbrock R, et al. Etomidate-analgesic combinations for the induction of anesthesia in cardiac patients. *Anaesthesist.* 1982;31:213–220.
115. Sprung J, Ogletree-Hughes ML, Moravec CS. The effects of etomidate on the contractility of failing and nonfailing human heart muscle. *Anesth Analg.* 2000;91:68–75.
116. Choi SD, Spulding BC, Gross JB, et al. Comparison of the ventilatory effects of etomidate and methohexital. Anesthesiology. 1985;62:442–447.
117. Doenicke AW, Roizen MF, Kugler J, et al. Reducing myoclonus after etomidate. *Anesthesiology.* 1999;90:113–119.
118. Laughlin TP, Newberg LA. Prolonged myoclonus after etomidate anesthesia. *Anesth Analg.* 1985;64:80–82.
119. Fragen RJ, Shanks CA, Molteni A, et al. Effects of etomidate on hormonal responses to surgical stress. *Anesthesiology.* 1984;61: 652–656.
120. Wagner RL, White PF, Kan PB, et al. Inhibition of adrenal steroidogenesis by the anesthetic etomidate. *N Engl J Med.* 1984;310: 1415–1421.
121. Owen H, Spence AA. Etomidate. *Br J Anaesth.* 1984;56:555–557.
122. Longnecker DE. Stress free: to be or not to be? *Anesthesiology.* 1984;61:643–644.
123. Duthie DJR, Fraser R, Nimmo WS. Effect of induction of anaesthesia with etomidate on corticosteroid synthesis in man. *Br J Anaesth.* 1985;57:156–159.
124. Wagner CE, Bick JS, Johnson D, et al. Etomidate use and postoperative outcomes among cardiac surgery patients. *Anesthesiology.* 2014;120:579–589.
125. Komatsu R, You J, Mascha EJ, et al. Anesthetic induction with etomidate, rather than propofol, is associated with increased 30-day mortality and cardiovascular morbidity after noncardiac surgery. *Anesth Analg.* 2013;117:1329–1337.
126. Pejo C, Santer P, Jeffrey S, et al. Analogues of etomidate: modifications around etomidate's chiral carbon and the impact on in vitro and in vivo pharmacology. *Anesthesiology.* 2014;121:290–301.
127. Watkins JA. Etomidate: an "immunologically safe" anaesthetic agent. *Anaesthesia.* 1983;34:208–210.
128. Ashton A. Guidelines for the rational use of benzodiazepines: when and what to use. *Drugs.* 1994;48:25–40.
129. Ghoneim MM, Mewaldt SP. Benzodiazepines and human memory: a review. *Anesthesiology.* 1990;72:926–938.
130. Nowell PD, Mazumdar S, Buysse DJ, et al. Benzodiazepines and zolpidem for chronic insomnia: a meta-analysis of treatment efficacy. *JAMA.* 1997;278:2170–2177.
131. Goodchild CS. GABA receptors and benzodiazepines. *Br J Anaesth.* 1993;71:127–133.
132. Mohler H, Richards JG. The benzodiazepine receptor: a pharmacological control element of brain function. *Eur J Anaesthesiol Suppl.* 1988;2:15–24.
133. Low K, Crestani F, Keist R, et al. Molecular and neuronal substrate for the selective attenuation of anxiety. *Science.* 2000;290:131–134.

134. McKernan RM, Rosahl TW, Reynolds DS, et al. Sedative but not anxiolytic properties of benzodiazepines are mediated by GABAA receptor alpha1 subtype. *Nat Neurosci.* 2000;3:587–592.
135. Seubert CN, Morey TE, Martynuk AE, et al. Midazolam selectively potentiates the A2a- but not the A1-receptor–mediated effects of adenosine. *Anesthesiology.* 2000;92:567–577.
136. Morris HH, Estes ML. Traveler's amnesia. Transient global amnesia secondary to triazolam. *JAMA.* 1987;258:945–946.
137. Gear RW, Miaskowski C, Heller PH, et al. Benzodiazepine mediated antagonism of opioid analgesia. *Pain.* 1997;71:25–29.
138. Gross JB, Blouin RT, Zandsberg S, et al. Effect of flumazenil on ventilatory drive during sedation with midazolam and alfentanil. *Anesthesiology.* 1996;85:713–720.
139. Petraglia F, Bakalakis S, Facchinetti F, et al. Effects of sodium valproate and diazepam on beta-endorphin, beta-lipotropin and cortisol secretion induced by hypoglycemic stress in humans. *Neuroendocrinology.* 1986;44:320–325.
140. Kalogeras KT, Calogero AE, Kuribayiashi T, et al. In vitro and in vivo effects of the triazolobenzodiazepine alprazolam on hypothalamic-pituitary adrenal function: pharmacological and clinical implications. *J Clin Endocrinol Metab.* 1990;70:1462–1471.
141. Kudoh A, Takase H, Takahira Y, et al. Postoperative confusion increases in elderly long-term benzodiazepine users. *Anesth Analg.* 2004;99:1674–1678.
142. Sheu JR, Hsiao G, Luk HN, et al. Mechanisms involved in the antiplatelet activity of midazolam in human platelets. *Anesthesiology.* 2002;96:651–658.
143. Rysler C, Stoffel N, Buser A, et al. Effect of beta-blockers, Ca^{2+} antagonists, and benzodiazepines on bleeding incidence in patients with chemotherapy induced thrombocytopenia. *Platelets.* 2010;21:77–83.
144. Reves JG, Fragen RJ, Vinik HR, et al. Midazolam: pharmacology and uses. *Anesthesiology.* 1985;62:310–324.
145. Greenblatt DJ, Abernathy DR, Locniskar A, et al. Effect of age, gender, and obesity on midazolam kinetics. *Anesthesiology.* 1984; 61:27–35.
146. Johnson TN, Rostami-Hodjegan A, Goddard JM, et al. Contribution of midazolam and its 1-hydroxy metabolite to preoperative sedation in children: a pharmacokinetic-pharmacodynamic analysis. *Br J Anaesth.* 2002;89:428–437.
147. Bauer TM, Ritz R, Haberthur C, et al. Prolonged sedation due to accumulation of conjugated metabolites of midazolam. *Lancet.* 1995;346:145–150.
148. Hiller A, Olkkola KT, Isohanni P, et al. Unconsciousness associated with midazolam and erythromycin. *Br J Anaesth.* 1990;65: 826–828.
149. Hase I, Oda Y, Tanaka K, et al. I.V. fentanyl decreases the clearance of midazolam. *Br J Anaesth.* 1997;79:740–743.
150. Vinik HR, Reves JG, Greenblatt DJ, et al. The pharmacokinetics of midazolam in chronic renal failure patients. *Anesthesiology.* 1983;59:390–394.
151. Veselis RA, Reinsel RA, Beattie BJ, et al. Midazolam changes regional cerebral blood flow in discrete brain regions: an H215O positron tomography study. *Anesthesiology.* 1997;87:1106–1117.
152. Papazian L, Albanese J, Thirion X, et al. Effect of bolus doses of midazolam on intracranial pressure and cerebral perfusion pressure in patients with severe head injury. *Br J Anaesth.* 1993;71: 267–271.
153. Giffin JP, Cottrell JE, Shwiry B, et al. Intracranial pressure, mean arterial pressure, and heart rate following midazolam or thiopental in humans with brain tumors. *Anesthesiology.* 1984;60:491–494.
154. Bergman I, Steeves M, Burckart G, et al. Reversible neurologic abnormalities associated with prolonged intravenous midazolam and fentanyl administration. *J Pediatr.* 1991;119:644–649.
155. Thurston TA, Williams CGS, Foshee SL. Reversal of a paradoxical reaction to midazolam with flumazenil. *Anesth Analg.* 1996;83:192.
156. Forster A, Gardaz JP, Suter PM, et al. Respiratory depression of midazolam and diazepam. *Anesthesiology.* 1980;53:494–499.
157. Gross JB, Zebroski ME, Carel WD, et al. Time course of ventilatory depression after thiopental and midazolam in normal subjects and in patients with chronic obstructive pulmonary disease. *Anesthesiology.* 1983;58:540–544.
158. Kanto J, Sjovall S, Buori A. Effect of different kinds of premedication of the induction properties of midazolam. *Br J Anaesth.* 1982;54:507–511.
159. Bailey PL, Pace NL, Ashburn MA, et al. Frequent hypoxemia and apnea after sedation with midazolam and fentanyl. *Anesthesiology.* 1990;73:826–830.
160. Gauthier RA, Dyck B, Chung F, et al. Respiratory interaction after spinal anesthesia and sedation with midazolam. *Anesthesiology.* 1992;77:909–914.
161. Samuelson PN, Reves JG, Kouchoukos NT, et al. Hemodynamic responses to anesthetic induction with midazolam or diazepam in patients with ischemic heart disease. *Anesth Analg.* 1981;60:802–809.
162. Lebowitz PW, Cote ME, Daniels AL, et al. Comparative cardiovascular effects of midazolam and thiopental in healthy patients. *Anesth Analg.* 1982;61:661–665.
163. Adams P, Gelman S, Reves JG, et al. Midazolam pharmacodynamics and pharmacokinetics during acute hypovolemia. *Anesthesiology.* 1985;63:140–146.
164. Cote CJ, Cohen IT, Suresh S, et al. A comparison of three doses of a commercially prepared oral midazolam syrup in children. *Anesth Analg.* 2002;94:37–43.
165. McMillan CO, Spahr-Schopfer IA, Sikich N, et al. Premedication of children with oral midazolam. *Can J Anaesth.* 1992;39:545–550.
166. Kain ZN, Hofstadter MB, Mayes LC et al. Midazolam. Effects on amnesia and anxiety in children. *Anesthesiology.* 2000;93:676–684.
167. Jacobs JR, Reves JG, Marty J, et al. Aging increases pharmacodynamic sensitivity to the hypnotic effects of midazolam. *Anesth Analg.* 1995;80:143–148.
168. Sarnquist FH, Mathers WD, Brock-Utne J, et al. A bioassay of a water-soluble benzodiazepine against sodium thiopental. *Anesthesiology.* 1980;52:149–153.
169. Jensen S, Schou-Olesen A, Huttel MS. Use of midazolam as an induction agent: comparison with thiopental. *Br J Anaesth.* 1982; 54:605–607.
170. Barr J, Zomorodi K, Bertaccini E, et al. A double-blind, randomized comparison of IV lorazepam vs. midazolam for sedation of ICU patients via a pharmacologic model. *Anesthesiology.* 2001;95:286–291.
171. Roberts KW, Crnkovic A, Steiniger JR. Post-anesthesia paradoxical vocal cord motion successfully treated with midazolam. *Anesthesiology.* 1998;89:517–519.
172. Dawes GS. The distribution and action of drugs on the fetus in utero. *Br J Anaesth.* 1973;45:766–769.
173. Greenblatt DJ, Koch-Weser J. Clinical toxicity of chlordiazepoxide and diazepam in relation to serum albumin concentration: a report from the Boston Collaborative Drug Surveillance Program. *Eur J Clin Pharmacol.* 1974;7:259–262.
174. Eustace PW, Hailey DM, Cox AG, et al. Biliary excretion of diazepam in man. *Br J Anaesth.* 1975;47:983–985.
175. Klotz U, Avant GR, Hoyumpa A, et al. The effects of age and liver disease on the disposition and elimination of diazepam in adult man. *J Clin Invest.* 1975;55:347–359.
176. Braunstein MC. Apnea with maintenance of consciousness following intravenous diazepam. *Anesth Analg.* 1979;58:52–53.
177. Gross JB, Smith L, Smith TC. Time course of ventilatory response to carbon dioxide after intravenous diazepam. *Anesthesiology.* 1982;57;18–21.
178. McCammon RL, Hilgenberg JC, Stoelting RK. Hemodynamic effects of diazepam-nitrous oxide in patients with coronary artery disease. *Anesth Analg.* 1980;59:438–441.
179. Marty J, Gauzit R, Lefevre P, et al. Effects of diazepam and midazolam on baroreflex control of heart rate and on sympathetic activity in humans. *Anesth Analg.* 1986;65:113–119.

180. Knapp RB, Dubow H. Comparison of diazepam with thiopental as an induction agent in cardiopulmonary disease. *Anesth Analg.* 1970;49:722–726.
181. Falk RB, Denlinger JK, Nahrwold ML, et al. Acute vasodilation following induction of anesthesia with intravenous diazepam and nitrous oxide. *Anesthesiology.* 1978;49:149–150.
182. Dretchen K, Ghoneim MM, Long JP. The interaction of diazepam with myoneural blocking agents. *Anesthesiology.* 1971;34:463–468.
183. De Jong RH, Heavner JE. Diazepam prevents and aborts lidocaine convulsions in monkeys. *Anesthesiology.* 1974;41:226–230.
184. Fragen RJ, Caldwell N. Lorazepam premedication: lack of recall and relief of anxiety. *Anesth Analg.* 1976;55:792–796.
185. Greenblatt DJ, Ehrenberg BL, Gunderman J, et al. Kinetic and dynamic study of intravenous lorazepam: comparison with intravenous diazepam. *J Pharmacol Exp Ther.* 1989;250:134–139.
186. Witte JL, Alegret C, Sessler DI, et al. Preoperative alprazolam reduces anxiety in ambulatory surgery patients: a comparison with oral midazolam. *Anesth Analg.* 2002;95:1601–1606.
187. Greenblatt DJ, Harmatz JS, Shapiro L, et al. Sensitivity to triazolam in the elderly. *N Engl J Med.* 1991;324:1691–1698.
188. Brogden RN, Goa KL. Flumazenil: a reappraisal of its pharmacological properties and therapeutic efficacy as a benzodiazepine antagonist. *Drugs.* 1991;42:1061–1089.
189. Ghoneim MM, Block RI, Ping Sum ST, et al. The interactions of midazolam and flumazenil on human memory and cognition. *Anesthesiology.* 1993;79:1183–1192.
190. Spivey WH. Flumazenil and seizures: analysis of 43 cases. *Clin Ther.* 1992;14:292–297.
191. White PF, Shafer A, Boyle WA, et al. Benzodiazepine antagonism does not provoke a stress response. *Anesthesiology.* 1989;70:636–639.
192. Kaukinen S, Kataja J, Kaukinen L. Antagonism of benzodiazepine-fentanyl anesthesia with flumazenil. *Can J Anaesth.* 1990;37:40–45.
193. Marty J, Nitenberg A, Philip I, et al. Coronary and left ventricular hemodynamic responses following reversal of flunitrazepam-induced sedation with flumazenil in patients with coronary artery disease. *Anesthesiology.* 1991;74:71–76.
194. Schwieger IM, Szlam F, Hug CC. Absence of agonistic or antagonistic effect of flumazenil (Ro 15-7088) in dogs anesthetized with enflurane, isoflurane, or fentanyl-enflurane. *Anesthesiology.* 1989;70:477–480.
195. Forster A, Crettenand G, Klopfenstein CE, et al. Absence of agonist effects of high-dose flumazenil on ventilation and psychometric performance in human volunteers. *Anesth Analg.* 1993;77:980–984.
196. Drover DR. Comparative pharmacokinetics and pharmacodynamics of short-acting hypnosedatives: zaleplon, zolpidem and zopiclone. *Clin Pharmacokinet.* 2004;43:227–238.
197. Bertisch SM, Herzig SJ, Winkelman JW, et al. National use of prescription medications for insomnia: NHANES 1999–2010. *Sleep.* 2014;37:343–349.
198. Huedo-Medina TB, Kirsch I, Middlemass J, et al. Effectiveness of non-benzodiazepine hypnotics in treatment of adult insomnia: meta-analysis of data submitted to the Food and Drug Administration. *BMJ.* 2012;345:e8343.
199. Woolston C. Death row incurs drug penalty. *Nature.* 2013;502:417–418.
200. Zeller A, Arras M, Jurd R, et al. Identification of a molecular target mediating the general anesthetic actions of pentobarbital. *Mol Pharmacol.* 2007;71:852–859.
201. Saidman LJ. Uptake, distribution, and elimination of barbiturates. In: Eger EI, ed. Anesthetic uptake and action. Baltimore, MD: Lippincott Williams & Wilkins; 1974.
202. Saidman LJ, Eger EI. The effect of thiopental metabolism on duration of anesthesia. *Anesthesiology.* 1966;27:118–126.
203. Sorbo S, Hudson RJ, Loomis JC. The pharmacokinetics of thiopental in pediatric surgical patients. *Anesthesiology.* 1984;61:666–670.
204. Manuli MA, Davies L. Rectal methohexital for sedation of children during imaging procedures. *AJR Am J Roentgenol.* 1993;160:577–580.
205. Liu LMP, Gaudreault P, Friedman PA, et al. Methohexital plasma concentrations in children following rectal administration. *Anesthesiology.* 1985;62:567–570.
206. Avram MJ, Krejcie TC, Henthorn TK. The relationship of age to the pharmacokinetics of early drug distribution: the concurrent disposition of thiopental and indocyanine green. *Anesthesiology.* 1990;72:403–411.
207. Stanski DR, Maitre PO. Population pharmacokinetics and pharmacodynamics of thiopental: the effect of age revisited. *Anesthesiology.* 1990;72:412–422.
208. Gin T, Mainland P, Chan MT, et al. Decreased thiopental requirements in early pregnancy. *Anesthesiology.* 1997;86:73–78.
209. Cote CJ, Petkau AJ. Thiopental requirements may be increased in children reanesthetized at least one year after recovery from extensive thermal injury. *Anesth Analg.* 1985;64:1156–1160.
210. Swerdlow BN, Holley FO, Maitre PO, et al. Chronic alcohol intake does not change thiopental anesthetic requirements, pharmacokinetics, or pharmacodynamics. *Anesthesiology.* 1990;72:455–461.
211. Ford FV, Morrell F, Whisler WW. Methohexital anesthesia in the surgical treatment of uncontrollable epilepsy. *Anesth Analg.* 1982;61:997–1001.
212. Rockoff MA, Goudsouzian NG. Seizures induced by methohexital. *Anesthesiology.* 1981;54:333–335.
213. Todd MM, Drummond JC, Sang H. The hemodynamic consequences of high-dose methohexital anesthesia in humans. *Anesthesiology.* 1984;61:495–501.
214. Bedford RF, Persing JA, Pobereskin L, et al. Lidocaine or thiopental for rapid control of intracranial hypertension. *Anesth Analg.* 1980;59:435–437.
215. Ward JD, Becker DP, Miller DJ, et al. Failure of prophylactic barbiturate coma in the treatment of severe head trauma. *J Neurosurg.* 1985;62:383–388.
216. Brain Resuscitation Clinical Trial I Study Group. Randomized clinical study of thiopental loading in comatose survivors of cardiac arrest. *N Engl J Med.* 1986;314:397–403.
217. Nussmeier NA, Arlund C, Slogoff S. Neuropsychiatric complications after cardiopulmonary bypass: cerebral protection by a barbiturate. *Anesthesiology.* 1986;64:165–170.
218. Todd MM, Chadwick HS, Shapiro HM, et al. The neurologic effects of thiopental therapy following experimental cardiac arrest in cats. *Anesthesiology.* 1982;57:76–86.
219. Filner BF, Karliner JS. Alterations of normal left ventricular performance by general anesthesia. *Anesthesiology.* 1976;45:610–620.
220. Drummond JC, Todd MM, U HS. The effect of high dose sodium thiopental on brain stem auditory and median nerve somatosensory evoked responses in humans. *Anesthesiology.* 1985;63;249–254.
221. Hirshman CA, Krieger W, Littlejohn G, et al. Ketamine-aminophylline-induced decrease in seizure threshold. *Anesthesiology.* 1982;56:464–467.
222. Etter MS, Helrich M, Mackenzie CF. Immunoglobulin E fluctuation in thiopental anaphylaxis. *Anesthesiology.* 1980;52:181–183.
223. Lilly JK, Hoy RH. Thiopental anaphylaxis and reagin involvement. *Anesthesiology.* 1980;53:335–337.
224. Clarke RSJ. Adverse effects of intravenously administered drugs in anaesthetic practice. *Drugs.* 1981;22:26–41.
225. Kohrs R, Durieux ME. Ketamine: teaching an old drug new tricks. *Anesth Analg.* 1998;87;1186–1193.
226. Reich DL, Silvay G. Ketamine: an update on the first twenty-five years of clinical experience. *Can J Anaesth.* 1989;36:186–197.
227. Kienbaum P, Heuter T, Paviakovic G, et al. S(+)-ketamine increases muscle sympathetic activity and maintains the neural response to hypotensive challenges in humans. *Anesthesiology.* 2001;94:252–258.

228. White PF, Ham J, Way WL, et al. Pharmacology of ketamine isomers in surgical patients. *Anesthesiology*. 1980;52:231–239.
229. Pfenninger EG, Durieux ME, Himmelseher S. Cognitive impairment after small-dose ketamine isomers in comparison to equianalgesic racemic ketamine in human volunteers. *Anesthesiology*. 2002;96:357–366.
230. Hirota K, Lambert DG. Ketamine: its mechanism(s) of action and unusual clinical uses. *Br J Anaesth*. 1996;77:441–444.
231. Wagner LE, Gingrich KJ, Kulli JC, et al. Ketamine blockade of voltage-gated sodium channels: evidence for a shared receptor site with local anesthetics. *Anesthesiology*. 2001;95:1406–1413.
232. Coates KM, Flood P. Ketamine and its preservative, benzethonium chloride, both inhibit human recombinant alpha7 and alpha4beta2 neuronal nicotinic acetylcholine receptors in *Xenopus* oocytes. *Br J Pharmacol*. 2001;134:871–879.
233. Weigand MA, Schmidt H, Zhao Q, et al. Ketamine modulates the stimulated adhesion molecule expression on human neutrophils in vitro. *Anesth Analg*. 2000;90:206–212.
234. Hurstveit O, Maurset A, Oye I. Interaction of the chiral forms of ketamine with opioid, phencyclidine, and muscarinic receptors. *Pharmacol Toxicol*. 1995;77:355–359.
235. Ho KK, Flood P. Single amino acid residue in the extracellular portion of transmembrane segment 2 in the nicotinic alpha7 acetylcholine receptor modulates sensitivity to ketamine. *Anesthesiology*. 2004;100:657–662.
236. Udesky JO, Spence NZ, Achiel R, et al. The role of nicotinic inhibition in ketamine-induced behavior. *Anesth Analg*. 2005;101:407–411.
237. White PF, Way WL, Trevor AJ. Ketamine: its pharmacology and therapeutic uses. *Anesthesiology*. 1982;56:119–136.
238. Demling RH, Ellerbee S, Jarrett F. Ketamine anesthesia for tangential excision of burn eschar: a burn unit procedure. *J Trauma*. 1978;18:269–270.
239. Himmelseher S, Durieux ME. Ketamine for perioperative pain management. *Anesthesiology*. 2005;102:211–220.
240. Subramaniam K, Balachundar S, Steinbrook RA. Ketamine as adjuvant analgesic to opioids: a quantitative and qualitative systematic review. *Anesth Analg*. 2004;99:482–495.
241. Liu H-T, Hollmann MW, Liu W-H, et al. Modulation of NMDA receptor function by ketamine and magnesium: part I. *Anesth Analg*. 2001;92:1173–1181.
242. Akamatsu TJ, Bonica JJ, Rhemet R. Experiences with the use of ketamine for parturition. I: primary anesthetic for vaginal delivery. *Anesth Analg*. 1974;53:284–287.
243. Janeczko GF, El-Etr AA, Youngest S. Low-dose ketamine anesthesia for obstetrical delivery. *Anesth Analg*. 1974;53:828–831.
244. Hodgkinson K, Marx GF, Kim SS, et al. Neonatal neurobehavioral tests following vaginal delivery under ketamine, thiopental, and extradural anesthesia. *Anesth Analg*. 1977;56:548–553.
245. Salt TE, Wilson DG, Prasad SK. Antagonism of N-methylaspartate and synaptic responses of neurones in the rat ventrobasal thalamus by ketamine and MK-801. *Br J Pharmacol*. 1988;94:443–448.
246. Sandler AN, Schmid R, Katz J. Epidural ketamine for postoperative analgesia. *Can J Anaesth*. 1998;45:99–102.
247. Waxman K, Shoemaker WC, Lippmann M. Cardiovascular effects of anesthetic induction with ketamine. *Anesth Analg*. 1980;59(5):355–358.
248. Guit JBM, Koning HM, Niemeijer RPE, et al. Ketamine as an analgesic for total intravenous anaesthesia with propofol. *Anaesthesia*. 1991;46:24–31.
249. Hirshman CA, Downes H, Farbood A, et al. Ketamine block of bronchospasm in experimental canine asthma. *Br J Anaesth*. 1979;51:713–718.
250. Dershwitz M, Sreter FA, Ryan JF. Ketamine does not trigger malignant hyperthermia in susceptible swine. *Anesth Analg*. 1989;69:501–503.
251. Eilers H, Philip LA, Bickler PE, et al. The reversal of fentanyl-induced tolerance by administration of "small-dose" ketamine. *Anesth Analg*. 2001;93:213–214.
252. Kudoh A, Takahira Y, Katagai H, et al. Small-dose ketamine improves the postoperative state of depressed patients. *Anesth Analg*. 2002;95:114–118.
253. Rodriguez CI, Kegeles L, Levinson A, et al. Randomized controlled crossover trial of ketamine in obsessive-compulsive disorder: proof of concept. *Neuropsychopharmacology*. 2013;38:2475–2483.
254. Kapur N, Friedman R. Oral ketamine: a promising treatment for restless legs syndrome. *Anesth Analg*. 2002;94:1558–1559.
255. Takeshita H, Okuda Y, Sari A. The effects of ketamine on cerebral circulation and metabolism in man. *Anesthesiology*. 1972;36:69–75.
256. Pfenninger E, Dick W, Ahnefeld FW. The influence of ketamine on both normal and raised intracranial pressure of artificially ventilated animals. *Eur J Anaesthesiol*. 1985;2:297–307.
257. Friesen RH, Thieme RE, Honda AT, et al. Changes in anterior fontanel pressure in preterm neonates receiving isoflurane, halothane, fentanyl, or ketamine. *Anesth Analg*. 1987;66:431–434.
258. Mayberg TS, Lam AM, Matta BF, et al. Ketamine does not increase cerebral blood flow velocity or intracranial pressure during isoflurane/nitrous oxide anesthesia in patients undergoing craniotomy. *Anesth Analg*. 1995;81:84–89.
259. Albanese J, Arnaud S, Rey M, et al. Ketamine decreases intracranial pressure and electroencephalographic activity in traumatic brain injury patients during propofol sedation. *Anesthesiology*. 1997;87:1328–1334.
260. Nagels W, Demeyere R, Van Hemelrijck J, et al. Evaluation of the neuroprotective effects of S(+)-ketamine during open-heart surgery. *Anesth Analg*. 2004;98:1595–1603.
261. Ferrer-Allado T, Brechner VL, Diamond A, et al. Ketamine-induced electroconvulsive phenomena in the human limbic and thalamic regions. *Anesthesiology*. 1973;38:333–344.
262. Celesia GG, Chen RC, Bamforth BJ. Effects of ketamine in epilepsy. *Neurology*. 1975;25:169–172.
263. Modica PA, Tempelhoff R, White PF. Pro- and anticonvulsant effects of anesthetics (part II). *Anesth Analg*. 1990;70:433–444.
264. Schubert A, Licine MG, Lineberry PJ. The effect of ketamine on human somatosensory evoked potentials and its modification by nitrous oxide. *Anesthesiology*. 1990;72:33–39.
265. Tweed WA, Minuck MS, Mymin D. Circulatory response to ketamine anesthesia. *Anesthesiology*. 1972;37:613–619.
266. Balfors E, Haggmark S, Nyhman H, et al. Droperidol inhibits the effects of intravenous ketamine on central hemodynamics and myocardial O2 consumption in patients with generalized atherosclerotic disease. *Anesth Analg*. 1983;62:193–197.
267. Hickey PR, Hansen DD, Cramoline GM, et al. Pulmonary and systemic hemodynamic responses to ketamine in infants with normal and elevated pulmonary vascular resistance. *Anesthesiology*. 1985;62:287–293.
268. Hoffman WE, Pelligrino D, Werner C, et al. Ketamine decreases plasma catecholamines and improves outcome from incomplete cerebral ischemia in rats. *Anesthesiology*. 1992;76:755–762.
269. Lundy PM, Lockwood PA, Thompson G, et al. Differential effects of ketamine isomers on neuronal and extraneuronal catecholamine uptake mechanisms. *Anesthesiology*. 1986;64:359–363.
270. Yli-Hankala A, Kirvela M, Randell T, et al. Ketamine anaesthesia in a patient with septic shock. *Acta Anaesthesiol Scand*. 1992;36:483–485.
271. Longnecker DE, Sturgill BC. Influence of anesthetic agents on survival following hemorrhage. *Anesthesiology*. 1976;45:516–521.
272. Weiskopf RB, Townley MI, Riordan KK, et al. Comparison of cardiopulmonary responses to graded hemorrhage during enflurane, halothane, isoflurane and ketamine anesthesia. *Anesth Analg*. 1981;60:481–492.

273. Koehntop DE, Liao JC, Van Bergen FH. Effects of pharmacologic alterations of adrenergic mechanisms by cocaine, tropolone, aminophylline and ketamine on epinephrine-induced arrhythmias during halothane nitrous oxide anesthesia. *Anesthesiology.* 1977;46:83–93.
274. Wong DHW, Jenkins LC. An experimental study of the mechanism of action of ketamine on the central nervous system. *Can Anaesth Soc J.* 1974;21:57–67.
275. Stanley TH. Blood pressure and pulse rate responses to ketamine during general anesthesia. *Anesthesiology.* 1973;39:648–649.
276. Traber DL, Wilson RD, Priano LL. Blockade of the hypertensive response to ketamine. *Anesth Analg.* 1970;49:420–426.
277. Baraka A, Harrison T, Kachachi T. Catecholamine levels after ketamine anesthesia in man. *Anesth Analg.* 1973;52:198–200.
278. Schwartz DA, Horwitz LD. Effects of ketamine on left ventricular performance. *J Pharmacol Exp Ther.* 1975;194:410–414.
279. Soliman MG, Brinale GF, Kuster G. Response to hypercapnia under ketamine anesthesia. *Can Anaesth Soc J.* 1975;22:486–494.
280. Taylor PA, Towey RM. Depression of laryngeal reflexes during ketamine anesthesia. *Br Med J.* 1971;2:688–689.
281. Sarma VJ. Use of ketamine in acute severe asthma. *Acta Anaesthesiol Scand.* 1992;36:106–107.
282. Laxenaire MC, Moneret-Vautrin D, Vervloet D. The French experience of anaphylactoid reactions. *Int Anesthesiol Clin.* 1985;23:145–160.
283. Nakagawa T, Hirakata H, Sato M et al. Ketamine suppresses platelet aggregation possibly by suppressed inositol triphosphate formation and subsequent suppression of cytosolic calcium increase. *Anesthesiology.* 2002;96:1147–1152.
284. Bowdle TA, Radant AD, Cowley DS, et al. Psychedelic effects of ketamine in healthy volunteers: relationship to steady-state plasma concentrations. *Anesthesiology.* 1998;88:82–88.
285. Fine J, Finestone SC. Sensory disturbances following ketamine anesthesia: recurrent hallucinations. *Anesth Analg.* 1973;52:428–430.
286. Meyers EF, Charles P. Prolonged adverse reactions to ketamine in children. *Anesthesiology.* 1978;49:39–40.
287. Modvig KM, Nielsen SF. Psychological changes in children after anesthesia: a comparison between halothane and ketamine. *Acta Anaesthesiol Scand.* 1977;21:541–544.
288. Moretti RJ, Hassan SZ, Goodman LI, et al. Comparison of ketamine and thiopental in healthy volunteers: effects on mental status, mood, and personality. *Anesth Analg.* 1984;63:1087–1096.
289. Cartwright PD, Pingel SM. Midazolam and diazepam in ketamine anaesthesia. *Anaesthesia.* 1984;59:439–442.
290. Toft P, Romer U. Comparison of midazolam and diazepam to supplement total intravenous anaesthesia with ketamine for endoscopy. *Can J Anaesth.* 1987;34:466–469.
291. Erbguth PH, Reiman B, Klein RL. The influence of chlorpromazine, diazepam and droperidol on emergence from ketamine. *Anesth Analg.* 1972;51:693–700.
292. Hejja P, Galloon S. A consideration of ketamine dreams. *Can Anaesth Soc J.* 1975;22:100–105.
293. Bidwai AV, Stanley HT, Graves CL, et al. The effects of ketamine on cardiovascular dynamics during halothane and enflurane anesthesia. *Anesth Analg.* 1975;54(5):588–592.
294. Fragen RJ, Avram MJ. Comparative pharmacology of drugs used for the induction of anesthesia. In: Stoelting RK, Barash PG, Gallagher TJ, eds. Advances in anesthesia. Chicago, IL: Year Book Medical Publishers; 1986:103–132.
295. Johnston RR, Miller RD, Way WL. The interaction of ketamine with d-tubocurarine, pancuronium, and succinylcholine in man. *Anesth Analg.* 1974;53:496–501.
296. Molojavyi A, Preckel B, Cofmere T, et al. Effects of ketamine and its isomers on ischemic preconditioning in the isolated rat heart. *Anesthesiology.* 2001;94:623–628.
297. Mullenheim J, Rulands R, Wietschorke T, et al. Late preconditioning is blocked by racemic ketamine, but not by S(+)-ketamine. *Anesth Analg.* 2001;93:265–270.
298. Bloor BC, Ward DS, Belleville JP, et al. Effects of intravenous dexmedetomidine in humans. II. Hemodynamic changes. *Anesthesiology.* 1992;77:1134–1142.
299. Sandler AN. The role of clonidine and alpha2-agonists for postoperative analgesia. *Can J Anaesth.* 1996;43:1191–1194.
300. Nelson LE, Lu J, Guo T, et al. The alpha2 adrenoreceptor agonist dexmedetomidine converges on an endogenous sleep-promoting pathway to exert its sedative effects. *Anesthesiology.* 2003;98:428–436.
301. Scheinin H, Aantaa R, Anttila M, et al. Reversal of the sedative and sympatholytic effects of dexmedetomidine with a specific alpha2 adrenoceptor antagonist atipamezole. A pharmacodynamic and kinetic study in healthy volunteers. *Anesthesiology.* 1998;89:574–584.
302. Shelly MP. Dexmedetomidine: a real innovation or more of the same? *Br J Anaesth.* 2001;87:677–678.
303. Buhrer M, Mappes A, Lauber R, et al. Dexmedetomidine decreases thiopental dose requirement and alters distribution pharmacokinetics. *Anesthesiology.* 1994;80:1216–1221.
304. Jalonen J, Hynynen M, Kuitunen A, et al. Dexmedetomidine as an anesthetic adjunct in coronary artery bypass grafting. *Anesthesiology.* 1997;86:331–345.
305. Kamibayashi T, Maze M. Clinical uses of alpha2-adrenergic agonists. *Anesthesiology.* 2000;93:1345–1349.
306. Segal IS, Vickery RG, Walton JK, et al. Dexmedetomidine diminishes halothane anesthetic requirements in rats through a postsynaptic alpha 2 adrenergic receptor. *Anesthesiology.* 1988;69:818–823.
307. Aantaa R, Maakola ML, Kallio A, et al. Reduction of the minimum alveolar concentration of isoflurane by dexmedetomidine. *Anesthesiology.* 1997;86:1055–1060.
308. Ramsay MAE, Luterman DL. Dexmedetomidine as a total intravenous anesthetic agent. *Anesthesiology.* 2004;101:787–790.
309. Levanen J, Makela ML, Scheinin H. Dexmedetomidine premedication attenuates ketamine-induced cardiostimulatory effects and postanesthetic delirium. *Anesthesiology.* 1995;82:1117–1125.
310. Memiş D, Turan A, Karamanlioğlu B, et al. Adding dexmedetomidine to lidocaine for intravenous regional anesthesia. *Anesth Analg.* 2004;98(3):835–840.
311. Talke P, Tayefeh F, Sessler DI, et al. Dexmedetomidine does not alter the sweating threshold, but comparably and linearly decreases the vasoconstriction and shivering thresholds. *Anesthesiology.* 1997;87:835–841.
312. Ingersoll-Weng E, Manecke GR, Thistlethwaite PA. Dexmedetomidine and cardiac arrest. *Anesthesiology.* 2004;100:738–739.
313. Hsu Y-W, Cortinez LI, Robertson KM, et al. Dexmedetomidine pharmacodynamics: part I. Crossover comparison of the respiratory effects of dexmedetomidine and remifentanil in healthy volunteers. *Anesthesiology.* 2004;101:1066–1076.
314. Venn RM, Bradshaw CJ, Spencer R, et al. Preliminary UK experience of dexmedetomidine, a novel agent for postoperative sedation in the intensive care unit. *Anaesthesia.* 1999;54:1136–1142.
315. Cortés R, Palacios JM. Muscarinic cholinergic receptor subtypes in the rat brain. I. Quantitative autoradiographic studies. *Brain Res.* 1986;362:227–238.
316. Putcha L, Cintrón NM, Tsui J, et al. Pharmacokinetics and oral bioavailability of scopolamine in normal subjects. *Pharm Res.* 1989;6:481–485.
317. Reis E. Scopolamine-morphine anesthesia. *Cal State J Med.* 1906;4:109–110.
318. Garde JF, Aston R, Endler GC, et al. Racial mydriatic response to belladonna premedication. *Anesth Analg.* 1978;57:572–576.

CHAPTER 6

Pain Physiology

Hui Yang • Bihua Bie • Mohamed A. Naguib

Pain is a complex phenomenon that includes both sensory-discriminative and motivational-affective components.[1] The sensory-discriminative component of pain depends on ascending projections of tracts (including the spinothalamic and trigeminothalamic tracts) to the cerebral cortex. Sensory processing at these higher levels results in the perception of the quality of pain (pricking, burning, aching), the location of the painful stimulus, and the intensity of the pain. The motivational-affective responses to painful stimuli include attention and arousal, somatic and autonomic reflexes, endocrine responses, and emotional changes. These account collectively for the unpleasant nature of painful stimuli.

The definition of pain as proposed by the International Association for the Study of Pain emphasizes the complex nature of pain as a physical, emotional, and psychological condition. It is recognized that pain does not necessarily correlate with the degree of tissue damage that is present. Failure to appreciate the complex factors that affect the experience of pain and reliance entirely on physical examination findings and laboratory tests may lead to misunderstanding and inadequate treatment of pain. Oversimplified anatomic concepts predispose to simplistic therapeutic interventions, such as neurectomy or rhizotomy, that may intensify pain or create new and often more distressing pain.

The nociceptive system is highly complex and adaptable. Sensitivity of most of its components can be reset by a variety of physiologic and pathologic conditions. Innovative medications are being developed that target the causes of pain by actions on pain transduction, transmission, interpretation, and modulation in both the peripheral nervous system (PNS) and the central nervous system (CNS).

Societal Impact of Pain

Pain is one of the most common reasons for visiting a physician. It is estimated that chronic pain may affect as many as 40% of the adult population.[2] The prevalence of low back pain ranges from 8% to 37% and is particularly prominent in patients between 45 and 60 years of age. It is estimated that 40 million persons experience musculoskeletal pain conditions.[3] Patients with malignant disease often experience increasing pain as their disease progresses. The costs to society related to chronic pain are immense with an estimate that the annual cost attributed to back pain, migraine headache, and arthritis of 40 billion dollars, excluding the costs of surgical procedures to treat pain and lost workdays.[1]

Neurobiology of Pain

The experience of pain involves a series of complex neurophysiologic processes, collectively termed ***nociception***, with four distinct components: transduction, transmission, modulation, and perception. Transduction is the process by which a noxious stimulus (e.g., heat, cold, mechanical distortion) is converted to an electrical impulse in sensory nerve endings. Transmission is the conduction of these electrical impulses to the CNS with the major connections for these nerves being in the dorsal horn of the spinal cord and thalamus with projections to the cingulate, insular, and somatosensory cortices. Modulation of pain is the process of altering pain transmission. It is likely that both inhibitory and excitatory mechanisms modulate pain (nociceptive) impulse transmission in the PNS and CNS. Pain perception is thought to be mediated through the thalamus acting as the central relay station for incoming pain signals and the primary somatosensory cortex serving for discrimination of specific sensory experiences.[1] Pain may occur in the absence of the occurrence of these four steps. For example, pain from trigeminal neuralgia occurs in the absence of transduction of a chemical stimulus at a nociceptor reflecting axonal discharges initiated at the site of a compressed or demyelinated nerve. Modulation of pain impulses may not occur if specific nervous system tracts are injured. For example, phantom limb pain occurs in the absence of nociception or nociceptors (pain receptors).

Peripheral Nerve Physiology of Pain

Nociceptors (Pain Receptors)

Nociceptors are a specialized class of primary afferents that respond to intense, noxious stimuli in skin, muscles, joints, viscera, and vasculature. Nociceptors are distinctive in that they typically respond to the multiple energy forms that produce injury (thermal, mechanical, and chemical stimuli) and provide information to the CNS regarding the location and intensity of noxious stimuli. In normal tissues, nociceptors are inactive until they are stimulated by sufficient energy to reach the stimulus (resting) threshold. Thus, nociceptors prevent random signal propagation (screening function) to the CNS for the interpretation of pain.

Specific types of nociceptors react to different types of stimuli. Generally, unmyelinated C-fiber afferents (conduction velocity <2 m per second) have receptive field of about 100 mm^2 in human and signal the burning pain from intense heat stimuli applied to the glabrous skin as well as the pain from sustained pressure. Usually, the receptive field of a C-fiber afferent is about near 100 mm^2 in human. Two types of myelinated A-fiber nociceptive afferents (conduction velocity >2 m per second) exist. Type I fibers (including Aβ and some Aδ fibers) are typically high-threshold mechanoreceptors and are usually responsive to heat and mechanical and chemical stimuli and may therefore be referred to as ***polymodal nociceptors***. Type II fibers (Aδ fibers with lower conduction velocity of about 15 m per second) have no demonstrable response to mechanical stimuli and are thought to signal first pain sensation from heat stimuli. Pain from both chemical and cold stimuli is transduced by nociceptors whose pain signals are conducted toward the CNS via both myelinated and unmyelinated nerve fibers.

Sensitization of Nociceptors

Sensitization of nociceptors refers to the increased responsiveness of peripheral neurons responsible for pain transmission to heat, cold, mechanical, or chemical stimulation. Sensitization of nociceptors frequently occurs and is attributable to the release of inflammatory mediators and adaptation of signaling pathways in primary sensory neurons induced by noxious stimuli. In the majority of cases of acute inflammation, the process naturally resolves as tissues heal and peripheral sensitization diminishes and nociceptors return to their original resting threshold. Chronic pain, however, occurs if the conditions associated with inflammation do not resolve, resulting in sensitization of peripheral and central pain signaling pathway and increased pain sensations to normally painful stimuli (***hyperalgesia***) and the perception of pain sensations in response to normally nonpainful stimuli (***allodynia***).

Numerous endogenous chemicals, neurotransmitters, peptides (such as substance P, calcitonin gene–related peptide or CGRP, bradykinin), eicosanoids and related lipids (prostaglandins, thromboxanes, leukotrienes, endocannabinoids), neurotrophins, cytokines, and chemokines, as well as extracellular proteases and protons, significantly contribute to the process of nociception and neuronal sensitization during peripheral inflammation and nerve injury.[4] Most of these mediators are not constitutively stored but rather are synthesized de novo at the site of injury. The agents contribute to pain via two principal mechanisms. Some of these agents (e.g., bradykinin, protons, prostaglandin E2, purines, and cytokines) can directly activate nociceptors and/or induce the sensitization of the nociceptor response to painful stimuli, whereas others (e.g., serotonin, histamine, arachidonic acid metabolites, and cytokines) may activate the inflammatory cells, which in turn release cytokines, thereby leading to sensitization. The variety of chemical mediators released during inflammation can potentiate nociceptor responses (Fig. 6-1).

A variety of receptors and ion channels have been identified on dorsal root ganglion neurons and on peripheral terminals of nociceptive afferent fibers. These receptors, including purinergic,[5] metabotropic glutamatergic, tachykinin,[6] TRPV1 receptor and neurotrophic receptors, and ion channels (e.g., Nav1.8) in primary sensory neurons may also undergo significant adaptation after noxious stimuli, significantly lowering the firing thresholds of nociceptors and critically contributing to the induction and maintenance of neuronal sensitization, which manifest as allodynia and hyperalgesia.[7]

Primary Hyperalgesia and Secondary Hyperalgesia

In general, tissue injury and inflammation may activate a cascade of events leading to enhanced pain in response to a given noxious stimulus, termed *hyperalgesia* (e.g., a mild pinprick causing severe pain). Hyperalgesia is defined as a leftward shift of the stimulus–response function that relates magnitude of pain to stimulus intensity. Hyperalgesia is a consistent feature that appears following somatic and visceral tissue injury and inflammation. Hyperalgesia at the original site of injury is termed ***primary hyperalgesia***, and hyperalgesia in the uninjured skin surrounding the injury is termed ***secondary hyperalgesia***. Primary hyperalgesia is usually manifested as decreased pain threshold, increased response to suprathreshold stimuli, spontaneous pain, and expansion of receptive field. Whereas primary hyperalgesia is characterized by the presence of enhanced pain from heat *and* mechanical stimuli, secondary hyperalgesia is characterized by enhanced pain response to *only* mechanical stimuli. It is usually accepted that interaction between the proinflammatory mediators and their receptors in nociceptors leads to the induction of primary hyperalgesia, and sensitization of central neuronal circuits

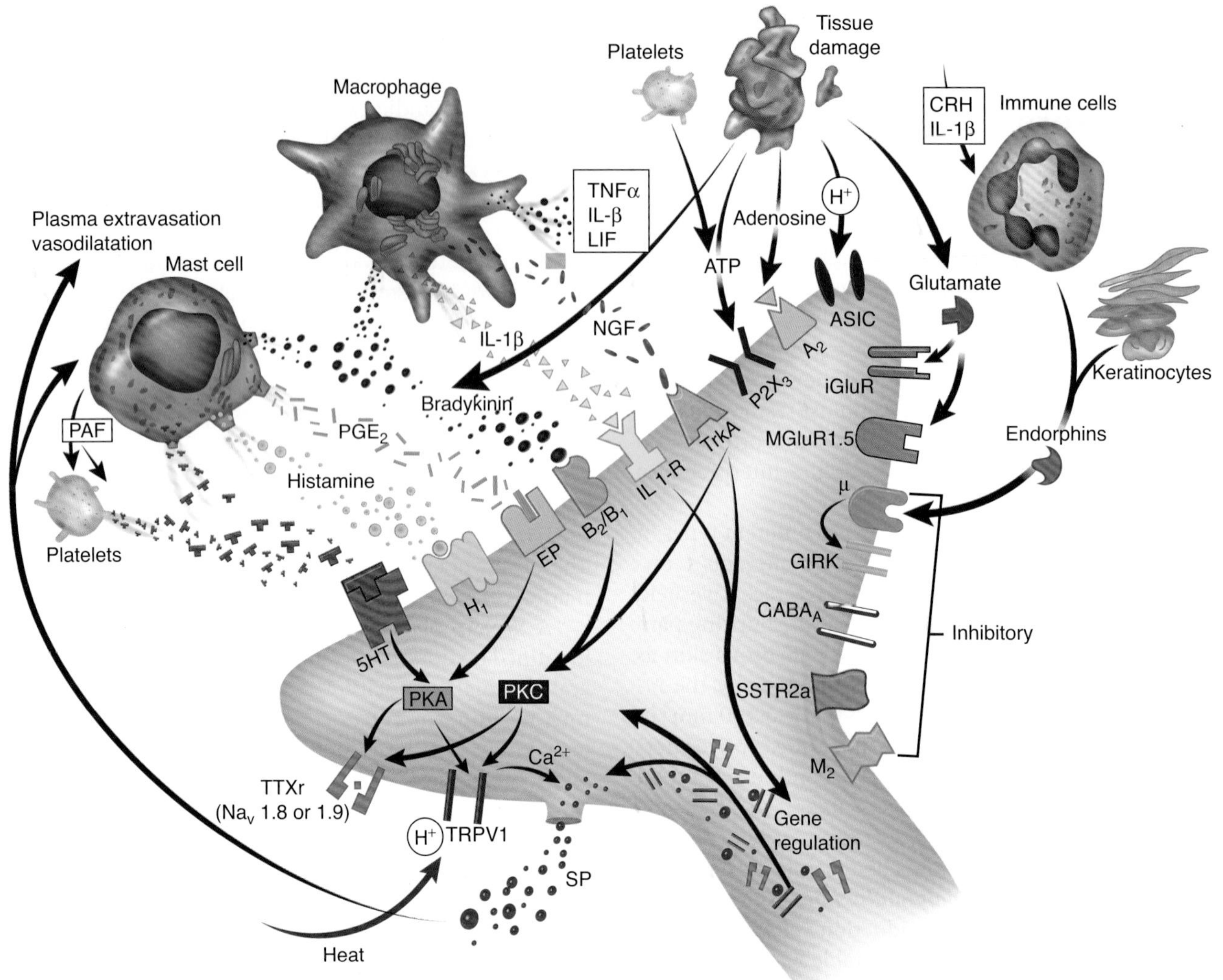

FIGURE 6-1 Cellular mechanism underlying nociceptor sensitization induced by peripheral inflammation. Activated immune cells (macrophages, mast cells, and other immune cells) and injured cells release numerous chemicals, which may directly or indirectly sensitize the peripheral nerve terminals. A_2, adenosine A_2 receptor; ASIC, acid-sensing ion channel; B_2/B_1, bradykinin receptor B_2/B_1; CRH, corticotrophin-releasing hormone; EP, E-prostanoid receptor; GIRK, G-protein-coupled inward rectifying potassium channel; H_1, histamine H_1 receptor; iGluR, ionotropic glutamate receptor; IL-1β, interleukin-1β; MGluR, metabotropic glutamate receptor; NGF, nerve growth factor; $P2X_3$, purinergic receptor P2X ligand-gated ion channel 3; PAF, platelet-activating factor; PGE_2, prostaglandin E_2; PKA, protein kinase A; PKC, protein kinase C; SP, substance P; SSTR2a, somatostatin receptor 2a; SP, substance P; TNFα, tumor necrosis factor alpha; TrkA, tyrosine kinase receptor A; TRPV1, transient receptor potential vanilloid receptor 1; TTXr, tetrodotoxin-resistant sodium channel; μ, μ opioid receptor; M_2, muscarinic receptor; 5HT, serotonin; LIF, leukemia inhibitory factor. (From McMahon S, Koltzenburg M. *Wall and Melzack's Textbook of Pain.* 5th ed. Philadelphia, PA: Churchill Livingstone; 2006.)

processing nociceptive information may account for the secondary hyperalgesia after tissue injury.

Central Nervous System Physiology

Pain transmission from peripheral nociceptors to the spinal cord and higher structures of the CNS is a dynamic process involving several pathways, numerous receptors, neurotransmitters, and secondary messengers. The spinal dorsal horn functions as a relay center for nociceptive and other sensory activity. The ascending pathways convey pain-related activity to the brainstem and forebrain in humans. Forebrain somatosensory cortex (SI and SII) accounts for the perception of sensory-discriminative of peripheral painful stimuli (i.e., the location and intensity of pain). Brain regions in the limbic cortex and thalamus account for the perception of motivational-affective components of pain. Descending projections originating from periaqueductal gray–rostral ventromedial medulla (PAG–RVM) system may either depress or facilitate the integration of painful information in the spinal dorsal horn (Fig. 6-2).

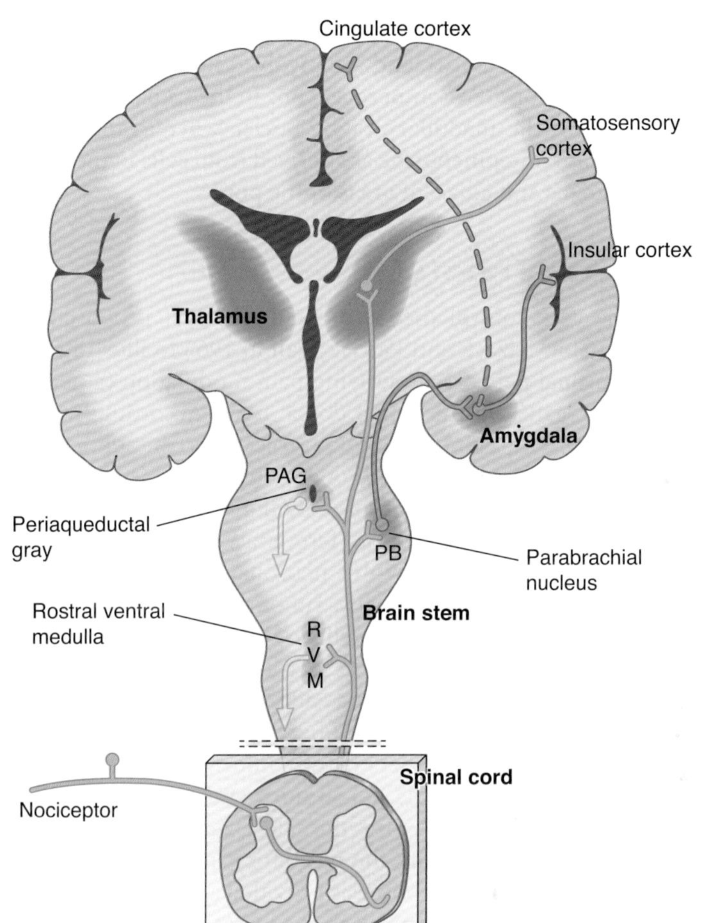

FIGURE 6-2 The projection pathway for the transmission of pain information to the brain. Primary afferent nociceptors convey noxious information to projection neurons within the dorsal horn of the spinal cord. A subset of these projection neurons transmits information to the somatosensory cortex via the thalamus, providing information about the location and intensity of the painful stimulus. Other projection neurons engage the cingulate and insular cortices via connections in the brainstem (parabrachial nucleus) and amygdala, contributing to the affective component of the pain experience. This ascending information also accesses neurons of the rostral ventral medulla and midbrain periaqueductal gray to engage descending feedback systems that modulate the transmission of nociceptive information through the spinal cord. (Modified from Basbaum AI, Bautista DM, Scherrer G, et al. Cellular and molecular mechanisms of pain. *Cell.* 2009;139[2]:267–284.)

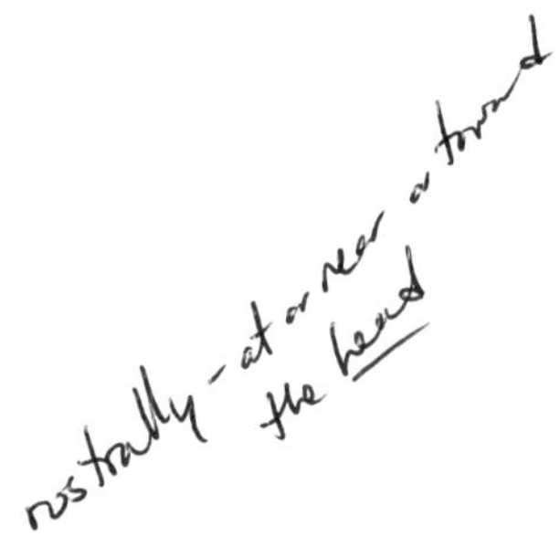

Dorsal Horn: The Relay Center for Nociception

Afferent fibers from peripheral nociceptors enter the spinal cord in the dorsal root, ascend or descend several segments in the Lissauer tract, and synapse with the dorsal horn neurons for the primary integration of peripheral nociceptive information. The dorsal horn contains four major neuronal components: the central terminals of primary afferent axons; intrinsic neurons, which terminate locally or extend into other spinal segments; projection neurons that pass rostrally in the white matter to reach various parts of the brain; and descending axons that extend caudally from several brain regions and terminate in the dorsal horn where they play an important role in modulating the integration of nociceptive information.

The central terminals of primary afferents occupy highly ordered spatial locations in the dorsal horn. The dorsal horn consists of six laminae (Fig. 6-3). Laminae I (marginal layer) and II (substantia gelatinosa) are often referred to as the ***superficial dorsal horn*** and are the primary regions where afferent C fibers synapse on

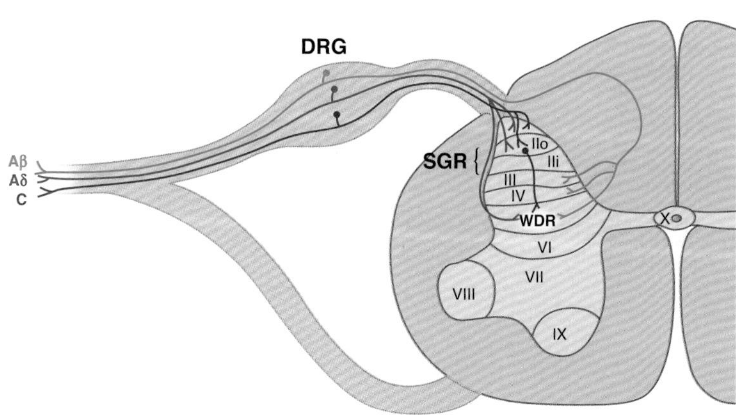

FIGURE 6-3 Schematic representation of the spinal projections of primary afferent fibers. In general, unmyelinated C fibers synapse with the interneurons in laminae I (marginal layer) and II (substantia gelatinosa of Rolando [SGR]). Cutaneous Aδ fibers usually project to laminae I, II, and V, and Aβ fibers primarily terminate in laminae III, IV, and V in dorsal horn. Large-diameter myelinated fibers innervating muscles, joint, and viscera may also terminate in laminae I, IV–VII, and the ventral horn. Second-order wide dynamic range (WDR) neurons are located in lamina V and receive input from nociceptive and nonnociceptive neurons. DRG, dorsal root ganglia.

second-order neurons. Lamina I contains both projection neurons and interneurons, and all of the neurons in lamina II are small interneurons. Lamina V is the site of second-order wide dynamic range (WDR) and nociceptive-specific (NS) neurons that receive input from nociceptive and nonnociceptive neurons. The NS neurons respond only to noxious stimuli in their peripheral environment, whereas WDR neurons respond to innocuous and noxious stimuli of many types, providing the neuronal mechanism for encoding of the intensity of stimuli. Both types of neurons are believed to be important in the perception of nociceptive information. Myelinated fibers innervating muscles and viscera terminate in laminae I, IV to VII, and the ventral horn, and the unmyelinated fibers from these organs mostly terminate in laminae I, II, and V as well as X.

Interneurons make up the great majority of the neuronal population throughout the dorsal horn. Many dorsal horn interneurons have axons that remain in the same lamina as the cell body, and they also give rise to axons that extend into other laminae. Interneurons in the dorsal horn can be divided into two main functional types: inhibitory cells, which use GABA and/or glycine as their principal transmitter, and excitatory glutamatergic cells. Interneurons in dorsal horn are important for integration and modulation of incoming nociceptive information.

Projection neurons with axons that project to the brain are present in relatively large numbers in lamina I and are scattered through the deeper part of the dorsal horn (laminae III to VI) and the ventral horn. Both the lamina I and the laminae III and IV projection neurons that express the NK1 receptor are heavily innervated by substance P–containing primary afferents. Those in lamina I, together with some of the projection cells in deeper laminae, have axons that cross the midline and ascend to a variety of supraspinal targets including the thalamus, the midbrain PAG, lateral parabrachial area of the pons, and various parts of the medullary reticular formation.

Two types of descending monoaminergic (serotoninergic and norepinephrinergic) axons project from the brain throughout the dorsal horn, mostly terminating in laminae I and II, and are involved in descending pain modulation. Serotoninergic axons in the spinal cord originate in the medullary raphe nuclei, whereas those that contain norepinephrine are derived from cells in the locus ceruleus and adjacent areas of the pons.

Gate Theory

The gate control theory of pain was first proposed by Ronald Melzack and Patrick Wall in 1965 to illustrate the neuronal network underlying pain modulation (a neurologic "gate") in the spinal dorsal horn. According to this theory, painful information is projected to the supraspinal brain regions if the gate is open, whereas painful stimulus is not felt if the gate is closed by the simultaneous inhibitory impulses (Fig. 6-4). Here is a commonly used example to describe how this neuronal network modulates pain transmission. Usually, rubbing the skin of painful area seems to somehow relieve the pain associated with a bumped elbow. In this case, rubbing the skin activates large-diameter myelinated afferents (Aβ), which are "faster" than Aδ fibers or C fibers conveying painful information. These Aβ fibers deliver information about pressure and touch to the dorsal horn and override some of the pain messages ("closes the gate") carried by the Aδ and C fibers by activating the inhibitory interneurons in the dorsal horn. This hypothesis provided a practical theoretical basis for some approaches such as massage, transcutaneous nerve stimulation, and acupuncture to effectively treat pain in clinical patients.

Central Sensitization of Dorsal Neurons

Peripheral inflammation and nerve injury could alter the synaptic efficacy and induce central sensitization in the dorsal horn neurons and is considered a fundamental mechanism underlying the induction and maintenance of chronic pain. This central sensitization takes a number of different and distinct forms.

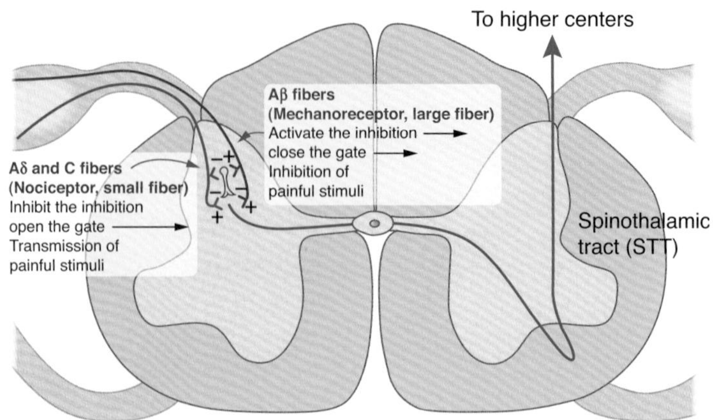

FIGURE 6-4 Illustration of gate theory for pain modulation in spinal dorsal horn. Lightly rubbing the skin of a painful, injured area seems to somehow relieve the painful sensation. Large-diameter myelinated afferents (Aβ) conveying pressure and touch information have "faster" conduction speed than Aδ fibers or C fibers conveying painful information to the dorsal horn. Thus, the application of light peripheral mechanical stimuli resulting in excitation of Aβ fibers can activate the inhibitory interneurons in the dorsal horn and thus close the "gate" to the simultaneous incoming pain signals carried by Aδ and C fibers. While the gate control theory is overly simplistic, it remains a valid conceptual framework for understanding pain and pain-related experiences.

One form of central sensitization is wind-up of dorsal horn neurons, an activity-dependent progressive increase in the response of neurons over the course of a train of inputs. Repetitive discharge of primary afferent nociceptors results in a co-release with glutamate of peptidergic neuromodulators such as substance P and CGRP from the nociceptor central terminals in dorsal horn. Temporal summation of these peptide-mediated slow excitatory postsynaptic potentials (EPSPs) may activate NMDA receptor, by removing Mg^{2+} suppression of the channel, and increase the excitability of dorsal horn neurons. A behavioral correlate of wind-up can be produced in humans by repeated peripheral noxious heat or mechanical stimuli, where the pain increases with each successive stimulus even though the stimulus intensity does not change.[8] After peripheral nerve injury, light touch can produce pain (allodynia) and repeated light touch can produce progressively increasing pain (summation).

The second form of central sensitization is a heterosynaptic activity-dependent plasticity that outlasts the initiating stimulus for tens of minutes. After the induction of this form of activity-dependent central sensitization by a brief (as short as 10 to 20 seconds), intense nociceptor-conditioning stimulus, normally, subliminal/subthreshold inputs begin to activate dorsal horn neurons as a result of an increase in synaptic efficacy. This NMDA receptor-mediated increase of synaptic efficacy occurs not only in those nociceptor central terminal synapses activated by the conditioning or initiating stimulus but also the synapses not activated by the conditioning or initiating stimulus (Fig. 6-5). For example, low-threshold sensory fibers activated by innocuous stimuli such as light touch can, after the induction of the heterosynaptic central sensitization, activate normally high–threshold nociceptive neurons, producing allodynia.

Other forms of central sensitization include long-term potentiation, transcription-dependent central sensitization, loss of inhibition, and rearrangement of synaptic contacts. The former refers to the fact that brief duration, high-frequency primary afferent stimulation does induce a potentiation of AMPA receptor–mediated responses at homosynapses on to second-order neurons. Peripheral noxious stimuli may produce transcriptional changes of several proteins critically involved in pain transmission (e.g., brain-derived neurotrophic factor [BDNF] and cytokines) in primary sensory and dorsal horn neurons, altering their function and facilitating pain transmission for prolonged periods. Activation of Aδ primary afferents may also induce long-term depression of transmission at primary afferent synapses on to inhibitory dorsal horn neurons, contributing to the augmentation of nociceptive information. Following a lesion to a peripheral nerve, the central axons of injured myelinated Aβ fibers sprout from their normal termination site in the deeper laminae (laminae II and IV) into lamina II of the dorsal horn, contributing to nerve injury–induced tactile allodynia.

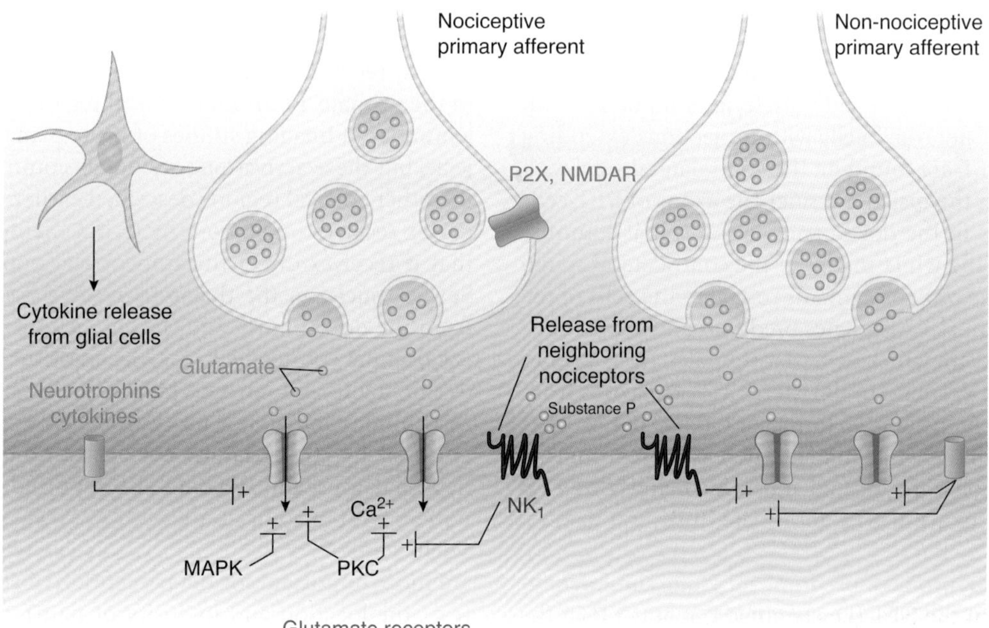

FIGURE 6-5 The synaptic mechanism underlying peripheral nociceptive stimuli-induced persistent heterosynaptic potentiation of dorsal horn neurons. Transmitters and mediators released from primary afferents and surrounding microglial cells, including substance P, neurotrophins, and cytokines, may act at a distance on dorsal horn neurons to produce long-lasting heterosynaptic potentiation of glutamatergic transmission. Note that both inputs from nociceptors and nonnociceptors may be potentiated. MAPK, mitogen-activated protein kinase; P2X, purinoreceptor; PKC, protein kinase C; NK_1, Neurokinin 1 (substance P receptor).

It is notable that accumulating evidence suggests that a critical role is played by microglia-mediated neuroinflammation in the dorsal horn plasticity that leads to neuropathic pain.[9]

Ascending Pathway for Pain Transmission

Ascending pathways from the spinal cord to sites in the brainstem and thalamus are important for the perception and integration of nociceptive information. The major ascending pathways important for pain include the spinothalamic tract (STT, direct projections to the thalamus), spinomedullary and spinobulbar projections (direct projections to homeostatic control regions in the medulla and brainstem), and spinohypothalamic tract (SHT, direct projections to the hypothalamus and ventral forebrain). Some indirect projections, such as the dorsal column system and the spinocervicothalamic pathway, also exist to forward nociceptive information to the forebrain through the brainstem. Similar pathways originating from the medulla trigeminal sensory nuclei also exist to process the nociceptive information from the facial structures.

Among these pathways, the STT is the most closely associated with pain, temperature, and itch sensation. Retrograde tracing studies demonstrate that the fibers traveling in the STT originate in the spinal dorsal horn neurons in lamina I (receiving input from small-diameter Aδ and C primary afferent fibers), laminae IV and V (receiving input primarily from large-diameter Aβ fibers from skin), and laminae VII and VIII (receiving convergent input from large-diameter skin and muscle, joint inputs). About 85% to 90% of neuronal cells with projections extending through the STT are found on the contralateral side, with 10% to 15% on the ipsilateral side. The axons of STT cells generally cross in the dorsal and ventral spinal commissures to reach the white matter of the contralateral spinal cord within one or two segments rostral to the cells of origin. The lateral STT originates predominantly from lamina I cells, and the anterior STT originates from deeper laminae V and VII cells. In the lateral STT, the axons from caudal body regions tend to be located more laterally (i.e., superficially) in the white matter, whereas those from rostral body regions are located more medially (closer to midline). The axons of STT terminate in several distinct regions of the thalamus.

Spinobulbar projections originate from similar neurons as those in the STT (i.e., laminae I, V, and VII in the spinal dorsal horn). Spinal projections to the medulla are bilateral, and those to the pons and mesencephalon have a contralateral dominance. Ascending spinobulbar projections terminate mainly in four major areas of the brainstem, including the regions of catecholamine cell groups (A1–A7), the parabrachial nucleus, PAG, and the brainstem reticular formation. Spinal projections to the brainstem are important for the integration of nociceptive activity with processes that subserve homeostasis and behavior.

The spinohypothalamic tract (SHT) originates bilaterally from cells in laminae I, V, VII, and X over the entire length of the spinal cord. The SHT axons often have connections with the contralateral diencephalon, decussate in the optic chiasm, and then descend ipsilaterally through the hypothalamus and as far as the brainstem. The SHT appears to be important for autonomic, neuroendocrine, and emotional aspects of pain.

Supraspinal Modulation of Nociception

Several brain areas have been recently defined using human brain imaging studies as key supraspinal regions involved in nociceptive perception. The most commonly activated regions during acute and chronic pain include SI, SII, anterior cingulate cortex (ACC), insular cortex (IC), prefrontal cortex, thalamus, and cerebellum (see Fig. 6-2). These brain regions form a cortical and subcortical network, which are critically involved in the formation of emotional aspects of pain and the central modulation of pain perception.

In primates, SI and SII receive noxious and innocuous somatosensory input from somatosensory thalamus.[10] Cingulate cortex receives input from medial thalamic nuclei that contain nociceptive neurons, including nucleus parafascicularis and the ventrocaudal part of nucleus medialis dorsalis, as well as from lateral thalamic regions. The IC also receives direct thalamocortical nociceptive input in the primate. Prefrontal cortical regions are activated in a number of imaging studies of acute pain in normal subjects, but these activations are not as common as those in the other cortical regions described earlier. The prefrontal cortex receives input from ACC, but there is no evidence that it receives direct thalamocortical nociceptive input. Several nuclei in the thalamus receive nociceptive input from the dorsal horn, and the cerebellum also has reciprocal spinal connectivity. Activation of the hypothalamus during acute and chronic pain is likely mediated by direct spinohypothalamic projections. Other subcortical regions, such as the striatum, nucleus accumbens, amygdala, hypothalamus, and PAG are also reported to be active in human pain imaging studies.

In general, somatosensory cortices (e.g., SI and SII) are more important for the perception of sensory features (e.g., the location and intensity of pain), whereas limbic and paralimbic regions (e.g., ACC and IC) are more important for the emotional and motivational aspects of pain.[11] Anesthetized humans, without conscious awareness of pain, still exhibit significant pain-evoked cerebellar activation, suggesting that pain-evoked cerebellar activity may be more important in regulation of afferent nociceptive activity than in the perception of pain.

Descending Pathways of Pain Modulation

The relationship between reported pain intensity and the peripheral stimulus that evokes the pain sensation depends on a host of variables, including the presence of other somatic stimuli and psychological factors such as arousal, attention, and expectation. Certain central mechanisms also exist to either impede or enhance the centripetal passage of nociceptive messages.[12] Evidence demonstrates that descending pathways originating from certain supraspinal regions may concurrently promote and suppress nociceptive transmission through the dorsal horn, termed the ***descending inhibition pathway*** (DI) and the descending facilitation pathway (DF).[12] Notably, there is no absolute, anatomic separation of substrates subserving these processes, and the stimulation of a single supraspinal structure may, via divergent actions of diverse transmitters and different receptor types, simultaneously trigger both DI and DF.

Electrical stimulation of the PAG and more rostral periventricular structures inhibits activity of nociceptive dorsal horn neurons and noxious stimulus-evoked reflexes and induces stimulation-evoked analgesia in rodents and humans. This establishes the PAG and the RVM regions of the brainstem as the critical brain regions underlying descending pain modulation (Fig. 6-6). PAG neurons receive direct or indirect inputs from several brain structures, including the amygdala, nucleus accumbens, hypothalamus and others, with ascending nociceptive afferents from the dorsal horn. The RVM includes the midline nucleus raphe magnus and the adjacent reticular formation that lies ventral to the nucleus reticularis gigantocellularis. The PAG and the adjacent nucleus cuneiformis are the major source of inputs to the RVM. The RVM receives input from serotonin-containing neurons of the dorsal raphe and neurotensinergic neurons of the PAG. The PAG–RVM connection is critical for pain modulation. The PAG projects only minimally to the spinal cord dorsal horn, and the pain-modulating action of the PAG on the spinal cord is relayed largely, if not exclusively, through the RVM.

Spinally projecting noradrenergic neurons of the pontine tegmentum contribute significantly to pain modulation. The locus ceruleus and the A5 and A7 noradrenergic cell groups are the major source of noradrenergic projections to the dorsal horn. Electrical stimulation in each of these regions produces behavioral analgesia and inhibition of dorsal horn neurons mediated by spinal α_2-adrenergic receptors.

The PAG–RVM system also contributes to hyperalgesia and allodynia in inflammatory and neuropathic models. Data clearly demonstrate that the PAG–RVM system can facilitate nociception in some but not all models. Discovering how this system is recruited to either inhibit

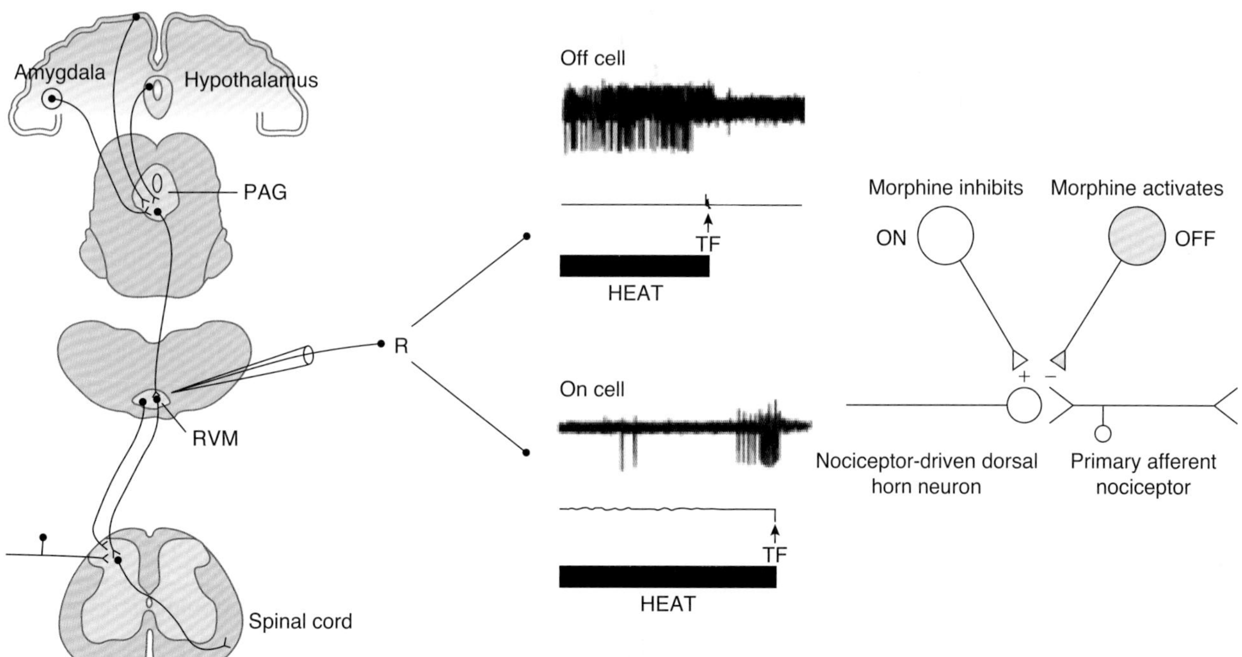

FIGURE 6-6 Properties of proposed medullary pain-modulating neurons. Single-unit extracellular recordings were performed by microelectrodes placed in the rostral ventromedial medulla (RVM) while peripheral noxious stimuli (heat) were applied. As shown by the oscilloscope sweeps, the firing of the off cell pauses just prior to the tail flick reflex (indicating pain sensation) in response to noxious heat, whereas the typical on-cell firing occurs before the tail flick. The right diagram illustrates that both on and off cells project to the spinal cord, where they exert bidirectional control over nociceptive dorsal horn neurons. (Modified from McMahon S, Koltzenburg M. *Wall and Melzack's Textbook of Pain*. 5th ed. Philadelphia, PA: Churchill Livingstone; 2006.)

or facilitate nociception under different conditions is an important challenge for our future understanding of descending modulation.

Electrical stimulation of the RVM at different currents can produce inhibition or facilitation of dorsal horn nociceptive processing, suggesting that there are parallel inhibitory and facilitatory output pathways from the RVM to spinal cord. In fact, there are three distinct populations of neurons in the RVM: those that discharge beginning just prior to the occurrence of withdrawal from noxious heat (on cells), those that stop firing just prior to a withdrawal reflex (off cells), and those that show no consistent changes in activity when withdrawal reflexes occur (neutral cells; see Fig. 6-6).[13] The on and off cells project specifically to laminae I, II, and V of the dorsal horn.[13] Activation of RVM neurons could inhibit nociceptive transmission in the dorsal horn via either direct inhibition of projection neurons or activation of inhibitory interneurons in dorsal horn. It is now clear that off cells exert a net inhibitory effect on nociception, and on cells exert a net facilitatory effect on nociception. Neutral cells are serotonergic neurons, and projections of neutral cells tonically release serotonin at the level of the dorsal horn and modulate the action of other descending pain modulation systems via 5-HT_3 receptor.[12]

It is also important to note that the PAG–RVM system serves as one of the major brain sites underlying opiate-induced analgesia. In the RVM, μ opioid receptors are primarily located on the on cells, and κ opioid receptor in the off cells. The μ opioid receptor agonists, including morphine and other opioid analgesics, produce a direct postsynaptic hyperpolarization by an increased K^+ conductance in RVM on cells.[14] These agents also act presynaptically to depress GABAergic synaptic transmission.[15] Activation of κ opioid receptors exhibits bidirectional pain modulation, either analgesia or antagonism of μ opioid receptor–mediated analgesia.[14,16] Chronic exposure to opiates induces emergence of functional δ opioid receptors in PAG–RVM system, which exhibit δ opioid receptor–mediated analgesia.[17]

Transition from Acute Pain to Chronic Pain

Acute pain is limited to the short-term, typically extending for days to weeks after injury. Acute pain provides an important protective mechanism, signaling the individual to protect the injured region from repeated injury, so that tissue healing can ensue. Under most circumstances, as tissue heals, the acute sensitization in the region surrounding the injury gradually subsides, and sensory thresholds revert to normal. Acute pain and the accompanying sensitization that accompany any injury do not typically persist after the initial injury has healed. In contrast, chronic pain is persistent pain that persists after all tissue healing appears to be complete and extends beyond the expected period of healing. In individuals with chronic pain, pain receptors continue to fire, even in the absence of tissue damage. There may no longer be a physically discernible tissue injury, yet the pain response persists. There is no clear delineation between when acute pain ends and chronic pain begins. Two common and practical cutoff points are often used, 3 months and 6 months after initial injury, as the likelihood that the pain will resolve diminishes with time and the likelihood that chronic pain will persist rises. Despite recent improvements in techniques for acute pain management, chronic pain persists in a significant proportion of patients following the most common surgical procedures.

While sensitization of peripheral and central nocisponsive neurons underlies the neurobiologic basis of the transition from acute pain to chronic pain, emerging evidence also suggests that an individual's psychologic response after injury as well as noxious stimuli–induced epigenetic modification[18,19] in the PNS and CNS are also critically involved in the induction and maintenance of chronic pain. Recent studies suggest that patients with subacute low back pain who are having negative affective experience (depression and poor adaptive skills) develop greater functional connectivity of nucleus accumbens with the prefrontal cortex, the brain regions processing emotion and reward, and these individuals are prone to develop persistent pain.[18,20]

Psychobiology of Pain

Unpleasant emotional experiences are an intrinsic and undesirable feature of painful experiences for the patients. Discomfort, fear of pain, and anxiety are the most common psychological responses observed in the patients with pain, although other adverse emotional responses, including depression, anger, disgust and guilt are not unusual in these patients.

Affective qualities of pain are transmitted and processed via the same pathways as those for the painful sensory transmission. Peripheral nociceptive information is delivered through spinoreticular pathways to diencephalic and telencephalic structures, including the medial thalamus, hypothalamus, amygdala, and limbic cortex. Central sensitization and adaptation of synaptic plasticity occur in these brain regions and contribute to the induction and maintenance of the emotional distress that often accompanies pain.[11]

Intrinsic interactions occur between the sensory and affective components of pain. Although the affective qualities of the painful experience vary from individual to individual, most patients experiencing acute or chronic pain display substantial emotional, behavioral, or social abnormalities. While these affective symptoms may gradually wane, a substantial proportion of patients with chronic pain experience debilitating depression, anxiety, cognitive deficits such as memory impairment, and other negative psychological components of pain. Similarly, emerging evidence suggests that severe emotional distress can trigger new pain or exacerbate ongoing pain in the patients with previous painful experiences.

Some Specific Types of Pain

Neuropathic Pain

Neuropathic pain is pain that persists after tissue injury has healed and is characterized by reduced sensory and nociceptive thresholds (allodynia and hyperalgesia). Injury of peripheral nerves by trauma, surgery, or diseases (e.g., diabetes) frequently results in the development of neuropathic pain. Cancer patients are at increased risk of neuropathic pain caused by radiotherapy or a variety of chemotherapeutic agents. Although acute and inflammatory pain are usually considered as an adaptive process of the pain system to provide warning and protection, neuropathic pain actually reflects a maladaptive (pathophysiologic) function of a damaged pain system. In many patients, neuropathic pain persists throughout life and negatively affects physical, emotional, and social quality of life.[19] Current treatments for neuropathic pain are only modestly effective, providing some symptomatic treatment for neuropathic pain. Opioids, gabapentin, amitriptyline, and medicinal cannabis preparations have been tried and shown to be only marginally effective.[21–23] The pathophysiologic processes that lead to neuropathic pain has the hallmarks of a neuroinflammatory response following innate immune system activation. Toll-like receptors 2 and 4 (TLR2 and TLR4) found on microglia appear to trigger glial activation, initiating proinflammatory and signal transduction pathways[24,25] that lead to the production of proinflammatory cytokines. Established mechanical allodynia can be reversed by intrathecally delivered TLR4 receptor antagonists,[26] preventing transcription factor NF-κB (nuclear factor kappa-light-chain-enhancer of activated B cells) activation and TNF-α (tumor necrosis factor-alpha) overproduction in the spinal cord after sciatic nerve injury.[27] Central cannabinoid receptor type 2 (CB_2) appears to play a protective role and administration of a CB_2 receptor agonist can blunt the neuroinflammatory response and prevent peripheral neuropathy through interference with specific signaling pathways.[28,29]

The common pathologic features of the neural damage include segmental abnormal myelination/demyelination and axonopathy, ranging from metabolic and axoplasmic transport deficits to frank transection of the axon (axotomy). After nerve injury occurs, the proximal stump of the axon seals off and forms a terminal swelling or "end bulb," and numerous fine processes ("sprouts") start to grow out from the end bulb within 1 or 2 days. These regenerating sprouts normally elongate within their original endoneurial tube and restore the normal sensation in appropriate peripheral targets. However, when the forward growth of the axon is blocked, such as after limb amputation, end bulbs and aborted sprouts form a tangled mass at the nerve end, a "nerve-end neuroma." Usually, the ectopic firing generated in end bulb and sprouts within the neuroma, as well as the cell bodies in DRG, significantly contribute to the nociceptive hypersensitivity and ectopic mechosensitivity that follow nerve injury.

Visceral Pain

While somatic pain is easily localized and characterized by distinct sensations, visceral pain is diffuse and poorly localized, typically referred to somatic sites (e.g., muscle and skin), and it is usually associated with stronger emotional and autonomic reactions. Visceral pain is often produced by stimuli different from those adequate for activation of somatic nociceptors. These features may be attributable to dual nerve innervation and the unique structure of visceral receptive endings.

Among all tissues in the body, the viscera are unique in that each organ receives innervation from two sets of nerves, either vagal and spinal nerves or pelvic and spinal nerves, and the visceral afferent innervation is sparse relative to somatic innervation. Spinal visceral afferent fibers have their cell bodies in dorsal root ganglia (DRG) and terminate in the spinal dorsal horn. The central termination of visceral afferents synapse spinal neurons in laminae I, II, V, and X over several segments and deliver the visceral sensory information through the contralateral spinothalamic tract or ipsilateral dorsal column to supraspinal brain sites. These spinal neurons also receive convergent input from somatic and other visceral structures, providing the structural basis for referred pain; for example, the left-sided jaw and arm pain that accompany myocardial ischemia are mediated by convergence of visceral and somatic sensory fields. Another nervous structure conveying pain information from organs in the thoracic and abdominal cavities is the vagus nerve, which has cell bodies in the nodose ganglion and central terminals in the nucleus tractus solitarii. The vagus afferent innervation plays an important role in the prominent autonomic and emotional reactions in visceral diseases associated with pain (Fig. 6-7). The majority of visceral afferent fibers are thinly myelinated Aδ fibers or unmyelinated C fibers with unencapsulated free nerve endings, with a small number of Aβ fibers associated with Pacinian corpuscles in the mesentery. Best characterized mechanosensitive endings in the viscera are the intraganglionic laminar endings (IGLEs) and intramuscular arrays associated with vagal afferent fibers that innervate the stomach. Most of these visceral sensory neurons contain substance P and/or CGRP, and they also express the high-affinity nerve growth factor receptor TrkA. These biomarkers significantly increase and the nociceptors become sensitized during visceral

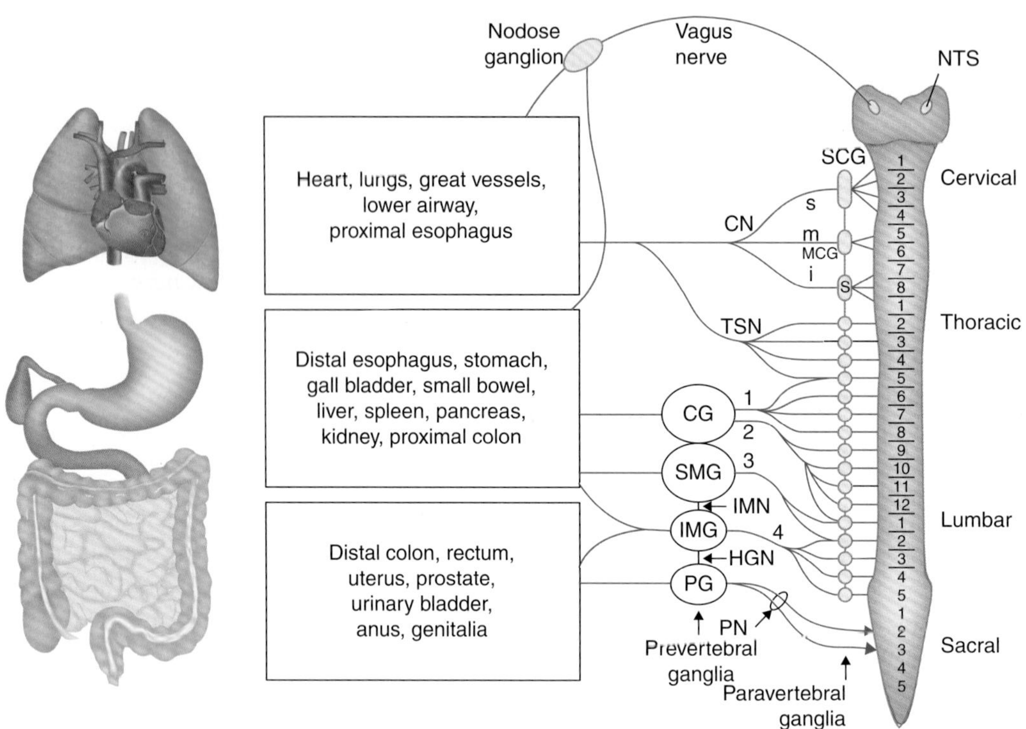

FIGURE 6-7 Visceral innervation. The vagus nerve, with cell bodies in the nodose ganglion and central terminals in the nucleus tractus solitarii (NTS), innervates organs in the thoracic and abdominal cavities. Afferent nerves with terminals in the spinal cord innervate the same thoracic and abdominal organs as well as those in the pelvic floor. Visceral spinal afferents pass through pre- and/or paravertebral ganglia en route to the spinal cord; their cell bodies are located in dorsal root ganglia (not illustrated). Prevertebral ganglia: CG, celiac ganglion; SMG, superior mesenteric ganglia; IMG, inferior mesenteric ganglia; and PG, pelvic ganglion. Paravertebral ganglia: SCG, superior cervical ganglia; MCG, middle cervical ganglia; and S, stellate ganglion. Nerves: CN, cardiac nerves (s, superior; m, middle; i, inferior);TSN, thoracic splanchnic nerves (1, greater; 2, lesser; 3, least; 4, lumbar splanchnic nerves); IMN, intermesenteric nerve; HGN, hypogastric nerve; and PN, pelvic nerve. (Modified from McMahon S, Koltzenburg M. *Wall and Melzack's Textbook of Pain.* 5th ed. Philadelphia, PA: Churchill Livingstone; 2006.)

inflammation. Unlike noxious stimuli to induce somatic pain, many damaging stimuli (cutting, burning, clamping) produce no pain when applied to visceral structures. Activation of visceral nociceptors is generally induced by ischemia, stretching of ligamentous attachments, spasm of smooth muscles, or distension of hollow structures such as the gallbladder, common bile duct, or ureter. These stimuli occur in many visceral pathologic processes, and the pain they induce may serve a survival function by promoting immobility.

Complex Regional Pain Syndromes

The International Association for the Study of Pain (IASP) *Classification of Chronic Pain* defines complex regional pain syndrome (CRPS) as "a variety of painful conditions following injury which appears regionally having a distal predominance of abnormal findings, exceeding in both magnitude and duration the expected clinical course of the inciting event often resulting in significant impairment of motor function, and showing variable progression over time." These chronic pain syndromes have different clinical features including spontaneous pain, allodynia, hyperalgesia, edema, autonomic abnormalities, active and passive movement disorders, and trophic changes of skin and subcutaneous tissues. Two types of CRPS, type I (reflex sympathetic dystrophy) and type II (causalgia), by the presence of a major identifiable nerve injury in the CRPS II and the absence of a major nerve injury in CRPS I. CRPS I develops more often than CRPS II, and females are more often affected than males (2:1 to 4:1). The incidence of CRPS I is 1% to 2% after fractures, 12% after brain lesions, and 5% after myocardial infarction, and the incidence of CRPS II in peripheral nerve injury varies from 2% to 14% in different series, with a mean around 4%.

The following IASP clinical criteria are applied to diagnose the CRPS. CRPS type I: (a) type I is a syndrome that develops after an initiating noxious event; (b) spontaneous pain or allodynia/hyperalgesia occurs, is not limited to the territory of a single peripheral nerve, and is disproportionate to the inciting event; (c) there is or has been evidence of edema, skin blood flow abnormality, or abnormal sudomotor activity in the region of the pain since the inciting event; and (d) this diagnosis is excluded by the existence of conditions that would otherwise account for the degree of pain and dysfunction. CRPS type II: (a) type II is a syndrome that develops after nerve injury; spontaneous pain or allodynia/hyperalgesia occurs and is not necessarily limited to the territory of the injured nerve; (b) there is or has been evidence of edema, skin blood flow abnormality, or abnormal sudomotor activity in the region of the pain since the inciting event; and (c) this diagnosis is excluded by the existence of conditions that would otherwise account for the degree of pain and dysfunction.

The mechanism underlying the pathogenesis of CRPS remains unclear, although it is recognized that CRPS is a neurologic disease including the autonomic, sensory, and motor systems as well as cortical areas involved in the processing of cognitive and affective information, and the inflammatory component appears to be particularly important in the acute phase of the disease. Effective, evidence-based treatment regimens for CRPS are lacking.

Pain in Neonate and Infant

Accumulating evidence overrides the outdated thought that young children do not feel pain due to the immaturity of the PNS and CNS. Reflex responses to somatic stimuli begin at 15 days (E15, where gestation is 21.5 days) in the rat fetus, and the human fetus develops pain perception by 23 weeks of gestation. Postnatal maturity of pain behavior develops quickly after birth. Usually, newborns and young children have significantly lower pain thresholds and exaggerated pain responses compared to adults.[30] Some clinical studies reveal the long-term effects of neonatal pain experience, which is affected by several confounding factors such as gestational age at birth, length of intensive care stay, intensity of the stimulus and parenting style. Toddlers and adolescents exhibit long-lasting hypersensitivity to painful stimuli after painful experiences as neonates. These observations highlight the clinical importance of optimal management of pain in neonates and infants.

Embryologic Origin and Localization of Pain

The position in the spinal cord to which visceral afferent fibers pass for each organ depends on the segment (dermatome) of the body from which the organ developed embryologically. This explains the phenomenon pain that is referred to a site distant from the tissue causing the pain (Fig. 6-8). For example, the heart originates in the neck and upper thorax such that visceral afferents enter the spinal cord at C3 to C5. As a result, the pain of myocardial ischemia is referred to the neck and arm. The gallbladder originates from the ninth thoracic segment, so visceral afferents from the gallbladder enter the spinal cord at T9. Skeletal muscle spasm caused by damage in adjacent tissues may also be a cause of referred pain. For example, pain from the ureter can cause reflex spasm of the lumbar muscles.

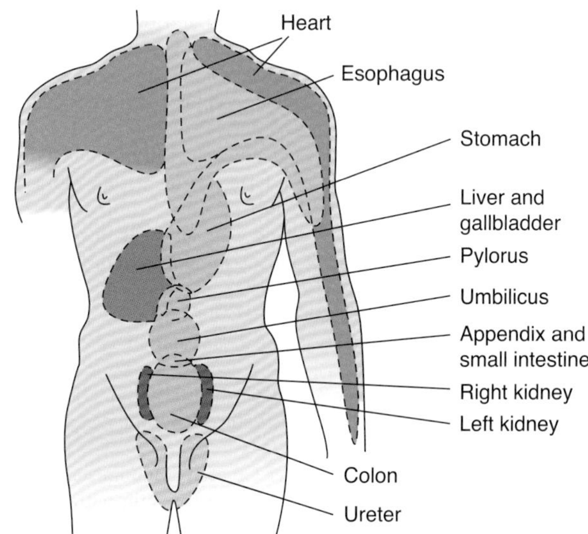

FIGURE 6-8 Surface area of referred pain from different visceral organs.

References

1. Anand KJ, Craig KD. New perspectives on the definition of pain. *Pain.* 1996;67:3–6; discussion 209–211.
2. Glajchen M. Chronic pain: treatment barriers and strategies for clinical practice. *J Am Board Fam Pract.* 2001;14:211–218.
3. Helmick CG, Lawrence RC, Pollard RA, et al. Arthritis and other rheumatic conditions: who is affected now, who will be affected later? National Arthritis Data Workgroup. *Arthritis Care Res.* 1995;8: 203–211.
4. Petho G, Reeh PW. Sensory and signaling mechanisms of bradykinin, eicosanoids, platelet-activating factor, and nitric oxide in peripheral nociceptors. *Physiol Rev.* 2012;92:1699–1775.
5. Chen Y, Zhang YH, Bie BH, et al. Sympathectomy induces novel purinergic sensitivity in sciatic afferents. *Acta Pharmacol Sin.* 2000;21: 1002–1004.
6. Bie B, Zhao ZQ. Peripheral inflammation alters desensitization of substance P-evoked current in rat dorsal root ganglion neurons. *Eur J Pharmacol.* 2011;670:495–499.
7. Basbaum AI, Bautista DM, Scherrer G, et al. Cellular and molecular mechanisms of pain. *Cell.* 2009;139:267–284.
8. Latremoliere A, Woolf CJ. Central sensitization: a generator of pain hypersensitivity by central neural plasticity. *J Pain.* 2009;10: 895–926.
9. Xu JT, Xin WJ, Wei XH, et al. p38 activation in uninjured primary afferent neurons and in spinal microglia contributes to the development of neuropathic pain induced by selective motor fiber injury. *Exp Neurol.* 2007;204:355–365.
10. Shi T, Apkarian AV. Morphology of thalamocortical neurons projecting to the primary somatosensory cortex and their relationship to spinothalamic terminals in the squirrel monkey. *J Comp Neurol.* 1995;361:1–24.
11. Bie B, Brown DL, Naguib M. Synaptic plasticity and pain aversion. *Eur J Pharmacol.* 2011;667:26–31.
12. Millan MJ. Descending control of pain. *Prog Neurobiol.* 2002;66: 355–474.
13. Fields HL, Heinricher MM. Anatomy and physiology of a nociceptive modulatory system. *Philos Trans R Soc Lond B Biol Sci.* 1985;308:361–374.
14. Pan ZZ, Tershner SA, Fields HL. Cellular mechanism for anti-analgesic action of agonists of the kappa-opioid receptor. *Nature.* 1997;389:382–385.

15. Vaughan CW, Ingram SL, Connor MA, et al. How opioids inhibit GABA-mediated neurotransmission. *Nature*. 1997;390:611–614.
16. Bie B, Pan ZZ. Presynaptic mechanism for anti-analgesic and anti-hyperalgesic actions of kappa-opioid receptors. *J Neurosci*. 2003;23: 7262–7268.
17. Ma J, Zhang Y, Kalyuzhny AE, et al. Emergence of functional delta-opioid receptors induced by long-term treatment with morphine. *Mol Pharmacol*. 2006;69:1137–1145.
18. Melloh M, Elfering A, Egli Presland C, et al. Predicting the transition from acute to persistent low back pain. *Occup Med (Lond)*. 2011;61:127–131.
19. Jensen MP, Chodroff MJ, Dworkin RH. The impact of neuropathic pain on health-related quality of life: review and implications. *Neurology*. 2007;68:1178–1182.
20. Baliki MN, Petre B, Torbey S, et al. Corticostriatal functional connectivity predicts transition to chronic back pain. *Nat Neurosci*. 2012;15:1117–1119.
21. Morello CM, Leckband SG, Stoner CP, et al. Randomized double-blind study comparing the efficacy of gabapentin with amitriptyline on diabetic peripheral neuropathy pain. *Arch Intern Med*. 1999;159:1931–1937.
22. Steinman MA, Bero LA, Chren MM, et al. Narrative review: the promotion of gabapentin: an analysis of internal industry documents. *Ann Intern Med*. 2006;145:284–293.
23. Phillips TJ, Cherry CL, Cox S, et al. Pharmacological treatment of painful HIV-associated sensory neuropathy: a systematic review and meta-analysis of randomised controlled trials. *PLoS One*. 2010;5:e14433.
24. Akira S, Takeda K. Toll-like receptor signalling. *Nat Rev Immunol*. 2004;4:499–511.
25. Lehnardt S, Massillon L, Follett P, et al. Activation of innate immunity in the CNS triggers neurodegeneration through a Toll-like receptor 4-dependent pathway. *Proc Natl Acad Sci U S A*. 2003;100: 8514–8519.
26. Hutchinson MR, Zhang Y, Brown K, et al. Non-stereoselective reversal of neuropathic pain by naloxone and naltrexone: involvement of toll-like receptor 4 (TLR4). *Eur J Neurosci*. 2008;28:20–29.
27. Bettoni I, Comelli F, Rossini C, et al. Glial TLR4 receptor as new target to treat neuropathic pain: efficacy of a new receptor antagonist in a model of peripheral nerve injury in mice. *Glia*. 2008;56: 1312–1319.
28. Naguib M, Diaz F, Xu J, et al. MDA7: a novel selective agonist for CB2 receptors that prevents allodynia in rat neuropathic pain models. *Br J Pharmacol*. 2008;155:1104–1116.
29. Naguib M, Xu JJ, Diaz P, et al. Prevention of paclitaxel-induced neuropathy through activation of the central cannabinoid type 2 receptor system. *Anesth Analg*. 2012;114:1104–1120.
30. Pan ZZ. A life switch in pain. *Pain*. 2012;153:738–739.

CHAPTER 7

Opioid Agonists and Antagonists

Kenneth Cummings III • Mohamed A. Naguib

Opioids remain the mainstay of modern perioperative care and pain management. The modern word ***opium*** is derived from the Greek word ***opion*** ("poppy juice"); the opium poppy (Papaver somniferum) is the source of 20 distinct alkaloids. Written mention of the medicinal use of poppy juice dates back to at least 300 BC, although religious use likely goes back much further.[1] Drugs derived from opium are referred to as ***opiates***. Morphine, the best-known opiate, was isolated in 1803, followed by codeine in 1832, and papaverine in 1848. Morphine can be synthesized but it is more easily derived from opium. The term ***narcotic*** is derived from the Greek word for stupor and traditionally has been used to refer to potent morphine-like analgesics with the potential to produce physical dependence. The development of synthetic drugs with morphine-like properties has led to the use of the term ***opioid*** to refer to all exogenous substances, natural and synthetic, that bind specifically to any of several subpopulations of opioid receptors and produce at least some agonist (morphine-like) effects. Opioids are unique in producing analgesia without loss of touch, proprioception, or consciousness. A convenient classification of opioids includes opioid agonists, opioid agonist–antagonists, and opioid antagonists (Table 7-1).

Chemical Structure of Opium Alkaloids

The active components of opium can be divided into two distinct chemical classes: phenanthrenes and benzylisoquinolines. The principal phenanthrene alkaloids present in opium are morphine, codeine, and thebaine (Fig. 7-1). The principal benzylisoquinoline alkaloids present in opium, which lack analgesic activity, are papaverine and noscapine. The three rings of the phenanthrene core are composed of 14 carbon atoms. The fourth piperidine ring includes a tertiary amine nitrogen and is present in most opioid agonists. At pH 7.4, the tertiary amine nitrogen is highly ionized, making the molecule water soluble. These are chiral molecules, with levorotatory isomers being biologically active at opioid receptors.

Semisynthetic Opioids

Simple modification of the morphine molecule yields many derivative compounds with differing properties. For example, substitution of a methyl group for the hydroxyl group on carbon 3 results in methylmorphine (codeine). Substitution of acetyl groups on carbons 3 and 6 results in diacetylmorphine (heroin). Thebaine has insignificant analgesic activity but serves as the precursor for etorphine (analgesic potency >1,000 times morphine).

Synthetic Opioids

Synthetic opioids contain the phenanthrene nucleus of morphine but are manufactured by synthesis rather than chemical modification of morphine. Morphine derivatives (levorphanol), methadone derivatives, benzomorphan derivatives (pentazocine), and phenylpiperidine derivatives (meperidine, fentanyl) are examples of groups of synthetic opioids. There are similarities in the molecular weights (236 to 326) and pKs of phenylpiperidine derivatives and amide local anesthetics.

Fentanyl, sufentanil, alfentanil, and remifentanil (Fig. 7-2) are synthetic opioids that are widely used to supplement general anesthesia or as primary anesthetic drugs in very high doses. There are important clinical differences between these opioids.[2–4] The major pharmacodynamic differences between these drugs are potency and rate of equilibration between the plasma and the site of drug effect (biophase).

Table 7-1

Classification of Opioid Agonists and Antagonists

Agonists	Agonists–Antagonists	Antagonists
Morphine	Pentazocine	Naloxone
Morphine-6-glucuronide	Butorphanol	Naltrexone
Meperidine	Nalbuphine	Nalmefene
Sufentanil	Buprenorphine	
Fentanyl	Nalorphine	
Alfentanil	Bremazocine	
Remifentanil	Dezocine	
Codeine	Meptazinol	
Hydromorphone		
Oxymorphone		
Oxycodone		
Hydrocodone		
Propoxyphene		
Methadone		
Tramadol		
Heroin		

Mechanism of Action

Opioids act as agonists at specific opioid receptors at presynaptic and postsynaptic sites in the central nervous system (CNS) (mainly the brainstem and spinal cord) as well as in the periphery.[5–7] These same opioid receptors normally are activated by three endogenous peptide opioid receptor ligands known as enkephalins, endorphins, and dynorphins. Opioids mimic the actions of these endogenous ligands by binding to opioid receptors, resulting in activation of pain-modulating (antinociceptive) systems.

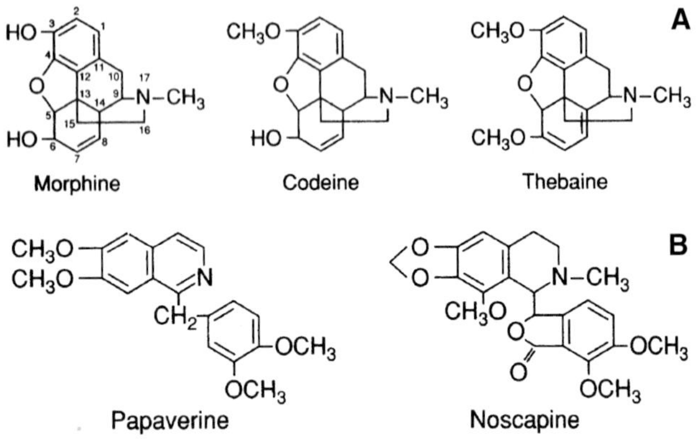

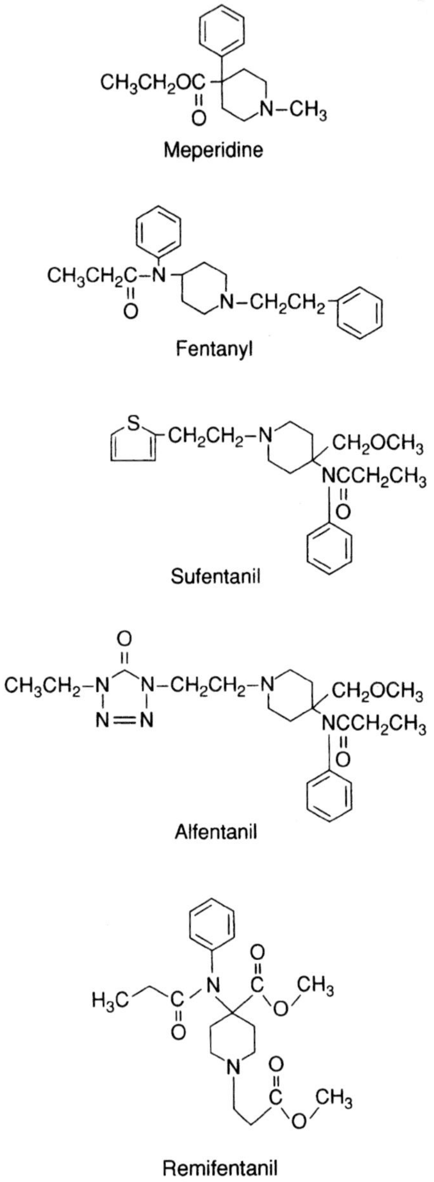

FIGURE 7-2 Synthetic opioid agonists.

FIGURE 7-1 Chemical structures of opium alkaloids. Phenanthrene **(A)** and benzylisoquinoline **(B)** alkaloids.

Existence of the opioid in the ionized state appears to be necessary for strong binding at the anionic opioid receptor site. Only levorotatory forms of the opioids exhibit agonist activity. Indeed, the naturally occurring form of morphine is the levorotatory isomer. The affinity of most opioid agonists for receptors correlates well with their analgesic potency.

The principal effect of opioid receptor activation is a decrease in neurotransmission.[8] This decrease in neurotransmission occurs largely by presynaptic inhibition of neurotransmitter release (acetylcholine, dopamine, norepinephrine, substance P), although postsynaptic inhibition of evoked activity may also occur. The intracellular biochemical events initiated by occupation of opioid receptors with an opioid agonist are characterized by increased potassium conductance (leading to hyperpolarization), calcium channel inactivation, or both, which produce an immediate decrease in neurotransmitter release.

All opioid receptor classes couple to intracellular guanine (G) proteins. Upon binding of an opioid agonist to the extracellular domain of the receptor, the receptor changes shape, which activates the G protein bound to its intracellular domain. The G protein replaces its bound guanine diphosphate (GDP) with guanine triphosphate (GTP) and dissociates into two active subunits. Subsequent mechanisms include inhibition of adenylate cyclase, decrease the conductance of voltage-gated calcium channels, or opening of inward-flowing potassium channels. Any of these effects ultimately results in decreased neuronal activity. Opioid receptors also modulate the phosphoinositide-signaling cascade and phospholipase C. The prevention of calcium ion inflow results in suppression of neurotransmitter release (substance P) in many neuronal systems. Hyperpolarization results from actions at potassium channels, thus preventing excitation or propagation of action potentials. Opioid receptors may regulate the functions of other ion channels including excitatory postsynaptic currents evoked by *N*-methyl-D-aspartate (NMDA) receptors.

Opioid receptor–mediated inhibition of adenylate cyclase is not responsible for an immediate effect but may have a delayed effect, possibly via a reduction in cyclic adenosine monophosphate (cAMP)–responsive neuropeptide genes and reduction in neuropeptide messenger RNA concentrations. Depression of cholinergic transmission in the CNS as a result of opioid-induced inhibition of acetylcholine release from nerve endings may play a prominent role in the analgesic and other side effects of opioid agonists. Opioids do not alter responsiveness of afferent nerve endings to noxious stimulation nor do they block conduction of nerve impulses along peripheral nerves (as opposed to local anesthetics).

Opioid Receptors

Opioid receptors are classified as μ, δ, and κ receptors[8,9] (Table 7-2). The names of the three subtypes developed from the ligands originally found to bind to them or their tissue of origin (mu—*m*orphine, kappa—*k*etocyclazocine, delta—isolated from mouse vas *d*eferens). These opioid receptors belong to a superfamily of seven transmembrane-segment G protein–coupled receptors that includes muscarinic, adrenergic, γ-aminobutyric acid, and somatostatin receptors. The opioid receptors have been cloned and their amino acid sequences defined.[10,11] A single μ-receptor gene has been identified and six distinct μ receptors subtypes have been characterized.

In the brain, opioid receptors are primarily found in the periaqueductal gray, locus ceruleus, and the rostral ventral medulla. In the spinal cord, opioid receptors are found both on interneurons and primary afferent

Table 7-2

Classification of Opioid Receptors

	Mu_1[a]	Mu_2[a]	Kappa	Delta
Effect	Analgesia (supraspinal, spinal)	Analgesia (spinal)	Analgesia (supraspinal, spinal)	Analgesia (supraspinal, spinal)
	Euphoria	Depression of ventilation	Dysphoria, sedation	Depression of ventilation
	Low abuse potential	Physical dependence	Low abuse potential	Physical dependence
	Miosis		Miosis	
		Constipation (marked)		Constipation (minimal)
	Bradycardia			
	Hypothermia			
	Urinary retention		Diuresis	Urinary retention
Agonists	Endorphins[b]	Endorphins[b]	Dynorphins	Enkephalins
	Morphine	Morphine		
	Synthetic opioids	Synthetic opioids		
Antagonists	Naloxone	Naloxone	Naloxone	Naloxone
	Naltrexone	Naltrexone	Naltrexone	Naltrexone
	Nalmefene	Nalmefene	Nalmefene	Nalmefene

[a]The existence of specific mu_1 and mu_2 receptors is not supported based on cloning studies of μ receptors.
[b]μ receptors seem to be a universal site of action for all endogenous opioid receptors.
Adapted from Atcheson R, Lambert DG. Update on opioid receptors. *Br J Anaesth*. 1994;73:132–134.

neurons in the dorsal horn. Consequently, direct application of opioid agonists to the spinal cord can produce intense analgesia.[12] Outside the CNS, opioid receptors are found on sensory neurons and immune cells. Immune cells recruited to sites of inflammation also secrete opioid peptides to provide local analgesia.[13] For example, intraarticular morphine is known to produce analgesia after knee surgery, presumably through action on peripheral nerves.[14]

The μ receptors are principally responsible for supraspinal and spinal analgesia. Theoretically, activation of a subpopulation of μ receptors (mu_1) is speculated to produce analgesia, whereas mu_2 receptors are responsible for hypoventilation, bradycardia, and physical dependence. Nevertheless, cloning of the μ receptors does not support the existence of separate mu_1 and mu_2 receptor subtypes.[9] It is possible that such subtypes result from posttranslational modification of a common precursor protein. Whether β-endorphins or even morphine itself is the endogenous ligand for μ receptors is unclear.[15] Endomorphins are peptides with high affinity and selectivity for μ receptors that are present in the brain.

Activation of κ receptors results in inhibition of neurotransmitter release via N-type calcium channels. Respiratory depression characteristic of μ receptor activation is less prominent with κ receptor activation, although dysphoria and diuresis may accompany activation of these receptors. κ receptor–mediated analgesia may be less effective for high-intensity painful stimulation than μ opioid–mediated. Opioid agonist–antagonists often act principally on κ receptors. δ receptors respond to the endogenous ligands known as ***enkephalins***, and these opioid receptors may serve to modulate the activity of the μ receptors.

Functional and physical interactions between these receptor subtypes have been noted.[16,17] Heteromerization between μ and δ opioid receptors leads to distinct receptor pharmacology in that doses of δ receptor ligands (agonists and antagonists) too low to trigger signaling can potentiate the binding and signaling of μ receptor agonists. Chronic, but not acute, morphine treatment results in an increase in μ-δ heteromers in key areas of the CNS that are implicated in pain processing.[18]

Endogenous Pain Modulating Mechanisms

The logical reason for the existence of opioid receptors and endogenous opioid agonists is to function as an endogenous pain suppression system. Once pain is consciously perceived, it has served its purpose and it is reasonable to posit that the ability to dampen this perception would have a survival benefit. Opioid receptors are located in areas of the brain (periaqueductal gray matter of the brainstem, amygdala, corpus striatum, and hypothalamus) and spinal cord (substantia gelatinosa) that are involved with pain perception, integration of pain impulses, and responses to pain (Fig. 7-3).[19] It is speculated that endorphins inhibit the release of excitatory neurotransmitters from terminals of nerves carrying nociceptive impulses. As a result, neurons are hyperpolarized, which suppresses spontaneous discharges and evoked responses. Analgesia induced by electrical stimulation of specific sites in the brain or mechanical stimulation of peripheral areas (acupuncture) most likely reflects release of endorphins.[20] Even the analgesic response to a placebo may also involve the release of endorphins. Sustained pain and stress induces the regional release of endogenous opioids interacting with μ opioid receptors in a number of cortical and subcortical brain regions. The activation of the μ opioid receptor system is associated with reductions in the sensory and affective ratings of the pain experience, with distinct neuroanatomic involvement.[21,22]

In addition, a recent study demonstrated that positive treatment expectancy substantially enhanced (doubled) the analgesic benefit of remifentanil, whereas negative treatment expectancy abolished remifentanil analgesia.[23] These subjective effects were substantiated by significant changes in the neural activity in brain regions involved with the coding of pain intensity. The positive expectancy effects were associated with activity in the endogenous pain modulation system, and the negative expectancy effects with activity in the hippocampus.[23] On the basis

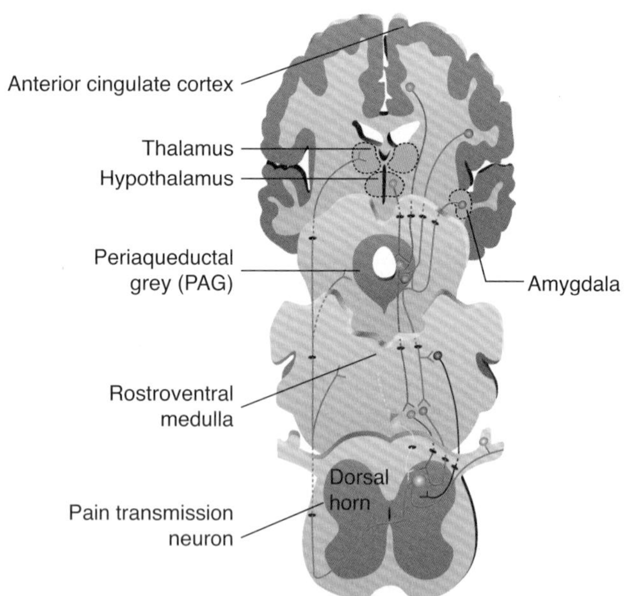

FIGURE 7-3 Opioid-sensitive pain modulation system. Limbic system areas project to the periaqueductal grey (PAG). The PAG in turn controls afferent pain transmission in the rostroventral medulla. This action can be both inhibitory *(red)* or facilitatory *(green)*. (From Fields H. State-dependent opioid control of pain. *Nat Rev Neurosci.* 2004;5[7]:565–575).

of subjective and objective evidence, we contend that an individual's expectation of a drug's effect critically influences its therapeutic efficacy and that regulatory brain mechanisms differ as a function of expectancy.

Common Opioid Side Effects

An ideal opioid agonist would have a high specificity for receptors, producing desirable responses (analgesia) and little or no specificity for receptors associated with side effects. To date, however, all opioids possess similar side effects that vary only in degree. Therefore, a focus on the effects of morphine provides a suitable starting point.

Cardiovascular System

Morphine, even in large doses, given to supine and normovolemic patients is unlikely to cause direct myocardial depression or hypotension. The same patients changing from a supine to a standing position, however, may manifest orthostatic hypotension and syncope, presumably reflecting morphine-induced impairment of compensatory sympathetic nervous system responses. For example, morphine decreases sympathetic nervous system tone to peripheral veins, resulting in venous pooling and subsequent decreases in venous return, cardiac output, and blood pressure.[24]

Morphine can also evoke decreases in systemic blood pressure due to drug-induced bradycardia or histamine release. Morphine-induced bradycardia results from increased activity of the vagal nerves, which probably reflects stimulation of the vagal nuclei in the medulla. Morphine may also exert a direct depressant effect on the sinoatrial node and acts to slow conduction of cardiac impulses through the atrioventricular node. These actions, may, in part, explain decreased vulnerability to ventricular fibrillation in the presence of morphine. Administration of opioids (morphine, fentanyl) in the preoperative medication or before the induction of anesthesia tends to slow heart rate during exposure to volatile anesthetics with or without surgical stimulation.[25]

Opioid-induced histamine release and associated hypotension are variable in both incidence and severity. The magnitude of morphine-induced histamine release and subsequent decrease in systemic blood pressure can be minimized by (a) limiting the rate of morphine infusion to 5 mg per minute intravenously (IV), (b) maintaining the patient in a supine to slightly head-down position, and (c) optimizing intravascular fluid volume. Conversely, administration of morphine, 1 mg/kg IV, over a 10-minute period produces substantial increases in the plasma concentrations of histamine that are paralleled by significant decreases in systemic blood pressure and systemic vascular resistance (Fig. 7-4).[26] It is important to recognize, however, that not all patients respond to this rate of morphine infusion with the release of histamine, emphasizing the individual variability associated with the

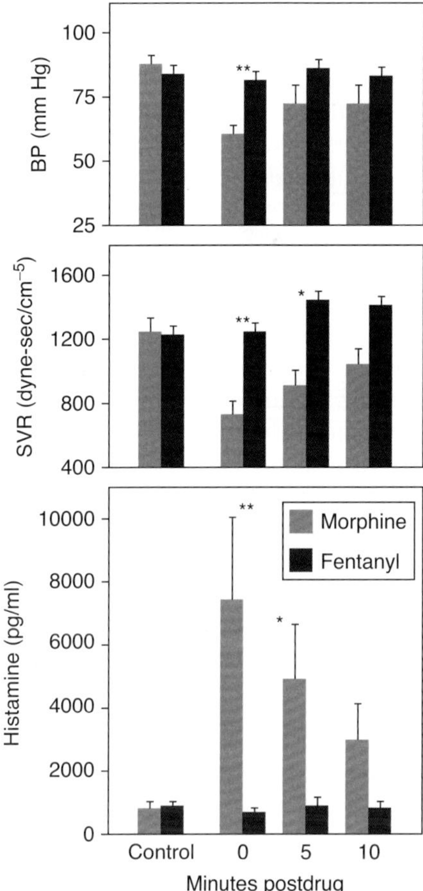

FIGURE 7-4 Morphine-induced decreases in systemic blood pressure (BP) and systemic vascular resistance (SVR) are accompanied by increases in the plasma concentration of histamine. Similar changes do not accompany the intravenous administration of fentanyl. (*$P < .05$; **$P < .005$; mean ± SE.) (From Rosow CE, Moss J, Philbin DM, et al. Histamine release during morphine and fentanyl anesthesia. *Anesthesiology.* 1982;56:93–96, with permission.)

administration of this drug. In contrast to morphine, the infusion of fentanyl 50 μg/kg IV over a 10-minute period does not cause release of histamine in any patient (see Fig. 7-4). Pretreatment of patients with H_1 and H_2 receptor antagonists does not alter release of histamine evoked by morphine but does prevent changes in systemic blood pressure and systemic vascular resistance.[27]

Morphine does not sensitize the heart to catecholamines or otherwise predispose to cardiac dysrhythmias as long as hypercarbia or arterial hypoxemia does not result from ventilatory depression. Tachycardia and hypertension that occur during anesthesia with morphine are not pharmacologic effects of the opioid but rather are responses to painful surgical stimulation that are not suppressed by morphine. Both the sympathetic nervous system and the renin-angiotensin axis contribute to these cardiovascular responses. Large doses of morphine or other opioid agonists may decrease the likelihood that tachycardia and hypertension will occur in response to painful stimulation, but once this response has occurred, administration of additional opioid is unlikely to be effective.

During anesthesia, however, opioids are commonly administered with inhaled or IV anesthetics to ensure amnesia. The combination of an opioid agonist such as morphine or fentanyl with nitrous oxide results in cardiovascular depression (decreased cardiac output and systemic blood pressure plus increased cardiac filling pressures), which does not occur when either drug is administered alone.[28] Likewise, decreases in systemic vascular resistance and systemic blood pressure may accompany the combination of an opioid and a benzodiazepine, whereas these effects do not accompany the administration of either drug alone (Fig. 7-5).[29]

Opioids have been increasingly recognized as playing a role in protecting the myocardium from ischemia. Through several mechanisms, most prominently though σ and κ receptors, opioids enhance the resistance of the myocardium to oxidative and ischemic stresses. Mitochondrial adenosine triphosphate (ATP)–regulated potassium channels (K_{ATP}) appear to be central to this signaling pathway.[30]

Ventilation

All opioid agonists produce dose-dependent and gender-specific depression of ventilation, primarily through an agonist effect at mu_2 receptors leading to a direct depressant effect on brainstem ventilation centers.[8] Because analgesic and ventilatory effects of opioids occur by similar mechanisms, it is assumed that equianalgesic doses of all opioids will produce some degree of ventilatory depression and reversal of ventilatory depression with an opioid antagonist always involves some reversal of analgesia. Opioid-induced depression of ventilation is characterized by decreased responsiveness of these ventilation centers to carbon dioxide as reflected by an increase in the resting $Paco_2$ and displacement of the carbon dioxide response curve to the right. Opioid agonists also interfere with pontine and medullary ventilatory centers that regulate the rhythm of breathing, leading to prolonged pauses between breaths and periodic breathing. It is possible that opioid agonists diminish sensitivity to carbon dioxide by decreasing the release of acetylcholine from neurons in the area of the medullary ventilatory center in response to hypercarbia. In this regard, physostigmine, which increases CNS levels of acetylcholine, may antagonize depression of ventilation but not analgesia produced by morphine.

Depression of ventilation produced by opioid agonists is rapid and persists for several hours, as demonstrated by decreased ventilatory responses to carbon dioxide. High doses of opioids may result in apnea, but the patient remains conscious and able to initiate a breath if asked to do so. Death from an opioid overdose is almost invariably due to depression of ventilation.

Clinically, depression of ventilation produced by opioids manifests as a decreased frequency of breathing that is often accompanied by a compensatory increase in tidal volume. The incompleteness of this compensatory

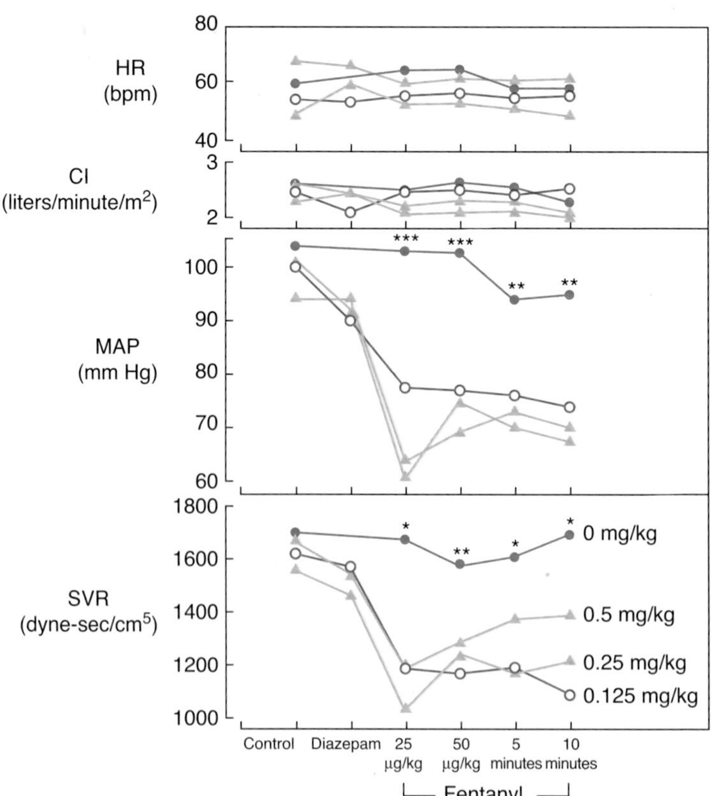

FIGURE 7-5 Administration of fentanyl (50 µg/kg IV at 400 µg per minute) after injection of diazepam (0.125 to 0.50 mg/kg IV) is associated with significant decreases in mean arterial pressure (MAP) and systemic vascular resistance (SVR), whereas heart rate (HR) and cardiac index (CI) do not change. Administration of fentanyl in the absence of prior injection of diazepam (0 mg/kg) is devoid of circulatory effects. (From Tomicheck RC, Rosow CE, Philbin DM, et al. Diazepam-fentanyl interaction: hemodynamic and hormonal effects in coronary artery surgery. *Anesth Analg.* 1983;62:881–884, with permission.)

increase in tidal volume is evidenced by predictable increases in the $Paco_2$. Many factors influence the magnitude and duration of depression of ventilation produced by opioid agonists. For example, advanced age and the occurrence of natural sleep increase the ventilatory depressant effects of opioids. Conversely, pain from surgical stimulation counteracts depression of ventilation produced by opioids. Likewise, the analgesic effect of opioids slows breathing that has been rapid and shallow due to pain.

Opioids produce dose-dependent depression of ciliary activity in the airways. Increases in airway resistance after administration of an opioid are probably due to a direct effect on bronchial smooth muscle and an indirect action due to release of histamine.

Cough Suppression

Opioids depress cough by effects on the medullary cough centers that are distinct from the effects of opioids on ventilation. The greatest cough suppression occurs with opioids that have bulky substitutions at the number 3 carbon position (codeine). One useful property of dextrorotatory isomers (such as dextromethorphan) is that they can suppress cough but do not produce analgesia or depression of ventilation. Thus, in some cases, opioids can be safely sold over-the-counter.

Central Nervous System

In the absence of hypoventilation, opioids decrease cerebral blood flow and possibly intracranial pressure (ICP). These drugs must be used with caution in patients with head injury because of their (a) associated effects on wakefulness, (b) production of miosis, and (c) depression of ventilation with associated increases in ICP if the $Paco_2$ becomes increased. Furthermore, head injury may impair the integrity of the blood–brain barrier, with resultant increased sensitivity to opioids.

The effect of morphine on the electroencephalogram (EEG) resembles changes associated with sleep. For example, there is replacement of rapid α waves by slower δ waves. Recording of the EEG fails to reveal any evidence of seizure activity after administration of large doses of opioids (see the section "Fentanyl"). Opioids do not alter the responses to neuromuscular blocking drugs. Skeletal muscle rigidity, especially of the thoracic and abdominal muscles, is common when large doses of opioid agonists are administered rapidly and intravenously.[31] Clonic skeletal muscle activity (myoclonus) occurring during administration of opioids may resemble grand mal seizures, but the EEG does not reflect seizure activity. Skeletal muscle rigidity may be related to actions at opioid receptors and involve interactions with dopaminergic and γ-aminobutyric acid–responsive neurons.

Miosis is due to an excitatory action of opioids on the autonomic nervous system component of the Edinger-Westphal nucleus of the oculomotor nerve. Tolerance to the miotic effect of morphine is not prominent. Miosis can be antagonized by atropine, and profound arterial hypoxemia in the presence of morphine can still result in mydriasis.

Rigidity

Rapid IV administration of large doses of an opioid (particularly fentanyl and its derivatives as used in cardiac surgery) can lead to generalized skeletal muscle rigidity. This can be severe enough to interfere with manual ventilation. Although generally termed ***chest wall*** rigidity, evidence supports the conclusion that the majority of resistance to ventilation is due to laryngeal musculature contraction. Inhibition of striatal release of γ-aminobutyric acid and increased dopamine production are the likely explanations for opioid-induced increased skeletal muscle tone .[32] The reported incidence of difficult ventilation after a moderate dose of sufentanil ranges from 84% to 100%.[33] Treatment is muscle relaxation with neuromuscular blocking drugs or opioid antagonism with naloxone.

Sedation

Postoperative titration of morphine frequently induces sedation that precedes the onset of analgesia.[34] The usual recommendation for morphine titration includes a short interval between boluses (5 to 7 minutes) to allow evaluation of its clinical effect. Sedation occurs in up to 60% of patients during morphine titration and represents a common reason to discontinue morphine titration for postoperative analgesia. The assumption that sleep occurs when pain is relieved is not necessarily accurate and morphine-induced sedation should not be considered as an indicator of appropriate analgesia during IV morphine titration.

Biliary Tract

Opioids can cause spasm of biliary smooth muscle, resulting in increases in biliary pressure that may be associated with epigastric distress or biliary colic. This pain may be confused with angina pectoris. Naloxone will relieve pain caused by biliary spasm but not myocardial ischemia. Conversely, nitroglycerin will relieve pain due to either biliary spasm or myocardial ischemia. Equal analgesic doses of fentanyl, morphine, meperidine, and pentazocine increase common bile duct pressure 99%, 53%, 61%, and 15% above predrug levels, respectively.[35] During surgery, opioid-induced spasm of the sphincter of Oddi may appear radiologically as a sharp constriction at the distal end of the common bile duct and be misinterpreted as a common bile duct stone. It may be necessary to reverse opioid-induced biliary smooth muscle spasm with naloxone so as to correctly interpret the cholangiogram. Glucagon, 2 mg IV, also reverses opioid-induced biliary smooth muscle spasm and, unlike naloxone, does not antagonize the analgesic effects of the opioid.[36] However, biliary muscle spasm does not occur in most patients who receive opioids. Indeed, the incidence of spasm of the sphincter of Oddi is about 3% in patients receiving fentanyl as a supplement to inhaled anesthetics.[37]

Contraction of the smooth muscles of the pancreatic ducts is probably responsible for increases in plasma amylase and lipase concentrations that may be present after the administration of morphine. Such increases may confuse the diagnosis when acute pancreatitis is a possibility.

Gastrointestinal Tract

Commonly used opioids such as morphine, meperidine, and fentanyl can produce spasm of the gastrointestinal smooth muscles, resulting in a variety of side effects including constipation, biliary colic, and delayed gastric emptying.

Morphine decreases the propulsive peristaltic contractions of the small and large intestines and enhances the tone of the pyloric sphincter, ileocecal valve, and anal sphincter. The delayed passage of intestinal contents through the colon allows increased absorption of water. As a result, constipation often accompanies therapy with opioids and may become a debilitating problem in patients who require chronic opioid therapy, as little tolerance develops to this effect. Of interest, opium was used to treat diarrhea before its use as an analgesic was popularized.

Increased biliary pressure occurs when the gallbladder contracts against a closed or narrowed sphincter of Oddi. Passage of gastric contents into the proximal duodenum is delayed because there is increased tone at the gastroduodenal junction. In this regard, preoperative medication that includes an opioid could slow gastric emptying (potentially increase the risk of aspiration) or delay the absorption of orally administered drugs. All these effects may be reversed or prevented by a peripheral-acting opioid antagonist (see the section "Methylnaltrexone").

Nausea and Vomiting

Opioid-induced nausea and vomiting are caused by direct stimulation of the chemoreceptor trigger zone in the floor of the fourth ventricle. This may reflect the role of opioid agonists as partial dopamine agonists at dopamine receptors in the chemoreceptor trigger zone. Indeed, apomorphine is a profound emetic and is also the most potent of the opioids at dopamine receptors. Stimulation of dopamine receptors as a mechanism for opioid-induced nausea and vomiting is consistent with the antiemetic efficacy of butyrophenones and phenothiazines. Morphine may also cause nausea and vomiting by increasing gastrointestinal secretions and delaying passage of intestinal contents toward the colon.

Morphine depresses the vomiting center in the medulla. As a result, IV administration of morphine produces less nausea and vomiting than the intramuscular (IM) administration of morphine, presumably because opioid administered IV reaches the vomiting center as rapidly as it reaches the chemoreceptor trigger zone. Nausea and vomiting are relatively uncommon in recumbent patients given morphine, suggesting that a vestibular component may contribute to opioid-induced nausea and vomiting.

Genitourinary System

Morphine can increase the tone and peristaltic activity of the ureter. In contrast to similar effects on biliary tract smooth muscle, the same opioid-induced effects on the ureter can be reversed by an anticholinergic drug such as atropine. Urinary urgency is produced by opioid-induced augmentation of detrusor muscle tone, but, at the same time, the tone of the urinary sphincter is enhanced, making voiding difficult.

Antidiuresis that accompanies administration of morphine to animals has been attributed to opioid-induced release of arginine vasopressin hormone (antidiuretic hormone). In humans, however, administration of morphine in the absence of painful surgical stimulation does not evoke the release of this hormone.[38] Furthermore, when morphine is administered in the presence of an adequate intravascular fluid volume, there is no change in urine output.

Cutaneous Changes

Morphine causes cutaneous blood vessels to dilate. The skin of the face, neck, and upper chest frequently becomes flushed and warm. These changes in cutaneous circulation are in part caused by the release of histamine. Histamine release probably accounts for urticaria and erythema commonly seen at the morphine injection site. In addition, morphine-induced histamine release probably accounts for conjunctival erythema and pruritus. Localized cutaneous evidence of histamine release, especially along the vein into which morphine is injected, does not represent an allergic reaction.

Placental Transfer

Opioids are readily transported across the placenta. Therefore, depression of the neonate can occur as a consequence of administration of opioids to the mother during labor. In this regard, maternal administration of morphine may produce greater neonatal depression than meperidine does.[39] This may reflect immaturity of the neonate's blood–brain barrier. Chronic maternal use of an opioid can result in the development of physical dependence in the fetus. Subsequent administration of naloxone to the neonate can precipitate neonatal abstinence syndrome.

Drug Interactions

The ventilatory depressant effects of some opioids may be exaggerated by amphetamines, phenothiazines, monoamine oxidase inhibitors, and tricyclic antidepressants. For example, patients receiving monoamine oxidase inhibitors may experience exaggerated CNS depression and hyperpyrexia after administration of an opioid agonist, especially meperidine. This exaggerated response may reflect alterations in the rate or pathway of metabolism of the opioid. Sympathomimetic drugs appear to enhance analgesia produced by opioids. The cholinergic nervous system seems to be a positive modulator of opioid-induced analgesia in that physostigmine enhances and atropine antagonizes analgesia.

Hormonal Changes

Prolonged opioid therapy may influence the hypothalamic-pituitary-adrenal axis and the hypothalamic-pituitary-gonadal axis, leading to endocrine and immune effects.[40,41] Morphine may cause a progressive decrease in plasma cortisol concentrations. The main effects of opioids on the hypothalamic-pituitary-gonadal axis involve modulation of hormone release including increased prolactin and decreased luteinizing hormone, follicle-stimulating hormone, testosterone, and estrogen concentrations.

Overdose

The principal manifestation of opioid overdose is depression of ventilation manifesting as a slow breathing frequency, which may progress to apnea. Pupils are symmetric and miotic unless severe arterial hypoxemia is present, which results in mydriasis. Skeletal muscles are flaccid, and upper airway obstruction may occur. Pulmonary edema commonly occurs, but the mechanism is not known. Hypotension and seizures develop if arterial hypoxemia persists. The triad of miosis, hypoventilation, and coma should suggest overdose with an opioid. Treatment of opioid overdose is mechanical ventilation of the patient's lungs with oxygen and administration of an opioid antagonist such as naloxone. Administration of an opioid antagonist to treat opioid overdose may precipitate acute withdrawal in dependent patients.

Provocation of Coughing

Paradoxically, preinduction administration of fentanyl, sufentanil, or alfentanil may be associated with significant reflex coughing.[42] The exact cause of opioid-induced cough is unclear but is thought to be due to imbalance between sympathetic and vagal innervation of the airways and/or stimulation of juxtacapillary irritant receptors.[43] Morphine and hydromorphone do not appear to cause this reaction.

Pharmacodynamic Tolerance and Physical Dependence

Pharmacodynamic tolerance and physical dependence with repeated opioid administration are characteristics of all opioid agonists and are among the major limitations of their clinical use. Cross-tolerance develops between all the opioids. Tolerance can occur without physical dependence, but the reverse does not seem to occur.

Tolerance is the development of the requirement for increased doses of a drug (in this case, an opioid agonist) to achieve the same effect previously achieved with a lower dose. Such acquired tolerance usually takes 2 to 3 weeks to develop with analgesic doses of morphine, although acute tolerance can develop much more quickly with highly potent opioids.[44] Tolerance develops to analgesic, euphoric, sedative, depression of ventilation, and emetic effects of opioids but not to their effects on miosis and bowel motility. The potential for physical dependence depends on the agonist effect of opioids. Indeed, physical dependence does not occur with opioid antagonists and is less likely with opioid agonist–antagonists. When opioid agonist actions predominate, there often develops, with repeated use, both psychological and physiologic need for the drug.

Physical dependence on morphine usually requires about 25 days to develop but may occur sooner in emotionally unstable persons. Some degree of physical dependence, however, occurs after only 48 hours of continuous medication. When physical dependence is established, discontinuation of the opioid agonist produces a typical withdrawal abstinence syndrome (Table 7-3).[45] Initial symptoms of withdrawal include yawning, diaphoresis, lacrimation, or coryza. Insomnia and restlessness are prominent. Abdominal cramps, nausea, vomiting, and diarrhea reach their peak in 72 hours and then decline over the next 7 to 10 days. During withdrawal, tolerance to morphine is rapidly lost, and the syndrome can be terminated by a modest dose of opioid agonist. The longer the period of abstinence, the smaller the dose of opioid agonist that will be required.

Pharmacodynamic tolerance has been related to neurologic changes that take place after long-term exposure to the opioid.[45] The classic explanation for tolerance to a receptor agonist involved changes occurring at the level of the receptors and involve receptor desensitization. Opioid receptors on the cell membrane surfaces become gradually desensitized by reduced transcription and subsequent decreases in the absolute numbers of opioid receptors (downregulation). A second mechanism proposed to explain pharmacodynamic tolerance involves upregulation of the cAMP system. Acutely, opioids inhibit functional activity of cAMP pathways by blocking adenylate cyclase, the enzyme that catalyzes the synthesis of cAMP. Long-term opioid exposure is associated with gradual recovery of cAMP pathways and tolerance develops. Increased

Table 7-3

Time Course of Opioid Withdrawal

Opioid	Onset	Peak Intensity	Duration
Meperidine	2–6 h	6–12 h	4–5 days
Fentanyl	2–6 h	6–12 h	4–5 days
Morphine	6–18 h	36–72 h	7–10 days
Heroin	6–18 h	36–72 h	7–10 days
Methadone	24–48 h	3–21 days	6–7 weeks

Adapted from Mitra S, Sinatra RS. Perioperative management of acute pain in the opioid-dependent patient. *Anesthesiology*. 2004;101:212–227.

synthesis of cAMP may be responsible for physical dependence and physiologic changes associated with withdrawal. Upregulation of cAMP has been most clearly demonstrated in the locus ceruleus of the brain. Clonidine, a centrally acting α_2-adrenergic agonist that diminishes transmission in sympathetic pathways in the CNS, is an effective drug in suppressing withdrawal signs in persons who are physically dependent on opioids. Tolerance is not due to enzyme induction, because no increase in the rate of metabolism of opioid agonists occurs.

Long-term pharmacodynamic tolerance characterized by opioid insensitivity may persist for months or years in some individuals and most likely represents persistent neural adaptation.[45] In this regard, NMDA glutamate receptors are important in the development of opioid tolerance and increased pain sensitivity. Prolonged exposure to opioids activates NMDA receptors via second messenger mechanisms and also downregulates spinal glutamate transporters. The resultant high synaptic concentrations of glutamate and NMDA receptor activation contribute to opioid tolerance and abnormal pain sensitivity (pronociceptive or sensitization process). The observation that treatment with small doses of ketamine (an NMDA receptor antagonist) abolishes the acute opioid tolerance seen with remifentanil supports this hypothesis.[46]

Opioid Agonists

Opioid agonists include but are not limited to morphine, meperidine, fentanyl, sufentanil, alfentanil, and remifentanil (see Table 7-1).[47] The most notable feature of the clinical use of opioids is the extraordinary variation in dose requirements for effective treatment of pain.[48] This interindividual variation emphasizes that usual doses of opioids may produce inadequate or excessive opioid effects. Opioid rotation may be useful when dose escalation is not effective in treating pain.

Morphine

Isolated in 1806 and named after Morpheus, the Greek god of dreams, morphine is the prototype opioid agonist to which all other opioids are compared. In humans, morphine produces analgesia, euphoria, sedation, and a diminished ability to concentrate. Other sensations include nausea, a feeling of body warmth, heaviness of the extremities, dryness of the mouth, and pruritus, especially in the cutaneous areas around the nose. The cause of pain persists, but even low doses of morphine increase the threshold to pain and modify the perception of noxious stimulation such that it is no longer experienced as pain. Continuous, dull pain is relieved by morphine more effectively than is sharp, intermittent pain. In contrast to nonopioid analgesics, morphine is effective against pain arising from the viscera as well as from skeletal muscles, joints, and integumental structures. Analgesia is most prominent when morphine is administered before the painful stimulus occurs.[49] In the absence of pain, however, morphine may produce dysphoria rather than euphoria.

Pharmacokinetics

Morphine is well absorbed after IM administration, with onset of effect in 15 to 30 minutes and a peak effect in 45 to 90 minutes. The clinical duration of action is about 4 hours. Morphine can be administered orally for treatment of chronic pain recognizing that absorption from the gastrointestinal is limited by significant first-pass metabolism in the liver, which limits the bioavailability of an orally administered dose to approximately 25% (1 mg of IV morphine ~4 mg of oral morphine). Morphine is usually administered IV in the perioperative period, thus eliminating the unpredictable influence of drug absorption. The peak effect (equilibration time between the blood and brain) after IV administration of morphine is delayed compared with opioids such as fentanyl and alfentanil, requiring about 15 to 30 minutes (Table 7-4).

Table 7-4

Pharmacokinetics of Opioid Agonists

	pK	Percent Nonionized (pH 7.4)	Protein Binding (%)	Clearance (mL/min)	Volume of Distribution (L)	Partition Coefficient	Elimination Half-Time (h)	Context Sensitive Half-Time: 4-Hour Infusion (min)	Effect-Site (Blood/Brain) Equilibration Time (min)
Morphine	7.9	23	35	1,050	224	1	1.7–3.3		
Meperidine	8.5	7	70	1,020	305	32	3–5		
Fentanyl	8.4	8.5	84	1,530	335	955	3.1–6.6	260	6.8
Sufentanil	8.0	20	93	900	123	1,727	2.2–4.6	30	6.2
Alfentanil	6.5	89	92	238	27	129	1.4–1.5	60	1.4
Remifentanil	7.3	58	66–93	4,000	30		0.17–0.33	4	1.1

Morphine inhaled as an aerosol from a nebulizer may act on afferent nerve pathways in the airways to relieve dyspnea as associated with lung cancer and associated pleural effusion.[50] However, profound depression of ventilation may follow aerosol administration of morphine.[51] The onset and duration of the analgesic effects of morphine are similar after IV administration or inhalation via a pulmonary drug delivery system that produces a fine aerosol.[52]

Plasma morphine concentrations after rapid IV injections do not correlate closely with the drug's pharmacologic activity, likely due to the delay in transit of morphine across the blood–brain barrier. Cerebrospinal fluid (CSF) concentrations of morphine peak 15 to 30 minutes after IV injection and decay more slowly than plasma concentrations (Fig. 7-6).[53] As a result, the analgesic and ventilatory depressant effects of morphine may not be evident during the initial high plasma concentrations after IV administration of the opioid. Likewise, these same drug effects persist despite decreasing plasma concentrations of morphine. Moderate analgesia probably requires maintenance of plasma morphine concentrations of at least 0.05 μg/mL.[54]

Only a small amount of administered morphine gains access to the CNS. For example, it is estimated that less than 0.1% of morphine that is administered IV has entered the CNS at the time of peak plasma concentrations. Reasons for poor penetration of morphine into the CNS include (a) relatively poor lipid solubility, (b) high degree of ionization at physiologic pH, (c) protein binding, and (d) rapid conjugation with glucuronic acid. Alkalinization of the blood, as produced by hyperventilation of the patient's lungs, will increase the nonionized fraction of morphine and thus enhance its passage into the CNS. Nevertheless, respiratory acidosis, which decreases the nonionized fraction of morphine, results in higher plasma and brain concentrations of morphine than are present during normocarbia (Fig. 7-7).[55] This suggests that carbon dioxide–induced increases in cerebral blood flow and enhanced delivery of morphine to the brain are more important than the fraction of drug that exists in either the ionized or nonionized fraction. In contrast to the CNS, morphine accumulates rapidly in the kidneys, liver, and skeletal muscles. Morphine, unlike fentanyl, does not undergo significant first-pass uptake into the lungs.[56]

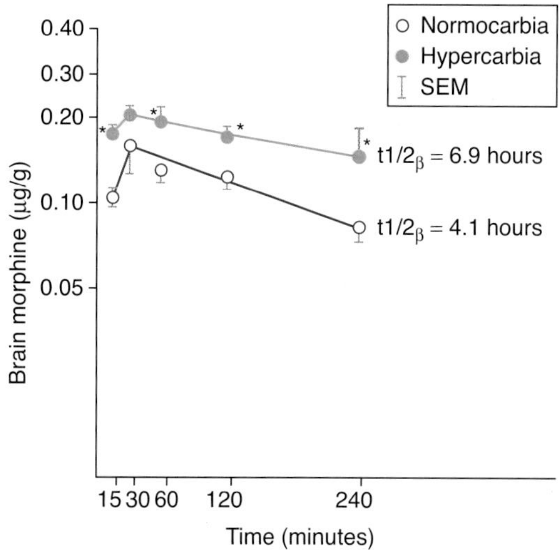

FIGURE 7-7 Hypercarbia, which decreases the nonionized fraction of morphine, results in a higher brain concentration and longer elimination half-time (t½β) than occurs in the presence of normocarbia. (*$P < .05$.) (From Finck AD, Ngai SH, Berkowitz BA. Antagonism of general anesthesia by naloxone in the rat. *Anesthesiology.* 1977;46:241–245, with permission.)

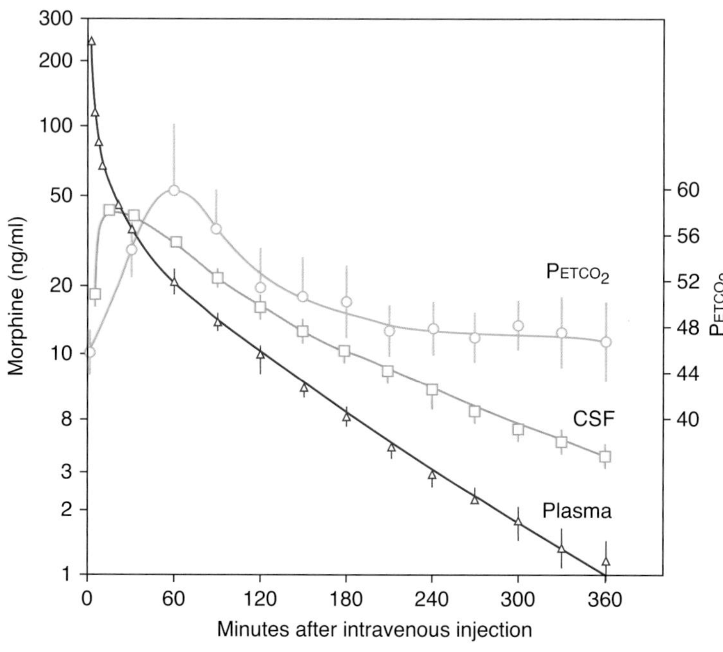

FIGURE 7-6 Cerebrospinal fluid (CSF) concentrations following intravenous administration of morphine decay more slowly than plasma concentrations. The end-tidal CO_2 concentration (P_{ETCO_2}) remains increased despite a decreasing plasma concentration of morphine. (Mean ± SE.) (From Murphy MR, Hug CC. Pharmacokinetics of intravenous morphine in patients anesthetized with enflurane-nitrous oxide. *Anesthesiology.* 1981;54:187–192, with permission.)

Metabolism

Metabolism of morphine is primarily conjugation with glucuronic acid in hepatic and extrahepatic sites, especially the kidneys. About 75% to 85% of a dose of morphine appears as morphine-3-glucuronide, and 5% to 10% as morphine-6-glucuronide (a ratio of 9:1). Morphine-3-glucuronide is detectable in the plasma within 1 minute after IV injection, and its concentration exceeds that of unchanged drug by almost 10-fold within 90 minutes (Fig. 7-8).[53] An estimated 5% of morphine is demethylated to normorphine, and a small amount of codeine may also be formed. Metabolites of morphine are eliminated principally in the urine, with only 7% to 10% undergoing biliary excretion. Morphine-3-glucuronide is detectable in the urine for up to 72 hours after the administration of morphine. A small fraction (1% to 2%) of injected morphine is recovered unchanged in the urine.

Morphine-3-glucuronide is pharmacologically inactive, whereas morphine-6-glucuronide produces analgesia and depression of ventilation via its agonist actions at μ receptors.[57] In fact, the ventilatory response to carbon dioxide is impacted similarly by morphine and morphine-6-glucuronide (Fig. 7-9).[58] The duration of action of morphine-6-glucuronide is greater than that of morphine, and it is possible that the majority of analgesic activity attributed to morphine is actually due to morphine-6-glucuronide, especially with long-term administration of morphine.[59] Morphine and morphine-6-glucuronide bind to μ opioid receptors with comparable affinity, whereas the analgesic potency of morphine-6-glucuronide is 650-fold higher than morphine.[60]

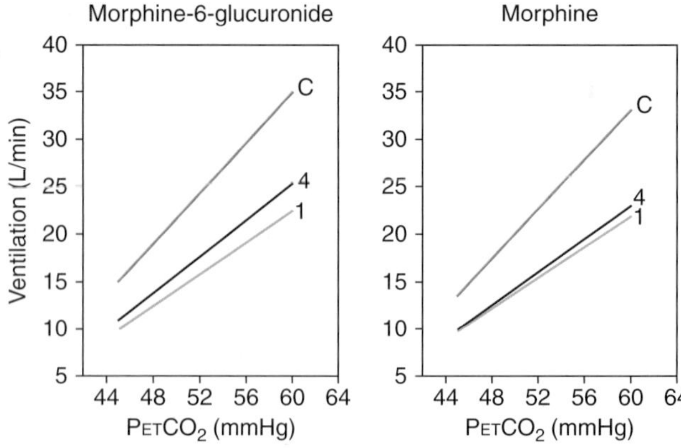

FIGURE 7-9 Influence of 0.2 mg/kg morphine-6-glucuronide IV and 0.13 mg/kg morphine IV on the ventilatory response to carbon dioxide. The effects of both opioids were similar over the 4-hour period of study. $P_{ET}CO_2$, end-tidal partial pressure of carbon dioxide. (From Romberg R, Olofsen E, Satron E, et al. Pharmacodynamic effect of morphine-6-glucuronide versus morphine on hypoxic and hypercapnic breathing in healthy volunteers. *Anesthesiology.* 2003;99:788–798, with permission.)

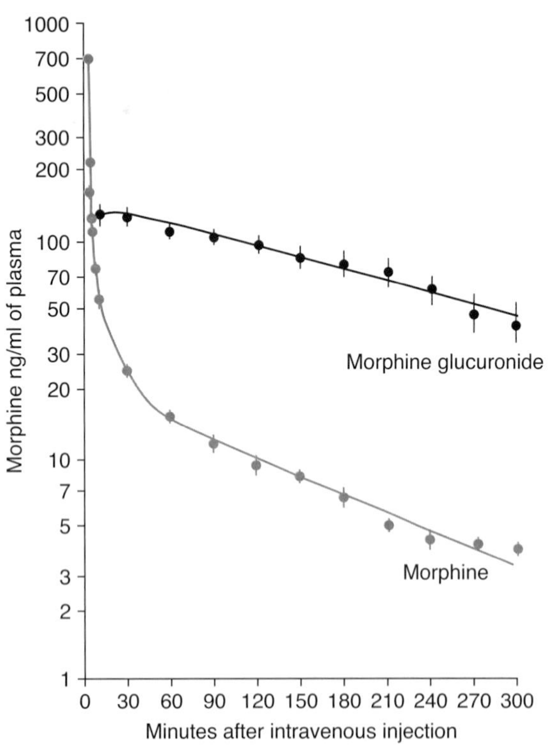

FIGURE 7-8 Morphine glucuronide is detectable in the plasma within 1 minute after intravenous injection, and its concentration exceeds that of unchanged morphine by almost 10-fold within 90 minutes. (Mean ± SE.) (From Murphy MR, Hug CC. Pharmacokinetics of intravenous morphine in patients anesthetized with enflurane-nitrous oxide. *Anesthesiology.* 1981;54:187–192., with permission.)

Renal metabolism makes a significant contribution to the total metabolism of morphine, which offers a possible explanation for the absence of any decrease in systemic clearance of morphine in patients with hepatic cirrhosis or during the anhepatic phase of orthotopic liver transplantation.[61]

Elimination of morphine glucuronides may be impaired in patients with renal failure, causing an accumulation of metabolites and unexpected ventilatory depressant effects of small doses of opioids (Fig. 7-10).[62] Indeed, prolonged depression of ventilation (>7 days) has been observed in patients in renal failure after administration of morphine.[63] Formation of glucuronide conjugates may be impaired by monoamine oxidase inhibitors, which is consistent with exaggerated effects of morphine when administered to patients being treated with these drugs.

Elimination Half-Time

After IV administration of morphine, the elimination of morphine-3-glucuronide is somewhat longer than for morphine (see Table 7-4 and Fig. 7-8).[53] The decrease in the plasma concentration of morphine after initial distribution of the drug is principally due to metabolism because only a small amount of unchanged opioid is excreted in the urine. Plasma morphine concentrations are higher in the elderly than in young adults (Fig. 7-11).[54] In the first 4 days of life, the clearance of morphine is decreased and its elimination half-time is prolonged compared with

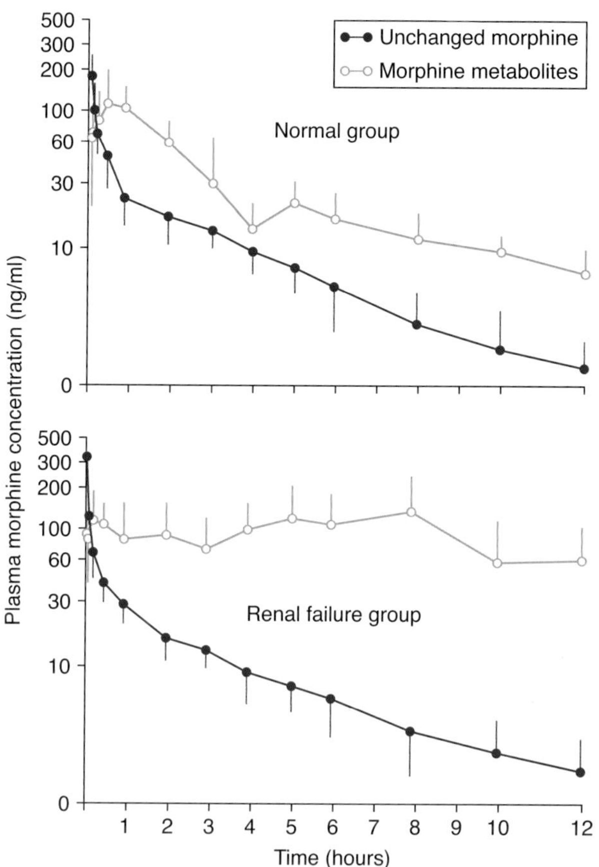

FIGURE 7-10 Plasma concentrations of unchanged morphine *(closed circles)* and morphine metabolites *(open circles)* in normal and renal failure patients. (From Chauvin M, Sandouk P, Scherrman JM, et al. Morphine pharmacokinetics in renal failure. *Anesthesiology.* 1987;66:327–331, with permission.)

that found in older infants.[64] This is consistent with the observation that neonates are more sensitive than older children to the respiratory depressant effects of morphine. Patients with renal failure exhibit higher plasma and CSF concentrations of morphine and morphine metabolites than do normal patients, reflecting a smaller volume of distribution (Vd).[65] Possible accumulation of morphine-6-glucuronide suggests the need for caution when administering morphine to patients with renal dysfunction. Concentrations of morphine in the colostrum of parturients receiving patient-controlled analgesia with morphine are low and it is unlikely that significant amounts of drug will be transferred to the breast-fed neonate.[66]

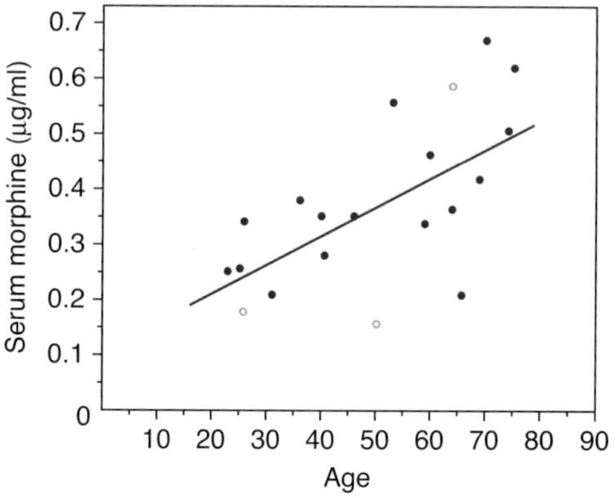

FIGURE 7-11 The plasma (serum) concentration of morphine increases progressively with advancing age. (From Berkowitz BA, Ngai SH, Yang JC, et al. The disposition of morphine in surgical patients. *Clin Pharmacol Ther.* 1975;17:629–635, with permission.)

Gender

Gender may affect opioid analgesia but the direction and magnitude of these differences depend on many interacting variables including the opioid used.[67] Morphine exhibits greater analgesic potency and slower speed of offset in women than men.[68] This observation is consistent with higher postoperative opioid consumption in men compared with women. Likewise, morphine decreases the slope of the ventilatory response to carbon dioxide in women, whereas in men, there was no significant effect.[69] Morphine has no demonstrated effect on the apneic threshold in women but causes an increase in men. Hypoxic sensitivity is decreased by morphine in women but not men.

Side Effects

Side effects described for morphine are also characteristic of other opioid agonists, although the incidence and magnitude may vary.

Meperidine

First synthesized in 1939, meperidine (also referred to as ***pethidine***) is a synthetic opioid agonist at μ and κ opioid receptors and is derived from phenylepiperidine (Fig. 7-2). There are several analogues of meperidine, including fentanyl, sufentanil, alfentanil, and remifentanil. Meperidine shares several structural features that are present in local anesthetics including a tertiary amine, an ester group, and a lipophilic phenyl group. Indeed, meperidine administered intrathecally blocks sodium channels to a degree comparable with lidocaine. Structurally, meperidine is similar to atropine, and it possesses a mild atropine-like antispasmodic effect on smooth muscle.

Pharmacokinetics

Meperidine is about one-tenth as potent as morphine. The duration of action of meperidine is 2 to 4 hours, making it a shorter acting opioid agonist than morphine. In equianalgesic doses, meperidine produces equivalent sedation, euphoria, nausea, vomiting, and depression of ventilation to morphine. Meperidine is absorbed from the gastrointestinal tract, but extensive first-pass hepatic metabolism (up to 80%) limits its oral usefulness.

Metabolism

Hepatic metabolism of meperidine is extensive, with about 90% of the drug initially undergoing demethylation to normeperidine and hydrolysis to meperidinic acid.[70]

Normeperidine subsequently undergoes hydrolysis to normeperidinic acid. Urinary excretion is the principal elimination route and is pH dependent. For example, if the urinary pH is <5, as much as 25% of meperidine is excreted unchanged. Indeed, acidification of the urine can be considered in an attempt to speed elimination of meperidine. Decreased renal function can predispose to accumulation of normeperidine.

Normeperidine has an elimination half-time of 15 hours (35 hours in patients in renal failure) and can be detected in urine for as long as 3 days after administration of meperidine. This metabolite is about one-half as active as meperidine as an analgesic. In addition, normeperidine produces CNS stimulation. Normeperidine toxicity manifesting as myoclonus and seizures is most likely during prolonged administration of meperidine as during patient-controlled analgesia, especially in the presence of impaired renal function.[70] Normeperidine may also be important in meperidine-induced delirium (confusion, hallucinations), which has been observed in patients receiving the drug for longer than 3 days, corresponding to accumulation of this active metabolite.

Elimination Half-Time

The elimination half-time of meperidine is 3 to 5 hours (see Table 7-4). Because clearance of meperidine primarily depends on hepatic metabolism, it is possible that large doses of opioid would saturate enzyme systems and result in prolonged elimination half-times. Nevertheless, elimination half-time is not altered by doses of meperidine up to 5 mg/kg IV. About 60% of meperidine is bound to plasma proteins. Elderly patients manifest decreased plasma protein binding of meperidine, resulting in increased plasma concentrations of free drug and an apparent increased sensitivity to the opioid. The increased tolerance of alcoholics to meperidine and other opioids presumably reflects an increased volume of distribution, resulting in lower plasma concentrations of meperidine for a given dose.

Clinical Uses

The clinical use of meperidine has declined greatly in recent years. Meperidine is the only opioid considered adequate for surgery when administered intrathecally, owing to its ability to block sodium channels in a way similar to local anesthetics in addition to its μ-mediated opioid acitivity.[71] An IM injection of meperidine for postoperative analgesia results in peak plasma concentrations that vary three- to fivefold as well as a time required to achieve peak concentrations that varies three- to sevenfold among patients.[72] The minimum analgesic plasma concentration of meperidine is highly variable among patients; however, in the same patient, differences in concentrations as small as 0.05 μg/mL can represent a margin between no relief and complete analgesia. A plasma meperidine concentration of 0.7 μg/mL would be expected to provide postoperative analgesia in about 95% of patients.[73] Normeperidine toxicity has been described in patients receiving meperidine for patient-controlled analgesia.[70] Therefore, because there are other effective agents, patient-controlled analgesia with meperidine cannot be recommended.

Meperidine may be effective in suppressing postoperative shivering that may result in detrimental increases in metabolic oxygen consumption. The antishivering effects of meperidine may reflect stimulation of κ receptors (estimated to represent 10% of its activity) and a drug-induced decrease in the shivering threshold (not present with alfentanil, clonidine, propofol, or volatile anesthetics).[74–76] In addition, meperidine is a potent agonist at α_2 receptors, which might contribute to antishivering effects.[77] Indeed, clonidine is even more effective than meperidine in reducing postoperative shivering. Butorphanol (a κ receptor agonist-antagonist) stops shivering more effectively than opioids with a predominant μ opioid receptor agonist effect. Evidence for a role of κ receptors in the antishivering effects of meperidine and butorphanol is the failure of naloxone to completely inhibit this drug-induced effect.

Unlike morphine, meperidine is not useful for the treatment of diarrhea and is not an effective cough suppressant. During bronchoscopy, the relative lack of antitussive activity of meperidine makes this opioid less useful. Meperidine is not used in high doses because of significant negative cardiac inotropic effects plus histamine release in a substantial number of patients.[78]

Side Effects

The side effects of meperidine generally resemble those described for morphine. Meperidine, in contrast to morphine, rarely causes bradycardia but instead may increase heart rate, reflecting its modest atropine-like qualities. Large doses of meperidine result in decreases in myocardial contractility, which, among opioids, is unique for this drug. Delirium and seizures, when they occur, presumably reflect accumulation of normeperidine, which has stimulating effects on the CNS.

Serotonin syndrome (autonomic instability with hypertension, tachycardia, diaphoresis, hyperthermia, behavioral changes including confusion and agitation, and neuromuscular changes manifesting as hyperreflexia) occurs when drugs capable of increasing serotonin administration are administered. In severe cases, coma, seizures, coagulopathy, and metabolic acidosis may develop. Administration of meperidine to patients receiving antidepressant drugs (monoamine oxidase inhibitors, fluoxetine) may elicit this syndrome.[79]

Meperidine readily impairs ventilation and may be even more of a ventilatory depressant than morphine. This opioid promptly crosses the placenta, and concentrations of meperidine in umbilical cord blood at birth may exceed maternal plasma concentrations.[39] Meperidine may produce less constipation and urinary retention than morphine. After equal analgesic doses, biliary tract spasm is less after meperidine injection than after morphine injection but greater than that caused by codeine.[35] Meperidine does not cause miosis but rather tends to cause mydriasis, reflecting its modest atropine-like actions. A dry mouth and an increase in heart rate are further evidence of the atropine-like effects of meperidine. Transient neurologic symptoms have been described following the administration of intrathecal meperidine for surgical anesthesia.[80]

The pattern of withdrawal symptoms after abrupt discontinuation of meperidine differs from that of morphine in that there are few autonomic nervous system effects. In addition, symptoms of withdrawal develop more rapidly and are of a shorter duration compared with those of morphine.

Fentanyl

Fentanyl is a phenylpiperidine-derivative synthetic opioid agonist that is structurally related to meperidine (see Fig. 7-2). As an analgesic, fentanyl is 75 to 125 times more potent than morphine. It was first synthesized by Janssen Pharmaceutica in 1960 during an assay of meperidine derivatives and subsequently released as the citrate salt under the trade name Sublimaze.[81]

Pharmacokinetics

A single dose of fentanyl administered IV has a more rapid onset and shorter duration of action than morphine. Despite the clinical impression that fentanyl produces a rapid onset, there is a distinct time lag between the peak plasma fentanyl concentration and peak slowing on the EEG. This delay reflects the effect-site equilibration time between blood and the brain for fentanyl, which is 6.4 minutes. The greater potency and more rapid onset of action reflect the greater lipid solubility of fentanyl compared with that of morphine, which facilitates its passage across the blood–brain barrier. Consequently, plasma concentrations of fentanyl (unlike morphine) correlate well with CSF concentrations. Likewise, the short duration of action of a single dose of fentanyl reflects its rapid redistribution to inactive tissue sites such as fat and skeletal muscles, with an associated decrease in the plasma concentration of the drug (Fig. 7-12).[82]

The lungs also serve as a large inactive storage site, with an estimated 75% of the initial fentanyl dose undergoing first-pass pulmonary uptake.[56] This nonrespiratory function of the lungs limits the initial amount of drug that reaches the systemic circulation and may play an important role in determining the pharmacokinetic profile of fentanyl. When multiple IV doses of fentanyl are administered or when there is continuous infusion of the drug, progressive saturation of these inactive tissue sites occurs. As a result, the plasma concentration of fentanyl does not decrease rapidly, and the duration of analgesia, as well as depression of ventilation, may be prolonged. Cardiopulmonary bypass causes clinically insignificant effects on the pharmacokinetics of fentanyl despite associated hemodilution, hypothermia, nonphysiologic blood flow and cardiopulmonary bypass–induced systemic inflammatory responses.[83]

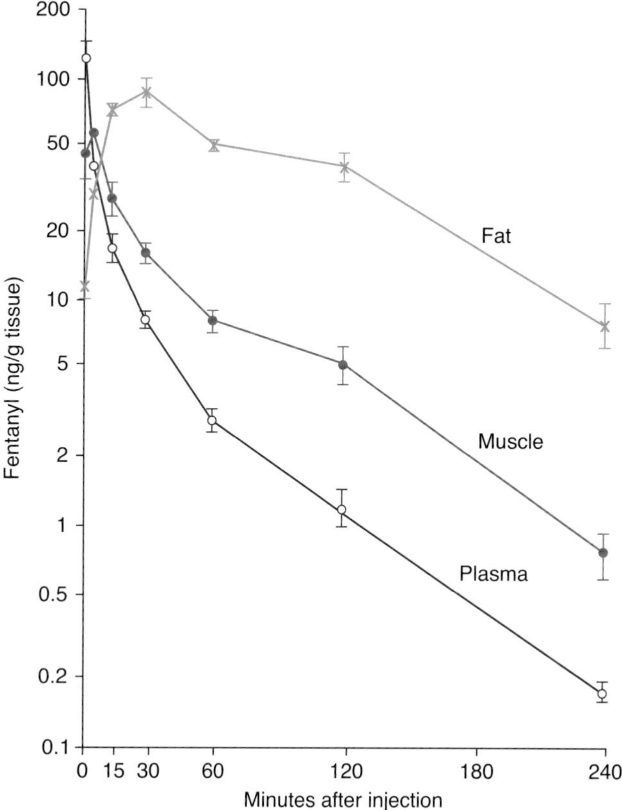

FIGURE 7-12 The short duration of action of a single intravenous dose of fentanyl reflects its rapid redistribution to inactive tissue sites such as fat and skeletal muscles, with associated decreases in the plasma concentration of drug. (Mean ± SE.) (From Hug CC, Murphy MR. Tissue redistribution of fentanyl and termination of its effects in rats. *Anesthesiology.* 1981;55:369–375, with permission.)

Metabolism

Fentanyl is extensively metabolized by *N*-demethylation, producing norfentanyl, hydroxyproprionyl-fentanyl, and hydroxyproprionyl-norfentanyl. Norfentanyl is structurally similar to normeperidine and is the principal metabolite of fentanyl in humans. It is excreted by the kidneys and can be detected in the urine for 72 hours after a single IV dose of fentanyl. Less than 10% of fentanyl is excreted unchanged in the urine. The pharmacologic activity of fentanyl metabolites is believed to be minimal.[84] Fentanyl is a substrate for hepatic P450 enzymes (CYP3A) and is susceptible to drug interactions that reflect interference with enzyme activity (less likely than with alfentanil).[85]

Elimination Half-Time

Despite the clinical impression that fentanyl has a short duration of action, its elimination half-time is longer than that for morphine (see Table 7-4). This longer elimination half-time reflects a larger Vd of fentanyl because clearance of both opioids is similar (see Table 7-4). The larger Vd of fentanyl is due to its greater lipid solubility and thus more rapid passage into tissues compared with the less lipid-soluble morphine. After an IV bolus, fentanyl distributes rapidly from the plasma to highly vascular tissues (brain, lungs, heart). More than 80% of the injected dose leaves the plasma in <5 minutes. The plasma concentrations of fentanyl are maintained by slow reuptake from inactive tissue sites, which accounts for persistent drug effects that parallel the prolonged elimination half time. In animals, the elimination half-time, Vd, and clearance of fentanyl are independent of the dose of opioid between 6.4 and 640 μg/kg IV.[86]

A prolonged elimination half-time for fentanyl in elderly patients is due to decreased clearance of the opioid because Vd is not changed in comparison with younger adults.[87] This change may reflect age-related decreases in hepatic blood flow, microsomal enzyme activity, or albumin production, as fentanyl is highly bound (79% to 87%) to protein. For these reasons, it is likely that a given dose of fentanyl will be effective for a longer period of time in elderly patients than in younger patients. A prolonged elimination half-time of fentanyl has also been observed in patients undergoing abdominal aortic surgery requiring infrarenal aortic cross-clamping.[88] Somewhat surprising, however, is the failure of hepatic cirrhosis to prolong significantly the elimination half-time of fentanyl.[89]

Context-Sensitive Half-Time

As the duration of continuous infusion of fentanyl increases beyond about 2 hours, the context-sensitive half-time of this opioid becomes greater than sufentanil (Fig. 7-13).[3,90] This reflects saturation of inactive tissue sites with fentanyl during prolonged infusions and return of the opioid from peripheral compartments to the plasma. This tissue reservoir of fentanyl replaces fentanyl eliminated by hepatic metabolism so as to slow the rate of decrease in the plasma concentration of fentanyl when the infusion is discontinued.

Cardiopulmonary Bypass

All opioids show a decrease in plasma concentration with initiation of cardiopulmonary bypass.[91] The degree of this decrease is greater with fentanyl because a significant proportion of the drug adheres to the surface of the cardiopulmonary bypass circuit. The decrease is least with opioids that have a large Vd such that the addition of prime volume is less important. In this respect, sufentanil and alfentanil may provide more stable plasma concentrations during cardiopulmonary bypass. Elimination of fentanyl and alfentanil has been shown to be prolonged by cardiopulmonary bypass.

Clinical Uses

Fentanyl is administered clinically in a wide range of doses. For example, low doses of fentanyl, 1 to 2 μg/kg IV, are injected to provide analgesia. Fentanyl, 2 to 20 μg/kg IV, may be administered as an adjuvant to inhaled anesthetics in an attempt to blunt circulatory responses to (a) direct laryngoscopy for intubation of the trachea, or (b) sudden changes in the level of surgical stimulation. Timing of the IV injection of fentanyl to prevent or treat such responses should consider the effect-site equilibration time, which for fentanyl is prolonged compared with alfentanil and remifentanil. Injection of an opioid such as fentanyl before painful surgical stimulation may decrease the subsequent amount of opioid required in the postoperative period to provide analgesia.[49] Administration of fentanyl 1.5 or 3 μg/kg IV 5 minutes before induction of anesthesia decreases the subsequent doses of isoflurane or desflurane with 60% nitrous oxide needed to block the sympathetic nervous system response to surgical stimulation (Fig. 7-14).[92] Large doses of fentanyl, 50 to

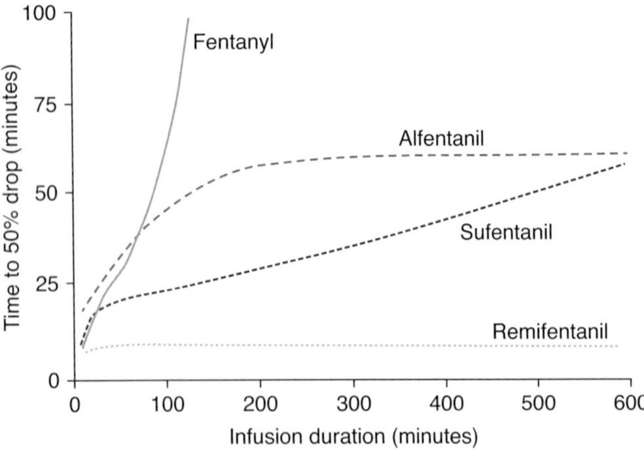

FIGURE 7-13 Computer simulation–derived context-sensitive half-times (time necessary for the plasma concentration to decrease 50% after discontinuation of the infusion) as a function of the duration of the intravenous infusion. (From Egan TD, Lemmens HJM, Fiset P, et al. The pharmacokinetics of the new short-acting opioid remifentanil [GI87084B] in healthy adult male volunteers. *Anesthesiology.* 1993;79: 881–892, with permission.)

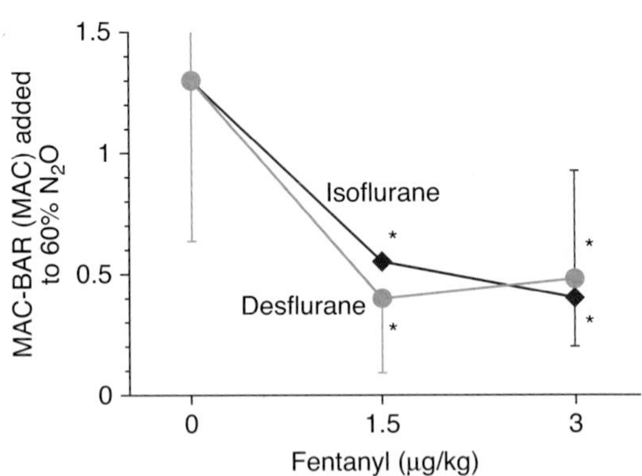

FIGURE 7-14 The anesthetic dose of desflurane and isoflurane required to block the adrenergic response (MAC-BAR) to incision in 50% of patients without and with fentanyl. There was no significant difference between the inhaled anesthetics at any fentanyl dose and both does of fentanyl significantly and similarly decreased MAC-BAR. (**P* <.05; mean ± SD.) (From Daniel M, Weiskopf RB, Noorani M, et al. Fentanyl augments the blockade of the sympathetic response to incision [MAC-BAR] produced by desflurane and isoflurane. Desflurane and isoflurane MAC-BAR without and with fentanyl. *Anesthesiology.* 1998;88:43–49, with permission.)

150 μg/kg IV, have been used alone to produce surgical anesthesia. Large doses of fentanyl as the sole anesthetic have the advantage of stable hemodynamics due principally to the (a) lack of direct myocardial depressant effects, (b) absence of histamine release, and (c) suppression of the stress responses to surgery. Disadvantages of using fentanyl as the sole anesthetic include (a) failure to prevent sympathetic nervous system responses to painful surgical stimulation at any dose, especially in patients with good left ventricular function; (b) unpredictable amnestic effects potentially leading to recall; and (c) postoperative depression of ventilation.[93–95] Intrathecal fentanyl (maximal benefit achieved with 25 μg) can produce rapid, profound analgesia for early labor with minimal side effects.[96]

Fentanyl may be administered as a transmucosal preparation (oral transmucosal fentanyl) in a delivery device (several formulations are available, including a lozenge mounted on a handle or a film or rapid-dissolving preparation applied to the buccal mucosa) designed to deliver 5 to 20 μg/kg of fentanyl. The goal is to decrease preoperative anxiety and facilitate the induction of anesthesia, especially in children.[97,98] In children 2 to 8 years of age, the preoperative administration of oral transmucosal fentanyl, 15 to 20 μg/kg 45 minutes before the induction of anesthesia, reliably induces preoperative sedation and facilitates induction of inhalation anesthesia.[99] These same patients, however, are likely to experience decreases in breathing frequency and arterial oxygenation and an increased incidence of postoperative nausea and vomiting that is not influenced by prophylactic administration of droperidol. In children 6 years of age and younger, the preoperative administration of oral transmucosal fentanyl, 15 μg/kg, is associated with an unacceptably high incidence of preoperative vomiting.[100] Conversely, another report did not observe an increased incidence of vomiting or arterial oxygen desaturation after premedication with oral transmucosal fentanyl.[101] For treatment of postoperative pain after orthopedic surgery, 1 mg of oral transmucosal fentanyl is equivalent to 5 mg of IV morphine.[102] Patients experiencing pain due to cancer may self-administer this opioid to the extent necessary to produce a desirable level of analgesia.

Transdermal fentanyl preparations delivering 75 to 100 μg per hour result in peak plasma fentanyl concentrations in about 18 hours that tend to remain stable during the presence of the patch, followed by a decreasing plasma concentration for several hours after removal of the delivery system, reflecting continued absorption from the cutaneous depot. These transdermal delivery systems were designed to produce stable, long-term fentanyl plasma concentrations in efforts to provide adequate, sustained analgesia for chronic, cancer-related pain. Each transdermal patch contains a depot of fentanyl that provides adequate drug to produce stable plasma fentanyl concentrations for 3 consecutive days. Transdermal fentanyl systems applied before the induction of anesthesia and left in place for 24 hours decrease the amount of parenteral opioid required for postoperative analgesia.[103] Acute toxic delirium has been observed in patients with chronic pain due to cancer being treated with transdermal fentanyl for prolonged periods of time.[104] It is possible that renal failure and accumulation of norfentanyl contributes to the possible toxic effects of prolonged use of transdermal fentanyl.

In dogs, maximal analgesic, ventilatory, and cardiovascular effects are present when the plasma concentration of fentanyl is approximately 30 ng/mL.[105] Thus, the analgesic actions of fentanyl cannot be separated from its effects on ventilation and heart rate. The fact that all receptor-mediated effects are similar at the same plasma concentration of fentanyl suggests saturation of the opioid receptors. Evidence of opioid overdose has been observed when an upper body warming blanket was placed intraoperatively and came into contact with the fentanyl patch and has been linked to increased dermal blood flow and resultant drug uptake caused by the warming.[106]

Side Effects

The side effects of fentanyl resemble those described for morphine. Persistent or recurrent depression of ventilation due to fentanyl is a potential postoperative problem.[107] Secondary peaks in plasma concentrations of fentanyl and morphine have been attributed to sequestration of fentanyl in acidic gastric fluid (ion trapping). Sequestered fentanyl could then be absorbed from the more alkaline small intestine back into the circulation to increase the plasma concentration of opioid and cause depression of ventilation to recur. This, however, may not be the mechanism for the secondary peak of fentanyl, because reabsorbed opioid from the gastrointestinal tract or skeletal muscles, as evoked by movement associated with transfer from the operating room, would be subject to first-pass hepatic metabolism. An alternative explanation for the secondary peak of fentanyl is washout of opioid from the lungs as ventilation to perfusion relationships are reestablished in the postoperative period.

Cardiovascular Effects

Unlike morphine, fentanyl, even in large doses (50 μg/kg IV), does not evoke the release of histamine (see Fig. 7-4).[26] As a result, dilatation of venous capacitance vessels leading to hypotension is unlikely. Carotid sinus baroreceptor reflex control of heart rate is markedly depressed by fentanyl, 10 μg/kg IV, administered to neonates (Fig. 7-15).[108] Therefore, changes in systemic blood pressure occurring during fentanyl anesthesia have to be carefully considered because cardiac output is principally rate dependent in neonates. Bradycardia is more prominent with fentanyl than morphine and may lead to occasional decreases in blood pressure and cardiac output.

Seizure Activity

Seizure-like activity has been described to follow rapid IV administration of fentanyl, sufentanil, and alfentanil.[109]

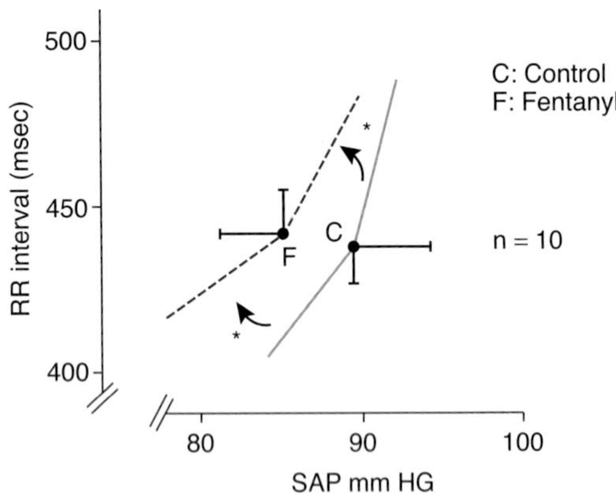

FIGURE 7-15 Fentanyl depresses the carotid sinus reflex–mediated heart rate response to changes in blood pressure in neonates. (*P <.02.) (From Murat I, Levron JB, Berg A, et al. Effects of fentanyl on baroreceptor reflex control of heart rate in newborn infants. *Anesthesiology.* 1988;68: 717–722, with permission.)

In the absence of EEG evidence of seizure activity, however, it is difficult to distinguish opioid-induced skeletal muscle rigidity or myoclonus from seizure activity. Indeed, recording of the EEG during periods of opioid-induced skeletal muscle rigidity fails to reveal evidence of seizure activity in the brain.[110] Even plasma concentrations as high as 1,750 ng/mL after rapid administration of fentanyl, 150 μg/kg IV, do not produce EEG evidence of seizure activity.[111] Conversely, opioids might produce a form of myoclonus secondary to depression of inhibitory neurons that would produce a clinical picture of seizure activity in the absence of EEG changes.

Somatosensory Evoked Potentials and Electroencephalogram

Fentanyl in doses exceeding 30 μg/kg IV produces changes in somatosensory evoked potentials that, although detectable, do not interfere with the use and interpretation of this monitor during anesthesia.[112] Opioids, including fentanyl, attenuate skeletal muscle movement at doses that have little effect on the EEG. This suggests that movement in response to surgical skin incision (used to measure minimum alveolar concentration [MAC]) primarily reflects the ability of a drug to obtund noxious reflexes and may not be the most appropriate measure for assessing consciousness or loss of consciousness.[113] This opioid effect confounds the use of bispectral analysis as a measure of anesthetic adequacy when lack of movement with surgical skin incision is used to define efficacy.[114]

Intracranial Pressure

Administration of fentanyl and sufentanil to head injury patients has been associated with modest increases (6 to 9 mm Hg) in ICP despite maintenance of an unchanged $Paco_2$.[115] These increases in ICP are typically accompanied by decreases in mean arterial pressure and cerebral perfusion pressure. In fact, increases in ICP do not accompany the administration of sufentanil when changes in mean arterial pressure are prevented (Fig. 7-16).[116] This suggests that increases in ICP evoked by sufentanil (and presumably fentanyl) may have been due to autoregulatory decreases in cerebral vascular resistance due to decreases in systemic blood pressure resulting in vasodilation, increased blood volume, and increased ICP. Nevertheless, opioid-induced increases in ICP are similar in the

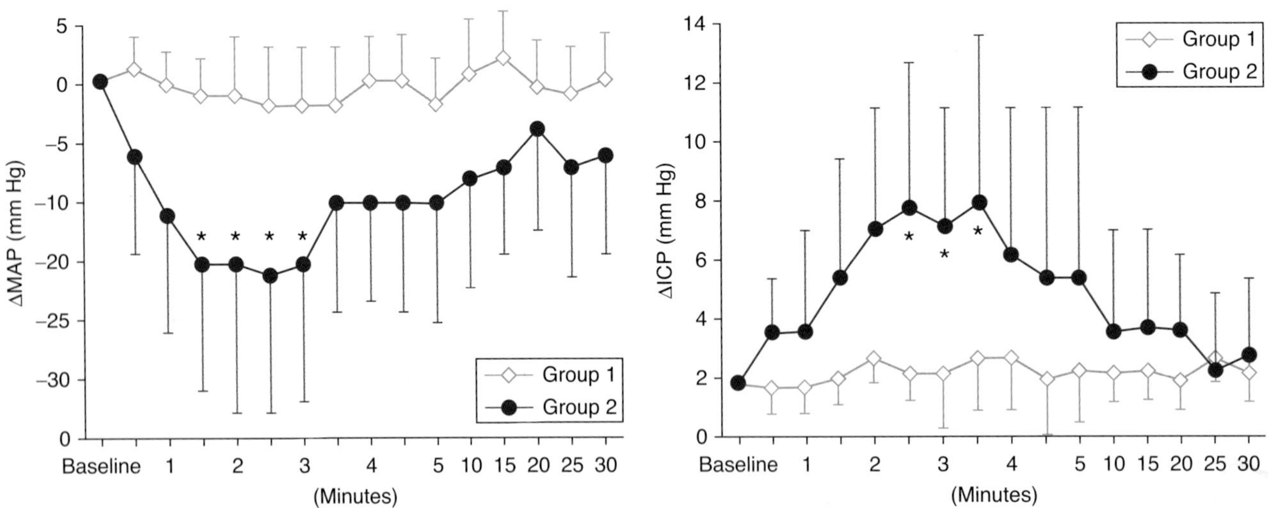

FIGURE 7-16 Changes in mean arterial pressure (MAP) and intracranial pressure (ICP) before and after administration of sufentanil, 3 μg/kg IV, to 30 patients with intracranial hypertension after severe brain trauma. ICP increased only in those patients who experienced a decrease in MAP after administration of sufentanil. (Mean ± SD; *P<.05 vs. group I.) (From Werner C, Kochs E, Bause H, et al. Effects of sufentanil on cerebral hemodynamics and intracranial pressure in patients with brain injury. *Anesthesiology.* 1995;83:721–726, with permission.)

presence of intact or impaired autoregulation, suggesting that mechanisms other than activation of the vasodilatory cascade need to be considered.[117]

Drug Interactions

Analgesic concentrations of fentanyl greatly potentiate the effects of benzodiazepines and decrease the dose requirements of propofol. The opioid-benzodiazepine combination displays marked synergism with respect to hypnosis and depression of ventilation.[118] In clinical practice, the advantage of synergy between opioids and benzodiazepines for the maintenance of patient comfort is carefully weighed against the disadvantages of the potentially adverse depressant effects of this combination.

Sufentanil

First synthesized in 1974, sufentanil is a thienyl analogue of fentanyl (see Fig. 7-2). The analgesic potency of sufentanil is 5 to 10 times that of fentanyl, which parallels the greater affinity of sufentanil for opioid receptors compared with that of fentanyl. Based on the plasma concentration necessary to cause 50% of the maximum slowing on the EEG (EC_{50}), sufentanil is 12 times more potent than fentanyl.[119] An important distinction from fentanyl is the 1,000-fold difference between the analgesic dose of sufentanil and the dose that produces seizures in animals. This difference is 160-fold for fentanyl and may be important when large doses of opioid agonists are used to produce anesthesia. Transient skeletal muscle spasm has been described after the accidental intrathecal injection of a large dose of sufentanil (40 μg), suggesting an irritative effect produced by the opioid.[120]

Pharmacokinetics

The elimination half-time of sufentanil is intermediate between that of fentanyl and alfentanil (see Table 7-4).[121] A single IV dose of sufentanil has a similar elimination half-time in patients with or without cirrhosis of the liver.[122] A prolonged elimination half-time has been observed in elderly patients receiving sufentanil for abdominal aortic surgery.[123] The Vd and elimination half-time of sufentanil is increased in obese patients, which most likely reflects the high lipid solubility of this opioid.[124]

A high tissue affinity is consistent with the lipophilic nature of sufentanil, which permits rapid penetration of the blood–brain barrier and onset of CNS effects (effect-site equilibration time of 6.2 minutes is similar to that of 6.8 minutes for fentanyl).[119] A rapid redistribution to inactive tissue sites terminates the effect of small doses, but a cumulative drug effect can accompany large or repeated doses of sufentanil. Sufentanil undergoes significant first-pass pulmonary uptake (approximately 60%) after rapid IV injection.[125] This pulmonary first-pass uptake is similar to fentanyl and greater than morphine (about 7%) and alfentanil (about 10%).

The extensive protein binding of sufentanil (92.5%) compared with that of fentanyl (79% to 87%) contributes to a smaller Vd, which is characteristic of sufentanil. Binding to α_1-acid glycoprotein constitutes a principal proportion of the total plasma protein binding of sufentanil. Levels of α_1-acid glycoprotein vary over a threefold range in healthy volunteers and are increased after surgery, which could result in a decrease in the plasma concentration of pharmacologically active unbound sufentanil. Lower concentrations of α_1-acid glycoprotein in neonates and infants probably account for decreases in protein binding of sufentanil in these age groups compared with that in older children and adults.[126] The resulting increased free fraction of sufentanil in the neonate might contribute to enhanced effects of this opioid. Indeed, fentanyl and its derivatives produce anesthesia and depression of ventilation at lower doses in neonates than in adults.[127]

Metabolism

Sufentanil is rapidly metabolized by *N*-dealkylation at the piperidine nitrogen and by O-demethylation. The products of *N*-dealkylation are pharmacologically inactive, whereas desmethyl sufentanil has about 10% of the activity of sufentanil. Less than 1% of an administered dose of sufentanil appears unchanged in urine. Indeed, the high lipid solubility of sufentanil results in maximal renal tubular reabsorption of free drug as well as its enhanced access to hepatic microsomal enzymes. Extensive hepatic extraction means that clearance of sufentanil will be sensitive to changes in hepatic blood flow but not to alterations in the drug-metabolizing capacity of the liver. Sufentanil metabolites are excreted almost equally in urine and feces, with about 30% appearing as conjugates. The production of a weakly active metabolite and the substantial amount of conjugated metabolite formation imply the possible importance of normal renal function for the clearance of sufentanil. Indeed, prolonged depression of ventilation in association with an abnormally increased plasma concentration of sufentanil has been observed in a patient with chronic renal failure.[128]

Context-Sensitive Half-Time

The context-sensitive half-time of sufentanil is actually less than that for alfentanil for continuous infusions of up to 8 hours in duration (see Fig. 7-13).[3] This shorter context-sensitive half-time can be explained in part by the large Vd of sufentanil compared to alfentanil. After termination of a sufentanil infusion, the decrease in the plasma drug concentration is accelerated not only by metabolism but also by continued redistribution of sufentanil into peripheral tissue compartments. Compared with alfentanil, sufentanil may have a more favorable recovery profile when used over a longer period of time. Conversely, alfentanil has a pharmacokinetic advantage for the treatment of discrete and transient noxious stimuli because its short effect-site equilibration time allows rapid access of the drug to the brain and facilitates titration.

Clinical Uses

In volunteers, a single dose of sufentanil, 0.1 to 0.4 μg/kg IV, produces a longer period of analgesia and less depression of ventilation than does a comparable dose of fentanyl (1 to 4 μg/kg IV).[129] Compared with large doses of morphine or fentanyl, sufentanil, 18.9 μg/kg IV, results in more rapid induction of anesthesia, earlier emergence from anesthesia, and earlier tracheal extubation.[130] As observed with other opioids, sufentanil causes a decrease in cerebral metabolic oxygen requirements and cerebral blood flow is also decreased or unchanged.[131] Bradycardia produced by sufentanil may be sufficient to decrease cardiac output. As observed with fentanyl, delayed depression of ventilation has also been described after the administration of sufentanil.[132]

Although large doses of sufentanil (10 to 30 μg/kg IV) or fentanyl (50 to 150 μg/kg IV) produce minimal hemodynamic effects in patients with good left ventricular function, the systemic blood pressure and hormonal (catecholamine) responses to painful stimulation such as median sternotomy are not predictably prevented.[133] It seems unlikely that any clinically useful dose of sufentanil or fentanyl will abolish such responses in all patients. Use of large doses of opioids, including sufentanil or fentanyl, to produce IV induction of anesthesia may result in rigidity of chest and abdominal musculature. This skeletal muscle rigidity makes ventilation of the patient's lungs with positive airway pressure difficult. Difficult ventilation during sufentanil-induced skeletal muscle rigidity may actually reflect obstruction at the level of the glottis or above, which can be overcome by tracheal intubation.[134]

Alfentanil

Alfentanil is an analogue of fentanyl that is less potent (one-fifth to one-tenth) and has one-third the duration of action of fentanyl (see Fig. 7-2). It was first synthesized in 1976. A unique advantage of alfentanil compared with fentanyl and sufentanil is the more rapid onset of action (rapid effect-site equilibration) after the IV administration of alfentanil. For example, the effect-site equilibration time for alfentanil is 1.4 minutes compared with 6.8 and 6.2 minutes for fentanyl and sufentanil, respectively (see Table 7-4).[4,135]

Pharmacokinetics

Alfentanil has a short elimination half-time compared with fentanyl and sufentanil (see Table 7-4). Cirrhosis of the liver, but not cholestatic disease, prolongs the elimination half-time of alfentanil.[136] Renal failure does not alter the clearance or elimination half-time of alfentanil.[137] The elimination half-time of alfentanil is shorter in children (4 to 8 years old) than adults, reflecting a smaller Vd in these younger patients.[138]

The rapid effect-site equilibration characteristic of alfentanil is a result of the low pK_a of this opioid such that nearly 90% of the drug exists in the nonionized form at physiologic pH. It is the nonionized fraction that readily crosses the blood–brain barrier. The rapid peak effect of alfentanil at the brain is useful when an opioid is required to blunt the response to a single, brief stimulus such as tracheal intubation or performance of a retrobulbar block.

The Vd of alfentanil is four to six times smaller than that of fentanyl (see Table 7-4).[139] This smaller Vd compared with that of fentanyl reflects lower lipid solubility and higher protein binding. Despite this lesser lipid solubility, penetration of the blood–brain barrier by alfentanil is rapid because of its large nonionized fraction at physiologic pH. Alfentanil is principally bound to α_1-acid glycoprotein, a protein whose plasma concentration is not altered by liver disease. Because protein binding is similar, it is likely that a decreased percentage of adipose tissue in children is responsible for the short elimination half-time.

Metabolism

Alfentanil is metabolized predominantly by two independent pathways, piperidine *N*-dealkylation to noralfentanil and amide *N*-dealkylation to *N*-phenylpropionamide. Noralfentanil is the major metabolite recovered in urine, with <0.5% of an administered dose of alfentanil being excreted unchanged. The efficiency of hepatic metabolism is emphasized by clearance of about 96% of alfentanil from the plasma within 60 minutes of its administration.

Attempts to develop reliable infusion regimens to attain and maintain specific plasma concentrations of alfentanil have been confounded by the wide interindividual variability in alfentanil pharmacokinetics. The most significant factor responsible for unpredictable alfentanil disposition is the 10-fold interindividual variability in alfentanil systemic clearance, presumably reflecting variability in hepatic intrinsic clearance. In this regard, it is likely that population variability in P450 3A4 (CYP3A4) activity (most abundant P450 hepatic enzyme and the major isoform of P450 responsible for alfentanil metabolism and clearance) is the mechanistic explanation for the interindividual variability in alfentanil disposition.[140] Alfentanil clearance is markedly influenced by CYP3A activity and alfentanil is a sensitive and validated probe for CYP3A activity.[85] Alterations in P450 activity may be responsible for the ability of erythromycin to inhibit the metabolism of alfentanil and a resulting prolonged opioid effect.[141]

Context-Sensitive Half-Time

The context-sensitive half-time of alfentanil is actually longer than that of sufentanil for infusions up to 8 hours in duration (see Fig. 7-13).[90] This phenomenon can be explained in part by the large Vd of sufentanil. After termination of a continuous infusion of sufentanil, the decrease in the plasma drug concentration is accelerated not only by metabolism but also by continued redistribution of sufentanil into peripheral compartments. Conversely, the

Vd of alfentanil equilibrates rapidly; therefore, peripheral distribution of drug away from the plasma is not a significant contributor to the decrease in the plasma concentration after discontinuation of the alfentanil infusion. Thus, despite the short elimination half-time of alfentanil, it may not necessarily be a superior choice to sufentanil for ambulatory sedation techniques.

Clinical Uses

Alfentanil has a rapid onset and offset of intense analgesia reflecting its very prompt effect-site equilibration. This characteristic of alfentanil is used to provide analgesia when the noxious stimulation is acute but transient as associated with laryngoscopy and tracheal intubation and performance of a retrobulbar block. For example, administration of alfentanil, 15 μg/kg IV, about 90 seconds before beginning direct laryngoscopy is effective in blunting the systemic blood pressure and heart rate response to tracheal intubation.[142] The catecholamine response to this noxious stimulation is also blunted by alfentanil, 30 μg/kg IV.[142] Alfentanil in doses of 10 to 20 μg/kg IV blunts the circulatory but not the catecholamine release response to the sudden exposure to high inhaled concentrations of desflurane.[143] Alfentanil, 150 to 300 μg/kg IV, administered rapidly, produces unconsciousness in about 45 seconds. After this induction, maintenance of anesthesia can be provided with a continuous infusion of alfentanil, 25 to 150 μg/kg/hour IV, combined with an inhaled anesthetic.[144] Unlike other opioids, supplemental doses of alfentanil seem to be more likely to decrease systemic blood pressure that is increased after painful stimulation. Alfentanil increases biliary tract pressures similarly to fentanyl. Alfentanil, compared with equipotent doses of fentanyl and sufentanil, is associated with a lower incidence of postoperative nausea and vomiting in outpatients.[145] Acute dystonia has been described after administration of alfentanil to a patient with untreated Parkinson's disease.[146] This may reflect an ability of opioids to decrease central dopaminergic transmission and suggests caution in administration of this opioid to patients with untreated Parkinson's disease.

Remifentanil

Remifentanil is a selective μ opioid agonist with an analgesic potency similar to that of fentanyl (15 to 20 times as potent as alfentanil) and a blood–brain equilibration (effect-site equilibration) time similar to that of alfentanil (see Table 7-4).[2,3,147–149] Although chemically related to the fentanyl family of short-acting phenylpiperidine derivatives, remifentanil is structurally unique because of its ester linkage (see Fig. 7-2). Remifentanil's ester structure renders it susceptible to hydrolysis by nonspecific plasma and tissue esterases to inactive metabolites.[3] This unique pathway of metabolism leads to (a) brief action, (b) precise and rapidly titratable effect due to its rapid onset and offset, (c) lack of accumulation, and (d) rapid recovery after discontinuation of its administration.

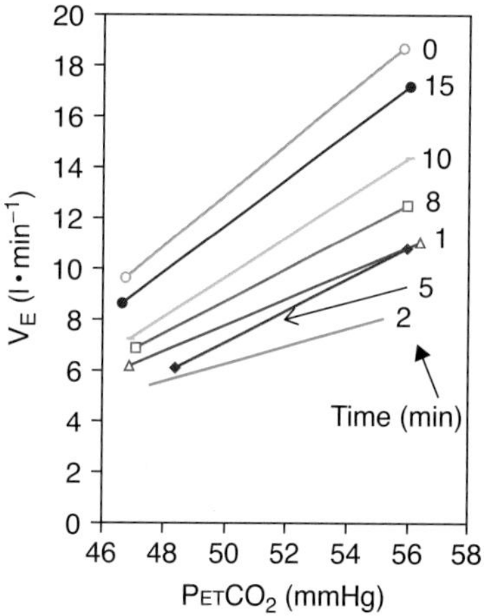

FIGURE 7-17 Carbon dioxide response curves before (time = 0) and at selected times after administration of 0.5 μg/kg IV remifentanil. (From Babenco HD, Conard PF, Gross JB. The pharmacodynamic effect of a remifentanil bolus on ventilatory control. *Anesthesiology.* 2000;92:393–398, with permission.)

Ventilation

After administration of 0.5 μg/kg IV remifentanil, there is a decrease in the slope and downward shift of the carbon dioxide ventilatory response curve that reaches its nadir after about 150 seconds following injection (Fig. 7-17).[150] Recovery after this small dose of remifentanil was complete within about 15 minutes. The combination of remifentanil and propofol is synergistic resulting in severe depression of ventilation (Fig. 7-18).[151]

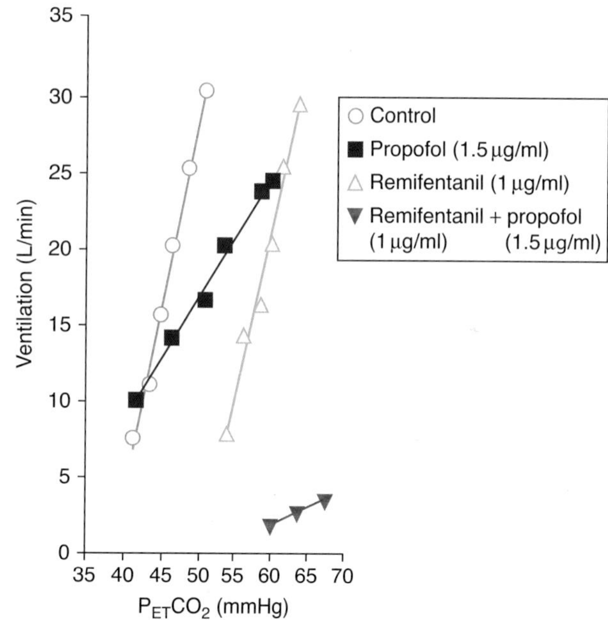

FIGURE 7-18 Ventilatory response curves from one individual. The combined administration of remifentanil and propofol decreased the slope of the carbon dioxide response curve and caused a rightward shift. (From Niewenhuijs DJF, Olofsen E, Romberd RR, et al. Response surface modeling of remifentanil-propofol interaction on cardiorespiratory control and bispectral index. *Anesthesiology.* 2003;98:312–322, with permission.)

Pharmacokinetics

The pharmacokinetics of remifentanil are characterized by small Vd, rapid clearance, and low interindividual variability compared to other IV anesthetic drugs. The rapid metabolism of remifentanil and its small Vd mean that remifentanil will accumulate less than other opioids. Because of its rapid systemic clearance, remifentanil provides pharmacokinetic advantages in clinical situations requiring predictable termination of drug effect. Remifentanil's pharmacokinetics is similar in obese and lean patients. Therefore, dosing regimens should be based on ideal (lean) body mass rather than total body weight.[152]

The most salient pharmacokinetic feature of remifentanil is the extraordinary clearance of nearly 3 L per minute, which is about eight times more rapid than that of alfentanil. Remifentanil has a smaller Vd than alfentanil. The combination of rapid clearance and small Vd produces a drug with a uniquely transient effect. In fact, the rate of decline (context-sensitive half-time) of the remifentanil plasma concentration will be nearly independent of the infusion duration (see Fig. 7-13).[2,3] The rapid effect-site equilibration means that a remifentanil infusion rate will promptly approach steady state in the plasma and its effect site. It is estimated that remifentanil plasma concentrations will reach a steady state within 10 minutes of beginning an infusion. The relationship between infusion rate and opioid concentration will be less variable for remifentanil than for other opioids. Furthermore, the rapid clearance of remifentanil, combined with the rapid blood–brain equilibration, means changes in infusion rates will be paralleled by prompt changes in drug effect.

Based on analysis of the EEG response, it is estimated that remifentanil is about 19 times more potent than alfentanil (EC_{50} for EEG depression 20 ng/mL vs. 376 ng/mL).[3] The effect-site equilibration time, however, is similar for both opioids, suggesting that remifentanil will have an alfentanil-like onset (see Table 7-4). For example, after a rapid IV injection, the peak effect-site concentration of remifentanil will be present within 1.1 minutes, compared with 1.4 minutes for alfentanil. The effect, however, will be more transient after administration of remifentanil than alfentanil.

Metabolism

Remifentanil is unique among the opioids in undergoing metabolism by nonspecific plasma and tissue esterases to inactive metabolites.[3] The principal metabolite, remifentanil acid, is 300 to 4,600-fold less potent than remifentanil as a μ agonist and is excreted primarily by the kidneys. *N*-dealkylation of remifentanil is a minor metabolic pathway in humans. Remifentanil does not appear to be a substrate for butyrylcholinesterases (pseudocholinesterase), and thus its clearance should not be affected by cholinesterase deficiency or anticholinergics.[2] Additionally, it is likely that remifentanil's pharmacokinetics will be unchanged by renal or hepatic failure because esterase metabolism is usually preserved in these states.[153] In this regard, the clearance of remifentanil is not altered during the anhepatic phase of liver transplantation. Hypothermic cardiopulmonary bypass decreases clearance of remifentanil by an average of 20%, presumably reflecting the effect of temperature on blood and tissue esterase activity. Esterase metabolism appears to be a very well-preserved metabolic system with little variability between individuals, which contributes to the predictability of drug effect associated with the infusion of remifentanil.

Elimination Half-Time

An estimated 99.8% of remifentanil is eliminated during the distribution (0.9 minute) and elimination (6.3 minutes) half-time. Clinically, remifentanil behaves like a drug with an elimination half-time of 6 minutes or less.

Context-Sensitive Half-Time

Context-sensitive half-time for remifentanil is independent of the duration of infusion and is estimated to be about 4 minutes.[2,3,154] This drug's rapid clearance is responsible for the lack of accumulation even during prolonged periods of infusion. In contrast, the context-sensitive half-times for sufentanil, alfentanil, and fentanyl are longer and depend significantly on the duration of the infusion (see Table 7-4 and Fig. 7-13).

Clinical Uses

The clinical uses of remifentanil reflect the unique pharmacokinetics of this drug, which allow rapid onset of drug effect, precise titration to the desired effect, the ability to maintain a sufficient effect-site concentration to suppress the stress response, and rapid recovery from the drug's effects. In cases where a profound analgesic effect is desired transiently (performance of a retrobulbar block), remifentanil may be useful. Prompt onset and short duration of action make remifentanil a useful selection for suppression of the transient sympathetic nervous system response to direct laryngoscopy and tracheal intubation in at-risk patients.[155] Intermittent remifentanil administered as patient-controlled analgesia is an effective and reliable analgesic during labor and delivery.[156] One additional benefit during labor would be rapid clearance from the neonatal circulation as well, thus reducing the risk of neonatal depression.[157] Conceivably, remifentanil could be used for long operations, when a quick recovery time is desired (neurologic assessment, wake-up test) but at a significantly higher cost than other opioids.

Anesthesia can be induced with remifentanil, 1 μg/kg IV administered over 60 to 90 seconds, or with a gradual initiation of the infusion at 0.5 to 1.0 μg/kg IV for about 10 minutes, before administration of a standard hypnotic prior to tracheal intubation.[158] The dose of hypnotic drug may need to be decreased to compensate for the synergistic effect with remifentanil. Remifentanil can be used as the analgesic component of a general anesthetic (0.25 to 1.00 μg/kg IV or 0.05 to 2.00 μg/kg/minute IV) or sedation techniques with the ability to rapidly recover from undesirable effects such as opioid-induced depression of ventilation or excessive sedation. Remifentanil, 0.05 to 0.10 μg/kg/minute, in combination with midazolam, 2 mg IV, provides effective sedation and analgesia during monitored anesthesia care in otherwise healthy adult patients.[159] Midazolam also produces a dose-dependent potentiation of remifentanil's depressant effect on breathing rate. Changes in remifentanil drug effect predictably follow changes in the infusion rate, making it possible to more precisely titrate to the desired response than with other opioids. Before cessation of the remifentanil infusion, a longer acting opioid should be administered to ensure analgesia when the patient awakens. The spinal or epidural administration of remifentanil is not recommended, as the safety of the vehicle (glycine, which acts as an inhibitory neurotransmitter) or opioid have not been determined.[2] Remifentanil, 100 μg IV, attenuates the acute hemodynamic responses to electroconvulsive therapy and does not alter the duration of electroconvulsive-induced seizure activity.[160]

Side Effects

The advantage of remifentanil possessing a short recovery period may be considered a disadvantage if the infusion is stopped suddenly, whether it be deliberate or accidental. It is important to administer a longer acting opioid for postoperative analgesia when remifentanil has been administered for this purpose intraoperatively. All fentanyl analogs, including remifentanil, have been reported to induce "seizure-like" activity.[161]

Nausea and vomiting, depression of ventilation, and mild decreases in systemic blood pressure and heart rate may accompany the administration of remifentanil. Depression of ventilation produced by remifentanil is not altered by renal or liver dysfunction. Histamine release does not accompany the administration of remifentanil. ICP and intraocular pressure are not changed by remifentanil.[162,163] High-dose remifentanil decreases cerebral blood flow and cerebral metabolic oxygen requirements without impairing cerebrovascular carbon dioxide reactivity.[164] Remifentanil delays drainage of dye from the gallbladder into the duodenum but the delay is shorter than with other opioids.[165]

Hyperalgesia

Postoperative analgesic requirements in patients receiving relatively large doses of remifentanil intraoperatively are often surprisingly high, suggesting remifentanil may be associated with acute opioid tolerance (Fig. 7-19).[166] In addition, delayed hyperalgesia may be produced by acute exposure to large doses of opioids. Tolerance to opioids is pharmacodynamic and tolerance is dose-dependent. Possible mechanisms for tolerance include alterations of the NDMA receptors and its intracellular second messenger systems. In this regard, NMDA receptor antagonists such as ketamine and magnesium block opioid tolerance.

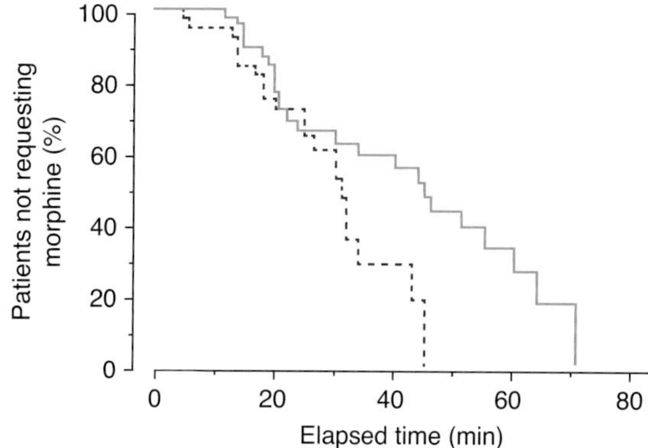

FIGURE 7-19 Cumulative curves for patients who did not request an additional morphine injection following discontinuation of remifentanil *(dashed line)* or desflurane *(solid line)*. (From Guignard B, Bossard AE, Coste C, et al. Acute opioid tolerance: intraoperative remifentanil increases postoperative pain and morphine requirement. *Anesthesiology.* 2000;93:409–417, with permission.)

Subanesthetic ketamine has been shown to decrease morphine requirements and the development of hyperalgesia after intraoperative remifentanil use (Fig. 7-20).[46,167] It is important to know that patients on chronic pain medication preoperatively would require higher doses of opioids postoperatively compared to naive patients and small doses ketamine would be an alternative therapeutic approach. However, those patients might be mistaken to have developed hyperalgesia to opioids.

A recent study in rodents has shown that morphine-induced hyperalgesia is associated with glial activation (indicating that this is not an acute phenomenon) and involved anion dysequilibrium potential between microglia and neuron pathway.[168]

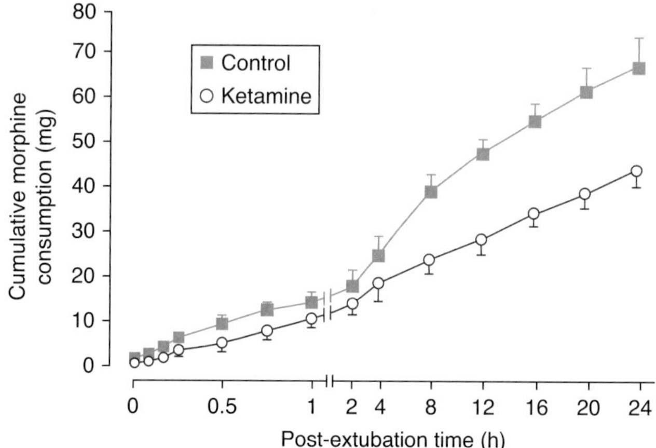

FIGURE 7-20 Cumulative postoperative morphine consumption in patients undergoing surgery with remifentanil infusions. Patients receiving subanesthetic ketamine infusions experienced less postoperative pain and required less morphine. (Reproduced from Guignard B, Coste C, Costes H, et al. Supplementing desflurane-remifentanil anesthesia with small-dose ketamine reduces perioperative opioid analgesic requirements. *Anesth Analg.* 2002;95[1]:103–108.)

Codeine

Codeine is the result of the substitution of a methyl group for the hydroxyl group on the number 3 carbon of morphine (see Fig. 7-1). The presence of this methyl group limits first-pass hepatic metabolism and accounts for the efficacy of codeine when administered orally. The elimination half-time of codeine after oral or IM administration is 3.0 to 3.5 hours. About 10% of administered codeine is demethylated in the liver to morphine, which may be responsible for the analgesic effect of codeine, although codeine-6-glucuronide may also exert an analgesic effect.[169] Consequently, interindividual variability in metabolism may lead to variable analgesic effect from codeine-containing drugs; some patients who claim that codeine is an ineffective drug for them may in fact poorly metabolize it to active forms. Any remaining codeine is demethylated to inactive norcodeine, which is conjugated or excreted unchanged by the kidneys.

Codeine is effective at suppressing cough at oral doses of 15 mg. Maximal analgesia, equivalent to that produced by 650 mg of aspirin, occurs with 60 mg of codeine. When administered IM, 120 mg of codeine is equivalent in analgesic effect to 10 mg of morphine. Most often, codeine is included in medications as an antitussive or is combined with nonopioid analgesics for the treatment of mild to moderate pain. The risk of physical dependence on codeine appears to be less than that of morphine and occurs only rarely after oral analgesic use. Codeine produces minimal sedation, nausea, vomiting, and constipation. Dizziness may occur in ambulatory patients. Even in large doses, codeine is unlikely to produce apnea. Administration of codeine IV is not recommended, because histamine-induced hypotension is likely.

Hydromorphone

First introduced in 1926, hydromorphone is a derivative of morphine that is about five times as potent as morphine but has a slightly shorter duration of action. It is less hydrophilic than morphine, leading to faster onset of analgesia. This opioid produces somewhat more sedation and evokes less euphoria than morphine. Because of rapid elimination and redistribution, oral dosing every 4 hours is needed to maintain adequate plasma concentrations for analgesia. Hydromorphone is an effective alternative to morphine in the treatment of opioid-responsive moderate to severe pain.[170] The uses and side effects of hydromorphone are the same as those of morphine, although histamine release is less prominent with hydromorphone. Similar to other opioids, large doses of hydromorphone have been reported to cause agitation and myoclonus.[171]

Oxymorphone

Oxymorphone is the result of the addition of a hydroxyl group to hydromorphone. It is about 10 times as potent as morphine and seems to cause more nausea and vomiting. The potential for physical dependence is great. An oral preparation of oxymorphone (immediate release) produces maximum plasma concentrations in 30 minutes with associated rapid onset of analgesia.[172]

Oxycodone

Oxycodone is commonly used orally for treating acute pain associated with illness or injury. This agent is about twice as potent as oral morphine and has a similar duration of analgesic action. Sustained-release oral oxycodone preparations provide stable plasma concentrations for the treatment of moderate to severe pain. Abuse potential is great including tampering (crushing and powdering) for IV or intranasal injection to obtain a rapid and powerful opioid effect. New, abuse-resistant formulations that are not easily solubilized for IV injection are now widely marketed.

Hydrocodone

Like oxycodone, hydrocodone is a commonly used oral opioid for treating acute pain associated with illness or injury. This agent is similar in potency to oral morphine and has a similar duration of analgesic action. A derivative of codeine, hydrocodone is a useful oral opioid, commonly combined with acetaminophen. The approval by the U.S. Food and Drug Administration of one extended release formulation (Zohydro) provoked much opposition due to its abuse potential and lack of abuse-deterrent features.[173] Originally classified as a schedule III drug (moderate abuse potential) in the United States, hydrocodone has subsequently been reclassified as schedule II (high abuse potential) due to increased reports of diversion and abuse.

Methadone

Methadone is a synthetic opioid agonist that produces analgesia in the setting of chronic pain syndromes and is highly effective by the oral route. The efficient oral absorption, prompt onset of action, and prolonged duration of action of methadone render this an attractive drug for suppression of withdrawal symptoms in physically dependent persons such as heroin addicts. Use of this agent is difficult, owing to the marked individual variation in both pharmacokinetic and pharmacodynamic effects. The long terminal elimination half-life of (mean of 26 hours) makes rapid titration impossible; indeed, altering the dose any more frequently than every 5 to 7 days is unwise in the chronic setting, as excess drug accumulation can lead to slow, delayed overdose, often appearing many days after the most recent dose change.

Opioid Withdrawal

Methadone can substitute for morphine at about one-fourth the dosage. Controlled withdrawal from opioids using methadone is milder and less acute than that from morphine. Methadone, 20 mg IV, produces postoperative analgesia lasting >24 hours, reflecting its prolonged (35 hours) elimination half-time. This drug is metabolized in the liver to inactive substances that are excreted in the urine and bile with small amounts of unchanged drug.

The side effects of methadone (depression of ventilation, miosis, constipation, biliary tract spasm) resemble those of morphine. Its sedative and euphoric actions are less than those produced by morphine. Methadone-induced miosis is less prominent than that caused by morphine, and complete tolerance to this action can develop.

Treatment of Chronic Pain

Methadone has been proposed as an alternative to slow-release formulations for treatment of chronic pain because of its low abuse potential. In addition, NMDA receptor antagonist activity may be useful in treatment of neuropathic pain and minimize the potential for development of tolerance. The principal disadvantage for use of methadone to treat chronic pain is its prolonged and unpredictable half-time. When methadone is administered more than once daily, as is common in treatment of chronic pain syndromes, the drug may accumulate and result in high plasma concentrations and associated depression of ventilation.[174] For this reason, slow-release formulations (such as oxycodone) may be preferable to methadone for the treatment of outpatient postoperative pain.

Propoxyphene

Propoxyphene is structurally similar to methadone. Oral doses of 90 to 120 mg of propoxyphene produce analgesia and CNS effects similar to those produced by 60 mg of codeine and 650 mg of aspirin. The only clinical use of propoxyphene is treatment of mild to moderate pain that is not adequately relieved by aspirin. Propoxyphene does not possess antipyretic or antiinflammatory effects, and antitussive activity is not significant.

Propoxyphene is completely absorbed after oral administration, but because of extensive first-pass hepatic metabolism (demethylation to norpropoxyphene), the systemic availability is limited. The elimination half-time after oral administration is about 14.5 hours. The most common side effects of propoxyphene are vertigo, sedation, nausea, and vomiting. Overdose is characterized by seizures, cardiac arrhythmias, and depression of ventilation.

Abrupt discontinuation of chronically administered propoxyphene results in a mild withdrawal syndrome. The incidence of abuse of propoxyphene is similar to that of codeine. Administration of this drug IV produces severe damage to veins and limits abuse by this route. Administration of propoxyphene in combination with alcohol and other CNS depressants may result in excessive drug-induced depression of ventilation.

Due to the unfavorable risk-benefit profile (and the availability of better alternatives), propoxyphene was voluntarily withdrawn from the United States market in 2010.

Tramadol

Tramadol is a centrally acting analgesic that has moderate affinity for μ receptors and weak κ and δ opioid receptor affinity but is 5 to 10 times less potent than morphine as an analgesic.[175] In addition to μ opioid agonist effects, tramadol enhances the function of the spinal descending inhibitory pathways by inhibition of neuronal reuptake of norepinephrine and 5-hydroxytryptamine (serotonin) as well as presynaptic stimulation of 5-hydroxytryptamine release. In volunteers, naloxone antagonized only an estimated 30% of the effect of tramadol.[176]

Tramadol is a racemic mixture of two enantiomers, one of which is responsible for inhibition of norepinephrine uptake, whereas the other is responsible for inhibition of 5-hydroxytryptamine reuptake and facilitation of its release, plus the actions of this drug at μ receptors. In this regard, tramadol may be an exception to the argument that chiral mixtures should be avoided when technology exists to prepare a single, pure isomer.[177] For example, the production of analgesia by tramadol with the absence of depression of ventilation and a low potential for the development of tolerance, dependence, and abuse may be a result of the complementary and synergistic antinociceptive interaction of the two enantiomers. Tramadol is metabolized by hepatic P450 enzyme systems to the major metabolite is O-desmethyltramadol, which also exerts modest stereoselective analgesic effects.

Tramadol 3 mg/kg administered orally, IM, or IV is effective for the treatment of moderate to severe pain. A marked decrease in postoperative shivering has been noted in treated patients and the minimal depressant effects on breathing are useful.[178] Tramadol slows gastric emptying although the effect is small compared with other opioids.[179] Tramadol is useful for the treatment of chronic pain because it is believed to be less likely to generate addiction and is not associated with major organ toxicity or significant sedative effects at standard doses. Toxicity from overdose can manifest as hypotension, bradycardia, seizures, coma, and rhabdomyolysis. Interestingly, IV lipid emulsion has also shown promise in reversing tramadol toxicity in a rabbit model.[180] Disadvantages of tramadol include its interaction with Coumadin anticoagulants (not all reports confirm this interaction) and the occurrence of drug-related seizures (avoid in patients with epilepsy or those being treated with drugs that lower the seizure threshold such as antidepressants).[181] A further drawback to the perioperative use of this drug as an analgesic is a high incidence of associated nausea and vomiting. Ondansetron may interfere with the analgesic component of tramadol that is due to effects on the reuptake and release of 5-hydroxytryptamine.

Heroin

Heroin (diacetylmorphine) is a synthetic opioid produced by acetylation of morphine. It was developed in 1898 and was originally claimed to have no addictive potential. When administered parenterally, heroin acts in a markedly different way than morphine. For example, there is rapid penetration of heroin into the brain, where it is hydrolyzed to the active metabolites monoacetylmorphine and morphine. The unique rapid entrance into the CNS is most likely caused by the lipid solubility and chemical structure of heroin. Compared with morphine, parenteral heroin has a (a) more rapid onset, (b) less opioid-induced nausea, and (c) greater potential for physical dependency. This greater liability for physical dependence is the reason that heroin is not available legally for clinical use in the United States.[182,183]

Opioid Agonist–Antagonists

Opioid agonist-antagonists include, but are not limited to, pentazocine, butorphanol, nalbuphine, buprenorphine, nalorphine, bremazocine, and dezocine (Fig. 7-21). These drugs bind to μ receptors, where they produce limited responses (partial agonists) or no effect (competitive antagonists). In addition, these drugs often exert partial agonist actions at other receptors, including κ and δ receptors. Antagonist properties of these drugs can attenuate the efficacy of subsequently administered opioid agonists. The side effects are similar to those of opioid agonists, and, in addition, these drugs may cause dysphoric reactions. The advantages of opioid agonist–antagonists are the ability to produce analgesia with limited depression of ventilation and a low potential to produce physical dependence. Furthermore, these drugs have a ceiling effect such that increasing doses do not produce additional responses. This ceiling effect on depression of ventilation, however, is often accompanied by an equally modest ability to decrease anesthetic requirements. In general, agonist-antagonist drugs should be reserved for patients who are unable to tolerate a pure agonist.

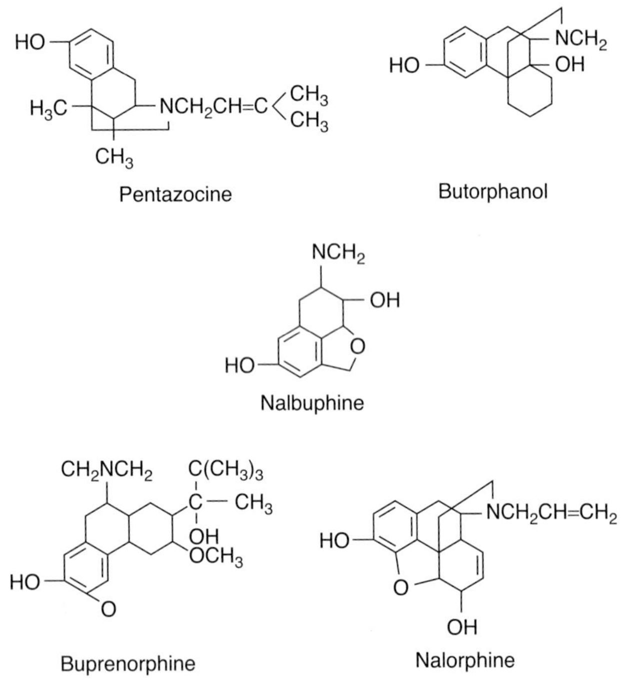

Pentazocine Butorphanol Nalbuphine Buprenorphine Nalorphine

FIGURE 7-21 Opioid agonist–antagonists.

Pentazocine

Pentazocine is a benzomorphan derivative that possesses opioid agonist actions as well as weak antagonist actions. It is presumed to exert its agonist effects at δ and κ receptors. Concomitant opioid antagonist activity is weak, being only about one-fifth as potent as nalorphine. Nevertheless, antagonist effects of pentazocine are sufficient to precipitate withdrawal symptoms when administered to patients who have been receiving opioids on a regular basis. The agonist effects of pentazocine are antagonized by naloxone. Indeed, physical dependence to pentazocine can be demonstrated by abrupt withdrawal precipitated by naloxone.

Pharmacokinetics

Pentazocine is well absorbed after oral or parenteral administration. First-pass hepatic metabolism is extensive, with only about 20% of an oral dose entering the circulation. Metabolism of pentazocine occurs by oxidation of terminal methyl groups, and resulting inactive glucuronide conjugates are excreted in the urine. An estimated 5% to 25% of an administered dose of pentazocine is excreted unchanged in the urine, and $<2\%$ undergoes biliary excretion. The elimination half-time is 2 to 3 hours.

Clinical Uses

Pentazocine, 10 to 30 mg IV or 50 mg orally, is used most often for the relief of moderate pain. An oral dose of 50 mg is equivalent in analgesic potency to 60 mg of codeine. Pentazocine is useful for treatment of chronic pain when there is a high risk of physical dependence. Placement in the epidural space produces a rapid onset of analgesia that is of shorter duration than that produced by morphine.

Side Effects

The most common side effect of pentazocine is sedation, followed by diaphoresis and dizziness. Sedation is prominent after epidural placement of pentazocine, presumably reflecting activation of κ receptors. Nausea and vomiting are less common than with morphine. Dysphoria, including fear of impending death, is associated with high doses of pentazocine. This tendency to dysphoria limits the physical dependence liability of pentazocine. Pentazocine produces an increase in the plasma concentrations of catecholamines, which may account for increases in heart rate, systemic blood pressure, pulmonary artery blood pressure, and left ventricular end-diastolic pressure that accompany administration of this drug. Pentazocine, 20 to 30 mg IM, produces analgesia, sedation, and depression of ventilation similar to 10 mg of morphine. Increasing the IM dose above 30 mg does not produce proportionate increases in these responses. The increase in biliary tract pressure is less than that produced by equal analgesic doses of morphine, meperidine, or fentanyl.[35] Pentazocine crosses the placenta and may cause fetal depression. In contrast to morphine, miosis does not occur after administration of pentazocine.

Butorphanol

Butorphanol is an agonist-antagonist opioid that resembles pentazocine. Compared with pentazocine, its agonist effects are about 20 times greater, whereas its antagonist actions are 10 to 30 times greater. It is speculated that butorphanol has a (a) low affinity for μ receptors to produce antagonism, (b) moderate affinity for κ receptors to produce analgesia and antishivering effects, and (c) minimal affinity for σ receptors, so the incidence of dysphoria is low.

Butorphanol is rapidly and almost completely absorbed after IM injection. In postoperative patients, 2 to 3 mg IM produces analgesia and depression of ventilation similar to 10 mg of morphine. Intranasal butorphanol has been used for the treatment of postoperative pain and migraine pain. The intraoperative use of butorphanol, like pentazocine, seems to be limited. The elimination half-time of butorphanol is 2.5 to 3.5 hours. Metabolism is principally to inactive hydroxybutorphanol, which is eliminated largely in the bile and to a lesser extent in the urine.

Side Effects

Common side effects of butorphanol include sedation, nausea, and diaphoresis. Dysphoria, reported frequently with other opioid agonist–antagonists, is infrequent after administration of butorphanol. Depression of ventilation is similar to that produced by similar doses of morphine. Like pentazocine, analgesic doses of butorphanol increase systemic blood pressure, pulmonary artery blood pressure, and cardiac output. Also, similar to pentazocine, the effects of butorphanol on the biliary and gastrointestinal tract seem to be milder than those produced by morphine. It may be difficult to use an opioid agonist effectively as an analgesic in the presence of butorphanol. This must be remembered when considering the use of butorphanol or any other opioid-agonist for preoperative medication. Withdrawal symptoms do occur after acute discontinuation of chronic therapy with butorphanol, but symptoms are mild.

Nalbuphine

Nalbuphine is an agonist-antagonist opioid that is related chemically to oxymorphone and naloxone. It is equal in potency as an analgesic to morphine and is about one-fourth as potent as nalorphine as an antagonist. Nalbuphine is metabolized in the liver and has an elimination half-time of 3 to 6 hours. Naloxone reverses the agonist effects of nalbuphine. Nalbuphine, 10 mg IM, produces analgesia with an onset of effect and duration of action similar to those of morphine. Depression of ventilation is similar to that of morphine until 30 mg IM of nalbuphine is exceeded, after which no further depression of ventilation occurs (ceiling effect).[184] Sedation is the most common side effect, occurring in about one-third of patients treated with nalbuphine. The incidence of dysphoria is less than that with pentazocine or butorphanol but is qualitatively similar and increases in frequency as the dose of nalbuphine is increased. In contrast to pentazocine and butorphanol, nalbuphine does not increase systemic blood pressure, pulmonary artery blood pressure, heart rate, or atrial filling pressures. For this reason, nalbuphine may be useful to provide sedation and analgesia in patients with heart disease, as during cardiac catheterization. Abrupt withdrawal of nalbuphine after chronic administration produces withdrawal symptoms that are milder than those of morphine and more severe than those of pentazocine. The abuse potential of nalbuphine is low.

The antagonist effects of nalbuphine are speculated to occur at μ receptors. As a result, the subsequent use of morphine-like drugs for anesthesia or postoperative analgesia after preoperative medication with nalbuphine may not provide adequate analgesia. Conversely, the antagonist effects of nalbuphine at μ receptors could be an advantage in the postoperative period to reverse lingering ventilatory depressant effects of opioid agonists while still maintaining analgesia. Nalbuphine, 10 to 20 mg IV, reverses postoperative depression of ventilation caused by fentanyl but maintains analgesia.[185] Evidence of recurrent hypoventilation often occurs 2 to 3 hours after administration of nalbuphine to antagonize the effects of fentanyl.

Buprenorphine

Buprenorphine is an agonist-antagonist opioid derived from the opium alkaloid thebaine. Its analgesic potency is great, with 0.3 mg IM being equivalent to 10 mg of morphine. After IM administration, the onset of buprenorphine effect occurs in about 30 minutes, and the duration of action is at least 8 hours. It is estimated that the affinity of buprenorphine for μ receptors is 50 times greater than that of morphine, and subsequent slow dissociation from these receptors accounts for its prolonged duration of action and resistance to antagonism with naloxone. After IM administration, nearly two-thirds of the drug appears unchanged in the bile and the remainder is excreted in urine as inactive metabolites.

Buprenorphine is effective in relieving moderate to severe pain such as that present in the postoperative period and that associated with cancer, renal colic, and myocardial infarction. Placed in the epidural space, the high lipid solubility (five times that of morphine) and affinity for opioid receptors limits cephalad spread and the likelihood of delayed depression of ventilation.[186] The antagonist effects of buprenorphine reflect the ability of this drug to displace opioid agonists from μ receptors.

Side Effects

The side effects of buprenorphine include drowsiness, nausea, vomiting, and depression of ventilation. These are similar in magnitude to the side effects of morphine but may be prolonged and resistant to antagonism with naloxone. Pulmonary edema has been observed after administration of buprenorphine.[187] In contrast to other opioid agonist-antagonists, dysphoria is unlikely to occur in association with administration of this drug. Because of its antagonist properties, buprenorphine can precipitate withdrawal in patients who are physically dependent on morphine. Conversely, withdrawal symptoms in patients who are physically dependent on buprenorphine develop slowly and are of lesser intensity than those associated with morphine. In this respect, withdrawal from buprenorphine resembles that from other opioid agonist–antagonists, and the risk of abuse is low.

Nalorphine

Nalorphine is equally potent with morphine as an analgesic but is not clinically useful because of a high incidence of dysphoria. The high incidence of dysphoria may reflect activity of this drug at σ receptors. The antagonist actions of nalorphine reflect its ability to displace opioid agonists from μ receptors.

Bremazocine

Bremazocine is a benzomorphan derivative that is twice as potent as morphine as an analgesic but, in animals, does not produce depression of ventilation or evidence of physical dependence. It is speculated that bremazocine interacts selectively with κ receptors. Failure of naloxone to reverse sedation produced by bremazocine is further evidence that this drug is acting at sites other than μ receptors.

Dezocine

Dezocine, 0.15 mg/kg IM, is an opioid agonist-antagonist with the analgesic potency, onset, and duration of action in the relief of postoperative pain comparable to morphine. Absorption of dezocine, 10 to 15 mg, after IM administration is rapid and complete, with analgesia occurring after about 30 minutes. After IV administration of dezocine, 5 to 10 mg, the onset of analgesia occurs in about 15 minutes. Elimination of dezocine is principally in the urine as a glucuronide conjugate. Like other opioid agonist–antagonists, dezocine exhibits a ceiling effect for depression of ventilation that parallels its analgesic activity.[188] Large doses of dezocine administered IV to humans do not produce significant changes in systemic blood pressure, pulmonary artery pressure, or cardiac output.

Dezocine has a high affinity for μ receptors and a moderate affinity for δ receptors. The interaction at δ receptors serves to facilitate the effect of agonist activity at μ receptors. The incidence of dysphoria is minimal after administration of dezocine, presumably reflecting the low affinity of this drug for σ receptors.

Meptazinol

Meptazinol is a partial opioid agonist with relative selectivity at mu_1 receptors. As a result, depression of ventilation does not occur with analgesic doses of meptazinol (100 mg IM is equivalent to morphine, 8 mg IM). The onset of analgesia is rapid, but the duration of action is <2 hours. Bioavailability after oral administration is <10%. Metabolism is to inactive glucuronide conjugates that are excreted by the kidneys. Protein binding is 20% to 25%, and the elimination half-time is about 2 hours. Physical dependence does not occur, miosis is slight, and constipation is absent. Nausea and vomiting are common side effects. Meptazinol cannot be substituted for an opioid agonist in patients physically dependent on opioids.

Opioid Antagonists

Minor changes in the structure of an opioid agonist can convert the drug into an opioid antagonist at one or more of the opioid receptor sites (Fig. 7-22).[189] The most common change is substitution of an alkyl group for a methyl group on an opioid agonist. For example, naloxone is the *N*-alkyl derivative of oxymorphone (see Fig. 7-21).

Naloxone, naltrexone, and nalmefene are pure μ opioid receptor antagonists with no agonist activity. The high affinity for opioid receptors characteristic of pure opioid antagonists results in displacement of the opioid agonist from μ receptors. After this displacement, the binding of the pure antagonist does not activate μ receptors and antagonism occurs.

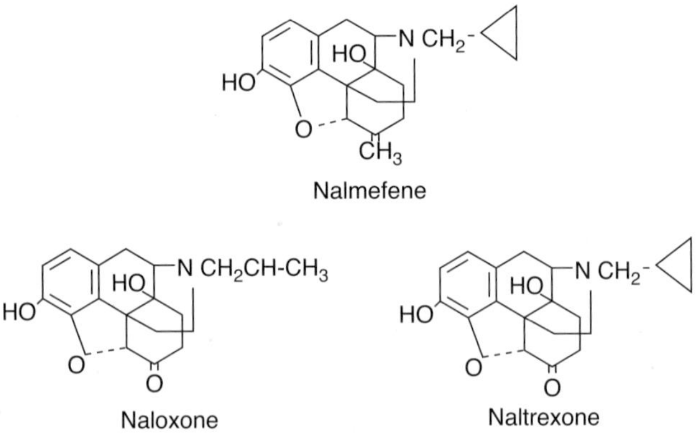

Nalmefene

Naloxone

Naltrexone

FIGURE 7-22 Opioid antagonists.

Naloxone

Naloxone is a nonselective antagonist at all three opioid receptors. Naloxone is selective when used to (a) treat opioid-induced depression of ventilation as may be present in the postoperative period, (b) treat opioid-induced depression of ventilation in the neonate due to maternal administration of an opioid, (c) facilitate treatment of deliberate opioid overdose, and (d) detect suspected physical dependence. Naloxone, 1 to 4 μg/kg IV, promptly reverses opioid-induced analgesia and depression of ventilation. The short duration of action of naloxone (30 to 45 minutes) is presumed to be due to its rapid removal from the brain. This emphasizes that supplemental doses of naloxone will likely be necessary for sustained antagonism of opioid agonists. In this regard, a continuous infusion of naloxone, 5 μg/kg/hour, prevents depression of ventilation without altering analgesia produced by neuraxial opioids.[190]

Naloxone is metabolized primarily in the liver by conjugation with glucuronic acid to form naloxone-3-glucuronide. The elimination half-time is 60 to 90 minutes. Naloxone is absorbed orally, but metabolism during its first pass through the liver renders it only one-fifth as potent as when administered parenterally.

Side Effects

Antagonism of opioid-induced depression of ventilation is accompanied by an inevitable reversal of analgesia. It may be possible, however, to titrate the dose of naloxone such that depression of ventilation is partially but acceptably antagonized to also maintain partial analgesia.

Nausea and vomiting appear to be closely related to the dose and speed of injection of naloxone. Administration of naloxone slowly over 2 to 3 minutes rather than as a bolus seems to decrease the incidence of nausea and vomiting. Awakening occurs either before or simultaneously with vomiting, which ensures that the patient's protective upper airway reflexes have returned and the likelihood of pulmonary aspiration is minimized.

Cardiovascular stimulation after administration of naloxone manifests as increased sympathetic nervous system activity, presumably reflecting the abrupt reversal of analgesia and the sudden perception of pain. This increased sympathetic nervous system activity may manifest as tachycardia, hypertension, pulmonary edema, and cardiac dysrhythmias.[191] Even ventricular fibrillation has occurred after the IV administration of naloxone and the associated sudden increase in sympathetic nervous system activity.[192]

Naloxone can easily cross the placenta. For this reason, administration of naloxone to an opioid-dependent parturient may produce acute withdrawal in the neonate.

Role in Treatment of Shock

Naloxone produces dose-related improvement in myocardial contractility and survival in animals subjected to hypovolemic shock and, to a lesser extent, in those subjected to septic shock.[193] The beneficial effects of naloxone in the treatment of shock occur only with doses >1 mg/kg IV, suggesting that the beneficial effects of this drug are not opioid receptor–mediated or, alternatively, are mediated by opioid receptors other than μ receptors—possibly δ and κ receptors.

Antagonism of General Anesthesia

The occasional observation that high doses of naloxone seem to antagonize the depressant effect of inhaled anesthetics may represent drug-induced activation of the cholinergic arousal system in the brain, independent of any interaction with opioid receptors.[194] A role of endorphins in the production of general anesthesia is not supported by data demonstrating a failure of naloxone to alter anesthetic requirements (MAC) in animals.

Naltrexone

Naltrexone, in contrast to naloxone, is highly effective orally, producing sustained antagonism of the effects of opioid agonists for as long as 24 hours. It has found a role in the treatment of alcoholism, possibly by reducing the pleasure associated with ethanol intoxication.[195]

Nalmefene

Nalmefene is a pure opioid antagonist that is a 6-methylene analogue of naltrexone (see Fig. 7-22).[196] Nalmefene is equipotent to naloxone. The recommended dose is 15 to 25 μg IV administered every 2 to 5 minutes until the desired effect is achieved, with the total dose not exceeding 1 μg/kg. Prophylactic administration of nalmefene significantly decreases the need for antiemetics and antipruritic medications in patients receiving IV patient-controlled analgesia with morphine.[197] The primary advantage of nalmefene over naloxone is its longer duration of action, which might provide a greater degree of protection from delayed depression of ventilation due to residual effects of the opioid as the antagonist is cleared. Compared with the brief elimination half-time of naloxone, the half-time of nalmefene is about 10.8 hours. This longer duration of action is likely due to the slower clearance of nalmefene compared with naloxone. Nalmefene is metabolized by hepatic conjugation, with <5% excreted unchanged in the urine. As with naloxone, acute pulmonary edema has occurred after the IV administration of nalmefene.[198]

Methylnaltrexone

Methylnaltrexone is a quaternary opioid receptor antagonist. The highly ionized quaternary methyl group limits the transfer of methylnaltrexone across the blood–brain barrier. As a result, methylnaltrexone is active at peripheral rather than central opioid receptors as demonstrated by its failure to penetrate the CNS sufficiently to promote withdrawal in morphine-dependent animals.

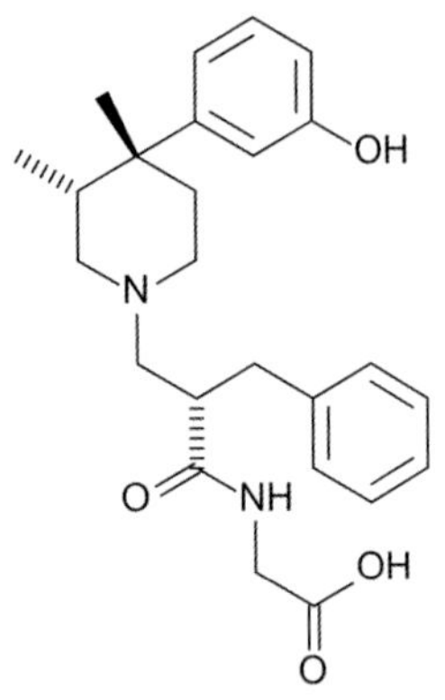

FIGURE 7-23 Chemical structure of alvimopan, a newer μ-selective oral peripheral opioid antagonist.

In humans, methylnaltrexone attenuates morphine-induced changes in the rate of gastric emptying and also decreases the incidence of nausea.[199] The attenuation of morphine-induced nausea may be due to antagonism of morphine at the chemoreceptor trigger zone (located outside the blood–brain barrier) or through limitation of the delay in gastric emptying, which, in itself, may cause nausea. Presumably, methylnaltrexone could prevent the undesirable effects of opioids on gastric emptying and possibly vomiting without altering centrally mediated analgesia.

Alvimopan

Alvimopan (Fig. 7-23) is a newer μ-selective oral peripheral opioid antagonist. Its oral bioavailability is approximately 6% and its metabolism also relies on gut flora.[200] It was approved by the U.S. Food and Drug Administration for treatment of postoperative ileus and has shown mixed results in subsequent clinical trials for treating ileus or opioid-induced constipation. Although likely safe in the acute setting, concern about a potential increase in cardiovascular events with long-term use has dampened enthusiasm for this drug.[201]

Tamper- or Abuse-Resistant Opioids

In recent years, prescribing of opioids for chronic noncancer pain has gained greater social acceptance. Correspondingly, the aggregate opioid consumption in the United States increased from 97 mg of morphine equivalents per person in 1997 to 710 mg in 2010.[202] Along with this increase in prescription use, there has been a dramatic rise in drug diversion and abuse, both of which have a significant human and economic cost.[203]

In an attempt to provide effective oral opioid analgesia with less potential for abuse, oral opioid formulations have been developed to reduce the ability to rapidly ingest the active ingredient (crushing, snorting, injecting) with subsequent euphoric effects.[204] Examples of this strategy include Suboxone (buprenorphine plus naloxone), Embeda (extended release morphine plus naltrexone), and OxyNal (oxycodone plus naltrexone). Convincing evidence of their efficacy is currently lacking, but they may prove to fill a useful role in chronic oral analgesic use by preventing opioid overdose due to crushing or injecting the extended-release opioid formulation.

Opioid Allergy

Although many patients claim "allergies" to opioids, true opioid allergy is rare. More often, predictable side effects of opioids such as localized histamine release, orthostatic hypotension, nausea, and vomiting are misinterpreted as an allergic reaction. Morphine contains a tertiary amine group, which causes nonimmune release of histamine. True allergic reactions to morphine are much rarer. Fentanyl is chemically dissimilar to morphine and, as such, does not cross-react with morphine derivatives.[205] To date, there have been only four reported cases of fentanyl-induced anaphylaxis [206–209], one of which was subsequently retracted due to an undiagnosed latex allergy.[210] In each of these cases, the reaction presented as hypotension and urticaria.

Opioid Immune Modulation

Opioid therapy may alter immunity through neuroendocrine effects or via direct effects on the immune system.[40,211] Opioid receptors are present on immune cells, including T and B lymphocytes, dendritic cells, neutrophils, macrophages, and microglia.[41] Prolonged exposure to opioids appears more likely than short-term exposure to produce immunosuppression especially in susceptible persons and abrupt withdrawal may also induce immunosuppression.

Of recent interest is the possible link between opioid-induced immunosuppression and cancer recurrence after resection.[212–215] Opioids alter the development, differentiation, and function of immune cells, and particularly seem to depress natural killer (NK) cell activity (Fig. 7-24).[216–218] NK cells are lymphoid lineage cells that induce apoptosis in target cells via mechanisms distinct from T lymphocytes and appear to be a major factor in tumor surveillance. Although immunosuppressant effects of opioids raise concerns, it is equally important to recognize that pain itself can impair immune function.

Anesthetic Requirements

The contribution of opioids to total anesthetic requirements can be estimated by determining the decrease in MAC of a volatile anesthetic in the presence of opioids.

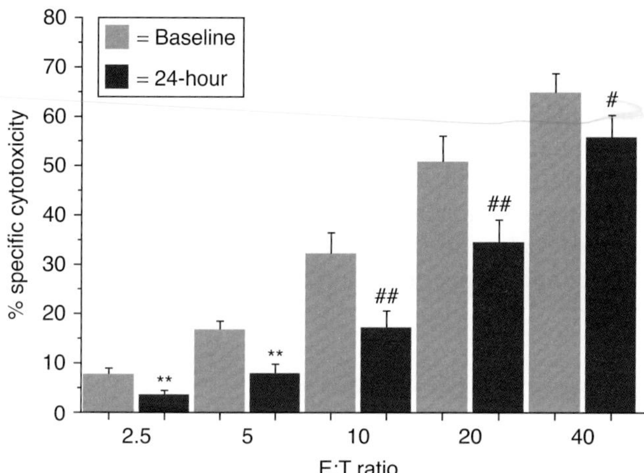

FIGURE 7-24 Depressed peripheral blood natural killer cell cytotoxicity immediately after a 24-hour high-dose morphine infusion in nine participants. Values are percent-specific cytotoxicity at each effector:target (E:T) ratio tested (mean plus/minus standard error). **, $P < .05$ versus baseline value; ##, $P < .005$ versus baseline value; #, $P < .01$ versus baseline value. (From Yeager M, Colacchio T, Yu C, et al. Morphine inhibits spontaneous and cytokine-enhanced natural killer cell cytotoxicity in volunteers. *Anesthesiology.* 1995;83[3]:500–508, with permission.)

In animals, morphine decreases the MAC of volatile anesthetics in a dose-dependent manner, but there appears to be a ceiling effect to the anesthetic-sparing ability of morphine, with a plateau at 65% MAC.[219] A single dose of fentanyl, 3 μg/kg IV 25 to 30 minutes before surgical incision, decreases isoflurane or desflurane MAC by about 50%.[220] In animals, sufentanil decreases enflurane MAC by 70% to 90%.[221] In patients, a sufentanil plasma concentration of 0.145 ng/mL produced a 50% decrease in isoflurane MAC, whereas plasma sufentanil concentrations of >0.5 ng/mL exhibited a ceiling effect.[222,223] As with other opioids, alfentanil administered to animals decreases MAC in a dose-dependent manner until a plateau is reached at about a 70% decrease in MAC. The decrease in MAC produced by remifentanil is similar to that produced by other opioids and ranges from 50% to 91%, depending on the plasma concentration of remifentanil.[224] These data cast serious doubt on the ability of opioid agonists to provide reliable amnesia during surgical procedures, even at extremely high doses.

Opioid agonist–antagonists are less effective than opioid agonists in decreasing MAC. For example, butorphanol, nalbuphine, and pentazocine maximally decrease MAC 11%, 8%, and 20%, respectively, even when the dose of these drugs is increased 40-fold.[225] The ceiling effect for MAC parallels the ceiling effect for depression of ventilation and is consistent with the clinical impression that even large doses of opioid agonist–antagonists do not produce unconsciousness or even prevent patient movement in response to painful stimulation. Thus, the intraoperative role for these drugs is minimal.

Patient-Controlled Analgesia

As an alternative to intermittent bolus dosing of medication, patients may be provided with a mechanism to address their own analgesic requirements. Termed ***patient-controlled analgesia*** (PCA), this most typically involves a programmable electronic pump, which delivers a prescribed dose of medication upon patient demand. The rationale of this technique is that, by using frequent, small doses of opioid, patients will have better control of their pain by keeping effect-site concentrations in the therapeutic range for a larger proportion of the time. Rather than wide swings between inadequate analgesia and oversedation, the PCA regimen is designed to allow patients to self-titrate their dosing to optimize their pain management (Fig. 7-25).

Proposed advantages of this technique include decreased health care provider workload, increased patient

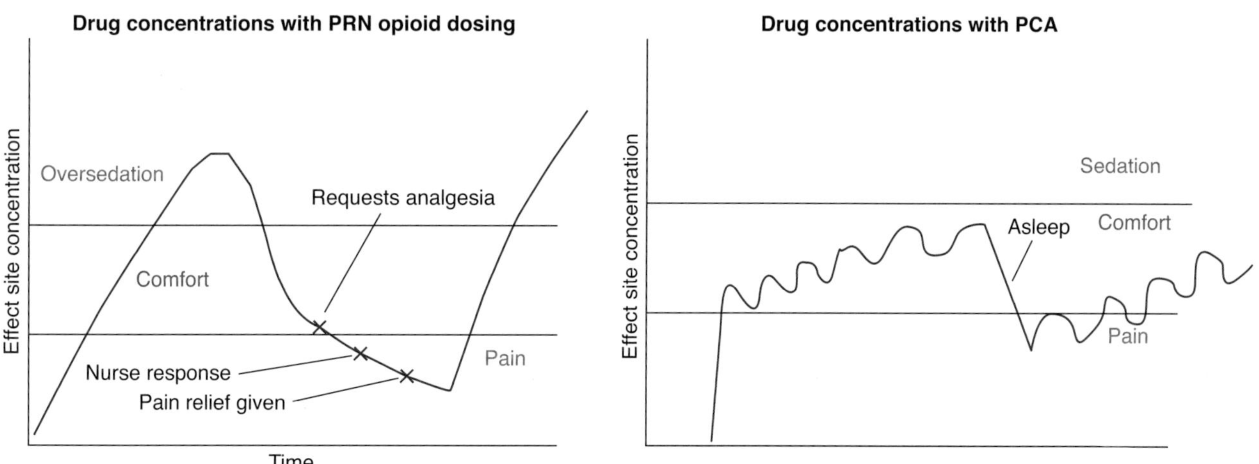

FIGURE 7-25 Effect site concentrations with traditional versus patient-controlled opioid dosing. After achieving effective concentrations, PCA allows patients to self-titrate opioid dosing to maintain effective analgesia.

Table 7-5

Suggested Starting Intravenous Patient-Controlled Analgesia Opioid Regimens

Drug	Basal Rate[a]	Bolus Dose	Bolus Interval (min)
Morphine	0–2 mg/h	1–2 mg	6–10
Hydromorphone	0–0.4 mg/h	0.2–0.4 mg	6–10
Fentanyl	0–60 μg/h	20–50 μg	5–10

[a]Basal infusions are not typically recommended for opioid-naive patients.

satisfaction, lower opioid consumption, and the inherent safety of needing a conscious patient to self-administer a dose of opioid.[226] Despite multiple studies, the most recent review by the Cochrane Collaboration suggests that PCA only provides marginally improved analgesia over conventional opioid therapy. Patient satisfaction, however, is higher with PCA.[227]

Typically, IV PCA opioids are used. Morphine, hydromorphone, and fentanyl are the most common choices. Suggested initial dosing regimens are listed in Table 7-5. Although PCA is usually used with IV opioids, there are a number of new technologies being evaluated, including transdermal fentanyl, sublingual sufentanil, oral opioids, intranasal opioids, and even inhaled opioids.[226] None are currently used clinically.

Owing to the unique pharmacokinetic profile of remifentanil, it has found a role in PCA for labor and delivery. Because remifentanil undergoes nonenzymatic hydrolysis in both the maternal and fetal circulations, it has minimal effects on the neonate. In cases where epidural analgesia is contraindicated, remifentanil PCA has shown to provide good analgesia during the first stage of labor.[228]

Neuraxial Opioids

Placement of opioids in the epidural or subarachnoid space to manage acute or chronic pain is based on the knowledge that opioid receptors (principally μ receptors) are present in the substantia gelatinosa of the spinal cord.[229] Analgesia produced by neuraxial opioids, in contrast to regional anesthesia with local anesthetics, is not associated with sympathectomy, sensory block, or weakness. Analgesia is dose related (epidural dose is 5 to 10 times the subarachnoid dose) and effective for visceral pain. Neuraxial morphine may decrease the MAC for volatile anesthetics, although not all investigators have demonstrated this effect.[230–232]

Analgesia that follows epidural placement of opioids reflects diffusion of the drug across the dura to gain access to μ opioid receptors in the spinal cord as well as systemic absorption to produce effects similar to those that would follow IV administration of the opioid. For example, the mechanism of postoperative analgesia produced by epidural administration of highly lipophilic opioids (fentanyl, sufentanil) is primarily a reflection of systemic absorption. In fact, it has been proposed that epidural administration of lipophilic opioids may offer no clinical advantages over IV administration.[233] Poorly lipid-soluble opioids such as morphine result in a slower onset of analgesia but a longer duration of action than lipid-soluble opioids when administered via the neuraxial route.

Pharmacokinetics

Opioids placed in the epidural space may undergo uptake into epidural fat, systemic absorption, or diffusion across the dura into the CSF.[234] Epidural administration of opioids produces considerable CSF concentrations of drug. Penetration of the dura is highly influenced by lipid solubility, but molecular weight may also be important. Fentanyl and sufentanil are, respectively, approximately 800 and 1,600 times as lipid soluble as morphine. After epidural administration, CSF concentrations of fentanyl peak in about 20 minutes and sufentanil in about 6 minutes. In contrast, CSF concentrations of morphine, after epidural administration, peak in 1 to 4 hours. Furthermore, only about 3% of the dose of morphine administered epidurally crosses the dura to enter the CSF.[235]

The epidural space contains an extensive venous plexus, and vascular absorption of opioids from the epidural space is extensive. After epidural administration, fentanyl blood concentrations peak in 5 to 10 minutes, whereas blood concentrations of the more lipid-soluble sufentanil peak even sooner.[236] In contrast, blood concentrations of morphine after epidural administration peak after 10 to 15 minutes. Epidural administration of morphine, fentanyl, and sufentanil produces opioid blood concentrations that are similar to those produced by an IM injection of an equivalent dose.[234] The addition of epinephrine to the solution placed into the epidural space decreases systemic absorption of the opioid but does not influence the diffusion of morphine across the dura into the CSF. The addition of epinephrine to intrathecal morphine solutions enhances postoperative analgesia compared with intrathecal morphine alone.[237] Vascular absorption after intrathecal administration of opioids is clinically insignificant.

Cephalad movement of opioids in the CSF principally depends on lipid solubility. For example, lipid-soluble opioids such as fentanyl and sufentanil are limited in their cephalad migration by uptake into the spinal cord, whereas less lipid-soluble morphine remains in the CSF for transfer to more cephalad locations. After lumbar intrathecal morphine administration, appreciable cervical CSF concentrations occur 1 to 5 hours after injection, whereas cervical CSF concentrations of highly lipid-soluble opioids are minimal after their epidural administration. The underlying cause of ascension of morphine is bulk flow of CSF. CSF ascends in a cephalad direction from the lumbar region, reaching the cisterna magna in 1 to 2 hours and the fourth and lateral ventricles by 3 to 6 hours.[234] Coughing or straining, but not body position, can affect movement of CSF. The elimination half-time of morphine in CSF is similar to that in plasma.[238]

Side Effects

Side effects of neuraxial opioids are caused by the presence of drug in either the CSF or systemic circulation.[234] In general, most side effects are dose dependent. Some side effects are mediated via interaction with specific opioid receptors, whereas others are nonspecific. Side effects are less common in patients chronically exposed to opioids. The four classic side effects of neuraxial opioids are pruritus, nausea and vomiting, urinary retention, and depression of ventilation.

Pruritus

Pruritus is the most common side effect with neuraxial opioids. It may be generalized but is more likely to be localized to the face, neck, or upper thorax. The incidence of pruritus varies widely and is often elicited only after direct questioning. Severe pruritus is rare, occurring in about 1% of patients. Pruritus is more likely to occur in obstetric patients, perhaps due to the interaction of estrogen with opioid receptors. The incidence may or may not be dose related. Pruritus usually occurs within a few hours of injection and may precede the onset of analgesia.

Although opioids may liberate the release of histamine from mast cells, this does not appear to be the mechanism for pruritus. Instead, pruritus induced by neuraxial opioids is likely due to cephalad migration of the opioid in CSF and subsequent interaction with opioid receptors in the trigeminal nucleus. An opioid antagonist such as naloxone is effective in relieving opioid-induced pruritus. Antihistamines may be an effective treatment for pruritus, but this is likely secondary to their sedative effect. Gabapentin, an anticonvulsant often used for treatment of neuropathic pain, has also shown some promise in the treatment of opioid-induced pruritus.[239,240]

Urinary Retention

The incidence of urinary retention varies widely and is most common in young males. Urinary retention with neuraxial opioids is more common than after IV or IM administration of equivalent doses of the opioid. The incidence of this side effect is not dose dependent or related to systemic absorption of the opioid. Urinary retention is most likely due to interaction of the opioid with opioid receptors located in the sacral spinal cord. This interaction promotes inhibition of sacral parasympathetic nervous system outflow, which causes detrusor muscle relaxation and an increase in maximum bladder capacity, leading to urinary retention. In humans, epidural morphine causes marked detrusor muscle relaxation within 15 minutes of injection that persists for up to 16 hours; it is readily reversed with naloxone.[190]

Depression of Ventilation

The most serious side effect of neuraxial opioids is depression of ventilation, which may occur within minutes of administration or may be delayed for hours. The incidence of ventilatory depression requiring intervention after conventional doses of neuraxial opioids is about 1%, which is the same as that after conventional doses of IV or IM opioids.[234]

Early depression of ventilation occurs within 2 hours of neuraxial injection of the opioid. Most reports of clinically important depression of ventilation involve epidural administration of fentanyl or sufentanil. This depression of ventilation most likely results from systemic absorption of the lipid-soluble opioid, although cephalad migration of opioid in the CSF may also be responsible. Clinically significant early depression of ventilation after intrathecal injection of morphine is unlikely.

Delayed depression of ventilation occurs more than 2 hours after neuraxial opioid administration and reflects cephalad migration of the opioid in the CSF and subsequent interaction with opioid receptors located in the ventral medulla. All reports of clinically significant delayed depression of ventilation involve morphine.[234] Delayed depression of ventilation characteristically occurs 6 to 12 hours after epidural or intrathecal administration of morphine. Clinically important depression of ventilation has not been described more than 24 hours after the epidural or intrathecal injection of morphine.

Factors that increase the risk of delayed depression of ventilation, especially concomitant use of any IV opioid or sedative, must be considered in determining the dose of neuraxial opioid (see Table 7-3).[234] Coughing may affect the movement of CSF and increase the likelihood of depression of ventilation. Obstetric patients appear to be at less risk for ventilatory depression, perhaps because of the increased stimulation to ventilation provided by progesterone.

Detection of depression of ventilation induced by neuraxial opioids may be difficult. Arterial hypoxemia and hypercarbia may develop despite a normal breathing rate (Fig. 7-26).[241] Pulse oximetry reliably detects opioid-induced arterial hypoxemia, and supplemental oxygen (2 L/min) is an effective treatment. The most reliable clinical sign of depression of ventilation, however, appears to be a depressed level of consciousness, possibly caused by hypercarbia.[234] In patients receiving supplemental oxygen, arterial hypoxemia is a very late sign of hypoventilation; thus, pulse oximetry is of limited value in detection of opioid-induced respiratory depression in these patients. Prophylactic infusions of naloxone are of variable efficacy in protecting against depression of ventilation.[190,242] Naloxone (0.25 μg/kg/hour IV) is effective in attenuating the side effects (nausea and vomiting, pruritus) associated with morphine-induced analgesia delivered by a patient-controlled IV delivery system.[243]

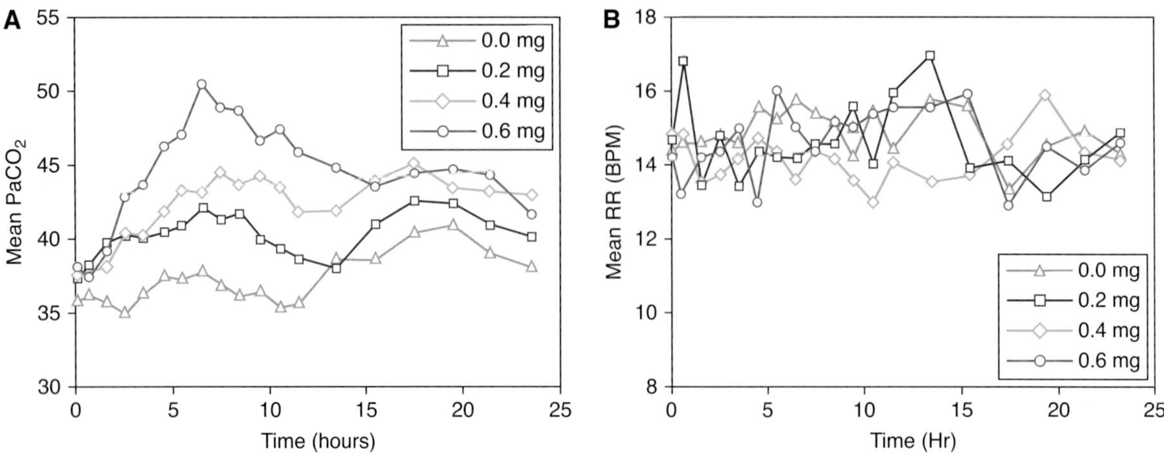

FIGURE 7-26 Mean respiratory rate (RR) **(A)** and mean arterial carbon dioxide partial pressure (mm Hg) **(B)** versus times before (time 0) and after three different doses of intrathecal morphine. (From Bailey PL, Rhondeau S, Schafer PG, et al. Dose-response pharmacology of intrathecal morphine in human volunteers. *Anesthesiology.* 1993;79:49–59, with permission.)

Sedation

Sedation after administration of neuraxial opioids appears to be dose related and occurs with all opioids but is most commonly associated with the use of sufentanil. When sedation occurs with neuraxial opioids, depression of ventilation must be considered. Mental status changes other than sedation may also occur with neuraxial opioids. Naloxone-reversible psychosis, catatonia, and hallucinations have been described.[234]

Central Nervous System Excitation

Tonic skeletal muscle rigidity resembling seizure activity is a well-known side effect of large IV doses of opioids, but this response is rarely observed after neuraxial administration. Myoclonic activity has been observed after neuraxial opioids and, in one report, progressed to a grand mal seizure.[244] Although large doses of opioids reliably produce seizures in animals, clinically relevant doses of IV or neuraxial opioids are unlikely to be associated with generalized cortical seizure activity in humans.[234] Cephalad migration of the opioid in CSF and subsequent interaction with nonopioid receptors in the brainstem or basal ganglia is the most likely explanation for opioid-induced CNS excitation. In this regard, opioids may block glycine or γ-aminobutyric acid–mediated inhibition.

Viral Reactivation

A link exists between the use of epidural morphine in obstetric patients and reactivation of herpes simplex labialis virus. Reactivation of the herpes virus occurs 2 to 5 days after epidural administration of the opioid.[245] Manifestation of symptoms of herpes labialis (cold sores) characteristically occurs in the same sensory innervation as the primary infection, which are usually facial areas innervated by the trigeminal nerve. The underlying mechanism causing herpes virus reactivation likely involves cephalad migration of opioid in CSF and subsequent interaction with the trigeminal nucleus.

Neonatal Morbidity

Systemic absorption after epidural administration of an opioid results in predictable blood levels of the drug in the neonate immediately after birth. Clinically important depression of ventilation has been observed in the newborns of mothers receiving epidural opioids.[234] The progress of labor in general does not seem to be adversely affected by neuraxial opioids.[246] After administration of epidural fentanyl or sufentanil to parturients, the concentration of opioid in breast milk is negligible. As a general rule, opioid analgesics should not be withheld from women recovering from cesarean delivery due to concerns of neonatal drug exposure in breast milk.

Miscellaneous Side Effects

Epidural morphine has been associated with sustained erection (priapism) and inability to ejaculate in male volunteers. Naloxone-reversible miosis, nystagmus, and vertigo may occur after neuraxial opioids, most commonly morphine. Neuraxial opioids may delay gastric emptying, most likely reflecting an interaction of the opioid with a spinal cord opioid receptor.[247] Neuraxial opioids, by inhibiting shivering, may cause decreased body temperature. Oliguria and water retention leading to peripheral edema have been reported after neuraxial opioid administration. Water retention is likely caused by release of vasopressin, stimulated by cephalad migration of the opioid in the CSF. Neuraxial opioids have been implicated as possible causes of spinal cord damage, especially following accidental use of opioids containing toxic preservatives.[234] Clinical manifestations in these patients include sensory and motor neurologic dysfunction, myoclonic spasms, paresis, and paralysis. On the other hand, neuraxial opioids have been administered chronically without adverse sequelae.

References

1. Brownstein MJ. A brief history of opiates, opioid peptides, and opioid receptors. *Proc Natl Acad Sci U S A*. 1993;90(12):5391–5393.
2. Burkle H, Dunbar S, Van Aken H. Remifentanil: a novel, short-acting, mu-opioid. *Anesth Analg*. 1996;83(3):646–651.
3. Egan TD, Lemmens HJ, Fiset P, et al. The pharmacokinetics of the new short-acting opioid remifentanil (GI87084B) in healthy adult male volunteers. *Anesthesiology*. 1993;79(5):881–892.
4. Shafer SL, Varvel JR. Pharmacokinetics, pharmacodynamics, and rational opioid selection. *Anesthesiology*. 1991;74(1):53–63.
5. Pleuvry BJ. Opioid receptors and their relevance to anaesthesia. *Br J Anaesth*. 1993;71(1):119–126.
6. Stein C. The control of pain in peripheral tissue by opioids. *N Engl J Med*. 1995;332(25):1685–1690.
7. Stein C. Peripheral mechanisms of opioid analgesia. *Anesth Analg*. 1993;76(1):182–191.
8. Atcheson R, Lambert DG. Update on opioid receptors. *Br J Anaesth*. 1994;73(2):132–134.
9. Lambert DG. Recent advances in opioid pharmacology. *Br J Anaesth*. 1998;81(1):1–2.
10. Li S, Zhu J, Chen C, et al. Molecular cloning and expression of a rat kappa opioid receptor. *Biochem J*. 1993;295(pt 3):629–633.
11. Chen Y, Mestek A, Liu J, et al. Molecular cloning and functional expression of a mu-opioid receptor from rat brain. *Mol Pharmacol*. 1993;44(1):8–12.
12. Yaksh TL. Pharmacology and mechanisms of opioid analgesic activity. *Acta Anaesthesiol Scand*. 1997;41(1, pt 2):94–111.
13. Rittner HL, Brack A, Machelska H, et al. Opioid peptide-expressing leukocytes: identification, recruitment, and simultaneously increasing inhibition of inflammatory pain. *Anesthesiology*. 2001; 95(2):500–508.
14. Heine MF, Tillet ED, Tsueda K, et al. Intra-articular morphine after arthroscopic knee operation. *Br J Anaesth*. 1994;73(3): 413–415.
15. Kosterlitz HW. Biosynthesis of morphine in the animal kingdom. *Nature*. 1987;330(6149):606.
16. Prinster SC, Hague C, Hall RA. Heterodimerization of g protein-coupled receptors: specificity and functional significance. *Pharmacol Rev*. 2005;57(3):289–298.
17. Milligan G. G protein-coupled receptor dimerisation: molecular basis and relevance to function. *Biochim Biophys Acta*. 2007; 1768(4):825–835.
18. Gupta A, Mulder J, Gomes I, et al. Increased abundance of opioid receptor heteromers after chronic morphine administration. *Sci Signal*. 2010;3(131):ra54.
19. Fields H. State-dependent opioid control of pain. *Nat Rev Neurosci*. 2004;5(7):565–575.
20. Pomeranz B, Chiu D. Naloxone blockade of acupuncture analgesia: endorphin implicated. *Life Sci*. 1976;19(11):1757–1762.
21. Bie B, Brown DL, Naguib M. Synaptic plasticity and pain aversion. *Eur J Pharmacol*. 2011;667(1–3):26–31.
22. Zubieta JK, Smith YR, Bueller JA, et al. Regional mu opioid receptor regulation of sensory and affective dimensions of pain. *Science*. 2001;293(5528):311–315.
23. Bingel U, Wanigasekera V, Wiech K, et al. The effect of treatment expectation on drug efficacy: imaging the analgesic benefit of the opioid remifentanil. *Sci Transl Med*. 2011;3(70):70ra14.
24. Lowenstein E, Whiting RB, Bittar DA, et al. Local and neurally mediated effects of morphine on skeletal muscle vascular resistance. *J Pharmacol Exp Ther*. 1972;180(2):359–367.
25. Cahalan MK, Lurz FW, Eger EI II, et al. Narcotics decrease heart rate during inhalational anesthesia. *Anesth Analg*. 1987;66(2): 166–170.
26. Rosow CE, Moss J, Philbin DM, et al. Histamine release during morphine and fentanyl anesthesia. *Anesthesiology*. 1982;56(2): 93–96.
27. Philbin DM, Moss J, Akins CW, et al. The use of H1 and H2 histamine antagonists with morphine anesthesia: a double-blind study. *Anesthesiology*. 1981;55(3):292–296.
28. Stoelting RK, Gibbs PS. Hemodynamic effects of morphine and morphine-nitrous oxide in valvular heart disease and coronary-artery disease. *Anesthesiology*. 1973;38(1):45–52.
29. Tomicheck RC, Rosow CE, Philbin DM, et al. Diazepam-fentanyl interaction—hemodynamic and hormonal effects in coronary artery surgery. *Anesth Analg*. 1983;62(10):881–884.
30. McPherson BC, Yao Z. Signal transduction of opioid-induced cardioprotection in ischemia-reperfusion. *Anesthesiology*. 2001; 94(6):1082–1088.
31. Bowdle TA, Rooke GA. Postoperative myoclonus and rigidity after anesthesia with opioids. *Anesth Analg*. 1994;78(4):783–786.
32. Costall B, Fortune DH, Naylor RJ. Involvement of mesolimbic and extrapyramidal nuclei in the motor depressant action of narcotic drugs. *J Pharm Pharmacol*. 1978;30(9):566–572.
33. Bennett JA, Abrams JT, Van Riper DF, et al. Difficult or impossible ventilation after sufentanil-induced anesthesia is caused primarily by vocal cord closure. *Anesthesiology*. 1997;87(5):1070–1074.
34. Paqueron X, Lumbroso A, Mergoni P, et al. Is morphine-induced sedation synonymous with analgesia during intravenous morphine titration? *Br J Anaesth*. 2002;89(5):697–701.
35. Radnay PA, Brodman E, Mankikar D, et al. The effect of equi-analgesic doses of fentanyl, morphine, meperidine and pentazocine on common bile duct pressure. *Anaesthesist*. 1980;29(1):26–29.
36. Jones RM, Fiddian-Green R, Knight PR. Narcotic-induced choledochoduodenal sphincter spasm reversed by glucagon. *Anesth Analg*. 1980;59(12):946–947.
37. Jones RM, Detmer M, Hill AB, et al. Incidence of choledochoduodenal sphincter spasm during fentanyl-supplemented anesthesia. *Anesth Analg*. 1981;60(9):638–640.
38. Philbin DM, Wilson NE, Sokoloski J, et al. Radioimmunoassay of antidiuretic hormone during morphine anaesthesia. *Can Anaesth Soc J*. 1976;23(3):290–295.
39. Way WL, Costley EC, Leongway E. Respiratory sensitivity of the newborn infant to meperidine and morphine. *Clin Pharmacol Ther*. 1965;6:454–461.
40. Ballantyne JC, Mao J. Opioid therapy for chronic pain. *N Engl J Med*. 2003;349(20):1943–1953.
41. Ninkovic J, Roy S. Role of the mu-opioid receptor in opioid modulation of immune function. *Amino Acids*. 2013;45(1):9–24.
42. Tweed WA, Dakin D. Explosive coughing after bolus fentanyl injection. *Anesth Analg*. 2001;92(6):1442–1443.
43. Cho HB, Kwak HJ, Park SY, et al. Comparison of the incidence and severity of cough after alfentanil and remifentanil injection. *Acta Anaesthesiol Scand*. 2010;54(6):717–720.
44. Duttaroy A, Yoburn BC. The effect of intrinsic efficacy on opioid tolerance. *Anesthesiology*. 1995;82(5):1226–1236.
45. Mitra S, Sinatra RS. Perioperative management of acute pain in the opioid-dependent patient. *Anesthesiology*. 2004;101(1): 212–227.
46. Joly V, Richebe P, Guignard B, et al. Remifentanil-induced postoperative hyperalgesia and its prevention with small-dose ketamine. *Anesthesiology*. 2005;103(1):147–155.
47. Cherny NI. Opioid analgesics: comparative features and prescribing guidelines. *Drugs*. 1996;51(5):713–737.
48. Aubrun F, Monsel S, Langeron O, et al. Postoperative titration of intravenous morphine in the elderly patient. *Anesthesiology*. 2002;96(1):17–23.
49. Woolf CJ, Wall PD. Morphine-sensitive and morphine-insensitive actions of C-fibre input on the rat spinal cord. *Neurosci Lett*. 1986; 64(2):221–225.
50. Tooms A, McKenzie A, Grey H. Nebulised morphine. *Lancet*. 1993;342(8879):1123–1124.
51. Lang E, Jedeikin R. Acute respiratory depression as a complication of nebulised morphine. *Can J Anaesth*. 1998;45(1):60–62.

52. Thipphawong JB, Babul N, Morishige RJ, et al. Analgesic efficacy of inhaled morphine in patients after bunionectomy surgery. *Anesthesiology*. 2003;99(3):693–700; discussion 6A.
53. Murphy MR, Hug CC Jr. Pharmacokinetics of intravenous morphine in patients anesthetized with enflurane-nitrous oxide. *Anesthesiology*. 1981;54(3):187–192.
54. Berkowitz BA, Ngai SH, Yang JC, et al. The diposition of morphine in surgical patients. *Clin Pharmacol Ther*. 1975;17(6):629–635.
55. Finck AD, Berkowitz BA, Hempstead J, et al. Pharmacokinetics of morphine: effects of hypercarbia on serum and brain morphine concentrations in the dog. *Anesthesiology*. 1977;47(5):407–410.
56. Roerig DL, Kotrly KJ, Vucins EJ, et al. First pass uptake of fentanyl, meperidine, and morphine in the human lung. *Anesthesiology*. 1987;67(4):466–472.
57. Vaughan CW, Connor M. In search of a role for the morphine metabolite morphine-3-glucuronide. *Anesth Analg*. 2003;97(2): 311–312.
58. Romberg R, Olofsen E, Sarton E, et al. Pharmacodynamic effect of morphine-6-glucuronide versus morphine on hypoxic and hypercapnic breathing in healthy volunteers. *Anesthesiology*. 2003; 99(4):788–798.
59. Hanna MH, Peat SJ, Woodham M, et al. Analgesic efficacy and CSF pharmacokinetics of intrathecal morphine-6-glucuronide: comparison with morphine. *Br J Anaesth*. 1990;64(5):547–550.
60. Paul D, Standifer KM, Inturrisi CE, et al. Pharmacological characterization of morphine-6 beta-glucuronide, a very potent morphine metabolite. *J Pharmacol Exp Ther*. 1989;251(2):477–483.
61. Sear JW. Drug biotransformation by the kidney: how important is it, and how much do we really know? *Br J Anaesth*. 1991;67(4): 369–372.
62. Chauvin M, Sandouk P, Scherrmann JM, et al. Morphine pharmacokinetics in renal failure. *Anesthesiology*. 1987;66(3):327–331.
63. Don HF, Dieppa RA, Taylor P. Narcotic analgesics in anuric patients. *Anesthesiology*. 1975;42(6):745–747.
64. Lynn AM, Slattery JT. Morphine pharmacokinetics in early infancy. *Anesthesiology*. 1987;66(2):136–139.
65. Hanna MH, D'Costa F, Peat SJ, et al. Morphine-6-glucuronide disposition in renal impairment. *Br J Anaesth*. 1993;70(5):511–514.
66. Baka NE, Bayoumeu F, Boutroy MJ, et al. Colostrum morphine concentrations during postcesarean intravenous patient-controlled analgesia. *Anesth Analg*. 2002;94(1):184–187, table of contents.
67. Kest B, Sarton E, Dahan A. Gender differences in opioid-mediated analgesia: animal and human studies. *Anesthesiology*. 2000; 93(2):539–547.
68. Sarton E, Olofsen E, Romberg R, et al. Sex differences in morphine analgesia: an experimental study in healthy volunteers. *Anesthesiology*. 2000;93(5):1245–1254; discussion 6A.
69. Dahan A, Sarton E, Teppema L, et al. Sex-related differences in the influence of morphine on ventilatory control in humans. *Anesthesiology*. 1998;88(4):903–913.
70. Stone PA, Macintyre PE, Jarvis DA. Norpethidine toxicity and patient controlled analgesia. *Br J Anaesth*. 1993;71(5):738–740.
71. Cozian A, Pinaud M, Lepage JY, et al. Effects of meperidine spinal anesthesia on hemodynamics, plasma catecholamines, angiotensin I, aldosterone, and histamine concentrations in elderly men. *Anesthesiology*. 1986;64(6):815–819.
72. Austin KL, Stapleton JV, Mather LE. Multiple intramuscular injections: a major source of variability in analgesic response to meperidine. *Pain*. 1980;8(1):47–62.
73. Austin KL, Stapleton JV, Mather LE. Relationship between blood meperidine concentrations and analgesic response: a preliminary report. *Anesthesiology*. 1980;53(6):460–466.
74. Alfonsi P, Sessler DI, Du Manoir B, et al. The effects of meperidine and sufentanil on the shivering threshold in postoperative patients. *Anesthesiology*. 1998;89(1):43–48.
75. Ikeda T, Sessler DI, Tayefeh F, et al. Meperidine and alfentanil do not reduce the gain or maximum intensity of shivering. *Anesthesiology*. 1998;88(4):858–865.
76. Kurz A, Ikeda T, Sessler DI, et al. Meperidine decreases the shivering threshold twice as much as the vasoconstriction threshold. *Anesthesiology*. 1997;86(5):1046–1054.
77. Takada K, Clark DJ, Davies MF, et al. Meperidine exerts agonist activity at the alpha(2B)-adrenoceptor subtype. *Anesthesiology*. 2002;96(6):1420–1426.
78. Flacke JW, Flacke WE, Bloor BC, et al. Histamine release by four narcotics: a double-blind study in humans. *Anesth Analg*. 1987; 66(8):723–730.
79. Tissot TA. Probable meperidine-induced serotonin syndrome in a patient with a history of fluoxetine use. *Anesthesiology*. 2003;98(6): 1511–1512.
80. Lewis WR, Perrino AC Jr. Transient neurological symptoms after subarachnoid meperidine. *Anesth Analg*. 2002;94(1):213–214, table of contents.
81. Stanley TH. The history and development of the fentanyl series. *J Pain Symptom Manage*. 1992;7(3)(suppl):S3–S7.
82. Hug CC Jr, Murphy MR. Tissue redistribution of fentanyl and termination of its effects in rats. *Anesthesiology*. 1981;55(4):369–375.
83. Hudson RJ, Thomson IR, Jassal R, et al. Cardiopulmonary bypass has minimal effects on the pharmacokinetics of fentanyl in adults. *Anesthesiology*. 2003;99(4):847–854.
84. Peng PW, Sandler AN. A review of the use of fentanyl analgesia in the management of acute pain in adults. *Anesthesiology*. 1999; 90(2):576–599.
85. Ibrahim AE, Feldman J, Karim A, et al. Simultaneous assessment of drug interactions with low- and high-extraction opioids: application to parecoxib effects on the pharmacokinetics and pharmacodynamics of fentanyl and alfentanil. *Anesthesiology*. 2003;98(4):853–861.
86. Murphy MR, Hug CC Jr, McClain DA. Dose-independent pharmacokinetics of fentanyl. *Anesthesiology*. 1983;59(6):537–540.
87. Bentley JB, Borel JD, Nenad RE Jr, et al. Age and fentanyl pharmacokinetics. *Anesth Analg*. 1982;61(12):968–971.
88. Hudson RJ, Thomson IR, Cannon JE, et al. Pharmacokinetics of fentanyl in patients undergoing abdominal aortic surgery. *Anesthesiology*. 1986;64(3):334–338.
89. Haberer JP, Schoeffler P, Couderc E, et al. Fentanyl pharmacokinetics in anaesthetized patients with cirrhosis. *Br J Anaesth*. 1982; 54(12):1267–1270.
90. Hughes MA, Glass PS, Jacobs JR. Context-sensitive half-time in multicompartment pharmacokinetic models for intravenous anesthetic drugs. *Anesthesiology*. 1992;76(3):334–341.
91. Gedney JA, Ghosh S. Pharmacokinetics of analgesics, sedatives and anaesthetic agents during cardiopulmonary bypass. *Br J Anaesth*. 1995;75(3):344–351.
92. Daniel M, Weiskopf RB, Noorani M, Eger EI II. Fentanyl augments the blockade of the sympathetic response to incision (MAC-BAR) produced by desflurane and isoflurane: desflurane and isoflurane MAC-BAR without and with fentanyl. *Anesthesiology*. 1998;88(1):43–49.
93. Hilgenberg JC. Intraoperative awareness during high-dose fentanyl—oxygen anesthesia. *Anesthesiology*. 1981;54(4):341–343.
94. Sprigge JS, Wynands JE, Whalley DG, et al. Fentanyl infusion anesthesia for aortocoronary bypass surgery: plasma levels and hemodynamic response. *Anesth Analg*. 1982;61(12):972–978.
95. Wynands JE, Townsend GE, Wong P, et al. Blood pressure response and plasma fentanyl concentrations during high- and very high-dose fentanyl anesthesia for coronary artery surgery. *Anesth Analg*. 1983;62(7):661–665.
96. Palmer CM, Cork RC, Hays R, et al. The dose-response relation of intrathecal fentanyl for labor analgesia. *Anesthesiology*. 1998; 88(2):355–361.
97. Macaluso AD, Connelly AM, Hayes WB, et al. Oral transmucosal fentanyl citrate for premedication in adults. *Anesth Analg*. 1996; 82(1):158–161.
98. Stanley TH, Leiman BC, Rawal N, et al. The effects of oral transmucosal fentanyl citrate premedication on preoperative behavioral responses and gastric volume and acidity in children. *Anesth Analg*. 1989;69(3):328–335.

99. Friesen RH, Lockhart CH. Oral transmucosal fentanyl citrate for preanesthetic medication of pediatric day surgery patients with and without droperidol as a prophylactic anti-emetic. *Anesthesiology.* 1992;76(1):46–51.
100. Epstein RH, Mendel HG, Witkowski TA, et al. The safety and efficacy of oral transmucosal fentanyl citrate for preoperative sedation in young children. *Anesth Analg.* 1996;83(6):1200–1225.
101. Dsida RM, Wheeler M, Birmingham PK, et al. Premedication of pediatric tonsillectomy patients with oral transmucosal fentanyl citrate. *Anesth Analg.* 1998;86(1):66–70.
102. Ashburn MA, Lind GH, Gillie MH, et al. Oral transmucosal fentanyl citrate (OTFC) for the treatment of postoperative pain. *Anesth Analg.* 1993;76(2):377–381.
103. Caplan RA, Ready LB, Oden RV, et al. Transdermal fentanyl for postoperative pain management. A double-blind placebo study. *JAMA.* 1989;261(7):1036–1039.
104. Kuzma PJ, Kline MD, Stamatos JM, et al. Acute toxic delirium: an uncommon reaction to transdermal fentanyl. *Anesthesiology.* 1995;83(4):869–871.
105. Arndt JO, Mikat M, Parasher C. Fentanyl's analgesic, respiratory, and cardiovascular actions in relation to dose and plasma concentration in unanesthetized dogs. *Anesthesiology.* 1984;61(4):355–361.
106. Frolich MA, Giannotti A, Modell JH. Opioid overdose in a patient using a fentanyl patch during treatment with a warming blanket. *Anesth Analg.* 2001;93(3):647–648.
107. Becker LD, Paulson BA, Miller RD, et al. Biphasic respiratory depression after fentanyldroperidol or fentanyl alone used to supplement nitrous oxide anesthesia. *Anesthesiology.* 1976;44(4):291–296.
108. Murat I, Levron JC, Berg A, et al. Effects of fentanyl on baroreceptor reflex control of heart rate in newborn infants. *Anesthesiology.* 1988;68(5):717–722.
109. Manninen PH. Opioids and seizures. *Can J Anaesth.* 1997;44(5, pt 1):463–466.
110. Smith NT, Benthuysen JL, Bickford RG, et al. Seizures during opioid anesthetic induction—are they opioid-induced rigidity? *Anesthesiology.* 1989;71(6):852–862.
111. Murkin JM, Moldenhauer CC, Hug CC Jr, et al. Absence of seizures during induction of anesthesia with high-dose fentanyl. *Anesth Analg.* 1984;63(5):489–494.
112. Schubert A, Drummond JC, Peterson DO, et al. The effect of high-dose fentanyl on human median nerve somatosensory-evoked responses. *Can J Anaesth.* 1987;34(1):35–40.
113. Glass PS, Bloom M, Kearse L, et al. Bispectral analysis measures sedation and memory effects of propofol, midazolam, isoflurane, and alfentanil in healthy volunteers. *Anesthesiology.* 1997;86(4): 836–847.
114. Sebel PS, Lang E, Rampil IJ, et al. A multicenter study of bispectral electroencephalogram analysis for monitoring anesthetic effect. *Anesth Analg.* 1997;84(4):891–899.
115. Albanese J, Durbec O, Viviand X, et al. Sufentanil increases intracranial pressure in patients with head trauma. *Anesthesiology.* 1993;79(3):493–497.
116. Werner C, Kochs E, Bause H, et al. Effects of sufentanil on cerebral hemodynamics and intracranial pressure in patients with brain injury. *Anesthesiology.* 1995;83(4):721–726.
117. de Nadal M, Munar F, Poca MA, et al. Cerebral hemodynamic effects of morphine and fentanyl in patients with severe head injury: absence of correlation to cerebral autoregulation. *Anesthesiology.* 2000;92(1):11–19.
118. Bailey PL, Pace NL, Ashburn MA, et al. Frequent hypoxemia and apnea after sedation with midazolam and fentanyl. *Anesthesiology.* 1990;73(5):826–830.
119. Scott JC, Cooke JE, Stanski DR. Electroencephalographic quantitation of opioid effect: comparative pharmacodynamics of fentanyl and sufentanil. *Anesthesiology.* 1991;74(1):34–42.
120. Malinovsky JM, Lepage JY, Cozian A, et al. Transient muscular spasm after a large dose of intrathecal sufentanil. *Anesthesiology.* 1996;84(6):1513–1515.
121. Bovill JG, Sebel PS, Blackburn CL, et al. The pharmacokinetics of sufentanil in surgical patients. *Anesthesiology.* 1984;61(5):502–506.
122. Chauvin M, Ferrier C, Haberer JP, et al. Sufentanil pharmacokinetics in patients with cirrhosis. *Anesth Analg.* 1989;68(1):1–4.
123. Hudson RJ, Bergstrom RG, Thomson IR, et al. Pharmacokinetics of sufentanil in patients undergoing abdominal aortic surgery. *Anesthesiology.* 1989;70(3):426–431.
124. Schwartz AE, Matteo RS, Ornstein E, et al. Pharmacokinetics of sufentanil in obese patients. *Anesth Analg.* 1991;73(6):790–793.
125. Boer F, Hoeft A, Scholz M, et al. Pulmonary distribution of alfentanil and sufentanil studied with system dynamics analysis. *J Pharmacokinet Biopharm.* 1996;24(2):197–218.
126. Meistelman C, Benhamou D, Barre J, et al. Effects of age on plasma protein binding of sufentanil. *Anesthesiology.* 1990;72(3):470–473.
127. Yaster M. The dose response of fentanyl in neonatal anesthesia. *Anesthesiology.* 1987;66(3):433–435.
128. Wiggum DC, Cork RC, Weldon ST, et al. Postoperative respiratory depression and elevated sufentanil levels in a patient with chronic renal failure. *Anesthesiology.* 1985;63(6):708–710.
129. Bailey PL, Streisand JB, East KA, et al. Differences in magnitude and duration of opioid-induced respiratory depression and analgesia with fentanyl and sufentanil. *Anesth Analg.* 1990;70(1):8–15.
130. Sanford TJ Jr, Smith NT, Dec-Silver H, et al. A comparison of morphine, fentanyl, and sufentanil anesthesia for cardiac surgery: induction, emergence, and extubation. *Anesth Analg.* 1986;65(3): 259–266.
131. Mayer N, Weinstabl C, Podreka I, et al. Sufentanil does not increase cerebral blood flow in healthy human volunteers. *Anesthesiology.* 1990;73(2):240–243.
132. Chang J, Fish KJ. Acute respiratory arrest and rigidity after anesthesia with sufentanil: a case report. *Anesthesiology.* 1985;63(6): 710–711.
133. Philbin DM, Rosow CE, Schneider RC, et al. Fentanyl and sufentanil anesthesia revisited: how much is enough? *Anesthesiology.* 1990;73(1):5–11.
134. Abrams JT, Horrow JC, Bennett JA, et al. Upper airway closure: a primary source of difficult ventilation with sufentanil induction of anesthesia. *Anesth Analg.* 1996;83(3):629–632.
135. Scott JC, Stanski DR. Decreased fentanyl and alfentanil dose requirements with age. A simultaneous pharmacokinetic and pharmacodynamic evaluation. *J Pharmacol Exp Ther.* 1987;240(1): 159–166.
136. Davis PJ, Stiller RL, Cook DR, et al. Effects of cholestatic hepatic disease and chronic renal failure on alfentanil pharmacokinetics in children. *Anesth Analg.* 1989;68(5):579–583.
137. Chauvin M, Lebrault C, Levron JC, et al. Pharmacokinetics of alfentanil in chronic renal failure. *Anesth Analg.* 1987;66(1):53–56.
138. Meistelman C, Saint-Maurice C, Lepaul M, et al. A comparison of alfentanil pharmacokinetics in children and adults. *Anesthesiology.* 1987;66(1):13–16.
139. Camu F, Gepts E, Rucquoi M, et al. Pharmacokinetics of alfentanil in man. *Anesth Analg.* 1982;61(8):657–661.
140. Kharasch ED, Russell M, Mautz D, et al. The role of cytochrome P450 3A4 in alfentanil clearance. Implications for interindividual variability in disposition and perioperative drug interactions. *Anesthesiology.* 1997;87(1):36–50.
141. Bartkowski RR, McDonnell TE. Prolonged alfentanil effect following erythromycin administration. *Anesthesiology.* 1990;73(3): 566–568.
142. Miller DR, Martineau RJ, O'Brien H, et al. Effects of alfentanil on the hemodynamic and catecholamine response to tracheal intubation. *Anesth Analg.* 1993;76(5):1040–1046.
143. Yonker-Sell AE, Muzi M, Hope WG, et al. Alfentanil modifies the neurocirculatory responses to desflurane. *Anesth Analg.* 1996;82(1):162–166.
144. Ausems ME, Hug CC Jr, de Lange S. Variable rate infusion of alfentanil as a supplement to nitrous oxide anesthesia for general surgery. *Anesth Analg.* 1983;62(11):982–986.

145. Langevin S, Lessard MR, Trepanier CA, et al. Alfentanil causes less postoperative nausea and vomiting than equipotent doses of fentanyl or sufentanil in outpatients. *Anesthesiology.* 1999;91(6):1666–1673.
146. Mets B. Acute dystonia after alfentanil in untreated Parkinson's disease. *Anesth Analg.* 1991;72(4):557–558.
147. Jhaveri R, Joshi P, Batenhorst R, et al. Dose comparison of remifentanil and alfentanil for loss of consciousness. *Anesthesiology.* 1997;87(2):253–259.
148. Rosow C. Remifentanil: a unique opioid analgesic. *Anesthesiology.* 1993;79(5):875–876.
149. Thompson JP, Rowbotham DJ. Remifentanil—an opioid for the 21st century. *Br J Anaesth.* 1996;76(3):341–343.
150. Babenco HD, Conard PF, Gross JB. The pharmacodynamic effect of a remifentanil bolus on ventilatory control. *Anesthesiology.* 2000;92(2):393–398.
151. Nieuwenhuijs DJ, Olofsen E, Romberg RR, et al. Response surface modeling of remifentanil-propofol interaction on cardiorespiratory control and bispectral index. *Anesthesiology.* 2003;98(2):312–322.
152. Egan TD, Huizinga B, Gupta SK, et al. Remifentanil pharmacokinetics in obese versus lean patients. *Anesthesiology.* 1998;89(3):562–573.
153. Hoke JF, Shlugman D, Dershwitz M, et al. Pharmacokinetics and pharmacodynamics of remifentanil in persons with renal failure compared with healthy volunteers. *Anesthesiology.* 1997;87(3):533–541.
154. Kapila A, Glass PS, Jacobs JR, et al. Measured context-sensitive half-times of remifentanil and alfentanil. *Anesthesiology.* 1995;83(5):968–975.
155. Thompson JP, Hall AP, Russell J, et al. Effect of remifentanil on the haemodynamic response to orotracheal intubation. *Br J Anaesth.* 1998;80(4):467–469.
156. Evron S, Glezerman M, Sadan O, et al. Remifentanil: a novel systemic analgesic for labor pain. *Anesth Analg.* 2005;100(1):233–238.
157. Kan RE, Hughes SC, Rosen MA, et al. Intravenous remifentanil: placental transfer, maternal and neonatal effects. *Anesthesiology.* 1998;88(6):1467–1474.
158. Hogue CW Jr, Bowdle TA, O'Leary C, et al. A multicenter evaluation of total intravenous anesthesia with remifentanil and propofol for elective inpatient surgery. *Anesth Analg.* 1996;83(2):279–285.
159. Avramov MN, Smith I, White PF. Interactions between midazolam and remifentanil during monitored anesthesia care. *Anesthesiology.* 1996;85(6):1283–1289.
160. Recart A, Rawal S, White PF, et al. The effect of remifentanil on seizure duration and acute hemodynamic responses to electroconvulsive therapy. *Anesth Analg.* 2003;96(4):1047–1450.
161. Haber GW, Litman RS. Generalized tonic-clonic activity after remifentanil administration. *Anesth Analg.* 2001;93(6):1532–1533.
162. Guy J, Hindman BJ, Baker KZ, et al. Comparison of remifentanil and fentanyl in patients undergoing craniotomy for supratentorial space-occupying lesions. *Anesthesiology.* 1997;86(3):514–524.
163. Warner DS, Hindman BJ, Todd MM, et al. Intracranial pressure and hemodynamic effects of remifentanil versus alfentanil in patients undergoing supratentorial craniotomy. *Anesth Analg.* 1996;83(2):348–353.
164. Klimscha W, Ullrich R, Nasel C, et al. High-dose remifentanil does not impair cerebrovascular carbon dioxide reactivity in healthy male volunteers. *Anesthesiology.* 2003;99(4):834–840.
165. Fragen RJ, Vilich F, Spies SM, et al. The effect of remifentanil on biliary tract drainage into the duodenum. *Anesth Analg.* 1999;89(6):1561–1564.
166. Guignard B, Bossard AE, Coste C, et al. Acute opioid tolerance: intraoperative remifentanil increases postoperative pain and morphine requirement. *Anesthesiology.* 2000;93(2):409–417.
167. Guignard B, Coste C, Costes H, et al. Supplementing desflurane-remifentanil anesthesia with small-dose ketamine reduces perioperative opioid analgesic requirements. *Anesth Analg.* 2002;95(1):103–108.
168. Ferrini F, Trang T, Mattioli TA, et al. Morphine hyperalgesia gated through microglia-mediated disruption of neuronal Cl(-) homeostasis. *Nat Neurosci.* 2013;16(2):183–192.
169. Vree TB, van Dongen RT, Koopman-Kimenai PM. Codeine analgesia is due to codeine-6-glucuronide, not morphine. *Int J Clin Pract.* 2000;54(6):395–398.
170. Angst MS, Drover DR, Lotsch J, et al. Pharmacodynamics of orally administered sustained-release hydromorphone in humans. *Anesthesiology.* 2001;94(1):63–73.
171. Thwaites D, McCann S, Broderick P. Hydromorphone neuroexcitation. *J Palliat Med.* 2004;7(4):545–550.
172. Gimbel J, Ahdieh H. The efficacy and safety of oral immediate-release oxymorphone for postsurgical pain. *Anesth Analg.* 2004;99(5):1472–1477.
173. Gershman JA, Fass AD. Hydrocodone rescheduling amendment and pipeline products on the horizon. *P T.* 2012;37(7):399–404.
174. Fishman SM, Wilsey B, Mahajan G, et al. Methadone reincarnated: novel clinical applications with related concerns. *Pain Med.* 2002;3(4):339–348.
175. Budd K, Langford R. Tramadol revisited. *Br J Anaesth.* 1999;82(4):493–495.
176. Collart L, Luthy C, Favario-Constantin C, et al. [Duality of the analgesic effect of tramadol in humans]. *Schweiz Med Wochenschr.* 1993;123(47):2241–2243.
177. Calvey TN. Chirality in anaesthesia. *Anaesthesia.* 1992;47(2):93–94.
178. Nieuwenhuijs D, Bruce J, Drummond GB, et al. Influence of oral tramadol on the dynamic ventilatory response to carbon dioxide in healthy volunteers. *Br J Anaesth.* 2001;87(6):860–865.
179. Crighton IM, Martin PH, Hobbs GJ, et al. A comparison of the effects of intravenous tramadol, codeine, and morphine on gastric emptying in human volunteers. *Anesth Analg.* 1998;87(2):445–449.
180. Vahabzadeh M, Moshiri M, Mohammadpour AH, et al. Promising effects of intravenous lipid emulsion as an antidote in acute tramadol poisoning. *Reg Anesth Pain Med.* 2013;38(5):425–430.
181. Kahn LH, Alderfer RJ, Graham DJ. Seizures reported with tramadol. *JAMA.* 1997;278(20):1661.
182. Angell M. Should heroin be legalized for the treatment of pain? *N Engl J Med.* 1984;311(8):529–530.
183. Mondzac AM. In defense of the reintroduction of heroin into American medical practice and H.R. 5290—the Compassionate Pain Relief Act. *N Engl J Med.* 1984;311(8):532–535.
184. Gal TJ, DiFazio CA, Moscicki J. Analgesic and respiratory depressant activity of nalbuphine: a comparison with morphine. *Anesthesiology.* 1982;57(5):367–374.
185. Bailey PL, Clark NJ, Pace NL, et al. Antagonism of postoperative opioid-induced respiratory depression: nalbuphine versus naloxone. *Anesth Analg.* 1987;66(11):1109–1114.
186. Lanz E, Simko G, Theiss D, et al. Epidural buprenorphine—a double-blind study of postoperative analgesia and side effects. *Anesth Analg.* 1984;63(6):593–598.
187. Gould DB. Buprenorphine causes pulmonary edema just like all other mu-opioid narcotics. Upper airway obstruction, negative alveolar pressure. *Chest.* 1995;107(5):1478–1479.
188. Gal TJ, DiFazio CA. Ventilatory and analgesic effects of dezocine in humans. *Anesthesiology.* 1984;61(6):716–722.
189. Glass PS, Jhaveri RM, Smith LR. Comparison of potency and duration of action of nalmefene and naloxone. *Anesth Analg.* 1994;78(3):536–541.
190. Rawal N, Schott U, Dahlstrom B, et al. Influence of naloxone infusion on analgesia and respiratory depression following epidural morphine. *Anesthesiology.* 1986;64(2):194–201.
191. Partridge BL, Ward CF. Pulmonary edema following low-dose naloxone administration. *Anesthesiology.* 1986;65(6):709–710.
192. Andree RA. Sudden death following naloxone administration. *Anesth Analg.* 1980;59(10):782–784.

193. Faden AI. Opiate antagonists and thyrotropin-releasing hormone. I. Potential role in the treatment of shock. *JAMA*. 1984; 252(9):1177–1180.
194. Kraynack BJ, Gintautas JG. Naloxone: analeptic action unrelated to opiate receptor antagonism? *Anesthesiology*. 1982;56(4): 251–253.
195. Srisurapanont M, Jarusuraisin N. Naltrexone for the treatment of alcoholism: a meta-analysis of randomized controlled trials. *Int J Neuropsychopharmacol*. 2005;8(2):267–280.
196. Dougherty TB, Porche VH, Thall PF. Maximum tolerated dose of nalmefene in patients receiving epidural fentanyl and dilute bupivacaine for postoperative analgesia. *Anesthesiology*. 2000;92(4): 1010–1016.
197. Joshi GP, Duffy L, Chehade J, et al. Effects of prophylactic nalmefene on the incidence of morphine-related side effects in patients receiving intravenous patient-controlled analgesia. *Anesthesiology*. 1999;90(4):1007–1011.
198. Henderson CA, Reynolds JE. Acute pulmonary edema in a young male after intravenous nalmefene. *Anesth Analg*. 1997;84(1):218–219.
199. Foss JF, O'Connor MF, Yuan CS, et al. Safety and tolerance of methylnaltrexone in healthy humans: a randomized, placebo-controlled, intravenous, ascending-dose, pharmacokinetic study. *J Clin Pharmacol*. 1997;37(1):25–30.
200. Holzer P. Opioid antagonists for prevention and treatment of opioid-induced gastrointestinal effects. *Curr Opin Anaesthesiol*. 2010;23(5):616–622.
201. Bream-Rouwenhorst HR, Cantrell MA. Alvimopan for postoperative ileus. *Am J Health Syst Pharm*. 2009;66(14):1267–1277.
202. Manchikanti L, Helm S II, Fellows B, et al. Opioid epidemic in the United States. *Pain Physician*. 2012;15(3)(suppl):ES9–ES38.
203. Strassels SA. Economic burden of prescription opioid misuse and abuse. *J Manag Care Pharm*. 2009;15(7):556–562.
204. Lourenco LM, Matthews M, Jamison RN. Abuse-deterrent and tamper-resistant opioids: how valuable are novel formulations in thwarting non-medical use? [Review]. *Exp Opin Drug Deliv*. 2013; 10(2):229–240.
205. Hepner DL, Castells MC. Anaphylaxis during the perioperative period. *Anesth Analg*. 2003;97:1381–1395.
206. Bennett MJ, Anderson LK, McMillan JC, et al. Anaphylactic reaction during anaesthesia associated with positive intradermal skin test to fentanyl. *Can J Anaesth*. 1986;33:75–78.
207. Fukuda T, Dohi S. Anaphylactic reaction to fentanyl or preservative. *Can J Anaesth*. 1986;33:826–827.
208. Zucker-Pinchoff B, Ramanathan S. Anaphylactic reaction to epidural fentanyl. *Anesthesiology*. 1989;71:599–601.
209. Cummings KC III, Arnaut KA. Case report: Fentanyl-associated intraoperative anaphylaxis with pulmonary edema. *Can J Anaesth*. 2007;54(4):301–306.
210. Zucker-Pinchoff B, Chandler MJ. Latex anaphylaxis masquerading as fentanyl anaphylaxis: Retraction of a case report. *Anesthesiology*. 1993;79:1153–1154.
211. Webster NR. Opioids and the immune system. *Br J Anaesth*. 1998; 81(6):835–836.
212. Biki B, Mascha E, Moriarty DC, et al. Anesthetic technique for radical prostatectomy surgery affects cancer recurrence: a retrospective analysis. *Anesthesiology*. 2008;109(2):180–187.
213. Buggy DJ, Smith G. Epidural anaesthesia and analgesia: better outcome after major surgery? Growing evidence suggests so. *BMJ*. 1999;319(7209):530–531.
214. Exadaktylos AK, Buggy DJ, Moriarty DC, et al. Can anesthetic technique for primary breast cancer surgery affect recurrence or metastasis? *Anesthesiology*. 2006;4:660–664.
215. Cummings KC III, Xu F, Cummings LC, et al. A comparison of epidural analgesia and traditional pain management effects on survival and cancer recurrence after colectomy: a population-based study. *Anesthesiology*. 2012;116(4):797–806.
216. Beilin B, Shavit Y, Hart J, et al. Effects of anesthesia based on large versus small doses of fentanyl on natural killer cell cytotoxicity in the perioperative period. *Anesth Analg*. 1996;82(3): 492–497.
217. Shavit Y, Ben-Eliyahu S, Zeidel A, et al. Effects of fentanyl on natural killer cell activity and on resistance to tumor metastasis in rats. Dose and timing study. *Neuroimmunomodulation*. 2004;11(4): 255–260.
218. Yeager MP, Colacchio TA, Yu CT, et al. Morphine inhibits spontaneous and cytokine-enhanced natural killer cell cytotoxicity in volunteers. *Anesthesiology*. 1995;83(3):500–508.
219. Steffey EP, Eisele JH, Baggot JD, et al. Influence of inhaled anesthetics on the pharmacokinetics and pharmacodynamics of morphine. *Anesth Analg*. 1993;77(2):346–351.
220. Sebel PS, Glass PS, Fletcher JE, et al. Reduction of the MAC of desflurane with fentanyl. *Anesthesiology*. 1992;76(1):52–59.
221. Hall RI, Murphy MR, Hug CC Jr. The enflurane sparing effect of sufentanil in dogs. *Anesthesiology*. 1987;67(4):518–525.
222. Schwartz JG, Garriott JC, Somerset JS, et al. Measurements of fentanyl and sufentanil in blood and urine after surgical application. Implication in detection of abuse. *Am J Forensic Med Pathol*. 1994;15(3):236–241.
223. Brunner MD, Braithwaite P, Jhaveri R, et al. MAC reduction of isoflurane by sufentanil. *Br J Anaesth*. 1994;72(1):42–46.
224. Lang E, Kapila A, Shlugman D, et al. Reduction of isoflurane minimal alveolar concentration by remifentanil. *Anesthesiology*. 1996; 85(4):721–728.
225. Murphy MR, Hug CC Jr. The enflurane sparing effect of morphine, butorphanol, and nalbuphine. *Anesthesiology*. 1982;57(6): 489–492.
226. Palmer PP, Miller RD. Current and developing methods of patient-controlled analgesia. *Anesthesiol Clin*. 2010;28(4):587–599.
227. Hudcova J, McNicol E, Quah C, et al. Patient controlled opioid analgesia versus conventional opioid analgesia for postoperative pain. *Cochrane Database Syst Rev*. 2006;4:CD003348.
228. Hinova A, Fernando R. Systemic remifentanil for labor analgesia. *Anesth Analg*. 2009;109(6):1925–1929.
229. Cousins MJ, Mather LE. Intrathecal and epidural administration of opioids. *Anesthesiology*. 1984;61(3):276–310.
230. Drasner K, Bernards CM, Ozanne GM. Intrathecal morphine reduces the minimum alveolar concentration of halothane in humans. *Anesthesiology*. 1988;69(3):310–312.
231. Licina MG, Schubert A, Tobin JE, et al. Intrathecal morphine does not reduce minimum alveolar concentration of halothane in humans: results of a double-blind study. *Anesthesiology*. 1991; 74(4):660–663.
232. Schwieger IM, Klopfenstein CE, Forster A. Epidural morphine reduces halothane MAC in humans. *Can J Anaesth*. 1992;39(9): 911–914.
233. de Leon-Casasola OA, Lema MJ. Postoperative epidural opioid analgesia: what are the choices? *Anesth Analg*. 1996;83(4): 867–875.
234. Chaney MA. Side effects of intrathecal and epidural opioids. *Can J Anaesth*. 1995;42(10):891–903.
235. Ionescu TI, Taverne RH, Drost RH, et al. Epidural morphine anesthesia for abdominal aortic surgery—pharmacokinetics. *Reg Anesth*. 1989;14(3):107–114.
236. Ionescu TI, Taverne RH, Houweling PL, et al. Pharmacokinetic study of extradural and intrathecal sufentanil anaesthesia for major surgery. *Br J Anaesth*. 1991;66(4):458–464.
237. Goyagi T, Nishikawa T. The addition of epinephrine enhances postoperative analgesia by intrathecal morphine. *Anesth Analg*. 1995;81(3):508–513.
238. Sjostrom S, Tamsen A, Persson MP, et al. Pharmacokinetics of intrathecal morphine and meperidine in humans. *Anesthesiology*. 1987;67(6):889–895.
239. Chiravanich W, Oofuvong M, Kovitwanawong N. Single dose of gabapentin for prophylaxis intrathecal morphine-induced pruritus in orthopedic surgery: a randomized controlled trial. *J Med Assoc Thai*. 2012;95(2):186–190.

240. Sheen MJ, Ho ST, Lee CH, et al. Preoperative gabapentin prevents intrathecal morphine-induced pruritus after orthopedic surgery. *Anesth Analg.* 2008;106(6):1868–1872.
241. Bailey PL, Rhondeau S, Schafer PG, et al. Dose-response pharmacology of intrathecal morphine in human volunteers. *Anesthesiology.* 1993;79(1):49–59; discussion 25A.
242. Morgan M. The rational use of intrathecal and extradural opioids. *Br J Anaesth.* 1989;63(2):165–188.
243. Gan TJ, Ginsberg B, Glass PS, et al. Opioid-sparing effects of a low-dose infusion of naloxone in patient-administered morphine sulfate. *Anesthesiology.* 1997;87(5):1075–1081.
244. Rozan JP, Kahn CH, Warfield CA. Epidural and intravenous opioid-induced neuroexcitation. *Anesthesiology.* 1995;83(4):860–863.
245. Crone LA, Conly JM, Storgard C, et al. Herpes labialis in parturients receiving epidural morphine following cesarean section. *Anesthesiology.* 1990;73(2):208–213.
246. Wong CA, Scavone BM, Peaceman AM, et al. The risk of cesarean delivery with neuraxial analgesia given early versus late in labor. *N Engl J Med.* 2005;352(7):655–665.
247. Kelly MC, Carabine UA, Hill DA, et al. A comparison of the effect of intrathecal and extradural fentanyl on gastric emptying in laboring women. *Anesth Analg.* 1997;85(4):834–838.

CHAPTER 8

Centrally Acting Nonopioid Analgesics

Hesham Elsharkawy • Mohamed A. Naguib

Opioid analgesics are widely used drugs for the management of both acute and chronic pain. Side effects of opioids often limit their dynamic range. The reality of drug dependence, misuse, and abuse makes consideration of in which populations they should be used and for which indications critical. There are several centrally acting nonopioid analgesic adjuvants whose efficacy is supported by scientific evidence. Adding nonnarcotic medications as part of multimodal analgesia is appealing. These agents relieve pain by mechanisms unrelated to opioid receptors; they do not cause respiratory depression, physical dependence, or abuse, and are not regulated under the Controlled Substances Act.

In order to minimize the adverse effects of opioid analgesic medications, anesthesiologists and surgeons are increasingly turning to nonopioid analgesic techniques as adjuvants for managing pain during the perioperative period. Neuraxial drug administration is a group of techniques that deliver drugs in close proximity to the spinal cord, that is, intrathecally into the cerebrospinal fluid (CSF) or epidurally into the fatty tissues surrounding the dura, by injection or infusion. The administration of centrally acting agents bypasses the blood–brain barrier resulting in much higher CSF concentrations while using reduced amounts of medication to achieve equipotent effect.

The addition of neuraxial nonopioid adjuvants to local anesthetics may improve the quality of analgesia. Nonopioid neuraxial adjuvants have a number of different mechanisms of action that are described in the paragraphs that follow. Potential advantages of these agents include a reduction in the dose of individual drugs, a reduction in opioid requirements, and potentially, a reduction in opioid-related side effects. However, the reduction in severe opioid-related side effects is seldom documented as the most severe side effects such as respiratory depression are rare. Adjuvant drugs have their own side effects which at best do not augment opioid side effects. Neuraxial administration of medications confers an inherent risk of injury to structures of the nervous system, not only by the needles and catheters used but also by neurotoxic effects of the compounds injected. Therefore, the potential neurotoxicity of any drug used in this setting requires careful study.[1]

In principle, any drug considered for intrathecal administration in humans requires histologic, physiologic, and behavioral testing in a number of animal species before clinical trials. Most drugs have not been sufficiently well studied to recommend their neuraxial use. Many drug preparations also contain antioxidants, preservatives, and excipients, which might contribute to neurotoxicity. *It is important to note that the U.S. Food and Drug Administration (FDA) has not approved neuraxial (epidural or subarachnoid) administration of most of the drugs listed in this chapter for routine clinical use. Nonetheless, many of these agents have undergone extensive study and in many cases that has included the requisite toxicity studies.*

α_2-Adrenergic Agonists

Epidural or intrathecal administration of α_2-adrenergic agonists provides analgesia by activating α_2-adrenergic receptors (G protein–coupled inhibitory receptors) on the sympathetic preganglionic neurons that mediate a reduction in norepinephrine release (via a negative feedback mechanism). Descending noradrenergic pathways, originating in nuclei A_5 and A_7 in the pons and midbrain appear to play a major inhibitory role on sympathetic preganglionic neuron activity.[2] The overall effect is sympatholysis resulting in analgesia, hypotension, bradycardia, and sedation.[3,4]

Clonidine

Clonidine acts as a selective partial α_2 receptor agonist. Neuraxial clonidine has been shown to be an effective analgesic for chronic cancer and noncancer pain, as well as for postoperative pain. Clonidine has antihypertensive effects and it has been shown to potentiate postoperative analgesia induced by local anesthetics. Spinal clonidine causes a 30% prolongation of sensory and motor block of local anesthetics. Clonidine is commonly administered epidurally in doses ranging from 75 to 150 μg. The doses used for intrathecal (spinal) analgesia ranges from 10 to 50 μg. For caudal analgesia, clonidine is administered as 1 μg/kg dose.

Intrathecal administration of clonidine 37.5 to 150 μg with bupivacaine results in a dose-dependent increase in sensory blockade and more pain-free intervals in the postoperative period. An intrathecal dose of 150 μg was noted to be associated with motor blockade.[4] With combined spinal/epidural anesthesia, intrathecal clonidine doses as low as 15 μg resulted in an increased duration of anesthesia, analgesia, and motor blockade.

Epidural clonidine in the postoperative period reduced visual analog scale (VAS) score and also decreased morphine consumption. Addition of clonidine intrathecally or epidurally was associated with significant reduction of heart rate and blood pressure.[5] Epidural clonidine 1 μg/mL when added to morphine 0.1 mg/mL in 0.2% ropivacaine significantly reduced postoperative pain scores of total knee arthroplasty patients.

Neuraxially administered opioids and α_2 agonists exhibit synergism.[3] The addition of clonidine to opioids for postoperative analgesia as a continuous epidural infusion reduces opioid requirements by 20% to 60%.[6] The addition of 75 μg clonidine to epidural ropivacaine results in longer and more effective analgesia for cesarean delivery. Clonidine is a useful adjunct for labor epidural analgesia. It has been shown to reduce local anesthetic requirements and improve pain scores when combined with 0.125% bupivacaine with or without fentanyl 2 μg/mL. When used in a concentration of 1 to 2 μg/mL, clonidine has no significant effects on fetal heart rate, Apgar scores, or umbilical cord gases. Clonidine may also have additional beneficial effects in women with preeclampsia. However, the FDA has issued a ***black box warning*** concerning the use of neuraxial clonidine in obstetric anesthesia because of related maternal hemodynamic instability. The warning states, "Obstetrical, Postpartum, or Perioperative Use: weigh risk/benefit; epidural clonidine generally not recommended for obstetrical, postpartum, or perioperative pain management due to risk of hemodynamic instability, esp. hypotension and bradycardia." As such, the benefit of adjuvant analgesia and potentially favorable hemodynamic effects must be weighed against the risks for each individual patient.

Neuraxial clonidine is indicated for the treatment of intractable pain in cancer patients unresponsive to maximum doses of opioids. This formed the basis for the approval of epidural clonidine by the FDA.[7] Its use as an adjunct has been most widely accepted in pediatric anesthesia, as a means of increasing the duration of analgesia from caudal block, and to a lesser extent in obstetric anesthesia, to provide analgesia in labor.[8]

Intrathecal clonidine appears to have antihyperalgesic properties.[3,8–11] As hyperalgesia is the physiologic expression of central nervous system (CNS) sensitization, it may be useful in preventing the increased risk or central sensitization and development of persistent pain after surgery in patients with severe postoperative pain.[12]

A recent systematic review aimed to quantify beneficial and harmful effects of clonidine when used as an adjuvant to intrathecal local anesthetics for surgery concluded that clonidine prolongs the regression of the sensory block in a dose-dependent manner, prolongs the time to the first request of an analgesic, and the duration of complete motor block, with weak evidence of dose-responsiveness. In addition, clonidine decreases the risk of intraoperative pain and increases the risk of arterial hypotension, without evidence of dose-responsiveness. Finally, clonidine has no relevant impact on the time to achieve complete sensory or motor block, on the extent of the cephalad spread of the sensory block, or on the risk of bradycardia.[13]

Dexmedetomidine

Dexmedetomidine has a higher affinity for α_2 receptors than clonidine and is associated with a fewer hemodynamic and systemic side effects at equivalent doses. Evidence indicates that neuraxial administration of dexmedetomidine produces spinal analgesia as efficiently as clonidine.[14–16] A dose of 3 μg of intrathecal dexmedetomidine was found to be equipotent with 30 μg of clonidine.[17] Intrathecal dexmedetomidine 5 μg and fentanyl 25 μg were compared for vaginal surgeries with bupivacaine anesthesia. Dexmedetomidine caused significantly longer sensory and motor blockade.[18]

Epidural dexmedetomidine exhibits synergism with local anesthetics, increasing the density of motor block, prolonging the duration of both sensory and motor block, and improving postoperative analgesia. Clinical studies exhibit potentiation of neuraxial local anesthetics, decrease in intraoperative anesthetic requirements with prevention of intraoperative awareness, and improved postoperative analgesia when epidural dexmedetomidine was used in conjunction with general anesthesia.[7,14–16,19,20] The addition of 2 μg/kg dexmedetomidine epidurally prolongs the duration of analgesia and decreases the requirement for rescue analgesics in patients undergoing lower limb orthopedic surgery, abdominal surgeries, and cesarean section which was associated with a significant fall in heart rate and mean arterial blood pressure. In thoracic surgery, the use of epidural dexmedetomidine decreases the anesthetic requirements, prevents awareness during anesthesia, and improves intraoperative oxygenation and postoperative analgesia.[21] Caudal dexmedetomidine in a dose of 2 μg/kg with bupivacaine used in pediatric patients undergoing hernia repair or orchiopexy was found to cause more sedation, prolonged analgesia, less anesthetic consumption, and less irritability. There were no hemodynamic differences when compared to patients who had received only bupivacaine.[22–24]

No neurotoxicity has been reported to date in studies in both humans and animals during intrathecal or epidural administration of dexmedetomidine. However, there is some evidence from animal studies of demyelination of the oligodendrocytes in the white matter, suggesting harmful effects on the myelin sheath when administered via the epidural route. Advanced pathologic investigations are required to establish the safety of α_2-adrenergic agonists. Nevertheless, the major side effects of α_2-adrenergic agonists are limited to hemodynamic effects (i.e., bradycardia and hypotension).

Neostigmine

Neostigmine acts by inhibiting acetylcholinesterase and preventing the breakdown of acetylcholine. Naguib and Yaksh[3,25] demonstrated that the intrathecal administration of cholinesterase inhibitors (neostigmine or edrophonium) produces a dose-dependent antinociceptive activity in rats (Fig. 8-1). These antinociceptive effects are independent of opioid and α_2-receptor systems and are primarily due to stimulation of muscarinic (but not nicotinic) cholinergic receptors. The use of intrathecal acetylcholinesterase inhibitors, such as neostigmine, results in analgesia in both preclinical and clinical models. Neostigmine is a hydrophilic molecule, like morphine, and when applied to the epidural space, it requires time for diffusion through the dura mater into the subarachnoid space.[26,27]

Intrathecal neostigmine has been used as an adjunct to intrathecal local anesthetic or opioid to prolong regional analgesia and improve hemodynamic stability, with variable results. Escalating doses of intrathecal neostigmine (10 to 100 μg) followed by 2% epidural lidocaine resulted in improved analgesia in a dose-independent manner after cesarean delivery.[28] The reduction in morphine requirements lasted up to 10 hours without adverse fetal effects, but the incidence of nausea varied from 50% to 100% in patients. In another study, intrathecal neostigmine (10 μg) alone was ineffective for labor pain relief, but when combined with intrathecal sufentanil, reduced the ED_{50} of sufentanil by approximately 25%.[29]

Epidural administration of neostigmine (100 to 200 μg) appears to avoid these clinically troublesome adverse effects while still improving local anesthetic-induced analgesia.[30,31] Combinations of epidural neostigmine with local anesthetics, opioids, or clonidine for labor analgesia displayed analgesic effectiveness, potentiating the analgesic effect of opioids and clonidine.[32–34] Epidural neostigmine does not affect motor blockade. Higher doses of intrathecal neostigmine can cause mild sedation.[27,35]

A meta-analysis evaluated the effectiveness and side effects of intrathecal neostigmine in the perioperative and peripartum settings. The authors concluded that adding intrathecal neostigmine to other spinal medications improves perioperative and peripartum analgesia marginally when compared with placebo. It is associated with significant side effects and the disadvantages outweigh the minor improvement in analgesia achieved.[36] Nausea and vomiting were seen less frequently in epidural neostigmine studies. This is thought to be due to the lower amount of neostigmine that reaches the CSF and the absence of cephalic distribution.[37] Neostigmine stimulates muscarinic receptors in the bronchial smooth muscles and leads to bronchospasm. In intrathecal neostigmine studies, except at very high doses (e.g., 750 μg), no change has been detected in oxyhemoglobin saturation and in end-tidal carbon dioxide levels.[38]

Intrathecal neostigmine at a dose of 1 μg/kg has been used in pediatric lower abdominal and urologic surgeries where it was found to increase analgesia.[39,40] Adverse gastrointestinal effects have made neostigmine an unpopular choice for neuraxial adjuvant therapy. Unlike intrathecal neostigmine, epidural neostigmine is not associated with an increased risk of nausea and vomiting; however, doses greater than 100 μg have been associated with sedation. It does not cause respiratory depression or pruritus either alone or in combination with neuraxial opioids.

Ketamine

Anesthetic and subanesthetic doses of ketamine have analgesic properties as a result of noncompetitive antagonism of *N*-methyl-D-aspartate (NMDA) receptors. With prolonged, repetitive nociceptive stimulation, NMDA receptors are activated, releasing excitatory neurotransmitters glutamate, aspartate, and neurokinin.[41] Its primary analgesic effect is mediated by antagonizing NMDA

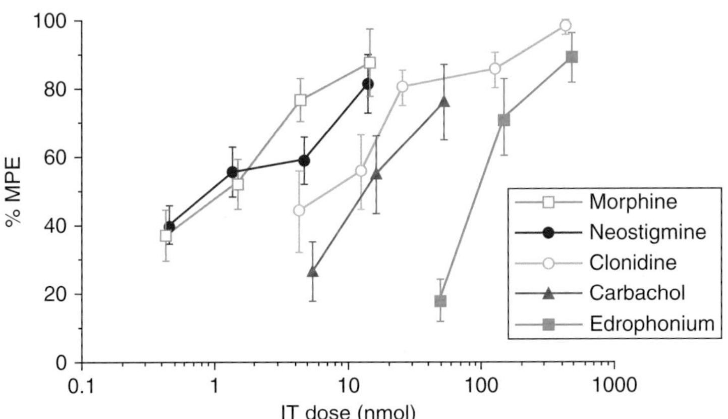

FIGURE 8-1 Log dose-response curves for the effects of intrathecally administered morphine, neostigmine, clonidine, carbachol, and edrophonium on the thermal nociceptive threshold. The response is presented as maximal possible effect (%MPE) versus log dose in nanomoles. Each point on the graph represents the mean ± standard error of the mean. (Reproduced from Naguib M, Yaksh TL. Antinociceptive effects of spinal cholinesterase inhibition and isobolographic analysis of the interaction with mu and alpha 2 receptor systems. *Anesthesiology.* 1994;80[6]:1338–1348, with permission).

receptors located on secondary afferent neurons in the dorsal horn of the spinal cord thus preventing enhancement of excitatory neurotransmission. These neurotransmitters are associated with many activities including central sensitization, wind-up, and the plasticity of various systems such as memory, vision, motor function, and spinal sensory transmission.

Neuraxial ketamine must be administered in a preservative-free solution to avoid neurotoxic effects.[42–45] Naguib et al.[46] studied epidural doses of 10 mg and 30 mg of ketamine and found that a 30-mg dose produced excellent postoperative pain relief. A low dose of ketamine at 4, 6, and 8 mg epidurally was found to be ineffective for postoperative analgesia.[47,48] Caudally administered ketamine 0.5 mg/kg along with 0.175% levobupivacaine 1 mL/kg has been used successfully without adverse effects in children for lower abdominal and urologic surgeries.[49] Epidural infusion of 0.25 mg/kg per hour of S(+)-ketamine during thoracic surgery provides better postoperative analgesia than epidural 0.25% ropivacaine (Fig. 8-2).[50] Both epidural infusions were started before skin incision and were run at

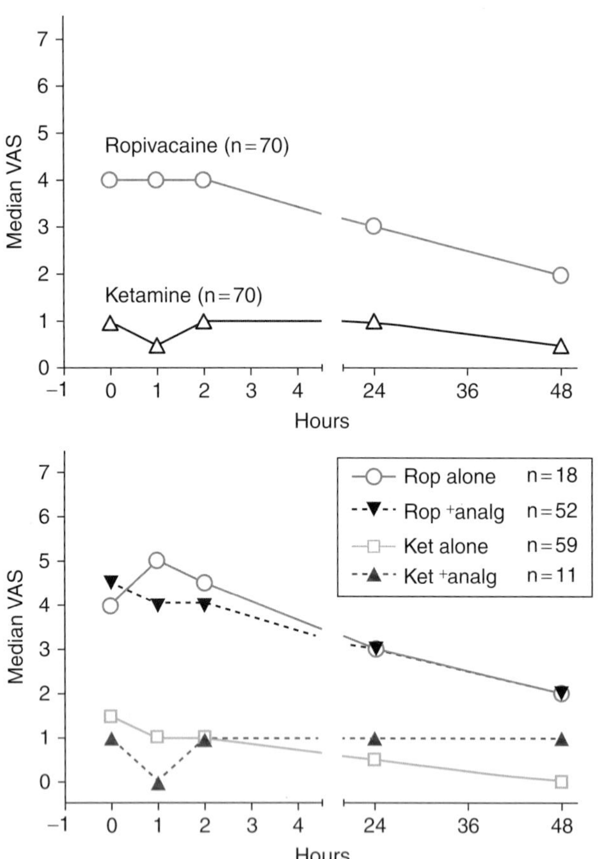

FIGURE 8-2 Postoperative median time courses of visual analog scale (VAS) scores in the ketamine and ropivacaine groups *(upper panel)* and in relation to analgesic consumption in the two groups *(lower panel)*. Open symbols, no analgesics required; closed symbols, analgesics added. (From Feltracco P, Barbieri S, Rizzi S, et al. Brief report: perioperative analgesic efficacy and plasma concentrations of S+ -ketamine in continuous epidural infusion during thoracic surgery. *Anesth Analg.* 2013;116[6]:1371–1375, with permission).

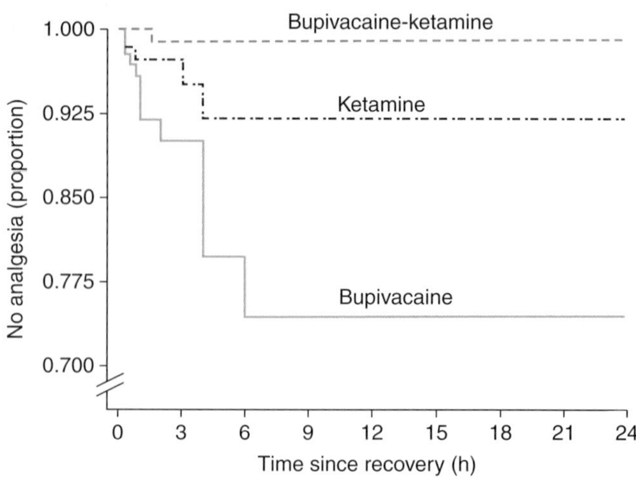

FIGURE 8-3 "Survival" curves for the bupivacaine, bupivacaine-ketamine, and ketamine groups. Proportion of patients in each group who had not required any analgesia since recovery from anesthesia. The bupivacaine-ketamine mixture provided better analgesia than the bupivacaine solution alone. Side effects such as motor weakness or urinary retention were not observed in the ketamine group. (From Naguib M, Sharif AM, Seraj M, et al. Ketamine for caudal analgesia in children: comparison with caudal bupivacaine. *Br J Anaesth.* 1991;67[5]:559–564, with permission).

6 mL per hour for the duration of surgical procedure in the previously cited studies.

Combination of epidural ketamine with local anesthetic and/or opioid infusions results in improved analgesia without significantly increasing adverse effects.[1,51,52] A bupivacaine-ketamine mixture provided better analgesia than bupivacaine alone (Fig. 8-3).[51] Side effects such as motor weakness or urinary retention were not observed in the ketamine group.[51] Adding low-dose ketamine to a multimodal epidural analgesia regimen provides better postoperative analgesia and reduces morphine consumption in thoracic, upper abdominal surgery, and lower abdominal surgeries.[50] Ketamine acts synergistically with opioid, dopaminergic, serotoninergic, and α-amino-3-hydroxy-5-methyl-4-isoxazolepropionic acid (AMPA) receptor agonists to produce dissociation between the thalamocortical and limbic systems. AMPA is a non-NMDA-type ionotropic glutamate receptor that mediates fast synaptic transmission in the CNS. Ketamine has also shown efficacy in the management of neuropathic pain, and it is believed to work through one or more of these mechanisms. In high doses, ketamine may have additional minor analgesic effects by modulating descending inhibitory pathways through inhibition of reuptake of neurotransmitters.

Reported side effects of epidural ketamine include sedation, headache, and transient burning back pain during injection with doses greater than 0.5 mg/kg. There has been no reported respiratory depression, hallucinations, cardiovascular instability, bladder dysfunction, or neurologic deficit with epidural doses up to 1 mg/kg. The incidence of nausea, vomiting, and pruritus when combined with neuraxial opioids is similar to that reported with neuraxial opioid alone.

There are limited human studies on the use of intrathecal ketamine due to the potential risk of neurotoxicity from its preservative benzalkonium chloride. Intrathecal ketamine has been shown to decrease morphine requirements in patients with terminal cancer and is useful in opioid-tolerant patients. The intrathecal administration of ketamine, however, did not prolong or improve the quality of anesthesia from bupivacaine, but increased adverse effects.[41] Ketamine has been administered intrathecally to 16 patients with war injuries of the lower limbs in varying doses from 5 to 50 mg in a volume of 3 mL of 5% dextrose.[53] In these doses, intrathecal ketamine resulted in a distinct sensory level in all patients and satisfactory surgical analgesia. Central effects (drowsiness, dizziness, and nystagmus) occurred in nine patients, but they remained conscious throughout; one patient experienced no central effects, and one patient developed dissociative anesthesia. Ketamine alone did not produce motor block, but addition of epinephrine resulted in complete motor block and may have intensified sensory blockade.[53]

The advantage of intrathecal ketamine is the lack of cardiovascular effects and respiratory depression. The main drawbacks of intrathecal ketamine are the potential for psychomimetic reactions, inadequate motor blockade, and short duration of action. Clinical manifestations of myelopathy suggestive of spinal cord injury were observed in a terminally ill cancer patient after continuous infusion intrathecal preservative-free ketamine at a rate of 5 mg per day for a duration of 3 weeks.[54]

Midazolam

Intrathecal midazolam produces analgesia by acting on γ-aminobutyric acid (GABA)-A receptors and reducing spinal cord excitability. GABA-A receptors are ligand-gated receptors located throughout the CNS and GABA is a major inhibitory neurotransmitter of the CNS, although glycine is prominent in the spinal cord. GABA binding results in a change of receptor configuration, causing an ion channel to open which allows chloride ions to flow down their electrochemical gradient into the cell. This results in hyperpolarization of the neuron and reduced action potential propagation.

A high density of benzodiazepine receptors (GABA-A) have been found in lamina II of the dorsal horn of the spinal cord, suggesting a possible role in pain modulation. Benzodiazepines have also been shown to act at opioid receptors.[55] The δ-selective opioid antagonist, naltrindole, suppresses the antinociceptive effect of intrathecal midazolam, suggesting that intrathecal midazolam is involved in the release of endogenous opioid acting at spinal δ receptors.[56] The substantia gelatinosa of the dorsal horn of the spinal cord contains a high density of GABA-A receptors. Benzodiazepines are likely to mediate their analgesic effect by increasing inhibition of nociceptive neurons in this area.

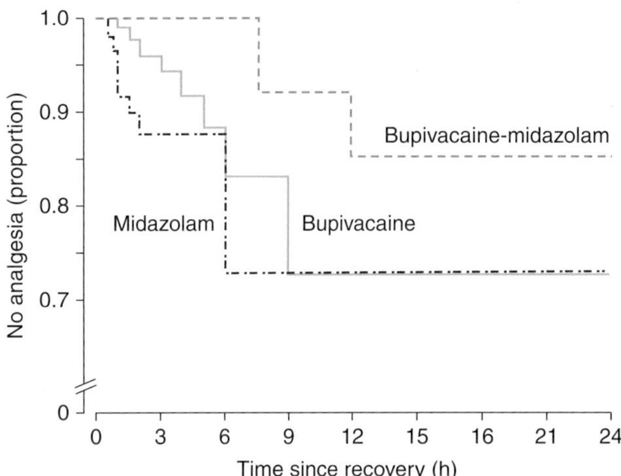

FIGURE 8-4 Caudal midazolam in a dose of 50 μg/kg provides equivalent analgesia to bupivacaine 0.25%, when administered postoperatively in a volume of 1 mL/kg for children following unilateral inguinal herniotomy. Survival curves for the bupivacaine, midazolam, and bupivacaine-midazolam groups. Proportion of patients in each group who had not required any analgesia since recovery from anesthesia. Times to first analgesic administration (paracetamol suppositories) were longer ($P < 0.001$) in the bupivacaine-midazolam group than in the other two groups. Side effects such as motor weakness, respiratory depression, or prolonged sedation were not observed in patients who received caudal epidural midazolam only. (From Naguib M, el Gammal M, ElhattabYS, et al. Midazolam for caudal analgesia in children: comparison with caudal bupivacaine. *Can J Anaesth.* 1995;42[9]:758–764, with permission).

Midazolam administered epidurally[57–61] or intrathecally[55,62–67] has been shown to have an analgesic effect (Fig. 8-4). Adding midazolam (10 to 20 mg for 12 hours) to continuous epidural infusion of bupivacaine (100 mg) for postoperative pain provided better analgesia than bupivacaine alone without sedative effects.[26,68,69]

Midazolam added to fentanyl-ropivacaine epidural analgesia was associated with a significant reduction in the incidence of postoperative nausea and vomiting compared with fentanyl-ropivacaine alone, and a significant decrease in the amount of patient-controlled epidural analgesia (PCEA) administered without a significant increase in adverse events in these patients who underwent subtotal gastrectomy and postcesarean delivery. The exact mechanism by which midazolam exerts its antiemetic action is not fully understood. Postulated mechanisms include glycine mimetic inhibitory effects, enhancement of the inhibitory effects of GABA, inhibition of dopamine release, and augmentation of adenosine-mediated inhibition of dopamine in the chemoreceptor trigger zone.[68–70] No sedation is observed at doses of 1 and 2 mg of epidural midazolam; however, sedation has been reported at higher doses.

Animal study has shown synergism between intrathecal midazolam and morphine.[71] Subsequent clinical studies have evaluated intrathecal and epidural midazolam for treatment of postoperative and chronic pain.[72] Intrathecal midazolam has also been investigated in combination with an opioid for labor analgesia.[64] These studies support the analgesic efficacy of intrathecal midazolam at doses <2 mg and in concentrations <1 mg/mL. Intrathecal midazolam is more effective for treatment of somatic pain than visceral pain.[72] The addition of intrathecal midazolam also decreases postoperative analgesic requirements. The incidence of postoperative nausea and vomiting is much less with intrathecal midazolam than that seen with intrathecal fentanyl.[73] Midazolam can be successfully combined with other drugs such as opioids and clonidine for additive effects[66] and has been used as a continuous infusion (12 mg per day) in patients with refractory pain.[62]

A serious risk of intrathecal drug administration is neurotoxicity and such neurotoxic effects have been demonstrated in animal studies. Most animal studies examining intrathecal administration of midazolam have demonstrated no neurotoxic effects, although two of the earliest studies reported signs of neurotoxicity. Current evidence suggests that the addition of midazolam in doses of 1 to 2 mg intrathecally is beneficial in the treatment of perioperative and chronic pain. Current evidence supports the use of midazolam in doses not exceeding 1 to 2 mg at concentrations not exceeding 1 mg/mL. Considerable experience in humans with the use of perioperative midazolam suggests no evident deleterious neurologic effects under these conditions.[63,74–76] The story of the experimental work on intrathecal midazolam in animals and humans is a cautionary tale in drug development. Investigators proceeded with clinical trials in humans at a time when the only available animal data suggested that intrathecal administration of midazolam might well be neurotoxic. Only after the human trials were performed did additional animal data emerge to support the lack of neurotoxicity,[74] raising significant ethical concerns about the progression of investigational work from animals to humans.

Tramadol

Tramadol is an analgesic combining mainly μ-opioid and monoaminergic activity through the inhibition of the neuronal uptake of serotonin and norepinephrine.[77] Animal studies have confirmed the analgesic effect of intrathecally administered tramadol. However, there is limited available data in humans. Epidural administration of tramadol has been the subject of some study[78–81] and did not demonstrate effective postoperative analgesia with epidural administration.[82,83]

The effect of intrathecal administration of tramadol to patients showed contradicting results.[84–86] Tramadol 1 to 2 mg/kg has also been administered caudally in children for postoperative analgesia.[87]

Droperidol

Epidural droperidol is effective for reducing pruritus and postoperative nausea and vomiting.[88] Long-term administration of intrathecal droperidol proved to be an excellent antiemetic in patients with nonmalignant pain.[89] It has been suggested that droperidol exerts direct actions on the brainstem chemoreceptor trigger zone. Although no side effects were observed, it is important to recognize the lack of laboratory data documenting the safety of neuraxial droperidol (including the potential for neurotoxicity).[90]

Adenosine

In the spinal cord, adenosine receptors are located in the superficial layers of the dorsal horn. Adenosine shows antinociceptive activity at adenosine A_1 receptors located in laminae I and II of the dorsal horn of the spinal cord.[91] Another proposed mechanism is enhancement of spinal norepinephrine release.[92]

Initial studies confirmed relative safety of intrathecal administration of adenosine in human volunteers with no reported clinical toxicity.[93,94] Intrathecal adenosine does not inhibit acute pain[95] but is effective in treating allodynia and hyperalgesia. Experimental hyperalgesia and allodynia is reduced by intrathecal adenosine in a non–dose-dependent fashion[96]; however, in clinical settings, it did not change the anesthetic requirement or postoperative analgesia.[97] Similarly, in combination with an opioid, intrathecal adenosine did not prolong analgesia during labor.[98]

Adenosine appears be effective in the treatment of neuropathic pain. Intrathecal adenosine is not associated with hypotension, motor blockade, or sedation. Following many clinical trials involving animal subjects, intrathecal adenosine 500 to 2,000 μg in human volunteers was shown to decrease allodynia in phase I clinical trials. The only side effect observed was transient lumbar pain after a dose of 2,000 μg.[99–101] The role of neuraxial adenosine in the armamentarium for treatment of acute or chronic pain awaits further delineation.

Conopeptides

Ziconotide

Ziconotide is a synthetic 25-amino acid, polybasic peptide with three disulfide bridges and is a derivative of an omega conotoxin found in the venom of the marine snail *conus magnus*. Ziconotide acts as a selective antagonist of neuronal (N-type) voltage-sensitive calcium channels within presynaptic neuronal terminals in the dorsal horn, thereby inhibiting nerve transmission. Ziconotide directly inhibits norepinephrine release and functions as a sympatholytic, resulting in decrease in mean and diastolic pressure, most profoundly when administered intravenously and normally negligible when dosed intrathecally.

Highly polar and water soluble, ziconotide is hypobaric at clinically useful concentrations and has a relatively large molecular weight. This agent has narrow therapeutic window, with neuropsychiatric side effects appearing in nearly all patients at higher doses or when dose escalation is too rapid. Initial infusion rates should be limited to 0.1 μg per hour with stepwise increase of this rate over time; CNS adverse effects are to be expected.[102–104] Ziconotide is the only FDA-approved, nonopioid approved for intrathecal administration for the treatment of neuropathic pain.

Ziconotide produces marked spinal antinociception in animal models of acute and persistent pain[105] and additional reports described its intrathecal administration to relieve severe neuropathic pain.[106–109] Following extensive demonstration of safety in animal models, clinical trials in humans suffering with poorly controlled pain associated with advanced illness demonstrated that side effects occurred in the majority of patients (92.9%).[110] Significant adverse events reported in the ziconotide group were dizziness, confusion, ataxia, abnormal gait, and memory impairment. Suicidality was increased with ziconotide as compared to placebo. Most of the side effects are self-limiting with cessation of therapy. The marked expense and nearly universal appearance of side effects in those receiving ziconotide have limited the use of this agent in clinical practice. A small number of patients with chronic pain gain significant, ongoing pain reduction with few or tolerable side effects when receiving intrathecal ziconotide infusions via chronic, implanted intrathecal drug delivery systems.

Other Investigational Conopeptides

Xen 2174

Xen 2174 is a conopeptide derived from a marine snail. The drug is found to inhibit norepinephrine transport and activate noradrenergic inhibitory pathways causing antihyperalgesic, antiallodynic, and antinociceptive effects.[111]

CGX-1160

CGX-1160 is a conopeptide that produces analgesia by activation of neurotensin receptor type 1 (NTR1). The drug has been found to be safe in a small number of patients with neuropathic pain related to spinal cord injury.[112]

The therapeutic index of these newer conopeptides may well be superior to that of ziconotide, but much additional investigational work is needed before they can reach clinical use. The promise of a novel nonopioid analgesic with significant efficacy in the treatment of neuropathic pain remains elusive but is the most alluring promise of this novel class of analgesics.

Octreotide

Octreotide is a synthetic octapeptide of the somatostatin derivative of human growth hormone. Octreotide administered spinally causes analgesia.[113,114] Intrathecal octreotide administered in an uncontrolled study to cancer patients for 5 years reduced pain without any adverse effects.[115] One prospective double-blind study involving 20 human subjects showed an absence of safety signals with intrathecal octreotide at a dose of 20 μg per hour.[116] The role of this agent in clinical practice remains undefined.

Baclofen

GABA acts as an inhibitory neurotransmitter in the CNS. Baclofen is an agonist of the GABA-B receptor. Baclofen suppresses neuronal transmission in the cerebral cortex, basal ganglia, thalamus, cerebellum, and spinal cord. The analgesic effects of baclofen are mediated postsynaptically via activating the G protein–linked GABA-B receptors in laminae II and III that result in increased potassium conductance and membrane hyperpolarization. Baclofen also acts presynaptically to inhibit Ca^{+2} conductance and, therefore, the release of glutamate and substance P, and postsynaptically to produce membrane hyperpolarization by increased potassium conductance through a G protein and second messenger system.[117]

Baclofen has low lipid solubility and low molecular weight makes it an appropriate candidate for spinal action when delivered by the epidural route, but there has been little meaningful study to date. Intrathecal baclofen has demonstrated efficacy in chronic pain syndromes associated with multiple sclerosis and complex regional pain syndrome (CRPS) type I. For somatic pain, intrathecal baclofen has been used for the treatment of low back pain with root compression syndromes.[118] Intrathecal baclofen is specifically used for spasticity and dystonia due to various conditions such as cerebral palsy and spastic posttraumatic spinal cord injury. Recent interest has also focused on its use as an analgesic.[117]

A typical intrathecal dose of baclofen is 25 to 200 μg per day through a programmable intrathecal pump. Intrathecal administration is superior to systemic administration with regard to efficacy and adverse effects.[119] Baclofen has also been observed to relieve central pain syndromes in patients with spasticity,[120] although it is uncertain whether this is primarily an effect on musculoskeletal pain because of reduced spasticity or a direct analgesic effect.[121] Some evidence suggests efficacy against nociceptive and neuropathic pain, particularly when used in combination with morphine and/or clonidine.

Baclofen has been investigated in the perioperative setting in a randomized, double-blind study for total knee arthroplasty as an adjuvant with spinal bupivacaine in a 100 μg single dose. The results showed a statistically significant reduction in opioid use in the postanesthesia care unit (PACU), lower pain scores for 48 to 72 hours postoperatively, and a lower severity of pain at 3 months after total knee arthroplasty in patients who received intrathecal baclofen compared to those who received spinal bupivacaine and saline.[122] Common side effects of baclofen include sedation, drowsiness, headache, nausea, and weakness. More serious side effects such as rhabdomyolysis and multiple organ failure have also been reported.[123,124] Like many of the other adjuvant analgesics discussed in this chapter, the role for intrathecal baclofen in the perioperative treatment of pain requires further study.

Calcitonin

Calcitonin is a naturally occurring hormone that has been recently demonstrated to reduce pain, independent of its peripheral action at bony sites. The epidural and intrathecal dose is 100 International Unit. There have been a few studies on its use as an analgesic in the literature.[125] Intrathecal administration of calcitonin is associated with side effects such as nausea and vomiting and nervousness; these were observed in a small number of calcitonin-treated patients. Postoperative nausea and vomiting occurred in 30% of patients who were provided with calcitonin mixed with bupivacaine.[126]

Cyclooxygenase Inhibitors

Ketorolac

Constitutive expression of cyclooxygenase (COX)-1 and COX-2 in the spinal cord, upregulation of cycloxygenase-1 and 2, and release and production of spinal prostaglandins occur after peripheral tissue injury. Intrathecal injection of prostaglandins causes hyperalgesia and allodynia.[127,128] Ketorolac is a COX inhibitor. The intrathecal delivery of COX inhibitors theoretically would reduce pain and central sensitization. Targeted inhibition of spinal COX may be a viable strategy for treating pain. This has led many investigators to postulate that neuraxial administration of nonsteroidal antiinflammatory drugs (NSAIDs) produces analgesia following excitatory input into the spinal cord.[129,130]

The pharmacokinetics of ketorolac in CSF obtained from dogs suggests rapid elimination and delayed tissue uptake; therefore, continuous infusion of intrathecal ketorolac may be a more effective strategy. Animal data appear promising and healthy volunteer studies have not identified any adverse neurologic side effects. Understanding the relevance of these observations to pain in humans has been hampered by lack of regulatory approval for intrathecal injection of these products.[74,76,101,131] Intrathecal injection of ketorolac was studied in humans in an open label, dose escalating safety study. Intrathecal ketorolac 0.25 to 2.0 mg was well tolerated, with the only adverse effect being a mild reduction in heart rate 15 to 60 minutes following injection.[127] Intrathecal ketorolac did not relieve chronic pain or extend anesthesia or analgesia from intrathecal bupivacaine administered at the beginning of surgery.[127]

These studies suggest that spinally produced prostaglandins may have a more limited role in pain and hypersensitivity in humans than predicted by animal studies, and intrathecal ketorolac may have limited analgesic effects in humans but could be active in states of central sensitization, including postoperative and chronic pain.

Gabapentin

Gabapentin acts on voltage-dependent calcium channels and inhibits glutamate release at the dorsal horn of the spinal cord. Oral gabapentin is approved as an anticonvulsant medication that demonstrated some efficacy in treating neuropathic pain.[132,133] Given the fact that gabapentin is not well absorbed from the gastrointestinal system and penetrates the blood–brain barrier poorly, its nonopioid properties and presumed spinal site of analgesic action made the study on intrathecal gabapentin attractive. However, a trial of extended (22 days) infusion of intrathecal gabapentin did not demonstrate statistically significant or clinically meaningful analgesic effects. Drug-related adverse events were similar to those for oral gabapentin.

Magnesium Sulfate

Magnesium has analgesic properties, primarily related to the regulation of calcium influx into cells[134] and antagonism of NMDA receptors in the CNS.[135–137] Several small trials investigating the analgesic efficacy of perioperative intravenous magnesium have been published, with conflicting results.[138–140] However, a meta-analysis of all available trials of systemically administered magnesium reported a reduction in postoperative opioid requirements approximately equal to that of ketorolac.[141] Animal studies have reported histologic neurotoxicity with weight-adjusted doses similar to those used in most human clinical trials to date,[142] whereas two case reports have described patients suffering from disorientation[143] and continuous periumbilical burning pain[144] following the injection of neuraxial magnesium.

An animal model showed that direct intrathecal administration of magnesium enhanced the antinociceptive effect of opioids for acute incisional pain[145] and suppressed nociceptive responses in neuropathic pain models.[146] The earliest clinical trials investigating intrathecal and epidural magnesium reported an increase in the median duration of analgesia[147] and decrease in opioid consumption by 25%,[148] respectively. The dose of neuraxial magnesium that confers optimal analgesia with the fewest possible side effects remains unclear.

The analgesic efficacy and safety of neuraxial magnesium for postoperative pain management has been assessed in a meta-analysis.[149] Intrathecal magnesium increased the time to first analgesic request, reduced morphine consumption at 24 hours postoperatively, and modestly reduced early postoperative pain scores. When administered in the epidural space, magnesium also increased the time to first analgesic request. These acute pain-related benefits reportedly occur without increased risk of hypotension, bradycardia, or sedation. The lack of reported complications associated with neuraxial magnesium must not be interpreted as an endorsement of its safety. Several animal studies have demonstrated that a risk of clinically relevant neurologic injury does exist.[150,151]

Conclusion

Neuraxial drug administration via the intrathecal and epidural route remains an important treatment option for the provision of anesthesia as well as analgesia in acute, cancer, and chronic pain. Additional dose-effect studies are needed for most agents to strengthen our understanding of the safety profile of these drugs when administered neuraxially before they become a part of routine clinical practice.

References

1. Walker SM, Goudas LC, Cousins MJ, et al. Combination spinal analgesic chemotherapy: a systematic review. *Anesth Analg.* 2002;95(3):674–715.
2. Coote JH. Noradrenergic projections to the spinal cord and their role in cardiovascular control. *J Auton Nerv Syst.* 1985;14(3):255–262.
3. Naguib M, Yaksh TL. Antinociceptive effects of spinal cholinesterase inhibition and isobolographic analysis of the interaction with mu and alpha 2 receptor systems. *Anesthesiology.* 1994;80(6):1338–1348.
4. Dobrydnjov I, Axelsson K, Gupta A, et al. Improved analgesia with clonidine when added to local anesthetic during combined spinal-epidural anesthesia for hip arthroplasty: a double-blind, randomized and placebo-controlled study. *Acta Anaesthesiol Scand.* 2005;49(4):538–545.
5. Huang YS, Lin LC, Huh BK, et al. Epidural clonidine for postoperative pain after total knee arthroplasty: a dose-response study. *Anesth Analg.* 2007;104(5):1230–1235.
6. Eisenach JC, DuPen S, Dubois M, et al. Epidural clonidine analgesia for intractable cancer pain. The Epidural Clonidine Study Group. *Pain.* 1995;61(3):391–399.
7. Kanazi GE, Aouad MT, Jabbour-Khoury SI, et al. Effect of low-dose dexmedetomidine or clonidine on the characteristics of bupivacaine spinal block. *Acta Anaesthesiol Scand.* 2006;50(2):222–227.
8. Eisenach JC, De Kock M, Klimscha W. alpha(2)-adrenergic agonists for regional anesthesia. A clinical review of clonidine (1984–1995). *Anesthesiology.* 1996;85(3):655–674.
9. De Kock M, Lavand'homme P, Waterloos H. The short-lasting analgesia and long-term antihyperalgesic effect of intrathecal clonidine in patients undergoing colonic surgery. *Anesth Analg.* 2005;101(2):566–572, table of contents.
10. Eisenach JC, Hood DD, Curry R. Intrathecal, but not intravenous, clonidine reduces experimental thermal or capsaicin-induced pain and hyperalgesia in normal volunteers. *Anesth Analg.* 1998;87(3):591–596.
11. Lavand'homme PM, Roelants F, Waterloos H, et al. An evaluation of the postoperative antihyperalgesic and analgesic effects of intrathecal clonidine administered during elective cesarean delivery. *Anesth Analg.* 2008;107(3):948–955.
12. Brennan TJ, Kehlet H. Preventive analgesia to reduce wound hyperalgesia and persistent postsurgical pain: not an easy path. *Anesthesiology.* 2005;103(4):681–683.
13. Elia N, Culebras X, Mazza C, et al. Clonidine as an adjuvant to intrathecal local anesthetics for surgery: systematic review of randomized trials. *Reg Anesth Pain Med.* 2008;33(2):159–167.
14. Eisenach JC, Shafer SL, Bucklin BA, et al. Pharmacokinetics and pharmacodynamics of intraspinal dexmedetomidine in sheep. *Anesthesiology.* 1994;80(6):1349–1359.
15. Fisher B, Zornow MH, Yaksh TL, et al. Antinociceptive properties of intrathecal dexmedetomidine in rats. *Eur J Pharmacol.* 1991;192(2):221–225.
16. Ishii H, Kohno T, Yamakura T, et al. Action of dexmedetomidine on the substantia gelatinosa neurons of the rat spinal cord. *Eur J Neurosci.* 2008;27(12):3182–3190.
17. Schnaider TB, Vieira AM, Brandao AC, et al. Intraoperative analgesic effect of epidural ketamine, clonidine or dexmedetomidine for upper abdominal surgery [in Portuguese]. *Rev Bras Anestesiol.* 2005;55(5):525–531.
18. Saadawy I, Boker A, Elshahawy MA, et al. Effect of dexmedetomidine on the characteristics of bupivacaine in a caudal block in pediatrics. *Acta Anaesthesiol Scand.* 2009;53(2):251–256.
19. Al-Mustafa MM, Abu-Halaweh SA, Aloweidi AS, et al. Effect of dexmedetomidine added to spinal bupivacaine for urological procedures. *Saudi Med J.* 2009;30(3):365–370.
20. Elhakim M, Abdelhamid D, Abdelfattach H, et al. Effect of epidural dexmedetomidine on intraoperative awareness and post-operative pain after one-lung ventilation. *Acta Anaesthesiol Scand.* 2010;54(6):703–709.
21. Hanoura S, Hassanin R, Singh R. Intraoperative conditions and quality of postoperative analgesia after adding dexmedetomidine to epidural bupivacaine and fentanyl in elective cesarean section using combined spinal-epidural anesthesia. *Anesth Essays Res.* 2013;7:168–172.
22. El-Hennawy AM, Abd-Elwahab AM, Abd-Elmaksoud AM, et al. Addition of clonidine or dexmedetomidine to bupivacaine prolongs caudal analgesia in children. *Br J Anaesth.* 2009;103(2):268–274.
23. Emery E. Intrathecal baclofen. Literature review of the results and complications [in French]. *Neurochirurgie.* 2003;49(2–3, pt 2):276–288.
24. Grewal A. Dexmedetomidine: new avenues. *J Anaesthesiol Clin Pharmacol.* 2011;27(3):297–302.
25. Naguib M, Yaksh TL. Characterization of muscarinic receptor subtypes that mediate antinociception in the rat spinal cord. *Anesth Analg.* 1997;85(4):847–853.
26. Congedo E, Sgreccia M, De Cosmo G. New drugs for epidural analgesia. *Curr Drug Targets.* 2009;10(8):696–706.
27. Hood DD, Eisenach JC, Tuttle R. Phase I safety assessment of intrathecal neostigmine methylsulfate in humans. *Anesthesiology.* 1995;82(2):331–343.
28. Krukowski JA, Hood DD, Eisenach JC, et al. Intrathecal neostigmine for post-cesarean section analgesia: dose response. *Anesth Analg.* 1997;84(6):1269–1275.
29. Nelson KE, D'Angelo R, Foss ML, et al. Intrathecal neostigmine and sufentanil for early labor analgesia. *Anesthesiology.* 1999;91(5):1293–1298.
30. Lauretti GR, de Oliveira R, Reis MP, et al. Study of three different doses of epidural neostigmine coadministered with lidocaine for postoperative analgesia. *Anesthesiology.* 1999;90(6):1534–1538.
31. Omais M, Lauretti GR, Paccola CA. Epidural morphine and neostigmine for postoperative analgesia after orthopedic surgery. *Anesth Analg.* 2002;95(6):1698–1701, table of contents.

32. Roelants F, Lavand'homme PM. Epidural neostigmine combined with sufentanil provides balanced and selective analgesia in early labor. *Anesthesiology*. 2004;101(2):439–444.
33. Roelants F, Lavand'homme PM, Mercier-Fuzier V. Epidural administration of neostigmine and clonidine to induce labor analgesia: evaluation of efficacy and local anesthetic-sparing effect. *Anesthesiology*. 2005;102(6):1205–1210.
34. Roelants F, Rizzo M, Lavand'homme P. The effect of epidural neostigmine combined with ropivacaine and sufentanil on neuraxial analgesia during labor. *Anesth Analg*. 2003;96(4):1161–1166, table of contents.
35. Harjai M, Chandra G, Bhatia VK, et al. A comparative study of two different doses of epidural neostigmine coadministered with lignocaine for post operative analgesia and sedation. *J Anaesthesiol Clin Pharmacol*. 2010;26(4):461–464.
36. Ho KM, Ismail H, Lee KC, et al. Use of intrathecal neostigmine as an adjunct to other spinal medications in perioperative and peripartum analgesia: a meta-analysis. *Anaesth Intensive Care*. 2005;33(1):41–53.
37. Kirdemir P, Ozkocak I, Demir T, et al. Comparison of postoperative analgesic effects of preemptively used epidural ketamine and neostigmine. *J Clin Anesth*. 2000;12(7):543–548.
38. Marucio RL, Luna SP, Neto FJ, et al. Postoperative analgesic effects of epidural administration of neostigmine alone or in combination with morphine in ovariohysterectomized dogs. *Am J Vet Res*. 2008;69(7):854–860.
39. Batra YK, Rajeev S, Panda NB, et al. Intrathecal neostigmine with bupivacaine for infants undergoing lower abdominal and urogenital procedures: dose response. *Acta Anaesthesiol Scand*. 2009;53(4):470–475.
40. Gabopoulou Z, Vadalouca A, Velmachou K, et al. Epidural calcitonin: does it provide better postoperative analgesia? An analysis of the haemodynamic, endocrine, and nociceptive responses of salmon calcitonin and opioids in epidural anesthesia for hip arthroplasty surgery. *Pain Pract*. 2002;2(4):326–331.
41. Kathirvel S, Sadhasivam S, Saxena A, et al. Effects of intrathecal ketamine added to bupivacaine for spinal anaesthesia. *Anaesthesia*. 2000;55(9):899–904.
42. Brock-Utne JG, Kallichurum S, Mankowitz E, et al. Intrathecal ketamine with preservative - histological effects on spinal nerve roots of baboons. *S Afr Med J*. 1982;61(12):440–441.
43. Borgbjerg FM, Svensson BA, Frigast C, et al. Histopathology after repeated intrathecal injections of preservative-free ketamine in the rabbit: a light and electron microscopic examination. *Anesth Analg*. 1994;79(1):105–111.
44. Errando CL, Sifre C, Moliner S, et al. Subarachnoid ketamine in swine—pathological findings after repeated doses: acute toxicity study. *Reg Anesth Pain Med*. 1999;24(2):146–152.
45. Rojas AC, Alves JG, Moreira ELR, et al. The effects of subarachnoid administration of preservative-free S(+)-ketamine on spinal cord and meninges in dogs. *Anesth Analg*. 2012;114(2):450–455.
46. Naguib M, Adu-Gyamfi Y, Absood GH, et al. Epidural ketamine for postoperative analgesia. *Can Anaesth Soc J*. 1986;33(1):16–21.
47. Kawana Y, Sato H, Shimada H, et al. Epidural ketamine for postoperative pain relief after gynecologic operations: a double-blind study and comparison with epidural morphine. *Anesth Analg*. 1987;66(8):735–738.
48. Locatelli BG, Frawley G, Spotti A, et al. Analgesic effectiveness of caudal levobupivacaine and ketamine. *Br J Anaesth*. 2008;100(5):701–706.
49. Yang CY, Wong CS, Chang JY, et al. Intrathecal ketamine reduces morphine requirements in patients with terminal cancer pain. *Can J Anaesth*. 1996;43(4):379–383.
50. Feltracco P, Barbieri S, Rizzi S, et al. Brief report: perioperative analgesic efficacy and plasma concentrations of S+ -ketamine in continuous epidural infusion during thoracic surgery. *Anesth Analg*. 2013;116(6):1371–1375.
51. Naguib M, Sharif AM, Seraj M, et al. Ketamine for caudal analgesia in children: comparison with caudal bupivacaine. *Br J Anaesth*. 1991;67(5):559–564.
52. Subramaniam K, Subramaniam B, Steinbrook RA. Ketamine as adjuvant analgesic to opioids: a quantitative and qualitative systematic review. *Anesth Analg*. 2004;99(2):482–495, table of contents.
53. Bion JF. Intrathecal ketamine for war surgery. A preliminary study under field conditions. *Anaesthesia*. 1984;39(10):1023–1028.
54. Karpinski N, Dunn J, Hansen L, et al. Subpial vacuolar myelopathy after intrathecal ketamine: report of a case. *Pain*. 1997;73(1):103–105.
55. Ho KM, Ismail H. Use of intrathecal midazolam to improve perioperative analgesia: a meta-analysis. *Anaesth Intensive Care*. 2008;36(3):365–373.
56. Goodchild CS, Guo Z, Musgreave A, et al. Antinociception by intrathecal midazolam involves endogenous neurotransmitters acting at spinal cord delta opioid receptors. *Br J Anaesth*. 1996;77(6):758–763.
57. Naguib M, el Gammal M, Elhattab YS, et al. Midazolam for caudal analgesia in children: comparison with caudal bupivacaine. *Can J Anaesth*. 1995;42(9):758–764.
58. Chakraborty S, Chakrabarti J, Bhattacharya D. Intrathecal tramadol added to bupivacaine as spinal anesthetic increases analgesic effect of the spinal blockade after major gynecological surgeries. *Indian J Pharmacol*. 2008;40(4):180–182.
59. Kumar P, Rudra A, Pan AK, et al. Caudal additives in pediatrics: a comparison among midazolam, ketamine, and neostigmine coadministered with bupivacaine. *Anesth Analg*. 2005;101(1):69–73, table of contents.
60. Nishiyama T, Matsukawa T, Hanaoka K. Continuous epidural administration of midazolam and bupivacaine for postoperative analgesia. *Acta Anaesthesiol Scand*. 1999;43(5):568–572.
61. Nishiyama T, Matsukawa T, Hanaoka K. Effects of adding midazolam on the postoperative epidural analgesia with two different doses of bupivacaine. *J Clin Anesth*. 2002;14(2):92–97.
62. Canavero S, Bonicalzi V, Clemente M. No neurotoxicity from long-term (>5 years) intrathecal infusion of midazolam in humans. *J Pain Symptom Manage*. 2006;32(1):1–3.
63. Hodgson PS, Neal JM, Pollock JE, et al. The neurotoxicity of drugs given intrathecally (spinal). *Anesth Analg*. 1999;88(4):797–809.
64. Tucker AP, Lai C, Nadeson R, et al. Intrathecal midazolam I: a cohort study investigating safety. *Anesth Analg*. 2004;98(6):1512–1520, table of contents.
65. Tucker AP, Mezzatesta J, Nadeson R, et al. Intrathecal midazolam II: combination with intrathecal fentanyl for labor pain. *Anesth Analg*. 2004;98(6):1521–1527, table of contents.
66. Yanez A, Peleteiro R, Camba MA. Intrathecal administration of morphine, midazolam, and their combination in 4 patients with chronic pain [in Spanish]. *Rev Esp Anestesiol Reanim*. 1992;39(1):40–42.
67. Johansen MJ, Gradert TL, Satterfield WC, et al. Safety of continuous intrathecal midazolam infusion in the sheep model. *Anesth Analg*. 2004;98(6):1528–1535.
68. Reid M, Herrera-Marschitz M, Hokfelt T, et al. Differential modulation of striatal dopamine release by intranigral injection of gamma-aminobutyric acid (GABA), dynorphin A and substance P. *Eur J Pharmacol*. 1988;147(3):411–420.
69. Splinter WM, MacNeill HB, Menard EA, et al. Midazolam reduces vomiting after tonsillectomy in children. *Can J Anaesth*. 1995;42(3):201–203.
70. Kohno T, Wakai A, Ataka T, et al. Actions of midazolam on excitatory transmission in dorsal horn neurons of adult rat spinal cord. *Anesthesiology*. 2006;104(2):338–343.
71. Yanez A, Sabbe MB, Stevens CW, et al. Interaction of midazolam and morphine in the spinal cord of the rat. *Neuropharmacology*. 1990;29(4):359–364.
72. Kim MH, Lee YM. Intrathecal midazolam increases the analgesic effects of spinal blockade with bupivacaine in patients undergoing haemorrhoidectomy. *Br J Anaesth*. 2001;86(1):77–79.

73. Boussofara M, Carles M, Raucoules-Aime M, et al. Effects of intrathecal midazolam on postoperative analgesia when added to a bupivacaine-clonidine mixture. *Reg Anesth Pain Med.* 2006; 31(6):501–505.
74. Yaksh TL, Allen JW. The use of intrathecal midazolam in humans: a case study of process. *Anesth Analg.* 2004;98(6):1536–1545, table of contents.
75. Cousins MJ, Miller RD. Intrathecal midazolam: an ethical editorial dilemma. *Anesth Analg.* 2004;98(6):1507–1508.
76. Yaksh TL, Allen JW. Preclinical insights into the implementation of intrathecal midazolam: a cautionary tale. *Anesth Analg.* 2004; 98(6):1509–1511.
77. Raffa RB, Friderichs E, Reimann W, et al. Opioid and nonopioid components independently contribute to the mechanism of action of tramadol, an 'atypical' opioid analgesic. *J Pharmacol Exp Ther.* 1992;260(1):275–285.
78. Baraka A, Jabbour S, Ghabash M, et al. A comparison of epidural tramadol and epidural morphine for postoperative analgesia. *Can J Anaesth.* 1993;40(4):308–313.
79. Delilkan AE, Vijayan R. Epidural tramadol for postoperative pain relief. *Anaesthesia.* 1993;48(4):328–331.
80. Fu YP, Chan KH, Lee TK, et al. Epidural tramadol for postoperative pain relief. *Ma Zui Xue Za Zhi.* 1991;29(3):648–652.
81. Pan AK, Mukherjee P, Rudra A. Role of epidural tramadol hydrochloride on postoperative pain relief in caesarean section delivery. *J Indian Med Assoc.* 1997;95(4):105–106.
82. Grace D, Fee JP. Ineffective analgesia after extradural tramadol hydrochloride in patients undergoing total knee replacement. *Anaesthesia.* 1995;50(6):555–558.
83. Wilder-Smith CH, Wilder-Smith OH, Farschtschian M, et al. Preoperative adjuvant epidural tramadol: the effect of different doses on postoperative analgesia and pain processing. *Acta Anaesthesiol Scand.* 1998;42(3):299–305.
84. Alhashemi JA, Kaki AM. Effect of intrathecal tramadol administration on postoperative pain after transurethral resection of prostate. *Br J Anaesth.* 2003;91(4):536–540.
85. Frikha N, Ellachtar M, Mebazaa MS, et al. Combined spinal-epidural analgesia in labor—comparison of sufentanil vs tramadol. *Middle East J Anesthesiol.* 2007;19(1):87–96.
86. Subedi A, Biswas BK, Tripathi M, et al. Analgesic effects of intrathecal tramadol in patients undergoing caesarean section: a randomised, double-blind study. *Int J Obstet Anesth.* 2013;22(4):316–321.
87. Ozcengiz D, Gunduz M, Ozbek H, et al. Comparison of caudal morphine and tramadol for postoperative pain control in children undergoing inguinal herniorrhaphy. *Paediatr Anaesth.* 2001; 11(4):459–464.
88. Lee IH, Lee IO. The antipruritic and antiemetic effects of epidural droperidol: a study of three methods of administration. *Anesth Analg.* 2007;105(1):251–255.
89. Ahmad-Sabry MH, Shareghi G. Long-term use of intrathecal droperidol as an excellent antiemetic in nonmalignant pain—a retrospective study. *Middle East J Anesthesiol.* 2012;21(6):857–862.
90. Grip G, Svensson BA, Gordh T Jr, et al. Histopathology and evaluation of potentiation of morphine-induced antinociception by intrathecal droperidol in the rat. *Acta Anaesthesiol Scand.* 1992;36(2): 145–152.
91. Poon A, Sawynok J. Antinociception by adenosine analogs and inhibitors of adenosine metabolism in an inflammatory thermal hyperalgesia model in the rat. *Pain.* 1998;74(2–3):235–245.
92. Gomes JA, Li X, Pan HL, et al. Intrathecal adenosine interacts with a spinal noradrenergic system to produce antinociception in nerve-injured rats. *Anesthesiology.* 1999;91(4):1072–1079.
93. Eisenach JC, Hood DD, Curry R. Phase I safety assessment of intrathecal injection of an American formulation of adenosine in humans. *Anesthesiology.* 2002;96(1):24–28.
94. Rane K, Segerdahl M, Goiny M, et al. Intrathecal adenosine administration: a phase 1 clinical safety study in healthy volunteers, with additional evaluation of its influence on sensory thresholds and experimental pain. *Anesthesiology.* 1998;89(5):1108–1115; discussion 9A.
95. Karlsten R, Gordh T Jr. An A1-selective adenosine agonist abolishes allodynia elicited by vibration and touch after intrathecal injection. *Anesth Analg.* 1995;80(4):844–847.
96. Eisenach JC, Curry R, Hood DD. Dose response of intrathecal adenosine in experimental pain and allodynia. *Anesthesiology.* 2002;97(4):938–942.
97. Rane K, Sollevi A, Segerdahl M. Intrathecal adenosine administration in abdominal hysterectomy lacks analgesic effect. *Acta Anaesthesiol Scand.* 2000;44(7):868–872.
98. Rane K, Sollevi A, Segerdahl M. A randomised double-blind evaluation of adenosine as adjunct to sufentanil in spinal labour analgesia. *Acta Anaesthesiol Scand.* 2003;47(5):601–603.
99. Eisenach JC, Hood DD, Curry R. Preliminary efficacy assessment of intrathecal injection of an American formulation of adenosine in humans. *Anesthesiology.* 2002;96(1):29–34.
100. Schug SA, Buerkle H, Moharib M, et al. New drugs for neuraxial blockade. *Curr Opin Anaesthesiol.* 1999;12(5):551–557.
101. Yaksh TL, Horais KA, Tozier N, et al. Intrathecal ketorolac in dogs and rats. *Toxicol Sci.* 2004;80(2):322–334.
102. McGivern JG. Ziconotide: a review of its pharmacology and use in the treatment of pain. *Neuropsychiatr Dis Treat.* 2007;3(1):69–85.
103. Schmidtko A, Lotsch J, Freynhagen R, et al. Ziconotide for treatment of severe chronic pain. *Lancet.* 2010;375(9725):1569–1577.
104. Wermeling DP. Ziconotide, an intrathecally administered N-type calcium channel antagonist for the treatment of chronic pain. *Pharmacotherapy.* 2005;25(8):1084–1094.
105. Bowersox SS, Gadbois T, Singh T, et al. Selective N-type neuronal voltage-sensitive calcium channel blocker, SNX-111, produces spinal antinociception in rat models of acute, persistent and neuropathic pain. *J Pharmacol Exp Ther.* 1996;279(3):1243–1249.
106. Brose WG, Gutlove DP, Luther RR, et al. Use of intrathecal SNX-111, a novel, N-type, voltage-sensitive, calcium channel blocker, in the management of intractable brachial plexus avulsion pain. *Clin J Pain.* 1997;13(3):256–259.
107. Penn RD, Paice JA. Adverse effects associated with the intrathecal administration of ziconotide. *Pain.* 2000;85(1–2):291–296.
108. Atanassoff PG, Hartmannsgruber MW, Thrasher J, et al. Ziconotide, a new N-type calcium channel blocker, administered intrathecally for acute postoperative pain. *Reg Anesth Pain Med.* 2000;25(3):274–278.
109. Wermeling D, Drass M, Ellis D, et al. Pharmacokinetics and pharmacodynamics of intrathecal ziconotide in chronic pain patients. *J Clin Pharmacol.* 2003;43(6):624–636.
110. Rauck RL, Wallace MS, Leong MS, et al. A randomized, double-blind, placebo-controlled study of intrathecal ziconotide in adults with severe chronic pain. *J Pain Symptom Manage.* 2006;31(5): 393–406.
111. National Institutes of Health Clinical Center. Resiniferatoxin to to treat severe pain associated with advanced cancer. http://clinicaltrials.gov/ct2/show/study/NCT00804154. Accessed April 1, 2014.
112. Kern SE, Allen J, Wagstaff J, et al. The pharmacokinetics of the conopeptide contulakin-G (CGX-1160) after intrathecal administration: an analysis of data from studies in beagles. *Anesth Analg.* 2007;104(6):1514–1520, table of contents.
113. Penn RD, Paice JA, Kroin JS. Intrathecal octreotide for cancer pain. *Lancet.* 1990;335(8691):738.
114. Penn RD, Paice JA, Kroin JS. Octreotide: a potent new non-opiate analgesic for intrathecal infusion. *Pain.* 1992;49(1):13–19.
115. Paice JA, Penn RD, Kroin JS. Intrathecal octreotide for relief of intractable nonmalignant pain: 5-year experience with two cases. *Neurosurgery.* 1996;38(1):203–207.
116. Deer TR, Kim CK, Bowman RG II, et al. The use of continuous intrathecal infusion of octreotide in patients with chronic pain of noncancer origin: an evaluation of side-effects and toxicity

in a prospective double-blind fashion. *Neuromodulation.* 2005; 8(3):171–175.
117. Slonimski M, Abram SE, Zuniga RE. Intrathecal baclofen in pain management. *Reg Anesth Pain Med.* 2004;29(3):269–276.
118. Vatine J, Magora F, Shochina M, et al. Effect of intrathecal baclofen in low back pain with root compression symptoms. *Pain Clin.* 1989; 2:207–217.
119. Hsieh JC, Penn RD. Intrathecal baclofen in the treatment of adult spasticity. *Neurosurg Focus.* 2006;21(2):e5.
120. Herman RM, D'Luzansky SC, Ippolito R. Intrathecal baclofen suppresses central pain in patients with spinal lesions. A pilot study. *Clin J Pain.* 1992;8(4):338–345.
121. Loubser PG, Akman NM. Effects of intrathecal baclofen on chronic spinal cord injury pain. *J Pain Symptom Manage.* 1996;12(4):241–247.
122. Sanders JC, Gerstein N, Torgeson E, et al. Intrathecal baclofen for postoperative analgesia after total knee arthroplasty. *J Clin Anesth.* 2009;21(7):486–492.
123. Broseta J, Garcia-March G, Sanchez-Ledesma MJ, et al. Chronic intrathecal baclofen administration in severe spasticity. *Stereotact Funct Neurosurg.* 1990;54–55:147–153.
124. Ochs GA. Intrathecal baclofen. *Baillieres Clin Neurol.* 1993;2(1): 73–86.
125. Donner B, Tryba M, Zenz M, et al. Intrathecal and epidural administration of non-opioid analgesics in acute and chronic pain treatment [in German]. *Schmerz.* 1994;8(2):71–81.
126. Rastogi V, dutta R, Kumar GP. A comparative study of premedication for prevention of vomiting induced by intrathecal calcitonin: a double blind study. *Internet J Anaesth.* 2008;16(2):3.
127. Eisenach JC, Curry R, Rauck R, et al. Role of spinal cyclooxygenase in human postoperative and chronic pain. *Anesthesiology.* 2010;112(5):1225–1233.
128. Eisenach JC, Curry R, Tong C, et al. Effects of intrathecal ketorolac on human experimental pain. *Anesthesiology.* 2010;112(5):1216–1224.
129. Malmberg AB, Yaksh TL. Hyperalgesia mediated by spinal glutamate or substance P receptor blocked by spinal cyclooxygenase inhibition. *Science.* 1992;257(5074):1276–1279.
130. Pellerin M, Hardy F, Abergel A, et al. Chronic refractory pain in cancer patients. Value of the spinal injection of lysine acetylsalicylate. 60 cases [in French]. *Presse Med.* 1987;16(30):1465–1468.
131. Eisenach JC, Curry R, Hood DD, et al. Phase I safety assessment of intrathecal ketorolac. *Pain.* 2002;99(3):599–604.
132. Morello CM, Leckband SG, Stoner CP, et al. Randomized double-blind study comparing the efficacy of gabapentin with amitriptyline on diabetic peripheral neuropathy pain. *Arch Intern Med.* 1999;159(16):1931–1937.
133. Steinman MA, Bero LA, Chren MM, et al. Narrative review: the promotion of gabapentin: an analysis of internal industry documents. *Ann Intern Med.* 2006;145(4):284–293.
134. Iseri LT, French JH. Magnesium: nature's physiologic calcium blocker. *Am Heart J.* 1984;108(1):188–193.
135. Feria M, Abad F, Sanchez A, et al. Magnesium sulphate injected subcutaneously suppresses autotomy in peripherally deafferented rats. *Pain.* 1993;53(3):287–293.
136. Tramer MR, Schneider J, Marti RA, et al. Role of magnesium sulfate in postoperative analgesia. *Anesthesiology.* 1996;84(2):340–347.
137. Woolf CJ, Thompson SW. The induction and maintenance of central sensitization is dependent on N-methyl-D-aspartic acid receptor activation; implications for the treatment of post-injury pain hypersensitivity states. *Pain.* 1991;44(3):293–299.
138. Jaoua H, Zghidi SM, Wissem L, et al. Effectiveness of intravenous magnesium on postoperative pain after abdominal surgery versus placebo: double blind randomized controlled trial [in French]. *Tunis Med.* 2010;88(5):317–323.
139. Tramer MR, Glynn CJ. An evaluation of a single dose of magnesium to supplement analgesia after ambulatory surgery: randomized controlled trial. *Anesth Analg.* 2007;104(6):1374–1379, table of contents.
140. Zarauza R, Saez-Fernandez AN, Iribarren MJ, et al. A comparative study with oral nifedipine, intravenous nimodipine, and magnesium sulfate in postoperative analgesia. *Anesth Analg.* 2000; 91(4):938–943.
141. De Oliveira G, Castro-Alves L, Khan J, et al. Perioperative systemic magnesium to minimize postoperative pain: a meta-analysis of randomized controlled trials. *Anesthesiology.* 2013;119(1): 178–190.
142. Saeki H, Matsumoto M, Kaneko S, et al. Is intrathecal magnesium sulfate safe and protective against ischemic spinal cord injury in rabbits? *Anesth Analg.* 2004;99(6):1805–1812, table of contents.
143. Goodman EJ, Haas AJ, Kantor GS. Inadvertent administration of magnesium sulfate through the epidural catheter: report and analysis of a drug error. *Int J Obstet Anesth.* 2006;15(1):63–67.
144. Dror A, Henriksen E. Accidental epidural magnesium sulfate injection. *Anesth Analg.* 1987;66(10):1020–1021.
145. Kroin JS, McCarthy RJ, Von Roenn N, et al. Magnesium sulfate potentiates morphine antinociception at the spinal level. *Anesth Analg.* 2000;90(4):913–917.
146. Xiao WH, Bennett GJ. Magnesium suppresses neuropathic pain responses in rats via a spinal site of action. *Brain Res.* 1994;666(2): 168–172.
147. Buvanendran A, McCarthy RJ, Kroin JS, et al. Intrathecal magnesium prolongs fentanyl analgesia: a prospective, randomized, controlled trial. *Anesth Analg.* 2002;95(3):661–666, table of contents.
148. Bilir A, Gulec S, Erkan A, et al. Epidural magnesium reduces postoperative analgesic requirement. *Br J Anaesth.* 2007;98(4): 519–523.
149. Albrecht E, Kirkham KR, Liu SS, et al. The analgesic efficacy and safety of neuraxial magnesium sulphate: a quantitative review. *Anaesthesia.* 2013;68(2):190–202.
150. Chanimov M, Cohen ML, Grinspun Y, et al. Neurotoxicity after spinal anaesthesia induced by serial intrathecal injections of magnesium sulphate. An experimental study in a rat model. *Anaesthesia.* 1997;52(3):223–228.
151. Simpson JI, Eide TR, Schiff GA, et al. Intrathecal magnesium sulfate protects the spinal cord from ischemic injury during thoracic aortic cross-clamping. *Anesthesiology.* 1994;81(6):1493–1499; discussion 26A–27A.

CHAPTER 9

Peripherally Acting Analgesics

Hesham Elsharkawy • Mohamed A. Naguib

An analgesic is any member of the group of drugs that are used to decrease pain sensation without loss of consciousness. The analgesic drugs may act on the peripheral nervous system and/or central nervous system (CNS). Peripheral analgesics act at the sensory input level by blocking transmission of the impulse to the brain. Their common feature was believed to be their site of action within the damaged tissues, and hence they were termed ***peripheral analgesics***. Experimental and clinical studies support the possibility of central site of action of many of these agents. In addition, peripheral administration of drugs can potentially optimize drug concentrations at the site of the origin of pain while leading to lower systemic levels and fewer adverse systemic effects and fewer drug interactions.

Recent efforts have been focused on peripherally selective compounds with limited ability to cross the blood–brain barrier (BBB). Nociceptive, inflammatory, and neuropathic pain all depend to some degree on the peripheral activation of primary sensory afferent neurons. A range of inflammatory mediators such as prostanoids, bradykinin, adenosine triphosphate (ATP), histamine, and serotonin can activate primary sensory afferent neurons. Inhibiting the actions of inflammatory mediators represents a strategy for the development of analgesics. Peripheral nerve endings also express a variety of inhibitory receptors such as opioid, α-adrenergic, cholinergic; adenosine and cannabinoid receptors, and agonists for these receptors also represent viable targets for drug development. The transmission of a pain signal from the periphery to the CNS is complex. Tissue damage results in peripheral release of endogenous mediators that can directly activate nociceptive afferent fibers, sensitize nociceptors, and/or cause increased local extravasation and vasodilatation. Nociceptive afferents have their neurons in the dorsal root ganglion and contact second-order neurons in the dorsal horn (for more details, see Chapter 6, Pain Physiology). Combinations of agents that act via different mechanisms may be particularly useful.

Nonsteroidal Antiinflammatory Drugs

The nonsteroidal antiinflammatory drugs (NSAIDs) are among the most commonly prescribed drugs in the world. This diverse class of drugs includes aspirin and several other selective and nonselective cyclooxygenase (COX) inhibitors with common analgesic, antiinflammatory, and antipyretic properties.[1] The COX pathway is shown in Figure 9-1. NSAIDs inhibit the biosynthesis of prostaglandins by preventing the substrate arachidonic acid from binding to the COX enzyme active site. The COX enzyme exist in two isoforms—COX-1 and COX-2 isoenzymes.[1]

COX-1 is constitutively expressed and catalyzes the production of prostaglandins that are involved in numerous physiologic functions, including maintenance of normal renal function in the kidneys, mucosal protection in the gastrointestinal tract, and production of proaggregatory thromboxane A_2 in the platelets. COX-2 expression can be induced by inflammatory mediators in many tissues and has a role in the mediation of pain, inflammation, and fever. There has been speculation on the existence of a third isoform, COX-3, which would explain the mechanism of action of acetaminophen, a poor inhibitor of COX-1 and COX-2, but appears to have little relevance in humans. Evidence indicates that, in addition to peripheral blockade of prostaglandin synthesis, central inhibition of COX-2 may play an important role in modulating nociception.

COX-2 selective inhibitors (known as the ***coxibs***) have less gastrointestinal toxicity than nonselective NSAIDs. However, increased cardiovascular risk has been associated with the use of this class of drugs.[2] They are used less frequently nowadays after withdrawal of rofecoxib and valdecoxib, following reports of excessive cardiac morbidity. Currently, celecoxib is the only COX-2 selective inhibitor available for clinical use. COX-2–selective inhibitors should be used cautiously in patients with underlying cardiovascular disease (see further discussion on "Cardiovascular Side Effects" section).

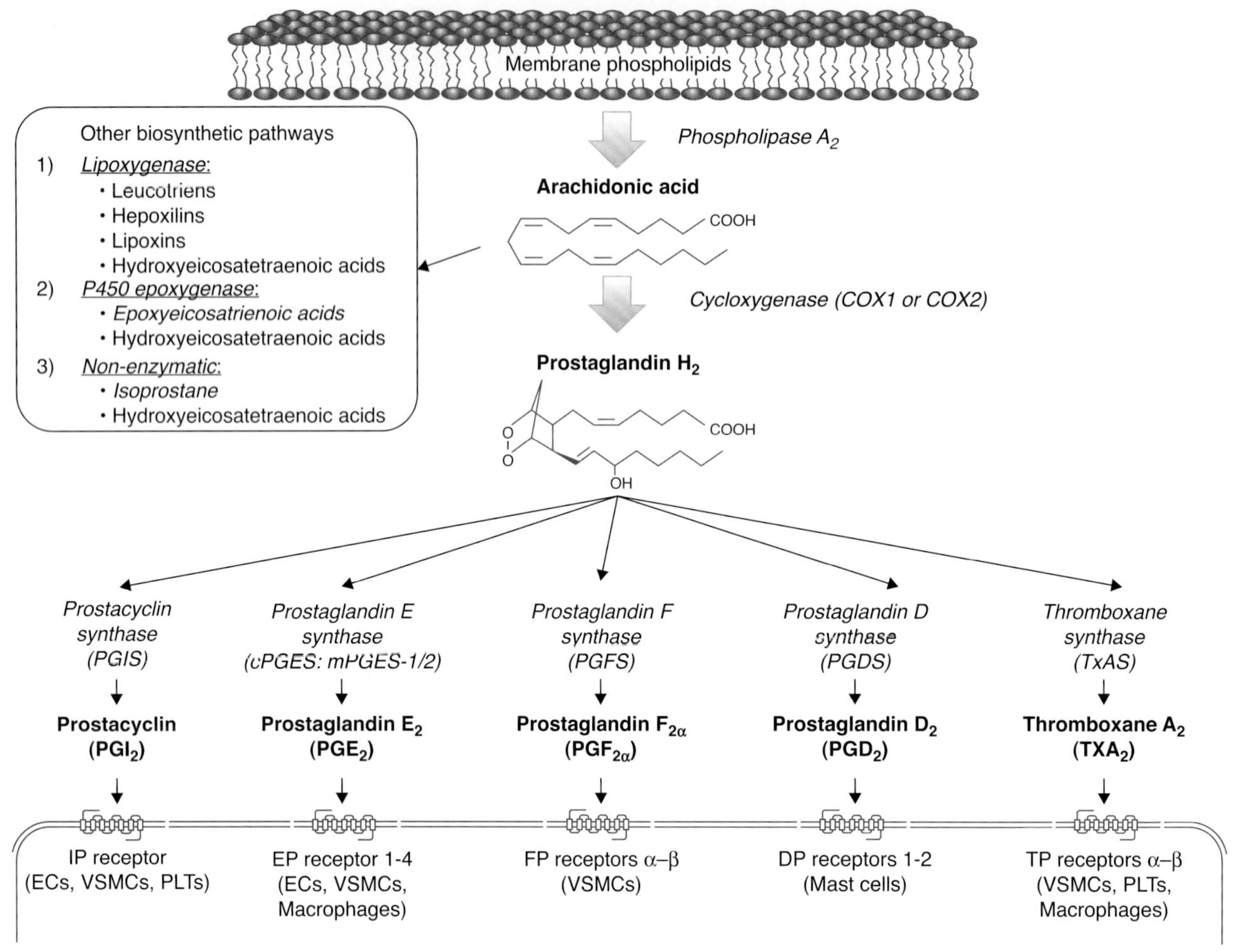

FIGURE 9-1 The cyclooxygenases pathway. ECs, endothelial cells; EP, PGE_2 receptor; DP, PGD_2 receptor; FP, $PGF_{2\alpha}$ receptor; IP, prostacyclin receptor; PLTs, platelets; TP, thromboxane receptor; VSMCs, vascular smooth muscle cells. (Reproduced from Cipollone F, Santovito D. EP receptors and coxibs: seeing the light at the end of the tunnel. *Circ Res.* 2013;113:91–93.)

Coxibs may be a safer alternative to NSAIDs in the perioperative settings. Although nonspecific NSAIDs provide analgesic efficacy similar to coxibs, their use has been limited in the perioperative setting because of platelet dysfunction and gastrointestinal toxicity. The potential benefits of coxibs include improved quality of analgesia, reduced incidence of gastrointestinal side effects versus conventional NSAIDs, and no platelet inhibition. NSAIDs can be classified according to numerous characteristics, including COX selectivity, and chemical and pharmacologic properties

NSAIDs belong to a number of chemical families including acetic acids, oxicams, propionic acids, salicylates, fenamates, furanones, and coxibs (Table 9-1). All NSAIDs are weakly acidic chemical compounds and share similarities in pharmacokinetic properties.[3] The volume of distribution of NSAIDs is low, ranging from 0.1 to 0.3 L/kg, suggesting minimal tissue binding. The plasma half-life of NSAIDs ranges from 0.25 to >70 hours, indicating wide differences in clearance rates. Hepatic or renal disease can alter NSAID protein binding and metabolism.[4]

Gastrointestinal absorption of NSAIDs occurs rapidly, usually within 15 to 30 minutes. After absorption, NSAIDs are more than 90% bound to albumin, which influences their distribution and drug-drug interaction potential. Hypoalbuminemia (e.g., due to alcoholic liver disease) can result in greater unbound drug and increased risk for NSAID-related adverse events.[4] The liver metabolizes most NSAIDs, with subsequent excretion into urine or bile. Enterohepatic recirculation occurs when a significant amount of an NSAID or its conjugated metabolites are excreted into the bile and then reabsorbed in the distal intestine. Hepatic NSAID elimination is dependent on the free fraction of NSAID within the plasma and the intrinsic enzyme activity of the liver. NSAIDs are primarily eliminated by renal and biliary excretion. Reduced renal function prolongs NSAID half-life, and the dose should be lowered proportionally in patients with impaired kidney

Table 9-1

Characteristics of Commonly Prescribed Nonsteroidal Antiinflammatory Drugs

Generic Name (Trade Name)	Dose[a] Available Dosages (mg)	Dose[a] Common Dosing Intervals	Pharmacokinetics Drug Metabolism	Pharmacokinetics Elimination Half-Life (h)
Nonselective NSAIDs				
Acetic Acid Group				
Diclofenac DR	25	BID-TID	Oxidation	1–2
(Voltaren)	50	QD-BID		
Diclofenac XR	75			
(Voltaren XR)	100			
Etodolac	200	BID-TID	Oxidation, conjugation	7
(Lodine)	300	QD		
Etodolac XL	400			
(Lodine XL)	500			
	400			
	500			
	600			
Ketorolac IM, IV injection *(generic)*	30	QD-QID	Conjugation	2.5–8.5
Indomethacin	25	BID-TID	Oxidation, conjugation	4.5–6
(Indocin)	50	QD-BID		
Indomethacin SR	75			
(Indocin SR)				
Nabumetone	500	QD-BID	Oxidation	22–30
(Relafen)	750			
Sulindac	150	BID	Oxidation, reduction	16
(Clinoril)	200			
Tolmetin	400	TID	Conjugation	5
(Tolectin)	600			
Oxicam Group				
Meloxicam	7.5	QD	Oxidation	13–20
(Mobic)	15			
Piroxicam	10	QD	Oxidation	30–86
(Feldene)	20			
Propionic Acid Group				
Fenoprofen	200	TID-QID	Glucuronidation	3
(Nalfon)	300			
Flurbiprofen	50	BID-QID	Oxidation	3–6
(Ocufen)	100			
Ibuprofen	400	TID-QID	Oxidation	2–2.5
(Motrin)	600			
	800			
Ketoprofen	50	TID-QID	Conjugation	2–4
	75	QD		3–7
Ketoprofen CR	100			
	150			
	200			

(continued)

Table 9-1

Characteristics of Commonly Prescribed Nonsteroidal Antiinflammatory Drugs *(continued)*

	Dose[a]		Pharmacokinetics	
Generic Name (Trade Name)	Available Dosages (mg)	Common Dosing Intervals	Drug Metabolism	Elimination Half-Life (h)
Naproxen	250	BID	Conjugation, oxidation	12–15
(Naprosyn)	375	QD		
(Naprelan)	500			
	375			
	500			
Oxaprozin *(Daypro)*	600	QD-BID	Oxidation, conjugation	50–60
Salicylate				
Aspirin	81	QD	Hydrolysis, conjugation, glucuronidation	0.25–0.5
(Ecotrin, Ascriptin)	325	BID-QID		
Choline magnesium	500	BID-TID		
	500			
Trisalicylate	750		Conjugation	2–12
(Trilisate)	1000			
Cyclooxygenase-2 Agents				
Coxib Group				
Celecoxib	100	QD-BID	Conjugation	11–16
(Celebrex)	200			

[a]A dosage range exists for each NSAID that must be individualized depending on patient characteristics and disease mechanism.

Reproduced from Vincent J-L, Abraham E, Moore FA, et al. *Textbook of Critical Care*. 6th ed. Philadelphia, PA: Elsevier Saunders; 2011:183, 1346–1353.

function.[3,4] Moderate to severe liver disease impairs NSAID metabolism, increasing the potential for toxicity.

Side Effects of Nonsteroidal Antiinflammatory Drugs

Platelet Function

Platelet aggregation and thus the ability to clot is primarily induced through an increase in thromboxane production following activation of platelet COX-1. There is no COX-2 isoenzyme in the platelet. NSAIDs and aspirin inhibit the activity of COX-1, but the COX-2–specific inhibitors (or COX-1–sparing drugs) have no effect on COX-1 and thus no effect on platelet function.[5]

Gastrointestinal Side Effects

NSAIDs are associated with a spectrum of upper gastrointestinal complications, ranging from endoscopic ulcers in 10% to 30% of patients to serious ulcer complications in 1% to 2% of patients, including perforation and bleeding.[6,7] Lower gastrointestinal tract complications are less well characterized.[8,9]

Risk factors for NSAID-associated gastrointestinal complications include high NSAID dose, older age, *Helicobacter pylori* infection, a history of prior ulcer, and concomitant use of low-dose aspirin, anticoagulants, or corticosteroids.[10,11] Therefore, it is generally recommended that patients with gastrointestinal risk factors should be treated with COX-2–selective agents or nonselective NSAIDs with gastrointestinal protective cotherapy.[12,13]

Cardiovascular Side Effects

NSAIDs are associated with an increased risk of cardiovascular adverse events such as myocardial infarction, heart failure, and hypertension. COX inhibition is likely to disturb the balance between COX-2–mediated production of proaggregatory thromboxane in platelets and antiaggregatory prostaglandin I_2 in endothelial cells. COX selectivity alone is not sufficient to define the risk of NSAID-associated cardiovascular complications. Based on two studies, the Vioxx Gastrointestinal Outcomes Research (VIGOR)[14] study and the Adenomatous Polyp Prevention on Vioxx (APPROVe) study,[15] rofecoxib was withdrawn from the market in 2004. Valdecoxib was subsequently withdrawn in 2005 due to a fourfold increase in the incidence of myocardial infarction.

The cardiovascular safety of nonselective NSAIDs has been under recent investigation. A meta-analysis of randomized trials found that high-dose ibuprofen and high-dose diclofenac were associated with a moderately increased risk of vascular events compared with placebo, similar to that observed with COX-2–selective agents; the risks associated with naproxen, although they cannot be completely excluded, appeared to be substantially lower.[16]

Studies are lacking on the long-term effects of nonselective NSAIDs on gastrointestinal and cardiovascular systems, which limit our understanding of the true benefits and risks of NSAIDs over the long term. To reduce the cardiovascular risks, the American Heart Association recommends that all NSAIDs should be used at their lowest effective dose. When NSAID therapy is required for patients at risk of cardiovascular complications, naproxen is recommended as the NSAID of choice.[17] A recent meta-analysis of the vascular and upper gastrointestinal effects of NSAIDs confirms that diclofenac and ibuprofen raise risk of major vascular events as much as coxibs. Naproxen has no effect on vascular outcomes but does increase upper gastrointestinal complications.[18]

Renal Side Effects

The effects of the NSAIDs on renal function include changes in the excretion of sodium, changes in tubular function, potential for interstitial nephritis, and reversible renal failure due to alterations in filtration rate and renal plasma flow. Prostaglandins and prostacyclins are important for maintenance of intrarenal blood flow and tubular transport. All NSAIDs, except nonacetylated salicylates, have the potential to induce reversible impairment of glomerular filtration rate; this effect occurs more frequently in patients with congestive heart failure; established renal disease with altered intrarenal plasma flow including diabetes, hypertension, or atherosclerosis; and with induced hypovolemia, salt depletion or significant hypoalbuminemia.[19,20] Avoiding perioperative use of NSAIDs in patients with hypovolemia from any cause is an important means of minimizing renal injury.

Liver Side Effects

The use of aspirin was associated with reduced risk of developing hepatocellular carcinoma and of death due to chronic liver disease, whereas non-aspirin NSAID use was only associated with reduced risk of death due to chronic liver disease.[21] Paradoxically, elevations in hepatic transaminase levels and liver failure have been reported with some of the NSAIDs.[22]

Pulmonary Side Effects

Many adverse reactions attributed to NSAIDs are due to inhibition of prostaglandin synthesis in local tissues. For example, patients with allergic rhinitis, nasal polyposis, and/or a history of asthma, in whom all NSAIDs effectively inhibit prostaglandin synthetase, are at increased risk for anaphylaxis.[23] The use of selective COX-2 inhibitors as an alternative to aspirin and other NSAIDs has been suggested for patients with aspirin-exacerbated respiratory disease. The highly selective COX-2 inhibitor etoricoxib has been shown to be tolerated in most but not all patients tested.[24] An oral provocation test is therefore recommended before prescribing etoricoxib for patients with aspirin-exacerbated respiratory disease.[24]

Hypersensitivity Reactions

Hypersensitivity reactions to NSAIDs do rarely occur, and they are more common in individuals with nasal polyps or asthma. Allergic reactions include bronchoconstriction, rhinitis, and urticaria. Recent data suggest a role of altered COX-2 regulation associated with the aspirin-intolerant asthma/rhinitis syndrome.[23] Because of the potential for cross-reactivity, avoidance of all NSAIDs is recommended. In rare cases, NSAIDs have been implicated in causing aseptic meningitis and, in children, Reye syndrome.[25]

Idiosyncratic Adverse Effects

Typical nonspecific reactions include skin rash and photosensitivity, aseptic meningitis, tinnitus, hearing loss, and neutropenia. The effect of prostaglandin inhibition may result in premature closure of the ductus arteriosus. Acetylsalicylic acid (ASA) has been associated with small for gestational age neonates and neonatal bruising; however, it has been used for many years in the treatment of patients who require NSAIDs while pregnant.[26] The most common toxicities associated with NSAIDs are gastrointestinal, cardiovascular, and renal and are related primarily to COX inhibition and decreased synthesis of prostaglandins.

Drug-Drug Interactions

Drug-drug interactions with NSAID therapy may result from their pharmacodynamic or pharmacokinetic interactions. Nonselective NSAIDs affect other antiplatelet agents via additive inhibition of platelet aggregation. The result is an increased bleeding risk with the concomitant use of NSAIDs and other antiplatelet agents.[25,27]

Significant drug-drug interactions have been documented with use of NSAIDs and lithium. NSAIDs decrease lithium clearance and increase serum lithium concentrations by inhibiting renal prostaglandin production and altering intrarenal blood flow.[25,27,28] Data are conflicting regarding the drug-drug interaction potential of angiotensin-converting enzyme (ACE) inhibitors and NSAIDs.[29]

Concurrent administration of digoxin and NSAIDs can decrease renal clearance of digoxin, increase plasma drug concentration, and potentiate digoxin toxicity. NSAIDs interact with anticonvulsant agents such as phenytoin and valproic acid by displacing the anticonvulsants from their protein-binding sites, which increases the free drug concentration. Combination use of corticosteroids and aspirin can increase renal clearance of salicylate and significantly decrease plasma salicylate concentrations.[27,28]

NSAIDs can be used in selected critically ill patients but should be used judiciously because of the potential for toxic adverse events, particularly renal toxicity in hypovolemic patients. The lowest effective dose of the NSAID should be used for the shortest duration indicated. Appropriate clinical and laboratory follow-up is necessary.

Acetaminophen

Acetaminophen (Tylenol, also known as paracetamol, *N*-acetyl-*p*-aminophenol, and nAPAP) is a popular antipyretic and analgesic found in many over-the-counter and prescription products. Acetaminophen is antipyretic and analgesic but has little, if any, antiinflammatory action. Acetaminophen is the leading cause of acute liver failure in the United States, and nearly half of acetaminophen-associated cases are due to unintentional overdose.

Acetaminophen has a central analgesic effect that is mediated through activation of descending serotonergic pathways. Debate exists about its primary site of action, which may be inhibition of prostaglandin synthesis. The mechanism of action has been debated. In animal models, it has been seen to inhibit COX-3. At the spinal cord level, it has been shown to antagonize neurotransmission by *N*-methyl-D-aspartate (NMDA), substance P, and nitric oxide pathways.

Oral acetaminophen has excellent bioavailability. Acetaminophen is suitable for analgesic or antipyretic uses; it is the first-line analgesic in osteoarthritis and particularly valuable for patients in whom aspirin is contraindicated (e.g., those with peptic ulcer disease, aspirin hypersensitivity, and children with febrile illness). The conventional oral dose of acetaminophen is 325 to 650 mg every 4 to 6 hours; total daily doses should not exceed 4,000 mg (2,000 mg per day for chronic alcoholics). In efforts to reduce the incidence of hepatotoxicity, a U.S. Food and Drug Administration (FDA) advisory panel recommended in 2009 a lower maximum daily dose of acetaminophen of 2,600 mg and a decrease in the maximum single dose from 1,000 mg to 650 mg.

An intravenous (IV) preparation of acetaminophen is currently available for clinical use. Optimal analgesia for moderate to severe postoperative pain cannot be achieved using a single agent alone.[30] IV paracetamol provides around 4 hours of effective analgesia for about 37% of patients with acute postoperative pain.[31] With its inherent safety and demonstrated efficacy, IV acetaminophen can prove to be an asset in managing perioperative pain.

Current evidence suggests that a combination of paracetamol and an NSAID may offer superior analgesia compared with either drug alone.[32]

Acetaminophen is well tolerated and has a low incidence of gastrointestinal side effects. However, acute overdosage can cause severe hepatic damage, and the number of accidental or deliberate poisonings with acetaminophen continues to grow. Chronic use of <2 g per day is not typically associated with hepatic dysfunction, but overuse of acetaminophen-containing narcotic and over-the-counter combination products marketed in the United States has led to heightened awareness of the possibility of toxicity.

The pharmacology of acetaminophen overdose, including its time course and treatment is interesting and important to understand. Damage to the liver results from one of acetaminophen's metabolites, *N*-acetyl-*p*-benzoquinoneimine (NAPQI). NAPQI leads to liver failure by depleting the liver's natural antioxidant glutathione and directly damaging liver cells, leading to liver failure. Treatment is aimed at removing the paracetamol from the body and replacing glutathione. Activated charcoal can be used to decrease absorption of acetaminophen in those who present, soon after ingestion of, an overdose. Acetylcysteine is administered as an antidote and acts as a precursor for glutathione and can neutralize NAPQI directly. Patients treated early after ingestion have a good prognosis.

Acetylsalicylic acid (Aspirin)

Aspirin is the oldest and most widely used medicinal compound in the world. It is considered separately from the NSAIDs due to its predominant use in the treatment of cardiovascular and cerebrovascular diseases. Aspirin is found in hundreds of over-the-counter medicines worldwide, and remains at the forefront of medicine, with newly discovered applications for the prevention and treatment of several life-threatening diseases. Aspirin is a derivative of salicylic acid. Aspirin and salicylate are rapidly metabolized in the plasma (e.g., by plasma esterases), erythrocyte, and liver, to salicylate in vivo.[33]

Aspirin has several different approved uses. Aspirin acts as a general analgesic by blocking the action of the COX enzymes and thus prevents the production of prostaglandins. Aspirin effectively treats headaches, back and muscle pain, and other general aches and pains. In addition, aspirin produces inhibition of COX and thus prostanoid synthesis[34] and also protein kinase.[35] However, these are not necessarily the most likely mechanisms.[36] Aspirin irreversibly inactivates COX, leading to prolonged inhibition of platelet aggregation.

Overdose

The mechanism of NSAID toxicity in overdose is related to both their acidic nature and their inhibition of prostaglandin production. The severity typically depends on

Table 9-2

Adverse Effects of Nonsteroidal Antiinflammatory Drugs

System	Adverse Effects
Cardiovascular	Hypertension, can exacerbate or induce heart failure, thrombotic events, possible increased risk of thrombotic/cardiovascular events with long-term use (use with caution in patients with preexisting disease; more likely with COX-2 inhibitors)
Respiratory	Nasal polyps, rhinitis, dyspnea, bronchospasm, angioedema, may exacerbate asthma
Hepatic	Hepatitis
Gastrointestinal	Gastropathy (can be asymptomatic), gastric bleeding, esophageal disease, pancreatitis
Hematologic	Increased intraoperative bleeding due to platelet inhibition/dysfunction (coxibs do not affect platelet function), will potentiate anticoagulation effect
Dermatologic	Urticaria, erythema multiforme, rash
Genitourinary	Renal insufficiency (use with caution in patients with preexisting renal disease), sodium/fluid retention, papillary necrosis, interstitial nephritis
Central nervous system	Headache, aseptic meningitis, hearing disturbances
Skeletal	Potential to inhibit bone growth/healing/formation
Pharmacologic interactions	NSAIDs displace albumin-bound drugs and can potentiate their effects (e.g., warfarin)

the dose ingested and the salicylate concentration that correlates with the degree of acid–base disturbance.[29,37] Salicylate levels of 300 to 600 mg/L are associated with mild toxicity, 600 to 800 mg/L with moderate toxicity, and greater than 800 mg/L with severe toxicity. For nonselective NSAIDs, plasma concentrations are not commonly measured because the half-life of many of these agents is relatively short.[37]

Symptoms include nausea, vomiting, abdominal pain, tinnitus, hearing impairment, and CNS depression (Table 9-2); with higher dose aspirin ingestion, metabolic acidosis, renal failure, CNS changes (e.g., agitation, confusion, coma), and hyperventilation with respiratory alkalosis due to stimulation of the respiratory center. The presence of acidemia permits more salicylic acid to cross the BBB.[38] With other nonselective NSAID ingestions, symptoms are similar.[37–39]

Management should be directed at symptomatic support, prevention of further absorption, and correction of acid–base imbalance.[37,38] There is no antidote for salicylate or NSAID poisoning. Appropriate hydration and activated charcoal should be considered within 1 hour after ingestion. Urine alkalinization increases salicylate elimination.[37] In severe cases of aspirin overdose, hemodialysis is effective at removing salicylate and correcting acid–base imbalances and has been shown to reduce morbidity and mortality.[38]

Steroids

Glucocorticoids have been used to reduce inflammation and tissue damage in a variety of conditions, including inflammatory bowel disease and rheumatoid arthritis. Its antiinflammatory action results in decreased production of various inflammatory mediators that play a major role in amplifying and maintenance of pain perception. Another proposed mechanism is by inhibition of phospholipase A_2 as well as changes in cell function induced by glucocorticoid receptor activation.

Glucocorticoids have the most powerful antiinflammatory characteristics of all steroids. Corticosteroids are a subgroup of compounds known as adrenocorticoids that are naturally secreted from the adrenal gland. The primary corticosteroid is hydrocortisone, which is the standard against which the pharmacologic properties of various synthetic corticosteroids are judged. Many synthetic agents that are more potent, have longer durations of action, have greater antiinflammatory activity, and generate fewer unwanted mineralocorticoid side effects than hydrocortisone have been developed. Mineralocorticoids are adrenal cortical steroid hormones that have a greater effect on water and electrolyte balance. The main endogenous hormone is aldosterone.

Different steroids vary with respect to their duration of action and relative corticosteroid and mineralocorticoid activity. Corticosteroids are divided into short, intermediate, and long-acting groups (Table 9-3). Short- and long-acting preparations cause less inhibition of the hypothalamic-pituitary-adrenal axis. Many of the unwanted side effects are related to the mineralocorticoid properties (Table 9-4).

Nearly all routes of administration can be used for corticosteroids. Although associated with significant toxicity when administered in large doses for long periods, adverse effects with a single dose of dexamethasone are minor.[40]

The use of corticosteroids for pain relief, although popular, has yet to gain wider acceptance because of concerns over side effects, such as adrenal suppression,

Table 9-3

Comparative Pharmacology of Endogenous and Synthetic Corticosteroids

	Antiinflammatory Potency	Sodium Retaining Potency	Equivalent Dose (mg)	Elimination Half-Time (h)	Duration of Action (h)	Route of Administration
Cortisol	1	1	20	1.5–3.0	8–12	Oral, topical, IV, IM, IA
Cortisone	0.8	0.8	25	0.5	8–36	Oral, topical, IV, IM, IA
Prednisolone	4	0.8	5	2–4	12–36	Oral, topical, IV, IM, IA
Prednisone	4	0.8	5	2–4	12–36	Oral
Methylprednisolone	5	0.5	4	2–4	12–36	Oral, topical, IV, IM, IA, epidural
Betamethasone	25	0	0.75	5	36–54	Oral, topical, IV, IM, IA
Dexamethasone	25	0	0.75	3.5–5.0	36–54	Oral, topical, IV, IM, IA
Triamcinolone	5	0	4	3.5	12–36	Oral, topical, IV, IM, epidural
Fludrocortisone	10	250	2	—	24	Oral, topical, IV, IM
Aldosterone	0	3,000				

IV, intravenous; IM, intramuscular; IA, intraarticular

Table 9-4

Potential Side Effects Associated with Corticosteroid Therapy

Dermatologic and Soft Tissue
- Skin thinning and purpura
- Cushingoid appearance
- Alopecia
- Acne
- Hirsutism
- Striae
- Hypertrichosis

Eye
- Posterior subcapsular cataract
- Elevated intraocular pressure/glaucoma
- Exophthalmos

Cardiovascular
- Hypertension
- Perturbations of serum lipoproteins
- Premature atherosclerotic disease
- Arrhythmias with pulse infusions

Gastrointestinal
- Gastritis
- Peptic ulcer disease
- Pancreatitis
- Steatohepatitis
- Visceral perforation

Renal
- Hypokalemia
- Fluid volume shifts

Genitourinary and reproductive
- Amenorrhea/infertility
- Intrauterine growth retardation

Bone
- Osteoporosis
- Avascular necrosis

Muscle
- Myopathy

Neuropsychiatric
- Euphoria
- Dysphoria/depression
- Insomnia/akathisia
- Psychosis
- Pseudo tumor cerebri

Endocrine
- Diabetes mellitus
- Hypothalamic-pituitary–adrenal insufficiency

Infectious disease
- Heightened risk of typical infections
- Opportunistic infections
- Herpes zoster

From: Saag KG, Furst D. Major side effects of glucocorticoids. In: Bose BD, editor. *UpToDate*. Wellesley, MA; UpToDate; 2004, with permission.

osteonecrosis, impaired wound healing, and concerns about efficacy. There is evidence supporting the use of corticosteroids in multimodal analgesia protocols to contribute to the postoperative recovery of the patient by minimizing opioid doses and therefore side effects. However, the optimal mode, dose, and timing of administration remain unclear.[41]

In recent meta-analysis,[42] patients treated with dexamethasone experienced less postoperative pain, required less postoperative opioids, had longer time to first analgesic dose, needed less rescue analgesia, and had shorter postanesthesia care unit (PACU) stays. Differences between the groups were however small and may not be clinically relevant. Perioperative dosing of dexamethasone had small but statistically significant analgesic benefits.[42] Investigators have begun to evaluate glucocorticoids as adjuvants for regional anesthesia. There is some evidence for an analgesic effect of local, spinal, and systemic corticosteroids in combination with bupivacaine.[43] Dexamethasone has been found to prolong local anesthetic block duration in animal and human studies, and adding methylprednisolone to local anesthetic increases the duration of axillary brachial block.[44]

Dexamethasone also prolongs the analgesia from interscalene blocks using ropivacaine or bupivacaine, with the effect being stronger with ropivacaine; the combined effect of dexamethasone and either drug produced nearly 22 hours of analgesia. Systemic glucocorticoids have also been shown to reduce postoperative pain. This raises the question whether the beneficial effects of adding glucocorticoid to a regional anesthetic is solely due to local effect or is mediated at least in part by systemic action.[45]

Steroids often administered to patients with arthritis and other chronic pain conditions, locally (e.g., intraarticularly) to limit the systemic side-effect profiles. Pain relief from glucocorticoid treatment has been reported to last for up to 3 weeks in osteoarthritis and 2 months in rheumatoid arthritis.[46]

Epidural injection of corticosteroids has been used to treat back pain (mainly due to nerve root irritation) in patients with a wide variety of spine pathologies including radiculopathy, spinal stenosis, disc-space narrowing, annular tears, spondylosis, spondylolisthesis, vertebral fractures, and postlaminectomy syndrome.[46] The only proven efficacy of epidural steroid injections is their ability to speed resolution of leg pain ("sciatica") in patients with acute intervertebral disc herniation and associated radicular pain.

Systemic Local Anesthetics

Lidocaine produces analgesia by suppressing the activity of sodium channels in neurons that respond to noxious stimuli, thereby preventing nerve conduction and pain transmission. Voltage-gated sodium channels (VGSCs) play a fundamental role in the control of neuronal excitability. Local anesthetics that block VGSCs have long been used to abolish pain temporarily by blocking nerve conduction.

Systemically administered local anesthetics such as IV lidocaine, oral mexiletine, and oral tocainide are effective in a number of chronic pain conditions. Early studies described successful treatment of acute pain syndromes such as postoperative pain,[47] burn pain,[48] and cancer pain.[49] Subsequent clinical reports have demonstrated the effectiveness in reducing pain associated with many chronic pain conditions.[50,51] Commonly used drugs include IV lidocaine and the orally active agents mexiletine and tocainide. The exact mechanism of action of systemic local anesthetics in pain control is unknown. Evidence suggests that the effect may involve selective blockade of pain fibers within the spinal cord or the dorsal root ganglia.[52]

Orally administered lidocaine has poor bioavailability. The elimination half-life is 1.5 to 2 hours and can increase in the event of decreased liver blood flow (e.g., congestive heart failure). Mexiletine has excellent oral bioavailability. The mean elimination half-life is 10 to 12 hours, which can increase to 25 hours with hepatic impairment. Only 10% of the drug is excreted unchanged by the kidney, and therefore renal impairment has minimal effect on half-life.[53]

At low doses, initial CNS symptoms include lightheadedness, dizziness, tinnitus, vertigo, blurred vision, and altered taste. Seizures occur at higher doses. Cardiovascular side effects include hypotension, bradycardia, and cardiovascular collapse, which can lead to cardiac arrest. In a meta-analysis, when used for treatment of neuropathic pain, lidocaine and mexiletine produced no major adverse events in controlled clinical trials, were superior to placebo to relieve neuropathic pain, and were as effective as other analgesics used for this condition; however, the long-term use of oral mexiletine is limited by the nearly universal appearance of nausea.[54]

Topical Application of 5% Lidocaine

The topical application of 5% lidocaine have been used in postherpetic neuralgia, the topical application of 5% lidocaine (as a gel or patch) has been demonstrated to significantly relieve pain and reduce pain intensity with a fast onset (within 30 minutes) and lasting for the duration of drug application.[55] Additionally, studies have also shown that lidocaine patches can provide pain relief in patients with various painful neuropathies.[56]

The use of a lidocaine patch 5% after different surgical procedures has been reported in several small studies.[57,58]

The most common adverse events generally involve mild skin reactions. There has been no reported drug-drug interaction in clinical trials. Recent evidence suggests that extended application does not result in Aβ-mediated sensory loss at the application site, which is particularly important in patients who already have a degree of sensory loss due to their underlying condition. The lidocaine patch provides a treatment option that carries a relatively low risk of systemic adverse effects and drug-drug interaction, even with continuous application of up to four patches per day. The efficacy of this approach alone would not be sufficient for providing adequate postoperative pain management.

Capsaicin

Capsaicin is a transient receptor potential vanilloid ($TRPV_1$) channels agonist.[59] $TRPV_1$ is a receptor that is markedly reduced in inflammatory conditions and is present on unmyelinated C fiber endings in the periphery. The activation of the TRPV receptors releases high-intensity impulses and releases the neurotransmitter substance P, which results in the initial phase of burning. Continued release of substance P in the presence of capsaicin leads to the depletion of capsaicin and a subsequent decrease in C fiber activation.[60] Capsaicin is the major pungent ingredient of hot chili peppers and other botanicals. Capsaicin 0.025%, 0.075%, and 0.25% creams and/or transdermal patches are available over-the-counter for the temporary relief of pain from arthritis, myalgias, arthralgias, and neuralgias. The FDA has granted capsaicin orphan drug status in the treatment of postherpetic neuralgia, intermetatarsal neuroma, erythromelalgia, and HIV-associated neuropathy. When used in the treatment of postherpetic neuralgia, a single treatment with the capsaicin 8% patch provided a pain intensity decrease of ≥30% for >35% of treated patients in weeks 2 through 12.[61] The FDA approved the prescription-only capsaicin 8% patch (Qutenza) for the management of neuropathic pain associated with postherpetic neuralgia. Topically applied capsaicin has moderate to poor efficacy in the treatment of chronic musculoskeletal or neuropathic pain.[62]

Ketamine

There has been a renewed interest in the use of subanesthetic doses of ketamine as an adjunct to provide postoperative pain relief in opioid-dependent patients.[63] NMDA receptor antagonists have been used in perioperative pain management. At low, subanesthetic doses (e.g., 0.15 to 1 mg/kg), ketamine exerts a specific NMDA blockade and, hence, modulates central sensitization induced both by the incision and tissue damage and by perioperative analgesics such as opioids.

There may be some role for ketamine in preventing opioid-induced hyperalgesia in patients receiving high doses of opioid for their postoperative pain relief.[64] However, clinical use of ketamine can be limited due to psychotomimetic adverse effects and other common adverse effects, including dizziness, blurred vision, and nausea and vomiting.[65] The usefulness of low-dose ketamine in the perioperative management of the opioid-tolerant patient is in need of further study.

Dexmedetomidine

Dexmedetomidine is a relatively new, highly selective, central α_2 agonist. Its sedative, pro-anesthetic, and pro-analgesic effects at 0.5 to 2 μg/kg given intravenously stem mainly from its ability to blunt the central sympathetic response by an as yet unknown mechanism. It also minimizes opioid-induced muscle rigidity, lessens postoperative shivering, causes minimal respiratory depression, and has hemodynamic stabilizing effects. Dexmedetomidine, when used as an adjunct, can reduce postoperative morphine consumption in various surgical settings.[66,67] A recent study has shown the analgesic efficacy of dexmedetomidine in postoperative pain relief. The authors of this study found that the addition of dexmedetomidine to IV PCA morphine resulted in superior analgesia, significant morphine sparing, and less morphine-induced nausea, while it was devoid of additional sedation and untoward hemodynamic changes

Clonidine

The use of low doses of clonidine proved to be a useful adjunct analgesic when given neuraxially and in combination with peripheral nerve blocks. Data from the systemic administration of clonidine also support the usefulness of low-dose IV administration as an adjunct for postoperative pain management.[68]

Opioids

Since the detection of morphine by the pharmacologist Friedrich Sertürner in 1806, opioids have been used as potent centrally acting analgesics. In addition to the central site of action, peripheral endogenous opioid analgesic systems have been extensively studied. The three classes of opioid receptors are widely distributed in addition to the CNS, in peripheral neurons, neuroendocrine organs (pituitary, adrenals), immune, and ectodermal cells. Opioid receptors are synthesized in the dorsal root ganglia (DRG) and transported centrally and peripherally to the nerve terminals.[69]

Efforts continue to develop opioid analgesics unable to cross the BBB, which act only peripherally, thus providing adequate analgesia without central side effects. Although peripheral opioid receptors are largely expressed by the primary sensory neurons, they are functionally inactive under most basal conditions.[70] The antinociceptive effect of systemic opioids is thought to be produced mainly at the central (particularly supraspinal) level,[71] although peripheral opioid receptors might also participate.[72,73]

Inflammation increases expression, transport, and accumulation of peripheral opioid receptors on peripheral terminals of sensory nerves but also triggers migration of opioid-containing immunocytes.[74] The peripheral effectiveness of opioids depends on the presence of inflammation, which triggers an enhanced expression of opioid receptors on primary afferents. Opioids were shown to have peripheral antinociceptive effects in inflammation.[72,73] Effective endogenous peripheral opioid analgesia requires an adequate number of functional opioid receptors on primary afferent neurons and a well-coordinated migration of opioid-secreting leukocytes out of the circulating blood to the inflamed site. Interestingly, this recruitment of opioid-containing cells to inflamed tissue has been shown to be suppressed by the administration of centrally acting opioids.[75] On the contrary, several studies indicate that a large portion of the analgesic effects produced by systemically administered opioids can be mediated by peripheral opioid receptors.[76] In an animal model of inflamed knee joint, intraarticular injection of μ and κ but not δ opioid agonists produced a dose-dependent blockade of autonomic response to a noxious stimulus.[77]

Opioids injected locally into soft tissues or joints produce potent analgesic effects that are mediated by peripheral (not central) opioid.[77] Pain relief has been reported after knee arthroscopy after intraarticular injection of morphine [78] and after submucosal injection of morphine in patients undergoing dental surgery.[79]

The role of the opioid receptor system in wound healing is another area of intense interest and study.[80] Peripherally acting opioids can reduce plasma extravasation, vasodilation, proinflammatory neuropeptides, immune mediators, and tissue destruction. Local administration of opioid agonists at low concentrations may offer a promising therapeutic strategy.[79,81]

There is strong evidence for a cardioprotective effect of both peripheral and central opioid receptors. The role of the different opioid receptor subtypes involved is still contradictory, but there is some evidence that opioids have infarct-sparing effects and facilitate ischemic preconditioning.[82] The endogenous opioid system is involved in the analgesic effect of the nonopioid analgesic celecoxib. There is evidence for both central[83] and peripheral[84] opioid receptor activation. In addition to this, there is animal evidence of the role of peripherally acting opioids in inflammatory arthropathy and inflammatory bowel disease.[85,86] These findings may guide the future development of novel peripherally restricted opioids.

Currently, there are no specific peripherally acting opioids available in the United States; investigators continue to work on developing novel potential agents. These peripheral opioid receptors play a critical role in modulating pain and inflammation. However, clinical data are still lacking.

References

1. Vane JR, Botting RM. Mechanism of action of nonsteroidal anti-inflammatory drugs. *Am J Med.* 1998;104:2S–8S; discussion 21S–22S.
2. Mukherjee D, Nissen SE, Topol EJ. Risk of cardiovascular events associated with selective COX-2 inhibitors. *JAMA.* 2001;286:954–959.
3. Davies NM, Skjodt NM. Choosing the right nonsteroidal anti-inflammatory drug for the right patient: a pharmacokinetic approach. *Clin Pharmacokinet.* 2000;38:377–392.
4. Needs CJ, Brooks PM. Clinical pharmacokinetics of the salicylates. *Clin Pharmacokinet.* 1985;10:164–177.
5. Dubois RN, Abramson SB, Crofford L, et al. Cyclooxygenase in biology and disease. *FASEB J.* 1998;12:1063–1073.
6. Silverstein FE, Graham DY, Senior JR, et al. Misoprostol reduces serious gastrointestinal complications in patients with rheumatoid arthritis receiving nonsteroidal anti-inflammatory drugs. A randomized, double-blind, placebo-controlled trial. *Ann Intern Med.* 1995;123:241–249.
7. Laine L. Nonsteroidal anti-inflammatory drug gastropathy. *Gastrointest Endosc Clin N Am.* 1996;6:489–504.
8. Chan FK, Lanas A, Scheiman J, et al. Celecoxib versus omeprazole and diclofenac in patients with osteoarthritis and rheumatoid arthritis (CONDOR): a randomised trial. *Lancet.* 2010;376:173–179.
9. Lanas A, Garcia-Rodriguez LA, Polo-Tomas M, et al. Time trends and impact of upper and lower gastrointestinal bleeding and perforation in clinical practice. *Am J Gastroenterol.* 2009;104:1633–1641.
10. Huang JQ, Sridhar S, Hunt RH. Role of Helicobacter pylori infection and non-steroidal anti-inflammatory drugs in peptic-ulcer disease: a meta-analysis. *Lancet.* 2002;359:14–22.
11. Gutthann SP, Garcia Rodriguez LA, Raiford DS. Individual nonsteroidal antiinflammatory drugs and other risk factors for upper gastrointestinal bleeding and perforation. *Epidemiology.* 1997;8:18–24.
12. Lanza FL, Chan FK, Quigley EM. Guidelines for prevention of NSAID-related ulcer complications. *Am J Gastroenterol.* 2009;104:728–738.
13. Chan FK, Abraham NS, Scheiman JM, et al. Management of patients on nonsteroidal anti-inflammatory drugs: a clinical practice recommendation from the First International Working Party on Gastrointestinal and Cardiovascular Effects of Nonsteroidal Anti-inflammatory Drugs and Anti-platelet Agents. *Am J Gastroenterol.* 2008;103:2908–2918.
14. Bombardier C, Laine L, Reicin A, et al. Comparison of upper gastrointestinal toxicity of rofecoxib and naproxen in patients with rheumatoid arthritis. VIGOR Study Group. *N Engl J Med.* 2000;343:1520–1528.
15. Bresalier RS, Sandler RS, Quan H, et al. Adenomatous Polyp Prevention on Vioxx Trial I: cardiovascular events associated with rofecoxib in a colorectal adenoma chemoprevention trial. *N Engl J Med.* 2005;352:1092–1102.
16. Kearney PM, Baigent C, Godwin J, et al. Do selective cyclo-oxygenase-2 inhibitors and traditional non-steroidal anti-inflammatory drugs increase the risk of atherothrombosis? Meta-analysis of randomised trials. *BMJ.* 2006;332:1302–1308.
17. Scheiman JM, Fendrick AM. Summing the risk of NSAID therapy. *Lancet.* 2007;369:1580–1581.
18. Coxib and Traditional NSAID Trialist's Collaboration. Vascular and upper gastrointestinal effects of non-steroidal anti-inflammatory drugs: meta-analyses of individual participant data from randomised trials. *Lancet.* 2013;382:769–779.
19. Whelton A. Renal and related cardiovascular effects of conventional and COX-2-specific NSAIDs and non-NSAID analgesics. *Am J Ther.* 2000;7:63–74.

20. Ong HT, Ong LM, Tan TE, et al. Cardiovascular effects of common analgesics. *Med J Malaysia.* 2013;68:189–194.
21. Sahasrabuddhe VV, Gunja MZ, Graubard BI, et al. Nonsteroidal anti-inflammatory drug use, chronic liver disease, and hepatocellular carcinoma. *J Natl Cancer Inst.* 2012;104:1808–1814.
22. Garcia Rodriguez LA, Williams R, Derby LE, et al. Acute liver injury associated with nonsteroidal anti-inflammatory drugs and the role of risk factors. *Arch Intern Med.* 1994;154:311–316.
23. Picado C, Fernandez-Morata JC, Juan M, et al. Cyclooxygenase-2 mRNA is downexpressed in nasal polyps from aspirin-sensitive asthmatics. *Am J Respir Crit Care Med.* 1999;160:291–296.
24. Koschel D, Weber CN, Hoffken G. Tolerability to etoricoxib in patients with aspirin-exacerbated respiratory disease. *J Investig Allergol Clin Immunol.* 2013;23:275–280.
25. Dabu-Bondoc S, Franco S. Risk-benefit perspectives in COX-2 blockade. *Curr Drug Saf.* 2008;3:14–23.
26. Nielsen GL, Sorensen HT, Larsen H, et al. Risk of adverse birth outcome and miscarriage in pregnant users of non-steroidal anti-inflammatory drugs: population based observational study and case-control study. *Br Med J.* 2001;322:266–270.
27. Verbeeck RK. Pharmacokinetic drug interactions with nonsteroidal anti-inflammatory drugs. *Clin Pharmacokinet.* 1990;19:44–66.
28. Brouwers JR, de Smet PA. Pharmacokinetic-pharmacodynamic drug interactions with nonsteroidal anti-inflammatory drugs. *Clin Pharmacokinet.* 1994;27:462–485.
29. Takkouche B, Etminan M, Caamano F, et al. Interaction between aspirin and ACE inhibitors: resolving discrepancies using a meta-analysis. *Drug Saf.* 2002;25:373–378.
30. Van Aken H, Thys L, Veekman L, et al. Assessing analgesia in single and repeated administrations of propacetamol for postoperative pain: comparison with morphine after dental surgery. *Anesth Analg.* 2004;98:159–165.
31. Tzortzopoulou A, McNicol ED, Cepeda MS, et al. Single dose intravenous propacetamol or intravenous paracetamol for postoperative pain. *Cochrane Database Syst Rev.* 2011;(10):CD007126.
32. Ong CK, Seymour RA, Lirk P, et al. Combining paracetamol (acetaminophen) with nonsteroidal antiinflammatory drugs: a qualitative systematic review of analgesic efficacy for acute postoperative pain. *Anesth Analg.* 2010;110:1170–1179.
33. Williams FM. Clinical significance of esterases in man. *Clin Pharmacokinet.* 1985;10:392–403.
34. Higgs GA, Moncada S, Vane JR. Eicosanoids in inflammation. *Ann Clin Res.* 1984;16:287–299.
35. Yuan M, Konstantopoulos N, Lee J, et al. Reversal of obesity- and diet-induced insulin resistance with salicylates or targeted disruption of Ikkbeta. *Science.* 2001;293:1673–1677.
36. Cronstein BN, Montesinos MC, Weissmann G. Salicylates and sulfasalazine, but not glucocorticoids, inhibit leukocyte accumulation by an adenosine-dependent mechanism that is independent of inhibition of prostaglandin synthesis and p105 of NFkappaB. *Proc Natl Acad Sci U S A.* 1999;96:6377–6381.
37. Bronstein AC, Spyker DA, Cantilena LR Jr, et al. 2011 Annual report of the American Association of Poison Control Centers' National Poison Data System (NPDS): 29th Annual Report. *Clin Toxicol (Phila).* 2012;50:911–1164.
38. Dargan PI, Wallace CI, Jones AL. An evidence based flowchart to guide the management of acute salicylate (aspirin) overdose. *Emerg Med J.* 2002;19:206–209.
39. Volans G, Hartley V, McCrea S, et al. Non-opioid analgesic poisoning. *Clin Med.* 2003;3:119–123.
40. McCormack K. The spinal actions of nonsteroidal anti-inflammatory drugs and the dissociation between their anti-inflammatory and analgesic effects. *Drugs.* 1994;47(suppl 5):28–45; discussion 46–47.
41. Salerno A, Hermann R. Efficacy and safety of steroid use for postoperative pain relief. Update and review of the medical literature. *J Bone Joint Surg Am.* 2006;88:1361–1372.
42. Waldron NH, Jones CA, Gan TJ, et al. Impact of perioperative dexamethasone on postoperative analgesia and side-effects: systematic review and meta-analysis. *Br J Anaesth.* 2013;110:191–200.
43. Mirzai H, Tekin I, Alincak H. Perioperative use of corticosteroid and bupivacaine combination in lumbar disc surgery: a randomized controlled trial. *Spine.* 2002;27:343–346.
44. Movafegh A, Razazian M, Hajimaohamadi F, et al. Dexamethasone added to lidocaine prolongs axillary brachial plexus blockade. *Anesth Analg.* 2006;102:263–267.
45. Cummings KC III, Napierkowski DE, Parra-Sanchez I, et al. Effect of dexamethasone on the duration of interscalene nerve blocks with ropivacaine or bupivacaine. *Br J Anaesth.* 2011;107:446–453.
46. Habib GS, Saliba W, Nashashibi M. Local effects of intra-articular corticosteroids. *Clin Rheumatol.* 2010;29:347–356.
47. Bartlett EE, Hutserani O. Xylocaine for the relief of postoperative pain. *Anesth Analg.* 1961;40:296–304.
48. Gordon RA. Intravenous Novocaine for analgesia in burns: (a preliminary report). *Can Med Assoc J.* 1943;49:478–481.
49. Gilbert CR, Hanson IR, Brown AB, et al. Intravenous use of xylocaine. *Curr Res Anesth Analg.* 1951;30:301–313.
50. Backonja MM. Local anesthetics as adjuvant analgesics. *J Pain Symptom Manage.* 1994;9:491–499.
51. Kastrup J, Angelo H, Petersen P, et al. Treatment of chronic painful diabetic neuropathy with intravenous lidocaine infusion. *Br Med J (Clin Res Ed).* 1986;292:173.
52. Woolf CJ, Wiesenfeld-Hallin Z. The systemic administration of local anaesthetics produces a selective depression of C-afferent fibre evoked activity in the spinal cord. *Pain.* 1985;23:361–374.
53. Labbe L, Turgeon J. Clinical pharmacokinetics of mexiletine. *Clin Pharmacokinet.* 1999;37:361–384.
54. Tremont-Lukats IW, Challapalli V, McNicol ED, et al. Systemic administration of local anesthetics to relieve neuropathic pain: a systematic review and meta-analysis. *Anesth Analg.* 2005;101:1738–1749.
55. Kwon YS, Kim JB, Jung HJ, et al. Treatment for postoperative wound pain in gynecologic laparoscopic surgery: topical lidocaine patches. *J Laparoendosc Adv Surg Tech A.* 2012;22:668–673.
56. Meier T, Wasner G, Faust M, et al. Efficacy of lidocaine patch 5% in the treatment of focal peripheral neuropathic pain syndromes: a randomized, double-blind, placebo-controlled study. *Pain.* 2003; 106:151–158.
57. Habib AS, Polascik TJ, Weizer AZ, et al. Lidocaine patch for postoperative analgesia after radical retropubic prostatectomy. *Anesth Analg.* 2009;108:1950–1953.
58. Saber AA, Elgamal MH, Rao AJ, et al. Early experience with lidocaine patch for postoperative pain control after laparoscopic ventral hernia repair. *Int J Surg.* 2009;7:36–38.
59. Tominaga M, Caterina MJ, Malmberg AB, et al. The cloned capsaicin receptor integrates multiple pain-producing stimuli. *Neuron.* 1998;21:531–543.
60. Wong GY, Gavva NR. Therapeutic potential of vanilloid receptor TRPV1 agonists and antagonists as analgesics: recent advances and setbacks. *Brain Res Rev.* 2009;60:267–277.
61. Mou J, Paillard F, Turnbull B, et al. Efficacy of Qutenza(R) (capsaicin) 8% patch for neuropathic pain: a meta-analysis of the Qutenza Clinical Trials Database. *Pain.* 2013;154:1632–1639.
62. Mason L, Moore RA, Derry S, et al. Systematic review of topical capsaicin for the treatment of chronic pain. *BMJ.* 2004;328:991.
63. Mitra S, Sinatra RS. Perioperative management of acute pain in the opioid-dependent patient. *Anesthesiology.* 2004;101:212–227.
64. Mitra S. Opioid-induced hyperalgesia: pathophysiology and clinical implications. *J Opioid Manag.* 2008;4:123–130.
65. Bell RF, Dahl JB, Moore RA, et al. Perioperative ketamine for acute postoperative pain. *Cochrane Database Syst Rev.* 2006;(1):CD004603.
66. Dholakia C, Beverstein G, Garren M, et al. The impact of perioperative dexmedetomidine infusion on postoperative narcotic use and duration of stay after laparoscopic bariatric surgery. *J Gastrointest Surg.* 2007;11:1556–1559.

67. Gurbet A, Basagan-Mogol E, Turker G, et al. Intraoperative infusion of dexmedetomidine reduces perioperative analgesic requirements. *Can J Anaesth.* 2006;53:646–652.
68. Habib AS, Gan TJ. Role of analgesic adjuncts in postoperative pain management. *Anesthesiol Clin North America.* 2005;23:85–107.
69. Rachinger-Adam B, Conzen P, Azad SC. Pharmacology of peripheral opioid receptors. *Curr Opin Anaesthesiol.* 2011;24:408–413.
70. Chen JJ, Dymshitz J, Vasko MR. Regulation of opioid receptors in rat sensory neurons in culture. *Mol Pharmacol.* 1997;51:666–673.
71. Khalefa BI, Shaqura M, Al-Khrasani M, et al. Relative contributions of peripheral versus supraspinal or spinal opioid receptors to the antinociception of systemic opioids. *Eur J Pain.* 2012;16:690–705.
72. Stein C, Millan MJ, Shippenberg TS, et al. Peripheral opioid receptors mediating antinociception in inflammation. Evidence for involvement of mu, delta and kappa receptors. *J Pharmacol Exp Ther.* 1989;248:1269–1275.
73. Shannon HE, Lutz EA. Comparison of the peripheral and central effects of the opioid agonists loperamide and morphine in the formalin test in rats. *Neuropharmacology.* 2002;42:253–261.
74. Mousa SA. Morphological correlates of immune-mediated peripheral opioid analgesia. *Adv Exp Med Biol.* 2003;521:77–87.
75. Heurich M, Mousa SA, Lenzner M, et al. Influence of pain treatment by epidural fentanyl and bupivacaine on homing of opioid-containing leukocytes to surgical wounds. *Brain Behav Immun.* 2007;21:544–552.
76. Labuz D, Mousa SA, Schafer M, et al. Relative contribution of peripheral versus central opioid receptors to antinociception. *Brain Res.* 2007;1160:30–38.
77. Nagasaka H, Awad H, Yaksh TL. Peripheral and spinal actions of opioids in the blockade of the autonomic response evoked by compression of the inflamed knee joint. *Anesthesiology.* 1996;85: 808–816.
78. Stein C, Hassan AH, Lehrberger K, et al. Local analgesic effect of endogenous opioid peptides. *Lancet.* 1993;342:321–314.
79. Likar R, Sittl R, Gragger K, et al. Peripheral morphine analgesia in dental surgery. *Pain.* 1998;76:145–150.
80. Stein C, Kuchler S. Targeting inflammation and wound healing by opioids. *Trends Pharmacol Sci.* 2013;34:303–312.
81. Bigliardi-Qi M, Gaveriaux-Ruff C, Zhou H, et al. Deletion of delta-opioid receptor in mice alters skin differentiation and delays wound healing. *Differentiation.* 2006;74:174–185.
82. Wong GT, Ling Ling J, Irwin MG. Activation of central opioid receptors induces cardioprotection against ischemia-reperfusion injury. *Anesth Analg.* 2010;111:24–28.
83. Rezende RM, Franca DS, Menezes GB, et al. Different mechanisms underlie the analgesic actions of paracetamol and dipyrone in a rat model of inflammatory pain. *Br J Pharmacol.* 2008;153: 760–768.
84. Francischi JN, Chaves CT, Moura AC, et al. Selective inhibitors of cyclo-oxygenase-2 (COX-2) induce hypoalgesia in a rat paw model of inflammation. *Br J Pharmacol.* 2002;137:837–844.
85. Walker JS. Anti-inflammatory effects of opioids. *Adv Exp Med Biol.* 2003;521:148–160.
86. Philippe D, Dubuquoy L, Groux H, et al. Anti-inflammatory properties of the mu opioid receptor support its use in the treatment of colon inflammation. *J Clin Invest.* 2003;111:1329–1338.

CHAPTER 10

Local Anesthetics

Kamal Maheshwari • Mohamed A. Naguib

Local anesthetics are used to provide analgesia and anesthesia for various surgical and nonsurgical procedures. These drugs are also used for acute and chronic pain management, to reduce perioperative stress, to improve perioperative outcomes, and to treat dysrhythmias. Local anesthetics produce reversible conduction blockade of impulses along central and peripheral nerve pathways. With progressive increases in concentrations of local anesthetics, the transmission of autonomic, somatic sensory, and somatic motor impulses is interrupted, producing autonomic nervous system blockade, sensory anesthesia, and skeletal muscle paralysis in the area innervated by the affected nerve.

Karl Koller introduced cocaine as the first local anesthetic in 1884, for use in ophthalmology. Halsted recognized the ability of injected cocaine to interrupt nerve impulse conduction, leading to the introduction of peripheral nerve block anesthesia and spinal anesthesia. Cocaine (an ester of benzoic acid) is present in large amounts in the leaves of *Erythroxylon coca*, a plant growing in the Andes Mountains, where its cerebral-stimulating qualities are well known. Another unique feature of cocaine is its ability to produce localized vasoconstriction, making it useful to shrink the nasal mucosa in rhinolaryngologic procedures and nasotracheal intubation. The first synthetic local anesthetic was the ester derivative procaine, introduced by Einhorn in 1905. Lidocaine was synthesized as an amide local anesthetic by Lofgren in 1943. It produces more rapid, intense, and longer-lasting conduction blockade than procaine. Unlike procaine, lidocaine is effective topically and is a highly efficacious cardiac antidysrhythmic drug. For these reasons, lidocaine is the standard to which all other anesthetics are compared.

Molecular Structure

Local anesthetics consist of a lipophilic and a hydrophilic portion separated by a connecting hydrocarbon chain (Fig. 10-1). The hydrophilic group is usually a tertiary amine, such as diethylamine, whereas the lipophilic portion is usually an unsaturated aromatic ring, such as paraaminobenzoic acid. The lipophilic portion is essential for anesthetic activity, and therapeutically useful local anesthetics require a delicate balance between lipid solubility and water solubility. In almost all instances, an ester(–CO–) or an amide (–NHC–) bond links the hydrocarbon chain to the lipophilic aromatic ring. The nature of this bond is the basis for classifying drugs that produce conduction blockade of nerve impulses as ester local anesthetics or amide local anesthetics (Fig. 10-2). The important differences between ester and amide local anesthetics relate to the site of metabolism and the potential to produce allergic reactions.

Local anesthetics are poorly soluble in water and therefore are marketed most often as water-soluble hydrochloride salts. These hydrochloride salt solutions are acidic (pH 6), contributing to the stability of the local anesthetic. An acidic pH is also important if epinephrine is present in the local anesthetic solution, because this catecholamine is unstable at an alkaline pH. Sodium bisulfite, which is strongly acidic, may be added to commercially prepared local anesthetic–epinephrine solutions (pH 4) to prevent oxidative decomposition of epinephrine.

Structure–Activity Relationships

Modifying the chemical structure of a local anesthetic alters its pharmacologic effects. For example, lengthening the connecting hydrocarbon chain or increasing the number of carbon atoms on the tertiary amine or aromatic ring often results in a local anesthetic with a different lipid solubility, potency, rate of metabolism, and duration of action (Table 10-1). Substituting a butyl group for the amine group on the benzene ring of procaine results in tetracaine. Compared with procaine, tetracaine is more lipid soluble, is 10 times more potent, and has a longer duration of action corresponding to a 4- to 5-fold decrease in the rate of metabolism. Halogenation of procaine to

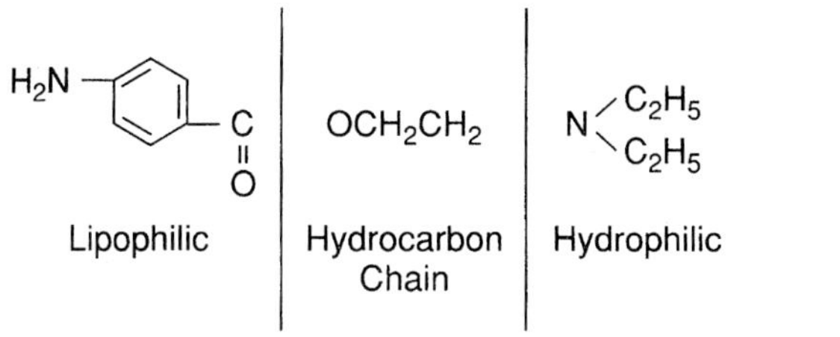

Lipophilic | Hydrocarbon Chain | Hydrophilic

FIGURE 10-1 Local anesthetics consist of a lipophilic and hydrophilic portion separated by a connecting hydrocarbon chain.

chloroprocaine results in a 3- to 4-fold increase in the hydrolysis rate of chloroprocaine by plasma cholinesterase. This rapid hydrolysis rate of chloroprocaine limits the duration of action and systemic toxicity of this local anesthetic. Etidocaine resembles lidocaine, but substituting a propyl group for an ethyl group at the amine end and adding an ethyl group on the alpha carbon of the connecting hydrocarbon chain produces a 50-fold increase in lipid solubility and a 2- to 3-fold increase in the duration of action.

Mepivacaine, bupivacaine, and ropivacaine are characterized as pipecoloxylidides (see Fig. 10-2). Mepivacaine has a methyl group on the piperidine nitrogen atom (amine end) of the molecule. Addition of a butyl group to the piperidine nitrogen of mepivacaine results in bupivacaine, which is 35 times more lipid soluble and has a potency and duration of action 3 to 4 times that of mepivacaine. Ropivacaine structurally resembles bupivacaine and mepivacaine, with a propyl group on the piperidine nitrogen atom of the molecule.

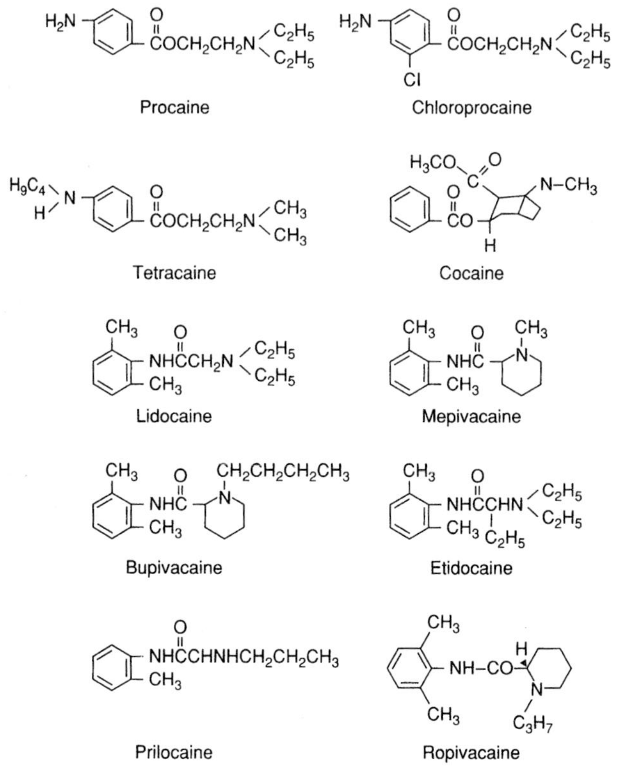

Procaine

Chloroprocaine

Tetracaine

Cocaine

Lidocaine

Mepivacaine

Bupivacaine

Etidocaine

Prilocaine

Ropivacaine

FIGURE 10-2 Ester and amide local anesthetics. Mepivacaine, bupivacaine, and ropivacaine are chiral drugs because the molecules possess an asymmetric carbon atom.

Racemic Mixtures or Pure Isomers

The pipecoloxylidide local anesthetics (mepivacaine, bupivacaine, ropivacaine, levobupivacaine) are chiral drugs because their molecules possess an asymmetric carbon atom (see Fig. 10-2). As such, these drugs may have a left- (S) or right- (R) handed configuration. Mepivacaine and bupivacaine are available for clinical use as racemic mixtures (50:50 mixture) of the enantiomers. The enantiomers of a chiral drug may vary in their pharmacokinetics, pharmacodynamics, and toxicity.[1] These differences in pharmacologic activity reflect the fact that individual enantiomers bind to receptors or enzymes that are chiral amino acids with stereoselective properties. The S enantiomers of bupivacaine and mepivacaine appear to be less toxic than the commercially available racemic mixtures of these local anesthetics.[2] In contrast to mepivacaine and bupivacaine, ropivacaine and levobupivacaine have been developed as a pure S enantiomers.[3] These S enantiomers are considered to produce less neurotoxicity and cardiotoxicity than racemic mixtures or the R enantiomers of local anesthetics, perhaps reflecting decreased potency at sodium ion channel.[4]

Liposomal Local Anesthetics

Various formulation and drug delivery system including liposomes, cyclodextrins, and biopolymers are studied to prolong the duration and to limit the toxicity of local anesthetics. The goal is to upload higher amount of local anesthetic into the molecule and to have a consistent release of local anesthetic in the tissues.[5] Liposomes, hydrophobic-based polymer particles such as Poly(lactic-co-glycolic acid) microspheres and solid polymers such as Poly(sebacic-co-ricinoleic acid) P(SA:RA) and their combination with synthetic and natural local anesthetic are examples of delivery systems currently in development or in clinical use.[6]

Drugs such as lidocaine, tetracaine, and bupivacaine have been incorporated into liposomes to prolong the duration of action and decrease toxicity.[7] Bupivacaine extended release liposome injection was recently approved by U.S. Food and Drug Administration (FDA) for local infiltration anesthesia for hemorrhoidectomy and bunionectomy.[8–10] Bupivacaine extended release liposome injection consists of microscopic, spherical, and multivesicular liposomes and each liposome particle is composed of a honeycomb-like structure of numerous

Table 10-1

Comparative Pharmacology of Local Anesthetics

Classification	Potency	Onset	Duration after Infiltration (min)	Maximum Single Dose for Infiltration (mg)	Toxic Plasma Concentration (μg/mL)	pK	Protein Binding (%)
Esters							
Procaine	1	Slow	45–60	500		8.9	6
Chloroprocaine	4	Rapid	30–45	600		8.7	
Tetracaine	16	Slow	60–180	100 (topical)		8.5	76
Amides							
Lidocaine	1	Rapid	60–120	300	>5	7.9	70
Prilocaine	1	Slow	60–120	400	>5	7.9	55
Mepivacaine	1	Slow	90–180	300	>5	7.6	77
Bupivacaine	4	Slow	240–480	175	>3	8.1	95
Levobupivacaine	4	Slow	240–480	175		8.1	>97
Ropivacaine	4	Slow	240–480	200	>4	8.1	94

Classification	Fraction Nonionized (%) at pH 7.4	Fraction Nonionized (%) at pH 7.6	Lipid Solubility	Volume of Distribution (L)	Clearance (L/min)	Elimination Half-Time (min)
Esters						
Procaine	3	5	0.6	65		9
Chloroprocaine	5	7		35		7
Tetracaine	7	11	80			
Amides						
Lidocaine	25	33	2.9	91	0.95	96
Prilocaine	24	33	0.9	191		96
Mepivacaine	39	50	1	84	9.78	114
Bupivacaine	17	24	28	73	0.47	210
Levobupivacaine	17	24		55		156
Ropivacaine	17			59	0.44	108

Adapted from Denson DD. Physiology and pharmacology of local anesthetics. In: Sinatra RS. *Acute pain: Mechanisms and management*. St. Louis, MO: Mosby; 1992:124; and Burm AG, van der Meer AD, van Kleef JW, et al. Pharmacokinetics of the enantiomers of bupivacaine following intravenous administration of the racemate. *Br J Clin Pharmacol*. 1994;38:125–129.

internal aqueous chambers. Lipid membranes separate these aqueous chambers, and the chambers contain encapsulated bupivacaine. Bupivacaine is released from the liposome particles by a complex mechanism over an extended period (up to 96 hours). In a randomized, double-blind, placebo-controlled, parallel-group study, bupivacaine extended release liposome injection demonstrated a statistically significant reduction in pain through 72 hours, decreased opioid requirements, delayed time to first opioid use, and improved patient satisfaction compared with placebo after hemorrhoidectomy[10] (Fig. 10-3). Bupivacaine extended release liposome injection has also been studied for use in nerve blocks,[11] intraoperative administration in ileostomy reversal,[12] but the results are inconclusive due to smaller sample size. At the time of this writing, bupivacaine extended release liposome injection has limited use, until more conclusive evidence is available for its clinical use.

Mechanism of Action

Local anesthetics bind to specific sites in voltage-gated Na^+ channels. They block Na^+ current, thereby reducing excitability of neuronal, cardiac or central nervous system tissue.[13] Local anesthetics prevent transmission of nerve impulses (conduction blockade) by inhibiting passage of sodium ions through ion-selective sodium channels in nerve membranes.[14] The sodium channel itself is a specific receptor for local anesthetic molecules. Failure of sodium ion channel permeability to increase slows the rate of depolarization such that threshold potential is not reached

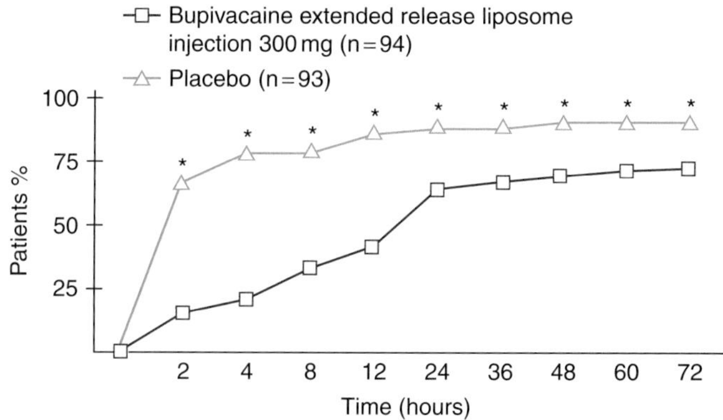

FIGURE 10-3 Time to first use of opioid rescue medication (percentage of patients) after surgery (full analysis set). *$P < .0001$. Bupivacaine extended-release liposome injection for prolonged postsurgical analgesia in patients undergoing hemorrhoidectomy: a multicenter, randomized, double-blind, placebo-controlled trial.[10]

and thus an action potential is not propagated (Fig. 10-4). Local anesthetics do not alter the resting transmembrane potential or threshold potential.

Sodium Channels

The sodium channel is a dynamic transmembrane protein consisting of the large sodium-conducting pore (α subunit) and varying numbers of adjacent smaller β subunits. Nine distinct functional subtypes of voltage-gated Na^+ channels are recognized, corresponding to nine genes for their pore-forming α subunits. These have different tissue distributions in the adult and are differentially regulated at the cellular level by receptor-coupled cell signaling systems.[15] Different isoforms of voltage-gated Na^+ channels, based on biophysical and pharmacologic studies, can provide distinct targets for interventions in various pain syndromes.[16] The large polypeptide that forms the α subunit is further divided into four subunits (DI to DIV) (Fig. 10-5). H is the α subunit that allows ion conduction and binds to local anesthetics. However, β subunits may modulate local

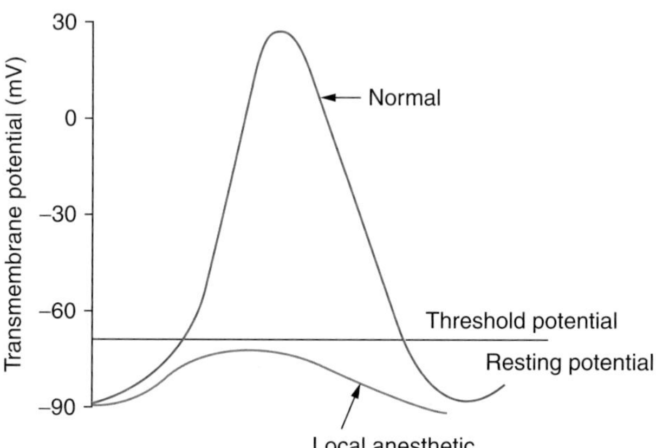

FIGURE 10-4 Local anesthetics slow the rate of depolarization of the nerve action potential such that the threshold potential is not reached. As a result, an action potential cannot be propagated in the presence of local anesthetic and conduction blockade results.

anesthetic binding to the α subunit. Binding affinities of local anesthetics to the sodium ion channels are stereospecific and depend on the conformational state of the sodium channel.[17] Sodium channels exist in activated-open, inactivated-closed, and rested-closed states during various phases of the action potential.[18] Voltage-gated Na^+ channels undergo fast and slow inactivation processes and this is critical for membrane excitability. The structural changes associated with the inactivation process are poorly understood.[19] In the resting nerve membrane, sodium channels are distributed in equilibrium between the rested-closed and inactivated-closed states. By selectively binding to sodium channels in inactivated-closed states, local anesthetic molecules stabilize these channels in this configuration and prevent their change to the rested-closed and activated-open states in response to nerve impulses. Sodium channels in the inactivated-closed state are not permeable to sodium, and thus conduction of nerve impulses in the form of propagated action potentials cannot occur. It is speculated that local anesthetics bind to specific sites located on the inner portion of sodium channels (internal gate or H gate) as well as obstructing sodium channels near their external openings to maintain these channels in inactivated-closed states.[14] This binding appears to be weak and to reflect a relatively poor fit of the local anesthetic molecule with the receptor. This is consistent with the broad variety of chemical structures that exhibit local anesthetic activity on sodium channels.[17]

Frequency-Dependent Blockade

Sodium ion channels tend to recover from local anesthetic–induced conduction blockade between action potentials. Additional conduction blockade is developed each time sodium channels open during an action potential (frequency-dependent blockade). Local anesthetic molecules can gain access to receptors only when sodium channels are in activated-open states and local anesthetic binds more strongly to inactivated state. For this reason, selective conduction blockade of nerve fibers by local anesthetics may be related to the nerve's characteristic frequencies of activity as well as to its anatomic properties

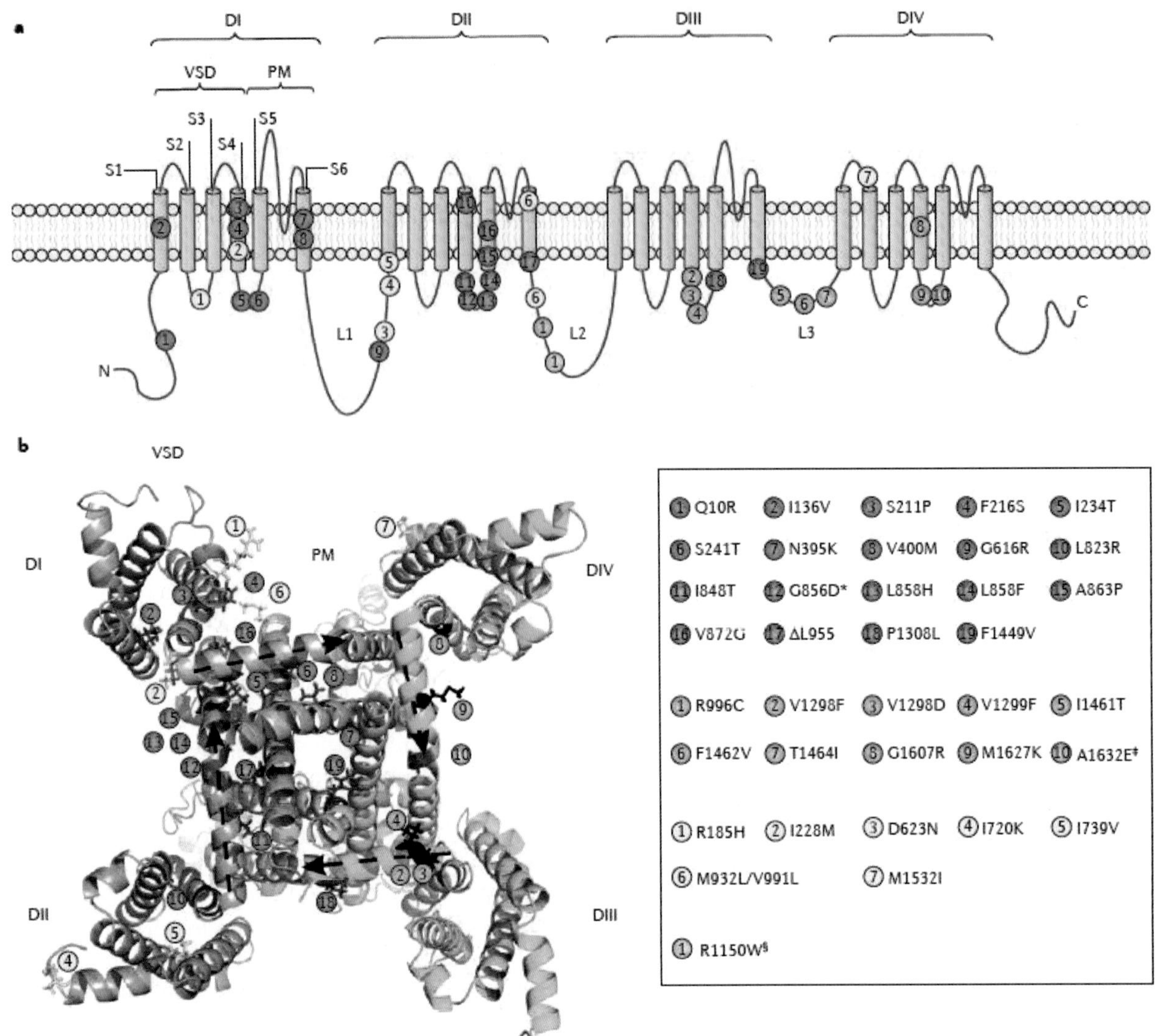

FIGURE 10-5 **A.** The sodium channel α subunit is a long polypeptide that folds into four homologous domains (DI–DIV), each of which consists of six transmembrane segments (S1–S6). The four domains are joined by three loops (L1–L3). Within each domain, S1–S4 comprise the voltage-sensing domain (VSD; S4, depicted in *green*, characteristically contains positively charged arginine and lysine residues), and S5–S6 and their extracellular linker comprise the pore module (PM). The linear schematic of the full-length channel shows the locations of amino acids affected by the gain-of-function *SCN9A* mutations that are linked to inherited erythromelalgia (IEM; *red symbols*), paroxysmal extreme pain disorder (PEPD; *grey symbols*), and small fiber neuropathy (SFN; *yellow symbols*). **B.** View of the folded $Na_V1.7$ from the intracellular side of the membrane based on the recently determined crystal structure of a bacterial sodium channel. The structure shows the central ion-conducting PM and four peripheral VSDs. Conformational changes in the VSDs in response to membrane depolarization are transmitted to the PMs through the S4–S5 linkers (identified by *arrows* through the helices). (From Dib-Hajj SD, Yang Y, Black JA, et al. The NaV1.7 sodium channel: from molecule to man. *Nat Rev Neurosci.* 2013;14:49–62, with permission.)

such as diameter. Indeed, a resting nerve is less sensitive to local anesthetic-induced conduction blockade than is a nerve that has been repetitively stimulated. The pharmacologic effects of other drugs, including anticonvulsants and barbiturates in addition to local anesthetics, may reflect frequency-dependent blockade.

Other Site of Action Targets

In addition to sodium ion channels, local anesthetics block voltage-dependent potassium ion channels. Compared with sodium ion channels, local anesthetics exhibit a much lower affinity for potassium channels. However, blockade of potassium ion channels might explain broadening of the action potential in the presence of local anesthetics. Considering the structural similarity between voltage-dependent calcium ion channels and sodium ion channels, it is not surprising that calcium ion currents (L-type is most sensitive) may also be blocked by local anesthetics.[20] Although local anesthetics are considered principally ion channel blockers, there is evidence that these drugs may also act on G protein–coupled receptors.[21]

Minimum Effective Concentration

The minimum concentration of local anesthetic necessary to produce conduction blockade of nerve impulses is termed the $\boldsymbol{C_m}$. The C_m is analogous to the minimum alveolar concentration (MAC) for inhaled anesthetics. Nerve fiber diameter influences C_m, with larger nerve fibers requiring higher concentrations of local anesthetic for production of conduction blockade. An increased tissue pH or high frequency of nerve stimulation decreases C_m.

Each local anesthetic has a unique C_m, reflecting differing potencies of each drug. The C_m of motor fibers is approximately twice that of sensory fibers; thus, sensory anesthesia may not always be accompanied by skeletal muscle paralysis. Despite an unchanged C_m, less local anesthetic is needed for subarachnoid anesthesia than for epidural anesthesia, reflecting greater access of local anesthetics to unprotected nerves in the subarachnoid space.

Peripheral nerves are composed of myelinated A and B fibers and unmyelinated C fibers. A minimal length of myelinated nerve fiber must be exposed to an adequate concentration of local anesthetic for conduction blockade of nerve impulses to occur. For example, if only one node of Ranvier is blocked (site of change in sodium permeability), the nerve impulse can jump (skip) across this node and conduction blockade does not occur. For conduction blockade to occur in an A fiber, it is necessary to expose at least two and preferably three successive nodes of Ranvier (approximately 1 cm) to an adequate concentration of local anesthetic. Both types of pain-conducting fibers (myelinated A-δ and unmyelinated C fibers) are blocked by similar concentrations of local anesthetics, despite the differences in the diameters of these fibers. Preganglionic B fibers are more readily blocked by local anesthetics than any fiber, even though these fibers are myelinated.

Differential Conduction Blockade

Differential conduction blockade is illustrated by selective blockade of preganglionic sympathetic nervous system B fibers using low concentrations of local anesthetics. Slightly higher concentrations of local anesthetics interrupt conduction in small C fibers and small- and medium-sized A fibers, with loss of sensation for pain and temperature. Nevertheless, touch, proprioception, and motor function are still present such that the patient will sense pressure but not pain with surgical stimulation. In an anxious patient, however, any sensation may be misinterpreted as failure of the local anesthetic.

Changes during Pregnancy

Increased sensitivity (more rapid onset of conduction blockade) may be present during pregnancy.[22] Alterations in protein-binding characteristics of bupivacaine may result in increased concentrations of pharmacologically active unbound drug in the parturient's plasma.[23] Nevertheless, progesterone, which binds to the same α_1-acid glycoprotein as bupivacaine, does not influence protein binding of this local anesthetic.[23] This evidence suggests that bupivacaine and progesterone bind to discrete but separate sites on protein molecules.

Pharmacokinetics

Local anesthetics are weak bases that have pK values somewhat above physiologic pH (see Table 10-1). As a result, <50% of the local anesthetic exists in a lipid-soluble nonionized form at physiologic pH. For example, at pH 7.4, only 5% of tetracaine exists in a nonionized form. Acidosis in the environment into which the local anesthetic is injected (as is present with tissue infection) further increases the ionized fraction of drug. This is consistent with the poor quality of local anesthesia that often results when a local anesthetic is injected into an acidic infected area. Local anesthetics with pKs nearest to physiologic pH have the most rapid onset of action, reflecting the presence of an optimal ratio of ionized to nonionized drug fraction (see Table 10-1).

Intrinsic vasodilator activity will also influence apparent potency and duration of action. For example, the enhanced vasodilator action of lidocaine compared with mepivacaine results in the greater systemic absorption and shorter duration of action of lidocaine. Bupivacaine and etidocaine produce similar vasodilation, but plasma concentrations of bupivacaine after epidural placement exceed those of etidocaine. Presumably, the greater lipid solubility of etidocaine results in tissue sequestration and less available drug for systemic absorption. Occasional prolonged sensory blockade after injection of etidocaine has been attributed to tissue sequestration.

Absorption and Distribution

Absorption of a local anesthetic from its site of injection into the systemic circulation is influenced by the site of injection and dosage, use of epinephrine, and pharmacologic characteristics of the drug (Fig. 10-6). The ultimate plasma concentration of a local anesthetic is determined by the rate of tissue distribution and the rate of clearance of the drug. For example, the infusion of lidocaine for 1 minute is followed by a rapid decrease in the drug's plasma concentration that is paralleled by an initial high uptake into the lungs and distribution of the local anesthetic to highly perfused tissues (brain, heart, and kidneys).[24] Lipid solubility of the local anesthetic is important in this redistribution, as well as being a primary determinant of intrinsic local anesthetic potency. After distribution to highly perfused tissues, the local anesthetic is redistributed to less well perfused tissues, including

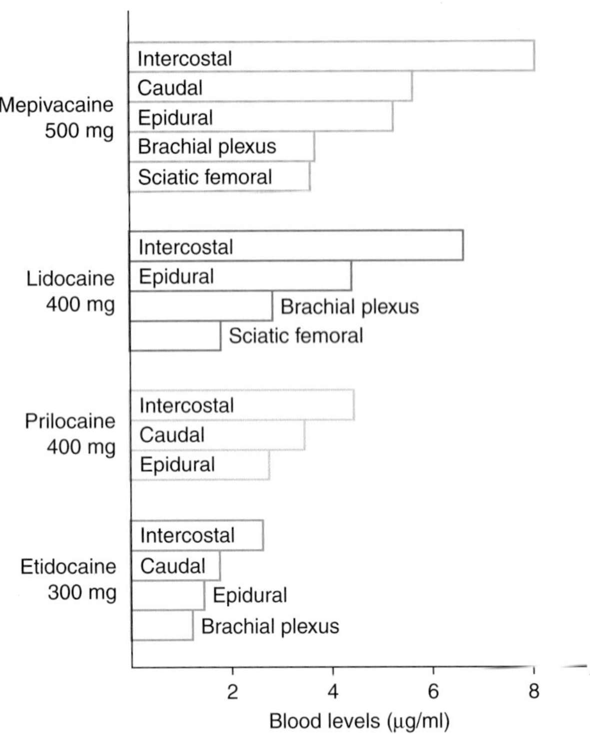

FIGURE 10-6 Peak plasma concentrations of local anesthetic are influenced by the site of injection for accomplishment of regional anesthesia. (From Covino BG, Vassallo HL. *Local Anesthetics: Mechanisms of Action and Clinical Use.* New York, NY: Grune & Stratton; 1976, with permission.)

skeletal muscles and fat. Consideration of cardiac output is important for describing the overall tissue distribution of local anesthetics and presumably their intercompartmental clearance.[25] Ultimately, the local anesthetic is eliminated from the plasma by metabolism and excretion.

In addition to the tissue blood flow and lipid solubility of the local anesthetic, patient-related factors such as age, cardiovascular status, and hepatic function will also influence the absorption and resultant plasma concentrations of local anesthetics. Protein binding of local anesthetics will influence their distribution and excretion. In this regard, protein binding parallels lipid solubility of the local anesthetic and is inversely related to the plasma concentration of drug (see Table 10-1) (Fig. 10-7).[26] Overall, after systemic absorption, amide local anesthetics are more widely distributed in tissues than ester local anesthetics.

Lung Extraction

The lungs are capable of extracting local anesthetics such as lidocaine, bupivacaine, and prilocaine from the circulation.[27] After rapid entry of local anesthetics into the venous circulation, this pulmonary extraction will limit the concentration of drug that reaches the systemic circulation for distribution to the coronary and cerebral circulations. For bupivacaine, this first-pass pulmonary extraction is dose dependent, suggesting that the uptake process becomes saturated rapidly.[28] Propranolol impairs bupivacaine extraction by the lungs, perhaps reflecting a common receptor site for the two drugs.[29] Furthermore, propranolol decreases plasma clearance of lidocaine and bupivacaine, presumably reflecting propranolol-induced decreases in hepatic blood flow or inhibition of hepatic metabolism.[30]

Placental Transfer

There may be clinically significant transplacental transfer of local anesthetics between the mother and fetus. Plasma protein binding influences the rate and degree of diffusion of local anesthetics across the placenta (see Table 10-1). Bupivacaine, which is highly protein bound (approximately 95%), has an umbilical vein–maternal arterial concentration ratio of about 0.32 compared with a ratio of 0.73 for lidocaine (approximately 70% protein bound) and a ratio of 0.85 for prilocaine (approximately 55% protein bound).[31] Ester local anesthetics, because of their rapid hydrolysis, are not available to cross the placenta in significant amounts. Acidosis in the fetus, which may occur during prolonged labor, can result in accumulation of local anesthetic molecules in the fetus (ion trapping) (Fig. 10-8).[32]

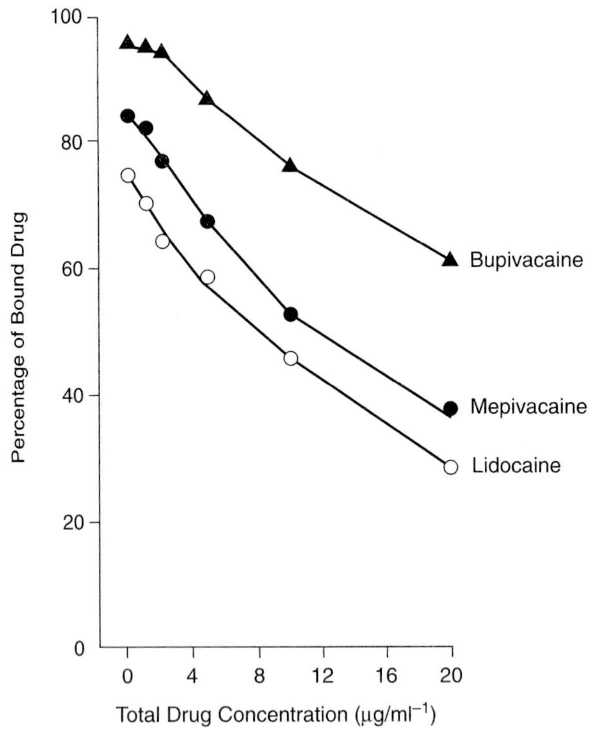

FIGURE 10-7 The percentage of local anesthetic bound to protein is inversely related to the plasma concentration of drug. (From Tucker GT, Boyes RN, Bridenbaugh PO, et al. Binding of anilide-type local anesthetics in human plasma: I. Relationships between binding, physiochemical properties, and anesthetic activity. *Anesthesiology.* 1970;33:287–293, with permission.)

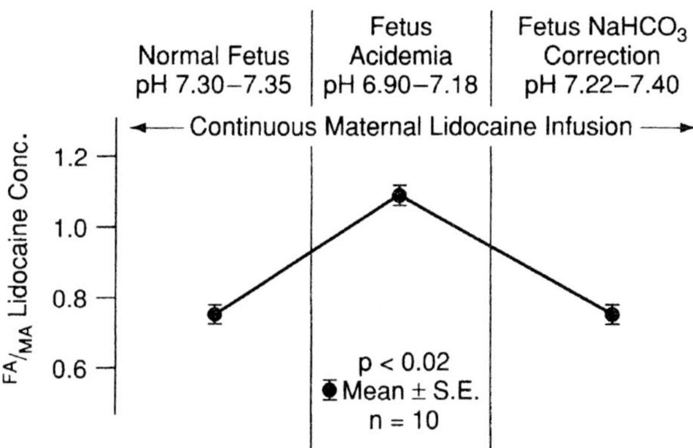

FIGURE 10-8 Fetal–maternal arterial (FA/MA) lidocaine ratios are greater during acidemia compared with a normal pH. (From Biehl D, Shnider SM, Levinson G, et al. Placental transfer of lidocaine: effects of fetal acidosis. *Anesthesiology.* 1978;48:409–412, with permission.)

Renal Elimination and Clearance

The poor water solubility of local anesthetics usually limits its renal excretion of unchanged drug to less than 5%.[33] The exception is cocaine, of which 10% to 12% of unchanged drug can be recovered in urine. Water-soluble metabolites of local anesthetics, such as paraaminobenzoic acid resulting from metabolism of ester local anesthetics, are readily excreted in urine. Clearance values and elimination half-times for amide local anesthetics probably represent mainly hepatic metabolism, because renal excretion of unchanged drug is minimal (see Table 10-1). Pharmacokinetic studies of ester local anesthetics are limited because of a short elimination half-time due to their rapid hydrolysis in the plasma and liver.

Metabolism of Amide Local Anesthetics

Amide local anesthetics undergo varying rates of metabolism by microsomal enzymes located primarily in the liver. Prilocaine undergoes the most rapid metabolism; lidocaine and mepivacaine are intermediate; and etidocaine, bupivacaine, and ropivacaine undergo the slowest metabolism among the amide local anesthetics. The initial step is conversion of the amide base to aminocarboxylic acid and a cyclic aniline derivative. Complete metabolism usually involves additional steps, such as hydroxylation of the aniline moiety and *N*-dealkylation of the aminocarboxylic acid.

Compared with that of ester local anesthetics, the metabolism of amide local anesthetics is more complex and slower. This slower metabolism means that sustained increases of the plasma concentrations of amide local anesthetics, and thus systemic toxicity, are more likely than with ester local anesthetics. Furthermore, cumulative drug effects of amide local anesthetics are more likely than with ester local anesthetics.

Lidocaine

The principal metabolic pathway of lidocaine is oxidative dealkylation in the liver to monoethylglycinexylidide followed by hydrolysis of this metabolite to xylidide. Monoethylglycinexylidide has approximately 80% of the activity of lidocaine for protecting against cardiac dysrhythmias in an animal model. This metabolite has a prolonged elimination half-time, accounting for its efficacy in controlling cardiac dysrhythmias after the infusion of lidocaine is discontinued. Xylidide has only approximately 10% of the cardiac antidysrhythmic activity of lidocaine. In humans, approximately 75% of xylidide is excreted in the urine as 4-hydroxy-2,6-dimethylaniline.

Hepatic disease or decreases in hepatic blood flow, which may occur during anesthesia, can decrease the rate of metabolism of lidocaine. For example, the elimination half-time of lidocaine is increased more than fivefold in patients with liver dysfunction compared with normal patients. Decreased hepatic metabolism of lidocaine should be anticipated when patients are anesthetized with volatile anesthetics. Maternal clearance of lidocaine is prolonged in the presence of pregnancy-induced hypertension, and repeated administration of lidocaine can result in higher plasma concentrations than in normotensive parturients.[34]

Prilocaine

Prilocaine is an amide local anesthetic that is metabolized to orthotoluidine. Orthotoluidine is an oxidizing compound capable of converting hemoglobin to its oxidized form, methemoglobin, resulting in a potentially life-threatening complication, methemoglobinemia (see the section "Methemoglobinemia"). When the dose of prilocaine is >600 mg, there may be sufficient methemoglobin present (3 to 5 g/dL) to cause the patient to appear cyanotic, and oxygen-carrying capacity is decreased. Methemoglobinemia is readily reversed by the administration of methylene blue, 1 to 2 mg/kg intravenously, over 5 minutes (total dose should not exceed 7 to 8 mg/kg). The ability of prilocaine to cause dose-related methemoglobinemia limits its clinical usefulness, with the exception of intravenous (IV) regional anesthesia. Prilocaine causes less vasodilation than other local anesthetics and thus can be utilized without epinephrine added to the local anesthetic solution.

Mepivacaine

Mepivacaine has pharmacologic properties similar to those of lidocaine, although the duration of action of mepivacaine is somewhat longer. Clearance of mepivacaine is decreased in neonates, leading to a prolonged elimination half-time. In contrast to lidocaine, mepivacaine lacks vasodilator activity. As such, mepivacaine is an alternate selection when addition of epinephrine to the local anesthetic solution is not recommended.

Bupivacaine

Possible pathways for metabolism of bupivacaine include aromatic hydroxylation, *N*-dealkylation, amide hydrolysis, and conjugation.[35] Only the *N*-dealkylated metabolite *N*-desbutylbupivacaine, has been measured in blood or urine after epidural or spinal anesthesia. The mean total urinary excretion of bupivacaine and its dealkylation and hydroxylation metabolites account for >40% of the total anesthetic dose.[35] α_1-Acid glycoprotein is the most important plasma protein-binding site of bupivacaine, and its concentration is increased in many clinical situations, including postoperative trauma.[36]

Ropivacaine

Ropivacaine is metabolized to 2,6-pipecoloxylidide and 3-hydroxyropivacaine by hepatic cytochrome P450 enzymes. Both metabolites have significantly less local anesthetic potency than ropivacaine. Because only a very small fraction of ropivacaine is excreted unchanged in the urine (about 1%) when the liver is functioning normally, dosage adjustments based on renal function do not seem necessary. However, in uremic patients, 2,6-pipecoloxylidide may accumulate and produce toxic effects.[37] Overall, clearance of ropivacaine is higher than that determined for bupivacaine, and its elimination half-time is shorter.[3] The higher clearance of ropivacaine may offer an advantage over bupivacaine in terms of systemic toxicity. The lipid solubility of ropivacaine is intermediate between lidocaine and bupivacaine. Ropivacaine is highly bound to α_1-acid glycoprotein.

Dibucaine

Dibucaine is a quinoline derivative with an amide bond in the connecting hydrocarbon chain. This local anesthetic is metabolized in the liver and is the most slowly eliminated of all the amide derivatives. Dibucaine is better known for its ability to inhibit the activity of normal butyrylcholinesterase (plasma cholinesterase) by more than 70%, compared with only approximately 20% inhibition of the activity of atypical enzyme. Atypical plasma cholinesterases account for prolonged effects and toxicity of drugs such as succinylcholine and chloroprocaine that are metabolized by this enzyme. Laboratory evaluation of patients suspected of having atypical pseudocholinesterase is facilitated by measurement of the degree of enzyme suppression by dibucaine, a test termed the ***dibucaine number***. See further discussion of dibucaine in Chapter 12, Neuromuscular Blocking Drugs and Reversal Agents.

Metabolism of Ester Local Anesthetics

Ester local anesthetics undergo hydrolysis by cholinesterase enzyme, principally in the plasma and to a lesser extent in the liver. The rate of hydrolysis varies, with chloroprocaine being most rapid, procaine being intermediate, and tetracaine being the slowest. The resulting metabolites are pharmacologically inactive, although paraaminobenzoic acid may be an antigen responsible for subsequent allergic reactions. The exception to hydrolysis of ester local anesthetics in the plasma is cocaine, which undergoes significant metabolism in the liver.

Systemic toxicity is inversely proportional to the rate of hydrolysis; thus, tetracaine is more likely than chloroprocaine to result in excessive plasma concentrations. Because cerebrospinal fluid contains little to no cholinesterase enzyme, anesthesia produced by subarachnoid placement of tetracaine will persist until the drug has been absorbed into the systemic circulation. Plasma cholinesterase activity and the hydrolysis rate of ester local anesthetics are slowed in the presence of liver disease or an increased blood urea nitrogen concentration. Plasma cholinesterase activity may be decreased in parturients and in patients being treated with certain chemotherapeutic drugs. Patients with atypical plasma cholinesterase may be at increased risk for developing excess systemic concentrations of an ester local anesthetic due to absent or limited plasma hydrolysis.

Procaine

Procaine is hydrolyzed to paraaminobenzoic acid, which is excreted unchanged in urine, and to diethylaminoethanol, which is further metabolized because only 30% is recovered in urine. Overall, <50% of procaine is excreted unchanged in urine. Increased plasma concentrations of paraaminobenzoic acid do not produce symptoms of systemic toxicity.

Chloroprocaine

Addition of a chlorine atom to the benzene ring of procaine to form chloroprocaine increases by 3.5 times the rate of hydrolysis of the local anesthetic by plasma cholinesterase, as compared with procaine. Resulting pharmacologically inactive metabolites of chloroprocaine are 2-chloro-aminobenzoic acid and 2-diethylaminoethanol. Maternal and neonatal plasma cholinesterase activity may be decreased up to 40% at term, but minimal placental passage of chloroprocaine confirms that even this decreased activity is adequate to hydrolyze most of the chloroprocaine that is absorbed from the maternal epidural space.[38,39]

Tetracaine

Tetracaine undergoes hydrolysis by plasma cholinesterase, but the rate is slower than for procaine.

Benzocaine

Benzocaine (ethyl aminobenzoate) is unique among clinically useful local anesthetics because it is a weak acid (pK_a 3.5), so that it exists predominantly in the nonionized form at physiologic pH. As such, benzocaine is ideally suited for topical anesthesia of mucous membranes prior to tracheal intubation, endoscopy, transesophageal echocardiography, and bronchoscopy. Onset of topical anesthesia is rapid and lasts 30 to 60 minutes. A brief spray of 20% benzocaine delivers the recommended dose of 200 to 300 mg. Systemic absorption of topical benzocaine is enhanced by defects in the skin and mucosa as well as from the gastrointestinal tract should any of the local anesthetic be swallowed. The product Cetacaine is marketed as a combination of 14% benzocaine, 2% tetracaine, and 2% butamben in a topical applicator that acts as an atomizer. Methemoglobinemia is a rare but potentially life-threatening complication following topical application of benzocaine, especially when the dose exceeds 200 to 300 mg (see the section "Methemoglobinemia").

Cocaine

Cocaine is metabolized by plasma and liver cholinesterases to water-soluble metabolites that are excreted in urine. Plasma cholinesterase activity is decreased in parturients, neonates, the elderly, and patients with severe underlying hepatic disease. Cocaine may be present in urine for 24 to 36 hours, depending on the route of administration and cholinesterase activity. Assays for the metabolites of cocaine in urine are useful markers of cocaine use or absorption (see the section "Cocaine Toxicity").

Alkalinization of Local Anesthetic Solutions

Alkalinization of local anesthetic solutions shortens the onset of neural blockade, enhances the depth of sensory and motor blockade, and increases the spread of epidural blockade.[40] The pH of commercial preparations of local anesthetic solutions ranges from 3.9 to 6.5 and is especially acidic if prepackaged with epinephrine (increased acidity prolongs the shelf life of epinephrine). The pK_a of local anesthetics used clinically is near 8, so that only a small fraction (about 3%) of the local anesthetic exists in the lipid-soluble form. Alkalinization increases the percentage of local anesthetic existing in the lipid-soluble form that is available to diffuse across lipid cellular barriers. Adding sodium bicarbonate will speed the onset of peripheral nerve block and epidural block by 3 to 5 minutes.

Adjuvant Mixed with Local Anesthetics

Dexmedetomidine has been used as an adjuvant in local anesthetic admixtures and a central effect is postulated for prolongation of the local anesthetic affect. IV dexmedetomidine, in a recent systematic review and meta-analysis, showed increased duration of motor and sensory block and also increased duration for first analgesic request after spinal anesthesia.[41] Magnesium has also shown promising initial results when introduced in to the intrathecal space as an addition to local anesthetic with or without opioids. Duration of spinal anesthesia was increased in magnesium group.[42] In pediatric patients, addition of clonidine and ketamine to the regional anesthesia showed good pharmacokinetic and pharmacodynamic profiles of efficacy and safety, improving and prolonging the action of associated local anesthetics.[43]

Combinations of Local Anesthetics

Local anesthetics may be combined in an effort to produce a rapid onset (chloroprocaine) and prolonged duration (bupivacaine) of action. Nevertheless, placement of chloroprocaine in the epidural space may decrease the efficacy of subsequent epidural bupivacaine-induced analgesia during labor. It is speculated that the low pH of the chloroprocaine solution could decrease the nonionized pharmacologically active fraction of bupivacaine. Tachyphylaxis to the local anesthetic mixture could also reflect local acidosis due to the low pH of the bathing solution. For these reasons, adjustment of the pH of the chloroprocaine solution with the addition of 1 mL of 8.4% sodium bicarbonate added to 30 mL of chloroprocaine solution just before placement into the epidural space may improve the efficacy of the chloroprocaine-bupivacaine combination.[44] Local anesthetic toxicity of combinations of drugs are additive rather than synergistic.[45]

Use of Vasoconstrictors

The duration of action of a local anesthetic is proportional to the time the drug is in contact with nerve fibers. For this reason, epinephrine (1:200,000 or 5 μg/mL) may be added to local anesthetic solutions to produce vasoconstriction, which limits systemic absorption and maintains the drug concentration in the vicinity of the nerve fibers to be anesthetized. Indeed, addition of epinephrine to a lidocaine or mepivacaine solution prolongs the duration of conduction blockade and decreases systemic absorption of local anesthetics by 20% to 30% (Fig. 10-9).[46,47] For bupivacaine, addition of epinephrine also increases the duration of conduction blockade but to a lesser degree and the reduction in systemic absorption is by 10% to 20%. Most local anesthetics, with the exception of ropivacaine, possess intrinsic vasodilator properties, and it is possible that epinephrine-induced vasoconstriction will slow clearance from the injection site, thus prolonging the time the drug is in contact with nerve fibers.

The impact of adding epinephrine to the local anesthetic solution is influenced by the specific local anesthetic selected and the level of sensory blockade required if a spinal or epidural anesthetic is chosen. For example, the impact of epinephrine in prolonging the duration of conduction blockade and decreasing systemic absorption of bupivacaine and etidocaine is less than that observed with lidocaine, presumably because the greater lipid solubility of bupivacaine and etidocaine causes them to bind avidly to tissues. The duration of sensory anesthesia in

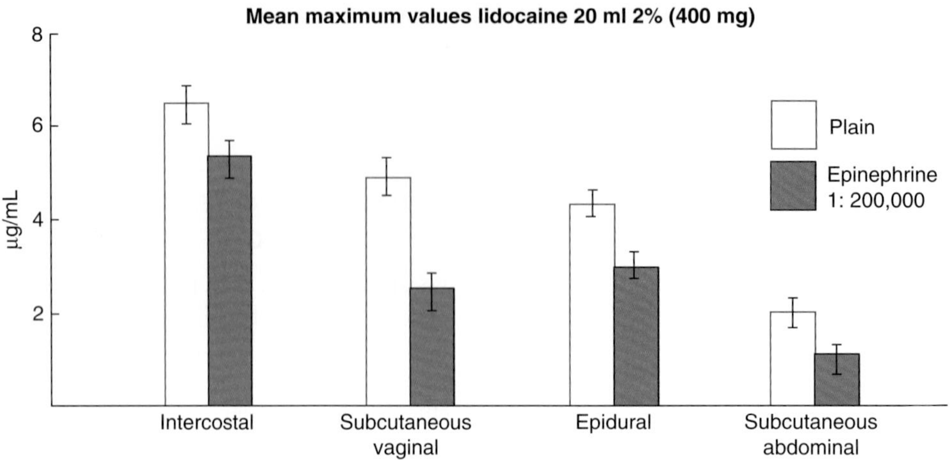

FIGURE 10-9 Addition of epinephrine to the solution containing lidocaine or prilocaine decreases systemic absorption of the local anesthetic by about one-third. (From Scott DB, Jebson PJR, Braid B, et al. Factors affecting plasma levels of lidocaine and prilocaine. *Br J Anaesth.* 1972;44:1040–1049, with permission.)

the lower extremities, but not the abdominal region, is extended when epinephrine (0.2 mg) or phenylephrine (2 mg) is added to local anesthetic solutions of bupivacaine or lidocaine placed into the subarachnoid space. Vasoconstrictors prolong the effect of tetracaine for spinal anesthesia. Epinephrine added to a low dose of tetracaine (6 mg) increases the success rate of spinal anesthesia, whereas the success rate is not altered by epinephrine when the subarachnoid dose of tetracaine is 10 mg.[48] In addition to decreasing systemic absorption to prolong conduction blockade, epinephrine may also enhance conduction blockade by increasing neuronal uptake of the local anesthetic. The α-adrenergic effects of epinephrine may be associated with some degree of analgesia that could contribute to the effects of the conduction blockade. The addition of epinephrine to local anesthetic solutions has little, if any, effect on the onset rate of local anesthesia.

Decreased systemic absorption of local anesthetic due to vasoconstriction produced by epinephrine increases the likelihood that the rate of metabolism will match that of absorption, thus decreasing the possibility of systemic toxicity. Whenever local anesthetic solutions containing epinephrine are administered in the presence of inhaled anesthetics, the possibility of enhanced cardiac irritability should be considered. Systemic absorption of epinephrine may accentuate systemic hypertension in vulnerable patients.

Adverse Effects of Local Anesthetics

The principal side effects related to the use of local anesthetics are allergic reactions and systemic toxicity due to excessive plasma and tissue concentrations of the local anesthetic. Systemic toxicity in association with regional anesthesia is estimated to result in seizures in 1 to 4 per 1,000 patient exposures to local anesthetics, with bupivacaine being the drug most likely to be associated with this adverse response.[49]

Allergic Reactions

Allergic reactions to local anesthetics are rare despite the frequent use of these drugs. It is estimated that less than 1% of all adverse reactions to local anesthetics are due to an allergic mechanism.[50] Instead, the overwhelming majority of adverse responses that are often attributed to an allergic reaction are instead manifestations of excess plasma concentrations of the local anesthetic.

Esters of local anesthetics that produce metabolites related to paraaminobenzoic acid are more likely than amide local anesthetics, which are not metabolized to paraaminobenzoic acid, to evoke an allergic reaction. An allergic reaction after the use of a local anesthetic may be due to methylparaben or similar substances used as preservatives in commercial preparations of ester and amide local anesthetics. These preservatives are structurally similar to paraaminobenzoic acid. As a result, an allergic reaction may reflect prior stimulation of antibody production by the preservative and not a reaction to the local anesthetic.

Cross-Sensitivity

Cross-sensitivity between local anesthetics reflects the common metabolite paraaminobenzoic acid. A similar cross-sensitivity, however, does not exist between classes of local anesthetics. Therefore, a patient with a known allergy to an ester local anesthetic can receive an amide local anesthetic without an increased risk of an allergic reaction. Likewise, an ester local anesthetic can be administered to a patient with a known allergy to an amide local anesthetic. It is important that the "safe" local anesthetic be preservative-free.

Documentation of Allergy

Documentation of allergy to a local anesthetic is based on the clinical history and perhaps the use of intradermal testing. The occurrence of rash, urticaria, and laryngeal edema, with or without hypotension and bronchospasm, is highly suggestive of a local anesthetic–induced allergic reaction. Conversely, hypotension associated with syncope or tachycardia when an epinephrine-containing local anesthetic solution is administered suggests an accidental intravascular injection of drug. Use of an intradermal test requires injection of preservative-free preparations of local anesthetic solutions to eliminate the possibility that the allergic reaction was caused by a substance other than the local anesthetic.

Local Anesthetic Systemic Toxicity

Local anesthetic systemic toxicity (LAST) is due to an excess plasma concentration of the drug. Plasma concentrations of local anesthetics are determined by the rate of drug entrance into the systemic circulation relative to their redistribution to inactive tissue sites and clearance by metabolism. Accidental direct intravascular injection of local anesthetic solutions during performance of peripheral nerve block anesthesia or epidural anesthesia is the most common mechanism for production of excess plasma concentrations of local anesthetics. A variety of factors influence the likelihood and severity of LAST, including individual patient risk factors, concurrent medications, location and technique of block, specific local anesthetic compound, total local anesthetic dose (the product of concentration and volume), timeliness of detection, and adequacy of treatment.[51] The magnitude of this systemic absorption depends on the (a) dose administered into the tissues, (b) vascularity of the injection site, (c) presence of epinephrine in the solution, and (d) physicochemical properties of the drug (see Table 10-1). For example, systemic absorption of local anesthetics is greatest after injection for an intercostal nerve bock, intermediate for epidural anesthesia, and least for a brachial plexus block.[52] Addition of 5 μg of epinephrine to every milliliter of local anesthetic solution (1:200,000 dilution) decreases systemic absorption of local anesthetics by approximately one-third[47] (see the section "Use of Vasoconstrictors"). Systemic toxicity of local anesthetics involves the central nervous system (CNS) and cardiovascular system.

Local anesthetics differ with regard to their CNS toxicity and cardiac toxicity. The cardiovascular/central nervous system (CV/CNS) ratio describes the dose required to produce CV arrhythmias versus that required to produce seizures.[53] If the ratio is lower, it implies a reduced safety margin for the local anesthetic compounds compared to the compound with higher ratio, to detect impending cardiotoxicity based on premonitory CNS signs. Bupivacaine is a more potent local anesthetic and generates arrhythmias at lower concentrations compared with lidocaine and mepivacaine. Also in animal studies (dogs), at comparable dosages, bupivacaine and etidocaine cause severe arrhythmias without decreased myocardial contractility, whereas lidocaine caused the opposite, that is, depressed myocardial contractility without arrhythmia.[54]

Central Nervous System Effects

Low plasma concentrations of local anesthetics are likely to produce numbness of the tongue and circumoral tissues, presumably reflecting delivery of drug to these highly vascular tissues (Table 10-2). As the plasma concentrations continue to increase, local anesthetics readily cross the blood–brain barrier and produce a predictable pattern of CNS changes. Restlessness, vertigo, tinnitus, and difficulty in focusing occur initially. Further increases in the CNS concentration of local anesthetic result in slurred speech and skeletal muscle twitching. Skeletal muscle twitching is often first evident in the face and extremities and signals the imminence of tonic-clonic seizures. Vivid fear of imminent death and a delusional belief of having died have been described in patients experiencing toxic reactions to local anesthetics administered for regional anesthesia and pain relief.[55]

Lidocaine and other amide local anesthetics may cause drowsiness before the onset of seizures. Seizures are classically followed by CNS depression, which may be accompanied by hypotension and apnea. The onset of seizures may reflect selective depression of inhibitory cortical neurons by local anesthetics, leaving excitatory pathways unopposed. An alternative explanation for seizures is local anesthetic–induced inhibition of the release of neurotransmitters, particularly γ-aminobutyric acid. The precise site of local anesthetic–induced seizures is not known, although it appears to be in the temporal lobe or the amygdala.

Table 10-2

Dose-Dependent Effects of Lidocaine

Plasma Lidocaine Concentration (μg/mL)	Effect
1–5	Analgesia
5–10	Circumoral numbness
	Tinnitus
	Skeletal muscle twitching
	Systemic hypotension
	Myocardial depression
10–15	Seizures
	Unconsciousness
15–25	Apnea
	Coma
>25	Cardiovascular depression

Plasma concentrations of local anesthetics producing signs of central nervous system (CNS) toxicity depend on the specific drug involved. Lidocaine, mepivacaine, and prilocaine demonstrate effects on the CNS at plasma concentrations of 5 to 10 μg/mL. The typical plasma concentration of bupivacaine associated with seizures is 4.5 to 5.5 μg/mL.[52] Ropivacaine and bupivacaine produce convulsions in awake animals at similar doses.[3] The threshold plasma concentration at which CNS toxicity occurs may be related more to the rate of increase of the serum concentration than to the total amount of drug injected.[33]

The active metabolites of lidocaine, including monoethylglycinexylidide, may exert an additive effect in causing systemic toxicity after epidural administration of lidocaine. For this reason, it has been recommended that the plasma venous concentration of lidocaine be monitored when the cumulative epidural dose of lidocaine is >900 mg.[56] The seizure threshold for lidocaine may be related to CNS levels of serotonin (5-hydroxytryptophan). For example, accumulation of serotonin decreases the seizure threshold of lidocaine and prolongs the duration of seizure activity.

There is an inverse relationship between the $Paco_2$ and seizure thresholds of local anesthetics, presumably reflecting variations in cerebral blood flow and resultant delivery of drugs to the brain. Increases in the serum potassium concentration can facilitate depolarization and thus markedly increase local anesthetic toxicity. Conversely, hypokalemia, by creating hyperpolarization, can greatly decrease local anesthetic toxicity. The threshold for neurotoxicity of lidocaine may be decreased when patients being treated with the antidysrhythmic drug mexiletine receive lidocaine during the perioperative period.[57]

Cardiovascular System Effects

The cardiovascular system is more resistant to the toxic effects of high plasma concentrations of local anesthetics than is the CNS. For example, lidocaine in plasma concentrations of <5 μg/mL is devoid of adverse cardiac effects, producing only a decrease in the rate of spontaneous phase 4 depolarization (automaticity). Nevertheless, plasma lidocaine concentrations of 5 to 10 μg/mL, and equivalent plasma concentrations of other local anesthetics, may produce profound hypotension due to relaxation of arteriolar vascular smooth muscle and direct myocardial depression (see Table 10-2). As a result, hypotension reflects both decreased systemic vascular resistance and decreased cardiac output.

Part of the cardiac toxicity that results from high plasma concentrations of local anesthetics occurs because these drugs also block cardiac sodium channels. At low concentrations of local anesthetics, this effect on sodium channels probably contributes to cardiac antidysrhythmic properties of these drugs. However, when the plasma concentrations of local anesthetics are excessive, sufficient cardiac sodium channels become blocked so that conduction and automaticity become adversely depressed. For example, excessive plasma concentrations of lidocaine may slow conduction of cardiac impulses through the heart, manifesting as prolongation of the P-R interval and QRS complex on the electrocardiogram. Effects of local anesthetics on calcium ion and potassium ion channels and local anesthetic-induced inhibition of cyclic adenosine monophosphate (cAMP) production may also contribute to cardiac toxicity.[58]

Selective Cardiac Toxicity

Accidental IV injection of bupivacaine may result in precipitous hypotension, cardiac dysrhythmias, and atrioventricular heart block.[59] After accidental IV injection, the protein-binding sites (α_1-acid glycoprotein and albumin) for bupivacaine are quickly saturated, leaving a significant mass of unbound drug available for diffusion into the conducting tissue of the heart. IV injection of bupivacaine or lidocaine to awake animals produces serious cardiac dysrhythmias only in animals receiving bupivacaine. Premature ventricular contractions, widening of the QRS complex, and ventricular tachycardia are the most common arrhythmias seen, though other arrhythmias including supraventricular tachycardia, atrioventricular heart block, and ST-T wave changes can also occur but are less common.[60] Cardiotoxic plasma concentrations of bupivacaine are 8 to 10 μg/mL.[61]

Physiologic changes and concomitant drug therapy may make patients more vulnerable to bupivacaine cardiac toxicity. For example, pregnancy may increase sensitivity to cardiotoxic effects of bupivacaine, but not ropivacaine, as emphasized by occurrence of cardiopulmonary collapse with a smaller dose of bupivacaine in pregnant compared with nonpregnant animals (Fig. 10-10).[3,62] The threshold for cardiac toxicity produced by bupivacaine may be decreased in patients being treated with drugs that inhibit myocardial impulse propagation (β-adrenergic blockers, digitalis preparations, calcium channel blockers).[63] Indeed, in the presence of propranolol, atrioventricular heart block and cardiac dysrhythmias occurred at plasma bupivacaine concentrations of 2 to 3 μg/mL.[61] This suggests that caution must be taken in the use of bupivacaine in patients who are on antidysrhythmic drugs or other cardiac medications known to depress impulse propagation. Epinephrine and phenylephrine may increase bupivacaine cardiotoxicity, reflecting bupivacaine-induced inhibition of catecholamine-stimulated production of cAMP.[64] The cardiac toxicity of bupivacaine in animals is enhanced by arterial hypoxemia, acidosis, or hypercarbia.

All local anesthetics depress the maximal depolarization rate of the cardiac action potential (V_{max}) by virtue of their ability to inhibit sodium ion influx via sodium channels. In isolated papillary muscle preparations, bupivacaine depresses V_{max} considerably more than lidocaine, whereas ropivacaine is intermediate in its depressant effect on V_{max} (Fig. 10-11).[3,65] The resulting slowed conduction of the cardiac action potential manifests on the

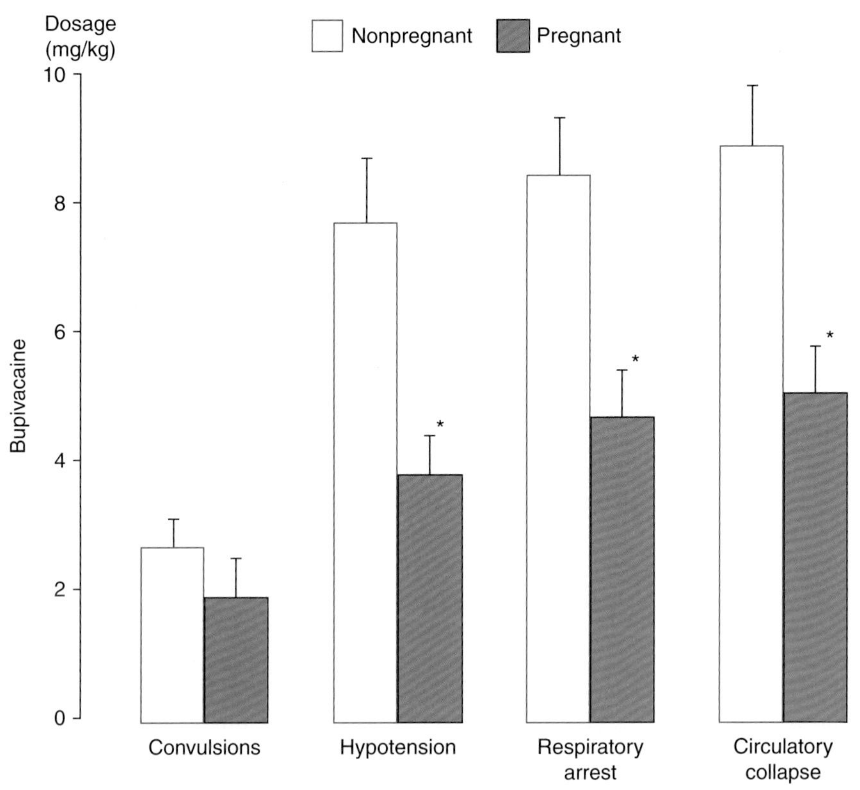

FIGURE 10-10 The dose of bupivacaine required to evoke toxic effects is less in pregnant than in nonpregnant ewes. (Mean ± SE; $*P < .05$.) (From Morishima HO, Pedersen H, Finster M, et al. Bupivacaine toxicity in pregnant and nonpregnant ewes. *Anesthesiology.* 1985;63:134–139, with permission.)

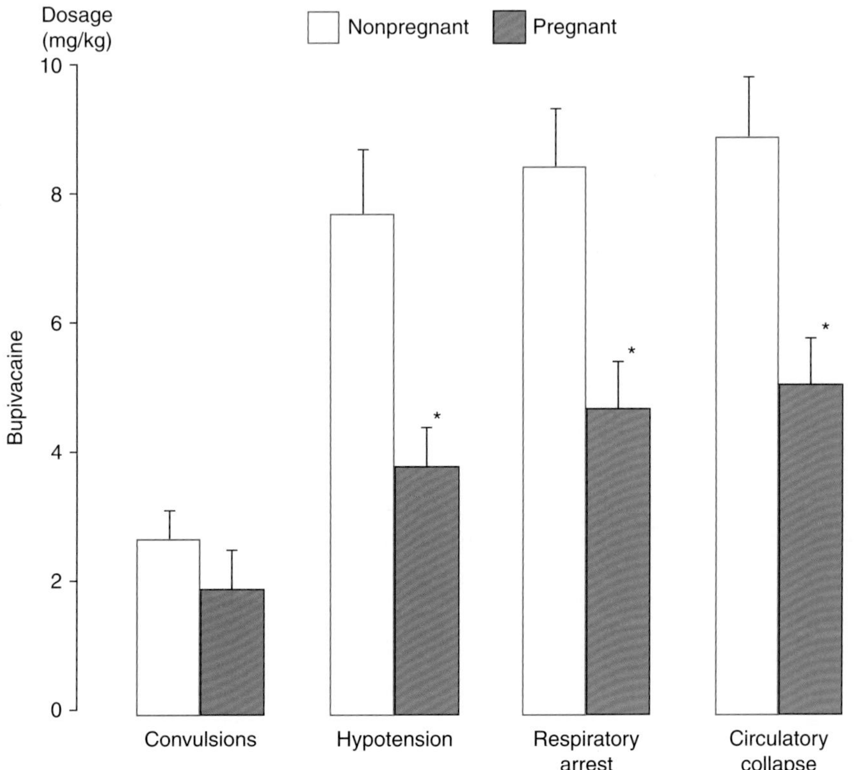

FIGURE 10-11 In an isolated papillary muscle preparation, V_{max} is depressed more by bupivacaine than by lidocaine ($*P < .05$; $**P < .01$). (From Clarkson CW, Hondeghem LM. Mechanism for bupivacaine depression of cardiac conduction: fast block of sodium channels during the action potential with slow recovery from block during diastole. *Anesthesiology.* 1985;62:396–405, with permission.)

electrocardiogram as prolongation of the P-R and QRS intervals and reentry ventricular cardiac dysrhythmias. Both bupivacaine and lidocaine block cardiac sodium ion channels during systole, whereas during diastole, highly lipid soluble bupivacaine dissociates off these channels at a slow rate compared with lidocaine, thus accounting for bupivacaine's persistent depressant effect on V_{max} and greater cardiac toxicity.[66] At normal heart rates, diastolic time is sufficiently long for lidocaine dissociation but bupivacaine block intensifies and depresses electrical conduction, causing reentrant-type ventricular dysrhythmias. Less lipid-soluble lidocaine dissociates rapidly from cardiac sodium channels and cardiac toxicity is low. Furthermore, high plasma concentrations of bupivacaine may cause ventricular cardiac dysrhythmias through a direct brainstem effect. The R enantiomer of bupivacaine is more toxic than the S enantiomer. For example, seizure activity following an interscalene block with levobupivacaine was not associated with cardiac dysrhythmias or other signs of cardiovascular toxicity.[67] In animals, levobupivacaine compared with bupivacaine was associated with a lower incidence of ventricular cardiac dysrhythmias, and successful resuscitation was more likely in the presence of levobupivacaine.[68,69] Ropivacaine is a pure S enantiomer that is less lipid soluble and less cardiotoxic than bupivacaine but more cardiotoxic than lidocaine.[70,71] Although, ropivacaine-induced cardiac arrest has been described following peripheral nerve block anesthesia, in contrast to bupivacaine, cardiac resuscitation is more likely to be successful.[72–74]

Tachycardia can enhance frequency-dependent blockade of cardiac sodium channels by bupivacaine, further contributing to the selective cardiac toxicity of this local anesthetic.[75] Conversely, a low degree of frequency-dependent blockade may contribute to the antidysrhythmic properties of lidocaine. In anesthetized dogs, bretylium, 20 mg/kg intravenously, reverses bupivacaine-induced cardiac depression and increases the threshold for ventricular tachycardia.[76] In an effort to decrease the potential for cardiotoxicity, in the event that accidental intravascular injection does occur, it may be prudent to limit the concentration of bupivacaine to be used for epidural anesthesia to 0.5%. In addition, slow or fractionated administration of all local anesthetics, but particularly bupivacaine, so as to detect systemic toxicity from accidental intravascular injection, should help decrease the risk of cardiotoxicity.[77]

Treatment of Local Anesthetic Systemic Toxicity

Treatment of LAST has undergone swift changes in last decade and includes prompt airway management, circulatory support, and mechanisms to remove local anesthetic from the receptor sites. Treatment should be instituted at the earliest suspicion of toxicity. Treatment of local anesthetic–induced seizures includes ventilation of the patient's lungs with oxygen because arterial hypoxemia and metabolic acidosis occur within seconds.[78] Equally important is the delivery of supplemental oxygen at the earliest sign of local anesthetic toxicity. IV administration of a benzodiazepine such as midazolam or diazepam is effective in suppressing local anesthetic–induced seizures. Propofol can be used for seizure treatment if hemodynamic stability is confirmed. For seizures that are not responsive to initial treatment, use of muscle relaxant such as succinylcholine or nondepolarizing blockers can help prevent acidosis and hypoxia associated with seizures. Early use of lipid emulsion for the treatment of local anesthetic toxicity is becoming standard of care. Multiple published cases have shown that intralipid can be successfully used for resuscitation, the mean total (bolus plus infusion) intralipid dose over the first 30 minutes was 3.8 mL/kg (range, 1.2 to 6.0 mL/kg). The American Society of Regional Anesthesia has published specific recommendations and checklist for treatment of LAST (Fig. 10-12).[51,79,80] Use of lipid emulsion is recommended at the earliest sign of toxicity after airway management. Initial bolus of 1.5 mL/kg 20% lipid emulsion followed by 0.25 mL/kg per minute of infusion, continued for at least 10 minutes after circulatory stability is attained is recommended. Epinephrine should be used at a lower than typical dose 10 to 100 μg during resuscitation, and vasopressin use is not recommended. Calcium channel blockers and β-blockers should be avoided. Nonresponse to treatment should prompt institution of cardiopulmonary bypass (CPB), whenever this modality is available. Prompt institution of CPB, with support of circulation while drug clearance proceeds, has been associated with full recovery from LAST in a number of case reports.

Neural Tissue Toxicity (Neurotoxicity)

Neurotoxicity from placement of local anesthetic–containing solutions into the epidural or subarachnoid space can lead to various complications. The spectrum of this neurotoxicity may range from patchy groin numbness and persistent isolated myotomal weakness to cauda equina syndrome.[81] Myofascial pain may be erroneously diagnosed as transient neurologic symptoms after intrathecal placement of local anesthetics.[82] Overall, permanent neurologic injury after regional anesthesia remains a very rare event.[83,84] Lidocaine-induced increases in intracellular calcium ion concentrations may be the mechanism for this toxicity.[85]

Transient Neurologic Symptoms

Transient neurologic symptoms (TNS) manifest as moderate to severe pain in the lower back, buttocks, and posterior thighs that appears within 6 to 36 hours after complete recovery from uneventful single-shot spinal anesthesia.[86] The etiology of transient neurologic symptoms is not known, but relief of pain with trigger point injections

A. If signs and symptoms of LAST occur, prompt and effective airway management is crucial to preventing hypoxia and acidosis, which are known to potentiate LAST.

B. If seizures occur, they should be rapidly halted with benzodiazepines. If benzodiazepines are not readily available, small doses of propofol or thiopental are acceptable.

C. Although propofol can stop seizures, large doses further depress cardiac function; propofol should be avoided when there are signs of CV compromise. If seizures persist despite benzodiazepines, small doses of succinylcholine or similar neuromuscular blocker should be considered to minimize acidosis and hypoxemia.

D. If cardiac arrest occurs, we recommend standard Advanced Cardiac Life Support with the following modifications:
- If epinephrine is used, small initial doses (10–100 μg boluses in the adult) are preferred.
- Vasopressin is not recommended.
- Avoid calcium channel blockers and β-adrenergic receptor blockers.
- If ventricular arrhythmias develop, amiodarone is preferred.

E. Lipid emulsion therapy
- Consider administering at the first signs of LAST, after airway management.
- Dosing:
  • 1.5 mL/kg 20% lipid emulsion bolus
  • 0.25 mL/kg per minute of infusion, continued for at least 10 minutes after circulatory stability is attained
  • If circulatory stability is not attained, consider rebolus and increasing infusion to 0.5 mL/kg per minute.
  • Approximately 10 mL/kg lipid emulsion for 30 minutes is recommended as the upper limit for initial dosing

F. Propofol is not a substitute for lipid emulsion.

G. Failure to respond to lipid emulsion and vasopressor therapy should prompt institution of cardiopulmonary bypass (CPB). Because there can be considerable lag in beginning CPB, it is reasonable to notify the closest facility capable of providing it when CV compromise is first identified during an episode of LAST.

FIGURE 10-12 American Society of Regional Anesthesia and Pain Medicine recommendations for managing local anesthetic systemic toxicity (LAST). CV, cardiovascular. (From Neal JM, Bernards CM, Butterworth JF IV, et al. ASRA practice advisory on local anesthetic systemic toxicity. *Reg Anesth Pain Med.* 2010;35:152–161.)

and nonsteroidal antiinflammatory drugs suggests a musculoskeletal component. In TNS, the sensory and motor neurologic examination is not abnormal and full recovery from symptoms usually occurs within 1 to 7 days.

The incidence of transient neurologic symptoms is greatest following the intrathecal injection of lidocaine (as high as 30%).[87] Initial reports of transient neurologic symptoms involved spinal anesthesia produced by hyperbaric 5% lidocaine, suggesting that the observed neurotoxicity might be, at least in part, concentration dependent. Nevertheless, the incidence of transient neurologic symptoms is similar after intrathecal placement of 1 mg/kg of either 5% or 2% lidocaine in 7.5% glucose.[88,89] For ambulatory patients undergoing arthroscopy, the incidence of transient neurologic symptoms is not altered by decreasing spinal lidocaine concentrations from 2% to 1% or 0.5% and are similar to the incidence of symptoms described with 5% lidocaine.[90] The risk of transient neurologic symptoms associated with bupivacaine, tetracaine, mepivacaine, prilocaine, or procaine is significantly less than with lidocaine.[91] In a recent Cochrane review, spinal anesthesia with lidocaine was associated with significantly higher incidence of TNS when compared to bupivacaine, prilocaine, or procaine.[92] Also, patients who experienced TNS were less satisfied and had more functional impairment compared to patients who did not experience TNS.

The lithotomy position,[93] early ambulation,[94] and the glucose concentration and osmolarity of the anesthetic solution do not influence the incidence of transient neurologic symptoms.[93] Vasoconstrictors can decrease blood supply to the nerve and there is evidence that adding phenylephrine to the local anesthetic solution increases the incidence of transient neurologic symptoms after spinal anesthesia with tetracaine.[93] There are some clinical data suggesting that addition of epinephrine to local anesthetic solutions does not alter the incidence of transient neurologic symptoms.[95]

Cauda Equina Syndrome

Cauda equina syndrome (CES) occurs when diffuse injury across the lumbosacral plexus produces varying degrees of sensory anesthesia, bowel and bladder sphincter dysfunction, and paraplegia. Cauda equina syndrome is most frequently associated with large central lumbar disc herniation, prolapse or sequestration with 50% to 60% patients having urinary retention on presentation.[96] In the regional anesthesia literature, initial reports of cauda equina syndrome were associated with the use of hyperbaric 5% lidocaine for continuous spinal anesthesia.[97,98]

In these cases, it was postulated that microcatheters used during continuous spinal anesthesia (28 gauge or smaller) contributed to inhomogeneous distribution of the local anesthetic solution, with pooling of high concentrations of the local anesthetic solution on certain dependent or stretched (lithotomy position) nerves. Nevertheless, this same complication has also been reported after intrathecal injection of 100 mg of 5% lidocaine through a 25-gauge needle.[99]

Anterior Spinal Artery Syndrome

Anterior spinal artery syndrome consists of lower extremity paresis with a variable sensory deficit that is usually diagnosed as the neural blockade resolves. The etiology of this syndrome is uncertain, although thrombosis or spasm of the anterior spinal artery is possible, as well as effects of hypotension or vasoconstrictor drugs. Although the addition of epinephrine to local anesthetic solutions has been implicated as a theoretical cause, spinal cord perfusion studies do not show a deleterious effect of the catecholamine.[100] Advanced age and the presence of peripheral vascular disease may predispose patients to development of anterior spinal artery syndrome. It may be difficult to distinguish symptoms due to anterior spinal artery syndrome from those caused by spinal cord compression produced by an epidural abscess or hematoma.

Methemoglobinemia

Methemoglobinemia is a rare but potentially life-threatening complication (decreased oxygen-carrying capacity) that may follow the administration of certain drugs or chemicals that cause oxidation of hemoglobin to methemoglobin more rapidly than methemoglobin is reduced to hemoglobin. Known oxidant substances include topical local anesthetics (prilocaine, benzocaine, and lidocaine), nitroglycerin, phenytoin, and sulfonamides.[101] Neonates may be at greater risk because of more readily oxidized fetal hemoglobin.

Methemoglobin cannot bind oxygen or carbon dioxide, resulting in loss of the hemoglobin molecule's transport function. Methemoglobin normally constitutes <1% of the total hemoglobin. Central cyanosis usually occurs when methemoglobin concentrations exceed 15%. The presence of methemoglobinemia is suggested by a difference between the calculated and measured arterial oxygen saturation. The diagnosis is confirmed by qualitative measurements of methemoglobin by cooximetry.

Methemoglobinemia is readily reversed by the administration of methylene blue, 1 to 2 mg/kg intravenously, over 5 minutes (total dose should not exceed 7 to 8 mg/kg). Methylene blue is reduced to leukomethylene blue, which then acts as an electron donor and nonenzymatically reduces methemoglobin to hemoglobin. Normal levels of methemoglobin should be achieved within 20 to 60 minutes after the administration of methylene blue. This therapeutic effect, however, is short-lived because methylene blue may be cleared before conversion of all the methemoglobin to hemoglobin. Furthermore, continued absorption of highly lipophilic local anesthetics such as benzocaine from adipose tissue stores may continue to occur after methylene blue plasma concentrations are no longer therapeutic.

Ventilatory Response to Hypoxia

Lidocaine at clinically useful plasma concentrations depresses the ventilatory responses to arterial hypoxemia.[102] In this regard, patients with carbon dioxide retention whose resting ventilation depends on hypoxic drive may be at risk of ventilatory failure when lidocaine is administered for treatment of cardiac dysrhythmias. Conversely, systemic absorption of bupivacaine, such as follows a brachial plexus block, stimulates the ventilatory response to carbon dioxide.

Hepatotoxicity

Continuous or intermittent epidural administration of bupivacaine to treat postherpetic neuralgia has been associated with increased plasma concentrations of liver transaminase enzymes that normalized when bupivacaine infusion was discontinued or lidocaine was substituted for bupivacaine.[103] The preservative present in both local anesthetics was the same. Drug-induced liver injury can be a direct toxic injury, an allergic reaction, or idiosyncratic metabolic abnormality. The hepatic dysfunction described seems most likely to represent an allergic reaction.[104]

Uses of Local Anesthetics

Local anesthetics are most often used to produce topical, infiltration, and regional anesthesia.[52,105] Less common reasons to select local anesthetics are to prevent or treat cardiac dysrhythmias, prevent or treat increases in intracranial pressure, provide analgesia, and treat grand mal seizures. Antiinflammatory effects of local anesthetics may be responsible for beneficial effects in the perioperative period that are attributed to spinal or epidural anesthesia.[106]

Regional Anesthesia

Regional anesthesia is classified according to the following six sites of placement of the local anesthetic solution: (a) topical or surface anesthesia, (b) local infiltration, (c) peripheral nerve block, (d) IV regional anesthesia (Bier block), (e) epidural anesthesia, and (f) spinal (subarachnoid) anesthesia (Table 10-3). Maximum doses of local anesthetics (based on body weight) as recommended

Table 10-3

Clinical Uses of Local Anesthetics

	Clinical Use	Concentration (%)	Onset	Duration (min)	Recommended Maximum Single Dose (mg)
Lidocaine	Topical	4	Fast	30–60	300
	Infiltration	0.5–1	Fast	60–240	300 or 500 with epinephrine
	IVRA	0.25–0.5	Fast	30–60	300
	PNB	1–1.5	Fast	60–180	300 or 500 with epinephrine
	Epidural	1.5–2	Fast	60–120	300 or 500 with epinephrine
	Spinal	1.5–5	Fast	30–60	100
Mepivacaine	Infiltration	0.5–1	Fast	60–240	400 or 500 with epinephrine
	PNB	1–1.5	Fast	120–240	400 or 500 with epinephrine
	Epidural	1.5–2	Fast	60–180	400 or 500 with epinephrine
	Spinal	2–4	Fast	60–120	100
Prilocaine	Infiltration	0.5–1	Fast	60–120	600
	IVRA	0.25–0.5	Fast	30–60	600
	PNB	1.5–2	Fast	90–180	600
	Epidural	2–3	Fast	60–180	600
Bupivacaine	Infiltration	0.25	Fast	120–480	175 or 225 with epinephrine
	PNB	0.25–0.5	Slow	240–960	175 or 225 with epinephrine
	Epidural	0.5–0.75	Moderate	120–300	175 or 225 with epinephrine
	Spinal	0.5–0.75	Fast	60–240	20
Levobupivacaine	Infiltration	0.25	Fast	120–480	150
	PNB	0.25–0.5	Slow	840–1,020	150
	Epidural	0.5–0.75	Moderate	300–540	150
	Spinal	0.5–0.75	Fast	60–360	20
Ropivacaine	Infiltration	0.2–0.5	Fast	120–360	200
	PNB	0.5–1	Slow	300–480	250
	Epidural	0.5–1	Moderate	120–360	200
	Spinal?				
Chloroprocaine	Infiltration	1	Fast	30–60	800 or 1,000 with epinephrine
	PNB	2	Fast	30–60	800 or 1,000 with epinephrine
	Epidural	2–3	Fast	30–60	800 or 1,000 with epinephrine
	Spinal	2–3	Fast	30–60	Preservative free[a]
Procaine	Spinal	10	Fast	30–60	1,000
Tetracaine	Topical	2	Fast	30–60	20
	Spinal	0.5	Fast	120–360	20
Benzocaine	Topical	Up to 20%	Fast	30–60	200
Cocaine	Topical	4–10	Fast	30–60	150

[a]Off-label use.

IVRA, intravenous regional anesthesia; PNB, peripheral nerve block.

Adapted from Covino BG, Wildsmith JAW. Clinical pharmacology of local anesthetic agents. In: Cousins MJ, Bridenbaugh PO, eds. *Neural Blockade in Clinical Anesthesia and Management of Pain*. Philadelphia, PA: Lippincott-Raven; 1998:97–128; Foster RH, Markham A. Levobupivacaine: a review of its pharmacology and use as a local anesthetic. *Drugs*. 2000;59:551–579.

for topical or peripheral nerve block anesthesia must be viewed as imprecise guidelines that often do not consider the pharmacokinetics of the drugs.[71]

Topical Anesthesia

Local anesthetics are used to produce topical anesthesia by placement on the mucous membranes of the nose, mouth, tracheobronchial tree, esophagus, or genitourinary tract. Cocaine (4% to 10%), tetracaine (1% to 2%), and lidocaine (2% to 4%) are most often used. It is estimated that topical cocaine anesthesia is used in >50% of rhinolaryngologic procedures performed annually in the United States.[107] (see the section "Cocaine Toxicity"). Cocaine's popularity for topical anesthesia reflects its unique ability to produce localized vasoconstriction, thus decreasing blood loss and improving surgical visualization. There is no difference between the intranasal anesthetic or vasoconstrictive effects of cocaine and those of a lidocaine-oxymetazoline or tetracaine-oxymetazoline mixture, emphasizing the usefulness of these combinations as substitutes for cocaine.[108] Procaine and chloroprocaine penetrate mucous membranes poorly and are ineffective for topical anesthesia.

Nebulized lidocaine is used to produce surface anesthesia of the upper and lower respiratory tract before fiberoptic laryngoscopy and/or bronchoscopy and as a treatment for patients experiencing intractable coughing.[109] The inhalation of local anesthetics by normal subjects does not alter airway resistance and may even produce mild bronchodilation.[110] In contrast, inhalation of nebulized lidocaine can cause bronchoconstriction in some patients with asthma, which may become an important consideration when bronchoscopy is planned in these patients.[109] Local anesthetics are absorbed into the systemic circulation after topical application to mucous membranes. Systemic absorption of tetracaine, and to a lesser extent lidocaine, after placement on the tracheobronchial mucosa produces plasma concentrations similar to those present after IV injection of the local anesthetic. For example, plasma lidocaine concentrations 15 minutes after laryngotracheal spray of the local anesthetic are similar to those concentrations present at the same time after an IV injection of a similar dose of lidocaine.[111] This systemic absorption reflects the high vascularity of the tracheobronchial tree and the injection of the local anesthetic as a spray that spreads the solution over a wide surface area.

Eutectic Mixture of Local Anesthetics

The keratinized layer of the skin provides an effective barrier to diffusion of topical drugs, making it difficult to achieve anesthesia of intact skin by topical application. A popular use of prilocaine is for topical anesthesia when used in a eutectic mixture. A 5% lidocaine–prilocaine cream (2.5% lidocaine and 2.5% prilocaine) allows the use of high concentrations of the anesthetic bases without concern about local irritation, uneven absorption, or systemic toxicity.[112,113] This combination of local anesthetics is considered a eutectic mixture of local anesthetics (EMLA), as the melting point of the combined drugs is lower than lidocaine or prilocaine alone. EMLA cream acts by diffusing through intact skin to block neuronal transmission from dermal receptors. Usually 1 to 2 g of EMLA cream are applied per a 10 cm^2 area of skin and covered with an occlusive dressing. The duration of application varies according to the type of procedure being undertaken and the site of application. For example, skin-graft harvesting requires 2 hours, whereas cautery of genital warts can be undertaken after only a 10-minute application. EMLA cream is effective in relieving the pain of venipuncture, arterial cannulation, lumbar puncture, and myringotomy in children and adults. Pain during circumcision in neonates is attenuated by this topical anesthetic.[113] Although 45 minutes has been suggested as the minimum effective onset time for decreasing the pain of IV cannulation, a significant decrease in pain scores may be noted after only 5 minutes. Low-frequency ultrasound pretreatment is effective in accelerating the onset of EMLA cream.[114] The addition of nitroglycerin ointment to EMLA cream increases the ease of venous cannulation by promoting venodilation.[115] If EMLA cream is used to anesthetize the skin before blood sampling, the results of the analyses of the blood are not distorted. However, the use of EMLA cream to prevent the pain of intradermal skin tests decreases the flare response and may lead to false-negative interpretation of weakly positive tests.

Skin blood flow, epidermal and dermal thickness, duration of application, and the presence of skin pathology are important factors affecting the onset, efficacy, and duration of EMLA analgesia. African Americans may be less responsive than Whites, presumably because of increased density of the stratum corneum.[116] Blanching of the skin may be seen after 30 to 60 minutes, probably due to vasoconstriction. Plasma levels of lidocaine and prilocaine are below toxic levels, although methemoglobin concentrations reflecting the metabolism of prilocaine may be increased in children <3 months of age, reflecting immature reductase pathways. The enzyme capacity for red blood cell methemoglobin reductase in children <3 months of age can be overloaded when EMLA cream is administered concurrently with other methemoglobin-inducing drugs (sulfonamides, acetaminophen, phenytoin, nitroglycerin, nitroprusside).[117] Likewise, EMLA cream should not be used in those rare patients with congenital or idiopathic methemoglobinemia. Local skin reactions, such as pallor, erythema, alterations in temperature sensation, edema, pruritus, and rash are common after EMLA cream application.

EMLA cream is not recommended for use on mucous membranes because of the faster absorption of lidocaine and prilocaine than through intact skin.[112] Similarly, EMLA cream is not recommended for skin wounds, and the risk of wound infection may be increased.[118] Patients being treated with certain antidysrhythmic drugs (mexiletine) may experience additive and potentially synergistic effects when exposed to EMLA cream. EMLA cream is contraindicated in patients with a known history of allergy to amide local anesthetics.

Other Topically Effective Local Anesthetics

Amethocaine, like EMLA cream, requires several minutes to become effective, and the cream must be covered with an occlusive dressing. A microemulsion of amethocaine increases skin penetration and shortens the time until cutaneous anesthesia is achieved.[119] New commercial preparations for topical anesthesia are being developed. Tetracaine in a 4% gel is used to provide topical anaesthesia for venous cannulation and a patch containing 7% lidocaine and 7% tetracaine has been developed to provide topical anesthesia by heat-assisted delivery. They provide comparable pain relief for venous cannulation in 90% of the patients.[120]

Local Infiltration

Local infiltration anesthesia involves extravascular placement of local anesthetic in the area to be anesthetized. Subcutaneous injection of the local anesthetic in the area to be traversed for placement of an intravascular cannula is one example. Lidocaine is the local anesthetic most often selected for infiltration anesthesia. Infiltration of 0.25% ropivacaine or bupivacaine is equally effective in the management of pain at an inguinal operative site.[121]

The duration of infiltration anesthesia can be approximately doubled by adding 1:200,000 epinephrine to the local anesthetic solution. Epinephrine-containing solutions, however, should not be injected intracutaneously or into tissues supplied by end arteries (fingers, ears, and nose) because resulting vasoconstriction can produce ischemia and may result in tissue necrosis.

Peripheral Nerve Block Anesthesia

Peripheral nerve block anesthesia is achieved by injection of local anesthetic solutions into tissues surrounding individual peripheral nerves or nerve plexuses such as the brachial plexus. When local anesthetic solutions are deposited in the vicinity of a peripheral nerve, they diffuse from the outer surface (mantle) toward the center (core) of the nerve along a concentration gradient.[122] Consequently, nerve fibers located in the mantle of the mixed nerve are anesthetized first. These mantle fibers usually are distributed to more proximal anatomic structures in contrast to distal structures innervated by nerve fibers near the core of the nerve. This explains the initial development of anesthesia proximally, with subsequent distal spread as local anesthetic solution diffuses to reach more central core nerve fibers. Conversely, recovery of sensation occurs in a reverse direction; nerve fibers in the mantle that are exposed to extraneural fluid are the first to lose local anesthetic, so that sensation returns initially to the proximal and last to the distal parts of the limb.

Skeletal muscle paralysis may precede the onset of sensory anesthesia if motor nerve fibers are distributed peripheral to sensory fibers in the mixed peripheral nerve.[122,123] Indeed, the sequence of onset and recovery from blockade of sympathetic, sensory, and motor nerve fibers in a mixed peripheral nerve depends as much on anatomic location of the nerve fibers within the mixed nerve as on their sensitivity to local anesthetics. This differs from results of in vitro studies on single nerve fibers, in which diffusion distance does not play a role. In an in vitro model, nerve fiber size is most important, with the onset of conduction blockade being inversely proportional to fiber size. For example, the smallest sensory and autonomic nervous system fibers are anesthetized first, followed by larger motor and proprioceptive axons.

The rapidity of onset of sensory anesthesia after injection of a local anesthetic solution into tissues around a peripheral nerve depends on the pK of the drug. The pK determines the amount of local anesthetic that exists in the active nonionized form at the pH of the tissue (see Table 10-1). For example, the onset of action of lidocaine occurs in approximately 3 minutes, whereas onset after injection of bupivacaine, levobupivacaine, or ropivacaine requires approximately 15 minutes, reflecting the greater fraction of lidocaine that exists in the lipid-soluble nonionized form. The onset and duration of sensory anesthesia for brachial plexus block produced by 0.5% bupivacaine, levobupivacaine, or ropivacaine is similar. Ropivacaine, 33 mL of a 0.5% solution used for performance of a subclavian perivascular block, produces a rapid onset of sensory anesthesia (about 4 minutes) with prolonged sensory (>13 hours) and motor blockade.[124] For ulnar nerve block, ropivacaine was found to be maximally effective at concentrations between 0.5% and 0.75%, and its onset and duration of action resembled those of bupivacaine.[125] Tetracaine, with a slow onset of anesthesia and a high potential to cause systemic toxicity, is not recommended for local infiltration or peripheral nerve block anesthesia.

Duration of peripheral nerve block anesthesia depends on the dose of local anesthetic, its lipid solubility, its degree of protein binding, and concomitant use of a vasoconstrictor such as epinephrine. The duration of action is prolonged more safely by epinephrine than by increasing the dose of local anesthetic, which also increases the likelihood of systemic toxicity. Bupivacaine combined with epinephrine may produce peripheral nerve block anesthesia lasting up to 14 hours. Conversely, not all reports document a prolongation of the duration of action when epinephrine is added to bupivacaine or ropivacaine.[126]

Continuous Peripheral Nerve Blocks

The modern practice of regional anesthesia has moved toward ultrasound (US)-guided peripheral nerve blocks and using perineural catheters for continuous infusions. Use of ultrasound guidance increases the chances for successful block, takes less time to perform, hastens onset, and prolongs block duration when compared to blocks performed with the guidance of peripheral nerve stimulation without ultrasound.[127] US guidance also decreased the risk of vascular puncture during block performance. Continuous nerve blocks have been shown to be associated with improved pain control, decreased need for opioid analgesics, less nausea, and greater patient satisfaction, when compared to single shot blocks.[128] Commonly used medications and their dosages are shown in Table 10-4. Midazolam, magnesium, dexmedetomidine, and ketamine have been used as additives to local anesthetic solutions for peripheral nerve blocks, but they cannot be routinely recommended due to a dearth of supportive data, modest efficacy, and (in the case of ketamine) significant adverse effects.[129]

Table 10-4

Dosage Chart for Common Continuous Nerve Blocks

Block Type	Local Anesthetic	Continuous Rate (mL/hr)	Bolus Dose (mL)	Lock Out Interval (min)	Number of Doses per Hour
Interscalene	0.25% Bupivacaine or 0.2% ropivacaine	8	12	60	1
Supraclavicular	0.25% Bupivacaine or 0.2% ropivacaine	8	12	60	1
Popliteal	0.25% Bupivacaine or 0.2% ropivacaine	8	12	60	1
Femoral[a]	0.12% Bupivacaine or 0.1% ropivacaine	8	0	—	—

[a]Lower concentration used for femoral block to reduce the chances of motor blockade and to prevent falls.

Intravenous Regional Anesthesia (Bier Block)

The IV injection of a local anesthetic solution into an extremity isolated from the rest of the systemic circulation by a tourniquet produces a rapid onset of anesthesia and skeletal muscle relaxation. This has been termed ***intravenous regional anesthesia***, often referred to as a ***Bier block*** after August Bier, who first described the use of local anesthetic in this manner to produce anesthesia of the limb. The duration of anesthesia is independent of the specific local anesthetic and is determined by how long the tourniquet is kept inflated. The mechanism by which local anesthetics produce IV regional anesthesia is unknown but probably reflects action of the drug on nerve endings as well as nerve trunks. Normal sensation and skeletal muscle tone return promptly on release of the tourniquet, which allows blood flow to dilute the concentration of local anesthetic.

Ester and amide local anesthetics produce satisfactory effects when used for IV regional anesthesia. Lidocaine is the most frequently selected amide local anesthetic for producing this type of regional anesthesia. Alternatives to lidocaine include prilocaine, mepivacaine, and ropivacaine. The onset, duration, and quality of IV regional anesthesia produced by 50 mL of a 0.5% solution of lidocaine or prilocaine are similar, but plasma concentrations of prilocaine are lower than those of lidocaine after tourniquet deflation (Fig. 10-13).[130] The associated degree of methemoglobinemia (3% of hemoglobin as methemoglobin) seen with prilocaine is far below the level needed to produce cyanosis (10% hemoglobin as methemoglobin). The significantly lower plasma prilocaine concentrations after tourniquet deflation may indicate a greater margin of safety for prilocaine compared to lidocaine in terms of potential systemic toxicity. Mepivacaine 5 mg/kg provided superior analgesia to lidocaine 3 mg/kg when utilized for IV regional anesthesia.[131] Plasma concentrations of lidocaine decreased significantly in the first 60 minutes following tourniquet deflation, whereas blood concentrations of mepivacaine remained below toxic concentrations. Ropivacaine, 1.2 mg/kg and 1.8 mg/kg compared with lidocaine 3 mg/kg produced comparable IV regional anesthesia but residual analgesia was longer lasting with ropivacaine.[132] Chloroprocaine is not selected for IV regional anesthesia because of a high incidence of thrombophlebitis. Bupivacaine is not recommended for IV regional anesthesia considering its greater likelihood than other local anesthetics for producing cardiotoxicity when the tourniquet is deflated at the conclusion of the anesthetic. Ropivacaine, although less likely to produce cardiotoxicity than bupivacaine, is not recommended for IV regional anesthesia over similar fears that its increased potency may lead to cardiotoxicity at the time of tourniquet release.

Epidural Anesthesia

Local anesthetic solutions placed in the epidural or sacral caudal space produce epidural anesthesia by two presumed mechanisms. First, local anesthetic diffuses across

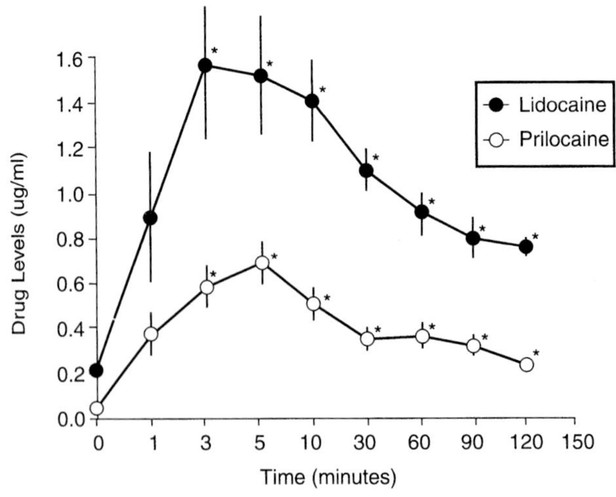

FIGURE 10-13 After tourniquet deflation, plasma concentrations of lidocaine exceed concentrations of prilocaine (mean ± SE; *$P < .05$). (From Bader AM, Concepcion M, Hurley RJ, et al. Comparison of lidocaine and prilocaine for intravenous regional anesthesia. *Anesthesiology.* 1988;69:409–412, with permission.)

the dura to act on nerve roots and the spinal cord as it does when injected directly into the lumbar subarachnoid space to produce spinal anesthesia. Second, local anesthetic also diffuses into the paravertebral area through the intervertebral foramina, producing multiple paravertebral nerve blocks. These slow diffusion processes account for the 15- to 30-minute delay in onset of sensory anesthesia after placement of local anesthetic solutions in the epidural space. Lidocaine is commonly used for epidural anesthesia because of its good diffusion through tissues. Despite a reasonable safety profile, bupivacaine is being replaced by levobupivacaine and ropivacaine, as these local anesthetics are associated with less risk for cardiac and central nervous system toxicity and are also less likely to result in unwanted postoperative motor blockade.

Bupivacaine and ropivacaine at similar concentrations (0.5% to 0.75%) produce similar prolonged sensory anesthesia (ropivacaine has a greater tendency to block A-δ and C fibers) when used for epidural anesthesia, but the motor anesthesia produced by ropivacaine is less intense and of shorter duration.[133,134] These characteristics of ropivacaine may be advantageous for obstetric patients in labor and for those experiencing acute and chronic pain. The addition of epinephrine 1:200,000 to 0.5% or 0.75% bupivacaine or ropivacaine does not appear to offer an advantage in terms of duration of action.[135] Use of 1% ropivacaine may provide longer sensory anesthesia than 0.75% bupivacaine, whereas the motor block is similar.[126,136] The lower systemic toxicity of ropivacaine compared with bupivacaine enables ropivacaine to be used for surgical anesthesia in concentrations up to 1%.[3] For postoperative analgesia, the epidural infusion of 0.2% ropivacaine at 6 to 10 mL per hour is effective.[137] Intermittent epidural bolus technique produces comparable results in analgesia, local anesthetic consumption and maternal satisfaction, when compared to continuous epidural infusion for epidural use in labor analgesia.[138]

In children, there is no difference with regard to postoperative analgesia provided by bupivacaine, levobupivacaine, or ropivacaine but unwanted motor blockade was more frequent in patients receiving bupivacaine (Fig. 10-14).[139] Epidural analgesia or anesthesia for labor or cesarean delivery is similar with 0.5% bupivacaine or ropivacaine but the duration of motor block is shorter in parturients receiving ropivacaine.[140] Likewise, 0.25% ropivacaine and 0.25% bupivacaine administered as intermittent doses into the epidural space are equally efficacious in providing relief of labor pain.[141] The conclusion is that ropivacaine and bupivacaine both provide excellent labor analgesia with no significant differences between the two drugs in the incidence of measured obstetric outcomes.[142] Increased plasma concentrations of local anesthetics after epidural anesthesia are of special importance when this technique is used to provide anesthesia to the parturient. Local anesthetics cross the placenta and may produce

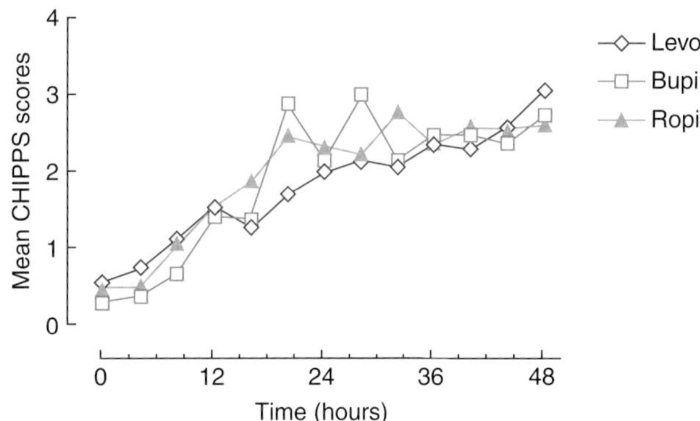

FIGURE 10-14 Mean postoperative pain scores (Children's and Infant's Postoperative Pain Score, CHIPPS) were similar in patients receiving epidural levobupivacaine (levo), bupivacaine (bupi) and ropivacaine (ropi) infusions. (From Negri PD, Ivani G, Tirri T, et al. A comparison of epidural bupivacaine, levobupivacaine, and ropivacaine on postoperative analgesia and motor blockade. *Anesth Analg*. 2004;99: 45–48, with permission.)

detectable, although not necessarily adverse, effects on the fetus for 24 to 48 hours. The fetus and neonate are less able to metabolize mepivacaine, resulting in a prolonged elimination half-time compared with that of adults. Use of a more lipid-soluble and protein-bound local anesthetic such as bupivacaine may limit passage across the placenta to the fetus. Even low doses of lidocaine, such as those used for spinal anesthesia during labor, result in some systemic absorption, as reflected by the presence of lidocaine and its metabolites in neonatal urine for >36 hours.[39] Conversely, bupivacaine is undetectable in neonatal plasma 24 hours after cesarean delivery using bupivacaine-induced spinal anesthesia.[143] Indeed, maternal plasma concentrations of bupivacaine in mothers of those neonates is approximately 5% of that level present after epidural anesthesia, and plasma umbilical vein concentrations are approximately 7% of those present after epidural anesthesia.

In contrast to spinal anesthesia, during epidural anesthesia, there often is not a zone of differential sympathetic nervous system blockade, and the zone of differential motor blockade may average up to four rather than two segments below the sensory level. Another difference from spinal anesthesia is the larger dose required to produce epidural anesthesia, leading to substantial systemic absorption of the local anesthetic. For example, peak plasma concentrations of lidocaine are 3 to 4 μg/mL after placement of 400 mg into the epidural space. Bupivacaine, 70 to 100 mg of 0.5% with 1:200,000 epinephrine placed in the epidural space, results in peak average plasma concentrations of 0.335 μg/mL occurring about 30 minutes after instillation of the local anesthetic.[144] Peak plasma concentrations of bupivacaine near 1 μg/mL occur when epinephrine is not added to the local anesthetic solution placed in the epidural space. Thus, addition of epinephrine to the local anesthetic solution may decrease systemic absorption of the local anesthetic by approximately one-third. The peak venous plasma concentration of ropivacaine is 1.3 μg/mL after epidural placement of 200 mg of the local anesthetic. Addition of 1:200,000 epinephrine solution decreases systemic absorption of ropivacaine by approximately one-third. Systemic absorption of epinephrine produces β-adrenergic stimulation characterized by peripheral vasodilation, with resultant decreases in systemic blood pressure, even though the inotropic and chronotropic effects of epinephrine increase cardiac output.

Addition of opioids to local anesthetic solutions placed in the epidural or intrathecal space results in improved analgesia.[145] An exception to this analgesic synergy is 2-chloroprocaine, which appears to decrease the effectiveness of epidural opioids when administered with local anesthetic solutions placed into the epidural space.[146] Combining local anesthetics and opioids for peripheral nerve blocks appears to be ineffective in altering the characteristics or results of the block.

Spinal Anesthesia

Spinal anesthesia is produced by injection of local anesthetic solutions into the lumbar subarachnoid space. Local anesthetic solutions placed into lumbar cerebrospinal fluid act on superficial layers of the spinal cord, but the principal site of action is the preganglionic fibers as they leave the spinal cord in the anterior rami. Because the concentration of local anesthetics in cerebrospinal fluid decreases as a function of distance from the site of injection, and because different types of nerve fibers differ in their sensitivity to the effects of local anesthetics, zones of differential anesthesia develop. Because preganglionic sympathetic nervous system fibers are blocked by concentrations of local anesthetics that are insufficient to affect sensory or motor fibers, the level of sympathetic nervous system denervation during spinal anesthesia extends approximately two spinal segments cephalad to the level of sensory anesthesia. For the same reasons, the level of motor anesthesia averages two segments below sensory anesthesia.

Dosages of local anesthetics used for spinal anesthesia vary according to the (a) height of the patient, which determines the volume of the subarachnoid space; (b) segmental level of anesthesia desired; and (c) duration of anesthesia desired. The total dose of local anesthetic administered for spinal anesthesia is more important than the concentration of drug or the volume of the solution injected. Tetracaine, lidocaine, bupivacaine, ropivacaine, and levobupivacaine are the local anesthetics most likely to be administered for spinal anesthesia.

Spinal anesthesia with lidocaine has been reported to produce a higher incidence of transient neurologic symptoms than spinal anesthesia produced by bupivacaine (see the section "Neural Tissue Toxicity [Neurotoxicity]"). For these reasons, bupivacaine has been proposed as an alternative local anesthetic to lidocaine for spinal anesthesia.[147,148] If lidocaine is selected, it may be prudent to limit the dose to 60 mg.[148] Bupivacaine used for spinal anesthesia is more effective than tetracaine in preventing lower extremity tourniquet pain during orthopedic surgery.[149] This effectiveness may reflect the ability of bupivacaine to produce greater frequency-dependent conduction blockade of fibers than does tetracaine. In parturients, the intrathecal placement of bupivacaine, 2.5 mg, plus sufentanil, 10 μg, provided labor analgesia and allowed the patients to continue to ambulate.[150] The addition of intrathecal fentanyl 5 μg provides a bupivacaine dose-sparing effect similar to that provided by 15 μg or 25 μg of IV fentanyl, resulting in less pruritus but a shortening of the duration of action.[151]

Ropivacaine, 3 mL of 0.5% or 0.75%, produces sensory anesthesia, although complete motor blockade was present in only about 50% of patients receiving the lower dose.[152] Ropivacaine is an acceptable local anesthetic to produce spinal anesthesia for cesarean section, and decreased lower extremity blockade compared with bupivacaine may be a desirable feature.[153,154] Levobupivacaine has equivalent clinical efficacy to bupivacaine for spinal anesthesia (Fig. 10-15).[155] Dibucaine is 1.5 to 2.0 times as potent as tetracaine when used for spinal anesthesia. In the past, chloroprocaine was not recommended for placement in the subarachnoid space because of potential neurotoxicity.[156–158] However, preservative-free 2-chloroprocaine solutions (2% and 3%) are available for intrathecal injection ("off-label use") and have been shown to produce reliable sensory and motor blockade with a short duration and little or no risk of transient neurologic symptoms, making this local anesthetic an attractive selection for outpatient surgical procedures performed under spinal anesthesia (Fig. 10-16).[159,160]

The specific gravity of local anesthetic solutions injected into the lumbar cerebrospinal fluid is important in determining spread of the drugs. Addition of glucose to local anesthetic solutions increases the specific gravity of local anesthetic solutions above that of cerebrospinal fluid (hyperbaric). Addition of distilled water lowers the specific gravity of local anesthetic solutions below that of cerebrospinal fluid (hypobaric). Cerebrospinal fluid does not contain significant amounts of cholinesterase enzyme; therefore, the duration of action of ester local anesthetics as well as amides placed in the subarachnoid space depends on systemic absorption of the drug.

Injected intrathecally, tetracaine produces a significant increase in spinal cord blood flow, an effect that can be prevented or reversed by epinephrine.[161] Vasodilation is less prominent with lidocaine, and bupivacaine produces vasoconstriction. Predictably, vasoconstrictors appear to be most effective in prolonging tetracaine-induced spinal anesthesia (up to 100%) and less effective at prolonging lidocaine spinal anesthesia, whereas the effect on bupivacaine spinal anesthesia remains controversial and is, at best, minimal.

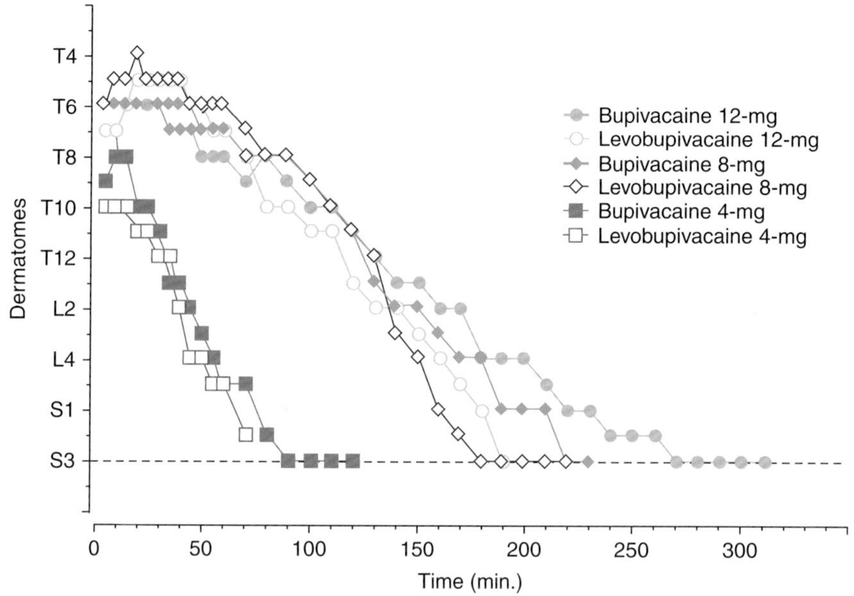

FIGURE 10-15 Recovery from sensory block occurs at a similar rate following spinal anesthesia produced with equipotent doses of bupivacaine and levobupivacaine. (From Alley EA, Kopacz DJ, McDonald SB, et al. Hyperbaric spinal levobupivacaine: a comparison to racemic bupivacaine in volunteers. *Anesth Analg.* 2002;94:188–193, with permission.)

Physiologic Effects

The goal of spinal anesthesia is to provide sensory anesthesia and skeletal muscle relaxation. It is the accompanying level of sympathetic nervous system blockade that produces physiologic alterations. Plasma concentrations of local anesthetics after subarachnoid injection are too low to produce physiologic changes.

Cardiac Arrest

Cardiac arrest may accompany hypotension and bradycardia associated with spinal anesthesia.[84,162,163] The incidence of hypotension is about 33%, and the incidence of bradycardia approximates 13% in nonobstetric populations. Risk factors for hypotension include sensory anesthesia above T5 and baseline systolic blood pressure of less than 120 mm Hg. Risk factors for bradycardia include sensory anesthesia above T5, baseline heart rate less than 60 beats per minute, prolonged P-R interval on the electrocardiogram, and concomitant treatment with β-blocking drugs. Common features of cardiac arrest in patients receiving spinal anesthesia have included administration of sedation to produce a sleeplike state without spontaneous verbalization and lack of early administration of epinephrine. Even when therapy is promptly administered, patients may be refractory to treatment, because local anesthetic-induced sympathetic nervous system blockade, which decreases circulating blood volume, may also cause a defective neuroendocrine response to stress. Even early administration of epinephrine in patients being previously monitored with pulse oximetry and capnography may not guarantee a good outcome following cardiac arrest during spinal anesthesia.[84]

Sympathetic nervous system blockade results in arteriolar dilatation, but systemic blood pressure does not decrease proportionally because of compensatory vasoconstriction in areas with intact sympathetic nervous

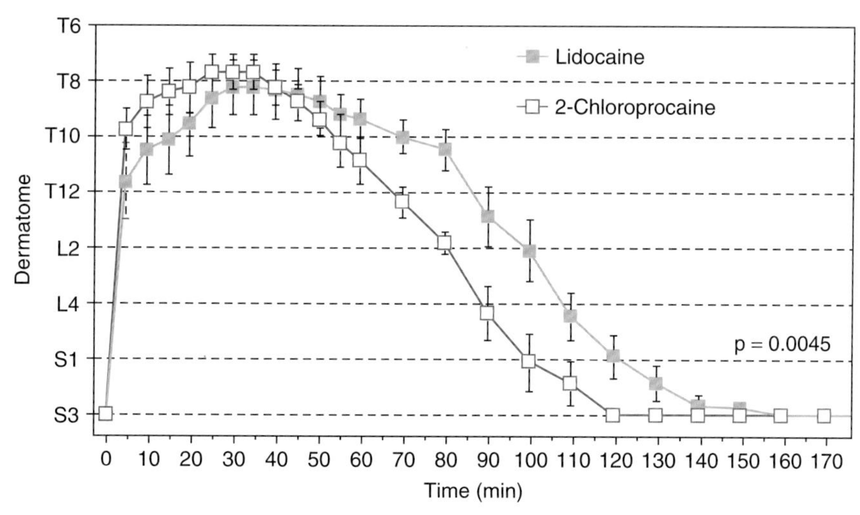

FIGURE 10-16 Recovery of sensory block is more rapid following spinal anesthesia produced with 2-chlorporocaine than with lidocaine. (From Kouri ME, Kopacz DJ. Spinal 2-chlorporcaine: a comparison with lidocaine in volunteers. *Anesth Analg.* 2004;98:75–80, with permission.)

system innervation. Compensatory vasoconstriction occurs principally in the upper extremities and does not involve the cerebral vasculature. Even with total sympathetic nervous system blockade produced by spinal anesthesia, the decrease in systemic vascular resistance is <15%. This change is minimal because smooth muscles of arterioles retain intrinsic tone and do not dilate maximally.

The most important cardiovascular responses produced by spinal anesthesia are those that result from changes in the venous circulation. Unlike arterioles denervated by sympathetic nervous system blockade, venules do not maintain intrinsic tone and thus dilate maximally during spinal anesthesia. The resulting increased vascular capacitance decreases venous return to the heart, leading to decreases in cardiac output and systemic blood pressure. The physiologic effect of spinal anesthesia on venous return emphasizes the risk of extreme systemic hypotension if this technique is instituted in hypovolemic patients. Blockade of preganglionic cardiac accelerator fibers (T1 to T4) results in heart rate slowing, particularly if decreased venous return and central venous pressure decrease the stimulation of intrinsic stretch receptors in the right atrium (Bezold Jarisch reflex). For example, heart rate will increase with a head-down position that increases venous return and central venous pressure so as to stimulate these receptors. During spinal anesthesia, myocardial oxygen requirements are decreased as a result of decreased heart rate, venous return, and systemic blood pressure.

Apnea

Apnea that occurs with an excessive level of spinal anesthesia probably reflects ischemic paralysis of the medullary ventilatory centers due to profound hypotension and associated decreases in cerebral blood flow. Concentrations of local anesthetics in ventricular cerebrospinal fluid are usually too low to produce pharmacologic effects on the ventilatory centers. Rarely is the cause of apnea due to phrenic nerve paralysis.

Analgesia

Lidocaine and procaine have been demonstrated to produce intense analgesia when injected intravenously. Use of local anesthetics for this purpose, however, is limited by the small margin of safety between IV analgesic doses and those that produce systemic toxicity. Nevertheless, continuous low-dose infusion of lidocaine to maintain a plasma concentration of 1 to 2 μg/mL decreases the severity of postoperative pain and decreases requirements for opioids without producing systemic toxicity.[164] Lidocaine administered intravenously also decreases anesthetic requirements for volatile drugs.[165] Lidocaine may also be administered intravenously in the perioperative period as a cough suppressant. In this regard, the cough reflex during intubation of the trachea is suppressed by plasma concentrations of lidocaine >2 μg/mL.[166] Stump pain (neuromas) but not phantom pain (cortical reorganization) following amputation is temporarily diminished by IV administration of lidocaine.[167]

Suppression of Ventricular Cardiac Dysrhythmias

In addition to suppressing ventricular cardiac dysrhythmias, the IV administration of lidocaine may increase the defibrillation threshold. Failure to recognize this effect could lead to unnecessary revision of the lead system of an implantable cardioverter defibrillator.[168]

Suppression of Grand Mal Seizures

Grand mal seizures have been suppressed by IV administration of low doses of lidocaine or mepivacaine. Presumably, these and perhaps other local anesthetics, when present at low plasma concentrations, are effective in suppressing seizures through initial depression of hyperexcitable cortical neurons. Nevertheless, inhibitory neurons are usually more sensitive to depressant actions of local anesthetics than are excitatory neurons, and excitatory phenomena predominate.

Antiinflammatory Effects

Local anesthetics modulate inflammatory responses and may be useful in mitigating perioperative inflammatory injury.[106] For example, overreactive inflammatory responses that destroy rather than protect are critical in the development of several perioperative phenomena including postoperative pain, adult respiratory distress syndrome, systemic inflammatory response syndrome, and multiple organ failure. Beneficial effects attributed to epidural anesthesia (e.g., pain relief, decreased thrombosis from hypercoagulability) may reflect antiinflammatory effects of local anesthetics. Adverse effects of local anesthetic–induced antiinflammatory effects include retardation of wound healing and increased risk of infection. Nevertheless, there is evidence that local anesthetics also possess significant antibacterial effects (tetracaine > bupivacaine > lidocaine).[169] IV lidocaine has been postulated to decrease perioperative stress and improve anesthetic depth. Effect on depth of anesthesia, of IV lidocaine, as measured by bispectral index (BIS) was studied in the presence or absence of midazolam. IV lidocaine decreased BIS by modulating the effect of midazolam, suggesting an increase in the depth of anesthesia.[170]

Mechanism

Antiinflammatory effects of local anesthetics are not dependent on the sodium ion channel blockade that is responsible for the anesthetic effects of these drugs. Local anesthetics may modulate inflammatory responses by inhibiting inflammatory mediator signaling. For example, local anesthetics inhibit platelet-activating factor (an inflammatory mediator), which is an established signaling mechanism in early acute respiratory distress syndrome, a typical postoperative inflammatory disorder.[171] Many of the mediators (thrombin, thromboxane, platelet-activating factor, and interleukins) of the inflammatory and hemostatic systems act through G protein–coupled receptors. Local anesthetics may inhibit G proteins, resulting in antiinflammatory effects.[172] In addition, local anesthetics inhibit neutrophil accumulation at sites of inflammation and impair free radical and mediator release.[173] Local anesthetics in clinically relevant concentrations inhibit superoxide anion production of platelet-activating factor–primed neutrophils.[171] Priming is the process whereby the response of neutrophils to a subsequent activating stimulus is potentiated. Levobupivacaine is more effective than bupivacaine and other local anesthetics in suppressing neutrophil priming.[174] Decreased generation of reactive oxygen radicals is associated with decreases in ischemic damage after myocardial infarction.

Bronchodilation

Inhaled lidocaine and ropivacaine attenuate histamine-induced bronchospasm and induce airway anesthesia. This response most likely reflects topical airway anesthesia, as bronchial reactivity is inhibited at plasma concentrations that are lower than those needed to attenuate bronchial reactivity. Nevertheless, dyclonine, a longer lasting and more potent local anesthetic, does not reliably attenuate bronchial hyperreactivity, suggesting that other properties of local anesthetics may be important.[175]

Tumescent Liposuction

The "tumescent" technique for liposuction is carried out via the subcutaneous infiltration of large volumes (5 or more liters) of solution containing highly diluted lidocaine (0.05% to 0.10%) with epinephrine (1:100,000). The taut stretching of overlying blanched skin by the large volume of solution and epinephrine-induced vasoconstriction is the origin of the term ***tumescent technique***.

The result is sufficient local anesthesia for the liposuction, virtually bloodless aspirates, and prolonged postoperative analgesia. Slow and sustained release of lidocaine into the circulation is associated with plasma concentrations <1.5 μg/mL that peak 12 to 14 hours after injection and then decline gradually over the next 6 to 14 hours.[176] Plasma concentrations of epinephrine peak at three to five times the upper normal limits approximately 3 hours following injection of the solution and return to normal after about 12 hours.[177] The recommended adult dose of lidocaine with epinephrine for regional anesthesia is about 7 mg/kg. When highly diluted lidocaine solutions are administered for tumescent liposuction, the dose of lidocaine may range from 35 to 55 mg/kg ("mega-dose lidocaine").[178] It is estimated that 1 g of subcutaneous tissue can absorb up to 1 mg of lidocaine ("tissue buffering system"). The injection of additional undiluted lidocaine for concomitant cosmetic procedures must be considered in estimating the likely plasma concentrations of lidocaine that will occur.

Tumescent liposuction is commonly used in aesthetic contouring of thigh, abdomen, hip and buttocks and its use is increasing in reconstructive plastic surgery procedures. Despite the popularity and presumed safety of tumescent liposuction, there are reports of increased mortality associated with this technique (greater than mortality associated with automobile accidents).[179] Causes of death may include lidocaine toxicity or local anesthetic–induced depression of cardiac conduction and contractility. Overall complication rate in a nationwide quality improvement study was 0.7% in which 0.57% was minor complications and 0.14% was major complications.[180,181]

Cocaine Toxicity

Cocaine abuse and intoxication is widespread across the globe. In the United States, 1.5 million (2010) adults use cocaine; in Europe, 4 million (2009) adults use cocaine.[182] Cocaine produces sympathetic nervous system stimulation by blocking the presynaptic uptake of norepinephrine and dopamine, thus increasing their postsynaptic concentrations. Because of this blocking effect, dopamine remains at high concentrations in the synapse and continues to affect adjacent neurons, producing the characteristic cocaine "high."[183,184] Chronic exposure to cocaine is postulated to affect adversely dopaminergic function in the brain due to dopamine depletion.

Pharmacokinetics

Once cocaine is absorbed, the pharmacokinetics, regardless of the route of administration, are similar.[185] Conversely, the route of administration is important in the rate of onset as well as the intensity and duration of cocaine's effects. For example, peak venous plasma concentrations of cocaine are achieved at approximately 30 to 40 minutes after intranasal administration and approximately 5 minutes after IV and smoked cocaine administration. The maximum physiologic effects of intranasal cocaine occur within 15 to 40 minutes, and the maximum subjective effects occur within 10 to 20 minutes. The duration of effects is approximately 60 minutes or longer after peak effects. The subjective effects occur within minutes of IV or smoked cocaine use, and the duration of effect is approximately 30 to 45 minutes. The elimination half-time of cocaine is 60 to 90 minutes, and metabolism is principally by plasma esterases (see the section "Metabolism of Ester Local Anesthetics"). Urinary excretion of unchanged cocaine (typically <1% of the total dose but may reach 10% to 12%) and metabolites (benzoylecgonine and ecgonine methyl ester representing about 65% of the dose) is similar regardless of the route of administration.

Adverse Physiologic Effects

Acute cocaine administration has local anesthetic, vasoconstrictive and sympathomimetic effects. Cardiac function is adversely affected and cocaine is known to cause coronary vasospasm, myocardial ischemia, myocardial infarction,

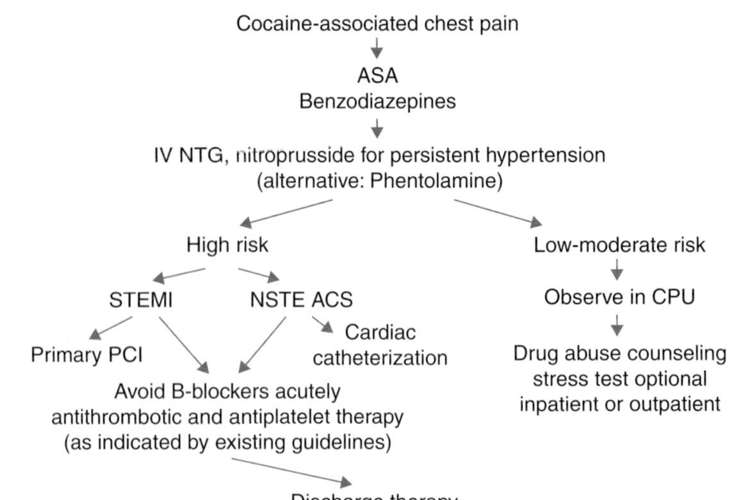

FIGURE 10-17 Therapeutic and diagnostic recommendations in cocaine-associated chest pain. ASA, acetylsalicylic acid; IV NTG, intravenous nitroglycerin; STEMI, ST-segment elevation myocardial infarction; NSTE ACS, Non–ST-segment elevation acute coronary syndrome; PCI, percutaneous coronary intervention; CPU, chest pain unit; ACE, angiotensin-converting enzyme.

and ventricular cardiac dysrhythmias, including ventricular fibrillation.[186] Associated hypertension and tachycardia further increase myocardial oxygen requirements at a time when coronary oxygen delivery is decreased by the effects of cocaine on coronary blood flow. Even remote cocaine use can result in myocardial ischemia and hypotension for as long as 6 weeks after discontinuing cocaine use.[187,188] Presumably, delayed episodes of myocardial ischemia are due to cocaine-induced coronary artery vasospasm. In animals, chronic cocaine exposure sensitizes the left anterior descending coronary artery to catecholamines, even in the absence of circulating cocaine. Excessive sensitivity of the coronary vasculature to catecholamines after chronic exposure to cocaine may be due in part to cocaine-induced depletion of dopamine activity. Cocaine-abusing parturients are at higher risk for interim peripartum events such as hypertension, hypotension, and wheezing episodes.[189] Cocaine produces dose-dependent decreases in uterine blood flow that result in fetal hypoxemia.[190]

Cocaine may produce hyperpyrexia, which could contribute to seizures. Unexpected patient agitation in the perioperative period may reflect the effects of cocaine ingestion.[191] There is a temporal relationship between the recreational use of cocaine and cerebrovascular accidents.[192] Administration of topical cocaine plus epinephrine, or the presence of volatile anesthetics that sensitize the myocardium, may exaggerate the cardiac-stimulating effects of cocaine. Cocaine should be used with caution, if at all, in patients with hypertension or coronary artery disease and in patients receiving drugs that potentiate the effects of catecholamines, such as monoamine oxidase inhibitors.

Treatment

Nitroglycerin has been used to treat cocaine-induced myocardial ischemia.[193] Although esmolol has been recommended to treat tachycardia due to cocaine overdose, there is also evidence that β-adrenergic blockade accentuates coronary artery vasospasm in the setting of acute cocaine overdose.[107,194] Whether β-adrenergic blockade is harmful for coronary vasospasm in the setting of chronic cocaine use is not known. Furthermore, administration of β-blocking drugs in the presence of catecholamine-induced hypertension and tachycardia has been associated with profound cardiovascular collapse and cardiac arrest that is unresponsive to aggressive cardiopulmonary resuscitation.[195] In this situation, administration of a vasodilating drug such as nitroprusside may be the safest intervention. α-Adrenergic blockade may be effective in treatment of coronary vasoconstriction due to cocaine, but in the presence of hypotension, this intervention is questionable.

In 2008, the American Heart Association published a statement for management of cocaine-associated chest pain and myocardial infarction[196] (Fig. 10-17). In addition to their beneficial effect in seizure control, benzodiazepines also help in acute coronary syndromes by relieving chest pain and improving hemodynamic profile. Nitroglycerin and phentolamine is useful in reversing coronary vasoconstriction.

References

1. Ehrlich GE. Racemic mixtures: harmless or potentially toxic? *Am J Hosp Pharm*. 1992;49:S15–S18.
2. Burm AG, Cohen IM, van Kleef JW, et al. Pharmacokinetics of the enantiomers of mepivacaine after intravenous administration of the racemate in volunteers. *Anesth Analg*. 1997;84:85–89.
3. McClure JH. Ropivacaine. *Br J Anaesth*. 1996;76:300–307.
4. Vladimirov M, Nau C, Mok WM, et al. Potency of bupivacaine stereoisomers tested in vitro and in vivo: biochemical, electrophysiological, and neurobehavioral studies. *Anesthesiology*. 2000; 93:744–755.

5. De Paula E, Cereda CM, Fraceto LF, et al. Micro and nanosystems for delivering local anesthetics. *Exp Opin Drug Deliv*. 2012;9: 1505–1524.
6. Weiniger CF, Golovanevski L, Domb AJ, et al. Extended release formulations for local anaesthetic agents. *Anaesthesia*. 2012;67: 906–916.
7. Mowat JJ, Mok MJ, MacLeod BA, et al. Liposomal bupivacaine. Extended duration nerve blockade using large unilamellar vesicles that exhibit a proton gradient. *Anesthesiology*. 1996;85:635–643.
8. Viscusi ER, Sinatra R, Onel E, et al. The safety of liposome bupivacaine, a novel local analgesic formulation. *Clin J Pain*. 2014; 30:102–110.
9. Candiotti K. Liposomal bupivacaine: an innovative nonopioid local analgesic for the management of postsurgical pain. *Pharmacotherapy*. 2012;32:19s–26s.
10. Barreveld A, Witte J, Chahal H, et al. Preventive analgesia by local anesthetics: the reduction of postoperative pain by peripheral nerve blocks and intravenous drugs. *Anesth Analg*. 2013;116:1141–1161.
11. Ilfeld BM, Malhotra N, Furnish TJ, et al. Liposomal bupivacaine as a single-injection peripheral nerve block: a dose-response study. *Anesth Analg*. 2013;117:1248–1256.
12. Marcet JE, Nfonsam VN, Larach S. An extended pain relief trial utilizing the infiltration of a long-acting multivesicular liposome formulation of bupivacaine, EXPAREL (IMPROVE): a phase IV health economic trial in adult patients undergoing ileostomy reversal. *J Pain Res*. 2013;6:549–555.
13. Nau C, Wang GK. Interactions of local anesthetics with voltage-gated Na+ channels. *J Membr Biol*. 2004;201:1–8.
14. Butterworth JF IV, Strichartz GR. Molecular mechanisms of local anesthesia: a review. *Anesthesiology*. 1990;72:711–734.
15. Docherty RJ, Farmer CE. The pharmacology of voltage-gated sodium channels in sensory neurones. *Handb Exp Pharmacol*. 2009;519–561.
16. Dib-Hajj SD, Yang Y, Black JA, et al. The NaV1.7 sodium channel: from molecule to man. *Nat Rev Neurosci*. 2013;14:49–62.
17. Lee-Son S, Wang GK, Concus A, et al. Stereoselective inhibition of neuronal sodium channels by local anesthetics. Evidence for two sites of action? *Anesthesiology*. 1992;77:324–335.
18. Bahring R, Covarrubias M. Mechanisms of closed-state inactivation in voltage-gated ion channels. *J Physiol*. 2011;589:461–479.
19. Payandeh J, Gamal El-Din TM, Scheuer T, et al. Crystal structure of a voltage-gated sodium channel in two potentially inactivated states. *Nature*. 2012;486:135–139.
20. Sugiyama K, Muteki T. Local anesthetics depress the calcium current of rat sensory neurons in culture. *Anesthesiology*. 1994;80: 1369–1378.
21. Hollmann MW, Wieczorek KS, Berger A, et al. Local anesthetic inhibition of G protein-coupled receptor signaling by interference with Galpha(q) protein function. *Mol Pharmacol*. 2001;59:294–301.
22. Datta S, Lambert DH, Gregus J, et al. Differential sensitivities of mammalian nerve fibers during pregnancy. *Anesth Analg*. 1983;62: 1070–1072.
23. Denson DD, Coyle DE, Thompson GA, et al. Bupivacaine protein binding in the term parturient: effects of lactic acidosis. *Clin Pharmacol Therapeut*. 1984;35:702–709.
24. Benowitz N, Forsyth FP, Melmon KL, et al. Lidocaine disposition kinetics in monkey and man. I. Prediction by a perfusion model. *Clin Pharmacol Ther*. 1974;16:87–98.
25. Kuipers JA, Boer F, de Roode A, et al. Modeling population pharmacokinetics of lidocaine: should cardiac output be included as a patient factor? *Anesthesiology*. 2001;94:566–573.
26. Tucker GT, Boyes RN, Bridenbaugh PO, et al. Binding of anilide-type local anesthetics in human plasma. I. Relationships between binding, physicochemical properties, and anesthetic activity. *Anesthesiology*. 1970;33:287–303.
27. Jorfeldt L, Lewis DH, Lofstrom JB, et al. Lung uptake of lidocaine in man as influenced by anaesthesia, mepivacaine infusion or lung insufficiency. *Acta Anaesthesiol Scand*. 1983;27:5–9.
28. Rothstein P, Cole J, Pitt B. Pulmonary extraction of bupivacaine is dose dependent. *Anesthesiology*. 1984;61:A236.
29. Rothstein P, Pitt B. Pulmonary extraction of bupivacaine and its modification by propranolol. *Anesthesiology*. 1983;59:A189.
30. Bowdle TA, Freund PR, Slattery JT. Propranolol reduces bupivacaine clearance. *Anesthesiology*. 1987;66:36–38.
31. Thomas J, Long G, Moore G, et al. Plasma protein binding and placental transfer of bupivacaine. *Clin Pharmacol Ther*. 1976;19: 426–434.
32. Biehl D, Shnider SM, Levinson G, et al. Placental transfer of lidocaine: effects of fetal acidosis. *Anesthesiology*. 1978;48:409–412.
33. Tucker GT, Mather LE. Clinical pharmacokinetics of local anaesthetics. *Clin Pharmacokinet*. 1979;4:241–278.
34. Ramanathan J, Bottorff M, Jeter JN, et al. The pharmacokinetics and maternal and neonatal effects of epidural lidocaine in preeclampsia. *Anesth Analg*. 1986;65:120–126.
35. Pihlajamaki K, Kanto J, Lindberg R, et al. Extradural administration of bupivacaine: pharmacokinetics and metabolism in pregnant and non-pregnant women. *Br J Anaesth*. 1990;64:556–562.
36. Dauphin A, Gupta RN, Young JE, et al. Serum bupivacaine concentrations during continuous extrapleural infusion. *Can J Anaesth*. 1997; 44:367–370.
37. Pere P, Salonen M, Jokinen M, et al. Pharmacokinetics of ropivacaine in uremic and nonuremic patients after axillary brachial plexus block. *Anesth Analg*. 2003;96:563–569, table of contents.
38. Kuhnert BR, Kuhnert PM, Philipson EH, et al. The half-life of 2-chloroprocaine. *Anesth Analg*. 1986;65:273–278.
39. Kuhnert BR, Philipson EH, Pimental R, et al. Lidocaine disposition in mother, fetus, and neonate after spinal anesthesia. *Anesth Analg*. 1986;65:139–144.
40. Curatolo M, Petersen-Felix S, Arendt-Nielsen L, et al. Adding sodium bicarbonate to lidocaine enhances the depth of epidural blockade. *Anesth Analg*. 1998;86:341–347.
41. Abdallah FW, Abrishami A, Brull R. The facilitatory effects of intravenous dexmedetomidine on the duration of spinal anesthesia: a systematic review and meta-analysis. *Anesth Analg*. 2013;117: 271–278.
42. Morrison AP, Hunter JM, Halpern SH, et al. Effect of intrathecal magnesium in the presence or absence of local anaesthetic with and without lipophilic opioids: a systematic review and meta-analysis. *Br J Anaesth*. 2013;110:702–712.
43. Mossetti V, Vicchio N, Ivani G. Local anesthetics and adjuvants in pediatric regional anesthesia. *Curr Drug Targets*. 2012;13: 952–960.
44. Chestnut DH, Geiger M, Bates JN, et al. The influence of pH-adjusted 2-chloroprocaine on the quality and duration of subsequent epidural bupivacaine analgesia during labor: a randomized, double-blind study. *Anesthesiology*. 1989;70:437–441.
45. Munson ES, Paul WL, Embro WJ. Central-nervous-system toxicity of local anesthetic mixtures in monkeys. *Anesthesiology*. 1977; 46:179–183.
46. Liu S. Local anesthetics and analgesia. In: Ashburn M, Rice L, eds. *The Management of Pain*. New York, NY: Churchill Livingstone; 1997:141–170.
47. Scott DB, Jebson PJ, Braid DP, et al. Factors affecting plasma levels of lignocaine and prilocaine. *Br J Anaesth*. 1972;44:1040–1049.
48. Carpenter RL, Smith HS, Bridenbaugh LD. Epinephrine increases the effectiveness of tetracaine spinal anesthesia. *Anesthesiology*. 1989;71:33–36.
49. Brown DL, Ransom DM, Hall JA, et al. Regional anesthesia and local anesthetic-induced systemic toxicity: seizure frequency and accompanying cardiovascular changes. *Anesth Analg*. 1995;81: 321–328.
50. Brown DT, Beamish D, Wildsmith JA. Allergic reaction to an amide local anaesthetic. *Br J Anaesth*. 1981;53:435–437.
51. Neal JM, Bernards CM, Butterworth JF IV, et al. ASRA practice advisory on local anesthetic systemic toxicity. *Reg Anesth Pain Med*. 2010;35:152–161.

52. Covino B, Wildsmith J. Clinical pharmacology of local anesthetic agents. In: Cousins M, Bridenbaugh P, eds. *Neural Blockade in Clinical Anesthesia and Management of Pain*. Philadelphia, PA: Lippincott-Raven; 1998:97–128.
53. Butterworth JF IV. Models and mechanisms of local anesthetic cardiac toxicity: a review. *Reg Anesth Pain Med*. 2010;35:167–176.
54. Feldman HS, Arthur GR, Covino BG. Comparative systemic toxicity of convulsant and supraconvulsant doses of intravenous ropivacaine, bupivacaine, and lidocaine in the conscious dog. *Anesth Analg*. 1989;69:794–801.
55. Marsch SC, Schaefer HG, Castelli I. Unusual psychological manifestation of systemic local anesthetic toxicity. *Anesthesiology*. 1998;88:531–533.
56. Inoue R, Suganuma T, Echizen H, et al. Plasma concentrations of lidocaine and its principal metabolites during intermittent epidural anesthesia. *Anesthesiology*. 1985;63:304–310.
57. Christie JM, Valdes C, Markowsky SJ. Neurotoxicity of lidocaine combined with mexiletine. *Anesth Analg*. 1993;77:1291–1294.
58. Butterworth J, James RL, Grimes J. Structure-affinity relationships and stereospecificity of several homologous series of local anesthetics for the beta2-adrenergic receptor. *Anesth Analg*. 1997;85:336–342.
59. Albright GA. Cardiac arrest following regional anesthesia with etidocaine or bupivacaine. *Anesthesiology*. 1979;51:285–287.
60. Kotelko DM, Shnider SM, Dailey PA, et al. Bupivacaine-induced cardiac arrhythmias in sheep. *Anesthesiology*. 1984;60:10–18.
61. Timour Q, Freysz M, Couzon P, et al. Possible role of drug interactions in bupivacaine-induced problems related to intraventricular conduction disorders. *Reg Anesth*. 1990;15:180–185.
62. Morishima HO, Pedersen H, Finster M, et al. Bupivacaine toxicity in pregnant and nonpregnant ewes. *Anesthesiology*. 1985;63:134–139.
63. Roitman K, Sprung J, Wallace M, et al. Enhancement of bupivacaine cardiotoxicity with cardiac glycosides and beta-adrenergic blockers: a case report. *Anesth Analg*. 1993;76:658–661.
64. Butterworth JF IV, Brownlow RC, Leith JP, et al. Bupivacaine inhibits cyclic-3′,5′-adenosine monophosphate production. A possible contributing factor to cardiovascular toxicity. *Anesthesiology*. 1993;79:88–95.
65. Clarkson CW, Hondeghem LM. Mechanism for bupivacaine depression of cardiac conduction: fast block of sodium channels during the action potential with slow recovery from block during diastole. *Anesthesiology*. 1985;62:396–405.
66. Atlee JL III, Bosnjak ZJ. Mechanisms for cardiac dysrhythmias during anesthesia. *Anesthesiology*. 1990;72:347–374.
67. Crews JC, Rothman TE. Seizure after levobupivacaine for interscalene brachial plexus block. *Anesth Analg*. 2003;96:1188–1190.
68. Groban L, Deal DD, Vernon JC, et al. Cardiac resuscitation after incremental overdosage with lidocaine, bupivacaine, levobupivacaine, and ropivacaine in anesthetized dogs. *Anesth Analg*. 2001;92:37–43.
69. Huang YF, Pryor ME, Mather LE, et al. Cardiovascular and central nervous system effects of intravenous levobupivacaine and bupivacaine in sheep. *Anesth Analg*. 1998;86:797–804.
70. Moller R, Covino BG. Cardiac electrophysiologic properties of bupivacaine and lidocaine compared with those of ropivacaine, a new amide local anesthetic. *Anesthesiology*. 1990;72:322–329.
71. Scott DB, Lee A, Fagan D, et al. Acute toxicity of ropivacaine compared with that of bupivacaine. *Anesth Analg*. 1989;69:563–569.
72. Chazalon P, Tourtier JP, Villevielle T, et al. Ropivacaine-induced cardiac arrest after peripheral nerve block: successful resuscitation. *Anesthesiology*. 2003;99:1449–1451.
73. Klein SM, Pierce T, Rubin Y, et al. Successful resuscitation after ropivacaine-induced ventricular fibrillation. *Anesth Analg*. 2003;97:901–903.
74. Polley LS, Santos AC. Cardiac arrest following regional anesthesia with ropivacaine: here we go again! *Anesthesiology*. 2003;99:1253–1254.
75. Kendig JJ. Clinical implications of the modulated receptor hypothesis: local anesthetics and the heart. *Anesthesiology*. 1985;62:382–384.
76. Kasten GW, Martin ST. Bupivacaine cardiovascular toxicity: comparison of treatment with bretylium and lidocaine. *Anesth Analg*. 1985;64:911–916.
77. Xuecheng J, Xiaobin W, Bo G, et al. The plasma concentrations of lidocaine after slow versus rapid administration of an initial dose of epidural anesthesia. *Anesth Analg*. 1997;84:570–573.
78. Moore DC, Crawford RD, Scurlock JE. Severe hypoxia and acidosis following local anesthetic-induced convulsions. *Anesthesiology*. 1980;53:259–260.
79. Weinberg GL. Treatment of local anesthetic systemic toxicity (LAST). *Reg Anesth Pain Med*. 2010;35:188–193.
80. Neal JM, Mulroy MF, Weinberg GL; American Society of Regional Anesthesia and Pain Medicine. American Society of Regional Anesthesia and Pain Medicine checklist for managing local anesthetic systemic toxicity: 2012 version. *Reg Anesth Pain Med*. 2012;37:16–18.
81. Horlocker TT, McGregor DG, Matsushige DK, et al. A retrospective review of 4767 consecutive spinal anesthetics: central nervous system complications. Perioperative Outcomes Group. *Anesth Analg*. 1997;84:578–584.
82. Naveira FA, Copeland S, Anderson M, et al. Transient neurologic toxicity after spinal anesthesia, or is it myofascial pain? Two case reports. *Anesthesiology*. 1998;88:268–270.
83. Eisenach JC. Regional anesthesia: vintage Bordeaux (and Napa Valley). *Anesthesiology*. 1997;87:467–469.
84. Lee LA, Posner KL, Domino KB, et al. Injuries associated with regional anesthesia in the 1980s and 1990s: a closed claims analysis. *Anesthesiology*. 2004;101:143–152.
85. Kuboyoma N, Nakoa S, Moriya Y, et al. Bupivacaine-included Ca2+ release on intracellular Ca2+ stores in rat DRG neurons. *Jpn J Pharmacol*. 1997;73:98–103.
86. Schneider M, Ettlin T, Kaufmann M, et al. Transient neurologic toxicity after hyperbaric subarachnoid anesthesia with 5% lidocaine. *Anesth Analg*. 1993;76:1154–1157.
87. Hodgson PS, Neal JM, Pollock JE, et al. The neurotoxicity of drugs given intrathecally (spinal). *Anesth Analg*. 1999;88:797–809.
88. Hampl KF, Schneider MC, Pargger H, et al. A similar incidence of transient neurologic symptoms after spinal anesthesia with 2% and 5% lidocaine. *Anesth Analg*. 1996;83:1051–1054.
89. Liu SS, Ware PD, Allen HW, et al. Dose-response characteristics of spinal bupivacaine in volunteers. Clinical implications for ambulatory anesthesia. *Anesthesiology*. 1996;85:729–736.
90. Pollock JE, Liu SS, Neal JM, et al. Dilution of spinal lidocaine does not alter the incidence of transient neurologic symptoms. *Anesthesiology*. 1999;90:445–450.
91. Schneider MC, Birnbach DJ. Lidocaine neurotoxicity in the obstetric patient: is the water safe? *Anesth Analg*. 2001;92:287–290.
92. Zaric D, Pace NL. Transient neurologic symptoms (TNS) following spinal anaesthesia with lidocaine versus other local anaesthetics. *Cochrane Database Syst Rev*. 2009;(2):CD003006.
93. Sakura S, Sumi M, Sakaguchi Y, et al. The addition of phenylephrine contributes to the development of transient neurologic symptoms after spinal anesthesia with 0.5% tetracaine. *Anesthesiology*. 1997;87:771–778.
94. Silvanto M, Tarkkila P, Makela ML, et al. The influence of ambulation time on the incidence of transient neurologic symptoms after lidocaine spinal anesthesia. *Anesth Analg*. 2004;98:642–646, table of contents.
95. Pollock JE, Neal JM, Stephenson CA, et al. Prospective study of the incidence of transient radicular irritation in patients undergoing spinal anesthesia. *Anesthesiology*. 1996;84:1361–1367.
96. Gardner A, Gardner E, Morley T. Cauda equina syndrome: a review of the current clinical and medico-legal position. *Eur Spine J*. 2011;20:690–697.
97. Lambert DH, Hurley RJ. Cauda equina syndrome and continuous spinal anesthesia. *Anesth Analg*. 1991;72:817–819.
98. Rigler ML, Drasner K, Krejcie TC, et al. Cauda equina syndrome after continuous spinal anesthesia. *Anesth Analg*. 1991;72:275–281.

99. Gerancher JC. Cauda equina syndrome following a single spinal administration of 5% hyperbaric lidocaine through a 25-gauge Whitacre needle. *Anesthesiology*. 1997;87:687–689.
100. Kozody R, Palahniuk RJ, Wade JG, et al. The effect of subarachnoid epinephrine and phenylephrine on spinal cord blood flow. *Can Anaesth Soc J*. 1984;31:503–508.
101. Nguyen ST, Cabrales RE, Bashour CA, et al. Benzocaine-induced methemoglobinemia. *Anesth Analg*. 2000;90:369–371.
102. Gross JB, Caldwell CB, Shaw LM, et al. The effect of lidocaine infusion on the ventilatory response to hypoxia. *Anesthesiology*. 1984;61:662–665.
103. Yokoyama M, Ohashi I, Nakatsuka H, et al. Drug-induced liver disease during continuous epidural block with bupivacaine. *Anesthesiology*. 2001;95:259–261.
104. Craft DV, Good RP. Delayed hypersensitivity reaction of the knee after injection of arthroscopy portals with bupivacaine (marcaine). *Arthroscopy*. 1994;10:305–308.
105. Foster RH, Markham A. Levobupivacaine: a review of its pharmacology and use as a local anaesthetic. *Drugs*. 2000;59:551–579.
106. Hollmann MW, Durieux ME. Local anesthetics and the inflammatory response: a new therapeutic indication? *Anesthesiology*. 2000;93:858–875.
107. Lange RA, Cigarroa RG, Flores ED, et al. Potentiation of cocaine-induced coronary vasoconstriction by beta-adrenergic blockade. *Ann Intern Med*. 1990;112:897–903.
108. Noorily AD, Noorily SH, Otto RA. Cocaine, lidocaine, tetracaine: which is best for topical nasal anesthesia? *Anesth Analg*. 1995;81:724–727.
109. McAlpine LG, Thomson NC. Lidocaine-induced bronchoconstriction in asthmatic patients. Relation to histamine airway responsiveness and effect of preservative. *Chest*. 1989;96: 1012–1015.
110. Kirkpatrick MB, Sanders RV, Bass JB Jr. Physiologic effects and serum lidocaine concentrations after inhalation of lidocaine from a compressed gas-powered jet nebulizer. *Am Rev Respir Dis*. 1987;136:447–449.
111. Viegas O, Stoelting RK. Lidocaine in arterial blood after laryngotracheal administration. *Anesthesiology*. 1975;43:491–493.
112. Gajraj NM, Pennant JH, Watcha MF. Eutectic mixture of local anesthetics (EMLA) cream. *Anesth Analg*. 1994;78:574–583.
113. Taddio A, Stevens B, Craig K, et al. Efficacy and safety of lidocaine-prilocaine cream for pain during circumcision. *N Engl J Med*. 1997;336:1197–1201.
114. Katz NP, Shapiro DE, Herrmann TE, et al. Rapid onset of cutaneous anesthesia with EMLA cream after pretreatment with a new ultrasound-emitting device. *Anesth Analg*. 2004;98:371–376, table of contents.
115. Teillol-Foo WL, Kassab JY. Topical glyceryl trinitrate and eutectic mixture of local anaesthetics in children. A randomised controlled trial on choice of site and ease of venous cannulation. *Anaesthesia*. 1991;46:881–884.
116. Hymes J, Spraker M. Racial differences in the effectiveness of a topically applied mixture of local anesthetics. *Reg Anesth*. 1986;11:11–13.
117. Jakobson B, Nilsson A. Methemoglobinemia associated with a prilocaine-lidocaine cream and trimetoprim-sulphamethoxazole. A case report. *Acta Anaesthesiol Scand*. 1985;29:453–455.
118. Powell DM, Rodeheaver GT, Foresman PA, et al. Damage to tissue defenses by EMLA cream. *J Emerg Med*. 1991;9:205–209.
119. Arevalo MI, Escribano E, Calpena A, et al. Rapid skin anesthesia using a new topical amethocaine formulation: a preclinical study. *Anesth Analg*. 2004;98:1407–1412, table of contents.
120. Ravishankar N, Elliot SC, Beardow Z, et al. A comparison of Rapydan® patch and Ametop® gel for venous cannulation. *Anaesthesia*. 2012;67:367–370.
121. Erichsen CJ, Vibits H, Dahl JB, et al. Wound infiltration with ropivacaine and bupivacaine for pain after inguinal herniotomy. *Acta Anaesthesiol Scand*. 1995;39:67–70.
122. Winnie AP, Tay CH, Patel KP, et al. Pharmacokinetics of local anesthetics during plexus blocks. *Anesth Analg*. 1977;56:852–861.
123. Winnie AP, La Vallee DA, Pe Sosa B, et al. Clinical pharmacokinetics of local anaesthetics. *Can Anaesth Soc J*. 1977;24:252–262.
124. Hickey R, Candido KD, Ramamurthy S, et al. Brachial plexus block with a new local anaesthetic: 0.5 per cent ropivacaine. *Can J Anaesth*. 1990;37:732–738.
125. Nolte H, Fruhstorfer H, Edstrom HH. Local anesthetic efficacy of ropivacaine (LEA 103) in ulnar nerve block. *Reg Anesth*. 1990;15: 118–124.
126. Niesel HC, Eilingsfeld T, Hornung M, et al. Ropivacaine 1% versus bupivacaine 0.75% without a vasoconstrictor. A comparative study of epidural anesthesia in orthopedic surgery [in German]. *Anaesthesist*. 1993;42:605–611.
127. Abrahams MS, Aziz MF, Fu RF, et al. Ultrasound guidance compared with electrical neurostimulation for peripheral nerve block: a systematic review and meta-analysis of randomized controlled trials. *Br J Anaesth*. 2009;102:408–417.
128. Bingham AE, Fu R, Horn JL, et al. Continuous peripheral nerve block compared with single-injection peripheral nerve block: a systematic review and meta-analysis of randomized controlled trials. *Reg Anesth Pain Med*. 2012;37:583–594.
129. Bailard NS, Ortiz J, Flores RA. Additives to local anesthetics for peripheral nerve blocks: Evidence, limitations, and recommendations. *Am J Health Syst Pharm*. 2014;71:373–385.
130. Bader AM, Concepcion M, Hurley RJ, et al. Comparison of lidocaine and prilocaine for intravenous regional anesthesia. *Anesthesiology*. 1988;69:409–412.
131. Prieto-Alvarez P, Calas-Guerra A, Fuentes-Bellido J, et al. Comparison of mepivacaine and lidocaine for intravenous regional anaesthesia: pharmacokinetic study and clinical correlation. *Br J Anaesth*. 2002;88:516–519.
132. Chan VW, Weisbrod MJ, Kaszas Z, et al. Comparison of ropivacaine and lidocaine for intravenous regional anesthesia in volunteers: a preliminary study on anesthetic efficacy and blood level. *Anesthesiology*. 1999;90:1602–1608.
133. Brown DL, Carpenter RL, Thompson GE. Comparison of 0.5% ropivacaine and 0.5% bupivacaine for epidural anesthesia in patients undergoing lower-extremity surgery. *Anesthesiology*. 1990; 72:633–636.
134. Feldman HS, Covino BG. Comparative motor-blocking effects of bupivacaine and ropivacaine, a new amino amide local anesthetic, in the rat and dog. *Anesth Analg*. 1988;67:1047–1052.
135. Cederholm I, Anskar S, Bengtsson M. Sensory, motor, and sympathetic block during epidural analgesia with 0.5% and 0.75% ropivacaine with and without epinephrine. *Reg Anesth*. 1994;19: 18–33.
136. Wood MB, Rubin AP. A comparison of epidural 1% ropivacaine and 0.75% bupivacaine for lower abdominal gynecologic surgery. *Anesth Analg*. 1993;76:1274–1278.
137. Erichsen CJ, Sjovall J, Kehlet H, et al. Pharmacokinetics and analgesic effect of ropivacaine during continuous epidural infusion for postoperative pain relief. *Anesthesiology*. 1996;84:834–842.
138. George RB, Allen TK, Habib AS. Intermittent epidural bolus compared with continuous epidural infusions for labor analgesia: a systematic review and meta-analysis. *Anesth Analg*. 2013;116: 133–144.
139. De Negri P, Ivani G, Tirri T, et al. A comparison of epidural bupivacaine, levobupivacaine, and ropivacaine on postoperative analgesia and motor blockade. *Anesth Analg*. 2004;99:45–48.
140. Alahuhta S, Rasanen J, Jouppila P, et al. The effects of epidural ropivacaine and bupivacaine for cesarean section on uteroplacental and fetal circulation. *Anesthesiology*. 1995;83:23–32.
141. Muir HA, Writer D, Douglas J, et al. Double-blind comparison of epidural ropivacaine 0.25% and bupivacaine 0.25%, for the relief of childbirth pain. *Can J Anaesth*. 1997;44:599–604.
142. Polley LS, Columb MO. Ropivacaine and bupivacaine: concentrating on dosing! *Anesth Analg*. 2003;96:1251–1253.

143. Kuhnert BR, Zuspan KJ, Kuhnert PM, et al. Bupivacaine disposition in mother, fetus, and neonate after spinal anesthesia for cesarean section. *Anesth Analg.* 1987;66:407–412.
144. Reynolds F. A comparison of the potential toxicity of bupivacaine, lignocaine and mepivacaine during epidural blockade for surgery. *Br J Anaesth.* 1971;43:567–572.
145. Solomon RE, Gebhart GF. Synergistic antinociceptive interactions among drugs administered to the spinal cord. *Anesth Analg.* 1994;78:1164–1172.
146. Coda B, Bausch S, Haas M, et al. The hypothesis that antagonism of fentanyl analgesia by 2-chloroprocaine is mediated by direct action on opioid receptors. *Reg Anesth.* 1997;22:43–52.
147. Carpenter RL. Hyperbaric lidocaine spinal anesthesia: do we need an alternative? *Anesth Analg.* 1995;81:1125–1128.
148. Drasner K. Lidocaine spinal anesthesia: a vanishing therapeutic index? *Anesthesiology.* 1997;87:469–472.
149. Stewart A, Lambert DH, Concepcion MA, et al. Decreased incidence of tourniquet pain during spinal anesthesia with bupivacaine. A possible explanation. *Anesth Analg.* 1988;67:833–837.
150. Campbell DC, Banner R, Crone LA, et al. Addition of epinephrine to intrathecal bupivacaine and sufentanil for ambulatory labor analgesia. *Anesthesiology.* 1997;86:525–531.
151. Stocks GM, Hallworth SP, Fernando R, et al. Minimum local analgesic dose of intrathecal bupivacaine in labor and the effect of intrathecal fentanyl. *Anesthesiology.* 2001,94:593–598; discussion 5A.
152. van Kleef JW, Veering BT, Burm AG. Spinal anesthesia with ropivacaine: a double-blind study on the efficacy and safety of 0.5% and 0.75% solutions in patients undergoing minor lower limb surgery. *Anesth Analg.* 1994; 78:1125–1130.
153. Halpern SH, Breen TW, Campbell DC, et al. A multicenter, randomized, controlled trial comparing bupivacaine with ropivacaine for labor analgesia. *Anesthesiology.* 2003;98:1431–1435.
154. Khaw KS, Ngan Kee WD, Wong EL, et al. Spinal ropivacaine for cesarean section: a dose-finding study. *Anesthesiology.* 2001;95: 1346–1350.
155. Alley EA, Kopacz DJ, McDonald SB, et al. Hyperbaric spinal levobupivacaine: a comparison to racemic bupivacaine in volunteers. *Anesth Analg.* 2002;94:188–193, table of contents.
156. Covino BG, Marx GF, Finster M, et al. Prolonged sensory/motor deficits following inadvertent spinal anesthesia. *Anesth Analg.* 1980;59:399–400.
157. Ravindran RS, Bond VK, Tasch MD, et al. Prolonged neural blockade following regional analgesia with 2-chloroprocaine. *Anesth Analg.* 1980;59:447–451.
158. Reisner LS, Hochman BN, Plumer MH. Persistent neurologic deficit and adhesive arachnoiditis following intrathecal 2-chloroprocaine injection. *Anesth Analg.* 1980;59:452–454.
159. Drasner K. Chloroprocaine spinal anesthesia: back to the future? *Anesth Analg.* 2005;100:549–552.
160. Kouri ME, Kopacz DJ. Spinal 2-chloroprocaine: a comparison with lidocaine in volunteers. *Anesth Analg.* 2004;98:75–80, table of contents.
161. Kozody R, Palahniuk RJ, Cumming MO. Spinal cord blood flow following subarachnoid tetracaine. *Can Anaesth Soc J.* 1985;32: 23–29.
162. Liu SS, McDonald SB. Current issues in spinal anesthesia. *Anesthesiology.* 2001;94:888–906.
163. Pollard JB. Cardiac arrest during spinal anesthesia: common mechanisms and strategies for prevention. *Anesth Analg.* 2001; 92:252–256.
164. Cassuto J, Wallin G, Hogstrom S, et al. Inhibition of postoperative pain by continuous low-dose intravenous infusion of lidocaine. *Anesth Analg.* 1985;64:971–974.
165. DiFazio CA, Neiderlehner JR, Burney RG. The anesthetic potency of lidocaine in the rat. *Anesth Analg.* 1976;55:818–821.
166. Yukioka H, Yoshimoto N, Nishimura K, et al. Intravenous lidocaine as a suppressant of coughing during tracheal intubation. *Anesth Analg.* 1985;64:1189–1192.
167. Wu CL, Tella P, Staats PS, et al. Analgesic effects of intravenous lidocaine and morphine on postamputation pain: a randomized double-blind, active placebo-controlled, crossover trial. *Anesthesiology.* 2002;96:841–848.
168. Peters RW, Gilbert TB, Johns-Walton S, et al. Lidocaine-related increase in defibrillation threshold. *Anesth Analg.* 1997;85: 299–300.
169. Pere P, Lindgren L, Vaara M. Poor antibacterial effect of ropivacaine: comparison with bupivacaine. *Anesthesiology.* 1999;91: 884–886.
170. Gottschalk A, McKay AM, Malik ZM, et al. Systemic lidocaine decreases the Bispectral Index in the presence of midazolam, but not its absence. *J Clin Anesth.* 2012;24:121–125.
171. Hollmann MW, Gross A, Jelacin N, Durieux ME. Local anesthetic effects on priming and activation of human neutrophils. *Anesthesiology.* 2001;95:113–122.
172. Hollmann MW, McIntire WE, Garrison JC, et al. Inhibition of mammalian Gq protein function by local anesthetics. *Anesthesiology.* 2002;97:1451–1457.
173. Kiefer RT, Ploppa A, Krueger WA, et al. Local anesthetics impair human granulocyte phagocytosis activity, oxidative burst, and CD11b expression in response to Staphylococcus aureus. *Anesthesiology.* 2003;98:842–848.
174. Hollmann MW, Kurz K, Herroeder S, et al. The effects of S(−)-, R(+)-, and racemic bupivacaine on lysophosphatidate-induced priming of human neutrophils. *Anesth Analg.* 2003;97:1053–1058, table of contents.
175. Groeben H, Grosswendt T, Silvanus MT, et al. Airway anesthesia alone does not explain attenuation of histamine-induced bronchospasm by local anesthetics: a comparison of lidocaine, ropivacaine, and dyclonine. *Anesthesiology.* 2001;94:423–428; discussion 5A-6A.
176. Klein JA. Tumescent technique for regional anesthesia permits lidocaine doses of 35 mg/kg for liposuction. *J Dermatol Surg Oncol.* 1990;16:248–263.
177. Burk RW III, Guzman-Stein G, Vasconez LO. Lidocaine and epinephrine levels in tumescent technique liposuction. *Plast Reconstr Surg.* 1996;97:1379–1384.
178. Ostad A, Kageyama N, Moy RL. Tumescent anesthesia with a lidocaine dose of 55 mg/kg is safe for liposuction. *Dermatol Surg.* 1996;22:921–927.
179. Rao RB, Ely SF, Hoffman RS. Deaths related to liposuction. *N Engl J Med.* 1999;340:1471–1475.
180. Hanke W, Cox SE, Kuznets N, et al. Tumescent liposuction report performance measurement initiative: national survey results. *Dermatol Surg.* 2004;30:967–977; discussion 978.
181. Svedman KJ, Coldiron B, Coleman WP III, et al. ASDS guidelines of care for tumescent liposuction. *Dermatol Surg.* 2006;32: 709–716.
182. Zimmerman JL. Cocaine intoxication. *Crit Care Clin.* 2012;28: 517–526.
183. Mendelson JH, Mello NK. Management of cocaine abuse and dependence. *N Engl J Med.* 1996;334:965–972.
184. Leshner AI. Molecular mechanisms of cocaine addiction. *N Engl J Med.* 1996;335:128–129.
185. Hatsukami DK, Fischman MW. Crack cocaine and cocaine hydrochloride. Are the differences myth or reality? *JAMA.* 1996;276:1580–1588.
186. Hollander JE, Hoffman RS, Burstein JL, et al. Cocaine-associated myocardial infarction. Mortality and complications. Cocaine-Associated Myocardial Infarction Study Group. *Arch Intern Med.* 1995;155:1081–1086.
187. Weicht GT, Bernards CM. Remote cocaine use as a likely cause of cardiogenic shock after penetrating trauma. *Anesthesiology.* 1996;85:933–935.
188. Nademanee K, Gorelick DA, Josephson MA, et al. Myocardial ischemia during cocaine withdrawal. *Ann Intern Med.* 1989;111: 876–880.

189. Kain ZN, Mayes LC, Ferris CA, et al. Cocaine-abusing parturients undergoing cesarean section. A cohort study. *Anesthesiology.* 1996;85:1028–1035.
190. Woods JR Jr, Plessinger MA, Clark KE. Effect of cocaine on uterine blood flow and fetal oxygenation. *JAMA.* 1987;257:957–961.
191. Bernards CM, Teijeiro A. Illicit cocaine ingestion during anesthesia. *Anesthesiology.* 1996;84:218–220.
192. Levine SR, Brust JC, Futrell N, et al. Cerebrovascular complications of the use of the "crack" form of alkaloidal cocaine. *N Engl J Med.* 1990;323:699–704.
193. Hollander JE, Hoffman RS, Gennis P, et al. Nitroglycerin in the treatment of cocaine associated chest pain—clinical safety and efficacy. *J Toxicol Clin Toxicol.* 1994;32:243–256.
194. Pollan S, Tadjziechy M. Esmolol in the management of epinephrine- and cocaine-induced cardiovascular toxicity. *Anesth Analg.* 1989;69:663–664.
195. Groudine SB, Hollinger I, Jones J, et al. New York State guidelines on the topical use of phenylephrine in the operating room. The Phenylephrine Advisory Committee. *Anesthesiology.* 2000;92:859–864.
196. McCord J, Jneid H, Hollander JE, et al; American Heart Association Acute Cardiac Care Committee of the Council on Clinical Cardiology. Management of cocaine-associated chest pain and myocardial infarction: a scientific statement from the American Heart Association Acute Cardiac Care Committee of the Council on Clinical Cardiology. *Circulation.* 2008;117:1897–1907.

CHAPTER 11

Neuromuscular Physiology

Mohamed A. Naguib

The mammalian neuromuscular junction is one of the most studied and best understood synapses.[1] The neuromuscular junction is a synapse that develops between a motor neuron and a muscle fiber and is made up of several components: the presynaptic nerve terminal, the postsynaptic muscle membrane, and the intervening cleft (or gap). In the 19th century and early years of the 20th century, there was broad support for the concept that impulses in nerves acted directly on muscle, resulting in muscular contraction—the "electrical theory." This theory was eventually refuted with the discovery of the role of acetylcholine in neuromuscular transmission,[2,3] and in 1936, the Nobel Prize in Physiology or Medicine was awarded to Sir Henry Hallett Dale and Otto Loewi "for their discoveries relating to chemical transmission of nerve impulses." This was followed by the discovery that a muscle membrane–bound allosteric protein, the nicotinic acetylcholine receptor.[4]

Muscle Types

Muscle is generally classified as skeletal, smooth, or cardiac. Both skeletal and cardiac muscles are striated muscles sharing a common basic organization of the contractile filaments. There are, however, distinct histologic and functional differences between these two muscles. Skeletal muscle cells are multinucleated and tubular in shape, whereas cardiac muscle cells may be mono- or binucleated and are branched and contain intercalated discs. Skeletal muscle is responsible for voluntary actions, whereas smooth muscle and cardiac muscle subserve functions related to the cardiovascular, respiratory, gastrointestinal, and genitourinary systems. Muscle composes 45% to 50% of total body mass, with skeletal muscles accounting for approximately 40% of body mass. An estimated 250 million cells are present in the more than 400 skeletal muscles of humans. Muscle cells are highly specialized cells for the conversion of chemical energy into mechanical energy. Inappropriate activity of smooth muscle is involved in many illnesses including hypertension, atherosclerosis, asthma, and disorders of the gastrointestinal tract.

Motor Units

Vertebrate skeletal muscles are innervated by large myelinated α motor neurons that originate from cell bodies located in the brainstem or ventral (anterior) horns of the spinal cord (Fig. 11-1).[5] The myelinated nerve axon reaches the muscle through mixed peripheral nerves. Motor nerves branch in the skeletal muscle with each nerve terminal innervating a single muscle cell.

The motor unit is the functional contractile unit and is composed of a single myelinated α motor neuron and all muscle fibers that receive innervation from this single neuron. Motor units vary in size. A large motor nerve innervates more muscle fibers than a smaller motor nerve does. In general, small motor units innervate the "red slow" muscle fibers, whereas large motor units innervate the "white or pale fast" muscle fibers. The slow muscle fibers appear red as a result of high contents of myoglobin, mitochondria, and capillaries compared with white muscle fibers. Unlike the white muscle fibers, the red fibers are resistant to fatigue.[6] Muscles contain a varying mixture of motor units depending on their function.

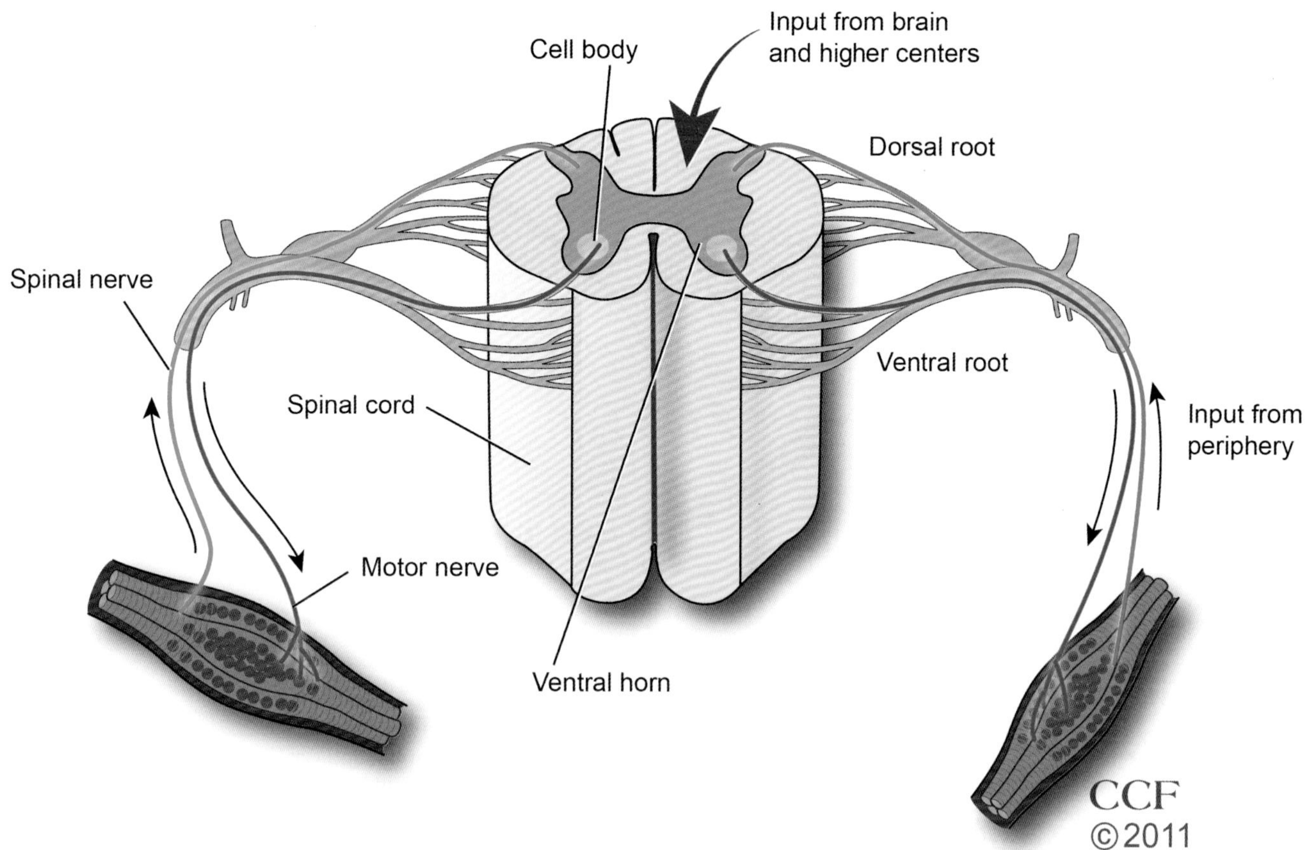

FIGURE 11-1 Schematic depiction of skeletal muscle innervation.

The Neuromuscular Junction

The neuromuscular junction (NMJ) or the endplate is a highly specialized synapse at which presynaptic motor nerve endings meet the postsynaptic membranes of skeletal muscles (motor endplates) (Fig. 11-2). The formation, differentiation, and function of the NMJ requires a proper interaction (cross-talk) between the nerve terminal and muscle cell (for a review, see Naguib et al.[1]). Failure of this cross-talk will result in a wide spectrum of neuromuscular disorders. It should be noted that in early postnatal period, muscle fibers receive multiple innervation. It has been shown in mice that on the second postnatal day, approximately 75% of muscle fibers are multiply innervated (>95% by two axons).[7] However, the transition from multiple to single innervation at the NMJ occurs within few days.[7] The motor nerve ending branches to form a complex of nerve terminals that invaginate into the skeletal muscle fiber but lie outside the sarcolemma. As each motor neuron approaches its target muscle fiber, it loses its myelin sheath and makes a contact with a single muscle fiber to form an NMJ. The naked motor nerve terminal that is not in contact with the muscle fiber is capped by Schwann cells. The importance of Schwann cells for development, survival, and repair of several aspects of NMJ is reviewed elsewhere.[1]

The NMJ is designed to transmit electrical impulses from the nerve terminal to the skeletal muscle via the chemical transmitter, acetylcholine (ACh). Structurally, the NMJ is consisted of a three components: (a) the *presynaptic* (or prejunctional) nerve terminal containing synaptic vesicles (filled with ACh) and mitochondria; (b) the *synaptic cleft* that contains basal lamina to which acetylcholinesterase enzyme responsible for hydrolysis of free ACh is attached; and (c) the *postsynaptic* (or postjunctional) muscle membrane that opposes the nerve terminal, which is highly infolded and these folds are called ***secondary folds*** (or secondary postsynaptic cleft). Membrane infoldings increase the surface area of the muscle plasma membrane in the postsynaptic region. Nicotinic acetylcholine receptors (nAChRs) are concentrated at the crests of these folds (directly opposing the *active zones* of the presynaptic membrane in which synaptic vesicles are clustered) and voltage-gated sodium channels (VGSC) are present in the troughs of the folds.

The plasticity of neuromuscular transmission is dependent on a highly orchestrated mechanism involving (a) synthesis, storage, and release of acetylcholine from the presynaptic region at the NMJ; (b) binding of acetylcholine to nicotinic receptors on the muscle membrane (postsynaptic region) and generation of action potentials; (c) rapid hydrolysis of acetylcholine by the enzyme acetylcholinesterase, which is present in the synaptic cleft; and (d) adaptation of the muscle contractile proteins to functional demands.[1] Synaptic plasticity is the "ability of

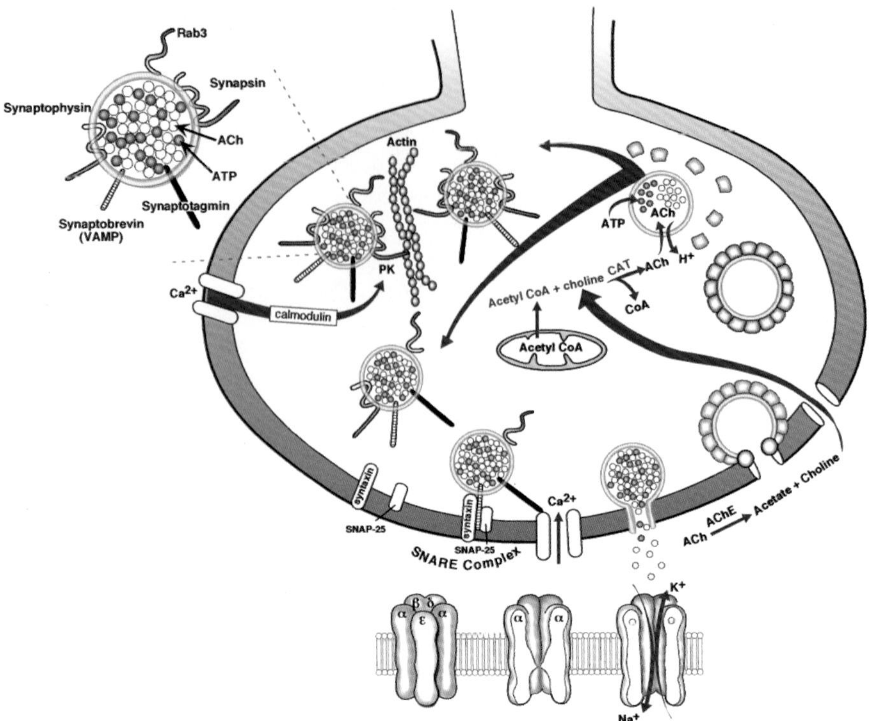

FIGURE 11-2 The synaptic vesicle exocytosis–endocytosis cycle. After an action potential and Ca^{2+} influx, phosphorylation of synapsin is activated by calcium-calmodulin activated protein kinases I and II. This results in the mobilization of synaptic vesicles (SVs) from the cytomatrix toward the plasma membrane. The formation of the SNARE complex is an essential step for the docking process. After fusion of SVs with the presynaptic plasma membrane, acetylcholine (ACh) is released into the synaptic cleft. Some of the released acetylcholine molecules bind to the nicotinic acetylcholine receptors (nAChRs) on the postsynaptic membrane while the rest is rapidly hydrolyzed by the acetylcholinesterase (AChE) present in the synaptic cleft to choline and acetate. Choline is recycled into the terminal by a high-affinity uptake system, making it available for the resynthesis of acetylcholine. Exocytosis is followed by endocytosis in a process dependent on the formation of a clathrin coat and of action of dynamin. After recovering of SV membrane, the coated vesicle uncoats and another cycle starts again. See text for details. Acetyl CoA, acetylcoenzyme A; CAT, choline acetyltransferase; PK, protein kinase. (From Naguib M, Flood P, McArdle JJ, et al. Advances in neurobiology of the neuromuscular junction: implications for the anesthesiologist. *Anesthesiology*. 2002;96:202–231.)

individual synaptic junctions to respond [i.e., to change in strength in response] to either use or disuse."[8]

Presynaptic Region

Synaptic Vesicles

Synaptic vesicles (SVs) are specialized secretory organelles (see Fig. 11-2). SVs are synthesized in the neuronal cell body in the endoplasmic reticulum and transported to the nerve terminal via the microtubule system. SVs are then loaded with ACh in the motor nerve endings. Acetylcholine is first synthesized in the cytoplasm of the nerve terminal from acetyl coenzyme A and choline in a reaction catalyzed by the soluble enzyme choline acetyltransferase. An energy-dependent "transporter" then accumulates acetylcholine within vesicles. Each vesicle appears to contain 5,000 to 10,000 molecules of acetylcholine. The acetylcholine contained in a single vesicle is often referred to as a "quantum" of transmitter. The synaptic vesicles possess a diverse set of specialized proteins that can be divided into two functional classes: proteins involved in the uptake of neurotransmitters (transport proteins) and proteins that mediate SV membrane traffic such as docking, fusion, and budding (for review, see Naguib et al.[1]). Ca^{2+} signal plays a pivotal role in the process of acetylcholine vesicles exocytosis (see Fig. 11-2). There are two pools of vesicles that differ in the probability of mobilization to the active site: a readily releasable store (active pool) and a reserve store. The active pool is aligned near the active zones.

The miniature endplate potential (MEPP) amplitude represents the depolarization of the postsynaptic membrane produced by the contents of a single vesicle. Endplate potential (EPP) results from summation of MEPP produced by ACh contents of ~50 to 300 SVs. Nearly 50% of the released acetylcholine is rapidly hydrolyzed by the acetylcholinesterase during the time of diffusion across the synaptic cleft before reaching nAChRs. The products of this hydrolysis are choline and acetate. Choline is recycled into the terminal by a high-affinity uptake system, making it available for the resynthesis of acetylcholine. The drug hemicholinium-3 inhibits the later mechanism. After exocytosis, the membrane components of the SVs are recovered by endocytosis and recycled for future use.

Synaptic Cleft

The synaptic cleft is ~20 to 50 nm wide. It separates nerve and muscle fiber plasma membranes and encompasses the synaptic basal lamina and is filled with extracellular fluid. Acetylcholinesterase enzyme is bound to the basal lamina at the cleft (Fig. 11-3).

Acetylcholinesterase ranks as one of the highest catalytic efficiencies known. The efficiency of acetylcholinesterase depends on its fast catalytic activity. It can catalyze acetylcholine hydrolysis (4,000 molecules of acetylcholine hydrolyzed per active site per second) at near diffusion-limited rates.[9] Acetylcholinesterase is highly concentrated at the NMJ but present in a lower concentration throughout the length of muscle fibers.[10] Acetylcholinesterase is regulated, in part, by muscle activity and by the spontaneous or nerve-evoked depolarization of the plasma membrane.[11] After denervation, there is a large decrease in the density of acetylcholinesterase molecules at the NMJ. In addition to hydrolysis of acetylcholine, acetylcholinesterase has other functions such as nerve growth–promoting activities[12] and modulation of nAChRs.

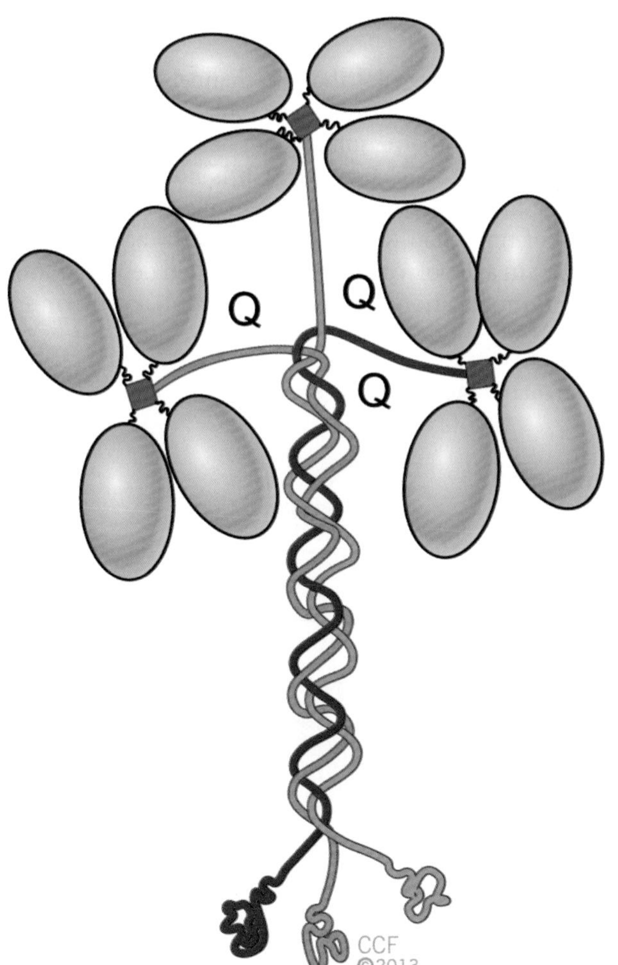

FIGURE 11-3 Structure of acetylcholinesterase.

The Nicotinic Acetylcholine Receptor at the Neuromuscular Junction

In the adult mammalian skeletal muscle the nicotinic acetylcholine receptor (nAChR) is a pentameric complex of two α subunits in association with a single β, δ, and ε subunit (Fig. 11-4). These subunits are organized to form a transmembrane pore (a channel) as well as the extracellular binding pockets for acetylcholine and other agonists or antagonists.[1] Each of the two α subunits has an acetylcholine-binding site. These sites are proteins located in pockets approximately 3.0 nm above the surface membrane at the interfaces of the α-ε and α-δ subunits.[13] The fetal nAChR contains a γ subunit instead of an ε adult subunit. The mature nAChR has shorter burst duration and a higher conductance to Na^+, K^+, and Ca^{2+} than the fetal nAChR.[1,14]

The fetal nAChR is a low-conductance channel in contrast to the high-conductance channel of the adult nAChR (Fig. 11-5). Thus acetylcholine release causes brief activation and reduced probability of channel opening.[1] Upregulation of nicotinic acetylcholine receptors (nAChRs), found in states of functional or surgical denervation, is characterized by the spreading of predominantly fetal type nAChRs. These receptors are resistant to nondepolarizing neuromuscular blockers and more sensitive to succinylcholine (SCh).[15] When depolarized, the immature isoform has a prolonged open channel time that exaggerates the K^+ efflux.[16]

Simultaneous binding of two acetylcholine molecules to the two α subunits of nAChRs initiates conformational changes that open a channel through the center of the receptor, allowing sodium and calcium ions to move into the skeletal muscle and potassium ions to leave. Each NMJ contains several million postjunctional receptors, and a burst of acetylcholine from the nerve ending opens at least 400,000 receptors. As a result, sufficient current flows through these open receptors to depolarize the endplate and create the action potential that triggers contraction of the skeletal muscle. It is the flow of ions that is the basis of normal neuromuscular transmission.

The two α subunits, in addition to being the binding sites for acetylcholine, are the sites occupied by neuromuscular blocking drugs. Nondepolarizing neuromuscular blocking drugs bind to one or both α subunits, but unlike acetylcholine, lack agonist activity (competitive blockade). As a result, conformational changes do not occur, and the receptor channel remains closed. Therefore, ions do not flow through these channels, and depolarization cannot occur at these sites. If enough channels remain closed, there is blockade of neuromuscular transmission. A nondepolarizing neuromuscular-blocking drug may show preference for one of the two α subunits. This may result in synergism if two nondepolarizing neuromuscular-blocking drugs with different selective preferences for each α subunit are administered simultaneously. The probability of binding is dependent on the concentration of acetylcholine and

FIGURE 11-4 Subunit composition of the nicotinic acetylcholine receptor (nAChR) in the endplate surface of adult mammalian muscle. The adult AChR is an intrinsic membrane protein with five distinct subunits (α2βδε). Each subunit contains four helical domains labeled M1 to M4. The M2 domain forms the channel pore. The *upper panel* shows a single α subunit with its N and C termini on the extracellular surface of the membrane lipid bilayer. Between the N and C termini, the α subunit forms four helices (M1, M2, M3, and M4), which span the membrane bilayer. The *lower panel* shows the pentameric structure of the nAChR of adult mammalian muscle. The N termini of two subunits cooperate to form two distinct binding pockets for acetylcholine. These pockets occur at the ε–α and the δ–α subunit interface. The M2 membrane spanning domain of each subunit lines the ion channel. The doubly liganded ion channel has equal permeability to Na^+ and K^+; Ca^{2+} contributes approximately 2.5% to the total permeability. (From Naguib M, Flood P, McArdle JJ, et al. Advances in neurobiology of the neuromuscular junction: implications for the anesthesiologist. *Anesthesiology*. 2002;96:202–231.)

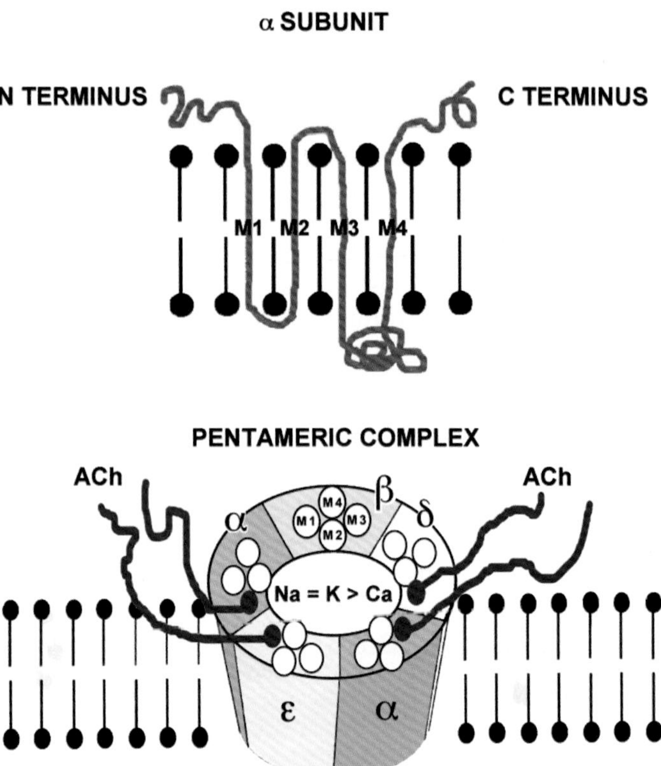

nondepolarizing neuromuscular-blocking drug at the receptor and the affinity of the receptor for the neurotransmitter or drug. When the neuromuscular-blocking drug diffuses from the nAChRs, the probability of receptor binding of acetylcholine increases, and the effect of the nondepolarizing neuromuscular-blocking drug decreases.

SCh, which is structurally two molecules of acetylcholine bound together, is a partial agonist at nAChRs and depolarizes (opens) the ion channels. This opening requires the binding of only one molecule of SCh to the α subunit. The other α subunit can be occupied by either acetylcholine or SCh. Because SCh is not hydrolyzed by acetylcholinesterase, the channel remains open for a longer period of time than would be produced by acetylcholine, resulting in a depolarizing block (sustained depolarization prevents propagation of an action potential). Furthermore,

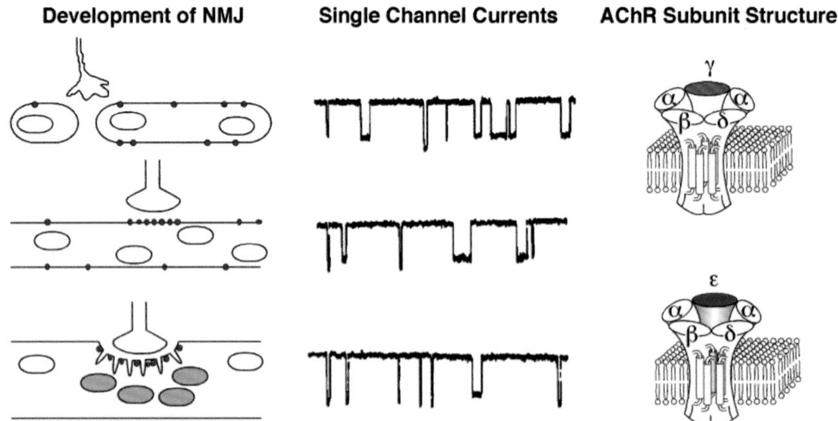

FIGURE 11-5 Development of the neuromuscular junction. **(Left)** Motor neuron growth cones contact myotubes as they fuse from myoblasts and express mostly fetal nicotinic acetylcholine receptors (nAChRs; marked in *blue*) in their surface membranes. In adult muscle, adult nAChRs (marked in *red*) predominate and are largely concentrated at the neuromuscular junction. **(Center)** Records of AChR channel openings from muscle membranes at different stages of neuromuscular development. Fetal *(top)* and adult nAChRs *(bottom)* are activated by acetylcholine to form ion channels of different conductance and gating properties. **(Right)** Subunit composition of fetal and adult AChR subtypes. Fetal and adult AChR subtypes are characterized by the presence of a γ and ε subunit, respectively. (From Naguib M, Flood P, McArdle JJ, et al. Advances in neurobiology of the neuromuscular junction: implications for the anesthesiologist. *Anesthesiology*. 2002;96:202–231.)

SCh can diffuse from nAChRs and repeatedly bind to other nAChRs until it is cleared from the area of the NMJ and is exposed to hydrolysis by plasma cholinesterase.

Large doses of nondepolarizing neuromuscular-blocking drugs may also prevent normal flow of ions by entering the channels formed by nAChRs to produce blockade within the channel. Similar blockade of sodium ion channels is produced by local anesthetics.

Neuromuscular Transmission and Excitation-Contraction Coupling

Motor Nerve

Depolarization of the motor nerve will open the voltage-gated Ca^{2+} channels that trigger both mobilization of synaptic vesicles and the fusion machinery in the nerve terminal to release acetylcholine.

Several forms of K^{+} channel present in the nerve terminal serve to limit the extent of Ca^{2+} entry and transmitter release (i.e., initiate repolarization of nerve terminal).[17]

Muscle

The released acetylcholine binds to α subunits of the nAChRs. These ligand-gated cation channels open almost instantaneously when two acetylcholine molecules bind cooperatively to sites on the extracellular surface of the protein, causing a conformational shift in the subunits. When the channel opens, sodium ions flow down their electrochemical gradient and into the muscle cell and depolarize the muscle cell membrane at the NMJ, whereas potassium simultaneously exits the cytosol of the fiber.[17,18] This depolarization activates voltage-gated sodium channels that present in the muscle membrane, which mediate the initiation and propagation of action potentials across the surface of the muscle membrane and into the transverse tubules (T-tubules) resulting in the upstroke of the action potential.[17–19]

There are two types of calcium channels, dihydropyridine receptor (DHPR) in the T-tubules and the ryanodine receptor (RyR1) in the sarcoplasmic reticulum (Fig. 11-6). The DHPRs act as "voltage sensors"[20,21] and are activated by membrane depolarization, which in turn activate RyR1 receptors. DHPR-RyR1 interaction[22] releases large amounts of Ca^{2+} from the sarcoplasmic reticulum that

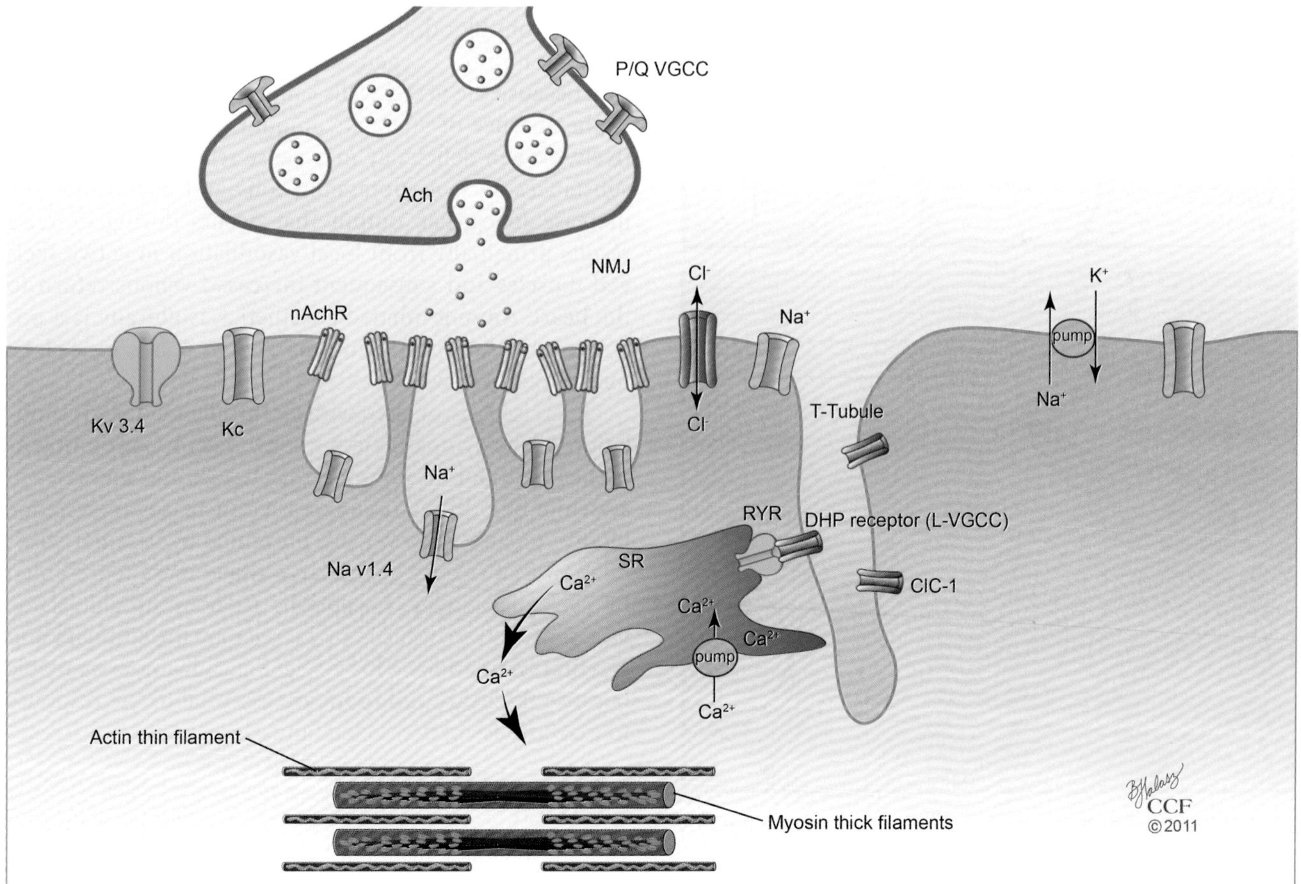

FIGURE 11-6 Neuromuscular transmission and excitation-contraction coupling. Ach, acetylcholine; VGCC (P/Q), voltage-gated calcium channel (P/Q type); nAchR, nicotinic acetylcholine receptor; NMJ, neuromuscular junction; RYR, the ryanodine receptor; DHP, dihydropyridine receptor; SR, sarcoplasmic reticulum; CIC, calcium-induced-calcium-release.

result in a transient increase in myoplasmic free Ca^{2+}, which binds to troponin C. This initiates movement of tropomyosin on the thin filament (actin) and allows cross bridges between the myosin with the binding sites on actin, which eventually result in force development. This process is known as excitation-contraction coupling (Fig. 11-7).[23] Shortly after releasing calcium, the sarcoplasmic reticulum begins to reaccumulate this ion by an active transport process (calcium pump). This transport mechanism can concentrate calcium up to 2,000-fold inside the sarcoplasmic reticulum. Adenosine triphosphate (ATP) provides the energy for calcium ion transport. Once the calcium concentration in the sarcoplasm has been lowered sufficiently, cross-bridging between myosin and actin ceases and the skeletal muscle relaxes. Failure of the calcium ion pump results in sustained skeletal muscle contraction and marked increases in heat production, leading to malignant hyperthermia. The gene for this calcium ion channel (ryanodine receptor) is on chromosome 19. A mutation in this gene is associated with malignant hyperthermia susceptibility in some patients.

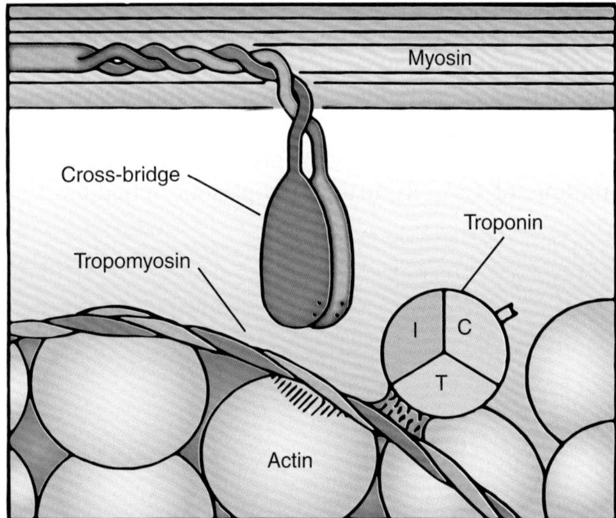

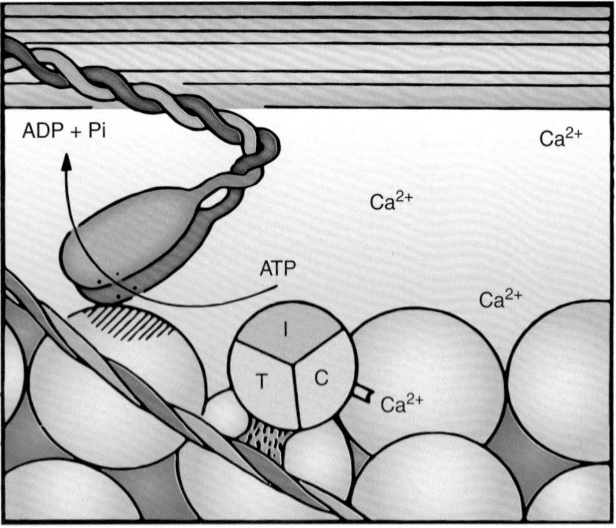

FIGURE 11-7 Contraction of skeletal muscle is initiated by attachment of calcium ions (Ca^{2+}) to troponin, leading to hydrolysis of adenosine triphosphate (ATP) and cross-bridging between actin and myosin. (From Ganong WF. *Review of Medical Physiology*. 21st ed. New York, NY: McGraw-Hill; 2003, with permission.)

Repolarization of the muscle membrane is initiated by the closing of the sodium channels and by the opening of potassium ion channel that conduct an outward K^+ current.[24] The return the muscle membrane potential to its resting level (approximately −70 to −90 mV) is achieved by allowing Cl^- to enter the cell through voltage-sensitive chloride channels.[17]

Blood Flow

Skeletal muscle blood flow can increase more than 20 times (a greater increase than in any other tissue of the body) during strenuous exercise. At rest, only 20% to 25% of the capillaries are open, and skeletal muscle blood flow is 3 to 4 mL/100 g per minute. During strenuous exercise, almost all skeletal muscle capillaries become patent. Opening of previously collapsed capillaries diminishes the distance that oxygen and other nutrients must diffuse from capillaries to skeletal muscle fibers and contributes an increased surface area through which nutrients can diffuse from blood. Presumably, exercise lowers the local concentration of oxygen, which in turn causes vasodilation because the vessel walls cannot maintain contraction in the absence of adequate amounts of oxygen. Alternatively, oxygen deficiency may cause release of vasodilator substances such as potassium ions and adenosine. The increase in cardiac output that occurs during exercise results principally from local vasodilation in active skeletal muscles and subsequent increased venous return to the heart. Among inhaled anesthetics, isoflurane is a potent vasodilator, producing marked increases in skeletal muscle blood flow.

Exercise is associated with a centrally mediated stimulation of the sympathetic nervous system manifesting as vasoconstriction in nonmuscular tissues and increases in systemic blood pressure. Excessive increases in systemic blood pressure, however, are prevented by vascular vasodilation that occurs in the large tissue mass represented by skeletal muscles. Exceptions to nonmuscular tissue vasoconstriction induced by exercise are the coronary and cerebral circulations. This is teleologically understandable because the heart and brain are essential to the response to exercise, as are the skeletal muscles.

Smooth Muscle

Smooth muscle is distinguished anatomically from skeletal and cardiac muscle because it lacks visible cross-striations (actin and myosin are not arranged in regular arrays). Smooth muscle is categorized as *multiunit* or *visceral* smooth muscle.

Multiunit smooth muscle contraction is controlled almost exclusively by nerve signals, and spontaneous contractions rarely occur. Examples of multiunit smooth muscles are the ciliary muscles of the eye, iris of the eye, and smooth muscles of many large blood vessels. Smooth muscle must develop force or shorten to provide motility or to alter the dimensions of an organ.

Smooth muscle cells lack T-tubules that provide electrical links to sarcoplasmic reticulum. However, the sarcolemma of smooth muscle contains saclike inpocketings (caveoli) that may be sites where calcium ions enter the cells through voltage-gated calcium ion channels. Calcium ions are released from the sarcoplasmic reticulum into the myoplasm when stimulatory neurotransmitters, hormones, or drugs bind to receptors on the sarcolemma. Calcium ion channels on the sarcoplasmic reticulum of smooth muscles includes ryanodine receptors (similar to that present in skeletal muscles) and inositol 1,4,5-triphosphate (IP_3)-gated calcium ion channels. Neurotransmitters or hormones that act via receptors in the sarcolemma can activate phospholipase C followed by the generation of the second messenger IP_3. IP_3 channels are activated when hormones bind to calcium-mobilizing receptors in the sarcoplasmic reticulum in smooth muscle cells.

Visceral smooth muscle is characterized by cell membranes that contact adjacent cell membranes, forming a functional syncytium that often undergoes spontaneous contractions as a single unit in the absence of nerve stimulation. These spontaneous action potentials are particularly prominent in tubular structures, accounting for peristaltic motion in sites such as the bile ducts, ureters, and gastrointestinal tract, especially when they are distended. Plateaus in the action potentials of visceral smooth muscle lasting up to 30 seconds may occur in the ureters and uterus. The normal resting transmembrane potential is approximately −60 mV, which is approximately 30 mV less negative than in skeletal muscles.

In addition to stimulation in the absence of extrinsic innervation, smooth muscles are unique in their sensitivity to hormones or local tissue factors. For example, smooth muscle spasm may persist for hours in response to norepinephrine or antidiuretic hormone, whereas local factors such as lack of oxygen or accumulation of hydrogen ions cause vasodilation. It is believed that local factors and hormones cause smooth muscle contraction by activating the calcium ion transport mechanism. Drugs relax smooth muscle by increasing the intracellular concentration of cyclic adenosine monophosphate or cyclic guanosine monophosphate.

Mechanism of Contraction

Smooth muscles contain both actin and myosin but, unlike skeletal muscles, lack troponin. In contrast to skeletal muscles, in which calcium binds to troponin to initiate cross-bridging, in smooth muscle the calcium-calmodulin complex activates the enzyme necessary for phosphorylation of myosin. This myosin has ATPase activity, and actin then slides on myosin to produce contraction.

The source of calcium in smooth muscle differs from that in skeletal muscle because the sarcoplasmic reticulum of smooth muscle is poorly developed. Most of the calcium that causes contraction of smooth muscles enters from extracellular fluid at the time of the action potential. The time required for this diffusion is 200 to 300 ms, which is approximately 50 times longer than for skeletal muscles. Subsequent relaxation of smooth muscles is achieved by a calcium ion transport system that pumps these ions back into extracellular fluid or into the sarcoplasmic reticulum. This calcium ion pump is slow compared with the sarcoplasmic reticulum pump in skeletal muscles. As a result, the duration of smooth muscle contraction is often seconds rather than milliseconds as is characteristic of skeletal muscles.

Smooth muscles, unlike skeletal muscles, do not atrophy when denervated, but they do become hyperresponsive to the normal neurotransmitter. This denervation hypersensitivity is a general phenomenon that is largely due to synthesis or activation of more receptors.

An NMJ similar to that present on skeletal muscles does not occur in smooth muscles. Instead, nerve fibers branch diffusely on top of a sheet of smooth muscle fibers without making actual contact. These nerve fibers secrete their neurotransmitter into an interstitial fluid space a few microns from the smooth muscle cells. Two different neurotransmitters, acetylcholine and norepinephrine, are secreted by the autonomic nervous system nerves that innervate smooth muscles. Acetylcholine is an excitatory neurotransmitter for smooth muscles at some sites and functions as an inhibitory neurotransmitter at other sites. Norepinephrine exerts the reverse effect of acetylcholine. It is believed that the presence of specific excitatory or inhibitory receptors in the membranes of smooth muscle fibers determines the response to acetylcholine or norepinephrine. When the neurotransmitter interacts with an inhibitory receptor instead of an excitatory receptor, the membrane potential of the smooth muscle fiber becomes more negative (hyperpolarized).

Uterine Smooth Muscle

Uterine smooth muscle is characterized by a high degree of spontaneous electrical and contractile activity. Unlike the heart, there is no pacemaker, and the contraction process spreads from one cell to another at a rate of 1 to 3 cm/s. Contractions of labor result in peak intrauterine pressures of 60 to 80 mm Hg in the second stage. Resting uterine pressure during labor is approximately 10 mm Hg. Movement of sodium ions appears to be the primary determinant in depolarization, whereas calcium ions are necessary for excitation-contraction coupling. Availability of calcium ions greatly influences the response of uterine smooth muscle to physiologic and pharmacologic stimulation or inhibition. Alpha excitatory and beta inhibitory receptors are also present in the myometrium.

References

1. Naguib M, Flood P, McArdle JJ, et al. Advances in neurobiology of the neuromuscular junction: implications for the anesthesiologist. *Anesthesiology*. 2002;96:202–231.
2. Loewi O. Über humorale Übertragbarkeit der Herznervenwirkung. *Pflugers Arch Gesamte Physiol Menschen Tiere*. 1921;189:239–242.
3. Dale HH, Feldberg W, Vogt M. Release of acetylcholine at voluntary motor nerve endings. *J Physiol*. 1936;86:353–380.
4. Changeux JP. The acetylcholine receptor: an "allosteric" membrane protein. *Harvey Lect*. 1981;75:85–254.
5. Berne RM, Levy MN, Koeppen BM, et al. *Physiology*. 5th ed. St Louis: Mosby; 2004.
6. Burke RE, Levine DN, Zajac FE III. Mammalian motor units: physiological-histochemical correlation in three types in cat gastrocnemius. *Science*. 1971;174:709–712.
7. Colman H, Nabekura J, Lichtman JW. Alterations in synaptic strength preceding axon withdrawal. *Science*. 1997;275:356–361.
8. Hughes JR. Post-tetanic potentiation. *Physiol Rev*. 1958;38:91–113.
9. Rosenberry TL. Acetylcholinesterase. *Adv Enzymol Relat Areas Mol Biol*. 1975;43:103–218.
10. Cresnar B, Crne-Finderle N, Breskvar K, et al. Neural regulation of muscle acetylcholinesterase is exerted on the level of its mRNA. *J Neurosci Res*. 1994;38:294–299.
11. Rossi SG, Vazquez AE, Rotundo RL. Local control of acetylcholinesterase gene expression in multinucleated skeletal muscle fibers: individual nuclei respond to signals from the overlying plasma membrane. *J Neurosci*. 2000;20:919–928.
12. Sung JJ, Kim SJ, Lee HB, et al. Anticholinesterase induces nicotinic receptor modulation. *Muscle Nerve*. 1998;21:1135–1144.
13. Machold J, Weise C, Utkin Y, et al. The handedness of the subunit arrangement of the nicotinic acetylcholine receptor from Torpedo californica. *Eur J Biochem*. 1995;234:427–430.
14. Villarroel A, Sakmann B. Calcium permeability increase of endplate channels in rat muscle during postnatal development. *J Physiol (Lond)*. 1996;496:331–338.
15. Martyn JA. Basic and clinical pharmacology of the acetylcholine receptor: implications for the use of neuromuscular relaxants. *Keio J Med*. 1995;44:1–8.
16. Kallen RG, Sheng ZH, Yang J, et al. Primary structure and expression of a sodium channel characteristic of denervated and immature rat skeletal muscle. *Neuron*. 1990;4:233–242.
17. Cooper EC, Jan LY. Ion channel genes and human neurological disease: recent progress, prospects, and challenges. *Proc Natl Acad Sci U S A*. 1999;96:4759–4766.
18. Jurkat-Rott K, Lerche H, Lehmann-Horn F. Skeletal muscle channelopathies. *J Neurol*. 2002;249:1493–1502.
19. Lehmann-Horn F, Jurkat-Rott K. Voltage-gated ion channels and hereditary disease. *Physiol Rev*. 1999;79:1317–1372.
20. Rios E, Pizarro G. Voltage sensor of excitation-contraction coupling in skeletal muscle. *Physiol Rev*. 1991;71:849–908.
21. Fill M, Copello JA. Ryanodine receptor calcium release channels. *Physiol Rev*. 2002;82:893–922.
22. MacKrill JJ. Protein-protein interactions in intracellular Ca2+-release channel function. *Biochem J*. 1999;337(pt 3):345–361.
23. Hoffman EP. Voltage-gated ion channelopathies: inherited disorders caused by abnormal sodium, chloride, and calcium regulation in skeletal muscle. *Annu Rev Med*. 1995;46:431–441.
24. Lehmann-Horn F, Jurkat-Rott K, Rudel R. Periodic paralysis: understanding channelopathies. *Curr Neurol Neurosci Rep*. 2002;2:61–69.

CHAPTER 12

Neuromuscular Blocking Drugs and Reversal Agents

Mohamed A. Naguib

The first successful administration of a neuromuscular blocker (curare) to produce surgical relaxation in an anesthetized patient occurred in 1912, when Arthur Läwen,[1] a German surgeon from Leipzig, used a partially purified preparation of the substance. Läwen's findings were subsequently ignored for nearly three decades until January 23, 1942, when Enid Johnson, following Harold Griffith's instructions, administered 5 mL of curare intravenously to a 20-year-old man who had been anesthetized with cyclopropane via a facemask for an appendectomy.[2] The use of neuromuscular blockers in clinical anesthesia has increased exponentially since that time.

Neuromuscular blockers that are currently available for clinical use are classified as (a) nondepolarizing neuromuscular blockers or (b) depolarizing neuromuscular blockers. Nondepolarizing neuromuscular blockers compete with acetylcholine for the active binding sites at the postsynaptic nicotinic acetylcholine receptor and are also called ***competitive antagonists***. Depolarizing neuromuscular blockers act as agonists (i.e., they are similar in structure to acetylcholine) at postsynaptic nicotinic acetylcholine receptors and cause prolonged membrane depolarization resulting in neuromuscular blockade. Succinylcholine is the only depolarizing neuromuscular blocker currently in clinical use.

Principles of Action of Neuromuscular Blockers at the Neuromuscular Junction

In the resting state, the ion channel of the acetylcholine receptor is closed (see Chapter 11). Simultaneous binding of two acetylcholine molecules to the α subunits[3] initiates conformational changes that open the channel.[4–6] On the other hand, binding of a single molecule of a nondepolarizing neuromuscular blocker (a competitive antagonist) to one α subunit is sufficient to produce neuromuscular block.[7]

Depolarizing neuromuscular blockers, such as succinylcholine, produce prolonged depolarization of the endplate region that results in desensitization of nicotinic acetylcholine receptors; inactivation of voltage-gated sodium channels at the neuromuscular junction; and increases in potassium permeability in the surrounding membrane. The end result is failure of action potential generation due to membrane hyperpolarization, and block ensues.

With respect to neuromuscular pharmacology, two enzymes of importance are known to hydrolyze choline esters: acetylcholinesterase and butyrylcholinesterase. Acetylcholinesterase (similar to red cell cholinesterase and also known as "true" cholinesterase) is present at the neuromuscular junction[8] and is responsible for the rapid hydrolysis of released acetylcholine to acetic acid and choline.[9] Butyrylcholinesterase (also known as plasma cholinesterase or pseudocholinesterase) is synthesized in the liver. Butyrylcholinesterase catalyzes the hydrolysis of succinylcholine, which occurs mainly in the plasma.

Structure of Neuromuscular Blocking Drugs

All neuromuscular blockers, being quaternary ammonium compounds, are structurally related to acetylcholine. The majority of neuromuscular blocking drugs currently available for clinical use are synthetic alkaloids. An exception is tubocurarine, which is extracted from plants. Although tubocurarine can be synthesized, it is less expensive to isolate this drug from the Amazonian vine *Chondodendron tomentosum*.

Characteristics of Nondepolarizing and Depolarizing Neuromuscular Block

During complete neuromuscular block, no response can be elicited by any pattern of nerve stimulation—single twitch, train-of-four (TOF) stimulation (four stimuli delivered every 0.5 second), or a tetanic stimulus. However, during partial neuromuscular block, the pattern of muscle response varies with the type of neuromuscular blocker administered and the degree of block.

Nondepolarizing Neuromuscular Block

Nondepolarizing neuromuscular block is characterized by (a) decrease in twitch tension, (b) fade during repetitive stimulation (TOF or tetanic), and (c) posttetanic potentiation (Fig. 12-1).

It is generally believed that twitch depression results from block of postsynaptic nicotinic acetylcholine receptors, whereas tetanic or TOF fade results from block of presynaptic nicotinic acetylcholine receptors.[10,11] Blockade of the presynaptic nicotinic acetylcholine receptors by neuromuscular blockers prevents acetylcholine from being made available (released from presynaptic nerve terminal) to sustain muscle contraction during high-frequency (tetanic or TOF) stimulation. Because the released acetylcholine does not match the demand, muscle fade is observed in response to stimulation.[12]

However, there is also strong contrary evidence indicating that fade could be simply a postjunctional (postsynaptic) phenomenon. This latter argument is supported by the fact that the snake toxin, α-bungarotoxin—which binds irreversibly to muscle (postjunctional) nicotinic acetylcholine receptors but does not bind to neuronal (prejunctional) nicotinic acetylcholine receptors—does produce fade.[13,14]

Depolarizing Neuromuscular Block

In the case of administration of a depolarizing neuromuscular blocking agent, such as succinylcholine, the muscle response that has been "classically" described is quite different. Depolarizing block (also called ***phase I block***) is often preceded by muscle fasciculation. During partial

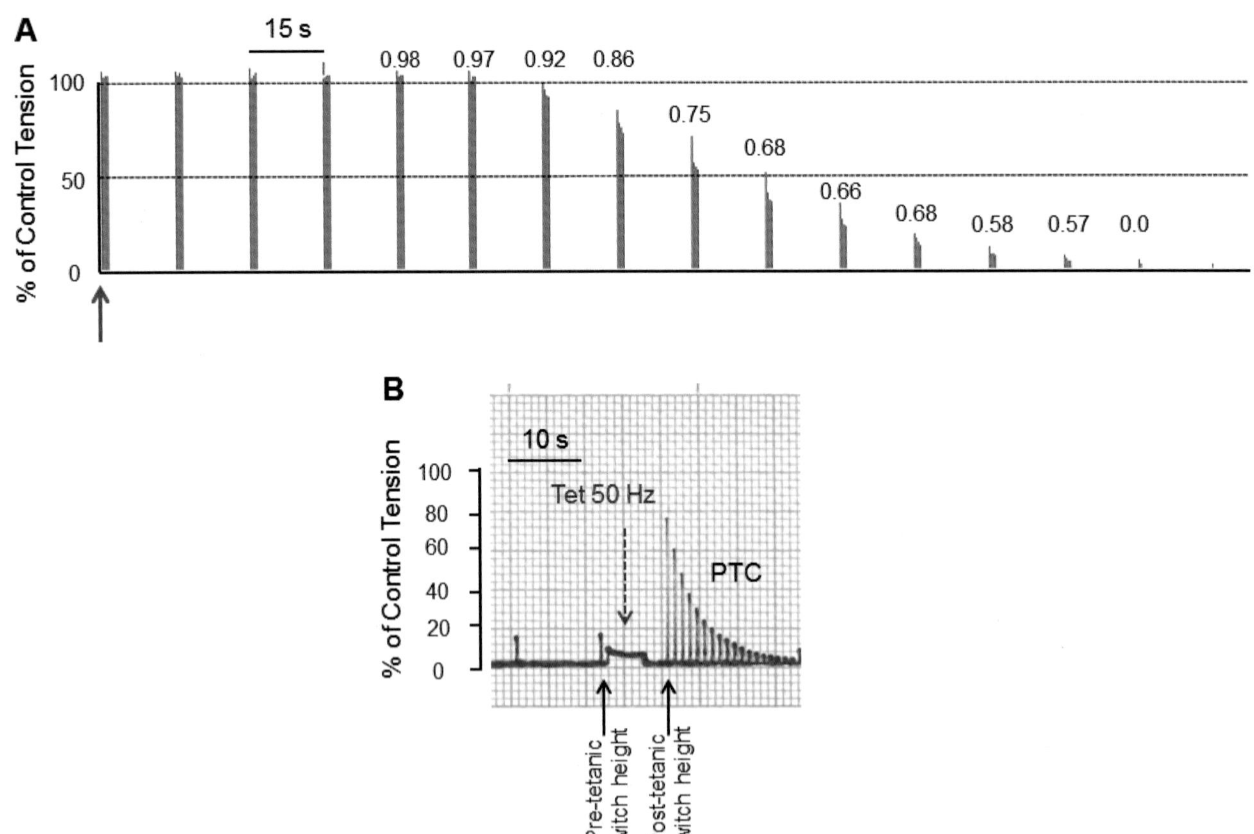

FIGURE 12-1 Acceleromyographic recording during the course of neuromuscular blockade induced by a nondepolarizing agent. **A:** Train-of-four (TOF) fade is noted during the onset of block. The *arrow* indicates the time of administration of a 2 × ED_{95} dose of the nondepolarizing neuromuscular blocking drug. The values corresponding to each TOF recording is the TOF ratio. **B:** Mechanomyographic recording during partial recovery from a nondepolarizing blockade. Tetanic fade and posttetanic potentiation are present after application of a 5-second, 50-Hz tetanic (Tet) stimulation (Tet 50 Hz). PTC, posttetanic count.

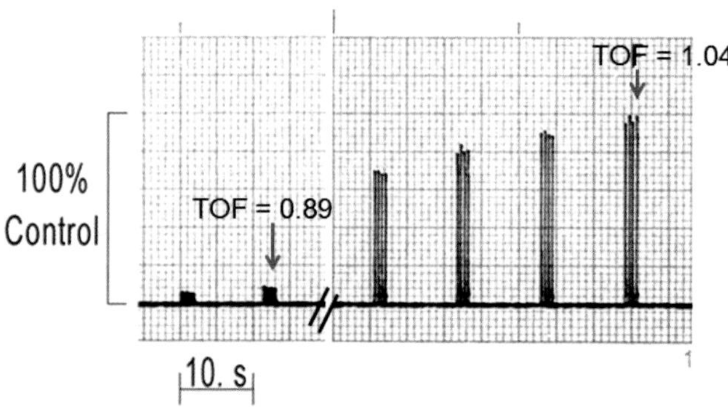

FIGURE 12-2 Mechanomyographic recording during recovery from 1.0 mg/kg succinylcholine. Note that there is no significant fade in the train-of-four (TOF) response during recovery. At 8% recovery of T1 (the first twitch in the train-of-four), the TOF ratio was 0.89, and at 96% recovery of T1, the TOF ratio was 1.04.

neuromuscular block, depolarizing block is characterized by (a) decrease in twitch tension, (b) no fade during repetitive stimulation (tetanic or TOF), and (c) no posttetanic potentiation (Fig. 12-2).

Pharmacology of Succinylcholine

Structure–Activity Relationships for Succinylcholine

Succinylcholine is a long, thin, flexible molecule composed of two molecules of acetylcholine linked through the acetate methyl groups (Fig. 12-3). Like acetylcholine, succinylcholine stimulates cholinergic receptors at the neuromuscular junction and at nicotinic (ganglionic) and muscarinic autonomic sites, opening the ionic channel in the acetylcholine receptor.

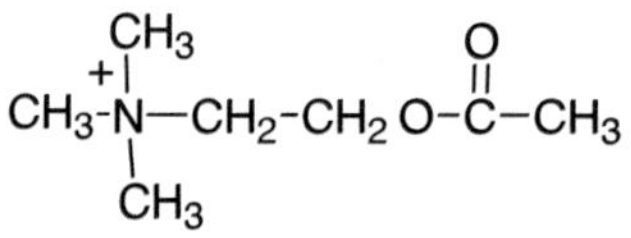

$CH_3-N^+(CH_3)_2-CH_2-CH_2-O-C(=O)-CH_3$

Acetylcholine

$CH_3-N^+(CH_3)_2-CH_2-CH_2-O-C(=O)-CH_2-CH_2-C(=O)-O-CH_2-CH_2-N^+(CH_3)_2-CH_3$

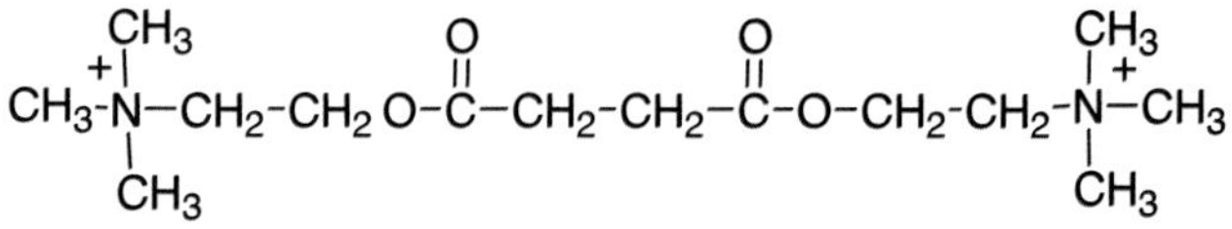

Succinylcholine

FIGURE 12-3 Structural relationship of succinylcholine, a depolarizing neuromuscular blocking agent, to acetylcholine. Succinylcholine consists of two acetylcholine molecules linked through the acetate methyl groups. Like acetylcholine, succinylcholine stimulates nicotinic receptors at the neuromuscular junction.

Pharmacokinetics, Pharmacodynamics, and Pharmacogenomics of Succinylcholine

Succinylcholine has an elimination half-life of 47 seconds (95% confidence interval of 24 to 70 seconds).[15] The elimination of succinylcholine appears to follow first-order kinetics.[15,16] The $t_{½}$ k_{e0} and Hill coefficient (after fitting two doses of 1 mg/kg succinylcholine) were 244 seconds (standard deviation 157) and 7.9 (standard deviation 3.3), respectively.[15] The dose of succinylcholine causing on average 95% suppression of twitch height (the ED_{95}) is approximately 0.3 mg/kg.[17,18]

The usual dose of succinylcholine required for tracheal intubation in adults is 1.0 mg/kg. Administration of 1 mg/kg succinylcholine results in complete suppression of response to neuromuscular stimulation in approximately 60 seconds. In patients with genotypically normal butyrylcholinesterase activity, time to recovery to 90% muscle strength following administration of 1 mg/kg succinylcholine ranges from 9 to 13 minutes.[19,20] In one study, administration of 0.6 mg/kg of succinylcholine resulted in acceptable intubating conditions at 60 seconds in 95% of patients.[21] The reported proportions of patients with acceptable intubating conditions after administration of 1.0 mg/kg succinylcholine varies from 91.8% to 97%.[22–24] It also appears that there are no advantages to using succinylcholine doses larger than 1.5 mg/kg in a rapid sequence induction of anesthesia. Paradoxically, succinylcholine doses as large as 2.0 mg/kg guaranteed excellent intubating conditions at 60 seconds in only 86.7% of patients.[25] It should be noted that the adequacy of intubating conditions is related not only to the use of a neuromuscular blocker but also to the depth of anesthesia, airway anatomy, and the experience of the laryngoscopist.

The short duration of action of succinylcholine is due to its rapid hydrolysis by butyrylcholinesterase (plasma cholinesterase) to succinylmonocholine and choline, such that only 10% of the administered drug reaches the neuromuscular junction.[26] Succinylmonocholine is a much weaker neuromuscular blocking agent than succinylcholine [27] and is metabolized much more slowly to succinic acid and choline.

There is little or no butyrylcholinesterase at the neuromuscular junction. Butyrylcholinesterase influences the onset and duration of action of succinylcholine by controlling the rate at which the drug is hydrolyzed in the plasma before it reaches, and after it leaves, the neuromuscular junction. Recovery from succinylcholine-induced blockade occurs as succinylcholine diffuses away from the neuromuscular junction, down a concentration gradient as the plasma concentration decreases.

Factors Affecting Butyrylcholinesterase Activity

Butyrylcholinesterase is synthesized by the liver and found in the plasma.[28,29] The elimination half-time of plasma cholinesterase is 8 to 16 hours, and levels of <75% are necessary for prolongation of succinylcholine effect. Butyrylcholinesterase is responsible for metabolism of succinylcholine, mivacurium, procaine, chloroprocaine, tetracaine, cocaine, and heroin. Neuromuscular block induced by succinylcholine or mivacurium is prolonged when there is a significant reduction in the concentration or activity of butyrylcholinesterase. The activity of the enzyme refers to the number of substrate molecules (μmol) hydrolyzed per unit of time, often expressed in International Units.

Factors that have been described as lowering butyrylcholinesterase activity are advanced liver disease,[30] advanced age,[31] malnutrition, pregnancy, burns, oral contraceptives, monoamine oxidase inhibitors, echothiophate, cytotoxic drugs, neoplastic disease, anticholinesterase drugs,[32,33] metoclopramide,[34] and bambuterol.[35,36] The β-blocker esmolol inhibits butyrylcholinesterase but causes only a minor prolongation of succinylcholine block.[37,38]

Neostigmine (and to a lesser degree edrophonium) causes a profound decrease in butyrylcholinesterase activity.[39] Even 30 minutes after administration of neostigmine, the butyrylcholinesterase activity remains about 50% of control values. Potent anticholinesterase drugs used in insecticides and occasionally in the treatment of glaucoma and myasthenia gravis, as well as chemotherapeutic drugs (nitrogen mustard and cyclophosphamide), may decrease butyrylcholinesterase activity so that prolonged neuromuscular blockade follows administration of succinylcholine. High estrogen levels, as observed in parturients at term, are associated with up to 40% decreases in butyrylcholinesterase activity. Paradoxically, the duration of action of succinylcholine-induced skeletal muscle paralysis is not prolonged, presumably reflecting an increased volume of distribution of the drug at term.

Genetic Variants of Butyrylcholinesterase

Neuromuscular block induced by succinylcholine or mivacurium can be significantly prolonged if the patient has an abnormal genetic variant of butyrylcholinesterase. Analysis of butyrylcholinesterase involves the determination of both enzyme activity and biochemical phenotypes. Phenotype is determined by the use of specific enzyme inhibitors (such as dibucaine or fluoride) that produce phenotype-specific patterns of dibucaine or fluoride numbers. Molecular genetic analyses can determine the true genotypes. For reviews, see Pantuck [40] and Goodall.[41]

It is important to recognize that the dibucaine number reflects quality of cholinesterase enzyme (ability to hydrolyze succinylcholine) and not the quantity of the enzyme that is circulating in the plasma. In case of the usual butyrylcholinesterase genotype ($E_1^uE_1^u$), the dibucaine number is 70 or higher, whereas in individuals homozygous for the atypical gene ($E_1^aE_1^a$) (frequency in general population of 1 in 3,500), the dibucaine number is less than 30. In individuals with the heterozygous atypical variant ($E_1^uE_1^a$) (frequency in general population of 1 in 480), the dibucaine number is in the range of 40 to 60.[42,43] In individuals with the homozygous atypical genotype ($E_1^aE_1^a$), the neuromuscular block induced by succinylcholine or mivacurium is prolonged to 4 to 8 hours, and in individuals with the heterozygous atypical genotype ($E_1^uE_1^a$), the period of neuromuscular block induced by succinylcholine or mivacurium is about 1.5 to 2 times that seen in individuals with the usual genotype ($E_1^uE_1^u$).[44] The longest period of apnea after the administration of succinylcholine was found in patients homozygous for the silent gene ($E_1^sE_1^s$).[44] In those patients, TOF stimulation will help in detecting the development of phase II block, a block that may appear after prolonged or repeated administration of succinylcholine and has characteristics similar to nondepolarizing neuromuscular blockers. The decision whether to attempt antagonism of a phase II block has always been controversial and the use edrophonium or neostigmine do not consistently result in adequate antagonism of neuromuscular blockade.[45] The alternative is to keep the patient adequately sedated and maintain artificial ventilation until the TOF ratio has recovered to 0.9 or more.

Fluoride-resistant butyrylcholinesterase variants have also been described. In case of the usual butyrylcholinesterase genotype ($E_1^uE_1^u$), the fluoride number is 60, whereas in individuals with the homozygous atypical genotype ($E_1^fE_1^f$), the fluoride number is 36.[44] Individuals with homozygous fluoride-resistant genotype exhibit mild to moderate prolongation of succinylcholine-induced paralysis. The heterozygous fluoride-resistant genotype usually produces clinically insignificant prolongation of succinylcholine block, unless accompanied by a second abnormal allele or by a coexisting acquired cause of butyrylcholinesterase deficiency.

Although the dibucaine or fluoride number indicates the genetic makeup of an individual with respect to butyrylcholinesterase, it does not measure the concentration of the enzyme in the plasma nor does it indicate the efficiency of the enzyme in hydrolyzing succinylcholine or mivacurium. Both of these latter factors are determined by measuring butyrylcholinesterase activity—which may be influenced by genotype.

Some rare butyrylcholinesterase variants are associated with increased enzyme activity (two to three times normal).[46] Resistance to succinylcholine[47] and mivacurium[48] as a result of increased butyrylcholinesterase activity has been described.

Side Effects of Succinylcholine

Cardiovascular Effects

Sinus bradycardia, junctional rhythm, and even sinus arrest may follow administration of succinylcholine. These cardiac effects reflect the actions of succinylcholine at cardiac muscarinic cholinergic receptors where the drug mimics the physiologic effects of acetylcholine. Cardiac dysrhythmias are most likely to occur when a second dose of succinylcholine is administered approximately 5 minutes after the first dose. Sinus bradycardia (resulting from stimulation of cardiac muscarinic receptors) is frequently seen in children[49] and in adults after a repeated dose of succinylcholine.[50] Atropine is effective in treating or preventing bradycardia.

In contrast to actions at cardiac muscarinic cholinergic receptors, the effects of succinylcholine at autonomic nervous system ganglia may produce ganglionic stimulation and associated increases in heart rate and systemic blood pressure. The ganglionic stimulation reflects an effect of succinylcholine on autonomic ganglia that resembles the physiologic effect of acetylcholine at these sites. Ventricular dysrhythmias after succinylcholine administration have been attributed to autonomic stimuli associated with laryngoscopy and tracheal intubation.[51]

Hyperkalemia

The administration of succinylcholine is associated with approximately 0.5 mEq/dL increase in the plasma potassium concentration in healthy individuals, which is well tolerated and generally does not cause dysrhythmias. Patients with renal failure are no more susceptible to an exaggerated hyperkalemic response to succinylcholine than are patients with normal renal function.[52,53]

Succinylcholine has been associated with severe hyperkalemia in patients with burn, severe abdominal infections,[54] severe metabolic acidosis,[55] closed head injury,[56] or conditions associated with upregulation of extrajunctional acetylcholine receptors (e.g., hemiplegia or paraplegia, muscular dystrophies, Guillain-Barré syndrome, and burn). For reviews, see Naguib et al.[8] and Martyn and Richtsfeld.[57] Because of the risk of massive rhabdomyolysis, hyperkalemia, and death in children with undiagnosed muscle disease, succinylcholine is not recommended for use in children except for emergency tracheal intubation.[58-60]

Myoglobinuria

Damage to skeletal muscles is suggested by the occurrence of myoglobinuria after administration of succinylcholine, especially to pediatric patients.[61] It is unlikely that succinylcholine-induced fasciculations could produce muscle damage resulting in myoglobinuria. Most of the patients with rhabdomyolysis and myoglobinuria were subsequently found to have malignant hyperthermia or muscular dystrophy.

Increased Intraocular Pressure

Succinylcholine usually causes an increase in intraocular pressure. The intraocular pressure peaks at 2 to 4 minutes after administration and returns to normal by 6 minutes.[62] This increase is likely the result of contraction of tonic myofibrils and/or transient dilatation of choroidal blood vessels. The use of succinylcholine is not widely accepted in open eye injury (when the anterior chamber is open) even though succinylcholine was shown to cause no adverse events in a series of 73 patients with penetrating eye injuries.[63] The efficacy of precurarization in attenuating increases in intraocular pressure following succinylcholine administration is controversial.[64-66]

Increased Intragastric Pressure

Administration of succinylcholine is associated with a variable increase in intragastric and lower esophageal sphincter pressures. The increase in intragastric pressure appears to be related to (a) the intensity of fasciculations of the abdominal skeletal muscles,[67] which could be prevented by prior administration of a nondepolarizing neuromuscular blocker; and (b) a direct increase in vagal tone. Administration of succinylcholine does not predispose to regurgitation in patients with an intact lower esophageal sphincter because the increase in intragastric pressure does not exceed the "barrier pressure."[68]

Increased Intracranial Pressure

Succinylcholine has the potential to increase intracranial pressure.[69] This increase can be attenuated or prevented by pretreatment with a nondepolarizing neuromuscular blocker.[70]

Myalgias

Postoperative skeletal muscle myalgia, which is particularly prominent in the skeletal muscles of the neck, back, and abdomen, can occur after administration of succinylcholine, especially to young adults undergoing minor surgical procedures that permit early ambulation. Myalgia localized to neck muscles may be perceived as pharyngitis ("sore throat") by the patient and attributed to tracheal intubation by the anesthesiologist. Muscle pain occurs more frequently in patients undergoing ambulatory surgery, especially in women, than in bedridden patients.[71] The incidence of muscle pain following administration of succinylcholine varies from 0.2% to 89%.[72] The mechanism of succinylcholine-induced myalgia appears to be complex and is not fully understood. One hypothesis proposes that myalgia is secondary to muscle damage by succinylcholine-induced fasciculations.[71] This hypothesis is supported by findings of myoglobinemia and increases in serum creatine kinase level following succinylcholine administration.[61,73,74] However, although prior administration of a small dose of a nondepolarizing neuromuscular blocker prevents fasciculations due to succinylcholine, this approach is not always effective in preventing succinylcholine-induced myalgia.[72,75] Another hypothesis suggests a possible role for prostaglandins and cyclooxygenases in succinylcholine-induced myalgias.[76,77] Pretreatment with a prostaglandin inhibitor (lysine acetylsalicylate or diclofenac) has been shown to be effective in decreasing the incidence of muscle pain after succinylcholine administration.[76,78] A meta-analysis showed that myalgia may best be prevented with muscle relaxants, lidocaine, or nonsteroidal antiinflammatory drugs.[79] It should be noted, however, that myalgias following outpatient surgery occur even in the absence of succinylcholine.[80,81]

Masseter Spasm

Succinylcholine is a known trigger agent for malignant hyperthermia. Although an increase in tone of the masseter muscle may be an early indicator of malignant hyperthermia,[82] it is not consistently associated with malignant hyperthermia.[83–85] It has been suggested that the high incidence of masseter spasm in children given succinylcholine may be due to inadequate succinylcholine dosage.[86]

Pharmacology of Nondepolarizing Neuromuscular Blockers

Available nondepolarizing neuromuscular blockers can be classified according to chemical class (the steroidal, benzylisoquinolinium, and other blockers) or according to rapidity of onset of action or duration of action (long-acting, intermediate-acting, or short-acting) of equipotent doses (Table 12-1). The pharmacodynamic and pharmacokinetic behaviors of currently used and new nondepolarizing neuromuscular blockers are shown in Tables 12-2 and 12-3, respectively.

Benzylisoquinolinium Compounds

The South American Indians' arrow poisons, known as curare, served as the basis for the development of the benzylisoquinoline-type relaxants. Tubocurarine, the most important curare alkaloid, was introduced as a neuromuscular blocking drug for use during surgical anesthesia.[1,2]

Tubocurarine

Tubocurarine is a monoquarternary, long-acting neuromuscular blocker (Fig. 12-4).[87] There is no active metabolism of tubocurarine. It is excreted unchanged in the urine, and the liver is probably a secondary route of elimination. Therefore, and because more suitable agents are available, tubocurarine is not indicated for use in patients with either renal[88] or hepatic failure. The onset of action of tubocurarine is slow, its duration of action is long, and its recovery is slow (see Table 12-2). The usual intubating dose is 0.5 to 0.6 mg/kg; maintenance doses are 0.1 to 0.2 mg/kg.

Atracurium

Atracurium consists of a racemic mixture of 10 stereoisomers.[89,90] These isomers have been separated into three geometrical isomer groups that are designated *cis-cis*, *cis-trans*, and *trans-trans* based on their configuration about the tetrahydroisoquinoline ring system.[89,90] The ratio of the *cis-cis*, *cis-trans*, and *trans-trans* isomers is approximately 10:6:1.[91]

Atracurium has been designed to undergo spontaneous degradation (Fig. 12-5) at physiologic temperature and pH by a mechanism called ***Hofmann elimination***, yielding laudanosine (a tertiary amine) and a monoquaternary acrylate as metabolites.[89,92] Furthermore, atracurium can undergo ester hydrolysis. Hofmann elimination is a purely

Table 12-1

Classification of Commonly Used and New Nondepolarizing Neuromuscular Blockers According to Duration of Action (Time to T1 = 25% of Control) after Administration of 2× ED_{95}[a]

	Duration of Action		
	Long (>50 min)	Intermediate (20–50 min)	Short (10–20 min)
Steroidal compounds	Pancuronium	Vecuronium Rocuronium	—
Benzylisoquinolinium compounds	Tubocurarine	Atracurium Cisatracurium	Mivacurium

ED_{95} is the dose that results in 95% depression of twitch height.

[a]The majority of nondepolarizing neuromuscular blockers are bisquaternary ammonium compounds. Tubocurarine, vecuronium, and rocuronium are monoquaternary compounds.

Table 12-2

Dose-Response Relationships and Pharmacodynamic Parameters for Nondepolarizing Neuromuscular Blocking Drugs in Human Subjects[a]

	ED_{50} (mg/kg)	ED_{95} (mg/kg)	CE_{50} (ng/mL)	K_{e0} (min^{-1})	Intubating Dose (mg/kg)	Maximum Block (%)	Time to Maximum Block (min)	Clinical Duration of Response[b] (min)
Long-acting								
d-Tubocurarine	0.23	0.48	370	0.13	0.6	97	5.7	81
Pancuronium	0.036	0.067	88	—	0.08	100	2.9	86
Intermediate-acting								
Rocuronium	0.147	0.305	3510	0.405	0.6	100	1.7	36
Vecuronium	0.027	0.043	92	0.17	0.1	100	2.4	44
Atracurium	0.12	0.21	449	0.13	0.5	100	3.2	46
Cisatracurium	0.026	0.04	126–158	0.07–0.09	0.1	100	5.2	45
Short-acting								
Mivacurium	0.039	0.067	79.9	0.18	0.15	100	3.3	16.8

ED_{50} and ED_{95} are the doses of each drug that produce, respectively, 50% and 95% decrease in the force of contraction or amplitude of the electromyogram of the adductor pollicis muscle following ulnar nerve stimulation.

CE_{50} is the neuromuscular junction concentration of each drug that produces a 50% decrease in the force of contraction or amplitude of the electromyogram of the adductor pollicis muscle following ulnar nerve stimulation.

k_{e0} is the rate constant for equilibration of drug between the plasma and the neuromuscular junction.

[a]Derived using simultaneous pharmacokinetic/pharmacodynamic modeling.

[b]Time from injection of the intubating dose to recovery of twitch to 25% of control.

Table 12-3

Pharmacokinetic Parameters of Neuromuscular Blocking Drugs

	Plasma Clearance (mL/kg/min)	Volume of Distribution (mL/kg)	Elimination Half-life (min)	Reference
Short-acting				
Mivacurium isomers				249
Cis-trans	106	278	2.0	
Trans-trans	57	211	2.3	
Cis-cis	3.8	227	68	
Intermediate-acting				
Atracurium	6.1	182	21	98
	10.9	280	17.3	250
Cisatracurium	5.2	31	—	106
Vecuronium	3.0	194	78	122
	5.3	199	53	251
Rocuronium	2.9	207	71	130
Long-acting				
d-Tubocurarine	2.4	250	84	252
Pancuronium	1.7	261	132	253

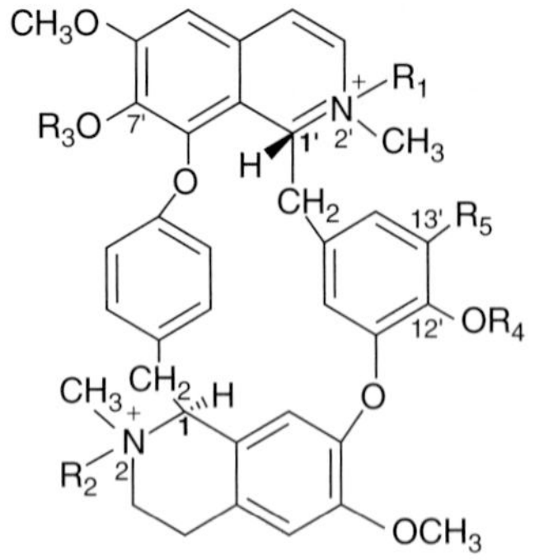

Cyclic benzylisoquinoline

Cyclic benzylisoquinoline derivatives

Name	R_1	R_2	R_3	R_4	R_5	1	1'
Tubocurarine	CH_3	H	H	H	H	*S*	*R*
Chondrocurine	CH_3	CH_3	H	H	H	*S*	*R*

R and *S* represent the stereochemical configuration about the designated carbon

FIGURE 12-4 Chemical structures of tubocurarine and chondrocurine.

chemical process that results in loss of the positive charges by molecular fragmentation to laudanosine and a monoquaternary acrylate.[93,94] Laudanosine depends on the liver for clearance, with approximately 70% excreted in the bile and the remainder in urine.[95] Hepatic cirrhosis in humans does not alter clearance of laudanosine, whereas excretion of this metabolite is impaired in patients with biliary obstruction.[96] Laudanosine easily crosses the blood–brain barrier, and it has central nervous system stimulating properties. The seizure threshold is not known in humans. In patients in the intensive care unit, blood levels of laudanosine can be as high as 5.0 to 6.0 μg/mL.[97] There is no evidence to suggest that prolonged administration of atracurium in the operating room or in the intensive care unit in patients with normal or impaired renal function is likely to result in concentrations of laudanosine capable of producing convulsions. The plasma elimination half-life of laudanosine is similar in patients with normal and impaired renal function—197 ± 38 and 234 ± 81 minutes, respectively.[98,99] Interestingly, laudanosine activates α4β2 nicotinic acetylcholine receptors and δ- and κ-opioid receptors. It has been suggested that this activation has neuroprotective effects.[100–103]

Cisatracurium

Cisatracurium is the 1R *cis*–1'R *cis* isomer of atracurium and represents about 15% of the marketed atracurium mixture by weight but more than 50% of the mixture in terms of potency or neuromuscular blocking activity (see Fig. 12-5). Like atracurium, cisatracurium is metabolized by Hofmann elimination to laudanosine and a monoquaternary alcohol metabolite.[104–106] There is no ester hydrolysis of the parent molecule.[104] Hofmann elimination accounts for 77% of the total clearance of 5 to 6 mL/kg per minute.[107] Twenty-three percent of the drug is cleared through organ-dependent means, with renal elimination accounting for 16% of this.[106] Because cisatracurium is about four to five times as potent as atracurium, about five times less laudanosine is produced, and accumulation of this metabolite is not thought to be of any consequence in clinical practice. Unlike atracurium, cisatracurium in the clinical dose range does not cause histamine release.[108,109] This indicates that the phenomenon of histamine release may be stereospecific.[108,110]

Mivacurium

Mivacurium is the only currently available short-acting neuromuscular blocker in the European Union, but its use in the United States has been discontinued by the manufacturer (see Table 12-2). Mivacurium consists of a mixture of three stereoisomers. Mivacurium is metabolized by butyrylcholinesterase at about 70% to 88% the rate of succinylcholine to a monoester, a dicarboxylic acid.[111,112] Mivacurium may produce histamine release, especially if administered rapidly.[113]

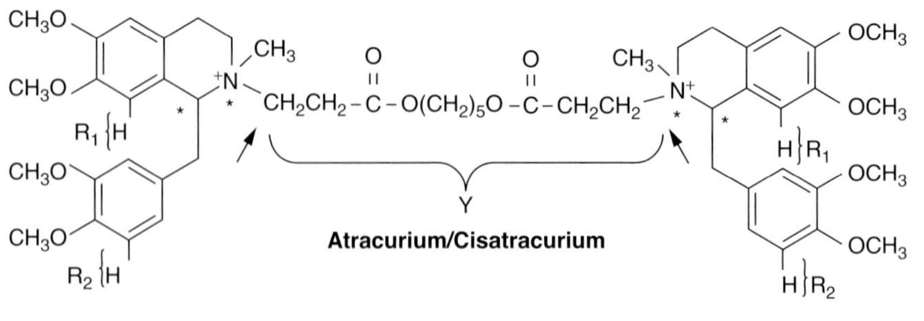

FIGURE 12-5 Chemical structures of atracurium, cisatracurium, and mivacurium. *Asterisk* indicates the chiral centers; *arrows* show cleavage sites for Hofmann elimination.

Atracurium/Cisatracurium

	Y	R_1	R_2
Mivacurium	$-(CH_2)_3O-C(=O)-(CH_2)_2CH{=}CH(CH_2)_2-C(=O)-O(CH_2)_3-$	$-OCH_3$	$-H$

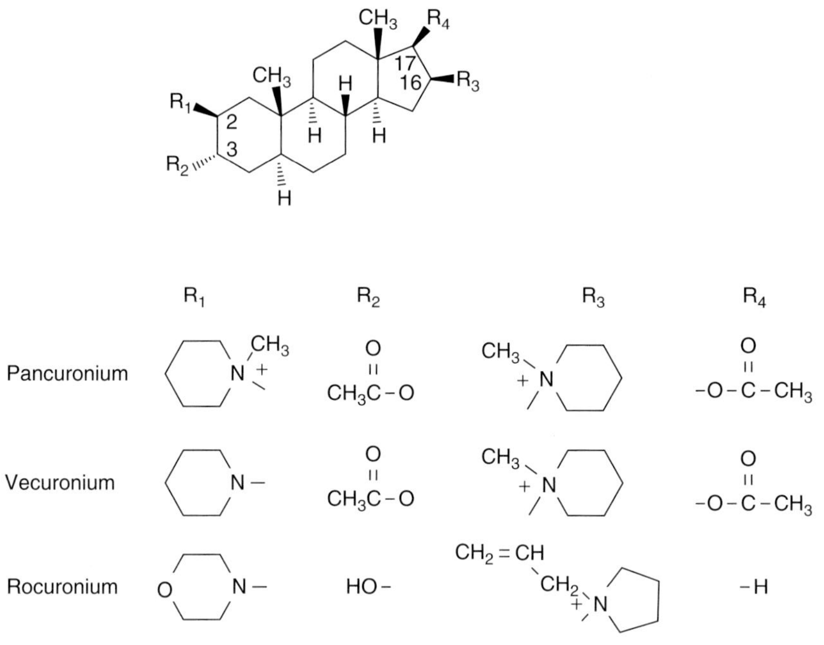

FIGURE 12-6 Chemical structures of the steroidal neuromuscular blockers pancuronium, vecuronium, and rocuronium.

Steroidal Compounds

The steroid skeleton possesses onium centers at different positions. In the steroidal compounds, it is probably essential that one of two nitrogen atoms in the molecule be quaternized.[114] The presence of acetyl ester (acetylcholine-like moiety) is thought to facilitate interaction of steroidal compounds with nicotinic acetylcholine receptors at the postsynaptic muscle membrane.[7,115]

Pancuronium

Pancuronium is a potent long-acting neuromuscular blocking drug with both vagolytic and butyrylcholinesterase-inhibiting properties (Fig. 12-6).[116] About 40% to 60% of pancuronium is cleared by the kidney[117] and 11% is excreted in the bile. A small amount (15% to 20%) is metabolized, mainly by deacetylation in the liver. The metabolites (3-OH, 17-OH, and 3,7-di-OH) are considerably less potent as neuromuscular blockers and are excreted in the urine.[118] Accumulation of the 3-OH metabolite is responsible for prolongation of the duration of block induced by pancuronium.

Vecuronium

Vecuronium is a monoquarternary neuromuscular blocker with an intermediate duration of action. Vecuronium is simply pancuronium without the quaternizing methyl group in the 2-piperidino substitution (see Fig. 12-6).[7,119] The minor molecular difference between vecuronium and pancuronium means that vecuronium is characterized by (a) a slight decrease in potency; (b) virtual loss of the vagolytic properties of pancuronium; (c) molecular instability in solution (this explains in part the shorter duration of action of vecuronium compared with pancuronium); and (d) increased lipid solubility, which results in a greater biliary elimination of vecuronium than pancuronium.[7,120]

The liver is the principal organ of elimination for vecuronium, and renal excretion accounts for excretion of approximately 30% of the administered dose. Approximately 30% to 40% of vecuronium is cleared in the bile as parent compound.[121] The duration of the vecuronium-induced neuromuscular block is therefore dependent primarily on hepatic function and, to a lesser extent, on renal function.[122,123] Vecuronium is metabolized in the liver by deacetylation into three possible metabolites: 3-OH, 17-OH, and 3,17-di-OH vecuronium. The 3-OH metabolite has 80% the neuromuscular blocking potency of vecuronium. Therefore, during prolonged administration of vecuronium, this metabolite may contribute to prolonged neuromuscular blockade.[124]

Vecuronium is prepared as a lyophilized powder because it is less stable in solution. Vecuronium cannot be prepared as a ready-to-use solution with a sufficient shelf life, even as a buffered solution. In pancuronium, the 2-piperidine is quaternized and no longer basic (charged). Thus, it does not participate in catalysis of the 3-acetate hydrolysis.

Rocuronium

Rocuronium (see Fig. 12-6) is an intermediately acting monoquaternary neuromuscular blocker with a fast onset of action than either pancuronium or vecuronium. Rocuronium is about six times less potent than vecuronium.[125,126] Rocuronium is primarily eliminated by the liver and excreted in bile. It is taken up into the liver by a carrier-mediated active transport system.[127] The putative metabolite, 17-desacetylrocuronium, has

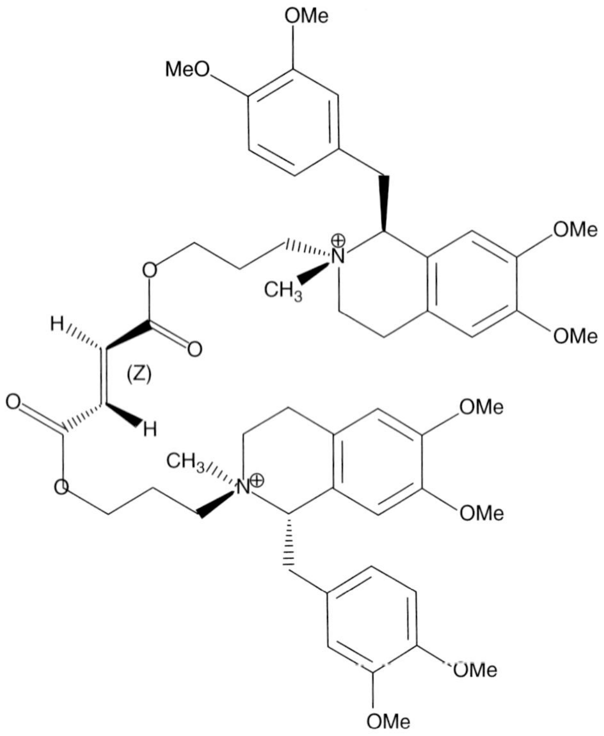

FIGURE 12-7 Chemical structure of CW002 (AV002).

not been detected in significant quantities. Approximately 30% of rocuronium is excreted unchanged in the urine.[128,129] At room temperature, rocuronium is stable for 60 days, whereas pancuronium is stable for 6 months.

Olefinic (Double-Bonded) Isoquinolinium Diester Compounds

CW002

CW002 (AV002), a benzylisoquinolinium fumarate ester-based compound, is an investigational neuromuscular blocking drug of intermediate duration of action (Fig. 12-7).[130] CW002 was designed to undergo cysteine adduction and possibly chemical hydrolysis more slowly than gantacurium. In dogs, administration of 0.08 mg/kg (10× ED_{95}) of CW002 resulted in a duration of action of 71 ± 4 minutes.[131] No signs of histamine release were observed in cats in doses up to 0.8 mg/kg (40× ED_{95}).

Potency of Nondepolarizing Neuromuscular Blockers

Drug potency is commonly expressed in terms of the dose-response relationship. The potency of neuromuscular blockers can be expressed as the dose of drug required to produce an effect—for example, 50% or 95% depression of twitch height, commonly expressed as ED_{50} and ED_{95}, respectively.[132] The neuromuscular blocking drugs have different potencies, as illustrated in Table 12-2. The dose-response curve for nondepolarizing neuromuscular blockers is sigmoidal, and different ED values have been derived in a variety of ways. The most commonly used technique is linear regression analysis after log-dose and probit- or logit-data transformation.

Recently, Kopman et al.[133] reported that the ED_{50} value is a very robust parameter and should be employed rather than the ED_{95} value when comparing the potency of neuromuscular blockers. They noted that the ED_{50} values calculated by different methods (nonlinear regression analysis, linear regression analysis, or Hill's equation) were interchangeable, and that the ED_{95} value was not a precise parameter because the confidence intervals of the ED_{95} were so wide.[133]

Factors that Increase the Potency of Nondepolarizing Neuromuscular Blockers

Inhalational anesthetics potentiate the neuromuscular blocking effect of nondepolarizing neuromuscular blockers. This potentiation results mainly in a decrease in the required dosage of neuromuscular blocker and prolongation of both the duration of action of the relaxant and recovery from neuromuscular block.[134] The magnitude of this potentiation depends on several factors, including the duration of inhalational anesthesia,[135–137] the specific inhalational anesthetic used,[138] and the concentration of inhalational agent used.[139] The rank order of potentiation is desflurane > sevoflurane > isoflurane > halothane > nitrous oxide–barbiturate–opioid or propofol anesthesia.[140–142] The mechanisms proposed for this potentiation include (a) a central effect on α motoneurons and interneuronal synapses,[143] (b) inhibition of postsynaptic nicotinic acetylcholine receptors,[144] and (c) augmentation of the antagonist's affinity at the receptor site.[145]

Some antibiotics can also potentiate neuromuscular blockade. The aminoglycoside antibiotics, the polymyxins, and lincomycin and clindamycin primarily inhibit the prejunctional release of acetylcholine and also depress postjunctional nicotinic acetylcholine receptor sensitivity to acetylcholine.[146] The tetracyclines, on the other hand, exhibit postjunctional activity only.[146]

Hypothermia or magnesium sulfate potentiates the neuromuscular blockade induced by nondepolarizing neuromuscular blockers.[147–150] The mechanism(s) underlying this potentiation may be pharmacodynamic, pharmacokinetic, or both.[149] High magnesium concentrations inhibit calcium channels at the presynaptic nerve terminals that trigger the release of acetylcholine.[8]

Most local anesthetics when given in large doses potentiate neuromuscular block; in smaller doses, no clinically significant potentiation occurs.[151] Antidysrhythmic drugs, such as quinidine, also potentiate neuromuscular block.[152]

Factors that Decrease the Potency of Nondepolarizing Neuromuscular Blockers

Resistance to nondepolarizing muscle blockers has been demonstrated in patients receiving chronic anticonvulsant therapy, as evidenced by accelerated recovery from neuromuscular blockade and the need for increased doses to achieve complete neuromuscular blockade. This resistance has been attributed to increased clearance,[153] increased binding of the neuromuscular blockers to α_1-acid glycoproteins, and/or upregulation of neuromuscular acetylcholine receptors.[154]

In hyperparathyroidism, hypercalcemia is associated with decreased sensitivity to atracurium and thus a shortened duration of neuromuscular blockade.[155] Increasing calcium concentrations also decreased the sensitivity to tubocurarine and pancuronium in a muscle-nerve model.[156]

Effect of Drug Potency on Speed of Onset

The speed of onset of action is inversely proportional to the potency of nondepolarizing neuromuscular blockers.[157,158] Low potency is predictive of rapid onset, and high potency is predictive of slow onset. Except for atracurium,[159] molar potency (the ED_{50} or ED_{95} expressed in μM/kg) is highly predictive of a drug's time to onset of effect (at the adductor pollicis muscle).[158] Rocuronium has a molar potency ($ED_{95} \approx 0.54$ μM/kg), which is about 13% that of vecuronium and only 9% that of cisatracurium. Thus, rapid onset of rocuronium is to be expected. It should be noted that a drug's measured molar potency is the end result of many contributing factors: the drug's intrinsic potency (the CE_{50}, the biophase concentration resulting in 50% twitch depression), the rate of equilibration between plasma and biophase (ke0), the initial rate of plasma clearance, and probably other factors as well.[160]

The influence of potency on speed of onset could be simply explained by the fact that, for an equipotent dose (e.g., a dose that results in 50% receptor occupancy), a low-potency drug (such as rocuronium) will have a higher number of molecules than a high-potency drug (such as tubocurarine). The higher number of drug molecules will result in a greater diffusion gradient of the low-potency drug from capillary to the neuromuscular junction (faster rate of drug transfer from plasma to biophase) and a greater biophase concentration of low-potency drug resulting in a fast onset.

The concept of "buffered diffusion" must be invoked to explain the slow recovery of long-acting neuromuscular blockers and to understand biophase kinetics.[161] Buffered diffusion is the process in which diffusion of a drug (e.g., diffusion of a neuromuscular blocker from the neuromuscular junction) is impeded because it binds to extremely high-density receptors within a restricted space (neuromuscular junction). This process is seen with high-potency but not low-potency drugs. Buffered diffusion causes repetitive binding to and unbinding from receptors, keeping potent drugs such as tubocurarine in the neighborhood of effector sites and potentially lengthening the duration of effect.[162,163]

Bevan[164] also proposed that rapid plasma clearance is associated with a rapid onset of action. The fast onset of succinylcholine is related to its rapid metabolism and plasma clearance.

Adverse Effects of Neuromuscular Blockers

Neuromuscular blocking agents seem to play a prominent role in adverse reactions that occur during anesthesia. The Committee on Safety of Medicines in the United Kingdom reported that 10.8% (218 of 2,014) of adverse drug reactions and 7.3% of deaths (21 of 286) were attributable to neuromuscular blocking drugs.[165]

Autonomic Effects

Neuromuscular blocking agents interact with nicotinic and muscarinic cholinergic receptors within the sympathetic and parasympathetic nervous systems and at the nicotinic receptors of the neuromuscular junction. Administration of tubocurarine is associated with marked ganglion blockade resulting in hypotension; in susceptible patients, manifestations of histamine release such as flushing, hypotension, reflex tachycardia, and bronchospasm can be seen. Pancuronium has a direct vagolytic effect. Pancuronium can block muscarinic receptors on sympathetic postganglionic nerve terminals,[166] resulting in inhibition of a negative-feedback mechanism whereby excessive catecholamine release is modulated or prevented.[167] Pancuronium may also stimulate catecholamine release from adrenergic nerve terminals.[168]

Histamine Release

Histamine release by benzylisoquinolinium compounds such as mivacurium, atracurium, and tubocurarine can cause skin flushing, decreases in blood pressure and systemic vascular resistance, and increases in pulse rate.[113,169–172] In contrast, steroidal neuromuscular blocking drugs are not associated with histamine release in typical clinical doses.[173–175] The clinical effects of histamine are seen when plasma concentrations increase to 200% to 300% of baseline values, especially if such concentrations are achieved quickly by rapid drug administration. The effect is usually of short duration (1 to 5 minutes), is dose related, and is clinically insignificant in healthy patients. Histamine has positive inotropic and chronotropic effects on the myocardial H_2 receptors, and there is some evidence that its chronotropic effect may result in part from the liberation of catecholamines.[176] While ganglionic block secondary to the administration of tubocurarine has been demonstrated to occur in various species,[177] the peripheral venous and arteriolar dilatation via stimulation of vascular H_1 and H_2 receptors can result in a significant degree of hypotension as well as carotid sinus–mediated reflex response to histamine-induced peripheral vasodilatation.[171] Other substances liberated by mast cell degranulation, such as tryptase or prostaglandins, may also play a role.[178] The serosal mast cell, located in the skin and connective tissue and near blood vessels and nerves, is principally involved in the degranulation process.[178]

For patients who may be compromised hemodynamically, selecting a drug with less or no histamine release (cisatracurium, vecuronium, or rocuronium) may be appropriate. Another strategy for maintaining cardiovascular stability involves slow administration of benzylisoquinolinium neuromuscular blocking drugs (over 60 seconds), or the prophylactic use of the combined histamine H_1- and H_2-receptor antagonists.

Respiratory Effects

The administration of benzylisoquinolinium neuromuscular blocking drugs (with the exception of cisatracurium) is associated with histamine release, which may result in increased airway resistance and bronchospasm in patients with hyperactive airway disease.

Allergic Reactions

Life-threatening anaphylactic (immune-mediated) or anaphylactoid reactions during anesthesia have been estimated to occur in 1 in 1,000 to 1 in 25,000 administrations and are associated with a mortality rate of about 5%.[179,180] In France, the most common causes of anaphylaxis in patients who experienced allergic reactions were reported to be neuromuscular blocking drugs (58.2%), latex (16.7%), and antibiotics (15.1%).[181] Anaphylactic reactions are mediated through immune responses involving immunoglobulin E antibodies fixed to mast cells. Anaphylactoid reactions are not immune mediated, and represent exaggerated pharmacologic responses in very sensitive individuals, who represent a very small proportion of the population. Cross-reactivity has been reported between neuromuscular blocking drugs and food, cosmetics, disinfectants, and industrial materials.[182]

Steroidal compounds (e.g., rocuronium, vecuronium, or pancuronium) result in no significant histamine release.[113,175] Nevertheless, in the aforementioned series from France, among cases of anaphylaxis due to neuromuscular blocking drugs, 43.1% were due to rocuronium and 22.6% to succinylcholine.[181] There are currently no standards regarding which diagnostic tests (skin prick test, interdermal test, or immunoglobulin E testing) should be performed to identify patients at risk.[183]

Treatment of anaphylactic reactions includes immediate administration of oxygen (100%) and intravenous epinephrine (10 to 20 μg/kg). Early tracheal intubation with a cuffed endotracheal tube should be considered in patients with rapidly developing angioedema. Fluids (crystalloid and/or colloid solutions) must be administered concurrently. Norepinephrine or a sympathomimetic drug (e.g., phenylephrine) may also be necessary to maintain perfusion pressure until the intravascular fluid volume can be restored. Dysrhythmias should be treated. The use of antihistamines and/or steroids is controversial.

Drugs for Reversal of Neuromuscular Blockade

Acetylcholinesterase at the Neuromuscular Junction

At the neuromuscular junction, acetylcholinesterase is the enzyme responsible for rapid hydrolysis of released acetylcholine.[9] Approximately 50% of the released acetylcholine is hydrolyzed during its diffusion across the synaptic cleft, before reaching nicotinic acetylcholine receptors. Acetylcholinesterase has one of the highest catalytic efficiencies known. It can catalyze acetylcholine hydrolysis at a rate of 4,000 molecules of acetylcholine hydrolyzed per active site per second, which is nearly the rate of diffusion.[9] Acetylcholinesterase is highly concentrated at the neuromuscular junction but is present in a lower concentration throughout the length of muscle fibers.[184]

Mechanisms of Action of Acetylcholinesterase Inhibitors

Recovery from muscle relaxation induced by nondepolarizing neuromuscular blockers ultimately depends on elimination of the neuromuscular blocker from the body. Acetylcholinesterase inhibitors (e.g., neostigmine, edrophonium, and less commonly, pyridostigmine) are used clinically to antagonize the residual effects of neuromuscular blockers and to accelerate recovery from nondepolarizing neuromuscular blockade. The acetylcholine that accumulates at the neuromuscular junction after administration of neostigmine competes with the residual molecules of the neuromuscular blocking drug for the available unoccupied nicotinic acetylcholine receptors at the neuromuscular junction. The clinical implication is that neostigmine has a ceiling effect on acetylcholinesterase. Once the inhibition of acetylcholinesterase is complete, administering additional doses of neostigmine will serve no useful purpose because the concentration of acetylcholine that can be produced at the neuromuscular junction is finite. "In practical terms, the maximum depth of block that can be antagonized approximately corresponds to the reappearance of the fourth response to TOF stimulation."[185] Because of their ceiling effect, the anticholinesterases cannot effectively antagonize profound or deep levels of neuromuscular blockade. Indeed, administering more neostigmine at this point may in fact worsen neuromuscular recovery.[186] This points to the limitations posed by the use of neostigmine in clinical practice and explains, in part, the high incidence of postoperative residual neuromuscular blockade.[187]

Antagonism of nondepolarizing neuromuscular blockade by acetylcholinesterase inhibitors depends primarily on five factors: (a) the depth of the blockade when reversal is attempted, (b) the anticholinesterase chosen, (c) the dose administered, (d) the rate of spontaneous clear of the neuromuscular blocker from plasma, and (e) the choice and depth of anesthetic agents administered.[188] For a detailed review, see Bevan and colleagues.[189,190] For neostigmine, the maximum effective dose is in the 60 to 80 μg/kg range,[191,192] and for edrophonium, it is in the 1.0 to 1.5 mg/kg range.[193,194] Antagonism of residual neuromuscular blockade induced by the various nondepolarizing neuromuscular blockers is similar (or possibly greater) in children and adults.[195] The potencies of different acetylcholinesterase inhibitors in antagonizing the currently available neuromuscular blockers (vecuronium, rocuronium, and cisatracurium) in different clinical scenarios have been reported by several groups of investigators.[196–198] Neostigmine is still the anticholinesterase agent most widely used by anesthesiologists worldwide.[199]

Clinical Pharmacology

Pharmacokinetics of Acetylcholinesterase Inhibitors

The elimination half-life of edrophonium is similar to those of neostigmine and pyridostigmine,[200] although that of pyridostigmine is somewhat longer.[201,202] Renal excretion accounts for about 50% of the excretion of neostigmine and about 75% of that of pyridostigmine and edrophonium. Renal failure decreases the plasma clearance of neostigmine, pyridostigmine, and edrophonium as much as, if not more than, that of the long-acting neuromuscular blockers.

Side Effects of Acetylcholinesterase Inhibitors

Inhibition of acetylcholinesterase not only increases the concentration of acetylcholine at the neuromuscular junction (nicotinic site) but also at all other synapses that use acetylcholine as a transmitter.

Cardiovascular Side Effects

Because only the nicotinic effects of acetylcholinesterase inhibitors are desired, the muscarinic effects must be blocked by atropine or glycopyrrolate.[7] To minimize the muscarinic cardiovascular side effects of acetylcholinesterase inhibitors, an anticholinergic agent should be coadministered with the acetylcholinesterase inhibitor. Atropine (7 to 10 μg/kg) matches the onset of action and pharmacodynamic profile of the rapid-acting edrophonium (0.5 to 1.0 mg/kg),[7] and glycopyrrolate (7 to 15 μg/kg) matches the slower acting neostigmine (40 to 70 μg/kg) and pyridostigmine.[203,204] In patients with preexisting cardiac disease, glycopyrrolate may be preferable to atropine,[205] and the acetylcholinesterase inhibitor and anticholinergic should be administered slowly (e.g., over 2 to 5 minutes). The hemodynamic effects of tracheal extubation are significantly greater than that following the coadministration of neostigmine and glycopyrrolate.

Pulmonary and Alimentary Side Effects

Administration of acetylcholinesterase inhibitors is associated with bronchoconstriction, increased airway resistance, increased salivation, and increased bowel motility (muscarinic effects). Anticholinergics tend to reduce this effect. Findings on whether neostigmine increases the incidence of postoperative nausea and vomiting are discrepant.[206,207] Neostigmine has been described as having antiemetic properties[208] and as having no effect on the incidence of postoperative nausea and vomiting.[207,209]

Monitoring of Neuromuscular Function

Monitoring of neuromuscular function after administration of a neuromuscular blocking drug serves at least two purposes in clinical settings. First, it allows the anesthesiologist to administer these agents with appropriate dosing; second, it ensures that the patient recovers adequately from residual effects of the neuromuscular blocker, thus guaranteeing patient safety. In the operating room, the depth of neuromuscular blockade is typically monitored by observing the response to stimulation of any superficial neuromuscular unit. Most commonly, contraction of the adductor pollicis muscle associated with stimulation of the ulnar nerve, either at the wrist or the elbow, is monitored. In certain circumstances, the peroneal nerve or the facial nerve may be monitored.

Clinical bedside criteria for tracheal extubation (such as a 5-second head lift, or ability to generate a peak negative inspiratory force of −25 to −30 cm H_2O) are insensitive indicators of the adequacy of neuromuscular recovery.[210] Kopman[211] noted that patients could sustain a 5-second head lift at a TOF ratio of <0.60. It is recommended that objective monitoring (e.g., digital display of the TOF ratio in real time) be used in the clinical setting. Subjective (visual or tactile) evaluation of the evoked muscular response to TOF stimulation is extremely inaccurate. Subjective evaluation of the evoked muscular response to TOF and tetanic stimulation are notoriously inaccurate as estimates of fade or postoperative residual neuromuscular blockade.[212,213] Depth of the blockade during maintenance of and recovery from the blockade should be monitored with repeated TOF stimuli.

Following administration of a nondepolarizing neuromuscular blocking agent, it is essential to ensure adequate return of normal neuromuscular function, to a TOF ratio of ≥0.9. A TOF ratio of <0.9 in unanesthetized volunteers has been associated with difficulty in speaking and swallowing, visual disturbances,[211] significant pharyngeal dysfunction resulting in a four- to fivefold increase in the risk of aspiration,[214,215] and decrease in hypoxic ventilatory drive.[216]

Perhaps the most convincing evidence that the use of an objective neuromuscular monitor (combined with a strong educational effort at the departmental level) can decrease the incidence of postoperative residual neuromuscular blockade comes from two studies by Baillard et al.[217,218] The first was a prospective study of the incidence of postoperative residual neuromuscular blockade following administration of vecuronium in 568 consecutive patients over a 3-month period in 1995. As was customary in the authors' department, no anticholinesterase antagonists were used in this series of patients, and peripheral nerve stimulatory devices were rarely used (<2.0%) intraoperatively. Postoperative residual neuromuscular blockade (indicated by an acceleromyographic TOF ratio of <0.70) was present in 42% of patients in the postanesthesia care unit. Of 435 patients who had been extubated in the operating room, the incidence of postoperative residual neuromuscular blockade was 33%.

As a result of these rather alarming findings, Baillard's department placed acceleromyographic monitors in all operating rooms a short time later. The department instituted a program of education about the use of neuromuscular monitoring and the indications for neostigmine administration. The authors' findings regarding the incidence of postoperative residual neuromuscular blockade were distributed to department staff. They then conducted repeat 3-month surveys of clinical practice in the years 2000 (n = 130), 2002 (n = 101), and 2004 (n = 218) to determine the success of their educational efforts. In the 9-year interval between the initial and the 2004 survey, the use of intraoperative monitoring of neuromuscular function rose from 2% to 60%, and reversal of residual antagonism increased from 6% to 42% of cases. One other notable change was in the choice of relaxant. In 1995, all patients received vecuronium, but this agent was gradually replaced by atracurium, which was used in 99% of cases in 2004. As a result of these changes in clinical practice, the incidence of postoperative residual neuromuscular blockade (acceleromyographic TOF ratio of <0.90) in Baillard's department decreased from 62% to <4%.

Although quantitative neuromuscular function monitoring is recommended, many anesthetics are given without such monitoring. Appropriate intraoperative use of a conventional nerve stimulator may decrease (but not eliminate) the incidence of postoperative residual neuromuscular blockade.[219] If neostigmine administration is timed at a TOF count of 4, then clinically significant postoperative residual neuromuscular blockade should be a rare event. Quantitative monitors (such as acceleromyography) should be seriously considered in two situations: (a) when no fade on TOF stimulation can be detected manually and the anesthesiologist is deciding not to reverse neuromuscular block or (b) when the anesthesiologist is attempting to reverse deep nondepolarizing block (TOF count ≤3).

Limitations of Acetylcholinesterase Inhibitors

As indicated in the previous sections, postanesthetic morbidity in the form of incomplete reversal and residual postoperative weakness is a frequent occurrence.[187,220–224] In 2003, for example, Debaene and colleagues[221] reported a 45% incidence of postoperative residual neuromuscular blockade in patients arriving in the postanesthesia care unit. Moreover, a recent survey indicated that most practitioners do not know what constitutes adequate recovery from neuromuscular blockade.[225] Although an argument can be made that these problems could be attributed to (a) lack of routine use of peripheral nerve stimulators (and more importantly, the quantitative ones) or (b) the ceiling effect of the reversal agents when administered at a deep level of neuromuscular blockade,[226,227] one study found that, despite both the use of nerve stimulators by clinicians with knowledge and expertise and administration of neostigmine, the incidence of critical respiratory events in the postoperative care unit remained a significant 0.8%.[222] Clearly, avoidance of critical respiratory events requires changes in clinical care.[224]

Nonclassic Reversal Drugs

Only a few studies have explored the potential of nonclassic reversal drugs that act independently of acetylcholinesterase inhibition. One such agent, purified human plasma cholinesterase, has been shown to be effective and safe in antagonizing mivacurium-induced neuromuscular blockade.[228] Similarly, cysteine has been shown to reverse the neuromuscular blocking effects of gantacurium.[229] Sugammadex, a novel selective relaxant-binding agent, is able to reverse both shallow and profound aminosteroid-induced neuromuscular blockade, and has a unique mechanism of action (see the following text) that distinguishes it from cholinesterase inhibitors.

Sugammadex: A Novel Selective Relaxant-binding Agent

Chemistry

Sugammadex is a modified γ-cyclodextrin (Fig. 12-8).[230–233] Cyclodextrins are cyclic dextrose units joined through one to four glycosyl bonds that are produced from starch or starch derivates using cyclodextrin glycosyltransferase. The three natural unmodified cyclodextrins consist of 6-, 7-, or 8-cyclic oligosaccharides and are called α-, β-, or γ-cyclodextrin, respectively. Their three-dimensional structures, which resemble a hollow, truncated cone or a doughnut, have a hydrophobic cavity and a hydrophilic

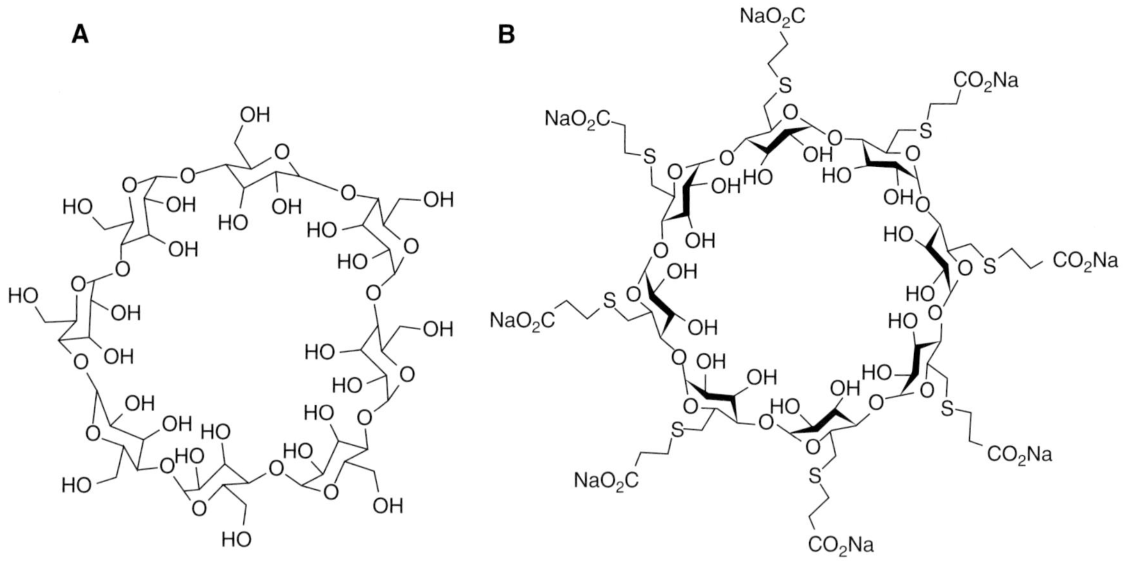

FIGURE 12-8 γ-Cyclodextrin **(A)** and sugammadex (modified γ-cyclodextrin) **(B)**.

exterior because of the presence of polar hydroxyl groups. Hydrophobic interactions trap the drug into the cyclodextrin cavity (the doughnut hole), resulting in formation of a water-soluble guest-host complex.

These modifications resulted in a sugammadex compound (with a molecular weight of 2,178) that is highly water soluble with a hydrophobic cavity large enough to encapsulate steroidal neuromuscular blocking drugs, especially rocuronium.[230–233] Sugammadex exerts its effect by forming very tight complexes at a 1:1 ratio with steroidal neuromuscular blocking agents (rocuronium > vecuronium >> pancuronium).[230–233] The intermolecular (van der Waals) forces, thermodynamic (hydrogen) bonds, and hydrophobic interactions of the sugammadex-rocuronium complex make it very tight.[230] The sugammadex-rocuronium complex has a very high association rate and a very low dissociation rate. It is estimated that for every 30 million sugammadex-rocuronium complexes, only one complex dissociates.

Sugammadex is the first selective relaxant-binding agent. It exerts no effect on acetylcholinesterases or on any receptor system in the body, thus eliminating the need for anticholinergic drugs and their undesirable adverse effects. Moreover, the unique mechanism of reversal by encapsulation is independent of the depth of neuromuscular block; thus, reversal can be accomplished even during profound neuromuscular block.

Pharmacokinetics and Metabolism

Sugammadex is biologically inactive and does not bind to plasma proteins.[234–236] Approximately 75% of the dose was eliminated through the urine. The mean percentage of the dose excreted in urine up to 24 hours after administration varied between 59% and 80%.[235] The kinetics of sugammadex appear to be dose dependent, in that clearance increased, and elimination half-life decreased, when the sugammadex dose was increased from 0.15 to 1.0 mg/kg.[235]

In the absence of sugammadex, rocuronium is eliminated mainly by biliary excretion (>75%) and to a lesser degree by renal excretion (10% to 25%). The plasma clearance of sugammadex alone is approximately three times lower than that of rocuronium alone.[237] In volunteers, the plasma clearance of rocuronium was decreased by a factor of >2 after administration of a ≥2.0 mg/kg dose of sugammadex.[235] This is because the biliary route of excretion becomes unavailable for the rocuronium-sugammadex complex, and rocuronium clearance decreases to a value approaching the glomerular filtration rate (120 mL per minute). As noted earlier, after administration of sugammadex, the plasma concentration of free rocuronium decreases rapidly, but the total plasma concentration of rocuronium (both free and that bound to sugammadex) increases.[238]

Because of the soluble nature of the sugammadex-rocuronium complex, urinary excretion of the complex is the major route of elimination of the rocuronium (65% to 97% of the administered dose is recovered in urine).[235,237] Excretion is rapid; approximately 70% of the administered dose is excreted within 6 hours and >90% within 24 hours. The renal excretion of rocuronium is increased by more than 100% after administration of 4 to 8 mg/kg of sugammadex.[237]

Sugammadex does not bind to human plasma proteins and erythrocytes to a significant extent. Metabolism of sugammadex is at most very limited, and the drug is predominantly eliminated unchanged by the kidneys. In patients with substantial renal impairment, clearances of sugammadex and rocuronium were decreased by a factor of 16 and 3.7, respectively, relative to that in healthy subjects, and the elimination half-lives were increased by a factor of 15 and 2.5, respectively. The effectiveness of dialysis in removing sugammadex and rocuronium from plasma was not demonstrated consistently. Therefore, sugammadex should be avoided in patients with a creatinine clearance of <30 mL per minute.

Pharmacodynamics

Sugammadex, used in appropriate doses, is capable of reversing any depth of neuromuscular blockade (profound or shallow) induced by rocuronium or vecuronium to a TOF ratio of ≥0.9 within 3 minutes.[224,239] During rocuronium- or vecuronium-induced neuromuscular blockade, intravenous administration of sugammadex results in rapid removal of free rocuronium or vecuronium molecules from the plasma. This creates a concentration gradient favoring movement of the remaining rocuronium or vecuronium molecules from the neuromuscular junction back into the plasma, where they are encapsulated by free sugammadex molecules. The latter molecules also enter the tissues and form a complex with the rocuronium or vecuronium. Therefore, the neuromuscular blockade of these agents is terminated rapidly by their diffusion away from the neuromuscular junction back into the plasma. This results in an increase in the total plasma concentration of rocuronium (both free and bound to sugammadex)[238] or vecuronium.

The efficacy of sugammadex in antagonizing different levels of rocuronium- or vecuronium-induced neuromuscular blockade has been demonstrated in several clinical studies.[237,240–245] At appropriate doses, no recurarization has been reported in human studies.

With profound block induced by rocuronium or vecuronium, larger doses of sugammadex (8 to 16 mg/kg) are required for adequate and rapid recovery. In Figure 12-9, the speed of recovery from 1.2 mg/kg rocuronium followed 3 minutes later by 16 mg/kg sugammadex is compared with the speed of spontaneous recovery from 1.0 mg/kg succinylcholine in surgical patients.[239] The total duration from administration of rocuronium until recovery of the TOF ratio (the ratio of the fourth to the first twitch height of the TOF) to ≥0.9 was shorter than the time needed for a similar degree of spontaneous recovery from 1.0 mg/kg succinylcholine-induced blockade. It should be noted, however, that all drugs behave in a dose-response manner.[246] A temporary decrease in TOF response was observed after reversal of muscle relaxation with an inadequate dose (0.5 mg/kg) of sugammadex administered 42 minutes after 0.9 mg/kg of rocuronium.[247]

Published data indicate that, if TOF count is 2 during recovery from rocuronium-induced neuromuscular

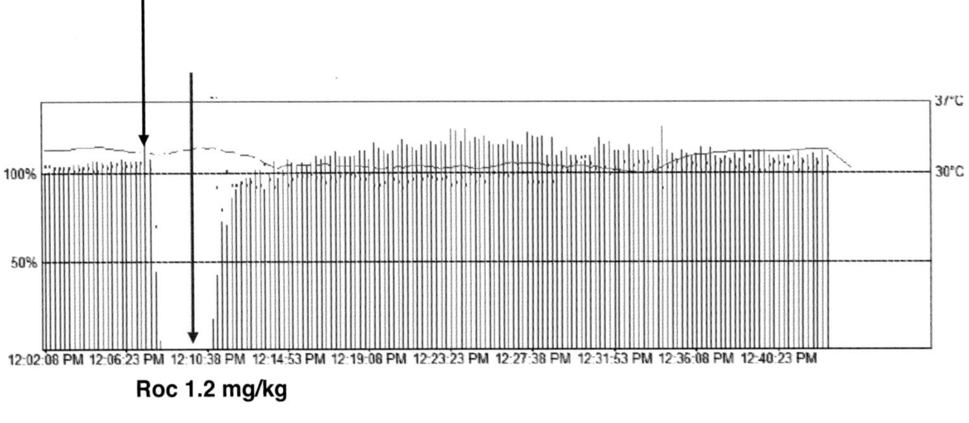

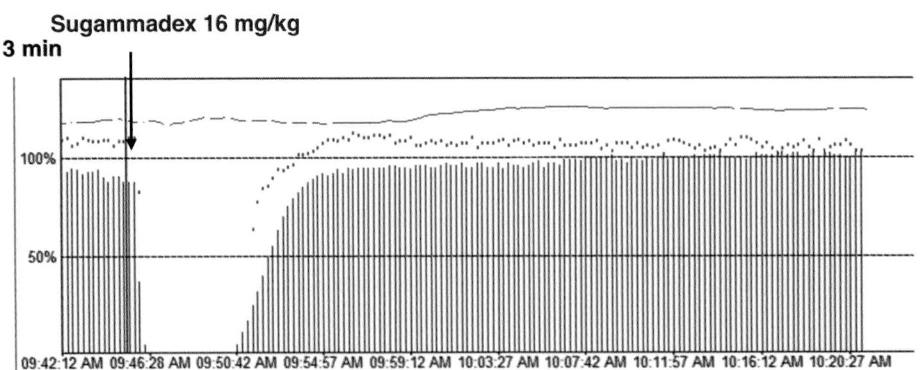

FIGURE 12-9 **Panel A** shows recovery of the twitch height and TOF ratio after administration of 1.2 mg/kg rocuronium, followed 3 minutes later by 16 mg/kg sugammadex, both given intravenously. Recovery to a first twitch height (T1) of 90% and a TOF ratio of 0.94 occurred 110 seconds later. The onset-offset time with this sequence (i.e., the time from the end of the injection of rocuronium to a T1 recovery to 90%) was 4 minutes 47 seconds. **Panel B** shows the effects of administering 1.0 mg/kg succinylcholine (Sch) with spontaneous recovery to a T1 of 90% occurring after 9 minutes 23 seconds. (Reproduced from Naguib M. Sugammadex: another milestone in clinical neuromuscular pharmacology. *Anesth Analg.* 2007;104:575–581, with permission.)

blockade, administering 2 mg/kg of sugammadex would be sufficient to produce adequate neuromuscular recovery (a TOF ratio of 0.9 or greater). Similarly, 4 mg/kg of sugammadex would be sufficient to produce adequate neuromuscular recovery from a deeper block at a 1 to 2 posttetanic count. A still more profound block would require a greater dose of sugammadex, in the range of 8 to 16 mg/kg.

Sugammadex is ineffective against succinylcholine and benzylisoquinolinium neuromuscular blockers such as mivacurium, atracurium, and cisatracurium because it cannot form inclusion complexes with these drugs.[248] Therefore, if neuromuscular blockade must be reestablished after using sugammadex, one of the benzylisoquinolinium neuromuscular blockers should be considered.

Safety and Tolerability

The U.S. Food and Drug Administration has expressed concerns about the safety of sugammadex, citing its possible association with allergic reactions and bleeding, and sugammadex has not been approved for clinical use in the United States. More than 5 million doses of sugammadex have been administered worldwide.

References

1. Läwen A. Über die Verbindung der Lokalanästhesie mit der Narkose, über hohe Extraduralanästhesie und epidurale Injektionen anästhesierender Lösungen bei tabischen Magenkrisen. *Beitr Klin Chir.* 1912;80:168–180.
2. Bodman RI, Gillies D. *Harold Griffith: The Evolution of Modern Anaesthesia.* Toronto, Canada: Hannah Institute & Dundurn Press; 1992.
3. Sine SM, Claudio T, Sigworth FJ. Activation of Torpedo acetylcholine receptors expressed in mouse fibroblasts. Single channel current kinetics reveal distinct agonist binding affinities. *J Gen Physiol.* 1990;96:395–437.
4. Devillers-Thiery A, Galzi JL, Eisele JL, et al. Functional architecture of the nicotinic acetylcholine receptor: a prototype of ligand-gated ion channels. *J Membr Biol.* 1993;136:97–112.
5. Grosman C, Zhou M, Auerbach A. Mapping the conformational wave of acetylcholine receptor channel gating. *Nature.* 2000;403:773–776.
6. Grosman C, Salamone FN, Sine SM, et al. The extracellular linker of muscle acetylcholine receptor channels is a gating control element. *J Gen Physiol.* 2000;116:237–240.
7. Bowman WC. *Pharmacology of Neuromuscular Function.* 2nd ed. London, United Kingdom: Wright; 1990.
8. Naguib M, Flood P, McArdle JJ, et al. Advances in neurobiology of the neuromuscular junction: implications for the anesthesiologist. *Anesthesiology.* 2002;96:202–231.
9. Rosenberry TL. Acetylcholinesterase. *Adv Enzymol Relat Areas Mol Biol.* 1975;43:103–218.
10. Bowman WC. Prejunctional and postjunctional cholinoceptors at the neuromuscular junction. *Anesth Analg.* 1980;59:935–943.
11. Prior C, Tian L, Dempster J, et al. Prejunctional actions of muscle relaxants: synaptic vesicles and transmitter mobilization as sites of action. *Gen Pharmacol.* 1995;26:659–666.
12. Faria M, Oliveira L, Timoteo MA, et al. Blockade of neuronal facilitatory nicotinic receptors containing alpha3beta2 subunits contribute to tetanic fade in the rat isolated diaphragm. *Synapse.* 2003;49:77–88.
13. Chang CC, Hong SJ. Dissociation of the end-plate potential run-down and the tetanic fade from the postsynaptic inhibition of acetylcholine receptor by alpha-neurotoxins. *Exp Neurol.* 1987;98: 509–517.
14. Nagashima M, Yasuhara S, Frick CG, et al. Alpha-bungarotoxin but not botulinum toxin causes fade during repetitive stimulation. In: *ASA Annual Meeting.* Orlando, FL: American Society of Anesthesiologists; 2008. A1399.
15. Torda TA, Graham GG, Warwick NR, et al. Pharmacokinetics and pharmacodynamics of suxamethonium. *Anaesth Intensive Care.* 1997;25:272–278.
16. Cook DR, Wingard LB, Taylor FH. Pharmacokinetics of succinylcholine in infants, children, and adults. *Clin Pharmacol Ther.* 1976;20:493–498.
17. Smith CE, Donati F, Bevan DR. Dose-response curves for succinylcholine: single versus cumulative techniques. *Anesthesiology.* 1988;69:338–342.
18. Kopman AF, Klewicka MM, Neuman GG. An alternate method for estimating the dose-response relationships of neuromuscular blocking drugs. *Anesth Analg.* 2000;90:1191–1197.
19. Viby-Mogensen J. Correlation of succinylcholine duration of action with plasma cholinesterase activity in subjects with the genotypically normal enzyme. *Anesthesiology.* 1980;53:517–520.
20. Katz RL, Ryan JF. The neuromuscular effects of suxamethonium in man. *Br J Anaesth.* 1969;41:381–390.
21. Naguib M, Samarkandi A, Riad W, et al. Optimal dose of succinylcholine revisited. *Anesthesiology.* 2003;99:1045–1049.
22. Blobner M, Mirakhur RK, Wierda JM, et al. Rapacuronium 2.0 or 2.5 mg kg-1 for rapid-sequence induction: comparison with succinylcholine 1.0 mg kg-1. *Br J Anaesth.* 2000;85:724–731.
23. Andrews JI, Kumar N, van den Brom RH, et al. A large simple randomized trial of rocuronium versus succinylcholine in rapid-sequence induction of anaesthesia along with propofol. *Acta Anaesthesiol Scand.* 1999;43:4–8.
24. Sparr HJ, Mellinghoff H, Blobner M, et al. Comparison of intubating conditions after rapacuronium (Org 9487) and succinylcholine following rapid sequence induction in adult patients. *Br J Anaesth.* 1999;82:537–541.
25. Naguib M, Samarkandi AH, El-Din ME, et al. The dose of succinylcholine required for excellent endotracheal intubating conditions. *Anesth Analg.* 2006;102:151–155.
26. Gissen AJ, Katz RL, Karis JH, et al. Neuromuscular block in man during prolonged arterial infusion with succinylcholine. *Anesthesiology.* 1966;27:242–249.
27. Foldes FF, McNall PG, Birch JH. The neuromuscular activity of succinylmonocholine iodide in man. *Br Med J.* 1954;1:967.
28. Lockridge O, Bartels CF, Vaughan TA, et al. Complete amino acid sequence of human serum cholinesterase. *J Biol Chem.* 1987;262:549–557.
29. Jensen FS, Schwartz M, Viby-Mogensen J. Identification of human plasma cholinesterase variants using molecular biological techniques. *Acta Anaesthesiol Scand.* 1995;39:142–149.
30. Foldes FF, Rendell-Baker L, Birch JH. Causes and prevention of prolonged apnea with succinylcholine. *Anesth Analg.* 1956;35:609.
31. Lepage L, Schiele F, Gueguen R, et al. Total cholinesterase in plasma: biological variations and reference limits. *Clin Chem.* 1985;31: 546–550.
32. Kopman AF, Strachovsky G, Lichtenstein L. Prolonged response to succinylcholine following physostigmine. *Anesthesiology.* 1978; 49:142–143.
33. Sunew KY, Hicks RG. Effects of neostigmine and pyridostigmine on duration of succinylcholine action and pseudocholinesterase activity. *Anesthesiology.* 1978;49:188–191.
34. Kao YJ, Tellez J, Turner DR. Dose-dependent effect of metoclopramide on cholinesterases and suxamethonium metabolism. *Br J Anaesth.* 1990;65:220–224.
35. Fisher DM, Caldwell JE, Sharma M, et al. The influence of bambuterol (carbamylated terbutaline) on the duration of action of

succinylcholine-induced paralysis in humans. *Anesthesiology.* 1988;69:757–759.
36. Bang U, Viby-Mogensen J, Wiren JE, et al. The effect of bambuterol (carbamylated terbutaline) on plasma cholinesterase activity and suxamethonium-induced neuromuscular blockade in genotypically normal patients. *Acta Anaesthesiol Scand.* 1990;34:596–599.
37. Barabas E, Zsigmond EK, Kirkpatrick AF. The inhibitory effect of esmolol on human plasmacholinesterase. *Can Anaesth Soc J.* 1986;33:332–335.
38. Murthy VS, Patel KD, Elangovan RG, et al. Cardiovascular and neuromuscular effects of esmolol during induction of anesthesia. *J Clin Pharmacol.* 1986;26:351–357.
39. Devcic A, Munshi CA, Gandhi SK, et al. Antagonism of mivacurium neuromuscular block: neostigmine versus edrophonium. *Anesth Analg.* 1995;81:1005–1009.
40. Pantuck EJ. Plasma cholinesterase: gene and variations. *Anesth Analg.* 1993;77:380–386.
41. Goodall R. Cholinesterase: phenotyping and genotyping. *Ann Clin Biochem.* 2004;41:98–110.
42. Kalow W, Staron N. On distribution and inheritance of atypical forms of human serum cholinesterase, as indicated by dibucaine numbers. *Can J Biochem Physiol.* 1957;35:1305–1320.
43. Kalow W, Genest K. A method for the detection of atypical forms of human serum cholinesterase: determination of dibucaine numbers. *Can J Biochem.* 1957;35:339.
44. Viby-Mogensen J, Hanel HK. Prolonged apnoea after suxamethonium: an analysis of the first 225 cases reported to the Danish Cholinesterase Research Unit. *Acta Anaesthesiol Scand.* 1978;22:371–380.
45. Ramsey FM, Lebowitz PW, Savarese JJ, et al. Clinical characteristics of long-term succinylcholine neuromuscular blockade during balanced anesthesia. *Anesth Analg.* 1980;59:110–116.
46. Yoshida A, Motulsky AG. A pseudocholinesterase variant (E Cynthiana) associated with elevated plasma enzyme activity. *Am J Hum Genet.* 1969;21:486–498.
47. Warran P, Theeman M, Bold AM, et al. Hypercholinesterasaemia and suxamethonium resistance. *Anaesthesia.* 1987;42:855–857.
48. Naguib M, Gomaa M, Samarkandi AH, et al. Increased plasma cholinesterase activity and mivacurium resistance: report of a family. *Anesth Analg.* 1999;89:1579–1582.
49. Craythorne NW, Turndorf H, Dripps RD. Changes in pulse rate and rhythm associated with the use of succinylcholine in anesthetized patients. *Anesthesiology.* 1960;21:465.
50. Stoelting RK, Peterson C. Heart-rate slowing and junctional rhythm following intravenous succinylcholine with and without intramuscular atropine preanesthetic medication. *Anesth Analg.* 1975;54:705–709.
51. Derbyshire DR, Chmielewski A, Fell D, et al. Plasma catecholamine responses to tracheal intubation. *Br J Anaesth.* 1983;55:855–860.
52. Walton JD, Farman JV. Suxamethonium hyperkalaemia in uraemic neuropathy. *Anaesthesia.* 1973;28:666–668.
53. Powell JN, Golby M. The pattern of potassium liberation following a single dose of suxamethonium in normal and uraemic rats. *Br J Anaesth.* 1971;43:662–668.
54. Kohlschutter B, Baur H, Roth F. Suxamethonium-induced hyperkalaemia in patients with severe intra-abdominal infections. *Br J Anaesth.* 1976;48:557–562.
55. Schwartz DE, Kelly B, Caldwell JE, et al. Succinylcholine-induced hyperkalemic arrest in a patient with severe metabolic acidosis and exsanguinating hemorrhage. *Anesth Analg.* 1992;75:291–293.
56. Stevenson PH, Birch AA. Succinylcholine-induced hyperkalemia in a patient with a closed head injury. *Anesthesiology.* 1979;51:89–90.
57. Martyn JA, Richtsfeld M. Succinylcholine-induced hyperkalemia in acquired pathologic states: etiologic factors and molecular mechanisms. *Anesthesiology.* 2006;104:158–169.
58. Rosenberg H, Gronert GA. Intractable cardiac arrest in children given succinylcholine. *Anesthesiology.* 1992;77:1054.
59. Morell RC, Berman JM, Royster RI, et al. Revised label regarding use of succinylcholine in children and adolescents. *Anesthesiology.* 1994;80:242–245.
60. Badgwell JM, Hall SC, Lockhart C. Revised label regarding use of succinylcholine in children and adolescents. *Anesthesiology.* 1994;80:243–245.
61. Ryan JF, Kagen LJ, Hyman AI. Myoglobinemia after a single dose of succinylcholine. *N Engl J Med.* 1971;285:824–827.
62. Pandey K, Badola RP, Kumar S. Time course of intraocular hypertension produced by suxamethonium. *Br J Anaesth.* 1972;44:191–196.
63. Libonati MM, Leahy JJ, Ellison N. The use of succinylcholine in open eye surgery. *Anesthesiology.* 1985;62:637–640.
64. Meyers EF, Krupin T, Johnson M, et al. Failure of nondepolarizing neuromuscular blockers to inhibit succinylcholine-induced increased intraocular pressure, a controlled study. *Anesthesiology.* 1978;48:149–151.
65. Konchigeri HN, Lee YE, Venugopal K. Effect of pancuronium on intraocular pressure changes induced by succinylcholine. *Can Anaesth Soc J.* 1979;26:479–481.
66. Miller RD, Way WL, Hickey RF. Inhibition of succinylcholine-induced increased intraocular pressure by non-depolarizing muscle relaxants. *Anesthesiology.* 1968;29:123–126.
67. Miller RD, Way WL. Inhibition of succinylcholine-induced increased intragastric pressure by nondepolarizing muscle relaxants and lidocaine. *Anesthesiology.* 1971;34:185–188.
68. Smith G, Dalling R, Williams TI. Gastro-oesophageal pressure gradient changes produced by induction of anaesthesia and suxamethonium. *Br J Anaesth.* 1978;50:1137–1143.
69. Minton MD, Grosslight K, Stirt JA, et al. Increases in intracranial pressure from succinylcholine: prevention by prior nondepolarizing blockade. *Anesthesiology.* 1986;65:165–169.
70. Stirt JA, Grosslight KR, Bedford RF, et al. "Defasciculation" with metocurine prevents succinylcholine-induced increases in intracranial pressure. *Anesthesiology.* 1987;67:50–53.
71. Waters DJ, Mapleson WW. Suxamethonium pains: hypothesis and observation. *Anaesthesia.* 1971;26:127–141.
72. Brodsky JB, Brock-Utne JG, Samuels SI. Pancuronium pretreatment and post-succinylcholine myalgias. *Anesthesiology.* 1979;51:259–261.
73. Maddineni VR, Mirakhur RK, Cooper AR. Myalgia and biochemical changes following suxamethonium after induction of anaesthesia with thiopentone or propofol. *Anaesthesia.* 1993;48:626–628.
74. McLoughlin C, Elliott P, McCarthy G, et al. Muscle pains and biochemical changes following suxamethonium administration after six pretreatment regimens. *Anaesthesia.* 1992;47:202–206.
75. Demers-Pelletier J, Drolet P, Girard M, et al. Comparison of rocuronium and d-tubocurarine for prevention of succinylcholine-induced fasciculations and myalgia. *Can J Anaesth.* 1997;44:1144–1147.
76. Naguib M, Farag H, Magbagbeola JA. Effect of pre-treatment with lysine acetyl salicylate on suxamethonium-induced myalgia. *Br J Anaesth.* 1987;59:606–610.
77. Jackson MJ, Wagenmakers AJ, Edwards RH. Effect of inhibitors of arachidonic acid metabolism on efflux of intracellular enzymes from skeletal muscle following experimental damage. *Biochem J.* 1987;241:403–407.
78. Kahraman S, Ercan S, Aypar U, et al. Effect of preoperative i.m. administration of diclofenac on suxamethonium-induced myalgia. *Br J Anaesth.* 1993;71:238–241.
79. Schreiber JU, Lysakowski C, Fuchs-Buder T, et al. Prevention of succinylcholine-induced fasciculation and myalgia: a meta-analysis of randomized trials. *Anesthesiology.* 2005;103:877–884.
80. Zahl K, Apfelbaum JL. Muscle pain occurs after outpatient laparoscopy despite the substitution of vecuronium for succinylcholine. *Anesthesiology.* 1989;70:408–411.
81. Smith I, Ding Y, White PF. Muscle pain after outpatient laparoscopy—influence of propofol versus thiopental and enflurane. *Anesth Analg.* 1993;76:1181–1184.

82. Donlon JV, Newfield P, Sreter F, et al. Implications of masseter spasm after succinylcholine. *Anesthesiology*. 1978;49:298–301.
83. Van der Spek AF, Fang WB, Ashton-Miller JA, et al. The effects of succinylcholine on mouth opening. *Anesthesiology*. 1987;67:459–465.
84. Leary NP, Ellis FR. Masseteric muscle spasm as a normal response to suxamethonium. *Br J Anaesth*. 1990;64:488–492.
85. Habre W, Sims C. Masseter spasm and elevated creatine kinase after intravenous induction in a child. *Anaesth Intensive Care*. 1996;24:496–499.
86. Meakin G, Walker RW, Dearlove OR. Myotonic and neuromuscular blocking effects of increased doses of suxamethonium in infants and children. *Br J Anaesth*. 1990;65:816–818.
87. Everett AJ, Lowe LA, Wilkinson S. Revision of the structures of (+)-tubocurarine chloride and (+)-chondocurine. *J Chem Soc*. 1970;D:1020–1021.
88. Miller RD, Matteo RS, Benet LZ, et al. The pharmacokinetics of d-tubocurarine in man with and without renal failure. *J Pharmacol Exp Ther*. 1977;202:1–7.
89. Stenlake JB, Waigh RD, Dewar GH, et al. Biodegradable neuromuscular blocking agents. Part 6—stereochemical studies on atracurium and related polyalkylene di-esters. *Eur J Med Chem*. 1984;19:441–450.
90. Tsui D, Graham GG, Torda TA. The pharmacokinetics of atracurium isomers in vitro and in humans. *Anesthesiology*. 1987;67:722–728.
91. Nehmer U. Simultaneous determination of atracurium besylate and its major decomposition products and related impurities by reversed-phase high-performance liquid chromatography. *J Chromatogr*. 1988;435:425–433.
92. Stenlake JB, Waigh RD, Urwin J, et al. Atracurium: conception and inception. *Br J Anaesth*. 1983;55(suppl 1):3S–10S.
93. Neill EA, Chapple DJ, Thompson CW. Metabolism and kinetics of atracurium: an overview. *Br J Anaesth*. 1983;55(suppl 1):23S–25S.
94. Chapple DJ, Clark JS. Pharmacological action of breakdown products of atracurium and related substances. *Br J Anaesth*. 1983;55(suppl 1):11S–15S.
95. Ward S, Weatherley BC. Pharmacokinetics of atracurium and its metabolites. *Br J Anaesth*. 1986;58(suppl 1):6S–10S.
96. Parker CJ, Hunter JM. Pharmacokinetics of atracurium and laudanosine in patients with hepatic cirrhosis. *Br J Anaesth*. 1989;62:177–183.
97. Yate PM, Flynn PJ, Arnold RW, et al. Clinical experience and plasma laudanosine concentrations during the infusion of atracurium in the intensive therapy unit. *Br J Anaesth*. 1987;59:211–217.
98. Fahey MR, Rupp SM, Fisher DM, et al. The pharmacokinetics and pharmacodynamics of atracurium in patients with and without renal failure. *Anesthesiology*. 1984;61:699–702.
99. Ward S, Boheimer N, Weatherley BC, et al. Pharmacokinetics of atracurium and its metabolites in patients with normal renal function, and in patients in renal failure. *Br J Anaesth*. 1987;59:697–706.
100. Zhang J, Haddad GG, Xia Y. delta-, but not mu- and kappa-, opioid receptor activation protects neocortical neurons from glutamate-induced excitotoxic injury. *Brain Res*. 2000;885:143–153.
101. Belluardo N, Mudo G, Blum M, et al. Central nicotinic receptors, neurotrophic factors and neuroprotection. *Behav Brain Res*. 2000;113:21–34.
102. Tassonyi E, Fathi M, Hughes GJ, et al. Cerebrospinal fluid concentrations of atracurium, laudanosine and vecuronium following clinical subarachnoid hemorrhage. *Acta Anaesthesiol Scand*. 2002;46:1236–1241.
103. Fodale V, Pratico C, Signer MR, et al. Perinatal neuroprotection by muscle relaxants against hypoxic-ischemic lesions: is it a possible hypothesis? *J Matern Fetal Neonatal Med*. 2005;18:133–136.
104. Welch RM, Brown A, Ravitch J, et al. The in vitro degradation of cisatracurium, the R, cis-R'-isomer of atracurium, in human and rat plasma. *Clin Pharmacol Ther*. 1995;58:132–142.
105. Lien CA, Schmith VD, Belmont MR, et al. Pharmacokinetics of cisatracurium in patients receiving nitrous oxide/opioid/barbiturate anesthesia. *Anesthesiology*. 1996;84:300–308.
106. Kisor DF, Schmith VD, Wargin WA, et al. Importance of the organ-independent elimination of cisatracurium. *Anesth Analg*. 1996;83:1065–1071.
107. Ornstein E, Lien CA, Matteo RS, et al. Pharmacodynamics and pharmacokinetics of cisatracurium in geriatric surgical patients. *Anesthesiology*. 1996;84:520–525.
108. Wastila WB, Maehr RB, Turner GL, et al. Comparative pharmacology of cisatracurium (51W89), atracurium, and five isomers in cats. *Anesthesiology*. 1996;85:169–177.
109. Lien CA, Belmont MR, Abalos A, et al. The cardiovascular effects and histamine-releasing properties of 51W89 in patients receiving nitrous oxide/opioid/barbiturate anesthesia. *Anesthesiology*. 1995;82:1131–1138.
110. Savarese JJ, Wastila WB. The future of the benzylisoquinolinium relaxants. *Acta Anaesthesiol Scand Suppl*. 1995;106:91–93.
111. Savarese JJ, Ali HH, Basta SJ, et al. The clinical neuromuscular pharmacology of mivacurium chloride (BW B1090U). A short-acting nondepolarizing ester neuromuscular blocking drug. *Anesthesiology*. 1988;68:723–732.
112. Head-Rapson AG, Devlin JC, Parker CJ, et al. Pharmacokinetics of the three isomers of mivacurium and pharmacodynamics of the chiral mixture in hepatic cirrhosis. *Br J Anaesth*. 1994;73:613–618.
113. Naguib M, Samarkandi AH, Bakhamees HS, et al. Histamine-release haemodynamic changes produced by rocuronium, vecuronium, mivacurium, atracurium and tubocurarine. *Br J Anaesth*. 1995;75:388–392.
114. Buckett WR, Hewett CL, Savage DS. Pancuronium bromide and other steroidal neuromuscular blocking agents containing acetylcholine fragments. *J Med Chem*. 1973;16:1116–1124.
115. Durant NN, Marshall IG, Savage DS, et al. The neuromuscular and autonomic blocking activities of pancuronium, Org NC 45, and other pancuronium analogues, in the cat. *J Pharm Pharmacol*. 1979;31:831–836.
116. Stovner J, Oftedal N, Holmboe J. The inhibition of cholinesterases by pancuronium. *Br J Anaesth*. 1975;47:949–954.
117. Agoston S, Vermeer GA, Kertsten UW, et al. The fate of pancuronium bromide in man. *Acta Anaesthesiol Scand*. 1973;17:267–275.
118. Miller RD, Agoston S, Booij LH, et al. The comparative potency and pharmacokinetics of pancuronium and its metabolites in anesthetized man. *J Pharmacol Exp Ther*. 1978;207:539–543.
119. Savage DS, Sleigh T, Carlyle I. The emergence of ORG NC 45, 1-[2 beta,3 alpha,5 alpha,16 beta,17 beta)-3, 17-bis(acetyloxy)-2-(1-piperidinyl)-androstan-16-yl]-1-methylpiperidinium bromide, from the pancuronium series. *Br J Anaesth*. 1980;52(suppl 1):3S–9S.
120. Hill SA, Scott RPF, Savarese JJ. Structure-activity relationships: from tubocurarine to the present day. *Bailliere's Clin Anesthesiol* 1994;8:317–348.
121. Lebrault C, Berger JL, D'Hollander AA, et al. Pharmacokinetics and pharmacodynamics of vecuronium (ORG NC 45) in patients with cirrhosis. *Anesthesiology*. 1985;62:601–605.
122. Fahey MR, Morris RB, Miller RD, et al. Pharmacokinetics of Org NC45 (norcuron) in patients with and without renal failure. *Br J Anaesth*. 1981;53:1049–1053.
123. Bencini AF, Scaf AH, Sohn YJ, et al. Disposition and urinary excretion of vecuronium bromide in anesthetized patients with normal renal function or renal failure. *Anesth Analg*. 1986;65:245–251.
124. Wright PM, Hart P, Lau M, et al. Cumulative characteristics of atracurium and vecuronium. A simultaneous clinical and pharmacokinetic study. *Anesthesiology*. 1994;81:59–68.
125. Wierda JM, Proost JH. Structure-pharmacodynamic-pharmacokinetic relationships of steroidal neuromuscular blocking agents. *Eur J Anaesthesiol Suppl*. 1995;11:45–54.

126. Naguib M, Samarkandi AH, Bakhamees HS, et al. Comparative potency of steroidal neuromuscular blocking drugs and isobolographic analysis of the interaction between rocuronium and other aminosteroids. *Br J Anaesth.* 1995;75:37–42.
127. Smit JW, Duin E, Steen H, et al. Interactions between P-glycoprotein substrates and other cationic drugs at the hepatic excretory level. *Br J Pharmacol.* 1998;123:361–370.
128. Khuenl-Brady K, Castagnoli KP, Canfell PC, et al. The neuromuscular blocking effects and pharmacokinetics of ORG 9426 and ORG 9616 in the cat. *Anesthesiology.* 1990;72:669–674.
129. Szenohradszky J, Fisher DM, Segredo V, et al. Pharmacokinetics of rocuronium bromide (ORG 9426) in patients with normal renal function or patients undergoing cadaver renal transplantation. *Anesthesiology.* 1992;899–904.
130. Savarese JJ, Belmont MR, Kraus K, et al. AV002: a promising cysteine-reversible intermediate duration neuromuscular blocker in rhesus monkeys. In: *ASA Meeting.* San Francisco, CA: American Society of Anesthesiologists; 2007. A986.
131. Sunaga H, Malhotora JK, Savarese JJ, et al. Dose response relationship for cysteine reversal of the novel muscle relaxant AV002 in dogs. In: *ASA Annual Meeting.* Orlando, FL: American Society of Anesthesiologists; 2008. A364.
132. Donlon JV Jr, Ali HH, Savarese JJ. A new approach to the study of four nondepolarizing relaxants in man. *Anesth Analg.* 1974;53:934–939.
133. Kopman AF, Lien CA, Naguib M. Determining the potency of neuromuscular blockers: are traditional methods flawed? *Br J Anaesth.* 2010;104:705–710.
134. Saitoh Y, Toyooka H, Amaha K. Recoveries of post-tetanic twitch and train-of-four responses after administration of vecuronium with different inhalation anaesthetics and neuroleptanaesthesia. *Br J Anaesth.* 1993;70:402–404.
135. Miller RD, Way WL, Dolan WM, et al. The dependence of pancuronium- and d-tubocurarine-induced neuromuscular blockades on alveolar concentrations of halothane and forane. *Anesthesiology.* 1972;37:573–581.
136. Miller RD, Crique M, Eger EI II. Duration of halothane anesthesia and neuromuscular blockade with d-tubocurarine. *Anesthesiology.* 1976;44:206–210.
137. Kelly RE, Lien CA, Savarese JJ, et al. Depression of neuromuscular function in a patient during desflurane anesthesia. *Anesth Analg.* 1993;76:868–871.
138. Rupp SM, Miller RD, Gencarelli PJ. Vecuronium-induced neuromuscular blockade during enflurane, isoflurane, and halothane anesthesia in humans. *Anesthesiology.* 1984;60:102–105.
139. Gencarelli PJ, Miller RD, Eger EI II, et al. Decreasing enflurane concentrations and d-tubocurarine neuromuscular blockade. *Anesthesiology.* 1982;56:192–194.
140. Miller RD, Way WL, Dolan WM, et al. Comparative neuromuscular effects of pancuronium, gallamine, and succinylcholine during forane and halothane anesthesia in man. *Anesthesiology.* 1971;35:509–514.
141. Wulf H, Ledowski T, Linstedt U, et al. Neuromuscular blocking effects of rocuronium during desflurane, isoflurane, and sevoflurane anaesthesia. *Can J Anaesth.* 1998;45:526–532.
142. Bock M, Klippel K, Nitsche B, et al. Rocuronium potency and recovery characteristics during steady-state desflurane, sevoflurane, isoflurane or propofol anaesthesia. *Br J Anaesth.* 2000;84:43–47.
143. Pereon Y, Bernard JM, Nguyen The Tich S, et al. The effects of desflurane on the nervous system: from spinal cord to muscles. *Anesth Analg.* 1999;89:490–495.
144. Franks NP, Lieb WR. Molecular and cellular mechanisms of general anaesthesia. *Nature.* 1994;367:607–614.
145. Paul M, Fokt RM, Kindler CH, et al. Characterization of the interactions between volatile anesthetics and neuromuscular blockers at the muscle nicotinic acetylcholine receptor. *Anesth Analg.* 2002;95:362–367.
146. Singh YN, Harvey AL, Marshall IG. Antibiotic-induced paralysis of the mouse phrenic nerve-hemidiaphragm preparation, and reversibility by calcium and by neostigmine. *Anesthesiology.* 1978;48:418–424.
147. Heier T, Caldwell JE, Sessler DI, et al. Mild intraoperative hypothermia increases duration of action and spontaneous recovery of vecuronium blockade during nitrous oxide-isoflurane anesthesia in humans. *Anesthesiology.* 1991;74:815–819.
148. Leslie K, Sessler DI, Bjorksten AR, et al. Mild hypothermia alters propofol pharmacokinetics and increases the duration of action of atracurium. *Anesth Analg.* 1995;80:1007–1014.
149. Caldwell JE, Heier T, Wright PM, et al. Temperature-dependent pharmacokinetics and pharmacodynamics of vecuronium. *Anesthesiology.* 2000;92:84–93.
150. Sinatra RS, Philip BK, Naulty JS, et al. Prolonged neuromuscular blockade with vecuronium in a patient treated with magnesium sulfate. *Anesth Analg.* 1985;64:1220–1222.
151. Usubiaga JE, Wikinski JA, Morales RL, et al. Interaction of intravenously administered procaine, lidocaine, and succinylcholine in anesthetized subjects. *Anesth Analg.* 1967;46:39–45.
152. Miller RD, Way WL, Katzung BG. The potentiation of neuromuscular blocking agents by quinidine. *Anesthesiology.* 1967;28:1036–1041.
153. Alloul K, Whalley DG, Shutway F, et al. Pharmacokinetic origin of carbamazepine-induced resistance to vecuronium neuromuscular blockade in anesthetized patients. *Anesthesiology.* 1996;84:330–339.
154. Kim CS, Arnold FJ, Itani MS, et al. Decreased sensitivity to metocurine during long-term phenytoin therapy may be attributable to protein binding and acetylcholine receptor changes. *Anesthesiology.* 1992;77:500–506.
155. Al-Mohaya S, Naguib M, Abdelatif M, et al. Abnormal responses to muscle relaxants in a patient with primary hyperparathyroidism. *Anesthesiology.* 1986;65:554–556.
156. Waud BE, Waud DR. Interaction of calcium and potassium with neuromuscular blocking agents. *Br J Anaesth.* 1980; 52:863–866.
157. Bowman WC, Rodger IW, Houston J, et al. Structure:action relationships among some desacetoxy analogues of pancuronium and vecuronium in the anesthetized cat. *Anesthesiology.* 1988;69:57–62.
158. Kopman AF, Klewicka MM, Kopman DJ, et al. Molar potency is predictive of the speed of onset of neuromuscular block for agents of intermediate, short, and ultrashort duration. *Anesthesiology.* 1999;90:425–431.
159. Kopman AF, Klewicka MM, Neuman GG. Molar potency is not predictive of the speed of onset of atracurium. *Anesth Analg.* 1999; 89:1046–1049.
160. Naguib M, Kopman AF. Low dose rocuronium for tracheal intubation. *Middle East J Anesthesiol.* 2003;17:193–204.
161. Adams PR. Drug interactions at the motor endplate. *Pflugers Arch.* 1975;360:155–164.
162. Donati F, Meistelman C. A kinetic-dynamic model to explain the relationship between high potency and slow onset time for neuromuscular blocking drugs. *J Pharmacokinet Biopharm.* 1991; 19:537–552.
163. Donati F. Onset of neuromuscular blockade: more than just the time to get there. *Anesth Analg.* 2013;117:757–759.
164. Bevan DR. The new relaxants: are they worth it? *Can J Anaesth.* 1999;46:R88–R100.
165. Anaesthetists and the reporting of adverse drug reactions. *Br Med J (Clin Res Ed).* 1986;292:949.
166. Vercruysse P, Bossuyt P, Hanegreefs G, et al. Gallamine and pancuronium inhibit pre- and postjunctional muscarine receptors in canine saphenous veins. *J Pharmacol Exp Ther.* 1979;209:225–230.
167. Savarese JJ, Lowenstein E. The name of the game: no anesthesia by cookbook. *Anesthesiology.* 1985;62:703–705.
168. Domenech JS, Garcia RC, Sastain JM, et al. Pancuronium bromide: an indirect sympathomimetic agent. *Br J Anaesth.* 1976;48:1143–1148.
169. Savarese JJ, Ali HH, Basta SJ, et al. The cardiovascular effects of mivacurium chloride (BW B1090U) in patients receiving nitrous oxide-opiate-barbiturate anesthesia. *Anesthesiology.* 1989;70:386–394.

170. Scott RP, Savarese JJ, Basta SJ, et al. Atracurium: clinical strategies for preventing histamine release and attenuating the haemodynamic response. *Br J Anaesth.* 1985;57:550–553.
171. Moss J, Rosow CE, Savarese JJ, et al. Role of histamine in the hypotensive action of d-tubocurarine in humans. *Anesthesiology.* 1981;55:19–25.
172. Basta SJ, Savarese JJ, Ali HH, et al. Histamine-releasing potencies of atracurium, dimethyl tubocurarine and tubocurarine. *Br J Anaesth.* 1983;55(suppl 1):105S–106S.
173. Naguib M, Abdulatif M, Absood A. Comparative effects of pipecuronium and tubocurarine on plasma concentrations of histamine in humans. *Br J Anaesth.* 1991;67:320–322.
174. Cannon JE, Fahey MR, Moss J, et al. Large doses of vecuronium and plasma histamine concentrations. *Can J Anaesth.* 1988;35: 350–353.
175. Levy JH, Davis GK, Duggan J, et al. Determination of the hemodynamics and histamine release of rocuronium (Org 9426) when administered in increased doses under N2O/O2-sufentanil anesthesia. *Anesth Analg.* 1994;78:318–321.
176. Moss J, Rosow CE. Histamine release by narcotics and muscle relaxants in humans. *Anesthesiology.* 1983;59:330–339.
177. Flacke W, Gillis RA. Impulse transmission via nicotinic and muscarinic pathways in the stellate ganglion of the dog. *J Pharmacol Exp Ther.* 1968;163:266–276.
178. Basta SJ. Modulation of histamine release by neuromuscular blocking drugs. *Curr Opinion Anaesth.* 1992;5:572.
179. Laxenaire MC, Moneret-Vautrin DA, Widmer S, et al. Anesthetics responsible for anaphylactic shock. A French multicenter study [in French]. *Ann Fr Anesth Reanim.* 1990;9:501–506.
180. Fisher MM, More DG. The epidemiology and clinical features of anaphylactic reactions in anaesthesia. *Anaesth Intensive Care.* 1981;9:226–234.
181. Mertes PM, Laxenaire MC, Alla F. Anaphylactic and anaphylactoid reactions occurring during anesthesia in France in 1999-2000. *Anesthesiology.* 2003;99:536–545.
182. Baldo BA, Fisher MM. Substituted ammonium ions as allergenic determinants in drug allergy. *Nature.* 1983;306:262–264.
183. Mertes PM, Moneret-Vautrin DA, Leynadier F, et al. Skin reactions to intradermal neuromuscular blocking agent injections: a randomized multicenter trial in healthy volunteers. *Anesthesiology.* 2007;107:245–252.
184. Cresnar B, Crne-Finderle N, Breskvar K, et al. Neural regulation of muscle acetylcholinesterase is exerted on the level of its mRNA. *J Neurosci Res.* 1994;38:294–299.
185. Beemer GH, Goonetilleke PH, Bjorksten AR. The maximum depth of an atracurium neuromuscular block antagonized by edrophonium to effect adequate recovery. *Anesthesiology.* 1995;82:852–858.
186. Payne JP, Hughes R, Al Azawi S. Neuromuscular blockade by neostigmine in anaesthetized man. *Br J Anaesth.* 1980;52:69–76.
187. Naguib M, Kopman AF, Ensor JE. Neuromuscular monitoring and postoperative residual curarisation: a meta-analysis. *Br J Anaesth.* 2007;98:302–316.
188. Naguib M, Lien CA. Pharmacology of muscle relaxants and their antagonists. In: Miller RD, Fleisher LA, Johns RA, et al, eds. *Miller's Anesthesia.* 6th ed. Philadelphia, PA: Elsevier Churchill Livingstone; 2005:481–572.
189. Bevan DR, Donati F, Kopman AF. Reversal of neuromuscular blockade. *Anesthesiology.* 1992;77:785–805.
190. Brull SJ, Kopman AF, Naguib M. Management principles to reduce the risk of residual neuromuscular blockade. *Curr Anesthesiol Rep.* 2013;3:130–138.
191. Magorian TT, Lynam DP, Caldwell JE, et al. Can early administration of neostigmine, in single or repeated doses, alter the course of neuromuscular recovery from a vecuronium-induced neuromuscular blockade? *Anesthesiology.* 1990;73:410–414.
192. Cronnelly R. Muscle relaxant antagonists. *Semin Anesth.* 1985;4:31.
193. Rupp SM, McChristian JW, Miller RD, et al. Neostigmine and edrophonium antagonism of varying intensity neuromuscular blockade induced by atracurium, pancuronium, or vecuronium. *Anesthesiology.* 1986;64:711–717.
194. Engbaek J, Ording H, Ostergaard D, et al. Edrophonium and neostigmine for reversal of the neuromuscular blocking effect of vecuronium. *Acta Anaesthesiol Scand.* 1985;29:544–546.
195. Fisher DM, Cronnelly R, Sharma M, et al. Clinical pharmacology of edrophonium in infants and children. *Anesthesiology.* 1984;61:428–433.
196. McCarthy GJ, Cooper R, Stanley JC, et al. Dose-response relationships for neostigmine antagonism of vecuronium-induced neuromuscular block in adults and the elderly. *Br J Anaesth.* 1992;69:281–283.
197. Naguib M, Abdulatif M, al-Ghamdi A. Dose-response relationships for edrophonium and neostigmine antagonism of rocuronium bromide (ORG 9426)-induced neuromuscular blockade. *Anesthesiology.* 1993;79:739–745.
198. Naguib M, Riad W. Dose-response relationships for edrophonium and neostigmine antagonism of atracurium and cisatracurium-induced neuromuscular block. *Can J Anaesth.* 2000;47: 1074–1081.
199. Suresh D, Carter JA, Whitehead JP, et al. Cardiovascular changes at antagonism of atracurium. Effects of different doses of premixed neostigmine and glycopyrronium in a ratio of 5:1. *Anaesthesia.* 1991;46:877–880.
200. Morris RB, Cronnelly R, Miller RD, et al. Pharmacokinetics of edrophonium in anephric and renal transplant patients. *Br J Anaesth.* 1981;53:1311–1314.
201. Cronnelly R, Stanski DR, Miller RD, et al. Renal function and the pharmacokinetics of neostigmine in anesthetized man. *Anesthesiology.* 1979;51:222–226.
202. Cronnelly R, Stanski DR, Miller RD, et al. Pyridostigmine kinetics with and without renal function. *Clin Pharmacol Ther.* 1980;28: 78–81.
203. Cronnelly R, Morris RB, Miller RD. Edrophonium: duration of action and atropine requirement in humans during halothane anesthesia. *Anesthesiology.* 1982;57:261–266.
204. Salem MG, Richardson JC, Meadows GA, et al. Comparison between glycopyrrolate and atropine in a mixture with neostigmine for reversal of neuromuscular blockade. Studies in patients following open heart surgery. *Br J Anaesth.* 1985;57:184–187.
205. van Vlymen JM, Parlow JL. The effects of reversal of neuromuscular blockade on autonomic control in the perioperative period. *Anesth Analg.* 1997;84:148–154.
206. Ding Y, Fredman B, White PF. Use of mivacurium during laparoscopic surgery: effect of reversal drugs on postoperative recovery. *Anesth Analg.* 1994;78:450–454.
207. Cheng C-R, Sessler DI, Apfel CC. Does neostigmine administration produce a clinically important increase in postoperative nausea and vomiting? *Anesth Analg.* 2005;101:1349–1355.
208. Boeke AJ, de Lange JJ, van Druenen B, et al. Effect of antagonizing residual neuromuscular block by neostigmine and atropine on postoperative vomiting. *Br J Anaesth.* 1994;72:654–656.
209. Hovorka J, Korttila K, Nelskyla K, et al. Reversal of neuromuscular blockade with neostigmine has no effect on the incidence or severity of postoperative nausea and vomiting. *Anesth Analg.* 1997;85:1359–1361.
210. Hutton P, Burchett KR, Madden AP. Comparison of recovery after neuromuscular blockade by atracurium or pancuronium. *Br J Anaesth.* 1988;60:36–42.
211. Kopman AF, Yee PS, Neuman GG. Relationship of the train-of-four fade ratio to clinical signs and symptoms of residual paralysis in awake volunteers. *Anesthesiology.* 1997;86:765–771.
212. Viby-Mogensen J, Jensen NH, Engbaek J, et al. Tactile and visual evaluation of the response to train-of-four nerve stimulation. *Anesthesiology.* 1985;63:440–443.
213. Dupuis JY, Martin R, Tetrault JP. Clinical, electrical and mechanical correlations during recovery from neuromuscular blockade with vecuronium. *Can J Anaesth.* 1990;37:192–196.

214. Eriksson LI, Sundman E, Olsson R, et al. Functional assessment of the pharynx at rest and during swallowing in partially paralyzed humans: simultaneous videomanometry and mechanomyography of awake human volunteers. *Anesthesiology*. 1997;87:1035–1043.
215. Sundman E, Witt H, Olsson R, et al. The incidence and mechanisms of pharyngeal and upper esophageal dysfunction in partially paralyzed humans: pharyngeal videoradiography and simultaneous manometry after atracurium. *Anesthesiology*. 2000;92:977–984.
216. Eriksson LI. The effects of residual neuromuscular blockade and volatile anesthetics on the control of ventilation. *Anesth Analg*. 1999;89:243–251.
217. Baillard C, Gehan G, Reboul-Marty J, et al. Residual curarization in the recovery room after vecuronium. *Br J Anaesth*. 2000;84: 394–395.
218. Baillard C, Clec'h C, Catineau J, et al. Postoperative residual neuromuscular block: a survey of management. *Br J Anaesth*. 2005;95:622–626.
219. Kopman AF, Ng J, Zank LM, et al. Residual postoperative paralysis. Pancuronium versus mivacurium, does it matter? *Anesthesiology*. 1996;85:1253–1259.
220. Viby-Mogensen J, Jorgensen BC, Ording H. Residual curarization in the recovery room. *Anesthesiology*. 1979;50:539–541.
221. Debaene B, Plaud B, Dilly MP, et al. Residual paralysis in the PACU after a single intubating dose of nondepolarizing muscle relaxant with an intermediate duration of action. *Anesthesiology*. 2003;98:1042–1048.
222. Murphy GS, Szokol JW, Marymont JH, et al. Residual neuromuscular blockade and critical respiratory events in the postanesthesia care unit. *Anesth Analg*. 2008;107:130–137.
223. Brull SJ, Naguib M, Miller RD. Residual neuromuscular block: rediscovering the obvious. *Anesth Analg*. 2008;107:11–4.
224. Naguib M, Brull SJ, Arkes HR. Reasoning of an anomaly: residual block after sugammadex. *Anesth Analg*. 2013;117:197–300.
225. Sorgenfrei IF, Viby-Mogensen J, Swiatek FA. Does evidence lead to a change in clinical practice? Danish anaesthetists' and nurse anesthetists' clinical practice and knowledge of postoperative residual curarization [in Danish]. *Ugeskr Laeger*. 2005;167:3878–3882.
226. Bartkowski RR. Incomplete reversal of pancuronium neuromuscular blockade by neostigmine, pyridostigmine, and edrophonium. *Anesth Analg*. 1987;66:594–598.
227. Beemer GH, Bjorksten AR, Dawson PJ, et al. Determinants of the reversal time of competitive neuromuscular block by anticholinesterases. *Br J Anaesth*. 1991;66:469–475.
228. Naguib M, el-Gammal M, Daoud W, et al. Human plasma cholinesterase for antagonism of prolonged mivacurium-induced neuromuscular blockade. *Anesthesiology*. 1995;82:1288–1292.
229. Belmont MR, Horochiwsky Z, Eliazo RF, et al. Reversal of AV430A with cysteine in rhesus monkeys. *Anesthesiology*. 2004;101:A1180.
230. Bom A, Bradley M, Cameron K, et al. A novel concept of reversing neuromuscular block: chemical encapsulation of rocuronium bromide by a cyclodextrin-based synthetic host. *Angew Chem Int Ed Engl*. 2002;41:266–270.
231. Adam JM, Bennett DJ, Bom A, et al. Cyclodextrin-derived host molecules as reversal agents for the neuromuscular blocker rocuronium bromide: synthesis and structure-activity relationships. *J Med Chem*. 2002;45:1806–1816.
232. Tarver GJ, Grove SJ, Buchanan K, et al. 2-O-substituted cyclodextrins as reversal agents for the neuromuscular blocker rocuronium bromide. *Bioorg Med Chem*. 2002;10:1819–1827.
233. Cameron KS, Clark JK, Cooper A, et al. Modified gamma-cyclodextrins and their rocuronium complexes. *Org Lett*. 2002;4: 3403–3406.
234. Zhang MQ. Drug-specific cyclodextrins: the future of rapid neuromuscular block reversal? *Drugs Future*. 2003;28:347–354.
235. Gijsenbergh F, Ramael S, Houwing N, et al. First human exposure of Org 25969, a novel agent to reverse the action of rocuronium bromide. *Anesthesiology*. 2005;103:695–703.
236. Sorgenfrei IF, Norrild K, Larsen PB, et al. Reversal of rocuronium-induced neuromuscular block by the selective relaxant binding agent sugammadex: a dose-finding and safety study. *Anesthesiology*. 2006;104:667–674.
237. Sparr HJ, Vermeyen KM, Beaufort AM, et al. Early reversal of profound rocuronium-induced neuromuscular blockade by sugammadex in a randomized multicenter study: efficacy, safety, and pharmacokinetics. *Anesthesiology*. 2007;106:935–943.
238. Epemolu O, Bom A, Hope F, et al. Reversal of neuromuscular blockade and simultaneous increase in plasma rocuronium concentration after the intravenous infusion of the novel reversal agent Org 25969. *Anesthesiology*. 2003;99:632–637.
239. Naguib M. Sugammadex: another milestone in clinical neuromuscular pharmacology. *Anesth Analg*. 2007;104:575–581.
240. Shields M, Giovannelli M, Mirakhur RK, et al. Org 25969 (sugammadex), a selective relaxant binding agent for antagonism of prolonged rocuronium-induced neuromuscular block. *Br J Anaesth*. 2006;96:36–43.
241. Suy K, Morias K, Cammu G, et al. Effective reversal of moderate rocuronium- or vecuronium-induced neuromuscular block with sugammadex, a selective relaxant binding agent. *Anesthesiology*. 2007;106:283–288.
242. Groudine SB, Soto R, Lien C, et al. A randomized, dose-finding, phase II study of the selective relaxant binding drug, sugammadex, capable of safely reversing profound rocuronium-induced neuromuscular block. *Anesth Analg*. 2007;104:555–562.
243. de Boer HD, Driessen JJ, Marcus MA, et al. Reversal of rocuronium-induced (1.2 mg/kg) profound neuromuscular block by sugammadex: a multicenter, dose-finding and safety study. *Anesthesiology*. 2007;107:239–244.
244. Puhringer FK, Rex C, Sielenkamper AW, et al. Reversal of profound, high-dose rocuronium-induced neuromuscular blockade by sugammadex at two different time points: an international, multicenter, randomized, dose-finding, safety assessor-blinded, phase II trial. *Anesthesiology*. 2008;109:188–197.
245. Flockton EA, Mastronardi P, Hunter JM, et al. Reversal of rocuronium-induced neuromuscular block with sugammadex is faster than reversal of cisatracurium-induced block with neostigmine. *Br J Anaesth*. 2008;100:622–630.
246. Naguib M. Sugammadex may replace best clinical practice: a misconception. *Anesth Analg*. 2007;105:1506-a–1507-a.
247. Eleveld DJ, Kuizenga K, Proost JH, et al. A temporary decrease in twitch response during reversal of rocuronium-induced muscle relaxation with a small dose of sugammadex. *Anesth Analg*. 2007; 104:582–584.
248. de Boer HD, van Egmond J, van de Pol F, et al. Sugammadex, a new reversal agent for neuromuscular block induced by rocuronium in the anaesthetized Rhesus monkey. *Br J Anaesth*. 2006;96: 473–479.
249. Head-Rapson AG, Devlin JC, Parker CJ, et al. Pharmacokinetics and pharmacodynamics of the three isomers of mivacurium in health, in end-stage renal failure and in patients with impaired renal function. *Br J Anaesth*. 1995;75:31–36.
250. Vandenbrom RH, Wierda JM, Agoston S. Pharmacokinetics and neuromuscular blocking effects of atracurium besylate and two of its metabolites in patients with normal and impaired renal function. *Clin Pharmacokinet*. 1990;19:230–240.
251. Lynam DP, Cronnelly R, Castagnoli KP, et al. The pharmacodynamics and pharmacokinetics of vecuronium in patients anesthetized with isoflurane with normal renal function or with renal failure. *Anesthesiology*. 1988;69:227–231.
252. Sheiner LB, Stanski DR, Vozeh S, et al. Simultaneous modeling of pharmacokinetics and pharmacodynamics: application to d-tubocurarine. *Clin Pharmacol Ther*. 1979;25:358–371.
253. Somogyi AA, Shanks CA, Triggs EJ. The effect of renal failure on the disposition and neuromuscular blocking action of pancuronium bromide. *Eur J Clin Pharmacol*. 1977;12:23–29.

CHAPTER 13

Antiepileptic and Other Neurologically Active Drugs

Pamela Flood • Mark Burbridge

Antiepileptic Drugs

Although 10% of people will report at least one seizure in their lifetime, it is estimated that 1% to 2% of the population worldwide meets the diagnostic criteria for epilepsy (Table 13-1).[1] ***Epilepsy*** is a collective term used to designate a group of chronic central nervous system (CNS) disorders characterized by the onset of sudden disturbances of sensory, motor, autonomic, or psychic origin. These disturbances are usually transient with the exception of status epilepticus and are almost always associated with abnormal discharges on the electroencephalogram. Only 30% of patients with seizures have an identifiable neurologic or systemic disorder.

The goal of pharmacologic treatment of epilepsy is to control seizures with minimal medication-related adverse effects. Approximately 70% of patients with epilepsy will become seizure-free using a single antiepileptic drug. For the remaining 30% of patients, further treatment options may include transitioning to another drug; combining the primary drug with an additional drug; or upon failure of medical therapy, progression to invasive procedures such as vagal nerve stimulator insertion or neurosurgical resection.[2] The antiepileptic drug selected to treat epilepsy is highly individualized and tailored to the individual patient, explaining the high interpatient variability in drug regimens. Criteria that must be considered in choosing an antiepileptic drug include efficacy for the characteristic seizures experienced by the patient, tolerability, safety, ease of use and frequency of administration, and pharmacokinetics (Table 13-2).[2] Over the last two decades, there has been a dramatic increase in drug choices, which offer markedly fewer side effects with often comparable efficacy to older drugs.[3] However, dose-related side effects can limit the use of any of the antiepileptic drugs (Table 13-3). Although side effects are normally associated with higher plasma levels of the drug, the specific concentration at which a patient develops toxicity varies considerably (Table 13-4).[4]

Pharmacokinetics

All antiepileptic drugs are administered once daily or more frequently. Sustained-release preparations are becoming increasingly available and preferred by patients. Absorption of these drugs from the gastrointestinal tract occurs slowly over a period of hours and may be incomplete, especially for gabapentin. Protein binding varies greatly (0% for gabapentin to 90% or greater for phenytoin). Hepatic and renal disease may necessitate dose adjustment. Medications that rely on renal excretion include gabapentin, pregabalin, levetiracetam, vigabatrin, and zonisamide and should be dosed according to renal function. The remaining drugs should be dosed according to the patient's degree of liver dysfunction.

Antiepileptic drug clearance and elimination half-time range from hours (carbamazepine, valproate, primidone, gabapentin) to days (phenytoin, lamotrigine, phenobarbital, zonisamide) (see Table 13-4). Because of their ability to induce or inhibit drug metabolism, all antiepileptic drugs, except gabapentin, levetiracetam, and vigabatrin, may be associated with pharmacokinetic drug interactions in which plasma drug concentrations and resulting pharmacologic effects of concomitantly administered drugs may be altered. Such drug interactions should be anticipated in all patients receiving antiepileptic drugs and subsequently receiving drugs for other purposes.

Drug Interactions Related to Protein Binding

Medications that compete for protein-binding sites of highly bound antiepileptic drugs (phenytoin, valproate, carbamazepine) can displace the bound drug and lead to increases in the plasma concentration of pharmacologically active antiepileptic drug. Commonly used medications that are highly protein bound include phenylbutazone, thyroxine, and salicylates. Albumin is the principal binding protein for antiepileptic drugs. Hypoalbuminemia, as may accompany renal or hepatic disease or malnutrition, can result in increased plasma

Table 13-1

Classification of Epileptic Seizures

Partial seizures (beginning locally)
- Simple partial seizures (consciousness not impaired)
- Complex partial seizures (consciousness impaired)
- Partial seizures evolving into secondary generalized seizures

Generalized seizures (convulsive or nonconvulsive)
- Absence seizures (petit mal)
- Myoclonic seizures
- Clonic seizures
- Tonic seizures
- Tonic-clonic seizures

Unclassified seizures

Adapted from Brodie MJ, Dichter MA. Antiepileptic drugs. *N Engl J Med.* 1996;334:168–175.

concentrations of unbound antiepileptic drug, resulting in toxicity despite therapeutic plasma concentrations. In pregnancy, hypoalbuminemia is due to a progressive increase in central volume which offsets the effect of hypoalbuminemia.

Drug Interactions Related to Accelerated Metabolism

Enzyme-inducing antiepileptic drugs that accelerate metabolism (carbamazepine, lamotrigine, oxcarbazepine, phenobarbital, phenytoin, topiramate, and primidone) may accelerate the metabolism of estrogen and progesterone and thus render oral contraceptives ineffective at usual doses. Patients being treated with antiepileptic drugs have increased dose requirements for thiopental, propofol, midazolam, opioids, and nondepolarizing neuromuscular blocking drug. Possible explanations for altered dose requirements for drugs administered during anesthesia include increased hepatic P450 enzyme activity as a result of enzyme-inducing effects of antiepileptic drugs, alterations in the number and/or responsiveness of receptors, and interactions with endogenous neurotransmitters.

Principles of Dosing

The initial dose is that which is high enough to expect clinical effect but low enough to avoid significant side effects (see Table 13-3). Gradual dose titration is recommended in all but emergency situations. The clinical response guides dose adjustment over time as there is significant variability in clinical response over a wide range of dosages. A common cause of medication ineffectiveness is failure to achieve a sufficiently high plasma concentration. Noncompliance is a particular concern in specific patient populations including adolescents and the elderly.[1,2,4]

To maintain plasma drug concentrations in a therapeutic range, equal doses of the antiepileptic drug are often administered at intervals equivalent to less than one elimination half-time of the drug (see Table 13-4). Dosing at one-half the drug's elimination half-time ensures that a single missed dose will not result in the plasma concentration decreasing below a therapeutic level.

Plasma Concentrations and Laboratory Testing

Phenytoin is the only agent for which monitoring is routinely recommended due to its nonlinear saturation dose kinetics. Routine laboratory monitoring of plasma concentrations for all other agents is not recommended.[2] For this reason, titration to clinical efficacy is recommended for guiding the dosages of antiepileptic drugs. Some patients may respond at low plasma concentrations, and some patients will not respond until high plasma concentrations are obtained. If a patient does not respond to a particular drug as expected, investigating the plasma drug concentration may aid in determining compliance and identifying potential pharmacokinetic interactions.[2,4]

Mechanism of Seizure Activity

Seizure activity in most patients with epilepsy has a localized or focal origin. The reason for the high frequency and synchronous firing in a seizure focus is usually unknown. Possible explanations include local biochemical changes, ischemia, loss of cellular inhibitory systems, infections, and head trauma.

Neurons in a chronic seizure focus exhibit a type of denervation hypersensitivity with regard to excitatory stimuli. The spread of seizure activity to neighboring normal cells is presumably restrained by normal inhibitory mechanisms. Factors such as changes in blood glucose concentrations, $Pa{O_2}$, $Pa{CO_2}$, pH, electrolyte balance, endocrine function, stress, and fatigue may facilitate the spread of a seizure focus into areas of the normal brain. If the spread is sufficiently extensive, the entire brain is activated and a tonic-clonic seizure with unconsciousness ensues. Conversely, if the spread is localized, the seizure produces signs and symptoms characteristic of the anatomic focus. Once initiated, a seizure is most likely maintained by reentry of excitatory impulses in a closed feedback pathway that may not even include the original seizure focus.

Mechanism of Drug Action

The mechanism of action of antiepileptic drugs is incompletely understood. It is commonly presumed that

Table 13-2

Antiepileptic Drugs Used to Treat Epilepsy

Drug	Principal Mechanism of Action	Targeted Seizure	Dosage Type
Carbamazepine	Sodium ion channel blockade	Partial seizures	10–40 mg/kg/day in two to three divided doses
Ethosuximide	T-type calcium ion change	Generalized seizures	15–40 mg/kg/day in two to three divided doses
Felbamate	Sodium ion channel blockade Glutamate antagonism Calcium ion channel blockade	Partial seizures Generalized seizures	15–45 mg/kg/day in two to three divided doses
Gabapentin	Unknown (? increases GABA release)	Partial seizures Generalized seizures	10–60 mg/kg/day
Lamotrigine	Sodium ion channel blockade Calcium ion channel blockade	Partial seizures Generalized seizures	200–500 mg/day in two divided doses
Levetiracetam	Unknown (? potassium and calcium ion channel blockade)	Partial seizures Generalized seizures	1,000–3,000 mg/day in two divided doses
Oxcarbazepine	Sodium ion channel blockade	Partial seizures Generalized seizures	900–2,400 mg/day in two divided doses
Phenobarbital	Chloride ion channels	Partial seizures Generalized seizures	2–5 mg/kg/day every day or in two divided doses
Phenytoin	Sodium ion channel blockade Calcium ion channels NMDA receptors	Partial seizures Generalized seizures	3–7 mg/kg/day in three divided doses
Primidone	Chloride ion channels GABA uptake	Partial seizures Generalized seizures	500–1500 mg/day in two to three divided doses
Tiagabine	Enhanced GABA activity Carbonic anhydrase inhibition	Partial seizures Generalized seizures	32–56 mg/kg/day in two to four divided doses
Topiramate	Sodium ion channel blockade Enhanced GABA activity Glutamate antagonism Calcium ion channel blockade	Partial seizures Generalized seizures	500–3,000 mg/day in two to four divided doses
Valproate	Sodium ion channel blockade Calcium ion channels	Partial seizures Generalized seizures	500–3,000 mg/day in two to four divided doses
Vigabatrin	GABA transaminase inhibition	Complex partial Infantile spasms	3,000 mg/day in two divided doses
Zonisamide	Sodium ion channel blockade Calcium ion channel blockade	Partial seizures Generalized seizures	200–600 mg/day in two to four divided doses

GABA, γ-aminobutyric acid; NMDA, *N*-methyl-D-aspartate.

antiepileptic drugs control seizures by decreasing neuronal excitability or enhancing inhibition of neurotransmission. This is achieved by altering intrinsic membrane ion currents (sodium, potassium, and calcium conductance) or by affecting activity of inhibitory neurotransmitters. Ion currents affected by antiepileptic drugs are primarily those involving the voltage-gated sodium and calcium ion channels. Drugs that delay reactivation of sodium channels (phenytoin, carbamazepine, primidone, valproate, and lamotrigine) during high frequency neuronal firing produce an inhibitory effect on creation of action potentials until neuronal discharge is blocked. Some drugs (phenytoin, carbamazepine, valproate, lamotrigine, and zonisamide) act at both sodium and calcium ion channels. Other drugs (ethosuximide and phenobarbital) act selectively at calcium ion channels. Ethosuximide selectively blocks the T-type calcium ion current, which is thought to act as a pacemaker for thalamic neurons and may be important in absence seizures. Drugs (phenobarbital and benzodiazepines) that alter synaptic function act primarily by enhancing γ-aminobutyric acid (GABA)–mediated neuronal inhibition. Benzodiazepines increase the frequency of GABA-mediated ion channel openings, whereas barbiturates increase the duration of ion channel openings. Tiagabine delays the reuptake of GABA from synaptic clefts, effectively enhancing GABA-mediated

Table 13-3

Side Effects of Antiepileptic Drugs

	Dose-Related	Idiosyncratic
Carbamazepine	Diplopia Vertigo Neutropenia Nausea Drowsiness Hyponatremia	Agranulocytosis Aplastic anemia Allergic dermatitis (rash) Stevens-Johnson syndrome Hepatotoxic effects Pancreatitis Teratogenicity
Ethosuximide	Nausea Anorexia Vomiting Agitation Headache Drowsiness	Agranulocytosis Aplastic anemia Allergic dermatitis (rash) Stevens-Johnson syndrome Lupus-like syndrome
Clonazepam	Sedation Vertigo Hyperactivity (children)	Allergic dermatitis (rash) Thrombocytopenia
Felbamate	Insomnia Anorexia Nausea Headache Irritability	Aplastic anemia Hepatotoxic effects
Gabapentin	Sedation Ataxia Vertigo Gastrointestinal disturbances	
Lamotrigine	Tremor Vertigo Diplopia Ataxia Headache Gastrointestinal disturbances	Stevens-Johnson syndrome
Levetiracetam	Sedation Anxiety Headache	Allergic dermatitis (rash)
Oxcarbazepine		Allergic dermatitis (rash)
Phenobarbital	Sedation Depression Hyperactivity (children)	Agranulocytosis Allergic dermatitis (rash) Stevens-Johnson syndrome Arthritic changes Hepatotoxic effects Teratogenicity
Phenytoin	Nystagmus Ataxia Nausea and vomiting Gingival hyperplasia Depression Megaloblastic anemia Drowsiness	Agranulocytosis Aplastic anemia Allergic dermatitis (rash) Stevens-Johnson syndrome Hepatotoxic effects Pancreatitis Acne Coarse facies Hirsutism Teratogenicity Dupuytren contracture

Table 13-3

Side Effects of Antiepileptic Drugs *(continued)*

	Dose-Related	Idiosyncratic
Primidone	Sedation	Rash Thrombocytopenia Agranulocytosis Lupus-like syndrome Teratogenicity
Tiagabine	Dizziness Aphasia Tremor	Allergic dermatitis (rash)
Topiramate	Sedation Ataxia Dizziness	Allergic dermatitis (rash)
Valproic acid	Tremor Weight gain Dyspepsia Nausea and vomiting Alopecia Peripheral edema Encephalopathy Teratogenicity Sedation	Agranulocytosis Aplastic anemia Allergic dermatitis (rash) Stevens-Johnson syndrome Hepatotoxic effects Pancreatitis
Vigabatrin	Anemia Sedation Permanent visual loss	
Zonisamide	Teratogenicity Dizziness Ataxia Nephrolithiasis Hyperactivity (children) Mania (adults)	Allergic dermatitis

Adapted in part from Brodie MJ, Dichter MA. Antiepileptic drugs. *N Engl J Med.* 1996;334:168–175; Dichter MA, Brodie MJ. New antiepileptic drugs. *N Engl J Med.* 1996;334:1583–1590.

neuronal inhibition after synaptic release of the neurotransmitter.

Major Antiepileptic Drugs

The principal antiepileptic drugs used to treat patients with epilepsy are carbamazepine, ethosuximide, pregabalin, gabapentin, clobazam, lamotrigine, levetiracetam, oxcarbazepine, phenobarbital, phenytoin, primidone, tiagabine, topiramate, valproate, and zonisamide (see Table 13-2). Since 2005, the number of agents has more than doubled, thereby offering broader therapeutic effectiveness with fewer drug interactions, broader spectrums of activity, and unique mechanisms of action (see Table 13-2) (Fig. 13-1).[5]

Benzodiazepines such as diazepam, lorazepam, and midazolam are used for short-term treatment of acute seizures or status epilepticus and are usually administered parenterally. Clonazepam can be used to treat epilepsy but most patients develop tolerance to its antiepileptic effects and sedation is a common side effect. Felbamate is reserved for use in selected patients with uncontrolled seizures due to its side effect profile. Clobazam, a benzodiazepine derivative, is a more recent addition to this class and is unique among other members of the class in that it does not induce significant levels of sedation and can be used for long-term therapy because tolerance is relatively uncommon.[6]

Drugs used in the treatment of partial seizures are carbamazepine, lamotrigine, oxcarbazepine, topiramate, zonisamide and phenytoin, which are highly effective and associated with an acceptable side effect profile (see Table 13-2). Valproate, lamotrigine, and topiramate are the antiepileptic drugs useful for treatment of patients with generalized seizures. Ethosuximide, lamotrigine, or valproate is effective in treatment of patients with generalized nonconvulsive seizures, especially absence seizures.

Table 13-4

Pharmacokinetics of Antiepileptic Drugs

	Plasma Therapeutic Concentration (μg/mL)	Protein Binding (%)	Elimination Half-Time (h)	Route of Elimination
Carbamazepine	6–12	70–80	8–24	Hepatic metabolism (active metabolite)
Clonazepam	0.02–0.08	80–90	30–40	Hepatic metabolism
Diazepam		95	20–35	Hepatic metabolism (active metabolites)
Ethosuximide	40–100	0	20–60	Hepatic metabolism (25% excreted unchanged)
Felbamate		22–25	20–23	Renal excretion
Gabapentin	2–20	0	6	Renal excretion
Lamotrigine		54	25	Hepatic metabolism
Lorazepam		80	14	Hepatic metabolism
Oxcarbazepine		40	8–10	Renal excretion
Phenobarbital	10–40	48–54	72–144	Hepatic metabolism (25% excreted unchanged)
Phenytoin	10–20	90–93	9–40	Saturable hepatic metabolism
Primidone	5–12	20–30	4–12	Hepatic metabolism to active metabolites of which 40% are excreted unchanged
Tiagabine		95	5–8	Hepatic metabolism
Topiramate		10	8–15	Renal excretion and hepatic metabolism
Valproic acid	50–100	88–92	7–17	Hepatic metabolism (active metabolites)
Zonisamide		50	50–70	Hepatic metabolism

Adapted in part from Brodie MJ, Dichter MA. Antiepileptic drugs. *N Engl J Med*. 1996;334:168–175; Dichter MA, Brodie MJ. New antiepileptic drugs. *N Engl J Med*. 1996;334:1583–1590.

Adverse Side Effects

Antiepileptic drugs may potentially produce numerous and varied adverse side effects. Newer agents have a significantly more favorable side effect profile. Some adverse side effects are dose-related (sedation, lethargy, neurotoxicity), whereas others are idiosyncratic (hypersensitivity, hepatotoxicity, aplastic anemia) (see Table 13-3).

Maternal Epilepsy

As previously mentioned, pregnancy can result from enzyme inducing antiepileptic drugs that render oral contraceptive pills less effective. Seizures during pregnancy can result in significant morbidity and mortality to both mother and fetus, making seizure control during this period imperative.[2] Monotherapy with the lowest dose possible is the guiding principle. Fetal organogenesis is largely complete by 8 weeks. Significant teratogenicity may occur during this period if pregnancy is not detected early enough to permit discontinuation of potentially teratogenic medications. Drug regimens in women of childbearing age should therefore be given special attention. In particular, parturients who take valproate and carbamazepine have more than double the risk of giving birth to a fetus with congenital malformations including neural tube defects such as spina bifida. Patients on lamotrigine have rates of congenital malformation comparable to the general population. Clobazam may be added as needed especially during labor. Conclusive data regarding other antiepileptic drugs during pregnancy is lacking, in part due to the ethical and regulatory difficulty of conducting randomized trials during pregnancy.[1]

Carbamazepine

Carbamazepine is an iminostilbenes derivative that is effective for suppression of nonconvulsive and convulsive partial seizures. In addition, this drug is useful in the management of patients with trigeminal neuralgia and glossopharyngeal neuralgia. Structurally, carbamazepine is related to the tricyclic antidepressant imipramine. Like phenytoin, carbamazepine alters ionic conductance and thus has a membrane-stabilizing effect.

Pharmacokinetics

This drug is available only as an oral preparation (see Table 13-4). Oral absorption is rapid, with peak plasma concentrations occurring 2 to 6 hours after ingestion. Plasma protein binding is 70% to 80%. The plasma elimination half-time is 8 to 24 hours. The principal metabolite of carbamazepine is an epoxide derivative that has antiseizure effects that may also be responsible for many of the dose-limiting side effects of this drug. Because this drug induces its own metabolism, many patients require a dosage increase in 2 to 4 weeks after initiation of therapy. The usual therapeutic plasma concentration of carbamazepine is 6 to 12 μg/mL.

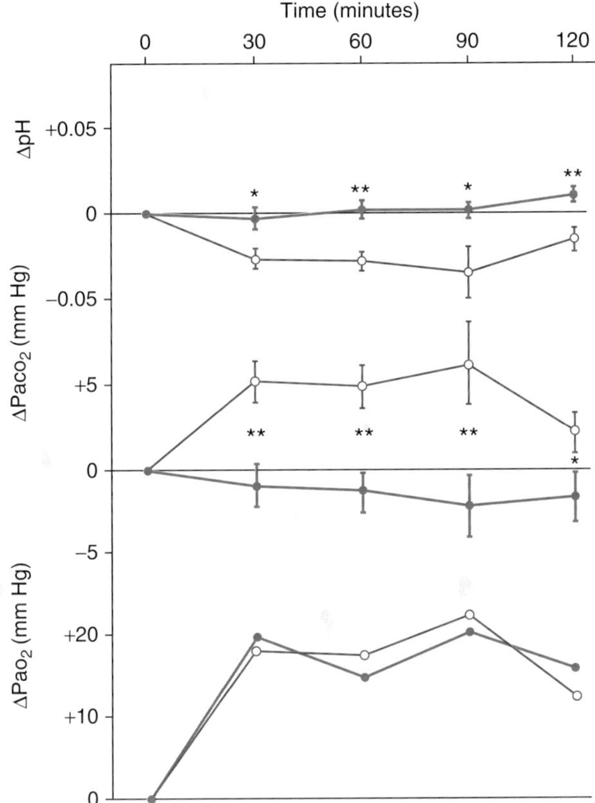

FIGURE 13-1 Doxapram, as a continuous infusion *(solid circles)*, may be used to maintain alveolar ventilation during administration of supplemental oxygen to patients with chronic obstructive airway disease. The *open circles* represent placebo. **P* <.05 compared with placebo infusion; ** *P*<.01 compared with placebo infusion. (From Moser KM, Luchsinger PC, Adamson JS, et al. Respiratory stimulation with intravenous doxapram in respiratory failure. *N Engl J Med.* 1973;288:428–431, with permission.)

Side Effects

The toxicity of carbamazepine is similar to that produced by phenytoin (see Table 13-3). Sedation, vertigo, diplopia, nausea, and vomiting are the most frequent side effects of this drug. Chronic diarrhea develops in some patients, whereas others experience the syndrome of inappropriate antidiuretic hormone secretion. Aplastic anemia, thrombocytopenia, hepatocellular and cholestatic jaundice, oliguria, hypertension, and cardiac dysrhythmias are rare but potentially life-threatening complications. Chronic suppression of white blood cell counts can occur. For these reasons, it may be prudent to monitor bone marrow, cardiac, hepatic, and renal function in patients being treated with carbamazepine. At high plasma concentrations, carbamazepine has an arginine vasopressin hormone-like action that may result in hyponatremia. Skin rash, often with other manifestations of drug allergy, occurs in approximately 10% of chronically treated patients.

In addition to inducing its own metabolism, carbamazepine can accelerate the hepatic oxidation and conjugation of other lipid-soluble drugs. The most common interaction is with oral contraceptive pills, and most women require an increase in the daily dose of estrogen. Carbamazepine also accelerates the metabolism of valproic acid, ethosuximide, corticosteroids, anticoagulants, and antipsychotic drugs. Drugs that inhibit the metabolism of carbamazepine sufficiently to cause toxic effects include cimetidine, propoxyphene, diltiazem, verapamil, isoniazid, and erythromycin.

Ethosuximide

Ethosuximide is the drug of choice for suppression of absence (petit mal) epilepsy in patients who do not also have tonic-clonic seizures. This drug acts by decreasing voltage-dependent calcium conductance in thalamic neurons. This is consistent with the speculated importance of the thalamocortical system in the etiology of absence seizures.

Pharmacokinetics

This drug is available only as an oral preparation (see Table 13-4). Peak plasma concentrations occur in 1 to 7 hours after oral administration. Ethosuximide is not significantly bound to albumin. Approximately 25% of the drug is excreted unchanged in urine, and the remainder is metabolized to inactive metabolites by hepatic microsomal enzymes. The elimination half-time is 20 to 60 hours. The usual maintenance dose of ethosuximide is 20 to 30 mg/kg. A plasma concentration of 40 to 100 μg/mL is required for satisfactory suppression of absence epilepsy.

Side Effects

Toxicity of ethosuximide is low, manifesting most often as gastrointestinal intolerance (nausea, vomiting) and CNS effects (lethargy, dizziness, ataxia, photophobia). There have been rare reports of bone marrow suppression.

Felbamate

Because of its potential to produce life-threatening side effects, felbamate is not used as a first-line drug for treatment of seizures but rather is reserved for patients with intractable epilepsy. Felbamate is used principally for poorly controlled partial and secondarily generalized seizures. It also decreases the frequency of seizures associated with the Lennox-Gastaut syndrome and myotonic and atonic forms of epilepsy.[7] The mechanism of action of felbamate is unknown but may involve action at voltage-gated sodium channels, NMDA and non-NMDA glutamate receptors, voltage-gated calcium currents, and GABA receptor modulation.[6]

Pharmacokinetics

Oral absorption is prompt and the elimination half-time is prolonged (see Table 13-4). Felbamate undergoes minimal metabolism with most of the drug being excreted unchanged by the kidneys.

Side Effects

Serious side effects include aplastic anemia and hepatotoxicity (see Table 13-3). Monitoring of treated patients with complete blood counts and liver function tests is indicated. Because felbamate is metabolized by hepatic cytochrome P450 enzymes, its metabolism is affected by concurrent administration of other drugs that are also metabolized by this system. In particular, concomitant administration of carbamazepine or phenytoin may decrease plasma concentrations of felbamate. Likewise, since felbamate is a potent inhibitor of P450 enzymes, it can slow the metabolism of phenytoin, phenobarbital, and valproic acid. In this regard, if a patient is receiving phenytoin, carbamazepine, or valproic acid and receives felbamate, the dose of these drugs should be decreased by 20% to 30% to prevent toxic effects.

Gabapentin

The pharmacokinetic considerations for gabapentin are discussed in detail in Chapter 8. Gabapentin is an analog of GABA that increases synaptic GABA considerations. Gabapentin induces dose-related sedation and it has efficacy in the treatment of anxiety, panic, and major depression.[8] Despite its multiple other uses, gabapentin has limited efficacy in the treatment of epilepsy.

Lamotrigine

Lamotrigine is a chemically novel anticonvulsant drug of the phenyltriazine class that most likely acts by stabilizing voltage-sensitive sodium ion channels, thus preventing release of aspartate and glutamate. This drug has a broad spectrum of activity and is effective when used alone or in combination in adults who have partial seizures or generalized seizures and in children with Lennox-Gastaut syndrome. When administered orally, lamotrigine is well absorbed and its plasma elimination half-time is about 25 hours (see Table 13-4). Drugs that induce hepatic microsomal enzymes (phenobarbital, phenytoin, and carbamazepine) decrease the elimination half-time of lamotrigine by about 50%, necessitating a higher dose. Conversely, valproic acid slows the metabolism of lamotrigine and extends its elimination half-time to about 60 hours. The most common side effects of lamotrigine are headache, nausea, vomiting, dizziness, diplopia, and ataxia (see Table 13-3). Tremor can be troublesome at higher doses. In approximately 5% of adults, a rash develops, which subsequently disappears in some patients, despite continued therapy. In a few patients, however, the rash is more serious, and fever, arthralgias, and eosinophilia occur. In rare cases, Stevens-Johnson syndrome has been reported.

Levetiracetam

Levetiracetam is effective in the management of partial-onset seizures in adults. Its mechanism of action is not fully known; however, it binds to certain presynaptic calcium channels, acting to reduce synaptic neurotransmitter release.[9] Side effects are considered minor and include sedation, asthenia, anxiety, and headache. The pharmacokinetic profile of levetiracetam is favorable, with the absence of hepatic metabolism and minimal protein binding. No significant drug interactions have been described with co-administration of other antiepileptic drugs.

Oxcarbazepine

Oxcarbazepine is a keto analogue of carbamazepine that provides equivalent seizure control but with fewer adverse side effects. After administration, oxcarbazepine acts as a prodrug that is converted to an active metabolite, 10-hydroxycarbazepine. Oxcarbazepine and its active metabolite do not induce hepatic microsomal enzymes nor does it displace other drugs from plasma protein-binding sites. As such, they are safer drugs to be used in combination therapy. Oxcarbazepine causes dose-dependent hyponatremia in up to half of patients, mandating monitoring of serum sodium levels at those receiving higher doses of this agent.

Phenobarbital

Phenobarbital is a long-acting barbiturate that is effective against all seizure types except nonconvulsive primary generalized seizures. Cognitive and behavioral side effects limit this drug's usefulness in the treatment of epilepsy. Because of these side effects, phenobarbital is considered a second-line drug in the treatment of epilepsy.

Phenobarbital appears to exert its antiepileptic properties partly through potentiation of the postsynaptic actions of the inhibitory neurotransmitter GABA and inhibition of the excitatory postsynaptic actions of glutamate. These drug-induced effects prolong the duration of chloride channel opening and thus limit the spread of seizure activity and increase the seizure threshold.

Pharmacokinetics

Oral absorption of phenobarbital is slow but nearly complete, with peak concentrations occurring 12 to 18 hours after a single dose (see Table 13-4). Plasma protein binding is 48% to 54%. Approximately 25% of phenobarbital is eliminated by pH-dependent renal excretion, with the remainder inactivated by hepatic microsomal enzymes. The principal metabolite is an inactive parahydroxyphenyl derivative that is excreted in urine as a sulfate conjugate. The elimination half-time of phenobarbital is prolonged.

The usual daily oral dose of phenobarbital is 60 mg in adults or 4 mg/kg in children. Plasma phenobarbital concentrations of 10 to 40 μg/mL are usually necessary for control of seizures. The value of measuring plasma phenobarbital concentrations is limited because the concentration associated with optimal control is highly variable among patients. In addition, the development of tolerance to the drug's CNS effects makes the toxic threshold imprecise.

Side Effects

Sedation in adults and children and irritability and hyperactivity in children are the most troublesome side effects when this drug is used to treat epilepsy (see Table 13-3). Tolerance to the sedative effects of phenobarbital may develop with chronic therapy. Depression develops in many adults taking phenobarbital, and confusion may occur in elderly patients. Cognitive effects include slowing of task processing. Scarlatiniform or morbilliform rash occurs in up to 2% of patients. Megaloblastic anemia that responds to folic acid administration and osteomalacia that responds to vitamin D therapy may occur during chronic phenobarbital therapy as well as during treatment with phenytoin. Nystagmus and ataxia are likely if the plasma phenobarbital concentration is >40 μg/mL. Abnormal collagen deposition manifesting as Dupuytren contracture may occur. Congenital malformations may occur when phenobarbital is administered chronically during pregnancy. Coagulation defects and hemorrhage in the neonate must be considered in the setting of fetal exposure. Interactions between phenobarbital and other drugs usually involve induction of hepatic microsomal enzymes. In this regard, phenobarbital is the classic example of a hepatic microsomal enzyme inducer that can accelerate the metabolism of many lipid-soluble drugs.

Phenytoin

Phenytoin is the prototype of the hydantoins and is effective for the treatment of partial and generalized seizures. Available in oral and intravenous (IV) preparations, phenytoin may be administered acutely to achieve effective plasma concentrations within 20 minutes. This drug has a high therapeutic index, and its administration is not accompanied by excessive sedation.

Mechanism of Action

Phenytoin regulates neuronal excitability and thus the spread of seizure activity from a seizure focus by regulating sodium and possibly calcium ion transport across neuronal membranes. This stabilizing effect on cell membranes is relatively selective for the cerebral cortex, although the effect also extends to peripheral nerves. In addition to the effect on ion fluxes, phenytoin acts on second messengers such as calmodulin and the cyclic nucleotides.

Pharmacokinetics

Phenytoin is a weak acid (pK 8.3) that is maintained in aqueous solutions as a sodium salt (see Table 13-4). The drug precipitates in solutions with a pH of <7.8. Its poor water solubility may result in slow and sometimes variable absorption from the gastrointestinal tract (30% to 97%). The initial daily adult oral dosage is 3 to 4 mg/kg. Doses of >500 mg daily are rarely tolerated. The long duration of action of phenytoin allows a single daily dosage, but gastric intolerance may necessitate divided dosage. After intramuscular (IM) injection, the drug precipitates at the injection site and is slowly absorbed. For this reason, IM administration is not recommended. The rate of IV administration of phenytoin should not exceed 50 mg per minute in adults and 1 to 3 mg/kg per minute (or 50 mg per minute, whichever is slower) in pediatric patients because of the risk of severe hypotension and cardiac arrhythmias.

Plasma Concentrations

Control of seizures is usually obtained when plasma concentrations of phenytoin are 10 to 20 μg/mL. In the control of digitalis-induced cardiac dysrhythmias, phenytoin, 0.5 to 1.0 mg/kg IV, is administered every 15 to 30 minutes until a satisfactory response is achieved or a maximum dose of 15 mg/kg is administered. A plasma phenytoin concentration of 8 to 16 μg/mL is usually sufficient to suppress cardiac dysrhythmias. Adverse side effects of phenytoin such as nystagmus and ataxia are likely when the plasma concentration of drug is >20 μg/mL. Nevertheless, the diagnosis of phenytoin toxicity should be made on the basis of clinical symptoms.

Protein Binding

Phenytoin is bound approximately 90% to plasma albumin. A greater fraction of phenytoin remains unbound in neonates, in patients with hypoalbuminemia, and in uremic patients.

Metabolism

Metabolism of phenytoin to inactive metabolites is by hepatic microsomal enzymes that are susceptible to stimulation or inhibition by other drugs. An estimated 98% of phenytoin is metabolized to the inactive derivative parahydroxyphenyl, which appears in urine as a glucuronide. Approximately 2% of phenytoin is recovered unchanged in urine.

When the plasma concentration of phenytoin is <10 μg/mL, metabolism follows first-order kinetics, and the elimination half-time averages 24 hours. At plasma concentrations of >10 μg/mL, the enzymes necessary for metabolism of phenytoin become saturated, and the elimination half-time becomes dose-dependent (zero-order kinetics). At this stage, relatively small increases in dose may result in dramatic increases in the plasma concentration of phenytoin. Zero-order kinetics in phenytoin metabolism resembles the metabolism of alcohol.

Side Effects

The side effects of phenytoin include CNS toxicity that manifests clinically as nystagmus, ataxia, diplopia, vertigo (cerebellar-vestibular dysfunction) and is likely when the plasma phenytoin concentration is >20 μg/mL. Peripheral neuropathy has been observed in up to 30% of chronically treated patients. Gingival hyperplasia occurs in approximately 20% of chronically treated patients and is probably the most common manifestation of phenytoin toxicity in children and adolescents. This complication is minimized by improved oral hygiene and does not necessarily require discontinuation of phenytoin therapy. Other reversible cosmetic side effects include acne, hirsutism, and facial coarsening. Administration of phenytoin during pregnancy may result in the fetal hydantoin syndrome, which manifests as wide-set eyes, broad mandible, and finger deformities.

Allergic reactions include morbilliform rash in 2% to 5% of patients. Hyperglycemia and glycosuria may reflect phenytoin-induced inhibition of insulin secretion. Megaloblastic anemia is rare and has been attributed to altered folic acid absorption but probably also involves altered folic acid metabolism. Phenytoin-induced hepatotoxicity, although rare, may occur in genetically susceptible persons who lack the enzyme phenytoin epoxide. This enzyme is necessary to convert an electrophilic intermediate formed after the oxidative metabolism of phenytoin to an inert and nontoxic product. Gastrointestinal irritation is due to alkalinity of the drug; this may be minimized by taking phenytoin after meals.

Phenytoin can induce the oxidative metabolism of many lipid-soluble drugs, including carbamazepine, valproic acid, ethosuximide, anticoagulants, and corticosteroids. Because its metabolism is saturable, inhibitory interactions are particularly likely to have neurotoxic effects. Interactions involving protein-binding displacement are not likely to be clinically significant.

Patients receiving phenytoin chronically have higher dose requirements for nondepolarizing neuromuscular blocking drugs such as vecuronium compared with untreated patients. Phenytoin induces hepatic enzymes and it is likely that metabolism and elimination of nondepolarizing neuromuscular blocking drugs is increased. Phenytoin may also produce mild blocking effects at the neuromuscular junction leading to upregulation of acetylcholine receptors.

Primidone

Primidone is metabolized to phenobarbital and another active metabolite, phenylethylmalonamide. The efficacy of this drug resembles that of phenobarbital, but it is less well tolerated. There is little to recommend this drug over phenobarbital for patients in whom treatment with a barbiturate is contemplated. Possible side effects include Dupuytren contracture, shortening of the QT segment, and coagulation defects. For this reason it is seldom prescribed.

Tiagabine

Tiagabine is a nipecotic acid moiety that is a potent inhibitor of GABA reuptake. This drug is utilized as adjunctive therapy for complex partial seizures. Possible side effects include dizziness, asthenia, aphasia, and tremor. Mental depression may accompany administration of tiagabine perhaps reflecting this drug's ability to increase GABA concentrations. Drug interactions are unlikely despite the high protein binding of tiagabine reflecting the small amount of drug needed to achieve clinical efficacy. Tiagabine has no effect on hepatic enzymes.

Topiramate

Topiramate is a broad-spectrum antiepileptic drug that is indicated as monotherapy or adjunctive therapy in children and adults for the control of partial, generalized tonic-clonic, and absence seizures. Efficacy in treatment of other neurologic and psychiatric disorders has been reported including bulimia, migraine headache, and essential tremor. Topiramate inhibits voltage-gated sodium ion channels, high-voltage activated calcium ion channels, and glutamate-mediated neurotransmission at specific receptor subtypes. It enhances chloride ion flux in $GABA_A$ receptors, and inhibition of. In addition, topiramate is a weak inhibitor of carbonic anhydrase. Minor side effects may include sedation, dizziness, and ataxia. Nephrolithiasis occurs in about 1.5% of treated patients perhaps reflecting this drug's action on carbonic anhydrase. Enzyme inducing drugs decrease plasma concentrations of topiramate, but topiramate does not affect hepatic P450 enzymes and undergoes minimal protein binding.

Valproic Acid

Valproic acid is a branched-chain carboxylic acid that is effective in the treatment of all primary generalized epilepsies and all convulsive epilepsies. It is somewhat less effective for the suppression of nonconvulsive partial seizures. This drug acts by limiting sustained repetitive neuronal firing through voltage-dependent sodium channels.

Pharmacokinetics

Valproic acid is available as a syrup and in an enteric-coated formulation, which is preferred because it decreases gastrointestinal side effects. After oral administration, absorption is prompt, with peak plasma concentrations of valproic acid occurring in 1 to 4 hours. Binding to plasma proteins is >80%. More than 70% of the drug can be recovered as inactive glucuronide conjugates. The elimination half-time is 7 to 17 hours. The usual daily dose of valproic acid is 1 to 3 g to achieve a therapeutic plasma concentration of 50 to 100 μg/mL. Nevertheless, the daily variation in plasma concentrations of valproic acid is great, and routine monitoring may not be helpful unless it is correlated with the patient's clinical condition.

Side Effects

Gastrointestinal side effects include anorexia, nausea, and vomiting. Weight gain is common in patients treated chronically with valproic acid. At higher doses, a fine distal tremor may develop. Thrombocytopenia is seen frequently at higher doses. The most serious side effect of valproic acid is hepatotoxicity occurring in about 0.2% of children younger than 2 years of age being treated chronically with this drug. The incidence of this potentially fatal hepatic necrosis decreases dramatically after 2 years of age. Approximately 20% of treated patients have hyperammonemia without hepatic damage. Sedation and ataxia are infrequent side effects of valproic acid.

Because valproic acid is partly eliminated as a ketone-containing metabolite, the urine ketone test may show false-positive results. Valproic acid can displace phenytoin and diazepam from protein-binding sites, resulting in increased pharmacologic effects produced by the displaced drug.

Valproic acid is an enzyme inhibitor. As a result of this enzyme inhibition, the metabolism of phenytoin is slowed by valproic acid. Valproic acid causes the plasma concentration of phenobarbital to increase almost 50%, presumably due to inhibition of hepatic microsomal enzymes. However, valproic acid does not interfere with the action of oral contraceptives.

Vigabatrin

Vigabatrin is used to treat refractory complex partial seizures. It may also be used as monotherapy to treat infantile spasms. Tablet and powder preparations are available and are bioequivalent. Its mechanism of action is imperfectly understood but is thought to involve irreversible inhibition of the GABA transaminase enzyme, thereby increasing the amount of GABA in the CNS. It is not protein bound and undergoes no significant metabolism. It is excreted unchanged in the urine. Dosage must therefore be adjusted if renal impairment is present. Significant side effects include permanent visual loss, anemia, somnolence, and fatigue.[10]

Zonisamide

Zonisamide is a broad-spectrum antiepileptic drug utilized as adjunctive therapy for management of partial and secondarily generalized seizures. Modulation of voltage-dependent calcium ion channels seems to be an important mechanism for this drugs ability to control seizures. In addition, zonisamide enhances GABA-mediated neuronal inhibition. Adverse side effects include sedation, dizziness, ataxia, anorexia, and behavioral disorders in children and manic responses in adults. Nephrolithiasis may occur in 3% of treated patients. Pharmacokinetic drug interactions are unlikely as zonisamide does not displace other drugs from protein-binding sites and effects on metabolism of other drugs are minimal.

Benzodiazepines

Benzodiazepines display anxiolytic, sedative, muscle-relaxant, and anticonvulsant effects (see Chapter 5). Benzodiazepine receptors in the brain are a subset of $GABA_A$ receptors. The binding of benzodiazepines to these receptors potentiates GABA-mediated neuronal inhibition, which increases chloride permeability and thereby leads to cellular hyperpolarization and inhibition of neuronal firing. In low doses, benzodiazepines suppress polysynaptic activity in the spinal cord and decrease neuronal activity in the mesencephalic reticular system.

Clonazepam

Clonazepam is generally added to other drug therapy and is used as a first-line drug only for myoclonic seizures.

Pharmacokinetics

Absorption of clonazepam after oral administration is rapid, with peak plasma concentrations occurring within 2 to 4 hours (see Table 13-4). IV administration of clonazepam results in rapid CNS effects. Approximately 50% of the drug is bound to plasma proteins. Clonazepam is extensively metabolized to inactive products, with <2% of an injected dose appearing unchanged in urine. The elimination half-time of this long-acting drug is 30 to 40 hours. The oral maintenance dose is unlikely to exceed 0.25 mg/kg. Therapeutic plasma concentrations of clonazepam are 0.02 to 0.08 μg/mL.

Side Effects

Sedation is present in approximately 50% of patients but tends to subside with chronic administration (see Table 13-3). Skeletal muscle incoordination and ataxia occur in approximately 30% of patients. Personality changes occur in approximately 25% of patients, manifesting as behavioral disturbances, including hyperactivity, irritability, and difficulty in concentration, especially in children. Elderly patients treated with clonazepam may experience depression. Increased salivary and bronchial secretions may be particularly prominent in children. Generalized seizure activity may be precipitated if the drug is discontinued abruptly.

Diazepam

Diazepam is a mainstay for the treatment of status epilepticus and local anesthetic–induced seizures. The typical approach is administration of 0.1 mg/kg IV every 10 to 15 minutes until seizure activity has been suppressed or a maximum dose of 30 mg has been administered (see Chapter 5). Diazepam has a long elimination half-time of 27 to 48 hours. Metabolism of diazepam results in active metabolites.

Lorazepam

Lorazepam has a shorter elimination half-time (8 to 25 hours) than diazepam but a longer duration of antiepileptic action because it is not rapidly redistributed. Lorazepam is metabolized in the liver and has no active metabolites. Lorazepam, which is available in parenteral and oral formulations, is used to treat status epilepticus and as intermittent therapy for seizure clusters.

Clobazam

Clobazam is used for complex partial, tonic-clonic, and myoclonic seizures primarily as a second-line agent. It is metabolized in the liver and has an active metabolite and is excreted by the kidneys. The elimination half-life is 16 to 18 hours. Its potential for sedation, lethargy, and loss of therapeutic effect is significantly lower than other benzodiazepines. Like other drugs of this class, significant withdrawal may occur if discontinuation is not gradual.[11]

Status Epilepticus

Status epilepticus is a medical emergency where the patient experiences prolonged or rapidly recurring convulsions for 5 minutes or more. The motor manifestations of convulsive status epilepticus may be symmetrical with tonic and then clonic activity. Rapid seizure control is associated with improved clinical outcome.[12]

Treatment

Treatment begins with ensuring a patent upper airway and administration of oxygen. Maintenance of ventilation may require tracheal intubation. IV access is obtained in anticipation of administering antiepileptic drugs. If hypoglycemia cannot be excluded, the patient is treated empirically with IV glucose (50 mL of 50% glucose for adults). Drug therapy of status epilepticus is typically with a benzodiazepine such as diazepam, lorazepam, or midazolam. In the absence of IV access, a rectal gel form of diazepam is available. Ventilatory depression necessitating support of ventilation may accompany administration of benzodiazepines. If benzodiazepines are not successful in extinguishing the seizure, other choices include fosphenytoin; phenytoin; phenobarbital; valproic acid; and continuous infusions of valproic acid, levetiracetam, and propofol. Hypotension and prolongation of the QT interval on the electrocardiogram may accompany administration of fosphenytoin necessitating a slowing in the rate of IV infusion.[12]

Drugs Used for Treatment of Parkinson's Disease

Parkinson's disease affects 1% of the population, predominantly in those older than 60 years of age although onset can occur significantly earlier. It is a chronically progressive neurodegenerative disease that results from the loss of dopaminergic neurons in the substantia nigra pars compacta region of the basal ganglia. The presence of Lewy bodies is also a consistent feature.[13] Dopamine is thought to act principally as an inhibitory neurotransmitter and acetylcholine as an excitatory neurotransmitter within the extrapyramidal system, and a proper balance is necessary for normal function. Approximately 80% of the dopamine in the brain is concentrated in the basal ganglia, mostly in the caudate nucleus and putamen. In patients with Parkinson's disease, the basal ganglia content of dopamine may be as low as 10% of normal. As a result, an excess of excitatory cholinergic activity manifesting as progressive tremor, skeletal muscle rigidity, bradykinesia, and disturbances of posture results.

The objective in treating Parkinson's disease is to treat debilitating symptoms. Currently, all approved medications offer only palliative relief, as they do not affect progression of the disease. Often, combinations of drugs with effects on the dopaminergic and cholinergic components of the extrapyramidal nervous system are used. Treatment regimens are selected based on the age of the patient as well as severity of symptoms. Pharmacologic treatment commences when motor symptoms become bothersome to the patient. Treatment strategies can be divided into those addressing motor symptoms; those addressing other adverse effects of the disease including nausea, depression, autonomic disturbances and cognitive impairment; and those addressing medication-related side effects.[13] Failure of pharmacologic therapy is an indication for deep brain stimulation, with the primary targets being the globus pallidus internus or subthalamic nucleus.[14]

Levodopa

Because dopamine does not readily cross the blood–brain barrier, the major approaches to therapy have involved the administration of its precursor, levodopa, or drugs that mimic the action of dopamine. Levodopa is the cornerstone of symptomatic therapy of Parkinson's disease and its efficacy is unsurpassed even by newer drugs. Levodopa crosses the blood–brain barrier and is converted to dopamine by aromatic-L-amino-acid decarboxylase (dopa decarboxylase enzyme), acting to replenish dopamine stores in the basal ganglia. Levodopa is usually administered with a peripheral decarboxylase inhibitor (carbidopa or benserazide) to maximize entrance of this precursor into the brain before it is converted to dopamine. Furthermore, side effects associated with increased peripheral concentrations of dopamine are less when it is combined with a decarboxylase inhibitor. Absorption of levodopa from the gastrointestinal tract is efficient, but the brief elimination half-time (1 to 3 hours) requires frequent dosing intervals to maintain a therapeutic concentration. An IV formulation of levodopa is not available.

The beneficial therapeutic response to levodopa typically diminishes after 5 to 10 years of treatment, presumably reflecting progression of the disease process and continuing loss of nigrostriatal neurons with a capacity to store dopamine. Abrupt discontinuation of levodopa therapy may result in a precipitous return of symptoms of Parkinson's disease and has been associated with a neuroleptic malignant-like syndrome. For this reason, levodopa should be continued throughout the perioperative period.

Metabolism

Approximately 95% of orally administered levodopa is rapidly decarboxylated to dopamine during the initial passage through the liver. The resulting dopamine cannot easily cross the blood–brain barrier to exert beneficial effects, whereas increased plasma concentrations of dopamine often lead to undesirable side effects. In this regard, inhibition of the peripheral activity of the decarboxylase enzyme greatly increases the fraction of administered levodopa that remains intact to cross the blood–brain barrier.

At least 30 metabolites of levodopa have been identified. Most of these metabolites are converted to dopamine, small amounts of which are subsequently metabolized to norepinephrine and epinephrine. Metabolism of dopamine yields 3,4-dihydroxyphenylacetic acid (homovanillic acid). Dietary methionine is necessary as a source of methyl donors to permit continued activity of catechol-*O*-methyltransferase (COMT), which is necessary for the metabolism of the excess amounts of dopamine that result from high doses of levodopa. Most metabolites of dopamine are excreted by the kidneys.

Side Effects

The most common side effects that occur during the first weeks of therapy with levodopa and dopamine agonists are nausea and hypotension. These side effects are associated with peak plasma concentrations of dopamine and may be minimized by taking medications after light meals or snacks. The most common problems that occur during long-term therapy are dyskinesias, fluctuations in mobility, increasing confusion, and psychosis. These problems become progressively more frequent after the first 3 years of therapy.

Gastrointestinal Dysfunction

Nausea and vomiting occur in about 80% of patients during the early period of treatment with levodopa. These responses reflect dopamine-induced stimulation of the chemoreceptor trigger zone which is not protected by the blood–brain barrier.[15] Nausea can be effectively treated with domperidone, which does not easily cross the blood–brain barrier and is therefore unlikely to exacerbate symptoms of Parkinson's disease. Domperidone inhibits dopamine-2 receptors in the chemoreceptor trigger zone of the medulla oblongata.[16] Trimethobenzamide can also be used and has a direct action on the chemoreceptor trigger zone and is devoid of dopaminergic action.[17] Dopamine-receptor antagonist antiemetics such as prochlorperazine, metoclopramide, promethazine must be avoided because they significantly worsen symptoms of Parkinson's disease. Gastrointestinal side effects tend to disappear with continuing therapy as tolerance develops.[13]

Cardiovascular Changes

Cardiovascular changes associated with levodopa most likely reflect α- and β-adrenergic responses evoked by increased plasma concentrations of dopamine and its metabolism to norepinephrine and epinephrine. Transient flushing of the skin is common during levodopa therapy.

Orthostatic Hypotension

Approximately 30% of patients develop orthostatic hypotension early in therapy. This can be due to autonomic dysfunction from the disease or as a result of levodopa treatment. It can be a significant problem in some patients and warrants continuous evaluation as it can result in syncopal episodes. Initial treatment consists of increased fluid and sodium intake, elevation of the head of the patient's bed, and compression stockings. If symptoms are persistent, administration of fludrocortisone, domperidone, or midodrine may be useful. Orthostatic hypotension becomes less prominent with continued therapy.[13,15]

Cardiac Dysrhythmias

Cardiac dysrhythmias, including sinus tachycardia, atrial and ventricular premature contractions, atrial fibrillation, and ventricular tachycardia, although rare, have been associated with levodopa therapy. Presumably, the potential β-adrenergic effects of dopamine and its metabolites on the heart contribute to cardiac dysrhythmias, although a cause-and-effect relationship has not been documented. Patients with preexisting disturbances of cardiac conduction or coronary artery disease are most likely to develop cardiac dysrhythmias in association with levodopa therapy. Propranolol is an effective treatment when cardiac dysrhythmias occur in these patients.[15]

Abnormal Involuntary Movements

Abnormal involuntary movements in the form of faciolingual tics; grimacing; and rocking movements of the arms, legs, or trunk are the most common side effects of chronic levodopa therapy, developing in about 50% of patients within 1 to 4 months after initiation of therapy. Rarely, exaggerated respiratory movements can produce an irregular gasping pattern, presumably reflecting dyskinesias of the diaphragm and intercostal muscles. Tolerance does not develop to abnormal involuntary movements.

Fluctuations in mobility are characterized by increasing bradykinesia at the end of an interval between doses. High-protein meals are avoided as a large influx of dietary amino acids can interfere with the transport of levodopa to the brain and result in sudden loss of mobility.

Psychiatric Disturbances

Confusion, visual hallucinations, and paranoia may reflect the natural disease process as well as its treatment. Elderly patients are particularly vulnerable to psychotic reactions, especially if treatment includes combinations of levodopa and anticholinergic drugs and the patient has a prior psychiatric history. Psychiatric disturbances usually begin as nocturnal phenomena, emphasizing the possible value of decreasing or discontinuing the last evening dose of levodopa. Neuroleptic drugs are not recommended for the treatment of psychiatric disturbances because these drugs may cause a protracted exacerbation of symptoms of Parkinson's disease. Quetiapine is a commonly prescribed medication as is clozapine. The routine laboratory monitoring with clozapine due to the risk of agranulocytosis often makes quetiapine a more attractive option.[13] Patients who develop drug-induced psychosis with no features of dementia may respond to electroconvulsive therapy.

Impulsive and compulsive behavior may also result from dopaminergic therapy. A history of obsessive compulsive disorder, addiction, or impulsive personality traits increases the likelihood. The development of these behaviors should be monitored regularly. Treatment is aimed at symptomatic relief primarily with dopamine agonists and less commonly with zonisamide, amantadine, topiramate, and valproate.[13,18]

Endocrine Changes

Dopamine inhibits the secretion of prolactin, presumably by stimulating the release of a prolactin inhibitory factor. The release of growth hormone that occurs in response to the administration of levodopa to normal patients is minimal or absent when levodopa is administered to patients with Parkinson's disease. Indeed, signs of acromegaly or diabetes mellitus do not occur in patients treated with levodopa. Large doses of levodopa may cause hypokalemia associated with increased plasma levels of aldosterone.

Laboratory Measurements

Urinary metabolites of levodopa cause false-positive tests for ketoacidosis. These metabolites also color the urine red and then black on exposure to air. Mild, transient increases in the blood urea nitrogen concentration may occur and can usually be controlled by increasing fluid intake. Increased liver transaminase concentrations occasionally occur. Positive Coombs' tests have been attributed to levodopa.

Drug Interactions

Drug interactions may occur in patients being treated with levodopa, resulting in increased or decreased therapeutic effects. Chronic treatment of animals with levodopa does not consistently change anesthetic requirements.

Antipsychotic Drugs

Antipsychotic drugs such as butyrophenones and phenothiazines can antagonize the effects of dopamine. For this reason, these drugs should not be administered to patients with known or suspected Parkinson's disease. Indeed, administration of droperidol to patients being treated with levodopa has produced severe skeletal muscle rigidity and even pulmonary edema, presumably reflecting sudden antagonism of dopamine. Droperidol has even produced a Parkinson's disease–like syndrome in otherwise healthy patients. Metoclopramide may also interfere with dopamine activity.

Monoamine Oxidase Inhibitors

Nonspecific monoamine oxidase inhibitors interfere with the inactivation of catecholamines, including dopamine, and are used in the treatment of atypical depression and Parkinson's disease. As a result, these drugs can exaggerate the peripheral nervous system and CNS effects of levodopa. Hypertension and hyperthermia are side effects associated with the concurrent administration of these drugs.

Anticholinergic Drugs

Anticholinergic drugs act synergistically with levodopa to improve certain symptoms of Parkinson's disease, especially tremor. Large doses of anticholinergics, however, can slow gastric emptying such that absorption of levodopa from the gastrointestinal tract is decreased.

Pyridoxine

Pyridoxine or vitamin B_6, in doses as low as 5 mg as present in multivitamin preparations, can abolish the therapeutic efficacy of levodopa by enhancing the activity of pyridoxine-dependent dopa decarboxylase and thus increasing the metabolism of levodopa in the circulation before it can enter the CNS.

Peripheral Decarboxylase Inhibitors

Levodopa is usually administered with a peripheral carboxylase inhibitor such as carbidopa or benserazide. As a result, more levodopa escapes metabolism to dopamine in the peripheral circulation and is available to enter the CNS. Furthermore, side effects related to high systemic concentrations of dopamine are decreased when levodopa is administered with a peripheral decarboxylase inhibitor. Nausea, vomiting, and cardiac dysrhythmias are diminished or absent. The incidence of abnormal involuntary movements and psychiatric disturbances is not altered by the combination of levodopa with a decarboxylase inhibitor.

Several combinations of levodopa and a peripheral carboxylase inhibitor are available as a levodopa augmentation strategy. Sinemet is composed of levodopa and carbidopa in a 10:1 or 4:1 ratio. Madopar is composed of levodopa and benserazide in a 4:1 ratio. Controlled-release preparations of levodopa and carbidopa provide a more constant therapeutic effect, but the onset of action is slower and the bioavailability is decreased compared with the standard combinations. Both carbidopa and benserazide are noncompetitive inhibitors of decarboxylase so there is no value in administering progressively higher doses of these enzyme inhibitors. Carbidopa and benserazide do not cross the blood–brain barrier and lack pharmacologic activity when administered alone.

Catechol-*O*-methyltransferase Inhibitors

COMT is partially responsible for the peripheral breakdown of levodopa. Accordingly, another levodopa augmentation strategy consists of blocking the COMT enzyme activity in the gastrointestinal tract with tolcapone or entacapone. Administration of either of these drugs slows the elimination of carbidopa-levodopa thus increasing the plasma concentrations by 10% to 15%. In patients treated with tolcapone, the daily dose of carbidopa-levodopa may need to be decreased by 10% to 30% to avoid dyskinesias or other hyperdopaminergic side effects.

Side Effects

Both tolcapone and entacapone worsen levodopa-induced dyskinesias and cause nausea and diarrhea. Tolcapone may cause hepatotoxicity in rare patients emphasizing the need to monitor liver function tests in treated patients. Rhabdomyolysis has been associated with tolcapone therapy. Entacapone can cause the patient's urine to appear orange. Both drugs can cause piloerection.

Synthetic Dopamine Agonists

Synthetic dopamine agonists require neither transformation nor facilitated transport across the blood–brain barrier. Available drugs include bromocriptine and pergolide (tetracyclic ergot alkaloids) and pramipexole, ropinirole, and rotigotine (nonergot alkaloids). After oral administration, the elimination half-time of bromocriptine and pergolide are longer than for levodopa. Absorption of bromocriptine from the gastrointestinal tract is rapid but incomplete. Extensive hepatic first-pass metabolism occurs and >90% of the metabolites are excreted in the bile, whereas <10% of the drug is excreted unchanged or as inactive metabolites in urine. Bromocriptine, 0.5 to 1.0 mg orally, is equivalent to levodopa, 100 mg in combination with either 25 mg of carbidopa or 25 mg of benserazide. The effectiveness of bromocriptine in the treatment of acromegaly reflects the paradoxical inhibitory effect of dopamine agonists on secretion of growth hormone. Bromocriptine also suppresses the excess prolactin secretion that is often associated with growth hormone secretion. A notable benefit of rotigotine is its antidepressant effects.

Side Effects

Visual and auditory hallucinations, hypotension, and dyskinesia occur more frequently in patients treated with bromocriptine than in those treated with levodopa. Synthetic dopamine agonists occasionally cause pleuropulmonary fibrosis, sometimes with pleural effusions. Depending on the severity of this side effect, the dose of agonist drug should be decreased or the drug discontinued. Another uncommon complication of dopamine agonist therapy is the development of erythromelalgia (red, edematous, tender extremities). If this complication occurs, it is usually necessary to discontinue the dopamine agonist. Asymptomatic increases of serum transaminase and alkaline phosphatase concentrations may occur. Vertigo and nausea are occasionally associated with bromocriptine therapy.

Nonergot alkaloids are supposed to cause less nausea and orthostatic hypotension than the ergot derivatives but this difference appears to be clinically insignificant. Nonergot alkaloids offer no advantage over ergot derivatives with respect to CNS side effects including confusion, hallucinations, and daytime sleep attacks that have been associated with motor vehicle accidents.

Anticholinergic Drugs

Anticholinergic drugs such as trihexyphenidyl and benztropine have modest effects on the clinical manifestations of Parkinson's disease. These drugs blunt the effects of the excitatory neurotransmitter acetylcholine, thus correcting the balance between dopamine and acetylcholine that is disturbed in the direction of cholinergic dominance. Anticholinergic drugs may help control the tremor and decrease the excess salivation associated with Parkinson's disease but seldom are useful for skeletal muscle rigidity and bradykinesia. Although the peripheral and CNS actions of these synthetic anticholinergic drugs are less prominent than those of atropine, side effects, including memory disturbances (especially in elderly patients), hallucinations, confusion, sedation, mydriasis, cycloplegia, adynamic ileus, and urinary retention, may still occur. The mydriatic effect could precipitate glaucoma in a susceptible patient. As more effective drugs have become available, the use of anticholinergic drugs to treat patients with Parkinson's disease has diminished.

Amantadine

Amantadine is an antiviral drug used for prophylaxis against infection with influenza A. This drug was discovered by chance to also produce symptomatic improvement in patients with Parkinson's disease. The mode of action of amantadine is not known, although it has been speculated that it facilitates the release of dopamine from dopaminergic terminals that remain in the nigrostriatum of patients with this disease. In addition, amantadine may delay uptake of dopamine back into nerve endings, exert anticholinergic effects, is a weak glutamate antagonist, and exhibits noncompetitive antagonist effects at *N*-methyl-D-aspartate (NMDA) receptors. Unlike anticholinergic drugs, amantadine may result in some improvement in skeletal muscle rigidity and bradykinesia. Amantadine is well absorbed after oral administration, and the elimination half-time is approximately 12 hours. More than 90% of the drug is excreted unchanged by the kidneys, necessitating dosage adjustments in patients with renal dysfunction. The side effects are similar to those produced by anticholinergic drugs but, in addition, chronic administration of amantadine tends to induce ankle edema and livedo reticularis of the legs with or without cardiac failure. In older patients, amantadine may aggravate confusion and psychosis.

Monoamine Oxidase Type B Enzyme Inhibitors

This category comprises two drugs, selegiline and rasagiline. Selegiline is a highly selective and irreversible inhibitor of monoamine oxidase type B enzyme (MAO-B) that has a weak antiparkinsonian effect when used alone and a moderate effect when used as an adjunct to carbidopa-levodopa. MAO-B enzyme activity is one of the principal catabolic pathways for dopamine in the CNS. Blocking MAO-B enzyme activity increases the intrasynaptic half-time of dopamine leading to improved motor fluctuations and tremor. In contrast to nonspecific monoamine oxidase inhibitors, selegiline does not result in life-threatening potentiation of the effects of catecholamines when administered concurrently with a centrally active amine. This reflects the fact that metabolism of norepinephrine in peripheral nerve endings is not altered by selegiline, which minimizes the likelihood of adverse responses during anesthesia in response to sympathomimetics. Insomnia is a significant side effect of selegiline. Other side effects of selegiline include confusion, hallucinations, mental depression, and paranoid ideation. Rasagiline has created enthusiasm as a potentially neuroprotective agent but this activity requires further evaluation.[19] It has action at both the MAO-A and MAO-B enzyme, but its affinity is up to 16 times greater for MAO-B. It is recommended both as monotherapy and adjunctive therapy.[20] Although a theoretical risk does exist for the precipitation of serotonin syndrome, this was not observed during clinical trials. Similarly, avoidance of tyramine is ideally recommended although no adverse reactions have been noted.[21]

Nonpharmacologic Treatment

Deep brain stimulation was approved to treat Parkinson's disease by the U.S. Food and Drug Administration (FDA) in 2002. Although not curative, it effectively controls symptoms resistant to medications or allows reduced reliance on drugs whose side effects have proven problematic. The mechanism of action of deep brain stimulation is unknown.[14] Other potential therapies under investigation include stem cell transplantation as well as transplantation of fetal mesencephalic tissue.

CENTRAL NERVOUS SYSTEM STIMULANTS

Analeptics are drugs that stimulate the CNS. These drugs were previously used in the treatment of generalized CNS depression accompanying deliberate drug overdoses, but this practice has been abandoned because these drugs lack specific antagonist properties and their margin of safety is narrow. The excitability of the CNS reflects a balance between excitatory and inhibitory influences that is normally maintained within relatively narrow limits. Analeptics can increase excitability either by blocking inhibition or by enhancing excitation.

Doxapram

Doxapram is an analeptic which acts centrally and at peripheral chemoreceptors to augment breathing efforts. The stimulus to ventilation produced by administration of doxapram, 1 mg/kg IV is similar to that produced by a PaO_2 of 38 mm Hg acting on the carotid bodies. An increase in tidal volume, more than an increase in breathing frequency, is responsible for the doxapram-induced increase in minute ventilation. Oxygen consumption is increased concomitantly with the increase in minute ventilation.

Doxapram has a large margin of safety as reflected by a 20- to 40-fold difference in the dose that stimulates ventilation and the dose that produces seizures. Nevertheless, continuous infusion of doxapram, as is required to produce a sustained effect on ventilation, often results in evidence of subconvulsive CNS stimulation (hypertension, tachycardia, cardiac dysrhythmias, vomiting, and increased body temperature). These changes are consistent with increased sympathetic nervous system outflow. Continuous infusion is also required because the duration of action of a single IV dose is relatively short at 5 to 10 minutes. It is metabolized extensively, and less than 5% is excreted unchanged in the urine.

Clinical Uses

Doxapram administered as a continuous infusion (2 to 3 mg per minute) has been used as a temporary measure to maintain ventilation during administration of supplemental oxygen to patients with chronic obstructive airway disease who otherwise depend on a hypoxic drive to maintain adequate minute ventilation. Its role in the postoperative period has been used in preventing the ventilatory depression produced by opioids without altering analgesia. It has also been shown to be useful in treating postoperative shivering. Its use with apneic neonates in intensive care units can often delay or prevent intubation and ventilation, thus reducing ventilator associated morbidity and mortality.

Methylphenidate

Methylphenidate is a mild CNS stimulant structurally related to amphetamine. Absorption after oral administration is rapid, and its low protein binding and high lipid solubility results in rapid uptake into the brain. Methylphenidate is useful in the treatment of attention deficit hyperactivity disorder in children and adults.[22] Hypertension, tachycardia, priapism, seizures, and serious cardiovascular events such as sudden cardiac death, stroke, and myocardial infarction have been described in patients treated with methylphenidate. Methylphenidate may also be effective in the treatment of narcolepsy, either alone or in combination with tricyclic antidepressants.[23]

Methylxanthines

Methylxanthines are represented by caffeine, theophylline, and theobromine. Solubility of methylxanthines is low and is enhanced by formation of complexes as represented by the combination of theophylline with ethylenediamine to form aminophylline. Methylxanthines have in common the ability to (a) stimulate the CNS, (b) produce diuresis, (c) increase myocardial contractility, and (d) relax smooth muscle, especially those in the airways.

Mechanism of Action

The best characterized cellular action of methylxanthines is antagonism of receptor-mediated actions of adenosine thus facilitating the release of catecholamines. Theophylline is more active than caffeine or theobromine as an antagonist at these receptors. At high concentrations, theophylline inhibits phosphodiesterase enzymes that are responsible for breakdown of cyclic adenosine monophosphate. Methylxanthines are completely absorbed after oral administration and eliminated primarily by metabolism in the liver. Unlike adults, premature infants metabolize theophylline in part to caffeine. Furthermore, the clearance of methylxanthines is greatly prolonged in the neonate compared with that in the adult.

Clinical Uses

Methylxanthines are used as analeptics to treat primary apnea of prematurity by stimulating medullary respiratory centers by increasing the sensitivity of these centers to carbon dioxide. The slowed metabolism of methylxanthines in neonates compared to adults is a consideration when using theophylline to stimulate ventilation in neonates. Smooth muscle relaxation and bronchodilation produced by theophylline may reflect a combination of effects including catecholamine release, phosphodiesterase inhibition, and inhibition of inflammation. The administration of theophylline during maintenance of anesthesia appears to have no added bronchodilator effect over that of the volatile anesthetic alone. Selective β_2-adrenergic agonists delivered by inhalation have largely replaced theophylline preparations in the treatment of bronchospasm associated with asthma.

Toxicity

A single oral dose of theophylline, 5 mg/kg, will produce a peak plasma concentration of 10 μg/mL in adults within 1 to 2 hours following ingestion. Increased levels of unbound drug may result in signs of toxicity despite therapeutic plasma concentrations of drug (10 to 20 μg/mL). Theophylline plasma concentrations, only slightly greater than the recommended therapeutic range, can produce evidence of CNS stimulation (nervousness, tremors), and at higher concentrations or with rapid IV administration, seizures are a possibility. Vomiting most likely reflecting CNS stimulation is common when plasma concentrations exceed 15 μg/mL. Tachycardia and cardiac dysrhythmias may appear most likely due to drug-induced release of catecholamines from the adrenal medulla.

Drug Interactions

Drugs may enhance (carbamazepine, rifampin) or inhibit (cimetidine, erythromycin) the hepatic metabolism of theophylline. Larger doses of benzodiazepines may be required in the presence of theophylline as benzodiazepines increase the CNS concentrations of adenosine, a potent CNS depressant, whereas theophylline is an adenosine receptor antagonist. Ketamine may decrease the seizure threshold for theophylline. Theophylline can partially antagonize the effects of nondepolarizing neuromuscular blocking drugs presumably by inhibition of phosphodiesterase.

Caffeine

Caffeine is a methylxanthine-derived phosphodiesterase inhibitor that is present in a variety of beverages and nonprescription medications. A prominent effect of caffeine is CNS stimulation. In addition, this substance acts as a cerebral vasoconstrictor and may cause secretion of acidic gastric fluid.

Pharmacologic uses of caffeine include administration to neonates experiencing apnea of prematurity.[24] Treatment of postdural puncture headache has historically been treated with doses ranging from 75 to 300 mg oral caffeine. Despite the limited evidence for this treatment, it continues to be a popular treatment modality.[25–27] Caffeine may be included in common cold remedies in an attempt to offset the sedating effects of certain antihistamines.[28]

Almitrine

Almitrine acts on the carotid body chemoreceptors to increase minute ventilation. It has been demonstrated to increase Pa_{O_2} and decrease Pa_{CO_2} in patients with chronic respiratory failure associated with obstructive pulmonary disease. Its mechanism of action has not been elucidated.[29] It is used as a measure to improve or prevent hypoxia during one-lung ventilation techniques, especially with IV anesthesia techniques.[30,31] IV administration of almitrine improves Pa_{O_2} in patients with acute lung injury but may also induce lactic acidosis and hepatic dysfunction.[32] Side effects of prolonged oral almitrine therapy include dyspnea and peripheral neuropathy which significantly limits its use.[33]

Modafinil

Modafinil is a wakefulness-promoting drug approved for patients with excessive daytime sleepiness associated with narcolepsy, obstructive sleep apnea, and shiftwork sleep disorder.[34,35] In addition, it may result in euphoria, as well as alteration in mood, affect, and thinking. Its mechanism of action is unknown. Its absorption is rapid and peak plasma concentrations are reached after 4 hours. It undergoes hepatic metabolism and its inactive metabolites are excreted by the kidneys. A feeling of fatigue and sedation following recovery from general anesthesia may be countered by administration of modafinil.[35]

CENTRALLY ACTING MUSCLE RELAXANTS

The primary indication for centrally acting muscle relaxants is spasticity, which may accompany pathologic conditions such as stroke, cerebral palsy, multiple sclerosis, amyotrophic lateral sclerosis, and injuries to the CNS. They act directly on the CNS or on skeletal muscles to relieve spasticity. Spasticity of skeletal muscles occurs when there is an abnormal increase in resistance to passive movement of a skeletal muscle group because of hyperactive proprioceptive or stretch reflexes.

Baclofen

Baclofen is the chlorophenol derivative of GABA that acts as an agonist at $GABA_B$ receptors in the dorsal horn of the spinal cord and is often administered for treatment of spastic hypertonia of cerebral and spinal cord origin. Baclofen relieves spasticity by activating G protein–linked presynaptic $GABA_B$ receptors that hyperpolarize muscle spindle afferent neurons, thereby decreasing the number and amplitude of excitatory postsynaptic potentials along the dendrites of motor neurons. This drug has no effect on the neuromuscular junction. Baclofen is particularly effective in the treatment of flexor spasms and skeletal muscle rigidity associated with spinal cord injury or multiple sclerosis. Intrathecal administration of baclofen may be an effective treatment of spinal spasticity that has not responded to oral administration of the drug.

Baclofen is rapidly and almost completely absorbed from the gastrointestinal tract. The elimination half-time is 3 to 6 hours, with approximately 80% of the drug excreted unchanged in urine, emphasizing the need to modify the dose in patients with renal dysfunction. Therapeutic plasma concentrations are 80 to 400 mg/mL.

Use of baclofen is limited by its side effects, which include sedation, skeletal muscle weakness, and confusion. Sudden discontinuation of chronic baclofen therapy may result in severe withdrawal reactions including evidence of multiple organ system failure, tachycardia, and both auditory and visual hallucinations. A case of cardiac arrest due to baclofen withdrawal has been reported. Vocal cord spasm has been described following abrupt discontinuation of an intrathecal baclofen infusion. Coma, depression of ventilation, and seizures may accompany an overdose of baclofen. The threshold for initiation of seizures may be lowered in patients with epilepsy. Mild hypotension may occur in awake patients being treated with oral baclofen, whereas bradycardia, hypotension, and delayed awakening have been observed when general anesthesia is induced in these patients. Hemodynamic instability and delayed awakening following general anesthesia have been described in a patient receiving an accidental intrathecal overdose of baclofen. A decrease in sympathetic nervous system outflow from the CNS mediated by a GABA-baclofen–sensitive system might contribute to this hemodynamic response. Rarely, increases in liver transaminases and blood glucose levels have occurred.

Benzodiazepines

Benzodiazepines are widely used as centrally acting skeletal muscle relaxants. Diazepam is the most widely prescribed of this class, followed by clonazepam. These drugs are particularly beneficial for spinal spasticity and have little effect on cerebral spasticity. Sedation may limit the efficacy of these drugs as muscle relaxants but may be useful for relief of spasms that limit sleep.[36]

Botulinum Toxin

Botulinum toxin causes irreversible inhibition of presynaptic acetylcholine release. Injections are made into spastic muscles, thereby causing weakening of muscle tone. Botulinum toxin is used in cases of central or peripheral spasticity, particularly when limited muscle groups are affected. It has been used for spasticity and to prevent contractures in cerebral palsy, multiple sclerosis, and after stroke. Focally, it can be used for blepharospasm, hemifacial spasm, and torticollis.[37]

Cyclobenzaprine

Cyclobenzaprine is related structurally and pharmacologically to the tricyclic antidepressants. Its anticholinergic effects are similar to those of tricyclic antidepressants and can include dry mouth, tachycardia, blurred vision, and sedation. The agent is commonly used in the short-term (1 to 2 weeks) management of lumbar sprain-strain injuries associated with painful muscle spasm. The mechanism of skeletal muscle relaxant effects produced by cyclobenzaprine is unknown. It must not be administered in the presence of monoamine oxidase inhibitors. In view of the potential adverse side effects of some tricyclic antidepressant drugs on the heart, the use of cyclobenzaprine may be questionable in patients with cardiac dysrhythmias or altered conduction of cardiac impulses.

Tizanidine

Tizanidine is a short acting α_2-adrenergic agonist whose structure is similar to clonidine. It reaches peak plasma levels at 2 hours after administration, and its clinical effect lasts only 6 hours, which necessitates repeated dosing if needed. Its absorption is highly variable depending on whether the patient has recently eaten or is fasted. Dosage adjustments must be made in patients with renal and hepatic dysfunction. Significant side effects include hypotension and care must be taken with patients who take antihypertensive agents. Significant sedation can also result, and there is an additive effect with other sedatives such as benzodiazepines. Discontinuation of therapy should be gradual as not to precipitate rebound hypertension, tachycardia, and/or hypertonia.

Dantrolene

Dantrolene exerts antispasmodic effects by inducing relaxation directly on muscle by decreasing calcium release from the sarcoplasmic reticulum. Its absorption from the gastrointestinal tract is slow and incomplete, and its half-life is 9 hours. The starting dose is usually 25 mg twice daily, and dosage can be increased up to 200 mg per day. Laboratory investigation for liver dysfunction should be undertaken prior to starting therapy as there is potential for hepatotoxicity especially in those patients with preexisting hepatic compromise.

References

1. Perucca E, Tomson T. The pharmacological treatment of epilepsy in adults. *Lancet Neurol.* 2011;10:446–456.
2. Elger CE, Schmidt D. Modern management of epilepsy: a practical approach. *Epilepsy Behav.* 2008;12:501–539.
3. Sirven JI, Noe K, Hoerth M, et al. Antiepileptic drugs 2012: recent advances and trends. *Mayo Clin Proc.* 2012;87(9):879–889.
4. Schmidt D. Drug treatment of epilepsy: options and limitations. *Epilepsy Behav.* 2009;15:56–65.
5. LaRoche SM, Helmers SL. The new antiepileptic drugs: clinical applications. *JAMA.* 2004;291(5):615–620.
6. Zupanc ML, Roell Werner R, Schwabe MS, et al. Efficacy of felbamate in the treatment of intractable pediatric epilepsy. *Pediatr Neurol.* 2010:42(6):396–403.
7. Dichter MA, Brodie MJ. New antiepileptic drugs. *N Engl J Med.* 1996;334:1583–1590.
8. Cavanna AE, Ali F, Rickards HE, et al. Behavioral and cognitive effects of anti-epileptic drugs. *Discov Med.* 2010;9:138–144.
9. Vogl C, Mochida S, Wolff C, et al. The synaptic vesicle glycoprotein 2A ligand levetiracetam inhibits presynaptic Ca^{2+} channels through an intracellular pathway. *Mol Pharmacol.* 2012;82:199–208.
10. Wild JM, Fone DL, Aljarudi S, et al. Modelling the risk of visual field loss arising from long-term exposure to the antiepileptic drug vigabatrin: a cross-sectional approach. *CNS Drugs.* 2013;27(10):841–849.
11. Klehm J, Sigride TS, Fernandez IS, et al. Clobazam: effect on frequency of seizures and safety profile in different subgroups of children with epilepsy. *Pediatr Neurol.* 2014:51(1):60–66.
12. Classen J, Silbergleit R, Weingart S, et al. Emergency neurological life support: status epilepticus. *Neurocrit Care.* 2012;17:S73–S78.
13. Connolly BS, Lang AE. Pharmacological treatment of Parkinson disease: a review. *JAMA.* 2014;311(16):1670–1683.
14. Follet K, Weaver F, Stern M, et al. Pallidal versus subthalmic deep-brain stimulation for Parkinson's disease. *N Eng J Med.* 2010;362: 2077–2091.
15. Calne DB. Treatment of Parkinson's disease. *N Engl J Med.* 1993; 329:1021–1027.
16. Braun M, Cawello W, Boekens, et al. Influence of domperidone on pharmacokinetics, safety, and tolerability of the dopamine agonist rotigotine. *Br J Clin Pharmacol.* 2009;67(2):209–215.
17. Gunzler SA. Apomorphine in the treatment of Parkinson disease and other movement disorders. *Expert Opin Pharmacother.* 2009;10(6):1027–1038.
18. Piray P, Zeighamy Y, Bahrami F, et al. Impulse control disorders in Parkinson's disease are associated with dysfunction in stimulus valuation but not action valuation. *J Neurosci.* 2014;34(23): 7814–7824.
19. Teo KC, Ho SL. Monoamine oxidase-B (MAO-B) inhibitors: implications for disease-modification in Parkinson's disease. *Transl Neurodegener.* 2013;2(1):2–19.
20. Lew MF. Rasagiline treatment effects on parkinsonian tremor. *Int J Neurosci.* 2013;123(12):859–865.
21. Chen JJ, Swope DM, Dashtipour K. Comprehensive review of rasagiline, a second generation monoamine oxidase inhibitor, for the treatment of Parkinson's disease. *Clin Ther.* 2007;29(9):1825–1849.
22. Wolraich ML, Doffing MA. Pharmacokinetic considerations in the treatment of attention-deficit hyperactivity disorder with methylphenidate. *CNS Drugs.* 2004;18(4):243–250.
23. Godfrey J. Safety of therapeutic methylphenidate in adults: a systematic review of the evidence. *J Psychopharmacol.* 2009;23(2): 194–205.
24. Schoen K, Yu T, Stockman C, et al. Use of methylxanthine therapies for the treatment and prevention of apnea of prematurity. *Pediatr Drugs.* 2014;16(2):169–177.
25. Baysinger CL, Pope JE, Lockhart EM, et al. The management of accidental dural puncture and postdural puncture puncture headache: a North American survey. *J Clin Anesth.* 2011;23(5):349–360.
26. Camman WR, Murray RS, Mushlin PS, et al. Effects of oral caffeine on postdural puncture headache. A double-blind, placebo-controlled trial. *Anesth Analg.* 1990;70:181–184.
27. Esmaoglu A, Akpinar H, Ugur F. Oral multidose caffeine-paracetamol combination is not effective for the prophylaxis of postdural puncture headache. *J Clin Anesth.* 2005;17:58–61.
28. Mitchell JL. Use of cough and cold preparations during breastfeeding. *J Hum Lact.* 1999;15(4):347–349.
29. Chen L, Miller FL, Malmkvist G, et al. Low-dose almitrine bismesylate enhances hypoxic pulmonary vasoconstriction in closed-chest dogs. *Anesth Analg.* 1990;71:475–483.
30. Bermejo S, Gallart L, Silva-Costa-Gomes T, et al. Almitrine fails to improve oxygenation during one-lung ventilation with sevoflurane anesthesia [ahead of print September 6, 2013]. *J Cardiothorac Vasc Anesth.* pii: S1053-0770(13)00163-8.
31. Dalibon N, Moutafis M, Liu N, et al. Treatment of hypoxemia during one-lung ventilation using intravenous almitrine. *Anesth Analg.* 2004;98:590–594.
32. B'chir A, Mebazaa A, Lossser M-R, et al. Intravenous almitrine bismesylate reversibly induces lactic acidosis and hepatic dysfunction in patients with acute lung injury. *Anesthesiology.* 1998;89: 823–830.
33. Howard P. Hypoxia, almitrine, and peripheral neuropathy. *Thorax.* 1999;44(4):247–250.
34. Launois SH, Tamisier R, Pepin JL. On treatment but still sleepy: cause and management of residual sleepiness in obstructive sleep apnea. *Curr Opin Pulm Med.* 2013;19(6):601–608.
35. Kumar R. Approved and investigational uses of modafinil: an evidence based review. *Drugs.* 2008;68(13):1803–1839.
36. Lapeyre E, Kuks JB, Meijler WJ. Spasticity: revisiting the role and the individual value of several pharmacological treatments. *Neurorehabilitation.* 2010;27(2):193–200.
37. Münchau A, Bhatia KP. Uses of botulinum toxin injection in medicine today. *BMJ.* 2000;320:161–165.

CHAPTER 14

Circulatory Physiology

Updated by: James Ramsay • Barrett Larson

Systemic Circulation

The systemic circulation supplies blood to all the tissues of the body except the lungs. Important considerations in understanding the physiology of the systemic circulation include the anatomic components of the systemic circulation, physical characteristics of the systemic circulation and of blood, determinants and control of tissue blood flow, regulation of systemic blood pressure, and regulation of cardiac output and venous return. In addition, the fetal circulation possesses many unique features, which distinguish it from the systemic circulation after birth.

Endothelial Function

The entire vascular system is lined by endothelial cells. Thus, the endothelium is a large and widely distributed structure. Indeed, it is estimated that the adult endothelium is composed of 10 trillion cells and weighs approximately 1 kg.[1] It is now widely appreciated that the endothelium is not simply an inert lining layer of the circulation but is an important "organ" that is involved in many physiologic processes in health and disease (Tables 14-1 and 14-2). The luminal side of the endothelium is lined with a "glycocalyx," a web of membrane-bound glycoproteins and proteoglycans, which plays an important role in transcapillary flow.[2] The healthy endothelium promotes vasodilation and confers antithrombotic and antiadhesive properties to the vessel wall; damage to the glycocalyx and endothelium result in increased vascular permeability and adherence of inflammatory mediators and cells. The endothelium also regulates smooth muscle proliferation and has an important role in the regulation of glucose and lipid metabolism. Endothelial dysfunction is an important element of cardiovascular disease and aging. Cardiovascular risk factors including smoking, diabetes mellitus, hyperlipidemia, obesity, and systemic hypertension are related to their adverse effects upon endothelial function.

Endothelial Function and Regulation of Vascular Tone

Endothelial synthesis and release of vasoactive mediators are important elements in the regulation of vascular tone. Substances are released by the endothelium in response to both mechanical and humoral stimuli and generally have an immediate effect upon the adjacent vascular smooth muscle tone. However, there may also be endothelium-induced long-term effects from vascular remodeling and smooth muscle hypertrophy. Under physiologic conditions, local vascular pressure and flow are the primary stimuli for endothelial vasoactive substance release. Nitric oxide and prostacyclin are powerful vasodilators released by endothelial cells and both also inhibit platelet aggregation and thrombosis. Continuous nitric oxide production maintains vascular tone in a normally low state. This minute-to-minute regulation of local vascular tone is controlled by type 3 constitutive nitric oxide synthase (cNOS). cNOS is a rapidly responding endothelial enzyme that catalyses the local conversion of L-arginine into small quantities of nitric oxide in response to endothelial shear stress during normal pulsatile flow. On the other hand, type 2 inducible NOS (iNOS) is a relatively slow-responding enzyme that catalyses the production of large amounts of nitric oxide in response to inflammatory cytokines. The widespread generation of large amounts of nitric oxide via iNOS is responsible for the low systemic vascular resistance and hypotension encountered in septic shock.[3] Endothelin-1 (ET-1) is a potent vasoactive compound released by the endothelium. Its predominant

Table 14-1

Physiologic Roles of Endothelial Function

Endothelial Function	Example
Regulation of vascular tone	Vasodilator release (nitric oxide, prostacyclin) Vasoconstrictor release (thromboxane A_2, leukotriene, endothelia, angiotensin-converting enzyme)
Regulation of coagulation	Procoagulant release Anticoagulant release
Vascular growth regulation (angiogenesis)	Growth factor synthesis and release
Lipid clearance	LDL receptor expression Lipoprotein lipase synthesis
Inflammatory regulation and defense	Inflammatory mediator synthesis and release
Vascular support matrix elaboration	Synthesis of collagen, laminin, fibronectin proteoglycans, proteases
Regulation of molecular transport	Transport of glucose, amino acid, and albumin

LDL, low-density lipoprotein.

effect is vasoconstriction via smooth muscle ET_A receptors. However, ET-1 can also cause vasodilation through its effect on endothelial ET_B receptors. ET-1 stimulates smooth muscle proliferation and is an important factor in the development of vascular structural changes in systemic and pulmonary hypertension.

Components of the Systemic Circulation

The components of the systemic circulation are the arteries, arterioles, capillaries, venules, and veins.

Table 14-2

Pathologic Processes Associated with Endothelial Dysfunction

Systemic hypertension
Pulmonary hypertension
Atherosclerosis
Sepsis and inflammation
Multisystem organ failure
Metastatic tumor spread
Thrombotic disorders

Arteries

The function of the arteries is to transport blood under high pressure to tissues. Therefore, arteries have strong vascular walls and blood flows rapidly through their lumens.

Arterioles

Arterioles are the last small branches of the arterial system, having diameters of less than 200 μm. Arterioles have strong muscular walls, which are capable of dilating or contracting and thus controlling blood flow into the capillaries. Indeed, blood flow to each tissue is controlled almost entirely by resistance to flow in the arterioles. Metarterioles arise at right angles from arterioles and branch several times, forming 10 to 100 capillaries which in turn connect with venules.

Capillaries

Capillaries are the sites for transfer of oxygen and nutrients to tissues and receipt of metabolic byproducts.

Venules and Veins

Venules collect blood from capillaries for delivery to veins, which act as conduits for transmitting blood to the right atrium. Because the pressure in the venous system is low, venous walls are thin. Nevertheless, walls of veins are muscular, which allows these vessels to contract or expand and thus store varying amounts of blood, depending on physiologic needs. As a result, veins serve an important storage function as well as being conduits to return blood to the right atrium. A venous pump mechanism is important for propelling blood forward to the heart.

Physical Characteristics of the Systemic Circulation

The systemic circulation contains about 80% of the blood volume, with the remainder present in the pulmonary circulation and heart (Fig. 14-1).[4] Of the blood volume in the systemic circulation, about 64% is in veins and 7% is in the cardiac chambers. The heart ejects blood intermittently into the aorta such that blood pressure in the aorta fluctuates between a systolic level of about 120 mm Hg and a diastolic level of about 80 mm Hg (Table 14-3) (Fig. 14-2).[4]

One of the primary responsibilities of the anesthesiologist is to maintain organ perfusion with oxygenated blood. Our standard physiologic monitors (heart rate, blood pressure, pulse oximetry, capnography) all serve as surrogate markers of organ perfusion and oxygenation. Currently, our standard monitoring techniques do not allow us to directly monitor the level of perfusion in specific organs or tissues. However, various techniques for monitoring end-organ perfusion are being explored and will likely be increasingly used in the years to come.

Progressive Declines in Systemic Blood Pressure

As blood flows through the systemic circulation, perfusion pressure decreases progressively to nearly 0 mm Hg

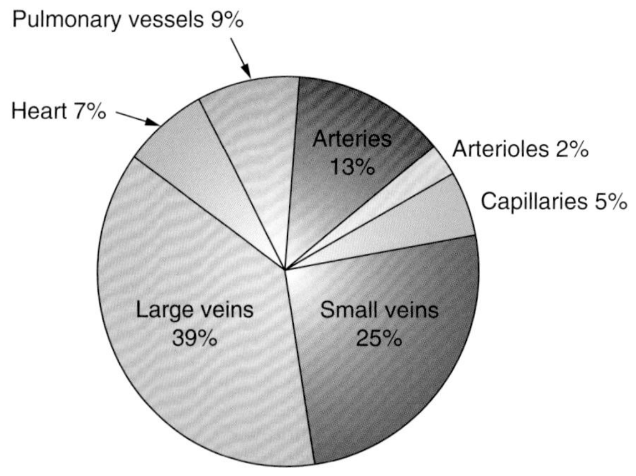

FIGURE 14-1 Distribution of blood volume in the systemic and pulmonary circulation. (From Guyton AC, Hall JE. *Textbook of Medical Physiology.* 10th ed. Philadelphia, PA: Saunders; 2000, with permission.)

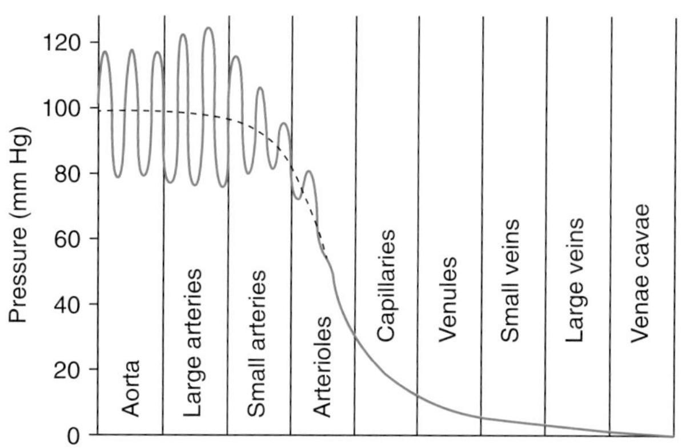

FIGURE 14-2 Systemic blood pressure decreases as blood travels from the aorta to large veins. (From Guyton AC, Hall JE. *Textbook of Medical Physiology.* 10th ed. Philadelphia, PA: Saunders; 2000, with permission.)

by the time blood reaches the right atrium (see Fig. 14-2).[4] The decrease in systemic blood pressure in each portion of the systemic circulation is directly proportional to the resistance to flow in the vessels. Resistance to blood flow in the aorta is minimal, and mean arterial pressure decreases only 3 to 5 mm Hg as blood travels into arteries as small as 3 mm in diameter. Resistance to blood flow begins to increase rapidly in small arteries, causing the mean arterial pressure to decrease to about 85 mm Hg at the beginning of the arterioles. It is in the arterioles that resistance to blood flow is the highest, accounting for about 50% of the resistance in the entire systemic circulation. As a result, systemic blood pressure decreases to about 30 mm Hg at the point where blood enters the capillaries. At the venous end of the capillaries, the intravascular pressure has decreased to about 10 mm Hg. The decrease in systemic blood pressure from 10 mm Hg to nearly 0 mm Hg as blood traverses veins indicates that these vessels impart far more resistance to blood flow than would be expected for vessels of their large sizes. This resistance to blood flow is caused by compression of the veins by external forces that keep many of them, especially the vena cava, partially collapsed.

Table 14-3

Normal Pressures in the Systemic Circulation

	Mean Value (mm Hg)	Range (mm Hg)
Systolic blood pressure[a]	120	90–140
Diastolic blood pressure[a]	80	70–90
Mean arterial pressure	92	77–97
Left ventricular end diastolic pressure	6	0–12
Left atrium		
a wave	10	2–12
v wave	13	6–20
Right atrium		
a wave	6	2–10
c wave	5	2–10
v wave	3	0–8

[a]Measured in the radial artery.

Pulse Pressure in Arteries

Pulse pressure reflects the intermittent ejection of blood into the aorta by the heart (see Table 14-3). The difference between systolic and diastolic blood pressure is the pulse pressure. A typical systemic blood pressure curve recorded from a large artery is characterized by a rapid increase in pressure during ventricular systole followed by a maintained high level of blood pressure for 0.2 to 0.3 second (Fig. 14-3). This plateau is followed by the dicrotic notch (incisura) at the end of systole and a subsequent, more gradual decrease of pressure back to the diastolic level.

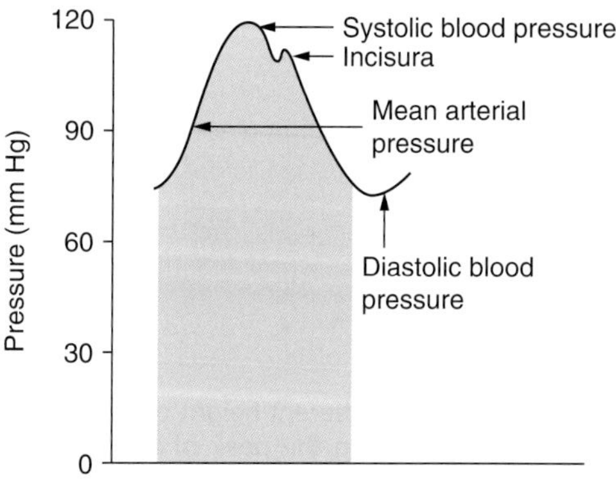

FIGURE 14-3 Schematic depiction of systemic blood pressure recorded from a large systemic artery. Mean arterial pressure is equal to the area under the blood pressure curve divided by the duration of systole.

The dicrotic notch reflects a decrease in the intraventricular pressure and a backflow of blood in the aorta, which causes the aortic valve to close.

Factors that Alter Pulse Pressure

The principal factors that alter pulse pressure in the arteries are the left ventricular stroke volume, velocity of blood flow, and compliance of the arterial tree. The larger the stroke volume, the greater the volume of blood that must be accommodated in the arterial vessels with each contraction resulting in an increased pulse pressure. Pulse pressure also increases when capacitance increases for outflow. When systemic vascular resistance decreases, flow of blood from arteries to veins is accelerated. Pulse pressure is also increased in the presence of patent ductus arteriosus and aortic regurgitation, reflecting rapid runoff of blood into the pulmonary circulation or left ventricle, respectively. In this regard, attempts have been made to predict systemic vascular resistance by the position of the dicrotic notch relative to the diastolic pressure. A controlled study, however, failed to confirm a correlation between the position of the dicrotic notch and the calculated systemic vascular resistance (Fig. 14-4).[5] An increase in heart rate while the cardiac output remains constant causes the stroke volume and pulse pressure to decrease. Pulse pressure is inversely proportional to the compliance (distensibility) of the arterial system. For example, with aging, the distensibility of the arterial walls often decreases (elastic and muscular tissues are replaced by fibrous tissue) and pulse pressure increases.

Transmission of the Pulse Pressure

There is often enhancement of the pulse pressure as the pressure wave is transmitted peripherally (Fig. 14-5).[4] Part of this augmentation results from the progressive decrease in compliance of the more distal portions of the large arteries. Second, pressure waves are reflected to some extent by the peripheral arteries. Specifically, when a pulsatile pressure wave enters the peripheral arteries and distends them, the pressure on these peripheral arteries causes the pulse wave to begin traveling backward. If the returning pulse wave strikes an oncoming wave, the two summate, causing a much higher pressure than would otherwise occur.

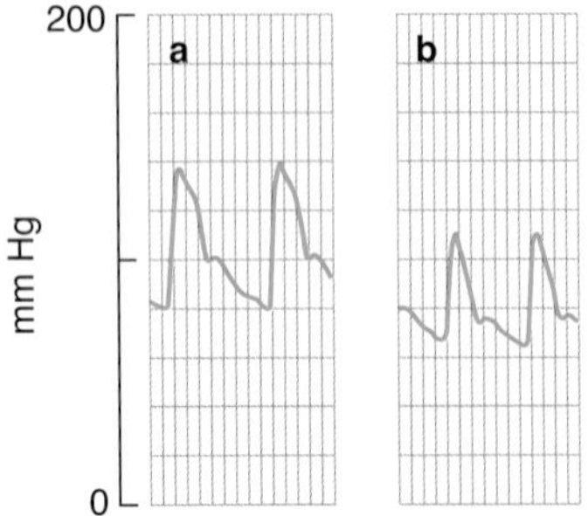

FIGURE 14-4 Despite a different height of the dicrotic notch (measured from baseline to the peak of the notch), the calculated systemic vascular resistance is similar for tracings *a* and *b*. (From Gerber MJ, Hines RL, Barash PG. Arterial waveforms and systemic vascular resistance: is there a correlation? *Anesthesiology*. 1987;66:823–825, with permission.)

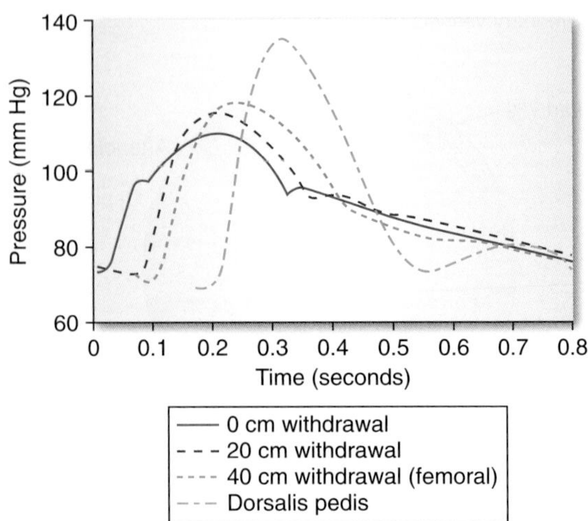

FIGURE 14-5 There is enhancement of the pulse pressure as the systemic blood pressure is transmitted peripherally. (From Guyton AC, Hall JE. *Textbook of Medical Physiology*. 10th ed. Philadelphia, PA: Saunders; 2000, with permission.)

These changes in the contour of the pulse wave are most pronounced in young patients, whereas in elderly patients with less compliant arteries, the pulse wave may be transmitted virtually unchanged from the aorta to peripheral arteries.

Augmentation of the peripheral pulse pressure must be identified whenever systemic blood pressure measurements are made in peripheral arteries. For example, systolic pressure in the radial artery is sometimes as much as 20% to 30% higher than that pressure present in the central aorta, and diastolic pressure is often decreased as much as 10% to 15%. Mean arterial pressures are similar regardless of the site of blood pressure measurement in a peripheral artery.

Pulse pressure becomes progressively less as blood passes through small arteries and arterioles until it becomes almost absent in capillaries (see Fig. 14-2).[4] This reflects the extreme distensibility of small vessels such that the small amount of blood that is caused to flow during a pulsatile pressure wave produces progressively less pressure increase in the more distal vessels. Furthermore, resistance to blood flow in these small vessels is such that flow of blood and, consequently, the transmission of pressure are greatly impeded.

Systemic Blood Pressure Measurement during and after Cardiopulmonary Bypass

Reversal of the usual relationship between aortic and radial artery blood pressures can occur during the late period of hypothermic cardiopulmonary bypass and in the early period after termination of cardiopulmonary bypass (Fig. 14-6).[6,7] One mechanism proposed for this

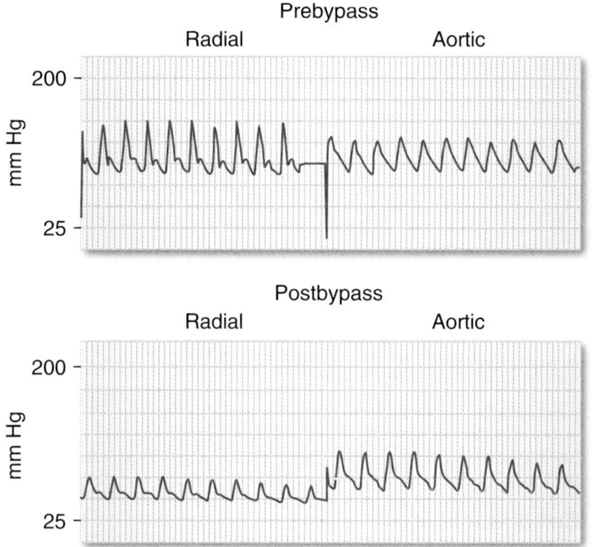

FIGURE 14-6 There may be a reversal of the usual relationship of simultaneous recordings of radial and aortic blood pressures (prebypass) in the early period after separation from cardiopulmonary bypass (postbypass). (From Stern DH, Gerson JI, Allen FB, et al. Can we trust the direct radial artery pressure immediately following cardiopulmonary bypass? *Anesthesiology.* 1985;62:557–561, with permission.)

unpredictable and transient disparity (usually persists for 10 to 60 minutes after discontinuation of cardiopulmonary bypass) is a high blood flow in the forearm and hand after rewarming on cardiopulmonary bypass, causing an increased pressure drop along the normal resistance pathway provided by the arteries leading to the radial site. Conversely, others describe the appearance of this gradient with initiation of cardiopulmonary bypass, suggesting that the etiology is associated with events such as cross-clamping of the aorta occurring during initiation of cardiopulmonary bypass rather than rewarming or discontinuing cardiopulmonary bypass (Fig. 14-7).[8,9] Failure

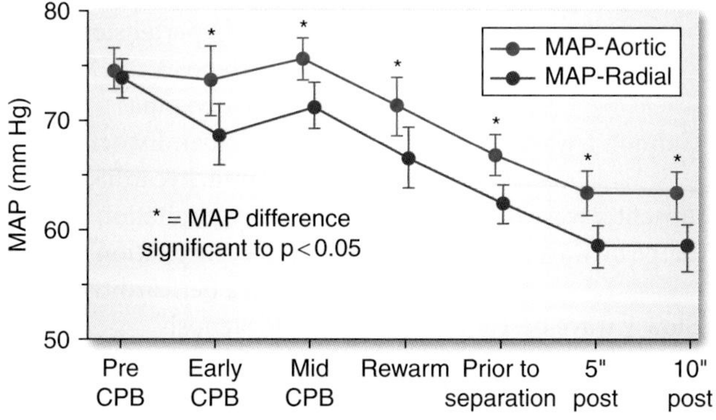

FIGURE 14-7 Comparison of mean arterial pressure (MAP) as measured from the aorta or radial artery before, during, and after cardiopulmonary bypass (CPB). (From Rich GF, Lubanski RE, McLoughlin TM. Differences between aortic and radial artery pressure associated with cardiopulmonary bypass. *Anesthesiology.* 1992;77:63–66, with permission.)

to recognize this disparity may lead to an erroneous diagnosis and unnecessary treatment. Systemic blood pressure measured in the brachial artery is more accurate and reliable during the periods surrounding cardiopulmonary bypass, which are most likely to be associated with disparities between the aortic and radial artery blood pressures.[10]

Pulsus Paradoxus

Pulsus paradoxus is an exaggerated decrease in systolic blood pressure (>10 mm Hg) during inspiration in the presence of increased intrapericardial pressures (cardiac tamponade). During normal inspiration, the decrease in intrathoracic pressure increases the compliance of the pulmonary vasculature, which leads to a relative decrease in pulmonary venous return to the left ventricle. The resultant reduction in left ventricular preload decreases the stroke volume, which manifests as a mildly decreased systolic blood pressure during inspiration (<10 mm Hg). Cardiac tamponade causes an exaggeration of this change in blood pressure with respiration.

Pulsus Alternans

Pulsus alternans is alternating weak and strong cardiac contractions causing a similar alteration in the strength of the peripheral pulse. A variety of physiologic conditions are associated with pulsus alternans. Digitalis toxicity, varying degrees of atrioventricular heart block, and left ventricular dysfunction are commonly associated with pulsus alternans. In the setting of left ventricular dysfunction, pulsus alternans is caused by cyclic alterations in the contractile state of the heart. A reduced stroke volume increases end diastolic volume, which results in increased myocardial contraction and therefore increased ventricular emptying and blood pressure (per the Frank-Starling law). During the subsequent cardiac cycle, the lower filling pressures in the left ventricle result in a decreased stroke volume and therefore decreased ventricular emptying and blood pressure.

Electrical Alternans

Electrical alternans is a phenomenon where the amplitude of the QRS complex changes between heart beats. This electrocardiographic finding is seen in cardiac tamponade and pericardial effusion, where the heart essentially moves within the fluid-filled pericardial sac during contraction.

Pulse Deficit

In the presence of atrial fibrillation or ectopic ventricular beats, two beats of the heart may occur so close together that the ventricle does not fill adequately and the second cardiac contraction ejects an insufficient volume of blood to create a peripheral pulse. In this circumstance, a second heart beat is audible with a stethoscope applied on the chest directly over the heart, but a corresponding pulsation in the radial artery cannot be palpated. This phenomenon is called a ***pulse deficit***.

Measurement of Blood Pressure by Auscultation

Measurement of blood pressure by auscultation uses the principle that blood flow in large arteries is laminar and not audible. If blood flow is arrested by an inflated cuff and the pressure in the cuff is released slowly, audible tapping sounds (Korotkoff's sounds) can be heard when the pressure of the cuff decreases just below systolic blood pressure and blood starts flowing in the brachial artery. These tapping sounds occur because flow velocity through the constricted portion of the blood vessel is increased, resulting in turbulence and vibrations that are heard through the stethoscope. Diastolic blood pressure correlates with the onset of muffled auscultatory sounds. The auscultatory method for determining systolic and diastolic blood pressure usually gives values within 10% of those determined by direct measurement from the arteries.

The width of the blood pressure cuff will affect measurements; ideally, the width of the blood pressure cuff should be 20% to 50% greater than the diameter of the patient's extremity. If the cuff is too narrow, the blood pressure will be overestimated. If the cuff is too large, the blood pressure may be underestimated.

Right Atrial Pressure

Right atrial pressure is regulated by a balance between venous return and the ability of the right ventricle to eject blood. Normal right atrial pressure is about 5 mm Hg, with a lower limit of about −5 mm Hg, which corresponds to the pressure in the pericardial and intrapleural spaces that surround the heart. Right atrial pressure approaches these low values when right ventricular contractility is increased or venous return to the heart is decreased by hemorrhage. Poor right ventricular contractility or any event that increases venous return (hypervolemia, venoconstriction) tends to increase right atrial pressure. Pressure in the right atrium is commonly designated the ***central venous pressure*** (CVP). Other factors that increase CVP include tension pneumothorax, heart failure, tamponade, pleural effusion, mechanical ventilation, positive end-expiratory pressure, Valsalva, pulmonary hypertension, and pulmonary embolism.

Jugular Venous Pressure

Jugular venous pressure or the pressure in the internal jugular vein mirrors the CVP. The normal jugular venous pressure reflects phasic changes in the right atrium and consists of three positive waves and three negative troughs (Fig. 14-8).[11] Abnormalities of these venous waveforms may be useful in the diagnosis of various cardiac conditions (Table 14-4).[11]

Peripheral Venous Pressure

Large veins offer little resistance to blood flow when they are distended. Most large veins, however, are compressed at multiple extrathoracic sites. For example, pressure in the external jugular vein is often so low that atmospheric

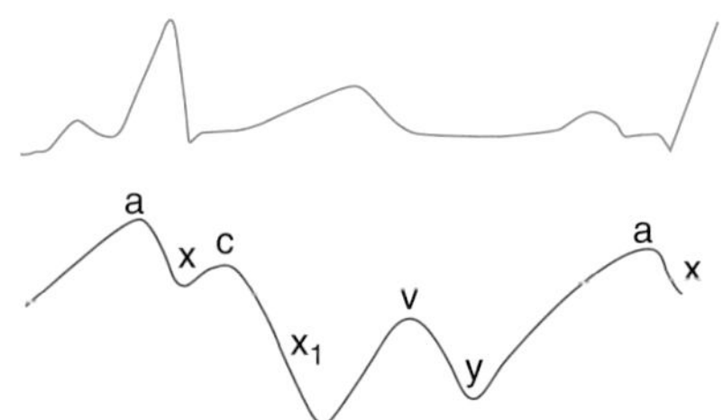

FIGURE 14-8 Simultaneous recording of the electrocardiogram *(top tracing)* and jugular venous pressure waves *(bottom tracing)*. (From Cook DJ, Simel DL. Does this patient have abnormal venous pressure? *JAMA*. 1996;275:630–634, with permission.)

pressure on the outside of the neck causes it to collapse. Veins coursing through the abdomen are compressed by intraabdominal pressure, which may increase 15 to 20 mm Hg as a result of pregnancy or ascites. When this occurs, pressure in leg veins must increase above abdominal pressure. It is important to recognize that veins inside the thorax are not collapsed because of the distending effect of negative intrathoracic pressure.

Effect of Hydrostatic Pressure

Pressure in veins below the heart is increased and that in veins above the heart is decreased by the effect of gravity

Table 14-4

Abnormalities of Jugular Venous Pressure Waveforms

Waveform	Cardiac Abnormality
Absent a wave	Atrial fibrillation Sinus tachycardia
Flutter waves	Atrial flutter
Prominent a waves	First-degree atrioventricular heart block
Large a wave	Tricuspid stenosis Pulmonary hypertension Pulmonic stenosis Right atrial myxoma
Cannon a waves	Atrioventricular dissociation Ventricular tachycardia
Absent x wave descent	Tricuspid regurgitation
Large cv waves	Tricuspid regurgitation Constrictive pericarditis
Slow y wave descent	Tricuspid stenosis Right atrial myxoma
Rapid y wave descent	Tricuspid regurgitation Atrial septal defect Constrictive pericarditis
Absent y wave descent	Cardiac tamponade

Adapted from Cook DJ, Simel DL. Does this patient have abnormal central venous pressure? *JAMA*. 1996;275:630–634.

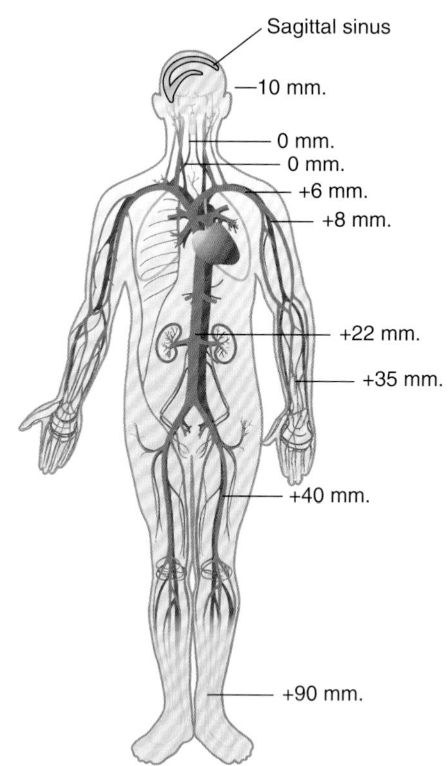

FIGURE 14-9 Effect of hydrostatic pressure on venous pressures throughout the body.

(Fig. 14-9).[4] As a guideline, pressure changes 0.77 mm Hg for every centimeter the vessel is above or below the heart. For example, in a standing human, pressure in the veins of the feet is 90 mm Hg because of the distance from the heart to the feet. Conversely, veins above the heart tend to collapse, with the exception being veins inside the skull, where they are held open by surrounding bone. As a result, negative pressure can exist in the dural sinuses and air can be entrained immediately if these sinuses are entered during surgery.

Hydrostatic pressure affects peripheral pressure in arteries and capillaries as well as veins. For example, a standing human who has a systemic blood pressure of 100 mm Hg at the level of the heart has a blood pressure of about 190 mm Hg in the feet.

Venous Valves and the Pump Mechanism

Valves in veins are arranged so that the direction of blood flow can be only toward the heart. In a standing human, movement of the legs compresses skeletal muscles and veins so blood is directed toward the heart. This venous pump or skeletal muscle pump is usually sufficient to maintain venous pressure below 25 mm Hg in a walking human. If an individual stands immobile, the venous pump does not function. As a result, pressures in the veins and capillaries of the legs can increase rapidly, resulting in leakage of fluid from the intravascular space. Indeed, as much as 15% of the blood volume can be lost from the intravascular space in the first 15 minutes of quiet standing.

Varicose Veins

Valves of the venous system can be destroyed when the veins are chronically distended by increased venous pressure as occurs during pregnancy or in an individual who stands most of the day. The end result is varicose veins characterized by bulbous protrusions of the veins beneath the skin of the legs. Venous and capillary pressures remain increased because of the incompetent venous pump, and this causes constant edema in the legs of these individuals. Edema interferes with diffusion of nutrients from the capillaries to tissues, so there is often skeletal muscle discomfort and the skin may ulcerate.

Reference Level for Measuring Venous Pressure

Hydrostatic pressure does not alter venous or arterial pressures that are measured at the level of the tricuspid valve. As a result, the reference point for pressure measurement is considered to be the level of the tricuspid valve. An appropriate external reference point for the level of the tricuspid valve in a supine individual is 5 cm posterior to the sternum at the level of the 4th intercostal space. A precise hydrostatic point to which pressures are referenced is essential for accurate interpretation of venous pressure measurements. For example, each centimeter below the hydrostatic point adds 0.77 mm Hg to the measured pressure, whereas 0.77 mm Hg is subtracted for each centimeter above this point. The potential error introduced by measuring pressures above or below the tricuspid valve is greatest with venous pressures that are normally low. For example, an error introduced by 5 cm of hydrostatic pressure has a much greater influence on the clinical interpretation of CVP than arterial pressure.

The reason for lack of hydrostatic effects at the tricuspid valve is the ability of the right ventricle to act as a regulator of pressure at this site. For example, if the pressure at the tricuspid valve increases, the right ventricle fills to a greater extent, thereby decreasing the pressure at the tricuspid valve toward normal. Conversely, if the pressure decreases at the tricuspid valve, the right ventricle does not fill optimally and blood pools in the veins until pressure at the tricuspid valve again increases to a normal value.

Measurement of right atrial pressure is accomplished by using a transducer or a fluid-filled manometer referenced to the level of the tricuspid valve. A venous pressure measurement in mm Hg can be converted to cm H_2O by multiplying the pressure by 1.36, which adjusts for the density of mercury relative to water (10 mm Hg equals 13.6 cm H_2O). Conversely, dividing the CVP measurement in cm H_2O by 1.36 converts this value to an equivalent pressure in mm Hg.

Blood Viscosity

Blood is a viscous fluid composed of cells and plasma. More than 99% of the cells in plasma are erythrocytes. As a result, leukocytes exert a minimal influence on the physical

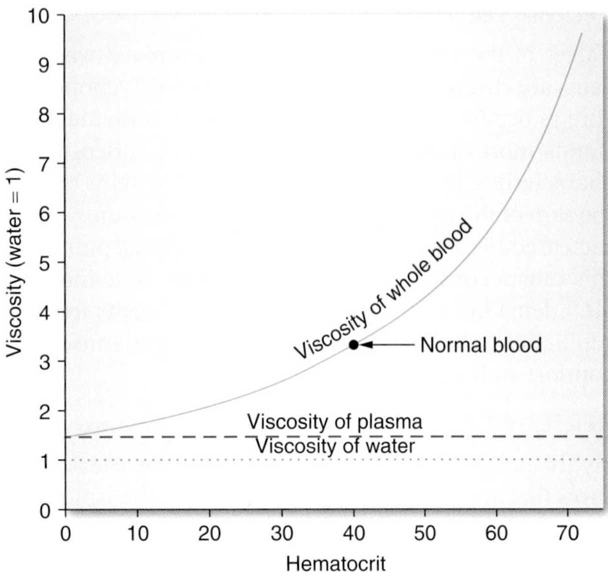

FIGURE 14-10 Hematocrit greatly influences the viscosity of blood. (From Guyton AC, Hall JE. *Textbook of Medical Physiology*. 10th ed. Philadelphia, PA: Saunders; 2000, with permission.)

characteristics of blood. The percentage of blood comprising erythrocytes is the hematocrit, which to a large extent determines the viscosity of blood (Fig. 14-10).[4] When the hematocrit increases to 60% to 70%, viscosity of blood is increased about 10-fold compared with water, and flow through blood vessels is greatly decreased. Plasma protein concentrations influence blood viscosity only minimally.

Viscosity exerts fewer effects on blood flow in capillaries than in larger vessels. This most likely reflects alignment of erythrocytes as they pass through small blood vessels rather than the random arrangement characteristic of flow through larger vessels. This alignment of erythrocytes, which greatly decreases the viscous resistance that occurs normally between cells, is largely offset by a decreased velocity of flow that greatly increases viscosity. The net effect may be that viscous effects in small blood vessels are similar to those that occur in large blood vessels.

Plasma is considered extracellular fluid that is identical to interstitial fluid except for the greater concentrations of proteins (albumin, globulin, fibrinogen) in plasma. These greater concentrations reflect the inability of plasma proteins to pass easily through capillaries into the interstitial spaces. The presence of albumin creates colloid osmotic pressure, which prevents fluid from leaving the capillaries.

Determinants of Tissue Blood Flow

Tissue blood flow is directly proportional to the pressure difference between two points (not absolute pressure) and inversely proportional to resistance to flow through the vessel. This relationship between flow, pressure, and resistance can be expressed mathematically as a variant of Ohm's law, in which blood flow (amperes) is directly proportional to the pressure drop across two points (voltage) and inversely proportional to resistance (Fig. 14-11). Rearrangement of this formula emphasizes that pressure is directly proportional to flow times resistance. Likewise, resistance is directly proportional to pressure and inversely proportional to flow. Furthermore, resistance is directly proportional to viscosity of blood and the length of the vessel and inversely proportional to the fourth power of the radius of the vessel (doubling the radius of the vessel or intravenous catheter size decreases resistance to flow 16-fold [Poiseuille's law]).

It is important to understand that resistance to blood flow cannot be measured but rather is a calculated value based on measurement of driving pressures and the cardiac output. For example, systemic vascular resistance is calculated as the difference between mean arterial pressure and right atrial pressure divided by cardiac output. Pulmonary vascular resistance is calculated as the difference between mean pulmonary artery pressure and left atrial pressure divided by the cardiac output. Resistance is expressed in dynes/s/cm^{-5} and is calculated by multiplying the equation for either systemic vascular resistance or pulmonary vascular resistance just described by a conversion factor of 80. Conductance is the reciprocal of resistance and is a measure of the amount of blood flow that can pass through a blood vessel in a given time for a given pressure gradient.

Vascular Distensibility

Blood vessels are distensible such that increases in systemic blood pressure cause the vascular diameter to increase, which in turn decreases resistance to blood flow. Conversely, decreases in intravascular pressure increase the resistance to blood flow. The ability of blood vessels to distend as intravascular pressure increases varies greatly in different parts of the circulation. Anatomically, the walls of arteries are stronger than those of veins. As a result, veins are 6 to 10 times as distensible as arteries. Systemic blood pressure can eventually decrease to a level where intravascular pressure is no longer capable of keeping the vessel open. This pressure averages 20 mm Hg and is defined as the ***critical closing pressure***. When the heart is abruptly stopped, the pressure in the entire circulatory system (mean circulatory pressure) equilibrates at about 7 mm Hg.

Vascular Compliance

Vascular compliance is defined as the increase in volume (capacitance) of a vessel produced by an increase in intra-

$$\text{Blood Flow (Q)} = \frac{\text{Pressure Difference Between Two Points (P)}}{\text{Resistance to Flow (R)}}$$

$$\Delta P = Q \times R$$

$$R = \Delta P / Q$$

FIGURE 14-11 The relationship between blood flow, pressure, and resistance to flow can be expressed as a variant of Ohm's law.

vascular pressure. The compliance of the entire circulatory system is estimated to be 100 mL for each 1 mm Hg increase in intravascular pressure.[4] The compliance of veins is much greater than that of arteries. For example, the volume of blood normally present in all veins is about 2,500 mL, whereas the arterial system contains only about 750 mL of blood when the mean arterial pressure is 100 mm Hg. Sympathetic nervous system activity can greatly alter the distribution of blood volume. Enhancement of sympathetic nervous outflow to the blood vessels, especially the veins, decreases the dimensions to the circulatory system, and the circulation continues to function almost normally even when as much as 25% of the total blood volume has been lost. ***Vasoconstriction*** or ***vasodilation*** refers to resistance changes in arterioles, whereas changes in the caliber of veins are described as ***venoconstriction*** or ***venodilation***.

Control of Tissue Blood Flow

Control of blood flow to different tissues includes local mechanisms, autonomic nervous system responses, and release of hormones. Total tissue blood flow or cardiac output is about 5 L per minute, with large amounts being delivered to the heart, brain, liver, and kidneys (Table 14-5).[4] In contrast, skeletal muscles represent 35% to 40% of body mass but receive only about 15% of the total cardiac output, reflecting the low metabolic rate of inactive skeletal muscles.

Local Control of Blood Flow

Local control of blood flow is most often based on the need for delivery of oxygen or other nutrients such as glucose or fatty acids to the tissues. The response to decreased oxygen delivery may reflect the local release of vasodilatory substances (adenosine, lactic acid, carbon dioxide, potassium ions), which results in increased tissue blood flow and oxygen delivery.

Table 14-5

Tissue Blood Flow

	Approximate Blood Flow		Cardiac Output
	(mL/min)	(mL/100 g/min)	(% of Total)
Brain	750	50	15
Liver	1,450	100	29
Portal vein	1,100		
Hepatic artery	350		
Kidneys	1,000	320	20
Heart	225	75	5
Skeletal muscles (at rest)	750	4	15
Skin	400	3	8
Other tissues	425	2	8
Total	5,000		100

Adapted from Guyton AC, Hall JE. *Textbook of Medical Physiology*. 10th ed. Philadelphia, PA: Saunders; 2000.

Autoregulation of Blood Flow

Autoregulation is a local mechanism that controls blood flow in which a specific tissue is able to maintain a relatively constant blood flow over a wide range of mean arterial pressures. When the mean arterial pressure increases, the associated increase in tissue blood flow causes the blood vessels to constrict, thereby limiting any increase in blood flow. Conversely, decreases in mean arterial pressure result in vasodilation, which maintains tissue blood flow. Autoregulatory responses to sudden changes in mean arterial pressure occur within 60 to 120 seconds. The ability of autoregulation to return local tissue blood flow to normal is incomplete.

Long-term Control of Blood Flow

Long-term regulatory mechanisms that return local tissue blood flow to normal involve a change in vascularity of tissues. For example, sustained increases in mean arterial pressure to specific tissues, as occurs above a coarctation of the aorta, is accompanied by a decrease in the size and number of blood vessels. Likewise, if metabolism in a tissue becomes chronically increased, vascularity increases, or, if metabolism is decreased, vascularity decreases. Indeed, inadequate delivery of oxygen to a tissue is the stimulus for the development of collateral vessels. Neonates exposed to increased concentrations of oxygen can manifest cessation of new vascular growth in the retina. Subsequent removal of the neonate from a high-oxygen environment causes an overgrowth of new vessels to offset the abrupt decrease in availability of oxygen. There may be so much overgrowth that the new vessels cause blindness (retrolental fibroplasia).

Autonomic Nervous System Control of Blood Flow

Autonomic nervous system control of blood flow is characterized by a rapid response time (within 1 second) and an ability to regulate blood flow to certain tissues at the expense of other tissues. The sympathetic nervous system is the most important component of the autonomic nervous system in the regulation of blood flow; sympathetic stimulation causes release of norepinephrine, which stimulates α-adrenergic receptors to produce vasoconstriction. Constriction of small arteries influences resistance to blood flow through tissues, whereas venoconstriction alters vascular capacitance and distribution of blood in the peripheral circulation. Sympathetic nervous system innervation is prominent in the kidneys and skin and minimal in the cerebral circulation.

Vasomotor Center

The vasomotor center, which is located in the pons and medulla, transmits sympathetic nervous system impulses through the spinal cord to all blood vessels. Evidence for a continuous, sustained state of partial vasoconstriction (vasomotor tone) is the abrupt decrease in systemic blood pressure that occurs when sympathetic nervous system innervation to the vasculature is abruptly interrupted, as by traumatic spinal cord transection or regional anesthesia. Activity of the vasomotor center can be influenced by impulses from a number of sites, including diffuse areas of the reticular activating system, hypothalamus, and cerebral cortex. Sympathetic nervous system impulses are transmitted to the adrenal medulla at the same time they are transmitted to the peripheral vasculature. These impulses stimulate the adrenal medulla to secrete epinephrine and norepinephrine into the circulation, where they act directly on adrenergic receptors in the walls of vascular smooth muscle.

The medial and lower portions of the vasomotor center do not participate in transmission of vasoconstrictor impulses but rather function as an inhibitor of sympathetic nervous system activity, which allows blood vessels to dilate. Conceptually, this portion of the vasomotor center is functioning as the parasympathetic nervous system.

Mass Reflex

The mass reflex is characterized by stimulation of all portions of the vasomotor center, resulting in generalized vasoconstriction and an increase in cardiac output in an attempt to maintain tissue blood flow. The alarm reaction resembles the mass reflex, but associated skeletal muscle vasodilation and psychic excitement are intended to prepare the individual to confront a life-threatening situation.

Syncope

Emotional fainting (vasovagal syncope) may reflect profound skeletal muscle vasodilation such that systemic blood pressure decreases abruptly and syncope occurs. Associated vagal stimulation results in bradycardia. This phenomenon may occur in patients who have an intense fear of needles, resulting in syncope during placement of an intravenous catheter.

Hormone Control of Blood Flow

Vasoconstrictor hormones that may influence local tissue blood flow include epinephrine, norepinephrine, angiotensin, and arginine vasopressin (formerly known as ***antidiuretic hormone***). Bradykinin, serotonin, histamine, prostaglandins, and low circulating concentrations of epinephrine are vasodilating substances. Local chemical factors, such as accumulation of hydrogen ions, potassium ions, and carbon dioxide, relax vascular smooth muscle and cause vasodilation. Carbon dioxide also has an indirect vasoconstrictor effect because it stimulates the outflow of sympathetic nervous system impulses from the vasomotor center.

Regulation of Systemic Blood Pressure

Systemic blood pressure is maintained over a narrow range by reciprocal changes in cardiac output and systemic vascular resistance. The autonomic nervous system and baroreceptors play a key role in moment-to-moment regulation of systemic blood pressure. Long-term regulation of blood pressure depends on control of fluid balance by the kidneys, adrenal cortex, and central nervous system.

Systolic, diastolic, and mean arterial pressure tends to increase progressively with age. Because a greater portion of the cardiac cycle is nearer the diastolic blood pressure, it follows that mean arterial pressure is not the arithmetic average of the systolic and diastolic blood pressures. Mean arterial blood pressure is the most important determinant of tissue blood flow because it is the average, tending to drive blood through the systemic circulation.

Rapid-Acting Mechanisms for the Regulation of Systemic Blood Pressure

Rapid-acting mechanisms for regulation of systemic blood pressure involve nervous system responses as reflected by the baroreceptor reflexes, chemoreceptor reflexes, atrial reflexes, and central nervous system ischemic reflex. These reflex mechanisms respond almost immediately to changes in systemic blood pressure. Furthermore, within about 30 minutes, these nervous system reflex responses are further supplemented by activation of hormonal mechanisms and shift of fluid into the circulation to readjust the blood volume. These short-term mechanisms can return systemic blood pressure toward but never entirely back to normal. Indeed, the impact of many of the rapid-acting regulatory mechanisms, such as the baroreceptor reflexes, diminishes with time as these mechanisms adapt to the new level of systemic blood pressure.

Baroreceptor Reflexes

Baroreceptors are nerve endings in the walls of large arteries in the neck and thorax, especially in the internal carotid arteries just above the carotid bifurcation and in the arch of the aorta (Fig. 14-12).[12] These nerve endings respond rapidly to changes in systemic blood pressure and are crucial for maintaining normal blood pressure when an individual changes from the supine to standing position. An increase in mean arterial pressure produces stretch of baroreceptor nerve endings, and increased numbers of nerve impulses are transmitted to the depressor portion of the vasomotor center, leading to a relative decrease in the central nervous system outflow of sympathetic nervous system (vasoconstrictive) impulses (Fig. 14-13).[12] The net effects are vasodilation throughout the peripheral circulation, decreased heart rate, and decreased myocardial contractility, which all act to decrease systemic blood pressure back toward normal. Conversely, decreases in systemic blood pressure reflexively produce changes likely to increase blood pressure. Baroreceptors adapt in 1 to 3 days to sustained changes in systemic blood pressure, emphasizing that these reflexes are probably of no importance in long-term regulation of blood pressure. Volatile anesthetics, particularly halothane, inhibit the

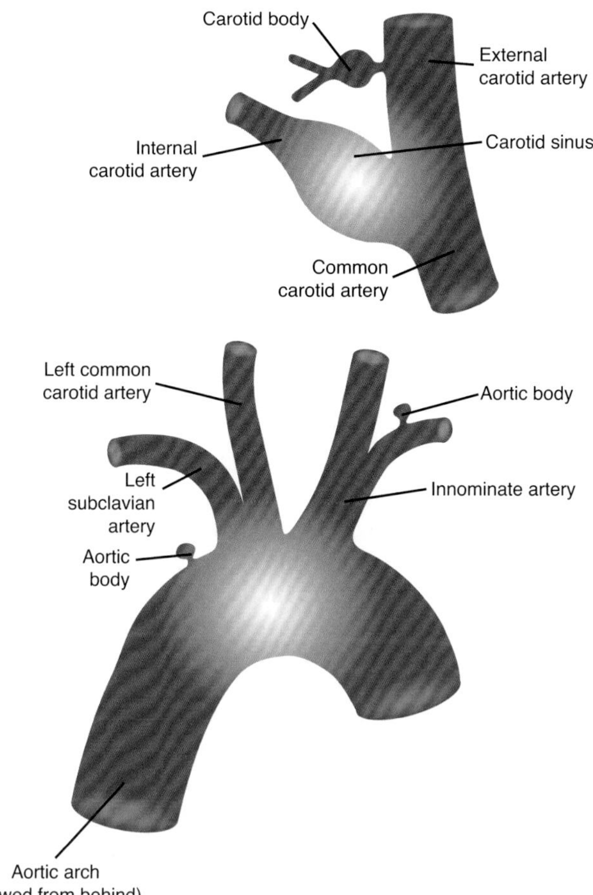

FIGURE 14-12 Baroreceptors are represented by the carotid sinus and receptors in the arch of the aorta. Chemoreceptors are located in the carotid and aortic bodies.

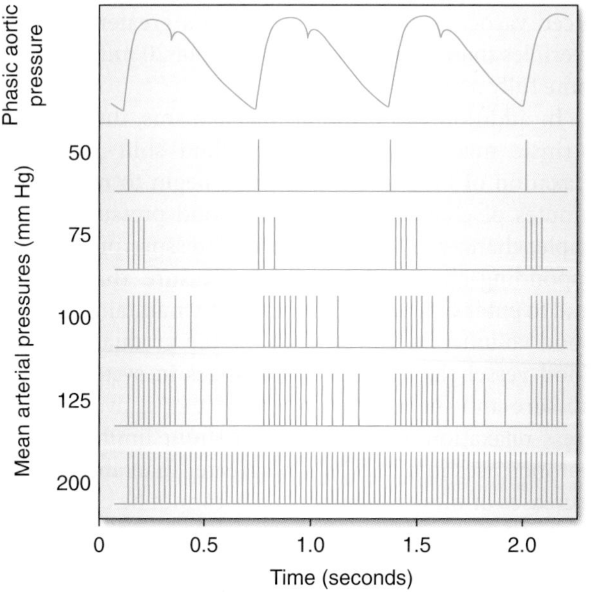

FIGURE 14-13 Discharges *(vertical lines)* in a single afferent nerve fiber from the carotid sinus at various arterial pressures, plotted against changes in aortic pressure with time. (From Ganong WF. *Review of Medical Physiology*. 21st ed. New York, NY: McGraw-Hill; 2003, with permission.)

heart rate response portion of the baroreceptor reflex that occurs in response to changes in systemic blood pressure (see Chapter 4).

Chemoreceptor Reflexes

Chemoreceptors are cells that transduce chemical signals into nerve impulses. There are chemoreceptors located in the carotid bodies and aortic body (see Fig. 14-12).[12] Each carotid or aortic body is supplied with an abundant blood flow through a nutrient artery so that the chemoreceptors are always exposed to oxygenated blood. When the systemic blood pressure, and thus the blood flow, decrease below a critical level, the chemoreceptors in the carotid body are stimulated by decreased availability of oxygen and also because of excess carbon dioxide and hydrogen ions that are not removed by the sluggish blood flow. Impulses from the chemoreceptors are transmitted to the vasomotor center, which results in reflex changes that tend to increase systemic blood pressure back toward the normal. Chemoreceptors do not respond strongly until systemic blood pressure decreases below 80 mm Hg. Chemoreceptors are more important in stimulating breathing when the $Pa{O_2}$ decreases below 60 mm Hg (ventilatory response to arterial hypoxemia). The ventilatory response to arterial hypoxemia is inhibited by subanesthetic concentrations of most of the volatile anesthetics (0.1 minimum alveolar concentration) as well as injected drugs such as barbiturates and opioids (see Chapters 4, 5, and 7).

Bezold-Jarisch Reflex

The Bezold-Jarisch reflex is a circulatory response whereby a decrease in left ventricular volume activates receptors that cause a paradoxical bradycardia. This compensatory decrease in heart rate allows for increased ventricular filling but may also exacerbate hypotension. The bradycardia and hypotension that can occur during spinal or epidural anesthesia have been attributed to this reflex.

Atrial Reflexes

The atria contain low-pressure atrial stretch receptors similar to baroreceptors in large arteries. Stretching of the atria evokes reflex vasodilation and decreases the systemic blood pressure back toward the normal level. An increase in atrial pressure also causes an increase in heart rate (Bainbridge reflex) due to a direct effect of the increased atrial volume on stretch of baroreceptors located in both atria at the venoatrial junctions. The increase in heart rate evoked by stretching of the atria prevents accumulation of blood in the atria, veins, or pulmonary circulation.

Central Nervous System Ischemic Reflex

The central nervous system ischemic reflex response occurs when blood flow to the medullary vasomotor center is decreased to the extent that ischemia of this vital center occurs. As a result of this ischemia, there is an intense outpouring of sympathetic nervous system activity, resulting in profound increases in systemic blood pressure. It is believed that this reflex response is caused by failure of slowly flowing blood to remove carbon dioxide from the vasomotor center. The central nervous system reflex response does not become highly active until mean arterial pressure decreases to less than 50 mm Hg and reaches its greatest degree of stimulation at systemic blood pressures of 15 to 20 mm Hg. This reflex response is not useful for regulation of normal blood pressure but rather acts as an emergency control system to prevent further decreases in systemic blood pressure when cerebral blood flow is dangerously decreased.

Cushing Reflex

The Cushing reflex is a central nervous system ischemic reflex response that results from increased intracranial pressure. When intracranial pressure increases to equal arterial pressure, the Cushing reflex acts to increase systemic blood pressure above intracranial pressure. Cushing's triad is defined as having (a) hypertension, (b) bradycardia, and (c) irregular respirations (due to brainstem dysfunction). The latter is not often seen in this era, as most patients with severe intracranial hypertension are now mechanically ventilated.

Respiratory Variations in Systemic Blood Pressure

Systemic blood pressure normally varies by 4 to 6 mm Hg in a wavelike manner during quiet spontaneous breathing. Systemic blood pressure is increased during end-inspiration and the beginning of exhalation and decreased during the remainder of the breathing cycle. This is due to increased venous return to the right heart during inspiration, which takes a few cardiac cycles to be transmitted to the left heart. Positive pressure ventilation of the lungs produces a reversed sequence of blood pressure change because the initial positive airway pressure simultaneously pushes more blood toward the left ventricle causing an increase in pressure; this is followed by a decrease in left ventricular filling due to the decrease in venous return to the right heart caused by the positive intrathoracic pressure.

Continuous or beat-to-beat monitoring of the changes in arterial blood pressure, pulse pressure, and stroke volume occurring during mechanical ventilation may provide an indication of the patient's ability to respond to volume administration with an increase in cardiac output or "fluid responsiveness." Respiratory variation in these parameters of more than 12% to 15% generally indicates fluid responsiveness. When the chest is closed and an adequate tidal volume is employed, "goal-directed" fluid resuscitation can be guided by such measurements.

Heart Rate Variability

Variations in heart rate occur during normal respiration, whereby inspiration increases heart rate and expiration decreases it. High-frequency heart rate variability is controlled by autonomic reflexes mediated by neural input to the heart supplied by the vagus nerve. Low-frequency heart rate variability results from the interaction between parasympathetic and sympathetic tone. Analysis of heart rate variability provides information regarding the integrity of the autonomic nervous system. High heart rate variability is a sign of good health and conversely, low heart rate variability can be a manifestation of disease (myocardial infarction, heart failure, neuropathy) and occurs universally following the denervation that occurs during cardiac transplantation.[13]

Systemic Blood Pressure Vasomotor Waves

Cyclic increases and decreases in systemic blood pressure lasting 7 to 10 seconds are referred to as ***vasomotor*** or ***Traube-Hering waves***. The presumed cause of vasomotor waves is oscillation in the reflex activity of baroreceptors. For example, increased systemic blood pressure stimulates baroreceptors, which then inhibit the sympathetic nervous system, causing a decrease in systemic blood pressure. Decreased systemic blood pressure decreases baroreceptor activity and allows the vasomotor center to become active once again, increasing the systemic blood pressure to a higher value.

Moderately Rapid-Acting Mechanisms for the Regulation of Systemic Blood Pressure

There are at least three hormonal mechanisms that provide either rapid or moderately rapid control of systemic blood pressure. These hormonal mechanisms are catecholamine-induced vasoconstriction, renin-angiotensin–induced vasoconstriction, and vasoconstriction induced by arginine vasopressin, all of which increase systemic blood pressure by increasing systemic vascular resistance. Circulating catecholamines may even reach parts of the circulation that are devoid of sympathetic nervous system innervation, such as metarterioles. Renin-angiotensin–induced vasoconstriction manifests to a greater degree on arterioles than veins and requires about 20 minutes to become fully active.

In addition to hormonal mechanisms, there are two intrinsic mechanisms (capillary fluid shift and stress-relaxation of blood vessels), which begin to react within minutes of changes in systemic blood pressure. For example, changes in systemic blood pressure produce corresponding changes in capillary pressure, thus allowing fluid to enter or leave the capillaries to maintain a constant blood volume. Stress-relaxation is the gradual change in blood vessel size to adapt to changes in systemic blood pressure and the amount of blood that is available. The stress-relaxation mechanism has definite limitations such that increases in blood volume greater than about 30% or decreases of more than about 15% cannot be corrected by this mechanism alone.

Long-term Mechanisms for the Regulation of Systemic Blood Pressure

Long-term mechanisms for the regulation of systemic blood pressure, unlike the short-term regulatory mechanisms, have a delayed onset but do not adapt, providing a sustained regulatory effect on systemic blood pressure. The renal–body fluid system plays a predominant role in long-term control of systemic blood pressure because it controls both the cardiac output and systemic vascular resistance. This crucial role is supplemented by accessory mechanisms, including the renin-angiotensin-aldosterone system and arginine vasopressin regulation.

Renal–Body Fluid System

Increased systemic blood pressure, as provoked by modest increases in blood volume, results in sodium ion and water excretion by the kidneys. The resultant decrease in blood volume leads to decreases in cardiac output and systemic blood pressure. After several weeks, the cardiac output returns toward normal, and systemic vascular resistance decreases to maintain the lower but more acceptable blood pressure. Conversely, a decrease in systemic blood pressure stimulates the kidneys to retain fluid. A special feature of this regulatory mechanism is its ability to return systemic blood pressure completely back to normal values. This contrasts with rapid-acting to moderately rapid-acting mechanisms, which cannot return systemic blood pressure entirely back to normal.

Renin-Angiotensin System

Aldosterone secretion that results from the action of angiotensin II on the adrenal cortex exerts a long-term effect on systemic blood pressure by stimulating the kidneys to retain sodium and water. The resulting increase in extracellular fluid volume causes cardiac output, and subsequently systemic blood pressure, to increase.

Regulation of Cardiac Output and Venous Return

Cardiac output is the amount of blood pumped by the left ventricle into the aorta each minute (product of stroke volume and heart rate), and venous return is the amount of blood flowing from the veins into the right atrium each minute. Because the circulation is a closed circuit, the cardiac output must equal venous return. Cardiac output for the average person weighing 70 kg and with a body surface area of 1.7 m^2 is about 5 L per minute. This value is about 10% less in women.

Determinants of Cardiac Output

Venous return is the main determinant of cardiac output. The metabolic requirements of tissues control cardiac output through alterations in resistance to tissue blood flow. For example, increased local metabolic needs lead to regional vasodilation, with a resulting increase in tissue blood flow and thus venous return. Cardiac output is increased by an amount equivalent to the venous return.

Any factor that interferes with venous return can lead to decreased cardiac output. Hemorrhage decreases blood volume such that venous return decreases and cardiac output decreases. Acute venodilation, such as that produced by spinal anesthesia and accompanying sympathetic nervous system blockade, can so increase the capacitance of peripheral vessels that venous return is reduced and cardiac output declines. Restoration of venous tone (with a vasoconstrictor) and/or administration of fluid can restore cardiac output. Positive pressure ventilation of the lungs, particularly in the presence of a decreased blood volume, causes a decrease in venous return and cardiac output.

Factors that increase cardiac output are associated with decreases in systemic vascular resistance. For example, anemia decreases the viscosity of blood, leading to a decrease in systemic vascular resistance and increase in venous return. An increased blood volume increases cardiac output by increasing the gradient for flow to the right atrium and by distending blood vessels, which decreases resistance to blood flow. Increased cardiac output caused by an increased blood volume lasts only 20 to 40 minutes because increased capillary pressures cause intravascular fluid to enter tissues, thereby returning blood volume to normal. Furthermore, increased pressure in veins caused by the increased blood volume causes the veins to distend (stress-relaxation). Cardiac output increases during exercise, in hyperthyroidism, and in the presence of arteriovenous shunts associated with hemodialysis, reflecting decreases in systemic vascular resistance.

Sympathetic nervous system stimulation increases myocardial contractility and heart rate to increase cardiac output beyond that possible from venous return alone. Maximal stimulation by the sympathetic nervous system can double cardiac output. Nevertheless, this sympathetic nervous system–induced increase of cardiac output is only transient, despite sustained increases in nervous system activity. A reason for this transient effect is autoregulation of tissue blood flow, which manifests as vasoconstriction to decrease venous return and thus decrease cardiac output back toward normal. In addition, increased systemic blood pressure associated with increases in the cardiac output causes fluid to leave the capillaries, thereby decreasing blood volume, venous return, and cardiac output.

An increase in myocardial contractility or inotropy can increase the stroke volume and thereby the cardiac output. Cardiac muscle is sensitive to calcium; most hormones and drugs which increase contractility augment intracellular calcium use. One newer agent available outside of the United States that is used to provide inotropic support in severe heart failure (levosimendan) sensitizes the myofibrils to calcium. Decreased contractility is caused by many anesthetic agents. Strictly speaking, changes in inotropic state should be defined in the absence of changes in preload and afterload; because many inotropic drugs affect these parameters as well, changes in cardiac output are not always due only to the inotropic activity.

Ventricular Function Curves

Ventricular function curves (Frank-Starling curves) depict the cardiac output at different atrial (ventricular end diastolic) filling pressures (Fig. 14-14). Clinically, ventricular function curves are used to estimate myocardial contractility. Improved cardiac function (sympathetic nervous system stimulation) is characterized by a shift of the cardiac output curve to the left of the normal curve (greater cardiac output for a given filling pressure), whereas a shift of the curve to the right of normal (myocardial infarction, cardiomyopathy) reflects decreased cardiac function. Even with a normal ventricular function curve, as preload is increased, a point is reached where further stretching of the cardiac muscle results in no further increase and eventually to a decrease in cardiac output.

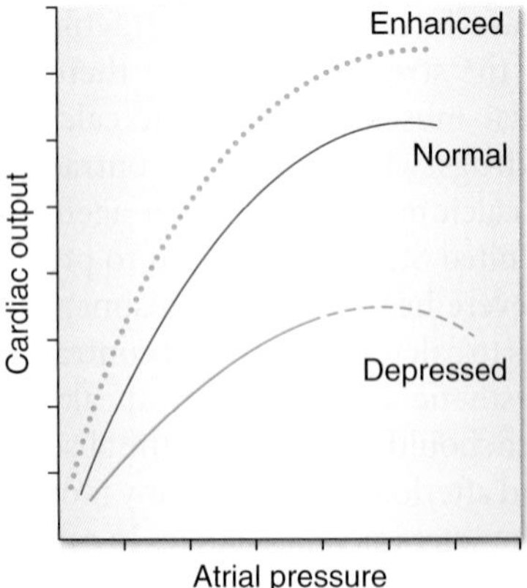

FIGURE 14-14 Ventricular function curves (Frank-Starling curves) depict the volume of forward ventricular ejection (cardiac output) at different atrial filling pressures and varying degrees of myocardial contractility.

Pressure–Volume Loops

Pressure–volume loops describe the dynamic characteristics of cardiac function (Fig. 14-15). If ventricular pressure is plotted against ventricular volume, each cardiac cycle can be depicted by a pressure–volume loop.

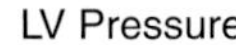

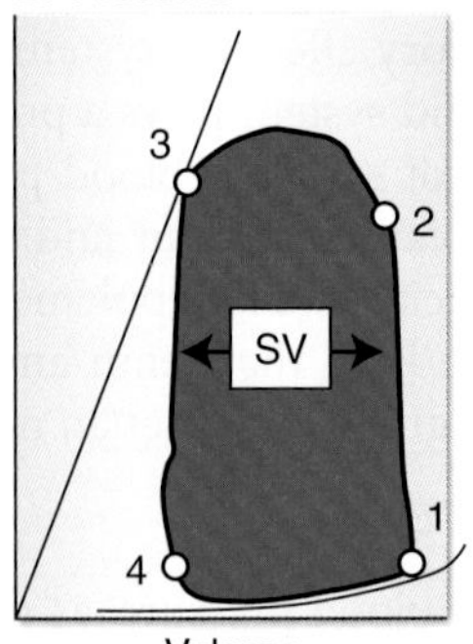

FIGURE 14-15 Pressure–volume loop representing the cardiac cycle. The end diastolic and the end systolic pressure–volume relationships represent the boundaries for the loops. The width of the pressure–volume loop represents the stroke volume (SV). Increases or decreases in myocardial contractility make the end systolic pressure volume relationship steeper or shallower. The four segments of the loop (isovolumic contraction, ejection, isovolumic relaxation, ventricular filling) for the left ventricle are depicted in succession by mitral valve closure *(1)*, aortic valve opening *(2)*, aortic valve closure *(3)*, and mitral valve opening *(4)*.

Shock Syndromes

Circulatory shock is characterized by inadequate tissue blood flow and oxygen delivery to cells resulting in generalized deterioration of cellular and organ function. Inadequate tissue flow is due to inadequate cardiac output and can result from decreased venous return, myocardial depression, or both. Cellular metabolism is depressed, and the amount of heat liberated is decreased resulting in a decreased body temperature particularly when the ambient environment is cold. In the early stages of shock, consciousness is usually maintained, although mental clarity may be impaired. Consciousness is likely to be lost as shock progresses. Low cardiac output greatly decreases urine output, eventually leading to anuria as glomerular pressure decreases below the critical value required for filtration of fluid into Bowman's capsule. Furthermore, the kidneys have such a high rate of metabolism that decreased renal blood flow may cause acute tubular necrosis (see Chapter 16). An important feature of persistent shock is eventual progressive deterioration of the heart. In addition to myocardial depression caused by decreased coronary artery blood flow, myocardial function can also be depressed by lactic acid, bacterial endotoxins, and myocardial depressant factor released from an ischemic pancreas.

Hemorrhagic Shock

Hemorrhage is the most common cause of shock due to decreased venous return. Any decrease in systemic blood pressure initiates powerful baroreceptor-mediated increases in sympathetic nervous system activity, manifesting as arterial constriction, venoconstriction, and direct myocardial stimulation. Venoconstriction is particularly important for sustaining venous return to the heart and, thus, maintaining cardiac output. Arterial constriction is responsible for initially maintaining systemic blood pressure despite decreases in cardiac output. This maintenance of systemic blood pressure sustains cerebral and coronary artery blood flow as significant vasoconstriction does not occur in these organs. In other organs, such as the kidneys, intense sympathetic nervous system–mediated vasoconstriction may decrease blood flow dramatically.

Nonhemorrhagic Hypovolemic Shock

Loss of plasma volume from the circulation can result in shock similar to that produced by hemorrhage. Intestinal obstruction results in fluid loss into the gastrointestinal tract and reduction in plasma volume. Severe burns may also be associated with sufficient loss of plasma volume to result in shock. Severe dehydration from any cause can also lead to hypovolemic shock due to reduction in plasma volume. Hypovolemic shock that results from a reduction in plasma volume has the same clinical characteristics as hemorrhagic shock except that selective reduction of the plasma volume greatly increases the viscosity of blood and exacerbates sluggish blood flow.

Neurogenic Shock

Neurogenic shock occurs in the absence of blood loss when vascular capacity increases so greatly that even a normal blood volume is not capable of maintaining venous return and cardiac output. Common causes of loss of vasomotor tone and subsequent neurogenic shock are traumatic transection of the spinal cord and acute blockade of the peripheral sympathetic nervous system by spinal or epidural anesthesia.

Septic Shock

Septic shock is characterized by profound peripheral vasodilation, increased cardiac output secondary to decreased systemic vascular resistance, increased vascular permeability with fluid loss from the vascular compartment, and development of disseminated intravascular coagulation. Septic shock is most commonly caused by gram-positive bacteria and less commonly by endotoxin-producing gram-negative bacteria. Endotoxins are bacterial membrane lipopolysaccharides that are made up of a toxic fatty acid (lipid A) core and a complex polysaccharide coat. Analogous molecules in the walls of gram-positive bacteria and fungi can also cause septic shock. The septic response is likely to reflect a systemic inflammatory response produced by exposure to bacterial cell products that ultimately lead to a progressively dysfunctional host response and multisystem organ failure. Elderly patients and those with immunosuppression are vulnerable to the development of sepsis and associated septic shock. The end stages of septic shock are not greatly different from the end stages of hemorrhagic shock, even though the initiating factors are markedly different. Mortality approaches 50% in septic shock despite significant improvements in supportive care.[14]

Measurement of Cardiac Output

The management of patients in the operating room and intensive care unit involves therapeutic interventions intended to optimize tissue oxygen delivery. Common interventions include fluid administration, blood transfusion, inotrope and vasoactive pharmacotherapy, heart rate and rhythm manipulation, mechanical assist devices, and mechanical ventilation. Ideally, these interventions should be guided by the measurement of cardiac output. However, cardiac output determination has traditionally required invasive techniques such as the insertion of pulmonary artery catheters. Recent advances in microprocessor technology, a greater awareness of the limitations and hazards of pulmonary artery catheter insertion, and a need to measure cardiac output in out of operating room settings such as the emergency department, have led to the development of newer monitoring techniques. The general trend has been to develop techniques that are less invasive and allow more frequent, or even continuous, measurement of cardiac output.[15] Nevertheless, the pulmonary artery thermodilution technique represents the clinical standard against which new techniques are compared.[16] Currently used methods of cardiac output measurement include Fick methods, indicator dilution methods, thermodilution, echocardiographic techniques, impedance cardiography, and pulse contour analysis.

Fick Method

Adolf Fick first described use of the "Fick principle" to estimate cardiac output in 1870. Cardiac output is estimated by dividing the oxygen consumption by the arteriovenous difference for oxygen (Fig. 14-16).[4] Oxygen consumption is usually measured by a respirometer containing a known oxygen mixture. The patient's exhaled gases are collected in a large inflatable reservoir (Douglas bag). The volume and oxygen concentrations of the exhaled gases are measured, allowing calculation of oxygen consumption. Venous blood used for calculation of oxygen content must be obtained from the right ventricle, or, ideally, the pulmonary artery, to ensure adequate mixing. Blood from the right atrium may not yet be adequately mixed to provide a true mixed venous sample. Blood used for determining the oxygen saturation in arterial blood can be obtained from any artery because all arterial blood is thoroughly mixed before it leaves the heart and therefore has the same concentration of oxygen.

The Fick principle can also be applied to carbon dioxide elimination from the lung.[17] The NICO (Novametrix Medical Systems, Inc., Wallingford, CT) is a continuous noninvasive monitor of cardiac output. By intermittently adding an additional dead space to the breathing circuit, CO_2 elimination is reduced thus increasing end-tidal CO_2. The change in end-tidal CO_2 is used to estimate the change in arterial CO_2 content. This proprietary system uses these data in a modified Fick equation to calculate cardiac output.

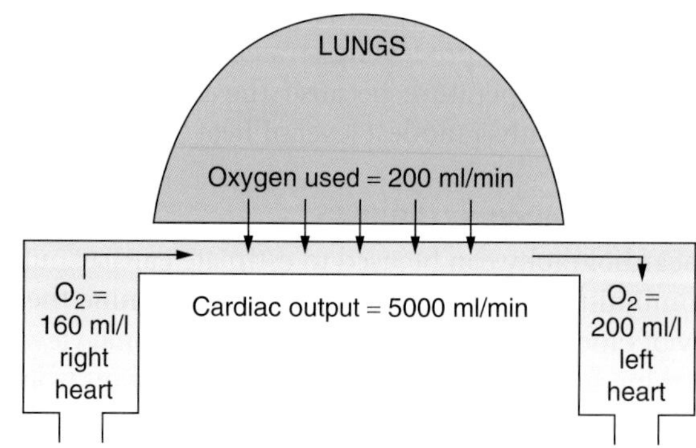

FIGURE 14-16 The Fick method calculates cardiac output as oxygen consumption divided by the arteriovenous difference for oxygen. (From Ganong WF. *Review of Medical Physiology*. 21st ed. New York, NY: McGraw-Hill; 2003, with permission.)

Indicator Dilution Method

In measuring the cardiac output by the indicator dilution method, a nondiffusible dye (indocyanine green) is injected into the right atrium (or central venous circulation), and the concentration of dye is subsequently measured continuously in the arterial circulation by a spectrophotometer. The area under the resulting time-concentration curve before recirculation of the dye occurs, combined with knowing the amount of dye injected, allows calculation of the pulmonary blood flow, which is the same as the cardiac output. It is necessary to extrapolate the dye curve to zero because recirculation of the dye occurs before the down slope of the curve reaches baseline. Early recirculation of the dye may indicate the presence of a right-to-left intracardiac shunt (foramen ovale), permitting direct passage of a portion of the dye to the left side of the heart without first passing through the lungs.

Thermodilution Method

A bolus of cold fluid may also be considered an indicator and used in the indicator dilution technique. A pulmonary artery catheter with ports in the right atrium and pulmonary artery and a temperature sensor on the distal port is used to measure thermodilution cardiac outputs. Thermodilution cardiac outputs are determined by measuring the change in blood temperature between two points (right atrium and pulmonary artery) after injection of a known volume of cold saline solution at the proximal right atrial port. The change in blood temperature as measured at the distal pulmonary artery port is inversely proportional to pulmonary blood flow (the extent to which the cold saline solution is diluted by blood), which is equivalent to cardiac output. The area under the temperature-time curve is converted to its equivalent in cardiac output. Advantages of this technique compared with the indicator dilution method include dissipation of cold in tissues so recirculation is not a problem, and safety of repeated and frequent measurements because saline is innocuous. Recent advances in thermodilution techniques include semicontinuous cardiac output determination using a heat-generating thermal filament incorporated into the pulmonary artery catheter. It is necessary to use sophisticated signal processing strategies to measure the downstream temperature because the thermal filament must generate only a modest level of heat for safety.

Echocardiographic Techniques

Echocardiography can be used to estimate cardiac output by combining the Doppler principle to determine the velocity of blood in the aorta with two-dimensional views to determine aortic diameter.[15] Conventional transesophageal or transthoracic echocardiographic techniques have the advantage that systolic and diastolic function, volume status, regional wall abnormalities, valve function, and the presence of pericardial effusion may also be evaluated. However, this technique requires significant operator expertise. More recently, Doppler techniques have been developed using transesophageal probes designed solely for the purpose of estimating cardiac output. Aortic dimensions are not measured but are estimated from age-, sex-, and body size–specific nomograms derived from large population studies. Transesophageal Doppler estimates of cardiac output require minimal operator training and allow rapid cardiac output estimation.

Impedance Cardiography

The thorax is a conductor whose impedance is altered by changes in blood volume and velocity with each cardiac cycle. Impedance cardiography is based on the principle of thoracic electrical bioimpedance and involves the placement of electrodes to allow the transmission of current and measurement of voltage across the chest.[18] Thus, thoracic electrical bioimpedance techniques can be used to noninvasively estimate cardiac output. However, the reliability of this technique is limited under several circumstances including patient movement, poor electrocardiogram signal quality, cardiac tachydysrhythmias, excessive thoracic fluid, and open chest wounds with metal retractors.

Pulse Contour Analysis

The first attempt to determine cardiac output from analysis of the pulse contour was made in 1904. The aortic pressure waveform is a function of the stroke volume and its interaction with the vascular tree. The arterial pulse contour can be modeled in a manner analogous to an electrical circuit that has specific values for resistance, compliance, and impedance.[17] Thus, the flow within that system can be estimated from the pressure waveform that is generated. The validity of this system is improved by calibration using a separate cardiac output estimation technique. However, in clinical practice, reliable use of this technique requires frequent recalibration because the peripheral circulation undergoes significant changes in arteriolar tone in response to physiologic and pharmacologic stimuli.

Microcirculation

The circulation exists to supply tissues with blood in amounts commensurate with their needs for oxygen and nutrients.[4] The microcirculation is defined as the circulation of blood through the smallest vessels of the body—arterioles, capillaries, and venules. Capillaries, whose walls consist of a single layer of endothelial cells, serve as the site for the rapid transfer of oxygen and nutrients to tissues and receipt of metabolic byproducts. There are an estimated 10 billion capillaries providing a total surface area that exceeds 6,300 m^2 for nutrient exchange. Capillary density varies from tissue to tissue. Capillaries are numerous in metabolically active tissues, such as cardiac and skeletal muscles, whereas in less active tissues, capillary density is low. Nevertheless, it is unlikely that any

Table 14-6

Anatomy of the Various Types of Blood Vessels

Vessel	Lumen Diameter	Approximate Cross-Sectional Area (cm^2)	Percentage of Blood Volume Contained
Aorta	2.5 cm	2.5	
Artery	0.4 cm	20	13
Arteriole	30 μm	40	1
Capillary	5 μm	2,500	6
Venule	20 μm	250	
Vein	0.5 cm	80	64[a]
Vena cava	3 cm	8	
Heart			7
Pulmonary circulation		18	9

[a]Blood volume contained in venules, veins, and vena cava.

functional cell is greater than 50 μm away from a capillary. The muscular arterioles serve as the major resistance vessels and regulate regional blood flow to the capillary beds. Venules act primarily as collecting channels and storage vessels.

Anatomy of the Microcirculation

Arterioles give rise to metarterioles, which give rise to capillaries (Table 14-6) (Fig. 14-17).[12] Other metarterioles serve as thoroughfare channels to the venules, bypassing the capillary bed. Capillaries drain via short collecting venules to the venules. Blood flow through capillaries is regulated by muscular precapillary sphincters present at the capillary opening. The arterioles, metarterioles, and venules contain smooth muscle. As a result, the arterioles serve as the major resistance vessels and regulate regional blood flow to the capillary beds, whereas the venules and veins serve primarily as collecting channels and storage or capacitance vessels.

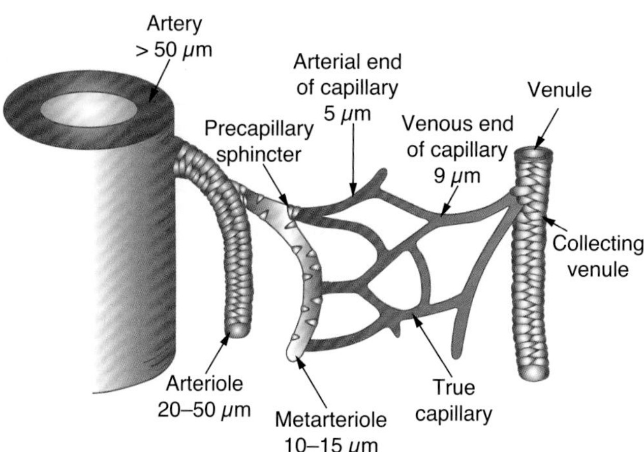

FIGURE 14-17 Anatomy of the microcirculation.

Capillary walls are about 1 μm thick, consisting of a single layer of endothelial cells surrounded by a thin basement membrane on the outside (Fig. 14-18).[12] The structure of the capillary wall varies from tissue to tissue, but in many organs, including those in skeletal, cardiac, and smooth muscle, the interdigitated junction between endothelial cells allows passage of molecules up to 10 nm in diameter. In addition, the cytoplasm of endothelial cells is attenuated to form gaps or pores that are 20 to 100 nm in diameter. These pores permit the passage of relatively large molecules. It also appears that plasma and its dissolved proteins are taken up by endocytosis, transported across endothelial cells, and discharged by exocytosis into

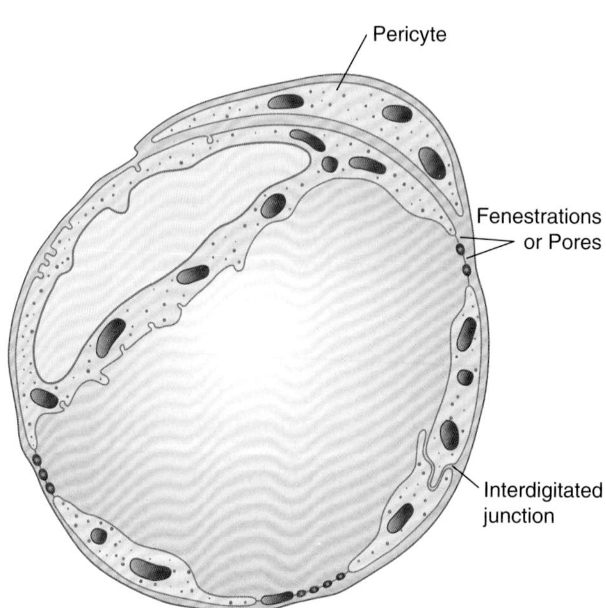

FIGURE 14-18 Capillaries include interdigitated junctions and pores to facilitate passage of lipid-insoluble ions and molecules.

the interstitial fluid. In the brain, the capillaries resemble those in skeletal muscles, except the interdigitated junctions between endothelial cells are tighter (blood–brain barrier), permitting passage of only small molecules.

The diameter of capillary pores is about 25 times the diameter of water molecules (0.3 nm), which are the smallest molecules that normally pass through capillary channels. Plasma proteins have diameters that exceed the width of capillary pores. Other substances, such as sodium, potassium, and chloride ions and glucose, have intermediate diameters (0.39 to 0.86 nm) such that permeability of capillary pores for different substances varies according to their molecular weights (Table 14-7). Oxygen and carbon dioxide are both lipid soluble and readily pass through endothelial cells.

True capillaries are devoid of smooth muscle and are therefore incapable of active constriction. Nevertheless, the endothelial cells that form them contain actin and myosin and can alter their shape in response to certain chemical stimuli. The diameter of capillaries (7 to 9 μm) is just sufficient to permit erythrocytes to squeeze through in single file. The thin walls of capillaries are able to withstand high intraluminal pressures because their small diameter prevents excessive wall tension (Laplace law).

Blood Flow in Capillaries

Blood flow in capillaries is approximately 1 mm per second and is intermittent rather than continuous. This intermittent blood flow reflects contraction and relaxation of metarterioles and precapillary sphincters in alternating cycles 6 to 12 times per minute.[19] The phenomenon of alternating contraction and relaxation is known as ***vasomotion***. Oxygen is the most important determinant of the degree of opening and closing of metarterioles and precapillary sphincters. A low Po_2 allows more blood to flow through capillaries to supply tissues. In this regard, the impact of oxygen on capillary blood flow provides a form of autoregulation of tissue blood flow.

In addition to nutritive blood flow through tissues that is regulated by oxygen, there is also nonnutritive (shunt) blood flow regulated by the autonomic nervous system. The nonnutritive blood flow is characterized by direct vascular connections between arterioles and venules. Some of these arteriovenous connections have muscular coverings so blood flow can be altered over a wide range. In some parts of the skin, these arteriovenous anastomoses provide a mechanism to permit rapid inflow of arterial blood to warm the skin and dissipate the heat.

Table 14-7

Permeability of Capillary Membranes

	Molecular Weight (Daltons)	Relative Permeability
Water	18	1.0
Sodium chloride	58.5	0.96
Glucose	180	0.6
Hemoglobin	66,700	0.01
Albumin	69,000	0.0001

Vasoactive Role of the Capillary Endothelium

The notion that the endothelium of capillaries is an inert single layer of cells serving only as a passive filter to permit passage of water and small molecules across the blood vessel wall is no longer considered valid.[20] Rather, the endothelium is now recognized as an important source of substances that cause contraction or relaxation of vascular smooth muscle.

One of these substances is prostacyclin that can relax vascular smooth muscle via an increase in cyclic adenosine monophosphate concentration. Prostacyclin is formed in the endothelium from arachidonic acid and the reaction is catalyzed by prostacyclin synthase. The principal function of prostacyclin is to inhibit platelet adherence to the endothelium and platelet aggregation and thus prevent intravascular clot formation.

The formation and release of nitric oxide (NO) is also important in the endothelium-mediated vascular dilation.[21] NO is released when endothelial cells are stimulated by acetylcholine or other vasodilator substances (adenosine triphosphate, bradykinin, serotonin, substance P, and histamine). NO release can be stimulated by the shear stress of blood flow on the endothelium. A vasoconstrictor peptide synthesized by the capillary endothelium is endothelin. Endothelin may affect vascular tone and blood pressure.

Fluid Movement across Capillary Membranes

Solvent and solute movement across capillary endothelial cells occurs by filtration, diffusion, and pinocytosis via endothelial vesicles.[22] Diffusion is the most important process for transcapillary exchange and pinocytosis is the least important. It is important to distinguish between filtration and diffusion through capillary membranes. Filtration is the net outward movement of fluid at the arterial end of capillaries. Diffusion of fluid occurs in both directions across capillary membranes.

Filtration

The four pressures that determine whether fluid will move outward across capillary membranes (filtration) or inward across capillary membranes (reabsorption) are capillary pressure, interstitial fluid pressure, plasma colloid osmotic pressure, and interstitial fluid colloid osmotic pressure. The net effect of these four pressures is a positive

Table 14-8

Filtration of Fluid at the Arterial Ends of Capillaries

Pressure favoring outward movement	
Capillary pressure	25 mm Hg
Interstitial fluid pressure	−6.3 mm Hg
Interstitial fluid colloid osmotic pressure	5 mm Hg
Total	36.3 mm Hg
Pressure favoring inward movement	
Plasma colloid osmotic pressure	28 mm Hg
Net filtration pressure	**8.3 mm Hg**

filtration pressure at the arterial end of capillaries, causing fluid to move outward across cell membranes into interstitial fluid spaces (Table 14-8). At the venous end of capillaries, the net effect of these four pressures is a positive reabsorption pressure causing fluid to move inward across capillary membranes into capillaries (Table 14-9). Overall, the mean values of the four pressures acting across capillary membranes are nearly identical such that the amount of fluid filtered nearly equals the amount reabsorbed (Table 14-10). Any fluid that is not reabsorbed enters the lymph vessels.

Traditionally, filtration has been considered to occur at the arterial end of the capillary and absorption to occur at the venous end because of the gradient of hydrostatic pressure along the capillary. Nevertheless, many capillaries only filter, whereas others only absorb. In some vascular beds such as the renal glomerulus, hydrostatic pressure in the capillary is high enough to cause filtration along the entire length of the capillary.

Capillary Pressure

Capillary pressure tends to move fluid outward across the arterial ends of capillary membranes. It is estimated that capillary pressure at the arterial end of capillaries is 25 mm Hg, whereas pressure at the venous end of capillaries is 10 mm Hg, corresponding to the pressure in venules. The mean capillary pressure is about 17 mm Hg. Changes in arterial pressure have little effect on capillary pressure and flow because of adjustments of precapillary resistance vessels. Autoregulation describes the maintenance of unchanged tissue blood flow despite changes in perfusion pressure.

Table 14-9

Reabsorption of Fluid at the Venous Ends of Capillaries

Pressure favoring outward movement	
Capillary pressure	10 mm Hg
Interstitial fluid pressure	−6.3 mm Hg
Interstitial fluid colloid osmotic pressure	5 mm Hg
Total	21.3 mm Hg
Pressure favoring inward movement	
Plasma colloid osmotic pressure	28 mm Hg
Net reabsorption pressure	**6.7 mm Hg**

Table 14-10

Mean Values of Pressures Acting across Capillary Membranes

Pressure favoring outward movement	
Capillary pressure	17 mm Hg
Interstitial fluid pressure	−6.3 mm Hg
Interstitial fluid colloid osmotic pressure	5 mm Hg
Total	28.3 mm Hg
Pressure favoring inward movement	
Plasma colloid osmotic pressure	28 mm Hg
Net overall filtration pressure	**0.3 mm Hg**

Interstitial Fluid Pressure

Interstitial fluid pressure tends to move fluid outward across capillary membranes. It is estimated that average interstitial fluid pressure is −6.3 mm Hg. This negative pressure acts as a vacuum to hold tissues together and maintain a minimal distance for diffusion of nutrients. Under normal conditions, almost all of the interstitial fluid is held in a gel that fills the spaces between cells. This gel contains large quantities of mucopolysaccharides, the most abundant of which is hyaluronic acid. Loss of negative interstitial fluid pressure allows fluid to accumulate in tissue spaces as edema.

Plasma Colloid Osmotic Pressure

Plasma proteins are principally responsible for the plasma colloid osmotic (oncotic) pressure that tends to cause movement of fluid inward through capillary membranes. Each gram of albumin exerts twice the colloid osmotic pressure of a gram of globulin. Because there is about twice as much albumin as globulin in the plasma, about 70% of the total colloid osmotic pressure results from albumin and only about 30% from globulin and fibrinogen.

A special phenomenon known as ***Donnan equilibrium*** causes the colloid osmotic pressure to be about 50% greater than that caused by proteins alone. This reflects the negative charge characteristic of proteins that necessitates the presence of an equal number of positively charged ions, mainly sodium ions, on the same side of the capillary membrane as the proteins. These extra positive ions increase the number of osmotically active substances and thus increase the colloid osmotic pressure. Indeed, about one-third of the normal plasma colloid osmotic pressure of 28 mm Hg is caused by positively charged ions held in the plasma by proteins. This is the reason that plasma proteins cannot be replaced by inert substances, such as dextran, without some decrease in plasma colloid osmotic pressure.

Interstitial Fluid Colloid Osmotic Pressure

Proteins present in the interstitial fluid are principally responsible for the interstitial fluid colloid osmotic pressure of about 5 mm Hg, which tends to cause movement of fluid outward across capillary membranes. Albumin, because of its small size, normally leaks 1.6 times as readily as globulins through capillaries, causing the proteins in interstitial fluids to have a disproportionately high albumin to globulin ratio. The total protein content of interstitial fluid is similar to the total protein content of plasma, but because the volume of the interstitial fluid is four times the volume of plasma, the average interstitial fluid protein content is only one-fourth that in plasma or about 1.8 g/dL. Interstitial fluid protein content also remains low because proteins cannot readily diffuse across capillary membranes, and any that crosses is likely to be removed by lymph vessels.

Diffusion

Diffusion is the most important mechanism for transfer of nutrients between the plasma and the interstitial fluid. Oxygen, carbon dioxide, and anesthetic gases are examples of lipid-soluble molecules that can diffuse directly through capillary membranes independently of pores. Sodium, potassium, and chloride ions and glucose are insoluble in lipid capillary membranes and therefore must pass through pores to gain access to interstitial fluids. The diffusion rate of lipid-soluble molecules across capillary membranes in either direction is proportional to the concentration difference between the two sides of the membrane. For this reason, large amounts of oxygen move from capillaries toward tissues, whereas carbon dioxide moves in the opposite direction. Typically, only slight partial pressure differences suffice to maintain adequate transport of oxygen between the plasma and interstitial fluid.

Pinocytosis

Pinocytosis is the process by which capillary endothelial cells ingest small amounts of plasma or interstitial fluid followed by migration to the opposite surface where the fluid is released. Transport of high-molecular-weight substances such as plasma proteins, glycoproteins, and polysaccharides (dextran) most likely occurs principally by pinocytosis.

Lymphatics

Lymph vessels represent an alternate route by which fluids flow from interstitial spaces into the blood. The most important function of the lymphatic system is return of proteins into the circulation and maintenance of a low-protein concentration in the interstitial fluid. The small amount of protein that escapes from the arterial end of the capillary cannot undergo reabsorption at the venous end of the capillary. If lymph vessels were not available, this protein would be progressively concentrated in the interstitial fluid, resulting in increases in interstitial fluid colloid osmotic pressure that, within a few hours, would produce life-threatening edema. Only cartilage, bone, epithelium, and tissues of the central nervous system are devoid of lymphatic vessels.

Anatomy

The major terminal lymph vessels are the thoracic duct and the right lymphatic duct (Fig. 14-19). The thoracic duct is the larger of the two (2 mm in diameter), entering the venous system in the angle of the junction of the left internal jugular and subclavian veins. The right lymphatic duct is not always present, and if it is, it rarely exists as such because the three vessels that occasionally unite to form it usually open separately into the right internal jugular, subclavian, and innominate veins. Damage (surgical or traumatic) to a thoracic duct can cause intrathoracic fluid accumulation.

Peripheral lymph vessels are small, difficult to identify, and contain flaplike valves between endothelial cells that open toward the interior, allowing the unimpeded entrance of interstitial fluid and proteins but preventing backflow.

Formation and Flow of Lymph

Lymph is interstitial fluid that flows into lymphatic vessels. The protein concentration of peripheral lymph is about 1.8 g/dL, whereas lymph from the gastrointestinal tract and liver contains two to three times this concentration of protein. The lymphatic system is one of the major

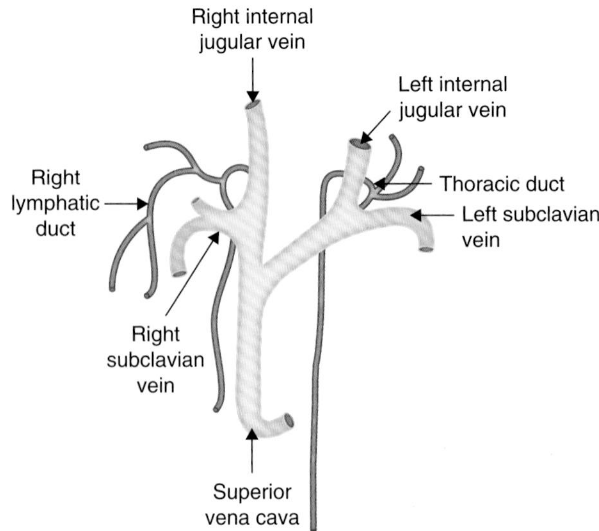

FIGURE 14-19 Depiction of the thoracic duct and right lymphatic duct as they enter the venous system.

channels for absorption of nutrients, especially fat, from the gastrointestinal tract. Bacteria that enter lymph vessels are removed and destroyed by lymph nodes.

Flow of lymph through the thoracic duct is about 100 mL per hour. A decrease in the normally negative value of interstitial fluid pressure increases the flow of interstitial fluid into terminal lymph vessels and consequently increases the rate of lymph flow. For example, at 0 mm Hg interstitial fluid pressure, the rate of lymph flow is increased 10 to 50 times compared with flow at an average interstitial fluid pressure of −6.3 mm Hg. Skeletal muscle contraction and passive movements of the extremities facilitate flow of lymph. For example, during exercise, lymph flow is increased up to 14 times that present at rest. Elevations in CVP can impair the return of lymph to the central circulation.

Edema

Edema is the presence of excess interstitial fluid in peripheral tissues that results from the inability of lymph vessels to adequately transport fluid. This may occur due to damage or obstruction of lymphatic vessels, excessive fluid administration, capillary fluid leakage due to increased permeability, low serum protein concentration, or elevated CVP. Peripheral edema most common in dependent areas may be accompanied by accumulation of fluid in potential spaces such as the pleural cavity, pericardial space, peritoneal cavity, and synovial spaces. Excessive fluid in the peritoneal space—one of the spaces most prone to develop edema fluid—is called ***ascites***. The peritoneal cavity is susceptible to the development of edema fluid because any increased pressure in the liver, such as occurs in cirrhosis or cardiac failure, causes transudation of protein-containing fluids from the surface of the liver into the peritoneal cavity.

Pulmonary Circulation

The pulmonary circulation is a low-pressure, low-resistance system in series with the systemic circulation. The volume of blood flowing through the lungs and systemic circulation is essentially identical. Blood passes through pulmonary capillaries in about 1 second, during which time it is oxygenated and carbon dioxide is removed.

Anatomy

Anatomically, the right ventricle is semilunar in shape, wrapped around the medial aspect of the left ventricle. The thickness of the right ventricle is one-third that of the left ventricle, as it normally generates pressures approximately 25% that of the left side.

The pulmonary artery extends only about 4 cm beyond the apex of the right ventricle before division into the right and left main pulmonary arteries. The pulmonary artery is a thin structure with a wall thickness about twice that of the vena cava and one-third that of the aorta. The large diameter and distensibility of the pulmonary arteries allows the pulmonary circulation to easily accommodate the stroke volume of the right ventricle. Pulmonary veins, like pulmonary arteries, are large in diameter and highly distensible. Pulmonary capillaries supply the estimated 300 million alveoli, providing a gas exchange surface of 70 m^2.

Pulmonary blood vessels are innervated by the sympathetic nervous system, but the density of these fibers is less than in systemic vessels. α-Adrenergic stimulation from norepinephrine produces vasoconstriction of the pulmonary vessels, whereas β-adrenergic stimulation, as produced by isoproterenol, results in vasodilation. Parasympathetic nervous system fibers from the vagus nerves release acetylcholine, which produces vasodilation of pulmonary vessels. Despite the presence of autonomic nervous system innervation, the resting vasomotor tone is minimal, and the larger pulmonary vessels are almost maximally dilated in the normal resting state. Indeed, overall regulation of pulmonary blood flow is passive, with local adjustments of perfusion relative to ventilation being determined by local oxygen tension.

The diameter of thin-walled alveolar vessels changes in response to alterations in the transmural pressure (intravascular pressure minus alveolar pressure). If alveolar pressure exceeds intravascular pressure as occurs in nondependent regions of the lungs during positive pressure ventilation, pulmonary capillaries collapse and blood flow ceases. The size of larger vessels embedded in the lung parenchyma (extraalveolar vessels) largely depends on lung volume. For example, resistance to flow through these vessels decreases as lung volumes increase because these vessels are tethered to the surrounding tissue (Fig. 14-20A,B). However, the largest pulmonary vessels, those at the hilum of the lung, vary in size in response to changes in intrapleural pressure.

Bronchial Circulation

Bronchial arteries from the thoracic aorta supply oxygenated blood to supporting tissues of the lungs, including connective tissue and airways. After bronchial arterial blood has passed through supporting tissues, the majority of it empties into pulmonary veins and enters the left atrium rather than passing back to the right atrium. The entrance of deoxygenated blood into the left atrium dilutes oxygenated blood and accounts for an anatomic shunt that is equivalent to an estimated 1% to 2% of the cardiac output. This anatomic shunt plus a part of coronary blood flow which drains directly into the left side of the heart are the reasons the cardiac output of the left ventricle slightly exceeds that of the right ventricle.

Pulmonary Lymph Vessels

Pulmonary lymph vessels extend from all the supportive tissues of the lung to the hilum of the lung and then to the thoracic duct. Pulmonary lymphatic flow facilitates the removal of edema fluid from alveolar spaces. Particulate

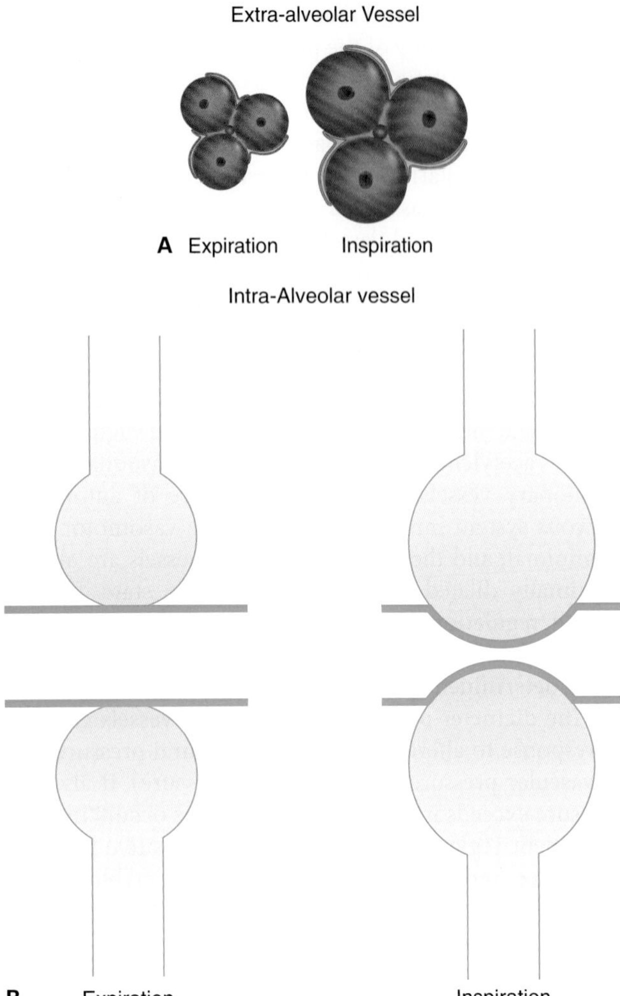

FIGURE 14-20 **A:** Schematic illustration of the effect of lung inflation on an extraalveolar vessel surrounded by three alveoli. Extraalveolar vessels are tethered by surrounding lung parenchyma and increase in caliber with lung inflation. **B:** Schematic illustration of an intraalveolar vessel adjacent to two alveoli. Intraalveolar vessels are compressed during lung inflation.

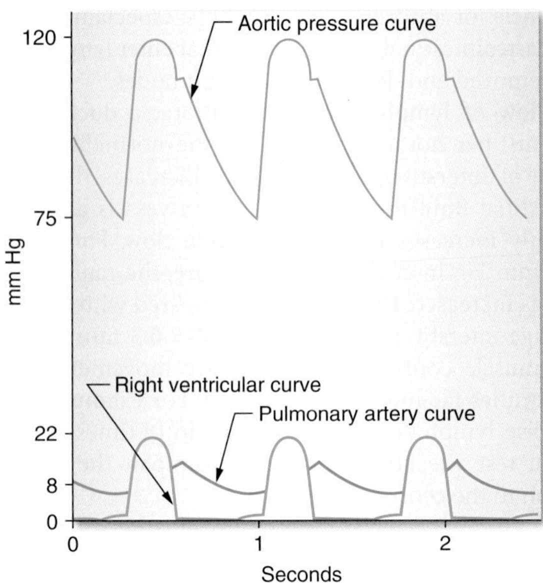

FIGURE 14-21 Comparison of intravascular pressures in the systemic and pulmonary circulations. (From Guyton AC, Hall JE. *Textbook of Medical Physiology.* 10th ed. Philadelphia, PA: Saunders; 2000, with permission.)

matter entering the alveoli is also eventually removed by lymph vessels.

Pulmonary Vascular Pressure

The normal pressure in the pulmonary artery is about 22/8 mm Hg, with a mean pulmonary artery pressure of 13 mm Hg (Fig. 14-21).[4] The mean pulmonary capillary pressure is about 10 mm Hg, and the mean pressure in the pulmonary veins is about 4 mm Hg, such that the pressure gradient across the pulmonary circulation is only 9 mm Hg. The resistance to blood flow in the pulmonary circulation is about one-tenth the resistance in the systemic circulation.

Pulmonary artery pressure is not typically influenced by left atrial pressures of less than 7 mm Hg. However, when left atrial pressure exceeds approximately 7 mm Hg, previously collapsed pulmonary veins are expanded, and pulmonary artery pressure increases in parallel with increases in left atrial pressure. In the absence of left ventricular failure, even marked increases in systemic vascular resistance do not cause the left atrial pressure to increase significantly. Consequently, the right ventricle continues to eject its stroke volume against a normal pulmonary artery pressure despite increased workloads imposed on the left ventricle. Accordingly, the right ventricular stroke volume is not measurably altered by changes in systemic vascular resistance unless the left ventricle fails.

Should the left ventricle fail, left atrial pressures can increase to greater than 15 mm Hg. Mean pulmonary artery pressures also increase, placing an increased workload on the right ventricle. If this occurs acutely, the right ventricle may also fail as it may not be able to generate an adequate stroke volume due to its structure (see earlier discussion). If pulmonary artery pressures rise gradually over time, the right ventricle may adapt with remodeling and dilation but will eventually begin to fail.

Measurement of Left Atrial Pressure

The left atrial pressure can be estimated by inserting a balloon-tipped catheter into a small pulmonary artery. When the balloon is temporarily inflated and the vessel is completely occluded, a stationary column of blood is created distal to the catheter tip. As a result, the pressure measured immediately distal to the balloon is equivalent to that downstream in the pulmonary veins. This measurement is termed the ***pulmonary artery occlusion pressure*** ("wedge" pressure although the catheter is not truly wedged) and is usually 2 to 3 mm Hg higher than left atrial pressure. If the balloon is deflated, flow will resume and the pulmonary artery end diastolic pressure can be measured. This measurement correlates with the pulmonary artery occlusion pressure in the absence of pulmonary hypertension.

Interstitial Fluid Space

The interstitial fluid space in the lung is minimal, and a continual negative pulmonary interstitial pressure of about −8 mm Hg dehydrates interstitial fluid spaces of the lungs and keeps the alveolar epithelial membrane in close approximation to the capillary membranes. As a result, the diffusion distance between gas in the alveoli and the capillary blood is minimal, averaging about 0.4 μm. Negative pressure in pulmonary interstitial spaces draws fluid from alveoli through alveolar membranes and into the interstitium, keeping the alveoli dry. Mean pulmonary capillary pressure is about 10 mm Hg, whereas plasma colloid osmotic pressure is about 28 mm Hg. This net pressure gradient of about 18 mm Hg discourages the movement of fluid out of capillaries, decreasing the likelihood of pulmonary edema.

Pulmonary Blood Volume

Blood volume in the lungs is about 450 mL. Of this amount, about 70 mL is in capillaries and the remainder is divided equally between pulmonary arteries and veins. Cardiac failure or increased resistance to flow through the mitral valve causes pulmonary blood volume to increase.

Cardiac output can increase nearly four times before pulmonary artery pressure becomes increased (Fig. 14-22).[4] This reflects the distensibility of the pulmonary arteries and opening of previously collapsed pulmonary capillaries. The ability of the lungs to accept greatly increased amounts of pulmonary blood flow, as during exercise, without excessive increases in pulmonary artery pressures is important in preventing development of pulmonary edema or right ventricular failure.

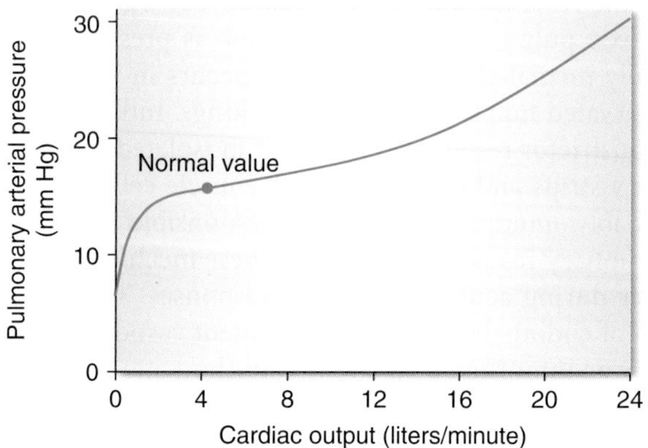

FIGURE 14-22 Cardiac output can increase nearly fourfold without greatly increasing the pulmonary arterial pressure. (From Guyton AC, Hall JE. *Textbook of Medical Physiology*. 10th ed. Philadelphia, PA: Saunders; 2000, with permission.)

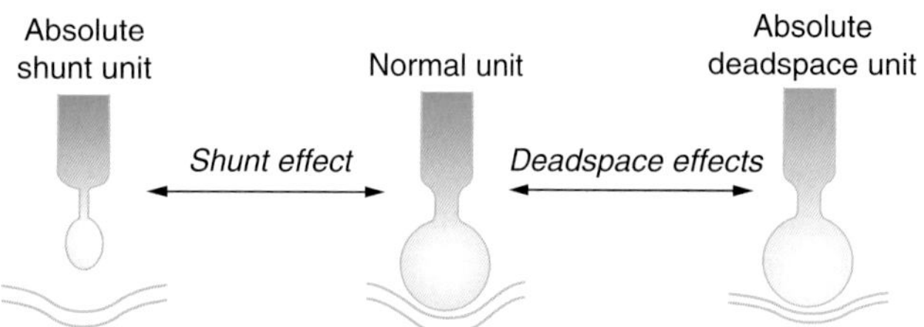

FIGURE 14-23 Gas exchange is maximally effective in normal lung units with optimal ventilation to perfusion (V/Q) relationships. The continuum of (V/Q) relationships is depicted by the ratios between normal and absolute shunt or dead space units.

Pulmonary blood volume can increase up to 40% when an individual changes from the standing to the supine position. This sudden shift of blood from the systemic circulation to pulmonary circulation is responsible for the decrease in vital capacity in the supine position and the occurrence of orthopnea in the presence of left ventricular failure.

Pulmonary Blood Flow and Distribution

Optimal oxygenation depends on matching ventilation to pulmonary blood flow.[23] Shunt occurs in lung areas that are perfused but inadequately ventilated, whereas dead space ventilation occurs in lung areas that are ventilated but inadequately perfused (Fig. 14-23). Although the lungs are innervated by the autonomic nervous system, it is doubtful that neural influences exert a major effect in the normal control of pulmonary blood flow. There is no doubt, however, that decreases in Pa_{O_2} cause increases in pulmonary artery and right ventricular pressures.

Clinically, segmental pulmonary blood flow can be studied by intravenous injection of radioactive xenon while monitoring is performed externally over the chest with radiation detectors. Xenon rapidly diffuses from capillaries into alveoli and radioactivity is detected early in well-perfused regions of the lung.

Endothelial Regulation of Pulmonary Blood Flow

Active vasodilation is crucial to the maintenance of the low resting tone of the normal pulmonary circulation. The pulmonary vascular endothelium is responsible for the synthesis and secretion of various compounds that regulate smooth muscle activity in the pulmonary circulation. The primary vasodilatory compounds are NO and prostacyclin. The predominant influence of a healthy pulmonary endothelium is to reduce pulmonary vascular tone. Endothelin is also released by the pulmonary endothelium and may have both a constrictive or dilatory effect depending on the circumstances. There are several negative feedback mechanisms in effect that regulate vascular tone. The synthesis and release of NO, prostacyclin, ET-1, and other vasoactive compounds are integrated into a system that optimizes pulmonary vascular tone and facilitates local control of ventilation to perfusion (V/Q) matching. Therapeutically, inhaled NO, intravenous and inhaled prostacyclin, and oral endothelin antagonists are used to treat pulmonary hypertension.

Nitric Oxide

NO is synthesized in endothelial cells by NO synthase (NOS). There are several isoforms of NOS, but it is likely that cNOS (also termed ***endothelial NOS*** or ***eNOS***) is responsible for the normal regulation of pulmonary vascular tone. The activity of cNOS is rapidly up- or downregulated and produces picomolar amounts of NO in response to stimuli such as shear stress and local oxygen tension. In pathologic states, another NOS isoform, iNOS, produces considerably larger quantities of NO but takes longer to upregulate and downregulate. iNOS is located in vascular smooth muscle cells and inflammatory macrophages. Inflammatory mediators are potent upregulators of iNOS activity. NO diffuses from its site of production, usually endothelial cells, into adjacent pulmonary vascular smooth muscle cells. NO induces vasorelaxation by stimulating the production of cyclic guanosine monophosphate (cGMP) by the enzyme guanylate cyclase. cGMP is promptly metabolized by phosphodiesterases. Increased cGMP production appears to stimulate phosphodiesterase upregulation, thus causing accelerating cGMP clearance. Indeed, phosphodiesterase upregulation may be partly responsible for suboptimal responses to inhaled NO and for rebound pulmonary hypertension after NO withdrawal. Type V phosphodiesterase is the predominant enzyme type in the pulmonary circulation. Selective inhibitors of type V phosphodiesterase such as sildenafil can both selectively decrease pulmonary vascular resistance when given alone and significantly potentiate the effects of iNOS and prostacyclin.

Endothelin

ET-1 is a potent endogenous peptide vasoconstrictor that also promotes smooth muscle proliferation. Endothelin has been implicated in the pathogenesis of some types of pulmonary hypertension because some patients have both increased expression and reduced clearance of ET-1 in lung tissue and plasma. There are two endothelin receptors: vascular smooth muscle endothelin A and endothelial endothelin B. Smooth muscle endothelin A receptor stimulation causes vasoconstriction, whereas endothelial endothelin B receptor stimulation causes both vasoconstriction and relaxation. ET-1 release is increased as part of the inflammatory response to cardiopulmonary bypass, thereby increasing the potential for pulmonary hypertension after cardiovascular surgery. Exposure to inhaled NO significantly increases ET-1 levels, suggesting that ET-1 may be partly responsible for rebound pulmonary hypertension after withdrawal of inhaled NO. Endothelin antagonists may prove to be useful in the treatment of pulmonary hypertension. Bosentan is an oral, nonselective endothelin antagonist that is used in the treatment of pulmonary hypertension.

Prostacyclin

Prostacyclin is a potent vasodilatory prostaglandin released by the pulmonary endothelium. Other prostaglandins, such as thromboxane A_2, have potent vasoconstrictive effects. Pulsatile flow and local shear stress are important stimuli for prostacyclin release. Prostacyclin receptor binding causes the activation of adenylate cyclase, thereby increasing local adenosine-3,5 cyclic monophosphate release. The adenyl cyclase pathway, regulated by prostacyclin, and the guanylate cyclase pathway, regulated by NO, are parallel pathways that converge to reduce vascular smooth muscle tone. Prostacyclin is also an extremely potent inhibitor of platelet aggregation and vascular smooth muscle proliferation. The chronic intravenous administration of prostacyclin is an established treatment for pulmonary hypertension and was first described more than 20 years ago. However, intravenous prostacyclin is not a selective pulmonary vasodilator and can cause significant systemic side effects, including hypotension, and will worsen V/Q matching in the pulmonary circulation. Both the positive and negative hemodynamic effects of prostacyclin are potentiated by the coadministration of phosphodiesterase inhibitors. Of particular interest to anesthesiologists are the encouraging findings with the inhaled aerosolized prostacyclin analogues iloprost and treprostinil. These drugs have physical characteristics that make them better suited to nebulization and have longer duration of action than intravenous prostacyclin.

Hypoxic Pulmonary Vasoconstriction

Alveolar hypoxia (Pao_2 <70 mm Hg) evokes vasoconstriction in the pulmonary arterioles supplying these alveoli. The net effect is to divert blood flow away from poorly ventilated alveoli. As a result, the shunt effect is minimized, and the resulting Pao_2 is maximized. The mechanism for hypoxic pulmonary vasoconstriction is presumed to be locally mediated, as this response occurs in isolated and denervated lungs as well as intact lungs. Indeed, this vasoconstrictor response is apparent in isolated pulmonary artery strips and isolated smooth muscle cells. There are probably multiple mechanisms responsible for hypoxic pulmonary vasoconstriction and these mechanisms likely differ during acute and chronic responses. The suppression of endothelial release of the potent vasodilator NO is likely an important element of both the acute and chronic response. A crucial component of the acute response is the inhibition of potassium channels that leads to membrane depolarization. Membrane depolarization increases calcium influx, which in turn activates the intracellular contractile response. Chronic vascular responses to hypoxia may be, in part, mediated by endothelin release and eventually involve vascular remodeling, eventually leading to irreversible increases in pulmonary vascular resistance (pulmonary hypertension).

Drug-induced inhibition of hypoxic pulmonary vasoconstriction could result in unexpected decreases in Pa_{O_2} in the presence of lung disease. Potent vasodilating drugs such as nitroprusside and nitroglycerin may be accompanied by decreases in Pa_{O_2} attributed to this effect.[24] Although animal studies suggest that potent inhaled anesthetic agents inhibit hypoxic vasoconstriction in a dose-dependent manner, in clinically relevant concentrations, these findings have not been supported by clinical studies in patients (Fig. 14-24).[25,26] The present consensus is that potent volatile anesthetics are acceptable choices for thoracic surgery requiring one-lung ventilation, particularly in view of the beneficial effects of these drugs on bronchomotor tone and their high potency that permits delivery of maximal concentrations of oxygen.[27]

Effect of Breathing

During spontaneous respiration, venous return to the heart is increased due to contraction of the diaphragm and abdominal muscles, which decreases intrathoracic pressure. The resulting augmented blood flow to the right atrium increases right ventricular stroke volume. In contrast to spontaneous breathing, positive pressure ventilation increases intrathoracic pressure and thus impedes venous return to the heart and decreases right ventricular stroke volume.

Regional Blood Flow in the Lungs

Although traditional teaching has focused on the gravitational effect of blood flow within the lungs, more recent work has demonstrated that the gravitational "zone"[28] (Fig. 14-25) has a relatively minor role in blood flow distribution. On average, pulmonary blood flow is greater in areas of the lung below the heart as compared to those above the heart,[29] but measurements have demonstrated greater variation from spot to spot in any isogravitational plane than there is on average from the top of the lung to the bottom. Indeed, only 25% of the variability in pulmonary blood flow is accounted for by gravitational effects. Furthermore, the local differences in flow at any isogravitational level are fairly constant over time, suggesting that approximately 75% of the distribution of pulmonary blood flow is determined by the branching structure of the pulmonary vascular tree.

Pulmonary Circulatory Pathology

Pulmonary Edema

Pulmonary edema is present when there are excessive quantities of fluid either in pulmonary interstitial spaces or in alveoli. Mild degrees of pulmonary edema may be limited to only an increase in the interstitial fluid volume. The alveolar epithelium, however, is not able to withstand more than a modest increase in interstitial fluid pressure before fluid spills into alveoli. Dehydrating forces of the colloid osmotic pressure of the blood in the lungs provide

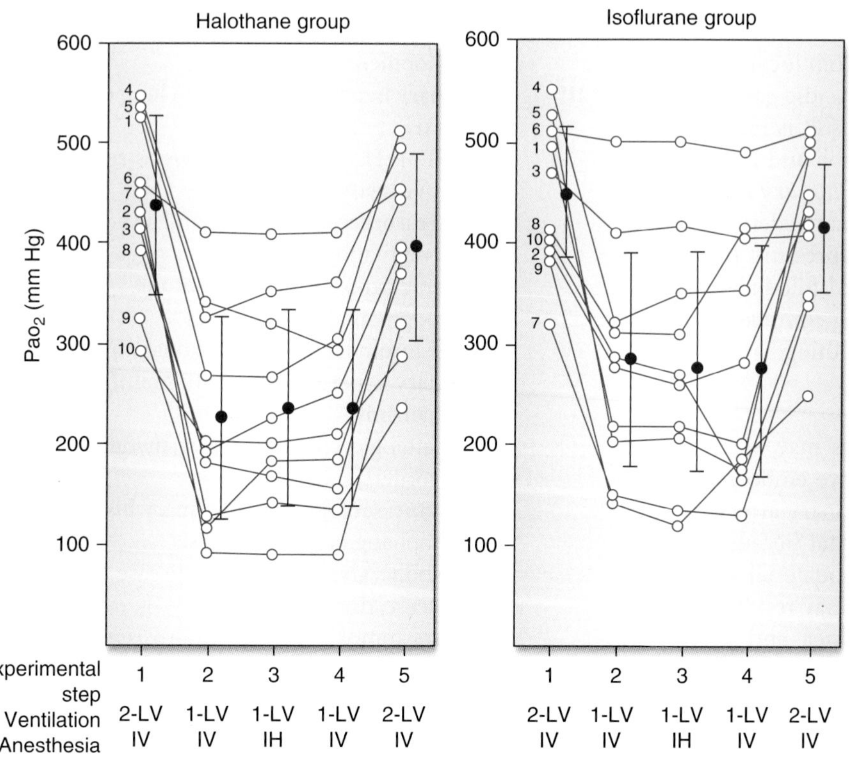

FIGURE 14-24 Pa_{O_2} was measured during two-lung ventilation (2-LV) and then during one-lung ventilation (1-LV) in patients anesthetized with fentanyl and diazepam without halothane or isoflurane (experimental steps 2 and 4) and with halothane or isoflurane (experimental step 3). Addition of halothane or isoflurane (about 1.2 minimum alveolar concentration) does not alter the Pa_{O_2}, suggesting these drugs do not inhibit hypoxic pulmonary vasoconstriction. Clear circles are individual patient data and closed circles are mean ± SD for each group. (From Rogers SN, Benumof JL. Halothane and isoflurane do not decrease Pa_{O_2} during one-lung ventilation in intravenously anesthetized patients. *Anesth Analg.* 1985;64:946–954, with permission.)

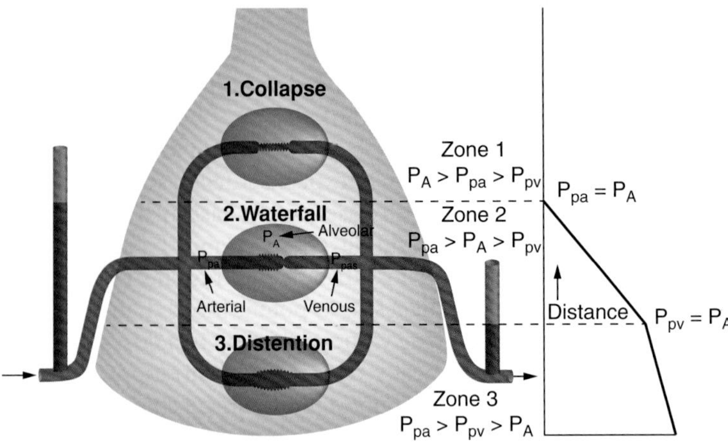

FIGURE 14-25 The lung is divided into three pulmonary blood flow zones reflecting the impact of alveolar pressure (P_A), pulmonary artery pressure (P_{pa}), and pulmonary venous pressure (P_{pv}) on the caliber of pulmonary blood vessels. (From West JB, Dollery CT, Naimark A. Distribution of blood flow in isolated lung: relation to vascular and alveolar pressures. *J Appl Physiol.* 1964;19:713–718, with permission.)

a large safety factor against development of pulmonary edema. In humans, plasma colloid osmotic pressure is about 28 mm Hg, so pulmonary edema rarely develops below a pulmonary capillary pressure of 30 mm Hg. The most common cause of acute pulmonary edema is greatly increased pulmonary capillary pressure resulting from left ventricular failure, and the lymphatic flow cannot adequately remove the increased fluid.

During chronic increases of left atrial pressure, pulmonary edema may not occur despite pulmonary capillary pressures as high as 45 mm Hg. Enlargement of the pulmonary lymph vessels allowing lymph flow to increase up to 20 times is the most likely reason pulmonary edema does not occur in the presence of chronically increased left atrial pressures. At the other end of the spectrum, a transplanted lung does not have any lymphatic drainage and is acutely sensitive to fluid overload or increased in left atrial pressure.

Pulmonary edema can also result from local capillary damage that occurs with inhalation of acidic gastric fluid or irritant gases, such as smoke. The result is rapid transudation of fluid and proteins into alveoli and interstitial spaces. This is called ***permeability pulmonary edema*** to distinguish it from "hydrostatic" pulmonary edema, which is due to increased pulmonary capillary pressure. In either case, increased interstitial fluid and fluid-filled alveoli interfere with gas exchange, decrease lung compliance, and result in an increase in the work of breathing.

Pulmonary Embolism

Embolism of venous clots to the lungs may be chronic with small emboli or acute with massive embolus. Total blockage of a major branch of a pulmonary artery by an embolus is usually not immediately fatal because other lung regions may be able to accommodate all the pulmonary blood flow, but major emboli may result in right ventricular strain and failure. Tachypnea and dyspnea are characteristic responses in awake patients experiencing pulmonary embolism; in the anesthetized patient, an acute decrease in end-tidal CO_2 may occur due to a sudden increase in dead space (loss of perfusion but not

Table 14-11

Classification of Pulmonary Hypertension

I	Pulmonary arterial hypertension (PAH)
	Idiopathic PAH (majority) and heritable PAH
	Drug- and toxin-induced PAH
	Connective tissue disease–associated PAH
	HIV-associated PAH
	Portal hypertension–associated PAH
	Congenital heart diseases
	Schistosomiasis
II	Pulmonary hypertension due to left heart disease
	LV systolic and diastolic dysfunction
	Valvular disease
	Congenital/acquired left heart inflow/outflow tract obstruction
	Developmental lung diseases
III	Pulmonary hypertension dues to lung diseases or hypoxia
	COPD, ILD, mixed restrictive/obstructive pattern disease
	Sleep disordered breathing and alveolar hypoventilation disorders
	Chronic exposure to high altitude
	Developmental lung diseases
IV	Chronic thromboembolic pulmonary hypertension
V	Pulmonary hypertension due to multifactorial mechanisms
	Hematologic: chronic anemia, myoproliferative disorders, splenectomy
	Systemic: sarcoidosis, pulmonary histiocytosis, lymphangioleiomyomatosis
	Metabolic: glycogen storage disease, Gaucher's disease, thyroid disease
	Others: tumor obstruction, fibrosis mediastinitis

From Simonneau G, Gatzoulis MA, Adatia I, et al. Updated clinical classification of pulmonary hypertension. *J Am Coll Cardiol.* 2013;62(25)(suppl):D34–D41.

ventilation to major part of the lung). Depending on the circumstance, anticoagulation, thrombolysis, or pulmonary embolectomy may be indicated.

Pulmonary Hypertension

The World Health Organization has classified pulmonary hypertension according to etiology (Table 14-11)[30] but the hemodynamic diagnosis in all causes is made when the sustained mean pulmonary artery pressure is above 25 mm Hg. The cause may be "primary" or idiopathic (type 1) or in association with other disease (other types). As mentioned earlier, gradual increases in pulmonary artery pressure may be tolerated by the right heart, but with progressive increases in pressure, right ventricular failure will eventually occur. In addition, many of the causes of pulmonary hypertension are associated with the development of hypoxemia. Treatment of the underlying cause, where possible, is of course more effective than treatment of the result, that is, oxygen for hypoxemia and pulmonary vasodilators; the pulmonary dilators mentioned earlier may not be effective or be associated with intolerable side effects. Lung transplant or in the case of right ventricular failure, heart–lung transplant may be required.

References

1. Galley HF, Webster NR. Physiology of the endothelium. *Br J Anaesth.* 2004;93:105–113.
2. Myburgh JA, Mythen MG. Resuscitation fluids. *N Engl J Med.* 2013;369:1243–1251.
3. Young JD. The heart and circulation in severe sepsis. *Br J Anaesth.* 2004;93:114–120.
4. Guyton AC, Hall JE. *Textbook of Medical Physiology.* 10th ed. Philadelphia, PA: Saunders; 2000.
5. Gerber MJ, Hines RL, Barash PG. Arterial waveforms and systemic vascular resistance: is there a correlation? *Anesthesiology.* 1987;66:823–825.
6. Pauca AL, Hudspeth AS, Wallenhaupt SL, et al. Radial artery-to-aorta pressure difference after discontinuation of cardiopulmonary bypass. *Anesthesiology.* 1989;70:935–941.
7. Stern DH, Gerson JI, Allen FB, et al. Can we trust the direct radial artery pressure immediately following cardiopulmonary bypass? *Anesthesiology.* 1985;62:557–561.
8. Baba T, Goto T, Yoshitake A, et al. Radial artery diameter decreases with increased femoral to radial arterial pressure gradient during cardiopulmonary bypass. *Anesth Analg.* 1997;85:252–258.
9. Rich GF, Lubanski RE, McLoughlin TM. Differences between aortic and radial artery pressure associated with cardiopulmonary bypass. *Anesthesiology.* 1992;77:63–66.
10. Bazaral MG, Welch M, Golding LAR, et al. Comparison of brachial and radial arterial pressure monitoring in patients undergoing coronary artery bypass surgery. *Anesthesiology.* 1990;73:38–45.
11. Cook DJ, Simel DL. Does this patient have abnormal central venous pressure? *JAMA.* 1996;275:630–634.
12. Ganong WF. *Review of Medical Physiology.* 21st ed. New York, NY: McGraw-Hill; 2003.
13. Cohen MA, Taylor JA. Short-term cardiovascular oscillations in man: measuring and modeling the physiologies. *J Physiol.* 2002;542(pt 3): 669–683.
14. Kaukonen KM, Bailey M, Suzuki S, et al. Mortality related to severe sepsis and septic shock among critically ill patients in Australia and New Zealand, 2000-2012. *JAMA.* 2014;311(13):1308–1316.
15. Tibby SM, Murdoch IA. Measurement of cardiac output and tissue perfusion. *Curr Opin Pediatr.* 2002;14:303–309.
16. Moise SF, Sinclair CJ, Scott DHT. Pulmonary artery blood temperature and the measurement of cardiac output by thermodilution. *Anaesthesia.* 2002;57:562–566.
17. Berton C, Cholley B. Equipment review: new techniques for cardiac output measurement–oesophageal Doppler, Fick principle using carbon dioxide, and pulse contour analysis. *Crit Care.* 2002;6:216–221.
18. Summers RL, Shoemaker WC, Peacock WF, et al. Bench to bedside: electrophysiologic and clinical principles of noninvasive hemodynamic monitoring using impedance cardiography. *Acad Emerg Med.* 2003;10:669–680.
19. Welsch DG, Segal SS. Endothelial and smooth muscle cell conduction in arterioles controlling blood flow. *Am J Physiol.* 1998;274:H323–H328.
20. Berne RM, Levy MN, Koeppen BM. *Physiology.* 5th ed. St Louis, MO: Mosby; 2004.
21. Feng Q, Hedner T. Endothelium-derived relaxing factor (EDRF) and nitric oxide. II. Physiology, pharmacology, and pathophysiological implications. *Clin Physiol.* 1990;10:503–510.
22. Michel CC, Neal CR. Openings through endothelial cells associated with increased permeability. *Microcirculation.* 1999;6:45–51.
23. West JB. Blood flow to the lung and gas exchange. *Anesthesiology.* 1974;41:124–138.
24. Colley PS, Cheney FW, Hlastala MP. Ventilation-perfusion and gas exchange effects of sodium nitroprusside in dogs with normal and edematous lungs. *Anesthesiology.* 1979;50:489–495.
25. Rogers SN, Benumof JL. Halothane and isoflurane do not decrease Pao_2 during one-lung ventilation in intravenously anesthetized patients. *Anesth Analg.* 1985;64:946–954.
26. Carlsson AJ, Bindsley L, Hedenstierna G. Hypoxia-induced pulmonary vasoconstriction in the human lung: the effect of isoflurane anesthesia. *Anesthesiology.* 1987;66:312–316.
27. Eisenkraft JB. Effects of anaesthetics on the pulmonary circulation. *Br J Anaesth.* 1990;65:63–78.
28. West JB, Dollery CT, Naimark A. Distribution of blood flow in isolated lung: relation to vascular and alveolar pressures. *J Appl Physiol.* 1964;19:713–718.
29. Glenny RW, Bernard S, Robertson HT, et al. Gravity is an important but secondary determinant of regional pulmonary blood flow in upright primates. *J Appl Physiol.* 1999;86:623–632.
30. Simonneau G, Gatzoulis MA, Adatia I, et al. Updated clinical classification of pulmonary hypertension. *J Am Coll Cardiol.* 2013;62(25) (suppl):D34–D41.

CHAPTER 15

Cardiac Physiology

Sumeet Goswami • Bessie Kachulis • Teresa A. Mulaikal • Jack S. Shanewise

The heart has four chambers and can be characterized as two pumps connected in series, each composed of an atrium and a ventricle. The atria function primarily as conduits to the ventricles, but they also contract weakly to facilitate movement of blood into the ventricles during the filling phase, diastole. The ventricles serve as pumps during systole to supply the main force that propels blood through the systemic and pulmonary circulations. Specialized excitatory and conductive fibers in the heart maintain cardiac rhythm and transmit action potentials through cardiac muscle to initiate contraction. Because the heart is coupled to two circulations in series, its function is influenced by the characteristics of both.

Cardiac Anatomy

Pericardium

The pericardium is a fibrous sac that contains the heart and the proximal portions of great vessels. It consists of two layers, the fibrous and serosal pericardium. The fibrous layer is fibrocollagenous and is continuous superiorly with the adventitia of the great vessels and the pretracheal fascia and inferiorly with the diaphragm. Anteriorly, the fibrous layer attaches to the sternum through the sternopericardial ligaments. The aorta, pulmonary arteries, and pulmonary veins also receive extensions from the fibrous pericardium. The serosal layer of the pericardium is enclosed within the fibrous pericardium and consists of a single, continuous membrane that is divided into two parts, the visceral and the parietal pericardium. The visceral layer surrounds the heart and the great vessels and is reflected on to the parietal layer that lines the inner surface of the fibrous pericardium.[1–3]

The potential space between visceral and parietal pericardium normally contains 15 to 35 mL of pericardial fluid. The inelastic nature of the pericardium limits acute dilation of the heart and enhances the resulting mechanical interaction of the four cardiac chambers. Acutely, the pericardium can only accommodate a small amount of pericardial fluid without changes in intrapericardial pressure. Once the amount of pericardial fluid exceeds a limited reserve capacity, the intrapericardial pressure increases steeply with small amounts of pericardial fluid, leading to tamponade physiology. Chronically, the pericardium can accommodate a large amount of fluid without causing tamponade because its size and compliance increase in compensation.[1–3]

Heart

The heart consists of four chambers. The right atrium receives deoxygenated blood from the superior vena cava, the inferior vena cava, the coronary sinus, and Thebesian cardiac veins. It pumps deoxygenated blood into right ventricle through the tricuspid valve. The right atrium is divided into three regions, the posteriorly located smooth-walled venous component, the anteriorly located vestibule of the tricuspid valve, and the right auricle. The venous component, or the sinus venosum, receives the vena cavae and the coronary sinus. The venous part of the atrium is separated from atrium proper and the auricle by a ridge of muscle called the ***crista terminalis***. The pectinate muscles are muscular trabeculae that extend anterolaterally from crista terminals into the auricle. Anterior to the orifice of inferior vena cava is the eustachian valve, which in the fetal circulation directs oxygen-rich blood from placenta into left atrium through the foramen ovale of atrial septum. The fossa ovalis is the thin part of the atrial septum, above and to the left of the orifice of inferior vena cava. The vestibule of the tricuspid valve is the anteroinferior portion of right atrium.[1,4]

The atrioventricular valvular complex, both on the right and the left side (tricuspid and mitral valve), consists of the annulus, the leaflets, the chordae tendineae, and the papillary muscles. The tricuspid valve is so named as it has three leaflets, one each located anterosuperiorly, septally, and inferiorly. The chordae tendineae are fibrous collagenous structures that support the leaflets of tricuspid and mitral valves during systole. True chordae arise usually from the papillary muscles or from the ventricular free wall and the septum. There are three papillary muscles in the right ventricle: two larger, located in the anterior and posterior positions of the right ventricle, and a smaller muscle arising from the ventricular septum.[1,4]

The right ventricle consists of the inlet adjacent to the tricuspid valve and the apex, both of which are trabeculated. The smooth-walled infundibulum or the outlet connects to the pulmonic valve. The inlet and outlet components are separated by a transverse ridge of muscle called the supraventricular crest or the crista supraventricularis. The many muscular ridges and protrusions into the inner surface of the inlet and apex are known as trabeculae carneae. The septal band or the septomarginal trabecula reinforces the septal surface; at the apex, it supports the anterior papillary muscle, from where it crosses to the parietal wall of the ventricle as the moderator band. The pulmonic valve is located at the distal end of the infundibulum and consists of three semilunar cusps, an anterior, a right, and a left cusp.[1,4]

The left atrium is normally smaller in size than the right but has thicker walls. The right atrium is anterior and somewhat to the right of the left atrium. The right and the left atrium are separated by the obliquely positioned atrial septum. The superior posterior aspect of the left atrium receives the pulmonary veins and forms the anatomic base of the heart. The left auricle is longer and narrower than the right auricle and is the only portion of the left atrium that is trabeculated.[1,4]

The mitral valve apparatus consists of an orifice with an annulus, anterior and posterior leaflets, many chordae tendineae, and two papillary muscles. The anterior and posterior leaflets converge at the anterolateral and posteromedial commissures, each of which is associated with a papillary muscle. The anterior leaflet is semicircular and occupies one-third of the circumference, whereas the posterior leaflet is elongated and narrow and is attached to the remaining two-thirds of the annulus. The posterior leaflet is divided into three parts based on the presence of two indentations: a lateral P1, a central P2, and a medial P3 scallop. The segments of anterior leaflet opposing the posterior leaflet are similarly designated as A1, A2, and A3 scallop (Fig. 15-1).[5]

The subvalvular apparatus consists of chordae tendineae and the papillary muscles. The chordae tendineae attach to the edges of mitral leaflets or to its ventricular surface. The left ventricle has two papillary muscles: the anterolateral papillary muscle and the posteromedial papillary muscle. The chordae tendineae arise from the papillary muscle and attach to the ipsilateral half of anterior and posterior mitral leaflets.[1,4]

The left ventricle is a cone-shaped structure that is longer and narrower than the right ventricle. In the long axis, it descends forward and to the left from its base at the atrioventricular groove to form the cardiac apex. Its walls are normally about two to three times thicker than the right ventricle. It consists of the inlet region, the apical trabecular component, and the smooth-walled outflow tract. Unlike the valvular orifices of the right ventricle, the orifices of the aortic and mitral valve are in fibrous continuity. The left ventricular outflow tract ends at the aortic valve. The aortic valve consists of three semilunar cusps that are supported within the three aortic sinuses of Valsalva. The cusps and the sinuses are called ***left***, ***right***, and ***noncoronary***.[1,4]

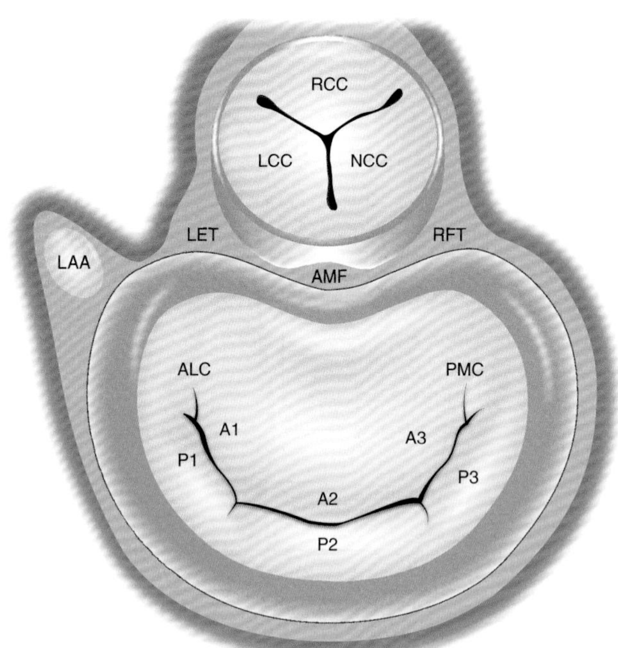

FIGURE 15-1 Representation of mitral valve anatomy.[5] Anterior mitral valve leaflet with scallops A1, A2, A3; posterior mitral valve leaflet with scallops P1, P2, P3; ALC, anterolateral commissure; AMF, aortic-mitral fibrosa; LAA, left atrial appendage; LCC, left coronary cusp of aortic valve; LFT, left fibrous trigone; NCC, noncoronary cusp of aortic valve; PMC, posteromedial commissure; RCC, right coronary cusp of aortic valve; RFT, right fibrous trigone. (From Debonnaire P, Palmen M, Marsan NA, et al. Contemporary imaging of normal mitral valve anatomy and function. *Curr Opin Cardiol.* 2012;27[5]:455–464.)

The Coronary Circulation

A unique feature of the coronary circulation is that the heart requires a continuous delivery of oxygen by coronary blood flow to function. At rest, the myocardium extracts about 75% of the oxygen delivered by coronary blood flow more than any other tissue in the body. So whenever myocardial oxygen demand increases, as with exercise, the coronary arteries must dilate to increase blood flow and oxygen delivery to meet the demand, or ischemia results. This coronary artery dilation is mediated through the local release of vasodilator substances within the myocardium.[6,7]

The right (RCA) and the left (LCA) coronary arteries arise respectively from the upper part of the right and the left coronary sinus of Valsalva and are the first branches of the aorta (Fig. 15-2). The RCA usually supplies the most of the right ventricle, a small part of the diaphragmatic

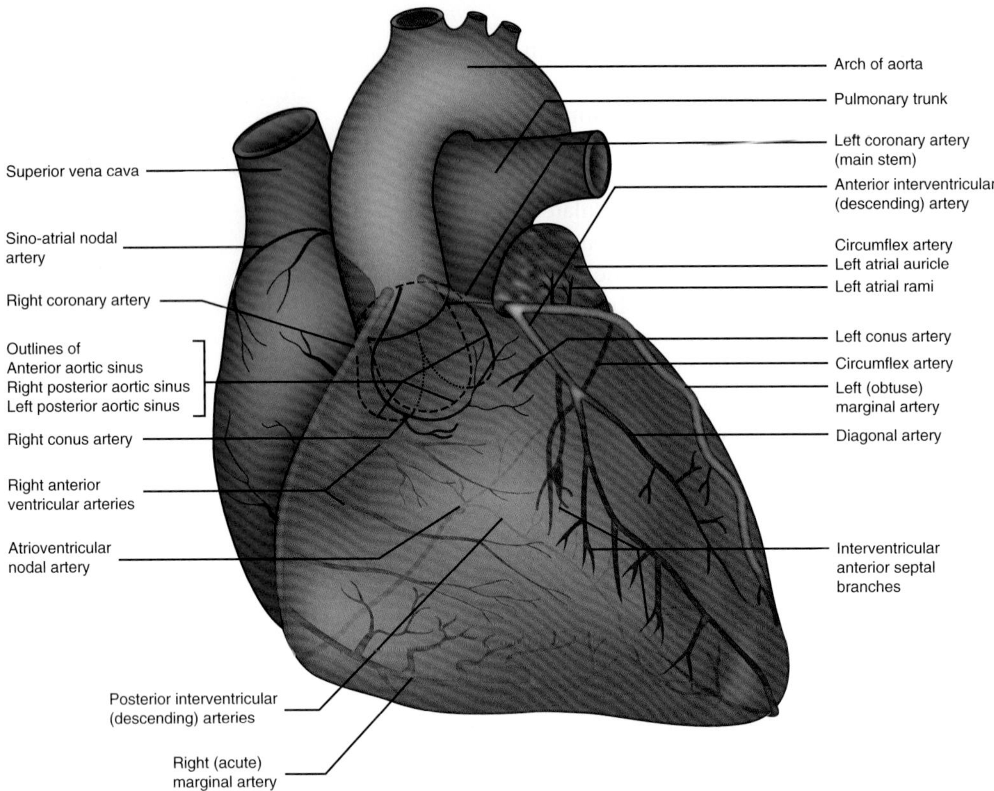

FIGURE 15-2 The coronary circulation.[1]

aspect of left ventricle, the right atrium, part of left atrium, and posteroinferior one-third of interventricular septum. The first segment of the RCA gives rise to right ventricular and atrial branches. The right ventricular branches are the right conus artery or the infundibular artery and the acute marginal arteries. The atrial branch in majority of the population is the artery to the sinoatrial node. The RCA passes directly into the right interventricular groove and descends to the right cardiac border, where it curves posteriorly and approaches the junction of interatrial and interventricular grooves (the crux of the heart) and gives rise to the posterior descending artery (PDA). Coronary artery dominance is defined by the artery that supplies the PDA. In 70% of the population, the PDA is supplied by the RCA, coronary circulation referred to as ***right dominant***. In 10% of the population, the PDA is supplied by circumflex artery (CxA) and is left dominant. In the remainder, the PDA is supplied by both the RCA and the CxA and the coronary circulation is considered codominant.[1,6]

The left main coronary artery usually supplies the free wall of the left ventricle, a narrow strip of the right ventricle anteriorly, the anterior two-thirds of ventricular septum, and most of left atrium. After arising from the left coronary sinus, the left main coronary artery passes to the left atrioventricular groove, where it branches into left anterior descending artery (LAD) and the CxA. The LAD, also known as ***anterior interventricular artery***, runs in the anterior interventricular groove and gives off right and left diagonal and septal branches. The right diagonal branches are small and rare; the left diagonal arteries can vary in number anywhere from two to nine and cross the anterior surface of the left ventricle. The septal branches supply most of the interventricular septum. The first septal branch is usually targeted for ablation in interventional treatment for hypertrophic cardiomyopathy. The CxA curves left in atrioventricular groove giving rise to obtuse marginal branches extending over the posterolateral wall toward the apex. The CxA continues into the posterior part of the atrioventricular groove, usually terminating prior to the crux of the heart, but in 10% of individuals, it continues to supply the PDA.[1,6]

The cardiac veins that run in atrioventricular and interventricular grooves drain a large part of coronary arterial blood into the right atrium via the coronary sinus (CS). The great cardiac vein that accompanies the LAD is joined by the oblique vein of the left atrium in the left atrioventricular groove to become the CS. Prior to draining into the right atrium, the middle cardiac vein that runs in the inferior interventricular groove and small cardiac vein that runs in right atrioventricular groove drain into the CS.[1,6]

The Cardiac Conduction System

The cardiac conduction system consists of the sinoatrial (SA) node, the atrioventricular (AV) node, the AV bundle also known as the ***bundle of His***, the bundle branches, and the Purkinje fibers (Fig. 15-3). The cardiac impulse is normally initiated by the SA node. This causes the atria to contract, first the right atrium followed by the left atrium. The blood supply to the SA node may be from either the RCA or the CxA.

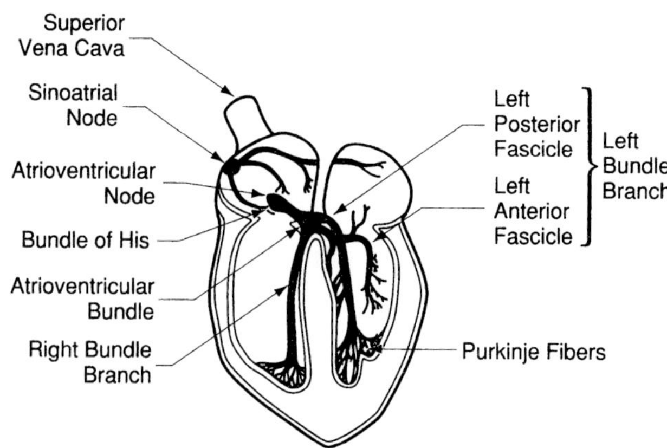

FIGURE 15-3 Cardiac conduction system.

From the SA node, the impulse is conducted to the AV node via the atrial myocardium. The AV node is located at the apex of region formed by the opening of the CS, the septal leaflet of the tricuspid valve, and the atrial septum, called the ***triangle of Koch***. The AV node is supplied by the RCA in a large majority of population, in the rest by the CxA. The cardiac electrical impulse is delayed in the AV node about a fifth of a second before being conducted to the bundle of His and on to the ventricles, so that the atria contract just before the ventricles to augment end diastolic filling. The bundle of His branches into right and left bundle branches. The left bundle splits further into anterior and posterior fascicles. The bundle branches descend through the ventricular septum, where they continue on as the Purkinje fibers that end up directly stimulating the myocardium to contract. The bundle of His and bundle branches are insulated from the myocardium by a fibrous sheath, thus forming specialized network of conduction tissue. This functional organization results in a coordinated, synchronized contraction of the atria and ventricles, improving the efficiency of the heart.[1,6,8,9]

Clinical Electrophysiology and Electrocardiogram

Body fluids are good electrical conductors, making it possible to record the sum of the action potentials of the cardiac cells on the surface of the body. Continuous monitoring of this electrocardiogram (ECG) during anesthesia is considered to be a standard of monitoring for all patients under the anesthesiologist's care. It is an essential tool for detecting myocardial ischemia, arrhythmias, and conduction system abnormalities.

Electrocardiogram Leads

The cardiac electrical activity is usually measured by electrodes placed on the skin. Bipolar leads consist of two electrodes, one positive and one negative. Unipolar leads consist of one positive electrode (exploring) and a composite pole that averages electrical activity from a number of other leads to zero potential, referred to as the ***indifferent electrode***. Depolarization directed toward the positive electrode produces a positive deflection, whereas directed away from it produces a negative deflection. When the depolarization wave is perpendicular to the lead, a biphasic deflection is recorded (Fig. 15-4). The 12-lead ECG consists of three bipolar standard limb leads, six unipolar precordial leads, and three unipolar augmented limb leads. The standard limb leads and the augmented limb leads record electrical impulses that flow in the frontal plane, whereas the precordial leads record impulses in the horizontal plane.

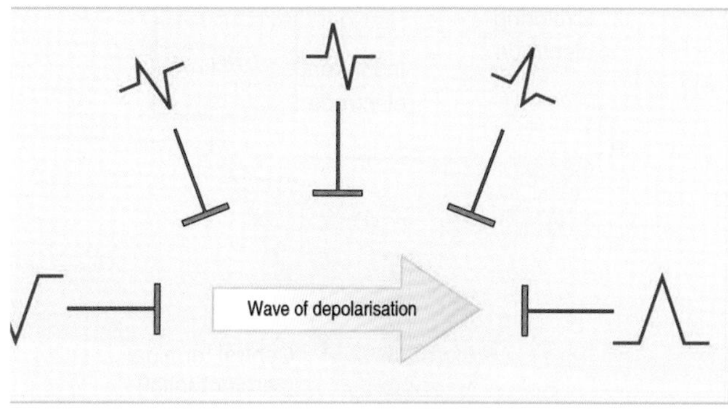

FIGURE 15-4 Wave of depolarization. Shape of QRS complex in any lead depends on orientation of that lead to vector of depolarization. (From Meek S, Morris F. Introduction. I—leads, rate, rhythm, and cardiac axis. *BMJ.* 2002;324[7334]:415–418.)

Standard Limb Leads

The standard limb leads, named I, II, and III, record the potential difference between two points of the body (Fig. 15-5). In lead I, the electrodes are placed on the left shoulder (positive) and right shoulder (negative). In lead II, the positive electrode is on the left leg and the negative is on the right shoulder. In lead III, the positive electrode is on the left leg and the negative on the left arm. The limb leads form the triangle of Einthoven, which is used together with the augmented limb leads to calculate the

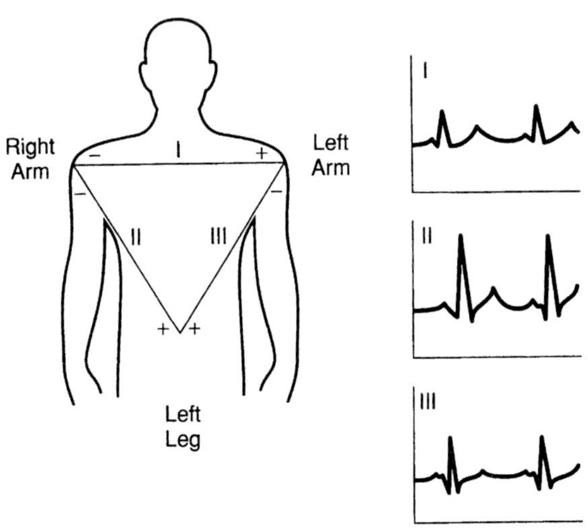

FIGURE 15-5 Standard limb leads of the electrocardiogram and typical recordings.

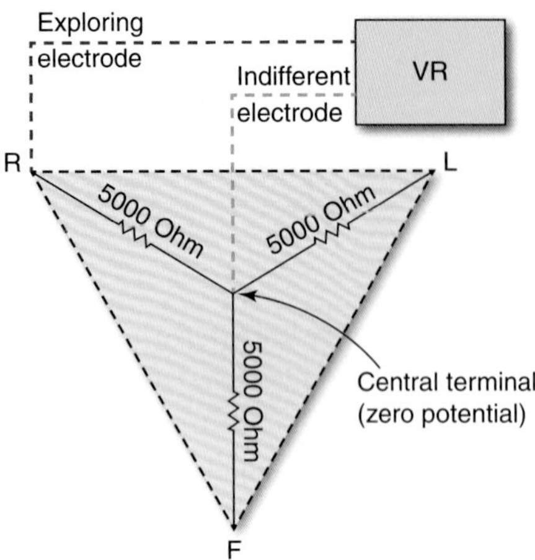

FIGURE 15-6 Unipolar limb lead circuit (VR).

electrical axis of the heart in the frontal axis. The direction of the depolarization of the atria parallels lead II, resulting in a prominent P wave in this lead.

Augmented Limb Leads

Augmented leads are similar to the standard limb leads but are unipolar. Linking the three limb leads through equal resistances (5,000 Ω), a central terminal is created with zero potential (Wilson's central terminal). This is based on Einthoven's theory that the R wave in lead II equals the sum of the R waves in leads I and III. The central terminal presents a stable reference potential point that is used to measure the varying potential at the exploring electrode (Fig. 15-6). Goldberger modified the central terminal by removing its link from the exploring electrode, achieving augmentation on the ECG deflections.[10] The positive (exploring) electrode for augmented voltage right arm (aVR) is on the right shoulder, for augmented voltage left arm (aVL) on the left shoulder, and for augmented voltage foot (aVF) on the left leg.

Precordial Leads

The precordial (V_1 to V_6) are unipolar leads that are placed on the chest wall, with the exploring electrode over one of six separate points (Table 15-1). The "indifferent" electrode is represented by the Wilson's central terminal, which is the average of the standard limb leads and normally has zero potential. The proximity of the heart surface to the electrode allows for detection of relatively small abnormalities in the ventricles without augmentation. Electric current flow is normally from the base to the apex of the heart. Therefore, leads V_1 and V_2, being near the base, record a negatively deflected QRS. Conversely, V_4 to V_6, being nearer the apex, record a positively deflected QRS.

Table 15-1

Placement of Precordial Leads

V_1	Fourth intercostal space at the right sternal border
V_2	Fourth intercostal space at the left sternal border
V_3	Equidistant between V_2 and V_4
V_4	Fifth intercostal space in the left midclavicular line
V_5	Fifth intercostal space in the left anterior axillary line
V_6	Fifth intercostal space in the left midaxillary line

Electrocardiographic Axis of the Heart

The axis represents the overall direction of the electric impulse in the heart and is created by averaging all the action potentials. It is biased toward the left because of the larger muscle mass of the left ventricle compared to the right. The standard limb leads combined with the augmented limb leads form the hexaxial diagram, which is used to calculate the electrical axis of the heart on the frontal plane (Fig. 15-7). This axis normally ranges between −30 and 90 degrees. Hypertrophy of the left ventricle shifts the axis to the left, and hypertrophy of the right shifts it to the right. Left axis deviation is defined as an axis less than −30 degrees and right axis deviation as more than 90 degrees. Abnormalities in the normal conduction pathway (blocks) in the heart also cause changes in the electrical axis.

Electrocardiogram Lead Systems

The three-lead system is the most basic ECG system. It consists of three electrodes, placed on the right arm, left arm, and left leg. It monitors electrical activity recorded by the bipolar standard limb leads (I, II, and II). Only one lead at a time is available. Two electrodes are used to form the selected lead and the third becomes the ground. Although the three-lead ECG provides adequate monitoring for arrhythmias, its use for detection of myocardial ischemia is limited.

In the modified three-lead bipolar standard limb lead system, the electrodes are placed in different locations on the chest wall. This allows for improved detection of arrhythmias (taller P waves) and monitoring for ischemia of the heart surface closer to each exploring pole. In the

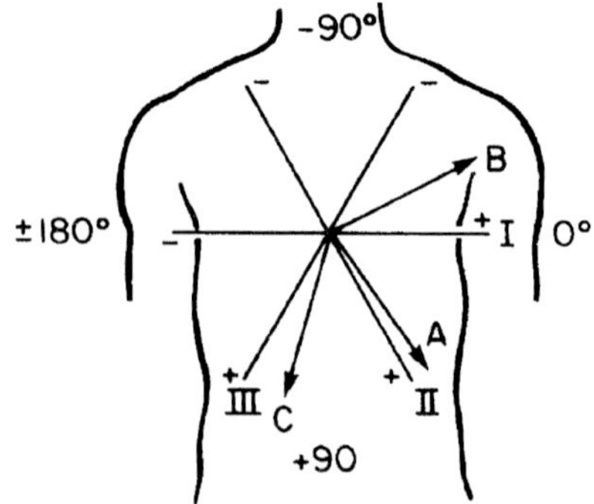

FIGURE 15-7 Electrical axis of the heart as determined from the standard limb leads of the electrocardiogram. In the normal heart, the electrical axis is approximately 59 degrees *(A)*. Left axis deviation shifts the electrical axis to less than 0 degrees *(B)*; right axis deviation is associated with an electrical axis of greater than 100 degrees.

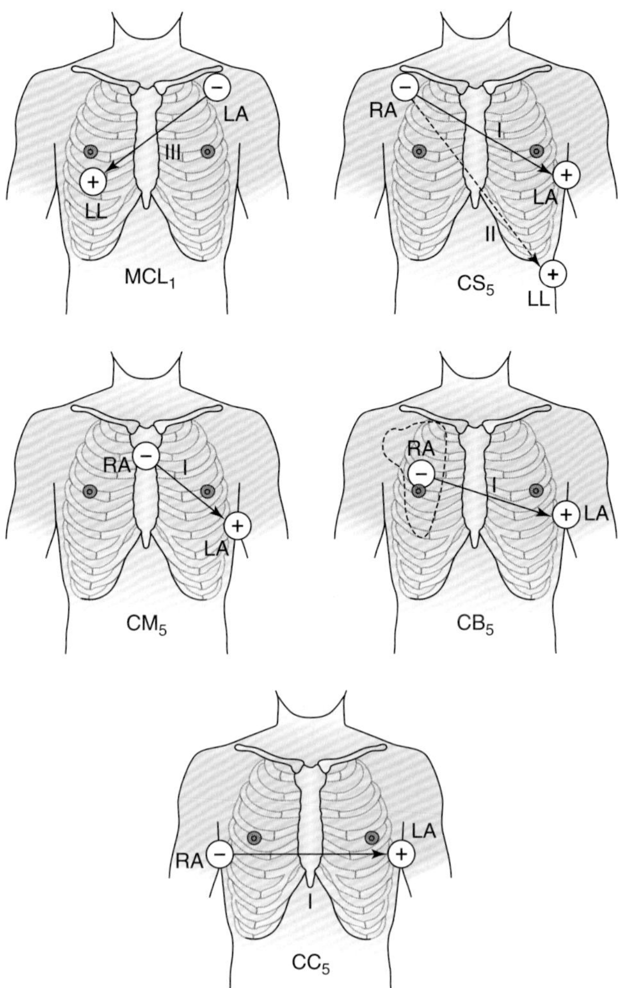

FIGURE 15-8 Modified bipolar standard limb lead system.

central subclavicular lead system (SC_5), one electrode is placed under the right clavicle, one in the V_5 position, and the ground electrode on the left leg. Other modified systems include the modified central leads (MCL), central manubrial (CM_5), central back (CB_5), and central cardiac 5 (V_5) lead systems (Fig. 15-8).

The five-lead system uses five electrodes placed on the right arm, right leg, left arm, left leg, and one on the chest wall in any one position from V_1 to V_6. Seven leads at a time may be monitored, six bipolar (I, II, III, aVR, aVL, aVF) and one unipolar (usually V_5.) The 10-lead system allows monitoring of 12 leads simultaneously, the 3 standard limb leads (I, II, III), the 3 augmented limb leads (aVR, aVL, aVF), and 6 precordial leads (V_1 to V_6). The electrodes are placed on the right arm and leg, left arm and leg, and on the anterior and anterolateral chest wall. This allows for monitoring of specific areas of the heart. Leads V_1 to V_4 monitor the anterior wall; leads I, aVL, V_5, and V_6, the lateral wall; and II, III, and aVF, the inferior wall.

London and colleagues[11] examined lead sensitivity for detecting intraoperative myocardial ischemia. They concluded that using single-lead monitoring, V_5 had the greatest sensitivity, 75%, whereas V_4 had 61%. V_4 and V_5 combined had 90%. Sensitivity for the standard combination used in the clinical setting, II and V_5, was 80%. Adding V_4 to II and V_5 increased the sensitivity to 96%. Although lead V_4 is more sensitive in detecting ischemia, lead II is superior in monitoring atrial arrhythmias.[11]

Invasive ECG may monitor the cardiac electrical activity using leads placed in the trachea, the esophagus, in the cardiac cavities, or the coronary vessels but are not used in the routine anesthesia practice. The His bundle ECG uses an electrode on a catheter in the heart placed near the tricuspid valve (Fig. 15-9). It records the activation of the AV node (A), the spreading of the electrical activity through the His bundle (H), and the ventricular depolarization (V). Information from the standard ECG and the His bundle ECG can be used to measure the time required for the impulse to travel between the sinus node and the AV node (AH) and through the AV node to the bundle of His and the ventricles. This allows detection of the site of a conduction delay, important for prognosis and treatment.

Decreased voltage on the ECG may be caused by multiple small myocardial infarcts, which prevent generation of large quantities of electrical currents or abnormal conditions around the heart that impede current conduction from the heart to the skin, such as pericardial fluid and pulmonary emphysema.

It is important to differentiate artifacts from real ECG findings. Artifacts may be caused by malfunctioning ECG system (cables, connections, etc.), improper skin preparation (oil, hair), lead misplacement/poor contact, patient's tremor/shivering, or muscular activity. External sources emitting electrical fields (electrocautery, 60 Hz power lines/light fixtures), cardiopulmonary bypass, somatosensory-evoked potential monitoring, and stimulators may also interfere with ECG recordings. All modern ECG monitors have incorporated filters for signal processing to minimize the presence of electrical artifacts.

Recording of the Electrocardiogram

The ECG is recorded on a graph paper consisting of 1-mm squares with every five squares separated by a darker line. Each 1-mm horizontal line represents 0.04 second and each 1-mm vertical line represents 0.1 mV, assuming proper calibration 1 cm/1 mV and standardized paper

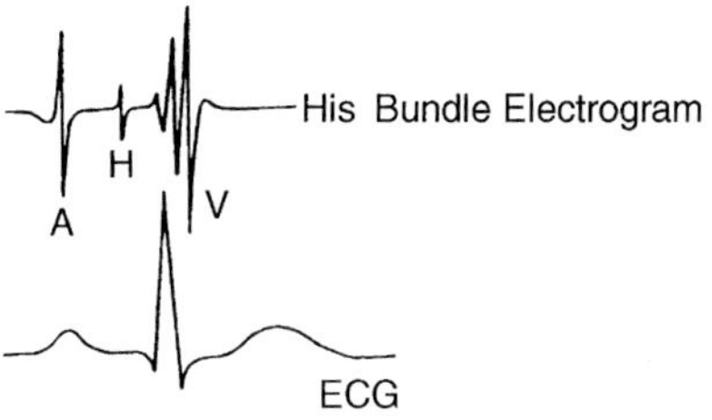

FIGURE 15-9 A normal His bundle electrogram and the corresponding electrocardiogram (ECG). (From Ganong WF. *Review of Medical Physiology*. 21st ed. New York, NY: McGraw-Hill; 2003.)

speed of 25 mm per second. Therefore, the distance between two darker lines represents 0.2 second and 0.5 mV on the horizontal and the vertical axes respectively. One minute (60 seconds) corresponds to 1,500 small or 300 big squares. The heart rate in beats per minute can be calculated by dividing 300 by the number of large boxes (or 1,500 by the number of small boxes) counted between two beats. Another method of calculating heart rate in beats per minute is to divide 60 by the number of seconds (= 0.04 second × number of small boxes) between two consecutive beats.

The electrical activity that activates the cardiac contraction is observed on a monitor display as a graph of voltage change through time. Modern monitors also have paper recorders allowing more thorough analysis of the ECG in complex situations. The Holter monitor is a small portable digital recorder that enables recording of the ECG for prolonged periods in ambulatory individuals to detect infrequent events.

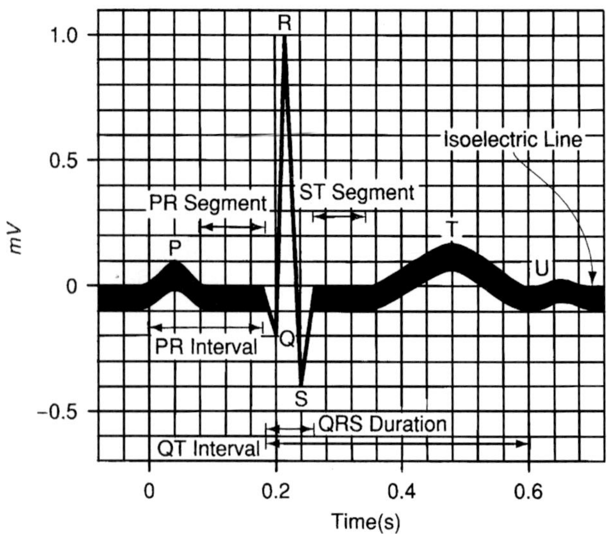

FIGURE 15-10 The normal waves and intervals on the electrocardiogram.

Normal Electrocardiographic Deflections

Normally, the cardiac electrical impulse is initiated at the SA node, which is located at junction of the superior vena cava to the right atrium. Any part of the conduction system can spontaneously depolarize and initiate an impulse, but the SA node normally has the highest rate of depolarization and is the pacemaker of the heart. The impulse is transmitted through the right and left intraatrial pathways to the AV node and then to the bundle of His and through the Purkinje fibers to the ventricular subendocardium, which causes the myocardium to depolarize from the endocardium to the epicardium. Repolarization happens in the reverse direction, from the epicardium to the endocardium. The speed of conduction is different between the various areas of the system, with the slowest through the AV node producing AV synchrony for optimal end diastolic filling from atrial contraction. The normal ECG consists of a P wave (atrial systole), a QRS complex (ventricular systole), and a T wave (ventricular repolarization). The atrial repolarization wave is obscured by the larger QRS complex (Fig. 15-10).

P Wave

The P wave represents the atrial depolarization and has a normal duration and amplitude of 0.08 to 0.12 second and less than 2.5 mm in the limb leads. Morphologically, it is positive in the standard limb leads and negative in aVR. Enlarged P wave signifies atrial enlargement.

P-R Interval

The P-R interval corresponds to the time from the beginning of the atrial depolarization to the beginning of the ventricular depolarization. It is measured from the start of the P wave to the start of the QRS and should not be confused with the PR segment, which is measured from the end of the P wave to the start of the QRS. The normal duration of the P-R interval is 0.12 to 0.2 second. Prolonged P-R interval is called first-degree AV block. In pericarditis, the P-R interval is depressed in most leads (whereas ST is elevated) and elevated in aVR (knuckle sign) (Fig. 15-11).

Q Wave

The Q wave is defined as an initial negative deflection of the QRS and is usually absent in leads aVR, V_1, and V_2. Normally, its duration is shorter than 0.04 second and its amplitude less than 0.4 to 0.5 mV. A Q wave whose amplitude is more than one-third of the corresponding R wave, duration is longer than 0.04 second, and depth is greater than 1 mm, is indicative of myocardial infarction (MI). The Q wave occurs because there is no electrical activity in the affected area. Therefore, the direction of the sum of the action potentials in the specific plane changes and is recorded accordingly. In the presence of anterior wall MI, Q waves develop in leads V_2 to V_4; in anteroseptal MI, in

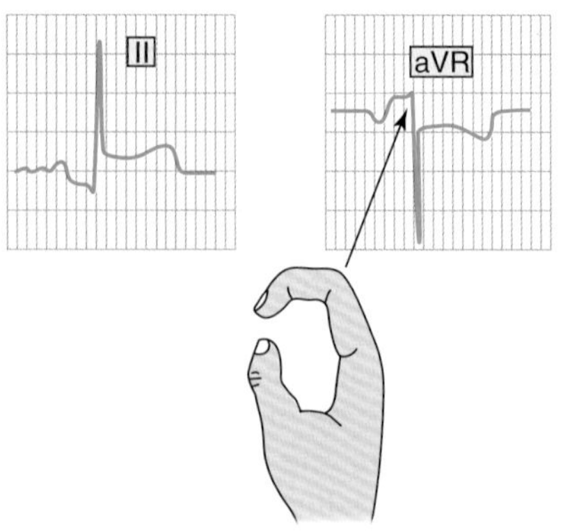

FIGURE 15-11 Acute pericarditis. Look for widespread ST segment elevation with concomitant PR depression in the same leads. The PR segment in aVR sticks above the baseline like a knuckle, reflecting atrial injury.

leads V_1 to V_3; in anterolateral MI, in leads V_4 to V_6 and I and aVL; in lateral MI, in leads V_5, V_6, I, and aVL; and in inferior MI, in leads II, III, and aVF.

QRS Complex

The QRS complex is caused by the depolarization of the ventricles and normally has a duration of less than 0.10 second. A prolonged QRS duration may be due to left ventricular hypertrophy (LVH), impaired ventricular conduction (bundle branch block), beats initiated outside the conduction system (ectopic or paced beats), and beats passing through abnormal conduction pathways (Wolff-Parkinson-White syndrome). Normally, the QRS amplitude gradually increases in the precordial leads from V_1 to V_5, a phenomenon called ***R wave progression***. The R wave is usually upright in the limb leads and downwardly deflected in aVR and V_1. Various criteria exist for defining LVH using the QRS amplitude. According to the Cornell criteria, LVH is present when the sum of the R wave in aVL and S wave in V_3 is greater than 28 mm in males and 20 mm in females. Based on the Sokolow-Lyon criteria, LVH is present when SV_1 + (R in V_5 or R in V_6) is greater than 35 mm or R in aVL is greater than 11 mm.

ST Segment

The ST segment starts when all myocardial cells are depolarized (end of QRS) and ends when ventricular repolarization begins (T wave). It is normally isoelectric and elevation or depression more than 1 mm from the baseline may indicate myocardial ischemia. Hyperkalemia and pericarditis may also cause ST elevation. J point elevation (where QRS and ST segment connect) and normal variants of early repolarization are nonpathologic findings that must be excluded (Fig. 15-12).

T Wave

The T wave is caused by the repolarization of the ventricles, and its normal amplitude is less than 10 mm in the precordial leads and 6 mm in the limb leads. Usually, in any lead, the T wave is deflected in the same directions as the QRS. Delay of conduction of cardiac impulses through the ventricles (prolonged depolarization), as occurs with myocardial ischemia, bundle branch blocks, or ectopic ventricular beats, may result in T-wave polarity opposite the QRS complex. Symmetrical or deeply inverted T waves may be indicative of myocardial ischemia. Inverted T waves in V_1 to V_3 in children (juvenile T waves) and occasionally in women can be a normal variant. Peaked T waves may be present in hyperkalemia, LVH, and intracranial bleeding.

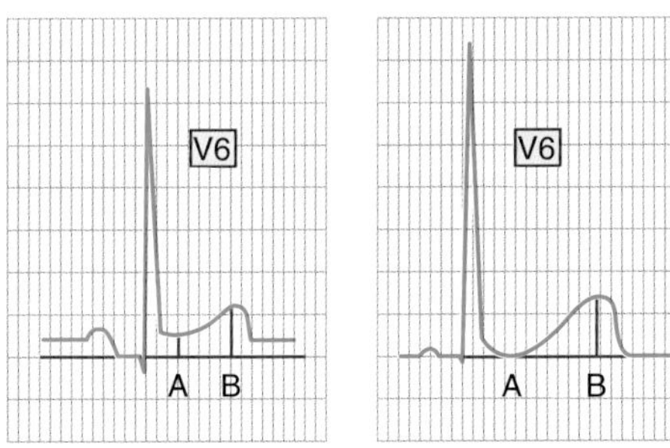

FIGURE 15-12 Differentiating pericarditis from early repolarization. Only lead V_6 is used. If A/B is greater than 25%, suspect pericarditis. If A/B is less than 25%, suspect early repolarization.

U Wave

The U wave, when present, follows the T wave and it probably represents part of the ventricular repolarization. It is most prominent in V_2 and V_3. Causes of increased U wave amplitude (>1.5 mm) include LVH, bradycardia, ischemia, electrolyte abnormalities (low potassium, magnesium, calcium), and medications.

QT Interval

The QT interval includes both ventricular depolarization and repolarization. It is measured from the beginning of the QRS to the end of the T wave and varies in duration according to heart rate. The QT interval corrected for heart rate (QTc) is calculated by dividing the QT interval by the squared root of the RR interval. Prolonged QTc (>0.44 second) may be associated with ventricular arrhythmias. Causes of prolonged QT include hypocalcemia, hypomagnesemia, medications, severe bradycardia, hypothermia, ischemia, intracranial hemorrhage, and myxedema of hypothyroidism.

Cardiac Physiology

Myocardium

The myocardium is the involuntary, striated muscle tissue in the heart between the epicardium and the endocardium; its cells are called ***cardiomyocytes***. The primary structural proteins of the cardiac muscle are actin and myosin filaments, which interdigitate and slide along each other during contraction in a manner similar to skeletal muscle. But unlike the skeletal muscle in which the actin and myosin filaments are linear and longitudinal, in cardiomyocytes, they are branched (Fig. 15-13).[12] Also, the cardiac T tubules are larger and broader and fewer in number than skeletal muscle. Cardiac muscle T tubules form diads with the sarcoplasmic reticulum intercalated discs with permeable junctions that allow rapid diffusion of ions so that action potentials travel easily from cell to cell. Thus, cardiomyocytes are functionally interconnected in a syncytium, so that activation of one cell results in the spread to all connected cells. The atrial syncytium is separated from the ventricular syncytium by the fibrous tissues around the AV valves, and the cardiac action potential is normally only conducted from the atria to the ventricles by a specialized conduction pathway through the AV node.[13]

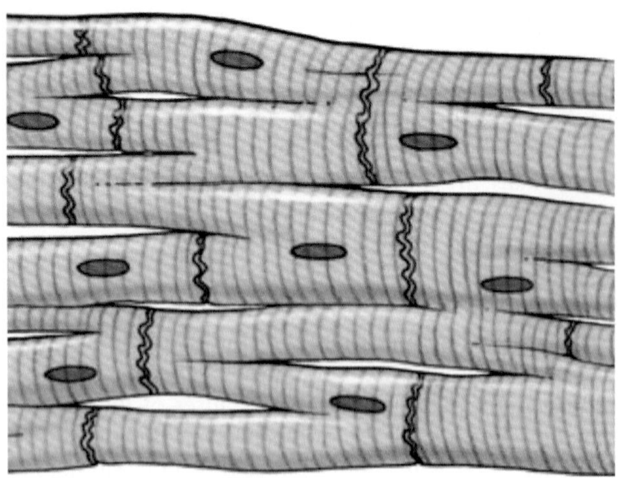

FIGURE 15-13 "Syncytial" interconnecting nature of cardiac muscle fibers.[21] (From Hall JE, Guyton AC. *Guyton and Hall Textbook of Medical Physiology.* 12th ed. Philadelphia, PA: Saunders/Elsevier; 2011.)

Cardiac Action Potential

At the initiation of an action potential in a cardiomyocyte, the cell membrane rapidly depolarizes as the transmembrane potential rises from −85 mV to +20 mV. The membrane remains depolarized for about 0.2 second, the plateau phase, which is then followed by rapid repolarization. This plateau causes the contraction of a cardiomyocyte to last much longer than a skeletal muscle cell and is due to the slow calcium channels, which open after the sodium channels and remain open several tenths of a second. Depolarization of the cardiomyocyte is also prolonged by a decrease in permeability of the potassium channels after initiation of the action potential, another difference from skeletal muscle. During the plateau phase, the cardiomyocyte cannot be restimulated for about 0.25 to 0.3 second, called the ***refractory period***. This is followed for additional 0.05 second by the relative refractory period, when the myocardium can only be stimulated by a strong excitatory signal.[12,14]

Excitation–Contraction Coupling

Excitation–contraction coupling in both cardiac and skeletal muscle occurs when the action potential spreads into the cell through transverse tubules (T tubules). Depolarization of the T tubule causes influx of calcium into the sarcoplasm, which binds to troponin activating the contraction of actin and myosin filaments. In the cardiomyocyte, however, the initial influx of calcium ions is just a small fraction of the amount needed for contraction, and it triggers an additional release of calcium from the sarcoplasmic reticulum into the sarcoplasm. The structural differences between cardiac and skeletal muscle reflect the difference in coupling mechanism. Myocardium has sparser and less developed sarcoplasmic reticulum and the T tubules are larger and store more calcium.[15,16]

Control of Cardiac Function

Neural Control

Heart function is controlled by the autonomic nervous system by both adrenergic and muscarinic acetylcholine receptors, modulating the cardiac output by influencing heart rate and myocardial contraction. The sympathetic nervous system, through adrenergic receptors with the neurotransmitter norepinephrine, has positive inotropic, chronotropic, and lusitropic effects on the heart. The parasympathetic nervous system, acting through muscarinic receptors with the neurotransmitter acetylcholine, has a more direct inhibitory effect on the heart through the vagal nerve reducing heart rate, AV node conduction, and cardiac contractility. The atria are innervated by both the sympathetic and parasympathetic nervous system, but the ventricles are supplied principally by the sympathetic nervous system (Fig. 15-14).[12,17]

Sympathetic nervous system fibers to the heart continually discharge at a slow rate maintaining a strength of ventricular contraction about 20% to 25% above the unstimulated state. Maximal sympathetic nervous system stimulation can increase cardiac output by about 100% above normal. Conversely, maximal parasympathetic nervous system stimulation decreases ventricular contractile strength only by about 30%, as the vagal innervation is sparse in the ventricles. Strong stimulation of the parasympathetic system can result in a period of asystole, followed by an escape rhythm between 20 and 40 beats per minute.[12,18]

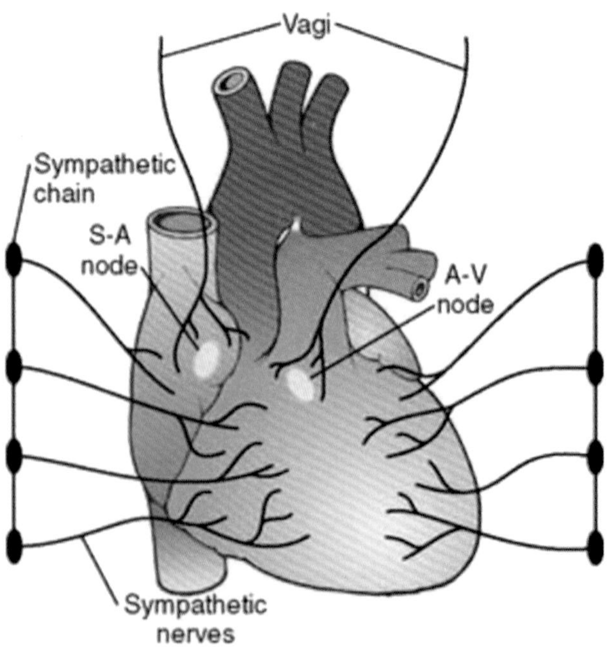

FIGURE 15-14 Cardiac sympathetic and parasympathetic nerves.[12] (From Hall JE, Guyton AC. *Guyton and Hall Textbook of Medical Physiology.* 12th ed. Philadelphia, PA: Saunders/Elsevier; 2011.)

Hormonal Control

Many hormones can have direct and indirect action on the heart during normal or pathophysiologic conditions. These hormones are produced within cardiomyocytes or by other tissues in the body. The hormones secreted by cardiomyocytes include natriuretic peptide, adrenomedullin, aldosterone, and angiotensin II.[19–21] Atrial (ANP) and B-type natriuretic protein (BNP) are released from atria and ventricle in response to increased stretch of the chamber wall. Both ANP and BNP participate in homeostasis of body fluids, in regulation of blood pressure, and in growth and development of cardiac tissue. In chronic heart failure, high ANP and BNP levels have been associated with increased mortality.[19] Adrenomedullin is a peptide hormone that increases level of cyclic adenosine monophosphate (cAMP) and has positive inotropic and chronotropic effects on the heart and is a vasodilator. The renin-angiotensin system is an important regulator of the cardiovascular system. Angiotensin II stimulates AT_1 receptors with positive inotropic and chronotropic effects. It also mediates cell growth and proliferation of cardiomyocytes, thus playing an important role in development of remodeling during cardiac hypertrophy and heart failure.[21]

Cardiac Cycle

Electrical and Mechanical Events

The cardiac cycle is a series of coordinated electromechanical events that result in the ejection of blood from the heart into the great vessels. Ventricular systole is defined as the period of myocardial contraction when the aortic and pulmonic valves are open and diastole as the period of relaxation and ventricular filling when the mitral and tricuspid valves are open. Each mechanical event is preceded by an electrical depolarization that generates an action potential and subsequent contraction.

Carl J. Wiggers[22] elegantly illustrated the mechanical, electrical, and acoustic events of the cardiac cycle. His diagram depicts the aortic, ventricular, and atrial pressure tracings with concomitant ECG, ventricular volume, and auscultatory findings[22] (Fig. 15-15). Systole begins with isometric contraction (A to C), followed by opening of the aortic valve and ejection of blood into the aorta, with a period of maximum ejection (C to D) and reduced ejection (D to F). Isometric contraction starts with closure of the mitral valve and ends with opening of the aortic valve, during which time no volume enters or leaves the ventricle. Approximately two-thirds of stroke volume is ejected during the period of maximum ejection and one-third during the period of reduced ejection. The ventricular volume curve that coincides with this event is inversely related to the aortic and ventricular pressure curves. Simultaneous electrical depolarization corresponds with the QRS complex of the ECG.

Diastole follows systole and is divided into prodiastole (F and G), isometric relaxation (G and H), rapid ventricular filling (H and I), diastasis (I and J), and filling by atrial contraction (J and K). During prodiastole, the semilunar, aortic, and pulmonic valves close. This is followed by isometric relaxation, the time between closure of the aortic valve and opening of the mitral valve. Ventricular filling depends on both the relaxation of the myocardium and chamber compliance.[23] There is a period of diastasis with minimal flow during which the ventricular volume remains relatively constant. This is followed by atrial contraction during late diastole, synchronous with the P wave of atrial depolarization on the ECG.

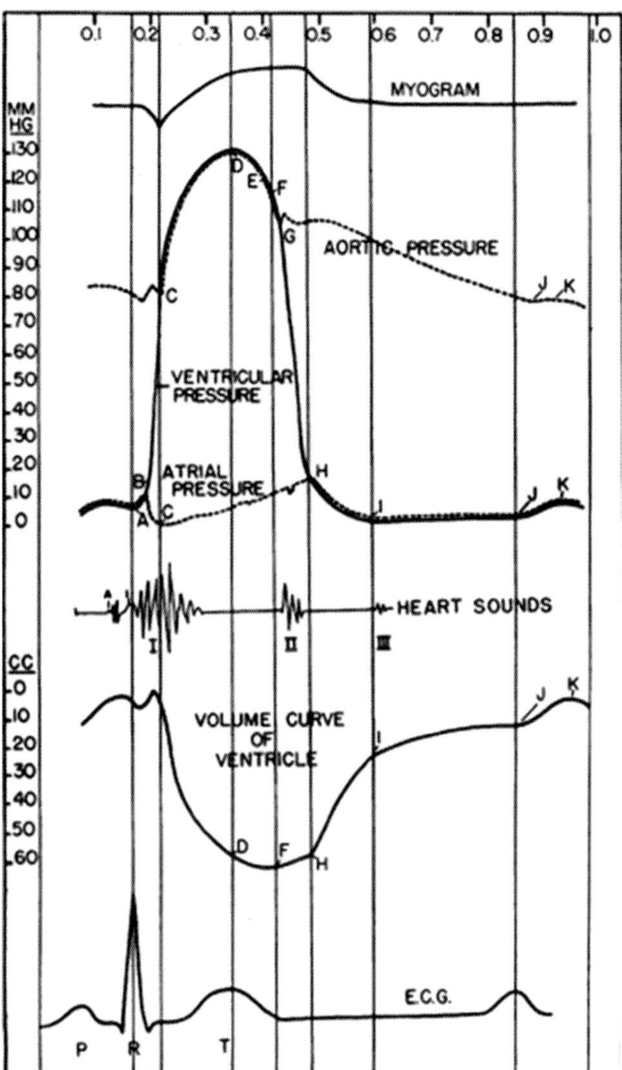

FIGURE 15-15 Cardiac cycle: mechanical, electrical, and acoustic events. (From Wiggers CJ. Dynamics of ventricular contraction under abnormal conditions. *Circulation.* 1952;5[3]: 321–348.)

The atrial pressure tracing, or central venous waveform, begins with an "a" wave that corresponds to atrial contraction at end diastole. The "c" wave represents ventricular systole during which time the right atrial pressure increases slightly as the right ventricle contracts against a closed tricuspid valve. The subsequent downward slope in the waveform, the "x descent," corresponds to atrial relaxation.

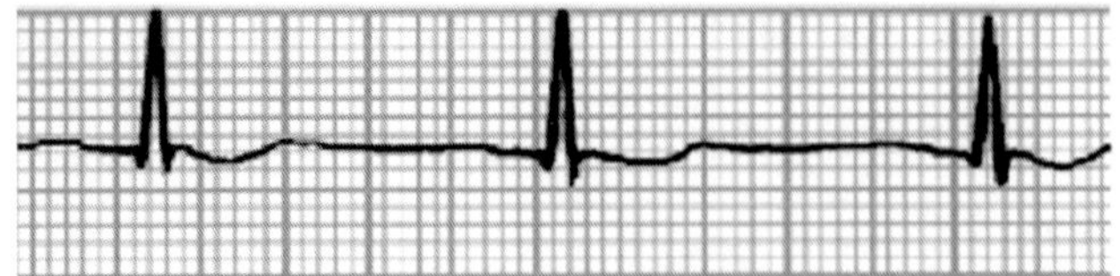

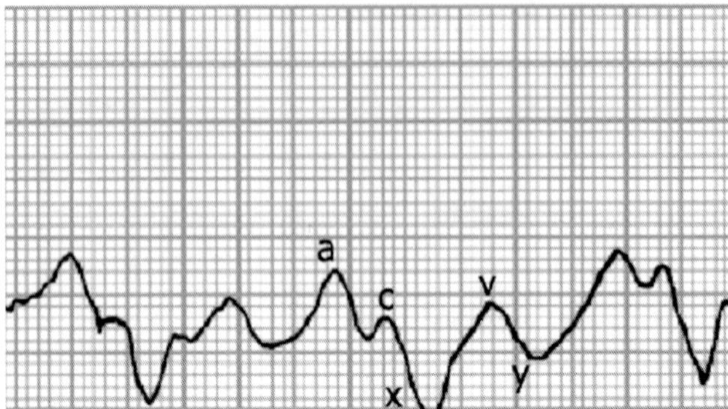

FIGURE 15-16 Central venous waveform. (From Pittman J, Ping JS, Mark JB. Arterial and central venous pressure monitoring. *Int Anesthesiol Clin.* 2004;42[1]:13–30.)

The "v" wave occurs during venous filling of the right atria towards the end of systole. The "y descent" represents a fall in right atrial pressures as the tricuspid valve opens and the right ventricle fills in diastole[24] (Fig. 15-16).

Myocardial Performance, Preload, and Afterload

In the early 1900s, Frank Otto and Ernest Henry Starling described what is known today as the Frank-Starling mechanism. In a series of publications, they demonstrated that myocardial stretch, called ***preload***, induced by increased venous return to the heart augments cardiac output,[25] and that increased end diastolic volume or right atrial pressure enhances myocardial contractility.[26,27]

In canine experiments, Arthur C. Guyton,[28] identified two factors affecting venous return or preload to the ventricle: right atrial pressure and mean circulatory filling pressure. Higher right atrial pressure diminishes venous return to the heart, whereas higher mean circulatory filling pressure, as measured by temporary cessation of cardiac output and equilibration of peripheral pressures, increases venous return. Increasing mean circulatory filling pressure, for example by transfusion, enhances venous return to the heart, thereby augmenting cardiac output without affecting contractility. He synthesized these findings with the Frank-Starling mechanism and graphically displayed superimposing cardiac response and venous return curves (Fig. 15-17).[28,29]

Afterload refers to the resistance or pressure against which the ventricle contracts. Mechanical obstruction such as aortic stenosis increases afterload and adversely affects myocardial performance. Pharmacologic interventions such as the administration of phenylephrine can increase afterload as well by increasing systemic vascular resistance. Afterload in its simplest interpretation often refers to the mean arterial pressure.

Left ventricular (LV) pressure–volume loops can be used to demonstrate how changes in preload and afterload affect stroke volume and end systolic and end diastolic pressure–volume relationships. The entire loop represents a single cardiac cycle with volume on the x-axis and pressure on the y-axis. The difference between end diastolic volume (EDV) and end systolic volume (ESV) equals stroke volume (SV). At end diastole, after closure of the mitral valve, isometric contraction increases the pressure in the LV cavity marking the beginning of systole. When

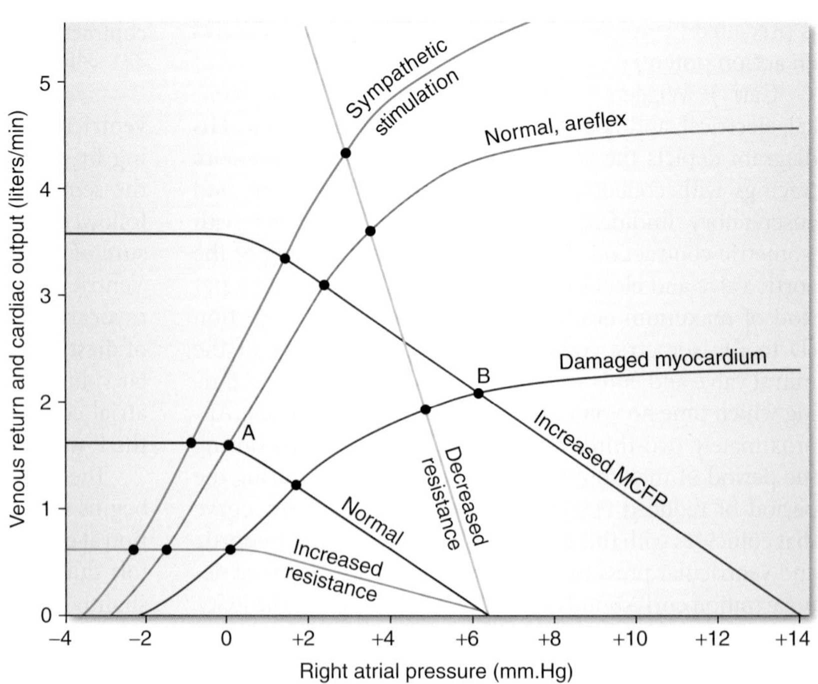

FIGURE 15-17 Determinants of cardiac output. (From Guyton AC. Determination of cardiac output by equating venous return curves with cardiac response curves. *Physiol Rev.* 1955;35[1]:123–129.)

the LV pressure exceeds that in the aorta, the aortic valve opens and ejection begins. After end systole and peak LV pressure, the aortic valve closes. This is followed by a brief period of isometric relaxation marking the beginning of diastole during which LV pressure falls and the LV volume does not change. Then the mitral valve opens, the LV fills accommodating the SV to be ejected during the subsequent cardiac contraction (Fig. 15-18A).

A drop in preload, for example with clamping of the inferior vena cava, will decrease SV, ESV, and EDV. The shape of the pressure–volume loop narrows, shortens, and shifts to the left[30] (Fig. 15-18B). An increase in afterload, for example with administration of phenylephrine, will cause end systolic pressure and volume to increase and SV to decrease, the loops get narrower and longer (Fig. 15-18C).[30] The slope of the end systolic pressure–volume relationship (ESPVR) is referred to as ***elastance*** and labelled "E_{es}" in the figures. It stays constant during changes in preload and afterload, is a measure of the strength of contraction, or contractility, and is steeper with increased contractility.[31,32]

Hemodynamic Calculations

Cardiac output (CO) is equal to heart rate multiplied by SV. As illustrated in the previous LV pressure–volume loops, SV = EDV − ESV. Mean arterial pressure (MAP) is two-third diastolic blood pressure plus one-third systolic blood pressure. MAP is also CO multiplied by systemic vascular resistance (Table 15-2).

There are several methods to measure CO, the volume of blood delivered by the heart to the body per minute, including thermodilution, the Fick method, and echocardiography. The thermodilution method uses a pulmonary artery (Swan-Ganz) catheter through which cool saline is injected into the right atrium. The cool saline mixes with warmer blood and the temperature change is recorded by a thermistor at the tip of the catheter, positioned in the main pulmonary artery. The CO is inversely proportional to the integral of the time-temperature curve.[33,34] Limitations of this method include tricuspid regurgitation and the presence of intracardiac shunts. Tricuspid regurgitation will underestimate the CO, as the cool injectate travels retrograde into the vena cava increasing the time it

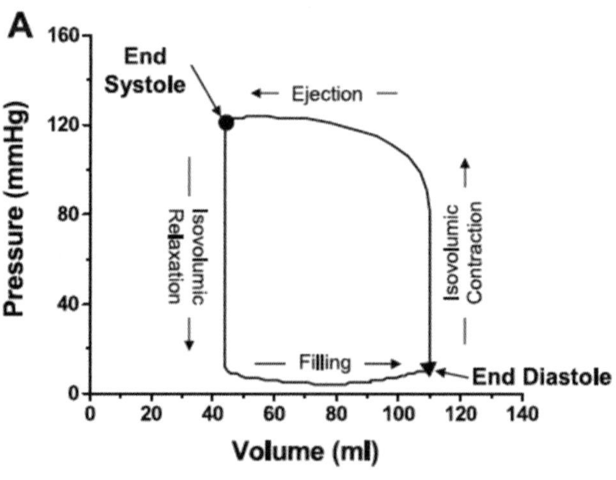

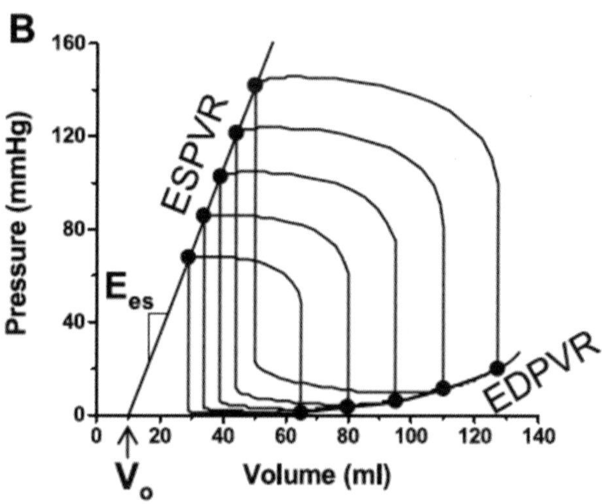

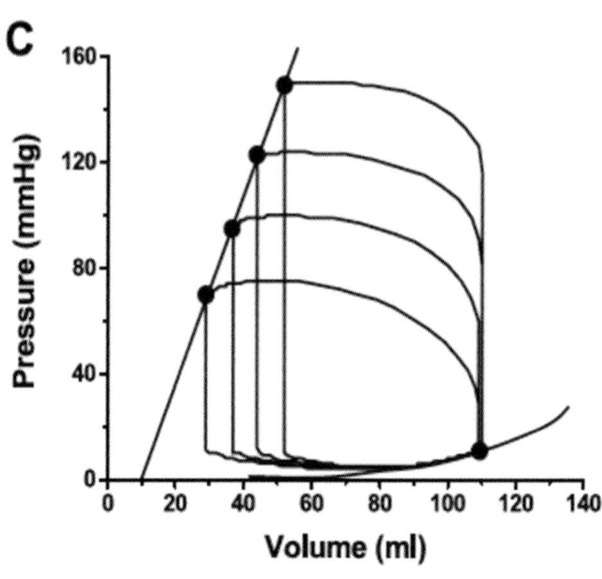

FIGURE 15-18 **A:** Pressure–volume loop of a single cardiac cycle. **B:** A reduction in ventricular filling pressure causes the loops to shift toward lower end systolic and end diastolic function. **C:** When afterload is increased, the loops get narrower and longer. EDPVR, end diastolic pressure–volume relationship; Ees, slope of linear ESPVR; ESPVR, end systolic pressure–volume relationship; Vo, volume axis intercept. (From Burkhoff D, Mirsky I, Suga H. Assessment of systolic and diastolic ventricular properties via pressure-volume analysis: a guide for clinical, translational, and basic researchers. *Am J Physiol Heart Circ Physiol.* 2005;289[2]:H501–512.)

Table 15-2

Hemodynamic Equations

CO = HR × SV
CI = CO / BSA
SV = EDV − ESV
MAP = CO × SVR
MAP = 2/3 diastolic pressure + 1/3 systolic pressure
SVR = [(MAP − CVP) / CO] × 80
PVR = [(mean PAP − wedge) / CO] × 80

CO, cardiac output; HR, heart rate; SV, stroke volume; CI, cardiac index; BSA, body surface area; EDV, end diastolic volume; ESV, end systolic volume; MAP, mean arterial pressure; SVR, systemic vascular resistance; CVP, central venous pressure; PVR, pulmonary vascular resistance; PAP, pulmonary artery pressure.

Table 15-3

Normal Hemodynamic Values

Cardiac index = 2.4 L/min
Cardiac output = 5–7 L/min
Stroke volume = 70–90 mL (1 mL/kg)
MAP = 60–90 mm Hg
CVP = 5–10 mm Hg
SVR = 800–1,200 dyne/s/cm^5
PVR = <250 dyne/s/cm^5
PAOP = 6–12 mm Hg
Mean PAP = 10–20 mm Hg

MAP, mean arterial pressure; CVP, central venous pressure; SVR, systemic vascular resistance; PVR, pulmonary vascular resistance; PAOP, pulmonary artery occlusion pressure; PAP, pulmonary artery pressure.

takes to reach the pulmonary artery. Conversely, intracardiac left to right shunts can falsely overestimate the CO.

CO can also be measured using the Fick method. Fick CO (liters per minute) = (oxygen consumption VO_2)/[(arteriovenous oxygen difference) × 10]. Oxygen consumption can be estimated based on a nomogram that accounts for patient age, sex, height, and weight. It can also be directly measured by exhaled breath analysis. The value 250 mL O_2 per minute is often used as a standardized reference. The difference in arterial versus venous oxygen content ($CaO_2 - CvO_2$) is calculated by the following formula:

$$(CaO_2 - CvO_2) = (1.34 \times Hgb \times SaO_2) - (1.34 \times Hgb \times SvO_2)$$

where SaO_2 is the arterial oxygen saturation and SvO_2 is the mixed venous oxygen saturation, that is, the saturation of pulmonary arterial blood. The arterial venous oxygen difference is inversely related to CO as long as the oxygen consumption of the body is constant.

Lastly, CO can be calculated by echocardiography. Pulsed wave doppler is used to record the velocity profile of flow in the left ventricular outflow tract (LVOT). Tracing this profile gives the velocity time integral (VTI) in centimeters. The LVOT VTI is multiplied by area of the LVOT in square centimeters to obtain the SV in milliliters. The LVOT is assumed to be circular in shape. The area of a circle is πr^2. The diameter of the LVOT is measured with two dimensional echocardiography and divided by two to obtain the radius in the area calculation. Therefore, SV = LVOT VTI × LVOT area (πr^2). A similar calculation can be made to obtain the SV through the right ventricular outflow tract (RVOT). The two numbers are identical provided there is no intracardiac shunt or regurgitation of the aortic or pulmonic valves. Multiplying the SV by the patient's heart rate yields CO.

After obtaining CO by one of these three methods, one can calculate systemic vascular resistance and pulmonary vascular resistance. Systemic vascular resistance (SVR) in Wood units is the MAP–central venous pressure divided by CO (see Table 15-2). To convert from Woods units to dynes/s/cm^5, the result is multiplied by 80. Similarly, to calculate pulmonary vascular resistance, the pulmonary artery occlusion pressure (PAOP) (a surrogate for the left atrial pressure) is subtracted from the mean pulmonary arterial pressure, and the result is divided by CO. The same conversion from Woods units applies. Obtaining CO and calculating SVR can often aid in narrowing a differential diagnosis in various types of shock. A mixed venous oxygen saturation (SvO_2) can also assist in narrowing the differential. Together, this information can guide therapeutic intervention toward inotropic support, volume administration, titration of vasopressors, or consideration of mechanical assist devices. In cardiogenic shock, for example, CO will be low, SVR high, and mixed venous saturation low. This is in contrast to vasodilatory or septic shock in which CO will be high, SVR low, and mixed venous saturation usually high. Normal hemodynamic values are listed in Table 15-3.

Pathophysiology

Ischemic Heart Disease

Ischemic heart disease refers to atherosclerosis of the coronary arteries that obstructs blood flow to the myocardium resulting in either stable symptoms, which can be medically managed, or unstable acute coronary syndromes, which may call for more invasive intervention such as revascularization by percutaneous coronary intervention (PCI) or coronary artery bypass graft (CABG) surgery. The development of atherosclerosis is an inflammatory process mediated by adherent leukocytes (phagocytes and T lymphocytes), cytokines, and smooth muscle cells that generate a lipid-rich necrotic plaque.[35–37] Risk factors for ischemic heart disease include hypertension, cigarette smoking, hyperlipidemia, and abdominal obesity.

Acute coronary syndromes include the following three entities: unstable angina, non–ST elevation myocardial infarction (NSTEMI), and ST elevation myocardial infarction (STEMI). All suspected patients are evaluated with a 12-lead ECG and biomarkers of myocardial injury, troponin and CK-MB. Those patients who show clinical, electrocardiographic, and laboratory evidence of MI are treated with heparin and evaluated with angiography for consideration of PCI or surgical intervention.[38,39]

Medical management of stable ischemic heart disease begins with risk factor reduction. β Blockade has been shown to confer a survival benefit in patients with prior MI or a low ejection fraction and decreases myocardial oxygen consumption. Oral or sublingual nitrates are effective in angina prophylaxis or during acute episodes. Antiplatelet agents such as aspirin are indicated unless bleeding precludes their use.[40–42] Statins are indicated for their lipid-lowering effects and antiinflammatory properties. Angiotensin-converting enzyme inhibitors assist in ventricular remodeling after MI. Diuretics optimize volume status and provide symptom relief in patients with heart failure.

Heart Failure

Heart failure is defined as "a complex clinical syndrome that results from any structural or functional impairment of ventricular filling or ejection of blood."[43] The underlying etiologies are numerous and include ischemia, hypertension, and diabetes. Other less common causes are valvular heart disease, infections such as viral myocarditis, toxins (alcohol, chemotherapeutic agents), and obesity.[44,45]

The American College of Cardiology/American Heart Association and the New York Heart Association functional classifications describe heart failure according to symptoms (Table 15-4). Heart failure can also be classified by ventricular function or ejection fraction. Heart failure with preserved ejection fraction, or diastolic heart failure, comprises those patients with an ejection fraction greater than 50% with echocardiographic evidence of abnormal diastolic function, an impairment in relaxation, and ventricular filling. The most important risk factor for diastolic heart failure is hypertension. Diastolic heart failure is more common in the elderly, female, and obese populations[45,46] and has now surpassed systolic heart failure as the leading class of heart failure.[47] Hospitalizations for heart failure with preserved ejection fraction are increasing over time, with minimal advancement in treatment modalities.[48] Risk factor modification including treatment of underlying hypertension is imperative.

Heart failure with reduced ejection fraction occurs in patients with an ejection fraction less than 40%. Patients often have concomitant diastolic dysfunction. One of the main risk factors for heart failure with reduced ejection fraction is coronary artery disease. Treatment modalities range from oral medication to intravenous inotropes to mechanical assist devices. Diuretics, angiotensin-converting enzyme inhibitors, and β blockers have been the foundation of medical management. Digoxin provides symptom relief and decreases hospital admissions, although it has no mortality benefit.[49] It can be useful in patients with associated atrial fibrillation to control heart rate. Patients with decompensated systolic heart failure may require acute positive inotropic therapy with milrinone, dobutamine, or

Table 15-4

ACCF/AHA Stages of Heart Failure and NYHA Functional Classification

ACCF/AHA Stages of HF	NYHA Functional Classification
A At high risk of HF but without structural heart disease or symptoms of HF	None
B Structural heart disease but without signs or symptoms of HF	I No limitation of physical activity. Ordinary physical activity does not cause symptoms of HF.
C Structural heart disease with prior or current symptoms of HF	I No limitation of physical activity. Ordinary physical activity does not cause symptoms of HF.
	II Slight limitation of physical activity. Comfortable at rest, but ordinary physical activity results in symptoms of HF.
	III Marked limitation of physical activity. Comfortable at rest, but less than ordinary activity causes symptoms of HF.
	IV Unable to carry on any physical activity without symptoms of HF or symptoms of HF at rest
D Refractory HF requiring specialized interventions	IV Unable to carry on any physical activity without symptoms of HF or symptoms of HF at rest

ACCF, American College of Cardiology Foundation; AHA, American Heart Association; HF, heart failure; NYHA, New York Heart Association.

From Yancy CW, Jessup M, Bozkurt B, et al. 2013 ACCF/AHA guideline for the management of heart failure: a report of the American College of Cardiology Foundation/American Heart Association Task Force on Practice Guidelines. *J Am Coll Cardiol*. 2013;62(16):e147–e239.

epinephrine. More invasive methods to support the failing ventricle include intraaortic balloon counterpulsation, ventricular assist devices, and cardiac transplantation.[50,51]

Valvular Heart Disease

Aortic Stenosis

Aortic stenosis is the most common valvular heart disease in elderly patients. It occurs as the trileaflet aortic valve calcifies with age, with congenitally bicuspid aortic valves in a younger patient population, or secondary to rheumatic heart disease. Symptoms usually develop when the valve area is less than 1 cm^2, considered within the severely stenotic range. The typical presentation is either chest pain, syncope, or dyspnea (i.e., heart failure) at which time patients are estimated to have a 5-, 3-, or 2-year 50% mortality, respectively.[52] Other conditions that may resemble aortic stenosis include hypertrophic cardiomyopathy, supravalvular stenosis, or subaortic membrane. The ventricle usually hypertrophies as a compensatory response to the increased afterload of the stenotic orifice, and diastolic dysfunction is a common finding. Even with normal coronary arteries, patients are at risk for subendocardial ischemia due to the severity of LVH. Hemodynamic optimization of these patients, especially during induction of anesthesia, includes maintaining adequate preload, a higher MAP, and lower heart rate. This allows more time for ventricular filling in the noncompliant heart while maintaining acceptable systemic perfusion to compensate for the increased transvalvular pressure gradient and relatively fixed CO.

Aortic Insufficiency

Aortic insufficiency can develop acutely or be more chronic in nature. Acute aortic insufficiency can be a result of trauma, endocarditis, or dissection. The pathophysiology of the two entities differs given that with chronic regurgitation, the ventricle has time to compensate by dilating and increasing diastolic compliance. This does not occur if the regurgitation occurs acutely. Aortic regurgitation in type A aortic dissection can be due to annular and aortic root dilation, asymmetric cusp coaptation due to pressure from a false lumen, flail aortic cusp due to annular disruption, or prolapse of the intimal flap through the valve (Fig. 15-19).[53] Acute, severe aortic insufficiency results in severe elevation in LV end diastolic pressure and can cause presystolic closure of mitral valve during diastole, diastolic mitral regurgitation, acute pulmonary edema, and heart failure.[53]

Chronic aortic insufficiency is characterized by volume and pressure overload of the left ventricle. Class I indications for surgery for severe aortic insufficiency include an ejection fraction of less than 50%, symptoms related to aortic insufficiency, and patients undergoing cardiac surgery for another reason.[54,55] Patients with chronic aortic insufficiency often have a dilated LV cavity as a result of volume overload, and surgery is a reasonable consideration in asymptomatic patients with an LV end diastolic dimension

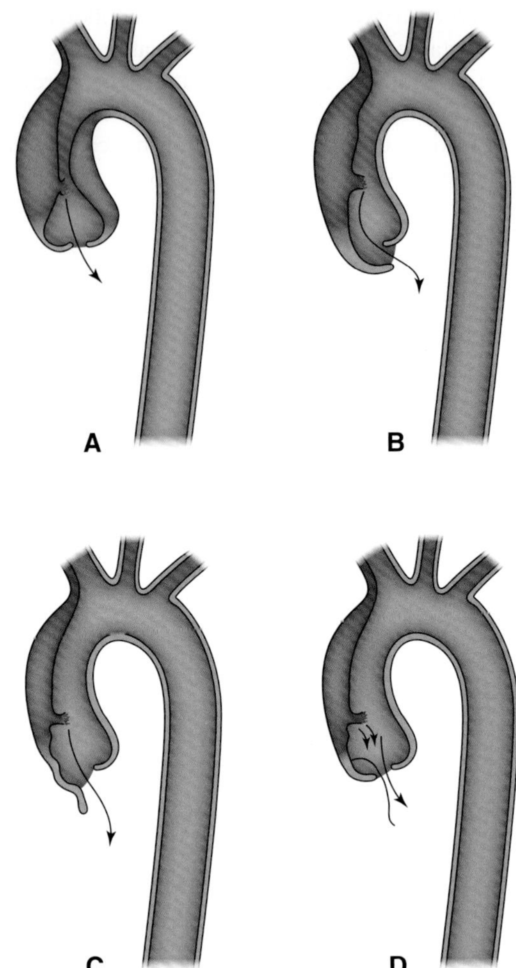

FIGURE 15-19 **A–D:** Mechanism of aortic regurgitation in proximal aortic dissection. (From Hamirani YS, Dietl CA, Voyles W, et al. Acute aortic regurgitation. *Circulation.* 2012;126:1121–1126.)

of greater than 65 mm or an LV end systolic dimension of greater than 50 mm (class II recommendation).[55]

Mitral Stenosis

Mitral stenosis is most often due to rheumatic heart disease, although it can be congenital or degenerative as well. With rheumatic mitral stenosis, thickening and fusion of the mitral commissures and leaflets and chordal thickening leads to a restricted orifice. Symptoms related to mitral stenosis are secondary to volume and pressure overload of the pulmonary circulation due to a fixed obstruction to LV filling. The LV end diastolic and ESVs are lower compared to a normal heart due to the left atrial–LV pressure gradient. Hemodynamic goals include avoiding tachycardia, which further decreases diastolic filling time. Any factors that further increase pulmonary hypertension should be avoided.

Mitral Regurgitation

Etiologies of mitral valve regurgitation include degenerative, rheumatic, congenital, and disorders related to coronary artery disease, endocarditis, or trauma. Characterizing the mechanism of mitral regurgitation, when severe, helps decide whether repair or replacement is feasible.[56] Mitral regurgitation can be a result of annular dilation, excessive leaflet motion (prolapse or flail), or restricted leaflet motion. The Carpentier classification describes the mechanisms of various types of mitral regurgitation.[57] Carpentier class I refers to functional mitral regurgitation related to a dilated annulus, class II refers to excessive leaflet motion in which the regurgitant jet is directed away from the degenerative leaflet, class III refers to restricted leaflet motion in which the regurgitant jet is ipsilateral to the effected leaflet or central in the case of bileaflet restriction (Fig. 15-20). Class IIIa is restricted leaflet motion involving the subvalvular apparatus (chordae and papillary muscles) seen in rheumatic heart disease. Class IIIb is restricted leaflet motion that often accompanies ischemic heart disease, in which the subvalvular apparatus is unaffected though ventricular wall motion may be compromised. Traditionally, mitral repair with preservation of the chordal apparatus has been favored over replacement, with evidence of decreased mortality and improvement of ejection fraction, although some more recent studies have suggested otherwise.[58–61]

Indications for surgical intervention in valvular heart disease include the following considerations: the presence of symptoms, the severity of the valvular lesion, the response of the ventricles to the volume and pressure overload, the effects of this overload on the pulmonary and systemic circulations, and the development of arrhythmias related to the lesions.[55] Patient comorbidities may make percutaneous procedures more favorable. The development and the transcatheter aortic valve implantation (TAVI) procedures, for example, offer an alternative to open heart surgery in those patients with aortic stenosis deemed to be high risk for operative intervention with similar mortality and reduction of symptoms.[62–65]

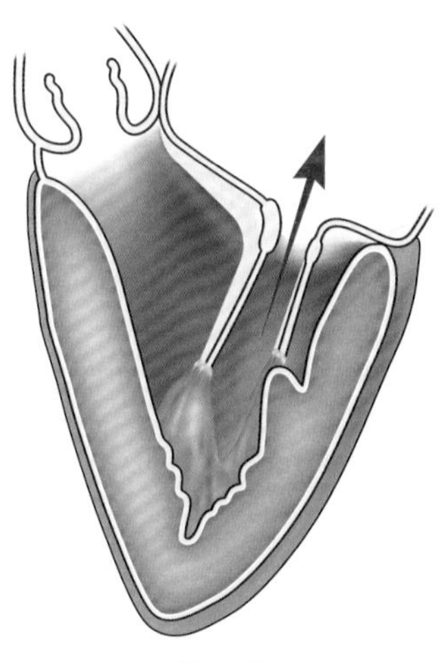

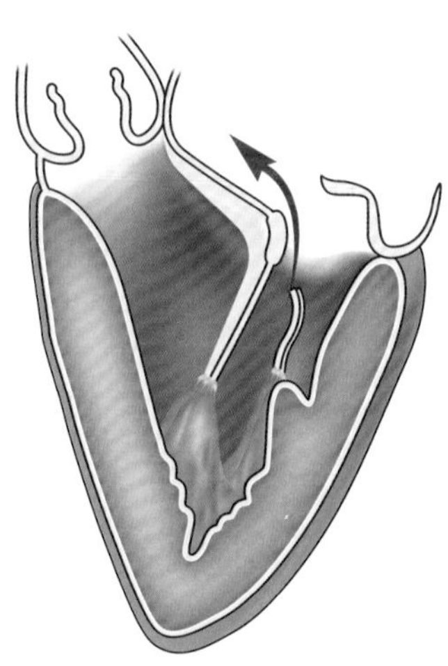

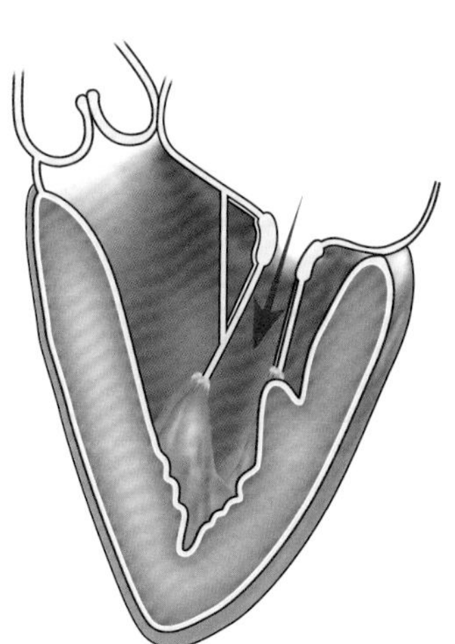

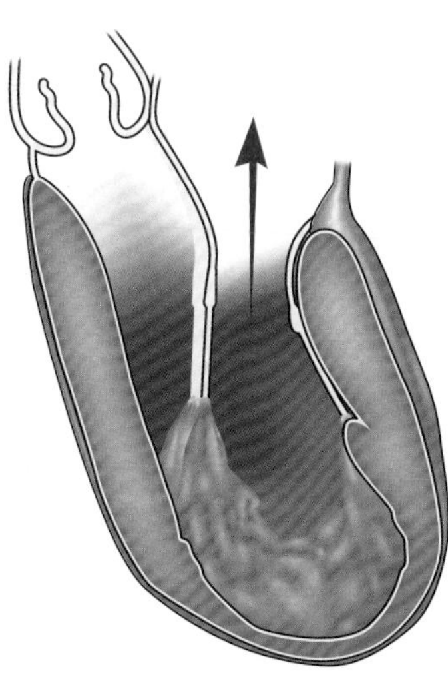

FIGURE 15-20 Carpentier classification of patients with mitral regurgitation (MR). Type I MR: normal leaflet length and motion but with annular dilation or leaflet perforation; type II MR: caused by leaflet prolapse, usually from myxomatous disease, papillary muscle rupture or elongation; type IIIa MR: rheumatic disease with subvalvular involvement; type IIIb MR: caused by ischemic or idiopathic cardiomyopathy causing tethering or restriction of leaflets. (From Fedak P, McCarthy PM, Bonow RO. Evolving concepts and technologies in mitral valve repair. *Circulation.* 2008;117:963–974.)

Cardiac Dysrhythmias

During the perioperative period, changes may take place that trigger cardiac dysrhythmias. It is important to monitor for arrhythmias throughout this time, as they may cause hemodynamic instability and increase morbidity and mortality. The incidence varies according to the type of surgery, morphology of arrhythmia, the form of monitoring (continuous vs. intermittent), and the patient's history. A multicenter study with 17,201 patients undergoing a variety of procedures concluded that 70.2% had dysrhythmias (bradycardia, tachycardia, other arrhythmias) and 1.6% of these needed treatment.[66] Bertrand et al.[67] reported an incidence of 84% and noted that arrhythmias presented more often during the endotracheal intubation and extubation phases. Atlee[68] reported in patients undergoing cardiothoracic surgery, the incidence of some arrhythmia may exceed 90% with continuous monitoring. Melduni et al.[69] reported it ranges from 4% to 20% for noncardiothoracic surgeries.

Etiology

Perioperative cardiac dysrhythmias are most likely to occur in patients with preexisting heart disease (coronary artery disease, valvular heart disease, or cardiomyopathies). Transient physiologic imbalances during the perioperative period make the heart more susceptible to abnormalities in the automaticity of pacemaker cells, the excitability of myocardial cells, and the conduction of the cardiac impulse.

Factors that may contribute to such imbalances include the following:

- Laryngoscopy, endotracheal intubation, ischemia, and release of catecholamines
- Electrolyte abnormalities, hypoxia, carbon dioxide levels, and pH changes
- Inhalation anesthetics, succinylcholine, anticholinesterase–anticholinergic combination reversal, most 5-HT_3 antagonists, droperidol, domperidone, and antiarrhythmics may prolong the QT interval and trigger arrhythmias.
- Extensive blockade of the sympathetic system by subarachnoid local anesthetics may produce bradyarrhythmias and prolong the QT interval.[70]
- Ketamine due to its cardiovascular-stimulating properties
- Direct stimulation of the heart during cardiothoracic procedures and catheter insertion or stimulation of the autonomic nervous system (vagal response)

Mechanisms of Arrhythmia

Automaticity

Automaticity of the heart is its ability to spontaneously generate an electrical impulse to initiate contraction. Any cell of the cardiac conduction system can trigger its own action potential and act as a pacemaker, including cells in the SA node, the AV node, and specialized conducting fibers of the atria and ventricles. Normally, the highest rate of spontaneous depolarization occurs in the SA node, making it the dominant pacemaker in the heart. Abnormal automaticity of any part of the conduction system can lead to arrhythmias.

The resting membrane potential of the pacemaker cells is −60 to −70 mV, whereas in the cardiac muscle cells, it is −90 mV. When the membrane voltage reaches this threshold negative charge, reduction of the potassium efflux and slow influx of sodium (funny current) and calcium (T-type calcium channels) occur. This leads to the initiation of spontaneous depolarization during phase 4 of the cardiac action potential. Because this phase corresponds to diastole, it is also called ***diastolic depolarization***. When the threshold potential is achieved (−40 mV), phase 0 is triggered mostly through activation of L-type calcium channels. Repolarization occurs during phase 3 when the potassium channels open and calcium channels close. Efflux of potassium causes the return to the resting membrane potential. Once a cell depolarizes, it is no longer excitable, being refractory to all stimuli. After this absolute refractory period, cardiac cells enter a relative refractory period during which only a greater than normal stimuli can cause cardiac cell membranes to depolarize (Fig. 15-21).

Excitability

Excitability is the ability of the cardiac cell to respond to a stimulus by depolarizing. A measure of excitability is the difference between the resting transmembrane potential and the threshold potential of the cell. The smaller the difference between these potentials, the more excitable or irritable is the cell. Therefore, enhanced automaticity occurs if the threshold potential becomes more negative or the

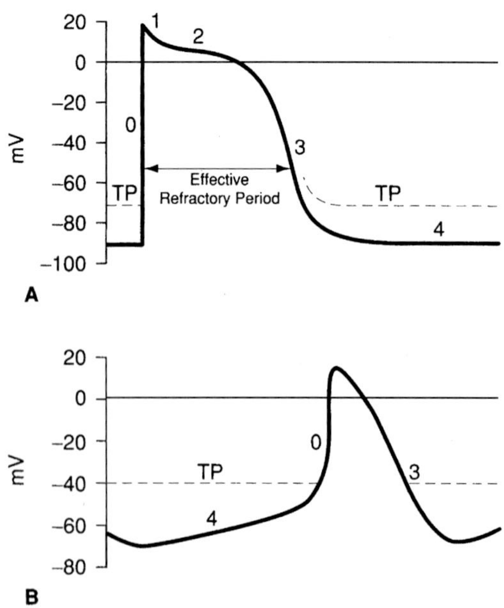

FIGURE 15-21 Cardiac action potential recorded from a ventricular contractile cell **(A)** or an atrial pacemaker cell **(B)**. TP, threshold potential.

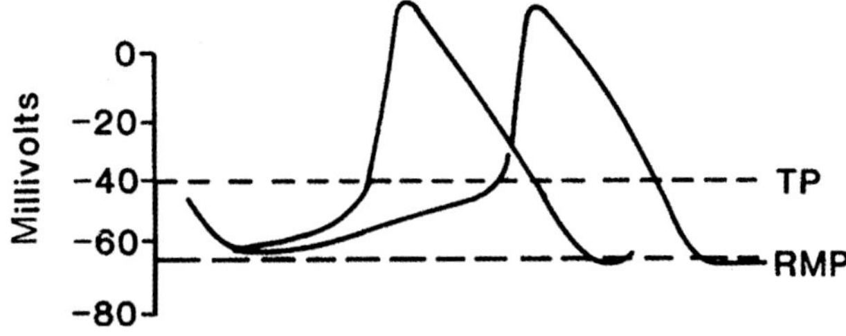

FIGURE 15-22 The rate of pacemaker discharge is dependent on the slope of spontaneous phase 4 depolarization, negativity of the threshold potential (TP), and negativity of the resting transmembrane potential (RMP).

resting membrane potential less negative. The opposite happens in hyperpolarization (Fig. 15-22). Acetylcholine released from M_2 receptors during parasympathetic stimulation increases the conductance of the slow potassium channels (the outward flux of potassium). This causes hyperpolarization of the resting membrane potential and increases the membrane potential difference necessary to overcome in order to reach the threshold potential, decreasing excitability. Acetylcholine also decreases the conductance of the sodium channels (influx of sodium), which leads to slower depolarization and decreased automaticity.[71] Sympathetic stimulation though β_1 receptors increases the conductance of the sodium channels resulting in the depolarization threshold potential being reached more quickly and increased heart rate.

Ectopic Pacemaker

An ectopic pacemaker (abnormal focus) manifests as a premature contraction of the heart that occurs between normal beats. A depolarization wave spreads outward from the ectopic pacemaker and initiates the premature contraction. The ectopic pacemaker may become persistent and assume the role of the dominant pacemaker in place of the SA node. The AV node and the bundle of His are the most common areas for the presence of an ectopic pacemaker. Impulses generated outside the SA node follow a different pathway in the conduction system (usually slower) generating a change in the configuration of the QRS wave on the ECG.

Types of Dysrhythmias

A systematic approach in reading the ECG is essential for accurate diagnosis and correct treatment. It is important to determine the rate and rhythm, the appearance of the P waves and their relation to the QRS, and the morphology of the QRS complex (Table 15-5).

Table 15-5

Diagnosis of Cardiac Dysrhythmias from the Electrocardiogram

- Are P waves present and what is their relationship to the QRS complexes?
- Are the amplitudes, durations, and contours of the P waves, P-R intervals, QRS complexes, and Q-T intervals normal?
- During tachycardia, is the R-P long and P-R interval short (or vice versa)?
- What are the atrial and ventricular discharge rates (same or different)?
- Are the P-P and R-R intervals regular or irregular?

Heart Block

Heart block may occur at the SA node, the AV node, or the bundle branches. Causes of heart block include ischemia, age-related degeneration of the conduction system, drug-induced depression of the impulse propagation (digitalis, β-adrenergic antagonists), excessive parasympathetic nervous system stimulation, pressure on the conduction system by atherosclerotic plaques, or direct stimulation of heart by devices, such wires and catheters.

First-degree AV heart block is considered to be present when there is still one-to-one AV conduction but the P-R interval is longer than 0.2 second at a normal heart rate (Fig. 15-23). Second-degree AV heart block is present when some AV conduction still is present but doesn't occur with every beat. It is classified as Mobitz type I (Wenckebach phenomenon) (Fig. 15-24) or Mobitz type II heart block (Fig. 15-25). Wenckebach phenomenon is characterized by a progressive beat to beat prolongation of the P-R interval until conduction of the cardiac impulse is completely interrupted and a P wave is recorded without a subsequent QRS complex. After this dropped beat, the cycle is repeated. Mobitz type II heart block is the occurrence of a nonconducted atrial impulse without a prior change in the P-R interval and is considered a higher degree of AV block than Mobitz type I.

Third-degree AV heart block is present when there is no conduction of beats from the atria to the ventricles. The P waves are dissociated from the QRS complexes and the heart rate depends on the intrinsic discharge rate of the ectopic pacemaker beyond the site of conduction block. If the ectopic pacemaker is near the AV node, the QRS complexes appear normal and the heart rate is typically 40 to 60 beats per minute (Fig. 15-26). When the site of the block is infranodal, the escape ventricular pacemaker often has a discharge rate of less than 40 beats per minute and the QRS complexes are wide, resembling a bundle branch block (Fig. 15-27).

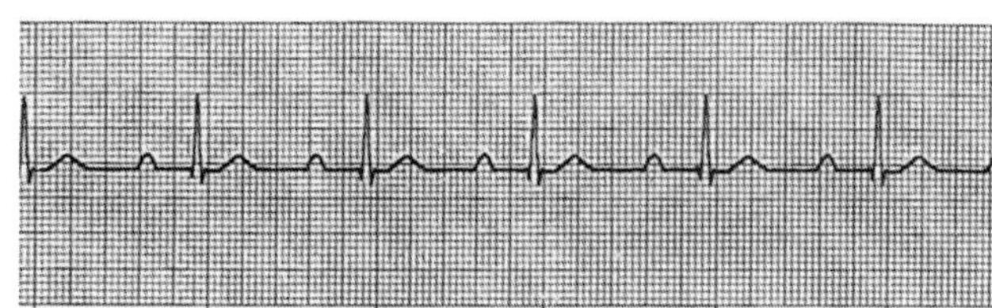

FIGURE 15-23 First-degree AV block.

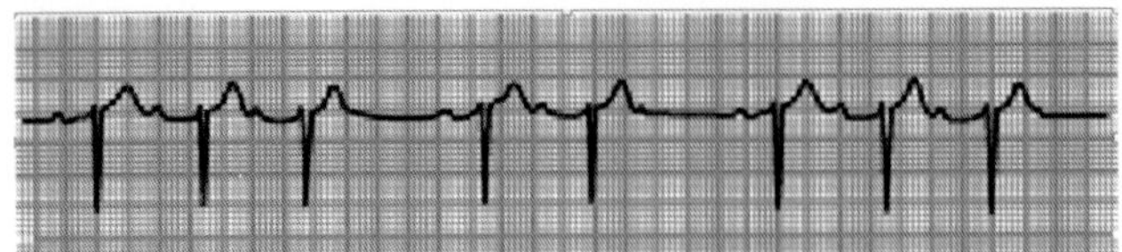

FIGURE 15-24 Mobitz type I (Wenckebach). (From Lange Instant Access EKG's and Cardiac Studies, Anil Patel.)

Patients may experience syncope (Stokes-Adams syndrome) at the onset of third-degree heart block, reflecting the 5- to 10-second period of asystole that may precede the initiation of an ectopic ventricular pacemaker. Occasionally, the interval of ventricular standstill at the onset of third-degree heart block is so long that death occurs. The treatment of patients with third-degree heart block usually requires insertion of a permanent artificial cardiac pacemaker. Temporary support may be provided with intravenous infusion of isoproterenol (chemical cardiac pacemaker) or a transvenous artificial cardiac pacemaker. The safe perioperative management of patients with implanted rhythm control devices such as pacemakers and implantable cardioverter defibrillators (ICD) requires a basic understanding of the classification, function, and emergency management of these devices.[72,73]

Bundle Branch Block

Blockage of the impulse conduction through the right or left bundle branches results in delay of activation of the corresponding ventricle, called ***bundle branch block***, which may be complete or incomplete. Hemiblock or fascicular block refers to the blockade of either the anterior or posterior fascicle of the left bundle branch. Left bundle branch block is clinically significant and cardiac disease must be ruled out. Right bundle branch is commonly seen in healthy individuals but may be caused by right heart enlargement from conditions such as atrial septal defect, chronic lung disease, or pulmonary embolism.

Electrocardiographic criteria for complete right bundle branch block (Fig. 15-28) include QRS duration longer than 120 milliseconds, "M-shaped" QRS complex in V_1 and V_2 (RSR'), and slurred S wave in I, aVL, and V_5 and V_6. Complete left bundle brunch block (LBBB) (Fig. 15-29) is characterized by QRS longer than 120 milliseconds, M-shaped QRS (RSR') complex in V_6, and QS or RS in V_1.

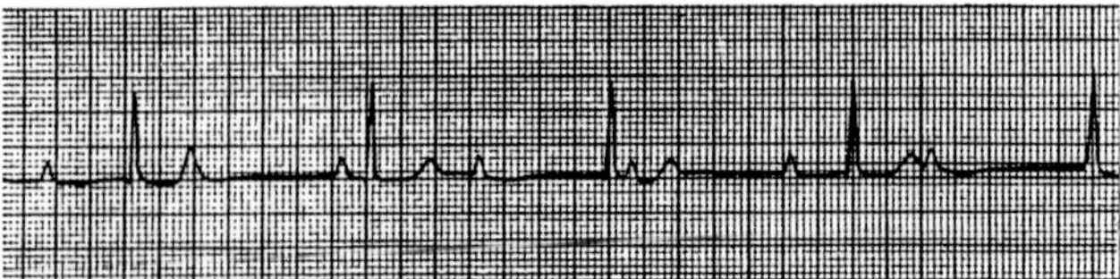

FIGURE 15-26 Third-degree atrioventricular heart block occurring at the level of the atrioventricular node (QRS complexes are narrow). There is no relation between the P waves and QRS complexes.

Reentry

A reentry circuit is the most likely mechanism for supraventricular tachycardia, atrial flutter, atrial fibrillation, premature ventricular contractions, ventricular tachycardia, and ventricular fibrillation. Reentry (circus movements) occurs when the same cardiac impulse returns to its site of initiation through a circuitous pathway and reexcites the cardiac tissue[74] (Fig. 15-30). This contrasts with automaticity, where each beat is initiated by a new impulse. Reentry circuits can develop at any place in the heart where there is an imbalance between conduction and refractoriness creating a slow and fast pathway. Causes of this imbalance include elongation of the conduction pathway such as occurs in dilated hearts (especially a dilated left atrium associated with mitral stenosis), decreased velocity of conduction of cardiac impulses as occurs with myocardial ischemia or hyperkalemia, and a shortened refractory period of cardiac muscle as produced by epinephrine or electric shock from an alternating current. Each of these conditions creates a situation in which cardiac impulses conducted by normal Purkinje fibers can return retrograde through abnormal Purkinje fibers that are not in a refractory state (a reentry circuit). Reentry circuits can be eliminated by speeding conduction through normal tissues so cardiac impulses reach their initial site of origin when the fibers are still refractory or by prolonging the refractory period of normal cells so the returning impulses cannot reenter.

Preexcitation Syndrome

A preexcitation syndrome is present when atrial impulses bypass the AV node through an abnormal conduction pathway to produce premature excitation of the ventricle. Normally, the ventricles are protected from rapid atrial rates by the refractory period of the AV node. The most common accessory conduction pathway producing a direct connection (anatomic loop) of the atrium to the

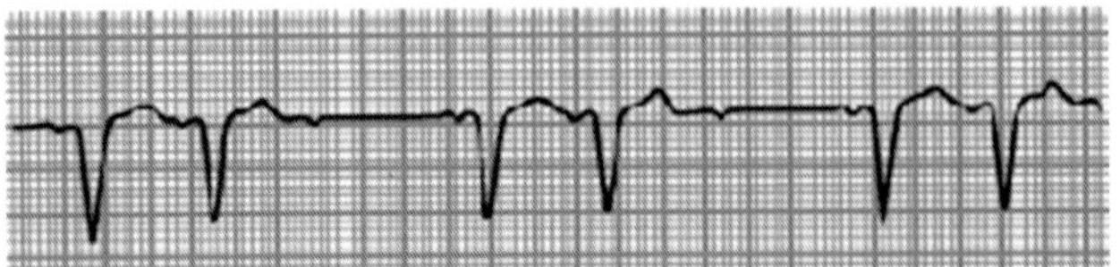

FIGURE 15-25 Mobitz type II. (From Lange Instant Access EKG's and Cardiac Studies, Anil Patel.)

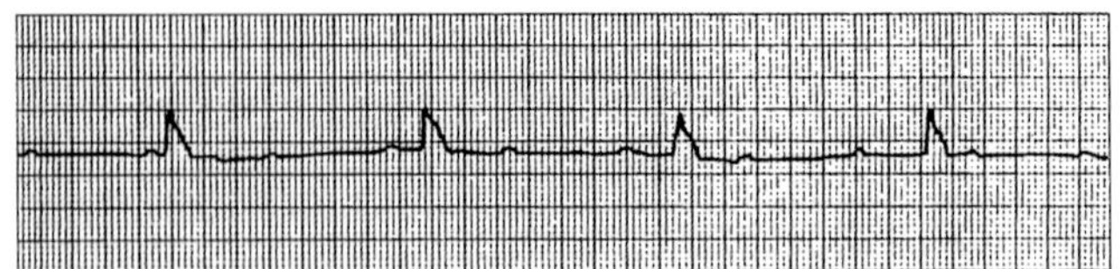

FIGURE 15-27 Third-degree atrioventricular heart block occurring at an infranodal level (QRS complexes are wide).

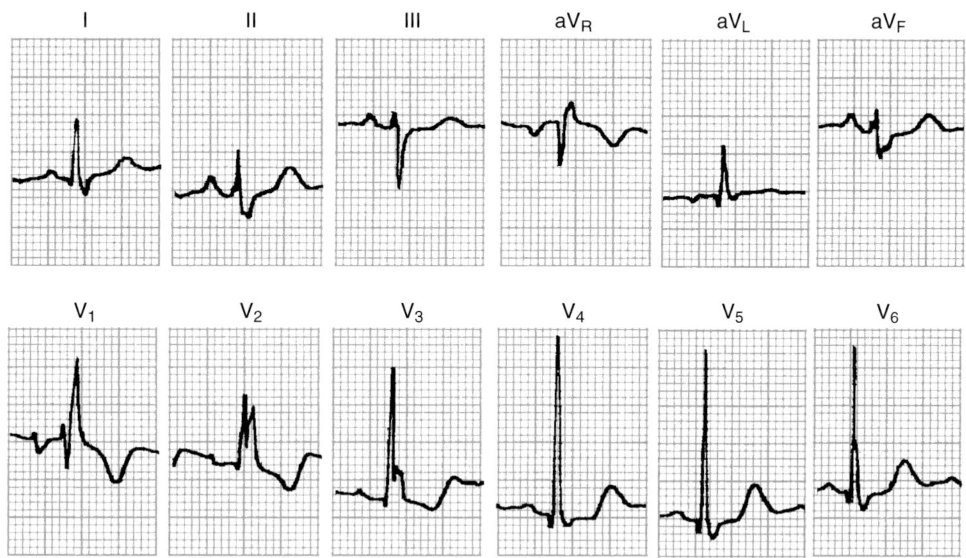

FIGURE 15-28 Right bundle branch block. (From Badescu GC, Sherman B, Zaidan JR, et al. Atlas of electrocardiography. In: Barash PG, Cullen BF, Stoelting RK, et al, eds. *Clinical Anesthesia*. 7th ed. Philadelphia, PA: Lippincott Williams & Wilkins; 2013:1701–1720.)

ventricle is known as ***Kent's bundle*** (usually left atrium to left ventricle) (Table 15-6).[75] Conduction via this accessory pathway produces the Wolff-Parkinson-White syndrome, most often manifesting as intermittent bouts of supraventricular tachyarrhythmias. Electrocardiographic features include short P-R interval (<0.12 second), slurring of the QRS (δ wave), and widening of the QRS (>0.12 second). Patients with preexcitation who are asymptomatic or have no history of tachyarrhythmia usually do not require treatment. According to the American College of

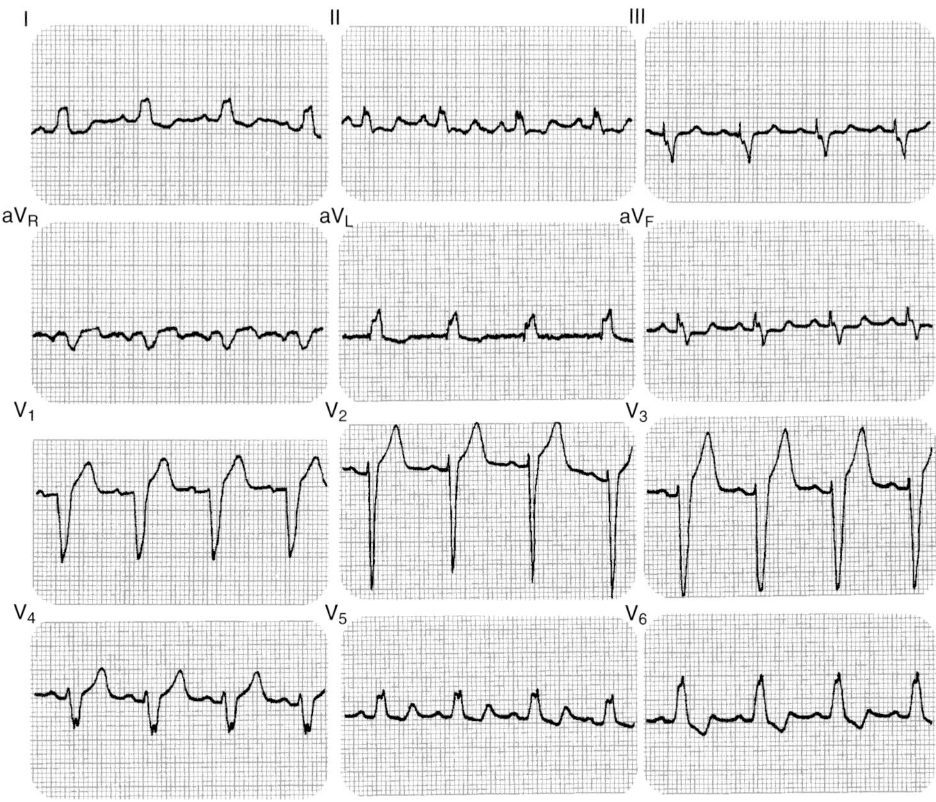

FIGURE 15-29 Left bundle branch block. (From Badescu GC, Sherman B, Zaidan JR, et al. Atlas of electrocardiography. In: Barash PG, Cullen BF, Stoelting RK, et al, eds. *Clinical Anesthesia*. 7th ed. Philadelphia, PA: Lippincott Williams & Wilkins; 2013:1701–1720.)

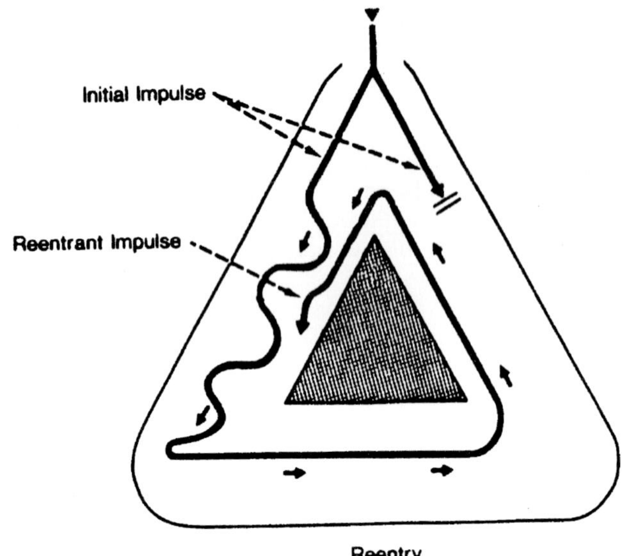

FIGURE 15-30 The essential requirement for initiation of a reentry circuit is a unilateral block that prevents uniform anterograde propagation of the initial cardiac impulse. This same cardiac impulse, under appropriate conditions, can traverse the area of block in a retrograde direction and become a reentrant cardiac impulse. (From Akhtar M. Management of ventricular tachyarrhythmias. JAMA. 1982;247:671–674, with permission.)

Cardiology, avoiding medications that block the conduction through the AV node is recommended, as this may lead to promote anterograde conduction through the accessory pathway.[76] Medications that slow the conduction down the pathologic pathway (procainamide, flecainide) are preferred. Elimination of the pathologic conduction pathway can be achieved with radiofrequency catheter ablation.[77]

Sinus Tachycardia

Sinus tachycardia is usually defined as a sinus rhythm with a resting heart rate of greater than 100 beats per minute (Fig. 15-31). A common cause of sinus tachycardia is sympathetic nervous system stimulation such as may occur during a noxious stimulus in the presence of low concentrations of anesthetic drugs. Hyperthermia increases heart rate approximately 18 beats per minute for every degree Celsius increase. Other important causes of sinus tachycardia include hypoxia, hypercarbia, hypovolemia, drugs, hormones, and intrinsic cardiac abnormalities.

Table 15-6

Accessory Pathways and Preexcitation Syndromes

	Connections
Kent's bundle	Atrium to ventricle
Mahaim bundle	Atrioventricular node to ventricle
Atriohisian fiber	Atrium to His bundle
James fiber	Atrium to atrioventricular node

Adapted from Atlee JL. Perioperative cardiac dysrhythmias: diagnosis and management. *Anesthesiology*. 1997;86:1397–1424.

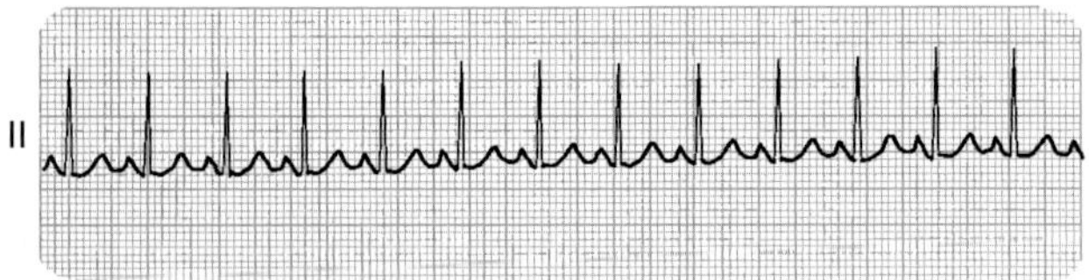

FIGURE 15-31 Sinus tachycardia. (From Badescu GC, Sherman B, Zaidan JR, et al. Atlas of electrocardiography. In: Barash PG, Cullen BF, Stoelting RK, et al, eds. *Clinical Anesthesia*. 7th ed. Philadelphia, PA: Lippincott Williams & Wilkins; 2013:1701–1720.)

Sinus Bradycardia

Sinus bradycardia is usually defined as a sinus rhythm with heart rate of less than 60 beats per minute (Fig. 15-32) and may be caused by parasympathetic nervous system (vagal) stimulation of the heart. Other causes may include hypoxia, medications, and cardiac conditions. Bradycardia that occurs in physically conditioned athletes reflects the ability of their hearts to eject a greater SV with each contraction compared with the less conditioned heart.

Sinus Dysrhythmias

Sinus dysrhythmia, normal variation in the SA node rate, is present during normal breathing with heart rate (R-R intervals) varying approximately 5% during various phases of the resting breathing cycle (Fig. 15-33). During inspiration, the heart rate increases and during expiration, it decreases. This variation may increase to 30% during deep breathing. These variations in heart rate with breathing most likely reflect baroreceptor reflex activity and changes in the negative intrapleural pressures that elicit a waxing and waning Bainbridge reflex. Variation in heart rate that is not related to breathing (nonphasic sinus dysrhythmia) is abnormal and may be a result of SA node dysfunction, aging, or digitalis intoxication. In perioperative settings, sinus dysrhythmia is usually transient and often caused by autonomic nervous system imbalance as the result of an intervention (spinal or epidural anesthesia, laryngoscopy, surgical stimulation) or by the effects of drugs on the SA node.

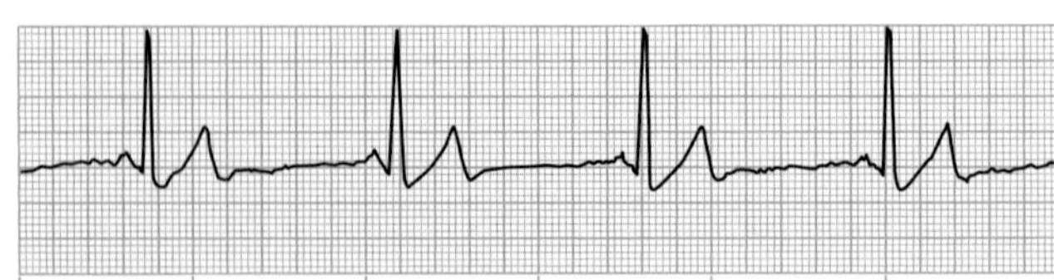

FIGURE 15-32 Sinus bradycardia. (From Badescu GC, Sherman B, Zaidan JR, et al. Atlas of electrocardiography. In: Barash PG, Cullen BF, Stoelting RK, et al, eds. *Clinical Anesthesia*. 7th ed. Philadelphia, PA: Lippincott Williams & Wilkins; 2013:1701–1720.)

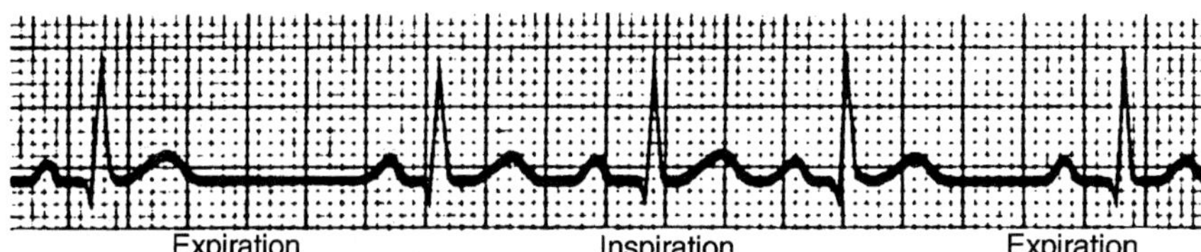

FIGURE 15-33 Sinus dysrhythmia reflecting changes in sinoatrial pacemaker activity with the breathing cycle.

Premature Atrial Contractions

Premature atrial contractions are recognized by an abnormal P wave and a shortened or prolonged P-R interval (Fig. 15-34). The QRS complex of the premature atrial contraction has a normal configuration. The interval between the premature atrial contraction and the succeeding contraction is not an exact multiple of the normal P-P interval (noncompensatory pause) because the SA node is reset. Premature atrial contractions are usually benign and often occur in individuals without heart disease.

Premature Nodal (Junctional) Contractions

Premature nodal contractions are characterized by the absence of normal P waves and P-R intervals preceding the QRS complexes (Fig. 15-35). The P wave may precede, follow, or be obscured by the QRS complex, as the cardiac impulse travels retrograde into the atria as it moves antegrade into the ventricles. Premature junctional contractions are less common than premature atrial and premature ventricular contractions and may be seen under normal conditions.

Nodal (Junctional) Paroxysmal Tachycardia

Nodal paroxysmal tachycardia resembles atrial paroxysmal tachycardia except P waves may precede, follow, or be obscured by the QRS complex (Fig. 15-36). It is common following heart surgery. Other causes include ischemia and digitalis intoxication.

Atrial Paroxysmal Tachycardia

Atrial paroxysmal tachycardia, which often occurs in otherwise healthy young individuals, is caused by rapid rhythmic discharges of impulses from an ectopic atrial pacemaker. The rhythm on the ECG is regular and the P waves are abnormal, often inverted, indicating a site of origin other than the SA node (Fig. 15-37). The QRS complex is narrow. The rapid discharge rate of this ectopic focus causes it to become the pacemaker. Typically, the onset of atrial paroxysmal tachycardia is abrupt and may end just as suddenly with the pacemaker shifting back to the SA node. Atrial paroxysmal tachycardia may be terminated by parasympathetic nervous system stimulation of the heart with drugs or by carotid sinus massage. Drugs that increase refractoriness of the AV node (adenosine, calcium channel blockers, β blockers) are preferred initial therapy for any narrow QRS paroxysmal supraventricular tachycardia.

Atrial Fibrillation

Atrial fibrillation is characterized by normal QRS complexes occurring at a rapid and irregularly irregular rate in the absence of identifiable P waves (Fig. 15-38). The irregular ventricular response reflects arrival of atrial impulses at the AV node at times that may or may not correspond to the refractory period of the node from a previous discharge. SV is decreased during atrial fibrillation due the loss of atrial contraction, which may contribute up to 30% to 40% in ventricular filling depending on the ventricular diastolic status and heart rate.

A pulse deficit (heart rate by palpation is less than that of the ECG) reflects the inability of each ventricular contraction to eject a sufficient SV to produce a detectable peripheral pulse. Etiology of atrial fibrillation includes autonomic nervous system stimulation, ischemia, electrolyte imbalance, atrial dilation, infiltration or fibrosis, hyperthyroidism, hypertension, and sleep apnea. There is an estimated 5% annual risk of thromboembolism in patients with atrial fibrillation who are not treated with anticoagulants. Treatment includes rate control therapy, direct current cardioversion, pharmacologic cardioversion (flecainide, dofetilide, propafenone, ibutilide, and amiodarone), catheter ablation, and surgical Maze procedure. Patients with persistent atrial fibrillation should be considered for anticoagulation to prevent left atrial clot and thromboembolism.[78,79] The following medications are used for rate control: β blockers, nondihydropyridine calcium channel antagonists (verapamil, diltiazem), digoxin, and amiodarone.

Atrial Flutter

Atrial flutter is a regular contraction of the atria at a rate of 250 to 300 beats per minute and on the ECG is characterized by 2:1, 3:1, or 4:1 conduction of atrial impulses to the

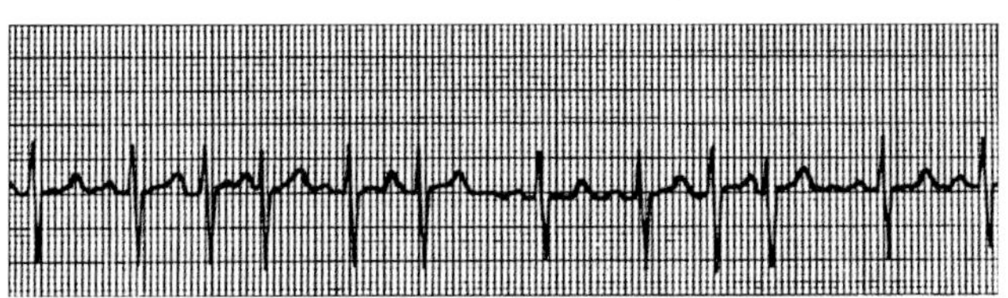

FIGURE 15-34 Premature atrial contractions resulting in an irregular rhythm.

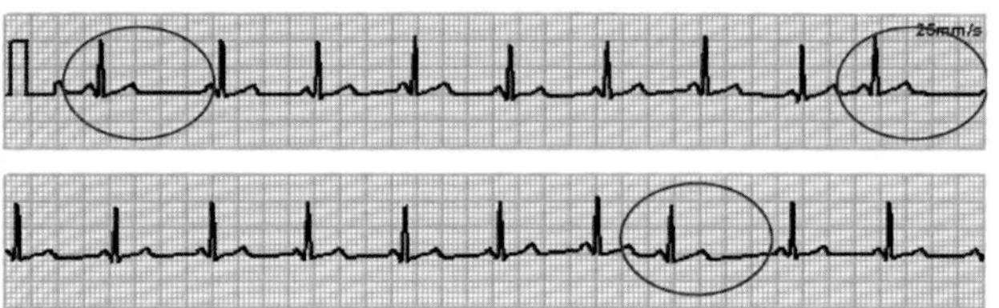

FIGURE 15-35 Premature nodal contractions. (From http://www.favoriteplus.com/blog/recognizing-ecg-irregularities/.) Accessed April 25, 2014.

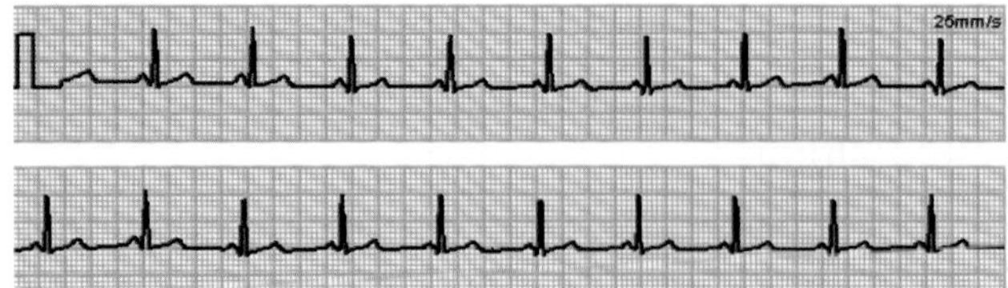

FIGURE 15-36 Nodal tachycardia. (From http://www.favoriteplus.com/blog/recognizing-ecg-irregularities/.) Accessed April 25, 2014.

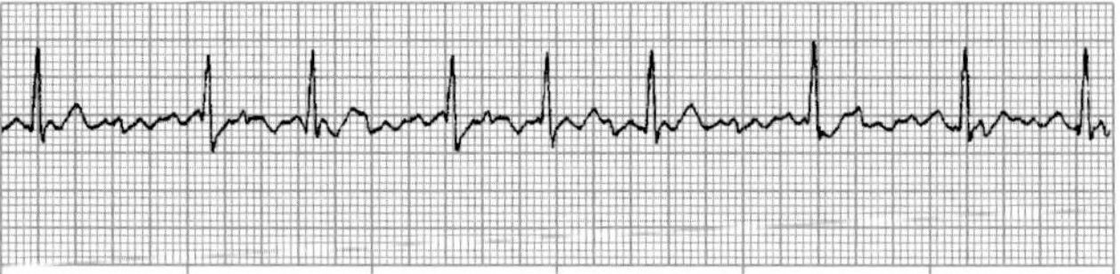

FIGURE 15-38 Atrial fibrillation. (From Badescu GC, Sherman B, Zaidan JR, et al. Atlas of electrocardiography. In: Barash PG, Cullen BF, Stoelting RK, et al, eds. *Clinical Anesthesia*. 7th ed. Philadelphia, PA: Lippincott Williams & Wilkins; 2013:1701–1720.)

ventricle (Fig. 15-39). This occurs because the functional refractory period of Purkinje fibers and ventricular muscle is such that no more than 200 impulses per minute can be transmitted to the ventricles. The P waves have a characteristic saw-toothed appearance, especially in leads II, III, aVF, and V_1. Atrial flutter is seen commonly in patients with chronic pulmonary disease, dilated cardiomyopathy, myocarditis, ethanol intoxication, and thyrotoxicosis. This dysrhythmia may last minutes to hours before changing to sinus rhythm or atrial fibrillation. Treatment is similar to that of atrial fibrillation.

Premature Ventricular Contractions

Premature ventricular contractions result from reentry or an ectopic pacemaker in the ventricles and are not preceded by a P wave. They are classified as unifocal or multifocal based on the morphology of the QRS depending on the number of sites of initiation. The QRS complex of the ECG is widened because the cardiac impulse is conducted through the slowly conducting muscle of the ventricle or an abnormal conduction pathway (Fig. 15-40). The voltage of the QRS complex of the premature ventricular contraction is increased, reflecting the absence of the usual neutralization that occurs when a normal cardiac impulse passes through both ventricles simultaneously. The T wave of premature ventricular contractions usually has an electrical potential opposite that of the QRS complex. A compensatory pause after a premature ventricular contraction occurs because the next impulse from the SA node reaches the ventricle during its refractory period. When a premature ventricular contraction occurs, the ventricle may not have adequately filled to produce a detectable pulse. The subsequent pulse, however, may be increased due to added ventricular filling that occurs during the compensatory pause that typically follows a premature ventricular contraction.

Premature ventricular contractions often reflect significant cardiac disease. For example, myocardial ischemia may be responsible for initiation of premature ventricular contractions from an irritable site in poorly oxygenated ventricular muscle. Other causes include valvular heart disease, high-catecholamine state, hypoxia, hypercapnia, cocaine, alcohol, caffeine, electrolyte abnormalities, and medications. Treatment of premature ventricular contractions includes removal of trigger factors, β blockers, calcium channel blockers, lidocaine, amiodarone, and radiofrequency ablation depending on the symptoms.

Ventricular Tachycardia

Ventricular tachycardia on the ECG resembles a series of ventricular premature contractions that occur at a rapid (200 to 300 beats per minute) and regular rate (Fig. 15-41). It is classified as monomorphic or polymorphic and predisposes to ventricular fibrillation. Common causes of ventricular tachycardia are myocardial ischemia, cardiomyopathies (dilated, hypertrophic, arrhythmogenic right ventricular cardiomyopathy), electrolyte abnormalities (potassium, magnesium, calcium), conditions that result in QT prolongation, drug toxicity, and congenital myocardial defects. SV is often severely depressed during ventricular tachycardia because the ventricles have insufficient time for cardiac filling. Presentation may include palpitations, shortness of breath, chest pain, presyncope, syncope, and sudden cardiac arrest causing death.[80]

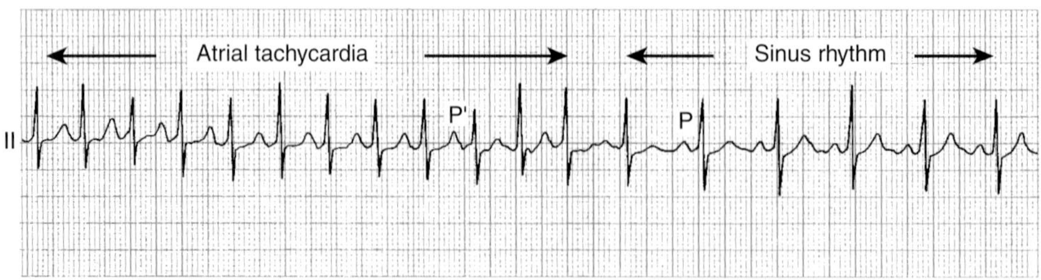

FIGURE 15-37 Atrial paroxysmal tachycardia. (From Badescu GC, Sherman B, Zaidan JR, et al. Atlas of electrocardiography. In: Barash PG, Cullen BF, Stoelting RK, et al, eds. *Clinical Anesthesia*. 7th ed. Philadelphia, PA: Lippincott Williams & Wilkins; 2013:1701–1720.)

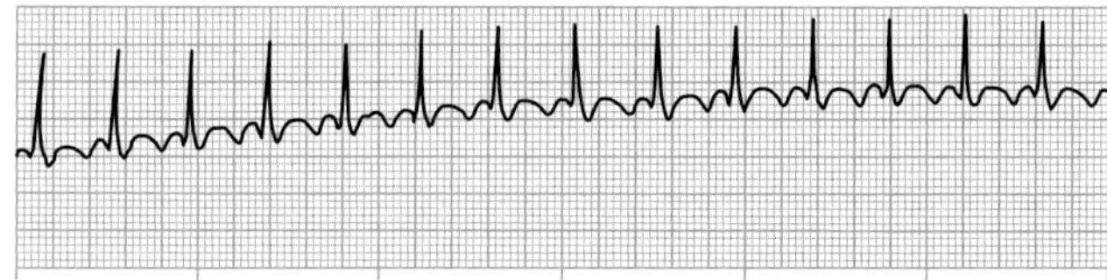

FIGURE 15-39 Atrial flutter. (From Badescu GC, Sherman B, Zaidan JR, et al. Atlas of electrocardiography. In: Barash PG, Cullen BF, Stoelting RK, et al, eds. *Clinical Anesthesia.* 7th ed. Philadelphia, PA: Lippincott Williams & Wilkins; 2013:1701–1720.)

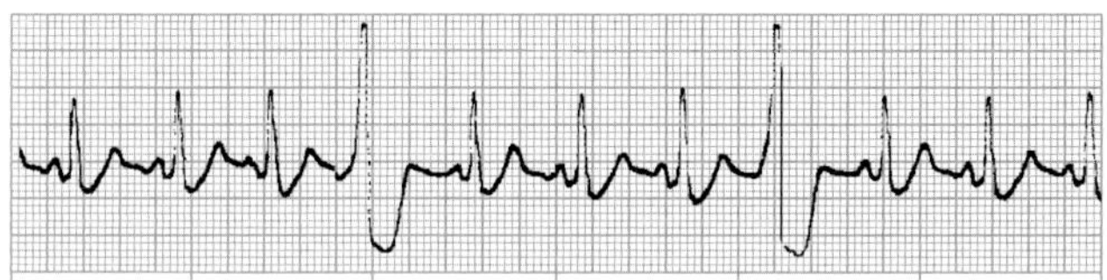

FIGURE 15-40 Multifocal premature ventricular contractions. (From Badescu GC, Sherman B, Zaidan JR, et al. Atlas of electrocardiography. In: Barash PG, Cullen BF, Stoelting RK, et al, eds. *Clinical Anesthesia.* 7th ed. Philadelphia, PA: Lippincott Williams & Wilkins; 2013:1701–1720.)

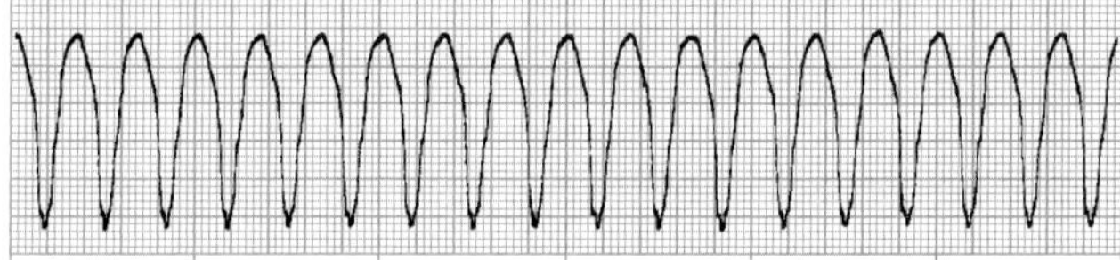

FIGURE 15-41 Ventricular tachycardia. (From Badescu GC, Sherman B, Zaidan JR, et al. Atlas of electrocardiography. In: Barash PG, Cullen BF, Stoelting RK, et al, eds. *Clinical Anesthesia.* 7th ed. Philadelphia, PA: Lippincott Williams & Wilkins; 2013:1701–1720.)

Coarse Ventricular Fibrillation

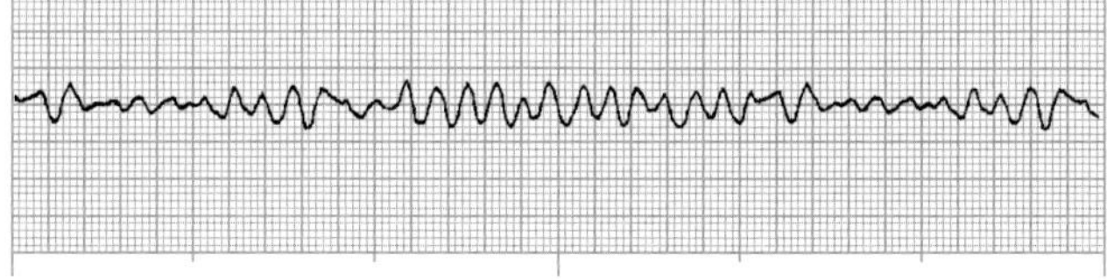

Fine Ventricular Fibrillation

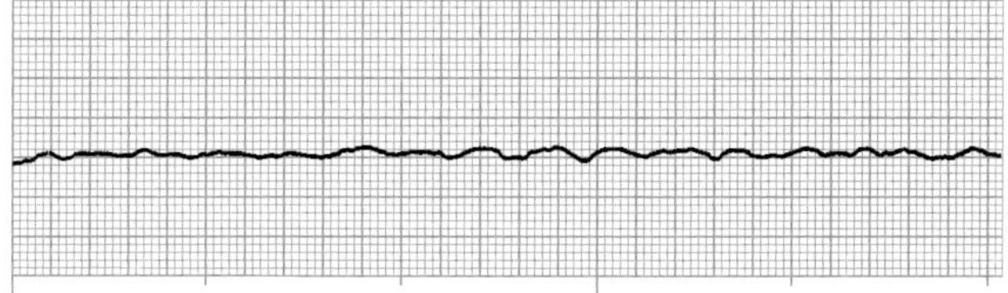

FIGURE 15-42 Ventricular fibrillation. (From Badescu GC, Sherman B, Zaidan JR, et al. Atlas of electrocardiography. In: Barash PG, Cullen BF, Stoelting RK, et al, eds. *Clinical Anesthesia.* 7th ed. Philadelphia, PA: Lippincott Williams & Wilkins; 2013:1701–1720.)

Nonsustained ventricular tachycardia may be defined as three or more consecutive ventricular beats at a rate greater than 100 beats per minute lasting less than 30 seconds and is usually asymptomatic.[81] Sustained ventricular tachycardia usually leads to hemodynamic instability and necessitates termination with electrical cardioversion. Therapies include correction of electrolyte abnormalities, ICD placement, β blockers (sotalol, amiodarone), ablation, and revascularization.[80]

Ventricular Fibrillation

Ventricular fibrillation is characterized on the ECG by an irregular wavy line with voltages that range from 0.25 to 0.5 mV (Fig. 15-42). There is total absence of coordinated contractions with cessation of any effective pumping activity and disappearance of detectable pulse and systemic blood pressure. Ventricular fibrillation is usually initiated by a reentry mechanism. The only effective treatment of ventricular fibrillation is the delivery of direct electric current through the ventricles (defibrillation), which simultaneously depolarizes all ventricular muscle. This depolarization allows the initiation of a cardiac pacemaker remote from the irritable focus responsible for the ventricular fibrillation. Cardiopulmonary resuscitation (CPR) must be initiated until a defibrillator becomes available. The survival rate of ventricular fibrillation may decrease by 7% to 10 % for every minute that defibrillation is delayed, depending on the CPR quality. If defibrillation is delayed for more than 12 minutes, the survival rate is less than 5%.[82] It is important to identify the patients at risk for ventricular fibrillation and place a prophylactic ICD.[80]

References

1. Strandring S, ed. *Gray's Anatomy: The Anatomical Basis of Clinical Practice.* 40th ed. Philadelphia, PA: Churchill Livingstone; 2008.
2. Peebles CR, Shambrook JS, Harden SP. Pericardial disease—anatomy and function. *Br J Radiol.* 2011;84(3, special issue): S324–S337.
3. Tabaksblat MH, Dan G, Argulian E, et al. *Anatomy and Physiology of the Pericardium.* New York, NY: Springer International Publishing; 2014.
4. Ho S, McCarthy KP, Josen M, et al. Anatomic-echocardiographic correlates: an introduction to normal and congenitally malformed hearts. *Heart.* 2001;86(suppl 2):II3–II11.
5. Debonnaire P, Palmen M, Marsan NA, et al. Contemporary imaging of normal mitral valve anatomy and function. *Curr Opin Cardiol.* 2012;27(5):455–464.
6. Anderson RH, Cook AC, Hlavacek AJ, et al. Normal cardiac anatomy. In: da Cruz EM, Ivy D, Jaggers J, eds. *Pediatric and Congenital Cardiology, Cardiac Surgery and Intensive Care.* London, United Kingdom: Springer-Verlag; 2014.
7. Tune JD, Gorman MW, Feigl EO. Matching coronary blood flow to myocardial oxygen consumption. *J Appl Physiol.* 2004;97(1):404–415.
8. Ho SY, McCarthy KP, Ansari A, et al. Anatomy of the atrioventricular node and atrioventricular conduction system. *Int J Bifurcat Chaos.* 2003;13(12):3665–3674.
9. Saremi F, Abolhoda A, Ashikyan O, et al. Arterial supply to sinuatrial and atrioventricular nodes: imaging with multidetector CT. *Radiol.* 2008;246(1):99–107; discussion 108–109.

10. Goldberger E. The aVL, aVR, and aVF leads: a simplification of standard lead electrocardiography. *Am Heart J.* 1942;24:378–396.
11. London MJ, Hollenberg M, Wong MG, et al. Intraoperative myocardial ischemia: localization by continuous 12-lead electrocardiography. *Anesthesiology.* 1988;69(2):232–241.
12. Hall JE, Guyton AC. *Guyton and Hall Textbook of Medical Physiology.* 12th ed. Philadelphia, PA: Saunders/Elsevier; 2011.
13. Cardiac muscle. Wikipedia: The Free Encyclopedia. http://en.wikipedia.org/wiki/Cardiac_muscle. Accessed June 21, 2014.
14. Bers DM. Cardiac excitation-contraction coupling. *Nature.* 2002; 415(6868):198–205.
15. Bers DM. Major cellular structures involved in excitation-contraction coupling. In: Bers DM, ed. *Excitation-Contraction Coupling and Cardiac Contractile Force.* 2nd ed. Kluwer Academic Publishers; 2001.
16. Fabiato A, Fabiato F. Calcium and cardiac excitation-contraction coupling. *Ann Rev Physiol.* 1979;41:473–484.
17. Mendelowitz D. Advances in parasympathetic control of heart rate and cardiac function. *News Physiol Sci.* 1999;14:155–161.
18. Brodde OE, Michel MC. Adrenergic and muscarinic receptors in the human heart. *Pharmacol Rev.* 1999;51(4):651–690.
19. Cameron VA, Ellmers LJ. Minireview: natriuretic peptides during development of the fetal heart and circulation. *Endocrinology.* 2003;144(6):2191–2194.
20. Schuijt MP, Danser AH. Cardiac angiotensin II: an intracrine hormone? *Am J Hypertens.* 2002;15(12):1109–1116.
21. Martinez A. Biology of adrenomedullin. Introduction. *Microsc Res Tech.* 2002;57(1):1–2.
22. Wiggers CJ. Dynamics of ventricular contraction under abnormal conditions. *Circulation.* 1952;5(3):321–348.
23. Khouri SJ, Maly GT, Suh DD, et al. A practical approach to the echocardiographic evaluation of diastolic function. *J Am Soc Echocardiogr.* 2004;17(3):290–297.
24. Pittman JA, Ping JS, Mark JB. Arterial and central venous pressure monitoring. *Int Anesthesiol Clin.* 2004;42(1):13–30.
25. Patterson SW, Starling EH. On the mechanical factors which determine the output of the ventricles. *J Physiol.* 1914;48(5):357–379.
26. Katz AM. Ernest Henry Starling, his predecessors, and the "Law of the Heart." *Circulation.* 2002;106(23):2986–2992.
27. Starling E. The Arris and Bale Lectures on some points in the pathology of heart disease. *Lancet.* 1897;149(3835):569–572.
28. Guyton AC. Determination of cardiac output by equating venous return curves with cardiac response curves. *Physiol Rev.* 1955;35(1): 123–129.
29. Henderson WR, Griesdale DE, Walley KR, et al. Clinical review: Guyton—the role of mean circulatory filling pressure and right atrial pressure in controlling cardiac output. *Crit Care.* 2010;14(6):243.
30. Burkhoff D, Mirsky I, Suga H. Assessment of systolic and diastolic ventricular properties via pressure-volume analysis: a guide for clinical, translational, and basic researchers. *Am J Physiol.* 2005;289(2):H501–H512.
31. Sagawa K. The end-systolic pressure-volume relation of the ventricle: definition, modifications and clinical use. *Circulation.* 1981; 63(6):1223–1227.
32. Sagawa K, Suga H, Shoukas AA, et al. End-systolic pressure/volume ratio: a new index of ventricular contractility. *Am J Cardiol.* 1977;40(5):748–753.
33. Swan HJ, Ganz W, Forrester J, et al. Catheterization of the heart in man with use of a flow-directed balloon-tipped catheter. *N Engl J Med.* 1970;283(9):447–451.
34. Ganz W, Donoso R, Marcus HS, et al. A new technique for measurement of cardiac output by thermodilution in man. *Am J Cardiol.* 1971;27(4):392–396.
35. Libby P, Theroux P. Pathophysiology of coronary artery disease. *Circulation.* 2005;111(25):3481–3488.
36. Libby P. Inflammation in atherosclerosis. *Nature.* 2002;420(6917): 868–874.
37. Libby P. Inflammation in atherosclerosis. *Arterioscler Thromb Vasc Biol.* 2012;32(9):2045–2051.
38. Jneid H, Anderson JL, Wright RS, et al; American College of Cardiology Foundation; American Heart Association Task Force on Practice Guidelines. 2012 ACCF/AHA focused update of the guideline for the management of patients with unstable angina/non–ST-elevation myocardial infarction (updating the 2007 guideline and replacing the 2011 focused update): a report of the American College of Cardiology Foundation/American Heart Association Task Force on Practice Guidelines. *Circulation.* 2012;126(7):875–910.
39. O'Gara PT, Kushner FG, Ascheim DD, et al. 2013 ACCF/AHA guideline for the management of ST-elevation myocardial infarction: a report of the American College of Cardiology Foundation/American Heart Association Task Force on Practice Guidelines. *Circulation.* 2013;127(4):e362–e425.
40. Fihn SD, Gardin JM, Abrams J, et al. 2012 ACCF/AHA/ACP/AATS/PCNA/SCAI/STS guideline for the diagnosis and management of patients with stable ischemic heart disease: a report of the American College of Cardiology Foundation/American Heart Association Task Force on Practice Guidelines, and the American College of Physicians, American Association for Thoracic Surgery, Preventive Cardiovascular Nurses Association, Society for Cardiovascular Angiography and Interventions, and Society of Thoracic Surgeons. *J Am Coll Cardiol.* 2012;60(24):e44–e164.
41. Fihn SD, Gardin JM, Abrams J, et al. 2012 ACCF/AHA/ACP/AATS/PCNA/SCAI/STS guideline for the diagnosis and management of patients with stable ischemic heart disease: a report of the American College of Cardiology Foundation/American Heart Association Task Force on Practice Guidelines, and the American College of Physicians, American Association for Thoracic Surgery, Preventive Cardiovascular Nurses Association, Society for Cardiovascular Angiography and Interventions, and Society of Thoracic Surgeons. *Circulation.* 2012;126(25):e354–e471.
42. Montalescot G, Sechtem U, Achenbach S, et al. 2013 ESC guidelines on the management of stable coronary artery disease: the Task Force on the management of stable coronary artery disease of the European Society of Cardiology. *Eur Heart J.* 2013;34(38): 2949–3003.
43. Yancy CW, Jessup M, Bozkurt B, et al. 2013 ACCF/AHA guideline for the management of heart failure: a report of the American College of Cardiology Foundation/American Heart Association Task Force on Practice Guidelines. *J Am Coll Cardiol.* 2013;62(16): e147–e239.
44. Kemp CD, Conte JV. The pathophysiology of heart failure. *Cardiovasc Pathol.* 2012;21(5):365–371.
45. Kenchaiah S, Evans JC, Levy D, et al. Obesity and the risk of heart failure. *N Engl J Med.* 2002;347(5):305–313.
46. Lee DS, Gona P, Vasan RS, et al. Relation of disease pathogenesis and risk factors to heart failure with preserved or reduced ejection fraction: insights from the Framingham Heart Study of the National Heart, Lung, and Blood Institute. *Circulation.* 2009;119(24): 3070–3077.
47. Bhuiyan T, Maurer MS. Heart failure with preserved ejection fraction: persistent diagnosis, therapeutic enigma. *Curr Cardiovasc Risk Rep.* 2011;5(5):440–449.
48. Steinberg BA, Zhao X, Heidenreich PA, et al. Trends in patients hospitalized with heart failure and preserved left ventricular ejection fraction: prevalence, therapies, and outcomes. *Circulation.* 2012;126(1):65–75.
49. Digitalis Investigation Group. The effect of digoxin on mortality and morbidity in patients with heart failure. *N Engl J Med.* 1997;336(8):525–533.
50. Pratt AK, Shah NS, Boyce SW. Left ventricular assist device management in the ICU. *Crit Care Med.* 2014;42(1):158–168.
51. Rose EA, Gelijns AC, Moskowitz AJ, et al. Long-term use of a left ventricular assist device for end-stage heart failure. *N Engl J Med.* 2001;345(20):1435–1443.
52. Turina J, Hess O, Sepulcri F, et al. Spontaneous course of aortic valve disease. *Eur Heart J.* 1987;8(5):471–483.
53. Hamirani YS, Dietl CA, Voyles W, et al. Acute aortic regurgitation. *Circulation.* 2012;126(9):1121–1126.

54. Bonow RO. Chronic mitral regurgitation and aortic regurgitation: have indications for surgery changed? *J Am Coll Cardiol.* 2013;61(7):693–701.
55. Nishimura RA, Otto CM, Bonow RO, et al. 2014 AHA/ACC guideline for the management of patients with valvular heart disease: a report of the American College of Cardiology/American Heart Association Task Force on Practice Guidelines. *Circulation.* 2014;129(23):e521–e643.
56. Fedak PW, McCarthy PM, Bonow RO. Evolving concepts and technologies in mitral valve repair. *Circulation.* 2008;117(7):963–974.
57. de Marchena E, Badiye A, Robalino G, et al. Respective prevalence of the different Carpentier classes of mitral regurgitation: a stepping stone for future therapeutic research and development. *J Card Surg.* 2011;26(4):385–392.
58. Acker MA, Parides MK, Perrault LP, et al. Mitral-valve repair versus replacement for severe ischemic mitral regurgitation. *N Engl J Med.* 2014;370(1):23–32.
59. Reece TB, Tribble CG, Ellman PI, et al. Mitral repair is superior to replacement when associated with coronary artery disease. *Ann Surg.* 2004;239(5):671–675; discussion 675–677.
60. Lee EM, Shapiro LM, Wells FC. Superiority of mitral valve repair in surgery for degenerative mitral regurgitation. *Eur Heart J.* 1997;18(4):655–663.
61. Rozich JD, Carabello BA, Usher BW, et al. Mitral valve replacement with and without chordal preservation in patients with chronic mitral regurgitation. Mechanisms for differences in postoperative ejection performance. *Circulation.* 1992;86(6):1718–1726.
62. Leon MB, Smith CR, Mack M, et al. Transcatheter aortic-valve implantation for aortic stenosis in patients who cannot undergo surgery. *N Engl J Med.* 2010;363(17):1597–1607.
63. Smith CR, Leon MB, Mack MJ, et al. Transcatheter versus surgical aortic-valve replacement in high-risk patients. *N Engl J Med.* 2011;364(23):2187–2198.
64. Makkar RR, Fontana GP, Jilaihawi H, et al. Transcatheter aortic-valve replacement for inoperable severe aortic stenosis. *N Engl J Med.* 2012;366(18):1696–1704.
65. Kodali SK, Williams MR, Smith CR, et al. Two-year outcomes after transcatheter or surgical aortic-valve replacement. *N Engl J Med.* 2012;366(18):1686–1695.
66. Forrest JB, Cahalan MK, Rehder K, et al. Multicenter study of general anesthesia. II. Results. *Anesthesiology.* 1990;72(2):262–268.
67. Bertrand CA, Steiner NV, Jameson AG, et al. Disturbances of cardiac rhythm during anesthesia and surgery. *JAMA.* 1971;216(10): 1615–1617.
68. Atlee JL. Perioperative cardiac dysrhythmias: diagnosis and management. *Anesthesiology.* 1997;86(6):1397–1424.
69. Melduni RM, Koshino Y, Shen WK. Management of arrhythmias in the perioperative setting. *Clin Geriatr Med.* 2012;28(4):729–743.
70. Staikou C, Stamelos M, Stavroulakis E. Impact of anaesthetic drugs and adjuvants on ECG markers of torsadogenicity. *Br J Anaesth.* 2014;112(2):217–230.
71. Razani B. Autonomic cardiac regulation. 2010–2014. http://www.pathwaymedicine.org/autonomic-cardiac-regulation. Accessed April 25, 2014.
72. Atlee JL, Bernstein AD. Cardiac rhythm management devices (part I): indications, device selection, and function. *Anesthesiology.* 2001;95(5):1265–1280.
73. Atlee JL, Bernstein AD. Cardiac rhythm management devices (part II): perioperative management. *Anesthesiology.* 2001;95(6): 1492–1506.
74. Akhtar M. Management of ventricular tachyarrhythmias. Part II. *JAMA.* 1982;247(8):1178–1181.
75. Wellens HJ, Brugada P, Penn OC. The management of preexcitation syndromes. *JAMA.* 1987;257(17):2325–2333.
76. Blomstrom-Lundqvist C, Scheinman MM, Aliot EM, et al. ACC/AHA/ESC guidelines for the management of patients with supraventricular arrhythmias—executive summary: a report of the American College of Cardiology/American Heart Association Task Force on Practice Guidelines and the European Society of Cardiology Committee for Practice Guidelines (writing committee to develop guidelines for the management of patients with supraventricular arrhythmias) developed in collaboration with NASPE-Heart Rhythm Society. *J Am Coll Cardiol.* 2003;42(8):1493–1531.
77. Kulig J, Koplan BA. Cardiology patient page. Wolff-Parkinson-White syndrome and accessory pathways. *Circulation.* 2010;122(15): e480–e483.
78. January CT, Wann LS, Alpert JS, et al. 2014 AHA/ACC/HRS guideline for the management of patients with atrial fibrillation: executive summary: a report of the American College of Cardiology/American Heart Association Task Force on Practice Guidelines and the Heart Rhythm Society [published online ahead of print March 28, 2014]. *J Am Coll Cardiol.*
79. Lip GY, Tse HF, Lane DA. Atrial fibrillation. *Lancet.* 2012;379(9816): 648–661.
80. Zipes DP, Camm AJ, Borggrefe M, et al. ACC/AHA/ESC 2006 guidelines for management of patients with ventricular arrhythmias and the prevention of sudden cardiac death: a report of the American College of Cardiology/American Heart Association Task Force and the European Society of Cardiology Committee for Practice Guidelines (writing committee to develop guidelines for management of patients with ventricular arrhythmias and the prevention of sudden cardiac death): developed in collaboration with the European Heart Rhythm Association and the Heart Rhythm Society. *Circulation.* 2006;114(10):e385–e484.
81. Katritsis DG, Camm AJ. Nonsustained ventricular tachycardia: where do we stand? *Eur Heart J.* 2004;25(13):1093–1099.
82. Samson R, Berg R, Bingham R; Pediatric Advanced Life Support Task Force, International Liaison Committee on Resuscitation. Use of automated external defibrillators for children: an update. An advisory statement from the Pediatric Advanced Life Support Task Force, International Liaison Committee on Resuscitation. *Resuscitation.* 2003;57(3):237–243.

CHAPTER 16

Renal Physiology

Updated by: Jonathan Hastie • Jack S. Shanewise

The kidneys play a central role in the maintenance of homeostasis of the body. The kidneys stabilize extracellular fluid electrolyte composition, maintain acid–base balance, regulate volume status and blood pressure, secrete erythropoietin and renin, and excrete toxins and metabolic waste. These functions involve complex interactions within the kidneys and with other organ systems and are frequently altered during anesthesia. Hence, a thorough understanding of kidney function is important for the anesthesiologist before, during, and after patients receive care in the operating room.

Kidney Structure and Function

Basic Anatomy of the Kidney

The kidneys are paired organs located below the diaphragm in the retroperitoneal space, weighing between 115 and 160 g each. Each kidney has an outer portion (cortex) and inner portion (medulla). The renal arteries arise from the abdominal aorta, and the renal veins direct blood flow into the inferior vena cava. The kidneys are prominently innervated by the sympathetic nervous system from T4 through T12.

The nephron is the functional unit of the kidney. (Fig. 16-1) A nephron is composed of a capillary bed called the ***glomerulus*** surrounded by epithelial cells called ***Bowman's capsule***. Bowman's capsule, in turn, is continuous with a long tubule that drains into the renal pelvis. Fluid is filtered through the glomerular capillaries and is converted, along the length of the renal tubule, into urine.[1] There are two types of nephrons: Juxtamedullary nephrons have tubules that descend into the renal medulla, whereas cortical nephrons are closer to the surface of the kidney.

The Glomerulus

Structure and Function of the Glomerulus

Glomeruli are found in the renal cortex and consist of a tuft of capillaries surrounded by Bowman's capsule, the dilated blind end of the renal tubule. Glomerular capillaries are uniquely interposed between two sets of arterioles. Blood flows from the afferent arterioles through the glomerular capillaries and then on to the efferent arterioles. Hence, pressure in the glomerular capillaries is a function of the vascular activity of both the afferent and efferent arterioles (Fig. 16-2): Afferent vasoconstriction lowers glomerular capillary pressure, whereas efferent arteriolar vasoconstriction raises glomerular capillary pressure. Glomerular capillary pressure causes water and low-molecular-weight substances to be filtered into Bowman's capsule and the renal tubule system.

Fluid that is filtered from the glomerular capillaries into the renal tubules is called ***glomerular filtrate***. Because the glomerular capillary membrane contains pores, its permeability is much greater than that of the typical tissue capillary. Fluid, amino acids, and ions are rapidly filtered, whereas higher molecular weight proteins are retained within the capillary. The composition of glomerular filtrate, then, is similar to plasma but without protein.

Glomerular Filtration Rate

The volume of collective glomerular filtrate formed over time is called the ***glomerular filtration rate*** (GFR). In a normal person, the GFR is approximately 125 mL per minute or 180 L per day. Because 99% of this 180 L of glomerular filtrate is reabsorbed, daily urine output is 1 to 2 L. As described earlier, glomerular capillary pressure leads to filtration into the renal tubule. The normal filtration pressure of approximately 10 mmHg is calculated as glomerular capillary pressure (60 mm Hg) minus colloid osmotic pressure (32 mm Hg) and pressure in Bowman's capsule (18 mm Hg) (Fig. 16-3). The filtration rate is influenced by several factors: Mean arterial pressure, cardiac output, and the sympathetic nervous system may each raise glomerular capillary pressure and increase the GFR.

The kidneys have an autoregulatory mechanism to modulate the effect of mean arterial pressure on the GFR.

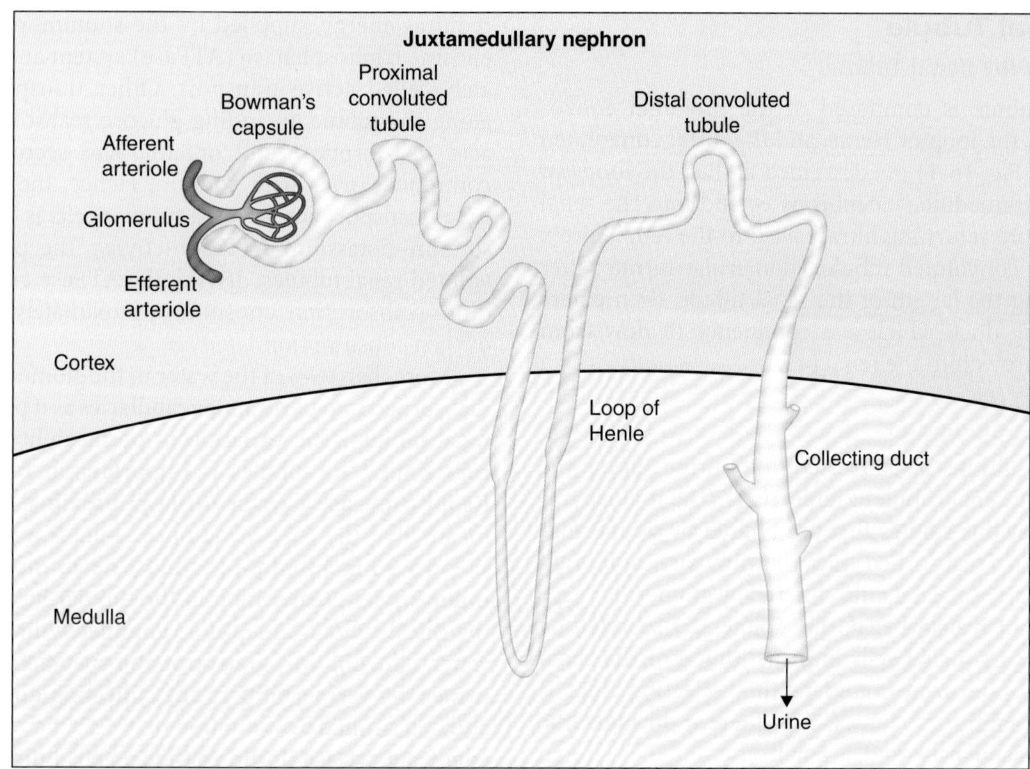

FIGURE 16-1 Schematic depiction of a juxtamedullary nephron.

This process of autoregulation involves feedback from the distal renal tubules to the glomerulus. Specialized cells in the distal renal tubules, called the ***macula densa***, signal the afferent or efferent renal arterioles to either vasoconstrict or vasodilate. Through the consequent adjustment of glomerular capillary pressure, a nearly constant filtration pressure leads to a consistent GFR across a range of mean arterial pressure, remaining relatively constant between mean arterial pressures of 60 and 160 mm Hg. Because even a small change in GFR can lead to wide variations in urine output, it is clear that tubule–glomerular feedback serves an important role in homeostasis.

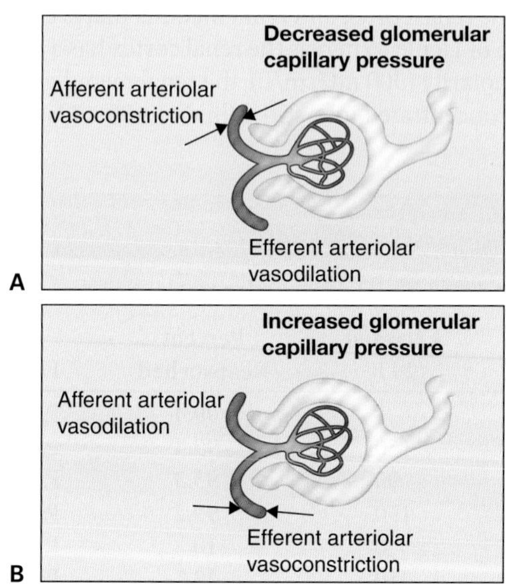

FIGURE 16-2 Glomerular filtration pressure. **A:** Afferent arteriolar vasoconstriction decreases glomerular capillary pressure and hence decreases GFR. **B:** Efferent arteriolar vasoconstriction increases glomerular capillary pressure and hence increases GFR.

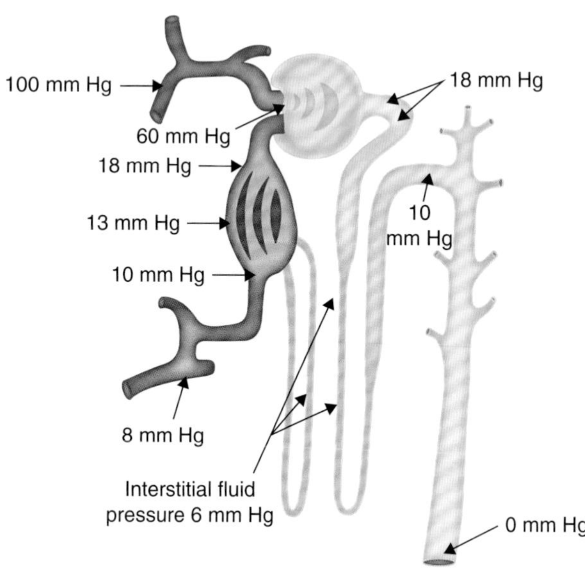

FIGURE 16-3 Intravascular pressures in the renal circulation. (From Guyton AC, Hall JE. *Textbook of Medical Physiology*. 10th ed. Philadelphia, PA: Saunders; 2000, with permission.)

The Renal Tubule

Structure of the Renal Tubule

The renal tubule is composed of the proximal convoluted tubule, the loop of Henle, and the distal convoluted tubule[1] (see Fig. 16-1). As described earlier, the loops of Henle in juxtamedullary nephrons extend into the renal medulla before returning filtrate back to the renal cortex in the distal convoluted tubule. Glomerular filtrate, after passing along the length of the renal tubule, then enters the collecting duct, which is a confluence of flow from several nephrons into the renal pelvis.

Renal Tubular Function

Glomerular filtrate is converted into urine along the course of the renal tubule[2] (Table 16-1). The majority of water and various solutes that are filtered by glomerular capillaries are reabsorbed into peritubular capillaries. Metabolic waste products, also filtered by glomerular capillaries, are not reabsorbed. Other solutes are secreted by renal tubular epithelial cells into the lumen of the renal tubule. Thus, the urine found in the collecting duct is composed mainly of substances filtered through the glomerular capillaries and a small amount of secreted substances. The process of reabsorption determines the volume of urine formed, whereas secretion is particularly important in determining the nature of the urine, such as concentration of potassium and hydrogen ions. Various portions of the renal tubule have differing roles in reabsorption and secretion[2] (see Table 16-1). Approximately two-thirds of all reabsorption and secretion in the renal tubules occurs in the proximal renal tubules. The most important factors influencing the reabsorption of sodium and water are aldosterone, arginine vasopressin (AVP), renal prostaglandins, and atrial natriuretic peptide.

Reabsorption of sodium involves moving this ion against a concentration gradient from the lumen of the proximal tubule into peritubular capillaries. This process requires energy, supplied by the sodium–potassium adenosine triphosphatase (ATPase) system and is appropriately called active transport. Other transport processes along the tubule, including glucose reabsorption, amino acid reabsorption, and organic acid secretion, share a common carrier with sodium. Hence, the great majority of transport across renal tubular cells is dependent on sodium–potassium ATPase activity. The proximal convoluted renal tubules, driving the ATPase enzyme for sodium reabsorption, consume approximately 80% of renal oxygen consumption.[3]

More than 99% of the water in the glomerular filtrate is reabsorbed into peritubular capillaries as it passes through renal tubules. The variation in permeability of epithelial cells lining the tubules is important in renal function. Rapid osmosis of water through proximal renal tubules means that the concentration of solutes on the capillary side of cell membranes is almost never more than a few milliosmoles greater than in the tubular lumen. However, the distal tubules are almost completely impermeable to water, allowing for control of the specific gravity of the urine. The permeability of the collecting ducts is variable and determined by the action of AVP. When AVP activates adenylate cyclase in the epithelial cells lining the collecting duct, the resulting cyclic adenosine monophosphate increases permeability of cell membranes to water. Hence, increased AVP leads to reabsorption of water from the collecting ducts, resulting in highly concentrated urine. Decreased AVP results in little water reabsorption and large amounts of dilute urine.

Countercurrent System

The ability of the kidneys to produce either dilute or concentrated urine depends on the gradient in osmolarity between the renal cortex and renal medulla that is created by the loop of Henle. Whereas the renal cortex has a relatively low osmolarity (300 mOsm/L), the renal medulla contains highly concentrated interstitial fluid (1,400 mOsm/L near

Table 16-1

Magnitude and Site of Solute Reabsorption or Secretion in the Renal Tubules

	Filtered (24 h)	Reabsorbed (24 h)	Secreted (24 h)	Excreted (24 h)	Percent Reabsorbed	Location
Water (L)	180	179		1	99.4	P,L,D,C
Sodium (mEq)	26,000	25,850		150	99.4	P,L,D,C
Potassium (mEq)	600	560	50	90	93.3	P,L,D,C
Chloride (mEq)	18,000	17,850		150	99.2	P,L,D,C
Bicarbonate (mEq)	4,900	4,900		0	10	P,D
Urea (mM)	870	460		410	53	P,L,D,C
Uric acid (mM)	50	49	4	5	98	P
Glucose (mM)	800	800		0	100	P

C, convoluted tubule; D, distal tubule; L, loop of Henle; P, proximal tubule.

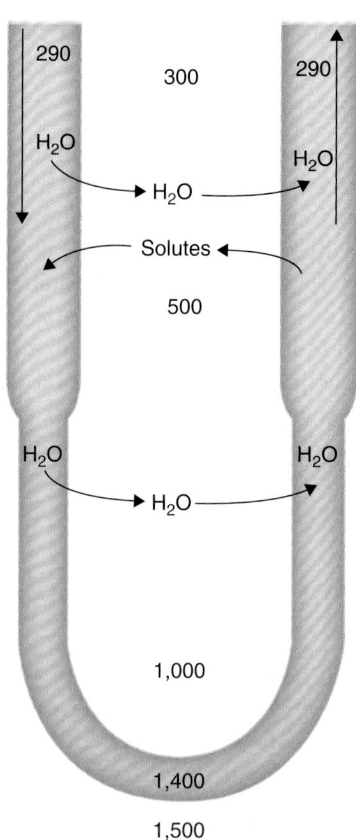

FIGURE 16-4 Countercurrent exchange of water and solutes in the vasa recta. (Adapted from Lote CJ, Harper L, Savage COS. Mechanisms of acute renal failure. *Br J Anaesth.* 1996;77:82–89, with permission.)

the renal pelvis) due to active reabsorption of solutes in the loop of Henle[3] (Fig. 16-4). The high medullary osmolarity is maintained in part by sluggish blood flow, preventing the removal of solutes.

Just as the juxtamedullary loops of Henle carry glomerular filtrate from the cortex into the renal medulla and back to the cortex, the vascular supply has a similar structure. The U-shaped arrangement of peritubular capillaries, known as the ***vasa recta***, parallels the loops of Henle. This forms a countercurrent system, in which capillary inflow runs parallel and in an opposite direction to capillary outflow.

Aquaporins

The high osmolarity in the renal medulla allows for the potential for quick reabsorption of water by osmosis as filtrate passes through the renal collecting ducts. This process is mediated by aquaporins, which are channels that facilitate rapid passage of water across lipid cell membranes at a velocity greater than possible by simple diffusion.[4–6] They are tetramer protein structures and are found in the kidneys, brain, salivary and lacrimal glands, and respiratory tract. Five aquaporins in the kidney have a role in water balance.[5] Aquaporin-1 is in the proximal renal tubules, while aquaporin-2 is found in the renal collecting ducts. In response to AVP, the channels in the tubular collecting duct edpithelium are opened, leading to reabsorption of water and formation of concentrated urine. In the absence of AVP, dilute urine traverses the collecting ducts without being affected by medullary osmolarity.

Tubular Transport Maximum

Tubular transport maximum (Tmax or T_{max}) is the maximum amount of a substance that can be actively reabsorbed from the lumens of renal tubules each minute. The Tm depends on the amounts of carrier substance and enzyme available to the specific active transport system in the lining epithelial cells of renal tubules.

The T_{max} for glucose is approximately 220 mg per minute. When the amount of glucose that filters through the glomerular capillary exceeds this amount, the excess glucose cannot be reabsorbed and passes into urine (Fig. 16-5). The usual amount of glucose in the glomerular filtrate entering proximal renal tubules is 125 mg per minute, and there is no detectable loss into urine. When the tubular load, however, exceeds approximately 220 mg per minute (threshold concentration), glucose begins to appear in urine. A blood glucose concentration of 180 mg/dL in the presence of a normal GFR results in delivery of 220 mg per minute of glucose into the renal tubular fluid. Loss of glucose in urine occurs at concentrations above the Tm for glucose. The presence of large amounts of unreabsorbed solutes in the urine such as glucose (or mannitol) produces osmotic diuresis by retaining water in the collecting system.

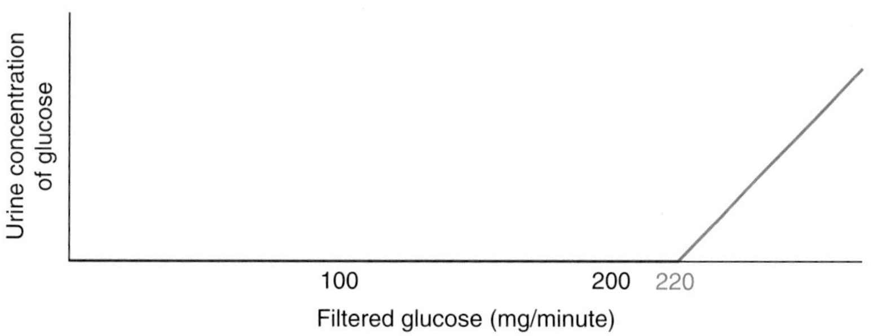

FIGURE 16-5 Transport maximum for glucose. Urinary concentration of glucose is negligible until the amount of filtered glucose exceeds the transport maximum.

Transport of Urine to the Bladder

From the collecting ducts, urine travels into the renal pelvis. A ureter arises from the pelvis of each kidney. At its distal end, the ureter penetrates the bladder obliquely such that pressure in the bladder compresses the ureter, thereby preventing reflux of urine into the ureter when bladder pressure increases during micturition.

Each ureter is innervated by the sympathetic and parasympathetic nervous system. As urine collects in the renal pelvis, the pressure in the pelvis increases and initiates a peristaltic contraction that travels downward along the ureter to force urine toward the bladder. Parasympathetic nervous system stimulation increases the frequency of peristalsis, whereas sympathetic nervous system stimulation decreases peristalsis.

Obstruction of a ureter by a stone causes intense reflex constriction and pain. In addition, pain elicits a sympathetic nervous system reflex (ureterorenal reflex) that causes vasoconstriction of the renal arterioles and a concomitant decrease in urine formation in the kidney when there is obstruction of the ureter.

As the bladder fills with urine, stretch receptors in the bladder wall initiate micturition contractions. Sensory signals are conducted to the sacral segments of the spinal cord through the pelvic nerves and then back again to the bladder through parasympathetic nervous system fibers. The micturition reflex is a completely automatic spinal cord reflex that can be inhibited (tonic contraction of the external urinary sphincter) or facilitated by centers in the brain. Spinal cord damage above the sacral region leaves the micturition reflex intact but is no longer controlled by the brain.

Renal Blood Flow

Although the kidneys represent about 0.5% of total body weight, their blood flow is disproportionately large at 20% to 25% of the cardiac output.[3] Renal blood flow is approximately 400 mL/100 g/minute, compared with 70 mL/100 g/minute for the heart and liver. The ability to autoregulate keeps renal blood flow relatively constant across a range of systemic mean arterial pressures. Because renal blood flow is large, the fraction of oxygen extraction is low despite high oxygen consumption, the PO_2 decreasing from 95 mm Hg in the renal artery only to about 70 mm Hg in the renal vein.

Approximately 90% of the renal blood flow is distributed to the renal cortex, with less than 10% of renal blood flow going to the medulla. The generous delivery of blood to the cortex supports flow-dependent functions such as glomerular filtration and tubular reabsorption processes of the cortex. By contrast, low blood flow in the medulla maintains a high interstitial fluid osmolarity, which in turn permits concentration of the urine.[7] Low blood flow also makes the medulla more susceptible to ischemia than the cortex.

Renal Cortex Blood Flow: Glomerular and Peritubular Capillaries

Blood enters the renal artery, whose branches ultimately supply the afferent arterioles of the glomeruli. As described earlier, afferent arterioles feed the glomerular capillary bed, out of which blood flows into the efferent arterioles[1] (see Fig. 16-1). The vascular resistance of the efferent arterioles raises glomerular capillary pressure, which promotes continuous filtration of fluid from glomerular capillaries into Bowman's capsule. Blood flows from the arterioles into a second capillary network called ***peritubular capillaries***. These capillaries have substantially lower pressure[8] (see Fig. 16-3), promoting reabsorption of fluid from the tubules into the peritubular capillaries.

Renal Medulla Blood Flow: The Vasa Recta

Capillaries that descend with the loops of Henle are referred to as the ***vasa recta***, which receive only 1% to 2% of renal blood flow. These capillaries, after descending into the renal medulla, return to the renal cortex and empty into veins. As described earlier, this countercurrent system minimizes the washout of solutes from the interstitial fluid of the medulla creating a high osmolarity that promotes the absorption of water from the collecting ducts and the formation of concentrated urine.

Autoregulation of Renal Blood Flow

Renal blood flow and GFR are kept relatively constant within a range of mean arterial pressure between approximately 60 and 160 mm Hg[8] (Fig. 16-6). Because the GFR parallels renal blood flow, cardiac output has an

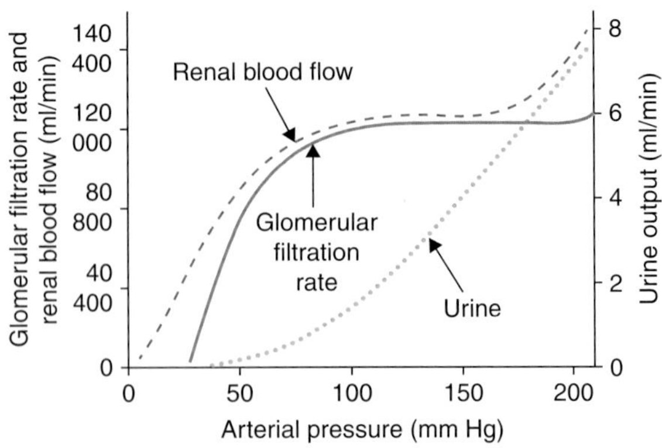

FIGURE 16-6 Autoregulation. Renal blood flow and glomerular filtration rate, but not urine output, are autoregulated between a mean arterial pressure of approximately 60 and 160 mm Hg. (From Guyton AC, Hall JE. *Textbook of Medical Physiology*. 10th ed. Philadelphia, PA: Saunders; 2000, with permission.)

important effect on the GFR. The mechanism for autoregulation is controversial.[9] One theory is a myogenic response, whereby increased perfusion pressure leads to an increased wall tension in the afferent arterioles, resulting in automatic contraction of the smooth muscle fibers in the vessel wall. This increases resistance keeping flow constant despite the increase in perfusion pressure.[3] An alternative hypothesis is that a tubuloglomerular feedback mechanism is responsible for autoregulation, whereby increased perfusion pressure will increase filtration, increasing the tubular fluid delivery to the macula densa, which then releases a factor or factors that cause vasoconstriction.

In the setting of decreased effective circulating volume, however, renal blood flow may be decreased despite adequate perfusion pressure. Activation of the sympathetic nervous system shunts cardiac output away from the kidneys. Hence, adequate systemic blood pressure does not necessarily indicate adequate renal perfusion in the presence of hypovolemia.

Juxtaglomerular Apparatus

The juxtaglomerular apparatus is where the distal renal tubule passes between the afferent and efferent arterioles. Epithelial cells of the distal renal tubules that contact these arterioles are called the ***macula densa***, whereas corresponding cells in the arterioles are known as ***juxtaglomerular cells***. In response to decreased renal blood flow, juxtaglomerular cells release renin into the circulation[3] (Fig. 16-7). Renin converts angiotensinogen to angiotensin I, which is then converted to angiotensin II by angiotensin-converting enzyme. Effects of angiotensin II include thirst, vasoconstriction, and salt and water reabsorption by the kidneys to maintain circulating volume and increase renal blood flow. Whether the initial cause of decreased renal blood flow is the result of hypovolemia, systemic hypotension, or sympathetic nervous system stimulation, the effect of renin is to maintain renal blood flow and GFR.

Regulation of Body Fluid

The kidneys have a primary role in the regulation of the amount and nature of body fluids. They control the following characteristics:

- Blood and extracellular fluid volume
- Osmolarity of body fluids
- Plasma concentration of ions and urea

Blood and Extracellular Fluid Volume

Blood volume is maintained over a narrow range despite large daily variations in fluid and solute intake or loss. The mechanism for control of blood volume also affects

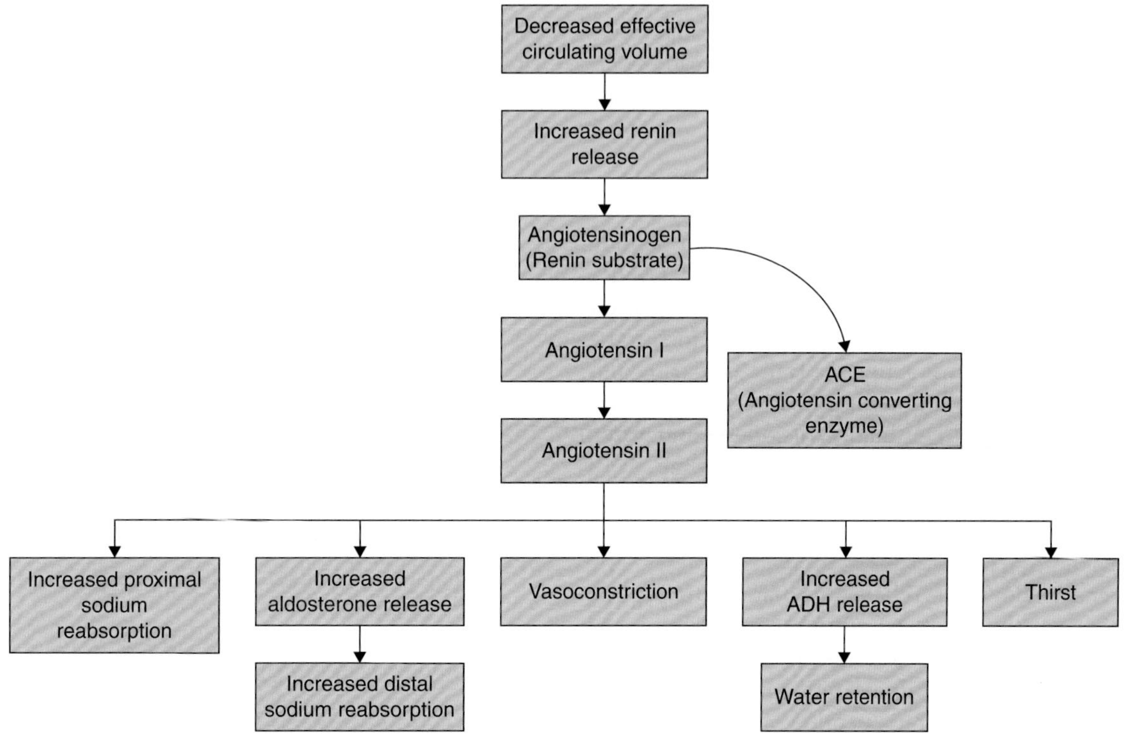

FIGURE 16-7 The role of the renin-angiotensin system in the maintenance of effective circulating volume. (From Lote CJ, Harper L, and Savage COS. Mechanisms of acute renal failure. *Br J Anaesth* 1996;77:82–89; with permission.)

systemic blood pressure and cardiac output, as these are interrelated. An increase in blood volume increases the cardiac output, which usually increases the systemic blood pressure. Increased cardiac output and systemic arterial pressure will increase renal blood flow and GFR, resulting in an increase in urine output. The negative feedback loop is completed by a consequent decrease in circulating blood volume.

This basic regulatory mechanism is augmented by other factors. In the setting of decreased blood volume, an increased circulating concentration of AVP will increase water reabsorption, whereas an increase in aldosterone promotes sodium reabsorption and thus an osmotic reabsorption of water. This decreases urine volume and restores blood volume. Another factor is mediated through atrial stretch receptors and atrial natriuretic peptide to be described in the next section.

Regulation of normal circulating blood volume is impaired by factors directly affecting vascular capacitance. Persistent vasoconstriction associated with essential hypertension or sympathetic nervous system stimulation (from pheochromocytoma, for example) results in a decrease in blood volume. Conversely, blood volume may be increased by chronic drug-induced vasodilation or the effects of severe varicose veins.

The regulation of extracellular fluid volume is controlled indirectly through the maintenance of circulating blood volume. An increase in blood volume leads to an increase in extracellular fluid volume, whereas decreased extracellular fluid volume accompanies reduced blood volume. Although these volumes move in the same direction, their proportional change is affected by capillary permeability, which is commonly influenced by perioperative factors. The extracellular fluid space may be considered as a reservoir for excess intravenous fluid administered during the perioperative period.

Atrial and Renal Natriuretic Factors

Cardiac atrial muscle synthesizes and secretes a peptide hormone known as ***atrial natriuretic peptide*** (ANP), which is released in response to increased right and left atrial pressure and volume. ANP binds to receptors in the renal collecting ducts and, acting via transcellular second messenger systems, inhibits sodium reabsorption. Hence, atrial "stretch" promotes elimination of sodium and water, and a subsequent decrease in circulating volume. ANP additionally has vasodilatory properties, thereby lowering systemic blood pressure and eliciting renal artery vasodilation.

The renal analogue of ANP is renal natriuretic peptide (urodilatin), which is synthesized in renal cortical nephrons. It is likely that ANP is primarily a cardiovascular regulator and relatively unimportant for sodium excretion, whereas renal natriuretic peptide participates in the intrarenal regulation of sodium excretion.[3,10] In mechanical ventilation, positive end-expiratory pressure reduces atrial distension and atrial transmural pressure. This reduces ANP release, which may contribute to sodium and water retention by the kidneys.

Osmolarity of Body Fluids

The primary determinant of body fluid osmolarity is the concentration of sodium in the extracellular fluid. Sodium ion concentration is largely controlled by two mechanisms: the osmoreceptor–AVP response and the thirst reflex. Aldosterone, by contrast, has a minimal role in the maintenance of sodium concentration and plasma osmolarity[8] (Fig. 16-8). Aldosterone-induced reabsorption of sodium is accompanied by reabsorption of water. For this reason, patients with primary hyperaldosteronism typically have increased extracellular fluid volume but nearly normal serum sodium levels.

Osmoreceptor–Arginine Vasopressin Hormone

In response to increased extracellular fluid osmolarity, osmoreceptors in the hypothalamus signal the posterior pituitary to increase the release of AVP. AVP is also secreted in the setting of water deprivation and hemorrhage. Circulating AVP causes collecting ducts to retain water and thus decreases serum sodium levels. Because sodium is the primary determinant of serum osmolality, this results in a decrease in osmolality. The inverse is also true. Abnormally low extracellular fluid osmolality will lead to a decrease in the release of AVP, thereby increasing the production of dilute urine. This increases serum sodium and osmolality toward normal. A small change in osmolality (as little as 1%) can produce a large change in circulating AVP concentration, producing tight regulation of serum osmolality.

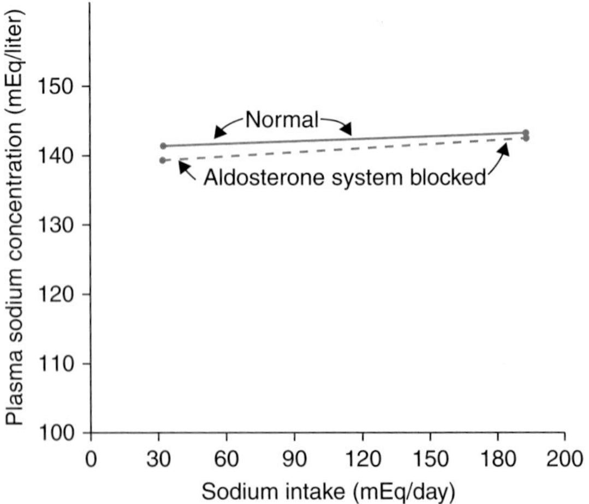

FIGURE 16-8 In the absence of aldosterone, the plasma concentration of sodium varies less than 2% over a sixfold range in sodium intake. (From Guyton AC, Hall JE. *Textbook of Medical Physiology*. 10th ed. Philadelphia, PA: Saunders; 2000, with permission.)

Thirst Reflex

The thirst reflex is primarily elicited by an increase in sodium concentration in the extracellular fluid. An increase in sodium as small as 2 mEq/L above normal (or an increase in osmolality of approximately 4 mOsm/L) will stimulate thirst, and water consumption decreases sodium concentration toward normal. In this way, extracellular fluid osmolality is maintained within a narrow range. In addition, angiotensin II promotes a thirst response, so circulatory changes that increase the production of angiotensin II, such as acute hemorrhage or congestive heart failure, will increase thirst.

Plasma Concentration of Ions and Urea

Sodium

The kidneys control the concentration of sodium through the process of reabsorption. As described earlier, active transport moves sodium ions from the tubular lumen into the peritubular capillaries. Two-thirds of the sodium in glomerular filtrate is reabsorbed in the proximal renal tubule, and less than 10% of sodium is expected to reach the distal renal tubule. The renin-angiotensin-aldosterone system modulates the sodium reabsorption by the renal tubules. Hypotension or decreased circulating blood volume leads to an increase in angiotensin, which is converted to angiotenin II in the lungs and ultimately results in increased sodium reabsorption. Angiotensin II leads to efferent arteriole vasoconstriction, increasing glomerular capillary pressure and GFR.

Lastly, angiotensin II increases secretion of aldosterone, which exerts its effect in the distal renal tubule. When aldosterone levels are increased, nearly all the remaining sodium is reabsorbed from the distal tubule, and urinary excretion of sodium is negligible. Typically, only 1% of the filtered sodium is excreted in the urine[2] (see Table 16-1).

Potassium

Potassium, after being filtered in the glomerulus, is then reabsorbed by the proximal tubule and loop of Henle. Potassium is either reabsorbed or secreted in the distal tubule and collecting duct, depending on the level of aldosterone. An increase in aldosterone increases potassium ion secretion into the renal tubules and consequently increases urinary potassium. The feedback mechanism allows for close regulation: Small changes in potassium concentration will lead to a substantial change in the concentration of aldosterone[8] (Fig. 16-9). When aldosterone activity is blocked by certain diuretics, plasma potassium concentration depends more on dietary intake of potassium, making hypokalemia or hyperkalemia more likely[8] (Fig. 16-10).

The regulation of sodium and hydrogen ion concentrations also has an effect on urinary excretion of potassium.

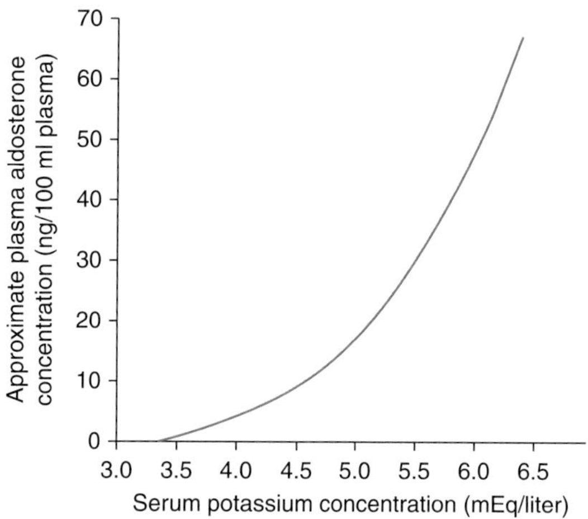

FIGURE 16-9 Small changes in the plasma concentrations of potassium evoke large changes in the plasma concentration of aldosterone. (From Guyton AC, Hall JE. *Textbook of Medical Physiology*. 10th ed. Philadelphia, PA: Saunders; 2000, with permission.)

Hydrogen ions compete with potassium for secretion into the renal tubules. In the presence of alkalosis (e.g., vomiting and loss of gastric acid), potassium is excreted in the urine in order to maintain acid–base balance. Conversely, a metabolic acidosis will lead to the secretion of hydrogen ions and retention of potassium, and plasma potassium concentration will increase. Sodium intake may influence plasma concentrations of potassium because sodium is transported through renal tubular epithelial cells in exchange for potassium.

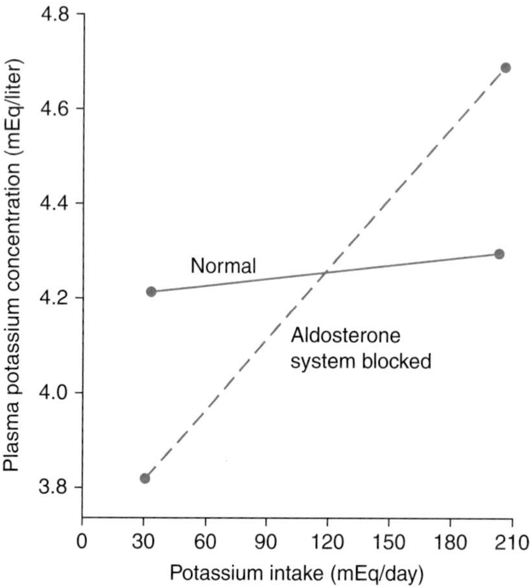

FIGURE 16-10 Plasma concentrations of potassium parallel intake when aldosterone activity is impaired. (From Guyton AC, Hall JE. *Textbook of Medical Physiology*. 10th ed. Philadelphia, PA: Saunders; 2000, with permission.)

Acid–Base Balance

The kidneys secrete excess hydrogen ions by exchanging a hydrogen ion for a sodium ion, thus acidifying the urine, and by the synthesis of ammonia, which combines with hydrogen to form ammonium. In the presence of hypovolemia, bicarbonate reabsorption by the kidneys will lead to acidification of the urine and a metabolic alkalosis.

Calcium and Magnesium

Calcium ion concentration is controlled principally by the effect of parathyroid hormone on bone reabsorption, which releases calcium. Additionally parathyroid hormone increases the reabsorption of calcium from the distal renal tubules and collecting ducts. Magnesium is reabsorbed by all portions of the renal tubules. Urinary excretion of magnesium parallels the plasma concentration of this ion.

Urea

Urea is the most abundant metabolic waste product. Without adequate clearance of urea, excessive accumulation in body fluids prevents normal function of multiple systems. Urea elimination depends on the plasma concentration of urea (blood urea nitrogen or BUN) and the GFR. Approximately 50% of the urea that is filtered into the renal tubules is eliminated in the urine; the remainder is reabsorbed. When the GFR is low, tubular filtrate flow is relatively slow, thus increasing the proportion of urea that is reabsorbed. This effectively increases the BUN by decreasing urinary elimination of urea. Conversely, when GFR increases, less urea is reabsorbed in the tubules, increasing its elimination in the urine, and BUN decreases.

Measuring Kidney Function

Formal measurement of kidney function requires labor-intensive studies such as collection of urine over time and measurement of blood and urine components. For clinical decision making, estimates of GFR are accessible and inexpensive, requiring only basic laboratory work. Serum creatinine (SCr), commonly used to measure changes in kidney function, is insensitive to small changes in GFR; GFR needs to decrease by about 50% before a rise in SCr is seen. For many years, the Cockcroft-Gault formula has been used to estimate GFR.[11]

$$GFR_{men} = (140 - \text{age}) \times \text{weight (kg)} / \text{serum creatinine (mg/dL)} \times 72$$

$$GFR_{women} = (140 - \text{age}) \times \text{weight (kg)} \times 0.85 / \text{serum creatinine (mg/dL)} \times 72$$

The difference in the formula between men and women accounts for the expected difference in muscle mass and creatinine production. The formula also takes into account the effect of age on GFR. Given an age-related decrease in muscle mass, GFR in an elderly person will typically be less than a younger person with the same weight and SCr.

The Modification of Diet in Renal Disease (MDRD) formula uses four variables to estimate GFR: age, SCr, ethnicity, and gender, and is independent of body weight.[12] Developed in a population of patients with chronic kidney disease in the United States, it has been widely adopted as a useful estimate of GFR, although questions remain concerning its applicability to other populations. Both Cockcroft-Gault and MDRD assume steady state conditions: balanced production and clearance of SCr leading to a consistent concentration. Because an acute reduction in GFR will result in a rise in SCr over many hours or days, these formulas are a poor measure of GFR in acute kidney injury.

Acute Kidney Injury

Acute kidney injury results in an abrupt reduction in the kidney's ability to eliminate nitrogenous waste products and maintain fluid and electrolyte homeostasis.[3,13] Despite the kidney's generous blood supply and large oxygen delivery, it remains at risk for ischemia in the perioperative period. Acute kidney injury may be classified by either the site of instigating pathology or the degree of injury sustained, as measured by changes in GFR and reduction in urine output. In light of the heterogeneous causes of acute kidney injury and the difficulty in comparing literature using disparate definitions,[13] there has been a great deal of recent interest in standardizing and streamlining the classification of acute kidney injury.

Classification

Acute kidney injury (AKI) has traditionally been classified by dividing the primary pathophysiology into prerenal, intrarenal, or postrenal causes[13] (Fig. 16-11).

Prerenal Azotemia

Abnormalities of the systemic circulation that lead to a decrease of renal blood flow have the potential to impair renal function. The term ***azotemia*** refers to any condition characterized by abnormally high levels of nitrogen-containing compounds, such as urea, creatinine, and other nitrogen-rich compounds, in the blood. Prerenal azotemia refers to decreases in renal function due to hypoperfusion in the setting of intact glomeruli and tubules. Correcting the underlying problems in circulation will improve renal function. Common causes of prerenal azotemia in hospitalized patients include septic shock, heart failure, liver failure, and perioperative hemodynamic changes that lead to decreased renal perfusion.[13] Medications may also be implicated in at-risk patients. Nonsteroidal antiinflammatory drugs (NSAIDs) are known to precipitate prerenal azotemia in hypovolemic patients or in patients with congestive heart failure.[13] Calcineurin

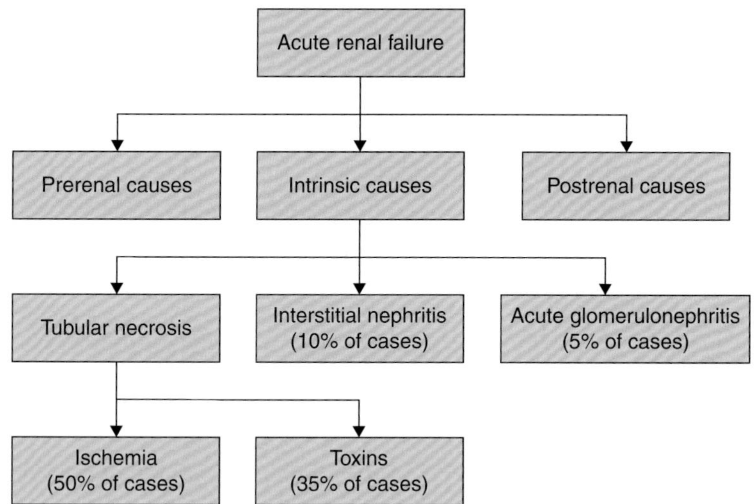

FIGURE 16-11 Classification of acute renal failure. (From Thadhani R, Pascual M, Bonventre JV. Acute renal failure. *N Engl J Med.* 1996;334:1448–1460, with permission.)

inhibitors, by causing vasoconstriction of afferent renal arteries, also reduce GFR and lead to prerenal azotemia.[14,15]

Intrinsic Causes of Acute Kidney Injury

The most common cause of intrinsic renal failure is acute tubular necrosis (ATN), caused by either ischemia or nephrotoxic agents. Less common causes seen perioperatively include acute glomerulonephritis and interstitial nephritis from such agents as β-lactam antibiotics and NSAIDs[8] (see Fig. 16-11). In cases of ATN secondary to ischemia, prolonged decreases in renal blood flow stimulate epithelial cells to reabsorb sodium to restore renal blood flow. This increase in active transport in the renal medullary tubules exacerbates the mismatch of oxygen supply and demand, leading to injury and the expression of proteins that regulate the response to hypoxia.[16,17] Thus, prerenal azotemia leads to ATN, and both entities may be considered to be on the continuum of ischemic renal disease.

Renal tubule cells are particularly susceptible to ischemia because of their transport-related oxygen requirements and the low baseline blood flow to the renal medulla. Injury is worsened both by hypoxemia and by endothelial cell swelling, which further decreases perfusion. Nephrotoxic agents such as aminoglycosides and iodinated radiocontrast media may also lead to ATN, either by direct injury to tubules or by processes mediated by free radicals.[13,18]

ATN secondary to renal medullary ischemia is the most common perioperative cause of AKI. In this setting, adequate urine output may be falsely reassuring. Ischemic ATN leads to failure of the sodium–potassium ATPase pump in the renal tubules; impairing their ability to concentrate urine. Thus, urine output does not correspond to the degree of cell damage or GFR in patients exposed to trauma, shock, or cardiovascular surgery.[19]

Postrenal Obstructive Nephropathy

Perioperative patients with AKI should also be evaluated for postrenal etiologies, particularly those with acute oliguria. Because the pathophysiology underlying this AKI involves hindrance to urine flow, this is also called ***obstructive nephropathy***. Causes include renal stones, prostatic hypertrophy, and mechanical obstruction of urinary catheters.

Acute Kidney Injury Diagnosis

Diagnostic Criteria

As recently as 2004, there was no widespread consensus definition of acute renal failure (ARF). Comparison of the literature was challenging as definitions and categories varied between studies. In 2004, the Acute Dialysis Quality Initiative group conducted a systematic review and consensus conference, which produced a five-tiered classification scheme for ARF, called ***RIFLE*** (risk, injury, failure, loss of kidney function, and end-stage kidney disease)[20] (Fig. 16-12). This scheme is based on easily measurable clinical variables and includes in its definition an accommodation for acute or chronic kidney disease.

The RIFLE classification includes three levels of renal dysfunction and two clinical outcomes. The degrees of renal dysfunction are defined either by (a) changes in SCr or estimated GFR (eGFR) or (b) oliguria. A patient may be categorized by meeting one definition, the other, or both. The criterion that leads to the worst classification should be used.[20]

- R—risk of renal dysfunction: increased SCr by 1.5-fold (GFR decrease by 25%) or urine output (UOP) less than 0.5 mL/kg/hour for 6 hours
- I—injury to the kidney: increased SCr by two-fold (GFR decrease by 50%) or UOP less than 0.5 mL/kg/hour for 12 hours
- F—failure of kidney function: increased SCr by three-fold (GFR decrease by 75%), SCr greater than 4 mg/dL, or UOP less than either 0.3 mL/kg/hour for 24 hours or anuria for 12 hours

RIFLE criteria		
	GFR criteria	Urine output criteria
Risk	Increased SCr by 1.5× or GFR decrease by 25%	UO < 0.5 ml/kg/h for six hours
Injury	Increased SCr by 2× or GFR decrease by 50%	UO < 0.5 ml/kg/h for twelve hours
Failure	Increased SCr by 3× or GFR decrease by 75% or SCr > 4 mg/dL	UO < 0.3 ml/kg/h for 24 hours or Anuria for 12 hours
Loss	Persistent acute renal failure (four weeks duration)	
ESKD	End stage kidney disease (greater than three months)	

FIGURE 16-12 RIFLE criteria. GFR, glomerular filtration rate; UO, urine output; SCr, serum creatinine; ESKD, end-stage kidney disease. (Adapted from Bellomo R, Ronco C, Kellum JA, et al; Acute Dialysis Quality Initiative Workgroup. Acute renal failure—definition, outcome measures, animal models, fluid therapy and information technology needs: the Second International Consensus Conference of the Acute Dialysis Quality Initiative [ADQI] Group. *Crit Care.* 2004;8[4]:R204–R212.)

Clinical outcomes include the following:

- L—Loss of kidney function is equivalent to persistent ARF, needing renal replacement therapy (RRT) for more than 4 weeks.
- E—end-stage kidney disease: need for dialysis for more than 3 months

Proposed modifications to the RIFLE criteria were made by the Acute Kidney Injury Network (AKIN) in 2007[21] (Fig. 16-13). The first three stages of RIFLE (risk, injury, and failure) correspond to the first three stages of injury in AKIN definitions. In addition, stage 1 AKI includes patients with a rise in SCr as little as 0.3 mg/dL, as even small increases in SCr are associated with worse outcomes.[21,22] AKIN further tightens the window to diagnosis of AKI by lab criteria or urine output to 48 hours as opposed to 7 days. Any patient with renal replacement therapy is included in stage 3, regardless of duration of therapy or concurrent urine output. Finally, "loss" and "end-stage kidney disease" have been removed, as they describe long-term

RIFLE criteria			Acute kidney injury network criteria		
	GFR criteria	Urine output criteria	Stage	Creatinine	Urine output criteria
Risk	Increased SCr by 1.5× or GFR decrease by 25%	UO < 0.5 ml/kg/h for six hours	1	1.5 to 2 times baseline or increase of 0.3 mg/dL	UO < 0.5 ml/kg/h for six hours
Injury	Increased SCr by 2× or GFR decrease by 50%	UO < 0.5 ml/kg/h for twelve hours	2	Increased 2 to 3 times baseline	UO < 0.5 ml/kg/h for twelve hours
Failure	Increased SCr by 3× or GFR decrease by 75% or SCr > 4 mg/dL	UO < 0.3 ml/kg/h for 24 hours or Anuria for 12 hours	3	>3 times baseline or SCr > 4.0 mg/dL with an acute increase of 0.5mg/dl	UO < 0.3 ml/kg/h for 24 hours or Anuria for 12 hours
Loss	Persistent acute renal failure (four weeks duration)				
ESKD	End stage kidney disease (greater than three months)				

FIGURE 16-13 RIFLE criteria compared to Acute Kidney Injury Network criteria. (Adapted from Mehta RL, Kellum JA, Shah SV, et al; Acute Kidney Injury Network. Acute Kidney Injury Network: report of an initiative to improve outcomes in acute kidney injury. *Crit Care.* 2007;11[2]:R31.)

outcomes rather than short-term categories. RIFLE and AKIN definitions have been compared and are in general concordance. It has been suggested that the AKIN definitions do not provide significant advantages, despite the increased sensitivity of stage 1 AKI.[23,24]

Biomarkers

As discussed earlier, the SCr and urine output are the most widely used diagnostic criteria to detect AKI. The use of SCr to estimate the GFR assumes steady-state conditions: Production of creatinine is equal to its clearance. It is therefore problematic to use SCr to estimate GFR in dynamic settings. Simply put, the rise in SCr lags an acute reduction in GFR. Furthermore, because even small changes in the GFR have significant impact on mortality and hospital length of stay,[22] the need for early detection of AKI has led to the pursuit for biomarkers that may give real-time information. The hope is that earlier detection of AKI could lead to therapeutic interventions that improve outcomes, and research in this area has been very active for some time.

Neutrophil gelatinase–associated lipocalin (NGAL) has been identified as an early marker of AKI.[25–27] Its expression is induced in renal tubular cells following ischemia-reperfusion injury, and it can be measured either in serum or urine soon after injury. Significant research has investigated this promising biomarker, although its clinical use has been slowed by a wide range of predictive value in various reports. An early meta-analysis suggested that NGAL is a useful predictor of early AKI across an array of clinical settings.[24] When using standardized assays, a generally agreed upon cutoff upper value of 150 ng/mL may be suggestive of AKI. Despite questions regarding appropriate cutoff values and assay technique, more recent reviews have reaffirmed NGAL's use in both the prediction of the presence and severity of AKI after cardiac surgery (AUC_{ROC} 0.82 to 0.83) and to predict delayed graft function after kidney transplantation (AUC_{ROC} 0.87).[28]

Other biomarkers of AKI are under ongoing investigation.[29] Cystatin-C, a cysteine proteinase inhibitor produced by all nucleated cells, is small in size and easily filtered in the glomerulus. Because it is metabolized in the proximal renal tubules, urinary concentrations are insignificant. Furthermore, its short half-life means serum levels will reflect GFR. Interleukin-18 (IL-18) is synthesized both in the proximal tubular cells and in cells that mediate inflammatory response. Elevated levels are seen in patients with ATN, although its role as a biomarker of AKI is confounded by evidence indicating it may represent more closely the presence of general inflammatory processes. Lastly, kidney injury molecule (KIM)-1 is a membrane protein expressed in injured proximal tubular epithelial cells. Although associated with ATN, its predictive value is still being defined.[29] Rather than relying on a single biomarker, a panel of biomarkers may be used in the future to predict AKI. Further research will also determine whether interventions in early AKI will affect clinical outcomes.

Anesthesia and the Kidneys

An understanding of kidney function is important for the anesthesiologist, as fundamental concepts of perioperative management include the maintenance of normal circulating volume, the regulation of electrolytes and acid–base status, and the clearance of metabolites and drugs. The perioperative time period is unique in that multiple potential insults, often concurrent or in rapid succession, challenge the kidney's functional ability. Perioperative AKI has an estimated overall incidence of 1% and is associated with an eightfold increase in risk of mortality.[30]

Anesthesia and Renal Blood Flow

Several perioperative factors affect renal blood flow either directly by hemodynamic effects or indirectly through actions of the sympathetic nervous system or AVP. Regardless of the immediate cause, a fall in renal blood flow tends to decrease the GFR by diminishing blood flow to the renal cortex. Likewise, decreased renal blood flow puts the renal medulla at risk for ischemia because the blood supply to this region is already low at baseline. The sum effect of these changes is conservation of sodium and water and, consequently, a decrease in urine output.

Many perioperative factors influence renal blood flow through changes in cardiac output or systemic arterial pressure. Anesthetic drugs commonly have significant direct hemodynamic effects, either by reducing systemic vascular resistance, depressing myocardial function, or decreasing effective preload. Likewise, perioperative hypovolemia (from preoperative fasting, bowel preparation, fluid shifts, acute hemorrhage, or any combination of factors) will decrease cardiac output and systemic arterial pressure, ultimately leading to a similar direct effect on renal blood flow.

Because the kidney has rich autonomic innervation, renal blood flow is also highly sensitive to the action of the sympathetic nervous system. Sympathetic stimulation leads to increased renal vascular resistance, which has two significant effects. First, blood is shunted away from the kidneys to other organs, preserving perfusion of critical organs such as the brain and heart. Second, constriction of the afferent renal arterioles lowers glomerular capillary pressure and decreases the GFR. Whether the root cause is pain, surgical stimulation, or exogenous catecholamines, excessive sympathetic stimulation can decrease glomerular blood flow to the point that urine output drops to nearly zero. Furthermore, painful stimuli elicit the release of AVP, which increases water absorption from the collecting ducts, resulting in concentrated urine. Retention of sodium and water caused by positive end-expiratory pressure is not associated with changes in the circulating plasma concentrations of AVP.[31]

These direct and indirect mechanisms altering renal blood flow are not mutually exclusive. Any factor that decreases the cardiac output will also lead to a release of AVP and an increase in the activity of both the sympathetic nervous system and the renin-angiotensin-aldosterone system. AVP and aldosterone tend to restore both normal circulating volume and normal renal blood flow by retaining sodium and water. Hypovolemia from acute hemorrhage also increases sympathetic tone, again reducing renal blood flow.

The autoregulation of renal blood flow may also be affected by perioperative factors. Although most anesthetic drugs do not abolish autoregulation, it is impaired in the following circumstances: severe sepsis, acute kidney failure, and cardiopulmonary bypass. Sustained changes in mean arterial pressure (greater than 10 minutes) are associated with a decreased ability to autoregulate renal blood flow. Autoregulation of GFR, by contrast, is sustained over longer periods of time. Thus, the GFR may remain near normal despite a marked reduction in renal blood flow.

It is important to remember that normal systemic arterial pressure does not ensure adequate renal blood flow and that renal ischemia may occur even in the absence of hypotension. Also, intraoperative urine output is a poor predictor of postoperative changes in renal function.[32] (Fig. 16-14). Hence, factors that commonly emerge in the perioperative setting including anesthetic agents, fluid shifts, stress response, changes in hemodynamics, and administration of catecholamines all have the potential to decrease renal blood flow and affect kidney function.

Perioperative Risk Assessment

An assessment of perioperative risk allows perioperative physicians to address this concern with patients and consultants, as well as to plan the anesthetic with the aim of avoiding AKI. In the patient population undergoing general surgery, the risk of AKI is believed to be about 1%. Patient risk factors include age older than 56 years, male gender, active congestive heart failure, ascites, diabetes, and hypertension (Table 16-2). Surgical factors increasing the likelihood of AKI are intraperitoneal surgery and emergent operations.[30] The risk of perioperative AKI remains a significant concern in vascular and cardiac surgery.[33–35] Sepsis and blood transfusions also increase the risk of AKI.

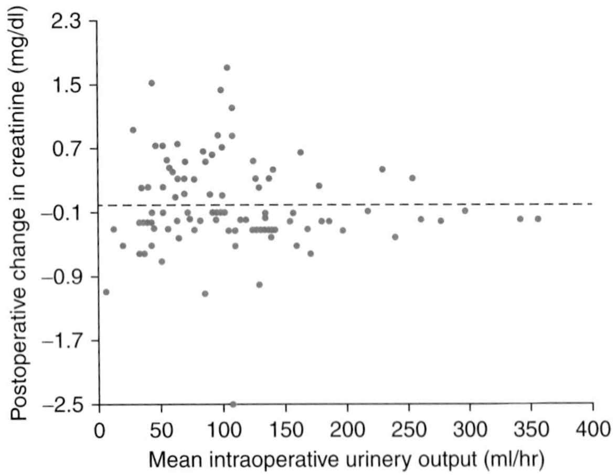

FIGURE 16-14 Intraoperative urine output. Mean intraoperative urine output does not correlate with postoperative changes in the plasma concentrations of creatinine. (From Alpert RA, Roizen MF, Hamilton WK, et al. Intraoperative urinary output does not predict postoperative renal function in patients undergoing abdominal aortic revascularization. *Surgery*. 1984;95:707–711, with permission.)

Table 16-2

Risk Factors for Perioperative Acute Kidney Injury

Patient Risk Factors	Surgical Risk Factors
Age >56 years	Intraperitoneal surgery
Male gender	Emergent operation
Active congestive heart failure	
Ascites	
Diabetes	
Hypertension	

Adapted from Kheterpal S, Tremper KK, Heung M, et al. Development and validation of an acute kidney injury risk index for patients undergoing general surgery: results from a national data set. *Anesthesiology*. 2009;110(3):505–515.

Patients undergoing cardiac surgery requiring cardiopulmonary bypass (CPB) are at particular risk. Alterations in renal blood flow, inflammatory response, microemboli, and direct toxicity are among the several mechanisms for kidney injury in these patients. Furthermore, clamping of the aorta in cardiac or major vascular surgery is associated with atheromatous emboli to the kidneys. Increased baseline SCr is the most significant risk factor for perioperative AKI after CPB. In patients with a baseline SCr between 2.0 and 4.0 mg/dL, the risk of AKI requiring dialysis is 10% to 20%. Other risk factors include ejection fraction less than 40% and preoperative use of an intraaortic balloon pump.[36] Patients undergoing valve surgery are at higher risk than those undergoing coronary artery bypass grafting alone.[37]

Intraoperative Management

Although the ability of the anesthesiologist to prevent AKI remains limited, general management principles include identifying potential causes of kidney injury (and mitigating their impact), minimizing exposure to nephrotoxic agents (NSAIDs and radiographic contrast) and the maintenance of renal blood flow. This can be accomplished by prompt correction of intravascular volume depletion and the maintenance of adequate systemic arterial pressure. Preoperative optimization of congestive heart failure, as well as maintaining normal cardiac output perioperatively, will help maintain renal blood flow. The judicious use of positive end-expiratory pressure and the avoidance of unnecessary increases in mean airway pressure will help maintain cardiac output and adequate renal blood flow. In laparoscopic surgery, using the lowest possible abdominal insufflation pressure will promote renal blood flow, although this must be balanced with operative needs. Adequate analgesia will minimize sympathetic nervous system-mediated decreases in renal blood flow. This may be a potential benefit of regional anesthesia. Agents used to promote afferent arteriolar dilation have not been shown to improve perioperative renal outcomes. Low-dose dopamine does not prevent AKI or improve morality.[38] Fenoldopam mesylate, a selective dopamine agonist, may reduce the risk of AKI in selected patient populations,[39,40] but further studies are needed to confirm this potential benefit.

References

1. Pitts RF. *Physiology of the Kidney and Body Fluids: An Introductory Text*. 3rd ed. Chicago, IL: Year Book Medical Publishers; 1974.
2. Ganong WF. *Review of Medical Physiology*. 21st ed. New York, NY: McGraw-Hill; 2003.
3. Lote CJ, Harper L, Savage CO. Mechanisms of acute renal failure. *Br J Anaesth*. 1996;77(1):82–89.
4. Agre P, King LS, Yasui M, et al. Aquaporin water channels—from atomic structure to clinical medicine. *J Physiol*. 2002;542(pt 1):3–16.
5. Kortenoeven MLA, Fenton RA. Renal aquaporins and water balance disorders. *Biochimica et Biophysica Acta*. 2014;1840:1533–1549.
6. Kozono D, Yasui M, King LS, et al. Aquaporin water channels: atomic structure molecular dynamics meet clinical medicine. *J Clin Invest*. 2002;109(11):1395–1399.
7. Epstein FH, Brezis M, Silva P, et al. Physiological and clinical implications of medullary hypoxia. *Artif Organs*. 1987;11(6):463–467.
8. Guyton AC, Hall JE. *Textbook of Medical Physiology*. 10th ed. Philadelphia, PA: W.B. Saunders; 2000.
9. Steinhausen M, Endlich K, Wiegman DL. Glomerular blood flow. *Kidney Int*. 1990;38(5):769–784.
10. Shirakami G, Segawa H, Shingu K, et al. The effects of atrial natriuretic peptide infusion on hemodynamic, renal, and hormonal responses during gastrectomy. *Anesth Analg*. 1997;85(4):907–912.
11. Cockcroft DW, Gault MH. Prediction of creatinine clearance from serum creatinine. *Nephron*. 1976;16(1):31–41.
12. Levey AS, Bosch JP, Lewis JB, et al; for Modification of Diet in Renal Disease Study Group. A more accurate method to estimate glomerular filtration rate from serum creatinine: a new prediction equation. *Ann Intern Med*. 1999;130(6):461–470.
13. Thadhani R, Pascual M, Bonventre JV. Acute renal failure. *N Engl J Med*. 1996;334(22):1448–1460.
14. Finn WF. FK506 nephrotoxicity. *Ren Fail*. 1999;21(3-4):319–329.
15. Kahan BD. Cyclosporine. *N Engl J Med*. 1989;321(25):1725–1738.
16. Byric RJ, Rose DK. Pathophysiology and prevention of acute renal failure: the role of the anaesthetist. *Can J Anaesth*. 1990;37(4)(pt 1): 457–467.
17. Conde E, Alegre L, Blanco-Sanchez I, et al. Hypoxia inducible factor 1-alpha (HIF-1 alpha) is induced during reperfusion after renal ischemia and is critical for proximal tubule cell survival. *PLoS One*. 2012;7(3):e33258.
18. Barrett BJ, Parfrey PS. Clinical practice. Preventing nephropathy induced by contrast medium. *N Engl J Med*. 2006;354(4):379–386.
19. Kellen M, Aronson S, Roizen MF, et al. Predictive and diagnostic tests of renal failure: a review. *Anesth Analg*. 1994;78(1):134–142.
20. Bellomo R, Ronco C, Kellum JA, et al; Acute Dialysis Quality Initiative Workgroup. Acute renal failure—definition, outcome measures, animal models, fluid therapy and information technology needs: the Second International Consensus Conference of the Acute Dialysis Quality Initiative (ADQI) Group. *Crit Care*. 2004;8(4): R204–R212.
21. Mehta RL, Kellum JA, Shah SV, et al; Acute Kidney Injury Network. Acute Kidney Injury Network: report of an initiative to improve outcomes in acute kidney injury. *Crit Care*. 2007;11(2):R31.
22. Chertow GM, Burdick E, Honour M, et al. Acute kidney injury, mortality, length of stay, and costs in hospitalized patients. *J Am Soc Nephrol*. 2005;16(11):3365–3370.
23. Bagshaw SM, George C, Bellomo R; ANZICS Database Management Committee. A comparison of the RIFLE and AKIN criteria for acute kidney injury in critically ill patients. *Nephrol Dial Transplant*. 2008;23(5):1569–1574.
24. Haase M, Bellomo R, Devarajan P, et al; NGAL Meta-analysis Investigator Group. Accuracy of neutrophil gelatinase-associated lipocalin (NGAL) in diagnosis and prognosis in acute kidney injury: a systematic review and meta-analysis. *Am J Kidney Dis*. 2009;54(6):1012–1024.
25. Mishra J, Ma Q, Prada A, et al. Identification of neutrophil gelatinase-associated lipocalin as a novel early urinary biomarker for ischemic renal injury. *J Am Soc Nephrol*. 2003;14(10):2534–2543.
26. Wagener G, Jan M, Kim M, et al. Association between increases in urinary neutrophil gelatinase-associated lipocalin and acute renal dysfunction after adult cardiac surgery. *Anesthesiology*. 2006;105(3):485–491.
27. Wagener G, Minhaz M, Mattis FA, et al. Urinary neutrophil gelatinase-associated lipocalin as a marker of acute kidney injury after orthotopic liver transplantation. *Nephrol Dial Transplant*. 2011;26(5):1717–1723.
28. Haase-Fielitz A, Haase M, Devarajan P. Neutrophil gelatinase-associated lipocalin as a biomarker of acute kidney injury: a critical evaluation of current status. *Ann Clin Biochem*. 2014;51(pt 3):335–351.
29. McIlroy DR, Wagener G, Lee HT. Biomarkers of acute kidney injury: an evolving domain. *Anesthesiology*. 2010;112(4):998–1004.
30. Kheterpal S, Tremper KK, Heung M, et al. Development and validation of an acute kidney injury risk index for patients undergoing general surgery: results from a national data set. *Anesthesiology*. 2009;110(3):505–515.
31. Payen DM, Farge D, Beloucif S, et al. No involvement of antidiuretic hormone in acute antidiuresis during PEEP ventilation in humans. *Anesthesiology*. 1987;66(1):17–23.
32. Alpert RA, Roizen MF, Hamilton WK, et al. Intraoperative urinary output does not predict postoperative renal function in patients undergoing abdominal aortic revascularization. *Surgery*. 1984;95(6): 707–711.
33. Loef BG, Epema AH, Smilde TD, et al. Immediate postoperative renal function deterioration in cardiac surgical patients predicts in-hospital mortality and long-term survival. *J Am Soc Nephrol*. 2005;16(1):195–200.
34. Thakar CV, Arrigain S, Worley S, et al. A clinical score to predict acute renal failure after cardiac surgery. *J Am Soc Nephrol*. 2005; 16(1):162–168.
35. Wijeysundera DN, Karkouti K, Beattie WS, et al. Improving the identification of patients at risk of postoperative renal failure after cardiac surgery. *Anesthesiology*. 2006;104(1):65–72.
36. Kumar AB, Suneja M. Cardiopulmonary bypass-associated acute kidney injury. *Anesthesiology*. 2011;114(4):964–970.
37. Haase M, Bellomo R, Matalanis G, et al. A comparison of the RIFLE and Acute Kidney Injury Network classifications for cardiac surgery-associated acute kidney injury: a prospective cohort study. *J Thorac Cardiovasc Surg*. 2009;138(6):1370–1376.
38. Bellomo R, Chapman M, Finfer S, et al. Low-dose dopamine in patients with early renal dysfunction: a placebo-controlled randomised trial. *Lancet* 2000;356(9248):2139–2143.
39. Landoni G, Biondi-Zoccai GG, Tumlin JA, et al. Beneficial impact of fenoldopam in critically ill patients with or at risk for acute renal failure: a meta-analysis of randomized clinical trials. *Am J Kidney Dis*. 2007;49(1):56–68.
40. Morelli A, Ricci Z, Bellomo R, et al. Prophylactic fenoldopam for renal protection in sepsis: a randomized, double-blind, placebo-controlled pilot trial. *Crit Care Med*. 2005;33(11):2451–2456.

CHAPTER 17

Intravenous Fluids and Electrolytes

Jessica Spellman • Jack S. Shanewise

Total body water and electrolytes are divided between the intracellular and extracellular compartments. The major electrolytes in the intracellular compartment are potassium, magnesium, calcium, and phosphate. The extracellular compartment consists of the interstitial, plasma, and transcellular fluid components, where sodium and chloride are the major electrolytes. Fluid movement between these spaces, and thus the effect of fluid therapies, depends on the levels of water, electrolytes, and colloid proteins among them and the composition and permeability of the membranes that separate them.

Total Body Fluid Composition

The adult body is composed of approximately 60% water, with some variation with age and gender, as well as significant variation among different tissues. For example, muscle is about 75% water, whereas adipose tissue only 10%. About two-thirds of total body fluid is intracellular and one-third extracellular (Fig. 17-1). The intracellular compartment is rich in potassium (the major cation), magnesium, calcium, phosphate (the major anion), and proteins. Extracellular volume (ECV) includes interstitial fluids (about 80% of the ECV), plasma (about 20%), and transcellular fluids, which are anatomically separate fluid spaces, such as the intraocular, gastrointestinal, and cerebrospinal fluids, and are not available for water and solute exchange with the remainder of the ECV. Extracellular fluids are rich in sodium (the major cation) and chloride (the major anion). These and other small ions move freely between plasma and interstitium in the extracellular compartment. The plasma also contains proteins, such as albumin and globulins, which create the colloid oncotic pressure. Plasma proteins are prevented from freely moving from vascular to interstitial space by the interplay of the vascular endothelial cells and the endothelial glycocalyx layer (EGL) coating the inside of the vascular space. Macromolecule movement out of the vascular space is dependent on the type of EGL pores and endothelial cell junctions, which have four phenotypes throughout the body. In the liver, spleen, and marrow, sinusoidal capillaries have large EGL pores and open fenestrations allowing macromolecules to pass between plasma and the interstitial space. The glomeruli have open capillary fenestrations with the effective pore size reduced by overlying EGL. Endocrine, choroid plexus, and gut mucosa vascular endothelial cells have inducible fenestrations. Nerve, muscle, connective tissue, and lung have nonfenestrated or continuous capillaries so that little transvascular filtration into the interstitium occurs in these tissues. In states of inflammation, changes in the endothelial cells and an increase in the number of large pores in the capillaries increase the amount of protein passing from vascular into interstitial spaces. The transcapillary escape rate of albumin to tissues is normally 5% per hour but can double during surgery and increase to 20% in sepsis.[1] Fluid in the interstitial space is returned to the circulation as lymph.[2] The cell membrane prevents sodium, the primary extracellular cation, from moving into the cell, except for a small amount by active pump transport, but isotonic fluids containing sodium added to the vascular space are distributed throughout the ECV so that only 20% of the volume infused remains in the plasma.[3]

Intravenous Fluid Types

Crystalloids

Crystalloids are fluid solutions containing ion salts and other low-molecular-weight substances. Crystalloids can be categorized based on their tonicity or osmotic pressure of the solution with respect to that of plasma. Examples are listed in Table 17-1. Administering large volumes of normal saline (NS) can result in hyperchloremic metabolic acidosis.[4] "Balanced" or "physiologic" crystalloid solutions contain a composition approximating that of extracellular fluid but are usually slightly hypotonic because of lower sodium concentration. Administering large volumes of balanced salt solutions can result in hyperlactatemia, metabolic alkalosis, hypotonicity, and cardiotoxicity

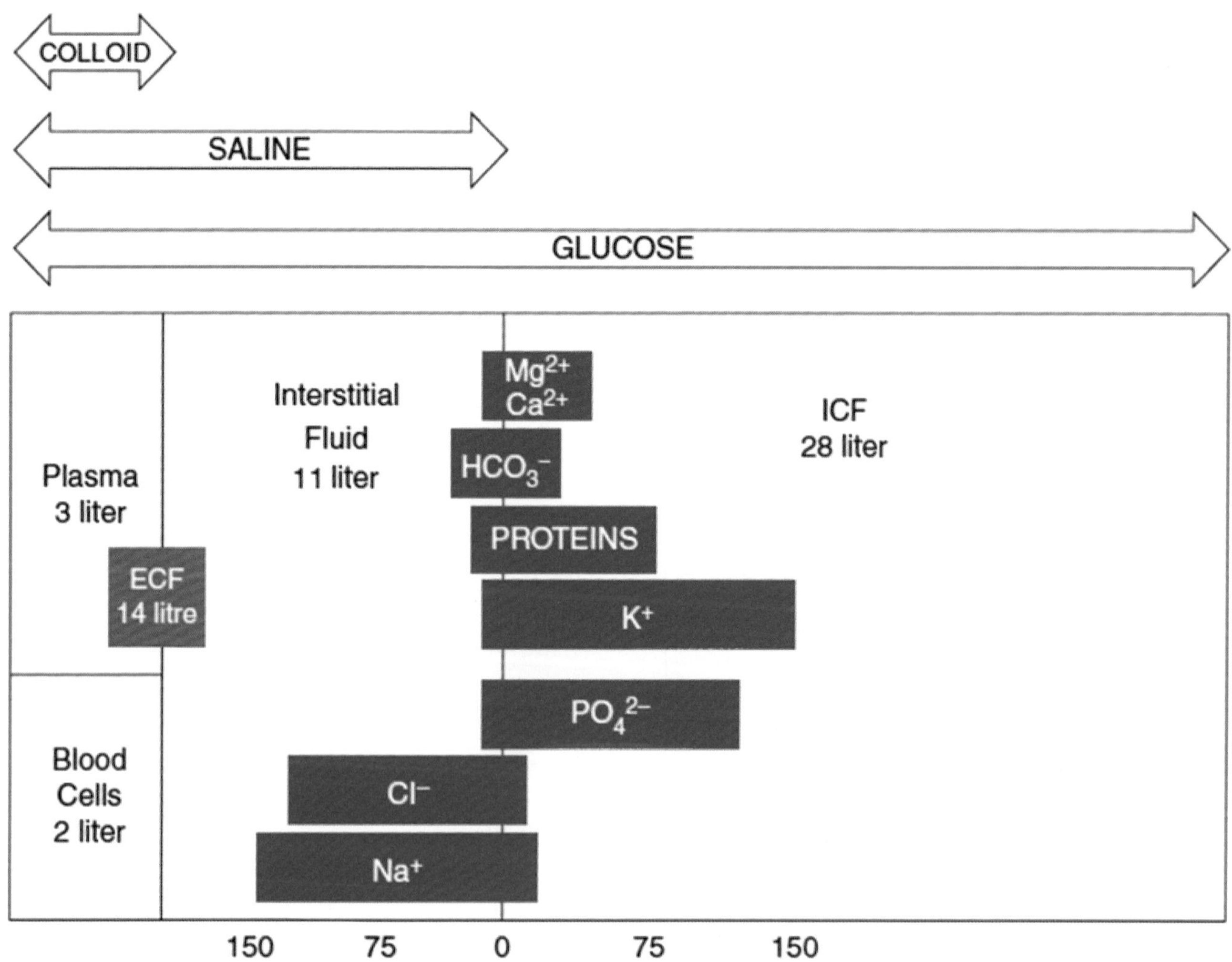

FIGURE 17-1 Body fluid compartments with main ion distribution. ECF, extracellular fluid; ICF, intracellular fluid. (Reused from Doherty M, Buggy DJ. Intraoperative fluids: how much is too much? *Br J Anaesth.* 2012;109:69–79, with permission.)

due to acetate. Calcium-containing balanced salt solution may cause formation of microthrombi when infused with citrate-containing banked blood.

Colloids

Colloid solutions contain macromolecules suspended in electrolyte solutions. These macromolecules, such as plant or animal polysaccharides or polypeptides, remain in the plasma compartment longer than crystalloid solutions; however, their distribution has been shown to be context sensitive, with larger percentages of the volume administered remaining intravascular in hypovolemic patients as compared to normovolemic patients.[3] Semisynthetic colloid solutions are metabolized and excreted and thus have a shorter duration of effect than human albumin solutions.[2] Examples are listed in Table 17-2.

Albumin (4% to 5%)

Albumin solution is produced from human blood and suspended in saline. It is heat-pasteurized at 60°C for 10 hours to reduce viral transmission. It is expensive to produce and distribute as compared to semisynthetic colloids and crystalloid solutions. The incidence of anaphylactoid reactions to albumin is 0.011%.[5]

The comparative effectiveness of fluid resuscitation with colloid versus crystalloid has been a long-standing controversy, which has been the subject of much recent clinical research. In the Saline versus Albumin Fluid Evaluation (SAFE) study, a multicenter, randomized, double-blind trial of 6,997 intensive care unit (ICU) patients, the effect of fluid resuscitation with albumin 4% or NS was evaluated. The primary outcome was death within 28 days. There was no significant increase in mortality (p = .87). The two groups also had similar rates of new single organ and multiple organ failure (p = .85), days spent in ICU (p = .44), days spent in hospital (p = .3), days of mechanical ventilation (p = .74), and days of renal replacement therapy (p = .41).[6] In a post hoc analysis of the SAFE study, of 460 patients with traumatic brain injury, the primary outcome of mortality was increased in the albumin-treated group (33.2%) versus the NS group

Table 17-1

Common Crystalloid Solutions

Solution	Osmolarity (mOsm/L)	Tonicity	pH	Calories (kcal/L)	Na^+ (mEq/L)	Cl^- (mEq/L)	K^+ (mEq/L)	Ca^{++} (mEq/L)	Mg^{++} (mEq/L)	Glucose (g/L)	Lactate (mEq/L)	Acetate (mEq/L)	Gluconate (mEq/L)
NS	308	Iso	5		154	154							
D5NS	560	Hyper	4	170	154	154				50			
D51/2NS	406	Hyper	4	170	77	77				50			
LR	273	Iso	6.5	9	130	109	4	3			28		
D5LR	525	Hyper	4.9	179	130	109	4	3		50	28		
Plasmalyte	294	Iso	140	21	140	98	5		3			27	23

D, dextrose; LR, lactated Ringer's; NS, normal saline.

From Warren BB, Durieux ME. Hydroxyethyl starch: safe or not? *Anesth Analg.* 1997;84:206–212.

Table 17-2

Common Colloid Solutions

Fluid	Trade Name	Source	Osmolarity (mOsm/L)	Na^+ (mmol/L)	Cl^- (mmol/L)	K^+ (mmol/L)	Ca^{++} (mmol/L)	Mg^{++} (mmol/L)	Lactate (mmol/L)	Acetate (mmol/L)	Octonate (mmol/L)	Malate (mmol/L)
Albumin 4%	Albumex	Human donor	250	148	128						6.4	
Albumin 5%		Human donor	309	154	154							
HES 10% (200/0.5)	Hemohes	Potato starch	308	154	154							
HES 6% (450/0.7)	Hextend	Maize starch	304	143	124	3	5	0.9	28			
HES 6% (130/0.4)	Voluven	Maize starch	308	154	154							
HES 6% (130/0.4)	Volulyte	Maize starch	286	137	110	4		1.5		34		
HES 6% (130/0.42)	Venufundin	Potato starch	308	154	154		2.5	1		24		
HES 6% (130/0.42)	Tetraspan	Potato starch	296	140	118	4						5

HES, hydroxyethyl starch.
From Myburgh JA, Mythen MG. Resuscitation fluids. *N Engl J Med.* 2013;369:1243–1251.

(20.4%, $p = .03$).[7] In an additional subgroup analysis of 1,218 patients with severe sepsis, albumin administration was associated with a decreased risk of death as compared to NS with an adjusted odds ratio of 0.71 (95% CI, 0.52–0.97; $p = .03$).[8] A more recent multicenter, open-label, randomized trial of 1,818 ICU patients with severe sepsis, the Albumin Italian Outcome Sepsis study, of 20% albumin and crystalloid versus crystalloid alone with primary outcome measure of death found no difference in survival at 28 or 90 days ($p = .29$).[9]

Semisynthetic Colloid Solutions

Solutions include hydroxyethyl starch (HES) solutions, succinylated gelatin, urea-linked gelatin–polygeline preparations, and dextran solutions. HES, the most commonly used semisynthetic colloid solutions, are created by attaching hydroxyethyl groups to carbons 2, 3, or 6 of the glucose moieties of starches of sorghum, maize, or potatoes. HES solutions vary with respect to HES concentrations (6% to 10%), molecular weights (70 to 670 kDa), molar substitution ratios (0.3 to 0.75), and crystalloid carrier solutions. The concentration influences the initial volume effect with 6% solutions being iso-oncotic and 10% solutions hyperoncotic. HES are polydisperse with particles in a wide range of molecular mass (dispersity is a measure of the heterogeneity of sizes of molecules or particles in a mixture); thus, the molecular weight is averaged by either weight or number, with high molecular weight preparations being associated with alterations in coagulation. The substitution ratio indicates the average fraction of glucose moieties bearing a hydroxyethyl group. HES can also be named hexa- (0.6), penta- (0.5), or tetra- (0.4) starches for this level of substitution. Substitution increases the solubility of the starch in water and inhibits the destruction of the starch by amylase, thus prolonging intravascular retention. HES can also be categorized with respect to the pattern of hydroxyethylation of the C_2 and C_6 carbon atoms. Hydroxyethyl groups in the C_2 position inhibit amylase access to the starch more effectively than hydroxyethyl groups at the C_6 position; thus, high C_2/C_6 ratios would be expected to hydrolyze more slowly. The maximum daily dose of HES is limited to 20 to 50 mL/kg of body weight/day but varies by solution.[10]

HES is removed from the circulation by redistribution and renal excretion. Redistribution of HES results in temporary storage in the skin, liver, and kidneys. Skin deposition results in non–histamine-associated pruritus. After 24 hours, 23% of the total dose is interstitial and at 26 weeks, trace amounts of HES are still detectable.[6] HES molecules with greater molecular weights and increased substitution ratios tend to be stored more than those with more rapid clearance and deposition appears to be dose-dependent.[10]

Renal excretion of HES occurs in two phases: immediate glomerular filtration of HES polymers less than 59 kDa and delayed glomerular filtration after HES metabolism by plasma α-amylase. This amylase functions as an endoamylase cleaving within the polyglucose chain instead of acting at the ends of the molecule, resulting in polydispersity and varying molecular weights of the remaining HES molecules in the plasma. Thus, pharmacokinetic parameters of plasma clearance and half-life will change over time, cannot be rigorously defined, and must not be interpreted as efficacy half-lives or contributing to the pharmacodynamics of volume effect of HES solutions.[11] Additionally, the hydroxyethyl groups retard hydrolysis of the compound by amylases, allowing longer presence in the plasma. Plasma levels of amylase are elevated after HES administration for 72 hours, without evidence of increased pancreatic production, owing to decreased renal elimination of amylase as it remains complexed to HES.[5] The pharmacokinetic profile of some HES solutions after single dose and multiple infusions in healthy volunteers is described in Tables 17-3[11] and 17-4,[11] and in impaired renal function in Table 17-5.[12]

HES compounds have effects on coagulation with reductions in factor VIII, von Willebrand factor, and platelet function, although the exact mechanisms are unclear. Coagulation effects are noted even when used below recommended maximum doses. Solutions with more rapid degradation are associated with less effects on coagulation.[10] The incidence of anaphylactoid reactions with HES use is 0.085%.[6]

HES solutions carry a U.S. Food and Drug Administration black box warning with the following recommendations: Do not use HES solutions in critically ill adult patients including those with sepsis and those admitted to the ICU; avoid use in patients with preexisting renal dysfunction; discontinue use of HES at the first sign of renal injury; need for renal replacement therapy has been reported up to 90 days after HES administration, continue to monitor renal function for at least 90 days in all patients; avoid use in patients undergoing open heart surgery in association with cardiopulmonary bypass due to excess bleeding; discontinue use of HES at first sign of coagulopathy.[13]

The Crystalloid versus Hydroxyethyl Starch Trial evaluated HES versus NS in a multicenter, prospective, blinded, parallel-group, randomized controlled trial of over 7,000 adult ICU patients.[14] Patients were randomized to receive either HES (6% [130/0.4] Voluven, Fresenius Kabi Norge AS, Halden, Norway) solution or NS until ICU discharge, death, or 90 days following randomization. Primary outcome was death 90 days after randomization, and secondary outcomes were acute kidney injury, failure, and treatment with renal replacement therapy. There was no significant difference in mortality during the study period (18% in the HES group and 17% in the NS group, $p = .26$) or renal failure (HES group 10.4% and 9.2% NS group, $p = .12$); however, significant differences in renal injury (34.6% HES group and 38% NS group, $p = .005$) and renal replacement therapy use (7% HES group, 5.8% NS group, $p = .04$) were found. Additionally, HES was associated with significantly more adverse events (0.3% vs. 2.8%, $p < .001$).

Table 17-3

Pharmacokinetic Parameters after a Single Dose of Different Hydroxyethyl Starch Types in Healthy Volunteers

HES Type (concentration)	Dose (g)	C_{max} (mg/mL)	$t_{½α}$ (h)	$t_{½β}$ (h)	$t_{½central}$ (h)	$AUC_∞$ (mg • h/mL)	CL (mL/min)	Infusion Time (min)
670/0.75 (6%)	0.6/kg	13	6.3[a]	46.4[b]	NA	926.0	0.98	20[c]
450/0.7[d] (6%)	30	7.8	NA	300[e]	NA	NA	NA	60
200/0.62 (6%)	30	5.2	5.08	69.7	44.42	NA	1.23	30
200/0.5 (10%)	50	8.0	3.35	30.6	7.12	NA	9.24	30
200/0.5 (6%)	30	6	NA	NA	NA	NA	4.88[f]	15[g]
200/0.5 (10%)	50	14	5.2	39.1	NA	NA	6.38[f]	15[g]
130/0.4 (6%)	26.3	3.7	1.39[h]	12.1[h]	1.55	14.3	31.4	30
130/0.4 (10%)	44.1	6.5	1.54[h]	12.8[h]	1.82	28.8	26.0	30

[a] Mean for 0–8 hours.
[b] Mean for 7–10 hours.
[c] Calculated for 70 kg body weight.
[d] Product label declaration, however *de facto* similar to 670/0.75.
[e] For days 7–28 post-treatment.
[f] Mean for 0–24 hours.
[g] BLood letting of 400 mL prior to infusion.
[h] Model independent.

$AUC_{0-∞}$, area under the plasma concentration-time curve from time zero to infinity; CL, total body clearance; C_{max}, maximum plasma concentration; NA, not available; $t_{½α}$, initial/distribution half-life; $t_{½β}$, terminal/elimination half-life; $t_{½central}$, elimination half-life from the central compartment.

From Jungheinrich C, Neff TA. Pharmacokinetics of hydroxyethyl starch. *Clin Pharmacokinet.* 2005;44:681–699.

Table 17-4

Pharmacokinetic Parameters and Residual Plasma Concentrations after Multiple Infusions of Different Types of Hydroxyethyl Starch in Healthy Volunteers

HES Type	Cumulative Dose (g)	Treatment Period	Plasma Concentration 24 h after Last Administration (mg/mL)	CL (mL/min)	$t_{½α}$ (h)	$t_{½β}$ (h)	$t_{½γ}$ (h)	AUC (mg • h/mL)	
								day 1	Last Day[a]
450/0.7	90	3 days (3 × 30 g)	9.6	<1	NA	NA	NA	NA	>>day1
200/0.62[b]	150	5 days (5 × 30 g)	7.8	0.983[c]	0.568	11.6	211	508	>>day1
200/0.5[b]	250	5 days (5 × 50 g)	3.4	4.86[c]	0.389	6.98	113	171	>>day1
200/0.5	250	5 days (5 × 50 g)	3.4	NA	NA	NA	NA	62.6	96.2
70/0.5	250	5 days (5 × 50 g)	3.0	NA	NA	NA	NA	NA	>>day1
130/0.4	500	10 days (10 × 50 g)	<0.5	22.8[d]	1.14[e]	9.1[e]	NA[f]	32.8	35.7

[a] Day 3, 5, or 10 according to length of treatment period.
[b] Three-compartment modelling.
[c] Taking days 1–5 into account.
[d] Day 1: 23.7; day 10: 21.8.
[e] Means from days 1 and 10.
[f] Not applicable for two-compartment modelling used; three-compartment modelling would yield a value of 33 hours.

AUC, area under the plasma concentration-time curve; CL, total body clearance; NA, not available; $t_{½α}$, initial/distribution half-life, $t_{½β}$, terminal/elimination half-life; $t_{½γ}$, terminal/elimination half-life in a three-compartment model; >>, indicates much greater than.

From Jungheinrich C, Neff TA. Pharmacokinetics of hydroxyethyl starch. *Clin Pharmacokinet.* 2005;44:681–699.

Table 17-5

Pharmacokinetic Parameters after a Single Dose of Hydroxyethyl Starch 6% (130/0.4) 500 mL in Different States of Renal Insufficiency

Variable	Renal Group[a]	Mean (CV %) (Geometric)	95% CI
$AUC_{(0-inf)}$ (mg • h/mL)	15– <30	41.1 (19.9)	(33.4, 50.6)
	30– <50	35.1 (13.9)	(28.1, 43.8)
	50– <80	20.0 (6.8)	(18.4, 21.8)
	80– <120	25.5 (21.3)	(18.3, 35.4)
	All subjects	29.8 (34.4)	(25.3, 35.0)
C_{max} (mg/mL)	15– <30	4.68 (17.4)	(3.90, 5.62)
	30– <50	4.37 (14.1)	(3.50, 5.46)
	50– <80	3.48 (12.5)	(2.99, 4.05)
	80– <120	5.11 (25.4)	(3.45, 7.57)
	All subjects	4.34 (21.9)	(3.91, 4.81)
Total plasma clearance (L/h)	15– <30	0.73 (20.3)	(0.59, 0.90)
	30– <50	0.85 (12.8)	(0.69, 1.05)
	50– <80	1.52 (6.9)	(1.40, 1.65)
	80– <120	1.19 (21.3)	(0.86, 1.65)
	All subjects	1.02 (34.9)	(0.87, 1.20)
Volume of distribution at steady state (L)	15– <30	14.2 (18.4)	(11.7, 17.2)
	30– <50	15.4 (12.7)	(12.7, 18.7)
	50– <80	27.1 (6.6)	(24.9, 29.5)
	80– <120	19.9 (23.1)	(13.8, 28.7)
	All subjects	18.4 (31.2)	(15.9, 21.3)
Terminal half-life (h)	15– <30	15.9 (8.8)	(14.5, 17.4)
	30– <50	15.5 (9.6)	(13.3, 18.0)
	50– <80	15.9 (5.4)	(14.8, 17.1)
	80– <120	17.2 (6.8)	(15.4, 19.2)
	All subjects	16.1 (8.1)	(15.5, 16.7)

HES, hydroxyethyl starch, CV, coefficient of variation, CI, confidence interval; AUC, area under the time concentration curve; C_{max}, peak concentration.

[a] Defined according to measurements of creatinine clearance (mL/min/1.73 m^2).

From Jungheinrich C, Scharpf R, Wargenau M, et al. The pharmacokinetics and tolerability of an intravenous infusion of the new hydroxyethyl starch 130/0.4 (6%, 500 mL) in mild-to-severe renal impairment. *Anesth Analg*. 2002;95:544–551.

HES (6% [130/0.42] Tetraspan, B. Braun Melsungen AG, Melsungen, Germany) has also been evaluated in a multicenter, parallel-group, blinded, randomized trial of 798 adult ICU patients with severe sepsis versus Ringer's acetate in the Scandinavian Starch for Severe Sepsis/Septic Shock trial. Primary outcomes measured were death or end-stage kidney failure at 90 days. Death was greater at 90 days in the HES group (51% vs. 43%, $p = .03$). One patient in each group had end-stage kidney failure; however, in the 90-day period, 22% of HES patients were treated with renal replacement therapy versus 16% in the Ringer's acetate group ($p = .04$).[15]

In the Efficacy of Volume Substitution and Insulin Therapy in Severe Sepsis multicenter, randomized trial evaluating adult ICU patients with severe sepsis, patients were randomized to receive either intensive insulin therapy or conventional insulin therapy in addition to either HES 10% pentastarch, HES 200/0.5, or lactated Ringer's for fluid resuscitation. Primary endpoints were death and mean score for organ failure. There were 537 patients who were evaluated and the trial was stopped early due to increased severe hypoglycemia events in the intensive insulin therapy group, but the comparison between HES and lactated Ringer's was continued with all patients receiving conventional insulin therapy. HES therapy was associated with higher rates of acute renal failure (34.9%, 22.8% in the lactated Ringer's group, $p = 0.002$) and renal replacement therapy than lactated Ringer's (18.3%, 9.2% lactated Ringer's group).[16]

Assessing Fluid Responsiveness

Fluid responsiveness may be defined as a 15% increase in cardiac output following a 500-mL IV fluid bolus, indicating that the patient is still on the ascending limb of the cardiac output/end diastolic volume curve, also referred to as the **cardiac function curve**[17] (Fig. 17-2). Fluid administration to a patient on the plateau part of the curve may be of little benefit and result in adverse effects. Filling pressure measures, particularly central venous pressure,

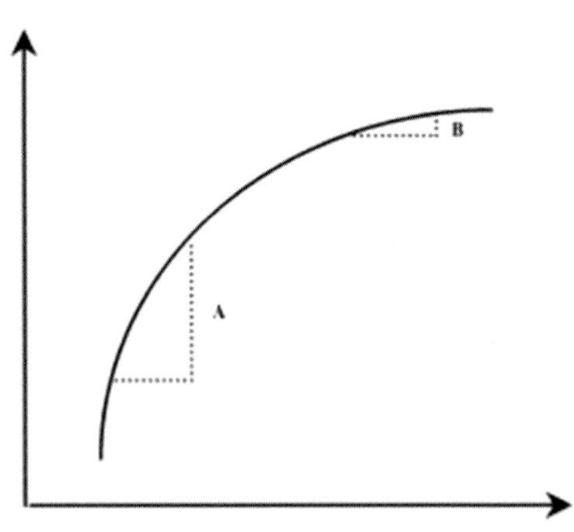

FIGURE 17-2 Schematic representation of Frank–Starling relationship between ventricular preload and stroke volume. A given change in preload induces a larger change in stroke volume when the ventricle operates on the ascending portion of the relationship (**A**, condition of preload dependence) than when it operates on the flat portion of the curve (**B**, condition of preload independence). (From Michard F, Teboul JL. Using heart-lung interactions to assess fluid responsiveness during mechanical ventilation. *Critical care*. 2000;4:282–289).

correlate poorly with blood volume, and changes in central venous pressure have been shown to poorly predict hemodynamic response to fluid challenge.[18] Stroke volume changes due to increases or decreases in right ventricular preload may be used to assess fluid responsiveness. Positive pressure ventilation decreases right ventricular stroke volume by decreasing venous return to the right heart and increasing right ventricular afterload. The decrease in right ventricular stroke volume is passed on to the left ventricle over subsequent cardiac cycles and if the left ventricle is preload dependent, decreases in the left ventricle stroke volume will cause a decrease in the arterial pulse pressure. These cyclic changes associated with positive airway pressure are greater when the ventricles are functioning on the steep, ascending portion of the cardiac function curve. Variation in the arterial pulse pressure (PPV) can be derived from analysis of the arterial pressure waveform and variation greater than 12% to 13% is predictive of volume responsiveness.[19] Other measures of these positive pressure–associated stroke volume changes include systolic pressure variation of the arterial waveform, stroke volume variation (SVV) derived from arterial pulse contour analysis, pleth variability index derived from pulse oximeter waveform analysis, inferior vena cava diameter variation measured by echocardiography, and descending aortic blood velocity measured by esophageal Doppler. Measures dependent on variations caused by positive pressure ventilation are limited by the presence of arrhythmia, spontaneous breathing, tidal volume settings (8 mL/kg ideal body weight minimum required for PPV and SVV),[19] low lung compliance (<30 mL/cm H_2O), increased abdominal pressure, and open chest surgery.[20]

The end-expiratory occlusion test is useful in ventilated patients with cardiac arrhythmias, mild amplitude spontaneous breathing activity, or low tidal volume positive pressure ventilation. The test assesses the effect of a 15-second interruption in the ventilation on cardiac preload. A 5% increase in pulse contour cardiac output (sensitivity 91%, specificity 100%) or pulse pressure (sensitivity 87%, specificity 100%) is suggestive of volume responsiveness.[21] Passive leg raising maneuvers (PLR) can be used to assess preload responsiveness in spontaneously breathing patients with arrhythmias but is limited in patients with intraabdominal hypertension. The test is performed in a supine patient by elevating the legs to 45 degrees while assessing cardiac output or stroke volume over 30 to 90 seconds. Cardiac output measures during PLR are more accurate in predicting fluid responsiveness than arterial pressure measurements during the maneuver.[22]

Important Fluid Constituents

Magnesium

Magnesium is almost all intracellular in bone (53%), muscle (27%), and soft tissues (19%), with less than 1% of total body magnesium in the extracellular fluid and only 0.3% in the plasma.[23] Most intracellular magnesium is bound to adenosine 5'-triphosphate and DNA, with less than 3% being in solution and ionized immediately available for intracellular magnesium homeostasis.[24] Plasma magnesium level is normally 1.7 to 2.4 mg/dL, where it is found in three states: ionized (62%), protein bound (33%), and complexed to anions (5%).[23] Given these distributions, plasma magnesium measurements may not be representative of total body magnesium stores. Also, magnesium measurements can be falsely elevated with hemolysis of the blood sample, which releases the intracellular electrolytes. Ingested magnesium is absorbed in the small intestines, primarily the ileum (75%),[24] via passive concentration effects and in the colon by active transcellular absorption.[25] Excretion occurs via the kidney with more than 95% of the filtered magnesium being reabsorbed in the renal tubules, with this mechanism effectively regulating the plasma level. Reabsorption occurs primarily (70%) in the ascending loop of Henle via passive mechanisms with a small amount occurring in both the proximal tubule via passive mechanisms and distal convoluted tubules via active mechanisms.[24] Bone, as the primary store of total body magnesium, provides a buffer for plasma magnesium levels through poorly understood mechanisms controlling magnesium incorporation into bone by osteoblasts and removal by osteoclasts.[25] Genetic mutations in colon transport channels[25] and loop of Henle junction proteins[24] can both result in hypomagnesemia.

Role of Magnesium

Magnesium plays a key role in many biologic processes including protein synthesis, neuromuscular function, and nucleic acid stability. It is involved in adenosine 5′-triphosphatase function, antagonizes *N*-methyl-D-aspartate (NMDA) glutamate receptors, inhibits catecholamine release, and is involved in the regulation of other electrolytes. For instance, magnesium antagonizes the uptake and distribution of calcium and modulates sodium and potassium currents thru nicotinic acetylcholine receptors, NMDA receptors, and ion pumps, thus affecting membrane potentials. Magnesium has antiarrhythmic properties related to calcium channel antagonism.[24] Intravenous (IV) magnesium administration can exert muscle-relaxing effects, enhance nondepolarizing neuromuscular blockers, attenuate muscle fasciculations and potassium release with administration of succinylcholine, and precipitate skeletal muscle weakness in patients with Lambert-Eaton syndrome and myasthenia gravis. It has been used to reduce anesthetic requirements and attenuate cardiovascular effects of laryngoscopy and intubation. Magnesium has been shown to vasodilate blood vessels in many vascular beds (mesenteric, skeletal muscle, uterine, cerebral, coronary, and the aorta). It also decreases blood–brain barrier disruption and limits cerebral edema formation after brain injury.[26] Side effects of IV administration include burning or pain on injection, drowsiness, nausea, headache, dizziness, muscle weakness, hypotension, and bradycardia.

Hypomagnesemia

Hypomagnesemia may result from dietary deficiency (as seen in chronic alcoholism), gastrointestinal malabsorption or secretion (diarrhea, vomiting, laxative use), renal losses (medication effects, nephrotoxic agents, endocrine disease, diabetic nephropathy), and chelation (citrate binding in the case of massive transfusion).[24] It is seen in as many as 11% of hospitalized patients and 65% of patients in the ICU. Clinical manifestations of hypomagnesemia result in cardiac and neuromuscular disorders and include symptoms of nausea, vomiting, weakness, convulsions, tetany, fasciculations, as well as electrocardiogram (ECG) abnormalities (prolonged PR and QT intervals, diminished T-wave morphology, torsades de pointes, and others) and accompanying hypokalemia and hypocalcemia.

Hypermagnesemia

Hypermagnesemia is rare and most commonly occurs with excessive administration of magnesium for therapeutic purposes. Clinical manifestations include QRS widening, hypotension, narcosis, diminution of deep tendon reflexes, respiratory depression from paralysis of muscles of ventilation, heart block, and cardiac arrest. Immediate treatment of life-threatening hypermagnesemia is with calcium gluconate, 10 to 15 mg/kg IV, followed by diuretics or dialysis, along with appropriate respiratory and circulatory support.

Preeclampsia

Magnesium appears to improve the clinical symptoms of preeclampsia by causing systemic, vertebral, and uterine vasodilation via direct effects on vessels as well as by increasing concentrations of endogenous vasodilators (endothelium-derived relaxing factor and calcitonin gene–related peptide) and attenuating endogenous vasoconstrictors (endothelin-1). Suggested dosing regimens of magnesium sulfate based on randomized trial data are 4 g IV loading dose over 10 to 15 minutes followed by infusion of 1 g per hour for 24 hours or 4 g IV loading dose with 10 g intramuscular (IM) followed by 5 g IM every 4 hours for 24 hours. Many other dosing regimens exist.[27] Infusions or repeat dosing should be combined with clinical monitoring of urine output, respiratory rate, and deep tendon reflexes. Serum monitoring of magnesium levels should be performed for signs of toxicity or renal impairment. Magnesium crosses the placenta and may result in neonatal lethargy, hypotension, and respiratory depression if administered for prolonged duration (more than 48 hours).[24] In a Cochrane Summaries review, magnesium was shown to decrease the risk of progression to eclampsia (RR, 0.41; CI, 0.29–0.58), decrease the risk of placental abruption (RR, 0.64; CI, 0.5–0.83), and increase caesarean section (RR, 1.05; CI, 1.01–1.1) but does not clearly affect maternal morbidity, stillbirth, or neonatal death or neurosensory disability at age 18 months. Reductions in maternal death were found to be nonsignificant.[28]

Cardiac Dysrhythmias

Excess magnesium blocks myocardial calcium influx resulting in decreased sinus node activity, prolonged atrioventricular (AV) conduction time, and increased AV node refractoriness. Arrhythmias associated with hypomagnesemia are often[29] accompanied by hypokalemia. Normalization of both electrolytes is recommended.[23] Magnesium administration may decrease the incidence of severe arrhythmia after myocardial infarction but use is limited by the incidence of hypotension.[24] There is no evidence that magnesium infusion during human cardiopulmonary resuscitation increases survival to hospital discharge; however, magnesium is recommended for patients with polymorphic wide complex tachycardia associated with familial or acquired long QT syndrome (torsades de pointes).[30] For digoxin-induced tachyarrhythmias in hypomagnesemic patients, magnesium should be administered while awaiting digoxin antibodies.[24] Prophylactic administration of magnesium during cardiopulmonary bypass has been shown to decrease the incidence of postoperative atrial fibrillation after coronary artery bypass graft surgery.

Analgesia

Magnesium has antinociceptive effects when administered IV or intrathecally, possibly due to inhibition of calcium influx, antagonism of NMDA receptors, or prevention of NMDA signaling. Data to support the use of magnesium as an analgesic or for preventative analgesia at this point is conflicting.[24]

Asthma

Magnesium causes bronchodilatation via inhibition of calcium-mediated smooth muscle contraction, inhibition of histamine release from mast cells, and inhibition of nicotinic acetylcholine release. IV magnesium (not inhaled) has been reported to improve bronchodilatation when standard therapies have failed; however, responses are variable.[23,31]

Pheochromocytoma

Magnesium's arteriolar-dilating effects combined with reduction in catecholamine release may be beneficial in the management of patients with pheochromocytoma prior to tumor excision and in hemodynamic catecholamine crisis.[32,33]

Calcium

As an important component of the skeleton, there is more calcium in the body than any other mineral. The plasma concentration of calcium is maintained between 4.5 and

5.5 mEq/L (8.5 to 10.5 mg/dL) by an endocrine control system involving vitamin D, parathyroid hormone, and calcitonin, which regulate intestinal absorption, renal reabsorption, and bone turnover. Total plasma calcium consists of calcium bound to albumin and proteins (40%), calcium complexed with citrate and phosphorus ions (9%), and freely diffusible ionized calcium (51%).[34] It is the ionized fraction of calcium that produces physiologic effects and is normally 2 to 2.5 mEq/L. The ionized concentration of calcium depends on arterial pH, with acidosis increasing and alkalosis decreasing the concentration. Additionally, plasma albumin binds nonionized calcium, thus, in low albumin states, less nonionized calcium is protein bound making more available to return to storage sites, such as bone and teeth. This may decrease the total plasma calcium, but symptoms of hypocalcemia do not occur unless the ionized calcium concentration is also decreased. Thus, nonionized plasma calcium levels must be interpreted with knowledge of the plasma albumin concentration and can be corrected according to the following formula: corrected Ca^{++} (mg/dL) = measured Ca^{++} (mg/dL) + [0.8 × (4.0 − albumin (mg/dL)].[35] However, calculations to correct serum nonionized calcium for hypoalbuminemia may not be reliable in critically ill patients.[36]

Role of Calcium

The majority of total body calcium (>99%) is present in bone and provides the skeleton with strength and a reservoir to maintain the intracellular and extracellular calcium concentrations. Calcium is important for neuromuscular transmission, skeletal muscle contraction, cardiac muscle contractility, blood coagulation, and intracellular signaling in its function as a second messenger. In cardiac myocytes, calcium regulates contraction, relaxation, and electrical signals that determine rhythm and triggers hypertrophy via calcineurin mechanisms.[37] In vascular smooth muscle, calcium induces a change in contractile state, increasing and decreasing vessel diameter.[38]

Hypocalcemia

Hypocalcemia can result from decreased plasma concentration of albumin, hypoparathyroidism, acute pancreatitis, vitamin D deficiency, chronic renal failure associated with hyperphosphatemia, citrate binding of calcium (in the case of transfused blood, particularly in hepatic failure and reduced citrate metabolism[39,40] or use of citrate in dialysis or plasmapheresis[41]), sepsis, and critical illness.[41] Malabsorptive states rarely result in hypocalcemia as serum levels are maintained by bone calcium stores. Symptoms of hypocalcemia include neuromuscular excitability, including muscle twitching, spasms, tingling, numbness, carpopedal spasm, tetany, seizures, and cardiac dysrhythmias.[42] Calcium can be administered by oral or IV route. IV preparations include calcium chloride which provides 27 mg of elemental calcium/mL and calcium gluconate which provides 9 mg.[41] IV calcium chloride may cause local irritation and necrosis if extravasated into the subcutaneous tissues and therefore is best administered centrally.

Hypercalcemia

Hyperparathyroidism is the most important cause of hypercalcemia and may be primary from parathyroid adenoma (85%), parathyroid hyperplasia (10%) which may be associated with multiple endocrine neoplasia syndromes, or, rarely (<1%), parathyroid carcinoma. Secondary hyperparathyroidism results from abnormal feedback loops present in renal failure and tertiary hyperparathyroidism from overactive responses to normal negative feedback mechanisms. Malignancies, such as squamous cell lung, breast, prostate, colon, adult T-cell, and multiple myeloma, may result in release of parathyroid hormone–related peptide from tumor cells, resulting in inappropriate hypercalcemia.[41] Malignancy-related hypercalcemia may also result from osteolytic activity at sites of skeletal metastases commonly seen in breast cancer, multiple myeloma, and lymphoma, and, rarely, malignancy-related hypercalcemia may result from tumor release of vitamin D.[35] Hypercalcemia may be associated with benign familial hypocalciuric hypercalcemia syndrome resulting from a mutation in calcium-sensing receptors. Hypercalcemia is also associated with granulomatous diseases such as sarcoidosis, tuberculosis, leprosy, coccidioidomycosis, and histoplasmosis and may result from excessive dietary supplement or medication side effects as a result of diuretic or lithium administration. Symptoms of hypercalcemia result from smooth muscle relaxation in the gut (constipation, anorexia, nausea, vomiting), decreased neuromuscular transmission (lethargy, hypotonia, confusion), renal effects (polyuria, dehydration, nephrolithiasis), cardiac rhythm abnormalities (QTc shortening, J waves following QRS complex), as well as pancreatitis.[41]

Treatment of hypercalcemia depends on the exact etiology but usually includes promoting renal excretion of calcium with IV fluids and loop diuretics while avoiding dehydration that would worsen any renal injury. Medications contributing to hypercalcemia should be discontinued and parathyroidectomy performed if indicated. Corticosteroids can be used to lower excessive calcium levels by inhibiting the effects of vitamin D, reducing intestinal absorption, and increasing renal excretion. Hydrocortisone 200 to 400 mg IV per day for 3 to 5 days[41] or prednisone 40 to 100 mg per day orally are recommended treatments for hypercalcemia associated with lymphoma and myeloma.[35] IV bisphosphonates to inhibit osteoclast bone resorption may be useful: pamidronate 60 to 90 mg IV or zoledronate 4 mg IV. Gallium nitrate 100 to 200 mg/mL/day IV infusion for 5 days is used to inhibit osteoclastic bone resorption for paraneoplastic hypercalcemia refractory to bisphosphonate therapy.[35] Calcitonin 4 to 8 International Units/kg subcutaneously or IM every

12 hours is less effective than bisphosphonates[35] or gallium nitrate[41] and works by inhibiting bone resorption and increasing renal calcium excretion. Mithramycin 25 μg/kg IV blocks bone resorption by inhibiting osteoclast RNA synthesis, but its use is limited by frequent dosing and toxicity (renal, hepatic, and hematologic).[35] Hemodialysis may also be used to treat acute, severe hypercalcemia.

Bone Composition

Bone is composed of an organic matrix that is strengthened by deposits of calcium salts. The organic matrix is greater than 90% collagen fibers, and the remainder is a homogeneous material called ***ground substance***. Ground substance is composed of proteoglycans that include chondroitin sulfate and hyaluronic acid. Salts deposited in the organic matrix of bone are composed principally of calcium and phosphate ions in a combination known as ***hydroxyapatites***.

The initial stage of bone production is the secretion by osteoclasts of collagen and ground substance. Calcium salts precipitate on the surfaces of collagen fibers, forming nidi that grow into hydroxyapatite crystals. Bone is continually being deposited by osteoblasts and is constantly being absorbed where osteoclasts are active. The bone-absorptive activity of osteoclasts is regulated by the parathyroid gland. Except in growing bones, the rate of bone deposition and absorption are equal, so the total mass of bone remains constant.

Because physical stress stimulates new bone formation, calcium is deposited by the osteoblasts in proportion to the compression load that the bone must carry. The deposition of bone at points of compression may be caused by small electrical currents induced by stress, called the ***piezoelectric effect***, stimulating osteoblastic activity at the negative end of current flow. Osteoblasts are maximally activated at a bone fracture, the resulting bulge of osteoblastic tissue and new bone matrix being known as ***callus***.

Osteoblasts secrete large amounts of alkaline phosphatase when they are actively depositing bone matrix. As a result, the rate of new bone formation is reflected by elevation of plasma concentration in alkaline phosphatase. Alkaline phosphatase concentrations are also increased by any disease process that causes destruction of bone (e.g., metastatic cancer, osteomalacia, and rickets).

Calcium salts almost never precipitate in normal tissues other than bone. A notable exception, however, is atherosclerosis, in which calcium precipitates in the walls of large arteries. Calcium salts are also frequently deposited in degenerating tissues or in old blood clots.

Bisphosphonates

Bisphosphonates are drugs with a phosphorus-carbon-phosphorus (P-C-P) chemical structure that resemble inorganic pyrophosphate (Fig. 17-3).[43] Inorganic pyrophosphate is involved in regulation of bone mineralization by binding hydroxyapatite crystals, inhibiting calcification. The phosphate groups of bisphosphonates, like inorganic pyrophosphate, bind hydroxyapatite crystals and become incorporated into sites of active bone remodeling, thus inhibiting calcification. The hydroxyl group attached to the central carbon further increases bisphosphonate's ability to bind calcium, and the final structural grouping is attached to the central carbon to determine the bisphosphonate's potency for inhibition of bone resorption. First-generation bisphosphonates (etidronate, clodronate, tiludronate), similar to inorganic pyrophosphate, become incorporated into adenosine triphosphate (ATP) by class II aminoacyl-transfer RNA synthetases after osteoclast-mediated uptake from bone and mineral surface. This abnormal ATP cannot be hydrolyzed, accumulates, and is believed to be cytotoxic to osteoclasts. Second- and third-generation bisphosphonates (alendronate, risedronate, ibandronate, pamidronate, and zoledronic acid) contain nitrogen or amino groups in this position, which increases the antiresorptive potency by binding and inhibiting farnesyl pyrophosphate synthase, leading to osteoclast apoptosis. Second- and third-generation bisphosphonate–induced osteoclast apoptosis can be detected by a reduction in biochemical markers of bone resorption; maximum suppression occurs within 3 months of initiation of oral therapy. Suppression is noted to be more rapid following IV administration. Duration of effect is a function of potency for mineral matrix binding, with zolendronic acid suppressing biochemical markers of bone resorption for up to 1 year in women with postmenopausal osteoporosis.

Clinical Uses

Bisphosphonates are useful in treating clinical conditions characterized by increased osteoclast-mediated bone resorption, for example: osteoporosis, Paget disease of bone, osteogenesis imperfecta, hypercalcemia, and malignant bony metastasis.

Pharmacokinetics

Oral bioavailability of bisphosphonates is low as they are hydrophilic with less than 1% absorbed after an oral dose. About 50% of the absorbed drug is retained in the skeleton, depending on renal function, rate of bone turnover, and binding site availability, and the remainder of drug is eliminated unchanged in the urine.[43,44]

Side Effects

Hypocalcemia may follow IV bisphosphonate infusion; treatment is supportive with calcium and vitamin D supplementation. Ten percent to 42% of patients receiving nitrogen-containing bisphosphonates IV may experience an acute phase reaction[44] with fever, myalgias, arthralgias, headaches, and influenza-like symptoms. The incidence of this reaction decreases with each subsequent infusion; pretreatment with antihistamines and antipyretics[44] can reduce the incidence and severity of symptoms. Severe musculoskeletal pain may occur at any point after initiating

A Inorganic pyrophosphate Bisphosphonate

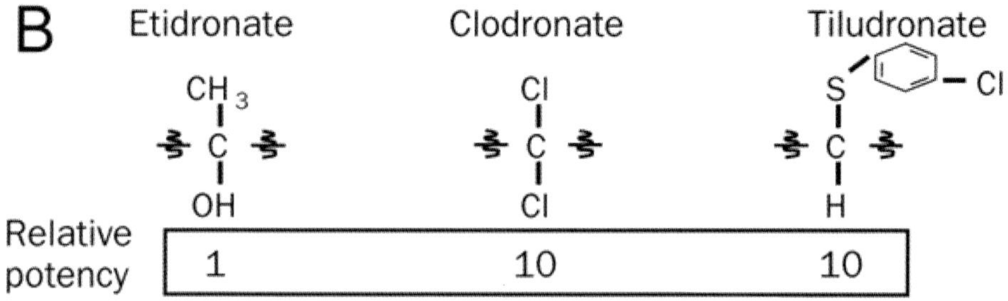

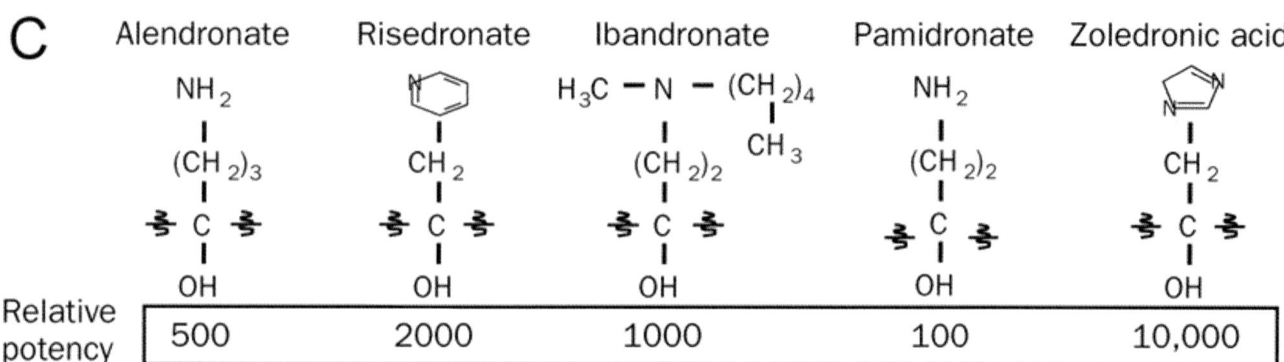

FIGURE 17-3 Inorganic pyrophosphate (PPi) and bisphosphonates. (Reused from Drake MT, Clarke BL, Khosla S. Bisphosphonates: mechanism of action and role in clinical practice. *Mayo Clin Proc.* 2008;83:1032–1045, with permission.)

bisphosphonates. Ocular inflammation (conjunctivitis, uveitis, episcleritis, scleritis) has been associated with both oral and IV bisphosphonate. Symptoms resolve within a few weeks of discontinuation. Esophageal irritation and erosion can occur with oral bisphosphonate therapy, particularly in the presence of gastroesophageal reflux disease or esophageal stricture; thus, it is often recommended that upright posture be maintained for 30 minutes after ingestion and that oral preparations be taken with a full glass of water.[44] Osteonecrosis of the jaw is associated with high-dose IV bisphosphonate use, primarily zoledronic acid and pamidronate, for oncologic conditions with an incidence of 1 to 10 per 100 patients. Associated risk factors for this complication include poor oral hygiene, history of recent dental procedures, denture use, and prolonged exposure to high IV bisphosphonate doses. The condition is rare for oral therapy of osteoporosis (1 in 10,000 to 1 in 100,000).[43,44] Bisphosphonate dosing should be adjusted in patients with renal insufficiency, and its use is cautioned in patients with creatinine clearance less than 30 mL per minute because IV therapy may lead to rapid deterioration of renal function. Serious atrial fibrillation (life-threatening or resulting in hospitalization or disability) occurred more often in patients treated with zoledronic acid than placebo (1.3% vs. 0.5%, $p < .001$) in the Health Outcomes and Reduced Incidence with Zoledronic Acid Once Yearly trial; however, there was no difference in the overall number of atrial fibrillation events in the two groups, and post hoc analysis of other trials have not yielded an association.[44] Hepatotoxicity has been reported with alendronate and zolendronate.[44]

Denosumab

Denosumab is another antiresorptive therapy for metabolic bone diseases. It is a human monoclonal antibody against RANKL, a receptor activator required to differentiate and activate osteoclasts. Denosumab is reversible, administered biannually via subcutaneous route, and is not eliminated by the kidneys. Like the bisphosphonates, it is also associated with osteonecrosis of the jaw.[45]

Potassium

Potassium is the second most common cation in the body and the principal intracellular cation. Approximately 3,500 mEq of potassium are present in the body of a 70-kg patient (40 to 50 mEq/kg). With 98% of the body's potassium being intracellular,[46] the concentration in the extracellular fluid is about 4 mEq/L, and the intracellular concentration is 150 mEq/L. Because of this huge difference in concentration, estimation of total body potassium content from serum potassium values is inaccurate, even though the vast majority of potassium (>90%) is readily exchangeable between the intra- and extracellular compartments.

Role of Potassium

Potassium has an important influence on the control of osmotic pressure and is a catalyst of numerous enzymatic reactions. It is involved in the function of excitable cell membranes (nerves, skeletal muscles, cardiac muscle) and is directly involved in the function of the kidneys. In cardiac cells, potassium decreases action potential duration, electrical inhomogeneity, and risk of digoxin toxicity. Potassium is an endothelial-dependent vasodilator; it decreases vascular smooth muscle cell proliferation and inhibits thrombus formation and platelet activation.[46] Disturbances of potassium homeostasis contribute to cardiac dysrhythmias, skeletal muscle weakness, and acid–base disturbances.

The kidney is the principal organ involved in body potassium homeostasis, primarily through control of active potassium secretion in the urine. This is different from most other electrolytes, which are regulated by control of reabsorption in the distal tubule. A number of hormones influence renal potassium secretion including aldosterone, glucocorticoids, catecholamines, and arginine vasopressin. Aldosterone acts at the renal collecting duct to increase reabsorption of sodium ions, which favors potassium secretion. Arginine vasopressin also increases secretion of potassium at the distal collecting tubule. Glucocorticoids influence renal potassium secretion by a direct action in the renal parenchyma. Catecholamines decrease renal secretion of potassium by an effect on the distal collecting system. Acidosis opposes and alkalosis favors potassium secretion. When uremia develops, gastrointestinal secretion of potassium increases, and when creatinine clearance is less than 20% of normal, gastrointestinal potassium loss can approach 20% of uptake.

Drugs Causing Hypokalemia

Diuretics that induce renal potassium loss are probably the most common cause of hypokalemia, but there are a number of other drugs that may result in this condition. Catecholamines shift potassium intracellularly, predominantly into the liver and skeletal muscle cells, and administration of β-adrenergic agonists in the treatment of bronchial asthma or premature labor may cause hypokalemia; in fact, β agonists may be useful in the treatment of hyperkalemia. Theophylline also causes potassium to move into cells, and hypokalemia should be anticipated in the presence of theophylline toxicity. Insulin induces potassium to move into cells and is used to treat severe hyperkalemia. Hypokalemia is caused by gastrointestinal losses of potassium from chronic laxative abuse or overaggressive bowel preparation for abdominal surgery. Large doses of penicillin and its synthetic derivatives increase excretion of potassium in the urine, and the direct nephrotoxicity of aminoglycoside antibiotics can also lead to excessive potassium loss.

Drugs Causing Hyperkalemia

Drugs that increase serum potassium concentrations do so by redistribution, suppression of aldosterone secretion, inhibition of potassium secretion in the distal collecting duct, or by direct cell destruction. Extracellular movement of potassium can result in plasma hyperkalemia without an increase in total body potassium. For example, succinylcholine causes a release of potassium from skeletal muscle cells, resulting in an increase of the serum potassium concentration by as much as 0.5 mEq/L. Digitalis toxicity can cause hyperkalemia by preventing potassium entry into cells. β-Adrenergic antagonists can cause a modest increase in the serum potassium concentration by virtue of an extracellular shift. Nonsteroidal antiinflammatory drugs may cause hyperkalemia by preventing aldosterone release. Potassium-sparing diuretics such as spironolactone inhibit the secretion of potassium in the distal collecting duct and can cause clinical hyperkalemia. Abrupt cell lysis from chemotherapy for acute blood cell proliferative malignancies can cause hyperkalemia through the release of intracellular potassium.

Hypokalemia

Skeletal muscle weakness and a predisposition to cardiac dysrhythmias are the most prominent symptoms of clinically significant hypokalemia. At the cellular level, hypokalemia causes hyperpolarity, increases resting potential, hastens depolarization, and increases automaticity and excitability of cardiac cells,[47] predisposing to tachydysrhythmias, including torsade de pointes[48] and atrial fibrillation[47], and sudden cardiac death particularly in the setting of acute myocardial infarction.[46] Potassium depletion also produces diastolic dysfunction of the myocardium.[46]

Treatment

It is important to determine the cause of hypokalemia before aggressive potassium replacement is initiated. For example, if serum potassium concentrations are acutely decreased due to intracellular redistribution and potassium therapy is initiated, potentially serious hyperkalemia could occur. If total body depletion is the cause of hypokalemia, the amount of increase in the plasma concentration of potassium produced by supplementation may be small due to rapid redistribution into intracellular sites.

Life-threatening hypokalemia, presenting as malignant cardiac dysrhythmias, acute digitalis intoxication, or extreme neuromuscular collapse, requires supplemental IV potassium administration. The rate of potassium infusion depends on the urgency of the indication, with a common recommendation being administration of IV potassium no greater than 10 mEq per hour peripherally and 20 mEq per hour centrally in adults. Morbidity associated with supplemental potassium therapy is not trivial. Patients with diminished internal potassium regulation, especially diabetics and renal failure patients, are at risk for accidental treatment-induced hyperkalemia.

Hyperkalemia

The earliest sign of hyperkalemia is peaked T waves on ECG, which typically occurs when the serum potassium concentration reaches 6 mEq/L. As the extracellular concentration increases further, the transmembrane gradient is decreased, with prolongation of the P-R interval and QRS widening on the ECG. At this point, the risk of asystole or ventricular fibrillation due to cardiac conduction blockade increases dramatically. Asystole may also occur due to decreased automaticity in the sinoatrial node. Occasionally, hyperkalemia presents with neuromuscular symptoms such as paresthesias and skeletal muscle weakness.

Treatment

The decision to treat hyperkalemia, in contrast to hypokalemia, is based on the degree of increase in the serum potassium concentration and the symptoms and signs that are present. If ECG changes other than peaked T waves occur, or if the serum potassium concentration is greater than 6.5 mEq/L, the incidence of serious cardiac compromise is high and rapid intervention is indicated.

Calcium is administered to rapidly offset the adverse effects of potassium on cardiac conduction and contractility. Calcium activates calcium ion channels so that ion flux through these channels generates an action potential and restores myocardial contractility, effectively antagonizing the adverse cardiac effects of hyperkalemia. The IV administration of 10 to 20 mL of a 10% calcium chloride solution restores myocardial contractility in 1 to 2 minutes and lasts for 15 to 20 minutes. Some prefer calcium gluconate over the chloride form because it induces more potassium secretion by the renal tubules. The IV administration of calcium must be slower in patients on digitalis preparations because acute hypercalcemia can precipitate digitalis toxicity. Serum potassium concentrations are not significantly changed by IV administration of calcium.

Other measures to treat hyperkalemia include IV administration of sodium bicarbonate, glucose-insulin mixtures, and β agonists to shift extracellular potassium ions into the cells. Alkalization of the blood with sodium bicarbonate, 0.5 to 1.0 mEq/kg IV, rapidly moves potassium into cells, decreasing the serum potassium level for as long as the arterial pH is increased. Glucose-insulin infusion (50 mL of 50% glucose plus 10 units of regular insulin) produces a sustained transfer of extracellular potassium into cells, resulting in a 1.5 to 2.5 mEq/L decrease in the serum potassium concentration after approximately 30 minutes. Sodium polystyrene sulfonate (Kayexalate) is an orally or rectally administered sodium exchange resin used to remove extracellular potassium in exchange for sodium in the large intestine. Potassium removal from the body also may be achieved by loop diuretics or, most rapidly and effectively, hemodialysis.

Phosphate

Phosphate is the major intracellular anion. The majority (85%) of total body phosphate is stored in the bone as hydroxyapatite crystals within the organic matrix. Most of the remainder is stored in soft tissue as phosphate, with only 1% located in the plasma.[49] The normal plasma concentration of phosphate is 3.0 to 4.5 mg/dL, accounting for both organic and inorganic forms.

Phosphate is important in energy metabolism, intracellular signaling (cyclic adenosine monophosphate and cyclic guanosine monophosphate), cell structure (phospholipids), oxygen delivery (2,3-disphosphoglycerate), regulation of the glycolytic pathway, the immune system, the coagulation cascade, and buffering to maintain normal acid–base balance. Phosphorus regulation is a result of the interplay of phosphate and calcium levels, vitamin D, and parathyroid hormone on gastrointestinal absorption, renal reabsorption, and bone storage. Phosphorous absorption from the gastrointestinal tract and reabsorption in the kidney proximal convoluted tubules is stimulated by Vitamin D, and renal reabsorption of phosphorous is inhibited by the effects of parathyroid hormone. Renal disease disrupts this regulation, and ectopic tissue calcification as well as hyperphosphatemia may result.[34]

A decrease in the plasma concentration of phosphate permits the presence of a higher plasma concentration of calcium and inhibits deposition of new bone salts. Hypophosphatemia (phosphorus concentration <1.5 mg/dL) causes a decrease in the concentration of ATP and 2,3-diphosphoglycerate in erythrocytes. Profound skeletal muscle weakness sufficient to contribute to hypoventilation may be caused by hypophosphatemia, as well as central nervous system dysfunction and peripheral neuropathy. Causes of hypophosphatemia include alcohol abuse; prolonged parenteral nutrition; medications such as acetazolamide, catecholamines, and theophylline; paracetamol overdose; large burns; recovery from hypothermia; hemodialysis; salicylate poisoning; and gram-negative bacteremia.[49]

Iron

Iron present in food is absorbed from the proximal small intestine, especially the duodenum, into the circulation, where it is bound to transferrin. Transferrin is a glycoprotein that delivers iron to specific receptors on cell membranes. Approximately 80% of the iron in plasma enters the bone marrow to be incorporated into new erythrocytes. In addition to bone marrow, iron is incorporated into reticuloendothelial cells of the liver and spleen. Iron is also an essential component of many enzymes necessary for energy transfer. A normal range for the plasma iron concentration is 50 to 150 μg/dL.

Iron that is stored in tissues is bound to protein as ferritin or in an aggregated form known as ***hemosiderin***. Hemoglobin synthesis is the principal determinant of the plasma iron turnover rate. When blood loss occurs, hemoglobin concentration is maintained by mobilization of tissue iron stores. Indeed, hemoglobin concentrations become chronically decreased only after these iron reserves are depleted. For this reason, the presence of a normal hemoglobin concentration is not a sensitive indicator of tissue iron stores. The infant, parturient, and menstruating female may have iron requirements exceeding amounts available in the diet and develop iron-deficiency anemia. Absorption of iron from the gastrointestinal tract is increased by ascorbic acid (vitamin C) or in the presence of iron deficiency. Antacids bind iron and impair its systemic absorption.

Iron Deficiency

Iron deficiency is estimated to be present in 20% to 40% of menstruating females but only about 5% of adult males and postmenopausal females. Attempts to prevent this deficiency of iron in large parts of the population include the addition of iron to flour, use of iron-fortified formulas for infants, and the prescription of iron-containing vitamin supplements during pregnancy.

Causes

Causes of iron-deficiency anemia include inadequate dietary intake of iron, increased iron requirements due to pregnancy or blood loss, or interference with absorption from the gastrointestinal tract. Most nutritional iron deficiency in the United States is mild. Severe iron deficiency is usually the result of blood loss, either from the gastrointestinal tract or, in females, from the uterus. Partial gastrectomy,[50] malabsorptive bariatric surgery,[51] and sprue are causes of inadequate iron absorption.

Diagnosis

Iron deficiency initially results in a decrease in iron stores and a parallel decrease in the erythrocyte content of iron. Depleted iron stores are indicated by decreased plasma concentrations of ferritin and the absence of reticuloendothelial hemosiderin in a bone marrow aspirate. Plasma ferritin concentrations of less than 12 μg/dL are diagnostic of iron deficiency. Iron-deficiency anemia is defined as depletion of total body iron associated with a decreased red cell hemoglobin concentration. The large physiologic variation in hemoglobin concentration, however, makes it difficult to reliably identify all individuals with iron-deficiency anemia. Because iron-deficiency anemia is so common in infants, menstruating females, and recent parturients, mild anemia in these patients is typically treated empirically with iron supplementation before pursuing a more exhaustive diagnostic workup. However, in males and postmenopausal females, iron deficiency is much less common so it is important to search for a cause of blood loss whenever anemia is present.

Treatment

Prophylactic use of iron preparations should be reserved for individuals at high risk for developing iron deficiency, such as pregnant and lactating females, low-birth-weight infants, and females with heavy menses. The inappropriate prophylactic use of iron should be avoided in adults because excessive accumulation of iron may damage tissues.

In iron-deficiency anemia, administration of medicinal iron increases the rate of erythrocyte production, resulting in a rise in hemoglobin concentration within 72 hours. If the concentration deficit of hemoglobin before treatment is more than 3 g/dL, therapeutic doses of oral or parenteral iron should increase the hemoglobin about 0.2 g/dL/day. An increase of 2 g/dL or more in the plasma concentration of hemoglobin within 3 weeks is evidence of a positive response to iron. If this response to iron therapy is not seen, other causes of anemia should be considered, such as the chronic blood loss, infectious process, or impaired gastrointestinal iron absorption.

There is no justification for continuing iron therapy beyond 3 weeks if a favorable response has not occurred. If a response to iron therapy is demonstrated, the iron should be continued until the hemoglobin concentration is normal and continued for 4 to 6 more weeks to reestablish iron stores. Full replenishment of tissue iron stores requires several months of therapy.

Oral Iron

Ferrous sulfate administered orally is the most frequent choice for the treatment of iron-deficiency anemia and is available as syrup, pills, or tablets. Ferric salts are less efficiently absorbed than ferrous salts from the gastrointestinal tract. Although other salts of the ferrous form of iron are available, they offer little or no advantage over sulfate preparations. The usual therapeutic dose of iron for adults to treat iron-deficiency anemia is 2 to 3 mg/kg (200 mg daily) in three divided doses. Prophylaxis and treatment of mild nutritional iron deficiency can be achieved with modest dosages of iron, such as 15 to 30 mg daily.

Nausea and upper abdominal pain are the most frequent side effects of oral iron therapy, particularly if the dosage is greater than 200 mg daily. Hemochromatosis is unlikely to result from oral iron therapy that is administered to treat nutritional anemia. Fatal poisoning from overdose of iron is rare, but children 1 to 2 years of age are most vulnerable. Symptoms of severe iron poisoning may occur within 30 minutes as vomiting, abdominal pain, and diarrhea. In addition, there may be sedation, hyperventilation due to acidosis, and cardiovascular collapse. Hemorrhagic gastroenteritis and hepatic damage are often prominent at autopsy in fatal iron toxicity. If iron overdose is suspected, a plasma concentration of greater than 0.5 mg/dL confirms the presence of a life-threatening situation, which should be treated with deferoxamine.

Parenteral Iron

Parenteral iron acts similarly to oral iron but should be used only if patients cannot tolerate or do not respond to oral therapy. In addition, tissue iron stores may be restored more rapidly with parenteral iron than oral therapy. There is no evidence, however, that the increase in hemoglobin is more prompt with parenteral iron than with oral iron.

Iron dextran injection contains 50 mg/mL of iron and is available for IM or IV use. After absorption, the iron must be split from the glucose molecule of dextran to become available to tissues. IM injection is painful, and there is concern about malignant changes at the injection site. For these reasons, IV administration of iron is preferred over IM injection. A dose of 500 mg of iron can be infused over 5 to 10 minutes.

The principal major adverse effect of parenteral iron therapy is the rare occurrence of a severe allergic reaction, presumably due to the presence of dextran. Less severe reactions include headache, fever, generalized lymphadenopathy, and arthralgias. Hemosiderosis is more likely to occur with parenteral iron therapy because it bypasses gastrointestinal absorptive regulatory mechanisms.

Copper

Copper is present in ceruloplasmin and is a constituent of other enzymes, including dopamine β-hydroxylase and cytochrome C oxidase. It is bound to albumin and is an essential component of several proteins. Copper is thought to act as a catalyst in the storage and release of iron from hemoglobin. It is believed to be essential for the formation of connective tissues, hematopoiesis, and function of the central nervous system. Copper deficiency is rare in the presence of an adequate diet. Supplements of copper should be given during prolonged hyperalimentation.

Zinc

Zinc is an enzymatic cofactor essential for cell growth and the synthesis of nucleic acid, carbohydrates, and proteins. Adequate zinc is provided by a diet containing sufficient animal protein. Diets in which protein is obtained primarily from vegetable sources may not supply adequate zinc. Zinc deficiency may occur in elderly or debilitated patients or during periods of increased requirements as in growing children, pregnancy, lactation, or infection. Severe zinc deficiency occurs most often in the presence of malabsorption syndromes. Symptoms of zinc deficiency include disturbances in taste and smell, suboptimal growth in children, hepatosplenomegaly, alopecia, cutaneous rashes, glossitis, and stomatitis.

Chromium

Chromium is important in a cofactor complex with insulin and thus is involved in normal glucose utilization. Deficiency has been accompanied by a diabetes-like syndrome, peripheral neuropathy, and encephalopathy.

Selenium

Selenium is a constituent of several metabolically important enzymes. A selenium-dependent glutathione peroxidase is present in human erythrocytes. There seems to be a close relationship between vitamin E and selenium. Deficiency of selenium has been associated with cardiomyopathy, suggesting the need to add this trace element to supplements administered during prolonged hyperalimentation.

Manganese

Manganese is concentrated in mitochondria, especially in the liver, pancreas, kidneys, and pituitary. It influences the synthesis of mucopolysaccharides, stimulates hepatic synthesis of cholesterol and fatty acids, and is a cofactor in many enzymes. Deficiency is unknown clinically, but supplementation is recommended during prolonged hyperalimentation.

Molybdenum

Molybdenum is an essential constituent of many enzymes. It is well absorbed from the gastrointestinal tract and is present in bones, liver, and kidneys. Deficiency is rare, whereas excessive ingestion has been associated with a gout-like syndrome.

References

1. Woodcock TE, Woodcock TM. Revised Starling equation and the glycocalyx model of transvascular fluid exchange: an improved paradigm for prescribing intravenous fluid therapy. *Br J Anaesth.* 2012;108;384–394.
2. Myburgh JA, Mythen MG. Resuscitation fluids. *N Engl J Med.* 2013;369:1243–1251.
3. Doherty M, Buggy DJ. Intraoperative fluids: how much is too much? *Br J Anaesth.* 2012;109:69–79.
4. Scheingraber S, Rehm M, Sehmisch C, et al. Rapid saline infusion produces hyperchloremic acidosis in patients undergoing gynecologic surgery. *Anesthesiology.* 1999;90:1265–1270.

5. Warren BB, Durieux ME. Hydroxyethyl starch: safe or not? *Anesth Analg*. 1997;84:206–212.
6. Finfer S, Bellomo R, Boyce N, et al. A comparison of albumin and saline for fluid resuscitation in the intensive care unit. *N Engl J Med*. 2004;350:2247–2256.
7. Myburgh J, Cooper DJ, Finfer S, et al. Saline or albumin for fluid resuscitation in patients with traumatic brain injury. *N Engl J Med*. 2007;357:874–884.
8. Finfer S, McEvoy S, Bellomo R, et al. Impact of albumin compared to saline on organ function and mortality of patients with severe sepsis. *Intens Care Med*. 2011;37:86–96.
9. Caironi P, Tognoni G, Masson S, et al. Albumin replacement in patients with severe sepsis or septic shock. *N Engl J Med*. 2014;370:1412–1521.
10. Westphal M, James MFM, Kozek-Langenecker S, et al. Hydroxyethyl starches. *Anesthesiology*. 2009;111:187–202.
11. Jungheinrich C, Neff TA. Pharmacokinetics of hydroxyethyl starch. *Clin Pharmacokinet*. 2005;44:681–699.
12. Jungheinrich C, Scharpf R, Wargenau M, et al. The pharmacokinetics and tolerability of an intravenous infusion of the new hydroxyethyl starch 130/0.4 (6%, 500 mL) in mild-to-severe renal impairment. *Anesth Analg*. 2002;95:544–551.
13. U.S. Food and Drug Administration. Hydroxyethyl starch solutions: FDA safety communication—boxed warning on increased mortality and severe renal injury and risk of bleeding. U.S. Food and Drug Administration Web site. http://www.fda.gov/Safety/MedWatch/SafetyInformation/SafetyAlertsforHumanMedicalProducts/ucm358349.htm. Accessed June 4, 2014.
14. Myburgh JA, Finfer S, Bellomo R, et al. Hydroxyethyl starch or saline for fluid resuscitation in intensive care. *N Engl J Med*. 2012;367:1901–1911.
15. Perner A, Haase N, Guttormsen AB, et al. Hydroxyethyl starch 130/0.42 versus Ringer's acetate in severe sepsis. *N Engl J Med*. 2012;367:124–134.
16. Brunkhorst FM, Engel C, Bloos F, et al. Intensive insulin therapy and pentastarch resuscitation in severe sepsis. *N Engl J Med*. 2008;358:125–139.
17. Garcia X, Pinsky MR. Clinical applicability of functional hemodynamic monitoring. *Ann Intens Care*. 2011;1:35.
18. Marik PE, Baram M, Vahid B. Does central venous pressure predict fluid responsiveness? A systematic review of the literature and a tale of seven mares. *Chest*. 2008;134:172–178.
19. Marik PE, Monnet X, Teboul JL. Hemodynamic parameters to guide fluid therapy. *Ann Intens Care*. 2011;1:1.
20. Monnet X, Teboul JL. Assessment of volume responsiveness during mechanical ventilation: recent advances. *Crit Care*. 2013;17:217.
21. Monnet X, Osman D, Ridel C, et al. Predicting volume responsiveness by using the end-expiratory occlusion in mechanically ventilated intensive care unit patients. *Crit Care Med*. 2009;37:951–956.
22. Cacallaro F, Sandroni C, Marano C, et al. Diagnostic accuracy of passive leg raising for prediction of fluid responsiveness in adults: systematic review and meta-analysis of clinical studies. *Intens Care Med*. 2010;36:1475–1483.
23. Fawcett WJ, Haxby EJ, Male DA. Magnesium: physiology and pharmacology. *Br J Anaesth*. 1999;83:302–320.
24. Herroeder S, Schonherr ME, DeHert SG, et al. Magnesium—essentials for anesthesiologists. *Anesthesiology*. 2011;114:971–993.
25. Alexander RT, Hoenderop JG, Bindels RJ. Molecular determinants of magnesium homeostasis: insights from human disease. *J Am Soc Nephrol*. 2008;19:1451–1458.
26. Euser AG, Cipolla NJ. Magnesium sulfate treatment for the prevention of eclampsia: a brief review. *Stroke*. 2009;40:1169–1175.
27. Duley L, Gulmezoglu AM, Henderson-Smart DJ, et al. Magnesium sulphate and other anticonvulsants for women with pre-eclampsia. *Cochr Database Syst Rev*. 2010:CD000025.
28. Duley L, Matar HE, Almerie MQ, et al. Alternative magnesium sulphate regimens for women with pre-eclampsia and eclampsia. *Cochr Database Syst Rev*. 2010:CD007388.
29. Alghamdi AA, Al-Radi OO, Latter DA. Intravenous magnesium for prevention of atrial fibrillation after coronary artery bypass surgery: a systematic review and meta-analysis. *J Cardiac Surg*. 2005;20(3):293–299.
30. Hazinski MF, Nolan JP, Billi JE, et al. Part 1: executive summary: 2010 International Consensus on Cardiopulmonary Resuscitation and Emergency Cardiovascular Care Science With Treatment Recommendations. *Circulation*. 2010;122:S250–S275.
31. Edwards L, Shirtcliffe P, Wadsworth K, et al. Use of nebulized magnesium sulphate as an adjuvant in the treatment of acute exacerbations of COPD in adults: a randomized double-blind placebo-controlled trial. *Thorax*. 2013;68:338–343.
32. Lord MS, Augoustides JGT. Perioperative management of pheochromocytoma: focus on magnesium, clevidipine, and vasopressin. *J Cardiothor Vasc Anesth*. 2012;26:526–531.
33. James MF, Cronje L. Pheochromocytoma crisis: the use of magnesium sulfate. *Anesth Analg*. 2004;99:680–686.
34. Peacock M. Calcium metabolism in health and disease. *Clin J Am Soc Nephrol*. 2010;5:S23–S30.
35. Pelosof LC, Gerber DE. Paraneoplastic syndromes: an approach to diagnosis and treatment. *Mayo Clin Proc*. 2010;85:838–854.
36. Calvi LM, Bushinsky DA. When is it appropriate to order an ionized calcium? *J Am Soc Nephrol*. 2008;19:1257–1260.
37. Marks AR. Calcium and the heart: a question of life and death. *J Clin Invest*. 2003;111:597–600.
38. Amberg GC, Navedo MF. Calcium dynamics in vascular smooth muscle. *Microcirculation*. 2013;20:281–289.
39. Meier-Kriesche HU, Finkel KQ, et al. Unexpected severe hypocalcemia during continuous venovenous hemodialysis with regional citrate anticoagulation. *Am J Kidney Dis*. 1999;33:E8.
40. Diaz J, Acosta F, Parrilla P, et al. Correlation among ionized calcium, citrate, and total calcium levels during hepatic transplantation. *Clin Biochem*. 1995;28:315–317.
41. Ariyan CE, Sosa JA. Assessment and management of patients with abnormal calcium. *Crit Care Med*. 2004;32:S146–S154.
42. Cooper MS, Gittoes NJL. Diagnosis and management of hypocalcaemia. *Br Med J*. 2008;336:1298–1302.
43. Drake MT, Clarke BL, Khosla S. Bisphosphonates: mechanism of action and role in clinical practice. *Mayo Clin Proc*. 2008;83:1032–1045.
44. Suresh E, Pazianas M, Abrahamsen B. Safety issues with bisphosphonate therapy for osteoporosis. *Rheumatology*. 2014;53:19–31.
45. Rachner TD, Khosla S, Hofbauer LC. New horizons in osteoporosis. *Lancet*. 2011;377:1276–1278.
46. Macdonald JE, Struthers AD. What is the optimal serum potassium level in our patients? *J Am Coll Cardiol*. 2004;43:155–161.
47. Auer J, Weber T, Berent R, et al. Serum potassium level and risk of postoperative atrial fibrillation in patients undergoing cardiac surgery. *J Am Coll Cardiol*. 2004;44:938–939.
48. Johnston J, Pal S, Nagele P. Perioperative torsade de pointes: a systematic review of published case reports. *Anesth Analg*. 2013;117:559–564.
49. Bugg NC, Jones JA. Hypophosphataemia: pathophysiology, effects, and management on the intensive care unit. *Anesthesiology*. 1998;53:895–902.
50. Beyan C, Beyan E, Kaptan K, et al. Post-gastrectomy anemia: evaluation of 72 cases with post-gastrectomy anemia. *Hematology*. 2007;12:81–84.
51. Gloy VL, Briel M, Bhatt DL, et al. Bariatric surgery versus non-surgical treatment for obesity: a systematic review and meta-analysis of randomised controlled trials. *Br Med J*. 2013;347:f5934.

CHAPTER 18

Sympathomimetic Drugs

Sansan S. Lo • Jack S. Shanewise

Naturally Occurring Catecholamines

Naturally occurring catecholamines are epinephrine, norepinephrine, and dopamine (see Table 18-1 and Fig. 18-1).

Epinephrine

Epinephrine is the prototype sympathomimetic. It is a circulating hormone synthesized, stored, and released from the adrenal medulla. Its natural functions upon release into the circulation include regulation of myocardial contractility, heart rate, vascular and bronchial smooth muscle tone, glandular secretions, and metabolic processes such as glycogenolysis and lipolysis. It is a potent activator of α-adrenergic receptors and also activates β_1 and β_2 receptors. Oral administration is not effective as epinephrine is rapidly metabolized in the gastrointestinal mucosa and liver. Therefore, epinephrine is administered subcutaneously, intravenously, or intramuscularly. Absorption after subcutaneous injection is slow because of local epinephrine–induced vasoconstriction. Epinephrine is poorly lipid soluble, preventing its ready entrance into the central nervous system (CNS) and accounting for the lack of cerebral effects.

Clinical Uses

Clinical uses of epinephrine include treatment of life-threatening allergic reactions/anaphylaxis, treatment of severe asthma and bronchospasm, administration during cardiopulmonary resuscitation as a vital therapeutic drug,[1] administration during periods of hemodynamic instability to promote myocardial contractility and increase vascular resistance, and continuous infusion for continuous support of myocardial contractility and vascular resistance. Epinephrine is used to promote inotropy during weaning from cardiopulmonary bypass. It is also used as a vasoconstrictor to increase oxygen delivery and increase cardiac output in sepsis.[2,3] Lastly, epinephrine is added to local anesthetic solutions to decrease systemic absorption prolonging the duration of action of the anesthetic for regional and local anesthesia. Epinephrine is used in local and field blocks to promote a bloodless surgical field.

Cardiovascular Effects

The cardiovascular effects of epinephrine result from stimulation of α- and β-adrenergic receptors (see Table 18-1).[4] Stimulation of α_1 receptors leads to arteriolar vasoconstriction and pulmonary artery vasoconstriction. α_1 Receptors are predominantly located in cutaneous, splanchnic, and renal vascular beds. Stimulation of α_2 receptors also leads to vasoconstriction. β_2 Receptor stimulation leads to vasodilation, predominantly in the skeletal muscles. The relative balance of α_1 and β_2 receptors in the vasculature of an organ determines epinephrine's overall effect on blood flow to the organ. The net effect of these changes in peripheral vascular tone is preferential distribution of cardiac output to skeletal muscles and increased systemic vascular resistance. Renal blood flow is substantially decreased by epinephrine, even in the absence of changes in systemic blood pressure. Epinephrine is estimated to be 2 to 10 times more potent than norepinephrine as a renal vasoconstrictor. In general, β_2 receptors are more sensitive to lower epinephrine doses while effects on α_1 receptors predominate at higher doses. At high doses, the predominant α activity and resultant vasoconstriction leads to increased afterload, which may impede increases in cardiac output. Initial tachycardia may be followed by heart rate decreases due to baroreceptor reflexes. Venous return is also enhanced by venoconstriction from the high density of α receptors in the venous vasculature system. Blood pressure is increased by an increase in cardiac index as well as an increase in systemic vascular resistance.

Epinephrine stimulates β_1 receptors causing an increase in heart rate, myocardial contractility, and cardiac output. There may be a mild decrease in diastolic blood pressure, reflecting vasodilation in skeletal muscle vasculature due to stimulation of β_2 receptors. The net effect of these systemic blood pressure changes is an increase in pulse pressure and a mild change in mean arterial pressure.

Table 18-1

Classification and Comparative Pharmacology of Sympathomimetics

	Receptors Stimulated				Cardiac Effects								
	α	β_1	β_2	Mechanism of Action	Cardiac Output	Heart Rate	Dysrhythmias	Peripheral Vascular Resistance	Renal Blood Flow	Mean Arterial Pressure	Airway Resistance	Central Nervous System Stimulation	Single Intravenous Dose (70-kg Adult)	Continuous Infusion Dose (70-kg Adult)
Natural catecholamines														
Epinephrine	+	++	++	Direct	++	++	+++	±	−−	+	−−	Yes	2–8 µg	1–20 µg/min
Norepinephrine	+++	++	+	Direct	−	−	+	+++	−−−	+++	NC	No	Not used	4–16 µg/min
Dopamine	++	++	+	Direct	+++	+	+	+	+++	+	NC	No	Not Used	2–20 µg/kg/min
Synthetic catecholamines														
Isoproterenol	0	+++	+++	Direct	+++	+++	+++	−−	−	±	−−−	Yes	1–4 µg	1–5 µg/min
Dobutamine	0	+++	+	Direct	+++	+	±	NC	++	+	NC		Not used	2–10 µg/kg/min
Synthetic noncatecholamines														
Ephedrine	++	+	+	Direct and indirect	++	++	++	+	−−	++	−−	Yes	10–25 µg	Not used
Phenylephrine	+++	0	+	Direct	−	−	NC	+++	−−−	+++	NC	No	50–100 µg	20–50 µg/min

0, none; +, minimal increase; ++, moderate increase; +++, marked increase; −, minimal decrease; −−, moderate decrease; −−−, marked decrease; NC, no change.

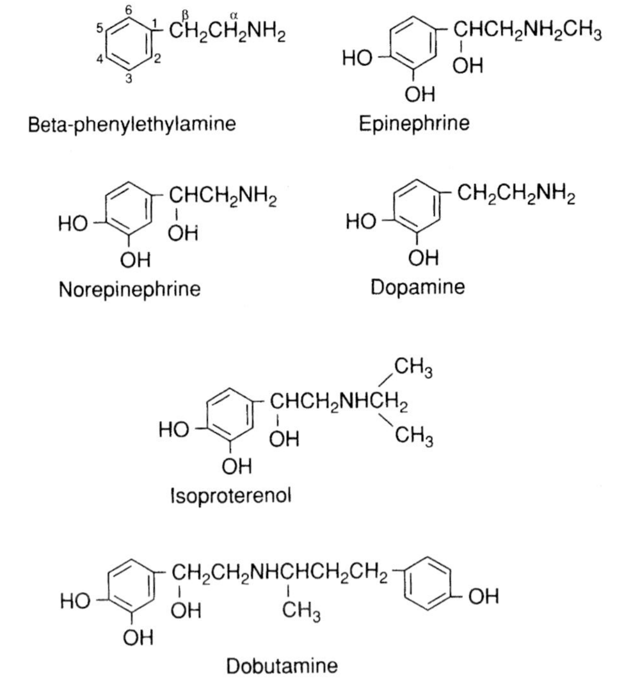

Beta-phenylethylamine

Epinephrine

Norepinephrine

Dopamine

Isoproterenol

Dobutamine

FIGURE 18-1 Sympathomimetics are derived from β-phenylethylamine, with a catecholamine being any compound that has hydroxyl groups on the 3 and 4 carbon positions of the benzene ring. The naturally occurring catecholamines are epinephrine, norepinephrine, and dopamine. Isoproterenol and dobutamine are synthetic catecholamines.

Epinephrine increases heart rate by accelerating the rate of spontaneous phase 4 depolarization, which also increases the likelihood of cardiac dysrhythmias. Epinephrine increases conduction velocity and decreases the refractory period in the atrioventricular node, bundle of His, Purkinje fibers, and ventricular muscle. It also may increase automaticity of latent pacemakers. Tachycardia, premature ventricular contraction, ventricular tachycardia, and ventricular fibrillation all may occur.

Increased cardiac output reflects epinephrine-induced increases in heart rate, myocardial contractility, and venous return. Repeated doses of epinephrine produce similar cardiovascular effects in contrast to the tachyphylaxis that accompanies administration of synthetic noncatecholamines that cause the release of norepinephrine, such as ephedrine. Myocardial oxygen consumption is increased with enhanced left ventricular preload, increased contractility, increased afterload, and tachycardia. Diastolic function is improved by increasing the rate of myocardial relaxation, and early left ventricular filling is enhanced.

Epinephrine stimulates renal β receptors, resulting in increased secretion of renin. In usual therapeutic doses, epinephrine has no significant vasoconstrictive effect on cerebral arterioles. Coronary blood flow is enhanced by epinephrine,[5] even at doses that do not alter systemic blood pressure.

Chronic increases in the plasma concentrations of epinephrine, as in patients with pheochromocytoma, result in a decrease of plasma volume because of a loss of protein-free fluid into the extracellular space. Arterial wall damage and local areas of myocardial necrosis may also accompany chronic circulating excesses of epinephrine. Conventional doses of epinephrine, however, do not produce these effects.

The hemodynamic effects of epinephrine are attenuated and can be blocked by prior administration of α- or β-adrenergic receptor antagonists.[4] Supratherapeutic doses of epinephrine may lead to acute heart failure, pulmonary edema, arrhythmias, hypertension, and myocardial ischemia.

Airway Smooth Muscle

Smooth muscles of the bronchi are relaxed by epinephrine-induced activation of β_2 receptors. By increasing intracellular concentrations of cyclic adenosine monophosphate (cAMP), β_2 stimulation decreases release of vasoactive mediators associated with symptoms of bronchial asthma. The bronchodilating effects of epinephrine are not seen in the presence of β-adrenergic blockade. In the presence of β-adrenergic blockade, epinephrine instead induces bronchoconstriction from stimulation of bronchial α receptors.

Metabolic Effects

Epinephrine has the most significant effect on metabolism of all the catecholamines.[6] β_1 Receptor stimulation due to epinephrine increases liver glycogenolysis and adipose tissue lipolysis, whereas α_1 receptor stimulation inhibits release of insulin. Liver glycogenolysis results from epinephrine-induced activation of hepatic phosphorylase enzyme. Lipolysis is due to epinephrine-induced activation of triglyceride lipase, which accelerates the breakdown of triglycerides to form free fatty acids and glycerol. Infusions of epinephrine usually increase plasma concentrations of glucose, cholesterol, phospholipids, and low-density lipoproteins. Release of endogenous epinephrine and the resulting glycogenolysis and inhibition of insulin secretion is the most likely explanation for perioperative hyperglycemia. In addition, epinephrine can inhibit peripheral glucose uptake, which is also due in part to inhibition of insulin secretion. Increased plasma concentrations of lactate presumably reflect epinephrine-induced glycogenolysis in skeletal muscles. Some studies demonstrate that epinephrine-induced hyperlactemia is primarily a transient phenomenon associated with inhibition of pyruvate dehydrogenase and has no relationship with cellular hypoxia and tissue perfusion or associated metabolic acidosis.[7]

Electrolytes

Selective β_2-adrenergic agonist effects of epinephrine are speculated to reflect activation of the sodium–potassium pump in skeletal muscles, leading to a transfer of potassium ions into cells (Fig. 18-2).[8] The observation that serum potassium measurements in blood samples obtained immediately before induction of anesthesia are lower than

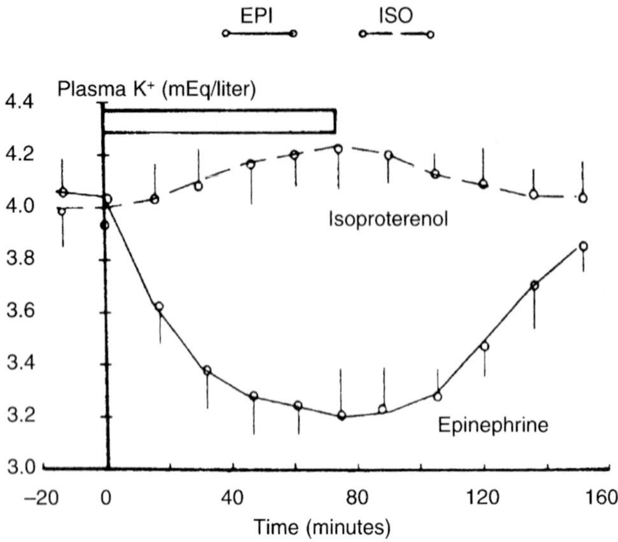

FIGURE 18-2 Selective β_2-adrenergic agonist effects of epinephrine are responsible for stimulating the movement of potassium ions (K^+) into cells, with a resulting decrease in the serum potassium concentration. (From Brown MJ, Brown DC, Murphy MB. Hypokalemia from beta2-receptor stimulation by circulating epinephrine. *N Engl J Med.* 1983; 309[23]:1414–1419, with permission.)

measurements 1 to 3 days preoperatively is presumed to reflect stress-induced release of epinephrine (Fig. 18-3).[9] The ability of a nonselective β_1 and β_2 antagonist (propranolol) but not a cardioselective β_1 antagonist (atenolol) to prevent "preoperative hypokalemia" is consistent for a β_2-adrenergic agonist effect as the explanation for potassium transfer (Fig. 18-4).[9] In making therapeutic decisions based on a preinduction serum potassium measurement, especially in patients without a reason to experience hypokalemia, one should consider the possible role of preoperative anxiety and the release of epinephrine.

Epinephrine-induced hypokalemia may contribute to cardiac dysrhythmias, which occasionally accompany stimulation of the sympathetic nervous system. Conversely, epinephrine may stimulate the release of potassium from the liver, tending to offset the decrease in extracellular concentration of this ion produced by entrance into skeletal muscles.

Ocular Effects

Epinephrine causes contraction of the radial muscles of the iris, producing mydriasis. Contraction of the orbital muscles produces an appearance of exophthalmos. Adrenergic receptors responsible for these ocular effects are likely α receptors as norepinephrine is less potent than epinephrine and isoproterenol has practically no ocular effects.

Gastrointestinal and Genitourinary Effects

Epinephrine, norepinephrine, and isoproterenol produce relaxation of gastrointestinal smooth muscle. Activation of β-adrenergic receptors relaxes the detrusor muscle of the bladder, whereas activation of α-adrenergic receptors contracts the trigone and sphincter muscles.

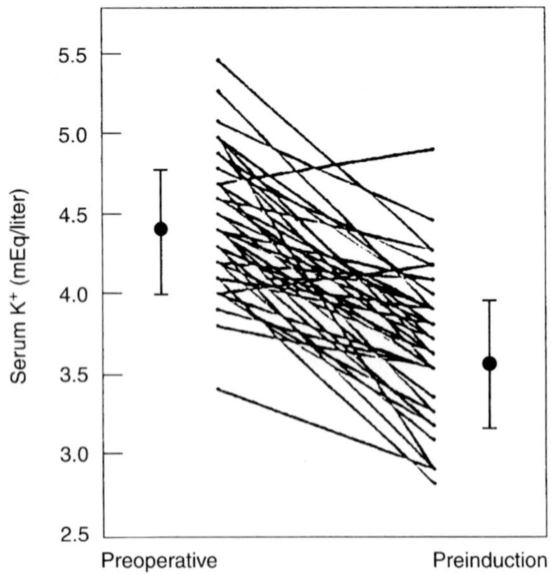

FIGURE 18-3 Individual and mean (± SD) plasma potassium (K^+) concentrations determined 1 to 3 days preoperatively and immediately before the induction (preinduction) of anesthesia. (From Kharasch ED, Bowdle TA. Hypokalemia before induction of anesthesia and prevention by beta 2 adrenoceptor antagonism. *Anesth Analg.* 1991;72[2]:216–220, with permission.)

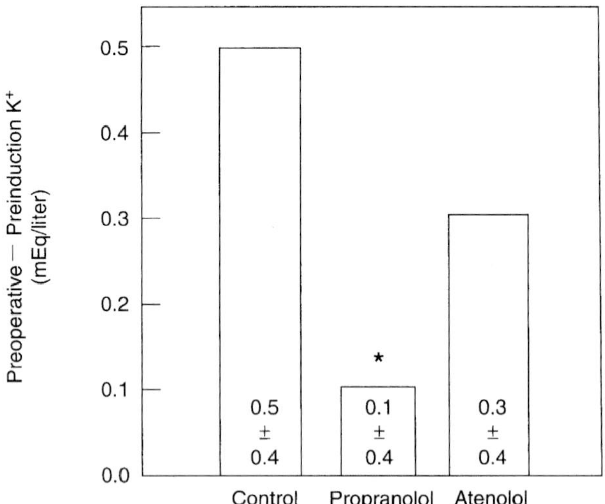

FIGURE 18-4 Propranolol, but not atenolol, was effective in blunting the difference between preoperative and preinduction serum potassium (K^+) concentrations compared with patients (controls) not receiving a β antagonist. Data are mean ± SD. The *asterisk* denotes a significant difference ($P < .02$) between controls and patients treated with propranolol. (From Kharasch ED, Bowdle TA. Hypokalemia before induction of anesthesia and prevention by beta 2 adrenoceptor antagonism. *Anesth Analg.* 1991;72[2]:216–220, with permission.)

Hepatosplanchnic vasoconstriction occurs as well as impaired renal blood flow as cardiac output is diverted to the dilated skeletal muscle vasculature.[10] This results in decreased hepatosplanchnic oxygen exchange and lactate clearance. The impairment of splanchnic circulation that occurs is greater than that associated with norepinephrine or dopamine.[11,12] It may be dependent on the severity of the shock state and the dose of epinephrine used.

Coagulation

Coagulation is accelerated by epinephrine. A hypercoagulable state present during the intraoperative and postoperative period may reflect stress-associated release of epinephrine. Epinephrine increases the total leukocyte count but causes eosinopenia. It is a potent inducer of platelet aggregation and increases factor V activity.

Norepinephrine

Norepinephrine is the endogenous neurotransmitter synthesized and stored in postganglionic sympathetic nerve endings and released with sympathetic nerve stimulation. It is the immediate precursor of epinephrine. Norepinephrine stimulates β_1- and α_1-adrenergic receptors. It is approximately equal in potency to epinephrine for stimulation of β_1 receptors but, unlike epinephrine, has minimal effect at β_2 receptors (see Table 18-1). Through its action on β_1 receptors, norepinephrine increases heart rate, conduction, and contractility. Norepinephrine is a potent α_1 agonist producing intense arterial and venous vasoconstriction in all vascular beds except for the coronary arteries.[13] Norepinephrine causes greater increase in systemic vascular resistance and diastolic blood pressure, mean arterial pressure, and systolic blood pressure than epinephrine. Venous vasoconstriction decreases venous capacitance, thereby increasing venous return to augment stroke volume and cardiac output. Heart rate changes may be minimal as baroreceptor reflexes triggered by arterial vasoconstriction are counteracted by β_1-mediated increases in heart rate. This is in contrast to epinephrine, which has a more significant chronotropic effect. Norepinephrine increases mean arterial pressure primarily by vasoconstriction and to lesser degree by increasing stroke volume and cardiac output. At higher doses, vasoconstriction predominates to an even greater extent. Norepinephrine and epinephrine increase total peripheral vascular resistance more than dobutamine (described in the following texts). Unlike epinephrine, norepinephrine has minimal metabolic effects. Hyperglycemia is unlikely to occur as a result of norepinephrine administration.

Intravenous administration of norepinephrine results in intense vasoconstriction in skeletal muscle, liver, kidneys, and skin vascular beds. Peripheral vasoconstriction may decrease tissue blood flow to the extent that metabolic acidosis occurs. Chronic infusion of norepinephrine or increased circulating concentrations of this catecholamine, as may be associated with pheochromocytoma, may cause precapillary vasoconstriction and loss of protein-free fluid into the extracellular space. Like epinephrine, norepinephrine dilates coronary arteries.[13]

A continuous infusion of norepinephrine, 2 to 16 μg per minute, may be used to treat refractory hypotension. Placement of norepinephrine in a 5% glucose solution provides sufficient acidity to prevent oxidation of the catecholamine. Extravasation during infusion can produce severe local vasoconstriction and possible necrosis; hence, administration should be via central venous access. Norepinephrine administration should be accompanied by invasive hemodynamic monitoring. The primary method of elimination is by reuptake into the adrenergic nerve endings where it is stored for subsequent release with only small amounts being metabolized.

Clinical Uses

The primary use of norepinephrine is as a potent vasoconstrictor to increase total peripheral vascular resistance and mean arterial pressure. It is a first-line agent in the treatment of refractory hypotension during severe sepsis.[2,3,14] Norepinephrine-induced vasoconstriction and redistribution of flow may increase splanchnic blood flow and urine output in severely hypotensive septic patients. Norepinephrine is also used for patients with low systemic vascular resistance after cardiopulmonary bypass. In patients with coronary artery disease, norepinephrine can be used to maintain perfusion pressure, although it should be balanced with the resultant increased afterload associated with high doses.

Side Effects

Norepinephrine should be used cautiously in patients with right ventricular failure. Norepinephrine increases venous return to the heart and also raises pulmonary artery pressures via stimulation of pulmonary vascular α_1-adrenergic receptors. Both of these may be poorly tolerated by patients with right heart failure.

The use of norepinephrine as an inotropic agent is limited by its action as a potent vasoconstrictor. The increased peripheral resistance and afterload may decrease cardiac output and increase the work of the left ventricle. Its use is also limited by the potential for tachycardia, although its arrhythmogenic potential is less than that of epinephrine.

One of the major concerns with norepinephrine use is organ ischemia. Excessive vasoconstriction and decreased perfusion of renal, splanchnic, and peripheral vascular beds may lead to end-organ hypoperfusion and ischemia. Renal arteriolar vasoconstriction may lead to oliguria and renal failure. However, when large doses of norepinephrine accompanied by adequate fluid volume resuscitation are used with caution to treat profound hypotension, perfusion pressure and renal blood flow may actually increase.

Dopamine

Dopamine is an endogenous catecholamine that is the immediate precursor of norepinephrine. Dopamine regulates cardiac, vascular, and endocrine function and is an important neurotransmitter in the central and peripheral nervous systems. The pharmacology of dopamine is complex as this catecholamine differentially stimulates a variety of dopaminergic as well as adrenergic receptors. It is a relatively nonspecific agonist at both dopamine$_1$ (D_1) and dopamine$_2$ (D_2) receptors and the α- and β-adrenergic receptors. D_1 receptors are located postsynaptically. When activated D_1 receptors elicit vasodilation in renal, mesenteric, coronary, and cerebral vascular beds and inhibition of sodium–potassium adenosine triphosphatase (Na^+–K^+ ATPase).[15] Activation of these receptors is mediated by adenylate cyclase stimulation. D_2 receptors are principally presynaptic and inhibit adenylate cyclase activity and release of norepinephrine in autonomic nervous system ganglia and adrenergic nerves (in renal and mesenteric vessels) leading to vasodilation.[16,17] D_2 receptors are also present in the pituitary gland, emetic center of the medulla, and kidney. Nausea and vomiting produced by dopamine probably reflect stimulation of D_2 receptors. Dopamine receptors may also be associated with the neural mechanism for "reward" that is associated with cocaine and alcohol dependence.

Traditionally, the pharmacokinetics of dopamine has been attributed to dose-dependent effects on varying receptors.[16] At low intravenous (IV) infusion rates (0.5 to 3 μg/kg/minute), dopamine primarily stimulates D_1 and D_2 receptors leading to vasodilation, decreased arterial blood pressure, and increased renal and splanchnic vascular blood flow. Diuresis and natriuresis also occur. The decrease in diastolic blood pressure might lead to a reflex increase in heart rate. At higher infusion rates (3 to 10 μg/kg/minute), dopamine primarily stimulates β_1-adrenergic receptors in the heart as well as α receptors in the peripheral vasculature. It also induces norepinephrine release from vascular sympathetic neurons. The activation of β receptors leads to increased cardiac output by increasing chronotropy and contractility along with vasodilation and afterload reduction. As the infusion rate is increased even further (>10 μg/kg/minute), dopamine predominantly stimulates α_1 receptors, acting similarly to a pure α agonist. The predominant stimulation of vascular smooth muscle α_1 receptors at these higher doses lead to arterial and venous vasoconstriction, increased systemic vascular resistance, and increased blood pressure attenuating further increases in cardiac output. Reflex bradycardia may also occur at this point.

This aforementioned dose-dependent model of dopamine's effects is too simplistic, even in healthy individuals. There are a wide range of clinical responses depending on individual variability in pharmacokinetics as well as other variables. For example, despite identical IV infusion rates, there may be a 10- to 75-fold variability in plasma dopamine concentrations produced even in healthy individuals with normal drug metabolism.[18] The etiology of the wide pharmacokinetic variability and variation in individual responses is likely multifactorial, reflecting differences in drug distribution, elimination, and endogenous levels, among other factors. Such differences may be even more profound in critically ill patients. Hence, the effects of dopamine cannot be predicted based on the dose,[19] and the drug must be titrated to effect.

Dopamine increases cardiac output by stimulation of β_1 receptors, increasing stroke volume. This increase in cardiac output is usually accompanied by only modest increases in heart rate, systemic blood pressure, and systemic vascular resistance. A portion of the effect of dopamine is also due to stimulation of endogenous norepinephrine release, which may predispose to the development of cardiac dysrhythmias. Nevertheless, dopamine is less dysrhythmogenic than epinephrine. The release of norepinephrine caused by dopamine may be an unreliable mechanism for increasing cardiac output when catecholamine stores are depleted, as occurs with patients in chronic cardiac failure. Dopamine increases myocardial oxygen consumption.

Dopamine causes both relaxation and contraction of vascular smooth muscle with the predominant effect varying by vascular bed, predominant receptor type, and dose administered. Dopamine's effect on pulmonary vascular resistance has not been well studied in humans, though there are some reports it may decrease pulmonary vascular resistance in patients with chronic obstructive pulmonary disease.

Rapid metabolism of dopamine with an elimination half-life of 1 to 2 minutes mandates its use as a continuous infusion (1 to 20 μg/kg/minute) to maintain therapeutic plasma concentrations. Dopamine should be dissolved in 5% glucose in water for IV administration to avoid the inactivation that may occur in alkaline solutions. Extravasation of dopamine, like norepinephrine, produces intense local vasoconstriction, which may be treated with local infiltration of phentolamine.[20] Dopamine is not effective orally and does not cross the blood–brain barrier in sufficient amounts to cause CNS effects. The immediate precursor of dopamine, L-dopa, is absorbed from the gastrointestinal tract and readily crosses the blood–brain barrier. Dopamine is partially protein bound. Approximately 25% is converted to norepinephrine. Dopamine undergoes metabolism in the liver with conjugation to sulfates and glucuronides, pulmonary endothelium by catechol-O-methyltransferase (COMT) and excretion by the kidneys.

Clinical Uses

Dopamine is used clinically to increase cardiac output in patients with decreased contractility, low systemic blood pressure, and low urine output as may be present after cardiopulmonary bypass or with chronic heart failure.[21] It is unique among the catecholamines in being able to simultaneously increase myocardial contractility, renal blood flow, glomerular filtration rate, excretion of sodium, and urine output.[22] Dopamine exerts its positive chronotropic, dromotropic, inotropic, and lusitropic (myocardial relaxant) effects via β_1-adrenergic receptors. Activation of arterial and venous α_1 receptors increases systemic vascular resistance, preload, and left ventricular afterload.[23] However, as dopamine increases pulmonary vascular resistance as well, it may not be the preferred inotropic agents in patients with pulmonary hypertension or right ventricular dysfunction.

The divergent pharmacologic effects of dopamine and dobutamine make their use in combination potentially useful. For example, infusions of dopamine and dobutamine in combination have been noted to produce a greater improvement in cardiac output, at lower doses, than can be achieved by either drug alone. Both are inotropic but each drug dilates different vascular beds such that the summation of afterload reduction by both drugs may produce a greater improvement in cardiac output than could be achieved by either drug alone. Dopamine may distribute the cardiac output to the renal and mesenteric vascular beds, whereas dobutamine may provide additional afterload reduction by dilating skin and skeletal muscle vascular beds. The objective of combination therapy is to increase coronary perfusion and cardiac output while decreasing afterload, similar to an intraaortic balloon pump.

Renal-Dose Dopamine

The term ***renal-dose dopamine*** or ***low-dose dopamine*** refers to the continuous infusion of small doses (1 to 3 μg/kg/minute) of dopamine to patients to promote renal blood flow. In healthy individuals, low-dose dopamine increases renal blood flow and induces natriuresis and diuresis. Theoretically, dopamine's renal vasodilating effects may be useful in patients with impaired renal function or in patients at risk of decreased renal perfusion as may occur with decreased cardiac output. Small doses of dopamine increase renal blood flow predominantly by D_1 receptors in the renal vasculature and possibly by D_2 receptors via inhibition of norepinephrine release. Larger doses predominantly increase renal blood flow by β-adrenergic–mediated increases in cardiac output. Higher doses of dopamine presumably stimulate α receptors to increase perfusion pressure. In addition, dopamine triggers natriuresis and diuresis through direct effect on tubular cell function. Dopamine binds to D_1 and D_2 receptors in the proximal tubule, thick ascending loop of Henle, and cortical collecting ducts inhibiting Na^+–K^+ ATPase activity, increasing Na+ excretion, inducing natriuresis and diuresis.[24] The activation of D_2 in inner medullary collecting ducts stimulates prostaglandin E_2 (PGE_2) production. This antagonizes the effects of antidiuretic hormone and results in increased free water clearance. PGE_2 enhances blood flow in the inner medulla. Inhibition of aldosterone also increases sodium excretion and diuresis. Hence, dopamine has direct and indirect effects on the renal vasculature in addition to functioning as a diuretic.

The term ***renal-dose*** or ***low-dose dopamine*** is misleading as dopamine has many effects at sites other than the kidneys, even at low doses. Dopamine's effects based on dose alone are unpredictable. Low-dose dopamine also implies an unproven beneficial effect on renal function.[25–27] In patients receiving dopamine before a "renal insult," there is a clear diuretic effect but none for improved creatinine clearance or decreased need for hemodialysis.[26] Despite drug-induced diuresis, there is no evidence that urine output in the presence of low cardiac output and/or hypovolemia protects renal function. The use of dopamine after the renal insult has occurred has not been shown to improve glomerular filtration rate. There is evidence that the beneficial effect of low-dose dopamine on renal blood flow and glomerular filtration rate observed in healthy individuals is due to drug-induced increases in cardiac output, and this benefit is lost in early renal failure.[27–29] No randomized controlled studies have demonstrated a decrease in the incidence of acute renal failure when dopamine is administered to patients considered to be at risk for developing acute renal failure in multiple patient populations (major vascular surgery,[30] cardiopulmonary bypass, intensive care,[31] heart failure, sepsis,[32] transplantation, patients exposed to nephrotoxic drugs[33]) confirming the results of two large retrospective studies[25,26] and two meta-analyses,[32,33] finding that dopamine does not prevent or reverse acute renal failure or improve outcome. Aside from one study demonstrating dopamine selectively increases renal blood flow in heart failure patients via dilation of both large conductance and small resistance renal blood vessels,[34] there exists no proven improvement in renal perfusion, creatinine clearance, or glomerular filtration rate and no alteration in the course of renal failure or the need for renal replacement therapy.

Dopamine leads to an increase in cortical and inner medullary blood flow, shunting flow from the outer medulla. It increases solute delivery to the distal tubular cells increasing medullary oxygen consumption. The outer medulla is highly metabolically active and highly susceptible to ischemic injury and acute renal failure. Dopamine can induce renal failure in both normo- and hypovolemic patients.

Low-dose dopamine is associated with multiple complications affecting the cardiovascular, pulmonary, gastrointestinal, endocrine, and immune systems. A multicenter observational study demonstrated that dopamine is an independent risk factor for death for patients with shock due to any cause.[35] In the absence of data confirming the efficacy of dopamine in preventing acute renal failure, renal-dose dopamine cannot be recommended.[25,36] In fact, not only does low-dose dopamine not confer any renal protective mechanism, it may in fact be detrimental.[27,37]

Cardiovascular Effects

Dopamine is associated more than dobutamine or epinephrine with dose-related sinus tachycardia and the potential to cause ventricular arrhythmias[23,38] and may predispose to myocardial ischemia by precipitating tachycardia, increasing contractility, increasing afterload, and precipitating coronary artery vasospasm. Dopamine increases peripheral vascular resistance and pulmonary artery pressures. Unlike dobutamine, dopamine does not inhibit hypoxic pulmonary vasoconstriction. Nevertheless, dopamine is not recommended for use in right heart failure.

Gastrointestinal Effects

Gastrointestinal mucosal ischemia and subsequent translocation of bacteria and bacterial toxins play an important role in the development of multiple organ dysfunction syndrome. Dopamine's effect on splanchnic blood flow and gastric intramucosal pH is controversial and inconsistent. There is no evidence that low-dose dopamine has beneficial effects on splanchnic function or reduces the progression to multiorgan failure in sepsis. Dopamine may increase flow to the muscular layer of the gut with decreased flow to the mucosal layer with detrimental effects and possibly gut ischemia. In septic patients, dopamine but not norepinephrine, as administered to maintain an acceptable mean arterial pressure, resulted in an uncompensated increase in splanchnic oxygen requirements. Although dopamine infusion in septic patients led to increased hepatosplanchnic perfusion, hepatosplanchnic oxygen uptake was reduced suggesting an impairment of hepatosplanchnic metabolism.[40] Most of these studies have looked at the effects of low-dose dopamine rather than doses used to treat hypotension.

D_2 receptors are also located in the enteric nervous system. Dopamine agonists interfere with gastrointestinal motility. Low-dose dopamine has been demonstrated to slow gastric motility in mechanically ventilated intensive care patients.[41]

Endocrine and Immunologic Effects

Dopamine disrupts metabolic and immunologic functions through its effects on hormones and lymphocyte function. The anterior pituitary plays a crucial role in metabolic and immunologic homeostasis. The initial stress response stimulates pituitary hormone release, whereas the chronic phase is associated with suppression of the hypothalamic-pituitary axis. In the acute phase of an illness, dopamine induces the pattern of hypopituitarism seen in prolonged critical illness and chronic stress. When dopamine is used in the chronic phase of illness, it further suppresses the circulating concentrations of pituitary hormones.[42]

Dopamine depresses the immune status by reducing serum prolactin levels. Prolactin is an immunoregulatory hormone affecting T and B lymphocytes. Dopamine inhibits lymphocyte proliferation, immunoglobulin synthesis, and cytokine production and promotes lymphocyte apoptosis. Dopamine also decreases the secretion of growth hormone, which has anabolic, lipolytic, and immune-stimulating properties. Growth hormone deficiency can contribute to impaired anabolism and a negative nitrogen balance. Dopamine's inhibition of thyrotropin-releasing hormone leads to "euthyroid sick syndrome." It also decreases dehydroepiandrosterone sulfate and may affect luteinizing hormone release. Dopamine's overall effect is to suppress the secretion and function of anterior pituitary hormones, aggravating catabolism and cellular immune function and inducing central hypothyroidism.[42]

Respiratory Effects

The infusion of low-dose dopamine in healthy subjects as well as heart failure patients interferes with the ventilatory response to arterial hypoxemia and hypercapnia, reflecting the role of dopamine as an inhibitory neurotransmitter at the carotid bodies.[43] The result is depression of ventilation in patients who are being treated with dopamine to increase myocardial contractility.[44] Dopamine also decreases arterial oxygen saturation by impairing regional ventilation/perfusion matching in the lungs.[45] Dose-dependent reductions in arterial Po_2 with increasing rates of dopamine in critically ill patients after major surgery have been demonstrated.[46] Arterial blood gases have been observed to deteriorate during infusion of dopamine.

One study demonstrated low-dose dopamine did not influence ventilation specifically in patients with chronic obstructive pulmonary disease either breathing spontaneously or being weaned from mechanical ventilation.[47] Dopamine may even decrease pulmonary vascular resistance in patients with chronic obstructive pulmonary disease. Other potential beneficial effects are improved respiratory muscle contraction, increased lung edema clearance, and inhibition of bronchoconstriction.[47,48] However, such reports are anecdotal or not tested in clinical studies.

Intraocular Pressure

Continuous infusions of dopamine to critically ill patients are associated with increases in intraocular pressure.[49] This may create a risk in patients with preexisting glaucoma especially if they are sedated and mechanically ventilated.

Synthetic Catecholamines

The two clinically useful synthetic catecholamines are isoproterenol and dobutamine (see Table 18-1 and Fig. 18-1).

Isoproterenol

Isoproterenol is the most potent activator of all the sympathomimetics with β_1 and β_2 receptor activity. It is two to three times more potent than epinephrine and at least 100 times more active than norepinephrine. In clinical doses, isoproterenol is devoid of α agonist effects and does not cause the vasoconstriction associated with the naturally occurring catecholamines.

The cardiovascular effects of isoproterenol reflect activation of β_1 receptors in the heart and β_2 receptors in skeletal muscle and to a lesser extent renal and splanchnic vascular beds. In an adult, continuous infusion of isoproterenol, 1 to 5 μg per minute, greatly increases heart rate, myocardial contractility, and cardiac automaticity, whereas vasodilation in skeletal muscles decreases systemic vascular resistance. Although cardiac output may increase thereby increasing systolic blood pressure, the mean arterial pressure may decrease due to decreases in systemic vascular resistance and associated decreases in diastolic blood pressure. Increases in cardiac output may be attenuated by impaired left ventricular filling due to tachycardia as well as decreased preload from venous vasodilation. There is preferential vasodilation in nonessential areas such as skeletal muscle. Decreased diastolic blood pressure, increased heart rate, and cardiac dysrhythmias may lead to a decrease in coronary blood flow at the same time that myocardial oxygen requirements are increased by tachycardia and increased myocardial contractility.[50] Compensatory baroreceptor-mediated reflex slowing of the heart rate does not occur during infusion of isoproterenol because mean arterial pressure is not increased. This combination of events may be deleterious in patients with coronary artery disease.

Compared to dobutamine, for a comparable increase in cardiac output, isoproterenol is associated with larger decreases in total peripheral vascular resistance and blood pressure. It is also associated with more tachycardia both from direct β effects as well as a reflex increase in heart rate with decreased vascular tone.

Metabolism of isoproterenol in the liver by COMT is rapid, necessitating a continuous infusion to maintain therapeutic plasma concentrations. Uptake of isoproterenol into postganglionic sympathetic nerve endings is minimal.

Clinical Uses

A continuous infusion of isoproterenol, 1 to 5 μg per minute, is effective in increasing the heart rate in adults in the presence of heart block. Isoproterenol is used to provide sustained increases in heart rate before insertion of a temporary or permanent cardiac pacemaker in the treatment of bradydysrhythmias. Isoproterenol's ability to decrease pulmonary vascular resistance may be useful in the management of pulmonary hypertension and right ventricular dysfunction.[51] The use of isoproterenol as an inotropic drug has decreased with the availability of inotropic agents such as dobutamine and phosphodiesterase inhibitors. Likewise, the use of isoproterenol as a bronchodilator has been supplanted by the availability of specific β_2 agonists.

Adverse Effects

Vasodilation and decreased blood pressure may limit the use of isoproterenol. In addition, it can lead to tachyarrhythmias. The combination of decreased diastolic blood pressure and increased heart rate and dysrhythmias may lead to myocardial ischemia.

Dobutamine

Dobutamine is a synthetic catecholamine derived from isoproterenol consisting of a 50:50 racemic mixture of two stereoisomers.[52] The (−) enantiomer is a potent α_1-adrenergic agonist as well as a weak β_1- and β_2-adrenergic agonist. The (+) enantiomer is a competitive antagonist at the α_1 receptor site as well as a potent β_1- and β_2-adrenergic agonist.[53] Dobutamine has potent β_1-adrenergic effects with weaker β_2-adrenergic activity. Its effect on α receptors increases at higher doses. Dobutamine's cardiovascular effects are a result of the combination of activity of its two stereoisomers.[53–56]

Dobutamine acts primarily as a positive inotropic agent. Dobutamine leads to an increase in intracellular cAMP, increasing calcium release from the sarcoplasmic reticulum to increase contractility. Cardiac output is increased primarily by an increase in stroke volume. Contractility is increased from its action on myocardial β_1 and α_1 receptors and, to a lesser extent, by decreased afterload from its effect on vascular smooth muscle β_2 receptors. Dobutamine has weak effects on vascular tone causing peripheral vasodilation. At higher doses, the (−) isomer stimulates α_1 receptors, limiting further vasodilation. Blood pressure usually is not significantly affected as α_1-mediated vasoconstriction by the (−) enantiomer is countered by α_1 antagonism by the (+) enantiomer and by its β_2 activity, although the latter may be unmasked by β blockade therapy.[53–56] In addition, there may be minimal effects on the mean arterial pressure as the increased cardiac output offsets the decrease in peripheral vascular resistance. Because dobutamine does not possess clinically important vasoconstrictor activity, it may be ineffective in patients who require increased systemic vascular resistance rather than augmentation of cardiac output to increase systemic blood pressure.

Dobutamine affects heart rate through its action on β_1-adrenergic receptors. Dobutamine stimulates sinoatrial node automaticity as well as atrioventricular nodal and ventricular conduction.[38] The chronotropic effects of dobutamine per unit gain in cardiac output are less than that of dopamine and isoproterenol but may be greater than that of epinephrine.[52,57,58] The increase in calcium that facilitates increased contractility also facilitates increased arrhythmias. At low doses, increases in heart rate may be minimal. However, high doses of dobutamine (>10 μg/kg/minute IV) may predispose the patient to tachycardia and cardiac dysrhythmias.

Dobutamine increases myocardial oxygen consumption by increasing tachycardia and myocardial contractility. Conversely, dobutamine-induced increases in cardiac output may indirectly lead to a decrease in heart rate in heart failure patients as sympathetic nervous system tone is reduced. Similarly, systemic vascular resistance may decrease by reflex withdrawal of sympathetic tone in addition to dobutamine's β_2 agonist effect. Myocardial oxygen consumption may also be reduced with improved contractility, decreased left ventricular end diastolic pressure (LVEDP), and decreased wall tension.

Dobutamine causes modest reductions in pulmonary arterial pressure and vascular resistance through its effects on β_2 receptors. In patients with increased pulmonary artery pressure after mitral valve replacement, an infusion of dobutamine (up to 10 μg/kg/minute) increases cardiac output and decreases systemic and pulmonary vascular resistance.[59] Dobutamine inhibits hypoxic pulmonary vasoconstriction. Pulmonary vasodilation may worsen ventilation/perfusion mismatching and may be associated with increased intrapulmonary shunt flow.[59]

Unlike dopamine, dobutamine does not act indirectly by stimulating the release of endogenous norepinephrine.[52] Dobutamine does not activate dopaminergic receptors to increase renal blood flow. Renal blood flow, however, may improve as a result of drug-induced increases in cardiac output.[60] Dobutamine but not dopamine is a coronary artery vasodilator. Redistribution of cardiac output in the presence of dobutamine may contribute to increased cutaneous heat loss manifesting as an additional decrease in body temperature.[61]

Rapid metabolism of dobutamine (half-life of 2 minutes) necessitates its administration as a continuous infusion of 2 to 10 μg/kg/minute to maintain therapeutic plasma concentrations. Tachyphylaxis may occur as it acts on β-adrenergic receptors. Like dopamine, dobutamine should be dissolved in 5% glucose in water for infusion to avoid inactivation of the catecholamine that may occur in an alkaline solution. Dobutamine undergoes biotransformation in the liver to inactive glucuronide conjugates and 3-0-methyldobutamine, most of which is excreted in the urine.[62]

Clinical Uses

Dobutamine produces potent β-adrenergic agonist effects at doses less than 5 μg/kg/minute IV increasing myocardial contractility (β_1 and α_1 receptors) and causing a modest degree of peripheral vasodilation (β_2 receptors). The levorotatory isomer of dobutamine stimulates α_1 receptors at higher doses (>5 μg/kg/minute) limiting further vasodilation. Individual variations exist with dose-dependent effects. Dobutamine is used to improve cardiac output in patients with congestive heart failure.[60,63] Dobutamine is also useful for weaning from cardiopulmonary bypass.[58] It may be of use in patients with pulmonary hypertension, although its effect on the pulmonary vasculature is less than that of the phosphodiesterase inhibitors. Combinations of drugs may be useful to increase the spectrum of activity and improve the distribution of cardiac output. For example, vasodilators may be combined with dobutamine or dopamine to decrease afterload, optimizing cardiac output in the presence of increased systemic vascular resistance. Most studies demonstrate minimal hemodynamic difference between dopamine and dobutamine use.[21] Dobutamine does not have significant venoconstrictor activity compared to dopamine, so increase in ventricular filling pressures may be seen at low doses.

When used in the context of ischemia as opposed to heart failure, the reduction in filling pressures and oxygen requirements from the increased contractility is not offset by the increased tachycardia. Myocardial oxygen consumption is increased by the increasing tachycardia and contractility, whereas coronary blood flow is decreased by vasodilation.[62] These properties make dobutamine useful for pharmacologic stress testing to detect potential areas of myocardial ischemia.

Adverse Effects

The use of dobutamine may be limited by the occurrence of tachyarrhythmias, although it is less likely than dopamine or isoproterenol. Sinus tachycardia occurs most commonly, although ventricular arrhythmias may also occur.[38] Tachyarrhythmias occur more frequently at higher dosages or in patients with underlying arrhythmias or heart failure. Also, prolonged continuous infusion of dobutamine associated with eosinophilic myocarditis and peripheral eosinophilia have been reported.

Synthetic Noncatecholamines

The commonly used noncatecholamine sympathomimetic drugs are ephedrine and phenylephrine (Fig. 18-5). These will be familiar to every reader.

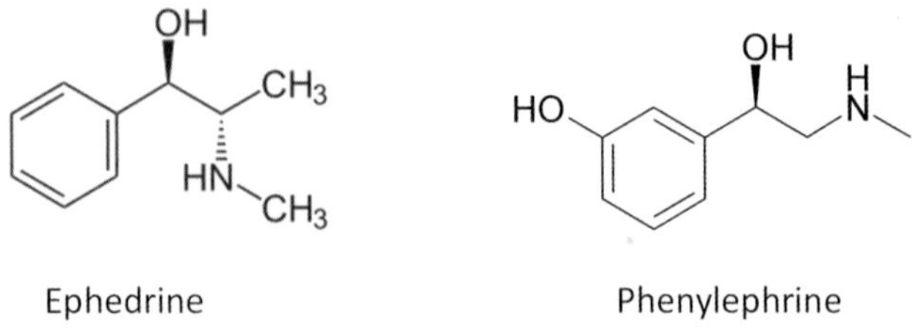

Ephedrine Phenylephrine

FIGURE 18-5 Synthetic noncatecholamine sympathomimetics.

Ephedrine

Ephedrine is an indirect-acting synthetic sympathomimetic that stimulates α- and β-adrenergic receptors. The pharmacologic effects of ephedrine are partly due to direct stimulation of adrenergic receptors (direct-acting)[64] and partly due to stimulation of release of endogenous norepinephrine (indirect-acting). Ephedrine is resistant to metabolism by monoamine oxidase (MAO) in the gastrointestinal tract, thus permitting unchanged drug to be absorbed into the circulation after oral administration. Intramuscular injection of ephedrine is clinically acceptable because drug-induced local vasoconstriction is insufficient to delay systemic absorption or lead to tissue injury.

Up to 40% of a single dose of ephedrine is excreted unchanged in urine. Some ephedrine is deaminated by MAO in the liver, and hepatic conjugation also occurs. The slow inactivation and excretion of ephedrine are responsible for the prolonged duration of action of this sympathomimetic.

Ephedrine, unlike epinephrine, does not produce marked hyperglycemia. Mydriasis accompanies the administration of ephedrine, and CNS stimulation does occur, although less than that produced by amphetamine.

Clinical Uses

Ephedrine, 5 to 10 mg IV administered to adults, is a commonly selected sympathomimetic to increase systemic blood pressure in the presence of sympathetic nervous system blockade produced by regional anesthesia or hypotension due to inhaled or injected anesthetics. In an animal model, ephedrine more specifically corrected the noncardiac circulatory changes produced by spinal anesthesia than did a selective α or β agonist drug.[65] Until recently, ephedrine was considered the preferred sympathomimetic for administration to parturients experiencing decreased systemic blood pressure owing to spinal or epidural anesthesia. Support for this practice was the observation in pregnant ewes that uterine blood flow was not greatly altered when ephedrine was administered to restore maternal blood pressure to normal after production of sympathetic nervous system blockade.[66,67] Recent reviews of trials of ephedrine versus phenylephrine have concluded that systemic blood pressure control is similar with both drugs but phenylephrine is associated with a higher umbilical artery pH at delivery than ephedrine.[68] Administration of phenylephrine by infusion during cesarean section to maintain maternal systolic blood pressure at baseline is associated with a lower incidence of fetal acidosis than is ephedrine.[69] Based on these data, it seems that α agonists such as phenylephrine may be preferable to ephedrine for treatment of maternal hypotension.

Ephedrine can be used as chronic oral medication to treat bronchial asthma because of its bronchodilating effects by activation of β_2-adrenergic receptors. Compared with epinephrine, the onset of action of ephedrine is slow, becoming complete only 1 hour or more after administration. A decongestant effect accompanying oral administration of ephedrine produces symptomatic relief from acute coryza. Ephedrine, 0.5 mg/kg intramuscularly, has an antiemetic effect similar to that of droperidol but with less sedation when administered to patients undergoing outpatient laparoscopy using general anesthesia.[70]

Cardiovascular Effects

The cardiovascular effects of ephedrine resemble those of epinephrine, but its systemic blood pressure–elevating response is less intense and lasts approximately 10 times longer. Intravenous ephedrine results in increases in systolic and diastolic blood pressure, heart rate, and cardiac output. Renal and splanchnic blood flows are decreased, whereas coronary and skeletal muscle blood flows are increased. Systemic vascular resistance may be altered minimally because vasoconstriction in some vascular beds is offset by vasodilation (β_2 stimulation) in other areas. These cardiovascular effects are due, in part, to α receptor–mediated peripheral arterial and venous vasoconstriction. The principal mechanism, however, for cardiovascular effects produced by ephedrine is increased myocardial contractility due to activation of β_1 receptors. In the presence of preexisting β-adrenergic blockade, the cardiovascular effects of ephedrine may resemble responses more typical of α-adrenergic receptor stimulation.

A second dose of ephedrine produces a less intense systemic blood pressure response than the first dose. This phenomenon, known as tachyphylaxis, occurs with many sympathomimetics. Tachyphylaxis to ephedrine appears to involve α receptor inhibition.[64]

Phenylephrine

Phenylephrine, 3-hydroxyphenylethylamine, is a synthetic noncatecholamine. Phenylephrine differs from epinephrine only in lacking a 4-hydroxyl group on the benzene ring. Clinically, phenylephrine mimics the effects of norepinephrine but is less potent and longer lasting. Phenylephrine principally stimulates α_1-adrenergic receptors by a direct effect, with only a small part of the pharmacologic response being due to its ability to evoke the release of norepinephrine (indirect-acting).[71] Phenylephrine exerts minimal effects on β-adrenergic receptors. The dose of phenylephrine necessary to stimulate α_1 receptors is far less than the dose that stimulates α_2 receptors. Phenylephrine primarily causes venoconstriction rather than arterial constriction. CNS stimulation is minimal.

Clinical Uses

Phenylephrine, 50 to 200 μg IV bolus, is often administered to adults to treat systemic blood pressure decreases that accompany sympathetic nervous system blockade produced by a regional anesthetic and peripheral vasodilation following administration of injected or inhaled anesthetics.[72] Phenylephrine is believed to be particularly useful in patients with coronary artery disease and in patients with aortic stenosis because it increases coronary perfusion pressure without chronotropic side effects, unlike most other sympathomimetics.

Phenylephrine has been used as a continuous infusion (20 to 100 μg per minute) in adults to maintain normal blood pressure during surgery. The reflex vagal effects produced by phenylephrine can be used to slow heart rate in the presence of hemodynamically significant supraventricular tachydysrhythmias.

Phenylephrine sufficient to increase systemic blood pressure in combination with inhaled nitric oxide results in a greater improvement in arterial oxygenation than with either drug alone.[73]

Topically applied, phenylephrine is a widely available nasal decongestant, usually with the brand name Neo-Synephrine. The nasal spray is a 1% solution, the same concentration as the *undiluted* phenylephrine ampule in the operating room. Intense nasal vasoconstriction precludes rapid absorption in awake subjects but must be used very cautiously if applied to the surgical field.[74]

Cardiovascular Effects

Rapid IV injection of phenylephrine to patients with coronary artery disease produces dose-dependent peripheral vasoconstriction and increases in systemic blood pressure, which are accompanied by decreases in cardiac output (Fig. 18-6).[75] Decreases in cardiac output may reflect increased afterload but more likely are due to baroreceptor-mediated reflex bradycardia in response to drug-induced increases in diastolic blood pressure. It is possible that decreases in cardiac output could limit the associated increases in systemic blood pressure. Rapid administration of phenylephrine, 1 μg/kg IV, to anesthetized patients with coronary artery disease causes a transient impairment of left ventricular global function.[76] Oral clonidine premedication augments the pressor response to phenylephrine, presumably due to clonidine-induced potentiation of α_1-mediated vasoconstriction.[77] Renal, splanchnic, and cutaneous blood flows are decreased but coronary blood flow is increased. Pulmonary artery pressure is increased by phenylephrine.

Metabolic Effects

Stimulation of α receptors by a continuous infusion of phenylephrine during acute potassium loading interferes with the movement of potassium ions across cell membranes into cells (Fig. 18-7).[78] Administration of phenylephrine in the absence of an acute potassium load does not change the plasma potassium concentration. This effect of α-adrenergic stimulation on movement of potassium ions across cell membranes is opposite to that produced by β_2 receptor stimulation (see Fig. 18-2).[8]

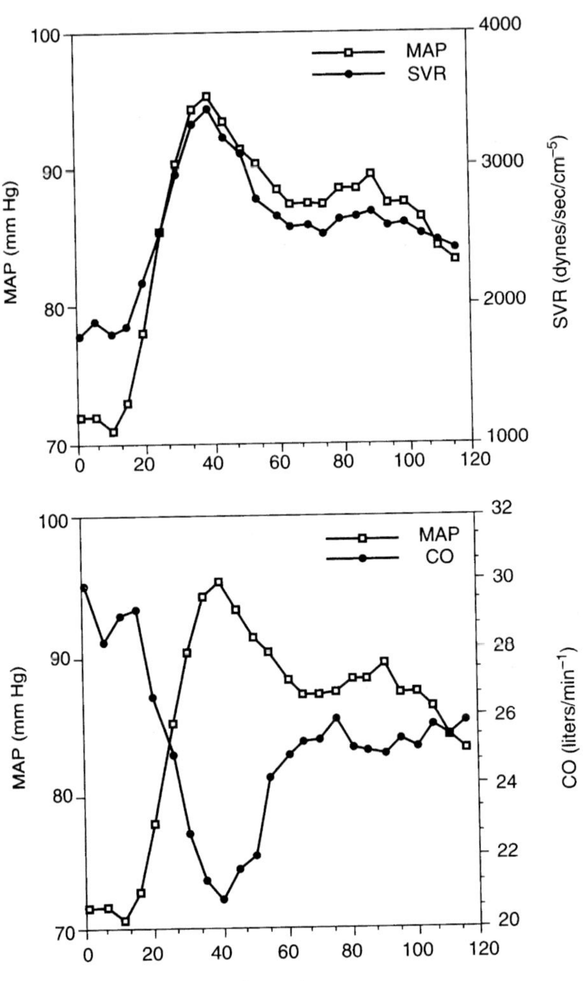

FIGURE 18-6 Hemodynamic response to rapid intravenous injection of phenylephrine in a single patient. Mean arterial pressure (MAP) and systemic vascular resistance (SVR) increase and cardiac output (CO) decreases in response to phenylephrine, with peak effects occurring 42 seconds after drug administration. (From Schwinn DA, Reves JG. Time course and hemodynamic effects of alpha-1-adrenergic bolus administration in anesthetized patients with myocardial disease. *Anesth Analg.* 1989;68[5]:571–578, with permission.)

Treatment of Overdose

Systemic manifestations of sympathetic nervous system activation (systemic hypertension, tachycardia, baroreceptor-mediated bradycardia) may accompany vascular absorption of α agonists (phenylephrine, epinephrine) when used as topical or injected vasoconstrictors in the surgical field.[74] Phentolamine, an α_1-adrenergic receptor antagonist, is an appropriate pharmacologic choice for phenylephrine toxicity.[79] β_2 receptor blockade increases peripheral vascular resistance. Additionally, phenylephrine overdose preferentially distributes blood to the pulmonary vascular beds. The natural protection of the pulmonary vascular overload is to maintain cardiac output. Since β_1 receptor blockades reduces cardiac output, treatment of phenylephrine-induced hypertensive crisis

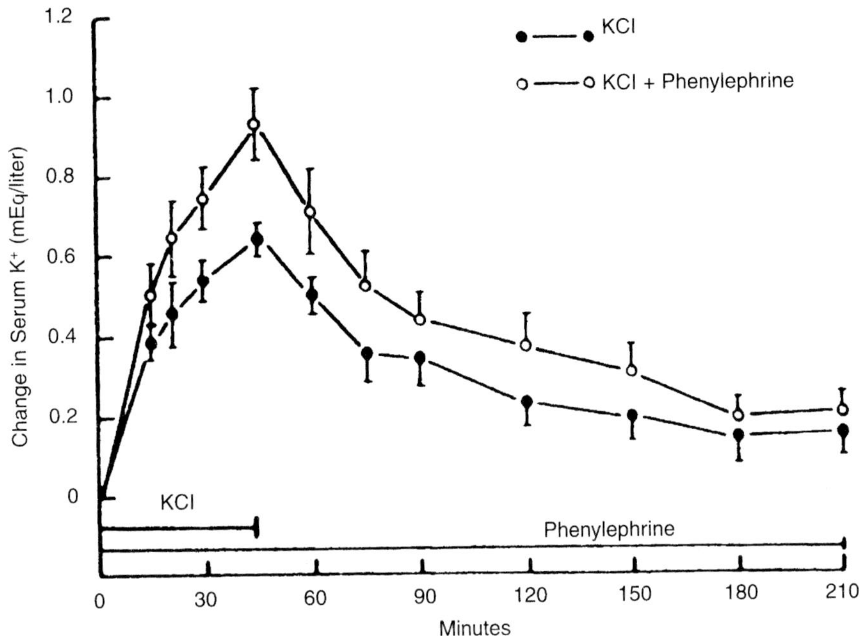

FIGURE 18-7 Plasma potassium (K^+) concentrations during the infusion of potassium chloride (KCl) increase more in patients also receiving phenylephrine. (From Williams ME, Rosa RM, Silva P, et al. Impairment of extrarenal potassium disposal by alpha-adrenergic stimulation. *N Engl J Med.* 1984;311[3]:145–149, with permission.)

with β-adrenergic blocking drugs is *contraindicated.* Case reports document that β-adrenergic blockade presages pulmonary edema and irreversible cardiovascular collapse in these cases.[74]

However, systemic hypertension induced by intravenously administered α agonists may not require treatment. The duration of action of IV phenylephrine and epinephrine is brief and hypertension may resolve spontaneously without pharmacologic interventions. Severe hypertension may require pharmacologic interventions but treatment must not decrease the ability of the stressed myocardium to increase contractility and heart rate. In this circumstance, vasodilating drugs such as nitroprusside or nitroglycerin may be helpful, along with phentolamine as noted earlier.

Selective β_2-Adrenergic Agonists

Selective β_2-adrenergic agonists relax bronchiole and uterine smooth muscle but in contrast to isoproterenol generally lack stimulating (β_1) effects on the heart. Nevertheless, high concentrations of these drugs are likely to cause stimulation of β_1 receptors. The chemical structure of selective β_2-adrenergic agonists (placement of hydroxyl groups on the benzene ring at sites different than the catecholamines) renders them resistant to methylation by COMT, thus contributing to their sustained duration of action. The commonly used β_2-adrenergic agonists are albuterol, metaproterenol, and terbutaline (Fig. 18-8) (Table 18-2).

Clinical Uses

β_2-Adrenergic agonists are the preferred treatment for acute episodes of asthma and the prevention of exercise-induced asthma.[80] Currently used β_2-adrenergic agonists may be divided into those with an intermediate duration of action (3 to 6 hours) and those that are long-acting (>12 hours).[80] Among the intermediate-acting drugs, there is little reason to choose one over the other. β_2-Adrenergic agonists are also used regularly in patients with chronic obstructive pulmonary disease, resulting in improved air flow and exercise tolerance. The long-acting β_2-adrenergic agonist salmeterol is highly lipophilic and has a high affinity for the β_2 receptor, resulting in prolonged activation at this site. In addition to the treatment

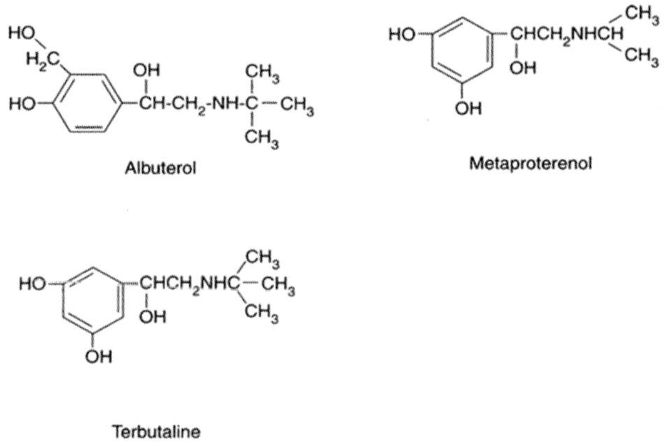

Albuterol

Metaproterenol

Terbutaline

FIGURE 18-8 Selective β_2-adrenergic agonists.

Table 18-2

Comparative Pharmacology of Selective β_2-Adrenergic Agonist Bronchodilators

	β_2 Selectivity	Peak Effect (min)	Duration of Action (h)	Concentration (μg per puff)	Method of Administration
Albuterol	High	30–60	4	90	MDI, oral
Metaproterenol	Moderate	30–60	3–4	200	Oral, subcutaneous
Terbutaline	High	60	4	200	MDI, oral, subcutaneous

MDI, metered-dose inhaler.

of bronchospasm, β_2-adrenergic agonists may also be administered as continuous infusions to stop premature uterine contractions (tocolytics).

Route of Administration

β_2-Adrenergic bronchodilators can be administered orally, by inhalation, subcutaneously, or via IV injection. The inhaled route is preferred because the side effects are fewer for any given degree of bronchodilation. Inhalation is as effective as parenteral administration for treating acute, severe attacks of asthma in most patients, although some who have severe bronchial obstruction may benefit initially from parenteral therapy.

Inhaled β_2-adrenergic agonists can be administered as an aerosol from a jet or ultrasonic nebulizer, or they can be administered from a metered-dose inhaler either as a propellant-generated aerosol or as a breath-propelled dry powder. With optimal inhalation technique (discharge the inhaler while taking a slow deep breath over 5 to 6 seconds, and then hold the breath at full inspiration for 10 seconds), approximately 12% of the drug is delivered from the metered-dose inhaler to the lungs; the remainder is deposited in the mouth, pharynx, and larynx.[80] The presence of an endotracheal tube decreases by approximately 50% to 70% the amount of drug delivered by a metered-dose inhaler that reaches the trachea.[81] Actuation of the metered-dose inhaler during a mechanically delivered inspiration increases the amount of drug that passes beyond the distal end of the tracheal tube. In general, the dose required in a nebulizer is 6 to 10 times that used in a metered-dose inhaler to produce the same degree of bronchodilation.

Side Effects

The widespread distribution of β_2-adrenergic receptors makes it likely that undesired responses may result when β_2-adrenergic agonists undergo systemic absorption. The ability to minimize these systemic side effects by decreasing plasma drug concentrations is an advantage of administering β_2-adrenergic bronchodilators by inhalation.

The principal side effect in awake subjects of β_2-adrenergic agonists treatment is tremor, which is caused by direct stimulation of β_2 receptors in skeletal muscles. Increased heart rate is less common with the selective β_2-adrenergic agonists, but even stimulation of β_2 receptors may result in vasodilation and reflex tachycardia. As there are β_2-adrenergic receptors in the heart, direct stimulation of the heart results from the use of selective β_2-adrenergic agonists. In patients with acute, severe asthma, β_2-adrenergic agonists may cause a transient decrease in arterial oxygenation presumed to reflect relaxation of compensatory vasoconstriction in areas of decreased ventilation. This is not a serious problem if supplemental oxygen is administered. Increased mortality in patients with severe asthma treated with β_2-adrenergic agonists is most likely a reflection of the severity of the asthma rather than a toxic effect of the drug therapy.[82,83]

Acute metabolic responses to β_2-adrenergic agonists include hyperglycemia, hypokalemia, and hypomagnesemia. Because these responses diminish with chronic administration, such changes are not important in patients receiving long-term therapy. Lactic acidosis may occur in association with β_2 agonist therapy, perhaps reflecting excess glycogenolysis and lipolysis from β_2 receptor activation.[84]

Albuterol

Albuterol, known as salbutamol outside the United States, is the preferred selective β_2-adrenergic agonist for the treatment of acute bronchospasm due to asthma. Administration is most often by metered-dose inhaler, producing about 100 μg per puff; the usual dose is two puffs delivered during deep inhalations 1 to 5 minutes apart. This dose may be repeated every 4 to 6 hours, not to exceed 16 to 20 puffs daily. Alternatively, 2.5 to 5 mg of albuterol (0.5 to 1 mL of 0.5% solution in 5 mL of normal saline) may be administered by nebulization every 15 minutes for three to four doses, followed by treatments hourly during the initial hours of therapy. The duration of action of an inhaled dose is about 4 hours, but significant relief of symptoms may persist up to 8 hours. The effects of albuterol and volatile anesthetics on bronchomotor tone are additive.[85]

Continuous nebulization of albuterol using a large reservoir system to deliver up to 15 mg per hour for 2 hours may be appropriate and necessary in the presence of life-threatening asthma. Tachycardia and hypokalemia may accompany these large doses of albuterol. Nevertheless, larger doses and more frequent dosing intervals for inhaled β-adrenergic agonist therapy are needed in acute severe asthma due to decreased deposition at the site of action (low tidal volumes and narrowed airways), alteration in the dose-response curve, and altered duration of activity. Inhaled albuterol (four puffs) blunts airway responses to tracheal intubation in asthmatic patients.[86]

Metaproterenol

Metaproterenol is a selective β_2-adrenergic agonist used to treat asthma. Administered by metered-dose inhaler, the daily dosage should not exceed 16 puffs, with each metered-aerosol actuation delivering approximately 650 μg. Oral administration is followed by excretion as conjugates of glucuronic acid.

Terbutaline

Terbutaline is a predominantly β_2-adrenergic agonist that may be administered orally, subcutaneously, or by inhalation to treat asthma. The subcutaneous administration of terbutaline (0.25 mg) produces responses that resemble those of epinephrine, but the duration of action is longer. The subcutaneous dose of terbutaline for children is 0.01 mg/kg. Administered by metered-dose inhaler, the daily dose should not exceed 16 to 20 puffs, with each metered-dose actuation delivering about 200 μg.

Digoxin

Digitoxin

Ouabain

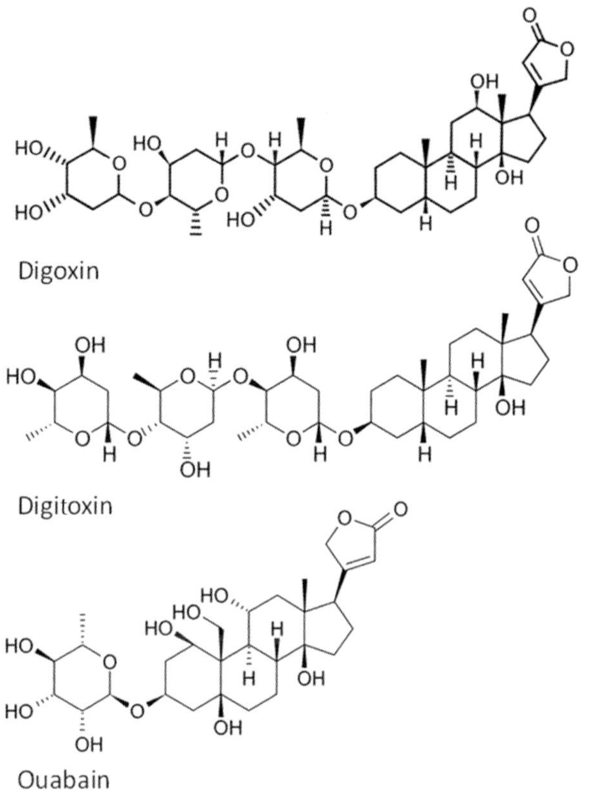

FIGURE 18-9 Cardiac glycosides.

Cardiac Glycosides

Digitalis is the term used for cardiac glycosides that occur naturally in many plants, including the foxglove plant. Digoxin, digitoxin, and ouabain are examples of clinically useful cardiac glycosides (Fig. 18-9). Of these, only digoxin remains commonly used.

Digoxin

Digoxin is used most often during the perioperative period for the management of supraventricular tachydysrhythmias (paroxysmal atrial tachycardia, atrial fibrillation, atrial flutter) associated with a rapid ventricular response rate based on the ability of these drugs to slow conduction of cardiac impulses through the atrioventricular node. The use of digoxin to treat acute decreases in left ventricular contractility is uncommon because of the availability of more potent and less toxic drugs. For example, patients treated with digoxin have a decreased risk of death from heart failure but an increased incidence of sudden death, presumably due to cardiac dysrhythmias (similar to increased risk of sudden death described for other positive inotropic drugs).[87,88] Based on this observation, digoxin may be selected only for treatment of symptoms that persist after administration of drugs (angiotensin-converting enzyme inhibitors, β-adrenergic antagonists) that do decrease overall mortality.[87] Nevertheless, digoxin continues to have an important therapeutic role in the treatment of chronic congestive heart failure. Digoxin may not be of benefit in high-output cardiac failure, such as that caused by hyperthyroidism or thiamine deficiency.

Intravenous administration of propranolol or esmolol combined with digoxin may provide more rapid control of supraventricular tachydysrhythmias and minimize the likelihood of toxicity by permitting decreases in the dose of both classes of drugs. Direct current cardioversion in the presence of digoxin may be hazardous because of increased risk of developing cardiac dysrhythmias, including ventricular fibrillation. In approximately 30% of patients with Wolff-Parkinson-White syndrome, digitalis decreases refractoriness in the accessory conduction pathway to the point that rapid atrial impulses can cause ventricular fibrillation. Digoxin may be harmful in patients with hypertrophic subaortic stenosis because increased myocardial contractility intensifies the resistance to ventricular ejection.

Pharmacokinetics

The bioavailability of oral digoxin is 60% to 80%.[89,90] In some patients, the digoxin levels may be reduced by up to 40% due to digestion by colonic bacteria (see product monograph). Peak plasma concentrations are observed 1 to 3 hours following oral administration. Following IV administration, the bioavailability is 100%, and peak plasma concentrations are observed immediately following administration as expected for all drugs. Digoxin is eliminated almost entirely by renal excretion, with a half-life of 1 to 2 days. The half-life is inversely proportional to glomerular filtration rate and thus increases with age or renal disease.

Figure 18-10 shows the plasma and effect site time course of 0.5 mg of digoxin, given either orally (Fig. 18-10A) or intravenously (Fig. 18-10B), based on the pharmacokinetic model of Jelliffe et al.[91] The time course of digoxin is reflected in the effect site concentration, shown in red, rather than the plasma concentration, shown in blue. The effect site is thought to include the myocardium, along with most other tissues.

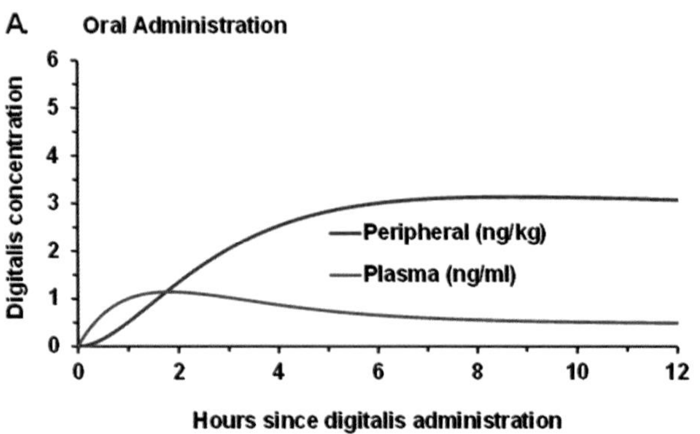

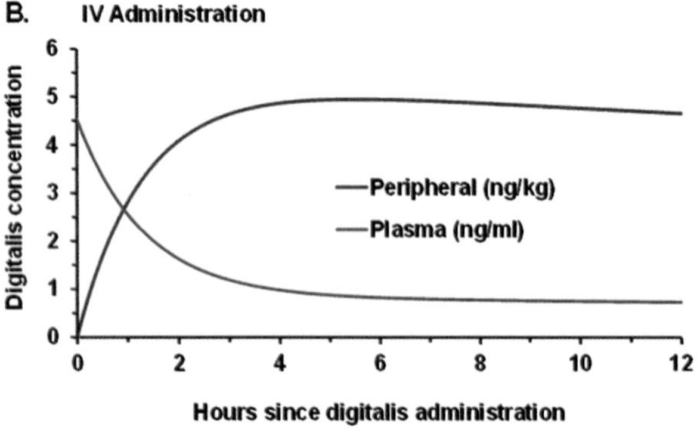

FIGURE 18-10 Simulated plasma *(blue line)* and peripheral *(red line)* concentrations of digoxin following a 0.5-mg oral **(A)** or intravenous **(B)** dose. The simulation is based on the pharmacokinetic model of Jelliffe RW, Milman M, Schumitzky A, et al. A two-compartment population pharmacokinetic-pharmacodynamic model of digoxin in adults, with implications for dosage. *Ther Drug Monit.* 2014;36(3):387–393.

The onset time for oral digoxin is 0.5 to 2 hours, with a peak effect about 6 hours after ingestion. With IV use, the onset time is 10 to 30 minutes, with a peak effect 2 to 4 hours after administration. After achievement of therapeutic plasma concentrations of digoxin by either the oral or IV route, the maintenance oral dose is adjusted according to the individual patient's response, the electrocardiogram (ECG), and the plasma concentration of digoxin.

Mechanism of Action

The complex mechanisms of the positive inotropic effect evoked by cardiac glycosides includes direct effects on the heart that modify its electrical and mechanical activity and indirect effects evoked by reflex alterations in autonomic nervous system activity. Cardiac glycosides selectively and reversibly inhibit the Na^+–K^+ ATPase ion transport system (sodium pump) located in the sarcolemma (cell wall) of cardiac cells. Cardiac glycosides bind to the α subunit on the extracellular surface of the ATPase enzyme, inducing a conformational change that interferes with outward transport of sodium ions across cardiac cell membranes. The result is an increase in intercellular sodium. A second transporter is the sodium–calcium exchanger, which transports calcium out of the cell in exchange for sodium. Intracellular sodium accumulates when the sodium–potassium exchanger is blocked by cardiac glycosides. The resulting increase in cellular sodium ion concentration in turn blocks the sodium–calcium exchanger and increases intracellular calcium. Increased intracellular calcium is the primary mechanism of inotropic action for digitalis and related cardiac glycosides. The positive inotropic effects produced by cardiac glycosides occur without changes in heart rate and are associated with decreases in left ventricular preload, afterload, wall tension, and oxygen consumption in the failing heart.[92]

The principal cardiovascular effect of digitalis glycosides administered to patients with cardiac failure is a dose-dependent increase in myocardial contractility that becomes significant with less than full digitalizing doses. The positive inotropic effect manifests as increased stroke volume, decreased heart size, and decreased LVEDP. Indeed, cardiac glycosides can double stroke volume from a failing and dilated left ventricle. The ventricular function curve (Frank-Starling curve) is shifted to the left (Fig. 18-11). Improved renal perfusion due to an overall increase in cardiac output favors mobilization and excretion of edema fluid, accounting for the diuresis that often accompanies the administration of cardiac glycosides to patients in cardiac failure. Excessive sympathetic nervous system activity that occurs as a compensatory response to cardiac failure is decreased with the improved circulation that accompanies administration of cardiac glycosides. The resulting decrease in systemic vascular resistance further enhances forward left ventricular stroke volume.

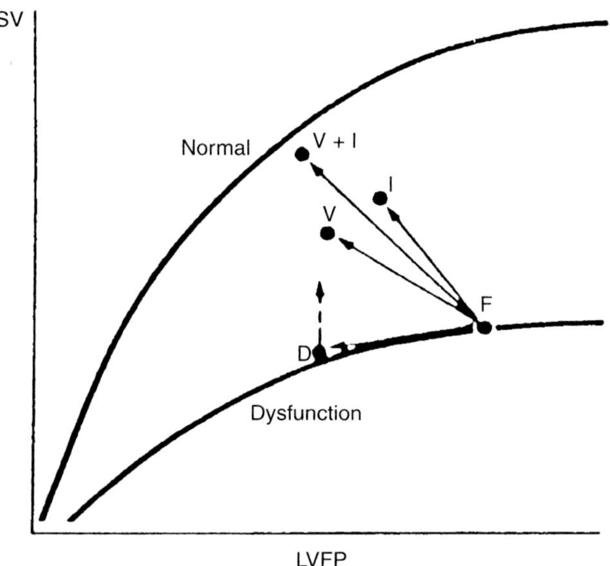

FIGURE 18-11 Cardiac glycosides shift the ventricular function curve of the failing myocardium to the left. LVFP, left ventricular filling pressure; SV, stroke volume.

Cardiac glycosides also increase myocardial contractility in the absence of cardiac failure. Nevertheless, the resulting tendency for cardiac output to increase may be offset by decreases in heart rate and direct vasoconstricting effects of cardiac glycosides on arterial, and to a lesser extent, venous smooth muscle. Indeed, cardiac output is often unchanged or even decreased when cardiac glycosides are administered to patients with normal hearts.

In addition to positive inotropic effects, cardiac glycosides enhance parasympathetic nervous system activity, leading to delayed conduction of cardiac impulses through the atrioventricular node and decreases in heart rate. The magnitude of this negative dromotropic and chronotropic effect depends on the preexisting activity of the autonomic nervous system. Increased parasympathetic nervous system activity decreases contractility in the atria, but direct positive inotropic effects of cardiac glycosides more than offset these nervous system–induced negative inotropic effects on the ventricles.

The electrophysiologic effects of therapeutic plasma concentrations of cardiac glycosides manifest on the ECG as (a) prolonged P-R intervals due to delayed conduction of cardiac impulses through the atrioventricular node, (b) shortened QTc intervals because of more rapid ventricular repolarization, (c) ST segment depression (scaphoid or scooped-out) due to a decreased slope of phase 3 depolarization of cardiac action potentials, and (d) diminished amplitude or inversion of T waves. The P-R interval is rarely prolonged to longer than 0.25 second, and the effect on the QTc interval is independent of parasympathetic nervous system activity. Changes in the ST segment and T wave do not correlate with therapeutic plasma concentrations of cardiac glycosides. Furthermore, ST-segment and T-wave changes on the ECG may suggest myocardial ischemia. When digitalis is discontinued, the changes on the ECG disappear in several weeks.

Toxicity

Cardiac glycosides have a narrow therapeutic range. Indeed, it is estimated that approximately 20% of patients who are being treated with cardiac glycosides experience some form of digitalis toxicity. The therapeutic effects of cardiac glycosides develop at approximately 35% of the fatal dose, and cardiac dysrhythmias typically manifest at approximately 60% of the fatal dose. The only difference between various cardiac glycosides when toxicity develops is the duration of adverse effects.

This increase in calcium responsible for the inotropic effects of digoxin are likely responsible for the arrhythmogenic effects as well.[93] The increased calcium is stored in the sarcoplasmic reticulum. In the setting of myocardial sarcoplasmic reticulum calcium overload, calcium may be released in waves from the sarcoplasmic reticulum, resulting in delayed afterdepolarizations. If strong enough, delayed afterdepolarizations may result in myocardial action potentials and arrhythmias.

The most frequent cause of digitalis toxicity in the absence of renal dysfunction is the concurrent administration of diuretics that cause potassium depletion. During anesthesia, hyperventilation of the patient's lungs can decrease the serum potassium concentration an average of 0.5 mEq/L for every 10 mm Hg decrease in $Paco_2$.[94] Hypokalemia probably increases myocardial binding of cardiac glycosides, resulting in an excess drug effect. Indeed, binding of cardiac glycosides to the Na^+–K^+ ATPase enzyme complex is inhibited by increases in the plasma concentration of potassium. Other electrolyte abnormalities that contribute to digitalis toxicity include hypercalcemia and hypomagnesemia. An increase in sympathetic nervous system activity as produced by arterial hypoxemia increases the likelihood of digitalis toxicity.

Elderly patients with decreased renal function are vulnerable to the development of digitalis toxicity if usual doses of digoxin are administered. Impaired renal function and electrolyte changes (hypokalemia, hypomagnesemia) that may accompany cardiopulmonary bypass could predispose the patient to the development of digitalis toxicity.

Diagnosis

Digoxin is often administered in situations where digitalis toxicity is difficult to distinguish from the effects of the cardiac disease. For this reason, determination of the plasma digoxin concentration may be used to indicate the likely presence of digitalis toxicity. A plasma digoxin concentration of less than 0.5 ng/mL eliminates the possibility of digitalis toxicity. Plasma concentrations between

0.5 and 2.5 ng/mL are usually considered therapeutic, and levels greater than 3 ng/mL are in a toxic range. Infants and children have an increased tolerance to cardiac glycosides, and their range of therapeutic concentrations for digoxin is 2.5 to 3.5 ng/mL.

Anorexia, nausea, and vomiting are early manifestations of digitalis toxicity. These symptoms, when present preoperatively in patients receiving cardiac glycosides, should arouse suspicion of digitalis toxicity.

There are no unequivocal features on the ECG that confirm the presence of digitalis toxicity.[95] Nevertheless, toxic plasma concentrations of digitalis typically cause atrial or ventricular cardiac dysrhythmias (increased automaticity) and delayed conduction of cardiac impulses through the atrioventricular node (prolonged P-R interval on the ECG), culminating in incomplete to complete heart block. Atrial tachycardia with block is the most common cardiac dysrhythmia attributed to digitalis toxicity. Activity of the sinoatrial node may also be directly inhibited by high doses of cardiac glycosides. Conduction of cardiac impulses through specialized conducting tissues of the ventricles is not altered, as evidenced by the failure of even toxic plasma concentrations of digoxin to alter the duration of the QRS complex on the ECG. Ventricular fibrillation is the most frequent cause of death from digitalis toxicity.

Treatment

Treatment of digitalis toxicity includes (a) correction of predisposing causes (hypokalemia, hypomagnesemia, arterial hypoxemia), (b) administration of drugs (phenytoin, lidocaine, atropine) to treat cardiac dysrhythmias, and (c) insertion of a temporary artificial transvenous cardiac pacemaker if complete heart block is present. Supplemental potassium decreases the binding of digitalis to cardiac muscle and directly antagonizes the cardiotoxic effects of cardiac glycosides. Serum potassium concentrations should be determined before treatment because supplemental potassium in the presence of a high preexisting plasma level of potassium will intensify atrioventricular block and depress the automaticity of ectopic pacemakers in the ventricles, leading to complete heart block. If renal function is normal and atrioventricular conduction block is not present, it is acceptable to administer potassium, 0.025 to 0.050 mEq/kg IV, to treat life-threatening cardiac dysrhythmias associated with digitalis toxicity, obviously with continuous ECG monitoring. Phenytoin (0.5 to 1.5 mg/kg IV over 5 minutes) or lidocaine (1 to 2 mg/kg IV) is effective in suppressing ventricular cardiac dysrhythmias caused by digitalis. Phenytoin is also effective in suppressing atrial dysrhythmias. Atropine, 35 to 70 μg/kg IV, can be administered to increase heart rate by offsetting excessive parasympathetic nervous system activity produced by toxic plasma concentrations of digitalis. Propranolol is effective in suppressing increased automaticity produced by digitalis toxicity, but its tendency to increase atrioventricular node refractoriness limits its usefulness when conduction blockade is present.

Life-threatening digitalis toxicity can be treated by administering digoxin antibodies,[96] decreasing the plasma concentration of digoxin. The digoxin–antibody complex is eliminated by the kidneys.

Drug Interactions

Quinidine produces a dose-dependent increase in the plasma concentration of digoxin that becomes apparent within 24 hours after the first dose. This effect of quinidine may be due to displacement of digoxin from binding sites in tissues.

Succinylcholine, or any other drug that can abruptly increase parasympathetic nervous system activity, could theoretically have an additive effect with cardiac glycosides. Cardiac dysrhythmias also could reflect succinylcholine-induced catecholamine release and resulting cardiac irritability. Despite these theoretical concerns, clinical experience does not support the occurrence of an increased incidence of cardiac dysrhythmias in patients being treated with cardiac glycosides and receiving succinylcholine.[97]

Sympathomimetics with β-adrenergic agonist effects may increase the likelihood of cardiac dysrhythmias in the presence of cardiac glycosides.[97] Intravenous administration of calcium may precipitate cardiac dysrhythmias in patients receiving cardiac glycosides. Any drug that facilitates renal loss of potassium increases the likelihood of hypokalemia and associated digitalis toxicity. The simultaneous administration of an oral antacid and digitalis decreases the gastrointestinal absorption of cardiac glycosides. Fentanyl, enflurane, and, to a lesser extent, isoflurane protect against digitalis-enhanced cardiac automaticity.[98]

Selective Phosphodiesterase Inhibitors

Phosphodiesterase inhibitors are a heterogeneous group of noncatecholamine nonglycoside compounds that exert a competitive inhibitory action on phosphodiesterase enzymes. Multiple types of phosphodiesterase enzymes exist in different tissues (cardiac muscle, vascular smooth muscle, platelets, liver, and lungs) possessing different cyclic nucleotide substrate specificity. Selective phosphodiesterase inhibitors exert different physiologic effects depending on their enzyme fraction specificity.[99] Selective inhibitors of phosphodiesterase fraction III (PDE III) (Fig. 18-12) decrease the hydrolysis of cAMP, leading to increased intracellular concentrations of cAMP in the myocardium and vascular smooth muscle. They

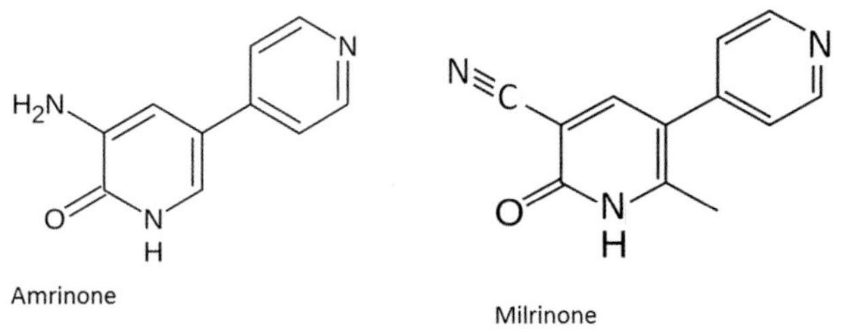

FIGURE 18-12 Selective inhibitors of phosphodiesterase subtype III, amrinone and milrinone.

also have an indirect effect on cyclic guanosine monophosphate–dependent protein kinase in vascular smooth muscle. In myocardium, increased intracellular cAMP concentrations result in stimulation of protein kinases that phosphorylate the sarcoplasmic reticulum, increasing inward calcium current, increasing intracellular calcium and contractility. In vascular smooth muscle, increased cAMP decreases calcium available for contraction by facilitating the uptake of calcium by the sarcoplasmic reticulum, leading to smooth muscle relaxation and vasodilation. Although PDE III isoenzymes exist in airway smooth muscle, bronchodilation is not a predominant clinical effect of the current cardiac-selective PDE III inhibitors.

The overall effect of selective PDE III inhibitors is to combine positive inotropic effects with smooth muscle relaxation in both arteriolar and venous beds. Hence, they have been termed ***inodilators***. Physiologic effects include increased contractility, increased cardiac output, and decreased LVEDP in addition to increased venous capacitance, decreased filling pressures (central venous pressure and pulmonary capillary wedge pressure), and decreased venous return to the heart. Mean pulmonary artery pressures and pulmonary and systemic vascular resistance are decreased. Selective PDE III inhibitors also improve the lusitropic state of the heart.[100] Diastolic relaxation is facilitated by enhanced calcium removal from the sarcoplasm, thereby improving ventricular filling.

Selective PDE III inhibitors have mild effects on heart rate and mean arterial pressure having association with rare arrhythmias and some decrease in mean arterial pressure. These inodilators decrease preload and afterload. Hence theoretically, wall tension and myocardial oxygen consumption should decrease, in contrast to dobutamine, which increases myocardial oxygen consumption as it increases contractility. Wall tension decreases with decreasing ventricular volume and with decreasing afterload, and myocardial oxygen consumption depends primarily on heart rate, contractility, and ventricular wall tension.

Selective PDE III inhibitors act independently of β-adrenergic receptors and will increase myocardial contractility in patients with myocardial depression from β receptor blockade and in patients who have down-regulation of β-adrenergic receptors and are refractory to catecholamine therapy. The effects of catecholamines, which also increase cAMP concentrations but through β-adrenergic stimulation, are potentially enhanced by PDE III inhibition. The hemodynamic response to selective PDE inhibitors exceeds that of cardiac glycosides and is synergistic to the actions of catecholamines. These drugs can be used in conjunction with digitalis without provoking digitalis toxicity. The PDE III inhibitors have their greatest clinical usefulness in patients who would benefit from combined inotropic and vasodilator therapy.

Amrinone (Inamrinone)

Amrinone is a bipyridine derivative that acts as a selective PDE III inhibitor and produces dose-dependent positive inotropic and vasodilator effects manifesting as increased cardiac output and decreased LVEDP.[101] The name amrinone was changed to inamrinone in the United States in 2000 to avoid confusion with amiodarone, much to the confusion of those accustomed to the name amrinone.

Amrinone increases cardiac index, left ventricular stroke index, and left ventricular ejection fraction, decreasing LVEDP, pulmonary capillary wedge pressure, pulmonary artery pressure, right atrial pressure, and systemic vascular resistance, with minimal effect on heart rate.[102] Depending on the cardiovascular status of the patient, amrinone may increase cardiac output either through its inotropic or vasodilating mechanisms.

Amrinone is subject to minimal protein binding and has a rapid distribution half-life of 1 to 2 minutes. The principal route of excretion is 26% to 40% unchanged drug in the urine with a large fraction undergoing N-acetylation and glucuronidation by the liver. The elimination half-time of amrinone in healthy patients is approximately 2.6 to 4.1 hours but may increase further in patients with severe heart failure.[102]

Amrinone is effective when administered orally as well as intravenously. However, oral administration is confounded by uncertainties in bioavailability as well as increased side effects with long-term oral use. Intravenous administration of a loading dose, 0.5 to 1.5 mg/kg, increases cardiac output within 5 minutes, with detectable positive inotropic effects persisting for approximately 2 hours. After the initial dose, a maintenance infusion of 2 to 10 μg/kg/minute produces positive inotropic effects that are maintained during the infusion (tachyphylaxis does not occur) and for several hours after discontinuation of the infusion. The recommended maximum daily dose is 10 mg/kg including the initial loading dose, which may be repeated 30 minutes after the first injection. Bolus administration should be administered slowly and carefully given the potential for hypotension.[102] The dose should be decreased in patients with severe renal dysfunction.

Patients who have failed to respond to catecholamines may respond to amrinone.

Side Effects

Hypotension from vasodilation, especially with rapid bolus administration, may occur and may be attenuated by slower administration or concomitant administration with vasopressors.

Dose-related thrombocytopenia may occur particularly with chronic oral therapy.[103] cAMP in platelets acts as intracellular messengers inhibiting the platelet activation sequence at several steps. Oral amrinone has been associated with accelerated peripheral platelet loss. Although the mechanism is unclear, it is thought to be a non–immune-mediated effect of amrinone or its metabolites.[104,105]

Phosphodiesterase inhibitors are thought to possess rare clinically significant dysrhythmogenic properties. Increased myocardial calcium is known to promote the development of cardiac arrhythmias. Amrinone increases atrioventricular nodal conduction and decreases atrial refractoriness.[38] It is difficult to assess in human studies whether arrhythmias are drug-induced or due to underlying ventricular dysfunction. Any proarrhythmic potential of amrinone appears to be dose-related and associated primarily with rapid IV administration.[38] Chronic oral amrinone has been associated with gastrointestinal intolerances in animals, as well as hepatic dysfunction.

Milrinone

Milrinone is a bipyridine derivative of amrinone with almost 30 times the inotropic potency of amrinone but less adverse side effects. Because of its reduced incidence of side effects, milrinone has replaced amrinone in clinical use. Cardiac output improves both as a result of increased inotropy as well as vascular smooth muscle relaxation of peripheral and pulmonary vessel.[106] Dose-dependent increases in cardiac index occur with minimal increases in myocardial oxygen consumption. Decreases in LVEDP, mean arterial pressure, central venous pressure, pulmonary artery occlusion pressure, pulmonary vascular resistance, and systemic vascular resistance occur as well as improvements in diastolic function.[107]

Milrinone is administered as an IV bolus of 50 μg/kg over 10 minutes followed by a continuous infusion of 0.375 to 0.75 μg/kg/minute to maintain plasma milrinone concentrations at or above therapeutic levels.[108] A bolus dose of 50 μg/kg was found to be as effective as a dose of 75 μg/kg with fewer side effects and more effective than a dose of 25 μg/kg.[109] The maximum daily dose of milrinone should not exceed 1.3 mg/kg/day. Approximately 70% of the drug in circulation is protein-bound. The elimination half-time is 2.7 hours and about 80% of the drug is excreted unchanged by the kidneys with a minor part undergoing glucuronide conjugation before excretion. The dose should be decreased in patients with severe renal dysfunction.

Clinical Uses

Milrinone may be useful in the management of acute left ventricular dysfunction such as after cardiac surgery. Successful weaning of high-risk patients from cardiopulmonary bypass may be enhanced by administration of milrinone.[107,109–111] Milrinone may potentiate the effects of adrenergic agents as well as help increase inotropy in chronic heart failure patients who have downregulation of β_1-adrenergic receptors. In patients with congestive heart failure, symptomatic and hemodynamic improvements as well as improvement in exercise have been reported, although milrinone use does not slow the natural progression of disease.[112] Routine short-term milrinone treatment for acute exacerbation of chronic heart failure without hypotension from a low cardiac output state is not supported,[113] although milrinone may be used as a bridge to orthotopic heart transplantation. It is particularly useful in the setting of pulmonary hypertension. Milrinone decreases pulmonary artery pressures more effectively than other positive inotropic agents, even dobutamine.[114,115] The inotropic effects of milrinone are reduced by acidosis, presumably reflecting decreased cAMP formation in acidotic muscle.[116]

Both milrinone and dobutamine improve cardiac index and decrease cardiac filling pressures although milrinone may be more effective for the latter with significant reductions in right and left heart filling pressures. Milrinone is associated with more vasodilation and greater decreases in systemic vascular resistance and blood pressure than dobutamine. Unlike dobutamine, milrinone rarely causes tachycardia. Both agents may increase myocardial oxygen consumption with milrinone doing so to a lesser extent. The choice between dobutamine and milrinone may be based on hemodynamic differences. Milrinone may be preferred in situations with high filling pressures, elevated pulmonary artery pressure, need for continued β blockade, decreased responsiveness to catecholamine therapy, and increased risk for tachyarrhythmias. Dobutamine may be preferred in situations with significant vasodilation or renal dysfunction.

Milrinone has the additional role of being able to reverse vasospasm in arterial grafts.[117] Milrinone is also thought to have antiinflammatory effects, and thus perioperative administration may dilate splanchnic vasculature and attenuate systemic inflammation in the acute phase response after cardiopulmonary bypass.[118,119]

Side Effects

Rapid administration of milrinone may decrease systemic vascular resistance, decrease venous return, and result in hypotension. The hypotension may be attenuated by slower bolus administration and concomitant administration with vasopressors.

Despite its beneficial hemodynamic actions, chronic oral therapy with milrinone may increase morbidity and mortality in patients with severe chronic heart failure and is not approved by the U.S. Food and Drug Administration

(FDA) for this indication.[112,120] The mechanism for this remains unknown although a proarrhythmic effect has been suggested. Rapid administration of large IV loading doses may also be associated with arrhythmias.[109] Enhanced atrioventricular nodal conduction is its major electrophysiologic effect. Milrinone may also increase ventricular automaticity in ischemic myocardium.[38] Ventricular and supraventricular arrhythmias have been reported with milrinone.[111–113]

Because of its higher potency, milrinone has less of an effect on platelets than amrinone. Although both agents inhibit in vitro platelet aggregation, short-term milrinone use did not cause significant changes in platelet number or function after cardiopulmonary bypass beyond the usual effects of cardiopulmonary bypass and cardiac surgery.[121]

Calcium

Calcium is present in the body in greater amounts than any other mineral. Calcium is important for (a) neuromuscular transmission, (b) skeletal muscle contraction, (c) cardiac muscle contractility, (d) blood coagulation, and (e) exocytosis necessary for release of neurotransmitters. In addition, calcium is the principal component of bone. The cytoplasmic concentration of ionized calcium is maintained at low levels by extrusion from the cells and sequestration of calcium ions within cellular organelles, particularly mitochondria, and in the sarcoplasmic reticulum of skeletal muscles. The large gradient for calcium across cell membranes is essential for calcium's role in transmembrane signaling in response to various electrical or chemical stimuli.

Calcium is a potent inotrope. Increasing the plasma concentrations of ionized calcium with exogenous administration of calcium chloride or calcium gluconate is commonly used to treat cardiac depression as may accompany delivery of volatile anesthetics, transfusion of citrated blood, and following termination of cardiopulmonary bypass. Calcium is necessary for excitation-contraction coupling in vascular smooth muscle and may result in a vasoconstricting effect on coronary arteries that impairs coupling of coronary blood flow to augment myocardial oxygen demand.[122]

Calcium Measurement

The plasma concentration of calcium is maintained between 4.3 and 5.3 mEq/L (8.5 to 10.5 mg/dL) by endocrine control of ion transport in the kidney, intestine, and bone, mediated by vitamin D, parathyroid hormone, and calcitonin.[123] Total plasma calcium consists of (a) calcium bound to albumin, (b) calcium complexed with citrate and phosphorus ions, and (c) freely diffusible ionized calcium. As would be expected, total plasma calcium decreases with low serum albumin and with hypophosphatemia.

It is the ionized calcium, and not the total plasma calcium, that produces the physiologic effects of calcium. Therefore, hypoalbuminemia and hypophosphatemia typically are not associated with signs of hypocalcemia. Conversely, large transfusions may be associated with acute hypocalcemia because of the binding of ionized calcium to the citrate anticoagulant.

Ionized calcium typically represents approximately 45% of the total plasma concentration. The ionized fraction of calcium changes with pH because calcium and hydrogen ions compete for the binding site on albumin. Acidosis increases ionized calcium, whereas alkalosis reduces ionized calcium.

Most laboratories now directly measure ionized calcium, the moiety of clinical interest.[124] A normal plasma ionized calcium concentration is 1 to 1.26 mmol/L[124,125] (2 to 2.5 mEq/L or 4 to 5 mg/dL).

Calcium Sensitizers

Levosimendan

Levosimendan is the first drug in a novel class of inotropes that increases contractility by increasing the sensitivity of the myocardium to calcium (Fig. 18-13). The inotropic enhancement is a result of binding of levosimendan to troponin C, increasing the sensitivity of troponin to calcium.[126,127] Levosimendan also activates adenosine triphosphate–regulated potassium channels (K_{ATP}),[128] causing vasodilation[129] and myocardial protection.[130] As a result, cardiac output is increased with decreased systemic vascular resistance and pulmonary vascular resistance. Oral bioavailability is 85%. Metabolism is largely hepatic with renal excretion.

Levosimendan was developed with an indication for the treatment of cardiogenic shock. A reduction in 180-day mortality has not been demonstrated compared to dobutamine in a meta-analysis performed by the Cochrane collaboration.[131] However, a more recent

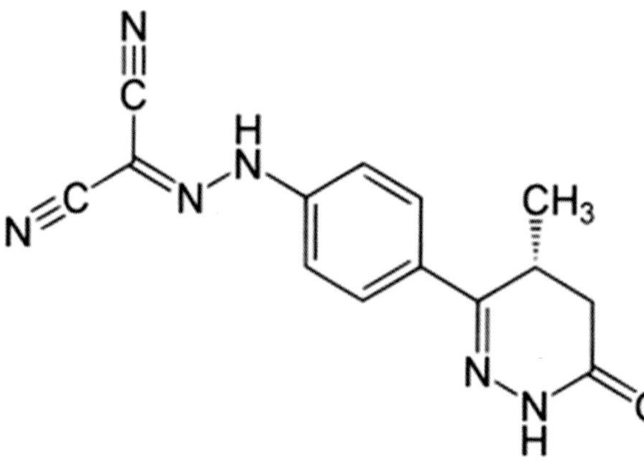

FIGURE 18-13 Levosimendan, the first of a new class of inotropes: calcium sensitizers.

meta-analysis suggested improved survival for patients with chronic heart failure.[132] There are also data suggesting that perioperative levosimendan reduces the risk of kidney injury following cardiac surgery.[133] Levosimendan is approved in many countries but is not currently approved by the FDA in the United States.

Pharmacokinetics

Levosimendan is available as a solution for IV administration. The IV loading dose is 6 to 12 μg/kg given over 10 minutes, followed by an infusion of 0.05 to 2 μg/kg/minute.[134] It has a half-life of about 1.5 hours. The clinical effects persist beyond the duration expected from the rapid half-life, likely the result of an active metabolite.[135] Oral bioavailability is about 84%.[136] Although oral administration has been studied, the drug is not available commercially in oral form.

References

1. Attaran RR, Ewy GA. Epinephrine in resuscitation: curse or cure? *Future Cardiol.* 2010;6(4):473–482.
2. Kellum JA, Pinsky MR. Use of vasopressor agents in critically ill patients. *Curr Opin Crit Care.* 2002;8(3): 236–241.
3. Myburgh JA. An appraisal of selection and use of catecholamines in septic shock—old becomes new again. *Crit Care Resusc.* 2006; 8(4):353–360.
4. Leenen FH, Chan YK, Smith DL, et al. Epinephrine and left ventricular function in humans: effects of beta-1 vs nonselective beta-blockade. *Clin Pharmacol Ther.* 1988;43(5):519–528.
5. Chilian WM, Layne SM, Eastham CL, et al. Effects of epinephrine on coronary microvascular diameters. *Circ Res.* 1987;61(5)(pt 2): II47–II53.
6. Trager K, Radermacher P. Catecholamines in the treatment of septic shock: effects beyond perfusion. *Crit Care Resusc.* 2003;5(4): 270–276.
7. Totaro RJ, Raper RF. Epinephrine-induced lactic acidosis following cardiopulmonary bypass. *Crit Care Med.* 1997;25(10): 1693–1699.
8. Brown MJ, Brown DC, Murphy MB. Hypokalemia from beta2-receptor stimulation by circulating epinephrine. *N Engl J Med.* 1983; 309(23):1414–1419.
9. Kharasch ED, Bowdle TA. Hypokalemia before induction of anesthesia and prevention by beta 2 adrenoceptor antagonism. *Anesth Analg.* 1991;72(2):216–220.
10. Levy B, Bollaert PE, Charpentier C, et al. Comparison of norepinephrine and dobutamine to epinephrine for hemodynamics, lactate metabolism, and gastric tonometric variables in septic shock: a prospective, randomized study. *Intensive Care Med.* 1997;23(3): 282–287.
11. De Backer D, Creteur J, Silva E, et al. Effects of dopamine, norepinephrine, and epinephrine on the splanchnic circulation in septic shock: which is best? *Crit Care Med.* 2003;31(6):1659–1667.
12. Meier-Hellmann A, Reinhart K, Bredle DL, et al. Epinephrine impairs splanchnic perfusion in septic shock. *Crit Care Med.* 1997; 25(3):399–404.
13. Sun D, Huang A, Mital S, et al. Norepinephrine elicits beta2-receptor-mediated dilation of isolated human coronary arterioles. *Circulation.* 2002;106(5):550–555.
14. Hollenberg SM. Vasoactive drugs in circulatory shock. *Am J Respir Crit Care Med.* 2011;183(7):847–855.
15. Goldberg LI, Rajfer SI. Dopamine receptors: applications in clinical cardiology. *Circulation.* 1985;72(2):245–248.
16. Goldberg LI. Cardiovascular and renal actions of dopamine: potential clinical applications. *Pharmacol Rev.* 1972;24(1):1–29.
17. Frishman WH, Hotchkiss H. Selective and nonselective dopamine receptor agonists: an innovative approach to cardiovascular disease treatment. *Am Heart J.* 1996;132(4):861–870.
18. MacGregor DA, Smith TE, Prielipp RC, et al. Pharmacokinetics of dopamine in healthy male subjects. *Anesthesiology.* 2000;92(2): 338–346.
19. Bailey JM. Dopamine: one size does not fit all. *Anesthesiology.* 2000;92(2):303–305.
20. Le A, Patel S. Extravasation of noncytotoxic drugs: a review of the literature. *Ann Pharmacother.* 2014;48(7):870–886.
21. Butterworth J. Selecting an inotrope for the cardiac surgery patient. *J Cardiothorac Vasc Anesth.* 1993;7(4)(suppl 2):26–32.
22. Vincent JL, Biston P, Devriendt J, et al. Dopamine versus norepinephrine: is one better? *Minerva Anestesiol.* 2009;75(5):333–337.
23. Goldberg LI. Dopamine—clinical uses of an endogenous catecholamine. *N Engl J Med.* 1974;291(14):707–710.
24. Seri I, Kone BC, Gullans SR, et al. Locally formed dopamine inhibits Na+-K+-ATPase activity in rat renal cortical tubule cells. *Am J Physiol.* 1988;255(4)(pt 2):F666–F673.
25. Kellum JA, M Decker J. Use of dopamine in acute renal failure: a meta-analysis. *Crit Care Med.* 2001;29(8):1526–1531.
26. Marik PE. Low-dose dopamine: a systematic review. *Intensive Care Med.* 2002;28(7):877–883.
27. Cottee DB, Saul WP. Is renal dose dopamine protective or therapeutic? No. *Crit Care Clin.* 1996;12(3):687–695.
28. Girbes AR, Lieverse AG, Smit AJ, et al. Lack of specific renal haemodynamic effects of different doses of dopamine after infrarenal aortic surgery. *Br J Anaesth.* 1996;77(6):753–757.
29. ter Wee PM, Smit AJ, Rosman JB, et al. Effect of intravenous infusion of low-dose dopamine on renal function in normal individuals and in patients with renal disease. *Am J Nephrol.* 1986;6(1):42–46.
30. Baldwin L, Henderson A, Hickman P. Effect of postoperative low-dose dopamine on renal function after elective major vascular surgery. *Ann Intern Med.* 1994;120(9):744–747.
31. Bellomo R, Chapman M, Finfer S, et al. Low-dose dopamine in patients with early renal dysfunction: a placebo-controlled randomised trial. *Lancet.* 2000;356(9248):2139–2143.
32. Marik PE, Iglesias J. Low-dose dopamine does not prevent acute renal failure in patients with septic shock and oliguria. *Am J Med.* 1999;107(4):387–390.
33. Chertow GM, Sayegh MH, Allgren RL, et al. Is the administration of dopamine associated with adverse or favorable outcomes in acute renal failure? *Am J Med.* 1996;101(1):49–53.
34. Elkayam U, Ng TM, Hatamizadeh P, et al. Renal vasodilatory action of dopamine in patients with heart failure: magnitude of effect and site of action. *Circulation.* 2008;117(2):200–205.
35. Sakr Y, Reinhart K, Vincent JL, et al. Does dopamine administration in shock influence outcome? Results of the Sepsis Occurrence in Acutely Ill Patients (SOAP) Study. *Crit Care Med.* 2006;34(3):589–597.
36. Debaveye YA, Van den Berghe GH. Is there still a place for dopamine in the modern intensive care unit? *Anesth Analg.* 2004;98(2): 461–468.
37. Schenarts PJ, Sagraves SG, Bard MR, et al. Low-dose dopamine: a physiologically based review. *Curr Surg.* 2006;63(3):219–225.
38. Tisdale JE, Patel R, Webb CR, et al. Electrophysiologic and proarrhythmic effects of intravenous inotropic agents. *Prog Cardiovasc Dis.* 1995;38(2):167–180.
39. Marik PE, Mohedin M. The contrasting effects of dopamine and norepinephrine on systemic and splanchnic oxygen utilization in hyperdynamic sepsis. *JAMA.* 1994;272(17):1354–1357.
40. Jakob SM, Ruokonen E, Takala J. Effects of dopamine on systemic and regional blood flow and metabolism in septic and cardiac surgery patients. *Shock.* 2002;18(1):8–13.

41. Dive A, Foret F, Jamart J, et al. Effect of dopamine on gastrointestinal motility during critical illness. *Intensive Care Med.* 2000;26(7):901–907.
42. Van den Berghe G, de Zegher F. Anterior pituitary function during critical illness and dopamine treatment. *Crit Care Med.* 1996;24(9):1580–1590.
43. Ward DS, Bellville JW. Reduction of hypoxic ventilatory drive by dopamine. *Anesth Analg.* 1982;61(4):333–337.
44. van de Borne P, Oren R, Somers VK. Dopamine depresses minute ventilation in patients with heart failure. *Circulation.* 1998;98(2):126–131.
45. Johnson RL Jr. Low-dose dopamine and oxygen transport by the lung. *Circulation.* 1998;98(2):97–99.
46. Shoemaker WC, Appel PL, Kram HB, et al. Comparison of hemodynamic and oxygen transport effects of dopamine and dobutamine in critically ill surgical patients. *Chest.* 1989;96(1):120–126.
47. Ciarka A, Rimacchi R, Vincent JL, et al. Effects of low-dose dopamine on ventilation in patients with chronic obstructive pulmonary disease. *Eur J Clin Invest.* 2004;34(7):508–512.
48. Ciarka A, Vincent JL, van de Borne P. The effects of dopamine on the respiratory system: friend or foe? *Pulm Pharmacol Ther.* 2007;20(6):607–615.
49. Brath PC, MacGregor DA, Ford JG, et al. Dopamine and intraocular pressure in critically ill patients. *Anesthesiology.* 2000;93(6):1398–1400.
50. Firth BG, Ratner AV, Grassman ED, et al. Assessment of the inotropic and vasodilator effects of amrinone versus isoproterenol. *Am J Cardiol.* 1984;54(10):1331–1336.
51. Daoud FS, Reeves JT, Kelly DB. Isoproterenol as a potential pulmonary vasodilator in primary pulmonary hypertension. *Am J Cardiol.* 1978;42(5):817–822.
52. Tuttle RR, Mills J. Dobutamine: development of a new catecholamine to selectively increase cardiac contractility. *Circ Res.* 1975;36(1):185–196.
53. Ruffolo RR Jr, Yaden EL. Vascular effects of the stereoisomers of dobutamine. *J Pharmacol Exp Ther.* 1983;224(1):46–50.
54. Ruffolo RR Jr. The pharmacology of dobutamine. *Am J Med Sci.* 1987;294(4):244–248.
55. Ruffolo RR Jr, Messick K. Systemic hemodynamic effects of dopamine, (+/−)-dobutamine and the (+)-and (−)-enantiomers of dobutamine in anesthetized normotensive rats. *Eur J Pharmacol.* 1985;109(2):173–181.
56. Ruffolo RR Jr, Spradlin TA, Pollock GD, et al. Alpha and beta adrenergic effects of the stereoisomers of dobutamine. *J Pharmacol Exp Ther.* 1981;219(2):447–452.
57. Butterworth JF IV, Prielipp RC, Royster RL, et al. Dobutamine increases heart rate more than epinephrine in patients recovering from aortocoronary bypass surgery. *J Cardiothorac Vasc Anesth.* 1992;6(5):535–541.
58. Tinker JH, Tarhan S, White RD, et al. Dobutamine for inotropic support during emergence from cardiopulmonary bypass. *Anesthesiology.* 1976;44(4):281–286.
59. Schwenzer KJ, Miller ED Jr. Hemodynamic effects of dobutamine in patients following mitral valve replacement. *Anesth Analg.* 1989;68(4):467–472.
60. Leier CV, Webel J, Bush CA. The cardiovascular effects of the continuous infusion of dobutamine in patients with severe cardiac failure. *Circulation.* 1977;56(3):468–472.
61. Shitara T, Wajima Z, Ogawa R. Dobutamine infusion modifies thermoregulation during general anesthesia. *Anesth Analg.* 1996;83(6):1154–1159.
62. Sonnenblick EH, Frishman WH, LeJemtel TH. Dobutamine: a new synthetic cardioactive sympathetic amine. *N Engl J Med.* 1979;300(1):17–22.
63. Jewitt D, Birkhead J, Mitchell A, et al. Clinical cardiovascular pharmacology of dobutamine. A selective inotropic catecholamine. *Lancet.* 1974;2(7877):363–367.
64. Liles JT, Dabisch PA, Hude KE, et al. Pressor responses to ephedrine are mediated by a direct mechanism in the rat. *J Pharmacol Exp Ther.* 2006;316(1):95–105.
65. Butterworth JF IV, Piccione W Jr, Berrizbeitia LD, et al. Augmentation of venous return by adrenergic agonists during spinal anesthesia. *Anesth Analg.* 1986;65(6):612–616.
66. Ralston DH, Shnider SM, DeLorimier AA. Effects of equipotent ephedrine, metaraminol, mephentermine, and methoxamine on uterine blood flow in the pregnant ewe. *Anesthesiology.* 1974;40(4):354–370.
67. McGrath JM, Chestnut DH, Vincent RD, et al. Ephedrine remains the vasopressor of choice for treatment of hypotension during ritodrine infusion and epidural anesthesia. *Anesthesiology.* 1994;80(5):1073–1081; discussion 28A.
68. Lee A, Ngan Kee WD, Gin T. A quantitative, systematic review of randomized controlled trials of ephedrine versus phenylephrine for the management of hypotension during spinal anesthesia for cesarean delivery. *Anesth Analg.* 2002;94(4):920–926, table of contents.
69. Cooper DW, Carpenter M, Mowbray P, et al. Fetal and maternal effects of phenylephrine and ephedrine during spinal anesthesia for cesarean delivery. *Anesthesiology.* 2002;97(6):1582–1590.
70. Rothenberg DM, Parnass SM, Litwack K, et al. Efficacy of ephedrine in the prevention of postoperative nausea and vomiting. *Anesth Analg.* 1991;72(1):58–61.
71. Thiele RH, Nemergut EC, Lynch C. The physiologic implications of isolated alpha(1) adrenergic stimulation. *Anesth Analg.* 2011;113(2):284–296.
72. Thiele RH, Nemergut EC, Lynch C. The clinical implications of isolated alpha(1) adrenergic stimulation. *Anesth Analg.* 2011;113(2):297–304.
73. Pearl RG. Phenylephrine and inhaled nitric oxide in adult respiratory distress syndrome. When are two better than one? *Anesthesiology.* 1997;87(1):1–3.
74. Groudine SB, Hollinger I, Jones J, et al. New York State guidelines on the topical use of phenylephrine in the operating room. The Phenylephrine Advisory Committee. *Anesthesiology.* 2000;92(3):859–864.
75. Schwinn DA, Reves JG. Time course and hemodynamic effects of alpha-1-adrenergic bolus administration in anesthetized patients with myocardial disease. *Anesth Analg.* 1989;68(5):571–578.
76. Goertz AW, Lindner KH, Seefelder C, et al. Effect of phenylephrine bolus administration on global left ventricular function in patients with coronary artery disease and patients with valvular aortic stenosis. *Anesthesiology.* 1993;78(5):834–841.
77. Inomata S, Nishikawa T, Kihara S, et al. Enhancement of pressor response to intravenous phenylephrine following oral clonidine medication in awake and anaesthetized patients. *Can J Anaesth.* 1995;42(2):119–125.
78. Williams ME, Rosa RM, Silva P, et al. Impairment of extrarenal potassium disposal by alpha-adrenergic stimulation. *N Engl J Med.* 1984;311(3):145–149.
79. Rhoney D, Peacock WF. Intravenous therapy for hypertensive emergencies, part 1. *Am J Health Syst Pharm.* 2009;66(15):1343–1352.
80. Nelson HS. Beta-adrenergic bronchodilators. *N Engl J Med.* 1995;333(8):499–506.
81. Crogan SJ, Bishop MJ. Delivery efficiency of metered dose aerosols given via endotracheal tubes. *Anesthesiology.* 1989;70(6):1008–1010.
82. Mullen M, Mullen B, Carey M. The association between beta-agonist use and death from asthma. A meta-analytic integration of case-control studies. *JAMA.* 1993;270(15):1842–1845.
83. Suissa S, Ernst P, Spitzer WO. Beta-agonist use and death from asthma. *JAMA.* 1994;271(11):821–822.
84. Liem EB, Mnookin SC, Mahla ME. Albuterol-induced lactic acidosis. *Anesthesiology.* 2003;99(2):505–506.
85. Tobias JD, Hirshman CA. Attenuation of histamine-induced airway constriction by albuterol during halothane anesthesia. *Anesthesiology.* 1990;72(1):105–110.

86. Maslow AD, Regan MM, Israel E, et al. Inhaled albuterol, but not intravenous lidocaine, protects against intubation-induced bronchoconstriction in asthma. *Anesthesiology*. 2000;93(5):1198–1204.
87. Packer M. End of the oldest controversy in medicine. Are we ready to conclude the debate on digitalis? *N Engl J Med*. 1997;336(8): 575–576.
88. Group DI. The effect of digoxin on mortality and morbidity in patients with heart failure. *N Engl J Med*. 1997;336(8):525–533.
89. Reuning RH, Sams RA, Notari RE. Role of pharmacokinetics in drug dosage adjustment. I. Pharmacologic effect kinetics and apparent volume of distribution of digoxin. *J Clin Pharmacol New Drugs*. 1973;13(4):127–141.
90. Sheiner LB, Rosenberg B, Marathe VV. Estimation of population characteristics of pharmacokinetic parameters from routine clinical data. *J Pharmacokinet Biopharm*. 1977;5(5):445–479.
91. Jelliffe RW, Milman M, Schumitzky A, et al. A two-compartment population pharmacokinetic-pharmacodynamic model of digoxin in adults, with implications for dosage. *Ther Drug Monit*. 2014; 36(3):387–393.
92. Kulick DL, Rahimtoola SH. Current role of digitalis therapy in patients with congestive heart failure. *JAMA*. 1991;265(22): 2995–2997.
93. Venetucci LA, Trafford AW, O'Neill SC, et al. The sarcoplasmic reticulum and arrhythmogenic calcium release. *Cardiovasc Res* 2008; 77(2):285–292.
94. Edwards R, Winnie AP, Ramamurthy S. Acute hypocapneic hypokalemia: an latrogenic anesthetic complication. *Anesth Analg* 1977; 56(6):786–792.
95. Atlee JL. Perioperative cardiac dysrhythmias: diagnosis and management. *Anesthesiology*. 1997;86(6):1397–1424.
96. Butler VP Jr, Chen JP. Digoxin-specific antibodies. *Proc Natl Acad Sci U S A*. 1967;57(1):71–78.
97. Bartolone RS, Rao TL. Dysrhythmias following muscle relaxant administration in patients receiving digitalis. *Anesthesiology*. 1983;58(6):567–569.
98. Ivankovich AD, Miletich DJ, Grossman RK, et al. The effect of enflurane, isoflurane, fluroxene, methoxyflurane and diethyl ether anesthesia on ouabain tolerance in the dog. *Anesth Analg*. 1976; 55(3):360–365.
99. Skoyles JR, Sherry KM. Pharmacology, mechanisms of action and uses of selective phosphodiesterase inhibitors. *Br J Anaesth*. 1992;68(3):293–302.
100. Monrad ES, McKay RG, Baim DS, et al. Improvement in indexes of diastolic performance in patients with congestive heart failure treated with milrinone. *Circulation*. 1984;70(6):1030–1037.
101. Benotti JR, Grossman W, Braunwald E, et al. Hemodynamic assessment of amrinone. A new inotropic agent. *N Engl J Med*. 1978; 299(25):1373–1377.
102. Levy JH, Bailey JM. Amrinone: pharmacokinetics and pharmacodynamics. *J Cardiothorac Anesth*. 1989;3(6)(suppl 2):10–14.
103. Ansell J, Tiarks C, McCue J, et al. Amrinone-induced thrombocytopenia. *Arch Intern Med*. 1984;144(5):949–952.
104. Ross MP, Allen-Webb EM, Pappas JB, et al. Amrinone-associated thrombocytopenia: pharmacokinetic analysis. *Clin Pharmacol Ther*. 1993;53(6):661–667.
105. Wilmshurst PT, Al-Hasani SF, Semple MJ, et al. The effects of amrinone on platelet count, survival and function in patients with congestive cardiac failure. *Br J Clin Pharmacol*. 1984;17(3):317–324.
106. Ludmer PL, Wright RF, Arnold JM, et al. Separation of the direct myocardial and vasodilator actions of milrinone administered by an intracoronary infusion technique. *Circulation*. 1986;73(1): 130–137.
107. Levy JH, Bailey JM, Deeb GM. Intravenous milrinone in cardiac surgery. *Ann Thorac Surg* 2002;73(1):325–330.
108. Bailey JM, Levy JH, Kikura M, et al. Pharmacokinetics of intravenous milrinone in patients undergoing cardiac surgery. *Anesthesiology*. 1994;81(3):616–622.
109. Butterworth JF IV, Hines RL, Royster RL, et al. A pharmacokinetic and pharmacodynamic evaluation of milrinone in adults undergoing cardiac surgery. *Anesth Analg*. 1995;81(4):783–792.
110. Feneck RO. Intravenous milrinone following cardiac surgery: II. Influence of baseline hemodynamics and patient factors on therapeutic response. The European Milrinone Multicentre Trial Group. *J Cardiothorac Vasc Anesth*. 1992;6(5):563–567.
111. Feneck RO. Intravenous milrinone following cardiac surgery: I. Effects of bolus infusion followed by variable dose maintenance infusion. The European Milrinone Multicentre Trial Group. *J Cardiothorac Vasc Anesth*. 1992;6(5):554–562.
112. DiBianco R, Shabetai R, Kostuk W, et al. A comparison of oral milrinone, digoxin, and their combination in the treatment of patients with chronic heart failure. *N Engl J Med*. 1989;320(11): 677–683.
113. Cuffe MS, Califf RM, Adams KF Jr, et al. Short-term intravenous milrinone for acute exacerbation of chronic heart failure: a randomized controlled trial. *JAMA*. 2002;287(12):1541–1547.
114. Feneck RO, Sherry KM, Withington PS, et al. Comparison of the hemodynamic effects of milrinone with dobutamine in patients after cardiac surgery. *J Cardiothorac Vasc Anesth*. 2001;15(3):306–315.
115. Eichhorn EJ, Konstam MA, Weiland DS, et al. Differential effects of milrinone and dobutamine on right ventricular preload, afterload and systolic performance in congestive heart failure secondary to ischemic or idiopathic dilated cardiomyopathy. *Am J Cardiol*. 1987;60(16):1329–1333.
116. Tanaka M, Ishikawa T, Nishikaawa T, et al. Influence of acidosis on cardiotonic effects of milrinone. *Anesthesiology*. 1998;88(3): 725–734.
117. Salmenpera M, Levy JH. The in vitro effects of phosphodiesterase inhibitors on the human internal mammary artery. *Anesth Analg*. 1996;82(5):954–957.
118. Hayashida N, Tomoeda H, Oda T, et al. Inhibitory effect of milrinone on cytokine production after cardiopulmonary bypass. *Ann Thorac Surg*. 1999;68(5):1661–1667.
119. Möllhoff T, Loick HM, Van Aken H, et al. Milrinone modulates endotoxemia, systemic inflammation, and subsequent acute phase response after cardiopulmonary bypass (CPB). *Anesthesiology*. 1999;90(1):72–80.
120. Packer M, Carver JR, Rodenheffer RJ, et al. Effect of oral milrinone on mortality in severe chronic heart failure. The PROMISE Study Research Group. *N Engl J Med*. 1991;325(21):1468–1475.
121. Kikura M, Lee MK, Safon RA, et al. The effects of milrinone on platelets in patients undergoing cardiac surgery. *Anesth Analg*. 1995;81(1):44–48.
122. Crystal GJ, Zhou X, Salem MR. Is calcium a coronary vasoconstrictor in vivo? *Anesthesiology*. 1998;88(3):735–743.
123. Bushinsky DA, Monk RD. Electrolyte quintet: calcium. *Lancet*. 1998;352(9124):306–311.
124. Moore EW. Ionized calcium in normal serum, ultrafiltrates, and whole blood determined by ion-exchange electrodes. *J Clin Invest*. 1970;49(2):318–334.
125. Larsson L, Ohman S. Serum calcium ion activity. Some aspects on methodological differences and intraindividual variation. *Clin Biochem*. 1979;12(4):138–141.
126. Haikala H, Linden IB. Mechanisms of action of calcium-sensitizing drugs. *J Cardiovasc Pharmacol*. 1995;26(suppl 1):S10–S19.
127. Sorsa T, Pollesello P, Solaro RJ. The contractile apparatus as a target for drugs against heart failure: interaction of levosimendan, a calcium sensitiser, with cardiac troponin c. *Mol Cell Biochem*. 2004;266(1–2):87–107.
128. Yokoshiki H, Katsube Y, Sunagawa M, et al. The novel calcium sensitizer levosimendan activates the ATP-sensitive K+ channel in rat ventricular cells. *J Pharmacol Exp Ther*. 1997;283(1): 375–383.
129. Pataricza J, Hõhn J, Petri A, et al. Comparison of the vasorelaxing effect of cromakalim and the new inodilator, levosimendan,

in human isolated portal vein. *J Pharm Pharmacol.* 2000;52(2): 213–217.
130. Kersten JR, Montgomery MW, Pagel PS, et al. Levosimendan, a new positive inotropic drug, decreases myocardial infarct size via activation of K(ATP) channels. *Anesth Analg.* 2000;90(1):5–11.
131. Unverzagt S, Wachsmuth L, Hirsch K, et al. Inotropic agents and vasodilator strategies for acute myocardial infarction complicated by cardiogenic shock or low cardiac output syndrome. *Cochrane Database Syst Rev.* 2014;1:CD009669.
132. Silvetti S, Greco T, Di Prima AL, et al. Intermittent levosimendan improves mid-term survival in chronic heart failure patients: meta-analysis of randomised trials. *Clin Res Cardiol.* 2014;103(7):505–513.
133. Niu ZZ, Wu SM, Sunn WY, et al. Perioperative levosimendan therapy is associated with a lower incidence of acute kidney injury after cardiac surgery: a meta-analysis. *J Cardiovasc Pharmacol.* 2014;63(2):107–112.
134. Figgitt DP, Gillies PS, Goa KL. Levosimendan. *Drugs.* 2001;61(5): 613–627; discussion 628–629.
135. Antoniades C, Antonopoulos AS, Tousoulis D, et al. Relationship between the pharmacokinetics of levosimendan and its effects on cardiovascular system. *Curr Drug Metab.* 2009;10(2):95–103.
136. Sandell EP, Hayha M, Antila S, et al. Pharmacokinetics of levosimendan in healthy volunteers and patients with congestive heart failure. *J Cardiovasc Pharmacol.* 1995;26(suppl 1):S57–S62.

CHAPTER 19

Sympatholytics

Steven Miller

α- and β-Adrenergic Receptor Antagonists

α- and β-Adrenergic receptor antagonists prevent the interaction of the endogenous neurotransmitter norepinephrine or sympathomimetics with the corresponding adrenergic receptors.[1] Interference with normal adrenergic receptor function attenuates sympathetic nervous system homeostatic mechanisms and evokes predictable pharmacologic responses. Presynapthic agonsim of α_2 receptors will result in a similar attenuation of sympathetic outflow.

α-Adrenergic Receptor Antagonists

α-Adrenergic receptor antagonists bind selectively to α-adrenergic receptors and interfere with the ability of catecholamines or other sympathomimetics to provoke α responses. Drug-induced α-adrenergic blockade prevents the effects of catecholamines and sympathomimetics on the heart and peripheral vasculature. The inhibitory action of epinephrine on insulin secretion is prevented. Orthostatic hypotension, baroreceptor-mediated reflex tachycardia, and impotence are invariable side effects of α-adrenergic blockade. Furthermore, absence of β-adrenergic blockade permits maximum expression of cardiac stimulation from norepinephrine, typically leading to tachycardia. These side effects prevent the use of nonselective α-adrenergic antagonists in the management of ambulatory essential hypertension.

Mechanism of Action

Phentolamine, prazosin, and yohimbine are competitive (reversible binding with receptors) α-adrenergic antagonists. In contrast, phenoxybenzamine binds covalently to α-adrenergic receptors to produce an irreversible and insurmountable type of α receptor blockade. Once α blockade has been established with phenoxybenzamine, even massive doses of sympathomimetics are ineffective until the effect of phenoxybenzamine is terminated by metabolism.

Phentolamine and phenoxybenzamine are nonselective α antagonists acting at postsynaptic α_1 receptors as well as presynaptic α_2 receptors. Prazosin is selective for α_1 receptors, whereas yohimbine is selective for α_2 receptors.

Phentolamine

Phentolamine is a substituted imidazoline derivative that produces transient nonselective α-adrenergic blockade (Fig. 19-1). Administered intravenously (IV), phentolamine produces peripheral vasodilation and a decrease in systemic blood pressure that manifests within 2 minutes and lasts 10 to 15 minutes. This vasodilation reflects α_1 receptor blockade and a direct action of phentolamine on vascular smooth muscle. Decreases in blood pressure elicit baroreceptor-mediated increases in sympathetic nervous system activity manifesting as cardiac stimulation. In addition to reflex stimulation, phentolamine-induced α_2 receptor blockade permits enhanced neural release of norepinephrine manifesting as increased heart rate and cardiac output. Indeed, cardiac dysrhythmias and angina pectoris may accompany the administration of phentolamine. Hyperperistalsis, abdominal pain, and diarrhea may be caused by a predominance of parasympathetic nervous system activity. Phentolamine undergoes principally hepatic metabolism and only about 10% of the drug is excreted unchanged in the urine.

Clinical Uses

The principal use of phentolamine is the treatment of acute hypertensive emergencies, as may accompany intraoperative manipulation of a pheochromocytoma or autonomic nervous system hyperreflexia. Administration of phentolamine, 30 to 70 μg/kg IV (1 to 5 mg), produces a prompt but transient decrease in systemic blood pressure. A continuous infusion of phentolamine (0.1 to 2 mg per minute) may be used to maintain normal blood pressure during the intraoperative resection of a pheochromocytoma. Local infiltration with a phentolamine-containing solution (5 to 15 mg in 10 mL of normal saline)

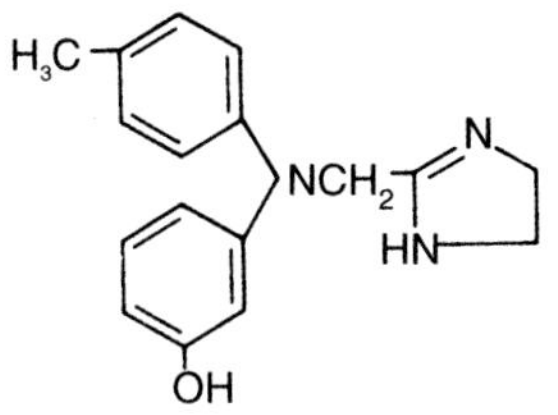

FIGURE 19-1 Phentolamine.

is appropriate when a sympathomimetic is accidentally administered extravascularly.

Phenoxybenzamine

Phenoxybenzamine is a haloalkylamine derivative that acts as a nonselective α-adrenergic antagonist by combining covalently with α-adrenergic receptors (Fig. 19-2). Blockade at postsynaptic α_1 receptors is more intense than at α_2 receptors.

Pharmacokinetics

Absorption of phenoxybenzamine from the gastrointestinal tract is incomplete. Onset of α-adrenergic blockade is slow, taking up to 60 minutes to reach peak effect even after IV administration. This delay in onset is due to the time required for structural modification of the phenoxybenzamine molecule, which is necessary to render the drug pharmacologically active. The elimination half-time of phenoxybenzamine is about 24 hours, emphasizing the likelihood of cumulative effects with repeated doses.

Cardiovascular Effects

Phenoxybenzamine administered to a supine, normovolemic patient in the absence of increased sympathetic nervous system activity produces little change in systemic blood pressure. Orthostatic hypotension, however, is prominent, especially in the presence of preexisting hypertension or hypovolemia. In addition, impairment of compensatory vasoconstriction results in exaggerated blood pressure decreases in response to blood loss or vasodilating drugs such as volatile anesthetics. Despite decreases in blood pressure, cardiac output is often increased and renal blood flow is not greatly altered unless preexisting renal vasoconstriction is present. Cerebral and coronary vascular resistances are not changed. α-Adrenergic blockade produced by maternal treatment may result in neonatal hypotension and respiratory distress in the first 72 hours of life.[2]

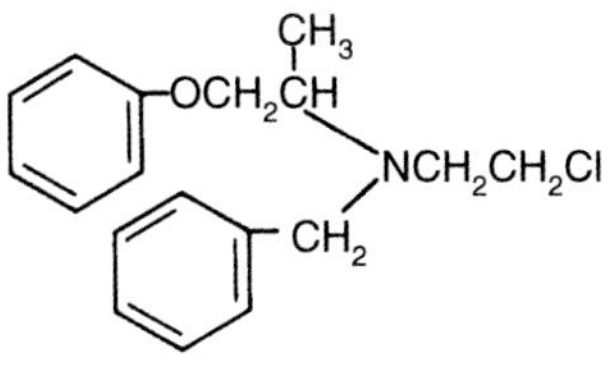

FIGURE 19-2 Phenoxybenzamine.

Noncardiac Effects

Phenoxybenzamine prevents the inhibitory action of epinephrine on the secretion of insulin. Catecholamine-induced glycogenolysis in skeletal muscles or lipolysis is not altered. Stimulation of the radial fibers of the iris is prevented, and miosis is a prominent component of the response to phenoxybenzamine. Sedation may accompany chronic phenoxybenzamine therapy. Nasal stuffiness is due to unopposed vasodilation in mucous membranes in the presence of α-adrenergic blockade.

Clinical Uses

Phenoxybenzamine, 0.5 to 1.0 mg/kg orally (prazosin is an alternative) is administered preoperatively to control blood pressure in patients with pheochromocytoma. Chronic α-adrenergic blockade, by relieving intense peripheral vasoconstriction, permits expansion of intravascular fluid volume as reflected by a decrease in the hematocrit. Excessive vasoconstriction with associated tissue ischemia, as accompanies hemorrhagic shock, may be reversed by phenoxybenzamine but only after intravascular fluid volume has been replenished.

Treatment of peripheral vascular disease characterized by intermittent claudication is not favorably influenced by α-adrenergic blockade because cutaneous rather than skeletal muscle blood flow is increased. The most beneficial clinical responses to α-adrenergic blockade are in diseases with a large component of cutaneous vasoconstriction, such as Raynaud's disease, where smaller arteries that supply blood to skin narrow, limiting blood circulation to affected areas.

Yohimbine

Yohimbine is a selective antagonist at presynaptic α_2 receptors, leading to enhanced release of norepinephrine from nerve endings. As a result, this drug may be useful in the treatment of the rare patient suffering from idiopathic orthostatic hypotension. In the past, impotence had been successfully treated with yohimbine in male patients with vascular, diabetic, and psychogenic origins. Yohimbine readily crosses the blood–brain barrier and may be associated with increased skeletal muscle activity and tremor. Excessive doses of yohimbine may produce tachycardia, hypertension, rhinorrhea, paresthesias, and dissociative states. Observations that α_2-adrenergic agonists can decrease anesthetic requirements by actions on presynaptic α_2 receptors in the central nervous system (CNS) suggest a possible interaction of yohimbine with volatile anesthetics.

Doxazosin

Doxazosin is approved for both treatment of hypertension and benign prostatic hypertrophy. It is a selective postsynaptic α_1 receptor antagonist that is 65% bioavailable with oral administration. Peak levels of doxazosin are seen 2 to 3 hours following oral administration and effectively relaxes prostatic and vascular smooth muscle. Doxazosin is primarily metabolized in the liver by O-demethylation and excreted in the feces. The terminal elimination life of doxazosin is 22 hours and is recommended as a single daily dose in the morning.

Prazosin

Prazosin is a selective postsynaptic α_1 receptor antagonist that leaves intact the inhibiting effect of α_2 receptor activity on norepinephrine release from nerve endings. As a result, prazosin is less likely than nonselective α-adrenergic antagonists to evoke reflex tachycardia. Prazosin dilates both arterioles and veins. Following oral administration, the onset of action is approximately 30 minutes and the duration of action is about 4 to 6 hours. Elimination of prazosin is principally by hepatic metabolism.

Terazosin

α Blocker therapy of benign prostatic hypertrophy is based on α_1-mediated innervation of prostatic smooth muscle that controls contraction of the prostate and obstruction of the bladder outlet. Terazosin is a long-acting orally effective α_1-adrenergic antagonist that may be useful in the treatment of benign prostatic hyperplasia by virtue of its ability to relax prostatic smooth muscle.

Tamsulosin

Tamsulosin is an orally effective α_{1a}-adrenergic antagonist that is indicated for the treatment of the signs and symptoms of benign prostatic hyperplasia. Side effects may include orthostatic hypotension, vertigo, and syncope. The clearance of tamsulosin is decreased in the presence of cimetidine.

Tolazoline

Tolazoline is a competitive nonselective α-adrenergic receptor antagonist. This drug has been used to treat persistent pulmonary hypertension of the newborn but its use for this purpose has been largely replaced by nitric oxide. Side effects of tolazoline include systemic hypotension with reflex tachycardia, cardiac dysrhythmias, and pulmonary and gastrointestinal hemorrhages. Tolazoline is excreted mainly unchanged by the kidneys.

α-Adrenergic Receptor Agonists

α_2-Adrenergic receptor agonists bind selectively to presynaptic α_2-adrenergic receptors and, by a negative feedback mechanism, decrease the release of norepinephrine from presynaptic nerve terminals and reduce sympathetic outflow with similar decreases in blood pressure as α_1 antagonists. Most α_2 receptors are found in the central nervous system especially in the brainstem and the locus ceruleus. Peripherial inhibition of α_2 receptors can result in inhibition of insulin release and induction of glucagon from the pancreas. Clinical pharmacologic effects include hypotension, bradycardia, and central sedation with some mild effects of analgesia all related to the sympatholytic effects.

Mechanism of Action

α_2-Adrenergic receptor agonists have selective affinity for α_2-adrenergic receptors and act competitively. Binding of α_2 agonists can be displaced from binding sites in the central nervous system resulting in reversal of the CNS effects. Withdrawal after even short-term use can result in a rebound effect with a dramatic increase in sympathetic outflow causing elevations in heart rate and hypertension to even dangerous levels.

Clonidine

Administration results in dose-dependent decreases in heart rate and blood pressure and is used clinically to treat resistant hypertension and tremors from central stimulant medications. Clonidine is a partial agonist of α_2 receptors with a 400:1 α_2:α_1 receptor preference. Clonidine is available in an intravenous, oral, and transdermal preparation and is metabolized in the liver but is excreted mostly unchanged in the urine and to a lesser extent in the bile and feces. Terminal half-life is approximately 12 to 16 hours but can be extremely variable with any liver or kidney dysfunction.

Dexmedetomidine

Dexmedetomidine is a selective α_2 agonist with a 1,600:1 preference for α_2 receptors. It is intravenously administered as an infusion from 0.1 to 1.5 μg/kg/minute with a terminal elimination half-life of 2 hours. Most often, this α_2 agonist is used in the intensive care and operating room settings as a sedative and analgesic due to its central sympatholytic effects. Dexmedetomidine undergoes extensive biotransformation in the liver and is excreted mostly in the urine; liver impairment can dramatically increase plasma levels and duration of action due to significantly decreased metabolism during infusion. It's potent binding and short half-life can induce physiologic dependence and result in the aforementioned withdrawal phenomenon after only days of administration resulting in tachycardia, hypertension, and anxiety. Interestingly, large intravenous boluses (0.25 to 1 μg/kg over 3 to 5 minutes) result in a paradoxical hypertension with a decrease in heart rate and resembles phenylephrine and is the resultant effect of crossover α_1 stimulation.

β-Adrenergic Receptor Antagonists

β-Adrenergic receptor antagonists bind selectively to β-adrenergic receptors and interfere with the ability of catecholamines or other sympathomimetics to provoke β responses. Drug-induced β-adrenergic blockade prevents the effects of catecholamines and sympathomimetics on the heart and smooth muscles of the airways and blood vessels. β Antagonist therapy should be continued throughout the perioperative period to maintain desirable drug effects and to avoid the risk of sympathetic nervous system hyperactivity associated with abrupt discontinuation of these drugs.

Propranolol is the standard β-adrenergic antagonist drug to which all other β-adrenergic antagonists are compared.

Mechanism of Action

β-Adrenergic receptor antagonists exhibit selective affinity for β-adrenergic receptors, where they act by competitive inhibition. Binding of antagonist drugs to β-adrenergic receptors is reversible such that the drug can be displaced from the occupied receptors if sufficiently large amounts of agonist become available. Competitive antagonism causes a rightward displacement of the dose-response curve for the agonist, but the slope of the curve remains unchanged, emphasizing that sufficiently large doses of the agonist may still exert a full pharmacologic effect. Chronic administration of β-adrenergic antagonists is associated with an increase in the number of β-adrenergic receptors.

β-Adrenergic receptors are G protein–coupled receptors and their occupancy by agonists (norepinephrine, epinephrine) stimulates G proteins that in turn activate adenylate cyclase to produce cyclic adenosine monophosphate (cAMP). Protein kinases are activated by cAMP, which phosphorylates proteins including L-type voltage-dependent calcium channels and troponin C in a variety of tissues (especially myocardium). The net effect of β-adrenergic stimulation in the heart is to produce positive chronotropic, inotropic, and dromotropic effects and these are the responses that are blunted by β-adrenergic receptor antagonists. It is estimated that about 75% of β receptors in the myocardium are β_1, whereas β_2 receptors account for about 20% of β receptors.

Structure–Activity Relationships

β-Adrenergic antagonists are derivatives of the β agonist drug isoproterenol (Fig. 19-3). Substitutions on the benzene ring determine whether the drug acts on β-adrenergic receptors as an antagonist or agonist. The levorotatory forms of β antagonists and agonists are more potent than the dextrorotatory forms. For example, the dextrorotatory isomer of propranolol has less than 1% of the potency of the levorotatory isomer for blocking β-adrenergic receptors.

Classification

β-Adrenergic receptor antagonists are classified as nonselective for β_1 and β_2 receptors (propranolol, nadolol, timolol, pindolol) and cardioselective (metoprolol, atenolol, acebutolol, betaxolol, esmolol, bisoprolol) for β_1 receptors (Tables 19-1 and 19-2). It is important to recognize that β receptor selectivity is dose dependent and is lost when large doses of the antagonist are administered. This emphasizes that selectivity should not be interpreted as specificity for a specific type of β-adrenergic receptor. β-Adrenergic antagonists are further classified as partial or pure antagonists on the basis of the presence or absence of intrinsic sympathomimetic activity (see Tables 19-1 and 19-2). Drugs that exhibit cardiac selectivity for β_1 receptors (cardioselective) are better suited for administration to patients with asthma and reactive airway disease. Theoretically, cardioselective drugs are better suited for treatment of patients with essential hypertension as these drugs lack inhibition of peripheral β_2 receptors that produce vasodilation.

β_1 Receptor blockade is associated with slowing of the sinus rate, slowing of conduction of cardiac impulses through the atrioventricular node, and a decrease in inotropy. These effects are relatively greater during activity than during rest. The result is a decrease in myocardial oxygen demand, with a subsequent decrease in the occurrence of myocardial ischemia during exercise. The decrease in heart rate also increases diastolic perfusion time, which may enhance myocardial perfusion. β_2 Receptor blockade increases the risk of bronchospasm in patients with reactive airway disease and may worsen the clinical symptoms of peripheral vascular disease.

β-Adrenergic antagonists may produce some degree of membrane stabilization in the heart (inhibition of propagation of action potentials across the cell membrane similar to sodium channel blockers that are class I antiarrhythmics) and thus resemble quinidine. This membrane stabilization effect, however, is detectable only at plasma concentrations that are far higher than needed to produce clinically adequate β-adrenergic blockade.

Pharmacokinetics

The principal difference in pharmacokinetics between all the β-adrenergic receptor antagonists is the elimination half-time ranging from brief for esmolol (about 10 minutes) to hours for the other drugs (see Table 19-1). Elimination half-time is considered in the perioperative period when redosing intervals are being developed or when conversion to another β-adrenergic receptor drug is planned. Among the β-adrenergic receptor antagonists, only propranolol is highly protein bound. The volume of distribution of these drugs is high and they are rapidly distributed following IV administration.

β-Adrenergic receptor antagonists are eliminated by several different pathways and this must be considered in the presence of renal and/or hepatic dysfunction (see Table 19-1). The therapeutic plasma concentration varies greatly among these drugs and between patients (interpatient variability). Explanations for interpatient variability include differences in basal sympathetic nervous system tone, flat dose-response curves for the drug so changes in plasma concentrations evoke minimal changes in pharmacologic effects, impact of active metabolites, and genetic differences in β-adrenergic receptors that influence how an individual patient responds to a given drug and plasma concentration.

Propranolol

Propranolol is a nonselective β-adrenergic receptor antagonist that lacks intrinsic sympathomimetic activity and thus is a pure antagonist (see Table 19-1). Antagonism

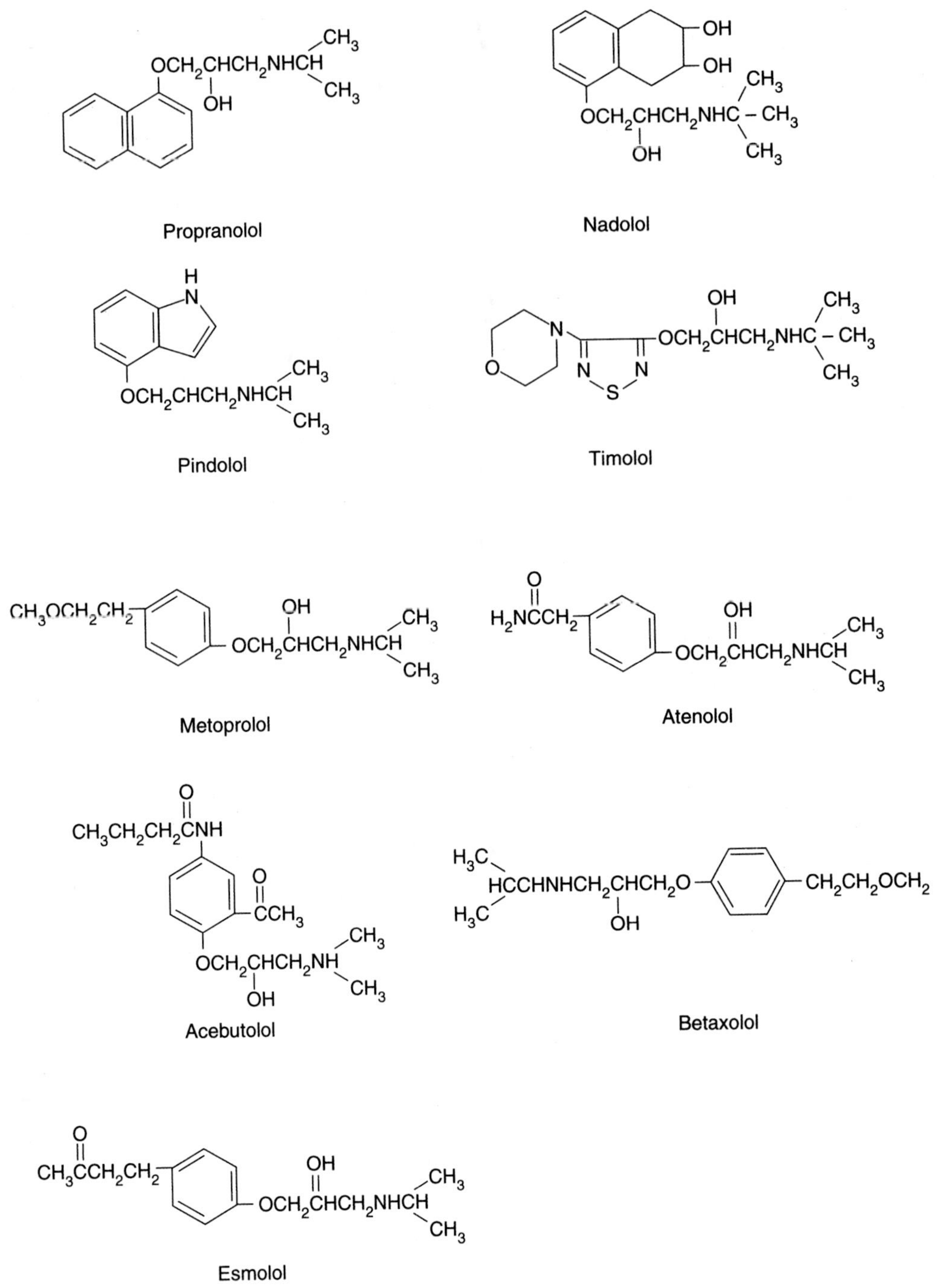

Propranolol

Nadolol

Pindolol

Timolol

Metoprolol

Atenolol

Acebutolol

Betaxolol

Esmolol

FIGURE 19-3 β-Adrenergic antagonists.

of β_1 and β_2 receptors produced by propranolol is about equal. As the first β-adrenergic antagonist introduced clinically, propranolol is the standard drug to which all β-adrenergic antagonists are compared. Typically, propranolol is administered in stepwise increments until physiologic plasma concentrations have been attained, as indicated by a resting heart rate of 55 to 60 beats per minute.

Cardiac Effects

The most important pharmacologic effects of propranolol are on the heart. Because of β_1-receptor blockade, propranolol decreases heart rate and myocardial contractility, resulting in decreased cardiac output. These effects on heart rate and cardiac output are especially prominent during exercise or in the presence of increased sympathetic nervous system activity. Heart rate slowing induced by propranolol lasts longer than the negative inotropic effects, suggesting a possible subdivision of β_1 receptors. Concomitant blockade of β_2 receptors by propranolol increases peripheral vascular resistance, including coronary vascular resistance. Although prolongation of systolic ejection and dilatation of the cardiac ventricles caused by propranolol increases myocardial oxygen requirements, the oxygen-sparing effects of decreased heart rate and

Table 19-1

Comparative Characteristics of β-Adrenergic Receptor Antagonists

	Propranolol	Nadolol	Pindolol	Timolol	Metoprolol	Atenolol	Acebutolol	Betaxolol	Esmolol
Cardiac selectivity	No	No	No	No	Yes	Yes	Yes	Yes	Yes
Partial agonist activity	No	No	Yes	No	No	No	Yes	No	No
Protein binding (%)	90–95	30	40–60	10	10	5	25		55
Clearance	Hepatic	Renal	Hepatic Renal	Hepatic	Hepatic	Renal	Hepatic Renal	Hepatic Renal	Plasma hydrolysis
Active metabolites	Yes	No	No	No	No	No	Yes		No
Elimination half-time (h)	2–3	20–24	3–4	3–4	3–4	6–7	3–4	11–22	0.15
First-pass hepatic metabolism (estimate) (%)	75	Minimal	10–15	50	60	10	60		
Blood level variability	+ + + +	+	+ +	+ + +	+ + + +	+	+ +		
Adult oral dose (mg)	40–360	40–320	5–20	10–30	50–400	50–200	200–800	10–20	
Adult intravenous dose (mg)	1–10		0.4–2	0.4–1	1–15	5–10	12.5–50		10–80 IV 50–300 μg/kg/min

+, minimal; + +, modest; + + +, moderate; + + + +, marked.

Table 19-2

Comparative Characteristics of β-Adrenergic Receptor Antagonists Effective in the Treatment of Congestive Heart Failure

	Metoprolol (Extended Release)	Carvedilol	Bisoprolol
Cardiac selectivity	Yes	No	Yes
Partial agonist activity	No	No	No
Initial oral dose[a]	6.25 mg twice daily	3.125 mg twice daily	1.25 mg daily
Desired dosage range[a]	50–150 mg daily	25–50 mg twice daily	5 mg daily

[a]Recommended doses for treatment of patients with mild to moderate congestive heart failure.

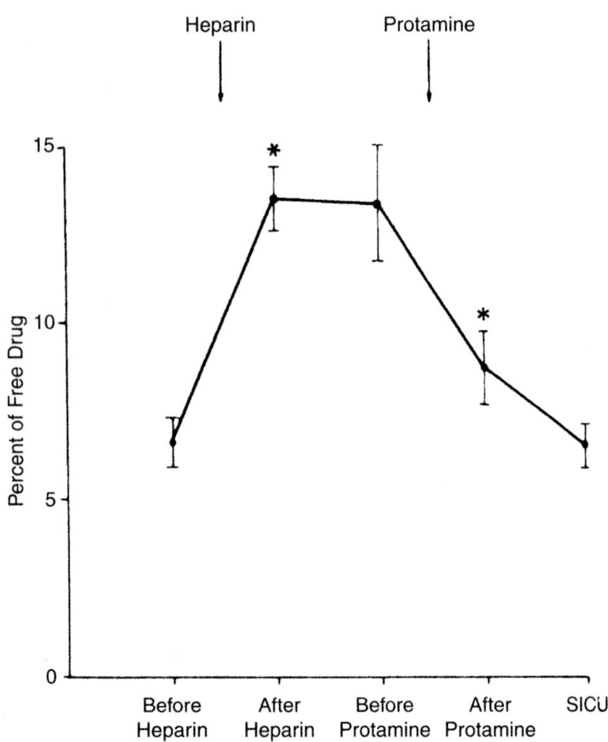

FIGURE 19-4 Heparin administration is associated with decreased plasma protein binding of propranolol manifesting as an increased plasma concentration of free (unbound) drug. (Mean ± SE; *P <.05.) SICU, surgical intensive care unit. (From Wood M, Shand DG, Wood AJ. Propranolol binding in plasma during cardiopulmonary bypass. *Anesthesiology*. 1979;51:512–516, with permission.)

myocardial contractility predominate. As a result, propranolol may relieve myocardial ischemia, even though drug-induced increases in coronary vascular resistance oppose coronary blood flow. Sodium retention associated with propranolol therapy most likely results from intrarenal hemodynamic changes that accompany drug-induced decreases in cardiac output.

Pharmacokinetics

Propranolol is rapidly and almost completely absorbed from the gastrointestinal tract, but systemic availability of the drug is limited by extensive hepatic first-pass metabolism, which may account for 90% to 95% of the absorbed dose. There is considerable individual variation in the magnitude of hepatic first-pass metabolism, accounting for up to 20-fold differences in plasma concentrations of propranolol in patients after oral administration of comparable doses.[3] Hepatic first-pass metabolism is the reason the oral dose of propranolol (40 to 800 mg per day) must be substantially greater than the IV dose (0.05 mg/kg given in increments of 0.5 to 1.0 mg every 5 minutes). Propranolol is not effective when administered intramuscularly.

Protein Binding

Propranolol is extensively bound (90% to 95%) to plasma proteins. Heparin-induced increases in plasma concentrations of free fatty acids due to increased lipoprotein lipase activity result in decreased plasma protein binding of propranolol (Fig. 19-4).[4] In addition, hemodilution that occurs when cardiopulmonary bypass is initiated may alter protein binding of drugs because of the nonphysiologic protein concentration in the pump prime.

Metabolism

Clearance of propranolol from the plasma is by hepatic metabolism. An active metabolite, 4-hydroxypropranolol, is detectable in the plasma after oral administration of propranolol. Indeed, cardiac β-blocking activity after equivalent doses of propranolol is greater after oral than after IV administration, presumably reflecting the effects of this metabolite, which is equivalent in activity to the parent compound. The elimination half-time of propranolol is 2 to 3 hours, whereas that of 4-hydroxypropranolol is even briefer. The plasma concentration of propranolol or the total dose does not correlate with its therapeutic effects. Furthermore, the assay for propranolol may not detect 4-hydroxypropranolol.

Elimination of propranolol is greatly decreased when hepatic blood flow decreases. In this regard, propranolol may decrease its own clearance rate by decreasing cardiac output and hepatic blood flow. Alterations in hepatic enzyme activity may also influence the rate of hepatic metabolism. Renal failure does not alter the elimination half-time of propranolol, but accumulation of metabolites may occur.

Clearance of Local Anesthetics

Propranolol decreases clearance of amide local anesthetics by decreasing hepatic blood flow and inhibiting metabolism in the liver.[5] For example, in humans, propranolol causes clearance to be decreased to a much greater extent (46%) than would be predicted from a maximum 25% decrease in hepatic blood flow, implying that drug metabolism in the liver has also been affected.[6] Bupivacaine clearance is relatively insensitive to changes in hepatic blood flow (low-extraction drug), suggesting that the 35% decrease in clearance of this local anesthetic reflects propranolol-induced decreases in metabolism (Fig. 19-5).[5] Because clearance of drugs with low extraction ratios is inversely related to plasma protein binding, an increase in bupivacaine binding to α_1-acid glycoprotein (responsible for 90% binding of bupivacaine) caused by propranolol could explain a decrease in clearance. Nevertheless, propranolol does not alter α_1-acid glycoprotein concentrations.[6] It is conceivable that systemic toxicity of bupivacaine could be increased by propranolol and presumably other β antagonists that interfere with the clearance of this and other amide local anesthetics.

Clearance of Opioids

Pulmonary first-pass uptake of fentanyl is substantially decreased in patients being treated chronically with propranolol.[7] As a result, two to four times as much injected fentanyl enters the systemic circulation in the time period immediately after injection. This response most likely reflects the ability of one basic lipophilic amine (propranolol) to inhibit the pulmonary uptake of a second basic lipophilic amine (fentanyl).

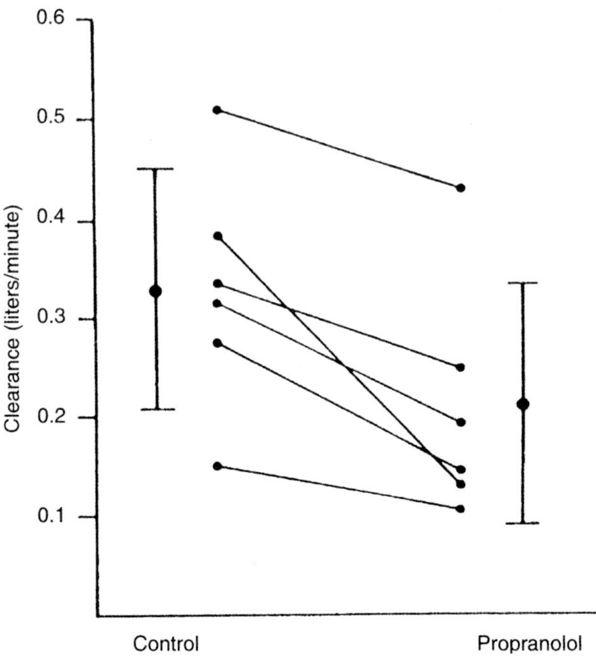

FIGURE 19-5 Bupivacaine clearance is decreased 35% in subjects treated with propranolol compared with control measurements. (From Bowdle TA, Freund PR, Slattery JT. Propranolol reduces bupivacaine clearance. *Anesthesiology.* 1987;66:36–38, with permission.)

Nadolol and Pindolol

Nadolol and pindolol are nonselective β-adrenergic receptor antagonists; nadolol is unique in that its long duration of action permits once daily administration.

Pharmacokinetics

Nadolol is slowly and incompletely absorbed (an estimated 30%) from the gastrointestinal tract. Metabolism does not occur, with about 75% of the drug being excreted unchanged in urine and the remainder in bile. Therefore, wide individual variations in plasma concentrations that occur with nadolol cannot be attributed to differences in metabolism, as occur with propranolol. The elimination half-time is 20 to 40 hours, accounting for the need to administer this drug only once a day. The elimination half-time of pindolol is 3 to 4 hours, and this is increased to longer than 11 hours in patients with renal failure.

Timolol

Timolol is a nonselective β-adrenergic receptor antagonist that is as effective as propranolol for various therapeutic indications. In addition, timolol is effective in the treatment of glaucoma because of its ability to decrease intraocular pressure, presumably by decreasing the production of aqueous humor. Timolol is administered as eyedrops in the treatment of glaucoma, but systemic absorption may be sufficient to cause resting bradycardia and increased airway resistance. Indeed, bradycardia and hypotension that are refractory to treatment with atropine have been observed during anesthesia in pediatric and adult patients receiving topical timolol with or without pilocarpine.[8] Timolol may be associated with impaired control of ventilation in neonates, resulting in unexpected postoperative apnea.[9] Immaturity of the neonate's blood–brain barrier may facilitate access of this drug to the CNS.

Pharmacokinetics

Timolol is rapidly and almost completely absorbed after oral administration. Nevertheless, extensive first-pass hepatic metabolism limits the amount of drug reaching the systemic circulation to about 50% of that absorbed from the gastrointestinal tract. Protein binding of timolol is not extensive. The elimination half-time is about 4 hours.

Metoprolol

Metoprolol is a selective β_1-adrenergic receptor antagonist that prevents inotropic and chronotropic responses to β-adrenergic stimulation. Conversely, bronchodilator, vasodilator, and metabolic effects of β_2 receptors remain intact such that metoprolol is less likely to cause adverse effects in patients with chronic obstructive airway disease or peripheral vascular disease and in patients vulnerable to hypoglycemia. It is important to recognize, however, that selectivity is dose related, and large doses of metoprolol are likely to become nonselective, exerting antagonist effects at β_2 receptors as well as β_1 receptors. Indeed, airway resistance may increase in asthmatic patients treated with metoprolol, although the magnitude of increase will be less than that evoked by propranolol. Furthermore, metoprolol-induced increases in airway resistance are more readily reversed with β_2-adrenergic agonists such as terbutaline.

Pharmacokinetics

Metoprolol is readily absorbed from the gastrointestinal tract, but this is offset by substantial hepatic first-pass metabolism such that only about 40% of the drug reaches the systemic circulation. Protein binding is low; it is estimated to account for about 10% of the drug. None of the hepatic metabolites have been identified as active. A small amount (<10%) of the drug appears unchanged in urine. There are two available oral formulation of metoprolol: metoprolol tartrate and metoprolol succinate. The elimination half-time of metoprolol tartrate is 2 to 3 hours and correlates to a need for at least a twice daily dosing strategy with a thrice daily or four times daily strategy providing a more reliable control of heart rate. Metoprolol succinate results in a significantly extended time to peak concentrations and overall decreased plasma concentrations compared to metoprolol tartrate at equal daily doses. Metoprolol succinate elimination half-time is 5 to 7 hours and can be used in once daily dosing regimens but in some patients can still result in β-blocker withdrawal tachycardia at 24 hours necessitating twice daily dosing. Overall, plasma concentrations of metoprolol do not correlate with therapeutic effects of the drug.

Atenolol

Atenolol is the most selective β_1-adrenergic antagonist that may have specific value in patients in whom the continued presence of β_2 receptor activity is desirable. In patients at risk for coronary artery disease who must undergo noncardiac surgery, treatment with IV atenolol before and immediately after surgery, followed by oral therapy during the remainder of the hospitalization, decreases mortality and the incidence of cardiovascular complications for as long as 2 years.[10] Perioperative administration of atenolol to patients at high risk for coronary artery disease significantly decreases the incidence of postoperative myocardial ischemia.[11]

The antihypertensive effect of atenolol is prolonged, permitting this drug to be administered once daily for the treatment of hypertension. Like nadolol, atenolol does not enter the CNS in large amounts, but fatigue and mental depression still occur. Unlike nonselective β-adrenergic antagonists, atenolol does not appear to potentiate insulin-induced hypoglycemia and can thus be administered with caution to patients with diabetes mellitus whose hypertension is not controlled by other antihypertensives.

Pharmacokinetics

About 50% of an orally administered dose of atenolol is absorbed from the gastrointestinal tract, with peak concentrations occurring 1 to 2 hours after oral administration. Atenolol undergoes little or no hepatic metabolism and is eliminated principally by renal excretion. The elimination half-time is 6 to 7 hours; this may increase to more than 24 hours in patients with renal failure. Therapeutic plasma concentrations of atenolol are 200 to 500 ng/mL.

Betaxolol

Betaxolol is a cardioselective β_1-adrenergic antagonist with no intrinsic sympathomimetic activity and weak membrane-stabilizing activity. High doses can be expected to produce some β_2-adrenergic antagonist effects on bronchial and vascular smooth muscle. Absorption after an oral dose is nearly complete. Its elimination half-time is 11 to 22 hours, making it one of the longest acting β-adrenergic antagonists. Clearance is primarily by metabolism, with renal elimination contributing less to overall removal of the drug from the plasma. A single oral dose daily is useful for the treatment of hypertension. A topical preparation is used as an alternative to timolol for treatment of chronic open-angle glaucoma. The risk of bronchoconstriction in patients with airway hyperreactivity may be less with betaxolol than with timolol.

Bisoprolol

Bisoprolol is a β_1 selective antagonist drug without significant intrinsic agonist activity. The elimination half-time is 9 to 12 hours. Bisoprolol is eliminated equally by renal and nonrenal mechanisms. Metabolites are pharmacologically inactive. The most prominent pharmacologic effect of bisoprolol is a negative chronotropic effect. Bisoprolol is useful in the treatment of essential hypertension and has been shown to improve survival in patients with mild to moderate congestive heart failure (see Table 19-2).

Nebivolol

Nebivolol is a very potent and selective β_1-antagonist drug[12] and is 3.5 times more selective than bisoprolol[13] without significant intrinsic agonist activity. Above doses of 10 mg, or in those patients with certain CYP polymorphisms, Nebivolol can exhibit low β_2 antagonism as well. With an elimination half-time of 12 to 19 hours, it is a once daily regimen that allows accidental delay in subsequent doses without withdrawal. Nebivolol is equally eliminated in the urine unchanged and in the feces as a inactive metabolite. The most prominent pharmacologic effect of bisoprolol is a negative chronotropic effect and is currently approved and useful in the treatment of essential hypertension.

Esmolol

Esmolol is a rapid-onset and short-acting selective β_1-adrenergic receptor antagonist that is administered only IV (see Fig. 19-3). After a typical initial dose of 0.5 mg/kg IV over about 60 seconds, the full therapeutic effect is evident within 5 minutes, and its action ceases within 10 to 30 minutes after administration is discontinued. These characteristics make esmolol a useful drug for preventing or treating adverse systemic blood pressure and heart rate increases that occur intraoperatively in response to noxious stimulation, as during tracheal intubation. For example, esmolol, 150 mg IV, administered about 2 minutes before direct laryngoscopy and tracheal intubation provides reliable protection against increases in both heart rate and systolic blood pressure, which predictably accompanies tracheal intubation (Fig. 19-6).[14]

Lidocaine or fentanyl is effective in blunting the increase in systolic blood pressure associated with laryngoscopy and tracheal intubation, but heart rate is not influenced (see Fig. 19-6).[14] Other reports describe prevention of perioperative tachycardia and hypertension with esmolol, 100 to 200 mg IV, administered over 15 seconds before the induction of anesthesia.[15,16] Prior administration of esmolol, 500 μg/kg/minute IV, to patients undergoing electroconvulsive therapy with anesthesia induced by methohexital plus succinylcholine results in attenuation of the heart rate increase and a decrease in the length of the electrically induced seizures.[17] Esmolol has been used during resection of pheochromocytoma and may be useful in the perioperative management of thyrotoxicosis, pregnancy-induced hypertension, and epinephrine- or cocaine-induced cardiovascular toxicity.[18–22] Conversely, treatment of excessive sympathetic nervous system activity produced by cocaine or systemic absorption of topical or subcutaneous epinephrine with β-adrenergic receptor antagonists has been associated with fulminant pulmonary edema and irreversible cardiovascular collapse.[23] It is possible that acute drug-induced β-receptor antagonism removes the ability of the heart to increase heart rate and myocardial contractility to compensate for catecholamine-induced increases in left ventricular afterload. In this regard, persistent symptomatic systemic hypertension owing to catecholamine-induced sympathetic nervous system stimulation is more safely treated with a peripheral vasodilator drug such as sodium nitroprusside or nitroglycerin. Detrimental effects of catecholamine release during anesthesia in patients with hypertrophic obstructive cardiomyopathy and in patients experiencing hypercyanotic spells associated with tetralogy of Fallot may be blunted by administration of esmolol.[24]

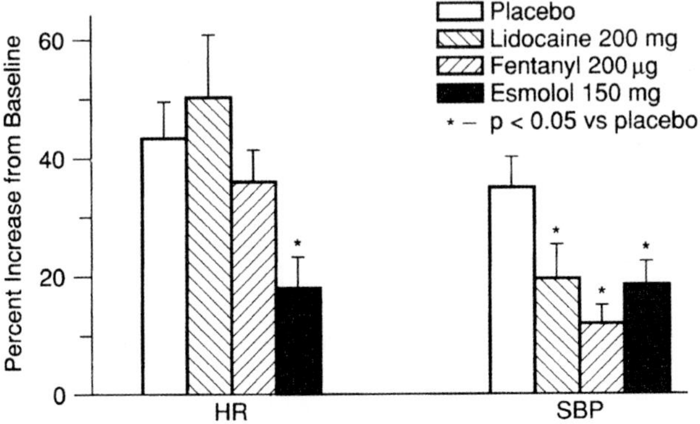

FIGURE 19-6 Maximum percent increases in heart rate (HR) and systolic blood pressure (SBP) after induction of anesthesia and direct laryngoscopy with tracheal intubation in patients pretreated with saline, lidocaine, fentanyl, or esmolol. All three drugs blunt the increase in SBP, but only esmolol is also effective in attenuating the increase in HR. (From Helfman SM, Gold MI, DeLisser EA, et al. Which drug prevents tachycardia and hypertension associated with tracheal intubation: lidocaine, fentanyl, or esmolol? *Anesth Analg.* 1991;72:482–486, with permission.)

The β_1 selectivity of esmolol may unmask β_2-mediated vasodilation by epinephrine-secreting tumors. Administration of esmolol to patients chronically treated with β-adrenergic antagonists has not been observed to produce additional negative inotropic effects.[25] The presumed reason for this observation is that esmolol, in the dose used, does not occupy sufficient additional β receptors to produce detectable increases in β blockade. Likewise, esmolol infused during cardiopulmonary bypass is not associated with adverse effects after discontinuation of cardiopulmonary bypass.[26]

Esmolol (1 mg/kg IV followed by 250 μg/kg/minute V) significantly decreases the plasma concentration of propofol required to prevent patient movement in response to a surgical skin incision.[27] This effect does not seem to be explained by a pharmacokinetic interaction between the two drugs.

Pharmacokinetics

Esmolol is available for IV administration only. The only other β-adrenergic antagonists that may be administered IV are propranolol and metoprolol. The commercial preparation of esmolol is buffered to pH 4.5 to 5.5, which may be one of the factors responsible for pain on injection. The drug is compatible with commonly used IV solutions and nondepolarizing neuromuscular blocking drugs. The elimination half-time of esmolol is about 9 minutes, reflecting its rapid hydrolysis in the blood by plasma esterases that is independent of renal and hepatic function.[28] Less than 1% of the drug is excreted unchanged in urine, and about 75% is recovered as an inactive acid metabolite. Clinically insignificant amounts of methanol also occur from the hydrolysis of esmolol. Plasma esterases responsible for the hydrolysis of esmolol are distinct from plasma cholinesterase, and the duration of action of succinylcholine is not predictably prolonged in patients treated with esmolol.[29] Evidence of the short duration of action of esmolol is return of the heart rate to predrug levels within 15 minutes after discontinuing the drug. Indeed, plasma concentrations of esmolol are usually not detectable 15 minutes after discontinuing the drug. Poor lipid solubility limits transfer of esmolol into the CNS or across the placenta.[19]

Side Effects

The side effects of β-adrenergic antagonists are similar for all available drugs, although the magnitude may differ depending on their selectivity and the presence or absence of intrinsic sympathomimetic activity. β-Adrenergic antagonists exert their most prominent pharmacologic effects as well as side effects on the cardiovascular system. These drugs may also alter airway resistance, carbohydrate and lipid metabolism, and the distribution of extracellular ions. β-Adrenergic antagonists may cause hypoglycemia.[30] Additive effects between drugs used for anesthesia and β-adrenergic antagonists may occur. β-Adrenergic antagonists penetrate the blood–brain barrier and cross the placenta. Gastrointestinal side effects include nausea, vomiting, and diarrhea. Fever, rash, myopathy, alopecia, and thrombocytopenia have been associated with chronic β-adrenergic antagonist treatment. β-Adrenergic antagonists have been reported to decrease plasma concentrations of high-density lipoproteins and to increase triglyceride and uric acid levels.

The principal contraindication to administration of β-adrenergic antagonists is preexisting atrioventricular heart block or cardiac failure not caused by tachycardia. Administration of β-adrenergic antagonists to hypovolemic patients with compensatory tachycardia may produce profound hypotension.[31] Nonselective β-adrenergic antagonists or high doses of selective β-adrenergic antagonists are not recommended for administration to patients with chronic obstructive airway disease. In patients with diabetes mellitus, there is the risk that β-adrenergic blockade may mask the signs of hyperglycemia and thus delay its clinical recognition.

Cardiovascular System

β-Adrenergic antagonists produce negative inotropic and chronotropic effects. In addition, the conduction speed of cardiac impulses through the atrioventricular node is slowed and the rate of spontaneous phase 4 depolarization is decreased. Preexisting atrioventricular heart block due to any cause may be accentuated by β-adrenergic antagonists.

The cardiovascular effects of β-adrenergic blockade reflect removal of sympathetic nervous system innervation to the heart (β_1 blockade) and not membrane stabilization, which occurs only at high plasma concentrations of the antagonist drug. In addition, nonselective β-adrenergic blockade resulting in β_2-adrenergic receptor antagonism may impede left ventricular ejection due to unopposed α-adrenergic receptor–mediated peripheral vasoconstriction. The magnitude of cardiovascular effects produced by β-adrenergic antagonists is greatest when preexisting sympathetic nervous system activity is increased, as during exercise or in patients in cardiac failure. Indeed, the tachycardia of exercise is consistently attenuated by β-adrenergic antagonists. Furthermore, administration of a β antagonist may precipitate cardiac failure in a patient who was previously compensated. Resting bradycardia is minimized and cardiac failure is less likely to occur when a partial β-adrenergic antagonist with intrinsic sympathomimetic activity is administered. Acute cardiac failure is rare with oral administration of β-adrenergic antagonists.

Classically, β-adrenergic antagonists prevent inotropic and chronotropic effects of isoproterenol as well as baroreceptor-mediated increases in heart rate evoked by decreases in systemic blood pressure in response to peripheral vasodilator drugs. Conversely, the influence of β-adrenergic antagonists on the cardiac-stimulating effects of calcium, glucagon, and digitalis preparations is not detectable. Likewise, β-adrenergic antagonists do not alter the response to α-adrenergic agonists such as epinephrine or phenylephrine. Indeed, the pressor effect of epinephrine is enhanced because the nonselective β antagonists prevent the β_2 vasodilating effect of epinephrine and leave unopposed its α-adrenergic effect. The presence of unopposed α-adrenergic–induced vasoconstriction may provoke paradoxical hypertension and may even precipitate cardiac failure in the presence of diseased myocardium that cannot respond to sympathetic nervous system stimulation because of β-adrenergic blockade. Unexpected hypertension has occurred in patients receiving clonidine who subsequently receive a nonselective β-adrenergic antagonist.[32] Presumably, blockade of the vasodilating effect normally produced by activity of β_2 receptors leaves unopposed α-adrenergic effects to provoke peripheral vasoconstriction with resulting hypertension.

Patients with peripheral vascular disease do not tolerate well the peripheral vasoconstriction associated with β_2 receptor blockade produced by nonselective β-adrenergic antagonists. Indeed, the development of cold hands and feet is a common side effect of β blockade. Vasospasm associated with Raynaud's disease is accentuated by propranolol.

The principal antidysrhythmic effect of β-adrenergic blockade is to prevent the dysrhythmogenic effect of endogenous or exogenous catecholamines or sympathomimetics. This reflects a decrease in sympathetic nervous system activity. Membrane stabilization is probably of little importance in the antidysrhythmic effects produced by usual doses of β-adrenergic antagonists.

Treatment of Excess Myocardial Depression

The usual clinical manifestations of excessive myocardial depression produced by β-adrenergic blockade include bradycardia, low cardiac output, hypotension, and cardiogenic shock.[33] Bronchospasm and depression of ventilation may also be associated with an overdose of β-adrenergic antagonist drugs. Seizures and prolonged intraventricular conduction of cardiac impulses are thought to be the result of local anesthetic properties of certain β-adrenergic antagonists (see Table 19-1). Hypoglycemia is a rare manifestation of β-adrenergic antagonist overdose.

Excessive bradycardia and/or decreases in cardiac output due to drug-induced β blockade should be treated initially with atropine in incremental doses of 7 μg/kg IV. Atropine is likely to be effective by blocking vagal effects on the heart and thus unmasking any residual sympathetic nervous system innervation. If atropine is ineffective, drugs to produce direct positive chronotropic and inotropic effects are indicated. For example, continuous infusion of the nonselective β-adrenergic agonist isoproterenol, in doses sufficient to overcome competitive β blockade, is appropriate. The necessary dose of isoproterenol may be 2 to 25 μg per minute IV (60 μg per minute IV was not effective in one report), which is 5 to 20 times the necessary dose in the absence of β blockade.[33] When a pure β-adrenergic antagonist is responsible for excessive cardiovascular depression, a pure β_1-adrenergic agonist such as dobutamine is recommended because isoproterenol, with β_1- and β_2-adrenergic agonist effects, could produce vasodilation before its inotropic effect develops. Dopamine is not recommended because α-adrenergic–induced vasoconstriction is likely to occur with the high doses required to overcome β blockade.

Glucagon administered to adults, 1 to 10 mg IV followed by 5 mg per hour IV, effectively reverses myocardial depression produced by β-adrenergic antagonists at normal doses because these drugs do not exert their effects by means of β-adrenergic receptors. For example, glucagon stimulates adenylate cyclase and increases intracellular cAMP concentrations independent of β-adrenergic receptors.[33] Calcium chloride, 250 to 1,000 mg IV, may also act independent of β-adrenergic receptors to offset excessive cardiovascular depression produced by β-adrenergic antagonists. Glucagon appears to be particularly effective in the presence of life-threatening bradycardia and has been described as the drug of choice to treat massive β-adrenergic antagonist overdose.[33]

In the presence of bradycardia that is unresponsive to pharmacologic therapy, it may be necessary to place a transvenous artificial cardiac pacemaker. Hemodialysis should be reserved to remove minimally protein-bound, renally excreted β-adrenergic antagonists in patients refractory to pharmacologic therapy.

Airway Resistance

Nonselective β-adrenergic antagonists such as propranolol consistently increase airway resistance as a manifestation of bronchoconstriction due to blockade of β_2 receptors. These airway resistance effects are exaggerated in patients with preexisting obstructive airway disease. Because bronchodilation is a β_2-adrenergic agonist response, selective β_1-adrenergic antagonists such as metoprolol and esmolol are less likely than propranolol to increase airway resistance.

Metabolism

β-Adrenergic antagonists alter carbohydrate and fat metabolism. For example, nonselective β-adrenergic antagonists such as propranolol interfere with glycogenolysis that ordinarily occurs in response to release of epinephrine during hypoglycemia. This emphasizes the need for β_2 receptor activity in glycogenolysis. Furthermore, tachycardia, which is an important warning sign of hypoglycemia in insulin-treated diabetics, is blunted by β-adrenergic antagonists. For this reason, nonselective β-adrenergic antagonists are not recommended for administration to patients with diabetes mellitus who may be at risk for developing hypoglycemia because of treatment with insulin or oral hypoglycemics. Altered fat metabolism is evidenced by failure of sympathomimetics or sympathetic nervous system stimulation to increase plasma concentrations of fatty-free acids in the presence of β-adrenergic blockade.

Distribution of Extracellular Potassium

Distribution of potassium across cell membranes is influenced by sympathetic nervous system activity as well as insulin. Specifically, stimulation of β_2-adrenergic receptors seems to facilitate movement of potassium intracellularly. As a result, β-adrenergic blockade inhibits uptake of potassium into skeletal muscles, and the plasma concentration of potassium may be increased. Indeed, increases in the plasma concentration of potassium associated with infusion of this ion are greater in the presence of β-adrenergic blockade produced by propranolol (Fig. 19-7).[34] In animals, increases in the plasma concentration of potassium after administration of succinylcholine last longer when β-adrenergic blockade is present.[35] In view of the speculated role of β_2 receptors in regulating plasma concentrations of potassium, it is likely that selective β_1-adrenergic antagonists would impair skeletal muscle uptake of potassium less than nonselective β-adrenergic antagonists.

Interaction with Anesthetics

Myocardial depression produced by inhaled or injected anesthetics could be additive with depression produced by β-adrenergic antagonists. Nevertheless, clinical experience and controlled studies in patients and animals have confirmed that additive myocardial depression with β-adrenergic antagonists and anesthetics is not excessive,

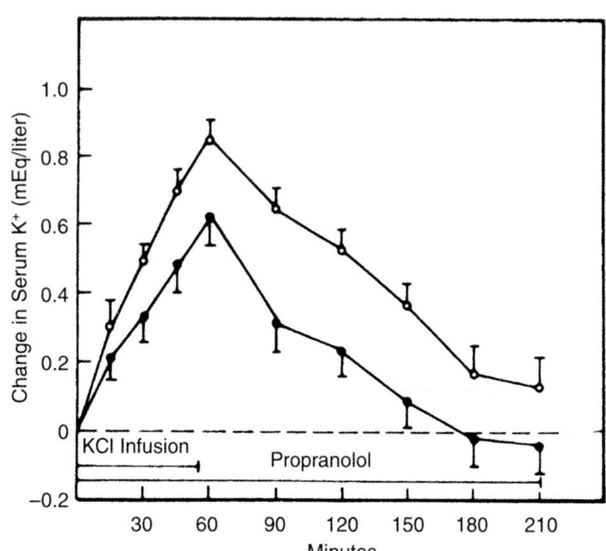

FIGURE 19-7 Increases in plasma (serum) potassium concentration (K^+) in response to infusion of potassium chloride (KCl) are greater in the presence of propranolol (*clear circles*) than in its absence (*solid circles*). Mean ± SE. (From Rosa RM, Silva P, Young JB, et al. Adrenergic modulation of extrarenal potassium disposal. *N Engl J Med.* 1980;302:431–434, with permission.)

and treatment with β-adrenergic antagonists may therefore be safely maintained throughout the perioperative period.[1] An exception may be patients treated with timolol in whom profound bradycardia has been observed in the presence of inhaled anesthetics.

Additive cardiovascular effects with inhaled anesthetics and β-adrenergic antagonists seem to be greatest with enflurane and least with isoflurane.[1] Sevoflurane and desflurane, like isoflurane, do not seem to be associated with significant additive cardiovascular effects when administered to patients being treated with β-adrenergic antagonists. Cardiac output and systemic blood pressure are similar with or without β-adrenergic blockade in the presence of one or two minimum alveolar concentration isoflurane.[36] Even acute hemorrhage does not alter the interaction between isoflurane and β-adrenergic antagonists.[37,38] In contrast, cardiac depression is more likely to occur in the presence of β blockade when acute hemorrhage occurs in animals anesthetized with enflurane.[39] Cardiovascular responses to even high doses of opioids such as fentanyl are not altered by preexisting β-adrenergic blockade. In the presence of anesthetic drugs that increase sympathetic nervous system activity (ketamine), or when excessive sympathetic nervous system activity is present because of hypercarbia, the acute administration of a β-adrenergic antagonist may unmask direct negative inotropic effects of concomitantly administered anesthetics, with resulting decreases in systemic blood pressure and cardiac output.[40]

Nervous System

β-Adrenergic antagonists may cross the blood–brain barrier to produce side effects. For example, fatigue and lethargy are commonly associated with chronic propranolol therapy. Vivid dreams are frequent, but psychotic reactions are rare. Memory loss and mental depression have been alleged to occur, although β-adrenergic antagonist therapy has not been shown to produce these effects.[41] Peripheral paresthesias have been described. Atenolol and nadolol are less lipid soluble than other β-adrenergic antagonists and thus may be associated with a lower incidence of CNS effects.

Fetus

β-Adrenergic antagonists can cross the placenta and cause bradycardia, hypotension, and hypoglycemia in newborn infants of mothers who are receiving the drug. Breast milk is also likely to contain β-adrenergic antagonists administered to the mother.

Withdrawal Hypersensitivity

Acute discontinuation of β-adrenergic antagonist therapy can result in excess sympathetic nervous system activity that manifests in 24 to 48 hours. Presumably, this enhanced activity reflects an increase in the number of β-adrenergic receptors (upregulation) during chronic therapy with β-adrenergic antagonists. Continuous infusion of propranolol, 3 mg per hour IV, is effective in maintaining therapeutic plasma concentrations in adult patients who cannot take drugs orally during the perioperative period.[42]

Clinical Uses

Clinical uses of β-adrenergic antagonists are multiple and in equivalent doses, all β-adrenergic antagonists seem to be equally effective in producing desired therapeutic effects (Table 19-3). It is accepted that patients being treated with β-adrenergic receptor antagonists should have their medication continued uninterrupted through the perioperative period. It is also recommended that patients at high risk for myocardial ischemia and presenting for major surgery should be treated with β-adrenergic receptor antagonists beginning preoperatively and continuing into the postoperative period.

Treatment of Essential Hypertension

Chronic therapy with β-adrenergic antagonists results in gradual decreases in systemic blood pressure. The antihypertensive effect of β-adrenergic blockade is largely dependent on decreases in cardiac output due to decreased heart rate. Large doses of β-adrenergic antagonists may decrease myocardial contractility as well. In many patients, systemic vascular resistance remains unchanged. An important advantage in the use of β-adrenergic antagonists for the treatment of essential hypertension is the absence of orthostatic hypotension. Often, a β-adrenergic antagonist is used in combination with a vasodilator to minimize reflex baroreceptor–mediated increases in heart rate and cardiac output produced by the vasodilator. All orally administered β-adrenergic antagonists appear to be equally effective antihypertensive drugs. Release of renin from the juxtaglomerular apparatus that occurs in response to stimulation of β_2 receptors is prevented by nonselective β-adrenergic antagonists such as propranolol. This may account for a portion of the antihypertensive effect of propranolol, especially in patients with high circulating plasma concentrations of renin. Because drug-induced decreases in secretion of renin will lead to decreased

Table 19-3

Clinical Uses of β-Adrenergic Blockers

Treatment of essential hypertension
Management of angina pectoris
Treatment of acute coronary syndrome
Perioperative β-adrenergic receptor blockade
Treatment of intraoperative myocardial ischemia
Suppression of cardiac dysrhythmias
Management of congestive heart failure
Prevention of excessive sympathetic nervous system activity
Preoperative preparation of hyperthyroid patients
Treatment of migraine headache

release of aldosterone, β-adrenergic antagonists will also prevent the compensatory sodium and water retention that accompanies treatment with a vasodilator.

Management of Angina Pectoris

Orally administered β-adrenergic antagonists are equally effective in decreasing the likelihood of myocardial ischemia manifesting as angina pectoris. This desirable response reflects drug-induced decreases in myocardial oxygen requirements secondary to decreased heart rate and myocardial contractility. The effective dose usually decreases resting heart rate to less than 60 beats per minute. A more important measure is the heart rate during exercise, which should not exceed 75% of the heart rate at which myocardial ischemia occurs.

The concept that β-adrenergic antagonists and calcium channel blockers act on different determinants of the myocardial oxygen supply-to-demand ratio suggests combined uses of these drugs would be beneficial in the management of patients with coronary artery disease. Nevertheless, the evidence from clinical studies suggests that patients managed with combined therapy do not experience greater beneficial therapeutic effects but may experience more adverse effects than if they had received optimal treatment with a single drug.[43]

Treatment of Acute Coronary Syndrome

It is recommended that all patients who experience an acute myocardial infarction receive IV β-adrenergic antagonists (assuming no contraindications are present) as early as possible, whether or not they receive reperfusion therapy. Treatment with β-adrenergic antagonists is contraindicated in the presence of severe bradycardia, unstable left ventricular failure, and atrioventricular heart block. Relative contraindications to treatment with β-adrenergic antagonists include asthma or reactive airway disease, mental depression, and peripheral vascular disease. Diabetes mellitus is not a contraindication to treatment with β-adrenergic antagonists recognizing that signs of hypoglycemia may be masked.

A growing body of literature is rising against the use of β blockers in patients who present with an acute coronary syndrome within the first 8 hours, especially if they present with ST elevation myocardial infarction (STEMI) or in cardiogenic shock.[44] STEMI patients had a greater risk of developing cardiogenic shock after β-blocker administration and those in shock had a greater risk of decompensating even further.[45] However, the incidence of nonfatal reinfarction and recurrent myocardial ischemia is decreased compared with patients in whom oral metoprolol was initiated 6 days following myocardial infarction.[46] β-Adrenergic antagonist prophylaxis after acute myocardial infarction is considered to be one of the most scientifically substantiated, cost-effective preventive medical treatments. Whether β-adrenergic antagonists can decrease mortality in patients with angina pectoris who have not yet experienced a myocardial infarction is unknown.

The cardioprotective effect of β-adrenergic antagonists is present with both cardioselective and nonselective drugs (see Tables 19-1 and 19-2). The mechanism of the cardioprotective effect is uncertain, but antidysrhythmic actions may be important. A nonselective β-adrenergic antagonist that prevents epinephrine-induced decreases in plasma potassium concentrations (a β_2-mediated response) may be useful in decreasing the incidence of ventricular dysrhythmias.

Perioperative β-Adrenergic Receptor Blockade

Perioperative β-adrenergic receptor blockade is recommended for patients considered at risk for myocardial ischemia (known coronary artery disease, positive preoperative stress tests, diabetes mellitus treated with insulin, left ventricular hypertrophy) during high-risk surgery (vascular surgery, thoracic surgery, intraperitoneal surgery, anticipated large blood loss).[47,48] The goal of preoperative therapy is a resting heart rate between 65 and 80 beats per minute.[49] All β-adrenergic receptor antagonists except those with intrinsic sympathetic nervous system activity decrease mortality. Perioperative myocardial ischemia is the single most important potentially reversible risk factor for mortality and cardiovascular complications after noncardiac surgery. Administration of atenolol for 7 days before and after noncardiac surgery in patients at risk for coronary artery disease may decrease mortality and the incidence of cardiovascular complications for as long as 2 years after surgery.[10] In another report, administration of atenolol IV before induction of anesthesia and every 12 hours after noncardiac surgery for 7 days to patients at high risk for coronary artery disease reduced the incidence of postoperative myocardial ischemia by 30% to 50%.[11] Decreases in perioperative myocardial ischemia are associated with reductions in the risk for death at 24 months. The incidence of bronchospasm, hypotension, bradycardia, and cardiac dysrhythmias was not increased in treated patients. The mechanism for the beneficial effects of perioperative β-adrenergic receptor blockade is not known but is most likely multifactorial (Table 19-4). It is not known if patients with cardiac risk factors but no signs of underlying coronary artery disease will benefit from perioperative administration of a β-adrenergic antagonist.[50]

Preoperatively, oral therapy can be initiated with atenolol 50 mg or bisoprolol 5 to 10 mg daily or metoprolol 25 to 50 mg twice daily. If the patient is seen the morning of surgery, atenolol 5 to 10 mg IV or metoprolol 5 to 10 mg IV can be titrated. Esmolol is an acceptable drug to achieve β-adrenergic receptor blockade during surgery and postoperatively in the intensive care unit where continuous IV infusions can be monitored. Alternatively, IV atenolol or metoprolol can be administered until the patient can take oral atenolol or bisoprolol. β-adrenergic receptor antagonists with sympathomimetic actions are not likely selections to produce perioperative β blockade. The Perioperative Ischemic Evaluation (POISE) trial has raised concerns over regimens that start β blockers in the acute preoperative setting due to an

Table 19-4

Possible Explanations for Cardioprotective Effects Produced by Perioperative β-Adrenergic Receptor Blockade

Decreased myocardial oxygen consumption and demand
Less stress on potentially ischemic myocardium owing to decreased heart rate and myocardial contractility
Attenuation of effects of endogenous catecholamines
Redistribution of coronary blood flow to ischemic areas
Increased coronary blood flow owing to increased diastolic time
Plaque stabilization owing to decrease in shear forces
Cardiac antidysrhythmic effects
Antiinflammatory effects (?)

all-cause increased mortality that is driven by an increase in cerebrovascular events. Criticisms of the POISE trial[51] point to its very aggressive escalation regimen (as much as 400 mg metoprolol succinate dosed in 24 hours) without regard to patient's baseline hemodynamics (systolic and mean pressure reductions of >30% below preoperative levels) which is well known to cause cerebrovascular hypoperfusion and infarction. This has prompted many practitioners to only start low-dose β-blocker regimens in the preoperative period or to hold initiation until postoperatively.

Treatment of Intraoperative Myocardial Ischemia

Appearance of evidence of myocardial ischemia on the electrocardiogram or as wall motion abnormalities on the transesophageal echocardiogram may benefit from treatment with a β-adrenergic receptor blocking drug, assuming the absence of contraindications (severe reactive airway disease, shock, left ventricular failure) and the presence of an adequate concentration of inhaled anesthetic drugs. The drug selected should be titrated IV to the desired heart rate (about 60 beats per minute) to attenuate myocardial ischemia. Treatment options include esmolol (1 to 1.5 mg/kg IV followed by a continuous infusion of 50 to 300 μg/kg/minute), metoprolol (5 mg IV), atenolol (5 to 10 mg IV), or propranolol (1 to 10 mg IV). The advantage of esmolol is the ability to titrate its effects to the desired heart rate. Nitroglycerin is often added to this treatment regimen.

Suppression of Cardiac Dysrhythmias

β-Adrenergic receptor blocking drugs are effective in the treatment of cardiac dysrhythmias as a result of enhanced sympathetic nervous system stimulation (thyrotoxicosis, pheochromocytoma, perioperative stress). Esmolol and propranolol are effective for controlling the ventricular response rate to atrial fibrillation and atrial flutter. These drugs are also effective for controlling atrial dysrhythmias following cardiac surgery. Propranolol may be effective for controlling torsades de pointes in patients with prolonged QTc intervals on the electrocardiogram. Acebutolol, metoprolol, atenolol, propranolol, and timolol are approved for prevention of sudden death following acute myocardial infarction.

Management of Congestive Heart Failure

Controlled studies have demonstrated that metoprolol, carvedilol, and bisoprolol improve ejection fraction and increase survival in patients in chronic heart failure (see Table 19-2). Sustained-release metoprolol is associated with improved survival.[52] Carvedilol, a nonselective β blocker with vasodilator and antioxidant properties, has been shown to decrease mortality associated with congestive heart failure.[53] When β blocking drugs are used to treat congestive heart failure, the initial doses of β blockers should be minimal and gradually increased.

Prevention of Excessive Sympathetic Nervous System Activity

β-Adrenergic blockade is associated with attenuated heart rate and blood pressure changes in response to direct laryngoscopy and tracheal intubation.[1,54] Hypertrophic obstructive cardiomyopathies are often treated with β-adrenergic antagonists. Tachycardia and cardiac dysrhythmias associated with pheochromocytoma and hyperthyroidism are effectively suppressed by propranolol. The likelihood of cyanotic episodes in patients with tetralogy of Fallot is minimized by β blockade. Propranolol has been used intraoperatively to prevent reflex baroreceptor–mediated increases in heart rate evoked by vasodilators administered to produce controlled hypotension. Even anxiety states as caused by public speaking have been treated with propranolol.

Preoperative Preparation of Hyperthyroid Patients

Thyrotoxic patients can be prepared for surgery in an emergency by IV administration of propranolol or esmolol or electively by oral administration of propranolol (40 to 320 mg daily).[55,56] Advantages of β-adrenergic antagonists include rapid suppression of excessive sympathetic nervous system activity and elimination of the need to administer iodine or antithyroid drugs.

Combined α- and β-Adrenergic Receptor Antagonists

Labetalol

Labetalol is a unique parenteral and oral antihypertensive drug that exhibits selective α_1- and nonselective β_1- and β_2-adrenergic antagonist effects (Fig. 19-8).[57,58] Presynaptic α_2 receptors are spared by labetalol such that released norepinephrine can continue to inhibit further release of catecholamines via the negative feedback mechanism resulting from stimulation of α_2 receptors. Labetalol is

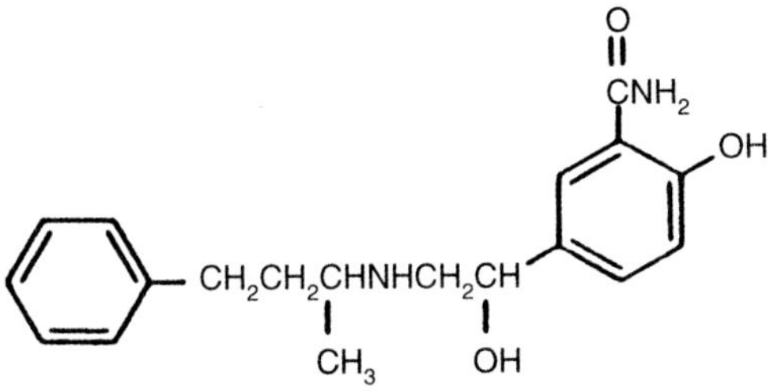

$$\text{C}_6\text{H}_5-\text{CH}_2\text{CH}_2\text{CH}(\text{CH}_3)\text{NHCH}_2\text{CH}(\text{OH})-\text{C}_6\text{H}_3(\text{OH})(\text{CNH}_2{=}\text{O})$$

FIGURE 19-8 Labetalol.

one-fifth to one-tenth as potent as phentolamine in its ability to block α receptors and is approximately one-fourth to one-third as potent as propranolol in blocking β receptors. In humans, the β to α blocking potency ratio is 3:1 for oral labetalol and 7:1 for IV labetalol.

Pharmacokinetics

Metabolism of labetalol is by conjugation of glucuronic acid, with 5% of the drug recovered unchanged in urine. The elimination half-time is 5 to 8 hours and is prolonged in the presence of liver disease and unchanged by renal dysfunction.

Cardiovascular Effects

Administration of labetalol lowers systemic blood pressure by decreasing systemic vascular resistance (α_1 blockade), whereas reflex tachycardia triggered by vasodilation is attenuated by simultaneous β blockade. Cardiac output remains unchanged. In addition to producing vasodilation by α_1 blockade, labetalol may cause vasodilation that is mediated by β_2-adrenergic agonist activity.[59] The maximum systemic blood pressure–lowering effect of an IV dose of labetalol (0.1 to 0.5 mg/kg) is present in 5 to 10 minutes.

Clinical Uses

Labetalol is a safe and effective treatment for hypertensive emergencies. For example, labetalol has been administered IV to control severe hypertension that may be associated with an epinephrine overdose as may occur during submucosal injection to produce surgical hemostasis.[60] Conversely, caution has been urged in using β-adrenergic blockers to treat phenylephrine and epinephrine overdose resulting from systemic absorption following topical application.[21] Large bolus doses of labetalol (2 mg/kg IV) administered to treat hypertensive emergencies may result in excessive decreases in blood pressure, whereas smaller doses (20 to 80 mg IV) are less likely to produce undesirable decreases in blood pressure.[61,62] Repeated doses of labetalol, 20 to 80 mg IV, may be administered about every 10 minutes until the desired therapeutic response is achieved.[62] Rebound hypertension after withdrawal of clonidine therapy and hypertensive responses in patients with pheochromocytoma can be effectively treated with labetalol. Labetalol is also effective in the treatment of angina pectoris. Availability of both an oral (100 to 600 mg twice a day) and IV preparation is useful for converting a patient with a hypertensive crisis to oral therapy after initial control with IV therapy.

Labetalol, 0.1 to 0.5 mg/kg IV, can be administered to anesthetized patients to attenuate increases in heart rate and blood pressure that are presumed to result from abrupt increases in the level of surgical stimulation. It is possible that existing depressant effects of the anesthetic drugs could accentuate the blood pressure–lowering properties of labetalol. In contrast to the results with nitroprusside, controlled hypotension produced with intermittent injections of labetalol, 10 mg IV, is not associated with increases in heart rate, intrapulmonary shunt, or cardiac output.[63]

Side Effects

Orthostatic hypotension is the most common side effect of labetalol therapy. Bronchospasm is possible in susceptible patients, reflecting the β-adrenergic antagonist effects of labetalol. Other adverse effects associated with β-adrenergic antagonists (congestive heart failure, bradycardia, heart block) are a potential risk of labetalol therapy, but the likely incidence and severity is substantially decreased. Incomplete α-adrenergic blockade in the presence of more complete β blockade could result in excessive α stimulation.[60] Fluid retention in patients treated chronically with labetalol is the reason for combining this drug with a diuretic during prolonged therapy.

Carvedilol

Carvedilol is a nonselective β-adrenergic receptor antagonist with α_1 blocking activity. This drug has no intrinsic β-adrenergic agonist effect. Following oral administration, carvedilol is extensively metabolized to products with pharmacologic activity possessing weak vasodilator actions. The elimination half-time is 7 to 10 hours and protein binding is extensive. Carvedilol is indicated for the treatment of mild to moderate congestive heart failure owing to ischemia or cardiomyopathy (see Table 19-2). This drug is also useful for the treatment of essential hypertension.

Calcium Channel Blockers

Calcium channel blockers (also known as ***calcium entry blockers*** and ***calcium antagonists***) are a diverse group of structurally unrelated compounds that selectively interfere with inward calcium ion movement across myocardial and vascular smooth muscle cells.[64,65] Calcium ions play a key role in the electrical excitation of cardiac cells and vascular smooth muscle cells.

Commercially available calcium channel blockers are classified based on chemical structure as phenylalkylamines, dihydropyridines, and benzothiazepines (Table 19-5 and Fig. 19-9). The phenylalkylamines and

Table 19-5

Classification of Calcium Channel Blockers

Phenylalkylamine
Verapamil
Dihydropyridines
Nifedipine
Nicardipine
Nimodipine
Isradipine
Felodipine
Amlodipine
Benzothiazepine
Diltiazem

benzothiazepines are selective for the atrioventricular node, whereas the dihydropyridines are selective for the arteriolar beds.[66] Common side effects of calcium channel blockers include systemic hypotension, peripheral edema, flushing, and headache. The various calcium channel blockers differ in terms of side effects, usual doses, metabolism, and duration of action (Tables 19-6 and 19-7).

Mechanism of Action

Calcium channel blockers bind to receptors on voltage-gated calcium ion channels (L, long-lasting; N, neural; and T, transient opening subtypes) resulting in maintenance of these channels in an inactive (closed) state. As a result, calcium influx is decreased and there is a reduction in intracellular calcium. The L-type channel (slow channel) has five subunits: α_1, α_2, β, γ, and δ. The α_1 subunit forms the central part of the channel and provides the main pathway for calcium ion entry into cells. All clinically used calcium channel blockers bind to a unique site on the α_1 subunit of the L-type calcium channels and thus diminish entry of calcium ions into cells. These structurally diverse drugs differ in their tissue selectivity, their binding site location on the α_1 subunit, and their mechanism of calcium blockade.

Voltage-gated calcium ion channels are present in the cell membranes of skeletal muscle, vascular smooth muscle, cardiac muscle, mesenteric muscle, glandular cells, and neurons (Fig. 19-10).[66] Calcium ion influx through L-type calcium channels is responsible for phase 2 of the cardiac action potential, which is important in excitation/contraction coupling in cardiac and vascular smooth muscle and depolarization in sinoatrial and atrioventricular nodal tissue. Thus, blockade of slow calcium channels by calcium channel blockers predictably results in slowing of the heart rate, reduction in myocardial contractility, decreased speed

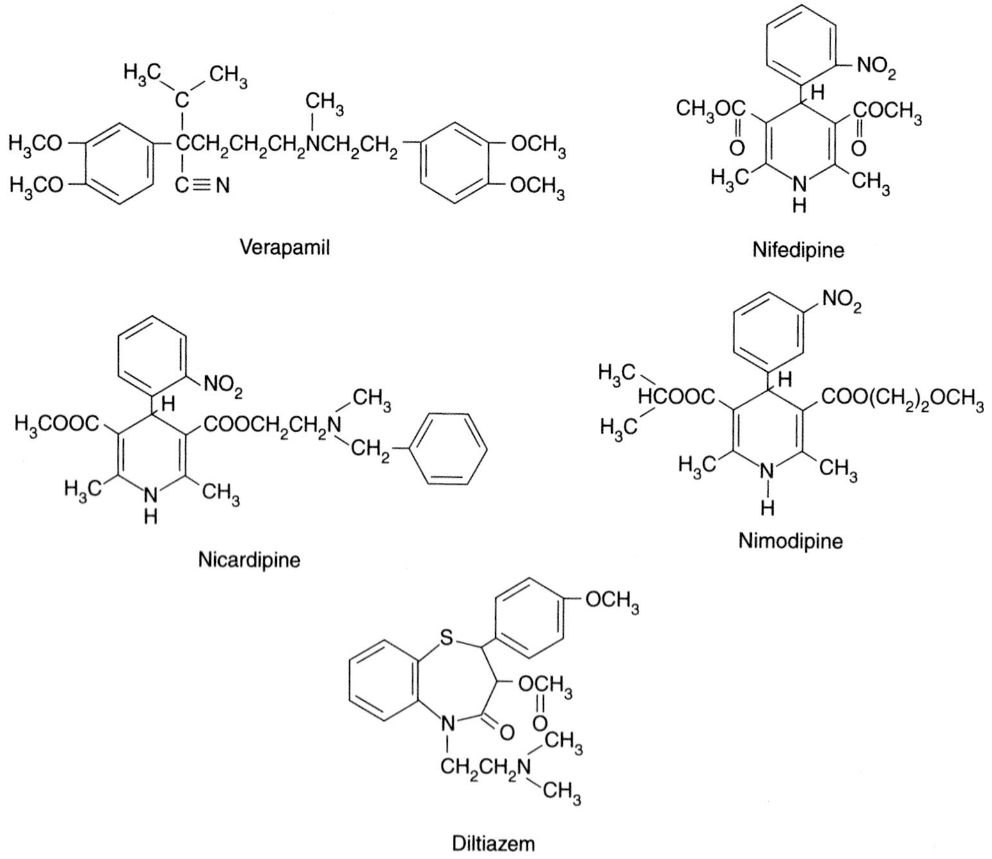

Verapamil

Nifedipine

Nicardipine

Nimodipine

Diltiazem

FIGURE 19-9 Calcium channel blockers.

Table 19-6

Comparative Pharmacologic Effects of Calcium Channel Blockers

	Verapamil	Nifedipine	Nicardipine	Diltiazem
Systemic blood pressure	Decrease	Decrease	Decrease	Decrease
Heart rates	Decrease	Increase to no change	Increase to no change	Decrease
Myocardial depression	Moderate	Moderate	Slight	Moderate
Sinoatrial node depression	Moderate	None	None	Slight
Atrioventricular node conduction	Marked	None	None	Moderate depression
Coronary artery dilation	Moderate	Marked	Greatest	Moderate
Peripheral artery dilation	Moderate	Marked	Marked	Moderate

of conduction of cardiac impulses through the atrioventricular node, and vascular smooth muscle relaxation.[67]

Direct activation of the vascular smooth muscle cell voltage-gated channels by neural impulses initiates an action potential, calcium ion influx, and myofilament contraction (see Fig. 19-10).[66] This process is known as ***excitation-contraction coupling***. The intracellular calcium combines with calmodulin, the calcium-binding protein, to form the calcium-calmodulin complex. This complex activates myosin and causes the formation of cross-bridges with actin. These cross-bridges begin the process of muscular contraction.

Pharmacologic Effects

The pharmacologic effects of calcium channel blockers may be predicted by considering the normal role of calcium ions in the production of action potentials, especially in cardiac cells. It is predictable that calcium channel blockers will produce decreased myocardial contractility, decreased heart rate, decreased activity of the sinoatrial node, decreased rate of conduction of cardiac impulses through the atrioventricular node, and vascular smooth muscle relaxation with associated vasodilation and decreases in systemic blood pressure.[67,68] Calcium channel

Table 19-7

Pharmacokinetics of Calcium Channel Blockers

	Verapamil	Nifedipine	Nicardipine	Nimodipine	Diltiazem
Dosage					
Oral	80–160 mg every 8 h	10–30 mg every 8 h	20 mg every 8 h	30–60 mg every 4–6 h	60–90 mg every 8 h
Intravenous	75–150 μg/kg	5–15 μg/kg		10 μg/kg	75–150 μg/kg
Absorption (%)					
Oral	>90	>90		>90	
Bioavailability (%)	10–20	65–70	30	5–10	40
Onset of effect (min)					
Oral	<30	<20	20–60	30–90	30
Sublingual		3			
Intravenous	1–3	1–3	1–3	1–3	
First-pass hepatic extraction after oral administration (%)	75–90	40–60	20–40	90	70–80
Protein binding (%)	83–93	92–98	95	99	98
Clearance					
Renal (%)	70	80	55	20	35
Hepatic (%)	15	<15	45	80	60
Active metabolites	Yes	No		Yes	
Therapeutic plasma concentration (ng/mL)	50–250	10–100	5–100	10–30	100–250
Elimination half-time (h)	3–7	3–7	3–5	2	4–6

From Reves JG, Kissin I, Lell WA, et al. Calcium entry blockers: uses and implications for anesthesiologists. *Anesthesiology*. 1982;57:504–518; Durand PG, Lehot JJ, Foex P. Calcium-channel blockers and anaesthesia. *Can J Anaesth*. 1991;38:75–89.

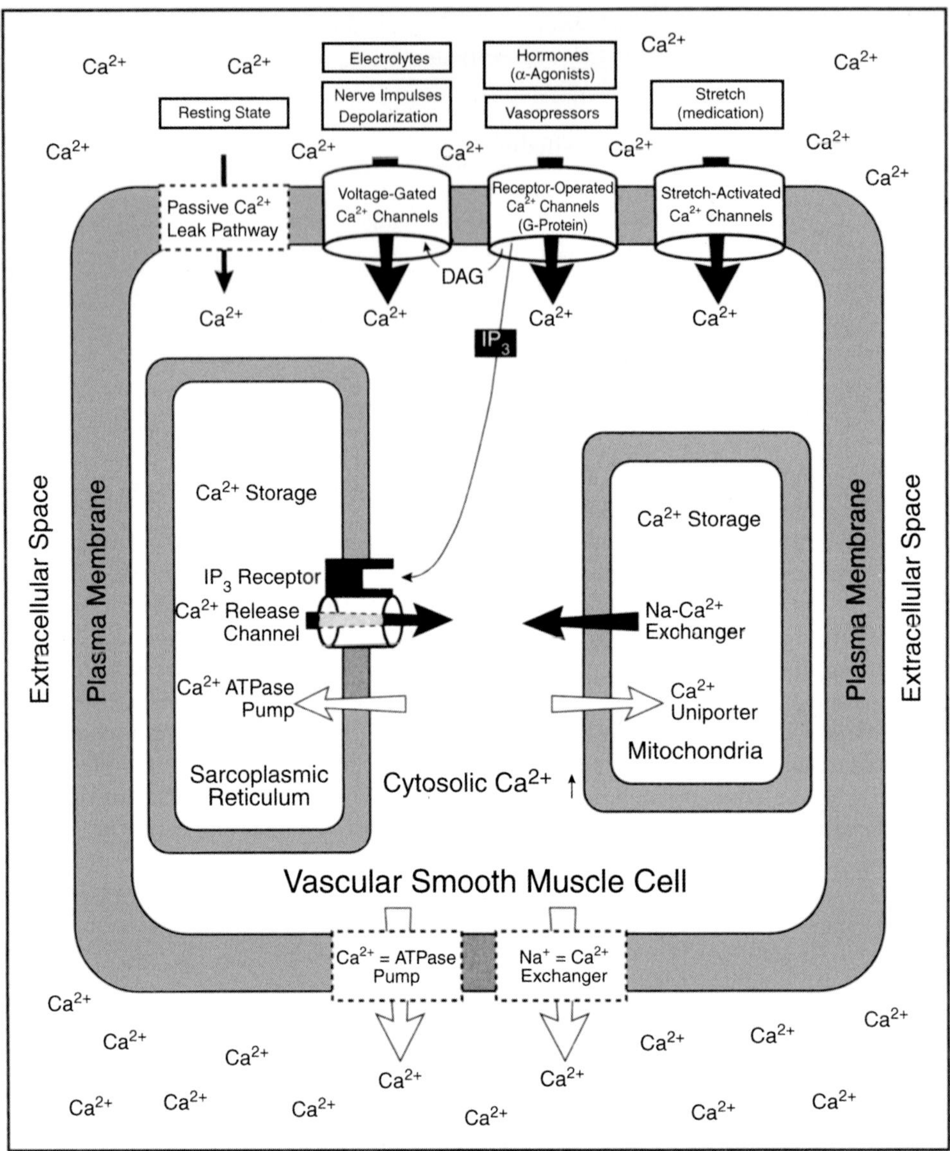

FIGURE 19-10 Calcium ion entry and exit from a vascular smooth muscle cell. Calcium enters the cytosol (*black arrows*) of the vascular smooth muscle cell either from the extracellular space through the plasma membrane (*top of diagram*) or from the intracellular storage areas. The primary entry sites for calcium ions are the voltage-gated channels. (From Kanneganti M, Halpern NA. Acute hypertension and calcium-channel blockers. *New Horiz.* 1996;4:19–25, with permission.)

blockers produce these effects to varying degrees (see Table 19-6).

All of the calcium channel blockers are effective for the treatment of coronary artery spasm. Calcium channel blockers decrease vascular smooth muscle contractility, thereby increasing coronary blood flow and causing peripheral vasodilation with reductions in systemic vascular resistance and systemic blood pressure. These drug-induced responses contribute to the antiischemic effects characteristic of calcium channel blockers. Because calcium channel blockers dilate the coronary arteries via a mechanism that is different from that of nitrates, the two classes of drugs complement each other in the treatment of coronary artery spasm. Calcium channel blockers are also effective for the treatment of chronic stable angina pectoris caused by fixed obstructive coronary artery lesions and for the treatment of unstable angina pectoris.

All calcium channel blockers exert negative inotropic effects, which are most significant with verapamil and diltiazem.

Phenylalkylamines

The phenylalkylamines bind to the intracellular portion of the L-type channel α_1 subunit when the channel is in an open state and conceptually occlude the channel (Fig. 19-11).[66]

Verapamil

Verapamil is a synthetic derivative of papaverine that is supplied as a racemic mixture. The dextroisomer of verapamil is

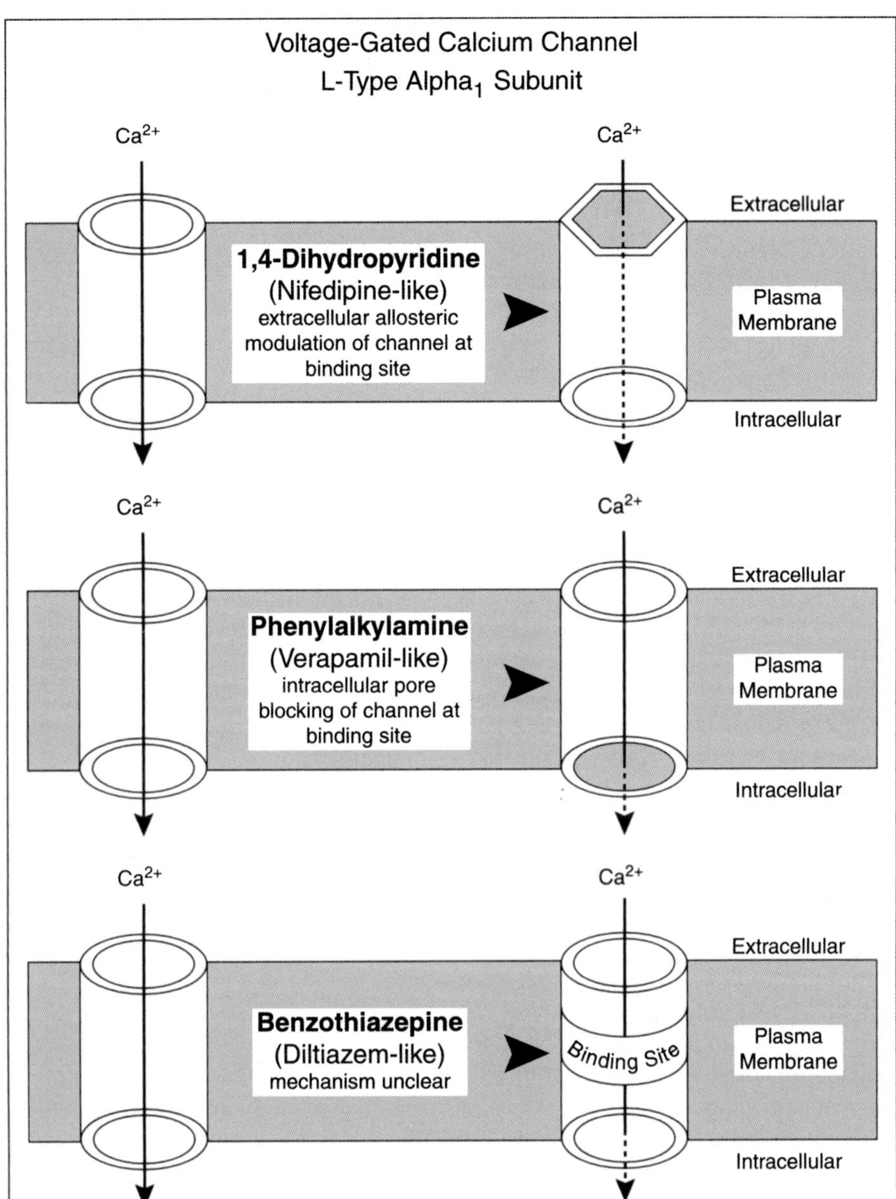

FIGURE 19-11 Mechanism of action of the three classes of calcium channel blockers. (From Kanneganti M, Halpern NA. Acute hypertension and calcium-channel blockers. *New Horiz.* 1996;4:19–25, with permission.)

devoid of activity at slow calcium channels and instead acts on fast sodium channels, accounting for the local anesthetic effects of verapamil (1.6 times as potent as procaine).[69] The levoisomer of verapamil is specific for slow calcium channels, and the predominance of this action accounts for the classification of verapamil as a calcium-blocking drug.

Side Effects

Verapamil has a major depressant effect on the atrioventricular node, a negative chronotropic effect on the sinoatrial node, a negative inotropic effect on cardiac muscle, and a moderate vasodilating effect on coronary and systemic arteries. The negative inotropic effects of verapamil seem to be exaggerated in patients with preexisting left ventricular dysfunction. For these reasons, verapamil should not be administered to patients in heart failure or patients with severe bradycardia, sinus node dysfunction, or atrioventricular nodal block. Likewise, this drug's negative inotropic and chronotropic effects may be enhanced in the presence of concomitant treatment with β-adrenergic antagonists. Isoproterenol may be useful to increase heart rate in the presence of drug-induced heart block. Verapamil may precipitate ventricular dysrhythmias in patients with Wolff-Parkinson-White syndrome.

Clinical Uses

Verapamil is effective in the treatment of supraventricular tachydysrhythmias, reflecting its primary site of action on the atrioventricular node (see Chapter 21). The mild vasodilating effects produced by verapamil make this drug useful in the treatment of vasospastic angina pectoris and essential hypertension. Indeed, calcium channel blockers are as effective as β blockers in relieving angina pectoris. Verapamil is not as active as nifedipine in its effects on vascular smooth muscle and therefore causes a less pronounced decrease in systemic blood pressure and less reflex peripheral sympathetic nervous system activity. Verapamil is effective in the treatment of symptomatic hypertrophic cardiomyopathy with or without left ventricular outflow obstruction.[70] Calcium channel antagonists should not be routinely administered for acute myocardial infarction as postinfarction mortality is not decreased.[71]

Verapamil may be useful in the treatment of maternal and fetal tachydysrhythmias as well as premature labor.[72] Administered IV to parturients, verapamil prolongs atrioventricular conduction of the fetus despite limited placental transport of the drug. Fetal hepatic extraction of verapamil is substantial, as evidenced by a plasma concentration in the fetal carotid artery that is less than that in the umbilical vein. Verapamil may decrease uterine blood flow, suggesting caution in the administration of this drug to parturients with impaired uteroplacental perfusion.[73]

Pharmacokinetics

Oral verapamil is almost completely absorbed, but extensive hepatic first-pass metabolism limits bioavailability to 10% to 20% (see Table 19-7). As a result, the oral dose (80 to 160 mg three times daily) is about 10 times the IV dose. The therapeutic plasma concentration of verapamil is 100 to 300 ng/mL. The activity of oral verapamil peaks in 30 to 45 minutes compared with about 15 minutes following IV administration. Pharmacologic effects following IV administration of verapamil appear within 2 to 3 minutes and may last 6 hours.

Demethylated metabolites of verapamil predominate, with norverapamil possessing sufficient activity to contribute to the antidysrhythmic properties of the parent drug. In view of the nearly complete hepatic metabolism of verapamil, almost none of the drug appears unchanged in the urine. Conversely, an estimated 70% of an injected dose of verapamil is recovered in urine as metabolites and about 15% is excreted via bile. Chronic oral administration of verapamil or the presence of renal dysfunction leads to the accumulation of norverapamil.

The elimination half-time of verapamil is 6 to 12 hours, and this may be prolonged in patients with liver disease. In this regard, chronic treatment with verapamil has rarely been associated with increased plasma concentrations of transaminase enzymes. Like nifedipine, verapamil is highly protein bound (90%), and the presence of other drugs (lidocaine, diazepam, propranolol) can increase the pharmacologically active, unbound portion of the drug.

Dihydropyridines

The dihydropyridines prevent calcium entry into the vascular smooth cells by extracellular allosteric modulation of the L-type voltage-gated calcium ion channels (see Fig. 19-11).[66] The primary affinity of the dihydropyridines nifedipine, nicardipine, isradipine, felodipine, and amlodipine is for the peripheral arterioles, whereas nimodipine favors cerebral vessels. The vasodilating effects of these drugs on venous capacitance vessels are minimal. As with other peripheral vasodilators, a reflex tachycardia attributed to sympathetic nervous system activity or baroreceptor reflexes may be observed with the acute administration of dihydropyridines.

Nifedipine

Nifedipine is a dihydropyridine derivative with greater coronary and peripheral arterial vasodilator properties than verapamil. There is minimal effect on venous capacitance vessels. Unlike verapamil, nifedipine has little or no direct depressant effect on sinoatrial or atrioventricular node activity. Peripheral vasodilation and the resulting decrease in systemic blood pressure produced by nifedipine activate baroreceptors, leading to increased peripheral sympathetic nervous system activity most often manifesting as an increased heart rate. This increased sympathetic nervous system activity counters the direct negative inotropic, chronotropic, and dromotropic effects of nifedipine. Nevertheless, nifedipine may produce excessive myocardial depression, especially in patients with preexisting left ventricular dysfunction or concomitant therapy with a β-adrenergic antagonist drug. The presence of aortic stenosis may also exaggerate the cardiac depressant effects of nifedipine.

Clinical Uses

Nifedipine is administered orally with a 10- to 30-mg dose producing an effect in about 20 minutes with a peak effect between 60 and 90 minutes. Nifedipine is used to treat patients with angina pectoris, especially that due to coronary artery vasospasm.

Pharmacokinetics

Absorption of an oral or sublingual dose of nifedipine is about 90%, with onset of an effect being detectable within about 20 minutes after administration (see Table 19-7). It is likely that most of the absorption of sublingual nifedipine is via the gastrointestinal tract from swallowed saliva. Protein binding approaches 90%. Hepatic metabolism is nearly complete, with elimination of inactive metabolites principally in urine (about 80%) and, to a lesser extent, in bile. The elimination half-time is 3 to 7 hours.

Side Effects

The side effects of nifedipine include flushing, vertigo, and headache. Less common side effects include peripheral edema (venodilation), hypotension, paresthesias, and skeletal muscle weakness. Glucose intolerance and hepatic dysfunction occur rarely. Nifedipine may induce renal dysfunction. Abrupt discontinuation of nifedipine has been associated with coronary artery vasospasm.

Nicardipine

Nicardipine lacks effects on the sinoatrial node and atrioventricular node and has minimal myocardial depressant effects. This drug has the greatest vasodilating effects of all the calcium entry blockers, with vasodilation being particularly prominent in the coronary arteries. Combination with a β-adrenergic antagonist for the treatment of angina is a consideration, as dihydropyridine calcium channel blockers do not significantly depress the sinoatrial node. Of all the antianginal drugs, the dihydropyridine calcium channel blockers produce the greatest dilatation of the peripheral arterioles. Therefore, either nifedipine or nicardipine may be particularly useful in patients who have residual hypertension despite β-adrenergic blockade.

Nicardipine is available in IV and oral preparations (other dihydropyridine calcium channel blockers are available only as oral preparations). A long elimination half-time is the basis for the recommendation that about 72 hours should elapse before increasing the oral dose. Nicardipine is metabolized in the liver and is highly protein bound (about 95%). The side effects of nicardipine are similar to nifedipine.

Clinical Uses

Nicardipine is used as a tocolytic drug having a similar tocolytic effect as salbutamol but with fewer side effects. When nicardipine is administered as a tocolytic, it binds to the inside of myometrial L-type voltage-dependent calcium ion channels, causing them to remain closed, and thus inhibits uterine contractility. Pulmonary edema associated with salbutamol used as a tocolytic has also been reported in a parturient treated with nicardipine.[74] Nicardipine, 40 μg/kg IV administered immediately before performing electroconvulsive therapy is effective in blunting acute hemodynamic responses to the treatment.[75]

Nimodipine

Nimodipine is a highly lipid-soluble analogue of nifedipine. Lipid solubility facilitates its entrance into the CNS, where it blocks the influx of extracellular calcium ions necessary for contraction of large cerebral arteries.

Clinical Uses

The lipid solubility of nimodipine and its ability to cross the blood–brain barrier is responsible for the potential value of this drug in treating patients with subarachnoid hemorrhage.

Cerebral Vasospasm

The vasodilating effect of nimodipine on cerebral arteries is uniquely valuable in preventing or attenuating cerebral vasospasm that often accompanies subarachnoid hemorrhage.[76] The initial event in the development of vasospasm may be an intracellular influx of calcium ions that cause contraction of smooth muscle cells in large cerebral arteries. Administration of nimodipine, 0.7 mg/kg orally as an initial dose followed by 0.35 mg/kg every 4 hours for 21 days, is associated with a decreased incidence of neurologic deficits due to cerebral vasospasm in patients who had experienced subarachnoid hemorrhage.[77] Blood and cerebrospinal fluid levels of nimodipine with this dosing regimen were 6.9 ng/mL and 0.77 ng/mL, respectively. In comatose patients who cannot take oral medications, the recommendation is to extract the contents of the nimodipine capsule into a syringe and administer the drug into a nasogastric tube. To ensure delivery of the drug into the stomach via a nasogastric tube, it is necessary to add up to 30 mL of saline to the nimodipine-containing solution.[78] Side effects have not been observed with the oral administration of nimodipine. Symptoms of excessive nimodipine effect would be expected to be related to cardiovascular effects such as peripheral vasodilation with associated systemic hypotension. Theoretically, drug-induced cerebral vasodilation could evoke increases in intracranial pressure, particularly in patients with preexisting decreases in intracranial compliance.

Cerebral Protection

Nimodipine has also been evaluated for cerebral protection after global ischemia as associated with cardiac arrest. The theoretical basis for considering calcium channel blockers for this purpose is the observation that lack of oxygen interferes with maintenance of the normal calcium ion gradient across cell membranes, leading to a massive increase (at least 200-fold) in the intraneuronal concentrations of this ion. In this regard, nimodipine is associated with improved neurologic outcome when administered to primates within 5 minutes after experiencing 17 minutes of cerebral ischemia.[79] The dose of nimodipine used (10 μg/kg IV followed by 1 μg/kg/minute IV) was associated with decreases in blood pressure that responded to infusion of fluids and/or dopamine.

Amlodipine

Amlodipine is a dihydropyridine derivative that is available for only oral administration (5 to 10 mg) resulting in a peak plasma concentration in 6 to 12 hours. Elimination half-time is 30 to 40 hours and about 90% of the drug undergoes hepatic metabolism to inactive products. Amlodipine appears to have minimal detrimental effects on myocardial contractility and provides antiischemic effects comparable to β blockers in patients with acute coronary syndrome.[71] The combination of amlodipine and β blockers may be more effective in the treatment of myocardial ischemia than either drug alone.

Benzothiazepines

Benzothiazepines act at the L-type channel α_1 subunit, although the mechanism of action is not well understood (see Fig. 19-11).[66] The benzothiazepine diltiazem may have two additional effects: It may act on the sodium–potassium pump, decreasing the amount of intracellular sodium available for exchange with extracellular calcium, and it may inhibit calcium-calmodulin binding.

Diltiazem

Diltiazem, like verapamil, blocks predominantly the calcium channels of the atrioventricular node and is therefore a first-line medication for the treatment of supraventricular tachydysrhythmias (see Chapter 21). It may also be used for the chronic control of essential hypertension. The effects of diltiazem on the sinoatrial and atrioventricular nodes and its vasodilating properties appear to be intermediate between those of verapamil and the dihydropyridines. Diltiazem exerts minimal cardiodepressant effects and is unlikely to interact with β-adrenergic blocking drugs to decrease myocardial contractility.[43]

Clinical Uses

The clinical use and drug interactions for diltiazem are similar to those of verapamil. Diltiazem is available as an oral capsule and can also be administered IV, especially for the management of angina pectoris. The recommended IV dose is 0.25 to 0.35 mg/kg over 2 minutes and is repeated in 15 minutes, if needed. After the initial IV dose, diltiazem can be given by continuous infusion of about 10 mg per hour for up to 24 hours.

Pharmacokinetics

Oral absorption of diltiazem is excellent with an onset of action in 15 minutes and a peak effect in about 30 minutes (see Table 19-7). The drug is 70% to 80% bound to proteins and is excreted as inactive metabolites principally in bile (about 60%) and, to a lesser extent, in urine (about 35%). Active metabolites of diltiazem include desacetyldiltiazem and desmethyldiltiazem. The elimination half-time for the parent drug is 4 to 6 hours and about 20 hours for metabolites. As with verapamil, liver disease may necessitate a decrease in the dosage of diltiazem.

Drug Interactions

The known pharmacologic effects of calcium channel blockers on cardiac, skeletal, and vascular smooth muscle, as well as on the conduction velocity of cardiac impulses, make drug interactions possible.[65] Verapamil and diltiazem have depressant effects on the generation of cardiac action potentials at the sinoatrial node and slow the movement of cardiac impulses through the atrioventricular node. Therefore, patients with preexisting cardiac conduction abnormalities may experience greater degrees of atrioventricular heart block with concurrent administration of β blockers or digoxin. Myocardial depression and peripheral vasodilation produced by volatile anesthetics could be exaggerated by similar actions of calcium channel blockers. Vasodilating effects of calcium channel blockers could result in exaggerated systemic hypotension should these drugs be administered to hypovolemic patients.

The likelihood of adverse circulatory changes due to interactions between calcium channel blockers and anesthetic drugs would seem to be greater in patients with preexisting atrioventricular heart block or left ventricular dysfunction. Nevertheless, treatment with calcium channel blockers can be continued until the time of surgery without risk of significant drug interactions, especially with respect to conduction of cardiac impulses.[80] Toxicity reflecting an overdose of calcium channel blockers may be partially reversed with IV administration of calcium or dopamine.

Anesthetic Drugs

Calcium channel blockers are vasodilators and myocardial depressants. In fact, the negative inotropic effects, depressant effects on sinoatrial node function, and peripheral vasodilating effects of these drugs and those of volatile anesthetics are similar, and there is evidence that volatile anesthetics have blocking effects on calcium channels.[81] For these reasons, calcium channel blockers must be administered with caution to patients with impaired left ventricular function or hypovolemia. Patients treated with a combination of β-adrenergic blockers and nifedipine tolerate high-dose fentanyl anesthesia and do not show evidence of additive depression of cardiac function when verapamil is infused.[82] Conversely, in anesthetized patients with preexisting left ventricular dysfunction, administration of verapamil is associated with myocardial depression and decreased cardiac output.[83] Furthermore, IV administration of verapamil or diltiazem during open chest surgery in patients with depressed ventricular function and anesthetized with a volatile anesthetic may be associated with further decreases in ventricular function.[81]

Treatment of cardiac dysrhythmias with calcium channel blockers in anesthetized patients produces only transient decreases in systemic blood pressure and infrequent prolongation of the P-R interval on the electrocardiogram. Because of the tendency to produce atrioventricular heart block, verapamil should be used cautiously in patients being treated with digitalis or β-adrenergic blocking drugs. Nevertheless, in patients with preoperative evidence of cardiac conduction abnormalities, the chronic combined administration of calcium channel blockers and β-adrenergic antagonists is not associated with cardiac conduction abnormalities in the perioperative period (Table 19-8).[80] β-Adrenergic agonists increase the number of functioning slow calcium channels in myocardial cell membranes through a cAMP mechanism and readily counter the effects of calcium channel blockers. Nevertheless, there is no evidence that patients being treated chronically with calcium channel blockers are at increased risk for anesthesia.

Neuromuscular Blocking Drugs

Calcium channel blockers alone do not produce a skeletal muscle relaxant effect (Fig. 19-12).[84] Conversely, these drugs potentiate the effects of depolarizing and nondepolarizing neuromuscular blocking drugs (see Fig. 19-12).[84,85] This potentiation resembles that produced by mycin antibiotics in the presence of neuromuscular blocking drugs. The local anesthetic effects of verapamil and diltiazem, reflecting inhibition of sodium ion flux via fast sodium channels, may also contribute to the potentiation of neuromuscular blocking drugs. Observations of skeletal muscle weakness after administration of verapamil to a patient with muscular dystrophy are inconsistent with diminished release of neurotransmitter.[86] Therefore, the neuromuscular effects of verapamil may be more likely to manifest in patients with a compromised margin of safety of neuromuscular transmission.

Table 19-8

Effect of Chronic Antianginal Therapy on Perioperative Heart Rate (beats per minute) and P-R Interval (ms)

	Before Induction	After Induction	10 min after Cardiopulmonary Bypass
Control			
Heart rate	72	71	87
P-R interval	160	156	164
Calcium channel blockers			
Heart rate	69	70	86
P-R interval	168	169	175
β-Adrenergic antagonists			
Heart rate	59	65	78
P-R interval	168	171	183
Nifedipine plus β-adrenergic antagonists			
Heart rate	67	69	86
P-R interval	175	177	186

From Henling CE, Slogoff S, Kodali SV, et al. Heart block after coronary artery bypass effect of chronic administration of calcium-entry blockers and β-blockers. *Anesth Analg.* 1984;63:515–520.

Antagonism of neuromuscular blockade may be impaired because of diminished presynaptic release of acetylcholine in the presence of a calcium channel blocker.[87] Indeed, calcium ions are necessary for the release of acetylcholine at the neuromuscular junction. In one report, edrophonium but not neostigmine was effective in antagonizing nondepolarizing neuromuscular blockade that was potentiated by verapamil.[88]

Local Anesthetics

Verapamil and diltiazem have potent local anesthetic activity, which may increase the risk of local anesthetic toxicity when regional anesthesia is administered to patients being treated with this drug.[89]

Potassium-Containing Solutions

Calcium channel blockers slow the inward movement of potassium ions. For this reason, hyperkalemia in patients being treated with verapamil may occur after much smaller amounts of exogenous potassium infusion as associated with the use of potassium chloride to treat hypokalemia or administration of stored whole blood.[90] In animals, however, pretreatment with verapamil does not alter the increases in plasma potassium concentrations that follow the administration of succinylcholine.[91]

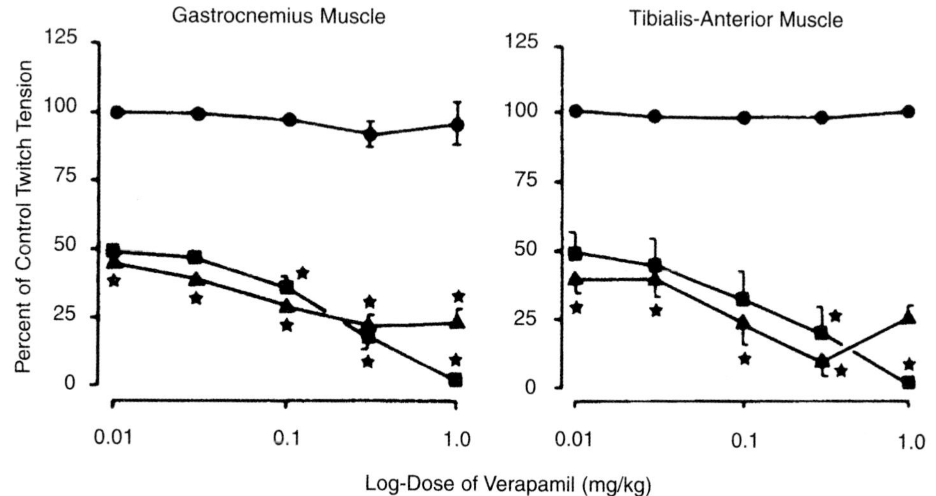

FIGURE 19-12 Infusion of verapamil in the absence of neuromuscular blocking drugs (*solid circles*) does not alter twitch height response (twitch tension) of indirectly stimulated rabbit skeletal muscle. When twitch tension is decreased to about 50% of control by the continuous infusion of pancuronium (*solid squares*) or succinylcholine (*solid triangles*), the addition of verapamil further decreases twitch tension. (The data points marked with "*" represent a statistically significant decrease in muscle twitch tension as compared to Verapamil alone. The errors represent the mean ± SE.) (From Durant NN, Nguyen N, Katz RL. Potentiation of neuromuscular blockade by verapamil. *Anesthesiology.* 1984;60:298–303, with permission.)

Dantrolene

The ability of both verapamil and dantrolene to inhibit intracellular calcium ion flux and excitation-contraction coupling would suggest this combination might be useful in the treatment of malignant hyperthermia. In swine, however, the administration of dantrolene in the presence of verapamil or diltiazem results in hyperkalemia and cardiovascular collapse (Fig. 19-13).[92] A patient receiving verapamil developed hyperkalemia and myocardial depression within 1.5 hours of being treated with dantrolene administered IV.[93] This same patient did not experience hyperkalemia when nifedipine was substituted for verapamil before pretreatment with dantrolene.

Whenever calcium channel blockers, especially verapamil or diltiazem, and dantrolene must be administered concurrently, invasive hemodynamic monitoring and frequent measurement of the plasma potassium concentration are recommended. It is speculated that verapamil alters normal homeostatic mechanisms for regulation of plasma potassium concentrations and may result in hyperkalemia from dantrolene-induced potassium release. Furthermore, there is evidence that verapamil does not influence the ability of known triggering drugs to evoke malignant hyperthermia in susceptible animals.[94]

Platelet Function

Calcium channel blockers may interfere with calcium-mediated platelet function.

Digoxin

Calcium channel blockers may increase the plasma concentration of digoxin, presumably by decreasing its plasma clearance.

H_2 Antagonists

Cimetidine and ranitidine by altering hepatic enzyme activity and/or hepatic blood flow may increase the plasma concentrations of calcium channel blockers.

Risks of Chronic Treatment

Despite the popularity of calcium channel blockers in the treatment of cardiovascular diseases (essential hypertension, angina pectoris), there is increasing concern about the long-term safety of these drugs, especially the short-acting dihydropyridine derivatives.[95] For example, the risk of developing cardiovascular complications has been described as being greater in patients treated with nifedipine compared with those receiving placebo or conventional therapy.[96] Increased perioperative bleeding and an increased incidence of gastrointestinal hemorrhage have been reported in patients receiving a dihydropyridine derivative.[97,98] The risk of developing cancer may be increased in those treated with calcium channel blockers compared with β-adrenergic antagonists or angiotensin-converting enzyme inhibitors.[99] For these reasons, treatment with calcium channel blockers, especially short-acting dihydropyridine derivatives, should generally be reserved for second-step rather than initial therapy.[95]

Cytoprotection

Drug-induced calcium channel blockade may provide cytoprotection against ischemic reperfusion injury. By decreasing calcium ion entry into cells and the conversion of xanthine dehydrogenase to xanthine oxidase (dependent

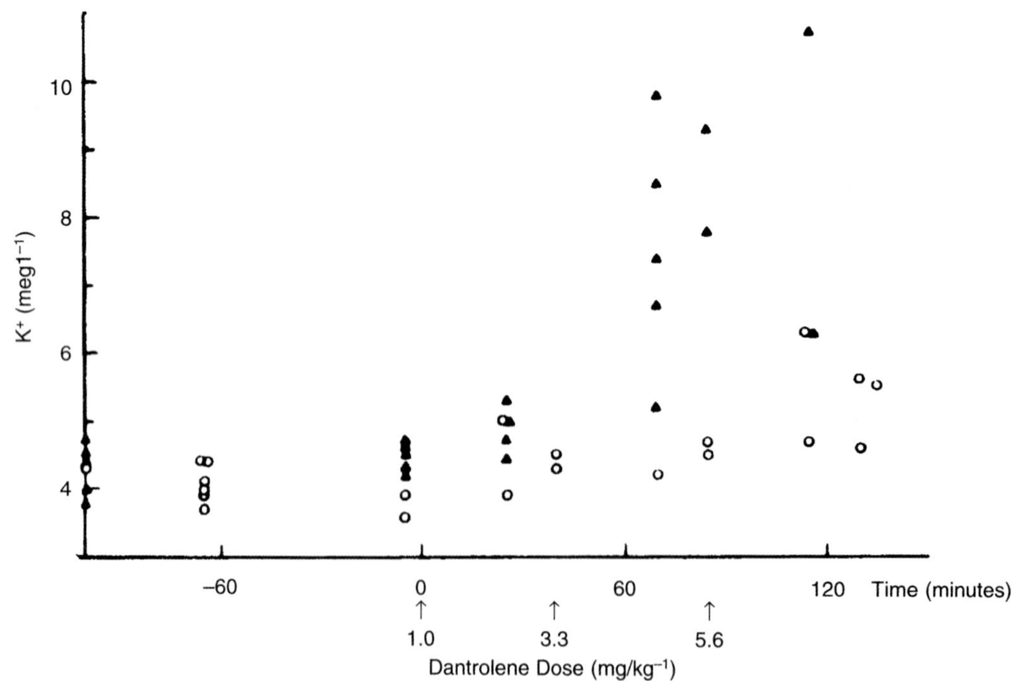

FIGURE 19-13 Administration of dantrolene to swine pretreated with verapamil (*solid triangles*) results in hyperkalemia compared with animals receiving only dantrolene (*open circles*). (From Saltzman LS, Kates RA, Corke BC, et al. Hyperkalemia and cardiovascular collapse after verapamil and dantrolene administration in swine. *Anesth Analg.* 1984;63:473–478, with permission.)

on the calcium-calmodulin complex), calcium channel blockers may limit the accumulation of oxygen free radicals. Calcium channel blockers may attenuate renal injury from nephrotoxic drugs such as cisplatinum and iodinated radiographic contrast media. The vasodilator effects of calcium channel blockers and resultant control of systemic hypertension may result in increases in renal blood flow and glomerular filtration rate, thus favoring natriuresis.

References

1. Foex P. A- and β-adrenoceptor antagonists. *Br J Anaesth.* 1984;56:751–765.
2. Aplin SC, Yee KF, Cole MJ. Neonatal effects of long-term maternal phenoxybenzamine therapy. *Anesthesiology.* 2004;100:1608–1610.
3. Shand DG. Drug therapy—propranolol. *N Engl J Med.* 1975;293:280–285.
4. Wood M, Shand DG, Wood AJ. Propranolol binding in plasma during cardiopulmonary bypass. *Anesthesiology.* 1979;51:512–516.
5. Bowdle TA, Freund PR, Slattery JT. Propranolol reduces bupivacaine clearance. *Anesthesiology.* 1987;66:36–38.
6. Conrad KA, Beyers JM, Finley PR, et al. Lidocaine elimination: effects of metoprolol and propranolol. *Clin Pharmacol Ther.* 1983;33:133–138.
7. Roerig DL, Kotryl KJ, Ahlf SB, et al. Effect of propranolol on the first pass uptake of fentanyl in the human and rat lung. *Anesthesiology.* 1989;71:62–68.
8. Mishra P, Calvey TN, Williams NE, et al. Intraoperative bradycardia and hypotension associated with timolol and pilocarpine eye drops. *Br J Anaesth.* 1983;55:897–899.
9. Bailey PL. Timolol and postoperative apnea in neonates and young infants. *Anesthesiology.* 1984;61:622.
10. Mangano DT, Layug EL, Wallace A, et al. Effect of atenolol on mortality and cardiovascular morbidity after noncardiac surgery. *N Engl J Med.* 1996;335:1713–1720.
11. Wallace A, Layug B, Tateo I, et al. Prophylactic atenolol reduces postoperative myocardial ischemia. *Anesthesiology.* 1998;88:7–17.
12. Nuttall SL, Routledge HC, Kendall MJ. A comparison of the beta1-selectivity of three beta1-selective beta-blockers. *J Clin Pharm Ther.* 2003:28(3):179–186.
13. Bundkirchen A, Brixius K, Bölck B, et al. Beta1-adrenoceptor selectivity of nebivolol and bisoprolol. A comparison of [3H]CGP 12.177 and [125I]iodocyanopindolol binding studies. *Eur J of Pharmacol.* 2003:460(1):19–26.
14. Helfman SM, Gold MI, DeLisser EA, et al. Which drug prevents tachycardia and hypertension associated with tracheal intubation: lidocaine, fentanyl, or esmolol? *Anesth Analg.* 1991;72:482–486.
15. Oxorn D, Knox JWD, Hill J. Bolus doses of esmolol for the prevention of perioperative hypertension and tachycardia. *Can J Anaesth.* 1990;37:206–209.
16. Sheppard S, Eagle CJ, Strunin L. A bolus dose of esmolol attenuates tachycardia and hypertension after tracheal intubation. *Can J Anaesth.* 1990;37:202–205.
17. Howie MB, Black HA, Zvara D, et al. Esmolol reduces autonomic hypersensitivity and length of seizures induced by electroconvulsive therapy. *Anesth Analg.* 1990;71:384–388.
18. Nicholas E, Deutschman CS, Allo M, et al. Use of esmolol in the intraoperative management of pheochromocytoma. *Anesth Analg.* 1988;67:1114–1117.
19. Ostman PL, Chestnut DH, Robillard JE, et al. Transplacental passage and hemodynamic effects of esmolol in the gravid ewe. *Anesthesiology.* 1988;69:738–741.
20. Pollan S, Tadjziechy M. Esmolol in the management of epinephrine and cocaine-induced cardiovascular toxicity. *Anesth Analg.* 1989; 69:663–664.
21. Thorne AC, Bedford RF. Esmolol for perioperative management of thyrotoxic goiter. *Anesthesiology.* 1989;71:291–294.
22. Zakowski M, Kaufman B, Berguson P, et al. Esmolol use during resection of pheochromocytoma: report of three cases. *Anesthesiology.* 1989;20:875–877.
23. Gourdine SB, Hollinger I, Jones J, et al. New York state guidelines on the topical use of phenylephrine in the operating room. *Anesthesiology.* 2000;92:859–864.
24. Ooi LG, O'Shea PJ, Wood AJ. Use of esmolol in the postbypass management of hypertrophic obstructive cardiomyopathy. *Br J Anaesth.* 1993;70:104–106.
25. de Bruijn NP, Croughwell N, Reves JG. Hemodynamic effects of esmolol in chronically β-blocked patients undergoing aortocoronary bypass surgery. *Anesth Analg.* 1987;66:137–141.
26. Cork RC, Kramer TH, Dreischmeier B, et al. The effect of esmolol given during cardiopulmonary bypass. *Anesth Analg.* 1995;80:28–40.
27. Johansen JW, Flaishon R, Sebel PS. Esmolol reduces anesthetic requirement for skin incision during propofol/nitrous oxide/morphine anesthesia. *Anesthesiology.* 1997;86:364–371.
28. Hall RI. Esmolol—just another β blocker? *Can J Anaesth.* 1992;39:757–764.
29. McCammon RL, Hilgenberg JC, Sandage BW, et al. The effect of esmolol on the onset and duration of succinylcholine-induced neuromuscular blockade. *Anesthesiology.* 1985;63:A317.
30. Brown DR, Brown MJ. Hypoglycemia associated with preoperative metoprolol administration. *Anesth Analg.* 2004;99:1427–1428.
31. Ramsey JG. Esmolol. *Can J Anaesth.* 1991;38:155–158.
32. Nies AS, Shand DG. Clinical pharmacology of propranolol. *Circulation.* 1975;52:6–15.
33. DeLima LGR, Kharasch ED, Butler S. Successful pharmacologic treatment of massive atenolol overdose: sequential hemodynamics and plasma atenolol concentrations. *Anesthesiology.* 1995;83:204–207.
34. Rosa RM, Silva P, Young JB, et al. Adrenergic modulation of extrarenal potassium disposal. *N Engl J Med.* 1980;302:431–434.
35. McCammon RL, Stoelting RK. Exaggerated increase in serum potassium following succinylcholine in dogs with β blockade. *Anesthesiology.* 1984;61:723–725.
36. Philbin DM, Lowenstein E. Lack of β-adrenergic activity of isoflurane in the dog: a comparison of circulatory effects of halothane and isoflurane after propranolol administration. *Br J Anaesth.* 1976;48:1165–1170.
37. Horan BF, Prys-Roberts C, Hamilton WK, et al. Haemodynamic responses to enflurane anaesthesia and hypovolaemia in the dog, and their modification by propranolol. *Br J Anaesth.* 1977;49:1189–1197.
38. Roberts JG, Foex P, Clarke TNS, et al. Haemodynamic interactions of high-dose propranolol pretreatment and anaesthesia in the dog. III. The effects of haemorrhage during halothane and trichloroethylene anaesthesia. *Br J Anaesth.* 1976;48:411–418.
39. Horan BF, Prys-Roberts C, Roberts JG, et al. Haemodynamic responses to isoflurane anaesthesia and hypovolaemia in the dog, and their modification by propranolol. *Br J Anaesth.* 1977;49:1179–1187.
40. Foex P, Ryder WA. Interactions of adrenergic β-receptor blockade (oxprenolol) and PCO_2 in the anesthetized dog: influence of intrinsic sympathomimetic activity. *Br J Anaesth.* 1981;53:19–26.
41. Bright RA, Everitt DE. β-blockers and depression: evidence against an association. *JAMA.* 1992;267:1783–1787.
42. Smulyan H, Weinberg SE, Howanitz PJ. Continuous propranolol infusion following abdominal surgery. *JAMA.* 1982;247:2539–2542.
43. Packer M. Combined β-adrenergic and calcium-entry blockade in angina pectoris. *N Engl J Med.* 1989;320:709–717.
44. Brandler E, Paladino L, Sinert R. Does the early administration of beta-blockers improve the in-hospital mortality rate of patients admitted with acute coronary syndrome? *Acad Emerg Med.* 2010:17(1)1–10.
45. Chen ZM, Pan HC, Chen YP, et al. Early intravenous then oral metoprolol in 45,852 patients with acute myocardial infarction: randomized placebo-controlled trial. *Lancet.* 2005: 366:1622–1632.
46. The TIMI Study Group. Immediate versus delayed catheterization and angioplasty following thrombolytic therapy for acute myocardial infarction. *JAMA.* 1988;260:2849–2856.
47. London MJ. Beta-adrenergic-receptor blockade and myocardial ischemia: something old, something new. *J Cardiothorac Vasc Anesth.* 2002;16(6):667–669.

48. Shjojania KG, Duncan BW, McDonald KM, et al. Safe but sound: patient safety meets evidence-based medicine. *JAMA*. 2002;288:508–513.
49. Auerbach AD, Goldman L. β-blockers and reduction of cardiac events in noncardiac surgery. *JAMA*. 2002;287:1435–1444.
50. Eagle KA, Froehlich JB. Reducing cardiovascular risk in patients undergoing noncardiac surgery. *N Engl J Med*. 1996;335:1761–1763.
51. Devereaux PJ, Yang H, Yusuf S, et al. Effects of extended-release metoprolol succinate in patients undergoing non-cardiac surgery (POISE trial): a randomised controlled trial. *Lancet*. 2008:371:1839–1847.
52. Hjalmarson A, Goldstein S, Gagerberg B, et al. Effects of controlled-release metoprolol on total mortality, hospitalizations, and well-being in patients with heart failure: the Metoprolol CR/XL Randomized Intervention Trial in Congestive Heart Failure (MERIT-HF). *JAMA*. 2000;283:1295–1302.
53. Colucci WS, Packer M, Bristow MR, et al. Carvedilol inhibits clinical progression in patients with mild symptoms of heart failure. *Circulation*. 1996;94:1199–1205.
54. Prys-Roberts C, Foex P, Biro GP, et al. Studies of anaesthesia in relation to hypertension. V. Adrenergic β-receptor blockade. *Br J Anaesth*. 1973;45:671–681.
55. Lee TC, Coffey RJ, Currier BM, et al. Propranolol and thyroidectomy in the treatment of thyrotoxicosis. *Ann Surg*. 1982;195:766–772.
56. Lennquits S, Jortso E, Anderberg B, et al. β blockers compared with antithyroid drug as preoperative treatment in hyperthyroidism: drug tolerance, complications, and postoperative thyroid function. *Surgery*. 1985;98:1141–1146.
57. MacCarthy EP, Bloomfield SS. Labetalol: a review of its pharmacology, pharmacokinetics, clinical uses and adverse effects. *Pharmacotherapy*. 1983;3:193–219.
58. Wallin JD, O'Neill WM. Labetalol: current research and therapeutic status. *Arch Intern Med*. 1983;143:485–490.
59. Baum T, Watkins RW, Sybertz EJ, et al. Antihypertensive and hemodynamic actions of SCH 19927, the R,R-isomer of labetalol. *J Pharmacol Exp Ther*. 1981;218:441–452.
60. Larsen LS. Labetalol in the treatment of epinephrine overdose. *Ann Emerg Med*. 1990;19:680–682.
61. Lebel M, Langlois S, Belleau LJ, et al. Labetalol infusion in hypertensive emergencies. *Clin Pharmacol Ther*. 1985;37:615–618.
62. Wilson DJ, Wallin JD, Vlachakis ND, et al. Intravenous labetalol in the treatment of severe hypertensive and hypertensive emergencies. *Am J Med*. 1983;75:95–102.
63. Goldberg ME, McNulty SE, Azad SS, et al. A comparison of labetalol and nitroprusside for inducing hypotension during major surgery. *Anesth Analg*. 1990;70:537–542.
64. Durand PG, Lehot JJ, Foex P. Calcium-channel blockers and anaesthesia. *Can J Anaesth*. 1991;38:75–89.
65. Kaplan NM. Calcium entry blockers in the treatment of hypertension: current status and future prospects. *N Engl J Med*. 1989;262:817–823.
66. Kanneganti M, Halpern NA. Acute hypertension and calcium-channel blockers. *New Horiz*. 1996;4:19–25.
67. Reves JG. The relative hemodynamic effects of calcium entry blockers. *Anesthesiology*. 1984;61:3–5.
68. Reves JG, Kissin I, Lell WA, et al. Calcium entry blockers: uses and implications for anesthesiologists. *Anesthesiology*. 1982;57:504–518.
69. Kraynack BJ, Lawson NW, Gintautas J. Local anesthetic effect of verapamil in vitro. *Reg Anesth*. 1982;7:114–117.
70. Spirito P, Seidman CE, McKenna WJ, et al. The management of hypertrophic cardiomyopathy. *N Engl J Med*. 1997;336:775–780.
71. Opie LH. First line drugs in chronic stable effort angina: the case for newer, longer-acting calcium channel blocking drugs. *J Am Coll Cardiol*. 2000;36:1967–1971.
72. Murad SHN, Tabsh KMA, Conklin KA, et al. Verapamil: placental transfer and effects on maternal and fetal hemodynamics and atrioventricular conduction in the pregnant ewe. *Anesthesiology*. 1985;62:49–53.
73. Murad SHN, Tabsh KMA, Shilyanski G, et al. Effects of verapamil on uterine blood flow and maternal cardiovascular function in the awake pregnant ewe. *Anesth Analg*. 1985;64:7–10.
74. Bal L, Thierry S, Brocas E, et al. Pulmonary edema induced by calcium-channel blockade for tocolysis. *Anesth Analg*. 2004;99:910–911.
75. Zhang Y, White PF, Thornton L, et al. The use of nicardipine for electroconvulsive therapy: a dose-ranging study. *Anesth Analg*. 2005;100(2):378–381.
76. Verma A. Opportunities for neuroprotection in traumatic brain injury. *J Head Trauma Rehabil*. 2000;15:1149–1156.
77. Allen GS, Ahn HS, Preziosi TJ, et al. Cerebral arterial spasm: a controlled trial of nimodipine in patients with subarachnoid hemorrhage. *N Engl J Med*. 1983;308:619–624.
78. Gelmers HJ, Gorter K, deWeerdt CJ, et al. A controlled trial of nimodipine in acute ischemic stroke. *N Engl J Med*. 1988;318:303–307.
79. Steen PA, Gisvold SE, Milde JH, et al. Nimodipine improves outcome when given after complete cerebral ischemia in primates. *Anesthesiology*. 1985;62:406–414.
80. Henling CE, Slogoff S, Kodali SV, et al. Heart block after coronary artery bypass—effect of chronic administration of calcium-entry blockers and β-blockers. *Anesth Analg*. 1984;63:515–520.
81. Merin RG. Calcium channel blocking drugs and anesthetics: is the drug interaction beneficial or detrimental? *Anesthesiology*. 1987;66:111–113.
82. Kapur PA, Norel EJ, Dajee H, et al. Hemodynamic effects of verapamil administration after large doses of fentanyl in man. *Can Anaesth Soc J*. 1986;33:138–144.
83. Chew CYC, Hecht HS, Collett JT, et al. Influence of severity of ventricular dysfunction on hemodynamic responses to intravenously administered verapamil in ischemic heart disease. *Am J Cardiol*. 1981;47:917–922.
84. Durant NN, Nguyen N, Katz RL. Potentiation of neuromuscular blockade by verapamil. *Anesthesiology*. 1984;60:298–303.
85. van Poorten JE, Chasmana KM, Kuypers SM, et al. Verapamil and reversal of vecuronium neuromuscular blockade. *Anesth Analg*. 1984;63:155–157.
86. Zalman F, Perloff JK, Durant NW, et al. Acute respiratory failure following intravenous verapamil in Duchenne's muscular dystrophy. *Am Heart J*. 1983;105:510–511.
87. Lawson NW, Kraynack BJ, Gintautas J. Neuromuscular and electrocardiographic responses to verapamil in dogs. *Anesth Analg*. 1983;62:50–54.
88. Jones RM, Cashman JN, Casson WR, et al. Verapamil potentiation of neuromuscular blockade: failure of reversal with neostigmine but prompt reversal with edrophonium. *Anesth Analg*. 1985;64:1021–1025.
89. Rosenblatt RM, Weaver JM, Want Y, et al. Verapamil potentiates the toxicity of local anesthetics. *Anesth Analg*. 1984;63:269.
90. Nugent M, Tinker JH, Moyer TP. Verapamil worsens rate of development and hemodynamic effects of acute hyperkalemia in halothane-anesthetized dogs. Effects of calcium therapy. *Anesthesiology*. 1984;60:435–439.
91. Roth JL, Nugent M, Gronert GA. Verapamil does not alter succinylcholine-induced increases in serum potassium during halothane anesthesia in normal dogs. *Anesth Analg*. 1985;64:1202–1204.
92. Saltzman LS, Kates RA, Corke BC, et al. Hyperkalemia and cardiovascular collapse after verapamil and dantrolene administration in swine. *Anesth Analg*. 1984;63:473–478.
93. Rubin AS, Zablocki AD. Hyperkalemia, verapamil, and dantrolene. *Anesthesiology*. 1987;66:246–249.
94. Gallant EM, Foldes FF, Rempel WE, et al. Verapamil is not a therapeutic adjunct to dantrolene in porcine malignant hyperthermia. *Anesth Analg*. 1985;64:601–606.
95. Chobanian AV. Calcium-channel blockers: lessons learned from MIDAS and other clinical trials. *JAMA*. 1996;276:829–830.
96. Furberg CD, Posaty BM, Meyer JV. Nifedipine: dose-related increase in mortality in patients with coronary heart disease. *Circulation*. 1995;92:1326–1331.
97. Pahor M, Guralnik JM, Furberg CD, et al. Risk of gastrointestinal hemorrhage with calcium antagonists in hypertensive patients over 67. *Lancet*. 1996;347:1061–1066.
98. Wagenknecht LE, Furberg CD, Hammon JW, et al. Surgical bleeding: unexpected effect of a calcium antagonist. *BMJ*. 1995;310:776–777.
99. Pahor M, Guralnik JM, Salive ME, et al. Do calcium-channel blockers increase the risk of cancer? *Am J Hypertens*. 1996;9:695–699.

CHAPTER 20

Vasodilators

Updated by: James Ramsay • Carter Peatross

As described in Chapter 14, control of vascular tone in the peripheral and pulmonary circulations is a complex interplay of local metabolism, endothelial function, and regulation by the sympathetic nervous and endocrine systems. This chapter deals with the anesthetic implications of preexisting conditions and medications patients may be receiving, which affect the vasculature, as well as medications given acutely in the perioperative period in order to reduce systemic and pulmonary vascular pressures.

Systemic Hypertension

Systemic hypertension is estimated to affect 30% of adults in the United States[1] and is defined as 150 to 159/90 to 99 mm Hg (stage 1) or greater than or equal to 160/100 mm Hg (stage 2).[2] By far, the most common type of hypertension is "essential" or "primary" for which there is no clear unifying pathophysiology despite decades of research. What is clear, however, is that hypertension is a major risk factor for cardiovascular disease including atherosclerosis, heart failure, stroke, renal disease, and overall decreased survival. "Secondary" hypertension is much less common and can be due to a variety of causes (Table 20-1). Antihypertensive medications are used to control both primary and secondary hypertension. If more than three medications are required for consistent control, a diagnosis of secondary hypertension should be strongly suspected.

Management of essential hypertension includes alteration in lifestyle and diet (smoking cessation, weight reduction, increased physical activity, salt restriction) and use of medications. Most commonly, a thiazide diuretic is the initial therapy as increased sodium excretion results in decreased blood pressure, and these medications are inexpensive and require infrequent dosing. However, their chronic use requires potassium monitoring and supplementation. Alternatively, monotherapy with a dihydropyridine calcium channel antagonist, such as amlodipine, or an angiotensin-converting enzyme (ACE) inhibitor or angiotensin II receptor blocker (ARB) may be used.

Calcium channel blockade offers a direct vasodilator effect without the requirement of salt restriction and is associated with relatively few side effects. Use of an ACE inhibitor or ARB targets the renin-angiotensin system, a major contributor to blood pressure control. Decreased renal perfusion and increased sympathetic nervous system activity cause the release of renin, which then acts on "renin substrate" or angiotensin I at various sites in the body to release angiotensin II, a potent vasocontrictor and promotor of sodium and water retention.[3] Inhibition of angiotensin II production (with ACE inhibitor) or blockade of its receptor (with ARB) causes a reliable and potent antihypertensive effect, with very few side effects. In addition, in patients with most types of cardiac disease, these drugs have a well-known survivial benefit. Although β-adrenergic blockade is also an option, these agents may be associated with inferior stroke protection (when compared to calcium channel blockade, ACE inhibitor, and ARB) in patients older than the age of 60 years[4] and have a greater potential for systemic side effects.

Specific Antihypertensive Drugs and Anesthesia

Hypertensive patients are likely to be receiving one or more of thiazide diuretics, calcium channel blockers, ACE inhibitors/ARB medications, and β-adrenergic blockers. Less commonly, patients may be receiving other drugs which antagonize the sympathetic nervous system (centrally acting α_2 agonist clonidine, peripheral α_1 antagonists, or α/β antagonists such as labetalol or carvedilol, nitrates, or hydralazine) (Table 20-2). Although many other drugs have been used in the past, they will not be discussed here. In general, antihypertensive therapy should be continued until the time of surgery, as managing poorly controlled hypertension is likely to be more difficult than managing the well-controlled hypertensive patient. Severe or poorly controlled hypertension is a relatively common

Table 20-1

Systemic Hypertension

Essential (primary)
Secondary
  Obstructive sleep apnea
  Renal disease
    Renal parenchymal disease
    Renal artery stenosis
  Endocrine disease
    Pheochromocytoma
    Primary aldosteronism
    Cushings's disease
    Hyperparathyroidism
    Hyper- and hypothyroidism
  Medications
    Oral contraceptives
    Chronic NSAID use
    Antidepressants
    Alcohol
  Aortic coarctation

NSAID, nonsteroidal antiinflammatory drug.

cause for postponement of surgery,[5] although evidence supporting this practice comes from small studies mostly more than 20 years old. Specific drugs and implications for perioperative management are discussed in the following text.

Sympatholytics

β-Adrenergic Blockers

As mentioned earlier, β blockers are less commonly used as first-line agents in hypertension as other agents may have a better safety profile for this indication in those older than the age of 60 years. In addition, β blockers have a potential side effect profile which limits their use in many patients including fatique, depression, and impotence. However, β blockers are indicated for long-term treatment of patients with coronary artery disease and heart failure and for their anthypertensive action in these patients.

Mechanism of Action

β Blockers can be classified according to whether they exhibit β_1 selective versus nonselective properties and whether they possess intrinsic sympathomimetic activity. A β blocker with selective properties binds primarily to β_1 (cardiac) receptors, whereas a β blocker with nonselective properties has equal affinity for β_1 and β_2 (vascular and bronchial smooth muscle, metabolic) receptors. The β blockers with intrinsic sympathomimetic activity tend to produce less bradycardia and thus are less likely to unmask left ventricular dysfunction. These drugs are also less likely to produce vasospasm and thus to exacerbate symptoms of peripheral vascular disease. The antihypertensive effect of β blockers and other vasodilators may be attenuated by nonsteroidal antiinflammatory drugs.[6]

Table 20-2

Intravenous Antihypertensive Drugs Commonly Used in the Perioperative Setting

DRUG Mechanism	DOSE Bolus Infusion	Onset	DURATION Plasma Half-life Clinical Effect[a]
Metoprolol β_1 Blocker	1–5 mg	1–5 min	Half-life: 3–7 h Clinical: 1–4 h
Labetalol $\alpha_1, \beta_1, \beta_2$ Blocker	5–20 mg 0.5–2 mg/min	1–5 min	Half-life: 6 h Clinical: 1–4 h
Esmolol Beta-1 blocker	50–300 μg/kg/min	1–2 min	Half-life: 9 min
Nicardipine Dihydropyridine Ca blocker	100 μg 5–15 mg/h	2–10 min	Half-life: 2–4 h Clinical: 30–60 min
Hydralazine Arteriolar dilator	5–20 mg	5–20 min	Half-life: 2–8 h Clinical: 1–8 h
Fenoldopam Dopamine type 1 agonist	0.05–1.6 μg/kg/min	5–10 min	Half-life: 5 min Clinical: 30–60 min
Nitroprusside NO donor	0.25–4 μg/kg/min	1–2 min	Half-life: <10 min Clinical: 1–10 min
Nitroglycerin NO donor	5–300 μg/kg/min	1–2 min	Half-life: 1–3 min Clinical: 5–10 min

[a]Clinical effect commonly seen after bolus dose or stopping infusion.
Ca, calcium; NO, nitric oxide.

In contrast to nonselective β blockers such as propranolol, cardioselective β_1 blockers (acebutolol, atenolol, metoprolol, bisoprolol) administered in low to moderate doses are unlikely to produce bronchospasm, decrease peripheral blood flow, or mask hypoglycemia. For these reasons, they are the preferred drugs for patients with pulmonary disease, insulin-dependent diabetes mellitus, or symptomatic peripheral vascular disease. The nonselective agent carvedilol which also has α_1 blocking action has been shown to improve survival in patients with systolic heart failure.[7] The cardioselective drugs metoprolol and bisoprolol have also been shown to provide a survival benefit in this population, although not as great as carvedilol. Labetalol is another nonselective β blocker which also has significant α_1 blocking action. The presence of α-adrenergic blocking properties results in less bradycardia and negative inotropic effects compared with "pure" β blockers. These α properties, however, may result in orthostatic hypotension. The incidence of bronchospasm is similar to that seen with atenolol or metoprolol. Intravenous (IV) labetalol is used in hypertensive emergencies and is particularly useful in managing patients with type B aortic dissections, facilitating conversion from IV to oral medications.

Side Effects

Treatment of hypertension with β blockers involves certain risks, including bradycardia and heart block, congestive heart failure, bronchospasm, claudication, masking of hypoglycemia, sedation, impotence, and when abruptly discontinued may precipitate angina pectoris or even myocardial infarction. Patients with any degree of congestive heart failure cannot generally tolerate more than modest doses of β blockers, yet it is clear that when dosage is slowly increased and the drugs are given chronically, the antiadrenergic effect provides a signficant benefit in chronic systolic heart failure. In patients with symptomatic asthma, β blockers should be avoided. β Blockers potentially increase the risk of serious hypoglycemia in diabetic patients because they blunt autonomic nervous system responses that would warn of hypoglycemia. Nevertheless, the incidence of hypoglycemia has not been shown to be increased in diabetic patients being treated with β-adrenergic antagonists to control hypertension.[8]

Intravenous β Blockers

IV β blockers available in North America include metoprolol, propranolol, labetalol (an α_1/nonselective β blocker), and esmolol, which is a very short-acting cardioselective agent, inactivated by plasma esterases. Perioperative β blockade can be used to continue preoperative therapy, but due to extensive first-pass activity for oral agents, the conversion to IV dosing is somewhat unpredictable. In the case of labetalol, its β:α ratio is 3:1 when taken orally and 7:1 when given IV.[9]

α_1 Receptor Blockers

Prazosin, terazosin, and doxazocin are oral, selective postsynaptic α_1-adrenergic receptor antagonists resulting in vasodilating effects on both arterial and venous vasculature. Absence of presynaptic α_2 receptor antagonism leaves intact the normal inhibitory effect on norepinephrine release from nerve endings. These drugs are unlikely to elicit reflex increases in cardiac output and renin release. In contrast, oral phenoxybenzamine and IV phentolamine are nonselective α blockers which also block presynaptic α_2 receptors. Both of these drugs are used almost exclusively in the management of pheochromocytoma and will not be discussed further. Urapidil is a potent α_1 antagonist and centrally acting serotonin antagonist which is available outside the United States in both oral and IV formulations.

In addition to treating essential hypertension, prazosin may be of value for decreasing afterload in patients with congestive heart failure. Prazosin may also be a useful drug for the preoperative preparation of patients with pheochromocytoma. This drug has been used to relieve the vasospasm of Raynaud's phenomenon. Another useful indication for prazosin in the treatment of essential hypertension is the presence of benign prostatic hypertrophy in older males, as this drug decreases the size of the gland.[10]

Pharmacokinetics

Prazosin is nearly completely metabolized, and less than 60% bioavailability after oral administration suggests the occurrence of substantial first-pass hepatic metabolism. The elimination half-time is about 3 hours and is prolonged by congestive heart failure but not renal dysfunction. The fact that this drug is metabolized in the liver permits its use in patients with renal failure without altering the dose.

Cardiovascular Effects

Prazosin decreases systemic vascular resistance without causing reflex-induced tachycardia or increases in renin activity as occurs during treatment with hydralazine or minoxidil. Failure to alter plasma renin activity reflects continued activity of α_2 receptors that normally inhibit the release of renin. Vascular tone in both resistance and capacitance vessels is decreased, resulting in decreased venous return and cardiac output.

Side Effects

The side effects of prazosin include vertigo, fluid retention, and orthostatic hypotension. Nonsteroidal antiinflammatory drugs may interfere with the antihypertensive effect of prazosin. Dryness of the mouth, nasal congestion, nightmares, urinary frequency, lethargy, and sexual dysfunction may accompany treatment with this drug. Hypotension during epidural anesthesia may be exaggerated in the presence of prazosin, reflecting drug-induced α_1 blockade that prevents compensatory vasoconstriction in the unblocked portions of the body.[11] The resulting decrease in systemic vascular resistance results in hypotension that may not be responsive to the usual clinical doses of an α_1-adrenergic agonist such as phenylephrine. In this situation, administration of epinephrine may be necessary to increase systemic vascular resistance and systemic blood pressure. Conceivably, the combination of prazosin and a β blocker could result in particularly refractory hypotension during regional anesthesia due to potentially blunted responses to β_1 as well as α_1 agonists.

α_2 Agonists

Clonidine is a centrally acting selective partial α_2-adrenergic agonist (220:1 α_2 to α_1 activity) that acts as an antihypertensive drug by virtue of its ability to decrease sympathetic output from the central nervous system (CNS). This drug has proved to be particularly effective in the treatment of patients with severe hypertension or renin-dependent disease. The usual daily adult dose is 0.2 to 0.3 mg orally. The availability of a transdermal clonidine patch designed for weekly administration is a more convenient formulation but is not useful in the acute setting as the onset is slow (hours). Another drug of the same class is IV dexmedetomidine, a much more α_2 selective drug which is approved for sedation rather than hypertension, although it does have a blood pressure–lowering action. Dexmedetomidine is discussed in Chapter 5.

Mechanism of Action

α_2-Adrenergic agonists produce clinical effects by binding to α_2 receptors of which there are three subtypes (α_{2A}, α_{2B}, α_{2C}) that are distributed ubiquitously, and each may be uniquely responsible for some, but not all, of the actions of α_2 agonists (Fig. 20-1).[12] α_{2A} Receptors mediate sedation, analgesia, and sympatholysis, whereas α_{2B} receptors mediate vasoconstriction and possibly antishivering effects. The startle response may reflect activation of α_{2C} receptors.

Clonidine stimulates α_2-adrenergic inhibitory neurons in the medullary vasomotor center. As a result, there is a decrease in sympathetic nervous system outflow from CNS to peripheral tissues. Decreased sympathetic nervous system activity is manifested as peripheral vasodilation and decreases in systemic blood pressure, heart rate, and cardiac output. The ability of clonidine to modify the function of potassium channels in the CNS (cell membranes become hyperpolarized) may be the mechanism for profound decreases in anesthetic requirements produced by clonidine and other even more selective α_2-adrenergic agonists such as dexmedetomidine. α_2 Receptors on blood vessels mediate vasoconstriction and on peripheral sympathetic nervous system nerve endings inhibit release of norepinephrine. Neuraxial placement of clonidine inhibits spinal substance P release and nociceptive neuron firing produced by noxious stimulation.

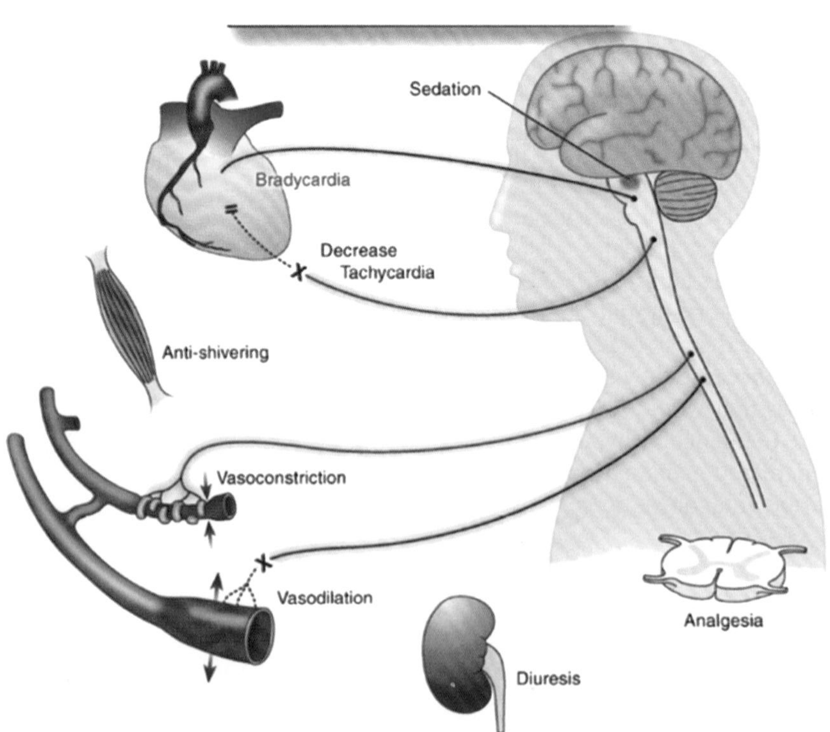

FIGURE 20-1 Schematic depiction of effects that are mediated by α_2-adrenergic receptors. The site for sedation is the locus ceruleus of the brainstem, whereas the principal site of analgesia is most likely the spinal cord. In the heart, the dominant effect of α_2 stimulation is attenuation of tachycardia through block of the cardioaccelerator nerves and bradycardia through vagal stimulation. In the peripheral vasculature, there are vasodilatory effects reflecting sympatholysis and vasoconstriction mediated by α_2 receptors in smooth muscle cells. (From Kamibayashi T, Maze M. Clinical uses of alpha$_2$-adrenergic agonists. *Anesthesiology*. 2000;93:1345–1349, with permission.)

Pharmacokinetics

Clonidine is rapidly absorbed after oral administration and reaches peak plasma concentrations within 60 to 90 minutes. The elimination half-time of clonidine is between 9 and 12 hours, with approximately 50% metabolized in the liver, whereas the rest is excreted unchanged in urine. The duration of hypotensive effect after a single oral dose is about 8 hours. The transdermal route requires about 48 hours to produce steady-state therapeutic plasma concentrations.

Cardiovascular Effects

The decrease in systolic blood pressure produced by clonidine is more prominent than the decrease in diastolic blood pressure. In patients treated chronically, systemic vascular resistance is little affected, and cardiac output, which is initially decreased, returns toward predrug levels. Homeostatic cardiovascular reflexes are maintained, thus avoiding the problems of orthostatic hypotension or hypotension during exercise. The ability of clonidine to decrease systemic blood pressure without paralysis of compensatory homeostatic reflexes is highly desirable. Renal blood flow and glomerular filtration rate are maintained in the presence of clonidine therapy.

Side Effects

The most common side effects produced by clonidine are sedation and xerostomia. Consistent with sedation and, perhaps more specifically, an agonist effect on postsynaptic α_2 receptors in the CNS are nearly 50% decreases in anesthetic requirements for inhaled anesthetics (minimum alveolar concentration) and injected drugs in patients pretreated with clonidine administered in the preanesthetic medication.[13] Patients pretreated with clonidine often manifest lower plasma concentrations of catecholamines in response to surgical stimulation and occasionally require treatment of bradycardia. As with other antihypertensive drugs, retention of sodium and water often occurs such that combination of clonidine with a diuretic is often necessary. Conversely, a diuretic effect during general anesthesia has been described after administration of oral clonidine, 2.5 to 5.0 μg/kg as preanesthetic medication.[14] Skin rashes are frequent, impotence occurs occasionally, and orthostatic hypotension is rare. Despite the fact that clonidine prevents opioid-induced skeletal muscle rigidity and produces skeletal muscle flaccidity, α_2 agonists have no effect on the responses evoked by neuromuscular blocking drugs.[15]

Rebound Hypertension

Abrupt discontinuation of clonidine therapy can result in rebound hypertension as soon as 8 hours and as late as 36 hours after the last dose.[16] Rebound hypertension is most likely to occur in patients who were receiving greater than 1.2 mg of clonidine daily. The increase in systemic blood pressure may be associated with a greater than 100% increase in circulating concentrations of catecholamines and intense peripheral vasoconstriction. Symptoms of nervousness, diaphoresis, headache, abdominal pain, and tachycardia often precede the actual increase in systemic blood pressure. β-Adrenergic blockade may exaggerate the magnitude of rebound hypertension by blocking the β_2 vasodilating effects of catecholamines and leaving unopposed their α vasoconstricting actions. Likewise, tricyclic antidepressant therapy may exaggerate rebound hypertension associated with abrupt discontinuation of clonidine therapy.[17] Tricyclic antidepressants can potentiate the pressor effects of norepinephrine.

Rebound hypertension can usually be controlled by reinstituting clonidine therapy or by administering a vasodilating drug such as hydralazine or nitroprusside. β-Adrenergic blocking drugs are useful but probably should be administered only in the presence of α-adrenergic blockade to avoid unopposed α vasoconstricting actions. In this regard, labetalol with α and β antagonist effects may be useful in the management of patients experiencing rebound hypertension. If oral clonidine therapy is interrupted because of surgery, use of transdermal clonidine provides a sustained therapeutic level of drug for as long as 7 days.[18] For a planned withdrawal, the clonidine dosage should be gradually decreased over 7 days or longer.

Rebound hypertension after abrupt discontinuation of chronic treatment with antihypertensive drugs is not unique to clonidine.[16] For example, abrupt discontinuation of β blocker therapy has been associated with clinical evidence of excessive sympathetic nervous system activity. Antihypertensive drugs that act independently of central and peripheral sympathetic nervous system mechanisms (direct vasodilators, ACE inhibitors) do not seem to be associated with rebound hypertension after sudden discontinuation of therapy.

Other Clinical Uses

α-Adrenergic agonists (clonidine and dexmedetomidine) induce sedation, decrease anesthetic requirements, and improve perioperative hemodynamic (attenuate blood pressure and heart rate responses to surgical stimulation) and sympathoadrenal stability.[12] Although a number of small studies have demonstrated these benefits, a recent large trial failed to demonstrate a cardioprotective effect when used perioperatively.[19] Both clonidine and dexmedetomidine have been used to help reduce the sympathetic nervous system hyperactivity associated with alcohol and opioid withdrawal. α_2 Receptors within the spinal cord modulate pain pathways resulting in analgesia, and intrathecal clonidine has been studied as an effective adjuvant to neuraxial blockade both enhancing and prolonging sensory and motor block.

Angiotensin-Converting Enzyme Inhibitors

ACE inhibitors represented a major advance in the treatment of all forms of hypertension because of their potency and minimal side effects, resulting in improved patient compliance.[20] These drugs are free of many of the CNS side effects associated with other antihypertensive drugs, including depression, insomnia, and sexual dysfunction. Other adverse effects, such as congestive heart failure, bronchospasm, bradycardia, and exacerbation of peripheral vascular disease, are not seen with ACE inhibitors either. Similarly, metabolic changes induced by diuretic therapy, such as hypokalemia, hyponatremia, and hyperglycemia, are not observed. Rebound hypertension, as seen with clonidine, has also not been observed with ACE inhibitors.

ACE inhibitors are most effective in treating systemic hypertension secondary to increased renin production. These drugs have been established as first-line therapy in patients with systemic hypertension, congestive heart failure, and mitral regurgitation. ACE inhibitors are more effective and possibly safer than other antihypertensive drugs in the treatment of hypertension in diabetics.[21] There is also evidence that ACE inhibitors delay the progression of diabetic renal disease.[22] As mentioned earlier, ACE inhibitors have been shown to provide a survival benefit in patients who have suffered a myocardial infarction and in patients with heart failure.[23]

Mechanism of Action

Angiotensin II normally binds to a specific cell membrane receptor (AT_1) that ultimately leads to increased release of calcium from sarcoplasmic reticulum to produce vasoconstriction. Decreased generation of angiotensin II due to the administration of an ACE inhibitor results in reduced vasoconstrictive effects. In addition, plasma concentrations of aldosterone are decreased resulting in less sodium and water retention. ACE inhibitors also block the breakdown of bradykinin, an endogenous vasodilator substance, which contributes to the antihypertensive effects of these drugs. ACE inhibitors, like statins, reduce activation of low-density lipoprotein (LDL) receptors and thus decrease plasma concentrations of LDL cholesterol. If the concentration of LDL cholesterol is already sufficiently low, ACE inhibitors may no longer be effective in reducing the rate of cardiovascular events.[24]

ACE inhibitors can be classified according to the structural element that interacts with the zinc ion of the enzyme as well as the form in which the drug is administered (prodrug or active form). Administration of ACE inhibitors as prodrugs increases oral bioavailability prior to their hepatic metabolism to the active drug. Enalapril is the prodrug of the active ACE inhibitor, enalaprilat, and conversion may be altered in patients with hepatic dysfunction. Captopril and lisinopril are not prodrugs. The major difference among clinically used ACE inhibitors is in duration of action.[25]

Side Effects

Cough, upper respiratory congestion, rhinorrhea, and allergic-like symptoms seem to be the most common side effects of ACE inhibitors.[26] It is speculated that these airway responses reflect potentiation of the effects of kinins due to drug-induced inhibition of peptidyl–dipeptidase activity and subsequent breakdown of bradykinin. If respiratory distress develops, prompt injection of epinephrine (0.3 to 0.5 mL of a 1:1,000 dilution subcutaneously) is advised. Angioedema is a potentially life-threatening complication of treatment with ACE inhibitors. Decreases in glomerular filtration rate may occur in patients treated with ACE inhibitors. For this reason, ACE inhibitors are used with caution in patients with preexisting renal dysfunction and are not recommended for patients with renal artery stenosis. Hyperkalemia is possible due to decreased production of aldosterone. The risk of hyperkalemia is greatest in patients with recognized risk factors (congestive heart failure with renal insufficiency).[28] Measurement of plasma concentrations of potassium may be indicated in these patients.

Preoperative Management

Adverse circulatory effects during anesthesia are recognized in patients chronically treated with ACE inhibitors leading some to recommend that these drugs be discontinued 12 to 24 hours before anesthesia and surgery.[29] A recent retrospective study of more than 75,000 patients (9,900 taking ACE inhibitors) suggested that although continuation of these drugs until the time of surgery is associated with more intraoperative hypotension, there were no adverse consequences.[30] The recent American College of Cardiology/American Heart Association guidelines for perioperative management suggests it is "reasonable" to continue these drugs until the time of surgery.[31] That being said, in small single center studies, the incidence of hypotension during induction of anesthesia in hypertensive patients chronically treated with ACE inhibitors was greater when ACE inhibitor therapy was continued until the morning of surgery compared with patients in whom therapy was discontinued at least 12 hours (captopril) or 24 hours (enalapril) preoperatively.[32] Exaggerated hypotension attributed to continued ACE inhibitor therapy has been responsive to crystalloid fluid infusion and/or administration of a catecholamine or vasopressin infusion. ACE inhibitors may increase insulin sensitivity and hypoglycemia, which is a concern when these drugs are administered to patients with diabetes mellitus. Nevertheless, there is no evidence that the incidence of hypoglycemia is greater in diabetics being treated with ACE inhibitors for control of hypertension.[8]

Specific Agents

Perioperative implications of different ACE inhibitors are similar; it is not clear that any one agent has more or less effect on perioperative blood pressure control. The only IV ACE inhibitor is enalaprilat; however, there is little published information to guide its use in this setting. It is not used as an infusion (i.e., dosing recommendations are for intermittent injection) and has a less predictable onset and duration of action as well as antihypertenisve action than short-acting direct vasodilators. Oral agents commonly seen are captopril, enalapril, lisinopril, and ramipril with the latter agents having a longer duration of action that captopril.

Angiotensin II Receptor Inhibitors

Angiotensin II receptor inhibitors produce antihypertensive effects by blocking the vasoconstrictive actions of angiotensin II without affecting ACE activity. Agents commonly used include losartan, candesartan, and valdesartan, all of which have a relatively long duration of action (one or twice daily dosing). There is no IV agent available. These agents have similar antihypertensive actions and benefits in patients with heart failure as ACE inhibitors, although the evidence is somewhat less robust. They also have similar side effect profile but do not inhibit breakdown of bradykinin, one of the benefits of ACE inhibitors and which may be a reason that ACE inhibitors are generally preferred as first-line therapy. A major difference between ACE inhibitors and ARBs is that ARBs do not cause cough, one of the reasons ACE inhibitors may not be tolerated (more than 10% of patients).

As with ACE inhibitors, hypotension following induction of anesthesia has been observed in patients being treated with ARBs causing some to recommend these drugs be discontinued on the day before surgery.[29]

Calcium Channel Blocking Drugs

Calcium channel blocking drugs used as antihypertensives inhibit calcium influx through the voltage-sensitive L-type calcium channels in vascular smooth muscle. They are arterial specific, with little effect on venous circulation. The calcium channel drugs are broadly categorized into drugs of the dihydropyridine class (nifedipine, amlodipine, nicardipine, clevidipine) and those of the nondihydropyridine class (verapamil and diltiazem). Verapamil and diltiazem are less potent vasodilators and both have negative inotropic and chronotropic activity limiting their use in patients with cardiac disease. In current practice, these drugs are more used for their antiarrhythmic action than antihypertensive action (see Chapter 21, Antiarrhythmic Drugs)

The dihydropyridines are potent vasodilators and are relatively safe to use in patients with heart failure and cardiac conduction defects, with the exception of large doses of short-acting nifedipine which may acutely lower the blood pressure and cause myocardial ischemia. As mentioned earlier, calcium channel blockers are particularly successful in treating hypertension in the elderly, African Americans, and salt-sensitive patients. The use of calcium channel blockers does not require concurrent sodium restriction, which makes these drugs unique antihypertensive drugs and perhaps the drugs of choice for patients who find sodium restriction unacceptable. The once-daily dosing of amlodipine is of particular appeal.

Nicardipine is available as an IV preparation for continuous infusion, and other shorter acting IV drugs such as clevidipine have been developed (clevidipine is broken down by plasma esterases). The use of IV nicardipine in the perioperative setting is well studied, and it also has been used in the treatment of hypertensive emergencies.[33] Clevidipine is also very effective in this setting but at the time of writing is not widely used in the United States.

Phosphodiesterase Inhibitors

The phosphodiesterases (PDEs) are a broad family of 11 isoenzymes which variably inhibit the breakdown of intracellular cyclic adenosine monophosphate (cAMP) and cyclic guanosine monophosphate (cGMP).[34] Although the many noncardiovascular actions of these enzymes are beyond the scope of this chapter, drugs of this class likely to be encountered by the anesthesiologist include the PDE3 inhibitors amrinone and milrinone and the PDE5 inhibitors sildenafil, tadalafil, and vardenafil. Inhibition of PDE causes vascular smooth muscle relaxation and, in the case of PDE III inhibitors, positive inotropy on intracellular calcium mobilization.

The IV PDE3 inhibitor milrinone has replaced amrinone due to its reduced side effect profile. Breakdown of both cAMP and cGMP are inhibited in myocardial cells and vascular smooth muscle by this enzyme. Its combined inotropic and vasodilator actions make it an ideal drug in the short-term treatment of heart failure, both in the intensive care and operative settings. An extensive literature documents its short-term hemodynamic benefits, whereas long-term oral use was associated with cardiovascular adverse effects and increased mortality. Although milrinone would not be a first-choice IV vasodilator in the absence of cardiac dysfunction, its vasodilation actions provide a significant benefit in the setting of heart failure.

The PDE5 inhibitors selectively inhibit the breakdown of cyclic cGMP, more in vascular smooth muscle than in other cardiovascular sites. Due to a high level of PDE5 in the lung, these drugs are effective pulmonary vasodilators, and they are also effective for erectile dysfunction. They are only available in oral formulations. Although peripheral (systemic) vascular effects are modest, when combined with other vasodilators, there can be significant lowering of blood pressure. Concurrent administration of nitroglycerin and erectile dysfunction drugs within 24 hours is not recommended as life-threatening hypotension from exaggerated systemic vasodilation may occur.[35]

Nitric Oxide and Nitrovasodilators

Nitric Oxide

Nitric oxide is recognized as a chemical messenger in a multitude of biologic systems, with homeostatic activity in the modulation of cardiovascular tone (see Chapter 14,

Circulatory Physiology), platelet regulation, and a neurotransmitter function in the CNS. In addition, it has roles in gastrointestinal smooth muscle relaxation and immune regulation. Therapeutically, nitric oxide (NO) is administered by inhalation (iNO) to produce relaxation of the pulmonary arterial vasculature.

Nitric oxide is synthesized in endothelial cells from the amino acid L-arginine by nitric oxide synthetase, a constitutively expressed enzyme. It then diffuses into precapillary resistance arterioles where it induces guanylate cyclase to increase the cGMP concentration, which in turn results in vasodilation. It is formerly known as "endothelial-derived relaxing factor." NO production has a large role in regulation of vascular tone throughout the body. There is evidence to support deficiency in NO production being related to various vascular diseases including essential hypertension. As a result of stress, an inducible form of NO synthetase can produce large amounts of NO contributing to excessive vasodilation. NO binds to the iron of heme-based proteins and thus is avidly bound and inactivated by hemoglobin leading to a half-time of less than 5 seconds under normal physiologic conditions.

As a therapeutic agent, inhaled NO affects the pulmonary circulation but not the systemic circulation due to its extremely rapid uptake by hemoglobin. Nitrovasodilators (nitrates and nitroprusside) work through generation of NO (see the following discussion) throughout the vasculature.

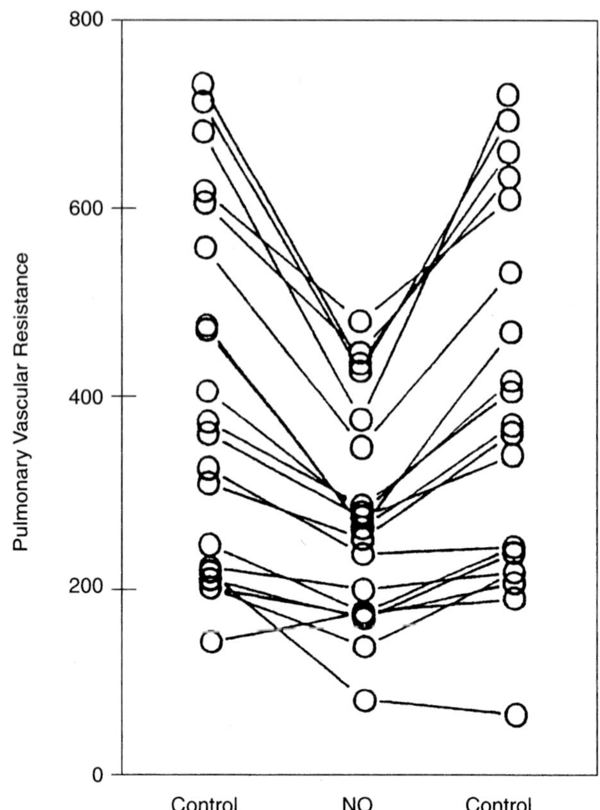

FIGURE 20-2 Inhalation of nitric oxide. Pulmonary vascular resistance (dyne/cm/s^{-5}) before, during, and after inhalation of nitric oxide (NO) for each patient before cardiopulmonary bypass. (From Rich GF, Murphy GD, Roos CM, et al. Inhaled nitric oxide: selective pulmonary vasodilation in cardiac surgical patients. *Anesthesiology.* 1993;78:1028–1035, with permission.)

Nitric Oxide as a Pulmonary Vasodilator

Inhaled NO causes pulmonary arterial vasodilation that is proportional to the degree of pulmonary vasoconstriction (Fig. 20-2). It has less effect on pulmonary vascular resistance if pulmonary vascular tone is not increased such as in types of pulmonary hypertension other than "primary." By dilating vessels in alveoli where it is locally delivered, iNO usually improves oxygenation by improving ventilation-perfusion matching.

In the United States, the only approved indication for inhaled NO is in pediatric lung injury. Inhaled NO, 10 to 20 ppm, has been used for therapy of persistent pulmonary hypertension of the newborn.[36,37] Inhalation of NO in premature infants with respiratory distress syndrome decreases the incidence of chronic lung disease and death.[38]

In the adult population, NO is used "off label" in managing severe pulmonary hypertension especially in the setting of acute right heart dysfunction or failure and in perioperative management of heart and lung transplant recipients. In acute lung injury and acute respiratory distress syndrome, inhaled NO will often provide a modest improvement in pulmonary hemodynamics and oxygenation, but clinical trials have failed to demonstrate an outcome benefit in this setting.

Toxicity

Inhaled NO increases methemoglobin levels as NO combines with hemoglobin. The increases in methemoglobin concentrations are usually modest. Life-threatening rebound arterial hypoxemia and pulmonary hypertension may accompany discontinuation of inhaled NO therapy.[39] Because of the variability in rebound pulmonary hypertension, it is important to wean patients from inhaled NO slowly. NO is oxidized to nitrogen dioxide (NO_2) especially in the presence of high concentrations of oxygen. NO_2 is a known pulmonary toxin ("silo-filler's disease") and is a possible product of the interaction of NO with oxygen. It is conceivable that NO_2 concentrations could produce pulmonary toxicity during treatment with NO. Continuous monitoring of inspired NO and NO_2 concentrations provided in the current delivery system is important to provide an early warning of possible pulmonary toxicity. In the presence of left heart dysfunction or failure, the increased pulmonary blood flow caused by iNO can precipitate acute left heart failure and pulmonary edema.

Nitrodilators

Sodium nitroprusside and IV nitroglycerin are historically the vasodilators most widely used by anesthesiologists. As described earlier, these agents work through the generation of NO, which then augments cyclic cGMP in vascular smooth muscle, both arteries and veins, leading to vasodilation. The more recent availability of IV nicardipine and other arterial-specific dilators such as clevidipine and fenoldopam has to some degree replaced the use of the nitrodilators, especially nitroprusside due to its potential toxicities discussed later.

Sodium Nitroprusside

Sodium nitroprusside (SNP) is a direct-acting, nonselective peripheral vasodilator that causes relaxation of arterial and venous vascular smooth muscle.[40] It is composed of a ferrous ion center complexed with five cyanide (CN^-) moieties and a nitrosyl group. The molecule is 44% cyanide by weight and is soluble in water. SNP lacks significant effects on nonvascular smooth muscle and on cardiac muscle. Its onset of action is almost immediate, equipotent on arteries and veins, and its duration is transient, requiring continuous IV administration to maintain a therapeutic effect. The extreme potency of SNP necessitates careful titration of dosage as provided by continuous infusion devices and frequent monitoring of systemic blood pressure, often by intraarterial monitoring.

Mechanism of Action

When infused IV, SNP interacts with oxyhemoglobin, dissociating immediately and forming methemoglobin while releasing cyanide and NO.[40] Once released, NO activates the enzyme guanylate cyclase present in vascular smooth muscle, resulting in increased intracellular concentrations of cGMP.[40] cGMP inhibits calcium entry into vascular smooth muscle cells and may increase calcium uptake by the smooth endoplasmic reticulum to produce vasodilation.[41] As such, NO is the active mediator responsible for the direct vasodilating effect of SNP. In contrast to the organic nitrates (nitroglycerin), which require the presence of thio-containing compounds to generate NO, SPN spontaneously generates this product, thus functioning as a prodrug.

Metabolism

Metabolism of SNP begins with the transfer of an electron from the iron of oxyhemoglobin to SNP, yielding methemoglobin and an unstable SNP radical.[40] This electron transfer is independent of electron activity. The unstable SNP radical promptly breaks down, releasing all five cyanide ions, one of which reacts with methemoglobin to form cyanomethemoglobin. The remaining free cyanide ions are available to rhodanese enzyme in the liver and kidneys for conversion to thiocyanate. Rhodanese uses thiosulfate ions as sulfur donors, and most adults can detoxify approximately 50 mg of SNP using existing sulfur stores. Normal adult methemoglobin concentrations (about 0.5% of all hemoglobin) are capable of binding the cyanide released from 18 mg of SNP. Cyanomethemoglobin remains in dynamic equilibrium with free cyanide and is nontoxic. The nonenzymatic release of cyanide from SNP is not inhibited by hypothermia as may be present during cardiopulmonary bypass, whereas enzymatic conversion of cyanide to thiocyanate may be delayed.[42]

Dose and Administration

Patients receiving SNP should have blood pressure monitored continuously via an arterial catheter. The recommended initial dose of SNP is 0.3 μg/kg/minute IV titrated to a maximum rate of 10 μg/kg/minute IV, with the maximum rate not to be infused longer than 10 minutes.[43] SNP infusion rates of greater than 2 μg/kg/minute IV result in dose-dependent accumulation of cyanide and the risk of cyanide toxicity must be considered. Therefore, as other less toxic drugs are widely available, a reasonable approach might be to change to a different medication if the required dose approaches 2 μg/kg/minute. Delivery of the SNP infusion as protected from light by aluminum foil is most often via an infusion pump.

Organ-Specific Effects

Cardiovascular

Baroreceptor-mediated reflex responses to SNP-induced decreases in systemic blood pressure manifest as tachycardia and increased myocardial contractility. These reflex-mediated responses may oppose the blood pressure–lowering effects of SNP. Although decreased venous return would tend to decrease cardiac output, the net effect is often an increase in cardiac output due to reflex-mediated increases in peripheral sympathetic nervous system activity combined with decreased impedance to left ventricular ejection. In the setting of left ventricular failure, SNP decreases systemic vascular resistance, pulmonary vascular resistance, and right atrial pressure, whereas the effect on cardiac output depends on the initial left ventricular end-diastolic pressure. There is no evidence that SNP exerts direct inotropic or chronotropic effects on the heart.

SNP may increase the area of damage associated with a myocardial infarction through a phenomenon called "coronary steal."[44] SNP dilates resistance vessels in non-ischemic myocardium, resulting in diversion of blood flow away from ischemic areas where collateral blood vessels are already maximally dilated. Decreases in diastolic blood pressure produced by SNP may also contribute to myocardial ischemia by decreasing coronary perfusion pressure and associated coronary blood flow.[45]

Renal

SNP-induced decreases in systemic blood pressure may result in decreases in renal function. Release of renin may accompany blood pressure decreases produced by SNP and contribute to blood pressure overshoots when the drug is discontinued.[46] Pretreatment with a competitive inhibitor of angiotensin II prevents blood pressure overshoots after discontinuation of SNP, thus confirming the participation of the renin-angiotensin system in this response.[47] Increased plasma concentrations of catecholamines also accompany hypotension produced by SNP.

Hepatic

In animals, SNP-induced decreases in systemic blood pressure do not result in hepatic hypoxia or changes in hepatic blood flow.[45] Furthermore, hepatic blood flow does not change when cardiac output is maintained in anesthetized patients, despite 20% to 60% decreases in systemic blood pressure produced by SNP.[48]

Cerebral

SNP increases cerebral blood flow and cerebral blood volume. In patients with decreased intracranial compliance, this may increase intracranial pressure (greater than the increase produced by nitroglycerin). It is likely that the rapidity of systemic blood pressure decrease produced by SNP exceeds the capacity of the cerebral circulation to autoregulate its blood flow such that intracranial pressure and cerebral blood flow change simultaneously but in opposite directions.[49] Nevertheless, increases in intracranial pressure produced by SNP are maximal during modest decreases (<30%) in mean arterial pressure. When SNP-induced decreases in mean arterial pressure are greater than 30% of the awake level, the intracranial pressure decreases to below the awake level.[50] Furthermore, decreasing blood pressure slowly over 5 minutes with SNP in the presence of hypocarbia and hyperoxia negates the increase in intracranial pressure that accompanies the rapid infusion of nitroprusside.[51] Patients with known inadequate cerebral blood flow as associated with dangerously increased intracranial pressure or carotid artery stenosis should probably not be treated with SNP. During cardiopulmonary bypass, SNP has been shown to have no direct effect on cerebral vasculature and autoregulation is preserved.[52] The potential adverse effects of SNP on intracranial pressure are not present if the drug is administered after the dura has been surgically opened.

Pulmonary

Decreases in the Pa_{O_2} may accompany the infusion of SNP and other peripheral vasodilators used to produce controlled hypotension. Attenuation of hypoxic pulmonary vasoconstriction by peripheral vasodilators is the presumed mechanism.[53] Addition of propranolol to the vasodilator regimen does not alter the magnitude of decrease in Pa_{O_2}.[54] Furthermore, peripheral vasodilator-induced decreases in blood pressure are more likely to increase the shunt fraction in patients with normal lungs than in those with chronic obstructive pulmonary disease.[55] It is speculated that hypotension in normal patients leads to decreased pulmonary artery pressure such that preferential perfusion of dependent but poorly ventilated alveoli occurs. In contrast, patients with chronic obstructive pulmonary disease may develop destructive vascular changes that prevent alterations in the distribution of pulmonary blood flow in response to vasodilation. The addition of positive end-expiratory pressure may reverse vasodilator-induced decreases in the Pa_{O_2}.[56]

Hematologic

Increased intracellular concentrations of cGMP, as produced by SNP and nitroglycerin, have been shown to inhibit platelet aggregation.[57] Infusion rates of SNP of greater than 3 μg/kg/minute may result in decreases in platelet aggregation and increased bleeding time.[58] The postoperative stress-induced increase in platelet aggregation is absent in SNP-treated patients.[59] Increased bleeding time could also be the result of vasodilation secondary to a direct effect of SNP on vascular tone. However, clinical measures of intraoperative bleeding are not increased in SNP-treated patients, suggesting that decreased ability of platelets to aggregate during and after controlled hypotension does not have an adverse clinical effect.[59]

Toxicity

Cyanide Toxicity

Clinical evidence of cyanide toxicity may occur when the rate of IV SNP infusion is greater than 2 μg/kg/minute or when sulfur donors and methemoglobin are exhausted, thus allowing cyanide radicals to accumulate. Because any free cyanide radical may bind inactive tissue cytochrome oxidase and prevent oxidative phosphorylation, increased cyanide concentrations may precipitate tissue anoxia, anaerobic metabolism, and lactic acidosis. Children may be less able to mobilize thiosulfate stores despite increasing cyanide concentrations, leading to accelerated toxicity.

Regardless of the SNP infusion rate or total administered dose, cyanide toxicity should be suspected in any patient requiring an increasing dose especially more than 2 μg/kg/minute or in a previously responsive patient who becomes less or unresponsive to the drug. Mixed venous P_{O_2} is increased in the presence of cyanide toxicity, indicating paralysis of cytochrome oxidase and inability of tissues to use oxygen. At the same time, metabolic acidosis (plasma lactate concentrations of >10 mM, which correlates with blood cyanide concentrations of >40 μM) develops as a reflection of anaerobic metabolism in the tissues. Decreased cerebral oxygen use is evidenced by the increased cerebral venous oxygen content. In awake patients, CNS dysfunction (mental status changes, seizures) may occur.

Treatment of Cyanide Toxicity

Appearance of tachyphylaxis in a previously sensitive patient in association with metabolic acidosis and increased mixed venous P_{O_2} mandates immediate discontinuation of SNP and administration of 100% oxygen despite normal oxygen saturation. Sodium bicarbonate is administered to correct metabolic acidosis. Sodium thiosulfate, 150 mg/kg IV administered over 15 minutes, is a recommended treatment for cyanide toxicity.[40] Thiosulfate acts as a sulfur donor to convert cyanide to thiocyanate. If cyanide toxicity is severe, with deteriorating hemodynamics and metabolic acidosis, the recommended treatment is slow IV administration of sodium nitrate, 5 mg/kg. Sodium nitrate converts hemoglobin to methemoglobin, which acts as an antidote by converting cyanide to cyanomethemoglobin. Alternatively, hydroxocobalamin (vitamin B_{12a}), which binds cyanide to form cyanocobalamin (vitamin B_{12}), can be administered (25 mg per hour IV to a maximum of 100 mg) to treat cyanide toxicity. In addition to being expensive, hydroxocobalamin may produce a reddish discoloration of the skin and mucous membranes.[60] Another treatment is methylene blue, 1 to 2 mg/kg IV, administered over 5 minutes, to facilitate the conversion of methemoglobin to hemoglobin.

Thiocyanate Toxicity

Thiocyanate is cleared slowly by the kidneys, with an elimination half-time of 3 to 7 days.[40] Clinical thiocyanate toxicity is rare, as thiocyanate is 100-fold less toxic than cyanide. In patients with normal renal function, 7 to 14 days of SNP infusion in the 2 to 5 μg/kg/minute range may be required to produce potentially toxic thiocyanate blood concentrations. SNP infusions for 3 to 6 days may result in thiocyanate toxicity in patients with chronic renal failure who are not undergoing periodic hemodialysis.

Nonspecific symptoms of thiocyanate toxicity include fatigue, tinnitus, nausea, and vomiting. Clinical evidence of neurotoxicity produced by thiocyanate includes hyperreflexia, confusion, psychosis, and miosis. Toxicity may progress to seizures and coma. Increased thiocyanate concentrations competitively inhibit uptake and binding of iodine in the thyroid gland, sometimes producing clinical hypothyroidism. Thiocyanate clearance can be facilitated by dialysis. Oxyhemoglobin can slowly oxidize thiocyanate back to sulfate and cyanide, but this is insufficient to cause cyanide toxicity.

Methemoglobinemia

Adverse effects from methemoglobinemia produced by SNP breakdown are unlikely even in patients with a congenital inability to convert methemoglobin to hemoglobin (methemoglobin reductase deficiency).[40] The total SNP dose required to produce 10% methemoglobinemia exceeds 10 mg/kg. Patients receiving such high doses of SNP who present with evidence of impaired oxygenation despite an adequate cardiac output and arterial oxygenation should have methemoglobinemia included in the differential diagnosis. Measurement of methemoglobin via cooximetry may be helpful in these patients.

Clinical Use

The use of SNP, as mentioned earlier, has significantly declined with the introduction of more selective arterial agents which have a greater margin of safety and much less or absent toxicity. In addition, selective arterial agents do not generally have such a dramatic or acute effect on blood pressure due to preservation of venous tone. Before the availability of these drugs, SNP was used widely and well studied in the settings of controlled hypotension, hypertensive emergencies, aortic and cardiac surgery, and heart failure. In this latter population, the combined preload and afterload effect is still a possible advantage but at the cost of blood pressure lability and systemic toxicity. It is likely the use of SNP will continue to decline as experience grows with the newer agents.

Nitrates

Nitroglycerin is an organic nitrate that acts principally on venous capacitance vessels and large coronary arteries to produce peripheral pooling of blood and decreased cardiac ventricular wall tension.[61,62] However, as the dose of nitroglycerin is increased, there is also relaxation of arterial vascular smooth muscle. Nitroglycerin can produce pulmonary vasodilation equivalent to the degree of systemic arterial vasodilation. The most common clinical use of nitroglycerin is sublingual or IV administration for the treatment of angina pectoris as a result of either atherosclerosis of the coronary arteries or intermittent vasospasm of these vessels. Controlled hypotension can also be achieved with the continuous infusion of nitroglycerin.

Mechanism of Action

Nitroglycerin, like SNP, generates NO, which stimulates production of cGMP to cause peripheral vasodilation (see earlier discussion). In contrast to SNP, which spontaneously produces NO, nitroglycerin requires the presence of thio-containing compounds. In this regard, the nitrate group of nitroglycerin is biotransformed to NO through a glutathione-dependent pathway involving both glutathione and glutathione S-transferase. Nitroglycerin is not recommended in patients with hypertrophic obstructive cardiomyopathy or in the presence of severe aortic stenosis, and venous pooling may be followed by syncope.

Route of Administration

Nitroglycerin is most frequently administered by the sublingual route, but it is also available as an oral tablet, a buccal or transmucosal tablet, a sublingual spray, and a transdermal ointment or patch. Sublingual administration of nitroglycerin results in peak plasma concentrations within 4 minutes. Only about 15% of the blood flow from the sublingual area passes through the liver, which limits the initial first-pass hepatic metabolism of nitroglycerin. In contrast, nitroglycerin is well absorbed after oral administration but it is largely inactive because of first-pass hepatic metabolism.

Transdermal absorption of nitroglycerin, 5 to 10 mg over 24 hours, provides sustained protection against myocardial ischemia. The plasma concentration resulting from transdermal absorption of nitroglycerin is low, but tolerance to the drug effect occurs when the patches are left in place for longer than 24 hours. It is possible that removing the patches after 14 to 16 hours will prevent the development of tolerance.

Continuous infusion of nitroglycerin, via special delivery tubing to decrease absorption of the drug into plastic, is a useful approach to maintain a constant delivered concentration of nitroglycerin.

Pharmacokinetics

Nitroglycerin has an elimination half-time of about 1.5 minutes.[62] There is a large volume of distribution, reflecting tissue uptake, and it has been estimated that only 1% of total body nitroglycerin is present in the plasma. For this reason, plasma nitroglycerin concentrations may vary widely because of differences in tissue binding.

Methemoglobinemia

The nitrite metabolite of nitroglycerin is capable of oxidizing the ferrous ion in hemoglobin to the ferric state with the production of methemoglobin.[63,64]

In particular, high doses of nitroglycerin may produce methemoglobinemia in patients with hepatic dysfunction. Treatment of methemoglobinemia is as discussed earlier with SNP toxicity.

Tolerance

A limitation to the use of all nitrates is the development of tolerance to their vasodilating effects. Tolerance is dose-dependent and duration-dependent, usually manifesting within 24 hours of sustained treatment. If ischemia occurs during continuous administration of nitroglycerin, responsiveness to the antiischemic effects of the nitrate can usually be restored by increasing the dose. The mechanism of tolerance is not well understood but may reflect a change in the vasculature that limits the vasodilating effects of the nitrates. A drug-free interval of 12 to 14 hours is recommended to reverse tolerance to nitroglycerin and other nitrates. Rebound myocardial ischemia may occur during the drug-free interval.

Clinical Use

Perioperatively, nitroglycerin in all its forms is used to treat suspected myocardial ischemia as well as volume overload in the setting of heart failure (preload reduction). As a systemic antihypertensive, both for treatment and achieving controlled hypotenion, nitroglycerin infusion can be effective but its preferential effect on veins rather than arteries can make it less effective in severe hypertension than drugs which preferentailly act on the arteries. Although nitroglycerin has no "toxicity" (other than possible methemoglobinemia with high doses), its use for hypertension has declined with the availability of IV nicardipine and fenoldopam.

Isosorbide Dinitrate

Isosorbide dinitrate is a commonly administered oral nitrate for the prophylaxis of angina pectoris and for preload reduction in patients with heart failure. Its effects are very similar to that of nitroglycerin but as an oral agent, isosorbide dinitrate is well absorbed from the gastrointestinal tract and it is not subject to the extensive first-pass metabolism that limits oral use of nitroglycerin. It exerts a physiologic effect lasting up to 6 hours when taken in large doses of 60 to 120 mg. The longer acting sustained release form provides a prolonged antianginal effect and improves exercise tolerance for up to 6 hours. Isosorbide dinitrate may also be administered sublingually, producing an effect lasting up to 2 hours. The metabolite of isosorbide dinitrate, isosorbide-5-mononitrate, is more active than the parent compound. Orthostatic hypotension accompanies acute administration of isosorbide dinitrate, but tolerance to this and other pharmacologic effects seems to develop with chronic therapy.

Hydralazine

Hydralazine is a direct systemic arterial vasodilator which both hyperpolarizes smooth muscle cells and activates guanylate cyclase to produce vasorelaxation.[65] Arterial vasodilation by hydralazine produce reflex sympathetic nervous system stimulation with resulting increases in heart rate and myocardial contractility so this drug is not generally recommended for patients with myocardial ischemia or coronary disease. It is an effective afterload-reducing agent and is still used in combination with nitrates for outpatient treatment of congestive heart failure and for intermittent IV dosing in the perioperative period or critical care setting. Although it has been widely used in hypertensive disorders associated with pregnancy, other agents may be associated with less adverse outcomes.[66] Long-term hydralazine is associated with a systemic lupus syndrome, limiting its widespread use. Acute IV administration has a slightly delayed onset making it less appealing than other immediate-onset medications.

Fenoldopam

Fenoldopam is a dopamine type 1 receptor agonist, causing systemic arterial dilation through increasing cyclic cAMP. It has a particular action of increasing renal blood flow and increasing urine output and also increasing splanchnic blood flow due to the density of dopamine type 1 receptors in these beds.[67] Because of this action, it has been viewed by some as a possible "new renal dopamine" which might have a renal protective effect, but evidence to support this hypothesis is weak. There is no question, however, that when compared to other IV antihypertensive drugs such as SNP or nicardipine, there is greater urine output with fenoldopam for the same degree of antihypertensive action. Fenoldopam is only available in an IV preparation, it has a rapid onset and 10-minute elimination half-life. As is the case with other arterial dilators, there is a baroreflex-mediated increase in heart rate and plasma catecholamine level associated with its use. Adverse effects are limited to an increase in intraocular pressure, making this drug unsuitable for patients with glaucoma.

Diuretics

As discussed earlier, diuretics continue to be first-line oral agents used for essential hypertension. Patients are most likely to be prescribed a thiazide drug, with more potent loop diuretics (furosemide, bumetanide) reserved for patients where thiazides are less effective such as patients with renal insufficiency or heart failure. Diuretics are not, strictly speaking, vasodilators although there is evidence for a venodilating effect of IV furosemide.[68]

Both thiazide and loop diuretics cause potassium loss and their use generally mandates supplementation with potassium and often magnesium. This is true both for oral outpatient use and acute IV dosing in the perioperative or critical care setting.

Aldosterone antagonists or "potassium-sparing" agents are less potent than loop diuretics but have a clear role in patients with heart failure where their addition to other antihypertensive drugs (e.g., ACE inhibitors) confers a survival benefit. This is possibly due to blocking aldosterone effects on the heart.

Drugs Not Discussed

The earlier discussion of antihypertensive drugs and vasodilators has not included a number of older agents which are rarely used now for this indication in clinical practice in North America. These include trimethaphan, diazoxide, alphmethyldopa, and adenosine. The reader is referred to old texts for a discussion of these agents.

References

1. Egan BM, Zhao Y, Axon RN. US trends in prevalence, awareness, treatment, and control of hypertension, 1988–2008. *JAMA*. 2010; 303:2043.
2. James PA, Oparil S, Carter BL, et al. 2014 evidence-based guideline for the management of high blood pressure in adults: report from the panel members appointed to the Eighth Joint National Committee (JNC 8). *JAMA*. 2014;311:507.
3. Ichihawi I, Harris RC. Angiotensin actions in the kidney: renewed insight into the old hormone. *Kidney Int*. 1991;40:583.
4. Wiyesonge CS, Bradley HA, Volmink J, et al. Beta-blockers for hypertension. *Cochrane Database Syst Rev*. 2012;11:CD002003.
5. Dix P, Howell S. Survey of cancellation rate of hypertensive patients undergoing anaesthesia and elective surgery. *Br J Anaesth*. 2001;86:789.
6. Polónia J. Interaction of antihypertensive drugs with anti-inflammatory drugs. Cardiology. 1997;88(suppl 3):47–51.
7. Packer M, Britow MR, Cohn JN, et al. The effect of carvedilol on morbidity and mortality in patients with chronic heart failure. *N Engl J Med*. 1996;334:1349.
8. Shorr RI, Ray WA, Daugherty JR, et al. Antihypertensives and the risk of serious hypoglycemia in older persons using insulin or sulfonylureas. *JAMA*. 1997;278:40–43.
9. MacCarthy EP, Bloomfield SS. Labetalol: a review of its pharmacology, pharmacokinetics, clinical uses and adverse effects. *Pharmacotherapy*. 1983:4:193–219.
10. Foglar R, Shibta K, Horie K, et al. Use of recombinant alpha-1 adrenoceptors to characterize subtype selectivity of drugs for the treatment of prostatic hypertrophy. *Eur J Pharmacol*. 1995;288:201–206.
11. Lydiatt CA, Fee MP, Hill GE. Severe hypotension during epidural anesthesia in a prazosin-treated patient. *Anesth Analg*. 1993;76: 1152–1153.
12. Kamibayashi T, Maze M. Clinical uses of alpha$_2$-adrenergic agonists. *Anesthesiology*. 2000;93:1345–1349.
13. Ghignone M, Calvillo O, Quintin L. Anesthesia and hypertension: the effect of clonidine on perioperative hemodynamics and isoflurane requirements. *Anesthesiology*. 1987;67:3–10.
14. Hamaya Y, Nishikawa T, Dohi S. Diuretic effect of clonidine during isoflurane, nitrous oxide, and oxygen anesthesia. *Anesthesiology*. 1994;81:811–819.
15. Talke PO, Caldwell JE, Richardson CA, et al. The effects of dexmedetomidine on neuromuscular blockade in human volunteers. *Anesth Analg*. 1999;88:633–639.
16. Husserl FE, Messerli FH. Adverse effects of antihypertensive drugs. *Drugs*. 1981;22:188–210.
17. Stiff JL, Harris DB. Clonidine withdrawal complicated by amitriptyline therapy. *Anesthesiology*. 1983;59:73–74.
18. White WB, Gilbert JC. Transdermal clonidine in a patient with resistant hypertension and malabsorption. *N Engl J Med*. 1985;313:1418.
19. Devereaux PJ, Mrkobrada M, Sessler DI, et al. Aspirin in patients undergoing noncardiac surgery. *N Engl J Med*. 2014;370:1494–1503.
20. Croog SH, Levine S, Testa MA, et al. The effects of antihypertensive therapy on the quality of life. *N Engl J Med*. 1986;314:1657–1661.
21. McDougall C, Marshall G, Brady A, et al. Should all diabetic patients receive an ace inhibitor? Results from recent trials. *Br J Cardiol*. 2005;12(2):130–134.
22. Hendry BM, Viberti GC, Hummel S, et al. Modelling and costing the consequences of using an ACE inhibitor to slow the progression of renal failure in type I diabetic patients. *Q J Med*. 1997;90:277–282.
23. Yancy CW, Jessup M, Bozkurt B, et al. 2013 ACCF/AHA guideline for the management of heart failure: executive summary: a report of the American College of Cardiology Foundation/American Heart Association Task Force on practice guidelines. *Circulation*. 2013;128:1810.
24. Pitt B. ACE inhibitors for patients with vascular disease without left ventricular dysfunction—may they rest in PEACE? *N Engl J Med*. 2004;351:2115–2117.
25. Mirenda JV, Grissom TE. Anesthetic implications of the renin-angiotensin system and angiotensin-converting enzyme inhibitors. *Anesth Analg*. 1991;72:667–683.
26. Israili ZH, Hall WD. Cough and angioneurotic edema associated with angiotensin-converting enzyme inhibitor therapy: a review of the literature and pathophysiology. *Ann Intern Med*. 1992;117:234–239.
27. Brown NJ, Snowden M, Griffin MR. Recurrent angiotensin-converting enzyme inhibitor-associated angioedema. *JAMA*. 1997;278:232–233.
28. Palmer BF. Managing hyperkalemia caused by inhibitors of the renin-angiotensin-aldosterone system. *N Engl J Med*. 2004;351:585–592.
29. Bertrand M, Godet G, Meersschaert K, et al. Should the angiotensin II antagonists be discontinued before surgery? *Anesth Analg*. 2001;92;26–30.
30. Tuan A, You J, Shiba A, et al. Angiotensin converting enzyme inhibitors are not associated with respiratory complications or mortality after noncardiac surgery. *Anesth Analg*. 2012;114:552–560.
31. Fleisher LA, Fleischmann LE, Auerbach AD, et al. 2014 ACC/ AHA guideline on perioperative cardiovascular evaluation and

management of patients undergoing noncardiac surgery [published online ahead of print August 1, 2014]. *Circulation*.
32. Coriat P, Richer C, Douraki T, et al. Influence of chronic angiotensin-converting enzyme inhibition on anesthetic induction. *Anesthesiology*. 1994;81:299–307.
33. Salgado DR, Silva E, Vincent J-L. Control of hypertension in the the critically ill: a pathophysiological approach. *Ann Intens Care*. 2013;3:17.
34. Keravis T, Lugnier C. Cyclic nucleotide phosphodiesterase (PDE) isozymes as targets of the intracellular signalling network: benefits of PDE inhibitors in various diseases and perspectives for future developments. *Br J Pharmacol*. 2012;165:1288–1305.
35. Cheitlin MD, Hutter AM, Brindis RG, et al. ACC/AHA expert consensus document: use of sildenafil (Viagra) in patients with cardiovascular disease. *J Am Coll Cardiol*. 1999;33:273–281.
36. Kinsella JP, Neish SR, Sheffer E, et al. Low-dose inhalational nitric oxide in persistent pulmonary hypertension of the newborn. *Lancet*. 1992;340:819–820.
37. Roberts JD, Fineman JR, Morin CF, et al. Inhaled nitric oxide and persistent pulmonary hypertension of the newborn. *N Engl J Med*. 1997;336:605–610.
38. Schreiber MD, Gin-Mestan K, Marks JD, et al. Inhaled nitric oxide in premature infants with respiratory distress syndrome. *N Engl J Med*. 2003;349:2099–2107.
39. Haddad E, Lowson SM, Johns RA, et al. Use of inhaled nitric oxide perioperatively and in intensive care patients. *Anesthesiology*. 2000; 92:1821–1825.
40. Friederich JA, Butterworth JF. Sodium nitroprusside: twenty years and counting. *Anesth Analg*. 1995;81:152–162.
41. Moncada S, Higgs A. The L-arginine-nitric oxide pathway. *N Engl J Med*. 1993;329:2002–2012.
42. Moore RA, Geller EA, Gallagher JD, et al. Effect of hypothermic cardiopulmonary bypass on nitroprusside metabolism. *Clin Pharmacol Ther*. 1985;37:680–683.
43. Food and Drug Administration. New labeling for sodium nitroprusside emphasized risk of cyanide toxicity. *JAMA*. 1991;265:487.
44. Becker LC. Conditions for vasodilator-induced coronary steal in experimental myocardial ischemia. *Circulation*. 1978;57:1103–1110.
45. Sivarajan M, Amory DW, McKenzie SM. Regional blood flows during induced hypotension produced by nitroprusside or trimethaphan in the rhesus monkey. *Anesth Analg*. 1985;64:759–766.
46. Khambatta HJ, Stone G, Khan E. Hypertension during anesthesia on discontinuation of sodium nitroprusside-induced hypotension. *Anesthesiology*. 1979;51:127–130.
47. Delaney TJ, Miller ED. Rebound hypertension after sodium nitroprusside prevented by saralism in rats. *Anesthesiology*. 1980;52:154–156.
48. Chauvin M, Bonnet F, Montembault C, et al. Hepatic plasma flow during sodium nitroprusside-induced hypotension in humans. *Anesthesiology*. 1985;63:287–293.
49. Rogers MC, Hamburger C, Owen K, et al. Intracranial pressure in the cat during nitroglycerin induced hypotension. *Anesthesiology*. 1979;51:227–229.
50. Turner JM, Powell D, Gibson RM. Intracranial pressure changes in neurosurgical patients during hypotension induced with sodium nitroprusside or trimethaphan. *Br J Anaesth*. 1977;49:419–424.
51. Marsh ML, Aidinis SJ, Naughton KVH, et al. The technique of nitroprusside administration modifies the intracranial pressure response. *Anesthesiology*. 1979;51:538–541.
52. Rogers AT, Prough DS, Gravlee GP, et al. Sodium nitroprusside infusion does not dilate cerebral resistance vessels during hypothermic cardiopulmonary bypass. *Anesthesiology*. 1991;74:820–826.
53. Colley PS, Cheney FW Jr, Hlastala MP. Ventilation-perfusion and gas exchange effects of sodium nitroprusside in dogs with normal and edematous lungs. *Anesthesiology*. 1979;50:489–495.
54. Miller JR, Benumof JL, Trousdale FR. Combined effects of sodium nitroprusside and propranolol on hypoxic pulmonary vasoconstriction. *Anesthesiology*. 1982;57:267–271.
55. Casthely PA, Lear S, Cottrell JE, et al. Intrapulmonary shunting during induced hypotension. *Anesth Analg*. 1982;61:231–235.
56. Berthelsen P, St. Haxholdt O, Husum R, et al. PEEP reverses nitroglycerin-induced hypoxemia following coronary artery bypass surgery. *Acta Anaesthesiol Scand*. 1986;30:243–246.
57. Brodde OE, Anlauf M, Graben N, et al. In vitro and in vivo down-regulation of human platelet alpha$_2$-adrenoreceptors by clonidine. *Eur J Clin Pharmacol*. 1982;23:403–409.
58. Hines R, Barash PG. Infusion of sodium nitroprusside induces platelet dysfunction in vitro. *Anesthesiology*. 1989;70:611–615.
59. Dietrich GV, Hessen M, Boldt J, et al. Platelet function, and adrenoceptors during and after induced hypotension using nitroprusside. *Anesthesiology*. 1996;85:1334–1340.
60. Hall AH, Rumack BH. Hydroxocobalamin/sodium thiosulfate as a cyanide antidote. *J Emerg Med*. 1987;5:115–121.
61. Kaplan JA, Finlayson DC, Woodward S. Vasodilator therapy after cardiac surgery: a review of the efficacy and toxicity of nitroglycerin and nitroprusside. *Can Anaesth Soc J*. 1980;27:154–158.
62. Parker JD, Parker JO. Nitrate therapy for stable angina pectoris. *N Engl J Med*. 1998;338:520–526.
63. Fibuch EE, Cecil WT, Reed WA. Methemoglobinemia associated with organic nitrate therapy. *Anesth Analg*. 1979;58:521–523.
64. Zurick AM, Wagner RH, Starr NJ, et al. Intravenous nitroglycerin, methemoglobinemia, and respiratory distress in a postoperative cardiac surgical patient. *Anesthesiology*. 1984;61:464–466.
65. Wei S, Kasuya Y, Yanagisawa M, et al: Studies on endothelium-dependent vasorelaxation by hydralazine in porcine coronary artery. *Eur J Pharmacol*. 1997;321:307–314.
66. MaGee LA, Cham C, Waterman EJ, et al: Hydralazine for treatment of severe hypertension in pregnancy: meta-analysis. *BMJ*. 2003;327: 955–960.
67. Murphy MB, Murray C, Shorten GD. Fenoldopam-a selective peripheral dopamine-receptor agonist for the treatment of severe hypertension. *N Engl J Med*. 2001;345:1548–1557.
68. Jhund PS, McMurray JJ, Davle AP. The acute vascular effects of frusemide in heart failure. *Br J Clin Pharmacol*. 2000;50:9–13.

CHAPTER 21

Antiarrhythmic Drugs

Updated by: James Ramsay • Nicholas Anast

Cardiac arrhythmias occur commonly in the perioperative period, most of which are relatively benign and are due to transient changes in physiology, surgical stimuli, or the effect of anesthetic agents. Arrhythmias that require treatment are most commonly supraventricular, with atrial fibrillation being especially common after cardiac surgery.[1,2] The chronic use of antiarrhythmic drugs for treatment and prevention of cardiac arrhythmias is limited by the potential for these drugs to depress left ventricular contractility and the triggering of new arrhythmias[3] (see the section "Proarrhythmic Effects"). Improved survival for patients receiving implantable cardiac defibrillator devices compared with antiarrhythmic drugs has altered the treatment paradigms for patients with ventricular arrhythmias.[4] Likewise, catheter ablation techniques are preferred treatments for many supraventricular arrhythmias including atrial and certain types of atrial fibrillation.[5] For these reasons, pharmacologic treatment of cardiac arrhythmias is principally used to suppress atrial fibrillation and atrial flutter that is not responsive to catheter ablation treatment and for patients with implantable cardioverter-defibrillator devices who are receiving frequent indicated electrical shocks.

Pharmacologic treatment of cardiac arrhythmias and disturbances of the conduction of cardiac impulses with antiarrhythmic drugs is based on an understanding of the electrophysiologic basis of the abnormality and the mechanism of action of the therapeutic drug to be administered.[1,6] The two major physiologic mechanisms that cause ectopic cardiac arrhythmias are reentry and enhanced automaticity. Factors encountered in the perioperative period that facilitate cardiac arrhythmias due to both mechanisms include hypoxemia, electrolyte and acid–base abnormalities, myocardial ischemia, altered sympathetic nervous system activity, bradycardia, and the administration of certain drugs. It is not commonly appreciated that alkalosis is even more likely than acidosis to trigger cardiac arrhythmias. Hypokalemia and hypomagnesemia predispose to ventricular arrhythmias and must be suspected in patients who are being treated with diuretics. Increased sympathetic nervous system activity lowers the threshold for ventricular fibrillation, a phenomenon that is attenuated by β blockade and vagal stimulation. Bradycardia predisposes to ventricular arrhythmias by causing a temporal dispersion of refractory periods among Purkinje fibers, creating an electrical gradient between adjacent cells. Enlargement of a failing left ventricle stretches individual myocardial cells and can thereby induce cardiac arrhythmias. Decreasing left ventricular volume with administration of digitalis, diuretics, or vasodilators helps to control cardiac arrhythmias that are precipitated by this mechanism.

In some patients, correction of identifiable precipitating events is not sufficient to suppress cardiac ectopic rhythms, and therefore, specific cardiac antiarrhythmic drugs may be indicated. Drugs administered for the chronic suppression of cardiac arrhythmias pose little threat to the uneventful course of anesthesia and should be continued up to the time of induction of anesthesia.[1,7] As mentioned earlier, the majority of cardiac arrhythmias that occur during anesthesia do not require therapy. Cardiac arrhythmias, however, do require treatment when hemodynamic function is compromised or the disturbance predisposes to more serious cardiac arrhythmias.

General anesthetic–related cardiac arrhythmias have been ascribed to abnormal pacemaker activity characterized by suppression of the sinoatrial node, with the emergence of latent pacemakers within or below the atrioventricular tissues.[6] Furthermore, development of reentry circuits is likely to be important in the mechanism of cardiac arrhythmias that occur during anesthesia. Certain anesthetics, particularly volatile drugs, may have effects on the specialized conduction system for cardiac impulses.

Mechanism of Action

Antiarrhythmic drugs produce pharmacologic effects by blocking passage of ions across sodium, potassium, and calcium ion channels present in the heart (Fig. 21-1). The cardiac action potential results from the interplay of multiple inward and outward currents via specific ion

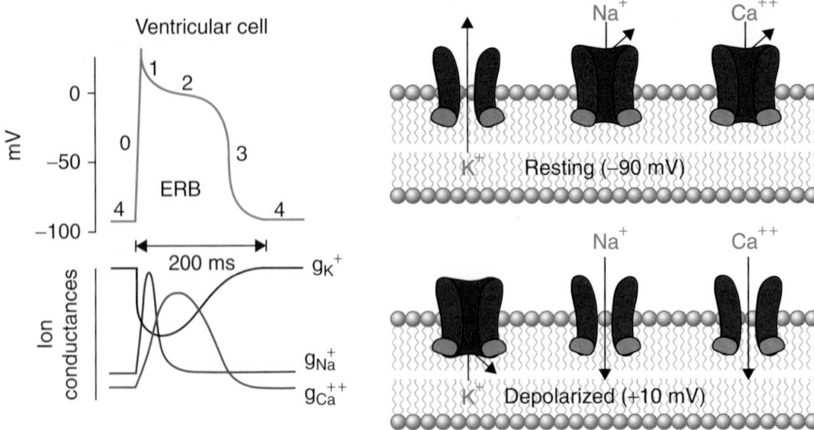

FIGURE 21-1 The physiologic basis of the cardiac action potential. Phase 0 represents rapid depolarization as a result of opening of Na^+ channels and closing of K^+ channels. Phase 1 is the period of initial repolarization that results from closure of Na^+ and opening of K^+ channels. Phase 2 is the plateau phase that results from the sustained Ca^{++} current that began with the initial depolarization. Phase 3 is repolarization due to opening of K^+ and closure of Ca^{++} channels. Phase 4 is the resting potential during which time K^+ channels are open and Na^+ and Ca^{++} channels are closed. The effective refractory period (ERP) is the time during which the cell cannot be depolarized again. (Adapted from Klabunde RE, ed. *Cardiovascular Physiology Concepts*. 2nd ed. Philadelphia, PA: Lippincott Williams & Wilkins; 2011.)

channels responsible for each of the five phases. The duration of each phase of the action potential differs in atrial compared with ventricular myocardium and the specialized systems for conduction of cardiac impulses differ in ion channel density. Ion channels are large membrane-bound glycoproteins that provide a pathway across cell membranes for the passage of ions. Ion channels exist in different states (open, inactivated, closed). In the inactivated state, the ion channel is unresponsive to a continued or new stimulus. The resting state is more prevalent during diastole, the active state occurs during the upstroke of the action potential, and the inactivated state occurs during the plateau phase of repolarization.

The effects of cardiac antiarrhythmic drugs on the action potential and effective refractory period of the cardiac action potential determine the clinical effect of these drugs. Drugs that primarily block inward sodium ion flow will slow conduction and result in suppression of the maximum upstroke velocity (V_{max}) of the cardiac action potential. Potassium channel blocking drugs prolong repolarization by increasing the duration of the cardiac action potential and the effective refractory period resulting in prolongation of the QTc interval on the electrocardiogram (ECG). Calcium channels are present in myocardial cells, and the α subunit of L and T calcium ion channels is the site of action of some cardiac antiarrhythmic drugs.

Classification

Cardiac arrhythmic drugs are most commonly classified into four groups based primarily on the ability of the drug to control arrhythmias by blocking specific ion channels and currents during the cardiac action potential (Tables 21-1 and 21-2).[8,9] Few cardiac antiarrhythmic drugs demonstrate

Table 21-1

Classification of Cardiac Antiarrhythmic Drugs

Class I (inhibit fast sodium ion channels)
Class IA
- Quinidine
- Procainamide
- Disopyramide
- Moricizine

Class IB
- Lidocaine
- Tocainide
- Mexiletine

Class IC
- Flecainide
- Propafenone

Class II (decrease rate of depolarization)
- Esmolol
- Propranolol
- Acebutolol

Class III (inhibit potassium ion channels)
- Amiodarone
- Sotalol
- Ibutilide
- Dofetilide
- Bretylium

Class IV (inhibit slow calcium channels)
- Verapamil
- Diltiazem

Table 21-2

Electrophysiologic and Electrocardiographic Effects of Cardiac Antiarrhythmic Drugs

	Class IA	Class IB	Class IC	Class II	Class III	Class IV
Depolarization rate (phase 0)	Decreased	No effect	Greatly decreased	No effect	No effect	No effect
Conduction velocity	Decreased	No effect	Greatly decreased	Decreased	Decreased	No effect
Effective refractory period	Greatly increased	Decreased	Increased	Decreased	Greatly increased	No effect
Action potential duration	Increased	Decreased	Increased	Increased	Greatly increased	Decreased
Automaticity	Decreased	Decreased	Decreased	Decreased	Decreased	No effect
P-R duration	No effect	No effect	Increased	No effect or increased	Increased	No effect or increased
QRS duration	Increased	No effect	Greatly increased	No effect	Increased	No effect
QTc duration	Greatly increased	No effect or decreased	Increased	Decreased	Greatly increased	No effect

completely specific effects on cardiac ion channels. Other characteristics including the impact of the drug on autonomic nervous system activity and myocardial contractility may be more important clinically. Antiarrhythmic drugs also differ in their pharmacokinetics and efficacy in treating specific types of arrhythmias (Tables 21-3 and 21-4).[7]

Class I Drugs

Class I drugs inhibit fast sodium channels during depolarization (phase 0) of the cardiac action potential with resultant decreases in depolarization rate and conduction velocity (see Fig. 21-1).[8]

Class IA Drugs

Class IA drugs (quinidine, procainamide, disopyramide, moricizine) lengthen both the action potential duration and the effective refractory period reflecting sodium channel inhibition and prolonged repolarization owing to potassium channel blockade.

Class IB Drugs

Class IB drugs (lidocaine, mexiletine, tocainide, phenytoin) are less powerful sodium channel blockers and, unlike class IA drugs, shorten the action potential duration and refractory period in normal cardiac ventricular

Table 21-3

Pharmacokinetics of Cardiac Antiarrhythmic Drugs

	Principal Clearance Mechanism	Protein Binding (%)	Elimination Half-Time (h)	Therapeutic Plasma Concentration
Quinidine	Hepatic	80–90	5–12	1.2–4.0 μg/mL
Procainamide	Renal/hepatic	15	2.5–5.0	4–8 μg/mL
Disopyramide	Renal/hepatic	15	8–12	2–4 μg/mL
Lidocaine	Hepatic	55	1.4–8.0	1–5 μg/mL
Tocainide	Hepatic/renal	10–30	12–15	4–10 μg/mL
Mexiletine	Hepatic	60–75	6–12	0.75–2.00 μg/mL
Flecainide	Hepatic	30–45	13–30	0.3–1.5 μg/mL
Propafenone	Hepatic	>95	5–8	
Propranolol	Hepatic	90–95	2–4	10–30 ng/mL
Amiodarone	Hepatic	96	8–107 d	1.5–2.0 μg/mL
Sotalol	Renal			
Verapamil	Hepatic	90	4.5–12.0	100–300 ng/mL

Table 21-4

Efficacy of Cardiac Antiarrhythmic Drugs

	Conversion of Atrial Fibrillation	Paroxysmal Supraventricular Tachycardia	Premature Ventricular Contractions	Ventricular Tachycardia
Quinidine	+	++	++	+
Procainamide	+	++	++	++
Disopyramide	+	++	++	++
Lidocaine	+	0	++	++
Tocainide	0	0	++	++
Mexiletine	0	0	++	++
Moricizine	0	0	++	++
Flecainide	0	+	++	++
Propafenone	0	+	++	++
Propranolol	+	++	+	+
Amiodarone	+	++	++	++
Sotalol	++	+	+	+
Verapamil	+	++	0	0
Diltiazem	+	++	0	0
Digitalis	++	++	0	0
Adenosine	0	++	0	0

0, no effect; +, effective; ++, highly effective.

muscle. In ischemic tissue, lidocaine may also block adenosine triphosphate (ATP)–dependent channels, thus preventing ischemia-mediated shortening of ventricular depolarization.

Class IC Drugs

Class IC drugs (flecainide, propafenone) are potent sodium channel blockers and markedly decrease the rate of phase 0 depolarization and speed of conduction of cardiac impulses. These drugs have little effect on the duration of the cardiac action potential and the effective refractory period in ventricular myocardial cells but do shorten the duration of the action potential in Purkinje fibers. This inhomogeneity of effects on the rate of cardiac depolarization plus the slowing of cardiac conduction may contribute to the proarrhythmic effects of these drugs.

Class II Drugs

Class II drugs are β-adrenergic antagonists. β-Adrenergic antagonists decrease the rate of spontaneous phase 4 depolarization resulting in decreased autonomic nervous system activity, which may be important in suppression of ventricular arrhythmia during myocardial ischemia and reperfusion. Drug-induced slowing of heart rate with resulting decreases in myocardial oxygen requirements is desirable in patients with coronary artery disease. β-Adrenergic antagonists slow the speed of conduction of cardiac impulses through atrial tissues resulting in prolongation of the P-R interval on the ECG, whereas the duration of action of the cardiac action potential in ventricular myocardium is not altered. These drugs are effective in decreasing the incidence of arrhythmia-related morbidity and mortality although the exact mechanism for this beneficial effect remains unclear.

Class III Drugs

Class III drugs (amiodarone, sotalol, bretylium) block potassium ion channels resulting in prolongation of cardiac depolarization, action potential duration, and the effective refractory period. These effects are beneficial in preventing cardiac arrhythmias by decreasing the proportion of the cardiac cycle during which myocardial cells are excitable and thus susceptible to a triggering event. Reentrant tachycardias may be suppressed if the action potential duration becomes longer than the cycle length of the tachycardia circuit.

In addition to class III effects, amiodarone exhibits sodium channel blockade (class I), β blockade (class II), and calcium channel blockade (class IV). Although this drug is U.S. Food and Drug Administration (FDA) approved for the treatment of refractory ventricular arrhythmias, it has become a widely used drug for the acute treatment and prevention of supraventricular and ventricular arrhythmias both in the operating room and the intensive care unit (see the following texts).

Sotalol is a long-acting, noncardioselective β-blocking drug consisting of a racemic mixture of levorotatory (L) and dextrorotatory (D) isomers that possess similar class III effects. The L isomer of sotalol acts as a β-adrenergic antagonist, whereas the D isomer may increase mortality in patients with ventricular dysfunction and recent myocardial infarction. The reduced incidence of proarrhythmia effects seen with amiodarone or racemic sotalol treatment may be related to beneficial class II effects.

Class IV Drugs

Class IV drugs are the calcium blockers verapamil and diltiazem, which act by inhibiting inward slow calcium ion currents that may contribute to the development of tachycardias. As such, these drugs may be useful in the treatment of both supraventricular tachyarrhythmias and idiopathic ventricular tachycardia. The dihydropyridine calcium blockers (nifedipine, nicardipine, nimodipine) do not have antiarrhythmic action.

Proarrhythmic Effects

Proarrhythmia effects describe bradyarrhythmias or tachyarrhythmias that represent new cardiac arrhythmias associated with antiarrhythmic drug treatment.[3] These include torsades de pointes (most common), incessant ventricular tachycardia, and wide complex ventricular rhythm.[8]

Torsades de Pointes

Torsades de pointes is triggered by early afterdepolarizations in a setting of delayed repolarization and increased duration of refractoriness manifesting as prolongation of the QTc interval on the ECG. Class IA (quinidine and disopyramide) and class III drugs (amiodarone) prolong the QTc interval by potassium channel blockade providing the setting for torsades de pointes. Drug-induced torsades de pointes is often associated with bradycardia because the QTc interval is longer at slower heart rates. Exacerbating factors such as hypokalemia, hypomagnesemia, poor left ventricular function, and concomitant administration of other QT-prolonging drugs are important predisposing factors in the development of this life-threatening rhythm.

Incessant Ventricular Tachycardia

Incessant ventricular tachycardia may be precipitated by drugs that slow conduction of cardiac impulses (class IA and class IC drugs) sufficiently to create a continuous ventricular tachycardia circuit (reentry). Incessant ventricular tachycardia is more likely to occur with high doses of class IC drugs and in patients with a prior history of sustained ventricular tachycardia and poor left ventricular function. Ventricular tachycardia due to this mechanism is generally slower because of the drug effect but may be resistant to drugs or electrical therapy. This rhythm is rarely associated with class IB drugs, which have a weaker blocking effect of sodium channels.

Wide Complex Ventricular Rhythm

Wide complex ventricular rhythm is usually associated with class IC drugs in the setting of structural heart disease. Excessive plasma concentrations of the drug or an abrupt change in the dose may result in this arrhythmia. Wide complex ventricular rhythm is thought to reflect a reentrant tachycardia and easily degenerates to ventricular fibrillation.

Efficacy and Results of Treatment with Cardiac Antiarrhythmic Drugs

Chronic suppression of ventricular ectopy with an antiarrhythmic drug other than amiodarone does not prevent future life-threatening arrhythmias and may increase mortality.[8] In fact, patients treated with class IC drugs experienced a higher incidence of sudden cardiac arrest reflecting the proarrhythmia effects of these drugs. Conversely, β-adrenergic antagonists that do not typically suppress ventricular arrhythmias appear to decrease mortality and the risk of life-threatening ventricular arrhythmias. In patients with a history of myocardial infarction and ventricular arrhythmias, mortality was increased in those who received class IA and class IC drugs, whereas mortality was decreased with amiodarone and β-adrenergic antagonists.[10] Survivors of cardiac arrest have a high risk of subsequent ventricular fibrillation and treatment of these patients with amiodarone results in fewer life-threatening cardiac events. The proarrhythmic and negative inotropic effects of class IA and class IC drugs precludes their administration to patients with congestive heart failure. In these patients, administration of amiodarone appears to be safe and effective.

Prophylactic Antiarrhythmic Drug Therapy

Although commonly used in the past, lidocaine is no longer recommended as prophylactic treatment for patients in the early stages of acute myocardial infarction and without malignant ventricular ectopy.[11] In fact, lidocaine does not decrease and may increase mortality because of an increase in the occurrence of fatal bradyarrhythmias and asystole.

Calcium channel antagonists are not recommended as routine treatment of patients with acute myocardial infarction because mortality is not decreased by these drugs. Calcium channel blockers may be administered to patients in whom myocardial ischemia persists despite treatment with aspirin, heparin, nitroglycerin, and β-adrenergic antagonists.

Magnesium is involved in many enzymatic reactions, produces systemic and coronary vasodilation, inhibits platelet aggregation, and decreases myocardial reperfusion injury. Data on the ability of magnesium to decrease mortality following myocardial infarction are conflicting.[12] Treatment with magnesium is indicated in patients following an acute myocardial infarction who develop torsades de pointes ventricular tachycardia.[13]

In patients with heart failure, amiodarone reduces the risk of sudden cardiac death by 29% and therefore represents a viable alternative in patients who are not eligible for or who do not have access to implanted cardiac defibrillator (ICD) therapy for the prevention of sudden cardiac death from arrhythmias.[14] Amiodarone can be considered as an adjuvant therapy to ICD in preventing recurrent shocks. However, amiodarone therapy is neutral with respect to all-cause mortality and is associated with a two- and fivefold increased risk of pulmonary and thyroid toxicity respectively.[14] Prophylactic dofetilide and azimilide did not demonstrate a mortality benefit either.[15] In summary, there is little role for prophylactic antiarrhythmic medications for the primary prevention of sudden cardiac death in patients with heart failure with the exception of amiodarone.

Atrial fibrillation after heart surgery is a common complication that has been associated with prolonged hospitalization and cardiovascular morbidity. Prophylactic therapy with amiodarone, β blockers, sotalol, and magnesium has been effective in reducing the occurrence of atrial fibrillation, length of hospital stay, and cost of hospital treatment and may be effective in reducing the risk of stroke.[16]

Decision to Treat Cardiac Arrhythmias

Drug treatment of cardiac arrhythmias is not uniformly effective and frequently causes side effects (see the section "Proarrhythmic Effects").[1,17] The benefit of antiarrhythmic drugs is clearest when it results in the immediate termination of a sustained tachycardia. There is no doubt that the termination of ventricular tachycardia by lidocaine or supraventricular tachycardia by adenosine or verapamil is a true benefit of antiarrhythmic therapy. Furthermore, when given for a limited period, side effects are less likely. Conversely, it has been difficult to demonstrate that antiarrhythmic drugs alleviate symptoms related to chronic cardiac arrhythmias, a situation in which the risk of side effects is greater. The increase in long-term mortality associated with certain drugs (Cardiac Arrhythmia Suppression Trial [CAST] and other trials) raises the possibility that some antiarrhythmics result in sensitization of the myocardium to concurrent triggering factors (myocardial ischemia, neurohumoral activation, myocardial stretch, slow healing process after a myocardial infarction) that then elicit cardiac arrhythmias.[17] The mechanism by which β-adrenergic antagonists decrease mortality after an acute myocardial infarction is not known.

The value of monitoring plasma drug concentrations in minimizing the risks associated with therapy is not established. In fact, many side effects appear to depend as much on the nature and extent of the underlying heart disease as on increased plasma drug concentrations.[17]

Antiarrhythmic Drug Pharmacology

Quinidine

Quinidine is a class IA drug that is effective in the treatment of acute and chronic supraventricular arrhythmias (Fig. 21-2).[18] Due to its side effect profile and low therapeutic index (see the following texts), and the availability of newer agents, quinidine is rarely used. It can prevent recurrence of supraventricular tachyarrhythmias or suppress premature ventricular contractions and can slow the ventricular rate in the presence of atrial fibrillation, and about 25% of patients with new-onset atrial fibrillation will convert to normal sinus rhythm when treated with quinidine. Supraventricular tachyarrhythmias associated with Wolff-Parkinson-White syndrome are effectively suppressed by quinidine.

Quinidine is most often administered orally in a dose of 200 to 400 mg four times daily. Oral absorption of quinidine is rapid, with peak concentrations in the plasma attained in 60 to 90 minutes and an elimination half-time of 5 to 12 hours. The therapeutic blood level of quinidine is 1.2 to 4.0 μg/mL. Intravenous (IV) quinidine is rarely used due to vasodilation and myocardial depression.

Mechanism of Action

Quinidine is the dextroisomer of quinine and, like quinine, has antimalarial and antipyretic effects. Unlike quinine, however, quinidine has intense effects on the heart. For example, quinidine decreases the slope of phase 4 depolarization, which explains its effectiveness in suppressing cardiac arrhythmias caused by enhanced automaticity.

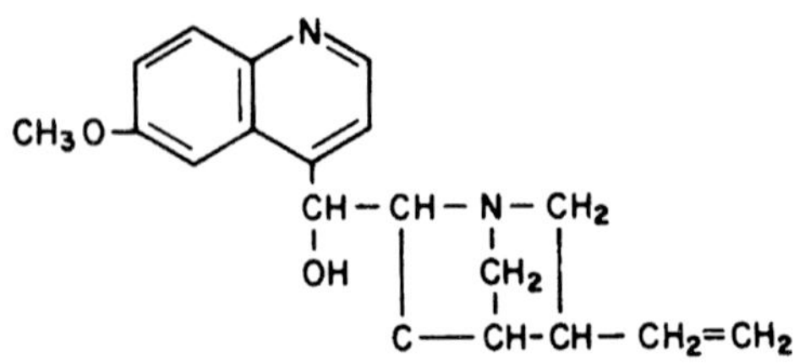

FIGURE 21-2 Quinidine.

Quinidine increases the fibrillation threshold in the atria and ventricles. Quinidine-induced slowing of the conduction of cardiac impulses through normal and abnormal fibers may be responsible for the ability of quinidine to occasionally convert atrial flutter or fibrillation to normal sinus rhythm. This drug can abolish reentry arrhythmias by prolonging conduction of cardiac impulses in an area of injury, thus converting one-way conduction blockade to two-way conduction blockade. A decrease in the atrial rate during atrial flutter or fibrillation may reflect slowed conduction velocity, a prolonged effective refractory period in the atria, or both.

Metabolism and Excretion

Quinidine is hydroxylated in the liver to inactive metabolites, which are excreted in the urine. About 20% of quinidine is excreted unchanged in the urine. Enzyme induction significantly shortens the duration of action of quinidine. The concurrent administration of phenytoin, phenobarbital, or rifampin may lower blood levels of quinidine by enhancing liver clearance. Because of its dependence on renal excretion and hepatic metabolism for clearance from the body, accumulation of quinidine or its metabolites may occur in the presence of impaired function of these organs. About 80% to 90% of quinidine in plasma is bound to albumin. Quinidine accumulates rapidly in most tissues except the brain.

Side Effects

Quinidine has a low therapeutic ratio, with heart block, hypotension, and proarrhythmia being potential adverse side effects. As the plasma concentration increases to more than 2 μg/mL, the P-R interval, QRS complex, and QTc interval on the ECG are prolonged. Patients with preexisting prolongation of the QTc interval or evidence of atrioventricular heart block on the ECG should not be treated with quinidine.

Patients in normal sinus rhythm treated with quinidine may show an increase in heart rate that is a result of presumably either an anticholinergic action and/or a reflex increase in sympathetic nervous system activity. This atropine-like action of quinidine opposes its direct depressant actions on the sinoatrial and atrioventricular nodes and is why digitalis is often given before quinidine therapy is initiated.

Allergic reactions may include drug rash or a drug fever that is occasionally associated with leukocytosis. Thrombocytopenia is a rare occurrence that is caused by drug–platelet complexes that evoke production of antibodies. Discontinuation of quinidine results in return of the platelet count to normal in 2 to 7 days. Nausea, vomiting, and diarrhea occur in about one-third of treated patients.

Like other cinchona alkaloids and salicylates, quinidine can cause cinchonism. Symptoms of cinchonism include tinnitus, decreased hearing acuity, blurring of vision, and gastrointestinal upset. In severe cases, there may be abdominal pain and mental confusion.

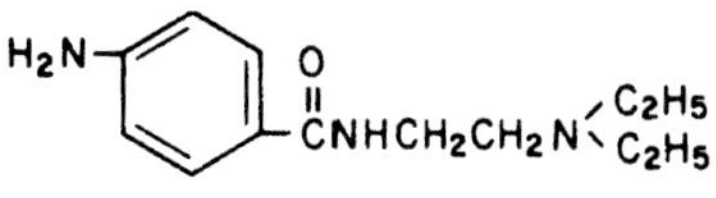

$H_2N-C_6H_4-C(=O)NHCH_2CH_2N(C_2H_5)_2$

FIGURE 21-3 Procainamide.

Because quinidine is an α-adrenergic blocking drug, it can interact in an additive manner with drugs that cause vasodilation. Quinidine also interferes with normal neuromuscular transmission and may accentuate the effect of neuromuscular blockings drugs. Recurrence of skeletal muscle paralysis in the immediate postoperative period has been observed in association with the administration of quinidine.[19]

Procainamide

Procainamide is as effective as quinidine for the treatment of ventricular tachyarrhythmias but less effective in abolishing atrial tachyarrhythmias (Fig. 21-3). Premature ventricular contractions and paroxysmal ventricular tachycardia are suppressed in most patients within a few minutes after IV administration, which is better tolerated than IV quinidine but may still cause hypotension. Procainamide can be administered IV at a rate not exceeding 100 mg every 5 minutes until the rhythm is controlled (maximum 15 mg/kg). When the cardiac arrhythmia is controlled, a constant rate of infusion (2 to 6 mg per minute) is used to maintain a therapeutic concentration of procainamide. The systemic blood pressure and ECG (QRS complex) are monitored continuously during infusion of this drug. The therapeutic blood level of procainamide is 4 to 8 μg/mL.

Mechanism of Action

Procainamide is an analogue of the local anesthetic procaine. Procainamide possesses an electrophysiologic action similar to that of quinidine but produces less prolongation of the QTc interval on the ECG. As a result, paradoxical ventricular tachycardia is a rare feature of procainamide therapy. Procainamide has no vagolytic effect and can be used in patients with atrial fibrillation to suppress ventricular irritability without increasing the ventricular rate. Like quinidine, procainamide may prolong the QRS complex and cause ST-T wave changes on the ECG.

Metabolism and Excretion

Procainamide is eliminated by renal excretion and hepatic metabolism. In humans, 40% to 60% of procainamide is excreted unchanged by the kidneys. The dose of procainamide must be decreased when renal function is abnormal. In the liver, procainamide that has not been excreted unchanged by the kidneys is acetylated to *N*-acetyl procainamide (NAPA), which is also eliminated by the kidneys. This metabolite is cardioactive and probably contributes to the antiarrhythmic effects of procainamide. In the presence of renal failure, plasma concentrations of NAPA may reach dangerous levels. Eventually, 90% of an administered dose of procainamide is recovered as unchanged drug or its metabolites.

The activity of the *N*-acetyltransferase enzyme response for the acetylation of procainamide is genetically determined. In patients who are rapid acetylators, the elimination half-time of procainamide is 2.5 hours compared with 5 hours in slow acetylators. The blood level of NAPA exceeds that of procainamide in rapid but not slow acetylators. Unlike its analogue, procaine, procainamide is highly resistant to hydrolysis by plasma cholinesterase. Evidence of this resistance is the fact that only 2% to 10% of an administered dose of procainamide is recovered unchanged in the urine as paraaminobenzoic acid.

Only about 15% of procainamide is bound to plasma proteins. Despite this limited binding in plasma, procainamide is avidly bound to tissue proteins with the exception of the brain.

Side Effects

Similar to quinidine, use of procainamide has dramatically decreased due to its side effect profile and availability of newer agents. Hypotension that results from procainamide is more likely to be caused by direct myocardial depression than peripheral vasodilation. Indeed, rapid IV injection of procainamide is associated with hypotension, whereas higher plasma concentrations slow conduction of cardiac impulses through the atrioventricular node and intraventricular conduction system. Ventricular asystole or fibrillation may occur when procainamide is administered in the presence of heart block, as associated with digitalis toxicity. Direct myocardial depression that occurs at high plasma concentrations of procainamide is exaggerated by hyperkalemia. As with quinidine, ventricular arrhythmias may accompany excessive plasma concentrations of procainamide.

Chronic administration of procainamide may be associated with a syndrome that resembles systemic lupus erythematosus. Serositis, arthritis, pleurisy, or pericarditis may develop, but unlike systemic lupus erythematosus, vasculitis is not usually present. Patients with this lupus-like syndrome often develop antinuclear antibodies (positive antinuclear antibody test). Slow acetylators are more likely than rapid acetylators to develop antinuclear antibodies. Symptoms disappear when procainamide is discontinued.

As with many drugs, procainamide may cause drug fever or an allergic rash. Although agranulocytosis is rare, leukopenia and thrombocytopenia may be seen after chronic use of procainamide, often in association with the lupus-like syndrome. The most common early, noncardiac complications of procainamide are gastrointestinal disturbances, including nausea and vomiting.

Disopyramide

Disopyramide is comparable to quinidine in effectively suppressing atrial and ventricular tachyarrhythmias

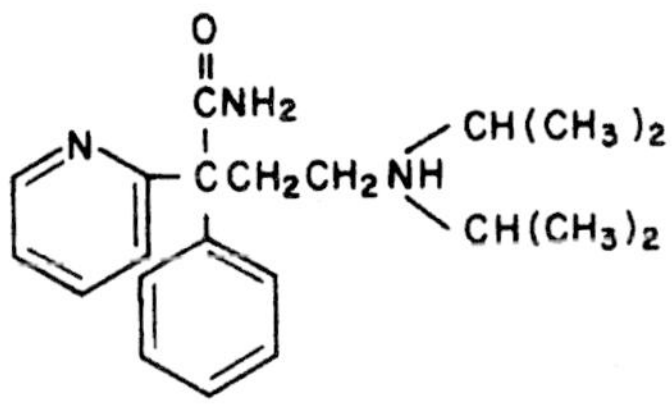

FIGURE 21-4 Disopyramide.

(Fig. 21-4). Absorption of oral disopyramide is almost complete, resulting in peak blood levels within 2 hours of administration. Therapeutic plasma concentrations of disopyramide are 2 to 4 μg/mL. About 50% of the drug is excreted unchanged by the kidneys. As a result, the typical elimination half-time of 8 to 12 hours is prolonged in the presence of renal dysfunction. A dealkylated metabolite with less antiarrhythmic and atropine-like activity than the parent drug accounts for about 20% of the drug's elimination. Disopyramide is not available in an IV formulation.

Side Effects

The most common side effects of disopyramide are dry mouth and urinary hesitancy, both of which are caused by the drug's anticholinergic activity. Some patients taking disopyramide also experience blurred vision or nausea. Prolongation of the QTc interval on the ECG and paradoxical ventricular tachycardia (similar to quinidine) may occur. For this reason, disopyramide should be administered cautiously if patients have known cardiac conduction effects. Disopyramide has significant myocardial depressant effects and can precipitate congestive heart failure and hypotension. The potential for direct myocardial depression, especially in patients with preexisting left ventricular dysfunction, seems to be greater with this drug than with quinidine and procainamide.

Moricizine

Moricizine is a phenothiazine derivative with modest efficacy in the treatment of sustained ventricular arrhythmias. In view of its proarrhythmic effects, this drug is reserved for the treatment of life-threatening ventricular arrhythmias when other drugs such as amiodarone are not available or contraindicated (e.g., allergy). It is not effective in the treatment of atrial arrhythmias. Moricizine decreases the fast inward sodium ion current and also decreases automaticity.

Side Effects

Proarrhythmic effects occur in 3% to 15% of patients treated chronically with moricizine. Patients with poor left ventricular function tolerate moricizine and small increases in systemic blood pressure and heart rate may accompany therapy. Plasma concentrations of theophylline may increase in patients treated with moricizine.

Lidocaine

Lidocaine is used principally for suppression of ventricular arrhythmias, having minimal if any effect on supraventricular tachyarrhythmias (see Chapter 10). This drug is particularly effective in suppressing reentry cardiac arrhythmias, such as premature ventricular contractions and ventricular tachycardia. The efficacy of prophylactic lidocaine therapy for preventing early ventricular fibrillation after acute myocardial infarction has not been documented and is no longer recommended (see earlier discussion).

In adult patients with a normal cardiac output, hepatic function, and hepatic blood flow, an initial administration of lidocaine, 2 mg/kg IV, followed by a continuous infusion of 1 to 4 mg per minute should provide therapeutic plasma lidocaine concentrations of 1 to 5 μg/mL. Decreased cardiac output and/or hepatic blood flow, as produced by anesthesia, acute myocardial infarction, or congestive heart failure, may decrease by 50% or more of the initial dose and the rate of lidocaine infusion necessary to maintain therapeutic plasma levels. Concomitant administration of drugs such as propranolol and cimetidine can result in decreased hepatic clearance of lidocaine. Advantages of lidocaine over quinidine or procainamide are the more rapid onset and prompt disappearance of effects when the continuous infusion is terminated, greater therapeutic index, and a much reduced side effect profile. Lidocaine for IV administration differs from that used for local anesthesia because it does not contain a preservative. Lidocaine is also well absorbed after oral administration but is subject to extensive hepatic first-pass metabolism. As a result, only about one-third of an oral dose of lidocaine reaches the circulation. Mexiletine (see the following texts) is an oral analogue of lidocaine. Intramuscular (IM) absorption of lidocaine is nearly complete. In an emergency situation, lidocaine, 4 to 5 mg/kg IM, will produce a therapeutic plasma concentration in about 15 minutes. This level is maintained for about 90 minutes.

Mechanism of Action

Lidocaine delays the rate of spontaneous phase 4 depolarization by preventing or diminishing the gradual decrease in potassium ion permeability that normally occurs during this phase. The effectiveness of lidocaine in suppressing premature ventricular contractions reflects its ability to decrease the rate of spontaneous phase 4 depolarization. The ineffectiveness of lidocaine against supraventricular tachyarrhythmias presumably reflects its inability to alter the rate of spontaneous phase 4 depolarization in atrial cardiac cells.

In usual therapeutic doses, lidocaine has no significant effect on either the QRS or QTc interval on the ECG or on atrioventricular conduction. In high doses, however, lidocaine can decrease conduction in the atrioventricular node as well as in the His–Purkinje system.

Metabolism and Excretion

Lidocaine is metabolized in the liver, and resulting metabolites may possess cardiac antiarrhythmic activity.

Side Effects

Lidocaine is essentially devoid of effects on the ECG or cardiovascular system when the plasma concentration remains less than 5 μg/mL. In contrast to quinidine and procainamide, lidocaine does not alter the duration of the QRS complex on the ECG, and activity of the sympathetic nervous system is not changed. Lidocaine depresses cardiac contractility less than any other antiarrhythmic drug used to suppress ventricular arrhythmias. Toxic plasma concentrations of lidocaine (>5 to 10 μg/mL) produce peripheral vasodilation and direct myocardial depression, resulting in hypotension. In addition, slowing of conduction of cardiac impulses may manifest as bradycardia, a prolonged P-R interval, and widened QRS complex on the ECG. Stimulation of the central nervous system (CNS) occurs in a dose-related manner, with symptoms appearing when plasma concentrations of lidocaine are greater than 5 μg/mL. Seizures are possible at plasma concentrations of 5 to 10 μg/mL. CNS depression, apnea, and cardiac arrest are possible when plasma lidocaine concentrations are greater than 10 μg/mL. The convulsive threshold for lidocaine is decreased during arterial hypoxemia, hyperkalemia, or acidosis, emphasizing the importance of monitoring these parameters during continuous infusion of lidocaine to patients for suppression of ventricular arrhythmias.

Mexiletine

Mexiletine is an orally effective amine analogue of lidocaine that is used for the chronic suppression of ventricular cardiac tachyarrhythmias. Combination with a β blocker or another antiarrhythmic drug such as quinidine or procainamide results in a synergistic effect that permits a decrease in the dose of mexiletine and an associated decrease in the incidence of side effects. Electrophysiologically, mexiletine is similar to lidocaine. The addition of the amine side group enables mexiletine to avoid significant hepatic first-pass metabolism that limits the effectiveness of orally administered lidocaine. The usual adult dose is 150 to 200 mg every 8 hours. As it is a lidocaine analog, mexiletine may be effective in decreasing neuropathic pain for patients in whom alternative pain medications have been unsatisfactory.[20]

Side Effects

Epigastric burning may occur and is often relieved by taking the drug with meals. Neurologic side effects include tremulousness, diplopia, vertigo, and occasionally slurred speech. Cardiovascular side effects resemble lidocaine. Increases in liver enzymes may occur especially in patients manifesting congestive heart failure. Blood dyscrasias occur rarely. Proarrhythmic effects may manifest in occasionally treated patients. Toxic effects may develop at plasma concentrations only slightly above therapeutic levels.

Tocainide

Tocainide, like mexiletine, is an orally effective amine analogue of lidocaine that was formerly used for the chronic suppression of ventricular cardiac tachyarrhythmias, but is no longer available in the United States. Its side effects resemble those of mexiletine, but in rare patients, this drug has caused severe bone marrow depression (leukopenia, anemia, thrombocytopenia) and pulmonary fibrosis.[20] The usual adult dose is 400 to 800 mg administered every 8 hours. As with mexiletine, the combination of tocainide with a β-adrenergic blocker or another antiarrhythmic drug has a synergistic effect.

Phenytoin

Phenytoin is particularly effective in suppression of ventricular arrhythmias associated with digitalis toxicity. This drug is effective, although to a lesser extent than quinidine, procainamide, and lidocaine, in the treatment of ventricular arrhythmias due to other causes. Phenytoin may be useful in the treatment of paradoxical ventricular tachycardia or torsades de pointes that is associated with a prolonged QTc interval on the ECG. Treatment of atrial tachyarrhythmias with phenytoin is not very effective.

Phenytoin can be administered orally or IV. Intramuscular administration is too unreliable to treat cardiac arrhythmias. The IV dose is 100 mg (1.5 mg/kg) every 5 minutes until the cardiac arrhythmia is controlled or 10 to 15 mg/kg (maximum 1,000 mg) has been administered. Because phenytoin can precipitate in 5% dextrose in water, it is preferable to give the drug via a delivery tubing containing normal saline. Slow IV injection into a large peripheral or central vein is recommended to minimize the likelihood of discomfort or thrombosis at the injection site. Therapeutic blood levels range from 10 to 18 μg/mL.

Mechanism of Action

The effects of phenytoin on automaticity and velocity of conduction of cardiac impulses resemble those of lidocaine. Phenytoin exerts a greater effect on the electrocardiographic QTc interval than does lidocaine and shortens the QTc interval more than any of the other antiarrhythmic drugs. Phenytoin has no significant effect on the ST-T waves or the QRS complex. It does not significantly depress the myocardium in usual doses but can cause hypotension when administered in high doses rapidly. Conduction of cardiac impulses through the atrioventricular node is improved, but activity of the sinus node may be depressed. The ability of some volatile anesthetics to depress the sinoatrial node is a consideration if administration of phenytoin during general anesthesia is planned.

Metabolism and Excretion

Phenytoin is hydroxylated and then conjugated with glucuronic acid for excretion in the urine. The elimination half-time is about 24 hours. Because phenytoin is metabolized by the liver, impaired hepatic function may result in higher than normal blood levels of the drug. Blood levels of phenytoin can be lowered by drugs, such as barbiturates, that enhance its rate of metabolism. Warfarin, phenylbutazone, and isoniazid may inhibit metabolism and increase phenytoin blood levels. Uremia increases the unbound fraction of phenytoin relative to the plasma-bound portion.

Side Effects

Phenytoin toxicity most commonly manifests as CNS disturbances, especially cerebellar disturbances. Symptoms include ataxia, nystagmus, vertigo, slurred speech, sedation, and mental confusion. Cerebellar symptoms correlate with phenytoin blood levels of greater than 18 μg/mL. Cardiac arrhythmias that have not been suppressed at this concentration are unlikely to respond favorably to further increases in the dosage of phenytoin. Phenytoin partially inhibits insulin secretion and may lead to increased blood glucose levels in patients who are hyperglycemic. Leukopenia, granulocytopenia, and thrombocytopenia may occur as a manifestation of drug-induced bone marrow depression. Nausea, skin rash, and megaloblastic anemia may occur.

Flecainide

Flecainide is a fluorinated local anesthetic analogue of procainamide that is more effective in suppressing ventricular premature beats and ventricular tachycardia than quinidine and disopyramide (Fig. 21-5). Flecainide is also effective for the treatment of atrial tachyarrhythmias. Because it delays conduction in the bypass tracts, flecainide can be effective for the treatment of tachyarrhythmias due to reentry mechanisms as associated with the Wolff-Parkinson-White syndrome. Chronic treatment of ventricular arrhythmias with flecainide after

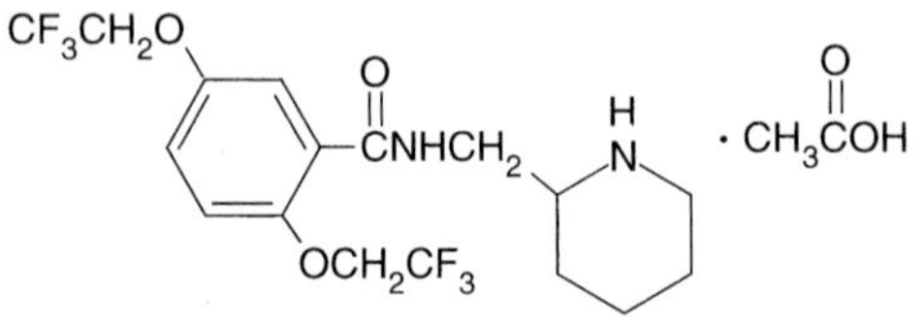

FIGURE 21-5 Flecainide.

myocardial infarction is not recommended due to an increased incidence of sudden death in treated patients.[21] Thus, flecainide should be reserved for the treatment of life-threatening arrhythmias.

Metabolism and Excretion

Oral absorption of flecainide is excellent, and a prolonged elimination half-time (about 20 hours) makes a twice daily dose of 100 to 200 mg acceptable. This drug is not available in an IV formulation. About 25% of flecainide is excreted unchanged by the kidneys, and the remainder appears as weakly active metabolites. Elimination of flecainide is decreased in patients with congestive heart failure or renal failure. Flecainide competes with metabolic pathways used by other drugs and as a result may increase the plasma concentrations of digoxin and propranolol. Coadministration of amiodarone and flecainide can double plasma flecainide concentrations. Phenytoin and other drugs that stimulate hepatic P450 enzymes may speed the elimination of flecainide. The therapeutic plasma concentration of flecainide ranges from 0.2 to 1.0 μg/mL. Flecainide has a moderate negative inotropic effect and a proarrhythmic effect, especially in patients with preexisting decreased left ventricular function. Vertigo and difficulty in visual accommodation are common dose-related side effects of flecainide therapy.

Side Effects

Proarrhythmic effects occur in a significant number of treated patients especially in the presence of left ventricular dysfunction. Flecainide prolongs the QRS complex by 25% or more and, to a lesser extent, prolongs the P-R interval on the ECG. These changes suggest the possibility of atrioventricular or infranodal conduction block of cardiac impulses. Flecainide may depress sinoatrial node function as do β-adrenergic antagonists and calcium channel blockers. For these reasons, flecainide is not administered to patients with second- and third-degree atrioventricular heart block. The most common noncardiac adverse effect of flecainide is dose-related blurred vision. Flecainide increases the capture thresholds of pacemakers. This is the amount of current required to electrically capture cardiac tissue. Therefore, capture thresholds should be remeasured in individuals with pacemakers after the steady-state flecainide dosage is changed.[22]

Propafenone

Propafenone, like flecainide, is an effective oral antiarrhythmic drug for suppression of ventricular and atrial tachyarrhythmias. This drug possesses weak β-adrenergic blocking and calcium blocking effects. Propafenone may be proarrhythmic, especially in patients with poor left ventricular function and sustained ventricular tachycardia.

Absorption after oral administration is excellent, and peak plasma levels occur in about 3 hours. The rate of metabolism is genetically determined with about 90% of patients able to metabolize propafenone efficiently in the liver. The principal metabolites in those who metabolize the drug rapidly are pharmacologically active and equivalent in antiarrhythmic potency to the parent drug. Because of extensive metabolism, the availability of propafenone increases significantly in the presence of liver disease.

Side Effects

Proarrrhythmic effects are more likely to occur in patients with preexisting ventricular arrhythmias. Propafenone depresses the myocardium and may cause conduction abnormalities such as sinoatrial node slowing, atrioventricular block, and bundle-branch block. Small doses of quinidine inhibit the metabolism of propafenone, whereas propafenone interferes with the metabolism of propranolol and metoprolol resulting in increased plasma concentrations of these β blockers. This drug also increases the plasma concentration of warfarin and may prolong the prothrombin time. Vertigo, disturbances in taste, and blurred vision are the common side effects. Nausea and vomiting may occur, and, rarely, cholestatic hepatitis or worsening of asthma manifests.

β-Adrenergic Antagonists

β-Adrenergic antagonists are effective for treatment of cardiac arrhythmias related to enhanced activity of the sympathetic nervous system (perioperative stress, thyrotoxicosis, pheochromocytoma). Propranolol and esmolol are effective for controlling the rate of ventricular response in patients with atrial fibrillation and atrial flutter. Multifocal atrial tachycardia may respond to esmolol or metoprolol but is best treated with amiodarone. Comparable doses of metoprolol (5 to 15 mg IV over 20 minutes, which lasts 5 to 7 hours) produces antiarrhythmic effects similar to those of propranolol, as well as the same potential side effects. Acebutolol is effective in the treatment of frequent premature ventricular contractions. β-Adrenergic antagonists, especially propranolol, may be effective in controlling torsades de pointes for patients with prolonged QTc intervals. Acebutolol, propranolol, and metoprolol are approved for prevention of sudden death following myocardial infarction. For example, in contrast to class I antiarrhythmic drugs, propranolol decreases sudden death as well as reinfarction rates in the first year after acute myocardial infarction.[11]

Mechanism of Action

The antiarrhythmic effects of β-adrenergic antagonists most likely reflect blockade of the responses of β receptors in the heart to sympathetic nervous system stimulation, as well as the effects of circulating catecholamines. As a result, the rate of spontaneous phase 4 depolarization and sinoatrial node discharge is decreased. The rate of conduction of cardiac impulses through the atrioventricular node is slowed as reflected by a prolonged P-R interval on the ECG. This drug has little effect on the ST-T wave, although it may shorten the overall QTc interval. β-Adrenergic antagonists can depress the myocardium not only by β blockade but also by direct depressant effects on cardiac muscle. In addition to β-adrenergic blockade, these drugs cause alterations in the electrical activity of myocardial cells. This cell membrane effect is probably responsible for some of the antidysrhythmic effects of β-adrenergic antagonists. Indeed, dextropropranolol, which lacks β-adrenergic antagonist activity, is an effective cardiac antiarrhythmic.

The usual oral dose of propranolol for chronic suppression of ventricular arrhythmias is 10 to 80 mg every 6 to 8 hours. The total daily dose is determined by the physiologic effects of propranolol on the heart rate and systemic blood pressure. Effective β blockade is usually achieved in an otherwise normal person when the resting heart rate is 55 to 60 beats per minute. For emergency suppression of cardiac arrhythmias in an adult, propranolol may be administered IV in a dose of 1 mg per minute (3 to 6 mg). The onset of action after IV administration is within 2 to 5 minutes, the peak effect at the atrioventricular node is within 10 to 15 minutes, and the duration of action is 3 to 4 hours. Administration at 1-minute intervals is intended to minimize the likelihood of excessive pharmacologic effects on the conduction of cardiac impulses. In patients with marginal systemic blood pressure or left ventricular dysfunction, the rate of administration may need to be slowed and the total dose limited to less than 3 mg.

Metabolism and Excretion

Orally administered propranolol is extensively metabolized in the liver, and a hepatic first-pass effect is responsible for the variation in plasma concentration; the therapeutic plasma concentration of propranolol may vary from 10 to 30 ng/mL. Propranolol readily crosses the blood–brain barrier. The principal metabolite of propranolol is 4-hydroxypropranolol, which possesses weak β-adrenergic antagonist activity. This active metabolite most likely contributes to the antiarrhythmic activity after the oral administration of propranolol. The elimination half-time of propranolol is 2 to 4 hours, although the antiarrhythmic activity usually persists for 6 to 8 hours.

Side Effects

Bradycardia, hypotension, myocardial depression, and bronchospasm are side effects of β-adrenergic antagonists that reflect the ability of these drugs to inhibit sympathetic nervous system activity. Patients with any degree of congestive heart failure are highly dependent on increased sympathetic nervous system activity as a compensatory mechanism. Attenuation of this compensatory response may accentuate congestive heart failure. In addition, the direct depressant effects of propranolol on myocardial contractility may further accentuate congestive heart failure. The use of propranolol in patients with preexisting atrioventricular heart block is not recommended. Propranolol may cause drug fever, an allergic rash, or nausea and may increase esophageal reflux. Cold extremities and worsening of Raynaud disease may occur. Interference with glucose metabolism may manifest as hypoglycemia in patients being treated for diabetes mellitus. The most common CNS side effects are mental depression and fatigue. Reversible alopecia may occur. Upregulation of β-adrenergic receptors occurs with chronic administration of β-adrenergic antagonists such that abrupt discontinuation of treatment may lead to supraventricular tachycardia that is particularly undesirable in patients with coronary artery disease. Slowly tapering the dose of β-adrenergic antagonist will prevent withdrawal responses.

Amiodarone

Amiodarone is a potent antiarrhythmic drug with a wide spectrum of activity against refractory supraventricular and ventricular tachyarrhythmias. In the presence of ventricular tachycardia or fibrillation that is resistant to electrical defibrillation, amiodarone 300 mg IV is recommended. Preoperative oral administration of amiodarone decreases the incidence of atrial fibrillation after cardiac surgery.[23] It is also effective for suppression of tachyarrhythmias associated with Wolff-Parkinson-White syndrome because it depresses conduction in the atrioventricular node and the accessory bypass tracts. Similar to β blockers and unlike class I drugs, amiodarone decreases mortality after myocardial infarction.[24]

After initiation of oral therapy, a decrease in ventricular tachyarrhythmias occurs within 72 hours. The maintenance dose can usually be gradually decreased to about 400 mg daily for suppression of ventricular tachyarrhythmias and 200 mg daily for suppression of supraventricular tachyarrhythmias. Administered IV over 2 to 5 minutes, a dose of 5 mg/kg produces a prompt antiarrhythmic effect that lasts up to 4 hours. Therapeutic blood concentrations of amiodarone are 1.0 to 3.5 μg/mL. After discontinuation of chronic oral therapy, the pharmacologic effect of amiodarone lasts for a prolonged period (up to 60 days), reflecting the prolonged elimination half-time of this drug.

Mechanism of Action

Amiodarone, a benzofurane derivative, is 37% iodine by weight and structurally resembles thyroxine (Fig. 21-6). It prolongs the effective refractory period in all cardiac tissues, including the sinoatrial node, atrium, atrioventricular node, His–Purkinje system, ventricle, and, in the case of Wolff-Parkinson-White syndrome, accessory bypass

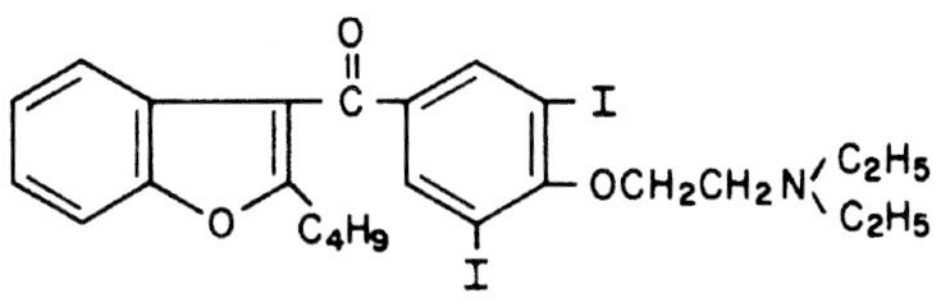

FIGURE 21-6 Amiodarone.

tracts. Amiodarone has an antiadrenergic effect (noncompetitive blockade of α and β receptors) and a minor negative inotropic effect, which may be offset by the drug's potent vasodilating properties.[25] Amiodarone acts as an antianginal drug by dilating coronary arteries and increasing coronary blood flow.

Metabolism and Excretion

Amiodarone has a prolonged elimination half-time (29 days) and large volume of distribution (Fig. 21-7).[26] This drug is minimally dependent on renal excretion as evidenced by an unchanged elimination half-time in the absence of renal function.[26] The principal metabolite, desethylamiodarone, is pharmacologically active and has a longer elimination half-time than the parent drug, resulting in accumulation of this metabolite with chronic therapy. Protein binding of amiodarone is extensive, and the drug is not easily removed by hemodialysis. There is an inconsistent relationship between the plasma concentration of amiodarone and its pharmacologic effects as the ultimate concentration of drug in the myocardium is 10 to 50 times that present in the plasma.

Side Effects

Side effects in patients treated chronically with amiodarone are common, especially when the daily maintenance dose exceeds 400 mg.[27] Screening tests, such as chest radiographs and tests for pulmonary function, thyroid-stimulating hormone, and liver function, are recommended. Other than the pulmonary function tests, these studies should be repeated at 3, 6, and 12 months and annually thereafter.[28]

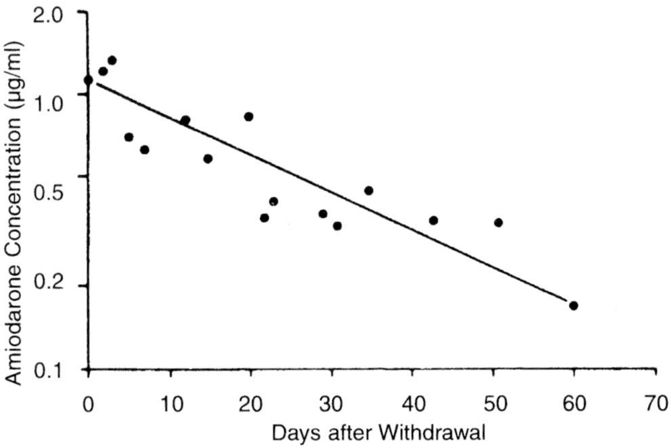

FIGURE 21-7 After discontinuation of amiodarone, the plasma concentration decreases slowly, resulting in a prolonged elimination half-time. (From Kannan R, Nademannee K, Hendrickson JA, et al. Amiodarone kinetics after oral doses. *Clin Pharmacol Ther.* 1982;31:438–444, with permission.)

Pulmonary Toxicity

The most serious side effect of amiodarone is pulmonary alveolitis (pneumonitis).[29,30] The overall incidence of amiodarone-induced pulmonary toxicity is estimated at 5% to 15% of treated patients, with a reported mortality of 5% to 10%. The cause of this drug-induced pulmonary toxicity is not known but may reflect the ability of amiodarone to enhance production of free oxygen radicals in the lungs that in turn oxidize cellular proteins, membrane lipids, and nucleic acids. It is suggested that high-inspired oxygen concentrations may accelerate these reactions.[31] For this reason, it may be prudent to restrict the inspired concentration of oxygen in patients receiving amiodarone and undergoing general anesthesia to the lowest level capable of maintaining adequate systemic oxygenation.[32] Indeed, postoperative pulmonary edema has been reported in patients being treated chronically with amiodarone.[32] Furthermore, there is evidence that patients with preexisting evidence of amiodarone-induced pulmonary toxicity are at increased risk for developing adult respiratory distress syndrome after surgery that requires cardiopulmonary bypass.[33,34] It must be recognized, however, that no animal model has established a cause-and-effect relationship between oral amiodarone administration and secondary oxygen-enhanced pulmonary toxicity.

There are two distinct types of presentation of patients with amiodarone-induced pulmonary toxicity.[30] The more common form of pulmonary toxicity consists of a slow insidious onset of progressive dyspnea, cough, weight loss, and pulmonary infiltrates on the chest x-ray. The second form of pulmonary toxicity has a much more acute onset of dyspnea, cough, arterial hypoxemia, and occasionally fever that may mimic an infectious pneumonia. Postoperative pulmonary edema attributed to amiodarone-induced pulmonary toxicity reflects this acute form of onset.

Cardiovascular

Like quinidine and disopyramide, amiodarone may prolong the QTc interval on the ECG, which may lead to an increased incidence of ventricular tachyarrhythmias, including torsades de pointes (proarrhythmic effect). Heart rate often slows and is resistant to treatment with atropine. Responsiveness to catecholamines and sympathetic nervous system stimulation is decreased as a result of drug-induced inhibition of α- and β-adrenergic receptors. Direct myocardial depressant effects are presumed to be minimal.[35] IV administration of amiodarone may result in hypotension, most likely reflecting the peripheral vasodilating effects of this drug. Atrioventricular heart block may also occur when the drug is administered IV. The negative inotropic effects of amiodarone may be enhanced in the presence of general anesthesia, β-adrenergic blockers, and calcium channel blockers.[36] Drugs that inhibit automaticity of the sinoatrial node (lidocaine) could accentuate the effects of amiodarone and increase the likelihood of sinus arrest. The potential need for a temporary artificial cardiac (ventricular) pacemaker and administration of a sympathomimetic such as isoproterenol may be a consideration in patients being treated with this drug and scheduled to undergo surgery.[37]

Ocular, Dermatologic, Neurologic, and Hepatic

Corneal microdeposits occur in most patients during amiodarone therapy, but visual impairment is unlikely. Optic neuropathy has been found in 1.8% of patients treated with amiodarone compared to 0.3% of the general population.[38] Optic neuropathy from amiodarone typically has a more insidious onset, milder degree of visual loss, longer duration of disc edema, and more often bilateral. Discontinuation often leads to slow improvement in visual acuity. Photosensitivity and rash develop in up to 10% of patients. Rarely, there may be a cyanotic discoloration (slate-gray pigmentation) of the face that persists even after the drug is discontinued. Neurologic toxicity may manifest as peripheral neuropathy, tremors, sleep disturbance, headache, or proximal skeletal muscle weakness.[39] Transient, mild increases in plasma transaminase concentrations may occur, and fatty liver infiltration has been observed.[39]

Pharmacokinetic

Amiodarone inhibits hepatic P450 enzymes resulting in increased plasma concentrations of digoxin, procainamide, quinidine, warfarin, and cyclosporine. Amiodarone also displaces digoxin from protein-binding sites. The digoxin dose may be decreased as much as 50% when administered in the presence of amiodarone. Amiodarone also increases the plasma concentrations of quinidine, procainamide, and phenytoin. The anticoagulant effects of warfarin are potentiated because amiodarone may directly depress vitamin K–dependent clotting factors.

Endocrine

Amiodarone contains iodine and has effects on thyroid metabolism, causing either hypothyroidism or hyperthyroidism in 2% to 4% of patients. Thyroid dysfunction may develop insidiously in these patients. Hyperthyroidism has occurred up to 5 months after discontinuation of amiodarone. Patients with preexisting thyroid dysfunction seem more likely to develop amiodarone-related alterations in thyroid function. Hyperthyroidism is best detected by finding an increased plasma concentration of triiodothyronine. Hypothyroidism is best detected by finding an increased plasma concentration of thyroid-stimulating hormone.

Amiodarone-induced hyperthyroidism reflecting the release of iodine from the parent drug is often refractory to conventional therapy. These patients may be intolerant of β-adrenergic blockade because of their underlying cardiomyopathies. When medical management fails, the performance of surgical thyroidectomy provides prompt metabolic control. Bilateral superficial cervical plexus blocks have been described for anesthetic management of subtotal thyroidectomy in these patients.[40]

Dronedarone

Dronedarone is a noniodinated benzofuran derivative of amiodarone that has been developed as an alternative for the treatment of atrial fibrillation and atrial flutter. Similar to amiodarone, dronedarone is a potent blocker of multiple ion currents. It is currently recommended for treatment of atrial fibrillation and atrial flutter in people whose hearts have either returned to normal rhythm or who undergo drug therapy or direct current cardioversion (DCCV) to maintain normal rhythm. Dronedarone reduced the rate of hospitalization in atrial fibrillation patients but did not demonstrate a reduction in mortality.[41] A trial of the drug in heart failure was stopped as an interim analysis showed a possible increase in heart failure deaths in patients with moderate to severe congestive heart failure.[42] As a result, the clinical utility of dronedarone is significantly limited by its efficacy and contraindication in patients with permanent atrial fibrillation or patients with advanced or recent congestive heart failure exacerbations.

Mechanism of Action

Dronedarone is a modified analogue of amiodarone and has the pharmacologic ability to block multiple ion channels, including the L-type calcium current, the inward sodium current, and multiple potassium currents. It also has sympatholytic effects.[43] However, it is a more potent blocker of peak sodium current and has stronger in vitro antiadrenergic effects compared with amiodarone.

Metabolism and Excretion

Dronedarone is well absorbed (70% to 94%) after oral administration, and absorption increases two- to threefold when it is taken with food. Dronedarone undergoes significant first-pass metabolism that reduces its net bioavailability to 15%. With sustained administration of 400 mg twice daily, steady-state plasma concentrations of 84 to 167 ng/mL are reached in 7 days. The clearance of dronedarone is principally nonrenal, with a terminal half-life of 20–40 hours. Dronedarone is a substrate for and a moderate inhibitor of CYP3A4. Consequently, dronedarone should not be coadministered with other CYP3A4 inhibitors such as antifungals, macrolide antibiotics, or protease inhibitors. When coadministered with moderate CYP3A4 inhibitors such as verapamil and diltiazem, lower doses of concomitant drugs should be used to avoid severe bradycardia and conduction block.[43]

Side Effects

The most frequently reported adverse effect of dronedarone is nausea and diarrhea. As compared to placebo, patients in the treatment group of the ATHENA trial had significantly increased rates of bradycardia, QT interval prolongation, diarrhea, nausea, and serum creatinine increase. In the ATHENA trial, patients in the treatment group did not have increased rates of interstitial lung disease, hyperthyroid, or hypothryroidism.[44]

Sotalol

Sotalol is a nonselective β-adrenergic antagonist drug at low doses, and at higher doses, it prolongs the cardiac action potential in the atria, ventricles, and accessory bypass tracts. Sotalol is administered for the treatment of sustained ventricular tachycardia or ventricular fibrillation.[45] This drug is also approved for the treatment of atrial tachyarrhythmia including atrial fibrillation as may follow cardiac surgery. Sotalol is not recommended in patients with asthma, left ventricular dysfunction, and cardiac conduction abnormalities including prolonged QTc intervals on the ECG. Because of its proarrhythmic effects, this drug is usually restricted for use in patients with life-threatening ventricular arrhythmias.

The daily oral dose of sotalol is 240 to 320 mg administered twice daily. Because sotalol is excreted mainly by the kidneys, the dosing intervals should be lengthened in patients with renal dysfunction. Sotalol does not bind to plasma proteins, is not metabolized, and it does not cross the blood–brain barrier to any extent. β-Adrenergic blocking effects of this drug primarily reflect activity of the levorotatory isomer.

Side Effects

The most dangerous side effect of sotalol is torsades de pointes, reflecting prolongation of the QTc interval on the ECG. Torsades de pointes is dose related, occurring in 0.5% of patients receiving 80 mg of sotalol daily and in 5.8% of patients receiving more than 320 mg daily. The β blocking effects of sotalol result in decreased myocardial contractility, bradycardia, and delayed conduction of cardiac impulses through the atrioventricular node. Other side effects of sotalol include fatigue, dyspnea, vertigo, and nausea.

Ibutilide

Ibutilide is effective for the conversion of recent onset atrial fibrillation or atrial flutter to normal sinus rhythm. Hepatic metabolism is extensive with production of inactive metabolites with the exception of hydroxy metabolites that possess weak antiarrhythmic effects. Polymorphic ventricular tachycardia with or without prolongation of the QTc interval on the ECG may occur during ibutilide treatment, especially in patient with predisposing factors (impaired left ventricular function, preexisting prolonged QTc intervals, hypokalemia, hypomagnesemia).

Dofetilide

Dofetilide is a potent, pure potassium channel blocking drug of the class III antiarrhythmic drugs. Dofetilide causes a dose-dependent prolongation of the action potential duration and hence, the QT interval. Dofetilide is effective for the conversion of recent onset atrial fibrillation or atrial flutter to normal sinus rhythm, as well as the maintenance of normal sinus rhythm in patients who have been successfully cardioverted. Oral absorption is greater than 90%, and 80% of the drug is excreted unchanged in the urine. The starting dose of 0.5 mg twice daily is the highest acceptable dose. Dosage adjustments are indicated based on renal function. Trimethoprim, cimetidine, and prochlorperazine can inhibit renal clearance of dofetilide. Proarrhythmic effects of dofetilide may occur when it is coadministered with calcium channel blocking drugs. Dofetilide does not depress myocardial contractility. Torsades de pointes occurs in a dose-related manner, especially in patients with preexisting left ventricular dysfunction. By FDA mandate, a patient must be admitted to a certified hospital for at least 72 hours for cardiac monitoring during initiation of dofetilide. Such monitoring is necessary to determine the presence of QT prolongation.

Bretylium

Bretylium is no longer recommended for treatment of ventricular fibrillation during cardiopulmonary resuscitation as it is less effective than amiodarone and has more side effects. It is no longer available in the United States and has been removed from advanced cardiac life support algorithms as it was found to be ineffective. This drug causes a direct early release of norepinephrine from adrenergic nerve endings, which can result in transient hypertension. Ultimately, the presence of bretylium in adrenergic nerve endings prevents the continued release of norepinephrine and may lead to orthostatic hypotension and bradycardia. Bretylium also potentiates the action of norepinephrine and epinephrine on adrenergic receptors by inhibiting the uptake of catecholamines.

Verapamil and Diltiazem

Among the calcium channel blockers, verapamil and diltiazem have the greatest efficacy for the treatment of cardiac arrhythmias.[1] Verapamil is highly effective in terminating paroxysmal supraventricular tachycardia, a reentrant tachycardia whose pathway usually includes the atrioventricular node. This drug also effectively controls the ventricular rate in most patients who develop atrial fibrillation or flutter. Verapamil, however, does not have a depressant effect on accessory tracts and thus will not slow the ventricular response rate in patients with Wolff-Parkinson-White syndrome. In fact, verapamil may cause reflex sympathetic nervous system activity that enhances conduction of cardiac impulses over accessory tracts and thus increases the ventricular response rate similar to digitalis. Verapamil has little efficacy in the therapy for ventricular ectopic beats.

The usual dose of verapamil for suppression of paroxysmal supraventricular tachycardia is 5 to 10 mg IV (75 to 150 μg/kg) over 1 to 3 minutes followed by a continuous infusion of about 5 μg/kg/minute to maintain a sustained effect. The administration of calcium gluconate, 1 g IV, approximately 5 minutes before administration of verapamil may decrease verapamil-induced hypotension without altering the drug's antiarrhythmic effects.[46] Chronic treatment with oral verapamil, 80 to 120 mg every 6 to 8 hours, may be useful for prevention of paroxysmal supraventricular tachycardia and for control of the ventricular response rate in atrial fibrillation or atrial flutter. Diltiazem, 20 mg IV, produces antiarrhythmic effects similar to those of diazepam, and the potential side effects are similar.

Mechanism of Action

Verapamil and the other calcium channel blockers inhibit the flux of calcium ions across the slow channels of vascular smooth muscle and cardiac cells. This effect on calcium ion flux manifests as a decreased rate of spontaneous phase 4 depolarization. Verapamil has a substantial depressant effect on the atrioventricular node and a negative chronotropic effect on the sinoatrial node. This drug exerts a negative inotropic effect on cardiac muscle and produces a moderate degree of vasodilation of the coronary arteries and systemic arteries.

Metabolism and Excretion

An estimated 70% of an injected dose of verapamil is eliminated by the kidneys, whereas up to 15% may be present in the bile. A metabolite, norverapamil, may contribute to the parent drug's antiarrhythmic effects. The need for a large oral dose is related to the extensive hepatic first-pass effect that occurs with the oral route of administration.

Side Effects

The side effects of verapamil used to treat cardiac arrhythmias reflect its effects on calcium ion flux into cardiac cells. Atrioventricular heart block is more likely in patients with preexisting defects in the conduction of cardiac impulses. Direct myocardial depression and decreased cardiac output are likely to be exaggerated in patients with poor left ventricular function. Peripheral vasodilation may contribute to hypotension. There may be potentiation of anesthetic-produced myocardial depression, and the effects of neuromuscular blocking drugs may be exaggerated.

By decreasing hepatic blood flow, cimetidine may increase the plasma concentration of verapamil. Verapamil, like quinidine, may increase the plasma concentration of digoxin by 50% to 75%. Excessive bradycardia has been observed when verapamil and propranolol are administered simultaneously.

Other Cardiac Antiarrhythmic Drugs

Digitalis

Digitalis preparations such as digoxin are effective cardiac antiarrhythmics for stabilization of atrial electrical activity and the treatment and prevention of atrial tachyarrhythmias. Because of their vagolytic effects, these drugs can also slow conduction of cardiac impulses through the atrioventricular node and thus slow the ventricular response rate in patients with atrial fibrillation. Conversely, digitalis preparations enhance conduction of cardiac impulses through accessory bypass tracts and can dangerously increase the ventricular response rate in patients with Wolff-Parkinson-White syndrome. The usual oral dose of digoxin is 0.5 to 1.0 mg in divided doses over 12 to 24 hours. Digitalis toxicity is a risk and may manifest as virtually any cardiac arrhythmia (most commonly atrial tachycardia with block).

Adenosine

Adenosine is an endogenous nucleoside that slows conduction of cardiac impulses through the atrioventricular node, making it an effective alternative to calcium channel blockers (verapamil) for the acute treatment of paroxysmal supraventricular tachycardia, including that due to conduction through accessory pathways in patients with Wolff-Parkinson-White syndrome.[47] This drug is not effective in the treatment of atrial fibrillation, atrial flutter, or ventricular tachycardia. The usual dose of adenosine is 6 mg IV followed, if necessary, by a repeat injection of 6 to 12 mg IV about 3 minutes later.

Adenosine receptors represent a logical target for treatment of pain. Adenosine agonists result in blockade of acute nociception and reduce hypersensitivity to thermal or mechanical stimuli in the presence of sensitization after peripheral inflammation or nerve injury. This response most likely reflects actions on extracellular G protein–coupled receptors present in the periphery and CNS, primarily in the spinal cord. Intrathecal administration of adenosine produces selective inhibition of hypersensitivity presumed to be due to central sensitization.[48]

Mechanism of Action

Adenosine has cardiac electrophysiologic effects similar to those of the calcium channel blockers verapamil and diltiazem.[1] It stimulates cardiac adenosine$_1$ receptors to increase potassium ion currents, shorten the action potential duration, and hyperpolarize cardiac cell membranes. In addition, adenosine decreases cyclic adenosine monophosphate concentrations. Its short-lived cardiac effects (elimination half-time 10 seconds) are due to carrier-mediated cellular uptake and metabolism to inosine by adenosine deaminase. Methylxanthines inhibit the actions of adenosine by binding to adenosine$_1$ receptors. Conversely, dipyridamole (adenosine uptake inhibitor) and cardiac transplantation (denervation hypersensitivity) potentiate the effects of adenosine.

Side Effects

The side effects associated with the rapid IV administration of adenosine include facial flushing, headache, dyspnea, chest discomfort, and nausea. Adenosine may produce transient atrioventricular heart block. Bronchospasm, although an uncommon complication, has been observed after the IV administration of adenosine, even in the absence of preexisting symptoms.[49,50] It is recommended that adenosine be used with caution, if at all, in patients known to have active wheezing. Several theories have been proposed to account for adenosine's bronchoconstrictor effect, including activation of adenosine receptors on the bronchial smooth muscle, mast cell degranulation, and stimulation of prostaglandin formation.[51] The pharmacologic effects of adenosine are antagonized by methylxanthines (theophylline, caffeine) and potentiated by dipyridamole.

Ranolazine

Although developed as treatment for angina, ranolazine has been noted to have efficacy in treatment of atrial arrhythmias and suppression of nonsustained ventricular tachycardia. Ranolazine is a piperazine derivative with a chemical structure similar to lidocaine. The cellular effects of ranolazine are attributed to binding at the local anesthetic binding site of the voltage-gated sodium channel. It is currently approved for the adjunctive treatment of chronic stable angina; however, multiple ongoing studies are evaluating the efficacy and safety of ranolazine in treatment of atrial fibrillation.

References

1. Atlee JL. Perioperative cardiac dysrhythmias: diagnosis and management. *Anesthesiology*. 1997;86:1397–1424.
2. Creswell LL, Schuessler RB, Rosenbloom M, et al. Hazards of postoperative atrial arrhythmias. *Ann Thorac Surg*. 1993;56:539–545.
3. Ben-David J, Zipes DP. Torsades de pointes and proarrhythmia. *Lancet*. 1993;341:1578–1583.
4. Zipes DP. Implantable cardioverter-defibrillator: a Volkswagen or Rolls Royce. *Circulation*. 2001;103:1372–1377.
5. Morady F. Radio-frequency ablation as treatment for cardiac arrhythmias. *N Engl J Med*. 1999;340:534–539.
6. Atlee JL, Bosnjak ZJ. Mechanisms of cardiac dysrhythmias during anesthesia. *Anesthesiology*. 1990;72:347–374.
7. Lucas WJ, Maccioli GA, Mueller RA. Advances in oral antiarrhythmic therapy: implications for the anaesthetist. *Can J Anaesth*. 1990;37:94–101.
8. Langberg JJ, DeLurgio DB. Ventricular arrhythmias. *Sci Am Med*. 1999;1(VI):1–12.
9. Williams VEM. Cardiac arrhythmias. In: Sandoe E, Fiensted-Jensen E, Olson KH, eds. *Symposium on Cardiac Arrhythmias*. Sodertalje, Sweden: AB Astra; 1970:449–472.
10. Kennedy HL, Brooks MM, Barker AH, et al. Beta blocker therapy in the Cardiac Arrhythmia Suppression Trial. CAST Investigators. *Am J Cardiol*. 1994;74:674–680.
11. Teo KK, Yusuf S, Furberg CD. Effects of prophylactic antiarrhythmic drug therapy in acute myocardial infarction: an overview of results from randomized controlled trials. *JAMA*. 1993;270:1589–1594.
12. Schechter M, Hod H, Chouraqui P, et al. Magnesium therapy in acute myocardial infarction when patients are not candidates for thrombolytic therapy. *Am J Cardiol*. 1995;75:321–328.
13. Ryan TJ, Antman EM, Brooks NH, et al. 1999 Update: ACC/AHA guidelines for the management of patients with acute myocardial infarction. *J Am Coll Cardiol*. 1999;34:890–899.
14. Piccini JP, Berger JS, O'Connor CM. Amiodarone for the prevention of sudden cardiac death: a meta-analysis of randomized controlled trials. *Eur Heart J*. 2009;30(10):1245–1253.
15. Torp-Renderson C, Moller M, Bloch-Thomsen PE, et al. Dofetilide in patients with congestive heart failure and left ventricular dysfunction. Danish investigations of arrhythmia and mortality on Dofetilide Study Group. *N Engl J Med*. 1999;341(12):857–865.
16. Arsenault KA, Yusuf AM, Crystal E, et al. Interventions for preventing post-operative atrial fibrillation in patients undergoing heart surgery. *Cochrane Database Syst Rev*. 2013;1:CD003611.
17. Roden DM. Risks and benefits of antiarrhythmic therapy. *N Engl J Med*. 1994;331:785–791.
18. Grace AA, Camm AJ. Quinidine. *N Engl J Med*. 1998;338:35–45.
19. Way WL, Katzung BG, Larson CP. Recurarization with quinidine. *JAMA*. 1967;200:163–164.
20. Chabal C, Jacobson L, Mariano A, et al. The use of oral mexiletine for the treatment of pain after peripheral nerve injury. *Anesthesiology*. 1992;76:513–517.
21. Echt DS, Liebson PR, Mitchell LB, et al. Mortality in patients receiving encainide, flecainide, or placebo: the Cardiac Arrhythmia Suppression Trial. *N Engl J Med*. 1991;324:781–788.
22. Fornieles-Perez H, Montoya-Garcia M, Levine PA, et al. Documentation of acute rise in ventricular capture thresholds associated with flecainide acetate. *Pacing Clin Electrophysiol*. 2002;25(5):871–872.
23. Daoud EG, Strickberger SA, Man KC, et al. Preoperative amiodarone as prophylaxis against atrial fibrillation after heart surgery. *N Engl J Med*. 1997;337:1785–1791.
24. Nadeemanee K, Singh BN, Stevenson WG, et al. Amiodarone and post-MI patients. *Circulation*. 1993;88:764–769.
25. Gottlieb SS, Riggio DW, Lauria S, et al. High dose oral amiodarone loading exerts important hemodynamic actions in patients with congestive heart failure. *J Am Coll Cardiol*. 1994;23:560–566.
26. Kannan R, Nademannee K, Hendrickson JA, et al. Amiodarone kinetics after oral doses. *Clin Pharmacol Ther*. 1982;31:438–444.
27. Mason JW. Amiodarone. *N Engl J Med*. 1987;316:455–463.
28. Ganjehei L, Massumi A, Nazeri A, et al. Pharmacologic management of arrhythmias. *Tex Heart Inst J*. 2011;38(4):344–349.
29. Dusman RE, Marshall SS, Miles WM, et al. Clinical features of amiodarone-induced pulmonary toxicity. *Circulation*. 1990;82:51–59.
30. Martin WJ, Rosenow EC. Amiodarone pulmonary toxicity: recognition and pathogenesis (part 1). *Chest*. 1988;93:1067–1075.
31. Kay GN, Epstein AE, Kirklin JK, et al. Fatal postoperative amiodarone pulmonary toxicity. *Am J Cardiol*. 1988;62:490–492.
32. Herndon JC, Cook AO, Ramsay AE, et al. Postoperative unilateral pulmonary edema: possible amiodarone pulmonary toxicity. *Anesthesiology*. 1992;76:308–312.
33. Kupferschmid JP, Rosengart TK, McIntosh CL, et al. Amiodarone-induced complications after cardiac operation for obstructive hypertrophic cardiomyopathy. *Ann Thorac Surg*. 1989;48:359–364.
34. Nalos PC, Kass RM, Gang ES, et al. Life-threatening postoperative pulmonary complications in patients with previous amiodarone pulmonary toxicity undergoing cardiothoracic operations. *J Thorac Cardiovasc Surg*. 1987;93:904–912.

35. MacKinnon G, Landymore R, Marble A. Should oral amiodarone be used for sustained ventricular tachycardia in patients requiring open-heart surgery? *Can J Surg*. 1983;26:355–357.
36. Teasdale S, Downar E. Amiodarone and anaesthesia. *Can J Anaesth*. 1990;37:151–155.
37. Navalgund AA, Alifimoff JK, Jakymec AJ, et al. Amiodarone-induced sinus arrest successfully treated with ephedrine and isoproterenol. *Anesth Analg*. 1986;65:414–416.
38. Feiner LA, Younge BR, Kazmier FJ, et al. Optic neuropathy and amiodarone therapy. *Mayo Clin Proc*. 1987;62(8):702–717.
39. Heger JJ, Prystowsky EN, Jackman WM, et al. Amiodarone: clinical efficacy and electrophysiology during long-term therapy for recurrent ventricular tachycardia or ventricular fibrillation. *N Engl J Med*. 1981;305:539–545.
40. Klein SM, Greengrass RA, Knudsen N, et al. Regional anesthesia for thyroidectomy in two patients with amiodarone-induced hyperthyroidism. *Anesth Analg*. 1997;85:22–24.
41. Zimetbaum PJ. Dronedarone for atrial fibrillation—an odyssey. *N Engl J Med*. 2009;360(18):1811–1813.
42. Kober L, Torp-Pendersen C, McMurray JJ, et al. Increased mortality after dronedarone therapy for severe heart failure. *N Engl J Med*. 2008;358(25):2678–2687.
43. Patel C, Yan GX, Kowey PR. Dronedarone. *Circulation*. 2009;120(7): 636–644.
44. Hohnloser SH, Crijns HJ, van Eickels M, et al. Effect of dronedarone on cardiovascular events in atrial fibrillation. *N Engl J Med*. 2009;360(7):668–678.
45. Hohnloser SH, Woosley RL. Sotalol. *N Engl J Med*. 1994;331: 31–37.
46. Salerno DM, Anderson B, Sharkey PJ, et al. Intravenous verapamil for treatment of multifocal atrial tachycardia with and without calcium pretreatment. *Ann Intern Med*. 1987;107:623–628.
47. Lerman BB, Belardinelli L. Cardiac electrophysiology of adenosine: basic and clinical concepts. *Circulation*. 1991;83:1449–1455.
48. Eisenach JC, Hood DD, Curry R. Preliminary efficacy assessment of intrathecal injection of an American formulation of adenosine in humans. *Anesthesiology*. 2002;96:29–34.
49. Aggarwal A, Farber NE, Warltier DC. Intraoperative bronchospasm caused by adenosine. *Anesthesiology*. 1993;79:1132–1135.
50. Bennett-Guerrero E, Young CC. Bronchospasm after intravenous adenosine administration. *Anesth Analg*. 1994;79:386–388.
51. Crimi N, Palermo F, Polosa R, et al. Effect of indomethacin on adenosine-induced bronchoconstriction. *J Allergy Clin Immunol*. 1989;83:921–925.

CHAPTER 22

Diuretics

Maya Jalbout Hastie • Jack S. Shanewise

Diuretics, drugs commonly used in the treatment of hypertension and heart failure, consist of a group of drugs with differing pharmacokinetic and pharmacodynamic properties. Their primary effect is to increase urine flow and to promote diuresis. Most diuretics produce their clinical effect by blocking sodium (Na^+) reabsorption in different locations of the nephron,[1] resulting in increased sodium ion delivery to the distal tubules. The normal driving force for potassium (K^+) excretion by distal renal tubules is the transtubular electrical potential difference created by sodium reabsorption. The presence of Na^+ in the distal tubules promotes its reabsorption in exchange for secretion of K^+ and results in hypokalemia. The sites of action of the different diuretics are illustrated in Figure 22-1. In general, diuretics with a site of action upstream of the collecting duct result in hyponatremia, hypokalemia, and metabolic alkalosis. In contrast, collecting duct diuretics result in hyperkalemia and metabolic acidosis.[2]

Carbonic Anhydrase Inhibitors

Acetazolamide is the prototype of a class of sulfonamide drugs that bind avidly to the enzyme carbonic anhydrase, producing noncompetitive inhibition of enzyme activity, principally in the proximal renal tubules as well as the collecting ducts (see Fig. 22-1; Table 22-1).[3] A Na^+-H^+ exchanger allows absorption of Na^+ in exchange for secretion of H^+ into the renal tubule. HCO_3^- and H^+ combine in the lumen of the proximal tubule to produce H_2CO_3. The enzyme carbonic anhydrase catalyzes the otherwise slow breakdown of H_2CO_3 into CO_2 and H_2O; CO_2 diffuses readily into the tubular cells, where cytoplasmic carbonic anhydrase catalyses the reverse reaction leading to HCO_3^-, which then follows an electrochemical gradient across the basal membrane into the interstitium. The net result is absorption of HCO_3^-. Inhibition of carbonic anhydrase in the proximal renal tubule by this class of diuretics results in decreased reabsorption of Na^+, HCO_3^-, and water.[1,3]

Pharmacokinetics and Pharmacodynamics

After oral administration, acetazolamide is excreted unchanged by the kidneys. The dose should be adjusted in patients with renal failure and the elderly.[4] Acetazolamide completely blocks membrane-bound and cytoplasmic carbonic anhydrase in the proximal tubule and to a lesser extent in the collecting ducts, preventing Na^+ and HCO_3^- absorption.[3] This increased excretion of HCO_3^- results in an alkaline urine and metabolic acidosis. Natriuresis associated with carbonic anhydrase inhibitors is modest, with an increase in fractional Na^+ excretion of up to 5%.[3] The increased delivery of Na^+ to the distal tubules leads to potassium loss. Most of the chloride is reabsorbed in the loop of Henle,[3] leading to the excretion of an alkaline urine in the presence of hyperchloremic metabolic acidosis.

Clinical Uses

In addition to its diuretic properties, acetazolamide is administered to decrease intraocular pressure in the treatment of glaucoma. There is a high concentration of the carbonic anhydrase enzyme in the ciliary processes; inhibition of the enzyme activity by acetazolamide results in decreased formation of aqueous humor and consequently a decrease in intraocular pressure.[2] Similarly, formation of cerebrospinal fluid is also inhibited by acetazolamide. Accordingly, acetazolamide has been used in the treatment of idiopathic intracranial hypertension.[2] Idiopathic intracranial hypertension, previously referred to as ***benign intracranial hypertension*** or ***pseudotumor cerebri***, is characterized by increased intracranial pressure (ICP) in the absence of tumors or other causes and manifests with headaches, pulsatile tinnitus, and papilledema and visual changes secondary to the elevated ICP, which can progress to vision loss. Women are more likely to be affected, especially obese women in their third decade of life. When treatment with acetazolamide fails, surgical placement of a ventriculoperitoneal shunt to reduce the elevated ICP is an option.

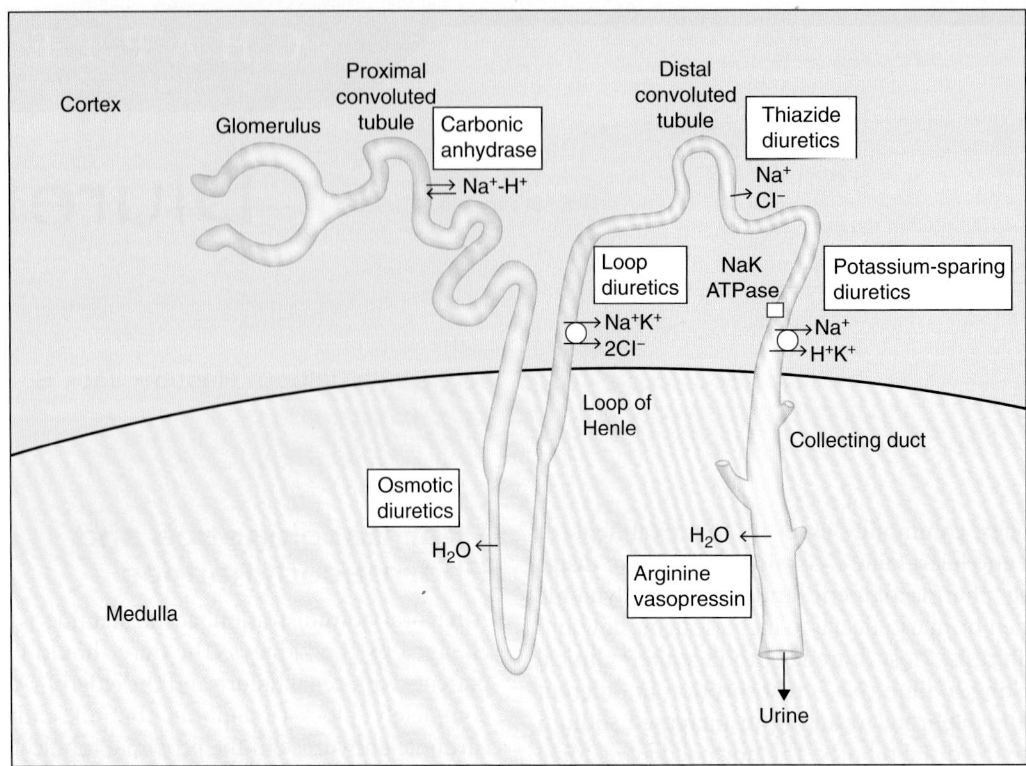

FIGURE 22-1 The sites of action of the different diuretics.

Lumbar punctures, in addition to being diagnostic by providing direct measurement of the elevated ICP, can provide symptomatic relief via removal of cerebrospinal fluid.

Acetazolamide may also be beneficial in the management of familial periodic paralysis because the drug-induced metabolic acidosis increases the local concentration of potassium in skeletal muscles.[2] Similarly, acetazolamide, by producing metabolic acidosis, may stimulate the respiratory drive in patients who are hypoventilating in a compensatory response to respiratory alkalosis, as occurs with altitude sickness. Altitude sickness, which can be prevented by a slow acclimatization process, develops following rapid ascent to high altitudes.[2] The hypoxia at high altitudes is counteracted by hyperventilation, which leads to respiratory alkalosis, which depresses ventilation. Acetazolamide-induced metabolic acidosis can reverse this hypoventilation.[2] Conversely, the loss of bicarbonate ions necessary to buffer carbon dioxide may result in the exacerbation of respiratory acidosis in patients with chronic obstructive airway disease, leading to central nervous system (CNS) depression.

Side Effects

There is a high incidence of systemic side effects associated with the use of acetazolamide such as fatigue, decreased appetite, depression, and paresthesias,[4] which could be secondary to the development of acidosis.[4] Acetazolamide dose should be reduced in patients with chronic renal insufficiency and avoided in patients with severe chronic renal insufficiency because of the increased risk of metabolic acidosis.[2]

Loop Diuretics

Furosemide, torasemide, azosemide, bumetanide, and ethacrynic acid are diuretics that inhibit reabsorption of sodium, potassium, and chloride by impairing activity of the Na^+-K^+-$2Cl^-$ transport protein in the medullary portions of the thick ascending limb of the loop of Henle. This area of the nephron is impermeable to water and accounts for the reabsorption of 20% to 30% of filtered Na^+.[1,2] Because of their site of action, loop diuretics are the most potent diuretics and have a dose-dependent response.[2] Diuretics in general and loop diuretics in particular are first-line therapy in patients with fluid retention resulting from heart failure.[2]

Pharmacokinetics and Pharmacodynamics

Ethacrynic Acid

Ethacrynic acid is no longer in clinical use because of its side effect profile. Ototoxicity, a common dose-dependent side effect of loop diuretics, is more common with ethacrynic acid.[2] Nausea is another common side effect.

Furosemide

Furosemide is effective when administered orally or intravenously (IV). However, absorption of orally administered furosemide varies between patients from 10% to 100%, with an average bioavailability of 50%.[2,5] Protein binding

Table 22-1

Diuretics and Their Sites of Action

	Receptors	Main Site of Action	Clinical Uses	Notable Side Effects
Carbonic anhydrase	Carbonic anhydrase	Proximal convoluted tubule	Altitude sickness Glaucoma	Metabolic acidosis
Loop diuretics	Na-K-2Cl cotransport	Medullary thick ascending loop of Henle	First-line diuretics in renal impairment	Ototoxicity Alkalosis Hypokalemia
Thiazides	Na-Cl cotransport	Cortical ascending loop of Henle	First-line therapy of hypertension	Alkalosis Hypokalemia Diabetes and dyslipidemia Hyperuricemia
Osmotic diuretics		Proximal convoluted tubule and loop of Henle	Increased intracranial pressure Oxygen free radical scavenging	Volume overload in CHF patients Hypokalemia, hyponatremia, hypomagnesemia
Potassium-sparing diuretics	Epithelial Na channel	Collecting duct	Adjuncts to loop diuretics or thiazides	Hyperkalemia
Aldosterone blockers	Na-K-ATPase	Collecting duct	Heart failure with low ejection fraction	Hyperkalemia
Dopamine and fenoldopam	D1	Proximal tubule and loop of Henle	Renal protection and hypertension treatment in critically ill patients	Effectiveness not substantiated
Brain natriuretic peptide	Na-K-ATPase	Collecting duct	Management of decompensated heart failure	
Vasopressin	V_2	Collecting duct	SIADH, CHF, cirrhosis	
Aquaporins	AQP	Collecting duct		

CHF, congestive heart failure; SIADH, syndrome of inappropriate antidiuretic hormone.

is extensive, with approximately 90% of the drug bound to albumin. Glomerular filtration and renal tubular secretion account for approximately 50% to 60% of furosemide excretion. The remaining 40% to 50% is conjugated to glucuronide in the kidneys.[2,5,6] The elimination half-life is 1 to 2 hours, resulting in the short duration of action. Furosemide has a rapid onset, producing diuresis within 5 to 10 minutes of administration, with a peak effect at 30 minutes and duration of action of 2 to 6 hours. In order to achieve natriuresis, furosemide needs to reach the site of action within the kidneys. In patients with normal renal function, 40 mg of IV furosemide will produce maximal natriuresis.[5] Because of decreased drug delivery to the tubule in chronic renal insufficiency, the dosing of loop diuretics should be increased in these patients.[2,5] Maximal diuresis can be achieved with an IV bolus of 160 to 200 mg, administered slowly to avoid the occurrence of tinnitus.[5] Doses larger than 200 mg will not result in increased natriuresis.[5] In addition, in patients with chronic renal insufficiency, a loading dose of furosemide followed by a continuous infusion may be used to achieve a sustained diuresis rather than repeated boluses.[1,5] More recently, the Diuretic Optimization Strategies Evaluation (DOSE) trial, a prospective randomized study of the use of loop diuretics in patients admitted with acute heart failure, did not find a significant difference in symptomatic relief or improvement of renal function with the use of high-dose diuretics or with continuous diuretic infusion, compared to low-dose or repeated diuretic boluses respectively.[7] The combination of furosemide with a different class of diuretic, such as a thiazide diuretic, may increase the response.[5]

Bumetanide and Torasemide

Bumetanide has a bioavailability of 80% to 100% after oral administration and can be administered orally, IV, or intramuscularly. It is 40 times more potent than furosemide except in its effect on potassium excretion.[2] Similar to bumetanide, torasemide's metabolism is mostly by the liver,[2] and in patients with liver failure, there is increased drug delivery to the kidneys.[5] Torasemide is twice as potent as furosemide and has a longer duration of action, with a plasma half-life of 3 to 4 hours[5] allowing for a once a day dosing regimen.[8]

Clinical Uses

Loop diuretics are not the first-line treatment for hypertension in patients with normal kidney function. However, they are first-line diuretics in patients with renal insufficiency.[1,5,8] The antihypertensive effect of loop diuretics is due to their ability to decrease intravascular fluid volume and eliminate salt. Compared to furosemide, the long-acting drug azosemide produces better blood pressure control, preserving the normal 10% decline in blood pressure in many individuals that occurs at night (nocturnal dipping) and is associated with better long-term outcomes.

Loop diuretics are commonly used in patients admitted with acute exacerbation of heart failure.[7,8] Diuresis leads to loss of water and salt with resulting decrease in intravascular volume thus lowering ventricular filling pressure and reducing pulmonary edema.[6] In addition, loop diuretics induce renal synthesis of vasodilatory prostaglandins, further enhancing their diuretic effects by increasing renal blood flow and leading to a redistribution of cortical blood flow.[6] Treatment with torasemide was found to decrease readmissions related to heart failure when compared to furosemide.[1]

Furosemide decreases ICP by inducing systemic diuresis and decreasing cerebrospinal fluid production. This diuretic-induced decrease in ICP is not accompanied by changes in cerebral blood flow or plasma osmolarity. Furosemide can be administered as single-drug therapy (0.5 to 1.0 mg/kg IV) or as a lower dose (0.1 to 0.3 mg/kg IV) in combination with mannitol. Alterations in the blood–brain barrier do not influence the immediate or subsequent effects of furosemide on ICP. This characteristic contrasts with that of mannitol, which may produce rebound intracranial hypertension if a disrupted blood–brain barrier allows mannitol to enter the CNS. A combination of furosemide and mannitol is more effective in decreasing ICP than either drug alone, but severe dehydration and electrolyte imbalance are also more likely.

In the presence of symptomatic hypercalcemia, furosemide may be used to lower the plasma concentration of calcium by stimulating urine output.

Side Effects

Side effects of loop diuretics most often manifest as abnormalities of fluid and electrolyte balance. They can lead to hypokalemia and increase the likelihood of digitalis toxicity. As with thiazide diuretics, loop diuretics may cause hyperuricemia, but this is rarely clinically significant. Likewise, hyperglycemia, although possible, is less likely to occur than with thiazide diuretics. Acute or chronic treatment of patients with diuretics, including loop diuretics, may result in tolerance to the diuretic effect ("braking phenomenon"). Acute tolerance is presumed to reflect activation of the renin-angiotensin system to retain sodium and water in the presence of a contracted extracellular fluid volume.[5] With chronic use of diuretics, there is evidence of a compensatory hypertrophy of those portions of the renal tubule (especially distal convoluted tubules) responsible for sodium retention, leading to decreased diuretic effectiveness.[5] When tolerance develops in a patient treated chronically with furosemide, it may be possible to reestablish a diuretic effect with the administration of a thiazide diuretic, which blocks the hypertrophied Na^+ reabsorption sites.[5]

Loop diuretics should only be administered to patients with a normal or increased intravascular fluid volume. Hypotension may result from administration of loop diuretics to hypovolemic patients exacerbating renal ischemic injury and concentrating nephrotoxins in the renal tubules. Accordingly, loop diuretics should be avoided in patients with acute renal insufficiency.[2,9]

Furosemide increases renal tissue concentrations of aminoglycosides and enhances the possible nephrotoxic effects of these antibiotics. Cephalosporin nephrotoxicity may also be increased by furosemide. In addition, loop diuretics potentiate nondepolarizing neuromuscular blockade.[2] Furosemide has been associated with an allergic interstitial nephritis similar to that occasionally produced by penicillin. Cross-sensitivity may exist when a patient allergic to other sulfonamides is given furosemide. The renal clearance of lithium is decreased in the presence of diuretic-induced decreases in sodium reabsorption, and plasma concentrations of lithium may be acutely increased by the IV administration of furosemide in the perioperative period.[10]

Ototoxicity, either transient or permanent, is a rare, dose-dependent complication associated with the use of loop diuretics. This side effect is most likely to occur with prolonged increases in the plasma concentration of these drugs in the presence of other ototoxic drugs such as aminoglycosides or in the presence of chronic renal insufficiency.[2]

Thiazide Diuretics

Thiazide diuretics are most often administered for long-term treatment of essential hypertension in which the combination of diuresis, natriuresis, and vasodilation are synergistic. Included in this class of drugs are hydrochlorothiazide and thiazide-like drugs, such as chlorthalidone and indapamide. Hydrochlorothiazide is the second most frequently prescribed antihypertensive medication, and thiazides are usually administered in combination with other antihypertensives.[11] Thiazide diuretics may also be used to mobilize edema fluid associated with renal, hepatic, or cardiac dysfunction. Less common uses of thiazide diuretics include management of diabetes insipidus and treatment of hypercalcemia.

Pharmacokinetics and Pharmacodynamics

Thiazide diuretics inhibit the Na^+-Cl^- cotransporter in the cortical portion of the ascending loop of Henle and the distal convoluted tubule, inhibiting reabsorption of 5% to 10% of the filtered sodium[2] (see Fig. 22-1). Enhanced distal delivery of Na^+ results in increased excretion of potassium into the renal tubules, resulting in an increase in the urinary excretion of sodium, chloride, and potassium ions. In addition, thiazide diuretics stimulate the reabsorption of calcium in the distal convoluted tube.[1]

Thiazide diuretics are readily absorbed when administered orally; hydrochlorothiazide has a 60% to 70% bioavailability, and they are extensively protein-bound.[8] Most thiazides are eliminated unchanged in the kidney; indapamide, however, is metabolized by the liver.[5] Thiazides' effectiveness markedly decreases in patients with renal insufficiency.[5] Thiazide diuretics have a long half-life of 8 to 12 hours, allowing for a convenient once-a-day dosing.[8] Chlorthalidone has the longest elimination half-life of 50 to 60 hours.[8] Indapamide, xipamide, and metolazone are structurally related to furosemide but share a thiazide-like mechanism of action with differences in their clinical effects.[2] When compared to hydrochlorothiazide, metolazone has a slow and unpredictable absorption and tends to accumulate because of its prolonged elimination half-life.[5] Thiazide diuretics, with the exception of metolazone, are ineffective in patients with severe renal insufficiency and the use of loop diuretics in these patients is recommended if diuresis is needed.[8]

Clinical Uses

Thiazide diuretics are recommended as first-line therapy for essential hypertension and the use of chlorthalidone specifically has been shown to decrease the risk of major cardiovascular events when compared to calcium channel blockers or angiotensin-converting enzyme inhibitors in a large randomized control trial, the Antihypertensive and Lipid-Lowering Treatment to Prevent Heart Attack Trial (ALLHAT).[12]

The antihypertensive effect of thiazide diuretics is due initially to a decrease in extracellular fluid volume, often with a decrease in cardiac output, which normalizes after several weeks.[1] The sustained antihypertensive effect of thiazide diuretics, however, is due to peripheral vasodilation, which requires several weeks to develop. It is unclear whether the resulting decrease in systemic vascular resistance after chronic thiazide therapy results from direct or indirect vasodilatory effect.[11]

Because they stimulate calcium reabsorption, thiazide diuretics are used in the treatment of calcium-containing renal calculi.[1] Although unlikely to cause hypercalcemia, thiazide diuretics should be used cautiously in patients with conditions that predispose to hypercalcemia, such as hyperparathyroidism and sarcoidosis.[2]

Chlorthalidone, a longer acting thiazide-like diuretic, is recommended for use in resistant hypertension, achieving better nighttime control of the blood pressure.[1] In addition, treatment with chlorthalidone resulted in decreased cardiovascular events when compared to treatment with lisinopril or amlodipine.[12]

Indapamide, a weak diuretic, decreases blood pressure by causing vasodilation.[2] In contrast, xipamide is a potent diuretic and kaliuretic, and frequent measurement of potassium levels is recommended when it is prescribed.[2] Metolazone can promote diuresis in patients with renal insufficiency, in whom the other thiazides effective, and is usually administered with a loop diuretic. Their concomitant use should be monitored closely because of their synergism and because of metolazone's propensity to accumulate due to its long elimination half-life.[2,5,8]

Side Effects

Thiazide diuretic–induced hypokalemic, hypochloremic, metabolic alkalosis is a common side effect when these drugs are administered chronically for maintenance treatment of essential hypertension. However, these side effects are usually well tolerated at low doses.[8] Hypokalemia may manifest as skeletal muscle weakness and gastrointestinal ileus and may increase the risk of developing digitalis toxicity. Depletion of sodium and magnesium ions may accompany kaliuresis. Cardiac dysrhythmias may occur as the result of diuretic-induced hypokalemia or hypomagnesemia. In addition, hypercalcemia may result, especially in patients receiving calcium supplements or vitamin D therapy.[2] The use of thiazide diuretics can potentiate nondepolarizing neuromuscular blockade by producing hypokalemia.[2] The effectiveness of thiazides is decreased in patients receiving nonsteroidal antiinflammatory drugs.[8] In addition, thiazide diuretics may promote lithium reabsorption in the proximal tubule by a compensatory mechanism, thereby potentiating toxicity in patients on lithium therapy.[2] Inhibition of renal tubular secretion of urate by thiazide diuretics can result in hyperuricemia in 50% of treated patients, and a small percentage of patients might develop clinical gout.[2,11]

Thiazide diuretics may cause glucose intolerance and aggravate glucose control in diabetic patients,[2] especially when used in combination with β blockers. The mechanism of hyperglycemia is unknown but may result from a drug-induced decrease of insulin release from the pancreas and peripheral resistance to the effects of insulin.[11] In addition, thiazide-induced hypokalemia may be associated with glucose intolerance and treating the hypokalemia may protect from developing diabetes.[8] Thiazide treatment may affect cholesterol and triglyceride levels, aggravating hyperlipidemia.[11] Intravascular fluid volume status should be considered in all patients treated with thiazide diuretics who are scheduled for surgery. The presence of orthostatic hypotension should arouse suspicion that intravascular fluid volume is decreased. Because of the structural similarities between sulfonamide antibiotics and thiazide and loop diuretics, it has been suggested that patients with sulfa allergy may demonstrate cross-reactivity to these classes of diuretics.[2]

Osmotic Diuretics

Osmotic diuretics such as mannitol, urea, isosorbide, and glycerin are inert substances that do not undergo metabolism and are filtered freely at the glomerulus. Their administration causes increased plasma and renal tubular fluid osmolality, with resulting osmotic diuresis.[3] Portions of the renal tubules that are highly permeable to water, namely, the proximal renal tubules and more importantly, the loop of Henle, represent the principal site of action of osmotic diuretics.[3]

Mannitol

Mannitol is the only osmotic diuretic in current use. Structurally, mannitol is a six-carbon sugar alcohol that does not undergo metabolism. It is not absorbed from the gastrointestinal tract, which necessitates its exclusive use by IV injection to achieve a diuretic effect. Mannitol does not enter cells, and its only means of clearance from the plasma is by glomerular filtration.

Pharmacokinetics and Pharmacodynamics

After administration, mannitol is completely filtered at the glomeruli, and none of the filtered drug is subsequently reabsorbed from the renal tubules.[3] By increasing tubular fluid osmolality, it decreases water reabsorption and promotes water diuresis.[2] Sodium is diluted in the retained water in the renal tubules, leading to less reabsorption of this ion. However, hypernatremia may result from the water diuresis.[2]

In addition to causing renal tubular effects, IV administration of mannitol also increases plasma osmolarity, thus drawing fluid from intracellular to extracellular spaces. This increased plasma osmolarity may result in an acute expansion of the intravascular fluid volume which could be poorly tolerated in patients with borderline cardiac function. Increased plasma osmolarity allows water to move along an osmotic gradient from tissues, including the brain, into the intravascular space, leading to decreased ICP. Mannitol is a scavenger of oxygen-free radicals, which may prevent cellular injury.

Clinical Uses

Mannitol is used primarily in the acute management of elevated ICP and in the treatment of glaucoma. Mannitol decreases ICP by increasing plasma osmolarity, which draws water from tissues, including the brain, along an osmotic gradient. Mannitol begins to exert an effect within 10 to 15 minutes, with a peak effect at 30 to 45 minutes and a duration of 6 hours.[13] The effect on ICP is dose-dependent within this dosing range and the larger dose may last longer. However, larger doses, up to 2 g/kg, and repeated administration can result in metabolic derangements. An intact blood–brain barrier is necessary for the cerebral effects of mannitol. If the blood–brain barrier is not intact, mannitol may enter the brain, drawing fluid with it and causing worsening of the cerebral edema. In addition, a rebound increase in ICP may occur following mannitol use.[13]

Mannitol has been used to prevent perioperative kidney failure in the setting of acute tubular necrosis. It is thought to provide renal protection via several mechanisms. As an osmotic diuretic, it is not reabsorbed by the tubules and results in osmotic diuresis that forces casts and necrotic debris out of the renal tubules. In addition, mannitol has been shown to cause vasodilation of vascular smooth muscle mediated by the release of prostaglandins,[13] which is dependent on the dose and rate of administration.[14] This vasodilation leads to improved renal blood flow, thereby protecting the kidneys from acute failure following renal tubular necrosis.[2,13] Mannitol also has free radical scavenging properties, which may protect transplanted kidneys following reperfusion.[2,13] Despite its common use during cardiac and major vascular surgery for renal protection, it has not been shown to prevent perioperative acute renal failure.[13]

Side Effects

The initial increase in intravascular volume associated with the administration of mannitol may be poorly tolerated in patients with left ventricular dysfunction, leading to pulmonary edema. For this reason, furosemide may be a preferred drug for treatment of increased ICP in patients with left ventricular dysfunction. In addition, in patients with renal insufficiency, mannitol is not filtered and will cause increase in the intravascular volume.[5] Prolonged use of mannitol may cause hypovolemia, electrolyte disturbances with hypokalemic hypochloremic alkalosis, and plasma hyperosmolarity due to excessive excretion of water and sodium.

Potassium-Sparing Diuretics

Potassium-sparing diuretics act on the collecting ducts and are grouped in two categories: pteridine analogs and aldosterone receptor blockers.[1] Pteridine analogs, such as triamterene and amiloride, prevent Na^+ reabsorption in the cortical collecting duct by blocking the epithelial Na^+ channels (ENa^+C), independent of aldosterone.

Aldosterone receptor blockers on the other hand, such as spironolactone and eplerenone, prevent the synthesis and the activation of the aldosterone-dependent basal cell Na^+-K^+-ATPase pump. Both mechanisms result in decreased Na^+ reabsorption without the increased K^+ secretion that would otherwise occur.[1] The collecting duct accounts for less than 3% of sodium reabsorption. Accordingly, potassium-sparing diuretics do not cause substantial diuresis and are not used as single antihypertensive therapy.[1,15] They are used in conjunction with thiazide diuretics to prevent the associated loss of potassium and magnesium.[8]

Pharmacokinetics and Pharmacodynamics

Oral absorption of amiloride and triamterene is limited (25% and 50%, respectively).[3] Amiloride is more potent than triamterene and is not metabolized but excreted unchanged in the kidneys.[5] Triamterene is a pteridine with a structural resemblance to folic acid. The metabolism of triamterene by the liver is extensive, and its metabolite, secreted into the renal tubule, has diuretic activity. Accordingly, both kidney and liver disease will affect the pharmacokinetics of triamterene.[5] The elimination half-time for triamterene is 4 hours and for amiloride is about 20 hours.[3]

Clinical Uses

Potassium-sparing diuretics are most often used in combination with loop diuretics or thiazide diuretics to augment diuresis and limit renal loss of potassium; they are rarely used as monotherapy.[15] Because cystic fibrosis is associated with increased sodium absorption across airway epithelium, aerosolized amiloride has been investigated in patients with cystic fibrosis. However, there is no evidence that topically administered amiloride causes any improvement in respiratory function or in mucus secretion in patients with cystic fibrosis.[16]

Side Effects

Hyperkalemia is the principal side effect of therapy with potassium-sparing diuretics, especially when combined with angiotensin-converting enzyme inhibitors or angiotensin II receptor blockers or in presence of nonsteroidal antiinflammatory drugs.[2,15] Although triamterene is a weak folic acid antagonist, it rarely causes megaloblastic anemia except in patients already at risk for folic acid deficiency.[15]

Aldosterone Antagonists

Spironolactone is a synthetic steroid analog and a nonspecific mineralocorticoid receptor antagonist.[8] This drug bears a close structural resemblance to aldosterone and results in potassium-sparing diuresis. Spironolactone binds to the cytoplasmic mineralocorticoid receptors in the collecting ducts, preventing Na^+ reabsorption via the Na^+-K^+ pump. Eplerenone is a selective aldosterone receptor blocker, has less affinity for other mineralocorticoid receptors, and is less potent than spironolactone.[15] It was previously believed that spironolactone effects were solely the result of competitive antagonism of aldosterone binding to the mineralocorticoid receptors. However, it has been shown that blocking the effects of other ligands, such as cortisol, on the mineralocorticoid receptors contributes to spironolactone and eplerenone clinical effects.[15] Conversely, blockade of aldosterone produces beneficial end-organ effects, independently of blood pressure control.[15] Spironolactone, when added to conventional therapy, was shown to effectively reduce morbidity and mortality in patients with heart failure with poor ejection fraction in the Randomized Aldactone Evaluation Study (RALES).[17] This is thought to be the result of prevention of aldosterone-induced cardiac remodeling and fibrosis.[15] However, spironolactone therapy was not found to significantly improve outcomes in patients with heart failure and preserved ejection fraction (diastolic heart failure).[18] Similarly, eplerenone, a selective mineralocorticoid receptor blocker, has been shown to improve morbidity and mortality compared to optimal medical treatment in patients with acute myocardial infarction and left heart failure in the Eplerenone in Acute Myocardial Infarction Heart Failure Efficacy and Survival Study (EPHESUS).[15,19]

Pharmacokinetics and Pharmacodynamics

Spironolactone and eplerenone exert their effect on the aldosterone receptor of the tubular cell and reach the tubular cells from the plasma, not from the tubular fluid.[2] They are the only diuretics that do not need to reach the renal tubule to exert their effect.[3] They provide competitive blockade of epithelial aldosterone receptors in the distal tubule and the collecting duct, preventing Na^+-K^+-ATPase activation and resulting in decreased sodium reabsorption and in decreased potassium excretion.[15] Oral absorption of spironolactone approaches 70% of the administered dose. Spironolactone undergoes extensive hepatic first-pass metabolism with multiple active metabolites,[5] which account for spironolactone's long half-life of 20 hours.[15] Spironolactone and its metabolites are extensively bound to plasma proteins and excreted by the kidneys. Similarly, eplerenone undergoes hepatic metabolism and its half-life is prolonged in the presence of CYTP3A4 inhibitors, such as ketoconazole and verapamil.[15]

Clinical Uses

Spironolactone and eplerenone are often prescribed for the treatment of essential hypertension, in combination with thiazides, particularly in patients with a low renin state (Black, the elderly, and diabetics) or patients with metabolic syndrome (the name for a group of risk factors that raises risk for heart disease and other health problems, such as diabetes and stroke).[15] Aldosterone antagonist diuretics are also used in patients with refractory hypertension, whose blood pressure remains difficult to control despite therapy with several medications, including a diuretic.[15] Furthermore, thiazide therapy might promote increased aldosterone levels because of decreased intravascular volume.[15] The combination of spironolactone with a thiazide diuretic results in improved diuresis and blood pressure control, in addition to prevention of the thiazide-induced hypokalemia and hypomagnesemia.[8]

In addition, spironolactone and eplerenone are used in the treatment of patients demonstrating "aldosterone escape," which results from incomplete aldosterone blockade during antihypertensive therapy with blockers of the renin-angiotensin-aldosterone system.[8,15] Aldosterone antagonists are used to promote diuresis in patients with edema and fluid overload associated with hyperaldosteronism, such as liver cirrhosis, nephrotic syndrome, and heart failure. Also, as discussed earlier, the administration of spironolactone along with an angiotensin-converting enzyme inhibitor in the treatment of patients with heart failure with poor ejection fraction results in a decrease in cardiovascular morbidity and mortality.[17]

Side Effects

Hyperkalemia, especially in the presence of impaired renal function, is the most serious side effect of treatment with spironolactone. In addition, the combination of spironolactone with angiotensin-converting enzyme inhibitors can exacerbate hyperkalemia in these patients.[2] Because it is a nonspecific mineralocorticoid receptor antagonist, spironolactone can block androgen and progesterone receptors, leading to gynecomastia and breast tenderness[8] that could prompt patients to seek cessation of therapy.[17]

Dopamine Receptor Agonists

Dopamine receptor agonists, such as dopamine and fenoldopam, result in natriuresis and increased renal blood flow via their actions on renal tubular dopamine-1 (D_1) receptors.

Pharmacokinetics and Pharmacodynamics

Endogenous dopamine is synthesized locally in the epithelial cells of the renal tubules and exerts its effect directly.[3] At low concentrations, dopamine produces its clinical effect via activation of dopamine receptors. Activation of D_1 receptors in the proximal renal tubule and in the loop of Henle increases cyclic adenosine monophosphate formation, resulting in inhibition of the Na^+-H^+ exchange and Na^+-K^+-ATPase pump.[3] In addition, D_1 receptors mediate an increase in renal blood flow leading to a small increase in glomerular filtration rate.[3] With increasing doses of dopamine, sympathetic activation begins to predominate. β activation results in increased inotropy, increased cardiac output, and elevation in systemic blood pressure. At even higher doses, α activation prevails, leading to vasoconstriction.

Fenoldopam is a fast-acting IV antihypertensive with a short half-life of 10 minutes,[3] used in the short-term treatment of patients with severe hypertension. Fenoldopam is a relatively selective D_1 receptor agonist with moderate affinity to α_2 receptors. It has no effect on D_2, β, or α_1 receptors.[3] Accordingly, it results in increased renal blood flow and decreased systemic vascular resistance.[20] Both dopamine and fenoldopam have poor availability after oral intake and are thus administered IV.

Clinical Uses

Dopamine is used to maintain renal blood flow in patients in cardiogenic shock with low or normal systemic vascular resistance.[3] Similarly, fenoldopam is used for its renal vasodilation properties and, even at higher doses it lacks sympathetic activity, thus it is used to treat resistant hypertension.[3] Both drugs have been used at very low doses to provide renal protection in high-risk patients, such as after cardiac or major vascular surgery, or following radioiodine contrast injection.[20] However, large randomized trials have not found a reduction in the incidence of perioperative acute renal failure with these drugs.[20,21,22]

Natriuretic Peptides

Atrial natriuretic peptide and brain natriuretic peptide are normally produced in the atria and ventricles of the heart, respectively, in response to myocardial wall stretch.[3] They exert their diuretic effect on the collecting duct of the kidneys by blocking the basal Na-K-ATPase channel. In the United States, nesiritide, a recombinant brain natriuretic peptide, is the only natriuretic peptide currently available. It is suggested in the management of patients with decompensated congestive heart failure,[23] although data on its effect on long-term morbidity and mortality are lacking.[24] It is administered IV as a continuous infusion and has a short half-life of 18 minutes.[3]

Vasopressin Receptor Antagonists

Vasopressin receptor antagonists, or vaptans, competitively inhibit V_2 receptor in the renal collecting duct, thereby leading to decreased water reabsorption. Currently, tolvaptan is the only U.S. Food and Drug Administration–approved selective V_2 receptor antagonist for the treatment of euvolemic and hypervolemic hyponatremia associated with syndrome of inappropriate antidiuretic hormone, congestive heart failure, or liver cirrhosis.[25]

Neprilysin Antagonists

Neprilysin (NEP) is a ubiquitous, membrane-bound metalloproteinase with greatest concentration in cardiovascular tissues and the kidneys.[26] The most important function of NEP appears to be the natriuretic peptides, including atrial natriuretic peptide, brain natriuretic peptide, and C-type natriuretic peptide. The natriuretic peptides are released by cardiac and renal tissues in response to increased cardiac wall stress and volume overload, as occurs in heart failure and hypertension. The natriuretic peptides stimulate renal secretion of water and are broken down by NEP. NEP activity is increased in heart failure, leading to accelerated breakdown of natriuretic peptides. Specific NEP inhibition has been shown to increase circulating levels of natriuretic peptides, promoting natriuresis; they have also been shown to reduce the cardiovascular remodeling that is inherent to end-stage heart failure. The NEP inhibitors, used alone or in combination with other agents, may well emerge as a novel group of agents for reducing morbidity and mortality associated with advanced heart failure.

Aquaporin Modulators

Aquaporins (AQP) are recently described membrane channels facilitating water movement across cells in response to osmotic gradient.[27] Subtypes of AQP respond to antidiuretic hormone (ADH) in the collecting duct of the kidney and mutations in those channels can result in hereditary nephrogenic diabetes insipidus.[2,27] Other subunits located in the cerebral perivascular astrocyte end foot may be involved in cerebral edema and in the pathogenesis of neuromyelitis optica.[2,27] Nephrogenic diabetes insipidus (NDI), which is characterized by polyuria and polydipsia, results from an inappropriate response to ADH. The most common form of NDI is acquired, usually secondary to lithium toxicity, hypercalcemia, or polycystic kidney disease. Hereditary NDI on the other hand is rare and can result either from an X-linked defect in V_2 receptors or from an autosomal recessive AQP_2 mutation.[27] Treatment with thiazide diuretics in these patients helps decrease the kidney's diluting ability.[27]

References

1. Roush GC, Kaur R, Ernst ME. Diuretics: a review and update. *J Cardiovasc Pharmacol Ther*. 2014;19(1):5–13.
2. Wile D. Diuretics: a review. *Ann Clin Biochem*. 2012;49(pt 5):419–431.
3. Goodman LS, Brunton LL, Chabner B, et al. *Goodman & Gilman's Pharmacological Basis of Therapeutics*. 12th ed. New York, NY: McGraw-Hill; 2011.
4. Yano I, Takayama A, Takano M, et al. Pharmacokinetics and pharmacodynamics of acetazolamide in patients with transient intraocular pressure elevation. *Eur J Clin Pharmacol*. 1998;54(1):63–68.
5. Brater DC. Diuretic therapy. *N Engl J Med*. 1998;339(6):387–395.
6. Leto L, Aspromonte N, Feola M. Efficacy and safety of loop diuretic therapy in acute decompensated heart failure: a clinical review. *Heart Fail Rev*. 2014;19(2):237–246.
7. Felker GM, Lee KL, Bull DA, et al; NHLBI Heart Failure Clinical Research Network. Diuretic strategies in patients with acute decompensated heart failure. *N Engl J Med*. 2011;364(9):797–805.
8. Ernst ME, Moser M. Use of diuretics in patients with hypertension. *N Engl J Med*. 2009;361(22):2153–2164.
9. Mehta RL, Pascual MT, Soroko S, et al; PICARD Study Group. Diuretics, mortality, and nonrecovery of renal function in acute renal failure. *JAMA*. 2002;288(20):2547–2553.
10. Havdal HS, Borison RL, Diamond BI. Potential hazards and applications of lithium in anesthesiology. *Anesthesiology*. 1979;50:534–537.
11. Duarte JD, Cooper-DeHoff RM. Mechanisms for blood pressure lowering and metabolic effects of thiazide and thiazide-like diuretics. *Expert Rev Cardiovasc Ther*. 2010;8(6):793–802.
12. ALLHAT Officers and Coordinators for the ALLHAT Collaborative Research Group. Major outcomes in high-risk hypertensive patients randomized to angiotensin-converting enzyme inhibitor or calcium channel blocker vs diuretic: the Antihypertensive and Lipid-Lowering Treatment to Prevent Heart Attack Trial (ALLHAT). *JAMA*. 2002;288(23):2981–2997.
13. Shawkat H, Westwood M-M, Mortimer A. Mannitol: a review of its clinical uses. *Contin Educ Anaesth Crit Care Pain*. 2012;12(2):82–85.
14. Ravissin P, Abou-Madi M, Archer D, et al. Changes in CSF pressure after mannitol in patients with and without elevated CSF pressure. *J Neurosurg*. 1988;69:869–876.
15. Epstein M, Calhoun DA. Aldosterone blockers (mineralocorticoid receptor antagonism) and potassium-sparing diuretics. *J Clin Hypertens*. 2011;13(9):644–648.
16. Burrows EF, Southern KW, Noone PG. Sodium channel blockers for cystic fibrosis. *Cochrane Database Syst Rev*. 2014;4:CD005087.
17. Pitt B, Zannad F, Remme WJ, et al. The effect of spironolactone on morbidity and mortality in patients with severe heart failure. *N Engl J Med*. 1999;341(10):709–717.
18. Pitt B, Pfeffer MA, Assmann SF, et al; TOPCAT Investigators. Spironolactone for heart failure with preserved ejection fraction. *N Engl J Med*. 2014;370(15):1383–1392.
19. Pitt B, Remme W, Zannad F, et al; Eplerenone Post-Acute Myocardial Infarction Heart Failure Efficacy and Survival Study Investigators. Eplerenone, a selective aldosterone blocker, in patients with left ventricular dysfunction after myocardial infarction. *N Engl J Med*. 2003;348(14):1309–1321.
20. Bove T, Landoni G, Calabro MG, et al. Renoprotective action of fenoldopam in high-risk patients undergoing cardiac surgery: a prospective, double-blind, randomized clinical trial. *Circulation*. 2005;111(24):3230–3235.
21. O'Hara JF Jr, Mahboobi R, Novak SM, et al. Fenoldopam and renal function after partial nephrectomy in a solitary kidney: a randomized, blinded trial. *Urology*. 2013;81(2):340–345.
22. Zangrillo A, Biondi-Zoccai GG, Frati E, et al. Fenoldopam and acute renal failure in cardiac surgery: a meta-analysis of randomized placebo-controlled trials. *J Cardiothorac Vasc Anesth*. 2012;26(3), 407–413.
23. Publication Committee for the VMAC Investigators. Intravenous nesiritide vs nitroglycerin for treatment of decompensated congestive heart failure: a randomized controlled trial. *JAMA*. 2002; 287(12):1531–1540.
24. Chen HH, Sundt TM, Cook DJ, et al. Low dose nesiritide and the preservation of renal function in patients with renal dysfunction undergoing cardiopulmonary-bypass surgery: a double-blind placebo-controlled pilot study. *Circulation*. 2007;116(11)(suppl):I-134–I-138.
25. Lehrich RW, Greenberg A. Hyponatremia and the use of vasopressin receptor antagonists in critically ill patients. *J Intensive Care Med*. 2012;27(4):207–218.
26. von Lueder TG, Atar D, Krum H. Current role of neprilysin inhibitors in hypertension and heart failure. *Pharmacol Ther*. 2014; 144(1):41–49.
27. Verkman AS, Anderson MO, Papadopoulos MC. Aquaporins: important but elusive drug targets. *Nat Rev Drug Discov*. 2014;13(4): 259–277.

CHAPTER 23

Lipid-Lowering Drugs

Sarah C. Smith • Jack S. Shanewise

Lipoprotein Metabolism

Lipoproteins are macromolecular lipid protein complexes responsible for the transport of lipids to and from the peripheral tissues. Lipoproteins are classified based on their relative density as (a) chylomicrons, (b) very-low-density lipoproteins (VLDLs), (c) intermediate-density lipoproteins (IDLs), (d) low-density lipoproteins (LDLs), and (e) high-density lipoproteins (HDLs) (Table 23-1). Lipoprotein metabolism can be divided into the exogenous and endogenous pathways (Fig. 23-1). The exogenous pathway refers to the processing of dietary fats, cholesterol, and lipid-soluble vitamins, whereas the endogenous pathway describes hepatic cholesterol synthesis and its distrubution to the peripheral tissues.

Exogenous Pathway

In the small intestine, bile emulsifies dietary fat and cholesterol, whereas lipase excreted by the pancreas hydrolyzes triglycerides. The intestinal endothelium takes up these products by endocytosis and packages lipids into large chylomicrons, which then enter the lymphatic system. After traveling through the thoracic duct, the chylomicrons enter the bloodstream where they interact with lipoprotein lipase (LPL) in vascular endothelial cells, yielding glycerol and free fatty acids, which can be utilized by the peripheral tissues for fuel or storage. During this process, the chylomicrons shrink and become chylomicron remnants. These remnants are transported to the liver where they are taken up by hepatocytes via endocytosis and subsequently hydrolyzed.

Endogenous Pathway

In the liver, hepatocytes synthesize cholesterol, lipids, and proteins, which are assembled into VLDL and excreted into the bloodstream. Similar to the processing of chylomicrons, endothelial cell LPL hydrolyzes the fats in VLDL particles, which then shrink to form IDL and LDL. LDL particles contain most of the cholesterol in plasma and are cleared from the blood by binding to LDL receptors (LDL-R) on hepatocytes. Apoproteins C and E are essential cofactors of the hydrolysis of VLDL and are contributed by HDL particles. HDL also transfers ApoC-II to chylomicrons in the exogenous pathway and is responsible for reverse cholesterol transport, in which excess cholesterol is delivered from the peripheral tissues to the liver for excretion in the bile.[1]

Lipid Disorders

A minority of lipid disorders arise from genetic defects in lipoprotein metabolism, which may present in the pediatric period or early adulthood. One such disorder, familial hypercholesterolemia, arises from a defect in the gene for LDL-R. Heterozygotes for this defect experience accelerated atherosclerosis and represent about 1 in 500 persons. Homozygotes are much more rare, have total and LDL cholesterol levels four times normal, and have an extreme propensity for atherosclerosis. Hyperlipidemia may also arise from secondary causes including obesity, diabetes, alcohol abuse, hypothyroidism, glucocorticoid excess, and hepatic or renal dysfunction.[1] Most cases of hyperlipidemia in adults arise from a combination of secondary causes, genetic predisposition, and environmental factors, including poor diet and a lack of exercise.[2]

It has been recognized for several decades that increased plasma concentrations of total and LDL cholesterol are associated with an increased risk of cardiovascular disease.[3,4] Conversely, higher HDL cholesterol levels appear to reduce the risk of atherosclerosis and cardiovascular events because of the critical role of HDL in reverse cholesterol transport.[5–7] Furthermore, lowering plasma concentrations of total and LDL cholesterol with pharmacologic agents decreases the risk of coronary events in patients with and without coronary artery disease.[8,9] Hypertriglyceridemia is known to cause pancreatitis, but its causal relationship to atherosclerosis is less well established.[2]

Table 23-1

Classification of Lipoproteins

Lipoprotein	Density (g/mL)	Diameter (nm)
Chylomicrons	<0.95	75–1,200
Very-low-density lipoproteins (VLDL)	0.95–1.006	30–90
Intermediate-density lipoproteins (IDL)	1.006–1.019	~30
Low-density lipoproteins (LDL)	1.019–1.063	~20
High-density lipoproteins (HDL)	1.063–1.21	8–12

From Jackson RL, Morrisett JD, Gotto AM Jr, et al. Lipoprotein structure and metabolism. *Physiol Rev.* 1976;56(2):259–316; Mahley RW, Innerarity TL, Rall SC Jr, et al. Plasma lipoproteins: apolipoprotein structure and function. *J Lipid Res.* 1984;25(12):1277–1294.

The safety and efficacy of 3-hydroxy-3-methylglutaryl coenzyme A reductase (HMG-CoA reductase) inhibitors, or statins, have been particularly well established,[9,10] as reflected in current guidelines issued by the the American College of Cardiology (ACC) and the American Heart Association (AHA). These guidelines advocate statin use in four high-risk groups (Table 23-2) for the primary or secondary prevention of atherosclerotic cardiovascular disease (ASCVD).[11] Based on these guidelines, about 56 million adults in the United States are eligible for statin therapy.[12] Therefore, anesthesiologists can expect to routinely encounter patients in the perioperative period taking statins for hyperlipidemia and the prevention of ASCVD. ACC/AHA guidelines no longer recommend target reductions of total or LDL cholesterol or the use of drugs other than statins for the treatment of hyperlipidemia.[11] However, alternative agents to statins are still used in clinical practice for the treatment of familial lipid disorders and for those who are intolerant of statins.

Drugs for Treatment of Hyperlipidemia

In the last several years, statins have become the mainstay of treatment for hyperlipidemia; however, there are multiple other agents used for patients intolerant of statins or those with genetic lipid disorders. The effects of these different classes of medications on LDL, HDL, and triglycerides are summarized in Table 23-3.

Statins

Statins are drugs that act as inhibitors of HMG-CoA reductase, the enzyme that catalyzes the rate-limiting step of cholesterol biosynthesis in which HMG-CoA is converted to mevalonate (see Fig. 23-1). Statins are structurally related to HMG-CoA and competitive inhibition of the enzyme causes an increase in hepatic LDL-R. The combined effect of decreased cholesterol synthesis and increased LDL uptake by the liver by statins results in a

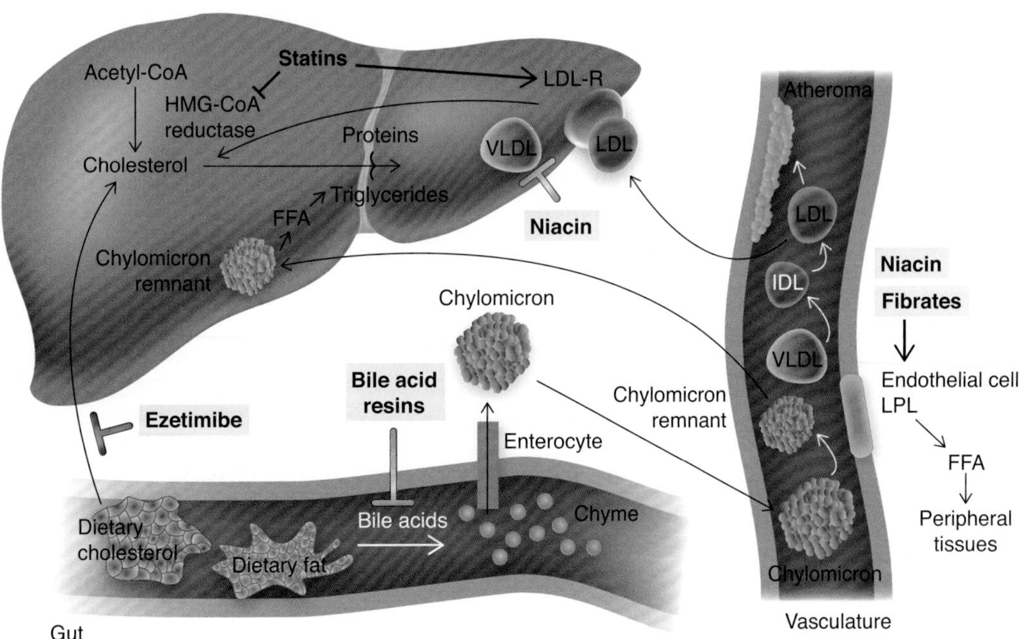

FIGURE 23-1 A diagrammatic representation of lipid metabolism. T-shaped markers indicate inhibition, arrow-shaped markers indicate enhancement.

Table 23-2

Statin Benefit Groups

1. Clinical evidence of ASCVD
2. LDL-C >190 mg/dL
3. Age 40–75 years with diabetes and an LDL-C 70–189 mg/dL
4. Age 40–75 years without diabetes, an LDL-C 70–189 mg/dL, and an estimated 10-year risk of ASCVD >7.5% (10-year risk of ASCVD based on Pooled Cohort Equations available at my.americanheart.org/cvriskcalculator)

ASCVD, atherosclerotic cardiovascular disease; LDL-C, low-density lipoprotein cholesterol.

Adapted from Stone NJ, Robinson JG, Lichtenstein AH, et al. 2013 ACC/AHA guideline on the treatment of blood cholesterol to reduce atherosclerotic cardiovascular risk in adults: a report of the American College of Cardiology/American Heart Association Task Force on Practice Guidelines. *Circulation.* 2014;63(25, pt B):2889–2934.

decrease in LDL concentration of 20% to 60%. Statins also increase HDL by approximately 10%, possibly from increased synthesis of apolipoprotein A-I. Plasma triglyceride concentrations decrease 10% to 20% in statin-treated patients, although this is usually insufficent as the sole treatment of hypertriglyceridemia.[2]

The drugs in this class (atorvastatin, fluvastatin, lovastatin, pravastatin, simvastatin, and rosuvastatin) are considered equivalent and relatively free of side effects. Randomized clinical trials have shown that statins lower cardiac events (total mortality, death from myocardial infarction, revascularization procedures, stroke, and peripheral vascular disease) in patients with or without atherosclerosis.[13,14] Furthermore, angiographic studies have shown benefit on coronary stenosis in native vessels or grafts in patients treated with statins as well as in patients experiencing acute coronary syndromes.[15] Early initiation of statin therapy following an acute myocardial infarction is recommended.[16,17]

The reduction in cardiac events observed with statin use may not be only secondary to the LDL lowering effects. Statins are thought to stabilize existing atherosclerotic plaques, and there is evidence that statins have many pleiotropic effects, including antiinflammatory, antioxidant, and vasodilatory properties. Reduced cardiac morbidity and mortality has even been reported following perioperative statin administration in high-risk groups, although this is not yet widely advocated.[18]

Origin and Chemical Structure

Lovastatin is a naturally occurring product isolated from a strain of *Aspergillus terreus.* Simvastatin and pravastatin are derived synthetically from a fermentation product of the same fungus, whereas atorvastatin, fluvastatin, and rosuvastatin are entirely synthetic compounds.[19]

Pharmacokinetics

Statins are variably absorbed from the gastrointestinal tract following oral ingestion. Bile acid–binding resins can decrease the absorption of these drugs. Lovastatin and simvastatin are prodrugs that require metabolism to the open β-hydroxy acid form to be pharmacologically active. Atorvastatin, fluvastatin, and pravastatin are administered as the active β-hydroxy acid form. Food intake increases plasma concentrations of lovastatin but has minimal effects on the other statins. All of the statins are highly protein bound with the exception of pravastatin. Except for pravastatin, all of the statins undergo extensive metabolism by hepatic P450 enzymes. Elimination half-times are 1 to 4 hours for all the statins except atorvastatin, which has an elimination half-time of 14 hours.

Despite the short elimination half-times, the duration of pharmacodynamic effects is about 24 hours. This is a consideration in the perioperative period when patients may not be able to ingest oral medications. Atorvastatin and fluvastatin undergo minimal renal excretion and probably do not require dosage adjustments in patients with renal insufficiency. Dosages of pravastatin and to a lesser degree lovastatin and simvastatin may need to be adjusted in patients with renal insufficiency. Statins are

Table 23-3

Drugs for Treatment of Hyperlipidemia

	LDL	HDL	Triglycerides
Diet change	↓10%–15%	Variable increase	↓10%–20%
Statins	↓20%–60%	↑10%–15%	↓10%–20%
Bile acid resins	↓15%–30%	↑3%–5%	No change or mild increase
Fibrates	↓5%–20% or increase	↑10%–35%	↓40%–50%
Ezetimibe	↓18%–22%	↑1%–3%	↓8%–12%
Niacin	↓15%–30%	↑20%–30%	↓20%–50%

teratogenic in animals and thus are not recommended for use during pregnancy.[20]

Side Effects

Statins are usually well tolerated with the most common complaints being gastrointestinal upset, fatigue, and headache. In clinical trials, less than 5% of patients treated with statins experienced adverse side effects, similar to the rate in placebo-treated groups. The incidence of side effects in the general population is thought to be higher.

Muscle-Related Adverse Effects

The most common adverse side effects from statins are skeletal muscle related. These can range in severity from simple myalgias to myositis with mild creatine kinase (CK) elevation to life-threatening rhabdomyolysis characterized by a greater than 10-fold elevation in CK. Myositis and rhabdomyolysis are quite rare and in clinical trials occur with similar frequency in placebo-treated groups. Conversely, myalgias are reported in as many as a third of statin-treated patients in clinical practice and more commonly in patients with certain risk factors (Table 23-4). The mechanisms underlying statin-related myotoxicity are incompletely understood. It is possible that by inhibiting HMG-CoA reductase, statins decrease not only cholesterol synthesis but also the formation of ubiquinone (otherwise known as coenzyme Q10), which is important for mitochondrial function and cell membrane integrity.[21] Alternatively, decreased cholesterol levels in skeletal muscle cell membranes may increase membrane fluidity, leading to unstable sarcolemma, myotonic discharges, and, in advanced but rare situations, rhabdomyolysis.[22]

Severe muscle-related adverse events associated with statin use are often secondary to drug interactions with agents that are also metabolized by the hepatocyte cytochrome P450 (CYP) system. Myopathy appears to be most frequent in patients treated with simvastatin and lovastatin, as these are metabolized by CYP3A4 and their concentrations are increased by CYP3A4 inhibitors, including Coumadin, protease inhibitors, macrolide antibiotics, and azole antifungals. Fluvastatin and rosuvastatin are metabolized by CYP2C9 and have the lowest rate of events. Drugs likely to be administered during anesthesia, including succinylcholine, have not been shown to increase the incidence of statin-induced myopathy.[21,23]

Table 23-4

Statin Myotoxicity Risk Factors

1. Age >80 years
2. Female sex
3. Asian ancestry
4. Renal/hepatic failure
5. Excessive alcohol use
6. History of prior muscle disease
7. Poorly controlled hypothyroidism

Hepatic Dysfunction

Persistent increases in plasma aminotransferase concentrations occur in 0.5% to 2% of treated patients and are dose-dependent. Discontinuation of the drug is recommended if plasma aminotransferase concentrations increase to more than three times normal. Progression to hepatic failure is extremely rare.[2]

Bile Acid Resins

Bile acid resins are effective for the treatment of lipid disorders in which the primary abnormality is an increased plasma LDL cholesterol concentration with a normal or near normal triglyceride level. The three drugs in this class, colesevelam, cholestyramine, and colestipol, have a low potential for toxicity and are well tolerated. Both drugs are available only as powders that must be hydrated before ingestion. There is no systemic absorption of these resins. Administered as monotherapy, bile acid–binding resins decrease plasma concentrations of LDL cholesterol by 15% to 30%. Plasma concentrations of triglycerides may increase 5% to 20% in treated patients owing to increased production of VLDLs.

Bile acid resins bind bile in the intestine, interrupting enterohepatic circulation and increasing fecal excretion that increases hepatic bile acid synthesis from cholesterol stores (see Fig. 23-1). This increases the production of hepatic LDL-R and increases the uptake of LDL cholesterol from blood, lowering plasma concentrations of LDL cholesterol. HMG-CoA reductase activity also increases.

Side Effects

Palatability and constipation are common complaints in patients being treated with cholestyramine. A high fluid intake is useful in minimizing constipation. Colesevelam has fewer gastrointestinal side effects and is approved for use in adolescents with familial hypercholesterolemia. There may be transient increases in the plasma concentrations of alkaline phosphatase and transaminases.

Because cholestyramine is a chloride form of an ion exchange resin, hyperchloremic acidosis can occur, especially in younger and smaller patients in whom the relative dose is larger. Absorption of fat-soluble vitamins as well as other pharmacologic agents may be impaired. For this reason, other drugs should be given at least 1 hour before or 4 hours after administration of cholestyramine.

Niacin

Niacin (nicotinic acid) is a water-soluble B complex vitamin that inhibits synthesis of VLDLs in the liver by an unknown mechanism (see Fig. 23-1). In addition, niacin inhibits release of free fatty acids from adipose tissue and increases the activity of lipoprotein lipase. The result of these effects is a dose-related 15% to 30% decrease in plasma LDL cholesterol concentrations, a 20% to 50% decrease in triglycerides, and a 20% to 30% increase in HDL. Niacin does not produce any detectable changes in synthesis of cholesterol nor does it alter excretion of bile acids.[24]

Pharmacokinetics

Niacin is readily absorbed from the gastrointestinal tract and undergoes extensive hepatic first-pass metabolism. The primary route of metabolism is methylation to *N*-methyl-nicotinamide. Niacin also undergoes conjugation with glycine to produce nicotinuric acid. Metabolites undergo renal excretion and at high doses, niacin undergoes renal excretion unchanged.

Side Effects

Niacin, unlike the resins and statins, has many side effects, which may limit its usefulness. The most common side effect is intense prostaglandin-induced cutaneous flushing that occurs in about 10% of patients. Aspirin administered 30 minutes before ingestion of niacin decreases flushing, whereas alcohol ingestion potentiates flushing. Abdominal pain, nausea and vomiting, diarrhea, and malaise are common complaints in treated patients. Hepatic dysfunction manifesting as increased plasma transaminase activity and cholestatic jaundice may be associated with large doses of niacin. Therefore, niacin is not recommended for administration to patients with liver disease. Hyperglycemia and abnormal glucose tolerance may occur in nondiabetic patients treated with niacin. Plasma concentrations of uric acid are increased, increasing the incidence of gouty arthritis. Niacin may exaggerate the orthostatic hypotension associated with antihypertensive drugs and the myopathy associated with statins. Peptic ulcer disease may be reactivated by niacin.

Fibrates

Fibrates are derivatives of fibric acid and are the most effective drugs for decreasing plasma concentrations of triglycerides. In the postoperative period, treatment with fibrates is restarted when the patient is well hydrated and able to ingest oral medications. There are three fibric acid derivatives commonly used for the treatment of hyperlipidemia: gemfibrozil, fenofibrate, and bezafibrate. Clofibrate was the original fibric acid derivative for treatment of increased plasma triglyceride concentrations. This drug is no longer considered the drug of choice, principally because of concern that noncardiovascular adverse events may be increased in treated patients.[25] Fibrates produce a dose-dependent 40% to 50% decrease in plasma triglycerides and 10% to 35% increase in HDL concentrations, whereas the effect on LDL concentrations is variable. Drug-induced increase in the activity of lipoprotein lipase is the likely mechanism for the triglyceride lowering effects of these drugs (see Fig. 23-1). This action of fibrates may reflect activation of specific transcription factors (peroxisome proliferator–activated receptors), which result in upregulation of genes for lipoprotein lipase and fatty acid oxidation. Induction of lipoprotein lipase contributes to lipolysis of triglyceride-rich lipoproteins, VLDL, and chylomicrons. When the LDL concentration increases, it is presumed to reflect improved catabolism of VLDLs and hence increased production of LDLs. Bezafibrate is also thought to improve insulin sensitivity.[26]

Pharmacokinetics

Gemfibrozil is well absorbed from the gastrointestinal tract following oral administration. Metabolism is by oxidation of a methyl group to form a hydroxymethyl and then a carboxyl metabolite. Protein binding is extensive. The elimination half-time of gemfibrozil is approximately 15 hours, with an estimated 70% of a single dose appearing unchanged in the urine. Fenofibrate is a prodrug that is hydrolyzed by esterases to the active metabolite, fenofibric acid. Fenofibric acid is metabolized by conjugation with glucuronic acid that undergoes extensive renal excretion. The elimination half-time of fenofibrate is about 20 hours. Absorption of fenofibrate is increased when the drug is administered with food. Protein binding is approximately 99%. Increased plasma concentrations of liver transaminase enzymes are more likely to occur with fenofibrate than with the other fibrates.

Side Effects

The most common side effects of the fibrates are gastrointestinal (abdominal pain, nausea) and headache. Gemfibrozil increases the cholesterol content of bile (lithogenicity) and may increase the formation of gallstones. The incidence of skeletal muscle myopathy and risk of rhabdomyolysis is increased when this drug is administered in combination with statins, especially lovastatin. The anticoagulant effect of warfarin is potentiated by gemfibrozil, presumably reflecting its displacement from binding sites on albumin. A mild increase in plasma transaminase enzymes may occur in treated patients. Considering the dependence on renal excretion for elimination and occasional increases in liver function tests, it may be prudent to avoid administration of this drug to patients with preexisting renal or hepatic disease. The increase in noncardiovascular mortality observed with clofibrate[25] may be due to low plasma cholesterol concentrations, which predispose patients to hemorrhagic stroke, particularly when systemic hypertension is present.[27] Nevertheless, much of the increased mortality at very low plasma concentrations of cholesterol may be attributable to specific diseases, which decrease cholesterol concentrations.

Ezetimibe

Ezetimibe is a relatively new agent for the treatment of hyperlipidemia that acts as a selective inhibitor of cholesterol absorption, which leads to a secondary upregulation of LDL-R (see Fig. 23-1). Cholesterol absorption is inhibited because of ezetimibe's ability to disrupt a complex between the annexin-2 and cavolin-1 proteins in the brush border of the small intestine. Used as monotherapy, ezetimibe decreases LDL cholesterol levels by 8% to 22% and it can potentiate the effect of statins by an additionl 17%. It modestly influences triglyceride levels and has a negligible effect on HDL cholesterol levels.[24] Clinical trials addressing the efficacy of ezetimibe in improving cardiovascular endpoints have been conflicting, with some showing a decreased risk of atherosclerotic events when used in conjunction with statins, whereas others have had negative results.[28,29]

Omega-3 Fatty Acids (Fish Oil)

One type of fat present in marine fish oils is highly unsaturated omega-3 fatty acid. The primary effect of this fatty acid is to decrease plasma concentrations of triglycerides, whereas the effect on the plasma LDL cholesterol concentrations is variable. It is not clear what dose is necessary to cause desirable effects on the plasma concentrations of triglycerides. Fish oil supplements are not regarded as drugs and thus are not regulated by the U.S. Food and Drug Administration. The long-term safety of taking fish oil capsules is not known, and there is no evidence that fish oil supplementation prevents heart disease.

Experimental and Emerging Agents

Lomitapide is an experimental inhibitor of microsomal triglyceride transfer protein, an intracellular lipid transport protein that is thought to be important for the production of chylomicrons in the intestine and VLDL by hepatocytes. Trials in patients with genetic lipid disorders have shown favorable reductions in LDL and triglycerides. The incidence of gastrointestinal side effects with lomitapide appears to be high, and elevation of liver enzymes has also been observed.

Mipomersen is an antisense oligopeptide that has been recently approved for the treatment of patients with homozygous familial hyperlipidemia. The antisense oligopeptide binds to mRNA molecules for apolipoprotein B-100, an important component of atherogenic lipoproteins. This binding interferes with translation of the mRNA and decreases apolipoprotein B-100 levels. Mipomersen is adminitered via weekly subcutaneous injection and leads to substantial decreases in non–HDL cholesterol and triglycerides. Like lomitapide, mipomersen frequently causes elevations in liver enzymes as well as steatosis.[23]

References

1. Longo DL, Harrison TR. *Harrison's Principles of Internal Medicine.* New York, NY: McGraw-Hill; 2012.
2. Brenner GM, Stevens CW. *Pharmacology.* Philadelphia, PA: Saunders/Elsevier; 2013.
3. Kannel WB, Castelli WP, Gordon T, et al. Serum cholesterol, lipoproteins, and the risk of coronary heart disease. The Framingham study. *Ann Intern Med.* 1971;74(1):1–12.
4. Keys A, Aravanis C, Blackburn H, et al. Probability of middle-aged men developing coronary heart disease in five years. *Circulation.* 1972;45(4):815–828.
5. Gordon T, Castelli WP, Hjortland MC, et al. High density lipoprotein as a protective factor against coronary heart disease. The Framingham study. *Am J Med.* 1977;62(5):707–714.
6. Castelli WP, Garrison RJ, Wilson PW, et al. Incidence of coronary heart disease and lipoprotein cholesterol levels. The Framingham study. *JAMA.* 1986;256(20):2835–2838.
7. Franceschini G. Epidemiologic evidence for high-density lipoprotein cholesterol as a risk factor for coronary artery disease. *Am J Cardiol.* 2001;88(12A):9N–13N.
8. Downs JR, Clearfield M, Weis S, et al. Primary prevention of acute coronary events with lovastatin in men and women with average cholesterol levels: results of AFCAPS/TexCAPS. Air Force/Texas Coronary Atherosclerosis Prevention Study. *JAMA.* 1998;279(20):1615–1622.
9. Mihaylova B, Emberson J, Blackwell L, et al; Cholesterol Treatment Trialists' Collaborators. The effects of lowering LDL cholesterol with statin therapy in people at low risk of vascular disease: meta-analysis of individual data from 27 randomised trials. *Lancet.* 2012;380(9841):581–590.
10. Baigent C, Blackwell L, Emberson J, et al; Cholesterol Treatment Trialists' Collaboration. Efficacy and safety of more intensive lowering of LDL cholesterol: a meta-analysis of data from 170,000 participants in 26 randomised trials. *Lancet.* 2010;376(9753):1670–1681.
11. Stone NJ, Robinson JG, Lichtenstein AH, et al. 2013 ACC/AHA guideline on the treatment of blood cholesterol to reduce atherosclerotic cardiovascular risk in adults: a report of the American College of Cardiology/American Heart Association Task Force on Practice Guidelines. *Circulation.* 2014;63(25, pt B):2889–2934.
12. Pencina MJ, Navar-Boggan AM, D'Agostino RB Sr, et al. Application of new cholesterol guidelines to a population-based sample. *N Engl J Med.* 2014;370(15):1422–1431.
13. Genser B, Marz W. Low density lipoprotein cholesterol, statins and cardiovascular events: a meta-analysis. *Clin Res Cardiol.* 2006; 95(8):393–404.
14. Taylor F, Huffman MD, Macedo AF, et al. Statins for the primary prevention of cardiovascular disease. *Cochrane Database Syst Rev.* 2013;1:CD004816.
15. Schwartz GG, Olsson AG, Ezekowitz MD, et al. Atorvastatin for acute coronary syndromes. *JAMA.* 2001;286(5):533–535.
16. Stenestrand U, Wallentin L. Early statin treatment following acute myocardial infarction and 1-year survival. *JAMA.* 2001;285(4): 430–436.
17. Bavry AA, Mood GR, Kumbhani DJ, et al. Long-term benefit of statin therapy initiated during hospitalization for an acute coronary syndrome: a systematic review of randomized trials. *Am J Cardiovasc Drugs.* 2007;7(2):135–141.
18. Chan WW, Wong GT, Irwin MG. Perioperative statin therapy. *Expert Opin Pharmacother.* 2013;14(7):831–842.
19. Schachter M. Chemical, pharmacokinetic and pharmacodynamic properties of statins: an update. *Fundam Clin Pharmacol.* 2005;19(1): 117–125.

20. Chong PH, Seeger JD, Franklin C, et al. Clinically relevant differences between the statins: implications for therapeutic selection. *Am J Med.* 2001;111(5):390–400.
21. Tompkins R, Schwartzbard A, Gianos E, et al. A current approach to statin intolerance. *Clin Pharmacol Ther.* 2014;96(1):74–80.
22. Graham DJ, Staffa JA, Shatin D, et al. Incidence of hospitalized rhabdomyolysis in patients treated with lipid-lowering drugs. *JAMA.* 2004;292(21):2585–2590.
23. Turan A, Mendoza ML, Gupta S, et al. Consequences of succinylcholine administration to patients using statins. *Anesthesiology.* 2011;115(1):28–35.
24. Gotto AM Jr, Moon JE. Pharmacotherapies for lipid modification: beyond the statins. *Nat Rev Cardiol.* 2013;10(10):560–570.
25. Gould AL, Rossouw JE, Santanello NC, et al. Cholesterol reduction yields clinical benefit. A new look at old data. *Circulation.* 1995;91(8):2274–2282.
26. Tenenbaum A, Fisman EZ. Fibrates are an essential part of modern anti-dyslipidemic arsenal: spotlight on atherogenic dyslipidemia and residual risk reduction. *Cardiovasc Diabetol.* 2012;11:125.
27. Law MR, Thompson SG, Wald NJ, et al. Assessing possible hazards of reducing serum cholesterol. *BMJ.* 1994;308(6925):373–379.
28. Rossebø AB, Pedersen TR, Boman K, et al. Intensive lipid lowering with simvastatin and ezetimibe in aortic stenosis. *N Engl J Med.* 2008;359(13):1343–1356.
29. Baigent C, Landray MJ, Reith C, et al. The effects of lowering LDL cholesterol with simvastatin plus ezetimibe in patients with chronic kidney disease (Study of Heart and Renal Protection): a randomised placebo-controlled trial. *Lancet.* 2011;377(9784):2181–2192.
30. Jackson RL, Morrisett JD, Gotto AM Jr, et al. Lipoprotein structure and metabolism. *Physiol Rev.* 1976;56(2):259–316.
31. Mahley RW, Innerarity TL, Rall SC Jr, et al. Plasma lipoproteins: apolipoprotein structure and function. *J Lipid Res.* 1984;25(12):1277–1294.

CHAPTER 24

Gas Exchange

Peter Slinger

The essentials of anesthesia are: applied physiology, pharmacology, and clinical monitoring with a little bit of internal medicine.
John Sandison, 1980.

Respiratory physiology is difficult; if the answer is simple you don't understand the question.
Peter Slinger, 2013.

During surgery, the anesthesiologist becomes, in part, an applied respiratory physiologist and an understanding of the physiology and pharmacology pertaining to the respiratory system is fundamental to anesthetic management. Understanding gas exchange is particularly challenging because respiratory physiology is not an exact science. Anesthesiologists work mainly with concepts that allow them to treat and predict the alterations in respiration associated with anesthesia and a variety of diseases. However, these concepts are all specific to the context of a patient's gas exchange at a specific time and in a specific situation and often cannot be extrapolated precisely to a situation of altered physiology. As will be discussed, even fundamental basics of respiratory physiology such as ***dead space*** and ***functional residual capacity*** are never absolute values but are dynamic and always changing.

Functional Anatomy

Upper Airway Anatomy and Gas Flow

Oropharynx and Nasopharynx

The air passages extending from the nares and lips through the nasopharynx and oropharynx, through the larynx to the cricoid cartilage make up the functional upper airway. The upper airway serves a host of functions; warming and humidifying passing air, filtering particulate matter, and preventing aspiration.[1]

During normal quiet breathing, air enters via the nose, a chamber separated in the midline along its entire length by a cartilaginous and bony septum. It is bounded laterally by the inferior, middle, and superior turbinates overlying the sinus ostia and inferiorly by the hard and soft palates and joining the nasopharynx posteriorly. The mucosa covering these structures is highly vascular and well innervated, facts that must be appreciated when performing nasopharyngeal intubation with endotracheal tubes, nasogastric sumps or feeding tubes, or fiberoptic bronchoscopes; this tissue is sensitive to even modest stimulation and is easily torn, leading to significant bleeding. The nasal passages represent a significant resistance to airflow, normally double that found in mouth breathing. Hence, normal subjects or patients will revert to mouth breathing during exercise or respiratory failure.

The pharynx is 12- to 15-cm long and is divided into the nasopharynx, the oropharynx, and the laryngopharynx (lying posterior to the larynx). The oropharynx is further subdivided into the velopharynx (posterior to the soft palate) and the retroglossal pharynx (posterior to the base of the tongue)[2] (Fig. 24-1). The supine position, sleep, and general anesthesia may promote obstruction of the oropharynx by the tongue, soft palate, and pharyngeal musculature as their tone decreases.[3] Flexion of the cervical spine generally increases upper airway resistance. During inspiration, a nonsedated spontaneously breathing patient dilates the oropharyngeal pharynx by contracting the genioglossus muscle and elevating the tongue off the pharyngeal wall in a coordinated reflex. This subconscious phasic inspiratory dilation opposes the tendency of

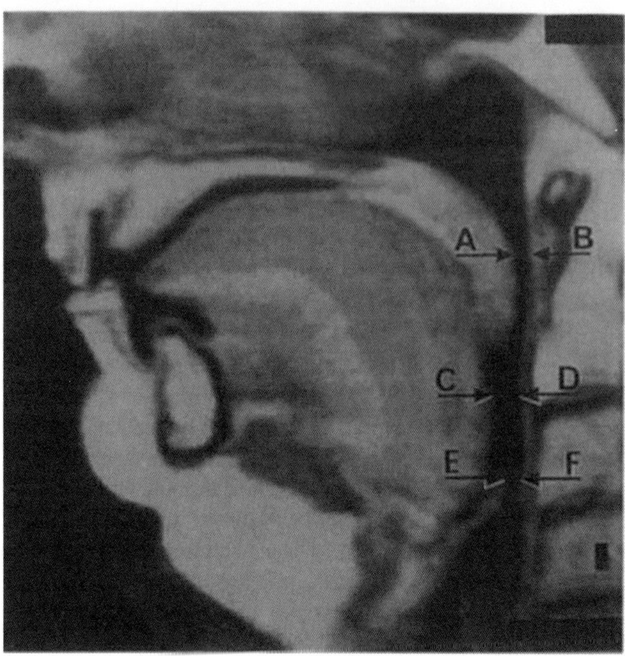

FIGURE 24-1 Sagittal MRI of the upper airway of an awake patient. *A-B* is the junction of nasopharynx with velopharynx, *C-D* is the retroglossal pharynx, *E-F* is the minimum anterior-posterior upper airway diameter at the tip of the epiglottis. The laryngopharynx extends downward from *E-F* to the cricoid cartilage. (From Shorten GD, Opie NJ, Graziotti P, et al. Assessment of the upper airway in awake, sedated and anaesthetized patients using magnetic resonance imaging. *Anaesth Intensive Care.* 1994;22:165–169, with permission.)

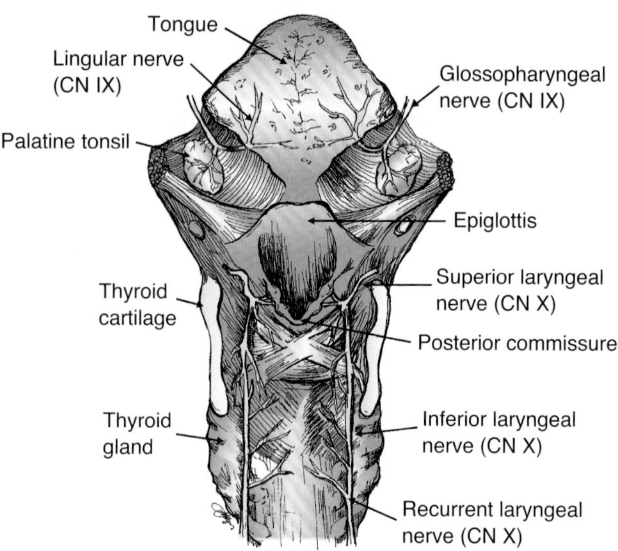

FIGURE 24-2 Diagram of the larynx from the base of the tongue to below the thyroid cartilage as viewed from its posterior aspect. Note the relationship of the superior laryngeal, inferior laryngeal, and recurrent laryngeal nerves and the posterior aspect of the larynx, thyroid, and trachea. Tracheal and thyroid surgery places these nerves at risk. (From Jaeger JM, Blank RS. Essential anatomy and physiology of the respiratory system and pulmonary circulation. In: Slinger P, ed. *Principles and Practice of Anesthesia for Thoracic Surgery.* New York, NY: Springer; 2011:51–69, with permission.)

the upper airway to collapse due to the negative airway pressure generated by the diaphragm during inspiration. Unfortunately, this reflex genioglossus activity is easily abolished by low doses of most anesthetics, with the exception of ketamine.[4]

Larynx

The larynx is a complex structure that lies anterior to the 4th to the 6th cervical vertebra and consists of several muscles, their ligaments, and associated cartilaginous structures (Fig. 24-2). The inlet of the larynx is bordered by the epiglottis, aryepiglottic folds, and the arytenoids. The larynx itself bulges into the pharynx posteriorly creating a deep pharyngeal recess anterolaterally on either side, the pyriform fossae. The pyriform fossae, which lie to each side of midline, are clinically relevant because of their tendency to trap food or foreign objects in the pharynx and as potential sites for the application of topical anesthesia to block the internal branch of the superior laryngeal nerve. The larynx serves as the organ of phonation, plays an important role in coughing, and in protection of the airway from entrainment of solids and liquids during swallowing.[5]

The primary support structure of the larynx is the thyroid cartilage that forms the point of articulation of the paired arytenoid cartilages with the vocal ligaments and their controlling musculature. Other essential structures include the hyoid bone and its attachments, the epiglottis, the cricoid cartilage, and the corniculate cartilages. The hyoid bone is a U-shaped bone that is attached directly to the stylohyoid ligament and muscle, to the mandible and tongue by the hyoglossus, mylohyoid, geniohyoid, and digastric muscles, and to the pharynx by the middle pharyngeal constrictor muscle. Beneath the hyoid bone is the remainder of the larynx suspended by its attachment, the thyrohyoid membrane and muscle. Although its function other than as a flexible anchor is unclear, it is possible to bisect its mandibular attachments ("suprahyoid release") and mobilize the larynx in order to facilitate its caudal displacement in tracheal resection procedures. The epiglottis is the midline elastic cartilage found inferior to the base of the tongue. It is anchored anteriorly to the hyoid bone and inferiorly to the inside of the anterior portion of the thyroid cartilage immediately above the vocal cords. Bilateral folds of the epiglottis curve posteriorly to form a mucosal ridge attached to the arytenoid cartilages sitting on top of the posterior lamina of the cricoid, the aryepiglottic folds. The epiglottis, aryepiglottic folds, and the corniculate tubercles form the inlet into the glottis below. The thyroid cartilage contains the larynx with its paired lamina fused anteriorly at the laryngeal prominence and extending posteriorly to terminate in superior and inferior horns or cornu. The thyroid cartilage serves as a stable point of attachment for numerous small muscles and ligaments which manipulate the vocal cords. The thyroid cartilage also has a mobile, membranous attachment to the cricoid ring.

The paired vocal cords attach posteriorly to the vocal process of each arytenoid and anteriorly meet at the junction of the thyroepiglottic ligament of the anterior portion of the thyroid cartilage. The triangular opening formed by the vocal ligaments is the glottis with its apex anteriorly (Fig. 24-3). The mean length of the relaxed open glottis is approximately 23 mm in males and 17 mm in females. The glottis at its widest (posterior) point is 6 to 9 mm but can be "stretched" to 12 mm.[6] It should be noted that the vocal cords are covered by a thin, adherent mucosa, producing a pearly white appearance. The absence of any submucosa implies that the vocal cords are unlikely to "swell" significantly as there is minimal space to accumulate edema fluid. However, the folds of mucosa and fibrous tissue lying parallel to the true vocal cords just superiorly in the glottis, the vestibular folds or "false vocal cords," can become edematous. The intrinsic laryngeal musculature functions to open the glottis during inspiration; close the glottis and constrict the superior structures during swallowing; and finely control abduction, adduction, and tension of the true vocal cords during phonation.

Pharyngeal Innervation

Innervation of the pharynx is supplied via sensory and motor branches of the glossopharyngeal nerve (CN IX) and vagus nerve (CN X) (external and internal branches of the superior laryngeal nerves, recurrent laryngeal nerves). The sensory innervation of the nasopharynx is derived from the maxillary division of the trigeminal nerve (CN V), whereas the oropharynx is diffusely innervated by sensory branches from the glossopharyngeal nerve (CN IX). The internal branch of the superior laryngeal nerve pierces the lateral aspect of the thyrohyoid membrane along with the superior laryngeal artery and vein to provide sensation for the base of the tongue, vallecula, epiglottis, aryepiglottic folds, pyriform recesses, and the superior aspect of the true vocal cords. The external branch of the superior laryngeal nerve provides motor to the cricothyroid muscle, a tensor of the true vocal cords. The recurrent laryngeal nerves supply sensation to the vocal cords and tracheobronchial tree as well as motor to all the remaining intrinsic musculature of the larynx. The right recurrent laryngeal nerve passes inferior to the right subclavian artery but the left originates at the level of the aortic arch and loops around the ligamentum arteriosum then both nerves ascend cephalad along the tracheoesophageal groove. This anatomy must be appreciated during esophageal and thyroid surgery and during both cervical and anterior mediastinoscopy, as these structures can be at risk. The larynx receives its blood supply from the superior and inferior laryngeal arterial branches of the superior and inferior thyroid arteries, respectively. These arteries follow the course of the superior and recurrent laryngeal nerves.

The major function of the upper airway is to provide a conduit for the initial inhalation then exhalation of gases to and from the lungs while contributing to multiple other functions (e.g., eating, drinking, speaking, etc). With respect to inhalation, the nasopharynx and posterior pharynx warm and humidify the inspired gas. This aids in maintaining core temperature and protects the more delicate epithelia lining the lower airways from desiccation. The airway epithelium secrets mucus, which coats the airway surface and maintains tissue hydration and also serves to trap particulate matter, bacteria, and viruses. Mucus also contains a number of enzymes with antioxidant, antiprotease, and antibacterial properties.[7]

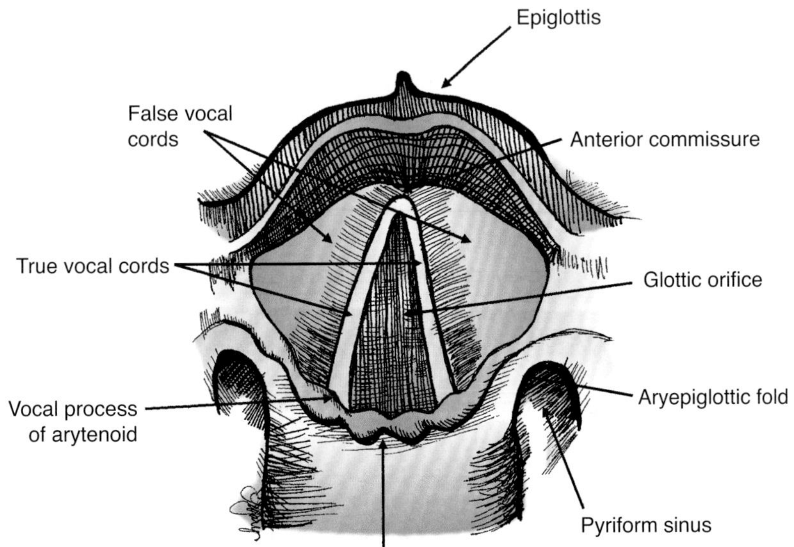

FIGURE 24-3 Diagram of the glottis as seen from above using a laryngoscope or fiberoptic bronchoscope. Note the triangular-shaped glottic introitus with its narrowest aspect at the anterior commissure. Passage of bronchoscopes, endotracheal tubes, and especially, double-lumen tubes should be directed posteriorly where the vocal cords will spread the widest. Note that the vocal process of the arytenoid cartilage pivots on a small point and can be traumatized and displaced with rough handling. (From Jaeger JM, Blank RS. Essential anatomy and physiology of the respiratory system and pulmonary circulation. In: Slinger P, ed. *Principles and Practice of Anesthesia for Thoracic Surgery*. New York, NY: Springer; 2011:51–69, with permission.)

Another important role of the airways and their mucus coat is the filtering of inhaled particulate matter by an elaborate defense system that takes advantage of the air-flow characteristics of the upper and lower airways and their associated epithelium. There are three mechanisms at work to produce mechanical filtering of inspired gases.[1] The first, inertial impaction, is capable of trapping particulates larger than 10 microns by virtue of the turbulent flow across the mucus lining the passageways. It accomplishes this task in minutes with mucus and saliva eventually swallowed. Gas flow slows within the bifurcating and branching tracheobronchial tree until it becomes more laminar. Particulates impact the airway wall according to particle size (sedimentation). Normally, the particles, including bacteria and similar-sized particles, are trapped in the mucus at this level of more proximal airways and are transported cephalad by the constant motion of the cilia, an apical feature of the respiratory epithelium, at a rate of approximately 2.5 mm per minute in the bronchi but over 5 mm per minute in the trachea. Lower airway mucus is usually cleared in about 24 hours although this can be drastically retarded in disease states such as cystic fibrosis or chronic bronchitis or conditions altering ciliary function or growth, such as tobacco smoking.[8] The filtering processes appear effective down to particles approximately 0.01 micron in diameter.

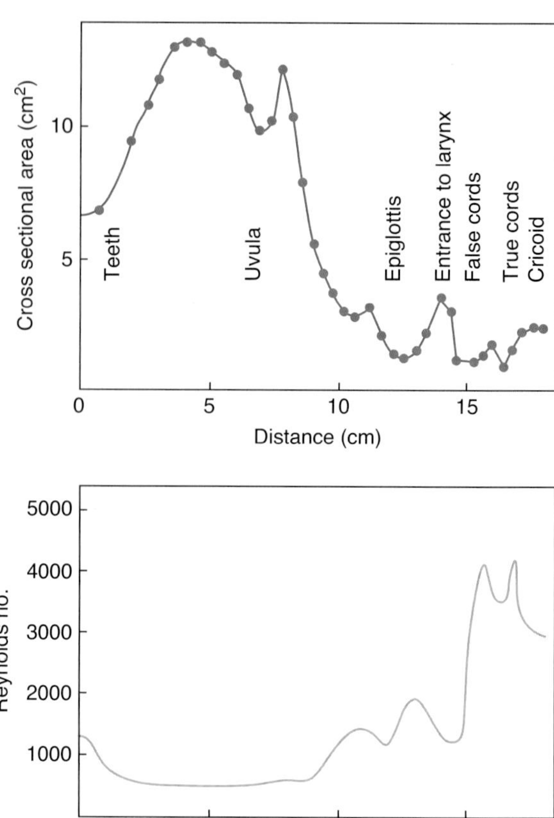

FIGURE 24-4 The cross-sectional area of the upper airway at various levels from the teeth to the cricoid cartilage *(top)* and the corresponding Reynolds numbers at each level *(bottom)* for air during a quiet inspiration (flow = 0.5l sec^{-1}). Flow will be laminar at Reynolds numbers <2,000 and turbulent at numbers >4,000. (From Burwell DR, Jones JG. The airways and anaesthesia. *Anaesthesia.* 1996;51:849–857, with permission.)

Upper Airway Gas Flow

Gas flow is directly proportional to the pressure gradient (ΔP) and inversely proportional to the resistance. When a gas (or liquid) flows through a straight unbranched tube, flow will usually be laminar and resistance is directly proportional to the viscosity of the gas and inversely proportional to the 4th power of the radius.

$$\text{Resistance} = 8 \times \text{length} \times (\text{viscosity}/\pi) \times (\text{radius})^4$$

However, at very high flow rates or when gas flows through an irregular tube or orifice, flow tends to become turbulent and resistance becomes proportional to the density of the gas and inversely proportional to the 5th power of the radius (i.e., changes in airway caliber affect resistance to turbulent flow more than laminar flow). Reynolds number is a dimensionless number that allows estimation of whether a flow is turbulent or laminar.[9]

$$\text{Reynolds number} = \text{velocity} \times \text{diameter} \times \text{density}/\text{viscosity}$$

In the airway, Reynolds numbers for air during quiet breathing are <2,000 throughout most of the upper and lower airway (Fig. 24-4). Reynolds numbers >4,000 are associated with turbulent flow and 2,000 to 4,000 is a mixture of laminar and turbulent flows. Helium is a gas with a low density compared to air or oxygen; however, the viscosity of the three is almost equal. A mixture of 80% helium/20% oxygen has a density approximately 0.33 that of air and 0.30 that of oxygen. In conditions of increased turbulent flow in large airways due to a mass or edema, breathing a mixture of helium and oxygen will decrease dyspnea for some patients (this is also why breathing helium changes phonation so that a person may imitate Donald Duck). This applies only to turbulent flows in large airways. Helium does not relieve dyspnea due to increased distal laminar airflow resistance such as in asthma or chronic obstructive pulmonary disease (COPD).

Tracheal and Bronchial Structure

The trachea originates at the cricoid cartilage (at the level of vertebra C6) and extends approximately 10 to 12 cm (females) and 12 to 14 cm (males) to terminate in a bifurcation (carina) at the T4/5 vertebral level (2nd intercostal space, the angle of Louis) (Fig. 24-5). The trachea is 22 ± 1.5 mm (males) to 19 ± 1.5 mm (females) in diameter and consists of 16 to 20 U-shaped cartilaginous rings that are closed posteriorly by fibrous tissue and a longitudinal smooth muscle band, the trachealis muscle.

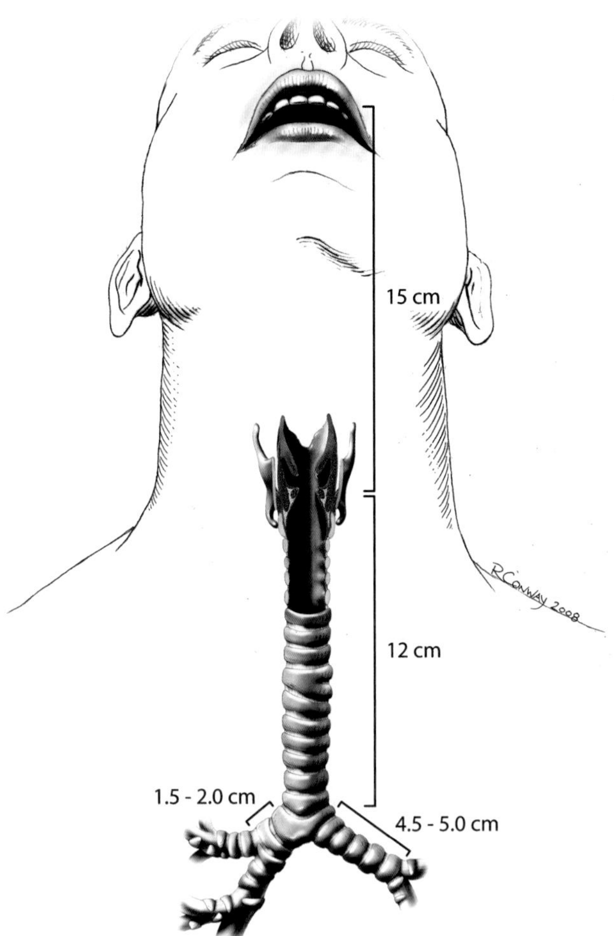

FIGURE 24-5 The average length from the incisors to the vocal cords is approximately 15 cm, and the distance from the vocal cords to the tracheal carina is 12 cm. The average distance from the tracheal carina to the take-off of the right upper bronchus is 2.0 cm in men and 1.5 cm in women. The distance from the tracheal carina to the take-off of the left upper and left lower lobe is approximately 5.0 cm in men and 4.5 cm in women. These anatomic distances apply to individuals with a height of 170 cm. (From Campos J. Lung isolation in patients with difficult airways. In: Slinger P, ed. *Principles and Practice of Anesthesia for Thoracic Surgery.* New York, NY: Springer; 2011:247–258, with permission.)

The right main bronchus is wider (16 vs. 13 mm), shorter (1.5 to 2.5 vs. 4.5 to 5.0 cm) and more vertical than the left. The right main bronchus gives off the upper lobar bronchus then continues as the bronchus intermedius giving off the right middle lobar bronchus and right lower lobar bronchus at the hilum of the lung at T5 (Fig. 24-6). The left main bronchus passes inferiorly and laterally below the aortic arch, anterior to the esophagus and descending thoracic aorta to reach the hilum of the left lung at T6. These dimensions can be quite variable among individuals and chest pathology can drastically change the anatomy.

The lobar bronchi (right upper, right middle, right lower and the left upper, left lower) extend into their segmental bronchi that can be readily visualized during flexible bronchoscopy. The right upper lobe bronchus gives off 3 segmental bronchi (apical, anterior, posterior) (Fig. 24-7), the right middle lobe bronchus splits into 2 segmental bronchi (lateral, medial), and the right lower lobe bronchus divides into a superior segment (directed posteriorly) and a basilar segmental bronchus which divides into 4 segments (medial basal, anterior basal, lateral basal, posterior basal) for a total of 10 segmental branches on the right. The left upper lobar bronchus splits into the superior division with "3" segments (a "fused" apical-posterior and an anterior) and the inferior division or lingual with 2 segments (superior and inferior). The left lower lobe bronchus branches into 4 lower segmental branches (superior, a "fused" anteromedial basal, lateral basal, and posterior basal) for a total of "10" segments on the left. An online interactive bronchoscopy simulator is available to demonstrate this anatomy (Fig. 24-8).

Respiratory Airways and Alveoli

The airways continue to divide into smaller diameter conduits until one arrives at the bronchioles with diameters less than 0.8 mm. At this level, the airways lose all remnants of cartilage and begin the transformation from purely conducting airways to those described as respiratory bronchioles. Respiratory bronchioles eventually divide into the final four generations of alveolar ducts, which then consist primarily of openings into the terminal alveolar sacs. In the descriptive model of Weibel[10] (Fig. 24-9A), the trachea branches into 23 generations of airways. The first 15 generations serve as conducting airways and the subsequent 8 generations become sufficiently thin-walled to allow some degree of gas exchange and are called ***acinar*** airways. One clinical aspect of this geometric progression of increasingly narrower airways (and blood vessels) by divergence and multiplication is that the overall cross-sectional area and therefore resistance to gas flow (or blood flow) becomes markedly less compared to the resistance of the proximal airway (or blood vessel) (Fig. 24-9B). This has an important impact on distribution of gas and blood flow, flow velocity, and, hence, transit time through key areas of gas exchange.

The interior of the trachea is lined with ciliated columnar epithelium, goblet cells (responsible for mucus production) (Fig 24-10), and with interspersed specialized chemical and tactile neuroreceptors. The lining of the airways transitions from pseudostratified columnar epithelia in the larger bronchi to a thinner cuboidal ciliated variety in the small bronchi. The airway epithelium and submucosa also contain lymphocytes, mast cells, and a variety of neuroendocrine cell types. The next layer consists of circumferential bands of smooth muscle cells and a connective tissue layer containing submucosal glands and plates of cartilage (replacing the solid cartilage rings in the very large airways) (Fig. 24-11). The outermost layer is a loose adventitial shell with lymphatic vessels,

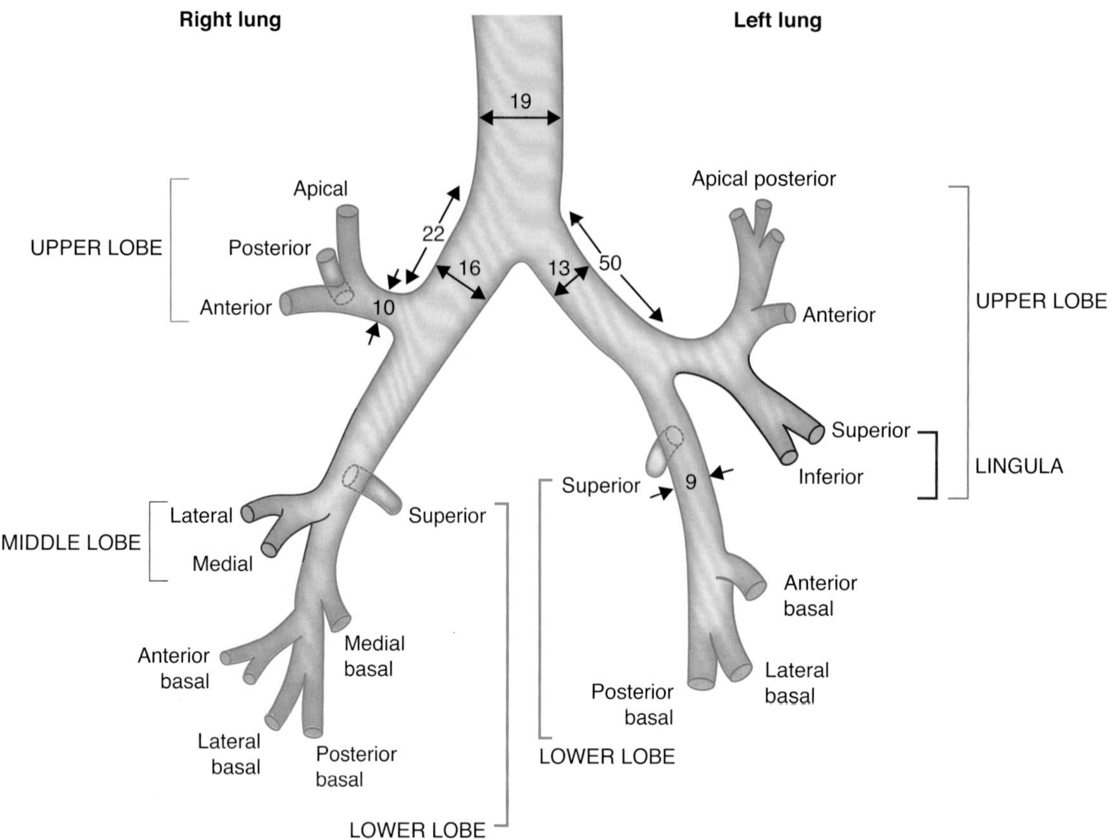

FIGURE 24-6 Diagram of the trachea, lobar, and segmental bronchi showing median lengths and diameters for a 170 cm height patient. The lengths and diameters of the bronchi vary considerably between individuals.

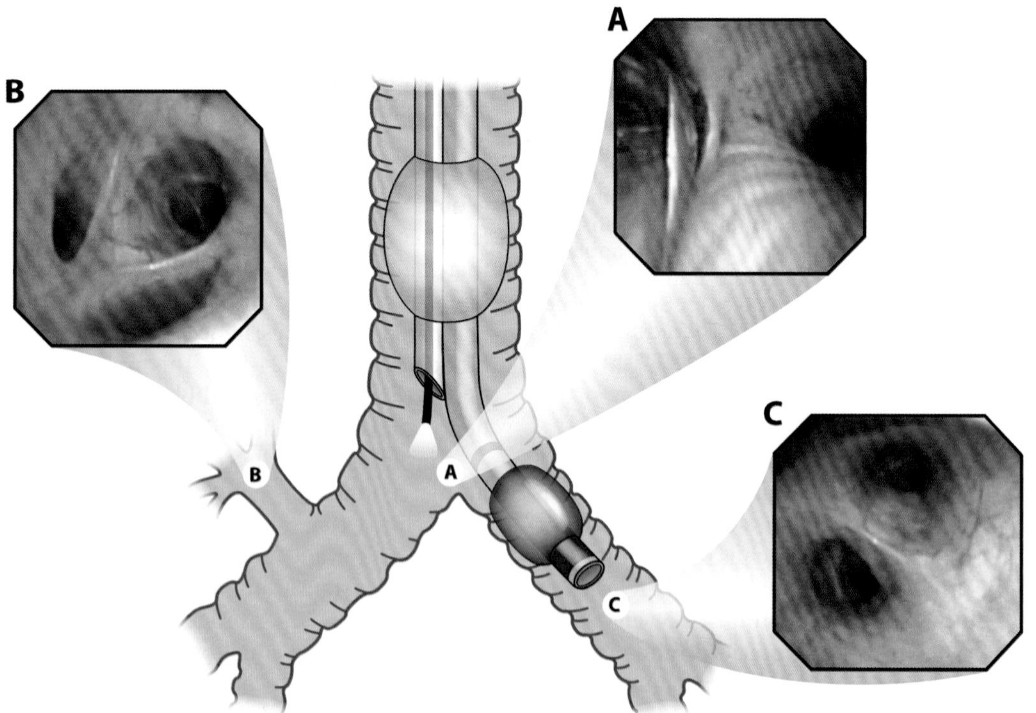

FIGURE 24-7 Bronchial anatomy as seen through a fiberoptic bronchoscope via a properly positioned left-sided double-lumen tube. *(A)* A view of the tracheal carina showing the orifice of the right mainstem bronchus and the bronchial lumen of the double-lumen tube in the left main bronchus. *(B)* The right upper bronchus showing the three segments (this trifurcation is unique in the bronchial tree and a useful landmark). *(C)* A view of the left mainstem bronchus showing the left upper *(top)* and lower *(bottom)* lobe bronchi. (From Campos J. Lung isolation in patients with difficult airways. In: Slinger P, ed. *Principles and Practice of Anesthesia for Thoracic Surgery*. New York, NY: Springer; 2011:227–246, with permission.)

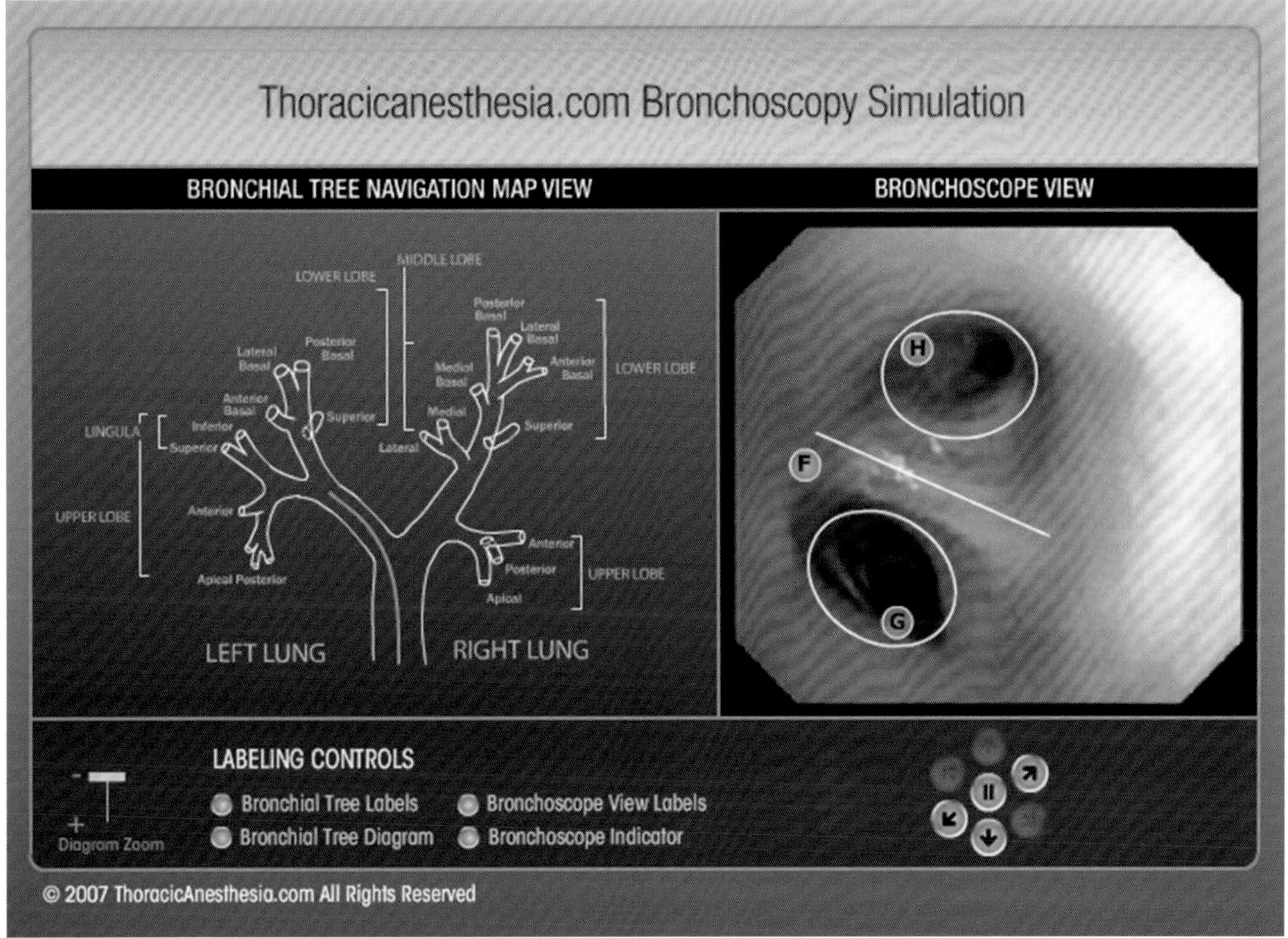

FIGURE 24-8 The free online bronchoscopy simulator at www.thoracicanesthesia.com. The user can navigate the tracheobronchial tree using real-time video by clicking on the lighted directional arrows under the "Bronchoscopic view" *(right)*. Clicking on the labels on the "Bronchoscopic view" gives details of the anatomy seen. The process is aided by the "Bronchial Tree Navigational Map View" *(left)*, which shows the simultaneous location of the bronchoscope as the *orange line* in the airway.

sympathetic and parasympathetic nerves, and nourishing blood vessels.

The respiratory bronchioles terminate in a pulmonary acinus, which has the appearance of a cluster of grapes on a network of stems. Each acinus may contain multiple alveolar ducts communicating with 2,000 alveoli arranged in a ring-like, honeycomb network. The alveolus is considered the primary site of gas exchange between the blood and gas in the lung. The alveolar septa are about 5 to 8 microns thick and are opposed by an alveolar surface on either side with the alveolar capillary bed sandwiched inside. The walls of the alveoli are extremely thin, between 0.1 and 0.2 microns, a feature that promotes rapid equilibration of gas by diffusion with the pulmonary capillary blood. In addition, gas can exchange between alveoli through pores of Kohn. There are approximately 300 million alveoli in the human lung, which provides an extraordinary surface area for gas exchange (e.g., 70 m^2).

There are three major cell types found in the alveolus: alveolar type I cells, alveolar type II cells, and alveolar macrophages. However, there are other cell types found under certain conditions in the lung (e.g., inflammation). Alveolar type I cells are squamous epithelial cells that cover most of the alveolar surface. These nucleated cells have few cytoplasmic organelles and a sparse cytoplasm splayed out in sheets over the alveolar surface forming a thin barrier between the air space and the pulmonary capillary endothelium. Alveolar type II cells are fewer in number, somewhat spherical, and coated on their apical surface with microvilli. In contrast to type I cells, alveolar type II cells possess many organelles including multilayered granular structures called ***lamellar bodies*** (Fig. 24-12). These lamellar bodies are the source of pulmonary surfactant, a lipoprotein coating the interior surface of the alveolus and capable of significantly reducing the surface tension of the alveolus air-surface interface. Surface tension reduction is considered an important physical mechanism to reduce any tendency for alveolar collapse at very low lung volumes.

The immune defenses of the lung are extremely important because of the direct exposure of this organ to the external environment via the airways. There are a

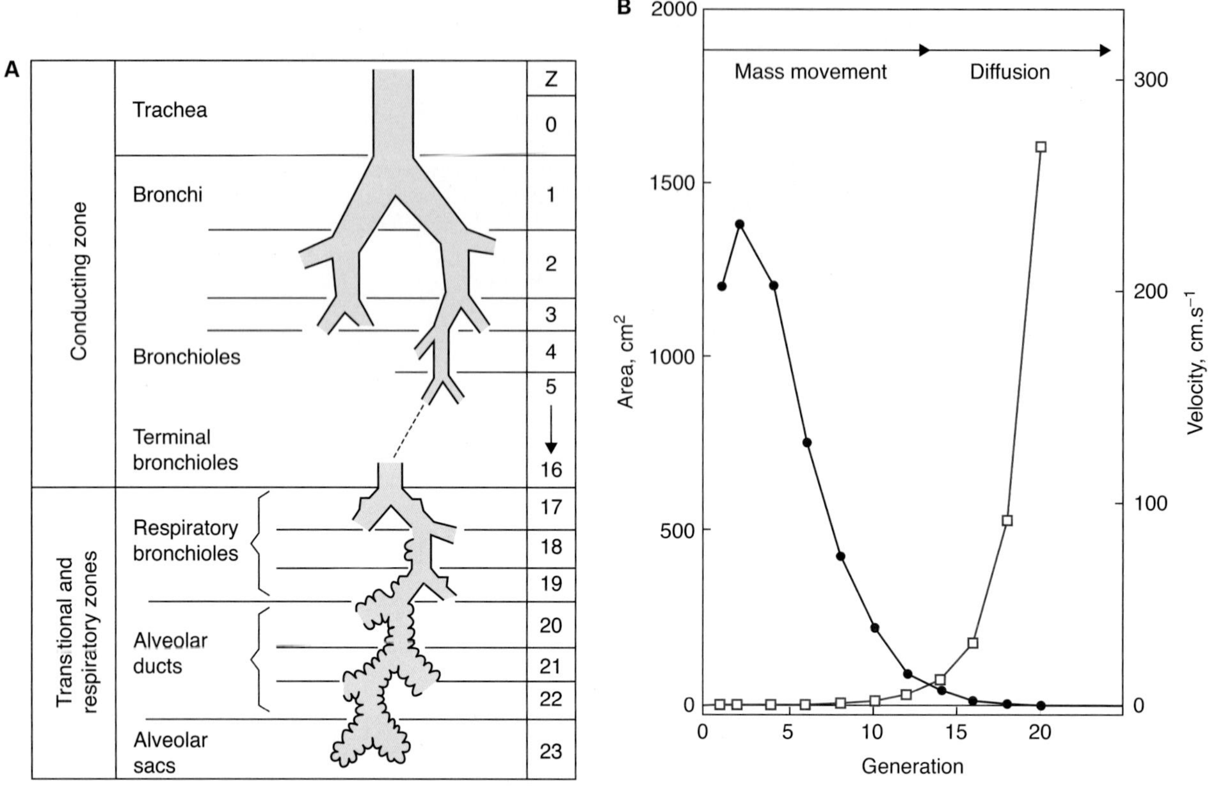

FIGURE 24-9 **A:** The symmetrical branching model of the tracheobronchial tree. **B:** The change in cross-sectional area *(open squares)* and gas velocities *(closed circles)* seen with normal quiet breathing. Mass movement of gas predominates down to the 14th/15th generation of bronchi below which diffusion becomes the predominant method of gas exchange. The airway dead space is the volume of the airways through which mass movement predominates. (From Burwell DR, Jones JG. The airways and anaesthesia. *Anaesthesia.* 1996:51:849–857, with permission.)

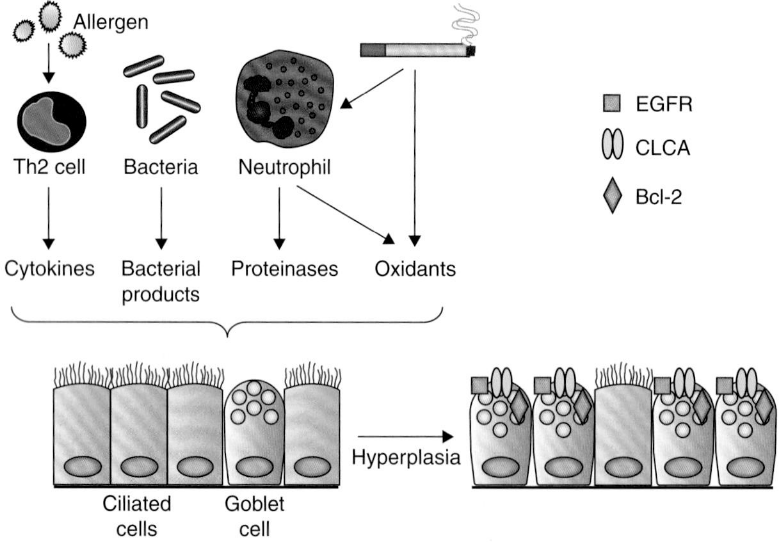

FIGURE 24-10 Normal respiratory epithelium *(bottom left)* has a predominance of ciliated to goblet cells. Goblet cell hyperplasia *(lower right)* occurs in response to chronic inflammatory stimuli *(upper left)*, which upregulate mucin production and/or induce goblet cell hyperplasia with associated increases in expression of epidermal growth factor receptors (EGFR), calcium-activated chloride channels (CLCA) and the antiapoptotic factor Bcl-2. (Modified from Yeazell L, Littlewood K. Nonrespiratory functions of the lung. In: Slinger P, ed. *Principles and Practice of Anesthesia for Thoracic Surgery.* New York, NY: Springer; 2011:103–119, with permission.)

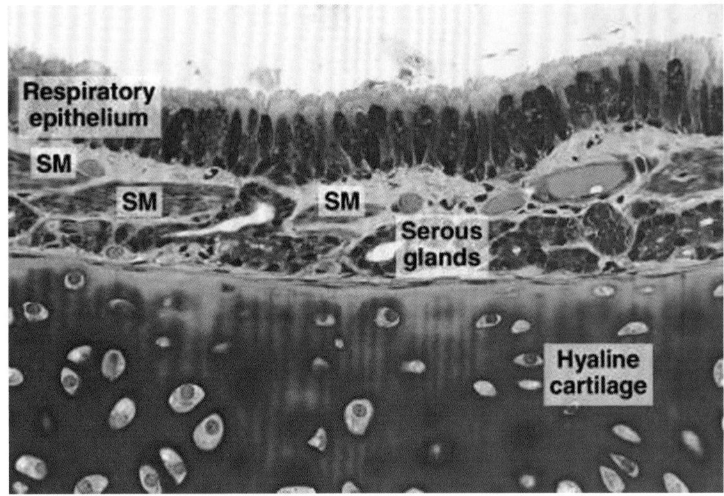

FIGURE 24-11 Microphotograph of a histologic section of the wall of an intrapulmonary bronchus. The mucosa, as in the trachea and extrapulmonary bronchi, consists of an epithelium (ciliated pseudostratified columnar with goblet cells), a basement membrane, and a lamina propria. The latter is rich in elastic fibers of the recoil mechanism. Unlike more proximal air passages, a muscularis is present and lies just external to the lamina propria. It is composed of two sets of smooth muscle (SM) fibers, which extend down the bronchial tree in a right and left spiral. The submucosa is a layer of loose connective tissue, which lies outside the muscularis. Bronchial glands are present in this layer and also extend into the intercartilaginous intervals. The cartilage-fibrous layer lies outside the submucosa. It contains discontinuous plates of hyaline cartilage and fibrous connective tissue. (From Junquiera LC, Carniero J. *Basic Histology Text and Atlas.* 10th ed. New York, NY: McGraw-Hill; 2003, with permission.)

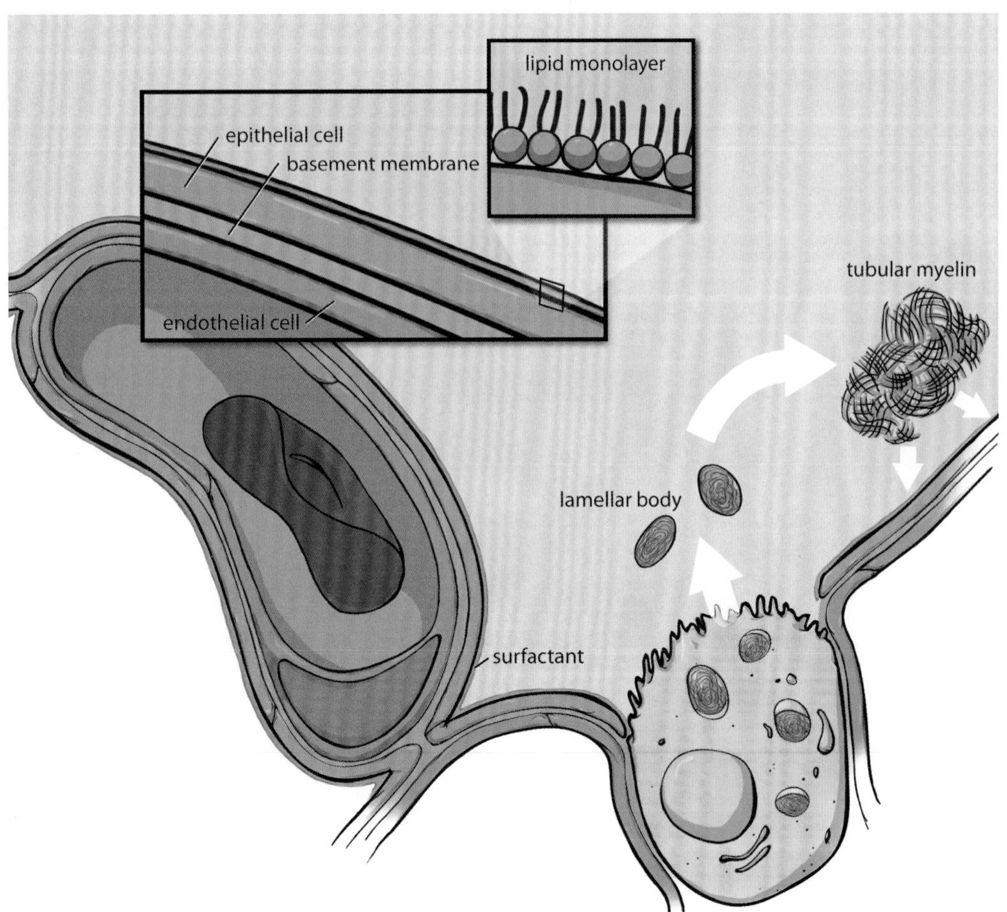

FIGURE 24-12 The diagram presents a scheme of the alveolar air-blood barrier, which consists of endothelial cells, epithelial cells (type I pneumocytes), and their common basement membrane. The large cuboidal cell *(bottom right)* is a type II pneumocyte producing surfactant, contained within its cytoplasm as lamellar bodies (onion-like structures), which are exocytosed into the alveolar lumen, then transform into tubular myelin and finally form surfactant (lipid monolayer) covering the surface of type I pneumocytes. The *upper left-hand side inset* shows details of the thin alveolar-capillary membrane, the *right-hand side inset* shows a scheme of the surfactant monolayer. (Modified from Wasowicz M. Anesthesia for combined cardiac and thoracic procedures. In: Slinger P, ed. *Principles and Practice of Anesthesia for Thoracic Surgery.* New York, NY: Springer; 2011:453–464, with permission.)

number of excellent reviews of the immune function of the lung but it is important to realize that there are many questions unanswered about how the lung responds to invasion and inflammation. Yet from a clinical standpoint, the pulmonary inflammatory response will greatly influence the perioperative management of the surgical patient. A few major defensive cell types residing in the alveolar spaces and interstitium are worth mentioning. Alveolar macrophages are derived from bone marrow monoblast precursor cells and migrate to the lung parenchyma (Fig. 24-13).[11] Alveolar macrophages are free to move over the surface of the alveolus and phagocytize foreign material that enters the alveolus including bacteria and particulates. Macrophages are cleared either through the lymphatics or are carried up and expelled via the airways. Lymphocytes, largely T lymphocytes, are widely distributed in the normal lung within paratracheal and hilar lymph nodes, in the interstitium of the bronchial tree as nodules or individual cells and in the alveolar walls. They play a critical role in the lung's primary immune response to inhaled antigens. Under some pathologic conditions in the lung, it is becoming apparent that an exaggerated inflammatory response and the activity of these cells and others may be harmful to the lung; the acute respiratory distress syndrome (ARDS) and emphysema are examples.

Pulmonary Circulation

Although the blood flow through the pulmonary circulation is normally equal to the blood flow though the sys-

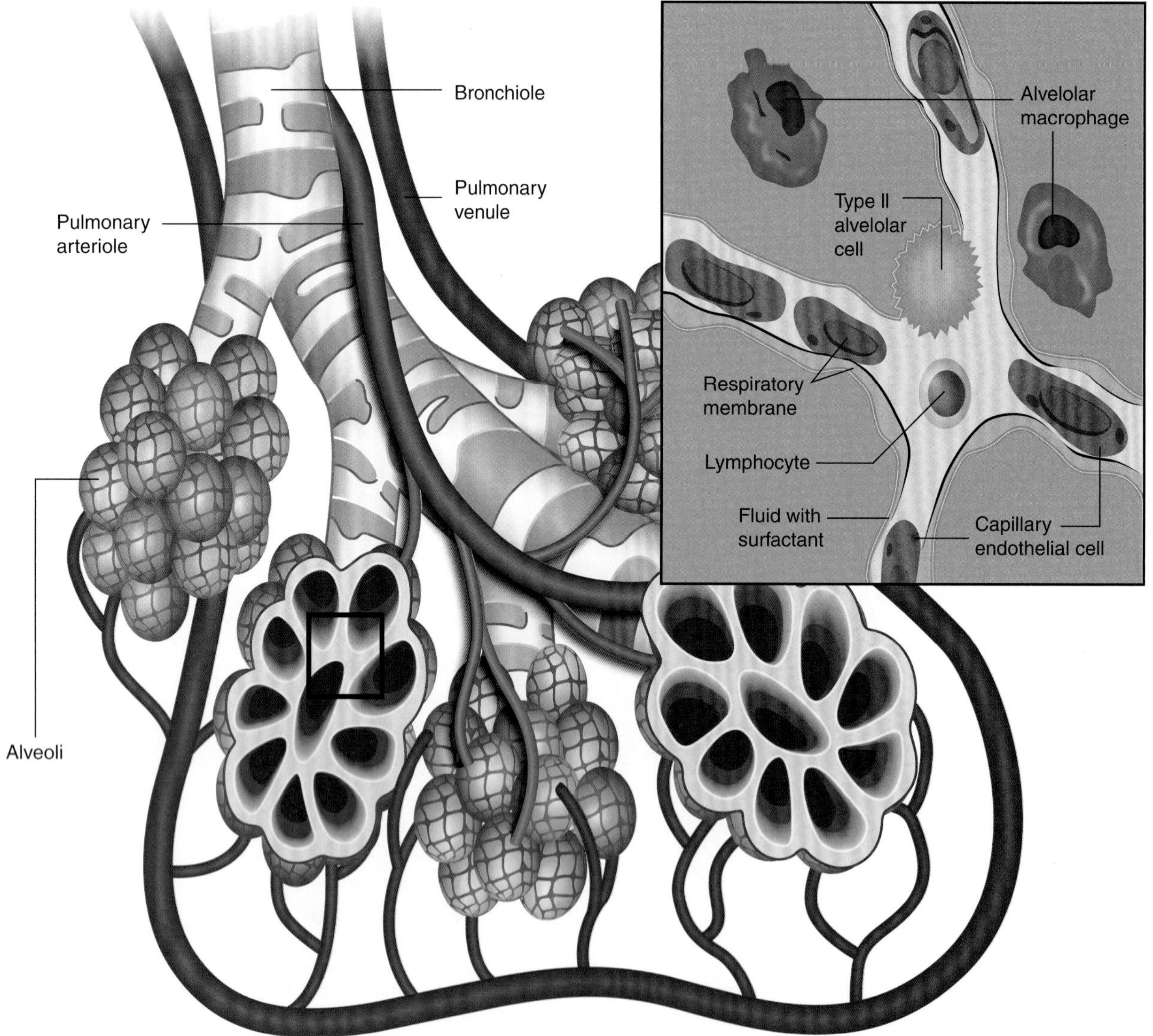

FIGURE 24-13 Diagram of a normal acinus of the lung showing the pulmonary capillaries. In the enlargement *(upper right)* the macrophages move freely into and out of the alveoli; however, the lymphocytes normally remain within the pulmonary capillaries. (From Duggan M, Kavanagh B. Pulmonary atelectasis. *Anesthesiology*. 2005;102:838–854, with permission.)

temic circulation (a major exception being intracardiac shunting when it exceeds systemic circulation), the pressures in the pulmonary circulation are normally lower than the systemic circulation because the pulmonary vascular resistance (PVR) is lower than the systemic resistance (approximately one-sixth of systemic resistance). This is because the pulmonary vessel walls contain less elastic and muscular tissue than systemic vessels of corresponding caliber. Pulmonary arterioles contract rapidly in response to hypoxemia in the alveolus and to a lesser extent to hypoxemia in mixed venous blood. This hypoxic pulmonary vasoconstriction (HPV) is unique to the pulmonary circulation (systemic arterioles dilate in response to hypoxia) and permits regional matching of perfusion to ventilation.

Like all endothelium, the vascular luminal wall of the pulmonary capillaries is lined by glycocalyx, a microcilial layer that acts as a molecular sieve.[12] This 0.1-micron layer prevents adhesion of platelets and leukocytes and is thought to trap larger molecules close to the endothelial membrane and locally increase the oncotic pressure. The glycocalyx covers the pores between endothelial cells and acts as a molecular sieve to control fluid flux. A healthy glycocalyx is important to prevent edema formation in the lung. However, the glycocalyx is damaged by inflammation and ischemia-reperfusion and this may contribute to the increased flux of fluid into the pulmonary extracellular matrix in these conditions.

The air passages receive their blood supply from systemic bronchial arteries down to the level of the respiratory bronchioles. Only one-third of the bronchial circulation returns to the systemic venous system, the remainder drains into the pulmonary veins and this constitutes the largest portion of the normal extrapulmonary venoarterial shunt. This bronchial shunt is less than 1% of the cardiac output in healthy individuals but may increase to 10% in bronchiectasis, emphysema, and some congenital cardiac conditions.

Thorax and Muscles of Respiration

The lungs are contained within the thorax. The bony thorax is composed of the 12 ribs, the sternum anteriorly and the thoracic vertebral column posteriorly. The caudal end of the thorax is formed by the diaphragm and the cranial end of the thorax is the thoracic inlet, within the ring formed by the first ribs, containing the trachea, esophagus, and the neurovascular supply to the head and arms. Bulk movement of air into and out of the lungs occurs as a result of changes in intrathoracic pressure created by rhythmic changes in the volume of the thorax. Expansion of the chest cavity occurs when three respiratory muscle groups work in concert. The diaphragm, intercostal muscles, and the accessory muscles (sternocleidomastoids, scalenes) are controlled by the respiratory centers of the brain to contract in a rhythmic pattern designed to match ventilation to gas exchange requirements. The abdominal musculature (rectus abdominis, external oblique, internal oblique, and transversus abdominis) can be recruited when more force is required for exhalation, although abdominal muscle tone may stabilize the rib cage during inspiration as well.[1]

Inspiration

The diaphragm is unique in that its muscle fibers radiate from a central tendinous structure to insert peripherally on the ventrolateral aspect of the first three lumbar vertebrae, the aponeurotic arcuate ligaments, the xiphoid process and the upper margins of the lower six ribs. Its motor innervation is solely from the right and left phrenic nerves, which originate from the 3rd, 4th, and 5th cervical spinal nerves. In the relaxed state, it forms a pronounced "dome" that closely apposes the chest wall for some distance before arching across. Contraction of the diaphragm causes a large caudal displacement of the central tendon resulting in a longitudinal expansion of the chest cavity. Simultaneously, its insertions on the costal margins cause the lower ribs to rise and the chest to widen. This diaphragmatic motion is responsible for the majority of quiet respiration. As the dome descends, it displaces the abdominal contents caudally. The fall in pleural pressure and accompanying lung expansion produce an increase in abdominal pressure and outward movement of the abdominal wall. The supine and Trendelenburg positions or surgical retractors can significantly interfere with this abdominal motion especially in the morbidly obese, necessitating controlled ventilation under anesthesia.

The intercostal muscles are thin sheet-like muscles with origins and insertions between the ribs. The internal intercostal muscles have their fibers oriented obliquely, caudally, and dorsally, from the rib above to the rib below. The external intercostal muscles have their fibers oriented obliquely, caudally, and ventrally, from the rib above to the rib below. All intercostals are innervated by the intercostal nerves running in the neurovascular bundle under the inferior lip of each rib. The contraction of the external intercostal muscles produces an inspiratory action by elevating the upper ribs to increase the anteroposterior dimensions of the chest in a "bucket-handle" motion. The lower ribs are also elevated by virtue of the force applied and their point of rotation to increase the transverse diameter of the thorax. The internal intercostals apply their force in such a direction as to rotate the ribs downward, decreasing the thoracic anteroposterior dimension to aid in active expiration (when required) and cough. In general, the intercostal muscles do not play a major role in quiet respiration but do in exercise or other conditions requiring high levels of ventilation.

The principal accessory respiratory muscles are the sternocleidomastoid and scalene muscles. The scalene muscles originate from the transverse processes of the 4th through the 8th cervical vertebrae and slope caudally to insert on the first two ribs. Their contraction during periods of high ventilatory demand, elevates and fixes the cephalad rib cage during inspiration. Similarly, the sternocleidomastoid muscles elevate the sternum and increase the longitudinal dimensions of the thorax.

Expiration

Expiration is a passive process in quiet breathing and is largely the response to relaxation of the inspiratory muscles and the balance of forces generated by the elastic recoil of the lungs and chest wall. When high levels of ventilation are required as in exercise or if airway resistance increases (as in exacerbations of asthma or COPD), the expiratory phase becomes an active process with forceful contraction of the rectus abdominis, the transverse abdominis, and the internal and external oblique muscles. The contraction of the abdominal musculature retracts the abdominal wall and pulls the lower ribs downward, which increases intraabdominal pressure and accelerates the cephalad displacement of the diaphragm during exhalation. The internal intercostal muscles depress the rib cage and provide a minor contribution to forced expiration. Innervation of the abdominal musculature is from thoracic nerves 7 through 12 and the 1st lumbar nerve.

Like most skeletal muscles, the diaphragm and intercostal muscles contain a heterogeneous mix of fiber types. The diaphragm has between 49% and 55% type I (slow-oxidative) fibers, the reminder a mix of the "faster high activity" types IIA and IIB fibers.[13] The types of skeletal muscle fibers are distributed fairly evenly throughout the diaphragm. Of note, the respiratory muscles retain the ability to adapt to stress and training. This includes responses to lung pathology which might seem maladaptive. Emphysema is a good example. The diaphragm undergoes changes at the sarcomere level, physically "losing" contractile units as hyperinflation of the lungs leads to increasing thoracic dimensions and "flattening" of the diaphragm.[14] Loss of sarcomeres in series with the central tendon may help to restore the mechanical advantage of the optimal length-tension relationship for the muscle.

Respiratory Mechanical Function

The basics of mechanical function of the respiratory system are the interaction of two opposing springs: the chest wall, which at rest is trying to expand, and the lungs, which at rest are trying to contract. (Fig. 24-14) The lungs and chest wall move together as a unit. This is made possible by the enclosed, air-tight thoracic cavity where the outer surface of the lungs and its visceral pleura are in close proximity to the parietal pleura covering the inner surface of the chest wall and the mediastinal structures. Changes in the intrathoracic volume are only possible because the inside of the lung is in continuity with the ambient atmosphere outside the thorax via the trachea and pharynx. The intimate contact between the layers of pleura is maintained by a negative intrapleural pressure generated in part by the intermolecular forces of the pleural fluid excluding gas from this space. This lubricating fluid allows freedom of the pleural layers to slide over one another but highly resists separation of the layers much like two panes of glass with a thin layer of water between them.

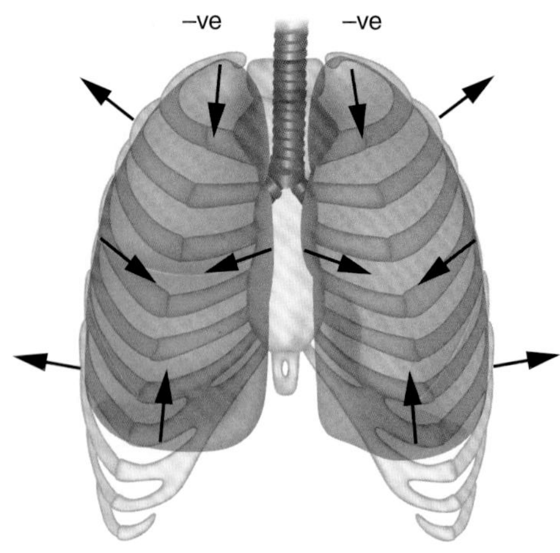

FIGURE 24-14 The respiratory system is at an elastic equilibrium at rest at functional residual capacity. The outward recoil of the chest wall is balanced by the inward recoil of the lungs. The opposing forces generate the negative intrathoracic pressure (mean approximately −5 cm H_2O) with a superior-inferior gradient due to gravitational effects on the lung parenchyma.

Normally, the intrapleural pressure is about −5 cm H_2O when the respiratory system is at equilibrium. Because of the deforming effect of gravity on the lung parenchyma, there is a vertical gradient of intrapleural pressure. This gradient is largest in the seated or upright position (Fig. 24-15). The volume of gas contained in the lungs at this resting point is termed ***functional residual capacity*** (FRC). For a healthy young adult male, total lung capacity (TLC) will be approximately 6 to 6.5 L and FRC will be 2.5 to 3 L. The oxygen contained in the FRC (500 to 600 mL) is the only reservoir of oxygen in the body.

Pathologic conditions such as the introduction of air or blood into the intrapleural space can rapidly disrupt this lung–chest wall interaction, leading to a compromise in respiratory function but also interfere with cardiovascular function. Examples of disruption of the intrapleural space would be a pneumothorax, empyema, pleural effusion, or bronchopleural fistula.

Lung Volumes and Spirometry

By convention, the static and dynamic subdivisions of gas contained within the lung are given a common nomenclature of volumes and capacities (Table 24-1 and Fig. 24-16). Volumes are most commonly measured by spirometry (Figs. 24-17 and 24-18) and capacities are then calculated as the sum of specific volumes. Simple spirometry can

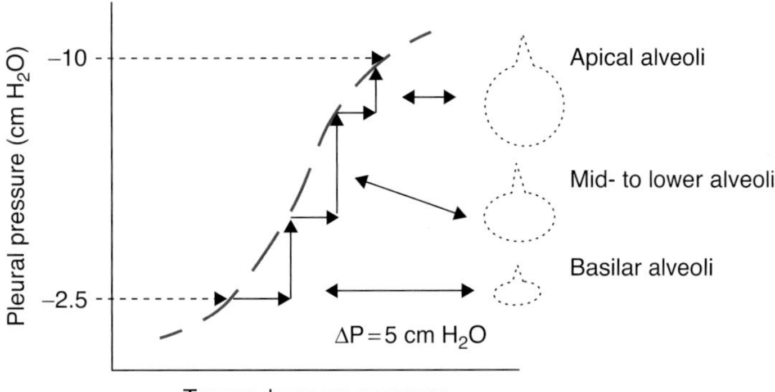

FIGURE 24-15 The static relationship between the transpulmonary pressure (alveolar pressure – pleural pressure) and the pressure in the pleural space results is a sigmoid curve of respiratory compliance. Pleural pressure is normally negative relative to atmospheric pressure. In the seated or upright position, the gradient is small at the base of the lung (intrapleural pressure [P_{PL}] least negative) but larger at the apex (P_{PL} most negative) because of the deforming effect of gravity on the lung parenchyma. This disparity results in larger alveoli at the apex then the dependent alveoli at the base. As a result of this sigmoid relationship, a given change in transpulmonary pressure produces the largest change in volume (and pleural pressure) where the alveoli are on the steepest portion of this curve (mid- to lower alveoli). (From Jaeger JM. Blank RS. Essential anatomy and physiology of the respiratory system and pulmonary circulation. In: Slinger P, ed. *Principles and Practice of Anesthesia for Thoracic Surgery.* New York, NY: Springer; 2011:51–69, with permission.)

Table 24-1

Lung Volumes and Capacities

Lung Volumes	Definition
Tidal volume (V_T)	Air volume inspired and expired during a relaxed breathing cycle
Residual volume (RV)	Volume remaining in the lung after a maximal expiratory effort
Expiratory reserve volume (ERV)	The volume of air that can be forcibly exhaled between the resting end-expiratory volume and RV
Inspiratory reserve volume (IRV)	The volume of air that can be inspired with maximal effort above the normal resting end-expiratory position of a V_T
Forced expiratory volume in 1 second (FEV_1)	The volume of air that can be exhaled in 1 second with maximal effort from the point of maximal inspiration
Lung Capacities	
Vital capacity (VC)	The amount of air that can be exhaled from the point of maximal inspiration to the point of maximal expiration (IRV + ERV)
Forced vital capacity (FVC)	The volume of air that can exhaled with maximal effort from TLC
Total lung capacity (TLC)	Total volume of air in the lungs after a maximal inspiration (IRV + ERV + RV)
Functional residual capacity (FRC)	Amount of air in the lung at the end of a quiet exhalation (ERV + RV)

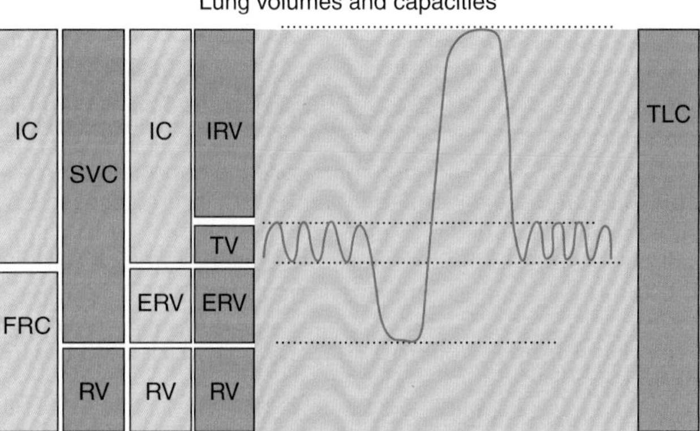

FIGURE 24-16 Complete pulmonary function testing will provide data on lung volumes and capacities to differentiate obstructive from restrictive lung diseases. IC, inspiratory capacity; RV, residual volume; SVC, slow vital capacity; ERV, expiratory reserve volume; TV, tidal volume; IRV, inspiratory reserve volume; TLC, total lung capacity. Functional residual capacity (FRC) = ERV + RV. Measuring closing volume and closing capacity requires insoluble gas washout techniques and is not included in routine pulmonary function testing. However, an appreciation of the variable relationship between closing capacity and FRC and the effects of anesthesia on FRC is essential for the anesthesiologist to understand the changes in gas exchange that occur during anesthesia. (From Slinger P, Darling G. Preanesthetic assessment for thoracic surgery. In: Slinger P, ed. *Principles and Practice of Anesthesia for Thoracic Surgery.* New York, NY: Springer; 2011:11–34, with permission.)

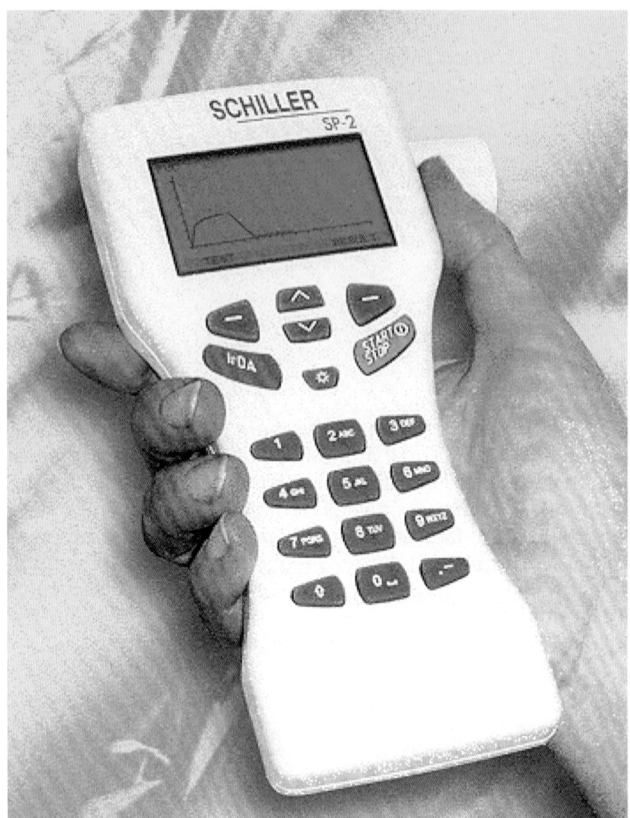

FIGURE 24-17 An example of a portable handheld spirometer that can be easily used in the preoperative assessment clinic or at the bedside to measure the majority of the clinically important lung volumes and capacities. (From Slinger P, Darling G. Preanesthetic assessment for thoracic surgery. In: Slinger P, ed. *Principles and Practice of Anesthesia for Thoracic Surgery*. New York, NY: Springer; 2011:11–34, with permission.)

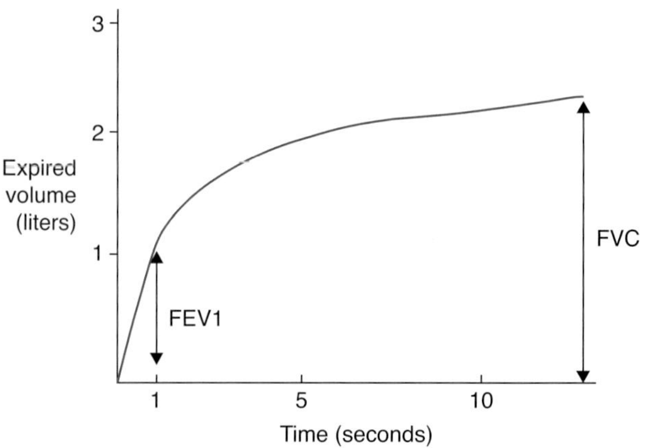

FIGURE 24-18 A simple spirogram. Expired volume is plotted against time. The total volume exhaled during a forced expiration from total lung capacity is the forced vital capacity (FVC). The fraction of the FVC that is exhaled in the first second is the forced expiratory volume in 1 second (FEV_1). These values are compared to normal data for age, sex, and height and given a percentage of predicted value (e.g., FEV_1%). (From Slinger P, Darling G. Preanesthetic assessment for thoracic surgery. In: Slinger P, ed. *Principles and Practice of Anesthesia for Thoracic Surgery*. New York, NY: Springer; 2011:11–34, with permission.)

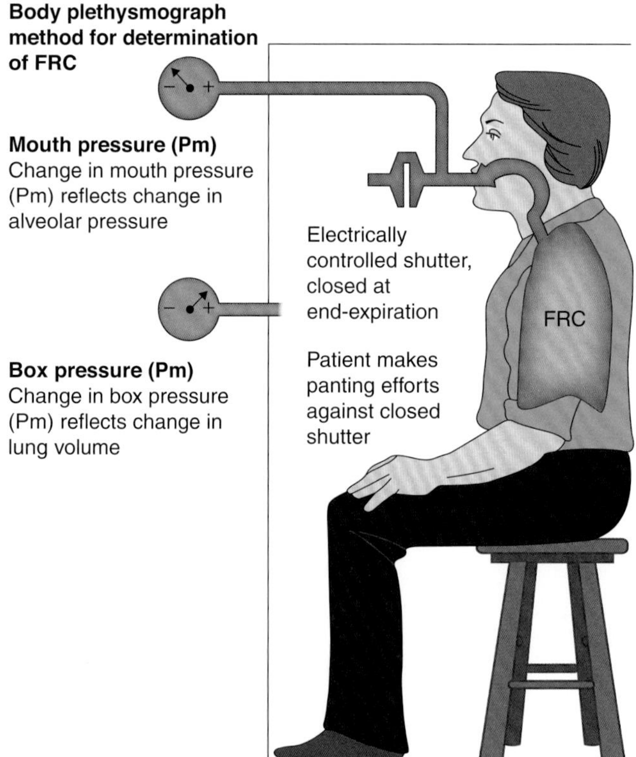

FIGURES 24-19 Complete measurement of lung volumes and capacities is commonly performed in the pulmonary function lab by whole-body plethysmography with the patient seated in an airtight box. Lung volumes can be calculated from changes in the airway and box pressure since the volume of the box is known. (From Slinger P, Darling G. Preanesthetic assessment for thoracic surgery. In: Slinger P, ed. *Principles and Practice of Anesthesia for Thoracic Surgery*. New York, NY: Springer; 2011:11–34, with permission.)

give all of the volumes and capacities listed in Table 24-1 except FRC, TLC, and residual volume (RV), all of which require a separate measurement of RV. RV can be measured by wash-in or washout dilution calculations using a relatively insoluble gas such as nitrogen or helium and a closed breathing circuit. In modern pulmonary function labs, these laborious techniques have largely been replaced by whole-body plethysmography, which is both simpler and more accurate (Fig 24-19), which measures FRC and this can be used to calculate RV by subtraction of expiratory reserve volume (ERV) measured by spirometry.

Spirometry measurements are commonly reported as "observed" (or measured) and "predicted" (Fig. 24-20). Predictions are based on population statistical means, which take into account age, sex, and height. For example, an observed forced expiratory volume in 1 second (FEV_1) of 1.0 L for an 85-year-old male, 152 cm in height (5-ft tall) is 85% predicted (within the normal range of 100% ± 20%) but and FEV_1 of 1.0 L for a 30-year-old male, 182 cm (6 ft) is 20% predicted, which would be consistent with severe end-stage lung disease. The FEV_1, forced vital capacity (FVC), and their ratio (FEV_1/FVC) are the most

Test performed			Pre BD		Post BD	
		Pred. val.	Obs.	%Pred. val	Obs.	%Pred. val
Total lung capacity	(TLC), L	4.2	**7.4**	**175**	----	----
Functional residual capacity	(FRC), L	2.6	**6.2**	**239**	----	----
Inspiratory capacity	(IC), L	1.6	**1.2**	**74**	----	----
Vital capacity	(VC), L	2.4	**1.5**	**63**	----	----
Residual volume	(RV), L	1.8	**5.9**	**322**	----	----
RV/TLC ratio	(RV/TLC), %	43	**80**	**184**	----	----
Forced vital capacity	(FVC), L	2.4	**1.5**	**62**	----	----
Forced exp. volume in 1 sec.	(FEV1), L	1.7	**0.6**	**34**	----	----
FEV1/FVC ratio	(FEV1/FVC), %	71	**39**	**55**	----	----
Max. Exp. flow @ 50% VC	(V50), L/sec	2.4	**0.17**	**7**	----	----
Max. Exp. flow @ 25% VC	(V25), L/sec	1.2	**0.07**	**6**	----	----
Mid expiratory flow 25-75%	(FEF 25-75), L/sec	2.0	**0.2**	**12**	----	----
Airway resistance	(Raw), cmH2O/L/sec	0.7	**2.5**	**387**		
Max. voluntary ventilation	(MVV), L/min	50	**----**	**----**		
Lung diffusion capacity	(DLco), ml/min/mmHg	12.6	**7.5**	**59**	*Normal limits: 75-125%*	
VA@BTPS from DLco	(VA@BTPS), L	4.2	**2.5**	**60**		

Note: %Pred. values are BOLD when outside of normal limits. (All except raw & DLco values.)

FIGURE 24-20 A copy of the pulmonary function laboratory test report for a patient with severe emphysema. Of the 15 different results in this report, the two results highlighted, the % predicted FEV_1 and DLCO, are the most useful tests for the anesthesiologist assessing a patient for possible pulmonary resection. This patient had taken a bronchodilator immediately before the test so the usual postbronchodilator (Post-BD) test was not repeated. Pred. val., predicted value corrected for the patient's age, sex, and height; Obs., patient's measured result; VA, the single-breath dilutional estimate of TLC from the DLCO. (From Slinger P, Darling G. Preanesthetic assessment for thoracic surgery. In: Slinger P, ed. *Principles and Practice of Anesthesia for Thoracic Surgery*. New York, NY: Springer; 2011:11–34, with permission.)

useful spirometry measurements for the anesthesiologist to assess the severity of a patient's lung disease or to evaluate a patient's operability for lung resection surgery.[15]

In addition, complete pulmonary function testing in the laboratory will commonly report measurements of volume ratios, flows, lung resistance, lung diffusion capacity for carbon monoxide (DLCO) and other measurements. The majority of these other values, although useful for distinguishing among different types and severities of pulmonary diseases in clinical chest medicine, are not commonly used in anesthesia. The exception is the DLCO which is a measurement of lung parenchymal function (i.e. alveolo-capillary gas transfer).

Closing Capacity and Closing Volume:

The key to understanding the complex changes which develop in the respiratory system during anesthesia is to appreciate the relationship between FRC and closing capacity (CC). CC is the sum of closing volume (CV) and RV. CV is the lung volume below which small airways begin to close (or at least cease to contribute expiratory gas) during expiration. Closure of small airways in the basal portions of the lung during deep expiration is a normal phenomenon due to the gravity-dependent increase in pleural pressure at the bases and due to the lack of parenchymal support in distal airways. CV and CC are not commonly measured in the pulmonary function lab. Measurement is either by a wash-in technique with a small bolus of an insoluble tracer gas such as ^{133}Xe slowly inhaled then exhaled from RV (Fig. 24-21) or by nitrogen washout after inspiration of a breath of oxygen from RV. Normal values for CC in seated healthy young adults are 15% to 20% of vital capacity (VC).[5] CC increases with age due to loss of structural parenchymal support tissue in the lung and an increase in RV. FRC increases slightly with age but the increase is greater for CC (Fig. 24-22).[16] CC changes very slowly over time. However, FRC changes on a minute-to-minute basis as the mechanical advantage of the two springs (lung and chest wall) which determine it change. CC exceeds FRC in the supine position at age 45 and in the upright position by age 65. During anesthesia, a decrease in the elastic recoil of the chest wall due to the muscle-relaxing effects of almost all general anesthetics (with the possible exception of ketamine) and neuromuscular blockers causes FRC to decrease and it will often fall below CC.[17] Similarly, an increase in elastic recoil of the lung due to fluid retention in the pulmonary parenchyma will lower the FRC. When an alveolar unit falls below its

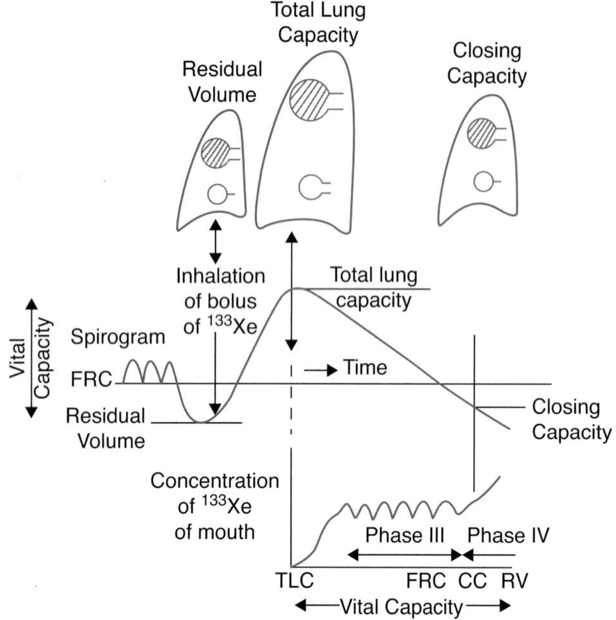

FIGURE 24-21 Measurement of closing capacity (CC) by the use of a tracer gas such as ^{133}Xe. The bolus of tracer gas is inhaled from residual volume and due to closure of some small airways is distributed only to those alveoli whose airways are still open (shown as the *shaded areas* in the diagram). During expiration, the concentration of the tracer gas becomes constant after the dead space is washed out. This plateau (phase III) gives way to a rising concentration of tracer gas (phase IV) when there is closure of the airways leading to the alveoli which did not receive the tracer gas. The measured volume from the onset of phase IV until the end of expiration (RV) is the closing volume (CV). CC is calculated as the sum of CV and RV (which is measured separately, see "Lung Volumes and Spirometry" in earlier discussion) (From Lumb AB, ed. *Nunn's Applied Respiratory Physiology*. 7th ed. Edinburgh, United Kingdom: Churchill Livingston Elsevier; 2010, with permission.)

CC, even for a brief period during one respiratory cycle, the concentration of oxygen (PA_{O_2}) in that unit falls slightly. This results in the increase of venoarterial admixture ("shunt"; see the following text) and decrease in arterial oxygen tension (Pa_{O_2}) seen in the elderly and during general anesthesia. When a region of the lung is kept below its CC, the loss in volume will eventually lead to atelectasis (Fig. 24-23) as the gas trapped in the alveoli is absorbed. A large part of the anesthesiologist's job in the perioperative period is restoring the balance between FRC and CC. Because CC cannot be changed, this involves improving FRC by a variety of techniques to improve the mechanical advantage of the chest wall. These techniques may include ensuring adequate reversal of neuromuscular blockers, upright positioning, regional analgesia and possibly the use of positive end-expiratory pressure (PEEP) or continuous positive airway pressure (CPAP). The physiologic differences between PEEP and CPAP are subtle. However, by common usage, when positive pressure is applied during expiration to the airway of a patient who is having positive pressure ventilation, this applied airway pressure is referred to as ***PEEP***. When a patient is breathing spontaneously, an applied airway pressure is referred to as ***CPAP***.

Compliance

Compliance is the change in lung volume for a given change in airway pressure. It is the reciprocal of "elastance." Monitoring changes in respiratory compliance is extremely important in ventilated patients as an early warning of changes in the lung or chest–abdominal wall complex that may negatively affect gas exchange. Compliance of the respiratory system (C_{RS}) is measured as the change in lung volume (ΔV) divided by the change in airway pressure (ΔP), this represents the difference between alveolar pressure, at a given lung volume, and ambient (atmospheric) pressure.

$$C_{RS} = \Delta V/\Delta P$$

The compliance of the respiratory system is dependent on the interaction of the compliance of the lung itself (C_L) and the compliance of the chest wall (C_{cw}). These two springs act similar to series capacitors in an electrical system, that is, storing energy, and the reciprocal of

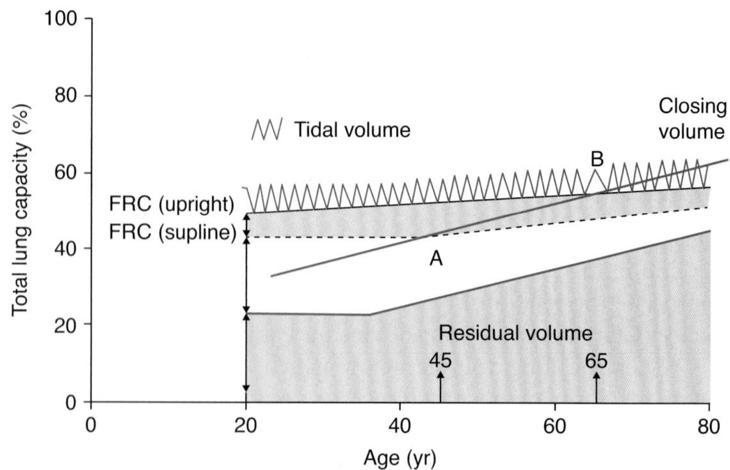

FIGURE 24-22 The effects of aging and position on closing volume, residual volume, and functional residual capacity (FRC) as a percent of total lung capacity. With aging, there is a slight increase in FRC but both closing volume and residual volume increase at a greater rate. (From Sprung J, Gajic O, Warner DO. Age related alterations in respiratory function-anesthetic consideration. *Can J Anaesth.* 2006;53:1244–1257, with permission.)

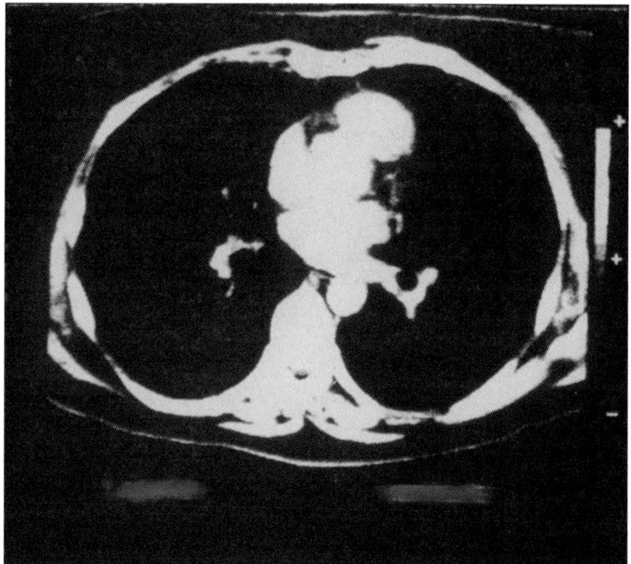

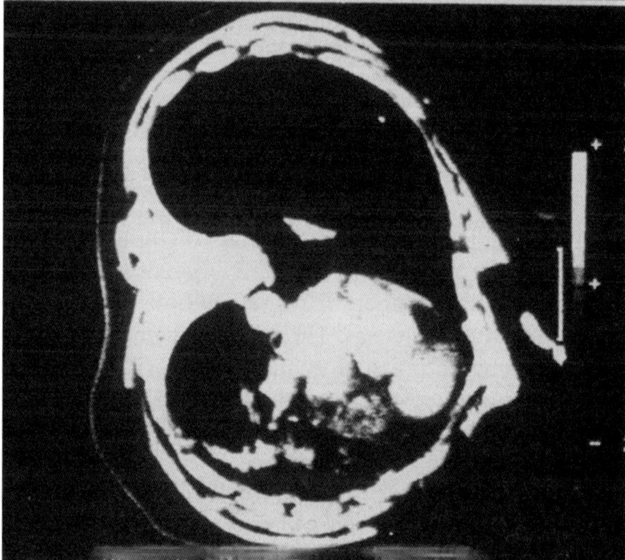

FIGURE 24-23 Thoracic CT scans of a patient awake *(top)* and then anesthetized and turned to the lateral position *(bottom)*. The dependent lung tends to fall below its closing capacity due to the effect of gravity and the compression of the mediastinum. This results in atelectasis, which can be seen developing in the dependent lung. (From Slinger P, Campos J. Anesthesia for thoracic surgery. In: *Miller's Anesthesia*. 7th ed. Philadelphia, PA: Churchill Livingstone Elsevier; 2010, with permission.)

respiratory compliance is the sum of the reciprocals of C_L and C_{cw}:

$$1/C_{RS} = 1/C_L + 1/C_{cw}$$

C_L is calculated as $\Delta V/\Delta P$, where ΔP = alveolar pressure − intrapleural ("transmural") pressure

C_{cw} is calculated as $\Delta V/\Delta P$, where ΔP = intrapleural pressure − ambient pressure

Intrapleural pressure is not easy to measure directly in the clinical setting. Esophageal pressure, from a balloon manometer, is commonly used as an approximation of intrapleural pressure in respiratory research. As the respiratory system inflates, both the lung and chest will produce their own unique compliance curves (Fig. 24-24).

Factors affecting C_L include the following:

1. Lung volume. Compliance is greatest at FRC and remains at this level until the lung inflates or deflates to approximately 15% of TLC above or below FRC, that is, the slope of C_{RS} is the steepest in this range, which includes the range of normal tidal volume breathing. Compliance is related to the normal FRC for a given lung and can be corrected for normal lung volume as the "specific compliance" (compliance/FRC), which is relatively constant at all ages.
2. Surface tension of the alveoli. This is probably the major factor determining lung recoil and C_L. A lung that is filled with water is actually more compliant than a normal lung because the air-fluid surface tension interaction is lost. Similarly, a lung that is depleted of surfactant is less compliant than normal. Without surfactant, the alveoli would be expected to behave like communicating bubbles and conform to the Laplace equation:

$$P = 2T/R$$

Where P is the gas pressure within a bubble, T is the surface tension of the wall, and R is the radius of the bubble. If the radius is decreased without a change in surface tension, the pressure will increase in the bubble and a small bubble will empty into a larger bubble (in the lung, this would lead to atelectasis). However, in the lung, surface tension decreases as the radius of the alveoli decreases and this opposes the collapse of smaller lung units. The exact mechanisms by which surfactant causes this effect are debated.[18] It could be related to a tighter packing of surfactant molecules as the radius decreases or the formation of surfactant multilayers. Other factors which affect the C_L include pulmonary blood volume and interstitial edema.

Factors affecting C_{cw} include posture, obesity, ossification of the costal cartilages, and scarring of the skin. The interaction of the compliances of these two springs produces the characteristic sigmoid pattern of the compliance curve of the respiratory system (see Fig. 24-24, *solid line*). At FRC, which is normally the relaxation volume of the respiratory system, the pull of the two springs in opposite directions balance one another. In a normal healthy individual, as the respiratory system inflates to 60% of TLC, the chest wall is aiding the muscles of respiration to inflate the lungs. However, as the lung inflates above this volume, the muscles of inspiration must work to distend both the lungs and the chest wall.

Dynamic compliance is the $\Delta V/\Delta P$ of the respiratory system measured at the instant gas flow. In a ventilated patient, this ΔP will = peak airway pressure − PEEP. This

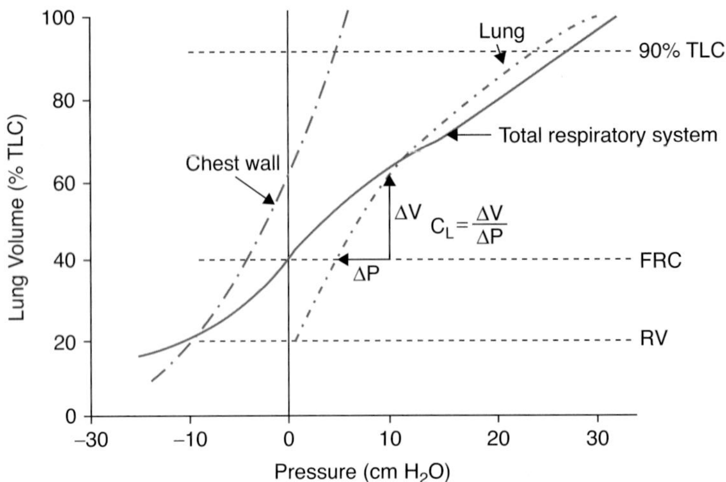

FIGURE 24-24 Static pressure-volume curves of the respiratory system. The isolated chest wall compliance curve (C_{cw}) *(large dash-dot line)* crosses the zero pressure or equilibrium point at approximately 60% of total lung capacity (TLC). The isolated lung compliance (C_L) *(small dash-dot line)* approaches its equilibrium point at about 20% TLC or residual volume (RV). The algebraic summation of the reciprocals of C_{cw} and C_L produce the compliance of the total respiratory system (C_{rs}) *(solid line)*. The outward recoil of the chest wall and the inward recoil of the lung will balance at functional residual capacity (FRC). Note that the chest wall will passively contribute to lung inflation up to 60%TLC above which the chest wall will oppose inflation and the compliance *(slope of the solid line)* will begin to decrease. (From Jaeger JM. Blank RS. Essential anatomy and physiology of the respiratory system and pulmonary circulation. In: Slinger P, ed. *Principles and Practice of Anesthesia for Thoracic Surgery*. New New York, NY: Springer; 2011:51–69, with permission.)

reflects the normal behavior of the respiratory system but will include the effects of airway resistance and the normal hysteresis of the lung parenchyma (hysteresis in this context refers to the tendency of an elastic material to resist change of shape both during stretch and contraction). Dynamic compliance will be affected by both the frequency of respiration and the velocity of gas flow.

Static compliance is the $\Delta V/\Delta P$ of the respiratory system measured at a point of no gas flow and when the pressure gradient has been allowed to equilibrate in the entire airway. This is difficult, but not impossible, to achieve in an awake subject by relaxing at end-inspiration against a closed airway. However, it is simple to measure in an anesthetized and paralyzed patient during ventilation in a volume-controlled mode (with a fixed inspiratory flow) by using an end-inspiratory pause. The ΔP for static compliance will = plateau airway pressure − PEEP.

Both static and dynamic compliances provide useful information for the anesthesiologist. The static compliance reflects more the actual distending pressure in the patient's alveoli. The difference between the two reflects the effects of airway resistance. During pressure-control ventilation, with a decreasing inspiratory airflow pattern, there will not be a discernible difference in the peak or plateau in the airway pressure so distinguishing between static and dynamic compliance is clinically difficult (Fig. 24-25). This negative, that is, loss of monitoring, aspect of pressure–control ventilation is largely compensated by the ability of pressure–control ventilation to more uniformly distribute gas flow in patients with COPD who have large differences in regional compliance within the lung (see the following text).

The inflation and deflation limbs of the compliance curve of the respiratory system are different (Fig. 24-26). For dynamic compliance, this is due to both airway resistance and lung hysteresis. These curves combine to produce the familiar "pressure-volume loop" (or "PV" or "ΔV/ΔP" or "compliance" curve) of the lung displayed by many modern anesthetic machines and its shape is determined mainly by the dynamic compliance of the respiratory system. The gap between the expiratory and inspiratory limbs of the combined curve will widen as tidal volume and respiratory rate increase. It is possible to generate a $\Delta V/\Delta P$ curve using static compliance if the lung is slowly inflated in a stepwise fashion. This curve will also show a gap between inspiration and expiration due mainly to lung hysteresis. This gap will be smaller than that for the dynamic $\Delta V/\Delta P$ curve.[19] An automated breath-by-breath calculation of compliance is displayed by the ventilation monitors of many modern anesthetic machines. It is difficult for these clinical monitors to measure at a true static "no flow" point at end-inspiration and therefore measured compliance changes may be truly due to increased tissue elastance (e.g., atelectasis or pulmonary edema) but may also be affected by changes in dynamic compliance (airway resistance), for example, bronchospasm or secretions.

Resistance

Respiratory system resistance is a complex and important topic. It is important because, in the perioperative period, complications such as bronchospasm or secretions in an endotracheal tube or partial circuit obstruction will present primarily as increased resistance. It is complex

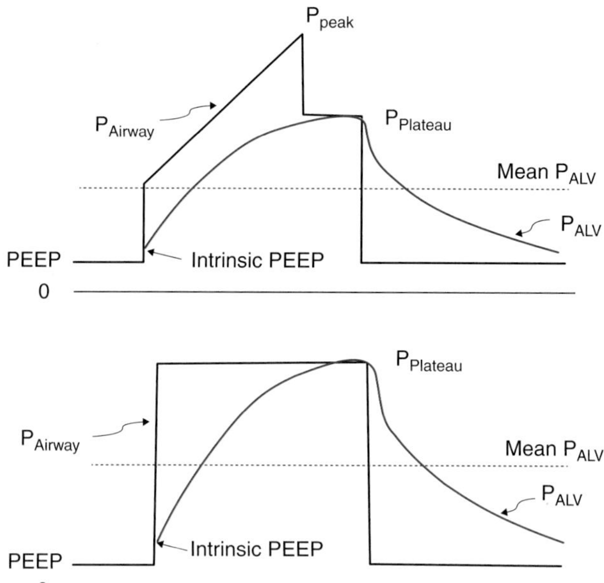

FIGURE 24-25 Comparison of the airway (P_{Airway}, *black line*) and alveolar (P_{ALV}, *red line*) pressures (vertical axis) for volume-control ventilation with an end-inspiratory hold (plateau) *(top)* and pressure-control ventilation *(bottom)* plotted against time (horizontal axis). For volume control ventilation the difference between the peak airway pressure (P_{Peak}) and the plateau pressure ($P_{Plateau}$) represents the resistance to gas flow. This is primarily due to the combined nonelastic resistance of the airway and circuit. This gas flow resistance cannot easily be monitored during pressure control ventilation, which has only a plateau pressure. Note that the mean alveolar pressure (mean P_{ALV}) in healthy individuals is approximately the same with the two methods of ventilation for the same tidal volumes. (From Ward D. Intraoperative ventilation strategies for thoracic surgery. In: Slinger P, ed. *Principles and Practice of Anesthesia for Thoracic Surgery.* New York, NY: Springer; 2011:297–308, with permission.)

because there are many types of resistance that contribute to the overall resistance of the respiratory system. When anesthesiologists think of respiratory resistance, they are mainly thinking of the nonelastic resistance to gas flow and they are primarily thinking of frictional airflow resistance. Nonelastic resistance is a major component of the work of breathing and because it cannot be stored, it is lost and dissipated as heat. Nonelastic resistance also includes the resistance of lung and chest wall tissue to deformation and compression of intrathoracic gas. Elastic resistance is the recoil of the lung and chest wall, and because it is recovered during expiration, it does not contribute to the work of breathing.

Respiratory resistance (R_{RS}) is calculated as the pressure gradient divided by the inspiratory flow. During a constant flow situation such as volume–control ventilation, this would be calculated from Figure 24-25 as:

$$R_{RS}\ (\text{cm } H_2O/\text{L per second}) = P_{Peak} - P_{Plateau}\ (\text{cm } H_2O)/\text{inspiratory gas flow (L per second)}$$

However, normal spontaneous ventilation and pressure–control ventilation have variable flow rates and a mean gas-flow rate approximation is necessary to calculate respiratory resistance. Airflow resistance in normal healthy individuals breathing spontaneously is approximately 1 cm H_2O/L per second. This can increase to 5 to 10 cm H_2O/L per second in COPD and asthma.[20] Breathing through an 8-mm internal diameter endotracheal tube at a flow of 1 L per second creates a resistance of approximately 5 cm H_2O/L per second and this increases to 8 cm H_2O/L per second for a 7-mm endotracheal tube.[21]

To quantitatively measure respiratory resistance in the operating room is not simple because it is difficult to separate respiratory system resistance from apparatus resistance. In the pulmonary function laboratory, this is done with plethysmography and a variety of flow-interrupter techniques. Fortunately, it is relatively simple to monitor changes in respiratory resistance in the operating room by following changes in dynamic compliance.

Gas flow during respiration is a mixture of turbulent and laminar flows and the turbulent/laminar interface moves in the air column during the respiratory cycle. Laminar flow occurs beyond the 11th generation airways. Turbulent flow in the larger conducting airways aids clearing of secretions by coughing. In a healthy person, frictional

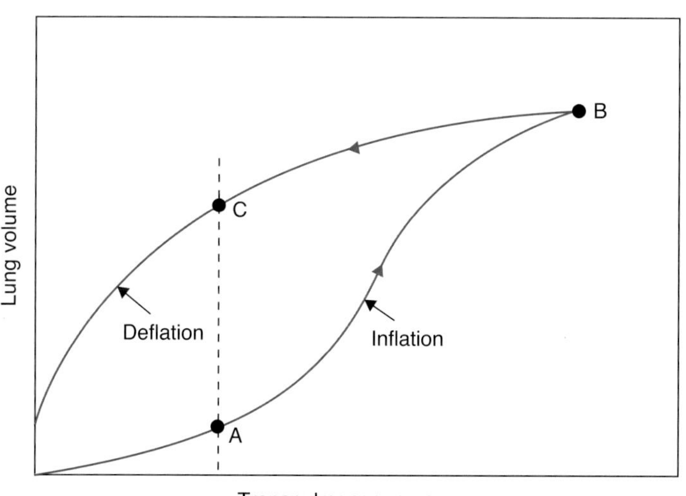

FIGURE 24-26 The pressure versus volume (PV) curve of the lung, often called the "compliance" curve. In this case, lung volume is plotted against transpulmonary pressure. Note that for the same pressure, the lung has a larger volume (i.e., is more compliant) during deflation than during inflation, as represented by the distance between points *A* and *C*. This is due to hysteresis of the lung tissue and is present whether the curves are measured dynamically (during a continuous flow) or statically (during interrupted flow). For a dynamic PV curve, the distance AC will be greater than for a static curve due to the additive effects of airflow resistance. The point of maximum slope of the inspiratory curve (inflation *arrow*) normally corresponds to FRC. If the lung is inflated starting at FRC, the "lower inflection point" of the curve *(point A)* is not seen.

airflow resistance is mainly due to larger airways: mouth and pharynx 40%, larynx and large airways 40%, small airways (<3-mm diameter) contribute 20%.[22] However, changes in airflow resistance are most commonly due to changes in the caliber of the small airways. Small airway caliber can be decreased by contraction of smooth muscle in the airway wall or by compression (due to reversal of the normal transluminal pressure gradient in the collapsible distal airways).

Airway resistance is inversely proportional to lung volume and increases exponentially as the lung deflates below FRC. The application of PEEP or CPAP to patients who have a decreased FRC will benefit their respiration not only by raising their FRC above CC but also by decreasing their respiratory resistance, and thus their work of breathing, at a higher lung volume.

An increase in resistance to inspiration is detected by the muscle spindles in the diaphragm and leads to an increased force of contraction. This spinal reflex is preserved during anesthesia. In the awake patient, this reflex is augmented by a conscious cortical response that also increases the force of inspiration.[23] Increased expiratory resistance does not normally initiate a response if the resistance is <10 cm H_2O. The FRC is increased passively by the increased resistance until the increased elastic recoil balances the increased work of expiration. However, the ensuing increased intrathoracic pressure may decrease venous return and cardiac output. Patients tolerate increased airway resistance by increasing the work of breathing and in the short term will usually maintain a normal arterial CO_2 ($Paco_2$). Eventually, a major increase in airway resistance may lead to respiratory muscle fatigue and the $Paco_2$ will start to rise. An elevated $Paco_2$ in a patient with increased respiratory resistance who has a normal baseline $Paco_2$ is an ominous sign of impending respiratory failure.

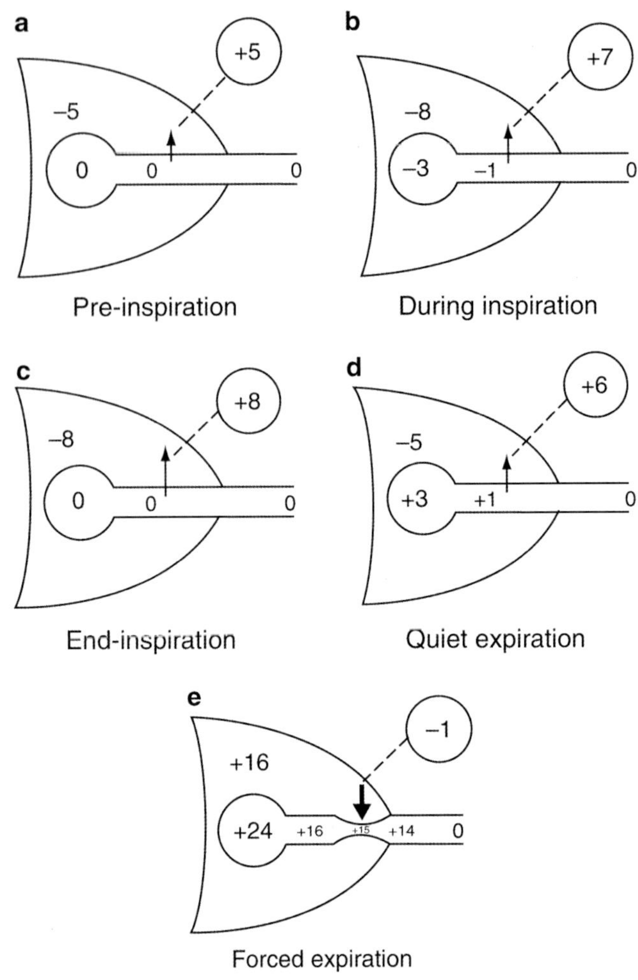

FIGURE 24-27 The effects of the intrapleural and alveolar pressures during quite breathing *(a–d)* and the creation of an equal pressure point in the airway of a normal patient during forced expiration *(e)*, see text for details. (From Ma M, Slinger P. Anesthesia for patients with end-stage lung disease. In: Slinger P, ed. *Principles and Practice of Anesthesia for Thoracic Surgery*. New York, NY: Springer; 2011:343–365, with permission.)

The Equal Pressure Point

Expiratory respiratory resistance will normally be lower than inspiratory resistance because the lung is at a larger volume at all stages of expiration than inspiration (see Fig. 24-26). However, there are situations when expiratory resistance exceeds inspiratory resistance, these include the following: during a forced expiration (or cough) in a normal patient, during quiet breathing in some patients with severe emphysema (see the following text), and during forced expiration in some patients with an intrathoracic tracheal tumor or tracheobronchial compression from a mediastinal mass. In these instances, where expiratory resistance exceeds inspiratory resistance, the underlying cause is dynamic airway compression, which creates a moving flow-limiting narrowing in the airway called the ***equal pressure point*** (EPP). In Figure 24-27 at FRC before inspiration, (a) airway pressure throughout is zero (no-flow situation) because the intrapleural (transpulmonary) pressure is −5 cm H_2O there is a net +5 cm H_2O pressure distending the airways and alveoli. As inspiration begins, (b) intrapleural and alveolar pressure falls by 3 cm H_2O and flow begins. Because of the pressure drop along the airway, the pressure will be negative in the airway but less than the alveolar pressure. This increases the distending pressure of the airways in this case from +5 to +6 cm H_2O. At end-inspiration, (c) the distending pressure in the no-flow condition is +8 cm H_2O and the pressure through the airway returns to zero. During quiet expiration, the recoil intrapleural pressure returns to −5 cm H_2O and this creates a net pressure in the alveolus of +3 cm H_2O, which diminishes proximally as air flows out the tracheobronchial tree. The downstream distending pressure falls along the airway (represented by +6 cm H_2O in Fig. 24-27D). Because this is a dynamic process, due to tissue resistance, the airway caliber will normally be larger at a given point for the same distending pressure during expiration than during inspiration. In a no-flow situation, the same distending pressure will result in equivalent airway diameters. During a forced expiration, (e) the airway pressures increase [in this case by 24 cm H_2O, resulting in a net intrapleural pressure of +16 cm H_2O for same lung volume as (c)] and a gradient is created along the expiratory air column. At the point where the intrapleural pressure equals the air column distending pressure (+16 cm H_2O), an EPP is created. The airway will narrow proximal to this point (+15) to the thoracic outlet (+14). This becomes the flow-limiting point of expiration and no amount of increased effort can increase the expiratory flow at a particular lung volume because the driving pressure is fixed by the difference between the alveolar and intrapleural pressures [8 cm H_2O in (e)]. This EPP allows the creation of a point of gas-flow acceleration and turbulence in the expiratory air column during normal coughing that has a Bernoulli effect (decreased lateral pressure in a region of increased flow velocity) to detach secretions from the tracheobronchial walls. During forced expiration, as lung volumes decrease and airway pressures decrease, intrapleural pressures are maintained and the EPP will move distally in the airway.[24]

During a maximal respiratory effort, the EPP is responsible for the difference in the shapes of the expiratory versus inspiratory limbs of the flow-volume curve (Fig. 24-28). The linear portion of the expiratory flow, after the initial peak flow, is caused by the EPP. The peak flow is effort-dependent but the linear portion of the expiratory flow is effort-independent (i.e., no amount of increased expiratory effort at a given lung volume can increase the maximal flow rate at that volume). During quiet breathing, the inspiratory and expiratory limbs of the flow-volume curve are mirror images due to the absence of an EPP. In the range of lung volumes used during quiet breathing, both inspiratory and expiratory flow normally can be increased approximately threefold by maximal effort if needed.

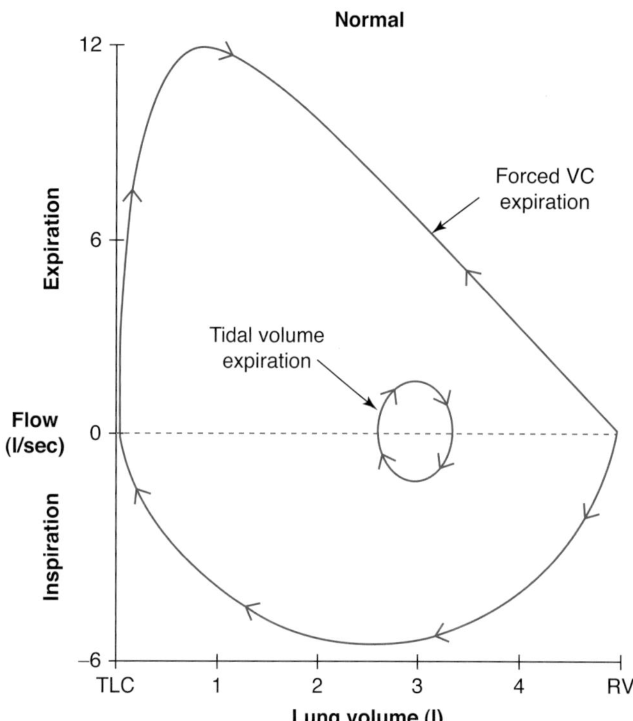

FIGURE 24-28 The air flow versus lung volume plot during maximal force inspiration and expiration of a normal individual *(outer curve)* from residual volume (RV) to total lung capacity (TLC). The *inner elliptical curve* "tidal volume" is during normal quiet breathing. During maximal inspiration, the curve is hyperbolic. During maximal expiration (forced VC expiration), after the initial peak, the curve becomes linear due to the formation of an equal pressure point in the airway.

Work of Breathing

Work is the product of *force* × *distance* or *pressure* × *volume*. Technically, ***work*** is calculated for a single event. However, the term ***work of breathing*** is commonly used to denote the ongoing energy expenditure required by the respiratory system. During normal quiet breathing, expiration is passive and does not require work. Half of the work of inspiration is stored in the deformation of the muscles of inspiration and the lung tissue. This potential energy provides the work necessary for expiration. The other half of the work of inspiration is dissipated as heat in overcoming the frictional forces of tissue and gas movement. The oxygen requirement for the work of breathing is less than 2% of the normal basal oxygen consumption (3 to 4 mL/kg per minute). In healthy individuals, the oxygen consumption of the muscles of respiration does not become important until rates of respiration approaching maximal minute ventilation (60 to 80 L per minute, i.e., 15 × basal ventilation) are reached. However, in patients with COPD, due to the mechanical inefficiency of the respiratory system, increasing the minute ventilation to 20 L per minute may increase the oxygen consumption of the muscles of respiration to levels of 200 mL per minute.[25]

The work performed against the elastic resistance of the lung and chest wall increases proportionally when breathing is slow and deep. Conversely, the work performed against air flow resistance increases when breathing is rapid and shallow. Each individual will have an optimal rate and tidal volume that minimizes the work of breathing depending on the compliance and resistance of their respiratory system. At rest, they will normally breathe at a rate that minimizes the oxygen consumption required for gas exchange. For normal adults, this usually corresponds to a resting respiratory rate of 15 to 16 breaths per minute. For patients with obstructive diseases, this rate will usually tend to be lower and higher for patients with restrictive lung diseases.[26]

Although the work of breathing is minimal for healthy individuals, it may represent a significant challenge for a patient with respiratory or cardiac failure who has diminished reserves. This always needs to be considered when weaning such a patient from mechanically assisted ventilation.

Respiratory Fatigue

Fatigue of the respiratory system may occur at any point from the central nervous system (CNS) to the muscles of respiration. The diaphragm is possibly the most fatigue-resistant skeletal muscle and can sustain resistive loads of up to 40% of maximal indefinitely. However, fatigue will occur with loads exceeding 40%. Because the oxygen supply requirement for the diaphragm is high in proportion to its mass, it is susceptible to hypoxia either due to decreased oxygen content of the arterial blood or due to decreased cardiac output.[27] The diaphragm can be rested for a short period by mechanical ventilation but histologic evidence of muscle fiber atrophy can be seen after as little as 18 hours of mechanical ventilation and clinical evidence of weakness is seen within days.[28] Ventilator-induced diaphragm dysfunction is characterized by atrophy of both type 1 and 2 fibers, with altered gene expression leading to an increase in proteolysis.[29]

Distribution of Ventilation

Initially, it is a difficult concept to grasp, but ventilation is preferentially distributed to the smaller alveoli close to the middle and lower portion of the lungs rather than to the larger alveoli in the more superior lung regions. This is because the lower alveoli are at a steeper portion of their compliance curve (see Fig. 24-15). The most frequent explanation for this nonuniformity is the effect of gravity on the lung parenchyma. In the upright posture, the greatest vertical height is attained by the lung. The tendency for the lung to retract away from the chest wall at its apex creates a more negative (subatmospheric) pleural pressure than the pleural pressure at the lower dependent portions of the lung where its weight reduces the magnitude of the negative pleural pressure. The gradient of pleural pressure from the lung apex to its base has been estimated at 0.4 cm H_2O per each centimeter of vertical height. Obviously, one might expect less of a transpulmonary pressure gradient from nondependent to dependent portions of the lung when supine or prone as compared to the upright position. In the upright individual, during a spontaneous breath, inspired gas will tend to preferentially enter those open alveoli near the base of the lung which are the most compliant. As the breath continues, the gas will enter the more apical, less compliant alveoli and any previously atelectatic basilar alveoli as they become recruited by the traction exerted by the remainder of the expanding lung. Also, the rate of inspiration directly impacts the homogeneity of gas distribution. At high inspiratory rates, air is distributed more evenly throughout the lung than at very slow rates.[30]

Pulmonary Circulation

The lung circulation is composed of two sources of blood flow: the pulmonary circulation from the main pulmonary artery and the smaller bronchial circulation arising from the aorta. The pulmonary circulation dominates, by volume, and serves to deliver the mixed venous blood to the alveolar capillaries to facilitate gas exchange and to act as a large, low-resistance reservoir for the entire cardiac output from the right ventricle. The bronchial circulation serves to provide nutritional support to the airways and their associated pulmonary blood vessels.[31] The bronchial circulation also provides a constant source of heat and moisture for warming and humidifying the inspired air.

Pulmonary Hemodynamics

Despite receiving all of the cardiac output from the right ventricle, the pulmonary vasculature maintains a relatively low pulmonary blood pressure. The normal adult mean pulmonary artery pressure (P_{PA}) is 9 to 16 mm Hg with systolic P_{PA} of 18 to 25 mm Hg. Several features enable the pulmonary circulation to maintain this high flow at such low pressures. First, the pulmonary vasculature is extremely thin-walled with far less arterial vascular smooth muscle than its systemic counterparts. The result is a highly compliant reservoir capable of accommodating an average 3.2 L/min/m^2 blood flow at rest or six to eight times that flow during exercise. Second, the total PVR is quite low, on the order of less than 250 dynes·sec·cm^{-5}. This minimizes the pressure work faced by the less robust right ventricle while still enabling the right ventricle to match the output of the left ventricle. PVR can change as a result of numerous factors, hypoxia, acidosis, mitral valve stenosis or regurgitation, left ventricular failure, primary pulmonary hypertension, or pulmonary emboli, to name just a few. PVR can be calculated using data from a pulmonary artery catheter as:

$$PVR = [(P_{PA} - PAOP) / CO] \times 79.9$$

where PAOP is the pulmonary artery catheter occlusion pressure, which is assumed to reflect the left atrial pressure, CO is cardiac output (L/min), and the factor, 79.9 converts from mm Hg/L per minute to units of absolute resistance (dynes·sec·cm^{-5}).

Distribution of Perfusion

There is a gradient of distribution of perfusion of the lung that is similar but not identical to the gradient of distribution of ventilation, with increased perfusion of regions in the central and lower regions compared to the upper regions. This perfusion gradient depends in part on the

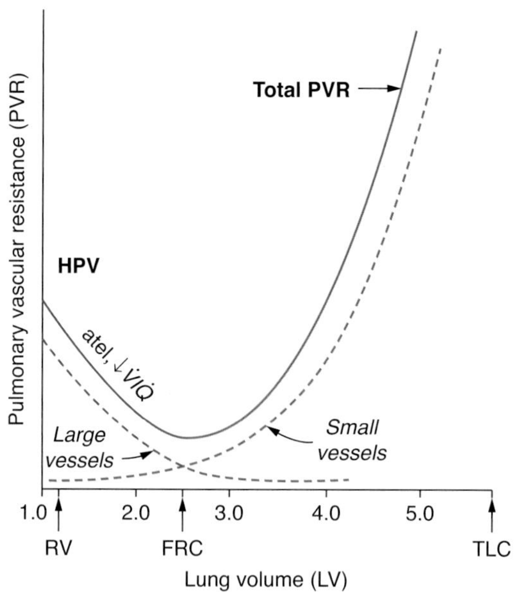

FIGURE 24-29 The relationship between pulmonary vascular resistance (PVR) and lung volume. PVR is lowest at functional residual capacity (FRC) and increases as the lung volume decreases toward residual volume (RV), owing primarily to the increase in resistance of large pulmonary vessels. PVR also increases as lung volume increases above FRC toward total lung capacity (TLC) because of an increase in resistance of small interalveolar lung vessels.

architecture of the lung and the resistance of the pulmonary vessels, which varies with lung volume and is lowest in the regions of the lung closest to FRC (Fig. 24-29). Gravity, posture, and alveolar pressure will also have effects on the distribution of pulmonary blood flow.[32]

Matching of Ventilation and Perfusion

Within certain limits, the lung attempts to match ventilation to perfusion. However, the matching is never ideal because the ventilation and perfusion gradients are not identical (Fig. 24-30). This matching is closer during spontaneous ventilation than during positive pressure ventilation. With positive pressure ventilation, the effects of alveolar pressure are increased and pulmonary blood flow distribution becomes less homogeneous. This led to the concept of perfusion zones of the lung as described by West[33] (Fig. 24-31A). In this concept, zone 1 (apical) is a region where alveolar pressure (P_A) exceeds both pulmonary arteriolar pressure (P_{PA}) and pulmonary venous pressure (P_{PV}); hence, this ventilated lung region has no perfusion. In zone 2 (transitional), P_{PA} exceeds P_A, which exceeds P_{PV} with partial limitation of pulmonary blood flow. In zone 3 (basilar), $P_{PA} > P_{PV} > P_A$, so there is unrestricted pulmonary blood flow. In zone 4 (atelectatic), a region of lung collapse, $P_{PA} >$ pulmonary interstitial fluid pressure (P_{ISF}) $> P_{PV} > P_A$, so again there is a limitation of pulmonary blood flow depending on the tissue pressure in the region of collapse. Although West's zones have been a useful concept to emphasize the effects of airway and alveolar pressure on pulmonary blood flow, these zones are an oversimplification. First, because alveolar pressure does not remain constant but varies throughout the respiratory cycle, more so during positive pressure than controlled ventilation. Thus, the boundaries between these zones are constantly moving. Also, it has been demonstrated by perfusion scanning that the distribution of blood flow in the lung is not actually in layers (like a cake) but in concentric spheres (like an onion) (Fig. 24-31B).

Dead Space

Like many concepts in respiratory physiology, dead space is crucially important in clinical practice and deceptively simple on the surface, but actually extremely complex. Any portion of an inspired breath, which does not enter gas exchanging lung units, is dead space (V_D). Minute ventilation (V_E) is the sum of alveolar ventilation (V_A) and dead space ventilation (V_D):

$$V_E = V_A + V_D$$

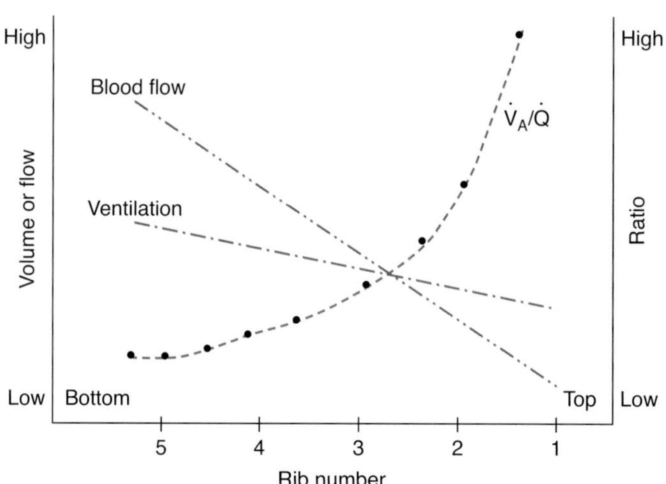

FIGURE 24-30 Distribution of blood flow (perfusion) and alveolar ventilation and the ventilation-to-perfusion ratio (V_A/Q) as a function of the distance from the base of the lung (to the left in the figure) to the apex (to the right). In the upright position, both ventilation and blood flow are greater at the base of the lung than at the apex. However, the gradient is steeper for blood flow than ventilation. Thus the V_A/Q ratio is higher at the apex than in the mid- or dependent lung regions. (Reproduced with permission from Slinger P. *Principles and Practice of Anesthesia for Thoracic Surgery*. New York, NY: Springer; 2011.)

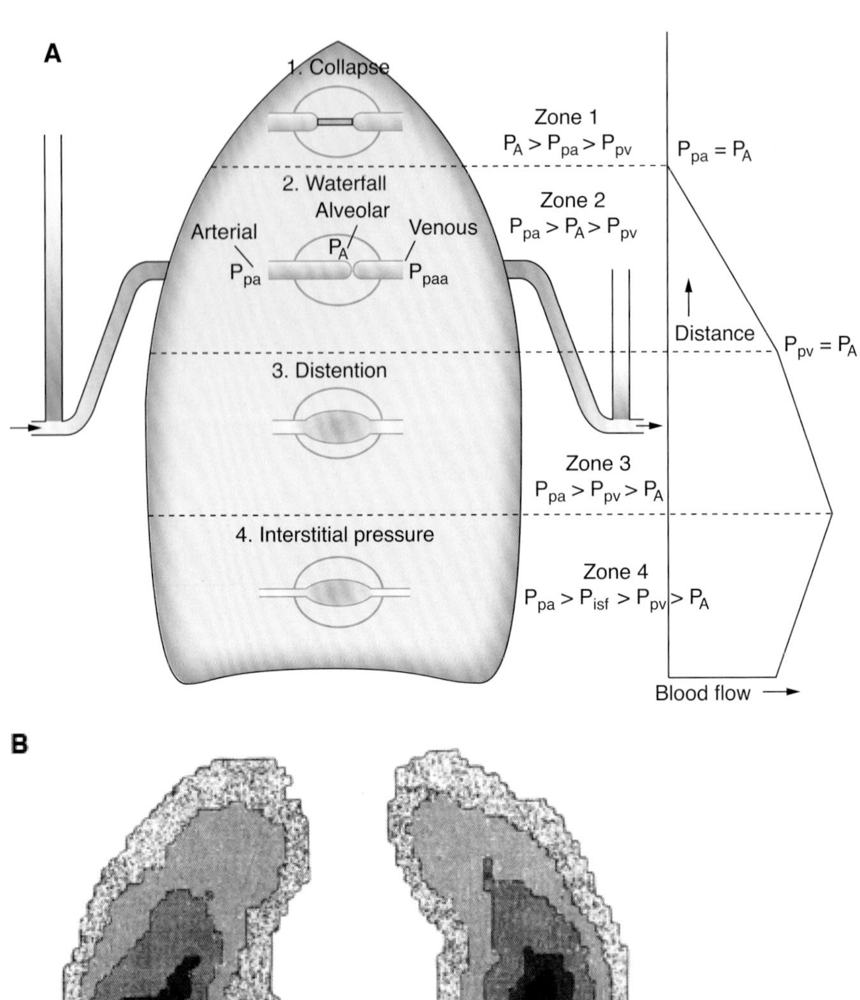

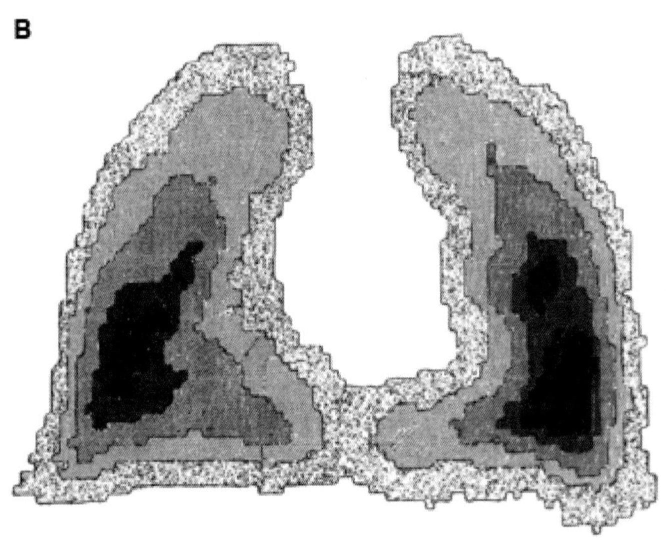

FIGURE 24-31 The distribution of pulmonary blood flow in the upright position. **A:** Pulmonary blood flow as affected by gravity and alveolar pressure. This classic description based on the work of West[33] divides pulmonary blood flow into four zones. P_A, alveolar pressure; P_{pa}, pulmonary arteriolar pressure; P_{pv}, pulmonary venous pressure, P_{isf}, pulmonary interstitial pressure. **B:** Subsequent investigations with lung scanning have shown that blood flow is actually distributed more in a central to peripheral pattern. (Reproduced with permission from Slinger P. *Principles and Practice of Anesthesia for Thoracic Surgery*. New York, NY: Springer; 2011.)

Dead space can be subdivided into two primary components: physiologic dead space and apparatus dead space. Apparatus dead space will only apply to patients attached to a breathing circuit. Physiologic dead space is further subdivided into airway dead space and alveolar dead space (Fig. 24-32). The airway dead space is the portion of a breath which goes to the mouth, pharynx, and tracheobronchial tree, but does not enter the alveoli. Airway dead space is also called ***anatomic*** dead space by some authors but this latter is a confusing term. Alveolar dead space is the portion of a breath that enters alveoli which are ventilated but not perfused (i.e., West's zone 1).

Airway dead space is relatively constant. However, it does vary directly with lung volume and bronchodilation increases airway dead space. As tidal volume (V_T) decreases, the portion of each breath that is dead space (V_D/V_T) ratio will increase. Airway dead space will decrease slightly, at lower lung volumes, but not enough to compensate for the fall in V_T. Airway dead space is decreased by endotracheal intubation, because much of the mouth and pharynx dead space is bypassed. However, the net effect on total dead space will depend on the additional equipment dead space of the circuit attached to the patient. For most correctly functioning modern anesthetic apparatus, equipment dead space is not clinically important.

A healthy person, breathing spontaneously, will have practically no alveolar dead space. Tidal volume breathing will usually result in a V_D/V_T ratio of approximately 0.3, entirely due to airway dead space. Alveolar dead space, however, becomes clinically important during positive pressure ventilation and in any condition of altered hemodynamics. Decreased cardiac output, pulmonary embolism, and changes in posture will all have clinically important effects on alveolar dead space, usually by

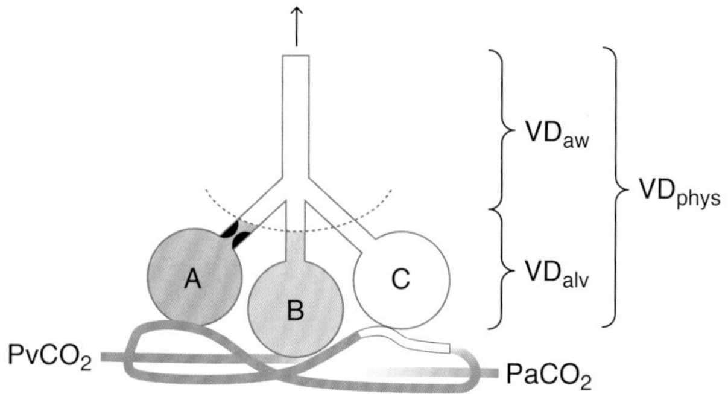

FIGURE 24-32 A simplified three-compartment model of the lung with *A* representing shunt; *B*, an ideal gas unit; and *C*, alveolar dead space (VD_{alv}). Physiologic dead space (VD_{phys}) is filled with air containing no CO_2, shown as the *white area*. VD_{phys} is the sum of airway dead space (VD_{aw}) and VD_{alv}. The airway-alveolar interface is demonstrated by the *dotted line*. (Reproduced with permission from Tusman G, Sipmann S, Bohm SH. Rationale of dead space measurement by volumetric capnography. *Anesth Analg.* 2012;114:866–874.)

increasing zone 1. These three components: apparatus, airway, and alveolar make up the total dead space.

Measurement of Dead Space

The measurement of dead space was described initially by Bohr.[34] Mixed expired gas is collected and CO_2 analyzed to give a mixed CO_2 tension (P_ECO_2) and the arterial blood gas ($Paco_2$) sampled. The Bohr equation is:

$$V_D/V_T = (Paco_2 - P_ECO_2)/Paco_2$$

The derived V_D/V_T ratio can be applied to minute ventilation or to a single breath. In a healthy person breathing spontaneously, because the alveolar dead space is very small, the end-tidal CO_2 tension (P_{ETCO_2}) can be substituted for $Paco_2$ in the Bohr equation to measure dead space. In the ventilated patient, alveolar dead space is often clinically significant and the absolute number calculated for dead space with this calculation will be falsely low. Similarly, P_{ETCO_2} can be substituted for P_ECO_2 to give an estimate of the alveolar dead space for a ventilated patient. This calculation is crude as an absolute measurement; however, the gradient $Paco_2$-P_{ETCO_2} is clinically an extremely useful trend. It is uncommon for airway dead space to change during the course of an anesthetic, so any increase in the $Paco_2$-P_{ETCO_2} gradient is most likely due to an increase in alveolar dead space. The $Paco_2$ is inversely related to the alveolar ventilation:

$$Paco_2 = (V_{CO2}/V_A) \times K$$

Where V_{CO2} is the total body production of CO_2 and V_A is the alveolar ventilation, and K is a constant. Because the patient's metabolic rate is usually constant during anesthesia (if body temperature is maintained), V_{CO2} is relatively constant. Changes of minute ventilation (tidal volume × respiratory rate) will usually cause a direct and inverse change in the $Paco_2$. However, this equation uses V_A (alveolar ventilation) not minute ventilation. If the dead space increases (e.g., decreased cardiac output) and minute ventilation is unchanged, alveolar ventilation will decrease and $Paco_2$ will rise.

Ventilation monitoring during anesthesia includes monitoring of expired CO_2. This is usually presented as time-based capnography. Volume-based capnography is similar but may allow for more accurate measurement of dead space and CO_2 production (Fig. 24-33).[35]

Shunt

Shunt or venous admixture is the portion of the venous blood returned to the heart that passes to the arterial circulation without being exposed to normally ventilated

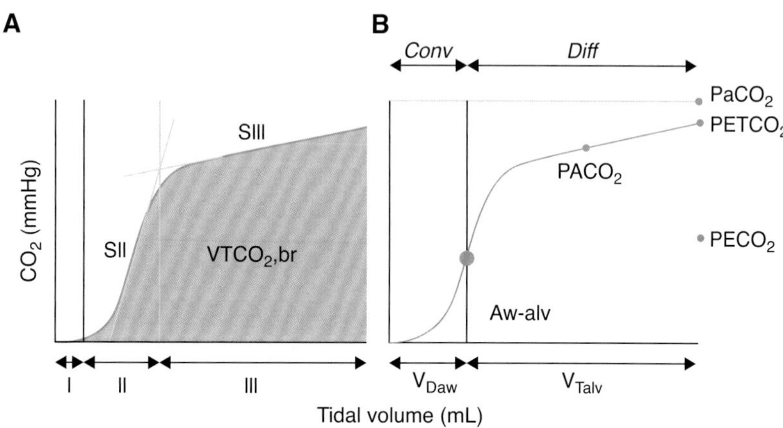

FIGURE 24-33 Capnometry. Expired CO_2 tension plotted here against tidal volume. CO_2 is most commonly displayed plotted against time. Integration of the expired gas flow and CO_2 signals allows calculation of CO_2 production ($VTCO_2$, br). The expired CO_2 curve has three phases (I, II, III) and two slopes (*S*II and *S*III). Airway dead space (V_{Daw}) can be measured from the midpoint of *S*II (Aw-alv) the airway-alveolar gas interface. The slope of *S*III increases with increased inequality of regional ventilation in the lung. V_{Talv}, alveolar tidal volume; $Paco_2$, arterial CO_2; P_{ACO_2}, mean alveolar CO_2; P_{ETCO_2}, end-tidal CO_2; P_ECO_2, mixed expired CO_2. (Reproduced with permission from Tusman G, Sipmann S, Bohm SH. Rationale of dead space measurement by volumetric capnography. *Anesth Analg.* 2012;114:866–874.)

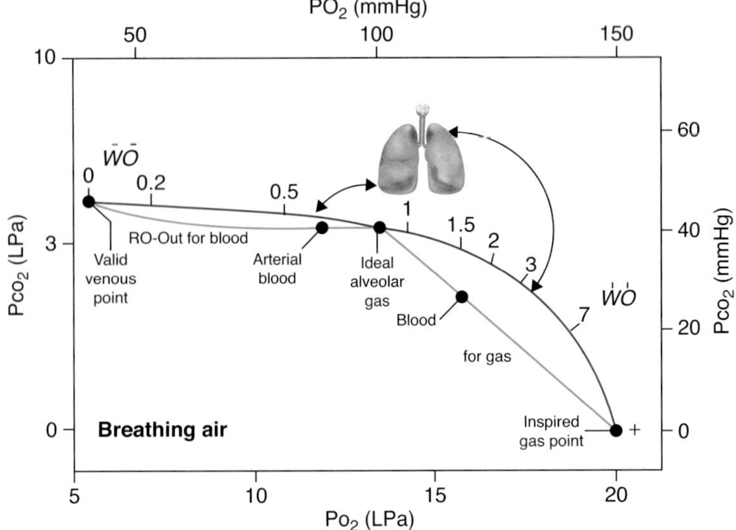

FIGURE 24-34 The *heavy line* indicated all possible values of alveolar O_2 (PAO_2) and CO_2 ($PACO_2$) with ventilation perfusion (V/Q) ratios ranging from zero (to the left, lung base) to infinity (to the right, lung apex) for a person breathing air. Mixed expired gas is a mixture of ideal alveolar gas and dead space. Arterial blood is a mixture of blood with the same gas tensions as ideal alveolar gas and shunt (mixed venous blood).

lung units. There are two major subdivisions of shunt: extrapulmonary and pulmonary. Extrapulmonary shunt is venous blood that does not pass through the lungs. There are two normal sources of this shunt: the thebesian veins in the left heart and the bronchial circulation. These normally represent <1% of the total cardiac output. Abnormal types of extrapulmonary shunt include congenital cardiac defects with right-left communications.

Pulmonary shunt is venous blood passing through lung regions with decreased or no alveolar ventilation. Figure 24-32*A* is an illustration of this concept in which shunt and dead space seem to be unrelated. However, like so much in respiratory physiology, Figure 24-32 is an oversimplification. Shunt and dead space are the extremes of the continuum of ventilation and perfusion matching (Fig. 24-34). Shunt has a large effect on Pao_2 but a limited effect on $Paco_2$. Shunt is the commonest cause of hypoxemia during anesthesia. Other causes are a low alveolar oxygen tension (e.g., hypoventilation or a low inspired O_2 concentration [FIO_2]) or a decreased mixed venous oxygen content (e.g., low cardiac output) (Fig. 24-35). The fraction of total cardiac output (Q_T) that is shunt (Q_S) can be calculated from the arterial (C_aO_2), pulmonary capillary ($C_{c'}O_2$) and mixed venous (pulmonary arterial) (CvO_2) oxygen contents. Calculation of blood oxygen contents will be discussed as follows.

$$Q_S/Q_T = C_{c'}O_2 - C_aO_2/C_{c'}O_2 - CvO_2$$

This can be remembered as the little step in oxygenation in Figure 24-35 ($C_{c'}O_2 - C_aO_2$) divided by the big step in oxygenation ($C_{c'}O_2 - C_vO_2$), so normally the shunt fraction (Q_S/Q_T) will be very small (<.05).

Alveolar–Arterial Oxygen Difference (A-aD_{O2})

Although the concept of shunt is extremely important and useful in anesthesia, it is uncommon to actually calculate the shunt fraction in patients. Similar to the calculation of the P_a-$ETCO_2$ gradient as a monitor of changes in dead space, the gradient of alveolar (PAO_2) to arterial oxygen (PaO_2) tension (A-aD_{O2}) can be used as a crude monitor of shunt. The A-aD_{O2} gradient is proportional to shunt but the absolute gradient increases as FIO_2 increases. However, if FIO_2 and PvO_2 (i.e., cardiac output and temperature) remain relatively constant, the trend of the A-aD_{O2} is a reasonably reliable monitor of changes in shunt. The PAO_2 is calculated from the theoretical "ideal" alveolar gas equation:

$$PAO_2 = P_IO_2 - PaCO_2/RQ$$

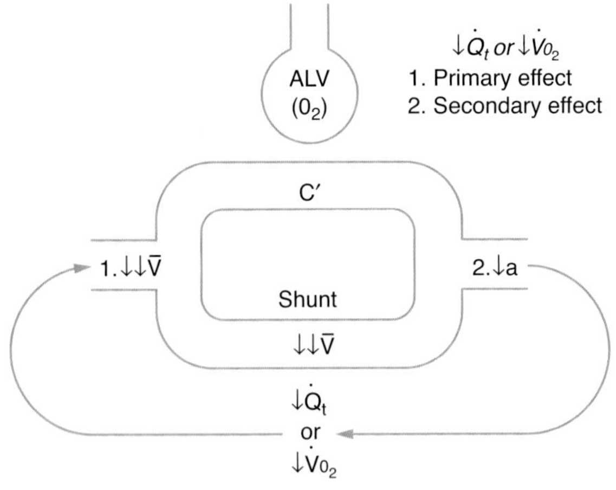

FIGURE 24-35 A simplified diagram of the effects of a decrease in mixed venous oxygen saturation *(v)* on arterial oxygenation *(a)*. Mixed venous blood passes either though ventilated lung regions (ALV), where it is oxygenated in the pulmonary capillaries *(c′)* or through nonventilated (shunt) lung regions. A decrease in mixed venous oxygen due to either a decrease in cardiac output (Qt) or an increase in oxygen consumption (V_{O2}) will pass thorough the pulmonary shunt and result in a fall in arterial oxygenation. (From *Nunn's Applied Respiratory Physiology*. 7th ed. Edinburgh, United Kingdom: Churchill Livingstone Elsevier; 2010, with permission.)

Because the volume of CO_2 produced is normally less than the volume of O_2 consumed, the $Paco_2$ cannot be substituted directly into the equation. In order to estimate the actual tension of oxygen in the ideal alveolus, the $Paco_2$ is divided by the respiratory quotient (RQ).

RQ (CO_2 production/O_2 consumption) is a dimensionless number which varies according to which substance is being consumed for fuel by the body. For carbohydrates, the approximate RQ = 1.0; for proteins, 0.9 to 0.8; and for fats, 0.7. A mixed value for RQ of 0.8 is commonly used in this equation.

The inspired PO_2 (P_IO_2) depends on the fractional concentration of inspired O_2 (Fio_2) and the barometric pressure (P_B) minus the saturated pressure of water vapor in the alveolus (P_{H2O}), which is 47 mm Hg:

$$P_IO_2 = F_{IO_2} \times (P_B - P_{H2O})$$

So the combined alveolar gas equation becomes:

$$P_{AO_2} = [F_{IO_2} \times (P_B - P_{H2O})] - Paco_2/RQ$$

For a person breathing air ($F_{IO_2} = 0.21$) at sea level (approximately $P_B = 760$ mm Hg) with a $Paco_2$ of 40 mm Hg, the ideal alveolar PO_2 calculation would be

$$P_{AO_2} = [0.21 \times (760 - 47)] - (40/0.8) = 100 \text{ mm Hg}$$

This is a simplified version of the equation which does not compensate for differences in the inspired and expired tidal volumes but is clinically useful for rapid calculation of the A-aDO_2.

Matching of Ventilation and Perfusion

Due to the combined effects of the architecture of the lung parenchyma and vasculature and gravity, there is a matching of ventilation and perfusion (V_A/Q) in the lung. Typical resting values in an adult are 4 and 5 L per minute for alveolar ventilation and cardiac output for a V_A/Q ratio of 0.8. As can be seen from Figure 24-34, this V_A/Q matching is optimal in central lung regions but becomes unequal at the apex and base of the lung. Positive pressure ventilation, decreased cardiac output, atelectasis, and many disease states will further interfere with normal V_A/Q matching.

Hypoxic Pulmonary Vasoconstriction

The lung has a unique reflex to try and minimize these perturbations in V_A/Q matching. This reflex is HPV. The pulmonary arterioles are unique in that they will respond to regional hypoxemia by constricting.[36] The arterioles in essentially all other tissues in the body vasodilate in response to hypoxemia. This reflex will tend to redirect blood flow from poorly or non-ventilated lung regions to better ventilated regions. The primary stimulus for HPV is alveolar hypoxia. HPV begins within seconds and is

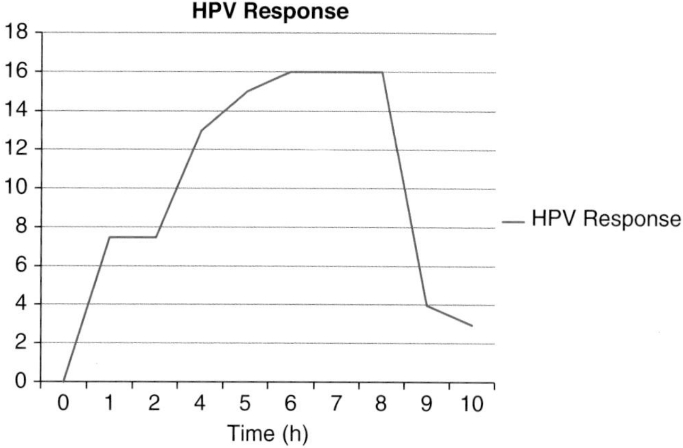

FIGURE 24-36 The relationship between hypoxic pulmonary vasoconstriction (HPV) (vertical axis) and time in hours (h) (horizontal axis) in humans exposed to isocapnic hypoxia (approximate inspired PO_2 60 mm Hg), beginning at 0h with a return to normoxia at 8h. HPV response was measured as the increase in echocardiographic right ventricular systolic pressure. Note the two-phase, rapid and slow, onset of HPV. Also note that after prolonged HPV, the pulmonary pressures do not return to baseline for several hours. (Based on data from Talbot NP, Balanos GM, Dorrington KL, et al. Two temporal components within the human pulmonary vascular response to 2h of isocapnic hypoxia. *J Appl Physiol.* 2005;98:1125–1139.)

biphasic with most of the rapid-phase response complete within 20 minutes. A slower phase begins after approximately 40 minutes and continues to increase over many hours (Fig. 24-36).[37] Of note, once the slow phase of HPV has started, the resolution of HPV will also be delayed. This has important implications for bilateral thoracic surgery cases involving sequential periods of alternating one-lung ventilation.

A low mixed venous PO_2 (PvO_2), and therefore low pulmonary artery PO_2, will augment the HPV response to a hypoxic F_{IO_2} but low PvO_2 alone has no effect.[38] As the size of the hypoxic lung segment increases, PVR increases, mixed venous oxygen tensions begin to fall, and the ability of HPV to shunt blood to the remaining well-ventilated lung becomes compromised. HPV remains intact despite chemical sympathectomy, bilateral vagotomy, and denervation of the carotid and aortic chemoreceptors.[39] Bilateral lung transplant recipients retain their hypoxic pulmonary vasoconstrictive responses.[40] HPV is augmented by conditions and chemicals which globally enhance PVR such as acidemia, hypercapnia, histamine, serotonin, and angiotensin II.

The actual cellular oxygen sensor for HPV has yet to be determined. Current research implicates the mitochondria of the pulmonary vascular smooth muscle cell as the main site. Numerous biochemical studies have indicated that selective interruption of the mitochondrial electron transport chain complexes can impair HPV. A unifying theme seems to be the hypoxia-induced change in the level of oxygen free radicals and hydrogen peroxide in the smooth muscle cell. These changes affect the release of calcium from the sarcoplasmic reticulum and the voltage-dependent membrane conductance to potassium resulting in depolarization and contraction of the smooth muscle, hence vasoconstriction.[41] The response may involve decreased production of nitric oxide by the pulmonary epithelium and endothelium.[42]

Oxygen Transport

Oxygen diffuses into the plasma of the pulmonary capillary blood, driven by its concentration gradient from the alveolus. This oxygen is then taken up by partially desaturated hemoglobin (Hb) molecules in the red blood cells of mixed venous blood to form oxyhemoglobin. Due to the high affinity of Hb for oxygen, a large proportion (normally >98%) of the total oxygen in arterial blood is carried within the red blood cells as oxyhemoglobin. Less than 2% is circulated as dissolved oxygen. However, it is actually the tension of the oxygen dissolved in plasma (PaO_2) that is measured in an arterial (or venous [PvO_2]) blood gas sample. There is a dynamic equilibrium between the oxygen dissolved in plasma and that bound to Hb within the red blood cells. The quantity of oxygen dissolved in blood is directly proportional to its partial pressure. For each mm Hg of PO_2, there is 0.003 mL of dissolved oxygen per 100 mL of blood. Thus, for a PaO_2 of 100 mm Hg, there will be 0.3 mL of dissolved O_2 in 100 mL of blood. This compares to approximately 20 mL of O_2 bound to Hb in the red cells and is usually not of clinical importance. However, this dissolved oxygen can approach 1.5 mL with an FIO_2 of 1.0 and can be clinically even more important in hyperbaric environments.

Normal adult hemoglobin (HbA) is a four-protein molecule with two α chains and two β chains. Each protein chain is attached to one heme unit (Fig. 24-37). Heme is an iron-porphyrin complex capable of reversible binding to one oxygen molecule at its ferrous (Fe^{++}) atom. As each of the four heme units binds an oxygen molecule, it causes a change in the shape of the Hb molecule which, in turn, causes the other heme units to be more exposed. The result is that each successive oxygen molecule is bound less (or more) tightly and released more (or less) easily. So the release of oxygen by Hb as the PO_2 in the surrounding plasma falls (and conversely the uptake of O_2 by Hb as the PO_2 rises) is not in a linear correlation with PO_2 but curvilinear producing the oxyhemoglobin saturation curve (or dissociation curve) (Fig. 24-38).

PO_2 values of 40, 50, and 60 will correspond (approximately) to saturations of 70%, 80%, and 90%.

The oxygen content of blood can be calculated if the PaO_2, the concentration of Hb in the blood, and the percent saturation of Hb is known. Pure HbO_2 will contain 1.39 mL/g. The saturation of the Hb in a blood sample is measured spectrophotometrically by comparing the absorption of two different wavelengths of near infrared light; one wavelength at which oxyhemoglobin (HbO_2) and deoxyhemoglobin have approximately the same absorbance (typically 940 nm) and one at which they differ widely (typically 660 nm). Pulse oximetry uses the same principle but corrects for the peak arterial phase of a capillary blood flow by subtracting for the baseline venous flow absorption. Modern rapid blood gas analyzers often estimate O_2 saturation based on measured PO_2 and standard oxyhemoglobin curves corrected for pH.

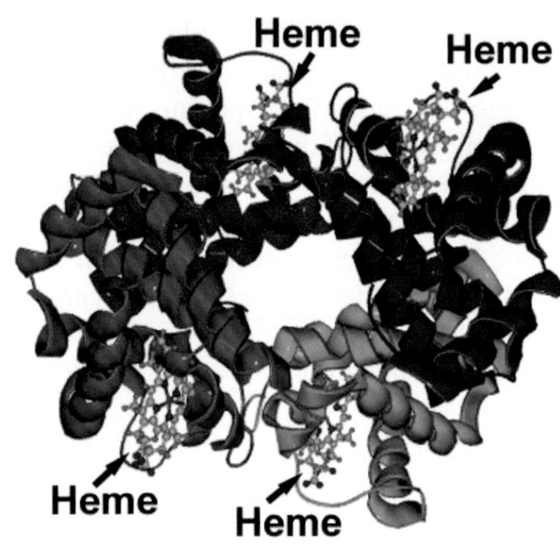

FIGURE 24-37 An oxyhemoglobin molecule is composed of two paired proteins, for hemoglobin A, these are two α chains and two β chains. Each globin chain is bound to a heme group capable of binding a single oxygen molecule.

$$\text{The content of oxygen in blood} = \text{dissolved } O_2 + O_2 \text{ bound as } HbO_2$$

$$\text{For 100 mL blood} = (PO_2 \times 0.003) + (\text{Hb concentration} \times \text{saturation}/100 \times 1.39)$$

For a patient with a Hb of 15 g/dL a PO_2 of 100 and saturation of 99% the blood, O_2 content would be = (100 × 0.003) + (15 × 0.99 × 1.39) = 0.3 + 20.6 = 20.9 mL O_2/100 mL blood. Mixed venous blood commonly has a saturation of approximately 70%, thus an O_2 content of 15 mL/100 mL.

Shifts of the Oxyhemoglobin Desaturation Curve

There are multiple different normal and abnormal variants of the Hb molecule. Each of these different Hb molecules has a different oxyhemoglobin desaturation curve (see Fig. 24-38). By convention, to compare these curves, the PO_2 at the point of 50% saturation (P_{50}) is used as a reference. For HbA, the P_{50} is 26 mm Hg. Fetal hemoglobin (HbF) has 2 α chains and 2 γ chains. It is the major form of Hb present at birth and is replaced by HbA over the first 6 months of life. HbF has a P_{50} of 19 so it is "left-shifted" from HbA. Because its affinity for O_2 is stronger than HbA, O_2 is preferentially drawn from the mother's

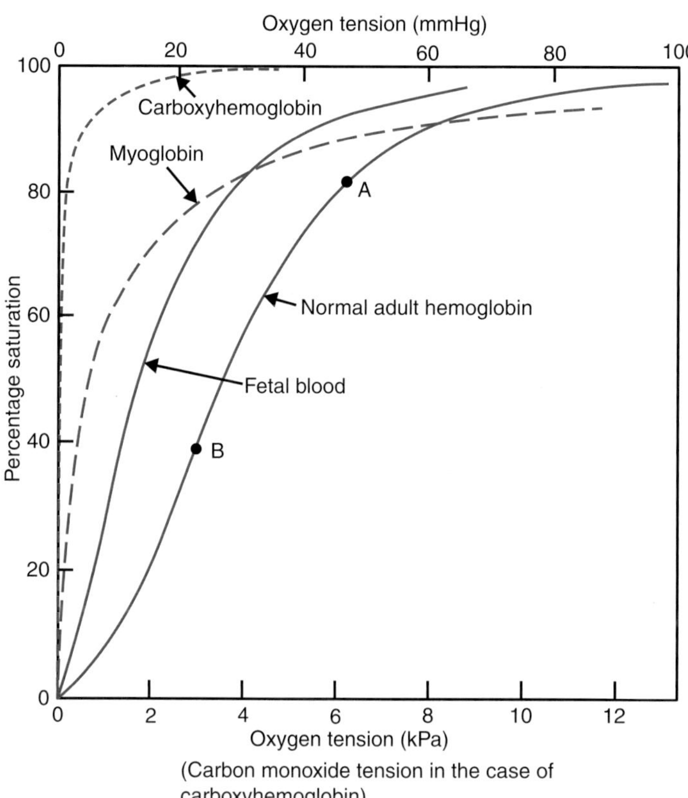

FIGURE 24-38 Dissociation curves of normal adult (HbA) and fetal (HbF) hemoglobin. Curves for myoglobin and carboxyhemoglobin are shown for comparison.

blood to that of the fetus. Carboxyhemoglobin (COHb) is an abnormal Hb formed when carbon monoxide binds with heme. Carbon monoxide displaces O_2 from heme and it shifts the oxyhemoglobin curve to the extreme left so that oxygen is not released to the tissues and cellular hypoxia results. The Fe^{++} atom in heme can be oxidized to Fe^{+++} by a variety of drugs and chemicals such as nitrates. This forms a type of Hb called methemoglobin and will not bind O_2.

The normal HbA oxygen saturation curve shifts to the left or right secondary to a variety of physiologic changes. An increase in hydrogen ion (H^+) concentration (i.e., a decrease in serum pH), an increase in body temperature (T) and an increase in 2,3-diphosphoglycerate (DPG) shift the curve to the right. 2,3-DPG is a compound normally present in red blood cells that tends to decrease the affinity of Hb for O_2. It is increased by exposure to a low environmental O_2 (e.g., at altitude) or in anemia. This can be remembered as DP**G**, **H+**, and **T** shift the Hb oxygen saturation curve to the right (ri**GHT**). And their converses (decrease DPG, alkalosis, hypothermia) shift the curve to the left. In most situations of physiologic stress (i.e., hypercarbia, acidosis, etc.), it is advantageous to have the HbO_2 curve shifted to the right and to increase oxygen unloading to the tissues.

There is normally no significant oxygen storage capacity in the body. This is unlike carbon dioxide, which has large stores in the body (see the following text). Oxygen is like rocket fuel and can be toxic to issues in excess over a prolonged period. An average-size adult's oxygen consumption is approximately 250 mL per minute. The total content of oxygen in their blood will be approximately 700 to 800 mL and in their FRC 500 mL (breathing air). Tissue hypoxia will begin very quickly if the oxygen supply is cut off. Washing out the FRC with an F_{IO_2} of 1.0 can potentially provide a reserve of 2,500 mL of O_2, a supply adequate for several minutes of apnea.

Carbon Dioxide Transport

Carbon dioxide (CO_2) is the main product of aerobic metabolism of proteins, fats, and carbohydrates. Carbon dioxide is moderately soluble in all body fluids (approximately 20 times more soluble than oxygen) and diffuses down its concentration gradient from its site of intracellular production into the capillary and venous blood. Similar to oxygen, the tension of dissolved CO_2 in blood is the portion measured in blood gas analysis. As can been seen in Figure 24-39, CO_2 transport is like an upside-down iceberg with the dissolved CO_2 as the only visible portion. But, this is only a small proportion of the total CO_2 in the blood. The majority of carbon dioxide is transformed to bicarbonate ion in the following reaction:

$$CO_2 + H_2O = H_2CO_3 = H^+ + HCO_3^-$$

The first step of this reaction is slow in plasma but progresses rapidly in the presence of the enzyme carbonic anhydrase, which is present in red blood cells. The majority of CO_2 in the blood follows this pathway and is transported in the blood as bicarbonate (HCO_3^-) after diffusion into

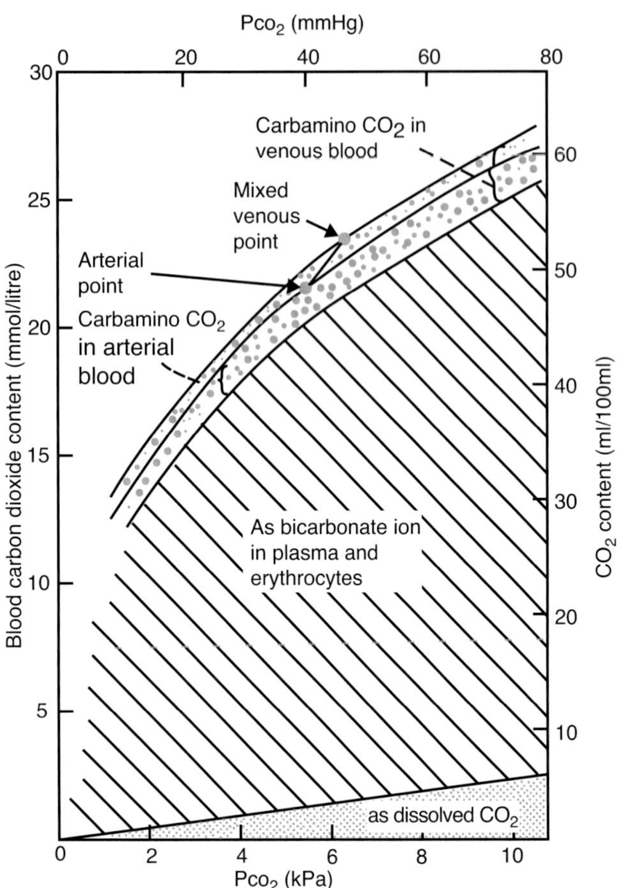

FIGURE 24-39 Transport of CO_2 in blood compared to the measured CO_2 tension. The tension dissolved CO_2 at the bottom is measured in blood gas analysis but it is only the tip of the upside-down iceberg. The majority of CO_2 is transported as dissolved bicarbonate in the plasma and red blood cells. These vary with PCO_2 but are little affected by the oxygenation of hemoglobin. Carbamino transport of CO_2 is strongly influenced by the oxygenation of Hb (the Haldane effect). (From *Nunn's Applied Respiratory Physiology*. 7th ed. Edinburgh, United Kingdom: Churchill Livingstone Elsevier; 2010, with permission).

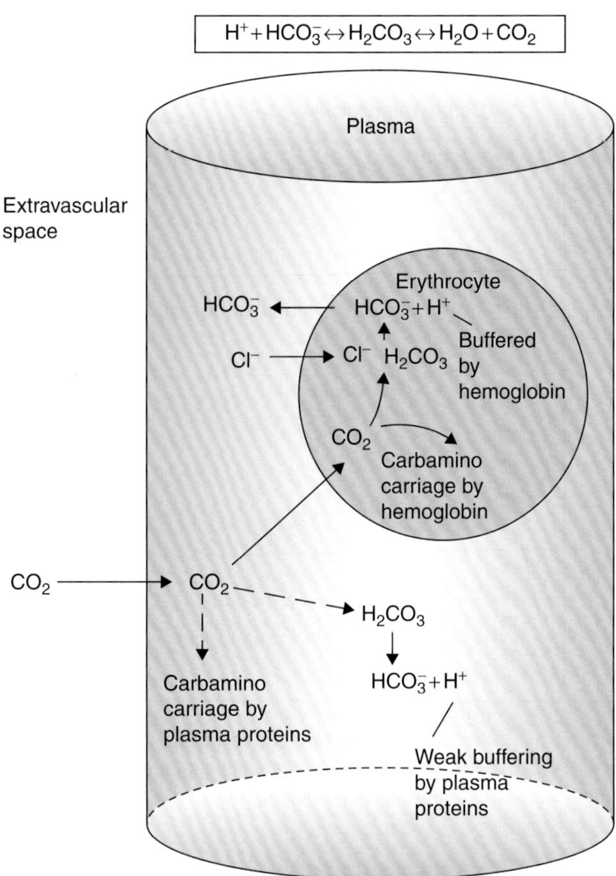

FIGURE 24-40 Carbon dioxide (CO_2) enters the plasma in molecular form from the tissues. The majority of CO_2 is transformed into bicarbonate (HCO_3^-) in the red blood cells; this reaction is catalyzed by carbonic anhydrase. A small proportion of plasma CO_2 is attached to plasma proteins as carbamino compounds or directly converted to HCO_3^- in the plasma. Some CO_2 in the red cell is also attached to hemoglobin as carbamino compounds. The excess hydrogen (H^+) ions generated in the red blood cell are transferred to the plasma in exchange for chloride ion (Cl^-) This is called the "chloride shift." (From *Nunn's Applied Respiratory Physiology*. 7th ed. Edinburgh, United Kingdom: Churchill Livingstone Elsevier; 2010, with permission).

red cells and enzymatic conversion (Fig. 24-40). A small portion of the CO_2 is transported in the blood combined to Hb as carbamino compounds. Blood with lower oxyhemoglobin saturation (i.e., venous blood) is capable of carrying more CO_2 than blood with well-saturated Hb (i.e., arterial). This is known as the Haldane effect. The Haldane effect is complicated and involves both increased carbamino-CO_2 carrying by desaturated Hb and also increased buffering of intracellular H+ by deoxygenated Hb, which is less acidic than oxygenated Hb.

There are two effects that are involved in the physiology of gas transport in the blood. They can be remembered as:

1. Shifts of the **OH**b curve due to changes in H^+, the Bohr effect: (b**OH**r)
2. Changes in CO_2 transport due to changes in oxygen saturation, the Haldane effect (the other one)

Because the volume of CO_2 in blood is large compared to the volume of O_2, for changes of approximately equal volumes of gas in the blood, the PCO_2 will change much less than the PO_2. For example, the volume production of CO_2 is approximately 0.8 of the oxygen consumption. However, the difference in PCO_2 between venous and arterial blood is normally only 5 mm Hg, whereas the difference between arterial and venous PO_2 is typically 60 mm Hg.

Respiratory Control

Central Nervous System

The stimulus for normal breathing is generated spontaneously by a combination of at least six groups of neurons in the medulla of the brainstem. Each neuronal group seems to be primarily responsible for one phase of the respiratory cycle: early inspiration, late inspiration, early expiration, etc. The function of these neuronal groups is primarily under the control of the central chemoreceptor area, also in the medulla. The central chemoreceptor increases or decreases minute ventilation according to the cerebral spinal fluid pH to maintain normocapnia[43] (Fig. 24-41).

Dissolved CO_2 in plasma diffuses easily across the blood–brain barrier into the cerebrospinal fluid (CSF) where it interacts with H_2O to form H^+ and HCO_3^-. The H^+ concentration in the CSF is the primary controller for normal minute ventilation. H^+ and HCO_3^- in plasma cross the blood–brain barrier very slowly. The brainstem central chemoreceptor is acutely sensitive to changes in pH. Normally, an awake individual's $Paco_2$ will vary less than 3 mm Hg. If the Pao_2 is normal, minute ventilation will increase 2 to 3 L per minute for each 1 mm Hg increase in $Paco_2$ to restore arterial and CSF pH to normal levels. Ventilation will increase in a linear fashion as $Paco_2$ rises until a maximal stimulation somewhere over a $Paco_2$ of 100 mm Hg is reached or until the respiratory mechanics will no longer permit an increase in minute ventilation. At levels over 100 mm Hg, dissolved CO_2 in the CSF begins to exert a narcotic effect on the CNS.

The central chemoreceptor is acutely sensitive to CNS depressants. Opioids, sedatives, and most general anesthetics decrease the respiratory response to hypercapnia.

Peripheral Chemoreceptors

The peripheral chemoreceptors are located primarily in the carotid bodies at the bifurcation of the carotid arteries and also in aortic bodies above and below the aortic arch. These receptors respond primarily to changes in Pao_2.[44] They function as a backup system and in the normal individual do not have a primary role in control of ventilation. The innervation of the carotid bodies is via the glossopharyngeal nerve (CN IX) and the aortic bodies via the vagus nerve (CN X). Although there is some tonic activity from these peripheral chemoreceptors, they do not normally stimulate ventilation until the Pao_2 falls to below a threshold of approximately 70 to 80 mm Hg. This threshold will be lowered in individuals who are adapted to altitude and in some chronic respiratory or congenital hypoxic cardiac diseases. The nerve stimulus from the peripheral chemoreceptors has two complementary actions

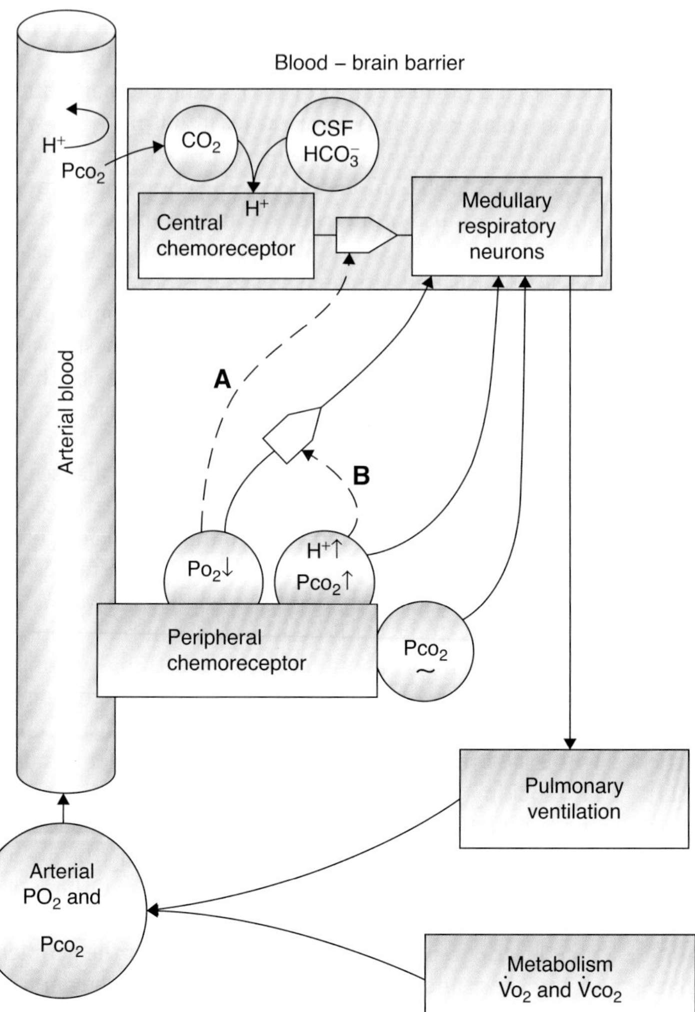

FIGURE 24-41 A diagram of the connections between individual components of the chemical and neural portions of the physiologic control of respiration (see text for details). (From *Nunn's Applied Respiratory Physiology*. 7th ed. Edinburgh, United Kingdom: Elsevier; 2010, with permission).

to increase ventilation. Primarily, there is a direct effect on the medullary respiratory neurons. Secondarily, there is an effect to increase the sensitivity to the stimulus of the central chemoreceptor to CSF pH (*dashed line A* in Fig. 24-41). The peripheral chemoreceptors also are sensitive to changes in arterial pH and $PaCO_2$, and acidosis will increase the hypoxic drive (*dashed line B* in Fig. 24-41). The hypoxic drive due to the peripheral chemoreceptors is decreased by volatile anesthetics, even in very low concentrations such as 0.1 minimum alveolar concentration (MAC), which are often present immediately after recovery from general anesthesia.[45] Although the hypercapnic response is also blunted in a dose-dependent fashion by volatile anesthetics, the response to hypoxemia is even more profoundly blocked.

Because of the combined effects of residual opioids on the central chemoreceptors and the blunting of hypoxic drive by trace amounts of volatile anesthetics, it is a common practice to initially administer supplemental oxygen to patients in the recovery room after general anesthesia then to follow the oxygen saturation using pulse oximetry as the supplemental oxygen is decreased prior to discharge. In the absence of shunt, with supplemental oxygen to raise the FIO_2 to 0.4, a patient's minute ventilation can fall temporarily to one-third of its normal value without significant hypoxemia (however, the $PaCO_2$ will rise and the pH will fall).

Other Neural Connections to the Medullary Respiratory Centers

The entire airway from the mucosal lining of the nose and mouth to the distal bronchi has both afferent and efferent neural connections to the central respiratory neurons. These connections are responsible for many of the normal respiratory reflexes such as the phasic inspiratory dilation of the upper airway during inspiration to maintain patency of the supra-glottic airway. This reflex activity is easily obtunded by CNS sedatives and anesthetics and is responsible for much of the upper airway obstruction seen during anesthesia and compounds the airway obstruction in patients with obstructive sleep apnea (OSA). Irritants in the airway trigger cough and sneeze reflexes via these neuronal connections.

The lung has stretch receptors that, in the nonsedated state, respond to regional changes in compliance associated with atelectasis by triggering a recruitment maneuver such as a sigh or a yawn (if you are yawning as you read this, hopefully it is to recruit your lungs and not because the content is boring). Passive stretching of the lungs can result in either inhibition of inspiration (Herring-Breuer reflex) or gasping (Heads reflex) depending on the clinical context.

The pulmonary capillaries are densely innervated by unmyelinated nerves (C fibers). This innervation is not important during normal ventilation but may be responsible for causing a sensation of dyspnea when the capillaries become engorged during congestive heart failure.

Abnormal Breathing Patterns

Abnormal patterns of breathing are rare. There are several recognized abnormal patterns which involve dysfunction of the central chemoreceptors. Primary alveolar hypoventilation syndrome (Ondine's curse) is a congenital insensitivity of the central chemoreceptor to changes in CSF pH. It results in apnea and hypoventilation, particularly during sleep. It can be treated with noninvasive ventilation and diaphragmatic pacing. Cheyne-Stokes respiration is a pattern of 10- to 20-second periods of apnea followed by periods of hyperventilation.[46] It is seen in some patients with CNS damage or severe illness and also during adaptation to altitude. It is caused by a delayed response interval in the central chemoreceptor. Cheyne-Stokes is the most severe form of periodic breathing, which is seen to some degree in neonates and the elderly and during sleep at all ages.

Altered Physiologic Conditions

Anesthesia

Nunn[47] showed that during anesthesia and spontaneous ventilation, gas exchange was altered by shunt and inhomogeneous V/Q ratios. He concluded from his observations that a normal range of PaO_2 could be maintained if the alveolar PO_2 (PAO_2) was at least 200 mm Hg, which would require an FIO_2 of at least 35%. Brismar and colleagues[48] in 1985 demonstrated using computed tomography that within 5 minutes of the induction of anesthesia, dependent regions of the lung developed an increase in density consistent with atelectasis. It is now accepted that this occurs in dependent lung regions in approximately 90% of patients who undergo general anesthesia using a wide variety of agents. Epidural anesthesia may be the one modality that appears to cause very little atelectasis and no change in V_A/Q matching or oxygenation.

The near universal finding of rapid lung collapse upon induction of anesthesia and the rapid reappearance after discontinuation of PEEP has led to the conclusion that atelectasis is due to compression of lung tissue rather than alveolar gas absorption behind occluded airways.[49] The fluoroscopic study by Froese and Bryan[50] of diaphragmatic motion of spontaneously breathing volunteers demonstrated that in the supine position the dependent portion of the diaphragm has the greatest displacement with each breath. Initiation of paralysis with neuromuscular blocking agents and positive pressure ventilation creates a reversal of this motion with the nondependent or superior aspect of the diaphragm undergoing the greatest displacement with each ventilated breath.[50] Others have confirmed and extended these observations using computed tomography.[51] It is now apparent that the geometry of the chest and diaphragm is altered under general anesthesia with relaxation of the chest wall and a marked cephalad displacement of the most dorsal portion of the diaphragm at end-expiration.

Absorption atelectasis can occur when the rate of gas uptake into the blood exceeds the rate of ventilation of the alveolus. The extreme condition is total occlusion of an airway which isolates the alveolar gas in the distal alveolar and respiratory airways. The gas pressure within this compartment initially is nearly at atmospheric pressure. However, given that mixed venous blood continues to perfuse this area, and the fact that the sum of the gas partial pressures within mixed venous blood is subatmospheric, gas uptake from the occluded compartment by blood continues and the alveoli collapses. Computer modeling has demonstrated that the rate of gas absorption from unventilated areas is dependent on the initial FIO_2.[52] However, in many clinical situations, the airway is not completely occluded but rather ventilation to an area becomes severely reduced. If the inspired V_A/Q ratio of a respiratory unit is reduced, a point is reached where the rate at which inspired gas enters the alveolus is exactly balanced by the gas uptake into the blood. If V_A/Q ratio drops below this critical equilibrium point, the volume of the alveolus declines and collapse ensues. Again, this process is augmented by the presence of a high PAO_2 and a rapid rate of gas uptake.

Loss of alveolar surfactant may play a role in alveolar instability at low alveolar volumes and collapse. The rapidity of alveolar collapse following alveolar recruitment maneuvers and discontinuation of PEEP has suggested that atelectasis per se may interfere with surfactant production. Therefore, atelectatic regions of the lung may be predisposed to recurrence of collapse because of reduced levels of surfactant, increased alveolar surface tension and, the aforementioned mechanisms, all contributing to reduced alveolar volumes. The effects of anesthetic drugs on HPV and ventilation/perfusion matching will be considered in the next chapter on Respiratory Pharmacology.

Position

In the spontaneously breathing patient, awake or during anesthesia, the majority of gas exchange is due to caudal displacement of the diaphragm, which occurs primarily in the dorsal portions of the thoraces. During deep anesthesia and paralysis, the diaphragm becomes relatively flaccid. The weight of the abdominal contents pushes cranially on the dorsal diaphragm and during inspiration, with positive pressure ventilation, gas preferentially distributes to the now more compliant ventral portions of the lungs.[53] The distribution of perfusion remains largely unchanged with predominance to the central and dependent portions of the lung. Thus, matching of ventilation/perfusion is decreased with induction of anesthesia and further decreased with paralysis and positive pressure ventilation. The addition of low levels of PEEP (<10 cm H_2O, after recruitment) will usually ameliorate this mismatch by slightly overdistending ventral lung regions but moving dependent lung regions to a more compliant portion of their pressure-volume curve.

During anesthesia and positive pressure ventilation in the prone position, the majority of diaphragm displacement during inspiration will remain in the dorsal (now the nondependent) portions of the thoraces and ventilation will be more homogeneously distributed in the lungs compared to the supine position. Matching of ventilation to perfusion will usually be superior in the prone position when compared with the supine position. However, unlike the supine position, the addition of PEEP in the prone position may lead to deterioration in ventilation/perfusion matching.[54] This applies to patients with normal lungs. This is unlike the situation in the patient with ARDS. In these patients in the supine position, pulmonary edema collects in the parenchyma of the dorsal portions of the lung. The combination of prone position and PEEP may lead to a more favorable matching of ventilation to perfusion, although this effect may be transient. The effects of the lateral position will be discussed in the "One-Lung Ventilation" section.

Obesity

The increased weight of the abdominal contents and chest wall impose a restrictive ventilatory pattern on the respiratory system with a decrease of all lung volumes but a preservation of the FEV_1/FVC ratio.[55] This is primarily important to the anesthesiologist because of the fall in FRC, which leads to increased venoarterial shunt and a tendency to desaturate during induction and maintenance of anesthesia and in the postoperative period. The FRC of an awake mildly obese patient of body mass index (BMI) 30 kg/m^2 will be 75% of predicted for a similar person but with a BMI of 20 and for a patient with a BMI >40 the FRC will be <66% predicted. Early studies of PEEP during anesthesia in obese patients showed mixed results in terms of improving oxygenation. This is due to the rapid development of atelectasis in these patients and the inability of PEEP, by itself, to correct atelectasis. As can be seen in Figure 24-42, the combination of a recruitment maneuver and 10 cm H_2O PEEP can eliminate atelectasis in a morbidly obese patient. The challenge in respiratory management of the obese patient perioperatively is to minimize the fall in FRC. This can be done with a variety of methods including the use of regional anesthesia/analgesia, avoiding long-acting muscle relaxants, positioning, and the use of postoperative CPAP.

Sleep-Disordered Breathing

Approximately 20% of the population has disorders of respiration during sleep ranging from simple snoring to OSA. These disorders all involve variable degrees of upper airway obstruction and apnea during normal sleep. OSA is defined by more than five episodes per hour of apnea, each >10 seconds. It is often combined with periods of hypopnea in the sleep apnea hypopnea syndrome (SAHS). OSA may be exacerbated by fluid shifts to the upper body

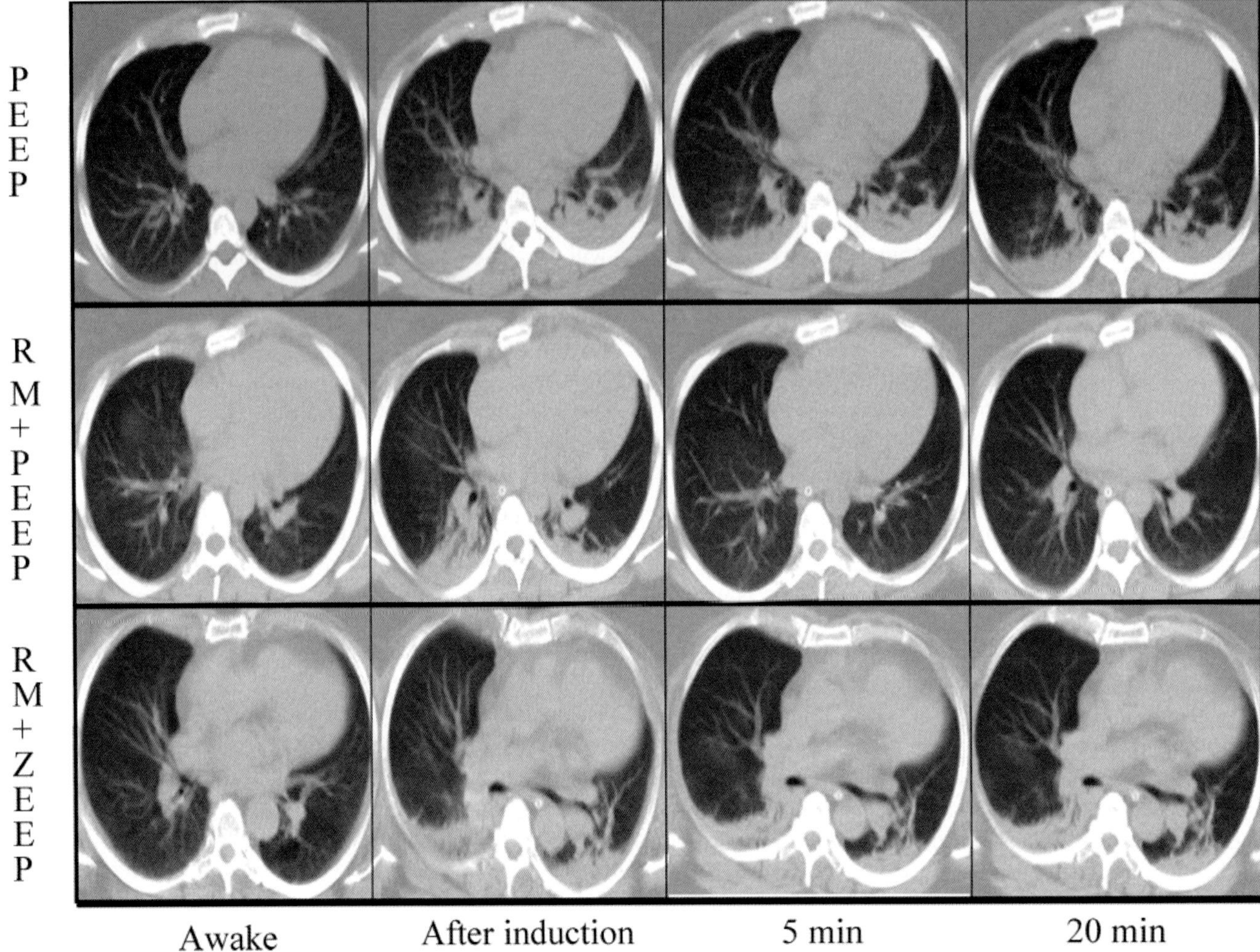

FIGURE 24-42 Each row is a representative computerized tomography scan 1 cm above the diaphragm in three different morbidly obese patients during anesthesia. The patient on the top row received 10 cm H_2O positive end-expiratory pressure (PEEP). The patient in the middle row received a recruitment maneuver (RM) (55 cm $H_2O \times 10$ seconds) after induction plus PEEP 10 cm H_2O. The patient in the bottom row received an RM and then zero end-expiratory pressure (ZEEP).

from the legs during sleep in patients with sedentary lifestyles.[56] The disturbance of normal sleep leads to daytime somnolence and the periods of hypoxia may contribute to cardiovascular morbidity. Treatments may include weight loss, CPAP devices, and upper airway surgery.[57] The obesity hypoventilation syndrome is a combination of obesity, hypoventilation, and severe OSA, which has been called the ***Pickwickian*** syndrome.[58]

Exercise

Normal oxygen consumption at rest is approximately 200 to 250 mL per minute (3 to 4 mL/kg per minute) for an adult; this is termed ***one metabolic equivalent*** (MET). Quick walking or climbing one flight of stairs requires 4 METs, bowling 8 METs, and competitive cross-country skiing 14 METs. Olympic rowers, skiers, and cyclists may exceed 80 mL/kg per minute oxygen consumption (20 METs).[59] To achieve this increase in oxygen consumption requires matching increases in minute ventilation and cardiac output. At a certain point, the increases in ventilation and cardiac output will not be able to supply adequate oxygen to the tissues for aerobic metabolism and further increase in muscle activity will require anaerobic metabolism producing lactic acid. This is called the ***anaerobic threshold***. It is most often the accumulation of lactate in tissues causing muscle dysfunction which limits prolonged exercise and not a limitation on minute ventilation or cardiac output. Exercise training raises the maximal oxygen consumption (VO_{2max}), the anaerobic threshold, and the tolerance for lactic acidosis. Exercise testing is an established medical procedure to measure a patient's VO_{2max} or to distinguish between respiratory and cardiac limitations in exercise capacity. VO_{2max} has been shown to be a useful preoperative test to identify patients at increased risk of complications from pulmonary resection surgery (preoperative VO_{2max} <15 to 20 mL/kg per minute) but has not been as well validated for other types of surgical procedure.[15] A useful estimate of a COPD patient's VO_{2max} can be made from the maximal distance they can walk in 6 minutes the "6-minute walk test" (6MWT). If the distance in meters is divided by 30, the result is an approximation of the VO_{2max} (e.g., 6MWT distance = 450 m, VO_{2max} = 450/30 = 15 mL/kg per minute).[60]

Altered Barometric Pressures

Altitude: The ambient PO_2 decreases proportionally as the barometric pressure falls with increases in altitude. The PO_2 is 149 mm Hg at sea level, 122 at 5,000 ft of elevation (e.g., Denver), and may be as low as 108 mm Hg in a commercial airliner pressurized to 8,000 ft (maximum permitted altitude-equivalent). For comparison, on the summit of Mount Everest, the PO_2 is 47 mm Hg (63,000 ft). There are both acute and chronic adaptations to the hypoxia associated with altitude. Primarily, the rapid adaptation involves hyperventilation, driven by the peripheral chemoreceptors to decrease the alveolar PCO_2 and thus increase the alveolar PAO_2. The secondary alkalinization of blood and CSF returns to normal after several days at altitude as bicarbonate is excreted. The increased pulmonary pressures due to HPV triggered by hypoxia can lead to high altitude pulmonary edema. This can be treated with oxygen, diuretics, and pulmonary vasodilators. Increased cerebral blood flow due to hypoxia is opposed in part by the cerebral vasoconstriction due to hypocapnia but may lead to cerebral edema. Chronic acclimatization to altitude involves a variety of cellular and metabolic changes such as a resetting of the peripheral chemoreceptors and polycythemia.

Anesthesia at mild elevations is generally uncomplicated as long as oxygen saturation is monitored and adequate supplemental oxygen is provided. This can be a problem with nitrous oxide. Most modern commercial vaporizers deliver reasonably accurate dosages of volatile anesthetics at modest elevations (<6,000 ft). Pressure in the air-filled cuff of an endotracheal tube or laryngeal mask airway will increase and decrease significantly with changes in ambient pressure, which may be associated with medical air transport.[61]

Hyperbaric oxygen in medical practice is delivered in a chamber pressurized to 2 to 3 times atmospheric pressure (ATM) (i.e., 1,400 to 2,100 mm Hg). Treatments are given with a high FIO_2, usually from a tight-fitting mask for several hours and repeated as required.[62] Indications include gas embolism, decompression sickness, necrotizing soft tissue infections, and carbon monoxide poisoning. At high FIO_2 levels, above 2 ATM, hyperoxia may cause convulsions. Prolonged exposure to a high PAO_2 causes pulmonary oxygen toxicity and a restrictive lung disease. A high PAO_2 in the neonate can cause retrolental fibroplasias, damaging the retinal of the eye.

Age

Infants and children: The overall compliance of the respiratory system is low in newborns and increases until late adolescence. Alveoli at birth have a lower amount of elastin than adults and a decreased amount of surfactant leading to decreased lung compliance. However, the compliance of the chest wall in newborns and infants is very high due to the absence of ossification of cartilages. This predisposes infants to a significant fall in FRC during anesthesia. In the awake state, FRC is maintained above CC in infants by a rapid respiratory rate. The respiratory muscles of infants have a lower percentage of fatigue-resistant type I fibers and they are more prone to respiratory fatigue. All airways are proportionately smaller in infants than adults and airway resistance is higher, resulting in increased work of breathing at rest and particularly during upper or lower airway infections (e.g., croup). The narrowest portion of the upper airway is at the cricoid cartilage until age 5 years.[63]

Control of breathing in the newborn is unique. Hypoxia initially causes increased ventilation, as in the adult, but then leads to a decrease in ventilation.[64] This is more exaggerated in preterm infants. Oxygen consumption is higher in newborns than adults (6 to 8 mL/kg/minute). HbF predominates at birth until 3 to 6 months of age. HbF hemoglobin has a low P_{50} (18 to 19 mm Hg), which increases oxygen loading in the placenta but decreases oxygen unloading in the tissues.

The elderly: changes in the respiratory system with age include decrease of muscle tone in the dilators of the pharynx, predisposing to upper airway obstruction during anesthesia.[65] There is a loss of the pulmonary vascular bed, which results in an increase of PVR and a 30% increase in mean pulmonary artery pressures and an increase in the alveolar dead space. The lung parenchyma loses elastic support tissue resulting in an increase of lung compliance, but the chest wall increases in stiffness so the net effect is an overall decrease in respiratory system compliance. With the loss of structural support of peripheral airways, the CC increases significantly; this is the change which has major anesthetic implications. The fall of FRC below CC leads to increased venoarterial shunt and is responsible for the decrease in PaO_2 with age. The mean PaO_2 of healthy patients will decline to approximately 80 mm Hg at age 70, after which it remains stable. The responsiveness of both central and peripheral chemoreceptors to hypercarbia and hypoxemia decreases with age.

Chronic Respiratory Disease

Chronic respiratory disease is commonly divided into two major categories: obstructive and restrictive. In obstructive disease, the FEV_1/FVC ratio is typically less than normal (<80%) with a decreased FEV_1. Restrictive disease typically has a normal FEV_1/FVC ratio and a decreased FEV_1. There is some overlap, with some patients (e.g., cystic fibrosis) showing a mixed obstructive/restrictive pattern. Severity of these diseases can be graded according to the FEV_1 as a percent of predicted values: mild, FEV_1 >70%; moderate, 50% to 70%; severe, 30% to 50%; and very severe <30%.

COPD incorporates three disorders: emphysema, peripheral airways disease, and chronic bronchitis. Any individual patient may have one or all of these conditions, but the dominant clinical feature is impairment of expiratory airflow. Life expectancy may be less than 3 years in severe COPD patients >60 years of age. Mild COPD patients should not have significant dyspnea, hypoxemia, or hypercarbia and other causes should be considered if these are present.[66]

Some moderate and severe COPD patients have an elevated $PaCO_2$ at rest. It is not possible to differentiate these "CO_2 retainers" from nonretainers on the basis of history, physical examination, or spirometric pulmonary function testing. This CO_2 retention seems to be related to an inability to maintain the increased work of respiration (Wresp) required to keep the $PaCO_2$ normal in patients with mechanically inefficient pulmonary function and not primarily due to an alteration of respiratory control mechanisms. The $PaCO_2$ rises in these patients when supplemental FIO_2 is administered due to a relative decrease in alveolar ventilation and an increase in alveolar dead space and shunt by the redistribution of perfusion away from lung areas of relatively normal V/Q matching to areas of very low V/Q ratio because regional HPV is decreased and also due to the Haldane effect.[67] However, supplemental oxygen must be administered to these patients postoperatively to prevent the hypoxemia associated with the unavoidable fall in FRC. The attendant rise in $PaCO_2$ should be anticipated and monitored. To identify these patients preoperatively, all moderate or severe COPD patients need an arterial blood gas analysis. Also, it is important to know the patient's baseline preoperative $PaCO_2$ to guide weaning if mechanical ventilation becomes necessary in the postoperative period.

COPD patients desaturate more frequently and severely than normal patients during sleep.[68] This is due to the rapid/shallow breathing pattern that occurs in all patients during REM sleep. In COPD patients breathing air, this causes a significant increase in the respiratory dead space/tidal volume (V_D/V_T) ratio and a fall in alveolar oxygen tension (PAO_2) and PaO_2. This is not the SAHS. There is no increased incidence of SAHS in COPD.

Right ventricular dysfunction occurs in up to 50% of moderate to severe COPD patients.[69] The dysfunctional right ventricle is poorly tolerant to sudden increases in afterload such as the change from spontaneous to controlled ventilation. Right ventricular function becomes critical in maintaining cardiac output as the pulmonary artery pressure rises. The right ventricular ejection fraction does not increase with exercise in COPD patients as it does in normal patients. Chronic recurrent hypoxemia is the cause of the right ventricular dysfunction and the subsequent progression to cor pulmonale. Patients who have episodic hypoxemia in spite of normal lungs (e.g., central alveolar hypoventilation, SAHS) develop the same secondary cardiac problems as COPD patients. The only therapy which has been shown to improve long-term survival and decrease right heart strain in COPD is supplemental oxygen. COPD patients who have resting PaO_2 less than 55 mm Hg should receive supplemental home oxygen and also those who desaturate to less than 44 mm Hg with exercise. The goal of supplemental oxygen is to maintain a PaO_2 60 to 65 mm Hg. Compared to patients with chronic bronchitis, emphysematous COPD patients tend to have a decreased cardiac output and mixed venous oxygen tension while maintaining lower pulmonary artery pressures.

Many patients with moderate or severe COPD will develop cystic air spaces in the lung parenchyma known as ***bullae*** (Fig. 24-43). These bullae will often be asymptomatic unless they occupy more than 50% of the hemithorax, in which case the patient will present with findings of restrictive respiratory disease in addition to their obstructive disease. A bulla is a localized area of loss of structural support tissue in the lung with elastic recoil of surrounding parenchyma (Fig. 24-44).[70] The pressure in a bulla is actually the mean pressure in the surrounding alveoli averaged over the respiratory cycle. This means that during normal spontaneous ventilation, the intra-bulla pressure is actually slightly negative in comparison to the surrounding parenchyma. However, whenever positive pressure ventilation is used, the pressure in a bulla will become positive in relation to the adjacent lung tissue and the bulla will expand with the attendant risk of rupture, tension pneumothorax, and bronchopleural fistula. Positive pressure ventilation can be used safely in patients with bullae provided the airway pressures are kept low and there is

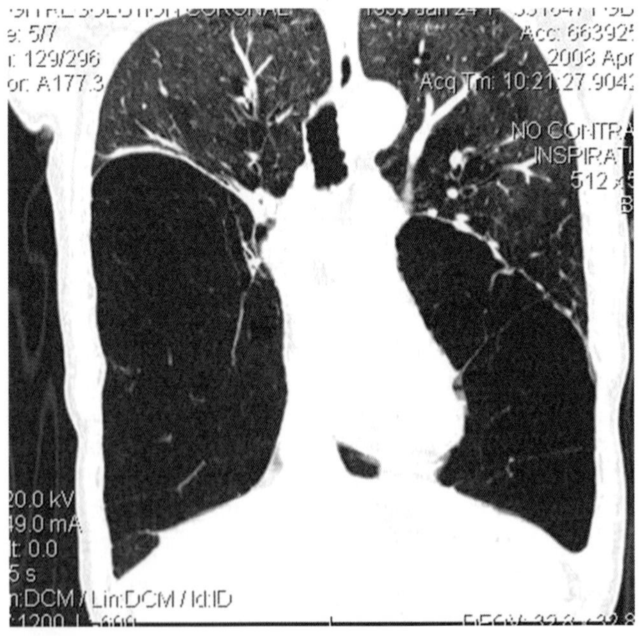

FIGURE 24-43 Coronal CT scan of a patient with bilateral giant lower lobe bullae. During positive pressure ventilation, the risk of bulla rupture and tension pneumothorax must always be kept in mind.

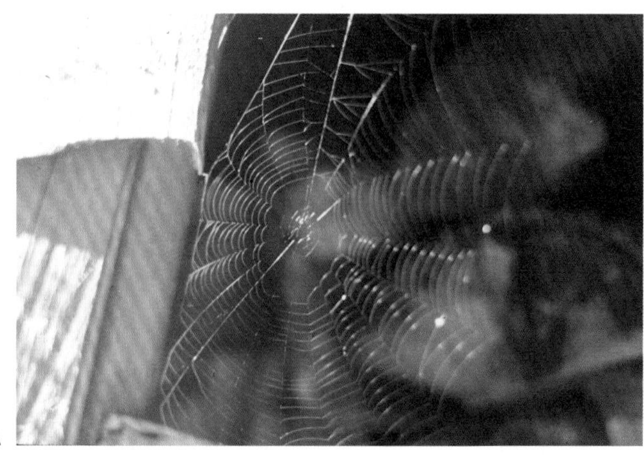

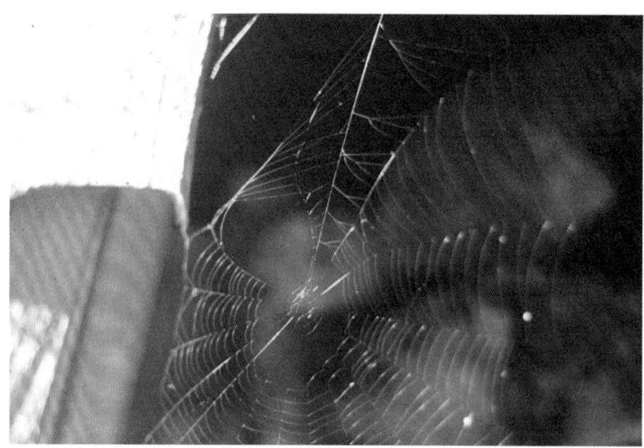

FIGURE 24-44 **A:** A spider's web seen on a woodbox on a sunny day as a lung model to demonstrate the pathophysiology of bullae. **B:** Breaking one septum of the spider's web causes a bulla to appear as elastic recoil pulls the web away from the area where structural support has been lost. Although the cells surrounding the bulla appear compressed, this is only due to redistribution of elastic forces. It is not positive pressure inside the bulla which causes this appearance of surrounding compression.

adequate expertise and equipment immediately available to insert a chest drain and obtain lung isolation if necessary. Due to the lower solubility of nitrogen in plasma compared to nitrous oxide, when a patient is converted from breathing air to breathing a mixture containing nitrous oxide during anesthesia, the nitrous oxide will diffuse into a bulla faster than the nitrogen can be absorbed and the bulla will increase in size with the attendant risk of rupture.

Severe COPD patients are often "flow-limited" even during tidal volume expiration at rest. Flow-limitation is present in normal patients only during a forced expiratory maneuver. Flow-limitation occurs when an EPP develops in the intrathoracic airways during expiration. During quiet expiration in the normal patient, the pressure in the lumen of the airways always exceeds the intrapleural pressure because of the upstream elastic recoil pressure, which is transmitted from the alveoli. The effect of this elastic recoil pressure diminishes as air flows downstream in the airway. With a forced expiration the intrapleural pressure may equal the intraluminal pressure at a certain point, the EPP, which then limits the expiratory flow (see Fig. 24-27). Then, any increase in expiratory effort will not produce an increase in flow at that given lung volume. Flow-limitation occurs particularly in emphysematous patients, who primarily have a problem with loss of lung elastic recoil and have marked dyspnea on exertion. Flow-limitation causes dyspnea because of stimulation of mechanoreceptors in the muscles of respiration, thoracic cage, and in the airway distal to the EPP. Any increase in the work of respiration will lead to increased dyspnea. This variable mechanical compression of airways by overinflated alveoli is the primary cause of the airflow obstruction in emphysema. Severely flow-limited patients are at risk for hemodynamic collapse with the application of positive pressure ventilation due to dynamic hyperinflation of the lungs. Even the modest positive airway pressures associated with manual ventilation with a bag/mask at induction can lead to hypotension because these patients have no increased resistance to inspiration but a marked obstruction of expiration. In some of these patients, this has contributed to the "Lazarus" syndrome in which patients have recovered from a cardiac arrest only after resuscitation and positive pressure ventilation were discontinued.[71]

Patients with severe COPD often breathe in a pattern that interrupts expiration before the alveolar pressure has fallen to atmospheric pressure. This incomplete expiration is due to a combination of factors which include flow-limitation, increased work of respiration and increased airway resistance. This interruption leads to an elevation of the end-expiratory lung volume above the FRC. This PEEP in the alveoli at rest has been termed ***auto-PEEP*** or ***intrinsic-PEEP***. During spontaneous respiration, the intrapleural pressure will have to be decreased to a level which counteracts auto-PEEP before inspiratory flow can begin. Thus, COPD patients can have an increased inspiratory load added to their already increased expiratory load.

Auto-PEEP becomes even more important during mechanical ventilation. It is directly proportional to tidal volume and inversely proportional to expiratory time. The presence of auto-PEEP is not detected by the manometer of standard anesthesia ventilators. It can be measured by end-expiratory flow interruption, a feature available on most intensive care ventilators. Auto-PEEP has been found to develop in most COPD patients during one-lung anesthesia.[72]

Restrictive lung diseases are often part of a multisystemic disease process such as connective tissue disorders. In a minority of patients, there is no other systemic disease (i.e., idiopathic pulmonary fibrosis). Patients are often more debilitated by their underlying disease (e.g., rheumatoid arthritis) than their lung disease. Patients with mild to moderate restrictive lung disease are, in general, less of a problem for the anesthesiologist to manage intraoperatively (compared to COPD) and more of a problem postoperatively. Due to the decrease in FRC in restrictive disease, these patients tend to develop an increased shunt during anesthesia and postoperatively. Restoration of the FRC postoperatively is commonly a problem and the use of regional anesthesia/analgesia, short-acting opioids and muscle relaxants, and noninvasive ventilation are often of benefit in the patient with restrictive disease.

One-Lung Ventilation

One-lung ventilation (OLV) is performed during thoracic surgery to facilitate the surgical exposure in the chest. OLV is commonly obtained by placement of a double-lumen endobronchial tube or a bronchial blocker with a standard endotracheal tube. During OLV, the anesthesiologist has the unique and often conflicting goals of trying to maximize atelectasis in the nonventilated lung to improve surgical access while trying to avoid atelectasis in the ventilated lung (usually the dependent lung) to optimize gas exchange. The gas mixture in the nonventilated lung immediately before OLV has a significant effect on the speed of collapse of this lung.[73] Because of its low blood-gas solubility, nitrogen (or an air-oxygen mixture) will delay collapse of this lung. This is particularly a problem at the start of minimally invasive thoracic surgery when surgical visualization in the operative hemithorax is limited and in patients with emphysema who have delayed collapse of the nonventilated lung due to decreased lung elastic recoil. It is important to thoroughly denitrogenate the operative lung, by ventilating with oxygen, immediately before it is allowed to collapse. Although nitrous oxide is even more effective than oxygen in speeding lung collapse (because of its solubility), it is not commonly used in thoracic anesthesia because many patients may have blebs or bullae. During the period of two-lung anesthesia before the start of OLV, atelectasis will develop in the dependent lung. It is useful to perform a recruitment maneuver to the dependent lung (similar to a Valsalva maneuver, holding the lung at an end-inspiratory pressure of 20 cm H_2O for 15 to 20 seconds) immediately after the start of OLV to decrease this atelectasis. Recruitment is important to maintain $Pa{O_2}$ levels during subsequent OLV.[74]

A major concern that influences anesthetic management for thoracic surgery is the occurrence of hypoxemia during OLV. There is no universally acceptable figure for the safest lower limit of oxygen saturation during OLV. A saturation greater than or equal to 90% ($Pa{O_2}$ >60 mm Hg) is commonly accepted, and for brief periods, a saturation in the high 80s may be acceptable in patients without significant comorbidity. However, the lowest acceptable saturation will be higher in patients with organs at risk of hypoxia due to limited regional blood flow (e.g., coronary or cerebrovascular disease) and in patients with limited oxygen transport (e.g., anemia or decreased cardiopulmonary reserve). Previously, hypoxemia occurred frequently during OLV. Reports for the period 1950 to 1980 describe an incidence of hypoxemia (arterial saturation <90%) of 20% to 25%. Current reports describe an incidence of less than 5%. This improvement is most likely due to several factors: improved lung isolation techniques, such as routine fiberoptic bronchoscopy to prevent lobar obstruction from double-lumen tubes; improved anesthetic agents, which cause less inhibition of HPV; and better understanding of the pathophysiology of OLV.

The pathophysiology of OLV is complex and involves the body's ability to redistribute pulmonary blood flow to the ventilated lung. Several factors aid and impede this redistribution and these are under the control of the anesthesiologist to a variable degree. These factors are illustrated in Figure 24-45. The anesthesiologist's goal during OLV is to maximize PVR in the nonventilated lung while minimizing PVR in the ventilated lung. PVR is lowest at FRC and increases as lung volume rises or falls above or below FRC. The anesthesiologist's aim, to optimize pulmonary blood flow redistribution during OLV, is to maintain the ventilated lung as close as possible to its FRC while facilitating collapse of the nonventilated lung to increase its PVR.[75] Most thoracic surgery is performed in the lateral position. Patients having OLV in the lateral position have significantly better $Pa{O_2}$ levels than patients

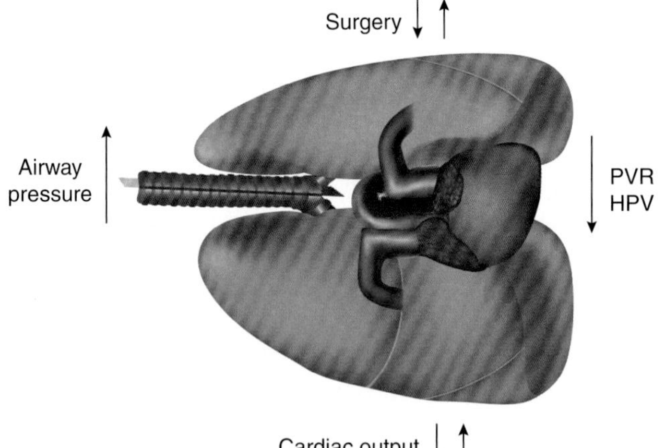

FIGURE 24-45 Factors affecting the distribution of pulmonary blood flow during one-lung ventilation. Hypoxic pulmonary vasoconstriction (HPV) and the collapse the nonventilated lung, which increase pulmonary vascular resistance (PVR), tend to distribute blood flow toward the ventilated lung. The airway pressure gradient between the ventilated and nonventilated thoraces tends to encourage blood flow to the nonventilated lung. Surgery and cardiac output can have variable effects either increasing or decreasing the proportional flow to the ventilated lung. Gravity will also increase the blood flow to the dependent lung.

during OLV in the supine position due to a preferential distribution of blood flow to the dependent lung caused by gravitational forces.

Extracorporeal Ventilatory Support

Various devices to supplement or replace the gas exchange function of the lung have been available clinically for the past several decades. These devices have been associated with a high incidence of complications, particularly cerebral hemorrhage and infarction, and have met with questionable outcome results in several studies. However, gradual progress in the technology has seen a resurgence of use of these devices.[76] Indications currently may include infant respiratory distress syndrome, adult respiratory distress syndrome, respiratory failure unresponsive to mechanical ventilation, and as a bridge to transplantation in end-stage lung diseases. During extracorporeal ventilation, less injurious mechanical ventilation strategies can be used on the native lungs with relatively normal FIO_2 and tidal volumes to allow some regression of the disease process in the lungs.

The options for extracorporeal ventilatory support include venovenous membrane oxygenation, with an oxygenator and a pump, indicated in primary respiratory failure; venoarterial membrane oxygenation, for combined respiratory and cardiac failure; and pumpless interventional lung assist, with a passive arterial-venous membrane gas-exchange device, which is primarily used in failure of CO_2 excretion with relatively maintained oxygenation.[77]

References

1. Jaeger JM. Blank RS. Essential anatomy and physiology of the respiratory system and pulmonary circulation. In: Slinger P, ed. *Principles and Practice of Anesthesia for Thoracic Surgery*. New York, NY: Springer; 2011:51–69.
2. Shorten GD, Opie NJ, Graziotti P, et al. Assessment of the upper airway in awake, sedated and anaesthetized patients using magnetic resonance imaging. *Anaesth Intens Care*. 1994;22:165–169.
3. Hudgel DW, Hendricks C. Palate and hypopharynx—sites of inspiratory narrowing of the upper airway during sleep. *Am Rev Respir Dis*. 1988;138:1542–1547.
4. Eikermann M, Grosse-Sundrup M, Zaremba S, et al. Ketamine activates breathing and abolishes the coupling between loss of consciousness and upper airway dilator muscle function. *Anesthesiology*. 2012;116:6–8.
5. Bartlett D. Respiratory function of the larynx. *Physiol Rev*. 1989;69:33–57.
6. Gal TJ. Anatomy and physiology of the respiratory system and the pulmonary circulation. In: Kaplan JA, Slinger PD, eds. *Thoracic Anesthesia*. 3rd ed. Philadelphia, PA: Churchill Livingstone; 2003:57–70.
7. Voynow JA, Rubin BK. Mucins, mucus, and sputum. *Chest*. 2009;135:505–512.
8. Gonda I. Particle deposition in the human respiratory tract. In: Crystal RG, West JB, Weibel ER, et al, eds. *The Lung: Scientific Foundations*. 2nd ed. Philadelphia, PA: Lippincott-Raven; 1997:2289–2308.
9. Lumb AB, ed. *Nunn's Applied Respiratory Physiology*, 7th ed. Edinburgh, United Kingdom: Churchill Livingstone Elsevier; 2010.
10. Burwell DR, Jones JG. The airways and anaesthesia. *Anaesthesia*. 1996;51:849–857.
11. Duggan M, Kavanagh B. Pulmonary atelectasis. *Anesthesiology*. 2005;102:838–854.
12. Chappell D, Jacob M, Hofman-Keifer K, et al. A rational approach to perioperative fluid management. *Anesthesiology*. 2008;109:723–724.
13. McKenzie DK, Gandevia SC. Skeletal muscle properties: diaphragm and chest wall. In: Crystal RG, West JB, Weibel ER, et al, eds. *The Lung: Scientific Foundations*. 2nd ed. Philadelphia, PA: Lipincott-Raven; 1997:981–991.
14. Levine S, Kaiser L, Leferovich J, et al. Cellular adaptations in the diaphragm in chronic obstructive pulmonary disease. *New Engl J Med*. 1997;337:1799–1806.
15. Lim E, Baldwin D, Beckles M, et al. Guidelines on the radical management of patients with lung cancer. *Thorax*. 2010;65(suppl 3):iii1–iii27.
16. Sprung J, Gajic O, Warner DO. Age related alterations in respiratory function-anesthetic consideration. *Can J Anaesth*. 2006;53:1244–1257.
17. Rothen HU, Sporre B, Engberg G, et al. Airway closure, atelectasis, and gas exchange during general anesthesia. *Br J Anaesth*. 1998;81:681–686.
18. Whitsett JA, Weaver TE. Hydrophobic surfactant proteins in lung function and disease. *N Engl J Med*. 2002;347:2141–2148.
19. Harris RS. Pressure-volume curves of the respiratory system. *Respir Care*. 2005;50:78–99.
20. Slats AM, Janssen K, van Schadewijk A, et al. Bronchial inflammation and responses to deep inspiration in asthma and chronic bronchitis. *Am J Respir Crit Care Med*. 2007;176:121–128.
21. Holst M, Striem J, Hedenstierna G. Errors in tracheal pressure recording in patients with a tracheostomy tube—a model study. *Intensive Care Med*. 1990;16:384–389.
22. Cotes JE, Chinn DJ, Miller MR. *Lung Function. Physiology, Measurement and Application in Medicine*. Oxford, United Kingdom: Blackwell Publishing; 2006.
23. Raux M, Starus C, Redolfi S, et al. Electroencephalographic evidence for pre-motor cortex activation during inspiratory loading in humans. *J Physiol*. 2007;578:569–578.
24. Ingram RH, McFadden ER. Localisation and mechanisms of airway responses. *N Engl J Med*. 1977;297:596–600.
25. Campbell EJM, Westlake EK, Cherniak RM. Simple methods of estimating oxygen consumption and the efficiency of the muscles of respiration. *J Appl Physiol*. 1957;11:303–308.
26. Lumb AB, ed. *Nunn's Applied Respiratory Physiology*. 7th ed. Edinburgh, United Kingdom: Churchill Livingstone Elsevier; 2010.
27. Fujii Y, Toyooka H, Amaha K. Diaphragmatic fatigue and its recovery are influenced by cardiac output. *J Anaesth*. 1991;5:17–23.
28. Levine S, Nguyen T, Taylor N, et al. Rapid disuse atrophy of diaphragm fibers in mechanically ventilated humans. *N Engl J Med*. 2008;358:1327–1355.
29. Goligher EC, Ferguson ND, Kavanagh BP. Ventilator induced diaphragm dysfunction. *Anesthesiology*. 2012;117:560–567.
30. Bake B, Wood L, Murphy B, et al. Effect of inspiratory flow rate on regional distribution of inspired gas. *J Appl Physiol*. 1974;37:8–17.
31. Widdicombe J. Anatomy and physiology of the airway circulation. *Am Rev Respir Dis*. 1992;146:S3–S7.
32. Clark AR, Tawhai MH, Hoffman EA, et al. The interdependent contributions of gravitational and structural features to perfusion distribution in a multiscale model of the pulmonary circulation. *J Appl Physiol*. 2011;110:943–955.
33. West J, Dollery C, Naimark A. Distribution of blood flow in isolated lung; relation to vascular and alveolar pressures. *J Appl Physiol*. 1964;19:713–724.
34. Bohr C. Uber die lugenathmung. *Skand Arch Physiol*. 1891;2:236.

35. Tusman G, Sipmann S, Bohm SH. Rationale of dead space measurement by volumetric capnography. *Anesth Analg*. 2012;114:866–874.
36. Sylvester JT, Shimoda LA, Aaronson PI, et al. Hypoxic pulmonary vasoconstriction. *Physiol Rev*. 2012;92:367–520.
37. Talbot NP, Balanos GM, Dorrington KL, et al. Two temporal components within the human pulmonary vascular response to 2h of isocapnic hypoxia. *J Appl Physiol*. 2005;98:1125–1139.
38. Domino KB, Wetstein L, Glasser SA, et al. Influence of mixed venous oxygen tension (PvO2) on blood flow to atelectatic lung. *Anesthesiology*. 1983;59:428–434.
39. Lejeune P, Vachiaery JL, Leeman M, et al. Absence of parasympathetic control of pulmonary vascular pressure-flow plots in hyperoxic and hypoxic dogs. *Respir Physiol*. 1989;78:123–133.
40. Robins ED, Theodore J, Burke CM, et al. Hypoxic vasoconstriction persists in the human transplanted lung. *Clin Sci*. 1987;72:283–287.
41. Evans AM, Dipp M. Hypoxic pulmonary vasoconstriction: cyclic adenosine diphosphate-ribose, smooth muscle Ca2+ stores and the endothelium. *Respir Physiol Neurobiol*. 2002;132:3–15.
42. Yamamoto Y, Nakano H, Ide H, et al. Role of airway nitric oxide on the regulation of pulmonary circulation by carbon dioxide. *J Appl Physiol*. 2001;91:1121–1130.
43. Gourine AV. On the peripheral and central chemoreception and control of breathing: an emerging role for ATP. *J Physiol*. 2005; 568:715–724.
44. Lopez-Barneo J, Ortega-Saenz P, Pardal R, et al. Carotid body oxygen sensing. *Eur Respir J*. 2008;32:1386–1398.
45. Knill RL, Manninen PH, Clement JL. Ventilation and chemoreflexes during enflurane sedation and anaesthesia in man. *Can Anaesth Soc J*. 1979;26:353–360.
46. Lorenzi-Filho G, Genta PR. A new straw in the genesis of Cheyne-Stokes respiration. *Chest*. 2008,134:7–9.
47. Nunn JF. Factors influencing the arterial oxygen tension during halothane anaesthesia with spontaneous respiration. *Br J Anaesth*. 1964;36:327–324.
48. Brismar B, Hedenstierna G, Lundquist H, et al. Pulmonary densities during anesthesia with muscular relaxation—a proposal of atelectasis. *Anesthesiology*. 1985;62:422–428.
49. Magnusson L, Spahn DR. New concepts of atelectasis during general anaesthesia. *Brit J Anaesth*. 2003;91:61–72.
50. Froese AB, Bryan AC. Effects of anesthesia and paralysis on diaphragmatic mechanics in man. *Anesthesiology*. 1974;41:242–255.
51. Reber A, Nylund U, Hedenstierna G. Position and shape of the diaphragm: implications for atelectasis formation. *Anaesthesia*. 1998;53:1054–1061.
52. Joyce CJ, Baker AB, Kennedy RR. Gas uptake from an unventilated area of the lung: computer model of absorption atelectasis. *J Appl Physiol*. 1993;74:1107–1116.
53. Gattinoni L, Caironi P. Prone positioning beyond physiology. *Anesthesiology*. 2010;113:1262–1264.
54. Petersson J, Ax M, Frey J, et al. Positive end-expiratory pressure redistributes regional blood flow and ventilation differently in supine and prone humans. *Anesthesiology*. 2010;113:1361–1369.
55. Jones RL, Nzekwu M-MU. The effects of body mass index on lung volumes. *Chest*. 2006;130:827–833.
56. Redolfi S, Yumino D, Ruttanaumpawan P. Relationship between overnight rostral fluid shift and obstructive sleep apnea in non-obese men. *Am J Resp Crit Care Med*. 2009;179:241–246.
57. Horner RL, Bradley TD. Update in sleep and control of ventilation 2008. *Am J Resp Crit Care Med*. 2009;179:528–532.
58. Mokhlesi B, Tulaimat A. Recent advances in the obesity hypoventilation syndrome. *Chest*. 2007;132:1322–1336.
59. Ainsworth BE, Haskell WL, Leon AS, et al. Compendium of physical activities: classification of energy costs of human physical activities. *Med Sci Sports Exerc*. 1993;25:71–80.
60. Carter R, Holiday DB, Stocks J, et al. predicting oxygen uptake for men and women with moderate to severe chronic obstructive pulmonary disease. *Arch Phys Med Rehab*. 2003;64:328–332.
61. Leissner KB, Mahmood FU. Physiology and pathophysiology at high altitude: considerations for the anesthesiologist. *J Anesth*. 2009;23: 534–553.
62. Tibbles PM, Eisenberg JS. Hyperbaric-oxygen therapy. *N Engl J Med*. 1993;334:1642–1648.
63. McNeice WL, Dierdorf SF. The pediatric airway. *Semin Pediatr Surg*. 2004;13:152–159.
64. Rigatto H, Brady J, Verduzco R. Chemoreceptor reflexes in preterm infants. *Pediatrics*. 1975:55:604–610.
65. Zaugg M, Lucchinetti E. Respiratory function in the elderly. *Anesthesiol Clin North America*. 2000;18:47–58.
66. American Thoracic Society. Standards for the diagnosis and care of patients with chronic obstructive pulmonary disease. *Am J Respir Crit Care Med*. 1995;152:s77–s121.
67. Simpson SQ. Oxygen-induced acute hypercapnia in chronic obstructive pulmonary disease: what's the problem? *Crit Care Med*. 2002;30:258–259.
68. Douglas NJ, Flenley DC. Breathing during sleep in patients with obstructive lung disease. *Am Rev Respir Dis*. 1990;141:1055–1057.
69. Schulman DS, Mathony RA. The right ventricle in pulmonary disease. *Cardiol Clin*. 1992;10:111–120.
70. Morgan MDL, Edwards CW, Morris J, et al. Origin and behavior of emphysematous bullae. *Thorax*. 1989;44:533–537.
71. Ben-David B, Stonebraker VC, Hershman R, et al. Survival after failed intraoperative resuscitation: a case of "Lazarus syndrome." *Anesth Analg*. 2001;92:690–695.
72. Slinger P, Hickey D. The interaction applied PEEP and auto-PEEP during one-lung ventilation. *J Cardiothorac Vasc Anesth*. 1998;12: 133–138.
73. Ko R, Kruger M, McRae K, et al. The use of air in the inspired gas mixture during two-lung ventilation delays lung collapse during one-lung ventilation. *Anesth Analg*. 2009;108:1092–1097.
74. Unzueta C, Tusman G, Suarez-Sipman F, et al. Alveolar recruitment improves ventilation during thoracic surgery: a randomized controlled trial. *Br J Anaesth*. 2012;108:517–524.
75. Slinger PD, Kruger M, McRae K, et al. The relation of the static compliance curve and PEEP to oxygenation during one-lung ventilation. *Anesthesiology*. 2001;95:1096–1102.
76. Peek GJ, Mugford M, Tiruvoipati R, et al. CESAR trial collaboration. Efficacy and economic assessment of conventional ventilatory support versus extracorporeal membrane oxygenation for severe adult respiratory failure (CESAR): a multicentre randomised controlled trial. *Lancet*. 2009;374:1351–1363.
77. Von Dossow-Hanfstingl V, Deja M, Zwisser B, et al. Post-operative management: extra-corporeal ventilatory therapy. In: Slinger P, ed. *Principles and Practice of Anesthesia for Thoracic Surgery*. New York, NY: Springer; 2011:647.

CHAPTER 25

Respiratory Pharmacology

Peter Slinger

This chapter will review the pharmacology of agents commonly encountered in anesthetic practice that are either administered to treat pulmonary diseases or administered into the airway or systemically for action at end organs other than the lung but have effects on the airway and the pulmonary circulation. The pharmacology of the airways will be considered first, then the pharmacology of the pulmonary circulation, and finally, the intrinsic action of the lungs on a variety of exogenous and endogenous substances.

Pharmacology of the Airways

Pharmacologic agents administered via the lungs take advantage of the interface between air and blood allowing for rapid uptake of drugs into the bloodstream or immediate use by cells that populate the airway.[1] The delivery of medications to the lungs can have systemic effects, direct effects on the airway, or both. For example, inhaled anesthetics are delivered via the lungs to act in the brain and have bronchodilatory effects. Conversely, β-adrenergic agonists delivered via aerosol exert direct effects on bronchial smooth muscle with few systemic effects. Drugs administered to the airway take advantage of the rapid exposure to blood and pulmonary parenchymal cells, making them advantageous for treating pulmonary parenchymal diseases such as asthma and chronic obstructive pulmonary disease (COPD).

Influence of the Autonomic Nervous System on the Airways

Traditionally, the autonomic nervous system (ANS) has been divided into two major parts, the parasympathetic and sympathetic nervous systems. The parasympathetic nervous system regulates airway caliber, airway glandular activity, and airway microvasculature.[2–4] The vagus nerve provides the preganglionic fibers, which synapse with postganglionic fibers in airway parasympathetic ganglia. Acetylcholine activates the muscarinic (M3) receptor of postganglionic fibers of the parasympathetic nervous system to produce bronchoconstriction.[5] Anticholinergics can provide bronchodilation even in the resting state because the parasympathetic nervous system produces a basal level of resting bronchomotor tone.[6]

Although the sympathetic nervous system plays no direct role in control of airway muscle tone, β_2-adrenergic receptors are present on airway smooth muscle cells and cause bronchodilation via stimulatory G mechanisms. The abundance of these receptors in the airway allows for pharmacologic manipulation of airway tone.[7]

The ANS also influences bronchomotor tone through the nonadrenergic noncholinergic (NANC) system.[8,9] The exact role of NANC in humans is not well defined; it has excitatory and inhibitory neuropeptides that influence inflammation and smooth muscle tone, respectively. Vasoactive intestinal peptide (VIP) and nitric oxide (NO) are the main inhibitory transmitters thought to be responsible for airway smooth muscle relaxation. Substance P (SP) and neurokinin A (NKA) are the main excitatory transmitters and have been shown to cause neurogenic inflammation, including bronchoconstriction. The precise role of NANC in healthy and diseased human lung is unclear.

Inhaled Adrenergic Agonists

The mainstay of therapy for bronchospasm, wheezing, and airflow obstruction is β-adrenergic agonists. β-adrenergic agonists used in clinical practice are typically delivered via inhalers or nebulizers, are β_2 selective, and are divided into short- and long-acting therapies.[10] Short-acting β_2 agonist therapy is effective for the rapid relief of wheezing, bronchospasm, and airflow obstruction. Longer acting β_2 agonists are used as maintenance therapy providing improvement in lung function and reduction in symptoms and exacerbations (Table 25-1).

Table 25-1

Pharmacologic Influence on the Autonomic Nervous System

Systemic Adrenergic Agonists	Inhaled Adrenergic Agonists	Inhaled Cholinergic Antagonists	Systemic Cholinergic Antagonists
	Short Acting	**Short Acting**	
Terbutaline	Albuterol	Ipratropium	Atropine
Epinephrine	Levalbuterol		Scopolamine
Albuterol	Metaproterenol		Glycopyrrolate
	Pirbuterol		
	Long Acting	**Long Acting**	
	Salmeterol	Tiotropium	
	Formoterol		
	Arformoterol		

From Wojciechowski P, Hurford W. Pharmacology of the airways. In: Slinger P, ed. *Principles and Practice of Anesthesia for Thoracic Surgery*. New York, NY: Springer; 2011:121–132, with permission.

Short-acting β_2 agonists bind to the β_2-adrenergic receptor located on the plasma membrane of smooth muscle cells, epithelial, endothelial, and many other types of airway cells.[11] This causes a stimulatory G protein to activate adenylate cyclase converting adenosine triphosphate (ATP) into cyclic adenosine monophosphate (cAMP). It is unknown precisely how cAMP causes smooth muscle relaxation; however, decreases in calcium release and alterations in membrane potential are the most likely mechanisms. Longer acting β_2 agonists have the same mechanism of action as short-acting β_2 agonists; however, they have unique properties that allow for a longer duration of action. For example, salmeterol has a longer duration of action because a side chain binds to the β_2-receptor and prolongs the activation of the receptor.[12] The lipophilic side chain of formoterol allows for interaction with the lipid bilayer of the plasma membrane and a slow, steady release prolonging its duration of action.

β_2 agonists have a central role in the management of obstructive airway diseases allowing for control of symptoms and improvement in lung function. Short-acting β_2 agonists such as albuterol, levalbuterol, metaproterenol, and pirbuterol are prescribed for the rapid relief of wheezing, bronchospasm, and airflow obstruction. Clinical effect is seen in a matter of minutes and lasts up to 4 to 6 hours. Scheduled, daily use of short-acting β_2 agonists has largely fallen out of favor and they are now used primarily as rescue therapy.[13–15] Long-acting β_2 agonists are prescribed for control of symptoms when rescue therapies (i.e., short-acting β_2 agonists) are used greater than two times per week.[16] Combination therapy including a long-acting β_2 agonist and an inhaled corticosteroid are effective in reducing symptoms, reducing the risk of exacerbation, and improving lung function while minimizing the dose of inhaled corticosteroid.[17]

Systemic absorption of inhaled β_2 agonists is responsible for a myriad of side effects, most of which are not serious. Most commonly, β_2 agonist therapy leads to tremors and tachycardia secondary to direct stimulation of the β_2-adrenergic receptor in skeletal muscle or vasculature, respectively.[18,19] In severe asthma, β_2 agonists may cause a temporary reduction in arterial oxygen tension of 5 mm Hg or more, secondary to β_2-mediated vasodilation in poorly ventilated lung regions.[20] Hyperglycemia, hypokalemia, and hypomagnesemia also can occur with β_2 agonist therapy but the severity of these side effects tends to diminish with regular use. Tolerance to β_2 agonists can occur with regular use over a period of weeks and, while not affecting peak bronchodilation, can be evidenced by a decrease in the duration of bronchodilation and the magnitude of side effects (tremor, tachycardia, etc.).[21,22] Tolerance likely reflects β_2-adrenergic receptor downregulation. β_2 agonist therapy withdrawal after regular use can produce transient bronchial hyperresponsiveness.

Evidence has associated the use of long-acting β_2 agonist therapy without concomitant use of a steroid inhaler with fatal and near-fatal asthma attacks.[23] In light of this evidence, it seems prudent to reserve long-acting β_2 agonists for patients that are poorly controlled on inhaled steroids alone or for those patients with symptoms sufficiently challenging to warrant the potential extra risk associated with use of the agents.

Systemic Adrenergic Agonists

Systemic administration of adrenergic agonists for asthma was used more frequently in the past. Oral, intravenous (IV), or subcutaneous administration of β-specific or nonspecific adrenergic agonists is now reserved for rescue therapy. The mechanism of action of systemically administered adrenergic agonists is the same as it is for inhaled agents. Binding of the drug to the β_2-adrenergic receptor on smooth muscle cells in the airway is responsible for the bronchodilatory effects. Specifically, β_2-receptor stimulation induces a stimulatory G protein to convert ATP to cAMP and in turn reduces intracellular calcium release and alters membrane potential.

Terbutaline can be given orally, subcutaneously, or intravenously, albuterol (salbutamol) can be given intravenously, and epinephrine is usually given subcutaneously or intravenously. Regardless of the route of administration, all three will produce bronchodilation. Comparison of IV and inhaled formulations of terbutaline failed to demonstrate any difference in bronchodilation and, with the propensity for IV formulations to cause side effects, inhaled therapy should be considered the first-line treatment.[24,25] This principle not only applies to terbutaline but all β-adrenergic agonists that are available in IV and inhaled forms. If inhaled therapy is not readily available or if inhaled therapy is maximized and symptoms persist, then subcutaneous epinephrine or terbutaline can be administered with improvement in symptoms and spirometry values.[26] In summary, subcutaneous or IV β agonists should be reserved only for rescue therapy.

The side effect profile of systemic adrenergic agonists is similar to the side effect profile for inhalational adrenergic agonists. The most common side effects are tremor and tachycardia. Arterial oxygen tension can be transiently decreased and hyperglycemia, hypokalemia, and hypomagnesemia can also be present. Escalating oral, subcutaneous, or IV doses can be associated with a greater incidence of side effects for the same degree of bronchodilation compared to inhaled β-adrenergic agonists.

Inhaled Cholinergic Antagonists

The use of anticholinergics for maintenance therapy and treatment of acute exacerbations in obstructive airway diseases is common. The parasympathetic nervous system is primarily responsible for bronchomotor tone and inhaled anticholinergics act on muscarinic receptors in the airway to reduce tone. The use of inhaled anticholinergics (see Table 25-1) in COPD as maintenance and rescue therapy is considered standard treatment.[27] Anticholinergics are not used for maintenance therapy in asthma and are only recommended for use in acute exacerbations.[28] The targets of therapy for anticholinergics are the muscarinic receptors located in the airway. There are three subtypes of muscarinic receptors found in the human airway.[29] Muscarinic 2 (M2) receptors are present on postganglionic cells and are responsible for limiting production of acetylcholine and protect against bronchoconstriction. M2 is not the target of inhaled anticholinergics but is antagonized by them. Muscarinic 1 (M1) and muscarinic 3 (M3) receptors are responsible for bronchoconstriction and mucus production and are the targets of inhaled anticholinergic therapy. Acetylcholine binds to the M3 and M1 receptors and causes smooth muscle contraction via increases in cyclic guanosine monophosphate (cGMP) or by activation of a G protein (Gq).[29] Gq activates phospholipase C to produce inositol triphosphate (IP3), which causes release of calcium from intracellular stores and activation of myosin light chain kinase causing smooth muscle contraction. Anticholinergics inhibit this cascade and reduce smooth muscle tone by decreasing release of calcium from intracellular stores.

There are two inhaled anticholinergics specifically approved for the treatment of obstructive airway diseases. Ipratropium is classified as a short-acting anticholinergic and is commonly used as maintenance therapy for COPD and as rescue therapy for both COPD and asthmatic exacerbations. It is not indicated for the routine management of asthma. Patients treated with ipratropium experience an increase in exercise tolerance, decrease in dyspnea, and improved gas exchange. Tiotropium is the only long-acting anticholinergic available for COPD maintenance therapy. Tiotropium has been shown to reduce COPD exacerbations, respiratory failure, and all-cause mortality.[30]

Inhaled anticholinergics are poorly absorbed and therefore serious side effects are uncommon. Most commonly, patients experience dry mouth, urinary retention, and can experience pupillary dilation and blurred vision if the eyes are inadvertently exposed to the drug. Some initial data suggested an increase in cardiovascular and stroke complications with tiotropium; however, additional studies did not consistently demonstrate these complications. In general, anticholinergics are safe and effective treatment for patients with obstructive airway diseases.

Systemic Cholinergic Antagonists

The systemically administered anticholinergics atropine and glycopyrrolate act via the same mechanisms as inhaled anticholinergics. While these anticholinergics can be administered by IV or inhalation, significant systemic absorption occurs and their use is generally limited by side effects. Atropine, in particular, is limited in use because of its tertiary ammonium structure. It has a tendency to cause tachycardia, gastrointestinal upset, blurred vision, dry mouth, and central nervous system effects secondary to its ability to cross the blood–brain barrier. Glycopyrrolate has a quaternary ammonium structure and is insoluble in lipids, similar to ipratropium and tiotropium, and has fewer systemic side effects than atropine. IV glycopyrrolate is also clinically limited in use secondary to side effects.[31] Glycopyrrolate has been studied as inhaled therapy, however, and is an effective bronchodilator with an intermediate duration of action.[32–35] Clinically, it has never been popular as a mainstay of therapy for obstructive airway diseases.

Influence of Inflammation on the Airway

Asthma and COPD, the most common obstructive airway diseases, have a component of inflammation as part of their pathogenesis. Although inflammation is a common pathogenesis, the characteristics and prominent cellular elements involved in the inflammatory process for each disease are distinct.[36] In COPD, neutrophils, macrophages, CD8+ T lymphocytes, and eosinophils are more prominent in the inflammatory composition. In asthma, eosinophils play a more prominent role followed by mast cells, CD 4+ T lymphocytes, and macrophages in the inflammatory composition. Inflammatory cell types present in sputum, biopsy specimens, and bronchoalveolar lavage fluid can help predict the response to antiinflammatory therapy. For example, eosinophilia in induced sputum of a patient presenting with a COPD exacerbation predicts an increase in steroid responsiveness.[37,38] Patients presenting to the operating room with obstructive airway diseases have a high likelihood of taking one of the antiinflammatory therapies in Table 25-2 for control of their disease.

Inhaled Corticosteroids

In the treatment of asthma, the use of inhaled corticosteroids (ICS) reduces the inflammatory changes associated with the disease, thereby improving lung function and reducing exacerbations that result in hospitalization and death.[39–41] On the contrary, the use of ICS as monotherapy in COPD is discouraged. In COPD, ICS are used as a part of combination therapy along with long-acting β-adrenergic agonists (LABA). The combination of drugs acts synergistically and is useful for reducing inflammation. Currently, combination therapy of ICS and LABA is recommended for use in severe to very severe COPD.[42] The glucocorticoid receptor alpha (GRα) located in the cytoplasm of airway epithelial cells is the primary target of ICS.[43,44] Passive diffusion of steroids into the cell allows for binding of the steroid ligand to GRα, dissociation of heat shock proteins, and subsequent translocation to the nucleus. The complex can bind to promoter regions of DNA sequences and either induce or suppress gene expression. Additionally, the steroid-receptor complex can interact with transcription factors already in place, such as the ones responsible for proinflammatory mediators, without binding to DNA and repress expression of those genes. The steroid-receptor complex also can affect chromatin structure by association with transcription factors that influence the winding of DNA around histones, reducing access of RNA polymerase and other transcription factors, and thus reducing expression of inflammatory gene products.

ICS are used in asthma as part of a multimodal treatment regimen and are added to a therapeutic regimen when there is an increase in severity or frequency of asthma exacerbations. There is good evidence to show that ICS can reduce both hospitalizations and death in asthma. The use of ICS in COPD is limited to use in severe to very severe COPD and in combination with LABA. Although no improvement in mortality has been consistently demonstrated with combination therapy (ICS/LABA), there are reported improvements in health status and lung function along with a reduction in exacerbations.

Side effects have been reported with the use of ICS in asthma and COPD. A meta-analysis reported an increase in pneumonia and serious pneumonia but not deaths when ICS was used in the treatment of COPD.[45] Other reported side effects in COPD and asthma include oropharyngeal candidiasis, pharyngitis, easy bruising, osteoporosis, cataracts, elevated intraocular pressure, dysphonia, cough, and growth retardation in children. As with any pharmacotherapy, the risks and benefits of therapy must be weighed, and the patient must be carefully monitored for adverse effects. This is especially true with the use of ICS in obstructive lung diseases.

Table 25-2

Pharmacologic Influence on Inflammation

Inhaled Corticosteroids	Leukotriene Modifiers	Mast Cell Stabilizers	Methylxanthines
Monotherapy	**Antagonists**		
Beclomethasone	Montelukast	Cromolyn Sodium	Theophylline
Budesonide	Zafirlukast	Nedocromil	Aminophylline
Ciclesonide	Pranlukast (not in U.S.)		
Flunisolide	**Inhibitors**		
Fluticasone	Zileuton		
Mometasone			
Triamcinolone			
Combination Therapy			
Budesonide/Formoterol			
Fluticasone/Salmeterol			

From Wojciechowski P, Hurford W. Pharmacology of the airways. In: Slinger P, ed. *Principles and Practice of Anesthesia for Thoracic Surgery*. New York, NY: Springer; 2011:121–132, with permission.

Systemic Corticosteroids

Systemic corticosteroids given in IV or oral form are used for treatment of asthma and COPD exacerbations. The mechanism of action is the same as it is for ICS, activation or suppression of gene products at a transcriptional level and alteration of chromatin structure. Patients that are hospitalized with a COPD exacerbation will typically receive IV corticosteroids to suppress any inflammatory component that may be contributing to the flare up. A study done at the Veterans Affairs medical centers in the United States published in 1999 reported that corticosteroid therapy shortened hospital length of stay and improved forced expiratory volume in 1 second versus placebo.[46] The study also compared a 2-week regimen versus an 8-week regimen of corticosteroids and found no difference, concluding that the duration of therapy should last only 2 weeks. In asthma, corticosteroids are recommended for exacerbations that are either severe, with a peak expiratory flow of less than 40% of baseline, or a mild to moderate exacerbation with no immediate response to short-acting β-adrenergic agonists. The recommended duration of therapy is 3 to 10 days without tapering. Alternatively, some patients with asthma and COPD will be receiving long-term oral corticosteroid therapy because their disease is difficult to manage. Side effects of systemic corticosteroids are well described and numerous. Hypertension, hyperglycemia, adrenal suppression, increased infections, cataracts, dermal thinning, psychosis, and peptic ulcers are reported complications of corticosteroid therapy.[47]

Leukotriene Modifiers

Leukotriene modifiers are used for the treatment of asthma. They are prescribed primarily for long-term control in addition to short-acting β-adrenergic agonists or in conjunction with ICS and short-acting β agonists. Leukotriene modifiers are taken by mouth, produce bronchodilatation in hours, and have maximal effect within days of administration. Their role in the management of COPD is not defined.[48] Arachidonic acid is converted to leukotrienes via the 5-lipoxygenase pathway.[49] Leukotrienes C_4, D_4, and E_4 are the end products of the pathway and cause bronchoconstriction, tissue edema, migration of eosinophils, and increased airway secretions. Leukotriene modifiers come in two different varieties, leukotriene receptor antagonists and leukotriene inhibitors.[49] The leukotriene inhibitor zileuton antagonizes 5-lipoxygenase inhibiting the production of leukotrienes.

Leukotriene modifiers improve lung function, reduce exacerbations, and are used as long-term asthma therapy.[50,51] Clinical trials have reported that ICS are superior to leukotriene modifiers for long-term control and should be the first-line choice.[52,53] Leukotriene modifiers provide an additional pharmacologic option for the control of asthma. Addition of leukotriene modifiers to ICS will improve control of symptoms of asthma as opposed to ICS alone.[54]

Leukotriene antagonists are usually well tolerated without significant side effects. Links between Churg-Strauss syndrome and the use of leukotriene antagonists have been reported, but it is not clear whether these reports reflect unmasking of a preexisting condition or whether there is a direct link between the two. Zileuton is known to cause a reversible hepatitis in 2% to 4% of patients.

Mast Cell Stabilizers

Cromolyn sodium and nedocromil are the two agents in this category that are used in the treatment of asthma. These agents are delivered by powder inhaler and are not first-line therapy for asthma. They do provide an alternative treatment when the control of asthma is not optimal on other conventional therapies. Cromolyn sodium and nedocromil stabilize submucosal and intraluminal mast cells.[55] These drugs interfere with the antigen-dependent release of mediators, such as histamine and slow-reacting substance of anaphylaxis, that cause bronchoconstriction, mucosal edema, and increased mucus secretion.

Systematic reviews of the available literature and consensus statements favor the use of ICS over cromolyn sodium or nedocromil as first-line agents to control symptoms of asthma.[56] Alternatively, cromolyn sodium and nedocromil may be used as preventative treatment before exercise or known allergen exposure causing symptoms of asthma. There are no major side effects reported with the use of cromolyn sodium and nedocromil. The most commonly reported side effects are gastrointestinal upset and coughing or irritation of the throat.

Methylxanthines

The role of theophylline, a methylxanthine, has changed since the introduction of ICS and LABA. Theophylline was a common choice for the control of asthma and COPD because of its bronchodilatory and antiinflammatory effects.[57] Currently, theophylline is recommended only as an alternative therapy and is not a first-line choice for asthma or COPD.[58,59] Theophylline acts via multiple pathways causing improvement in symptoms in obstructive lung diseases. Theophylline is a nonselective inhibitor of phosphodiesterase and increases levels of cAMP and cGMP causing smooth muscle relaxation. Antagonism of the A_1 and A_2 adenosine receptors also causes smooth muscle relaxation via inhibition of the release of histamine and leukotrienes from mast cells, another reported action of theophylline. In asthma, theophylline reduces the number of eosinophils in bronchial specimens and, in COPD, reduces the number neutrophils in sputum, having an antiinflammatory effect in both conditions. In addition, theophylline activates histone deacetylase and reduces the expression of inflammatory genes. Theophylline and aminophylline are reported to improve diaphragmatic function; however, data have not demonstrated this effect consistently.[60]

Theophylline has been relegated to an alternative therapy in both asthma and COPD. This has occurred largely because of its significant side effect profile and the subsequent need for monitoring of blood level. Patients that are already on an ICS and a LABA and still have symptoms may benefit from the addition of theophylline, especially if leukotriene modifiers and other alternatives are not tolerated. Theophylline can cause significant and life-threatening side effects if not dosed carefully and monitored appropriately. Side effects tend to be more prominent when blood levels exceed 20 mg/L. The most common side effects include headache, nausea, vomiting, restlessness, abdominal discomfort, gastroesophageal reflux, and diuresis. The most significant side effects include seizures, cardiac arrhythmias, and death. Adverse effects from theophylline may be avoided if the clinician follows the patient carefully, monitors blood levels regularly, and educates the patient on the signs and symptoms of overdose.

Influence of Anesthetics on the Airways

Volatile Anesthetics

Volatile anesthetics have a host of effects on the respiratory system. Volatile anesthetics reduce bronchomotor tone and all commonly used volatile anesthetics (Table 25-3), except desflurane, produce a degree of bronchodilatation that may be helpful in patients with obstructive lung disease or in patients that experience any degree of bronchoconstriction.[61] Rooke and colleagues[62] in 1997 reported that sevoflurane produced a greater reduction in respiratory system resistance than isoflurane or halothane. Volatile anesthetics likely induce bronchodilation by decreasing intracellular calcium, partly mediated by an increase in intracellular cAMP and by decreasing the sensitivity of calcium mediated by protein kinase C.[63] The effect is seen to a greater degree in distal airway smooth muscle secondary to the T-type voltage-dependent calcium channel, which is sensitive to volatile anesthetics.[64]

Volatile anesthetics are administered to provide amnesia and blunt the response to surgical stimulation but can be of use in patients that have obstructive airway diseases or experience bronchoconstriction in the operating room. Multiple case reports provide examples of how volatile agents were used solely for the treatment of status asthmaticus.[65–68] The main concern with the use of volatile anesthetics is the rare occurrence of malignant hyperthermia. Hypotension can also be a concern with volatile anesthetics; however, the blood pressure is usually easily restored with small amounts of vasopressors. Deep levels of anesthesia associated with high concentrations of volatile anesthetics may be undesirable, and prolonged administration outside the operating room is problematic.

Table 25-3

Anesthetics with a Favorable Influence on Bronchomotor Tone

Volatile Anesthetics	Intravenous Anesthetics
Isoflurane	Propofol
Sevoflurane	Ketamine
Halothane	Midazolam

From Wojciechowski P, Hurford W. Pharmacology of the airways. In: Slinger P, ed. *Principles and Practice of Anesthesia for Thoracic Surgery*. New York, NY: Springer; 2011:121–132, with permission.

Intravenous Anesthetics

IV anesthetics can decrease bronchomotor tone when used for induction or IV anesthesia in the operating room. Ketamine, propofol, and midazolam (see Table 25-3) have relaxant effects on airway smooth muscle.[69] Etomidate and thiobarbiturates do not affect bronchomotor tone to the same extent.[70] The choice of IV anesthetics for induction and maintenance of anesthesia may be important for a patient with reactive airway disease. The mechanism of reduction of bronchomotor tone for the IV anesthetics is largely unknown. Ketamine is thought to have a direct relaxant effect on smooth muscle.[71] Propofol is thought to reduce vagal tone and have a direct effect on muscarinic receptors by interfering with cellular signaling and inhibiting calcium mobilization.[72,73] The preservative metabisulfite in propofol prevents the inhibition of vagal-mediated bronchoconstriction.[74]

Choosing an agent such as propofol or ketamine can be beneficial in patients with bronchospasm or obstructive airway disease. The use of these IV agents for induction or maintenance of anesthesia over other agents can be useful in minimizing the intraoperative effects of bronchospasm. Although each of the IV anesthetics carries a unique side effect profile, the major effects are not related to the airway. The use of ketamine is associated with increased salivation and coadministration of a small dose of anticholinergic can attenuate secretion production. Propofol is associated with hypotension that usually is easily corrected with vasopressors.

Local Anesthetics

Local anesthetics are primarily used to suppress coughing and blunt the hemodynamic response to tracheal intubation.[75,76] Although animal models have demonstrated some ability of local anesthetics to relax bronchial smooth muscle, in clinical practice the use of local anesthetics as pure bronchodilators is limited by toxicity and the ready availability of more potent bronchodilators such as short-acting β-adrenergic agonists.

Influence of Adjunctive Agents on the Airway

Helium (administered as a mixture of helium and oxygen [heliox]) has the advantage of having a low Reynolds' number and less resistance during turbulent airflow especially in large airways (see Chapter 24). A trial in patients with COPD exacerbations failed to demonstrate a statistically significant reduction in the necessity for endotracheal intubation in patients treated with noninvasive ventilation and helium-oxygen mixtures.[77] Helium-oxygen mixtures may be useful as short-term temporizing therapy to decrease the work of breathing in patients with upper airway obstruction. The use of helium-oxygen mixtures is limited by a progressive reduction in efficacy at higher inspired oxygen concentrations.

Antihistamines: Histamine release from mast cells and basophils is responsible for airway inflammation and bronchoconstriction in asthma.[78] Antihistamines are not standard therapy for asthma, but the use of antihistamines and leukotriene modifiers for allergen-induced bronchoconstriction has shown promise for diminishing the early and late responses to allergens.[78,79] Patients that have allergen-induced asthma or patients that experience an allergic reaction in the operating room may benefit from antihistamines to attenuate the role that histamine plays in bronchoconstriction.

Magnesium sulfate is not standard therapy for asthma exacerbations. Magnesium sulfate is thought to produce additional bronchodilation when given in conjunction with standard therapy for asthma exacerbations. Currently, IV magnesium therapy is reserved as an alternative therapy when the patient has not responded to standard therapy.[80] The combination of nebulized magnesium sulfate and β-adrenergic agonists have also been studied and show potential benefit in asthma exacerbations.[81] Overall, magnesium sulfate, IV or nebulized, is not a first-line therapy for asthma exacerbations and should be reserved for situations when the patient is not responding to conventional therapy.

Pharmacology of the Pulmonary Circulation

Patients with pulmonary hypertension (PHTN) are high-risk candidates for both cardiac and noncardiac surgery. They have poor cardiorespiratory reserve and are at risk of having perioperative complications including pulmonary hypertensive crises with resultant heart failure, respiratory failure, and dysrhythmias.[82,83] Anesthetic management of these patients can be complex and challenging. Drugs affecting the pulmonary vascular bed are routinely administered during anesthesia, and their effects are of particular interest in patients with PHTN. Reducing the consequences of an elevated pulmonary vascular resistance and the resulting right ventricular dysfunction should be considered as the primary goal of therapy with pulmonary vasodilators. Owing to the contractile properties of the naive right ventricle, attempts at improving its contractility are generally not effective. Therefore, principles of management of PHTN center on reducing right ventricular afterload while preserving coronary perfusion by avoiding reductions in systemic blood pressure.[84]

Anesthetic Drugs

Evaluating the effects of anesthetic drugs on the pulmonary vasculature is challenging. In clinical practice and research, these drugs are rarely administered in isolation. Their administration can lead to concurrent changes in nonpulmonary hemodynamic parameters such as cardiac output (CO) that ultimately affect pulmonary artery pressure (PAP). An increase in PAP may be the result of increased pulmonary vascular resistance (PVR), increased CO, or an increase in left atrial pressure (LAP) (PAP = [PVR × CO] + LAP). In addition, general anesthesia involves manipulation of variables that affect PVR, including fraction of inspired oxygen ($F_{I}O_2$), carbon dioxide (CO_2), and positive pressure ventilation (PPV).

Ketamine

Historically, ketamine has occupied a controversial position in anesthesia for patients with PHTN. Despite its current widespread use in these challenging patients, it has been classically taught that ketamine causes pulmonary vasoconstriction and should be used with extreme caution in this group. The mechanism of action of ketamine is not fully elucidated. It is an *N*-methyl-D-aspartic acid (NMDA) receptor antagonist and also binds to opioid receptors and muscarinic receptors.[85] It appears to stimulate release as well as inhibit neuronal uptake of catecholamines which may account for its cardiostimulatory and bronchodilatory effects. Some animal studies have shown an endothelium-independent vasodilatory response to ketamine in the pulmonary bed.

The effects of ketamine on the human pulmonary vasculature appear to be complex and the clinical literature reveals a vast heterogeneity in regard to results. Factors known to affect pulmonary vasoreactivity such as $F_{I}O_2$, CO_2, presence of PHTN, and presence of premedicants are not reported or acknowledged in many studies. The hemodynamic effects of a bolus of ketamine can be attenuated or abolished with premedicants such as droperidol, dexmedetomidine, or benzodiazepines.[86] Early study of the drug's hemodynamic profile in adult patients showed increases of PAP and PVR in the range of 40% to 50%. This, combined with increases in variables contributing to myocardial oxygen consumption, raised concern about the use of ketamine in patients with coronary artery disease (CAD) and PHTN. More recently in the pediatric literature, Williams et al.[87] showed no change in PVR or mean pulmonary artery pressure (mPAP) after ketamine administration in spontaneously breathing children with severe PHTN undergoing cardiac catheterization. In another pediatric study, ketamine maintained pulmonary to systemic blood flow and did not affect pulmonary pressure or resistance in children with intracardiac shunt undergoing cardiac catheterization. Propofol, on the other hand, decreased systemic vascular resistance (SVR) leading to increased right to left shunting.[88] In adult patients undergoing one-lung ventilation (OLV) for lung resection, ketamine did not significantly increase PAP or PVR compared to enflurane. Other case reports highlight the value of the relative cardiostability of the drug in patients with minimal cardiorespiratory reserve.[89,90] Many clinicians incorporate this drug into their routine inductions for patients with severe PHTN (e.g., pulmonary endarterectomy or lung transplantation). The advantages, in particular maintenance of stable hemodynamics and coronary perfusion pressure, seem to outweigh the potential disadvantages.

Propofol

Propofol is commonly used in anesthesia, including for patients with PHTN. It is frequently used to maintain anesthesia during and after lung transplantation. The effects of propofol are thought to be primarily mediated by γ-aminobutyric acid (GABA) receptors. The concerning hemodynamic effect of propofol in the context of PHTN is a decrease in SVR, which can not only have effects on intracardiac shunting, if present, but can lead to decreased coronary artery perfusion of the right ventricle and resultant right ventricular dysfunction. In regard to direct effects on the pulmonary vasculature, animal studies have shown that during increased tone conditions in the pulmonary vasculature, propofol may act as a pulmonary vasoconstrictor.[91] Propofol has also been shown to interfere with acetylcholine-induced pulmonary vasodilation in dogs.[92] On the other hand, in isolated pulmonary arteries from human and chronically hypoxic rats, etomidate and to a lesser extent propofol showed vessel relaxation.[93] The clinical significance of these contradictory results is unknown.

Etomidate

Etomidate is an imidazole that mediates its clinical actions primarily at GABA A receptors. As mentioned earlier, it appears to have vasorelaxant properties in isolated pulmonary arteries. Its major attribute as an induction agent is its stable hemodynamic profile. In patients with cardiac disease, an induction dose of etomidate increased mean arterial pressure (MAP), decreased SVR, and decreased PAP.[94] In pediatric patients without PHTN presenting for cardiac catheterization, there was no significant change in any hemodynamic parameters after induction with etomidate.[95]

Opioids

Opioids seem to have little to no deleterious effects on the pulmonary vascular system. In anesthetized cats, administration of morphine, fentanyl, remifentanil, and sufentanil caused a vasodilatory response under elevated tone conditions in isolated lobar artery.[96] The mechanism seems to involve histamine- and opioid-mediated receptor pathways. Clinical experience would echo the cardiostability of judicious narcotic administration in hemodynamically fragile patients.

Volatile Anesthetics

At clinically relevant concentrations, modern volatile anesthetics likely have little to no direct vasodilating effect on the pulmonary vasculature. In pigs, sevoflurane administration depressed right ventricular function with no change in PVR.[97] This suggests that the decreases in PAP observed with volatile anesthetics may partially occur secondary to the decreases in CO seen with these agents. Nitrous oxide is typically avoided in patients with PHTN as it is believed to cause pulmonary vasoconstriction, perhaps via release of catecholamines from sympathetic nerves supplying the pulmonary vasculature. In patients with mitral stenosis and PHTN presenting for cardiac surgery, administration of nitrous oxide after fentanyl anesthesia (7.5 to 10 μg/kg) increased PVR, PAP, and cardiac index (CI).[98] However, a subsequent study showed that in the presence of high-dose fentanyl (50 to 75 μg/kg), 70% nitrous oxide is actually was associated with a decrease in PAP and CO in patients with secondary PHTN, with no echocardiographic changes in right ventricular function.[99]

Neuromuscular Blockers

Pancuronium increases PAP in dogs with lung injury.[100] It is theorized to do so indirectly by increases in CO and directly by increasing PVR, possibly by its antagonist actions at muscarinic receptors in the pulmonary vasculature. Rocuronium, cisatracurium, and vecuronium have little to no effect on most cardiac indices in patients undergoing coronary artery bypass graft (CABG).[101]

Magnesium

Magnesium is a vasodilator in both the systemic and pulmonary circulations. The mechanism of action of magnesium's effects on vasodilation is likely through its effects on membrane channels involved in calcium flux and through its action in the synthesis of cAMP. It would appear to be an important cofactor for endothelial-dependent pulmonary vasodilation. It has been used successfully to wean NO in PHTN.[102] Increasing doses of magnesium in piglets with acute embolic PHTN decreased mPAP, increased CO, and decreased PVR.[103] Magnesium has been used to treat persistent PHTN of the newborn, but controversy surrounds its use.

Regional Analgesia

Pain can increase PVR.[104] Perioperative thoracic epidural analgesia (TEA) is commonly used in abdominal and thoracic surgery. TEA may decrease PAP through decreases in CO or via attenuation of the pulmonary sympathetic outflow. In pigs, TEA depresses right ventricular function in acute PHTN.[105] Unilateral thoracic paravertebral block with lidocaine has been shown to decrease myocardial contractility up to 30% and significantly decrease systemic pressure; an effect that may be attenuated by epinephrine. In general, the potential benefits of regional anesthesia in thoracoabdominal surgery typically outweigh the risks of hypotension and right ventricular dysfunction. As with most anesthetic interventions in patients with PHTN, careful titration and monitoring is paramount. A few reports illustrate successful use of epidural analgesia in this patient population.[106]

Vasopressors and Inotropes

Vasopressors and inotropes are commonly required during anesthesia to counteract the effects of cardiodepressant and vasodilating drugs. Treatment of hypotension in these patients can be difficult to manage given the typical cautious fluid administration most patient populations.

The innervation and receptor content of the pulmonary vasculature is complex. Neurotransmitter receptors in this system include those from the adrenergic, cholinergic, and dopaminergic families as well as histamine, serotonin, adenosine, purines, and peptides. The pulmonary vasculature's response to sympathetic activation will generally result in an increase in PVR. In human pulmonary artery, administration of acetylcholine induces pulmonary relaxation.[107]

The response of the pulmonary system to exogenous vasopressor administration is dependent on the clinical situation. Consequently, results of studies are heterogeneous. In anesthetized dogs without PHTN, dopamine, epinephrine, norepinephrine, and phenylephrine all increase PAP to varying degrees by varying mechanisms but with no drug is there a significant increase in PVR.[108] Dopamine does not increase PVR after lung transplantation in pigs.[109] In anesthetized patients with chronic secondary PHTN undergoing cardiac surgery, both norepinephrine and phenylephrine increase PAP and PVRI with minimal change in CI.[110] Within the clinically relevant MAP target in this study, norepinephrine decreased the mPAP to MAP ratio, but phenylephrine did not, suggesting it may be a better choice in this patient cohort. In a dog model of acute PHTN, however, phenylephrine restored perfusion to the ischemic right ventricle and therefore increased CO.[111] This is a relevant observation, as it illustrates the importance of coronary artery perfusion in the setting of right ventricular strain and that maintenance of systemic pressure by whatever method may be the most important principle in this subset of patients.

Vasopressin has also been studied. In a chronic hypoxic rat model, vasopressin administration resulted in a V1 receptor–mediated pulmonary vasodilation.[112] In an acute PHTN model in dogs, vasopressin increased PVR and resulted in a substantial decrease in right ventricular contractility.[113] Human studies of effects of vasopressin on the pulmonary vasculature are limited. Vasopressin has been used successfully after cardiac surgery in patients with PHTN and resistant hypotension.[114] The use of vasopressin to treat acute right ventricular failure in patients with IPPH has been described in obstetric anesthesia.[115]

Pulmonary Vasodilators

Pulmonary vasodilators are typically employed to improve right ventricular function in the setting of PHTN or in an effort to enhance regional pulmonary blood flow and improve intrapulmonary shunt. In the acute care setting, however, it is these agent's pulmonary vasodilatory effects that are being exploited. In general, parenteral and oral vasodilators are hampered by their relatively nonselective actions in the pulmonary vascular bed. In addition to their hypotensive systemic hemodynamic effects, their use may also lead to perfusion of underventilated alveoli, worsen intrapulmonary shunt and, in turn, worsen oxygenation. The ideal pulmonary vasodilator should have a rapid onset of action, a short half-life, and produce regional pulmonary vasodilation. This would avoid systemic hypotension and the potential adverse effects on ventilation-perfusion matching that limit the use of systemic agents in critically ill patients. In this regard, inhaled vasodilators are attractive as they preferentially dilate ventilated alveoli and have less systemic effects.

Nitric Oxide

Inhaled nitric oxide (iNO) is preferentially delivered to ventilated lung units leading to improved perfusion to alveoli that are able to participate in gas exchange. This "selective effect" leads to a decrease in intrapulmonary shunt. Medical grade NO may be administered either noninvasively (via a face mask) or through a ventilator circuit. If administered through a circuit, a device is used that can regulate the concentration of NO and monitor levels of nitrogen dioxide—a by-product of NO when it combines with oxygen (Fig. 25-1). At present, iNO is only approved for infants with respiratory distress syndrome. This approval stems from large prospective placebo-controlled studies demonstrating that NO reduced the need for extracorporeal membrane oxygenation (ECMO) and reduced the requirement for oxygen therapy following intensive care unit (ICU) discharge.[116] Although there is controversy about a dose-response relationship for NO and pulmonary vasodilation, the typical dose ranges from 10 to 40 ppm. Methemoglobin levels need to be monitored when NO is administered for more than 24 hours. Heart and lung transplantation represent two distinct areas where acute pulmonary vasodilation has strong theoretic benefit as it relates to improving acute right ventricular failure and attenuating reperfusion injury, respectively. The acute right ventricular failure complicating heart transplantation may be attenuated with the use of a pulmonary vasodilator. Although several studies suggest

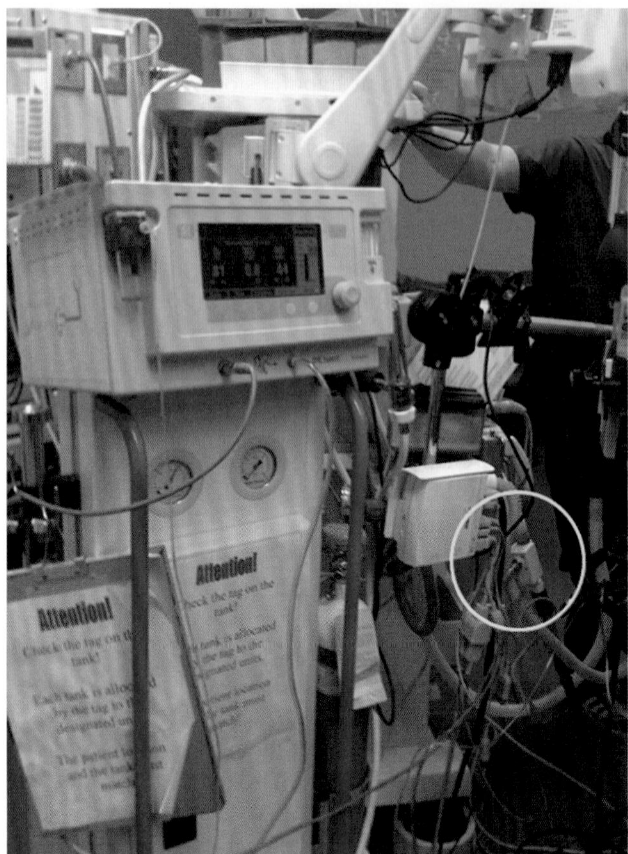

FIGURE 25-1 A commercial device for administration of nitric oxide (NO) via a ventilator circuit. NO is administered into the inspiratory limb of the anesthesia circuit close to the connection to the endotracheal tube. The concentration of the toxic metabolite nitrogen dioxide (NO_2) is monitored in the circuit via an attachment to the expiratory limb (*circled* in the photograph).

that NO may be useful preoperatively in risk-stratifying patients scheduled for cardiac transplant, only case series support the use of inhaled NO to reverse the right ventricular dysfunction following cardiac transplant. However, based on clinical experience, inhaled NO has become a standard of care in many transplant centers. The beneficial immune-modulating effects of inhaled NO in addition to its vasodilating properties were felt to be responsible for preliminary studies of using inhaled NO to prevent primary graft dysfunction (PGD) after lung transplantation.[117] Although a randomized clinical trial failed to show benefit in preventing PGD, it is commonly used to treat the hypoxemia and PHTN seen in established, severe PGD.[118] Owing to the inherent cost of using inhaled NO, other pulmonary vasodilators have been evaluated.

In nontransplant thoracic surgery, NO has been studied as a potential treatment for the gas exchange abnormalities associated with OLV. Its effects are controversial but it would appear that it exerts its maximal benefits in patients with elevated pulmonary vascular resistance index (PVRI) and the poorest gas exchange before administration.[119] NO can be quickly delivered via the circuit of an anesthetic or intensive care ventilator; however, it is expensive and not widely available.

Prostaglandins

Prostanoids induce relaxation of vascular smooth muscle, inhibit growth of smooth muscle cells and are powerful inhibitors of platelet aggregation.[120] Inhaled prostanoids involve an aerosol delivery mechanism that is attached by a nebulizer to the ventilator circuit (Fig. 25-2). Treatment may be limited by inefficiencies in aerosolization. Owing to the short half-life of epoprostenol, the drug must also be continuously nebulized.[121] As a result, changes of dose delivery with alterations in ventilator volumes, FIO_2, airway pressures, and solvent evaporation may be challenging. The synthetic prostanoids, treprostinil and iloprost, hold promise as inhaled vasodilators in that they may only require intermittent administration. When nebulized, prostanoids can lead to similar improvements in oxygenation and pulmonary pressures as compared to inhaled NO. A crossover study compared inhaled NO to inhaled prostaglandins in

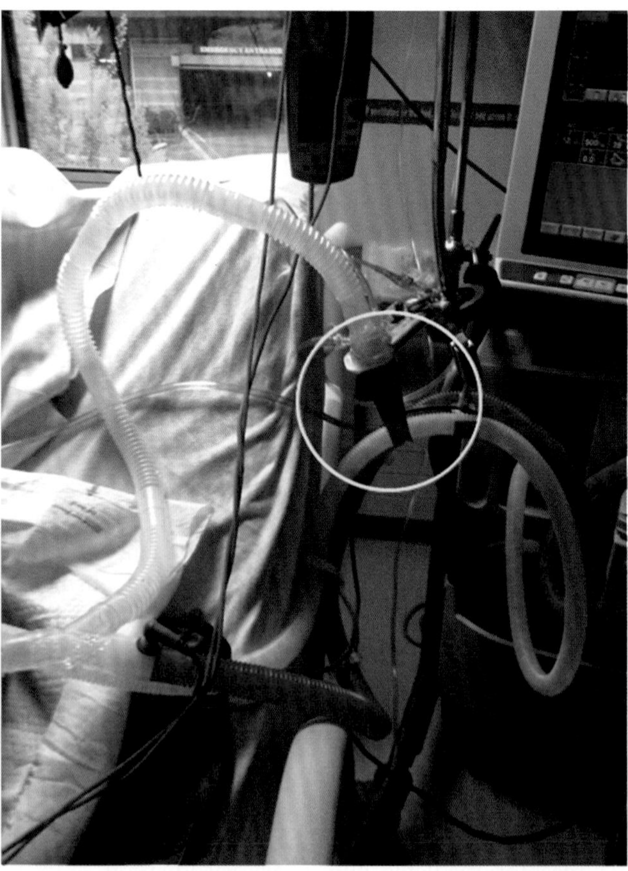

FIGURE 25-2 Prostacyclin can be delivered via continuous nebulization into an intensive care (pictured here) or an anesthesia ventilator circuit for specific pulmonary vasodilation.

patients after lung ($n = 19$) or heart ($n = 6$) transplant. In this acute hemodynamic study, there was no significant difference in hemodynamics or oxygenation between agents.[122] Prostacyclin can be delivered by nebulizer into a ventilator circuit at a starting dose of 50 ng/kg per minute and clinical effects should be evident within 10 minutes.[123]

Use of IV prostaglandins during OLV results in a decrease in both systemic and pulmonary pressures and either no change or a decrease in Pa_{O_2}. Selective infusion of prostaglandin into the pulmonary artery of the ventilated lung in a human model during OLV resulted in stable systemic pressure and a reduction in PVR and increase in Pa_{O_2}.[124] However, this route of administration is not practical in routine thoracic anesthesia practice. Inhaled prostacyclin decreases PVRI and PAP with maintenance of favorable systemic pressures but does not change Pa_{O_2} during OLV.[125]

Both iNO and prostaglandins have been shown to affect platelet function. This could theoretically contribute to perioperative bleeding during large surgeries such as lung transplantation and is a concern in regard to neuraxial analgesia. The clinical relevance of platelet inhibition with these inhaled agents is unknown. In cardiac surgery patients, laboratory confirmation of platelet dysfunction with inhaled prostacyclin did not correlate with chest tube losses.[126] Also, in an obstetrical patient with PHTN on IV prostacyclin, conversion to inhaled prostacyclin allowed for a successful labor epidural placement with no complications.[127]

Phosphodiesterase Inhibitors

Phosphodiesterase inhibitors prevent the degradation of cGMP and cAMP. cAMP and cGMP are activated by NO and are intermediaries in a pathway that leads to vasodilation via the activation of protein kinases and reduction in cytosolic calcium. Milrinone is an adenosine-3′, 5′-cAMP–selective phosphodiesterase enzyme (PDE) inhibitor. When nebulized, it has been shown to lead to a relative reduction in PVR compared to SVR.[128] The inhalation of milrinone selectively dilated the pulmonary vasculature without systemic effects. When milrinone is combined with inhaled prostacyclin, there appears to be a potentiation and prolongation of the pulmonary vasodilatory effect.[129]

Owing to the relatively higher expression of phosphodiesterase 5 (PDE5) in the pulmonary circulation relative to the systemic circulation, PDE5 inhibitors have a relative selective effect on PVR as opposed to SVR. In addition to their relatively selective pulmonary vasodilatory effects, their effects on smooth muscle proliferation and cellular apoptosis may be responsible for benefit of these agents when administered chronically in patients with idiopathic pulmonary arterial hypertension (PAH). A direct effect on the right ventricle has been postulated; however, the clinical relevance of this finding is uncertain.

Although the benefits of oral sildenafil and tadalafil in chronic PAH have been evaluated in prospective controlled trials, most of the acute applications for these agents have been described in case reports or small cohort studies and as such have not been approved for these indications. In the acute setting, sildenafil has been demonstrated to enhance the effects of inhaled NO and may also be useful in blunting the rebound in pulmonary pressures that occurs during weaning of inhaled NO.[130] The benefits of sildenafil in acute pulmonary embolism, cardiac transplantation, and in patients with PHTN being considered for pulmonary thromboendarterectomy have also been described.[131]

Hypoxic Pulmonary Vasoconstriction

IV anesthetic agents have no effect on hypoxic pulmonary vasoconstriction (HPV). All of the volatile anesthetics inhibit HPV in a dose-dependent fashion. Animal studies suggest that this inhibition is dependent on the agent: halothane > enflurane > isoflurane/desflurane/sevoflurane.[132] The older agents were potent inhibitors of HPV and this may have contributed to the high incidence of hypoxemia reported during OLV in the 1960s and 1970s (see earlier); many of these studies used 2 to 3 minimum alveolar concentration (MAC) doses of halothane during anesthesia.

In doses of less than or equal to 1 MAC, the modern volatile anesthetics (isoflurane, sevoflurane,[133] and desflurane[134]) are weak, and equipotent, inhibitors of HPV. The inhibition of the HPV response by 1 MAC of a volatile agent such as isoflurane is approximately 20% of the total HPV response, and this could account for only a net 4% increase in total arteriovenous shunt during OLV, which is a difference too small to be detected in most clinical studies.[135] In addition, volatile anesthetics cause less inhibition of HPV when delivered to the active site of vasoconstriction via the pulmonary arterial blood than via the alveolus. This pattern is similar to the HPV stimulus characteristics of oxygen. During established OLV, the volatile agent only reaches the hypoxic lung pulmonary capillaries via the mixed venous blood. No clinical benefit in oxygenation during OLV has been shown for total IV anesthesia above that seen with 1 MAC of the modern volatile anesthetics.[136] N_2O inhibits HPV. N_2O is usually avoided during thoracic anesthesia.

HPV is decreased by systemic vasodilators such as nitroglycerin and nitroprusside. In general, vasodilators can be expected to cause some deterioration in Pa_{O_2} during anesthesia. Thoracic epidural sympathetic blockade probably has little or no direct effect on HPV, which is a localized chemical response in the lung.[137] However, thoracic epidural anesthesia can have an indirect effect on oxygenation if it is allowed to cause hypotension and a fall in CO, thus decreasing mixed venous oxygen saturation.

Intrinsic Pharmacologic Effects of the Lungs

The lungs receive essentially the entire CO and the surface area of their vascular bed is enormous (70 to 100 m^2). The lungs contain nearly half of the body's endothelium and have an extraordinarily high perfusion of 14 mL/min/g tissue (as opposed to the next-highest renal perfusion of 4 mL/min/g tissue). Thus, there is ample blood-endothelial interface for surface enzyme activity as well as uptake and secretion.[138] The largest population of cells involved in pulmonary metabolism of blood-borne substances is, as might be expected, the pulmonary endothelium. Consistent with high metabolic activity, endothelial cells typically have both extensive cytoplasmic vesicles and prominent caveolae. The caveolae are tiny membrane invaginations and near-membrane vesicles similar to those found elsewhere in the body, measuring 50 to 100 nm, associated with caveolin proteins, and derived from lipid rafts within the membrane. The predominant activities of these caveolae, thought to include endocytosis and signal transduction, have not been fully delineated, and may be pleiotropic.[139] The endothelial cells structurally have large luminal projections and invaginations, providing an even greater interface area at the microscopic level.

Metabolism by the endothelial cell occurs either on the surface of the cell via enzymes associated with the membrane ("ectoenzymes") or by cytosolic processing after substances are taken up by the cell. Some surface enzymes are distributed along the luminal membrane, whereas others are associated exclusively with the caveolae. Figure 25-3 schematically depicts these processes with example substances and pathways. Metabolism may be further divided into exogenous versus endogenous substances as well as deactivated versus activated products. The terminology of pulmonary metabolism can be confusing and sometimes inconsistent. In general, "pulmonary uptake" (or "extraction") is simply used to describe transfer from blood to lung. It does not indicate whether the substance of interest is subsequently metabolized or returned back into the blood (with or without alteration). "First-pass" uptake is used to describe the amount of substance removed from the blood on the first cycle through the lungs. "Extraction" is also sometimes misused synonymously with first-pass uptake. "Clearance" may be used to describe a substance undergoing actual elimination, either in terms similar to renal clearance as volume of blood from which the substance would be completely removed (milliliters per minute or milliliters per kilogram per minute), or as a comparison of pulmonary arterial concentration versus systemic arterial concentration.

The lung has a pronounced impact on the blood concentration of substances even when it does not ultimately break them down or secrete them. This is because of simple uptake and retention of substances, often followed by release back into the blood. This "capacitor effect"[140] of the lungs in which any rapid rise or fall in concentration is attenuated is revisited in the following discussion regarding local anesthetic toxicity.

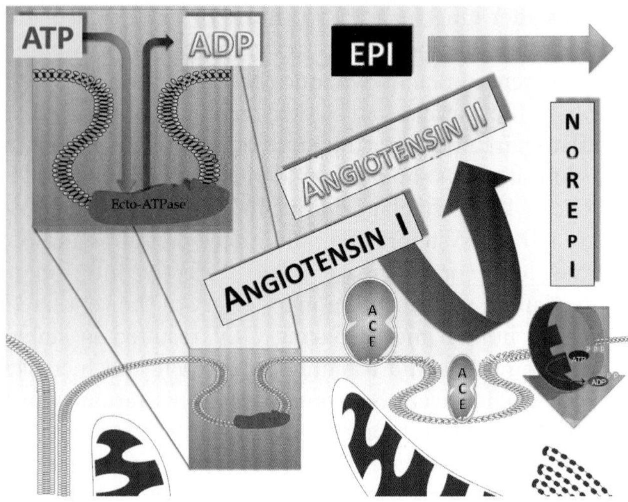

FIGURE 25-3 Schematic examples of pulmonary endothelial metabolism. Surface enzymes may be restricted to the caveolae (Ecto-ATPase in the *inset* above is an example), or present on both the luminal surface and caveola (e.g., angiotensin-converting enzyme [ACE]). Another characteristic of pulmonary endothelium is selective uptake, here exemplified by the ATP-dependent uptake of norepinephrine (NOR-EPI), while epinephrine (EPI) is not taken up. (From Yeazell L, Littlewood K. Nonrespiratory functions of the lungs. In: Slinger P, ed. *Principles and Practice of Anesthesia for Thoracic Surgery.* New York, NY: Springer; 2011:103–120, with permission.)

Exogenous Substances

Drugs

The cytochrome P450 monooxygenase enzyme systems are the most studied metabolic pathways for medications. The lungs have been found to have substantial concentrations of P450 isoenzymes, particularly within type II pneumocytes, Clara cells, and endothelial cells. While P450 and other enzyme systems have long been known to exist in the human lung, the actual activity of lung enzymes ranges from negligible to 33% of that of the liver.[141]

Opioids

Fentanyl has been shown to have a markedly variable first-pass uptake up to 90% in humans. The same investigators found that significant amounts of fentanyl then returned from the lungs into the blood with a biphasic pattern, equilibrating after about a minute in the fast phase and nearly 25 minutes for the slow phase. The uptake of fentanyl is higher than expected even for this basic and lipophilic drug. Active uptake of fentanyl has been demonstrated in human lung endothelial cells. Sufentanil demonstrates uptake that is a little more than half that of fentanyl. Morphine has a much lower uptake of about 10%.[142]

Local Anesthetics

For lidocaine, there is a first-pass uptake of approximately 50% with significant retention at 10 minutes.[143] The uptake of lidocaine has also been examined in a variety of physiologic circumstances. Under extremes of metabolic acidosis and alkalosis, lidocaine demonstrates increased uptake with higher blood pH. It is postulated that this finding is the consequence of increased drug lipophilicity because, in a less acidic environment, more of the drug is in its nonionized form. Bupivacaine has been investigated less extensively than lidocaine and with less consistent results. In most animal species, peak extraction has been reported as high with variable first-pass retention. In humans, however, the effective first-pass extraction appears to be lower when studied by epidural dosing.[144]

Two areas of interest in the practice of clinical anesthesia are intimately linked with the pulmonary uptake of local anesthetics. The first is the relative safety of levobupivacaine and ropivacaine in comparison to bupivacaine. These drugs have, in fact, been the subject of several investigations. Early animal studies suggested decreased toxicity of these newer preparations. However, a review of the pharmacodynamics and pharmacokinetics of local anesthetics[145] describes the challenges of comparing toxicities in clinical practice. A second area of interest is the treatment of local anesthetic toxicity with lipid emulsion. The issue of pulmonary uptake and delayed release of local anesthetics must be considered in the treatment of suspected local anesthetic toxicity with emulsified lipid.[146]

Hypnotics

Thiopental has been found to have nearly 15% first-pass uptake in humans[147] with little or no metabolism. The pulmonary uptake of ketamine was found to be slightly less than 10% without subsequent metabolism.[148] For propofol, most work shows about 30% first-pass uptake and negligible metabolism of propofol by the lungs.[149]

Endogenous Substances

Angiotensin-Converting Enzyme

The lung plays a critical role in the renin-angiotensin system because of the pulmonary endothelium's high concentration of angiotensin-converting enzyme (ACE). When the kidney responds to changes in physiologic parameters such as vascular volume, blood pressure, and adrenergic stimulation by the cleaving of prorenin, the resultant renin catalyzes the formation of angiotensin I from angiotensinogen. It is ACE that then converts angiotensin I to the critically important vasoconstrictor, angiotensin II. Although ACE can be found on vascular endothelium throughout the body as well as in the plasma, the pulmonary endothelium has an abundance of ACE as a surface or ectoenzyme on the vascular membrane[150] (Fig. 25-4). The newly formed angiotensin II is not taken up or further metabolized by the endothelial cell, but rather immediately returns to the blood. Clinically, ACE inhibitors have been useful drugs in the management of systemic hypertension.[151]

Bradykinin is a nine amino acid peptide produced in multiple sites throughout the body from kininogen through the action of plasma kallikrein. It is in turn metabolized by several peptidases. Bradykinin is degraded by ACE and more than 90% of bradykinin is eliminated on first-pass through the lungs.[152] Bradykinin's effects are wide-ranging, including antithrombotic and profibrinolytic activity in the coagulation system, as well as modulation of NO and prostacyclin release. Specific to the lung,

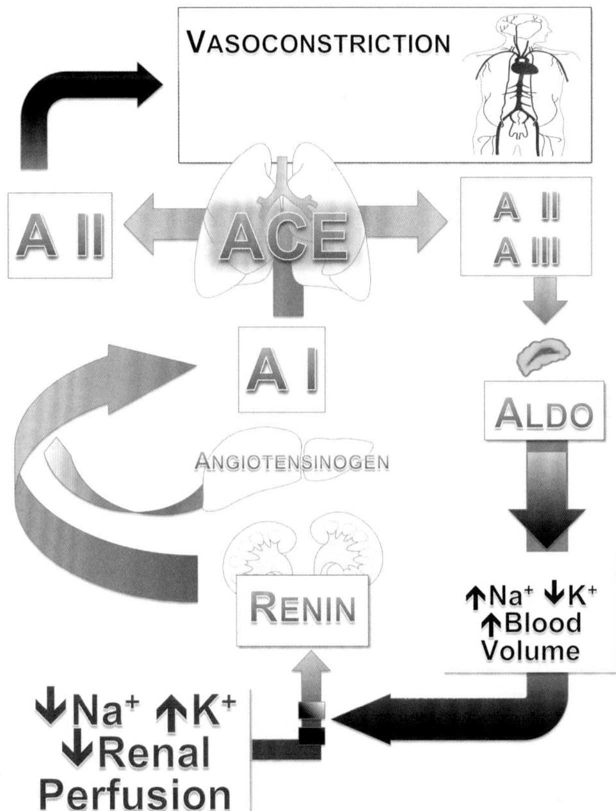

FIGURE 25-4 An example of the lung's central role in the body's endocrine processes, in this case the renin-angiotensin-aldosterone axis. In response to sodium, potassium, and renal perfusion changes, renin is secreted by the kidneys. Renin cleaves angiotensinogen (renin substrate) from the liver to form angiotensin I (AI). The lung then converts AI to AII through the action predominately of endothelium-associated angiotensin-converting enzyme (ACE). AII causes vasoconstriction and is involved in stimulation of aldosterone (ALDO) secretion by the adrenal gland, resulting in retention of sodium and volume by the kidney. (From Yeazell L, Littlewood K. Nonrespiratory functions of the lungs. In: Slinger P, ed. *Principles and Practice of Anesthesia for Thoracic Surgery*. New York, NY: Springer; 2011:103–120, with permission.)

bradykinin has vasodilating effects on normal pulmonary vessels but is vasoconstrictive when the pulmonary endothelium is destroyed in animal models.[153] Bradykinin is a bronchoconstrictor.[154] Some side effects of ACE inhibitors, such as angioedema and cough, and some of the beneficial impact, such as decreased myocardial infarctions and improved renal function, involve modification of bradykinin metabolism.

Biogenic Amines

Histamine; serotonin (5-hydroxytryptamine or 5-HT); and the three naturally occurring catecholamines dopamine, norepinephrine, and epinephrine comprise the group commonly termed biogenic amines. 5-HT is produced predominately by the gastrointestinal tract's chromaffin cells. Ingested tryptophan undergoes a two-step conversion first by tryptophan-5-hydroxylase and then by L-amino acid decarboxylase to serotonin. Mast cells and neuroendocrine cells in the lung are also capable of producing serotonin by uptake of tryptophan along the same enzymatic pathway. Once released from the gastrointestinal tract, there is avid uptake of 5-HT, particularly by nerve endings and platelets. These cells do not metabolize 5-HT to any great extent. The remainder of 5-HT is extracted by the lung and, to a lesser degree, the liver. In the case of these organs, the 5-HT is metabolized to 5-hydroxyindoleacetic acid (5-HIAA) by cytosolic monoamine oxidase (MAO) and aldehyde dehydrogenase. 5-HIAA is a useful marker of carcinoid syndrome with increased histamine turnover. MAO inhibitors block the cytosolic metabolism of 5-HT but not its uptake, whereas several drugs, including volatile anesthetic agents, block uptake but not intracellular metabolisms.[155]

Because it is not lipophilic, the pulmonary uptake of 5-HT is an active process, predominately via endothelial cells and with some variability between species. The pulmonary uptake of 5-HT by the lung is typically reported to be 90% or greater, meaning that little 5-HT reaches the systemic vasculature under normal circumstances. This model of production and uptake of 5-HT plays a pivotal role in several pathologic processes relevant to clinical anesthesiology. In carcinoid syndrome, the right heart receives a high concentration of 5-HT before being extracted and metabolized by the pulmonary circulation. This is thought to be the reason that the right heart shows the greatest myocardial and valvular injury in this syndrome.[156] The valvular injury of substances related to 5-HT such as methysergide and ergotamine, and those that increase 5-HT such as fenfluramine, and the recreational drug "ecstasy" (3,4-methylenedioxymethamphetamine), known to activate 5-HT receptors, are all similar to carcinoid cardiac disease. When an intracardiac right-to-left shunt is present in the carcinoid patient with a partial bypass of the pulmonary circulation, the left heart demonstrates valvular injury similar to that of the right heart.[157]

Pulmonary embolism presents another clinical situation pertinent to 5-HT activity. The mass effect of embolism does not, in itself, account for the typical cardiopulmonary consequences. The platelet aggregation and activation associated with acute pulmonary embolism results in degranulation with the release of 5-HT, well known to be a potent vasoconstrictor and to increase bronchial smooth muscle tone. This release of 5-HT and, perhaps, decreased local uptake of 5-HT are postulated to cause local and regional vascular changes. Other actions of elevated 5-HT, such as promotion of further platelet aggregation and inhibition of the vasodilating prostacyclin likely also play a role in the full response to pulmonary embolism.[158] Histamine, in contrast to 5-HT, has almost no uptake in the pulmonary circulation.

Just as the lung has the enzymes to metabolize both histamine and serotonin but the ability to take up only serotonin, its uptake of catecholamines also demonstrates marked selectivity. Norepinephrine demonstrates a 35% to 50% first-pass uptake with subsequent metabolism by catechol-*O*-methyltransferase (COMT), MAO, aldehyde reductase, and aldehyde dehydrogenase.[159] However, dopamine, isoproterenol, and epinephrine have essentially no uptake.

Arachidonic Acid Metabolites

Extensive production and metabolism of arachidonic acid derivatives occurs in the lung. The term eicosanoids refers to the 20-carbon carboxylic acids derived from the metabolism of the lipid membrane component icosatetraenoic acid, more commonly known as arachidonic acid. The action of phospholipase A_2 converts the esterified form, as found in the membrane, and releases arachidonic acid from structural glycerol. Once free, arachidonic acid may follow three main metabolic pathways in the lung: the lipoxygenase pathway produces leukotrienes, lipoxins, and some of the hydroxyeicosatetraenoic acids (HETEs); the cyclooxygenase (COX) pathway produces prostaglandins, thromboxane, and prostacyclin; and the cytochrome P450 monooxygenase system produces cis-epoxyeicosatrienoic acids and HETEs that are different than the products of the lipoxygenase pathway.

The leukotrienes promote inflammatory responses in the lung. They are responsible for bronchoconstriction and increased pulmonary vascular permeability, are chemotactic and chemokinetic for neutrophils, and facilitate eosinophil degranulation.[160] They are produced by activated inflammatory cells within the lung as well as those arriving in response to inflammation. The lipoxins have become identified as critical factors in the resolution of inflammation throughout the body.[161] They inhibit eosinophil and neutrophil chemotaxis and adhesion, as well as natural killer cell activation. They are endothelium-dependent vasodilators of both pulmonary and systemic vasculature.

COX catalyzes the cyclization and oxygenation of arachidonic acid, producing prostaglandin PGG_2 which is converted to PGH_2. There are subtypes of the COX enzyme, most notably COX-1 and COX-2. There has been great interest in COX-2 since its discovery in the 1990s because its inhibition was hoped to be more specific in controlling pain and inflammation without injury to the gastroduodenal mucosa. Although effective, the emergence of a small but real increase in cardiovascular risk of COX-2 inhibitors has tempered their use.[162] Complicating this issue further, many of the nonspecific COX inhibitors such as acetaminophen, salicylates, and the nonsteroidal antiinflammatory agents ibuprofen and naproxen show only slightly less COX-2 avidity than some of the newer COX-2–specific inhibitors. Following the production of PGH_2, the metabolic pathway divides into branches producing the various bioactive prostanoids; the enzymes of particular interest here are PGD synthase, PGE synthase, prostacyclin synthase, and thromboxane synthase. The final products of these pathways typically have opposed or balancing effects locally and regionally. Prostaglandin E_2 (PGE_2) and PGI_2 are bronchodilators, for example, whereas $PGF_{2\alpha}$, PGD_2, and thromboxane A_2 (TXA_2) cause bronchoconstriction. Similarly, PGD_2, PGE_2, $PGF_{2\alpha}$, and TXA_2 are potent vasoconstrictors, whereas PGE_1 and PGF_2 are vasodilators.

The cytochrome P450 monooxygenase system provides three pathways of arachidonic acid metabolism, which result in epoxyeicosatetraenoic acids (EETs), HETEs, or dihydroxyeicosatetraenoic acids (dHETEs). The HETEs and EETs have been shown experimentally to affect pulmonary vascular and bronchomotor tone. 20-HETE and 5-, 6-, 11-, and 12-EETs all have relaxing effects on both the lung vasculature and airways. They are further known to have general antiinflammatory effects, to modulate reperfusion injury, and to inhibit platelet aggregation. Within the lung, 15-HETE and 20-HETE may both modify hypoxic vasoconstriction.[163]

References

1. Wojciechowski P, Hurford W. Pharmacology of the airways. In: Slinger P, ed. *Principles and Practice of Anesthesia for Thoracic Surgery*. New York, NY: Springer; 2011:121–132.
2. Lewis MJ, Short AL, Lewis KE. Autonomic nervous system control of the cardiovascular and respiratory systems in asthma. *Respir Med*. 2006;100(10):1688–1705.
3. Burwell DR, Jones JG. The airways and anaesthesia—I. Anatomy, physiology and fluid mechanics. *Anaesthesia*. 1996;51(9):849–857.
4. Canning BJ, Fischer A. Neural regulation of airway smooth muscle tone. *Respir Physiol*. 2001;125(1–2):113–127.
5. Barnes PJ. Pharmacology of airway smooth muscle. *Am J Respir Crit Care Med*. 1998;158(5):S123–S132.
6. Lumb AB, Nunn JF. *Nunn's Applied Respiratory Physiology*. 6th ed. Philadelphia, PA: Elsevier Butterworth Heinemann; 2005.
7. Johnson M. The beta-adrenoceptor. *Am J Respir Crit Care Med*. 1998;158(5, pt 3):S146–S153.
8. Widdicombe JG. Autonomic regulation. i-NANC/e-NANC. *Am J Respir Crit Care Med*. 1998;158(5, pt 3):S171–S175.
9. Drazen JM, Gaston B, Shore SA. Chemical regulation of pulmonary airway tone. *Annu Rev Physiol*. 1995;57:151–170.
10. Fanta CH. Asthma. *N Engl J Med*. 2009;360(10):1002–1014.
11. Nelson HS. Beta-adrenergic bronchodilators. *N Engl J Med*. 1995; 333(8):499–506.
12. Johnson M, Butchers PR, Coleman RA, et al. The pharmacology of salmeterol. *Life Sci*. 1993;52(26):2131–2143.
13. Drazen JM, Israel E, Boushey HA, et al. Comparison of regularly scheduled with as-needed use of albuterol in mild asthma. Asthma Clinical Research Network. *N Engl J Med*. 1996;335(12):841–847.
14. Israel E, Chinchilli VM, Ford JG, et al. Use of regularly scheduled albuterol treatment in asthma: genotype-stratified, randomised, placebo-controlled cross-over trial. *Lancet*. 2004;364(9444): 1505–1512.
15. Israel E, Drazen JM, Liggett SB, et al. The effect of polymorphisms of the beta(2)-adrenergic receptor on the response to regular use of albuterol in asthma. *Am J Respir Crit Care Med*. 2000;162(1): 75–80.
16. National Asthma Education and Prevention Program Coordinating Committee, National Heart, Lung, and Blood Institute, U.S. Department of Health and Human Services. Expert Panel Report 3 (EPR-3): Guidelines for the diagnosis and management of asthma—summary report 2007. http://www.nhlbi.nih.gov/guidelines/asthma/asthsumm.pdf. Accessed January 7, 2010.
17. Gibson PG, Powell H, Ducharme FM. Differential effects of maintenance long-acting beta-agonist and inhaled corticosteroid on asthma control and asthma exacerbations. *J Allergy Clin Immunol*. 2007;119(2):344–350.
18. Bengtsson B. Plasma concentration and side-effects of terbutaline. *Eur J Respir Dis Suppl*. 1984;134:231–235.
19. Teule GJ, Majid PA. Haemodynamic effects of terbutaline in chronic obstructive airways disease. *Thorax*. 1980;35(7):536–542.
20. Wagner PD, Dantzker DR, Iacovoni VE, et al. Ventilation-perfusion inequality in asymptomatic asthma. *Am Rev Respir Dis*. 1978;118(3):511–524.
21. Repsher LH, Anderson JA, Bush RK, et al. Assessment of tachyphylaxis following prolonged therapy of asthma with inhaled albuterol aerosol. *Chest*. 1984;85(1):34–38.
22. Georgopoulos D, Wong D, Anthonisen NR. Tolerance to beta 2-agonists in patients with chronic obstructive pulmonary disease. *Chest*. 1990;97(2):280–284.
23. Nelson HS, Weiss ST, Bleecker ER, et al. The Salmeterol Multicenter Asthma Research Trial: a comparison of usual pharmacotherapy for asthma or usual pharmacotherapy plus salmeterol. *Chest*. 2006; 129(1):15–26.
24. Williams SJ, Winner SJ, Clark TJ. Comparison of inhaled and intravenous terbutaline in acute severe asthma. *Thorax*. 1981;36(8): 629–631.
25. Pierce RJ, Payne CR, Williams SJ, et al. Comparison of intravenous and inhaled terbutaline in the treatment of asthma. *Chest*. 1981;79(5):506–511.
26. Spiteri MA, Millar AB, Pavia D, et al. Subcutaneous adrenaline versus terbutaline in the treatment of acute severe asthma. *Thorax*. 1988;43(1):19–23.
27. Flynn RA, Glynn DA, Kennedy MP. Anticholinergic treatment in airways diseases. *Adv Ther*. 2009;26(10):908–919.
28. Karpel JP, Schacter EN, Fanta C, et al. A comparison of ipratropium and albuterol vs albuterol alone for the treatment of acute asthma. *Chest*. 1996;110(3):611–616.
29. Restrepo RD. A stepwise approach to management of stable COPD with inhaled pharmacotherapy: a review. *Respir Care*. 2009; 54(8):1058–1081.
30. Tashkin DP, Celli B, Senn S, et al. A 4-year trial of tiotropium in chronic obstructive pulmonary disease. *N Engl J Med*. 2008;359(15): 1543–1554.
31. Gal TJ, Suratt PM. Atropine and glycopyrrolate effects on lung mechanics in normal man. *Anesth Analg*. 1981;60(2):85–90.
32. Gal TJ, Suratt PM, Lu JY. Glycopyrrolate and atropine inhalation: comparative effects on normal airway function. *Am Rev Respir Dis*. 1984;129(5):871–873.
33. Villetti G, Bergamaschi M, Bassani F, et al. Pharmacological assessment of the duration of action of glycopyrrolate vs tiotropium and ipratropium in guinea-pig and human airways. *Br J Pharmacol*. 2006;148(3):291–298.

34. Haddad EB, Patel H, Keeling JE, et al. Pharmacological characterization of the muscarinic receptor antagonist, glycopyrrolate, in human and guinea-pig airways. *Br J Pharmacol.* 1999;127(2):413–420.
35. Tzelepis G, Komanapolli S, Tyler D, et al. Comparison of nebulized glycopyrrolate and metaproterenol in chronic obstructive pulmonary disease. *Eur Respir J.* 1996;9(1):100–103.
36. Sutherland ER, Martin RJ. Airway inflammation in chronic obstructive pulmonary disease: comparisons with asthma. *J Allergy Clin Immunol.* 2003;112(5):819–827; quiz 828.
37. Fujimoto K, Kubo K, Yamamoto H, et al. Eosinophilic inflammation in the airway is related to glucocorticoid reversibility in patients with pulmonary emphysema. *Chest.* 1999;115(3):697–702.
38. Pizzichini E, Pizzichini MM, Gibson P, et al. Sputum eosinophilia predicts benefit from prednisone in smokers with chronic obstructive bronchitis. *Am J Respir Crit Care Med.* 1998;158(5, pt 1): 1511–1517.
39. Chanez P, Bourdin A, Vachier I, et al. Effects of inhaled corticosteroids on pathology in asthma and chronic obstructive pulmonary disease. *Proc Am Thorac Soc.* 2004;1(3):184–190.
40. Suissa S, Ernst P, Benayoun S, et al. Low-dose inhaled corticosteroids and the prevention of death from asthma. *N Engl J Med.* 2000;343(5):332–336.
41. Donahue JG, Weiss ST, Livingston JM, et al. Inhaled steroids and the risk of hospitalization for asthma. *JAMA.* 1997;277(11):887–891.
42. Calverley PM, Anderson JA, Celli B, et al. Salmeterol and fluticasone propionate and survival in chronic obstructive pulmonary disease. *N Engl J Med.* 2007;356(8):775–789.
43. Barnes PJ. Molecular mechanisms of corticosteroids in allergic diseases. *Allergy.* 2001;56(10):928–936.
44. Pujols L, Mullol J, Torrego A, et al. Glucocorticoid receptors in human airways. *Allergy.* 2004;59(10):1042–1052.
45. Singh S, Amin AV, Loke YK. Long-term use of inhaled corticosteroids and the risk of pneumonia in chronic obstructive pulmonary disease: a meta-analysis. *Arch Intern Med.* 2009;169(3):219–229.
46. Niewoehner DE, Erbland ML, Deupree RH, et al. Effect of systemic glucocorticoids on exacerbations of chronic obstructive pulmonary disease. Department of Veterans Affairs Cooperative Study Group. *N Engl J Med.* 1999;340(25):1941–1947.
47. McEvoy CE, Niewoehner DE. Adverse effects of corticosteroid therapy for COPD. A critical review. *Chest.* 1997;111(3):732–743.
48. Usery JB, Self TH, Muthiah MP, et al. Potential role of leukotriene modifiers in the treatment of chronic obstructive pulmonary disease. *Pharmacotherapy.* 2008;28(9):1183–1187.
49. Drazen JM, Israel E, O'Byrne PM. Treatment of asthma with drugs modifying the leukotriene pathway. *N Engl J Med.* 1999;340(3): 197–206.
50. Reiss TF, Chervinsky P, Dockhorn RJ, et al. Montelukast, a once-daily leukotriene receptor antagonist, in the treatment of chronic asthma: a multicenter, randomized, double-blind trial. Montelukast Clinical Research Study Group. *Arch Intern Med.* 1998;158(11):1213–1220.
51. Israel E, Rubin P, Kemp JP, et al. The effect of inhibition of 5-lipoxygenase by zileuton in mild-to-moderate asthma. *Ann Intern Med.* 1993;119(11):1059–1066.
52. Brabson JH, Clifford D, Kerwin E, et al. Efficacy and safety of low-dose fluticasone propionate compared with zafirlukast in patients with persistent asthma. *Am J Med.* 2002;113(1):15–21.
53. Malmstrom K, Rodriguez-Gomez G, Guerra J, et al. Oral montelukast, inhaled beclomethasone, and placebo for chronic asthma. A randomized, controlled trial. Montelukast/Beclomethasone Study Group. *Ann Intern Med.* 1999;130(6):487–495.
54. Price DB, Hernandez D, Magyar P, et al. Randomised controlled trial of montelukast plus inhaled budesonide versus double dose inhaled budesonide in adult patients with asthma. *Thorax.* 2003;58(3): 211–216.
55. Bernstein IL. Cromolyn sodium. *Chest.* 1985;87(1)(suppl):68S–73S.
56. Guevara JP, Ducharme FM, Keren R, et al. Inhaled corticosteroids versus sodium cromoglycate in children and adults with asthma. *Cochrane Database Syst Rev.* 2006;(2):CD003558.
57. Barnes PJ. Theophylline: new perspectives for an old drug. *Am J Respir Crit Care Med.* 2003;167(6):813–818.
58. Global Intiative for Asthma. www.ginasthma.com. Accessed January 7, 2010.
59. Global Initiative for Chronic Obstructive Lung Disease. www.goldcopd.com. Accessed January 7, 2010.
60. Aubier M, De Troyer A, Sampson M, et al. Aminophylline improves diaphragmatic contractility. *N Engl J Med.* 1981;305(5):249–252.
61. Goff MJ, Arain SR, Ficke DJ, et al. Absence of bronchodilation during desflurane anesthesia: a comparison to sevoflurane and thiopental. *Anesthesiology.* 2000;93(2):404–408.
62. Rooke GA, Choi JH, Bishop MJ. The effect of isoflurane, halothane, sevoflurane, and thiopental/nitrous oxide on respiratory system resistance after tracheal intubation. *Anesthesiology.* 1997;86(6): 1294–1299.
63. Yamakage M. Direct inhibitory mechanisms of halothane on canine tracheal smooth muscle contraction. *Anesthesiology.* 1992; 77(3):546–553.
64. Yamakage M, Chen X, Tsujiguchi N, et al. Different inhibitory effects of volatile anesthetics on T- and L-type voltage-dependent Ca2+ channels in porcine tracheal and bronchial smooth muscles. *Anesthesiology.* 2001;94(4):683–693.
65. Gold MI, Helrich M. Pulmonary mechanics during general anesthesia: V. Status asthmaticus. *Anesthesiology.* 1970;32(5):422–428.
66. Parnass SM, Feld JM, Chamberlin WH, et al. Status asthmaticus treated with isoflurane and enflurane. *Anesth Analg.* 1987;66(2): 193–195.
67. Johnston RG, Noseworthy TW, Friesen EG, et al. Isoflurane therapy for status asthmaticus in children and adults. *Chest.* 1990;97(3): 698–701.
68. Schwartz SH. Treatment of status asthmaticus with halothane. *JAMA.* 1984;251(20):2688–2689.
69. Cheng EY, Mazzeo AJ, Bosnjak ZJ, et al. Direct relaxant effects of intravenous anesthetics on airway smooth muscle. *Anesth Analg.* 1996;83(1):162–168.
70. Eames WO, Rooke GA, Wu RS, et al. Comparison of the effects of etomidate, propofol, and thiopental on respiratory resistance after tracheal intubation. *Anesthesiology.* 1996;84(6):1307–1311.
71. Wanna HT, Gergis SD. Procaine, lidocaine, and ketamine inhibit histamine-induced contracture of guinea pig tracheal muscle in vitro. *Anesth Analg.* 1978;57(1):25–27.
72. Lin CC, Shyr MH, Tan PP, et al. Mechanisms underlying the inhibitory effect of propofol on the contraction of canine airway smooth muscle. *Anesthesiology.* 1999;91(3):750–759.
73. Brown RH, Wagner EM. Mechanisms of bronchoprotection by anesthetic induction agents: propofol versus ketamine. *Anesthesiology.* 1999;90(3):822–828.
74. Brown RH, Greenberg RS, Wagner EM. Efficacy of propofol to prevent bronchoconstriction: effects of preservative. *Anesthesiology.* 2001;94(5):851–855.
75. Yukioka H, Hayashi M, Terai T, et al. Intravenous lidocaine as a suppressant of coughing during tracheal intubation in elderly patients. *Anesth Analg.* 1993;77(2):309–312.
76. Hamill JF, Bedford RF, Weaver DC, et al. Lidocaine before endotracheal intubation: intravenous or laryngotracheal? *Anesthesiology.* 1981;55(5):578–581.
77. Maggiore SM, Richard JC, Abroug F, et al. A multicenter, randomized trial of noninvasive ventilation with helium-oxygen mixture in exacerbations of chronic obstructive lung disease. *Crit Care Med.* 2010;38(1):145–151.
78. Lordan JL, Holgate ST. H1-antihistamines in asthma. *Clin Allergy Immunol.* 2002;17:221–248.
79. Richter K, Gronke L, Janicki S, et al. Effect of azelastine, montelukast, and their combination on allergen-induced bronchoconstriction in asthma. *Pulm Pharmacol Ther.* 2008;21(1):61–66.
80. Rowe BH, Bretzlaff JA, Bourdon C, et al. Magnesium sulfate for treating exacerbations of acute asthma in the emergency department. *Cochrane Database Syst Rev.* 2000;(2):CD001490.

81. Blitz M, Blitz S, Hughes R, et al. Aerosolized magnesium sulfate for acute asthma: a systematic review. *Chest.* 2005;128(1):337–344.
82. Reimer C, Granton J. Pharmacology of the pulmonary circulation. In: Slinger P, ed. *Principles and Practice of Anesthesia for Thoracic Surgery.* New York, NY: Springer, 2011:133–142.
83. Lai HC, Wang KY, Lee WL, et al. Severe pulmonary hypertension complicates postoperative outcome of non-cardiac surgery. *Br J Anaesth.* 2007;99(2):184–190.
84. Strumpher J, Jacobsohn E. Pulmonary hypertension and right ventricular dysfunction: physiology and perioperative management. *J Cardiothorac Vasc Anesth.* 2011;25:687–704.
85. Hirota K, Lambert DG. Ketamine: its mechanism(s) of action and unusual clinical uses. *Br J Anaesth.* 1996;77(4):441–444.
86. Reich DL, Silvay G. Ketamine: an update on the first twenty-five years of clinical experience. *Can J Anaesth.* 1989;36(2):186–197.
87. Williams GD, Philip BM, Chu LF, et al. Ketamine does not increase pulmonary vascular resistance in children with pulmonary hypertension undergoing sevoflurane anesthesia and spontaneous ventilation. *Anesth Analg.* 2007;105(6):1578–1584.
88. Oklu E, Bulutcu FS, Yalcin Y, et al. Which anesthetic agent alters the hemodynamic status during pediatric catheterization? Comparison of propofol versus ketamine. *J Cardiothorac Vasc Anesth.* 2003;17(6):686–690.
89. Heller AR, Litz RJ, Koch T. A fine balance—one-lung ventilation in a patient with Eisenmenger syndrome. *Br J Anaesth.* 2004; 92(4):587–590.
90. Kopka A, McMenemin IM, Serpell MG, et al. Anaesthesia for cholecystectomy in two non-parturients with Eisenmenger's syndrome. *Acta Anaesthesiol Scand.* 2004;48(6):782–786.
91. Kondo U, Kim SO, Nakayama M, et al. Pulmonary vascular effects of propofol at baseline, during elevated vasomotor tone, and in response to sympathetic alpha- and beta-adrenoreceptor activation. *Anesthesiology.* 2001;94(5):815–823.
92. Kondo U, Kim SO, Murray PA. Propofol selectively attenuates endothelium-dependent pulmonary vasodilation in chronically instrumented dogs. *Anesthesiology.* 2000;93(2):437–446.
93. Ouedraogo N, Mounkaila B, Crevel H, et al. Effect of propofol and etomidate on normoxic and chronically hypoxic pulmonary artery. *BMC Anesthesiol.* 2006;6:2.
94. Colvin MP, Savege TM, Newland PE, et al. Cardiorespiratory changes following induction of anaesthesia with etomidate in patients with cardiac disease. *Br J Anaesth.* 1979;51(6):551–556.
95. Sarkar M, Laussen PC, Zurakowski D, et al. Hemodynamic responses to etomidate on induction of anesthesia in pediatric patients. *Anesth Analg.* 2005;101(3):645–650.
96. Kaye AD, Hoover JM, Kaye AJ, et al. Morphine, opioids, and the feline pulmonary vascular bed. *Acta Anaesthesiol Scand.* 2008;52(7):931–937.
97. Kerbaul F, Bellezza M, Mekkaoui C, et al. Sevoflurane alters right ventricular performance but not pulmonary vascular resistance in acutely instrumented anesthetized pigs. *J Cardiothorac Vasc Anesth.* 2006;20(2):209–216.
98. Schulte-Sasse U, Hess W, Tarnow J. Pulmonary vascular responses to nitrous oxide in patients with normal and high pulmonary vascular resistance. *Anesthesiology.* 1982;57(1):9–13.
99. Konstadt SN, Reich DL, Thys DM. Nitrous oxide does not exacerbate pulmonary hypertension or ventricular dysfunction in patients with mitral valvular disease. *Can J Anaesth.* 1990;37(6): 613–617.
100. Hemmerling TM, Russo G, Bracco D. Neuromuscular blockade in cardiac surgery: an update for clinicians. *Ann Card Anaesth.* 2008;11(2):80–90.
101. McCoy EP, Maddieneri VR, Elliott P, et al. Hemodynamic effects of rocuronium during fentanyl anesthesia. *Can J Anesth.* 1993; 40:703–708.
102. al-Halees Z, Afrane B, el-Barbary M. Magnesium sulfate to facilitate weaning of nitric oxide in pulmonary hypertension. *Ann Thorac Surg.* 1997;63(1):298–299.
103. Haas NA, Kemke J, Schulze-Neick I, et al. Effect of increasing doses of magnesium in experimental pulmonary hypertension after acute pulmonary embolism. *Intensive Care Med.* 2004; 30(11):2102–2109.
104. Houfflin Debarge V, Sicot B, Jaillard S, et al. The mechanisms of pain-induced pulmonary vasoconstriction: an experimental study in fetal lambs. *Anesth Analg.* 2007;104(4):799–806.
105. Rex S, Missant C, Segers P, at al. Thoracic epidural anesthesia impairs the hemodynamic response to acute pulmonary hypertension by deteriorating right ventricular-pulmonary arterial coupling. *Crit Care Med.* 2007;35(1):222–229.
106. Armstrong P. Thoracic epidural anaesthesia and primary pulmonary hypertension. *Anaesthesia.* 1992;47(6):496–499.
107. Barnes PJ, Liu SF. Regulation of pulmonary vascular tone. *Pharmacol Rev.* 1995;47(1):87–131.
108. Pearl RG, Maze M, Rosenthal MH. Pulmonary and systemic hemodynamic effects of central venous and left atrial sympathomimetic drug administration in the dog. *J Cardiothorac Anesth.* 1987;1(1):29–35.
109. Roscher R, Ingemansson R, Algotsson L, et al. Effects of dopamine in lung-transplanted pigs at 32 degrees C. *Acta Anaesthesiol Scand.* 1999;43(7):715–721.
110. Kwak YL, Lee CS, Park YH, et al. The effect of phenylephrine and norepinephrine in patients with chronic pulmonary hypertension*. *Anaesthesia.* 2002;57(1):9–14.
111. Vlahakes GJ, Turley K, Hoffman JI. The pathophysiology of failure in acute right ventricular hypertension: hemodynamic and biochemical correlations. *Circulation.* 1981;63(1):87–95.
112. Jin HK, Yang RH, Chen YF, et al. Hemodynamic effects of arginine vasopressin in rats adapted to chronic hypoxia. *J Appl Physiol.* 1989;66(1):151–160.
113. Leather HA, Segers P, Berends N, et al. Effects of vasopressin on right ventricular function in an experimental model of acute pulmonary hypertension. *Crit Care Med.* 2002;30(11):2548–2552.
114. Tayama E, Ueda T, Shojima T, et al. Arginine vasopressin is an ideal drug after cardiac surgery for the management of low systemic vascular resistant hypotension concomitant with pulmonary hypertension. *Interact Cardiovasc Thorac Surg.* 2007;6(6):715–719.
115. Price LC, Forrest P, Sodhi V, et al. Use of vasopressin after Caesarean section in idiopathic pulmonary arterial hypertension. *Br J Anaesth.* 2007;99(4):552–555.
116. Roberts JD Jr, Fineman JR, Morin FC III, et al. Inhaled nitric oxide and persistent pulmonary hypertension of the newborn. The Inhaled Nitric Oxide Study Group. *N Engl J Med.* 1997;336(9): 605–610.
117. Mosquera I, Crespo-Leiro MG, Tabuyo T, et al. Pulmonary hypertension and right ventricular failure after heart transplantation: usefulness of nitric oxide. *Transplant Proc.* 2002;34(1): 166–167.
118. Meade MO, Granton JT, Matte-Martyn A, et al. A randomized trial of inhaled nitric oxide to prevent ischemia-reperfusion injury after lung transplantation. *Am J Respir Crit Care Med.* 2003; 167(11):1483–1489.
119. Rocca GD, Coccia C, Pompei L, et al. Hemodynamic and oxygenation changes of combined therapy with inhaled nitric oxide and inhaled aerosolized prostacyclin. *J Cardiothorac Vasc Anesth.* 2001;15(2):224–227.
120. Vane JR, Botting RM. Pharmacodynamic profile of prostacyclin. *Am J Cardiol.* 1995;75(3):3A–10A.
121. Olschewski H, Simonneau G, Galie N, et al. Inhaled iloprost for severe pulmonary hypertension. *N Engl J Med.* 2002;347(5):322–329.
122. Khan TA, Schnickel G, Ross D, et al. A prospective, randomized, crossover pilot study of inhaled nitric oxide versus inhaled prostacyclin in heart transplant and lung transplant recipients. *J Thorac Cardiovasc Surg.* 2009;138(6):1417–1424.
123. Jerath A, Srinivas C, Vegas A, et al. The successful management of severe protamine-induced pulmonary hypertension using inhaled prostacyclin. *Anesth Analg.* 2010;110:365–369.

124. Chen TL, Lee YT, Wang MJ, et al. Endothelin-1 concentrations and optimization of arterial oxygenation and venous admixture by selective pulmonary artery infusion of prostaglandin E1 during thoracotomy. *Anaesthesia*. 1996;51:422–426.
125. Bund M, Henzler D, Walz R, et al. Aerosolized and intravenous prostacyclin during one-lung ventilation. Hemodynamic and pulmonary effects [in German]. *Anaesthesist*. 2004;53(7):612–620.
126. Haraldsson A, Kieler-Jensen N, Wadenvik H, et al. Inhaled prostacyclin and platelet function after cardiac surgery and cardiopulmonary bypass. *Intensive Care Med*. 2000;26(2):188–194.
127. Hill LL, De Wet CJ, Jacobsohn E, et al. Peripartum substitution of inhaled for intravenous prostacyclin in a patient with primary pulmonary hypertension. *Anesthesiology*. 2004;100(6):1603–1605.
128. Urdaneta F, Lobato EB, Beaver T, et al. Treating pulmonary hypertension post cardiopulmonary bypass in pigs: milrinone vs. sildenafil analog. *Perfusion*. 2008;23(2):117–125.
129. Lakshminrusimha S, Porta NF, Farrow KN, et al. Milrinone enhances relaxation to prostacyclin and iloprost in pulmonary arteries isolated from lambs with persistent pulmonary hypertension of the newborn. *Pediatr Crit Care Med*. 2009;10(1):106–112.
130. Atz AM, Wessel DL. Sildenafil ameliorates effects of inhaled nitric oxide withdrawal. *Anesthesiology*. 1999;91(1):307–310.
131. Dias-Junior CA, Vieira TF, Moreno H Jr, et al. Sildenafil selectively inhibits acute pulmonary embolism-induced pulmonary hypertension. *Pulm Pharmacol Ther*. 2005;18(3):181–186.
132. Lohser J. Evidence-based management of one-lung ventilation. *Anesth Clinics*. 2008;26:241–272.
133. Wang JY, Russel GN, Page RD, et al. A comparison of the effects of sevoflurane and isoflurane on arterial oxygenation during one-lung anesthesia. *Br J Anesth*. 2000;81:850–853.
134. Wang JY, Russel GN, Page RD, et al. A comparison of the effects of desflurane and isoflurane on arterial oxygenation during one-lung anesthesia. *Anaesthesia*. 2000;55:167–173.
135. Benumof J. Isoflurane anesthesia and arterial oxygenation during one-lung ventilation. *Anesthesiology*. 1986;64:419–422.
136. Reid CW, Slinger PD, Lewis S. Comparison of the effects of propofol-alfentanil versus isoflurane anesthesia on arterial oxygenation during one-lung anesthesia. *J Cardiothorac Vasc Anesth*. 1997;10:860–863.
137. Brimioulle S, Vachiery J-L, Brichant J-F, et al. Sympathetic modulation of hypoxic pulmonary vasoconstriction in intact dogs. *Cardiovasc Res*. 1997;34:384–392.
138. Yeazell L, Littlewood K. Nonrespiratory functions of the lungs. In: Slinger P, ed. *Principles and Practice of Anesthesia for Thoracic Surgery*. New York, NY: Springer; 2011:103–120.
139. Parat M, Kwang WJ. The biology of caveolae: achievements and perspectives. *Int Rev Cell Mol Biol*. 2009;273:117–162.
140. Upton RN, Doolette DJ. Kinetic aspects of drug disposition in the lungs. *Clin Exp Pharmacol Physiol*. 1999;26(5–6):381–391.
141. Pacifici GM, Franchi M, Bencini C, et al. Tissue distribution of drug-metabolizing enzymes in humans. *Xenobiotica*. 1988;18(7): 849–856.
142. Waters CM, Krejcie TC, Avram MJ. Facilitated uptake of fentanyl, but not alfentanil, by human pulmonary endothelial cells. *Anesthesiology*. 2000;93(3):825–831.
143. Krejcie TC, Avram MJ, Gentry WB, et al. A recirculatory model of the pulmonary uptake and pharmacokinetics of lidocaine based on analysis of arterial and mixed venous data from dogs. *J Pharmacokinet Biopharm*. 1997;25(2):169–190.
144. Sharrock NE, Mather LE, Go G, et al. Arterial and pulmonary arterial concentrations of the enantiomers of bupivacaine after epidural injection in elderly patients. *Anesth Analg*. 1998;86(4):812–817.
145. Mather LE, Copeland SE, Ladd LA. Acute toxicity of local anesthetics: underlying pharmacokinetic and pharmacodynamic concepts.[see comment]. *Reg Anesth Pain Med*. 2005;30(6):553–566.
146. Marwick PC, Levin AI, Coetzee AR. Recurrence of cardiotoxicity after lipid rescue from bupivacaine-induced cardiac arrest. *Anesth Analg*. 2009;108(4):1344–1346.
147. Roerig DL, Kotrly KJ, Dawson CA, et al. First-pass uptake of verapamil, diazepam, and thiopental in the human lung. *Anesth Analg*. 1989;69(4):461–466.
148. Henthorn TK, Krejcie TC, Niemann CU, et al. Ketamine distribution described by a recirculatory pharmacokinetic model is not stereoselective. *Anesthesiology*. 1999;91(6):1733–1743.
149. Upton RN, Ludbrook G. A physiologically based, recirculatory model of the kinetics and dynamics of propofol in man. *Anesthesiology*. 2005;103(2):344–352.
150. Orfanos SE, Langleben D, Khoury J, et al. Pulmonary capillary endothelium-bound angiotensin-converting enzyme activity in humans. *Circulation*. 1999;99(12):1593–1599.
151. Muntner P, Krousel-Wood M, Hyre AD, et al. Antihypertensive prescriptions for newly treated patients before and after the main antihypertensive and lipid-lowering treatment to prevent heart attack trial results and seventh report of the joint national committee on prevention, detection, evaluation, and treatment of high blood pressure guidelines. *Hypertension*. 2009;53(4):617–623.
152. Skidgel RA. Bradykinin-degrading enzymes: structure, function, distribution, and potential roles in cardiovascular pharmacology. *J Cardiovasc Pharmacol*. 1992;20(suppl 9):S4–S9.
153. Skidgel RA, Erdos EG. Angiotensin converting enzyme (ACE) and neprilysin hydrolyze neuropeptides: a brief history, the beginning and follow-ups to early studies. *Peptides*. 2004;25(3):521–525.
154. Suguikawa TR, Garcia CA, Martinez EZ, et al. Cough and dyspnea during bronchoconstriction: comparison of different stimuli. *Cough*. 2009;5:6.
155. Cook DR, Brandom BW. Enflurane, halothane, and isoflurane inhibit removal of 5-hydroxytryptamine from the pulmonary circulation. *Anesth Analg*. 1982;61(8):671–675.
156. Shah PM, Raney AA. Tricuspid valve disease. *Curr Probl Cardiol*. 2008;33(2):47–84.
157. Mizuguchi KA, Fox AA, Burch TM, et al. Tricuspid and mitral valve carcinoid disease in the setting of a patent foramen ovale. *Anesth Analg*. 2008;107(6):1819–1821.
158. Stratmann G, Gregory GA. Neurogenic and humoral vasoconstriction in acute pulmonary thromboembolism [see comment]. *Anesth Analg*. 2003;97(2):341–354.
159. Philpot RM, Andersson TB, Eling TE. Uptake, accumulation, and metabolism of chemicals by the lung. In: Bakhle YS, Vane JR, eds. *Metabolic Functions of the Lung*. New York, NY: Marcel Dekker; 1977:123–171.
160. Haeggstrom JZ, Kull F, Rudberg PC, et al. Leukotriene A4 hydrolase. *Prostaglandins Other Lipid Mediat*. 2002;68–69:495–510.
161. Romano M, Recchia I, Recchiuti A. Lipoxin receptors. *ScientificWorldJournal*. 2007;7:1393–1412.
162. Funk CD, FitzGerald GA. COX-2 inhibitors and cardiovascular risk. *J Cardiovasc Pharmacol*. 2007;50(5):470–479.
163. Jacobs ER, Zeldin DC. The lung HETEs (and EETs) up. *Am J Physiol Heart Circ Physiol*. 2001;280(1):H1–H10.

CHAPTER 26

Acid–Base Disorders

Peter Slinger

The management of acid–base disorders requires establishing the cause(s) of the disorder and then treating the underlying physiologic derangement. The treatment of acid–base disturbances is complex for a variety of reasons including the fact that the laboratory information on which we make decisions is rarely complete. This is because we often do not have access to all the data which influence a patient's acid–base status (e.g., serum phosphate, sulfate, etc.). The acid–base disturbance is often evolving rapidly (e.g., ischemia, shock, etc.) and there is a delay getting laboratory results. The algorithms which have been designed to help us understand acid–base therapy are based on steady-state conditions and the terminology that we use to describe acid–base chemistry is not intuitive (Table 26-1). However, with just blood gas and common serum biochemistry data, we can manage the majority of clinical acid–base disorders.

The central focus of treating acid–base disturbances is the understanding of the biochemistry of the hydrogen ion. Hydrogen ion concentrations in the various body fluid compartments are precisely regulated in the face of enormous variations in local production and clearance. Deviations in hydrogen ion concentrations from the normal range can cause marked alterations in protein structure and function, enzyme activity, and cellular function. Although hydrogen ions are continuously produced in the hydrolysis of adenosine triphosphate, the largest contribution of metabolic acids arises from the oxidation of carbohydrates, principally glucose, to produce carbon dioxide (volatile acid, approximately 24,000 mEq per day). By comparison, the average net production of nonvolatile metabolic acid, such as lactate, is relatively small (approximately 60 mEq per day).

The hydrogen ion concentration is regulated to maintain the arterial blood pH between 7.35 and 7.45. However, expression of the hydrogen ion concentration as pH masks large variations in hydrogen ion concentration despite small changes in pH. For example, a pH range of 7.0 to 7.7 is associated with a fivefold change (100 nmol/L to 20 nmol/L) in hydrogen ion concentration. The pH of venous blood and interstitial fluid is lower than that of arterial blood (approximately 7.35).

Mechanisms for Regulation of Hydrogen Ion Concentration

Regulation of pH over a narrow range depends on (a) buffer systems, (b) ventilatory responses, and (c) renal responses. The buffer system mechanism is local and immediate, but incomplete. Ventilatory responses are slower (minutes) and usually incomplete. Renal responses develop very slowly (hours) but can produce nearly complete pH correction.

Buffer Systems

Body fluids contain acid–base buffer systems that immediately combine with acid or alkali to prevent excessive changes in the hydrogen ion concentration. This ability to neutralize excess protons maintains the local pH near 7.4 in the face of continuous acid generation. The most important buffer systems are (a) bicarbonate and carbonic acid in plasma, interstitial and intracellular fluid, and bone; (b) hemoglobin and other proteins in intracellular fluid; (c) plasma proteins; and (d) phosphates in intracellular and extracellular fluid and the kidney (Fig. 26-1).

Bicarbonate Buffering System

The bicarbonate buffering system consists of carbonic acid (H_2CO_3) and sodium bicarbonate ($NaHCO_3$). Bicarbonate buffer is primarily a product of the approximately 200 mL of carbon dioxide produced per minute, of which considerably less than 1% dissolves to become carbonic acid. Carbonic acid is a weak acid because of its limited degree of dissociation (<5% at physiologic pH) into hydrogen and bicarbonate ions (Fig. 26-2). Most carbonic acid in solution almost immediately dissociates into carbon dioxide and water, the net result being a very high concentration of dissolved carbon dioxide compared to the concentration of bicarbonate ions. This relationship is

Table 26-1

Basic Definitions

p: a mathematical notation for a concentration expressed as the −log to the base 10, useful to describe substances present in the plasma in very low concentrations
pH: the concentration of free hydrogen ions (H^+) in a solution. The pH of water is 7.0 at 25°C and 6.8 at 37°C. The normal pH of most body fluids is 7.4 (range 7.35–7.45). This means that there are 40 nmol/L of H^+ in plasma (for comparison, there are 140 million nmol/L of Na^+ [140 mmol/L] in plasma).
pH_i: intracellular pH
Acid: a substance that increases the hydrogen ion concentration of a fluid (proton donor)
Alkali (or base): a substance that decreases the hydrogen ion concentration of a fluid (proton acceptor)
Buffer: a substance which reduces the change of pH in a solution when amounts of acid or base are added
K_a: the dissociation constant for a dissolved acid (HA), that is, the eqilibrium ratio: $[H^+]$ $[A^-]/[HA]$
pK_a: the −log of K_a for a given acid, for example, for carbonic acid (H_2CO_3), $pK_a = 6.2$. By convention, "strong" acids (e.g., HCl) have a $pK_a < -2$ (more free H^+ at equilibrium) and "weak" acids (e.g., H_2CO_3) have a pK_a −2 to +12 (this is confusing, but due to the negative logarithmic notation, a smaller number indicates a higher concentration of free H^+)
Anions: a negative ionized particle (e.g., HCO_3^-, Cl^-), that is, an excess of electrons vs. protons
Cations: a positively charged particle (e.g., Na^+, K^+), that is, an excess of protons vs. electrons
Strong ions: the ions of substances which are completely dissociated in body fluids (e.g., Na^+, Cl^-, K^+, SO_4^{2-}, Mg^{2+}, Ca^{2+})
Mole (mol): a fixed number [6.022×10^{23}(Avogadro's number)] of elementary entities (atoms, molecules, ions, electrons, etc.)
Molecular weight (MW) (actually, the "molecular mass"): the mass of 1 mole of a specific entity
Equivalent (Eq): the amount of a substance that will supply or react with 1 mole of H^+ ions (in acid–base reactions) or supply 1 mole of electrons (in oxidation–reduction reactions) mmol = mol/1,000, mEq = Eq/1,000. For singly charged particles (e.g., Na^+), 1 mmol/L = 1 mEq/L; for doubly changed particles (e.g., Mg^{2+}), 1 mmol/L = 2 mEq/L
Mole day: an informal annual holiday based on Avogadro's number on October 23 (10/23) from 6:02 AM to 6:02 PM

described mathematically by the Henderson-Hasselbalch equation, which can be used to calculate the pH of a solution if the concentration of bicarbonate ions and dissolved carbon dioxide is known (Fig. 26-3).

The addition of a strong acid such as hydrochloric acid to the bicarbonate buffering system results in conversion of the strong acid to weak carbonic acid (Fig. 26-4). Therefore, a strong acid lowers the pH of body fluids only slightly. The addition of a strong base, such as potassium hydroxide, to the bicarbonate buffering system results in the formation of a weak base and water. Buffers are most effective when they operate at a pH that is close to their pK_a (under these circumstances, the buffer system is approximately 50% dissociated). The bicarbonate buffering system is not a powerful buffer because its pK_a of 6.1 differs greatly from the normal pH of 7.4. Physiologically, buffers are most effective when their pK_a is equal to normal pH. However, the bicarbonate system is important because (a) bicarbonate is present in significant quantities in nearly all fluid compartments, (b) the concentration of its components is ultimately regulated by the lungs and kidneys, and (c) in severe acidosis the pH approaches the pK_a of the bicarbonate system thus increasing its efficiency.

The bicarbonate buffer system accounts for >50% of the total buffering capacity of blood. Approximately one-third of the bicarbonate buffering capacity of blood occurs within erythrocytes. The electrical charge of bicarbonate ions limits their diffusion into cells other than erythrocytes.

Hemoglobin Buffering System

Hemoglobin is a particularly effective buffer because it is localized in quantity in erythrocytes; it has a pK_a of 6.8 and has a buffering capacity that varies with oxygenation. The imidazole ring of the amino acid histidine has a pK_a that is close to the physiologic pH. Thus, hemoglobin and other histidine-containing proteins are excellent physiologic buffers. Furthermore, deoxygenated hemoglobin is a

$$HHb \rightleftharpoons H^+ + Hb^-$$

$$HProt \rightleftharpoons H^+ + Prot^-$$

$$H_2PO_4^- \rightleftharpoons H^+ + HPO_4^{2-}$$

$$H_2CO_3 \rightleftharpoons H^+ + HCO_3^-$$

FIGURE 26-1 Buffering systems present in the body. Hb, hemoglobin; Prot, protein.

$$CO_2 + H_2O \rightleftharpoons H_2CO_3 \rightleftharpoons HCO_3^- + H^+$$

FIGURE 26-2 Hydration of carbon dioxide results in carbonic acid (H_2CO_3), which can subsequently dissociate into bicarbonate and hydrogen ions.

$$pH = 6.10 + \log \frac{HCO_3^-}{Paco_2\ (0.03)}$$

FIGURE 26-3 The Henderson-Hasselbalch equation can be used to calculate the pH of a solution from the concentration of bicarbonate and the Pco_2.

weaker acid (better proton acceptor) than oxyhemoglobin. Thus, in the systemic capillaries, dissociation of oxyhemoglobin to deoxyhemoglobin facilitates the binding of hydrogen ions produced by the dissociation of carbonic acid. This situation is reversed in the pulmonary circulation where the conversion of deoxyhemoglobin to oxyhemoglobin facilitates the release of hydrogen ions.

Protein Buffering System

Like hemoglobin, other histidine-containing proteins are important intracellular buffers. Proteins are localized in high concentrations within the cell where it is estimated that approximately 75% of all the buffering of body fluids occurs, mostly by proteins. Of particular importance is the local buffering of hydrogen ions by proteins in the mitochondria. Although the relatively low concentration of plasma proteins limits their role as extracellular buffers, hypoproteinemia will further reduce buffering capacity, especially in the critically ill patient.

Phosphate Buffering System

The phosphate buffering system is important in most fluid compartments but is especially important in renal tubules, where phosphate is concentrated. Renal tubular fluid is more acidic than extracellular fluid, bringing the pH of renal tubular fluid closer to the pK_a (6.8) of the phosphate buffering system. Phosphate is a very important intracellular buffer because it is the most abundant intracellular anion. Furthermore, the relatively acidic pH of intracellular fluid is closer to the pK_a of the phosphate buffering system than is the pH of extracellular fluid.

Intracellular pH Regulation

Although blood pH is commonly measured clinically, it is the intracellular pH (pH_i) that is of functional importance. The routine measurement and manipulation of pH_i is not possible in current practice. Indeed, during hypothermic cardiopulmonary bypass and hibernation, the pH_i in heart and brain tissue appears to be highly regulated despite significant deviations in systemic pH. Cellular metabolism, transmembrane transport, membrane potential generation, cell growth and division, cytoskeletal structure, and contractile function are processes that are crucially dependent on pH_i (Table 26-2). Furthermore, the optimal function of several organelles, including lysosomes and mitochondria, require that their local pH is significantly different from the general pH_i. Thus there are highly regulated mechanisms to maintain local pH_i including intracellular buffer systems and membrane-bound proton transporters. Indeed, the pH_i (7.0) is higher than is predicted by the −90mV transmembrane potential (pH 6.8). As in the extracellular compartment, intracellular protons are rapidly bound to weak acids and bases resulting in a low free proton concentration.

$$HCL + NaHCO_3 \longrightarrow H_2CO_3 + NaCl$$

FIGURE 26-4 The addition of a strong acid (hydrochloric acid [HCl]) to the bicarbonate buffering system results in the formation of weak carbonic acid (H_2CO_3).

Table 26-2

Intracellular Functions Affected by Local pH

Cellular metabolism
Cytoskeletal structure
Muscle contractility
Cell–cell coupling
Membrane conductance
Intracellular messengers
Cell activation, growth, and proliferation
Cell volume regulation
Intracellular membrane flow

Ventilatory Responses

Ventilation is quantitatively the most important mechanism of acid removal, given the enormous daily production of volatile acid compared to nonvolatile acid. Ventilatory responses cannot return pH to 7.4 when a metabolic abnormality is responsible for the acid–base disturbance. This reflects the fact that the intensity of the stimulus responsible for increases or decreases in alveolar ventilation will begin to diminish as pH returns toward 7.4. As a "buffer," ventilatory responses are able to buffer up to twice the amount of acids or bases as all the chemical buffers combined. However, compensation for extreme metabolic acidosis imposes a significant respiratory burden. If the bicarbonate (HCO_3^-) is reduced to 10 mmol/L, the carbon dioxide tension must be reduced to 15 mm Hg in order to normalize the pH. Most patients cannot hyperventilate to below 20 mm Hg. Further, it is likely that the insult causing severe metabolic acidosis will also adversely affect respiratory muscle function, thus compromising the respiratory response.

Renal Responses

The day-to-day renal contribution to acid–base regulation is directed toward the conservation of bicarbonate and the excretion of hydrogen ions. Plasma bicarbonate is freely filtered at the glomerulus. Almost all filtered bicarbonate must be reabsorbed from the glomerular filtrate to maintain the normal plasma bicarbonate concentration

(25 mEq/L) and plasma pH. Most bicarbonate reabsorption occurs in the proximal convoluted tubule and is facilitated by the presence of carbonic anhydrase in the luminal fluid and is driven by the sodium-potassium-ATPase pump in the peritubular cell membrane. Active sodium ion extrusion from the renal tubular cell into the peritubular circulation favors sodium diffusion from the tubular lumen into the tubular cell in exchange for hydrogen ions. Hydrogen in the renal tubular fluid then combines with filtered bicarbonate to form carbonic acid. Carbonic anhydrase facilitates the dissociation of carbonic acid into water and carbon dioxide that both enter the renal tubular cell. Carbon dioxide and water generate bicarbonate, which enters the peritubular circulation accompanied by sodium. The remaining hydrogen ions are secreted into the lumen in exchange for sodium (Fig. 26-5). Inhibition of carbonic anhydrase by acetazolamide interferes with the reabsorption of bicarbonate ions from renal tubular fluid. As a result, excess bicarbonate ions are lost in the urine and the plasma bicarbonate concentration is decreased.

Hydrogen ions are secreted into renal tubules by epithelial cells lining proximal renal tubules, distal renal tubules, and collecting ducts. At the same time, sodium ions are reabsorbed in exchange for the secreted hydrogen ions and combine with bicarbonate ions in the peritubular capillaries. This process is facilitated by aldosterone. As a result, the amount of sodium bicarbonate in the plasma is increased during the secretion of hydrogen ions into renal tubules. Active hydrogen ion transport is inhibited when the urinary pH drops below 4.0. Thus, hydrogen ions must combine with ammonia and phosphate buffers in the renal tubular lumen to prevent the pH from decreasing below

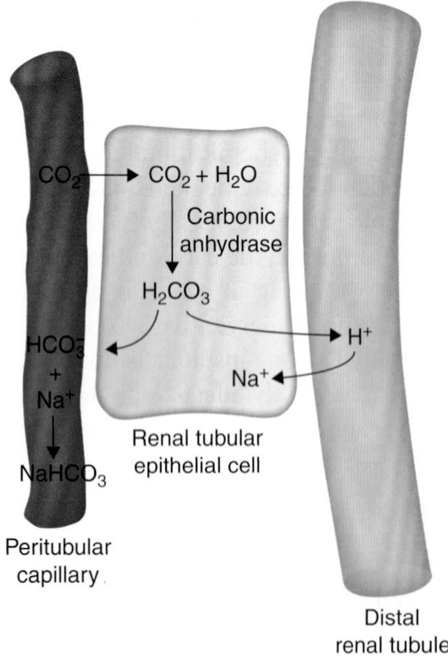

FIGURE 26-5 Schematic depiction of the renal tubular secretion of hydrogen ions, which are formed from the dissociation of carbonic acid in renal tubular epithelial cells.

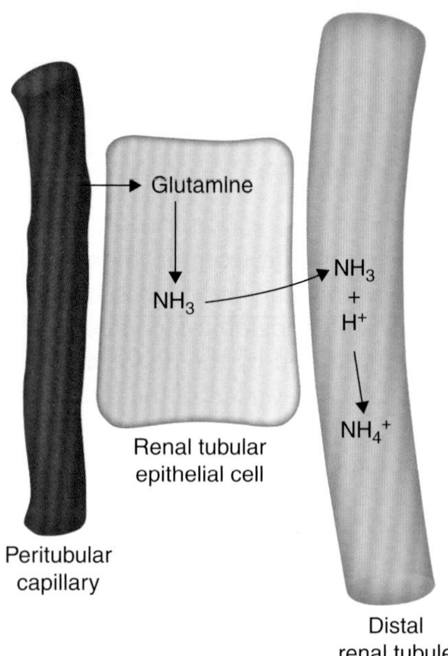

FIGURE 26-6 Ammonia formed in renal tubular epithelial cells combines with hydrogen ions in the renal tubules to form ammonium.

this critical level. Ammonia is generated in the mitochondria of the proximal tubule. Ammonia (NH_3) combines with hydrogen ions to form ammonium (NH_4^+), which is excreted in the urine in combination with chloride ions as the weak acid ammonium chloride (Fig. 26-6). In renal insufficiency, the capacity to generate urinary ammonia is impaired, thus reducing hydrogen ion excretion.

Renal responses that regulate hydrogen ion concentrations do so by acidification or alkalinization of the urine. In the presence of acidosis, the rate of hydrogen ion secretion exceeds the net loss of bicarbonate ion into the renal tubules. As a result, an excess of hydrogen ions is excreted into the urine. In the presence of alkalosis, the effect of the titration process in the renal tubules is to increase the number of bicarbonate ions filtered into the renal tubules relative to the secretion of hydrogen ions. Excess bicarbonate ions are excreted into the urine accompanied by cations, most often sodium.

Extracellular fluid is electroneutral such that the sum of the positive charges of all cations must equal the sum of negative charges of all anions. In the process of altering the plasma concentration of bicarbonate ions, it is mandatory to remove some other anion each time the concentration of bicarbonate ions is increased or to increase some other anion when the bicarbonate concentration is decreased. Typically, the anion that follows changes in the concentration of bicarbonate ions is chloride. As the most abundant extracellular anion, physiologic manipulation of chloride appears to be an important element of pH control. Conceptually, when bicarbonate ions are replaced by chloride ions, the pH will generally tend to decrease as a weak acid (carbonic acid) is replaced by a strong acid (hydrochloric acid).

The value of renal regulation of hydrogen ion concentration is not its rapidity but instead its ability to nearly completely neutralize any excess acid or alkali that enters the body fluids. Ordinarily, the kidneys can remove up to 500 mmol of acid or alkali each day. If greater quantities than this are generated, the kidneys are unable to maintain normal acid–base balance, and acidosis or alkalosis occurs. Even when the plasma pH is 7.4, a small amount of acid is still lost each minute. This reflects the daily production of 50 to 80 mmol of more acid than alkali. Indeed, the normal urine pH of approximately 6.4 is due to the presence of this excess acid in the urine.

Classification of Acid–Base Disturbances

Acid–base disturbances are categorized as respiratory or metabolic acidosis (pH <7.35) or alkalosis (pH >7.45) (Table 26-3).[1] An acid–base disturbance that results primarily from changes in alveolar ventilation is described as respiratory acidosis or alkalosis. An acid–base disturbance unrelated to changes in alveolar ventilation is designated as metabolic acidosis or alkalosis. Compensation describes the secondary renal or ventilatory responses that occur as a result of the primary acid–base disturbance.

The principal manifestation of severe respiratory or metabolic acidosis is depression of the central nervous system. For example, coma is a characteristic of severe diabetic acidosis or renal dysfunction leading to uremia. The principal manifestation of respiratory or metabolic alkalosis is increased excitability of the peripheral nervous system and central nervous system. As a result, there may be repetitive stimulation, causing skeletal muscles to undergo sustained contraction known as tetany. Tetany of respiratory muscles may interfere with adequate ventilation of the lungs. Central nervous system excitability may manifest as seizures.

Table 26-3

Distinguishing Respiratory and Metabolic Acidosis versus Alkalosis

	pH	$PaCO_2$	Bicarbonate
Respiratory acidosis			
Acute	↓↓	↑↑↑	↑
Chronic	NC	↑↑↑	↑↑
Respiratory alkalosis			
Acute	↑↑	↓↓↓	↓
Chronic	NC	↓↓↓	↓↓
Metabolic acidosis			
Acute	↓↓↓	↓	↓↓↓
Chronic	↓	↓↓↓	↓↓↓
Metabolic alkalosis			
Acute	↑↑↑	↑	↑↑↑
Chronic	↑↑	↑↑	↑↑↑

↑, increase; ↓, decrease; NC, no change from normal.

Respiratory Acidosis

Any event (drug or disease) that decreases alveolar ventilation results in an increased concentration of dissolved carbon dioxide in the blood (increased $PaCO_2$), which in turn leads to formation of carbonic acid and hydrogen ions. By convention, carbonic acid resulting from dissolved carbon dioxide is considered a respiratory acid, and respiratory acidosis is present when the pH is <7.35 and $PaCO_2$ is >45 mm Hg. It is important to note that although an increase in dissolved carbon dioxide generates an equivalent increase in both the hydrogen ion and bicarbonate ion concentrations, the pH will fall. This is because the relative increase in hydrogen ions is significantly greater than the relative increase in bicarbonate ions since the plasma concentration of H^+ is far lower than the concentration of HCO_3^-. An increase in carbon dioxide sufficient to reduce the pH from 7.4 to 7.1 will essentially double the hydrogen ion concentration from 40 to 79 nmol/L, compared to an increase in the bicarbonate ion concentration only from 24.000000 to 24.000039 mmol/L.

Acidosis, respiratory or metabolic, often has profound effects on many drug and enzyme interactions in the body, which function optimally only within normal pH ranges. Of particular importance to the anesthesiologist is the clinical scenario of increasing respiratory acidosis due to inadequate reversal of muscle relaxants and the interaction between anticholinesterases and the enzyme acetylcholinesterase. The commonest method to reverse the muscle relaxant effects of nondepolarizing neuromuscular blocker agents (NMBAs) is by administering an anticholinesterase, such as neostigmine. Anticholinesterases inhibit normal acetylcholinesterase, increasing the concentration of acetylcholine in the synaptic clefts of the neuromuscular junction and thus antagonizing the neuromuscular block. The concentration of NMBAs remains essentially unchanged at the time of reversal. If the reversal is inadequate due to an excess of NMBAs or due to the limited duration of action of the anticholinesterase (e.g., 20 to 30 minutes for neostigmine) then inadequate alveolar minute ventilation can lead to progressive respiratory acidosis, which will potentiate the NMBAs and weaken the effects of the anticholinesterase. This clinical picture of increasing muscle weakness after a seemingly appropriately reversed neuromuscular block has been termed "recurarization."[2] Although this was more of a clinical problem with the older longer acting NMBAs (e.g., pancuronium), it can still occur with the newer shorter acting drugs (e.g., rocuronium).

Respiratory Alkalosis

Respiratory alkalosis is present when increased alveolar ventilation removes sufficient carbon dioxide from the body to decrease the hydrogen ion concentration to the extent that pH becomes >7.45. A physiologic cause of respiratory alkalosis is hyperventilation due to stimulation of chemoreceptors by a low Po_2 associated with ascent to altitude. Kidneys compensate with time for this loss of carbon dioxide by excreting bicarbonate ions in association with sodium and potassium ions. This renal compensation is evident in individuals residing at altitude who have a nearly normal pH despite a low $Paco_2$. A frequent cause of acute respiratory alkalosis is iatrogenic hyperventilation of the lungs as during anesthesia. Tetany that accompanies alkalosis reflects hypocalcemia due to the greater affinity of plasma proteins for calcium ions in an alkaline, compared with an acidic, solution.

Metabolic Acidosis

The most common and most confusing acid–base disorder that clinicians are required to manage is metabolic acidosis. Any acid formed in the body other than carbonic acid from carbon dioxide is considered a metabolic acid, and its accumulation results in metabolic acidosis. Acidosis impairs myocardial contractility and the responses to endogenous or exogenous catecholamines.[3] Hemodynamic deterioration is usually minimal (in the awake state) when the pH remains >7.2 due to compensatory increases in sympathetic nervous system activity. Of great clinical importance are the accentuated detrimental effects of metabolic acidosis in individuals with underlying left ventricular dysfunction or myocardial ischemia or in those in whom sympathetic nervous system activity may be impaired, as by drug-induced β-adrenergic blockade or general anesthesia. Respiratory acidosis may produce more rapid and profound myocardial dysfunction than does metabolic acidosis, reflecting the ability of carbon dioxide to freely diffuse across cell membranes and exacerbate intracellular acidosis.

Acute metabolic acidosis has been treated with intravenous administration of an exogenous buffer, usually sodium bicarbonate, in the hope that normalizing pH will attenuate the detrimental effects of acidosis. The effectiveness of the use of sodium bicarbonate to treat metabolic acidosis is debatable.[4] Sodium bicarbonate administration increases the carbon dioxide load to the lungs, leading to further increases in arterial and intracellular Pco_2 if alveolar ventilation is not concomitantly increased. It is estimated that 1 mEq/kg sodium bicarbonate, given intravenously, produces approximately 180 mL of carbon dioxide and necessitates a transient doubling of alveolar ventilation to prevent hypercarbia. In the presence of increased dead space ventilation, even greater increases in alveolar ventilation are required for carbon dioxide elimination to equal production. Even if $Paco_2$ is maintained normal, it is possible that tissue pH_i and the risk of ventricular fibrillation will not be altered by administration of sodium bicarbonate during cardiopulmonary resuscitation. Also, the standard formulation of sodium bicarbonate, 8.4%, is hypertonic and this will have a plasma-expanding effect that contributes to dilutional acidosis (see the following text). However, if alveolar ventilation can be increased to deal with the increased carbon dioxide load from administration of sodium bicarbonate (initial bolus dose 0.5 to 1 mEq/kg), then it can be useful as a temporizing measure to help restore hemodynamic stability in shock combined with severe metabolic acidosis.[5]

Lactic Acidosis

Under normal circumstances, lactate is produced at a rate of approximately 1 mmol/kg per hour. Normal clearance of lactate maintains its serum concentration between 0.5 and 1.0 mmol/L. Most lactate is cleared by the liver, where it undergoes oxidation, gluconeogenesis, and eventual conversion to bicarbonate. Lactate undergoes both passive diffusion and active transport into the liver via a monocarboxylate transporter. However, active transport becomes saturated at serum lactate concentrations that exceed 2.5 mmol/L. Severe reductions in hepatic blood flow, which occur during shock, will decrease hepatic lactate clearance. Lactic acid is a strong acid and therefore dissociates almost completely under physiologic conditions into the lactate anion and a hydrogen ion. Although lactate accumulation has classically been taught to occur mainly during anaerobic glycolysis, it is now clear that significant lactate generation occurs under normoxic conditions. Indeed, lactate is an important gluconeogenic precursor and is involved in cell-to-cell signaling. However, in the critically ill patient, lactate production may increase while lactate clearance is impaired and lactic acidosis may occur. Point-of-care testing allows almost instantaneous lactate determinations to be performed in the operating room and intensive care unit. A serum lactate >1.5 mmol/L upon admission is an independent predictor of mortality in critically ill patients. Furthermore, failure to decrease lactate concentration to ≤1.0 mmol/L 24 hours after admission is also associated with significant mortality.

The investigational drug dichloroacetate (DCA) decreases lactate concentration in cardiogenic shock, burns, diabetic ketoacidosis, and malaria. DCA activates the mitochondrial pyruvate dehydrogenase complex, thus accelerating the irreversible oxidation of lactate via pyruvate to acetyl CoA, which then enters the Krebs cycle. The buffer tris(hydroxymethyl)aminomethane (THAM) can be used to treat metabolic acidosis and does not generate carbon dioxide. It may be particularly useful, as an alternative to sodium bicarbonate, to treat metabolic acidosis in patients who are hypernatremic.[6]

Dilutional Acidosis

Because the pH of water at 37°C is 6.8, any increase in the free-water volume of the body will contribute to acidosis (e.g., administration of 5% dextrose). Dilutional acidosis also occurs when the plasma pH is decreased by extracellular volume expansion with chloride-containing solutions such as normal saline. Clinically, a hyperchloremic metabolic acidosis may accompany large-volume infusion of

Table 26-4

Electrolytes in Plasma and Commonly Available Crystalloid Solutions

	Na	Cl	K	Ca	Mg	Lactate	Acetate			
Solution	(mEq/L)							Gluconate	pH	mOsm
Plasma	144	107	5	2	1.5				7.4	290
NS	154	154							5.5	308
RL	130	109	4	3		28			6.5	273
Plasmalyte	140	98	5		3		27	23 (mmol)	7.4	294
Ionolyte	137	110	4		1.5		34		7.4	287

mOsm, osmolarity; NS, normal saline; RL, Ringer's lactate.

isotonic saline.[7] Normal saline is commonly thought of as being a "physiologic" solution because it has an osmolarity close to plasma and does not lyse red blood cells. However, it has a pH (5.7) that is more acidic than plasma and contains significantly more chloride (154 vs. 100 mmol/L) and slightly more sodium (154 vs. 140 mmol/L) (Table 26-4). Thus, infusion of a large volume of normal saline will increase plasma chloride concentration to a relatively greater degree than sodium concentration. Chloride can be thought of as a strong acid, (hydrochloric acid-proton donor), just as sodium can be thought of as a strong base (sodium hydroxide-hydroxyl donor).[8]

Other Causes of Metabolic Acidosis

Renal failure prevents excretion of acids formed by normal metabolic processes, and metabolic acidosis occurs. Severe diarrhea and associated loss of sodium bicarbonate rapidly leads to metabolic acidosis, especially in the pediatric age group. Lack of insulin secretion (diabetes mellitus) or starvation impairs glucose utilization, forcing tissues to metabolize fat to meet energy needs. As a result, the plasma concentration of ketones such as acetoacetic acid may increase sufficiently to cause metabolic acidosis.

Differential Diagnosis of Metabolic Acidosis

Several different methods have been developed over the past 60 years to help clinicians in the differential diagnosis and treatment of acid–base disturbances, particularly relating to metabolic acidosis. All of these methods have their strengths and their weaknesses because they are based on theoretical stable states. In clinical practice, these methods have been made less relevant by the ability to get rapid laboratory or point-of-care results for several plasma values such as lactate.

Base Excess

The concept of base excess (BE) and its converse base-deficit were developed in the 1940s. This is defined as the amount of strong acid or base to return the plasma pH to 7.4 assuming $Paco_2$ 40 mm Hg and normothermia. The BE is calculated (not measured) by modern blood gas analyzers from an algorithm based on measured HCO_3^- and pH. In isolated acute respiratory acidosis or alkalosis, the BE should not change (normal value = 0). BE remains useful to alert the clinician to the presence of a concurrent metabolic acidosis (BE < 0) in the presence of a respiratory acidosis (pH <7.35, $Paco_2$ >45 mm Hg) or to the presence of an underlying metabolic alkalosis (BE $>$ 0). Mixed respiratory and metabolic acidosis is a common clinical problem. Also, it alerts the physician to the severity of the metabolic derangement, which can then be used as a guide to the initial therapy. The weakness of the BE measurement is that it does not distinguish among the possible causes of metabolic acidosis.

Anion Gap

Calculation of the anion gap may assist in the evaluation of acid–base disorders. The anion gap is a derived value based on the principle of electrochemical neutrality such that the sum of the positive (cationic) charges in a solution must equal the sum of the negative (anionic) charges. The major extracellular anions are chloride and bicarbonate. Other significant anions include proteins, phosphate, sulfate, and organic acids (including lactate). The latter are less commonly measured in routine practice and are referred to as "unmeasured anions." The predominant extracellular cation is sodium. Although potassium is now routinely measured, its inclusion in the anion gap calculation is inconsistent and varies from institution to institution. Potassium is often grouped with the other "unmeasured cations," calcium, and magnesium. Under normal circumstances, the concentration of the predominant cation (sodium) exceeds that of the combined predominant anions (chloride and bicarbonate) [anion gap = $Na^+ - (HCO_3^- + Cl^-)$] by 9 to 13 mEq/L. For electroneutrality to occur, the concentration of the combined unmeasured anions must therefore exceed that of the unmeasured cations by the same amount. The term "anion gap" refers solely to the difference in concentration between the traditionally measured anions and cations. The anion gap does not imply a true discrepancy between the total positive and negative charges in physiologic solution where the total anion charge must equal the total cation charge.

Table 26-5

Causes of Metabolic Acidosis

Increased Anion Gap	Normal Anion Gap
• Lactic acidosis • Ketoacidosis • Chronic renal failure (accumulation of sulfates, phosphates, urea) • Intoxication: organic acids (salicylates, ethanol, methanol, formaldehyde, ethylene glycol, paraldehyde), INH, sulfates, metformin • Massive rhabdomyolysis	• Hyperchloremic acidosis (excess saline administration) • Diarrhea (long-standing bicarbonate loss) • Pancreatic fistula • Renal tubular acidosis • Intoxication: ammonium chloride, acetazolamide, toluene

Metabolic acidosis is most often associated with an increase in the anion gap (Table 26-5). An increase in the concentration of unmeasured anions (or a decrease in the concentration of unmeasured cations) will increase the anion gap. Lactic acidosis, ketoacidosis, and renal failure increase the concentration of unmeasured endogenous anions. Exogenous anions will also increase the concentration of unmeasured anions (salicylate toxicity, ethylene glycol, and methanol ingestion). Hyperchloremic acidosis and renal tubular acidosis (bicarbonate loss) will have a normal anion gap. The weaknesses of the anion gap concept include that it does not differentiate between the causes of increased anion gap metabolic acidosis; it does not correct for pH changes due to free-water volume increase or decreases; and it does not correct for changes in serum albumin and phosphate, which have an effect on acid–base balance.

Strong Ion Gap

The strong ion gap (SIG) method is also based on the concept of electroneutrality of plasma.[9] The SIG compares the excess measured serum concentrations of strong cations (Na^+, K^+, Mg^{2+}, Ca^{2+}) to the calculated total of measurable anions (Cl^-, HCO_3^-, albumin, phosphate); the normal gap is 6 to 10 mEq/L. The SIG can be corrected for changes in plasma free-water volume and may be more useful in combined causes of metabolic acidosis, which are common in clinical practice. Measurement of the plasma lactic acid concentration and calculation of the anion gap from sodium, chloride, and bicarbonate permits differentiation of dilutional acidosis from acidosis due to tissue hypoperfusion.

Simplified Approach to Metabolic Acidosis of Uncertain Etiology

When the cause of a metabolic acidosis is unclear, measure the serum lactate, blood urea nitrogen (BUN), creatinine, and glucose. If this does not identify the etiology of the acidosis, then send serum for toxicology to measure salicylates, methanol, ethylene glycol, etc.

Metabolic Alkalosis

Metabolic alkalosis is commonly iatrogenic. Causes include vomiting with excess loss of hydrochloric acid, nasogastric suction, chronic administration of diuretics, hypoalbuminemia, and excess secretion of aldosterone. Excess administration of sodium bicarbonate may be an iatrogenic cause of metabolic alkalosis. A loss of free water (pH 6.8) will cause a volume-contraction alkalosis. Treatment involves treating the underlying cause.

Compensation for Acid–Base Disturbances

Respiratory acidosis is compensated for within 6 to 12 hours by increased renal secretion of hydrogen ions, with a resulting increase in the plasma bicarbonate concentration. After a few days, the pH will be normal despite persistence of an increased $Paco_2$. Sudden correction of chronic respiratory acidosis, by iatrogenic hyperventilation, may result in acute metabolic alkalosis because increased plasma bicarbonate is not promptly eliminated by the kidneys.

Respiratory alkalosis is compensated for by decreased reabsorption of bicarbonate ions from renal tubules. As a result, more bicarbonate ions are excreted in the urine, which decreases the plasma concentration of bicarbonate and returns the pH toward normal despite persistence of a decreased $Paco_2$.

Metabolic acidosis stimulates alveolar ventilation, which causes rapid removal of carbon dioxide from the body and decreases the hydrogen ion concentration toward normal. This respiratory compensation for metabolic acidosis, however, is only partial because pH remains somewhat below normal.

Metabolic alkalosis diminishes alveolar ventilation, which in turn causes accumulation of carbon dioxide and a subsequent increase in hydrogen ion concentration. As with metabolic acidosis, the respiratory compensation for metabolic alkalosis is only partial. Renal compensation for metabolic alkalosis is increased by reabsorption of hydrogen ions.

This metabolic compensation is limited by the availability of sodium, potassium, and chloride ions. During prolonged vomiting, there may be excessive loss of chloride ions along with sodium and potassium. When this occurs, the kidneys preferentially conserve sodium and potassium ions and the urine becomes paradoxically acidic. Indeed, the presence of paradoxical aciduria indicates electrolyte depletion.

Effects of Temperature on Acid–Base Status

Temperature changes have several effects on blood and tissue pH and P_{CO_2}. As blood is cooled, carbon dioxide becomes more soluble. Therefore, for a given carbon dioxide content, the partial pressure will decrease as the temperature falls. The magnitude of this change is approximately 4.5% per degree Celsius and will tend to increase the pH. The blood pH is further increased as the dissociation of water into protons and hydroxyl ions decreases with cooling, thus decreasing hydrogen ion concentration. In addition, proton buffering by hemoglobin α-imidazole groups is enhanced by hypothermia. The sum of these effects is an increase of 0.015 pH units per degree Celsius decrease in temperature. These changes are probably insignificant within the physiologic temperature range but are important when interpreting blood-gas and acid–base data during induced cooling during cardiopulmonary bypass. If the blood temperature is decreased by 10°C to 27°C, the pH will increase to 7.6. Two alternate blood-gas management strategies, "α-stat" and "pH-stat" are utilized during hypothermia in the operating room (Table 26-6).

pH-Stat Management

During hypothermic conditions, blood pH is increased and P_{CO_2} is decreased. The pH-stat strategy seeks to return the pH and P_{CO_2} of hypothermic blood to normal. During hypothermic cardiopulmonary bypass, this strategy usually involves the addition of carbon dioxide via the oxygenator. A purported advantage of this strategy is that cerebral blood flow will be increased because carbon dioxide is a potent cerebral vasodilator. However, delivery of microemboli to the brain may also be increased. Temperature correction of blood gas samples is required to interpret the values obtained from a hypothermic patient but measured at 37°C. The pH-stat strategy is used more often in surgery for pediatric congenital heart disease, especially during cooling and deep hypothermic circulatory arrest.[10] Under these circumstances, enhanced cerebral perfusion that facilitates brain cooling is thought to be desirable. Cerebral injury secondary to global hypoperfusion is thought to be a greater threat than delivery of microemboli in this patient population. Hypothermia, hypocarbia (via the Bohr effect), and alkalosis, all shift the oxyhemoglobin dissociation curve to the left and impair tissue oxygen delivery. The addition of carbon dioxide during pH-stat management will counter these effects and facilitate oxygen unloading from hemoglobin.

Table 26-6

α-Stat versus pH-Stat Management during Hypothermia

	α Stat	pH Stat
Carbon dioxide added to oxygenator	No	Yes
Enzyme function	Near normal	Decreased
Cerebral blood flow	Normal	Increased
Blood gas temperature correction required	No	Yes
Hb-O_2 dissociation curve	Marked left shift	Less marked left shift

α-Stat Management

The α-stat strategy seeks to replicate the alkalinization of blood that occurs during cooling in poikilothermic mammals (e.g., naked mole rat). This strategy seeks to optimize enzyme function during hypothermia. The α of α-stat refers to the charged portion of the histidine imidazole residue. The objective is to maintain biologic neutrality by preserving the α-imidazole and protein charge state, the OH^-/H^+ ratio, and therefore enzyme function, even though the pH will increase. This strategy is most often used during adult cardiopulmonary bypass and does not generally encourage the delivery of microemboli to the brain because supplemental carbon dioxide is not generally administered. This strategy does not require temperature correction of blood gas results.

There are examples of both strategies in nature. Homeotherms (e.g., humans) have homeostatic mechanisms for maintaining the temperature of the internal environment within very narrow limits. Homeotherms and hibernating animals hypoventilate in order to maintain blood pH at 7.4 as their body temperature decreases (pH-stat). pH_i is low in most tissues under these circumstances and suppresses metabolism and conserves energy stores in nonfunctioning tissues. However, the brain and heart of these animals employ α-stat strategies to maintain pH_i at α-stat values and to maintain near normal function. Poikilotherms (e.g., snakes) have not developed mechanisms for regulating the temperature of their internal environment that changes with that of the external environment. Poikilotherms use the α-stat strategy and allow their blood pH to increase and P_{CO_2} to decrease with cooling in order to preserve cellular and enzyme function over wide temperature ranges.

References

1. Black RM. Disorders of acid-base and potassium balance. In: *ACP Medicine*. Danbury, CT: WebMD Professional Publishing; 2001.
2. Srivastava A, Hunter J. Reversal of neuromuscular blockade. *Br J Anaesth*. 2009;103:115–129.

3. Hindman BJ. Sodium bicarbonate in the treatment of subtypes of acute lactic acidosis: physiologic considerations. *Anesthesiology.* 1990;72:1064–1066.
4. Graf H, Leach W, Arieff AI. Metabolic effects of sodium bicarbonate in hypoxic lactic acidosis in dogs. *Am J Physiol.* 1985;249:F630–F635.
5. Forsythe SM, Schnmidt GM. Sodium bicarbonate for treatment of lactic acidosis. *Chest.* 2000;117:260–267.
6. Hoste EA, Colpaert K, Vanholder RC, et al. Sodium bicarbonate versus THAM in ICU patients with mild metabolic acidosis. *J Nephrol.* 2005;18:303–307.
7. Moritz ML, Ayus JC. Water water everywhere: standardized postoperative fluid therapy with 0.9% normal saline. *Anesth Analg.* 2010;110:293–295.
8. Levetown M. Saline-induced hyperchloremic metabolic acidosis. *Crit Care Med.* 2002;30:259–261.
9. Story DA, Morimatsu H, Bellomo R. Strong ions, weak ions and base excess. *Br J Anaesth.* 2004;92:54–60.
10. Abdul Aziz KA, Meduoye A. Is pH-stat or alpha-stat the best technique to follow in patients undergoing deep hypothermic circulatory arrest? *Interact Cardiovasc Thorac Surg.* 2010;10:271–282.

CHAPTER 27

Physiology of Blood and Hemostasis

Jerrold H. Levy

Understanding the physiology of blood and its interactions for hemostasis is a critical aspect of managing perioperative bleeding. With the ever increasing application of anticoagulation therapies for cardiovascular diseases, patients also present with multiple underlying acquired coagulation abnormalities. Further, in an acutely bleeding and hemorrhagic patient, additional coagulation changes occur that are covered in the chapter on physiology and management of massive transfusion. Understanding the physiology of coagulation and blood interactions is important in determining the preoperative bleeding risk of patients and in managing hemostatic therapy perioperatively.

At the center of hemostasis is the ability to generate thrombin, a serine protease. Thrombin plays pivotal roles in the activation of additional coagulation factors as shown in Figures 27-1 and 27-2.[1] Most coagulation factors circulate in the body as inactive enzymatic precursors that are called ***zymogens***.[1] However, there are multiple critical steps in clot formation that involve additional cofactors, humoral proteins, cellular components, and cell surface receptors. Following tissue injury, thrombin is generated in a highly regulated way that keeps the effects of this activation local to the site of injury and prevents uncontrolled systemic thrombosis. In surgical patients, multiple perturbations occur, and the hemostatic and inflammatory systems are closely related and have significant cross talk. Managing perioperative hemostasis also requires consideration of the postoperative hypercoagulability that may follow, and important advances have been made as new pharmacologic strategies are available and used to treat both procoagulation states and cardiovascular disease. This chapter will review the physiology of hemostasis, clot formation, and thrombin generation.

Hemostasis and History

The term ***hemostasis*** essentially means to stop bleeding and refers to the physiologic process that keeps blood within damaged blood vessels, the opposite of hemorrhage. Multiple mechanisms are involved in hemostasis, a process critical for survival. The elucidation of models to explain the molecular and cellular interactions of the clotting cascade continue to evolve over time. The best understood clotting cascade is the Waterfall/Cascade model that most clinicians learned in medical school and was developed about 50 years ago but is still used as an educational tool.[1] However, this acellular model does not tell the entire story and has been further refined by Hoffman and Monroe[2] in their cell-based model that focuses on both cellular and humoral interactions and (see Fig. 27-1). Hemostasis is also a complex inflammatory response that provides host defense mechanisms to prevent exsanguination following injury, trauma, and/or surgery. Many of the hemostatic factors have complex inflammatory signaling properties that orchestrate further host defense mechanisms, healing, and a multitude of

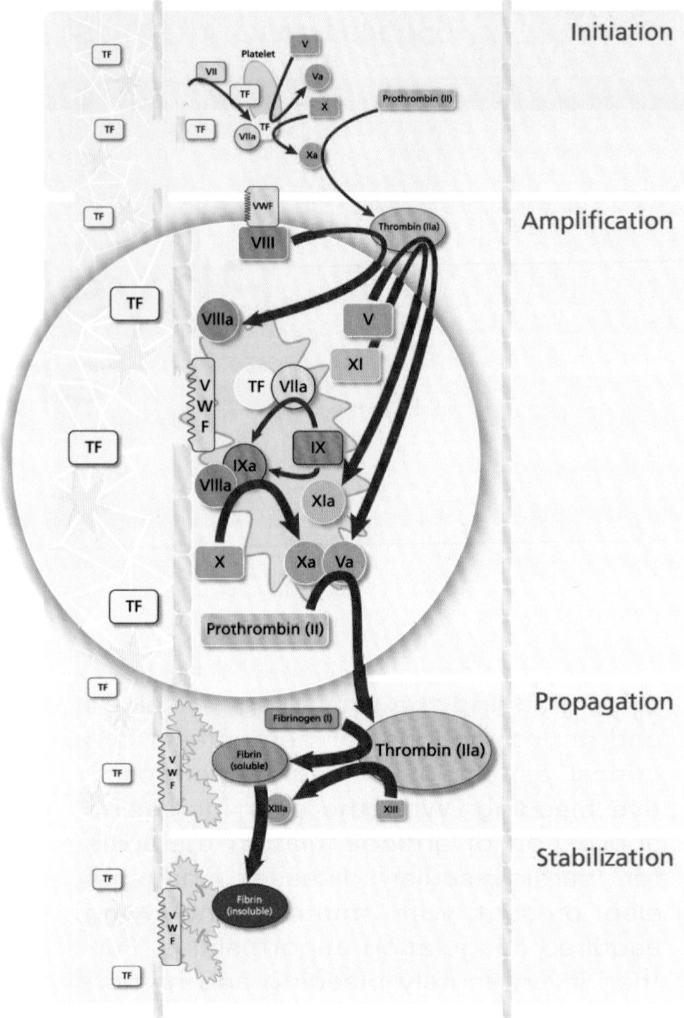

FIGURE 27-1 Initiation, amplification, propagation, and stabilization of hemostasis and clot formation. This describes the complexity of the clotting process and illustrates the interaction between coagulation factors and the cell surfaces of platelets in what has been described as the cellular model of hemostasis. Four sequential and interrelated stages include initiation, amplification, propagation, and stabilization as shown. This model also combines multiple aspects of the classic waterfall/cascade model, and further explains additional aspects of hemostasis that the classic acellular model does not. (Modified from Monroe DM, Hoffman M. What does it take to make the perfect clot? *Arterioscler Thromb Vasc Biol.* 2006;26:41–48.)

other functions. There are multiple aspects of the physiology of hemostasis and clot formation that will be considered separately.

Initiation of Coagulation

Initiation of coagulation by procoagulant activities has been traditionally separated into extrinsic, intrinsic, and common pathways. However, a better understanding of the complex interactions has created a better conceptual integration of these pathways. Following tissue injury and vascular endothelial disruption, activation of hemostasis occurs by tissue factor (TF) expression on the subendothelial vascular basement of the blood vessel as shown in Figures 27-1 and 27-2.[1-3] TF is a transmembrane receptor expressed by perivascular/vascular cells that binds factor VIIa.[4] Vascular injury with loss of normal endothelial function allows for expression of extravascular TF and initiation of clotting.[4] TF is also present in the circulation as microparticles that are small membrane vesicles that appear following cellular injury or death and may contribute to thrombosis with sepsis or other procoagulant states. Activated factor VII (factor VIIa), a serine protease that circulates in blood in low concentrations, allows for formation of the factor VIIa/TF complex, and conversion of factor X to factor Xa.[1,3] Subsequently, factor Xa (also a serine protease) generates trace amounts (0.1–1 nM) of thrombin.[1,3] Thrombin generation is subsequently amplified by other coagulation factors from the intrinsic cascade that includes factors XI, IX, and VIII dependent activities, although both the extrinsic (factor VIIa/TF) and intrinsic (factors IXa/VIIIa) tenase complexes produce factor Xa, which is also an important target form many anticoagulation agents. "Tenase" is a contraction of the words "ten" and the suffix "-ase" and refers to these factor complexes which activate inactive factor X through enzymatic cleavage. Multiple factors influence the degree of activation including the local TF concentration and type of cell surface supporting enzyme/cofactor complex assembly as platelets also will contribute to this response.[1,3] The interaction of both cellular and plasma-dependent mechanisms generates the prothrombinase complex (factors Xa, Va, and prothrombin) assembly

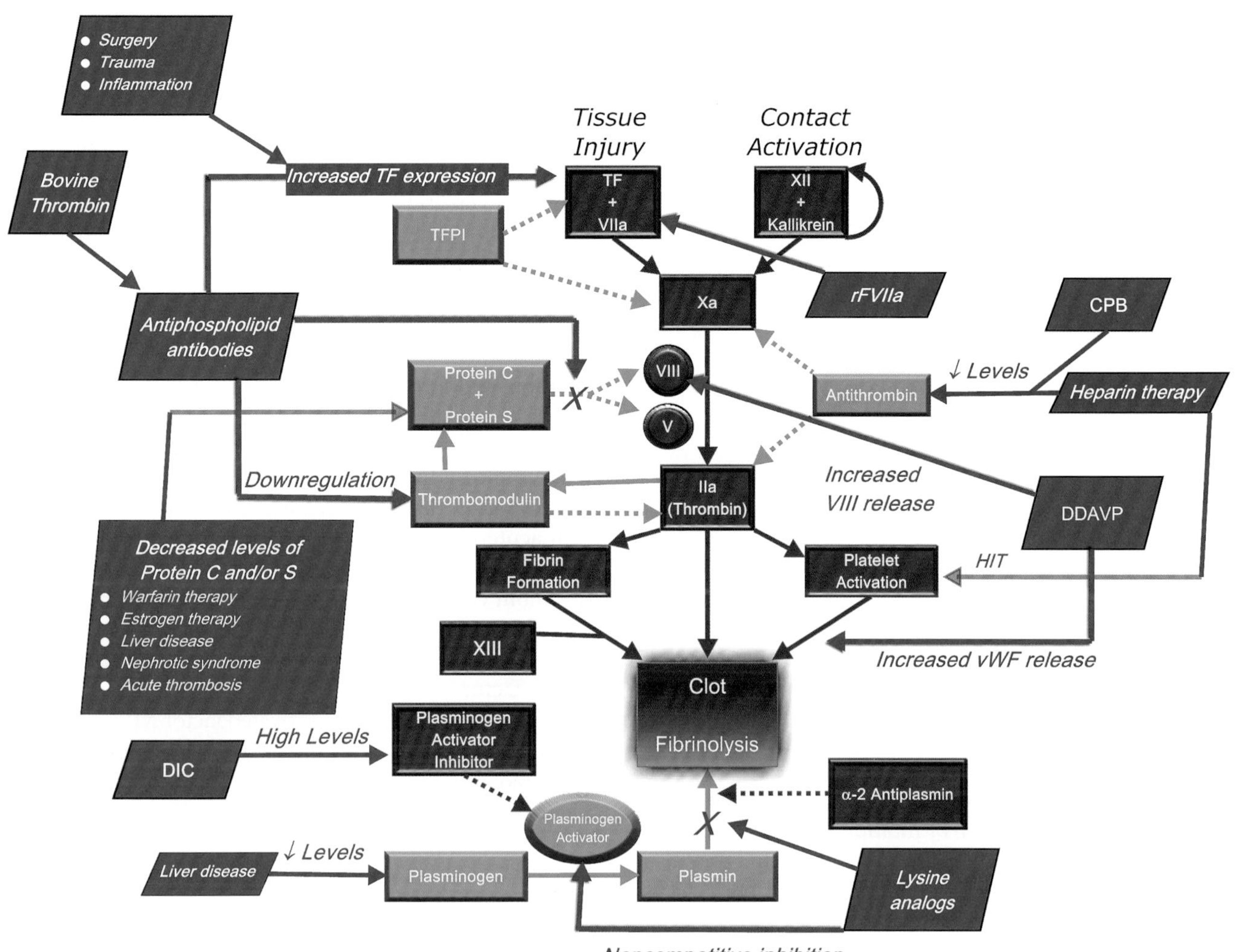

FIGURE 27-2 Procoagulant forces *(red)* and natural anticoagulant/fibrinolytic forces *(green)* and diagrammed. Dashed lines indicated an inhibitory effect. Acquired risk factors are presented in blue boxes with white lettering and arrows indicating the mechanism for the hypercoagulable effect. "X's" denote a specific block in a pathway. Note that some acquired risk factors have multiple effects; see text for full details. CPB, cardiopulmonary bypass; DDAVP, desmopressin; DIC, disseminated intravascular coagulation;TF, tissue factor;TFPI, tissue factor pathway inhibitor. (Modified from Sniecinski RM, Hursting MJ, Paidas MJ, et al. Etiology and assessment of hypercoagulability with lessons from heparin-induced thrombocytopenia. *Anesth Analg.* 2010;112:46–58)

that enzymatically cleaves prothrombin to produce thrombin, another critical factor targeted in anticoagulation therapy. The orchestration of hemostasis and factors influencing its balance are shown in Figures 27-1 and 27-2.

As part of the activation, there are also checks and balances in the system to prevent an over exuberant prothrombotic effect from occurring and regulate thrombin generation to localize clot at the site of vascular injury as shown in Figure 27-2. Tissue factor pathway inhibitor (TFPI) neutralizes factor Xa when it is in a complex with TF-factor VIIa.[1,3] The other regulator of TF-trigger procoagulant response is antithrombin (AT, formerly called antithrombin III; a serine protease inhibitor; SERPIN), which circulates at a high concentration (150 μg/mL, ~2.7 μM) and neutralizes the initially formed factor Xa and thrombin.[1,3] Overall factor VIIa patrols the circulation in search of sites of vascular injury where TF is exposed, and trace quantities of factor Xa and thrombin initiate a procoagulant response. Plasma levels of the different coagulation proteins are listed in Table 27-1.

Propagation of Coagulation

Platelets further amplify or potentially initiate clot formation at the site of vascular injury. Inflammatory cells all contain adhesion molecules to facilitate binding in the rapid flow of blood vessels as shown in Figure 27-1. Following vascular injury and exposure of the subendothelial vascular basement membrane, von Willebrand factor (vWF) that circulates in a multimeric form binds to the damaged blood vessel. Platelets then adhere to subendothelial collagen-vWF via their glycoprotein (GP) Ib receptors and are activated. Thrombin generation that also occurs locally is a potent activator/agonist for platelets by stimulating protease activated receptor

Table 27-1

Plasma Levels, Half-lives of Coagulation Factors

Factor	Level (μM)	Half-life (h)
Fibrinogen	7.6	72–120
Prothrombin	1.4	72
Factor V	0.03	36
Factor VII	0.01	3–6
Factor VIII	0.00003	12
Factor IX	0.09	24
FX	0.17	40
Factor XI	0.03	80
Factor XIII	0.03	120–200
vWF	0.03	10–24
Protein C	0.08	10
Protein S	0.14	42
Antithrombin	2.6	48–72

vWF, von Willebrand factor.
Modified from Tanaka KA, Key NS, Levy JH. Blood coagulation: hemostasis and thrombin regulation. *Anesth Analg.* 2009;108:1433–1446.

(PAR)-1 and PAR-4.[1,3] Thrombin activation of platelets further amplifies clot formation by multiple mechanisms. Platelet glycoprotein Ib receptors bind to factor XI, and they also localize factor VIII to the site of endothelial disruption via its carrier protein vWF.[5] Also, factor V is released from platelet α-granules upon platelet activation, and factors XI, VIII, and V further amplify and sustain procoagulant responses (the "intrinsic pathway") after thrombin-mediated activation. The serine protease factor XIa mediates the activation of factor IX to factor Xa, and factor VIIIa serves as a cofactor to factor IXa. Factor IXa, a serine protease, activates factor X to factor Xa, and factor Va serves as a cofactor to factor Xa.[1,3] In the absence of factor VIIIa or factor IXa, as is clinically observed in hemophilia A or B, the initiation of coagulation is normal, but amplification/propagation is altered. Patients with hemophilia clot, but they develop bleeding in muscle and joints due to low TF expression.

Tissue Factor, Thrombin, and Fibrin(ogen) in Clot Formation and Stability

When generated, thrombin facilitates the proteolytic conversion of circulating, soluble fibrinogen to an insoluble fibrin meshwork. This complex mechanism involves the cleavage of *N*-terminal peptides from fibrinogen, end-to-end polymerization of fibrin monomers to protofibrils, and lateral aggregation of protofibrils to fibers.[1,3] Fibrin's biophysical characteristics provide extensive structural support to the clot; individual fibers can be strained >330% without rupturing. The fibrin network that forms can be influenced by many different factors including fibrin(ogen)-binding proteins (e.g., factor XIII), thrombin, and fibrinogen present during fibrin formation.

Role of Fibrinogen

Fibrinogen is a critical protein for clot formation, and has a critical role in hemostasis.[6] Fibrinogen is critical for clot formation and creating the dense lattice structure as shown in Figure 27-3. Fibrinogen also binds to platelet glycoprotein IIb/IIIa receptors to facilitate clot formation and is affected by many antiplatelet agents. In addition, fibrinogen facilitates the cross-linking and network formation for clot and the subsequent fibrin polymerization that is catalyzed by thrombin and thrombin-activated factor XIII that locally at the site of activation. Of all the coagulation factors, fibrinogen circulates at the highest concentration (7.6 μM, ~200 to 400 mg/dL). In pregnancy and during acute inflammatory responses that often occur postoperatively, fibrinogen is an acute-phase reactant.[6] Platelets that are activated by multiple agonists express glycoprotein IIb/IIIa receptors. Thrombin catalyzes the conversion of fibrinogen to fibrin monomers after thrombin cleaves the fibrinopeptides from the fibrinogen Aa and B3 chains. Platelets that are activated release factor XIII A subunits that further polymerize fibrin monomers into fibrin. Activated factor XIII also cross-links a2-antiplasmin to fibrin, making fibrin more resistant to degradation. Thrombin released locally modulates the thickness and the fibrinolytic resistance of fibrin fibers.

Thrombin generation is critical to clot formation, platelet activation, and fibrinogen cross linking.[1,3] With normal hemostatic function, the peak thrombin level reaches 200 to 500 nM, facilitating the formation of a dense

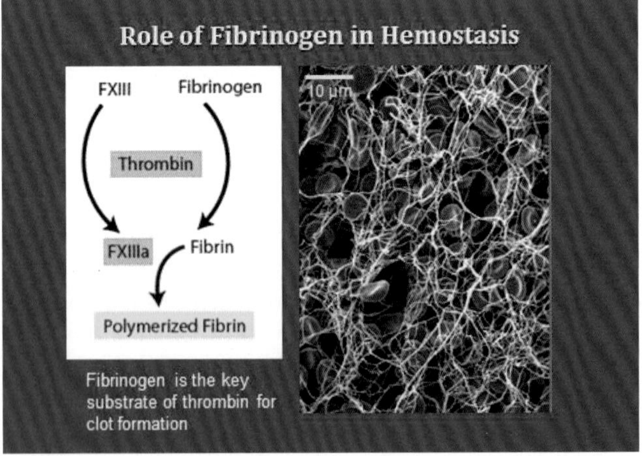

FIGURE 27-3 Fibrinogen is converted to fibrin that polymerizes by the action of thrombin. The electron micrograph shows a fibrin clot with red blood cells trapped. Platelets also are critical to fibrin formation, but they are 8 to 10 microns and not visible in the photo. Fibrinogen receptors on the platelet surface (called ***IIb/IIIa receptors***) facilitate the lattice network of fibrin formation. Factor XIII, a transglutamase, is also important for cross-linking the fibrin clot to create a stronger clot that is resistant to fibrinolysis. (Modified from Tanaka KA, Key NS, Levy JH. Blood coagulation: hemostasis and thrombin regulation. *Anesth Analg.* 2009;108:1433–1446.)

fibrin network for normal clot function and hemostasis. However, in patients with hemophilia and other bleeding abnormalities, lower levels of thrombin generation occur and as a result clot formation is altered, thus hemophiliacs commonly bleed into joints. Thrombin generation at the junction of the injured vasculature and subendothelial basement membrane is amplified by platelet activation and release of procoagulant microparticles.[1,3] Thrombin has a complex effect of releasing tissue plasminogen activator (t-PA) to simultaneously initiate fibrinolysis. This occurs by binding to thrombomodulin but also by activated factor XIII and activation of thrombin-activatable fibrinolysis inhibitor (also called TAFI). Fibrin polymerization, thrombin, and activated factor X generated at the site of vascular injury site are released systemically.

Critical Factor Levels for Hemostasis

A critical question is what levels of fibrinogen, platelets, and other coagulation proteins are necessary to optimize hemostasis in the surgical patients. Many blood bank experts as well as older guidelines only recommended treating fibrinogen levels if they have decreased below ~1.0 g/L (100 mg/dL), a level similar to the management of congenital afibrinogenemia.[6] There is increasing data about the critical role of fibrinogen and current European guidelines recommend higher fibrinogen levels of 1.5 to 2.0 g/L for treating coagulopathy. Recent studies have demonstrated the critical role of fibrinogen for aortic surgery, postpartum hemorrhage, cardiac surgery, and cystectomy. Of note is that studies suggest that further normalization of fibrinogen to levels more consistent with normal circulating concentrations of 2 to 3 g/L may be important for adequate hemostasis.

Role of Factor XIII

Factor XIII plays a major role in the terminal phase of the clotting cascade that promotes formation of cross-linked fibrin polymers and generation of a stable hemostatic plug.[7] Factor XIII exists as a tetrameric precursor (zymogen) of 2 A and 2 B subunits and is converted into an active transglutaminase (factor XIIIa) by thrombin and calcium.[7] In this activated form, factor XIIIa mechanically stabilizes fibrin and protects it from fibrinolysis. As a result, patients with a deficiency in factor XIII develop a rare but severe bleeding disorder.[8,9] A congenital deficiency in factor XIII is clinically defined as a plasma level of less than 5% of the protein.[7] Most cases of factor XIII deficiency are due to lack of the A subunit with less than 1% factor XIII activity. Congenital factor XIII deficiency is inherited as an autosomal recessive disease and was first reported in Switzerland in 1960.[10] The incidence of factor XIII deficiency is currently estimated as one in 3 to 5 million births in the United States.[11] An acquired deficiency in factor XIII can arise from the development of antibodies against factor XIII. We have also studied factor XIII repletion, and although it did not decrease bleeding or transfusion requirement in cardiac surgery, levels of >50% to 60% may to reduce bleeding in surgical patients with low fibrinogen levels (<1.5 g/L).[7]

Role of Platelets and von Willebrand Factor

Platelets adhere to sites of vascular injury and to each other by direct and indirect effects that are part of a complex cellular mechanism required for hemostasis. Although platelet aggregation is mediated in part by bridging/binding of the integrin glycoprotein IIb/IIIa on platelet surfaces by the adhesive protein fibrinogen, this process is far more complex than simple interactions and the lattice formation of the two elements.

There are multistep adhesion processes involving distinct receptors and adhesive ligands that are also dependent on flow conditions, especially with the critical role of platelet function in arterial hemostatic mechanisms. Thus, following vascular injury, the subendothelial surface is exposed which then binds to vWF that is synthesized in the endothelium and critical for platelet adhesion in arteries and arterioles that have high shear rates.

vWF is critical to facilitate platelet adhesion in rapid blood flow environments. vWF binds to an adhesion ligand, its platelet membrane receptor, GPIb-IX-V. Once platelets adhere, they are activated by a complex series of steps including release of adenosine diphosphate (ADP) and thromboxane A_2, agonists that activate additional platelets and bind P2Y12 receptors and express IIb/IIIa receptors. These important receptors are the target of common pharmacologic agents including clopidogrel, prasugrel, and ticagrelor. Platelets provide a catalytic membrane surface for further thrombin generation and clot formation and mediate additional platelet and leukocyte recruitment by mechanisms that include release of microparticles that mediate leukocyte-leukocyte and leukocyte–endothelial cell interactions. When activated, platelets may also form occlusive thrombi in cardiovascular diseases that result in myocardial infarction, stroke, or other acute ischemic syndromes of other organs.

Endothelial Regulation of Coagulation

The vascular endothelium provides an extensive interface that is critical for both anticoagulant and procoagulants functions as shown in Figure 27-2.[12–15] Increased shear forces and flow across the endothelium release important anticoagulation agents (Table 27-2) that include a diverse series of molecules, including nitric oxide, prostacyclin, and ecto-ADPase that degrade the platelet agonist ADP. Additionally, endothelium-derived TFPI is localized on the surface of vascular endothelium, and reduces the procoagulant activities of the TF–factor VIIa initiation step.[1,3] Heparin sulfate is located on endothelial surfaces and binds antithrombin in the circulation to further provide anticoagulant activity on the vascular surface. Thrombin is

Table 27-2

Endothelial Proteins and Mediators of Hemostasis

ADAMTS-13
Endothelial protein C receptor
Glycocalyx
Heparan sulfate
Nitric oxide
Plasminogen activator inhibitor-1
Prostacyclin
Protein C
Protein S
Thrombomodulin
Tissue factor
Tissue factor pathway inhibitor
Tissue-type plasminogen activator
von Willebrand factor

ADAMTS-13, *a* disintegrin *and* metalloprotease with a *t*hrombo*s*pondin type 1 motif, member *13*.

scavenged to keep thrombin activity local at the site of vascular injury by another endothelium-bound protein called ***thrombomodulin***.[1,3] Thrombomodulin is used clinically in Japan for DIC and is currently being studied for treatment of sepsis in the United States. Endothelial activation also provides anticoagulation by releasing t-PA from the endothelial stores of the Weibel-Palade bodies. t-PA activates plasmin from plasminogen which, in turn, promotes fibrinolysis, a critical component of vascular patency.[1,3]

The endothelium is critical for procoagulant effects as well.[12–15] Endothelial damage following vascular injury or inflammatory responses initiates an array of procoagulant responses that include release of TF, vWF, plasminogen activator inhibitor (PAI)-1, and PARs. TF as discussed is critical for initiation of clot formation and thrombin generation. vWF allows for platelets to bind and activate locally at the site of vascular injury. PAI-1 prevents plasmin generation and fibrinolysis, or clot cleavage. PARs further signal platelet and a host of other responses by thrombin and other inflammatory mediators.[12–15]

This complex equilibrium of hemostasis continues and is constantly scavenged by many of these important mechanisms to localize hemostasis to the site of vascular injury through this multitude of regulatory mechanisms. Thrombin that is scavenged and bound to thrombomodulin is an important step in the generation of the anticoagulant protein C and TAFI.[12–15] Activated protein C has multiple antiinflammatory and cytoprotective functions by modulating endothelial protein C receptor (EPCR) and PAR-1 (thrombin receptor).[16–18] TAFI also exerts antiinflammatory effects by cleaving bradykinin and C5a. Activated protein C has also seen therapeutic use as a therapy in sepsis, along with antithrombin.

Other important factors in hemostatic regulation include the circulating release of vWF that circulates as a multimer complex and is a key adhesive protein for platelets as further discussed in the following text. vWF is also increased during inflammation and is downregulated by ADAMTS-13 (***A*** ***D***isintegrin ***a***nd ***M***etalloprotease with a ***T***hrombo***S***pondin type 1 motif, member ***13***), which is also synthesized by endothelial cells.[19] In addition to vWD, other vWF abnormalities can occur due to increased degradation that occurs with ventricular assist devices or aortic stenosis, or decreased regulation due to lack of the cleaving enzyme that can occur with hemolytic uremic syndrome or thrombotic thrombocytopenic purpura.

Antithrombin and Proteins C and S

As discussed earlier, thrombin generation for hemostasis is localized because anticoagulant activities of endothelial cells modulate thrombin and other procoagulant proteases as shown in Figure 27-2.[20] Other proteins including antithrombin, protein C, and protein S are also important serine proteases that exert anticoagulant and antiinflammatory activities. Protein C circulates in the inactive state in plasma at concentrations of 4 to 5 μg/mL (~0.08 μM) and is proteolytically activated by thrombin to activated protein C.[20] Thrombin is again scavenged by binding to endothelial thrombomodulin, activating protein C. Activated protein C binds protein S, and together they function as a critical anticoagulant by inhibiting factor Va and factor VIIIa, two cofactors in thrombin generation and clot formation (see Fig. 27-2). Activated protein C has been studied in sepsis but is no longer available for that indication.

Inflammation and Coagulation: An Important Link

Coagulation is closely linked to inflammatory responses through complex networks of plasma and cellular components including proteases of the clotting and fibrinolytic cascades.[21,22] Hemostatic initiation, contact activation, and other pathways amplify inflammatory responses and can collectively produce end-organ damage in the process of their normal function as host defense mechanisms. Coagulation is activated as a central element of both a local and a systemic response to inflammation.[22] Surgical injury and additional activation that can occur following cardiopulmonary bypass produces inflammatory responses initiated by contact of blood with the damaged vasculature and other nonendothelial extracorporeal circuits. In vascular surgical and trauma patients, ischemia-reperfusion injury of organs can also occur.[23] TF has important proinflammatory effects mediated by thrombin, plasmin, and other proteases.[21,22,24]

Coagulation Testing

The two tests most frequently used in the perioperative setting, other than blood counts, include the prothrombin time used to evaluate the extrinsic coagulation cascade and the activated partial thromboplastin time, used to evaluate the intrinsic pathway of the classic coagulation system. The prothrombin time is affected by reductions of factors VII, X, V, and prothrombin and is used to measure the effect of warfarin and other agents with vitamin K antagonist activity or the consequences of decreased synthetic activity resulting from hepatic dysfunction. Although prothrombin time is used commonly for perioperative coagulation screening, its use and target values are still controversial and often based on consensus rather than supportive data. Clinical hemostasis may not be adequately evaluated with prothrombin times alone as is apparent in patients with hemophilia who have isolated factor VIII or IX deficiency despite normal prothrombin times.

The partial thromboplastin time is another widely used coagulation test that assesses the intrinsic coagulation cascade. Most partial thromboplastin times are activated using an agent such as ellagic acid, kaolin, or celite.[25] The partial thromboplastin time is used to monitor lower doses of unfractionated heparin (up to ~1.0 unit/mL), argatroban, and bivalirudin. At higher heparin concentrations used during cardiac surgery the activated clotting time is used.

Although these coagulation tests are used to evaluate bleeding, they only examine specific components of the overall coagulation cascade and may not be useful to determine the exact cause of the coagulopathy. As should be apparent from the discussion in this chapter, multiple factors influence normal coagulation and lead to coagulopathy in a perioperative setting including hemorrhage and dilution, fibrinolysis, hypothermia, and vascular injury .[26,27] These in vitro laboratory tests do not include the important interaction of platelets with coagulation factors or measurement of the stability of a hemostatic plug as these tests actually measure initial clot formation alone.

Whole blood viscoelastic tests including thromboelastography and thromboelastometry provide multiple insights in to coagulation factor interaction and allow assessment of individual characteristics of either individual limbs of hemostasis or global monitoring of coagulation, and they have been widely used in the perioperative and trauma setting. The commonly used thromboelastometric variables include coagulation time (in seconds), clot formation time (in seconds), angle (in degrees), maximum clot firmness (in millimeters), and lysis time (in seconds). Coagulation time represents the onset of clotting, whereas clot formation time and angle both represent the initial rate of fibrin polymerization. Maximal clot firmness is a measure of the maximal viscoelastic strength of clot. Lysis time is used for the diagnosis of premature lysis or hyperfibrinolysis.

Perioperative Changes in Coagulation

In surgical patients, there are multiple perioperative events that influence hemostatic function and produce coagulopathy. Vascular and tissue injury are important contributors to bleeding, but with significant hemorrhage and resuscitation with crystalloids/colloids, a dilutional coagulopathy can occur resulting from significant reductions in platelet counts/dilutional thrombocytopenia and factor deficiencies. The end result is a multifactorial reduction of thrombin generation, hypofibrinogenemia, and lack of other factors that reduce clot formation and this state is accompanied by increased fibrinolysis. The poorly formed fibrin clot contributes to bleeding, and increasing hemodilution simultaneously leads to a reduction in important proteins that balance hemostasis and anticoagulation, including antithrombin, TFPI, protein C, protein S, and thrombomodulin.[20] These complex hemostatic changes also contribute to the coagulopathic state.

Hemostatic Therapy

When perioperative bleeding occurs, we use red blood cells and hemostatic factors that include plasma/fresh frozen plasma, platelet concentrates, and cryoprecipitate (see further discussion in Chapter 28, Blood Products and Blood Components and Chapter 29, Procoagulants). Postoperatively, an important anabolic state occurs that increases hemostatic factors for several days. Many of the factors that modulate this acute inflammatory response postoperatively will increase cytokines and other important signaling molecules that will increase cellular and protein synthesis. These changes will increase bone marrow production of red blood cells and platelets; increase fibrinogen and vWF; and create a hypercoagulable, procoagulant response. This is important and also integral to the current practice of use of anticoagulation for postoperative venous thromboembolic prophylaxis because of the increased thrombotic potential postoperatively.

Postoperative Hypercoagulability

The complex balance in hemostatic function can be readily altered in the postoperative setting. Because of loss of vascular endothelial function and other prohemostatic changes, venous and arterial thromboembolic events increase with age.[20] Acute myocardial infarction and thrombotic stroke can occur following disruption of atheromatous plaques in coronary and cerebral arteries. The rupture of a lipid core expresses multiple procoagulant molecules that expose TF, lead to thrombin generation, and activate platelets, all leading to coagulation. Embolic and other thrombotic events occurring locally at the site of an atherosclerotic plaque can result in myocardial infarction and ischemic stroke. Additional abnormalities present in cancer patients can also initiate coagulation and other prothrombotic events that increase the risk of venous thromboembolic events.

Congenital coagulation factor deficiencies or polymorphisms of critical proteins including hemophilia A or B, vWF, antithrombin, protein C, protein S, factor V Leiden, and prothrombin (polymorphisms) are more uncommon in the perioperative period but do occur and often require specific management strategies—these conditions can present with either bleeding or thrombosis. Acquired or congenital absence of the anticoagulant proteins reduces normal clot formation and regulation, and untreated patients are at an increased risk for venous thromboembolic problems, including pulmonary embolism. A more common occurrence is the antiphospholipid syndrome that is caused by the lupus anticoagulant, which is a phospholipid binding antibody. Of note is that patients may present with prolonged prothrombin times and partial thromboplastin times, but they are actually hypercoagulable.[20]

Disseminated Intravascular Coagulation

Disseminated intravascular coagulation (DIC) is a coagulation disorder that occurs when pathologic activation of the hemostatic systems occurs following major tissue injury associated with trauma, sepsis due to bacterial, fungal, or viral causes, or other complex occurrences of vasculopathy that occurs in eclampsia.[28,29] Activation of the coagulation system occurs; however, the multiple endothelial and circulating anticoagulation mechanisms that are part of hemostatic mechanisms are unable to inhibit systemic thrombin formation. The pathophysiologic changes of DIC include hemostatic activation characterized by microvascular deposition of clot/fibrin and thrombotic microangiopathy. Platelets are also activated and are sequestered into the pulmonary, renal, hepatic, and other organs, depleting platelets, fibrinogen, antithrombin, and other hemostatic factors. The end result is an imbalance, resulting in either a hemorrhagic coagulopathy or procoagulant state. The diagnosis of DIC is based on clinical and laboratory findings that follow.

Thrombocytopenia occurs in DIC due to the mechanisms described; however, in the perioperative setting and in critically ill patients, thrombocytopenia is common. The most common cause of perioperative thrombocytopenia is the dilutional effect following volume resuscitation; nonetheless, current strategy is to treat massive transfusion coagulopathy in the setting of trauma and surgery, and this strategy includes the administration of platelets and other clotting factors (platelets, fresh frozen plasma, and/or cryoprecipitate). Coagulation factors are also decreased in DIC, and this presents clinically with prolonged prothrombin times or activated partial thromboplastin times. In DIC and other similar syndromes, such as thrombotic thrombocytopenic purpura and hemolytic uremic syndrome, decreased levels of the protease ADAMTS-13 can occur. This protease converts ultra-large von Willebrand multimers in plasma that are otherwise prothrombotic. The uncleaved multimers increase vascular platelet sequestration and the subsequent development of thrombotic microangiopathy and organ dysfunction.[29] Fibrinogen levels are also used in diagnosing DIC but, despite consumption, plasma levels are affected by multiple factors and may only detect severe cases of DIC.[29] D-dimers are also used in the diagnosis of DIC and are fragments of cross-linked fibrinogen that are cleaved by fibrinolysis. D-dimer levels are increased in DIC but also with venous thromboembolism and following any recent trauma or surgery, thus they may not be helpful in the surgical patient. Finally, antithrombin levels decrease in DIC, and have been suggested as a therapeutic target to replete. Overall, in DIC, removal of the underlying source of the problem, treatment with antibiotics for infections, and perhaps instituting anticoagulation in efforts to reduce further consumption of coagulation factors are critical considerations.[30]

Conclusion

The physiology of coagulation and hemostatic regulation are critical homeostatic mechanisms that are critical to survival. The interaction of the vasculature with both circulating plasma proteins and platelets is important for understanding the physiology of the hemostatic system, and the ability to modulate hemostasis and respond to vascular injury. Multiple disease states including atherosclerosis, acquired coagulation deficiencies, and the pharmacologic effects of many therapies used for atherosclerotic vascular disease may contribute to the problems of perioperative hemostatic management. Our goal is to reduce bleeding without the adverse effects of thrombosis. This concern is complicated by the interaction of coagulation and subsequent inflammatory responses. As discussed in the other chapters on coagulation that follow pharmacologic interventions, based on the authors' understanding of the physiology of hemostasis, it is critical for the perioperative management and further discussed in other chapters.

References

1. Tanaka KA, Key NS, Levy JH. Blood coagulation: hemostasis and thrombin regulation. *Anesth Analg*. 2009;108:1433–1446.
2. Hoffman M, Monroe DM. Coagulation 2006: a modern view of hemostasis. *Hematol Oncol Clin North Am*. 2007;21:1–11.
3. Tanaka KA, Levy JH. Regulation of thrombin activity—pharmacologic and structural aspects. *Hematol Oncol Clin North Am*. 2007;21:33–50.
4. Mackman N. The role of tissue factor and factor VIIa in hemostasis. *Anesth Analg*. 2009;108:1447–1452.
5. Lane DA, Philippou H, Huntington JA. Directing thrombin. *Blood*. 2005;106:2605–2612.
6. Levy JH, Welsby I, Goodnough LT. Fibrinogen as a therapeutic target for bleeding: a review of critical levels and replacement therapy. *Transfusion*. 2014;54(5):1389–1405.
7. Levy JH, Greenberg C. Biology of factor XIII and clinical manifestations of factor XIII deficiency. *Transfusion*. 2013;53:1120–1131.
8. Hsieh L, Nugent D. Factor XIII deficiency. *Haemophilia*. 2008;14:1190–1200.
9. Ichinose A, Souri M, Izumi T, et al. Molecular and genetic mechanisms of factor XIII A subunit deficiency. *Semin Thromb Hemost*. 2000;26:5–10.
10. Schroeder V, Durrer D, Meili E, et al. Congenital factor XIII deficiency in Switzerland: from the worldwide first case in 1960 to its molecular characterisation in 2005. *Swiss Med Wkly*. 2007;137:272–278.

11. Warkentin TE, Greinacher A. Heparin-induced thrombocytopenia and cardiac surgery. *Ann Thorac Surg*. 2003;76:638–648.
12. Aird WC. Endothelium as an organ system. *Crit Care Med*. 2004;32: S271–S279.
13. Aird WC. Coagulation. *Crit Care Med*. 2005;33:S485–S487.
14. Aird WC. Mechanisms of endothelial cell heterogeneity in health and disease. *Circ Res*. 2006;98:159–162.
15. Aird WC. Vascular bed-specific thrombosis. *J Thromb Haemost*. 2007;5(suppl 1):283–291.
16. Esmon CT. The protein C pathway. *Chest*. 2003;124:26S–32S.
17. Ludeman MJ, Kataoka H, Srinivasan Y, et al. PAR1 cleavage and signaling in response to activated protein C and thrombin. *J Biol Chem*. 2005;280:13122–13128.
18. Mosnier LO, Zlokovic BV, Griffin JH. The cytoprotective protein C pathway. *Blood*. 2007;109:3161–3172.
19. Sadler JE. Von Willebrand factor, ADAMTS13, and thrombotic thrombocytopenic purpura. *Blood*. 2008;112:11–18.
20. Sniecinski RM, Hursting MJ, Paidas MJ, et al. Etiology and assessment of hypercoagulability with lessons from heparin-induced thrombocytopenia. *Anesth Analg*. 2010;112:46–58.
21. Levi M, van der Poll T, Buller HR. Bidirectional relation between inflammation and coagulation. *Circulation*. 2004;109:2698–2704.
22. Esmon CT. The impact of the inflammatory response on coagulation. *Thromb Res*. 2004;114:321–327.
23. Mojcik CF, Levy JH. Aprotinin and the systemic inflammatory response after cardiopulmonary bypass. *Ann Thorac Surg*. 2001;71: 745–754.
24. Mackman N. The role of the tissue factor-thrombin pathway in cardiac ischemia-reperfusion injury. *Semin Vasc Med*. 2003;3:193–198.
25. White GC II. The partial thromboplastin time: defining an era in coagulation.[see comment]. *J Thromb Haemost*. 2003;1:2267–2270.
26. Despotis GJ, Filos KS, Zoys TN, et al. Factors associated with excessive postoperative blood loss and hemostatic transfusion requirements: a multivariate analysis in cardiac surgical patients. *Anesth Analg*. 1996;82:13–21.
27. Carroll RC, Chavez JJ, Snider CC, et al. Correlation of perioperative platelet function and coagulation tests with bleeding after cardiopulmonary bypass surgery. *J Lab Clin Med*. 2006;147:197–204.
28. Levi M, Toh CH, Thachil J, et al. Guidelines for the diagnosis and management of disseminated intravascular coagulation. British Committee for Standards in Haematology. *Br J Haematol*. 2009;145:24–33.
29. Levi M, Meijers JC. DIC: which laboratory tests are most useful. *Blood Rev*. 2011;25:33–37.
30. Hotchkiss RS, Levy JH, Levi M. Sepsis-induced disseminated intravascular coagulation, symmetrical peripheral gangrene, and amputations. *Crit Care Med*. 2013;41:e290–e291.
31. Monroe DM, Hoffman M. What does it take to make the perfect clot? *Arterioscler Thromb Vasc Biol*. 2006;26:41–48.

CHAPTER 28

Blood Products and Blood Components

Jerrold H. Levy

Millions of blood components are transfused annually, especially in surgical and trauma patients. While blood transfusions are considered to be standard of care in perioperative management, overall data supporting their efficacy has never been demonstrated in a prospective controlled clinical trial in the manner that drugs are approved for use. Currently, the relative benefit/risk of transfusions has become part of informed consent. Overall, blood products should be considered in the same manner and scientific perspective as we consider drugs and pharmacologic therapies. Important in the use of blood products as drugs is the fact that transfusions have important risks, costs, and supply/inventory considerations.

A pivotal study of transfusion fatalities by the Serious Hazards of Transfusion (SHOT) scheme in the United Kingdom and the U.S. Food Drug Administration (FDA) Center for Biologics Evaluation and Research (CBER) in the United States suggest that transfusion-related deaths appear to be declining.[1,2] The development of specific hemovigilance networks in France in 1994 and SHOT in the United Kingdom in 1996 led to reports that transfusion-related acute lung injury (TRALI) has been the most common cause of mortality and morbidity associated with transfusion. In the United States, TRALI was the cause of reported fatalities in 43% of patients who received transfusion, followed by hemolytic transfusion reactions (23%). TRALI will be covered in more detail later in this chapter. Of note is that both known risks and ongoing potential for new viral contaminants (unknown risks) are likely associated with transfusion.

Despite our extensive use of transfusions in the perioperative setting, they have been associated with a complex series of adverse events including infections, stroke, renal failure, multiorgan failure, and increased hospital and intensive care unit (ICU) length of stay (LOS). Most data and studies evaluating transfusions have been from retrospective studies and include *observational* data from patients already predestined to suffer adverse outcomes. Other important issues that transfusions pose in addition to the risks are the costs and blood inventory required for managing patients. *Patient Blood Management* initiatives have evolved from ongoing work by many different interests to develop evidence-based transfusion practices and strategies to reduce bleeding and the need for allogeneic transfusions. In the perioperative setting, multiple specialties and health care providers influence the decision to transfuse a patient. Further, most work has focused on red blood cells (RBCs) and hemoglobin concentrations, with far less emphasis on coagulation factors whose effects are more difficult to measure. Because the decision to transfuse a patient is complex, rarely can a single laboratory value be an absolute indicator of the need for transfusion. Decisions to transfuse require multiple clinical considerations including risk factors, comorbidities, hemodynamic stability, and the rate of bleeding, especially in hemorrhagic shock, a common perioperative emergency.

The appropriate use of blood products, including RBCs, fresh frozen plasma (FFP), cryoprecipitate, or platelet transfusions, continues to be defined in surgical patients. Further, in some countries, purified protein concentrates are used instead of transfusion factors, as in the case of fibrinogen concentrates instead of cryoprecipitate. Guidelines and transfusion algorithms for the management of bleeding in surgical patients are available.[3,4] Multiple risk factors are important when considering patients at risk for bleeding (Table 28-1).

Blood products are administered as therapeutic agents in perioperative management. Despite guidelines, most physicians either have not read the guidelines or have difficulty following them. Clinicians often resort to empiric therapy because laboratory tests are difficult to obtain, take too long, do not determine platelet defects, or because they have concerns about later getting blood products from the blood bank in a timely fashion for high-risk patients. Of note is that transfusions are important for massive bleeding following trauma and transfusion under these conditions will be considered in a separate chapter. In a critically ill patient, the importance of a multimodality approach is important rather than focusing on the individual transfused components.

Table 28-1

Predictors of Postoperative Bleeding: Cardiothoracic Surgery

Advanced age
Small body size or preoperative anemia (low RBC volume)
Antiplatelet and antithrombotic drugs
Prolonged operation (CPB time)—high correlation with OR type
Emergency operation
Other comorbidities (CHF, COPD, HTN, PVD, renal failure)

RBC, red blood cell; CPB, cardiopulmonary bypass; CHF, congestive heart failure; COPD, chronic obstructive pulmonary disease; HTN, hypertension; OR, operating room; PVD, peripheral vascular disease.
From Ferraris VA, Ferraris SP, Saha SP, et al. Perioperative blood transfusion and blood conservation in cardiac surgery: the STS and the SCA Clinical Practice Guideline. *Ann Thorac Surg.* 2007;83:S27–S86.

The American Society of Anesthesiologists established the Task Force on Blood Component Therapy to develop evidence-based guidelines for transfusing RBCs, platelets, FFP, and cryoprecipitate in perioperative settings. Specific guidelines were developed according to a defined methodology.[5] The recommendations of the task force were reported and can be found at http://www.asahq.org/publicationsAndServices/transfusion.pdf (Table 28-2). Although these guidelines are reported as recommendations, there are also other important considerations regarding the use of specific blood units in surgical patients that need to be considered. The rationale for transfusion of individual blood components will also be considered.

Transfusion Therapy for Bleeding

Volume replacement in the perioperative setting when there is critical bleeding requires the use of replacement therapy. Although crystalloid, colloid, and RBCs are used initially, none provide coagulation factors or platelets and thus their use can exacerbate coagulopathy. Severe bleeding requires use of FFP, platelets, cryoprecipitate, and factor concentrates (e.g., fibrinogen and prothrombin complex concentrates) to restore circulating levels of hemostatic factors. Following massive transfusion therapy, hypothermia and acidosis frequently occur, further complicating bleeding. Thus, temperature and pH must be monitored and corrected during any ongoing transfusion effort.

Red Blood Cells

There is no single minimum acceptable hemoglobin level that can be applied to all patients when deciding when to transfuse RBCs. Chronic anemia is better tolerated than acute anemia. However, with acute anemia, compensatory mechanisms that increase cardiac output and improve oxygen transport depend on the patient's cardiovascular reserve. In surgical patients with heart failure and/or flow-restricting lesions, compensation during acute anemia may be limited. Multiple factors should be considered

Table 28-2

Evidence-Based Indications for Transfusing Red Blood Cells, Platelets, Fresh Frozen Plasma, and Cryoprecipitate in Perioperative Settings Guidelines

1. The risks of bleeding in surgical patients are determined by the extent and type of surgery, the capacity to control bleeding, the expected rate of bleeding, and the outcomes of uncontrolled bleeding.
2. RBC transfusions should not be dictated by a single hemoglobin "trigger" but instead should be based on each individual patient's risks of developing complications of inadequate oxygenation. RBC transfusions are rarely indicated when the hemoglobin concentration is >10 g/dL and are nearly always indicated when it is <6 g/dL. The indications for autologous transfusion may be more liberal than for allogeneic transfusion.
3. Prophylactic platelet transfusion is ineffective when thrombocytopenia is due to increased platelet destruction. Surgical patients with microvascular bleeding usually need platelet transfusion if the platelet count is <50,000 platelets/μL and rarely platelet transfusion if the platelet count is >100,000 platelets/μL.
4. Fresh frozen plasma (FFP) is indicated for urgent reversal of warfarin therapy, correction of known coagulation factor deficiencies for which specific concentrates are unavailable, and correction of microvascular bleeding when prothrombin and partial thromboplastin times are >1.5 times normal. FFP is not indicated for increasing plasma volume or albumin concentration.
5. Cryoprecipitate should be considered for patients with von Willebrand's disease unresponsive to desmopressin, bleeding patients with von Willebrand's disease, and bleeding patients with fibrinogen levels <80–100 mg/dL.

RBC, red blood cell.
Practice guidelines for perioperative blood transfusion and adjuvant therapies: an updated report by the American Society of Anesthesiologists Task Force on Perioperative Blood Transfusion and Adjuvant Therapies. *Anesthesiology.* 2006;105:198–208.

including intravascular volume, whether the patient is actively bleeding, and the need for improvement in oxygen transport. For instance, the patient receiving multiple inotropes and requiring an intraaortic balloon pump who is anemic following surgery may need RBC transfusion at a higher hemoglobin level than an otherwise healthy and hemodynamically stable patient. The decision to transfuse must weigh the risks of transfusion against the need for improved oxygen-carrying capacity in recovery from trauma, surgery, or illness.[5] The American Society of Anesthesiologists Task Force on Perioperative Blood Transfusion noted in its recommendations that transfusion of RBCs should usually be administered when the hemoglobin concentration is low (e.g., <6 g/dL in a young, healthy patient), especially when the anemia is acute. RBCs are usually unnecessary when the hemoglobin concentration is more than 10 g/dL. These conclusions may be altered in the presence of anticipated blood loss or active critical (i.e., myocardium, central nervous system or renal) or target organ ischemia. Determining whether intermediate hemoglobin concentrations (i.e., 6 to 10 g/dL) justify or require RBC transfusion should be based on any ongoing indication of organ ischemia, potential or actual ongoing bleeding (rate and magnitude), the patient's intravascular volume status, and the patient's risk factors for complications of inadequate oxygenation. These risk factors include a low cardiopulmonary reserve and high oxygen consumption."[5] Hemoglobin triggers for transfusion are not to be taken as absolute; patients with significant cardiac disease should be transfused if signs or symptoms of inadequate myocardial oxygenation appear.

One important aspect of adverse events associated with RBC transfusion relates to the age of RBCs transfused and changes that occur in stored RBCs as they age (the so-called storage lesion).[6–8] Although RBCs are stored for up to 42 days after donation, biochemical changes occur in RBCs as they age. Studies suggest that RBC units stored for long periods (often described as >14 to 21 days) may lead to adverse effects. The mechanisms for these adverse events include senescent RBC fragments, impaired nitric oxide production, and increased nitric oxide scavenging by stored RBCs, together with reduced nitric oxide synthesis by dysfunctional endothelial cells. However, many of the studies demonstrating adverse outcomes are from large retrospective studies with all of the inherent problems associated with retrospective analyses and not all studies are in agreement.

Red Blood Cell Storage Lesions

RBCs develop a complex series of biochemical and metabolic changes during storage in the blood bank that include depletion of adenosine triphosphate (ATP) and of 2,3-diphosphoglycerate (2,3-DPG); membrane phospholipid vesiculation and shedding, protein oxidation, and lipid peroxidation of the cell membrane. As the blood ages, RBCs undergo shape changes with increased fragility that may impair microcirculatory flow. Because of increased red cell–endothelial cell interaction, bioreactive lipids and other substances are released that may initiate inflammatory responses leading to TRALI, as described in more detail in the following text. These complex changes can also decrease oxygen delivery and increase hemolysis. When free hemoglobin is released from the RBC, it binds to nitric oxide and this nitric oxide scavenging causes endothelial dysfunction and additional proinflammatory events including generation of oxygen free radicals.

Red Blood Cell Storage and Tissue Oxygenation Parameters

Transfusion of RBCs is used therapeutically to increase the oxygen-carrying capacity of blood and thereby improve oxygen delivery to tissues. Multiple retrospective studies have attempted to evaluate the clinical outcomes of critically ill patients receiving fresh compared to older blood. There are multiple analysis in the literature that examine the clinical effect of blood storage in multiple patient groups including trauma patients, ICU patients, and patients undergoing cardiac surgery or those with acute heart disease with variable effects. Most of the studies are observational based and there is clinical equipoise regarding results. Currently, a randomized study is underway to address this issue as will be described later. As they also note, previous systematic reviews and a meta-analysis conducted in critically ill patients have been inconclusive.

Current studies underway include the Red Cell Storage Duration Study (RECESS: NCT00991341), a prospective, randomized clinical trial (RCT). The National Heart, Lung and Blood Institute (NHLBI)–funded RECESS is a multicenter RCT. Complex cardiac surgical procedures are being randomized to receive RBC units stored for 10 days or fewer versus RBCs stored for at least 21 days and will include approximately 1,434 patients. Outcomes being evaluated include multiple organ dysfunction score, all-cause mortality, and other measures of organ dysfunction will be evaluated. Other clinical studies include The Canadian Age of Blood Evaluation (ABLE) study (trial of the resuscitation of critically ill patients: ISRCTN44878718) is currently being conducted in ICU patients. It will enroll a total of 2,510 patients in Canada, France, and the United Kingdom and will compare 90-day mortality between patients transfused with fresh RBC (storage <8 days) compared to current practices. The TRANSFUSE trial (ACTRN12612000453886) started in 2012 in Australia and New Zealand is a large (5,000 patients) pivotal, multicenter, randomized, controlled trial in critically ill patients to determine whether, compared with standard care, transfusion of the freshest available RBC decreases patient mortality. Completion is expected in 2015.

The true impact of the age of stored RBC on patient outcomes remains in question but an answer should emerge from these ongoing clinical trials. Although RBC transfusions are used extensively in the perioperative setting, all transfusions can be associated with adverse events. Multiple factors are responsible for the storage lesion that is specific to RBCs, and current studies will further resolve the questions.

Plasma/Fresh Frozen Plasma

Plasma is transfused for multiple indications, especially in surgical and trauma patients. Plasma use has increased with the increasing understanding of its role in managing the coagulopathy associated with massive transfusion (massive transfusion is covered in detail in a separate chapter). Currently, plasma and FFP are used to replace volume and coagulation factors during massive transfusion, to treat or prevent future bleeding during surgery and invasive procedures, to reverse warfarin therapy in patients, and for treatment of coagulation factor abnormalities where specific concentrates are not available. FFP is plasma frozen within 8 hours of collection. However, many plasma units transfused in the United States are actually frozen within 24 hours after phlebotomy (FP24). The difference is that cryoprecipitate can be obtained from FFP but not FP24; nonetheless, experts agree that FFP and FP24 can be transfused interchangeably and most clinicians refer to both products as FFP, despite this subtle distinction. Thawed plasma (either FFP of FP24) stored for up to 5 days before administration is also commonly used for transfusion. Plasma is used throughout the text to refer to FFP, FP24, or thawed plasma, as most scientific evidence supporting and distinctions among different plasma transfusion practices is limited.

Following collection of a unit of blood, FFP is the plasma that remains after RBC and platelet removal and contains blood coagulation factors, fibrinogen, and other plasma proteins in a volume of 170 to 250 mL that is then frozen and can be stored for up to 1 year. Most plasma administered in perioperative settings is actually FP24. Before administration, the plasma must be thawed in a water bath at 37°C, which takes about 30 minutes. After thawing, the units of FFP are stored at 1°C to 6°C and are transfused within 24 hours. FFP should be administered through a component administration set with a 170-micron filter. If not used within 24 hours, it can be relabeled as "thawed plasma" and stored at 1°C to 6°C for an additional 4 days. Thawed plasma maintains normal levels of all factors except factor V which falls to 80% of normal and factor VIII which falls to 60% of normal during storage.[9] Because these levels are above the in vivo threshold for normal hemostatic function for these factors and factor VIII is an acute phase reactant, thawed plasma can be used as a substitute for FFP.[9]

FFP is used for treating bleeding because of coagulopathies that are associated with a prolongation of either the activated partial thromboplastin time (aPTT) or prothrombin time (PT)/international normalized ratio (INR) greater than 1.5 times normal, or a specific coagulation factor assay of less than 25%.[5] FFP is often used to reverse the effect of warfarin before surgery or during active bleeding episodes (see prothrombin complex concentrates later in this chapter and chapter 29). When FFP is indicated, it should be administered in a dose calculated to achieve a minimum of 30% of plasma factor concentration. Ten to 15 mL/kg of FFP will generally result in a rise of most coagulation proteins by 25% to 30% (or increases in 0.25 to 0.3 U/mL), although a dose of 5 to 8 mL/kg may be adequate to urgently reverse warfarin anticoagulation but varies based on the initial levels of the vitamin K–dependent coagulation factors.[5] FFP is also an important part of a transfusion algorithm for posttraumatic bleeding that is covered in more detail in the chapter on massive transfusion.

Guidelines exist in many countries for the use of plasma and include active bleeding preoperatively, invasive procedures in patients with acquired coagulation abnormalities, immediate correction of vitamin K antagonists (e.g., warfarin), thrombotic thrombocytopenic purpura, and patients with a congenital coagulation factor deficiency where specific factor concentrates are not available. Published plasma transfusion indications are listed in Table 28-3.

Table 28-3

Plasma Transfusion Indications

1. Management of bleeding or to prevent bleeding prior to an urgent invasive procedure in patients requiring replacement of multiple coagulation factors
2. Massively transfused patients who have clinically significant coagulation deficiencies and hypovolemia
3. Patients on warfarin therapy with bleeding or that need to undergo an invasive procedure before vitamin K could reverse the effects of warfarin or who need only transient reversal of warfarin effects
4. For transfusion or plasma exchange in patients with thrombotic thrombocytopenic purpura (TTP) and some cases of hemolytic uremic syndrome (HUS)
5. Management of patients with selected coagulation factor deficiencies, congenital or acquired, for which no specific coagulation concentrates are available
6. Management of patients with rare specific plasma protein deficiencies, when recombinant products or purified products are unavailable
7. Fresh frozen plasma (FFP) is the product of choice for patients specifically requiring replacement of the labile clotting factors or other proteins with poor storage stability because the other plasma products may be deficient in these factors during liquid storage; deficiencies due to consumption/hemodilution rarely fall to levels that are inadequately treated with non-FFP plasma components; consultation with a hematologist or transfusion medicine physician is recommended for assistance with indications

Plasma is overused in surgery, most often because of the empirical nature of transfusion therapy. The most common cause of bleeding after surgery is platelet dysfunction. Further, the PT and partial thromboplastin times (PTT), which are widely used to evaluate bleeding, have never been demonstrated to accurately reflect the cause of bleeding in surgical patients. Indeed, the PT and PTT can be abnormal in patients who are not bleeding. Despite the widespread use of plasma, there is little evidence for its effectiveness outside of trauma patients requiring massive transfusion.[10,11] Analyses of randomized controlled trials have been unable to demonstrate consistent evidence of benefit for plasma in most clinical scenarios.[10–12] The use of plasma in many situations to treat elevated INRs, especially when the INR is less than 1.7 is problematic, as these patients may not be at risk of bleeding and the lowest INR obtainable with plasma is approximately 1.5 because that is the INR of plasma/FFP.[13] A recent survey evaluating approximately 5,000 plasma transfusions reported that 43% were administered in the absence of bleeding in efforts to correct abnormal coagulation tests preoperatively or before invasive procedures, and in 31% of cases where plasma was given the INR was 1.5 or less.[14]

Plasma transfusions, like all blood products, have the potential for adverse effects. A recent study reported a 6% incidence of transfusion-associated circulatory overload (TACO) in ICU patients, which can occur when patients with heart failure/ventricular dysfunction are given as little as 2 to 4 units of plasma.[15] TRALI is a major cause of mortality and morbidity from blood transfusion, although its incidence has declined with the use of plasma from male donors or female donors who have no history of pregnancy.[16,17] TRALI and TACO will be considered in more detail later.

Solvent/Detergent–Treated Plasma

Human pooled plasma that has been solvent/detergent (S/D) treated is now available commercially in a sterile, frozen solution of pooled human plasma from donors that has been treated with an S/D process. This method of preparation kills certain viruses and minimizes the risk of serious virus transmission but also removes other agents, including cellular debris and lipid contaminants. This process is thought to reduce the risk of TRALI. The plasma used to manufacture this product is collected from specific pools of U.S. donors who have been screened and tested for diseases transmitted by blood, and determined to be suitable donors. Collected donor pools include approximately 500 to 1,600 donors. This product is used extensively in Europe and other countries and approximately 13 million have been administered outside of the United States. In the United States, this product is indicated for replacement of multiple coagulation factors in patients with acquired deficiencies due to liver disease, those undergoing cardiac surgery and liver transplantation, and for plasma exchange in patients with thrombotic thrombocytopenic purpura. Administration is based on ABO blood group compatibility.

The collection and testing process for this pooled and treated plasma is extensive; unlike other blood products, it is extensively purified and tested. The product is manufactured from U.S. plasma donations that are extensively tested for viral markers with each pool limited to 630 to 1,520 individual donors. Frozen plasma units are thawed, pooled, filtered through a 1-μm pore membrane, then treated with S/D reagents (1% tri[n-butyl] phosphate [TNBP] and 1% octoxynol for 1 to 1.5 hours at +30°C [86°F]) to inactivate enveloped viruses. The S/D reagents are removed by sequential oil and solid phase extraction procedures that also remove prions. After sterile filtration, the product is filled into blood bags, labeled, deep-frozen, and stored at 4°F. The S/D treatment step has been shown to effectively inactivate relevant pathogenic and enveloped viruses.

Leukocyte antibodies are not detected in S/D plasma because the process dilutes white blood cell antibodies and soluble human leukocyte antigens (HLAs) are present in the product, neutralizing the antibodies. This pooled and treated plasma product has not been associated with TRALI, with more than 13 million units transfused to date.

Cryoprecipitate

In the early 1960s, attempts to create an improved factor VIII concentrate led to the development of cryoprecipitate. Cryoprecipitate forms when frozen plasma is allowed to thaw slowly at 1°C to 10°C; cryoprecipitate is rich in fibrinogen, factor VIII, and factor XIII but also contains other factors. This product was introduced as a therapy for patients with hemophilia A[18,19]; however, its major use today is to replete fibrinogen levels during coagulopathies. Cryoprecipitate contains fibrinogen and high concentrations of factor VIII, von Willebrand factor, and factor XIII.

Cryoprecipitate is composed of the insoluble proteins that precipitate when FFP is thawed and is named for that process. The residual volume of cryoprecipitate (~15 mL) is refrozen and stored. Cryoprecipitate contains therapeutic amounts of factor VIII:C, factor XIII, von Willebrand factor, and fibrinogen. Each bag of cryoprecipitate contains 80 to 100 units of factor VIII:C, 150 to 200 mg of fibrinogen, significant amounts of factor XIII, and von Willebrand factor, including the high-molecular-weight multimers. Cryoprecipitate is used not only to increase fibrinogen levels depleted because of massive hemorrhage or coagulopathy but also for the treatment of congenital or acquired factor XIII deficiency. For fibrinogen replacement therapy, in Europe, specific fibrinogen concentrates are available (see the following text); however, 1 unit of cryoprecipitate per 10 kg body weight increases plasma fibrinogen by roughly 50 to 70 mg/dL in the absence of continuing consumption or massive bleeding.[20] The minimum hemostatic level of fibrinogen is traditionally suggested to be around 100 mg/dL but normal fibrinogen levels are 200 mg/dL and higher, and higher levels of fibrinogen may be important for clot formation (see "Fibrinogen Concentrates" section). Because cryoprecipitate does not contain factor V, it should not be the sole replacement therapy for disseminated intravascular coagulopathy (DIC), which is almost always associated with a variety of factor deficiencies and thrombocytopenia. Because fibrinogen is an important determinant of hemostatic function and clot strength, fibrinogen levels should be routinely evaluated in bleeding patients especially following multiple transfusions. Hypofibrinogenemia itself can cause a prolonged PT and PTT, and FFP transfusion alone may not provide sufficient repletion. Cryoprecipitate is likely underused in cardiac surgical patients who are bleeding and "refractory" to standard FFP and platelets.

Cryoprecipitate has been withdrawn from many European countries due to safety concerns, primarily the transmission of pathogens. Instead, commercial fibrinogen preparations are available for fibrinogen replacement therapy. The fibrinogen concentrates used for repleting fibrinogen levels are free of known pathogens, stored as a lyophilized product, and can be readily administered when required. Nevertheless, cryoprecipitate remains available for hemostatic therapy in several countries, including the United States, Canada, and the United Kingdom. An adult dose of cryoprecipitate is ~10 units obtained from 10 different donors, and is equivalent to ~2 g fibrinogen.

Platelet Concentrates

Platelets that are used clinically are either pooled random-donor platelet concentrates or single-donor apheresis and can be stored for up to 5 days. In medical patients, a platelet count of 10,000/μL is a typical threshold for prophylactic platelet transfusion (normal platelet count ranges from 150,000 to 400,000 platelets per μL), but the optimal platelet count or dose is still being evaluated. Consensus descriptions suggest the platelet count for therapeutic transfusions to control or prevent bleeding with trauma or surgical procedures requires a higher transfusion trigger of 100,000/μL for neurosurgical procedures and between 50,000/μL and 100,000/μL for other invasive procedures or trauma. Many transfused products, including platelets, undergo leukoreduction to reduce alloimmunization rates, cytomegalovirus (CMV) transmission, and febrile transfusion reactions. Whether leukoreduction reduces immunomodulatory effects of transfusion (i.e., decreases infection rates and cancer recurrence) is still controversial, as is the use of universal leukoreduction as the procedure, is associated with significant cost.

Platelet concentrates can be prepared either from whole blood or by apheresis. For many years, the use of platelet concentrates was the standard for platelet administration, and this required exposure to multiple donors, as 10 units of platelets required 10 different donors. An important advantage of platelets collected by apheresis is that a sufficient enough number can be collected from a single donor while an equivalent number of platelets require pooling of at least 4 to 6 whole blood–derived platelets concentrates. Reducing donor exposures by using apheresis platelets also has the potential advantages of reducing transfusion-transmitted infections and platelet alloimmunization where antibodies form because platelets have many antigens besides ABO.[21,22] Testing has reduced the infectious risk to low levels. The quality of apheresis platelets is similar to pooled random-donor platelets concentrates, these two products can be used interchangeably based on availability and cost considerations.[21,22]

There remains significant risk of bacterial infection with platelet administration, because they are stored at 22°C rather than at the 4°C storage used for red cell storage; storage at 22°C is permissive for bacterial growth. Some studies have suggested a reduction in bacterial transmission by transfusion with the use of single-donor platelets.[21,22] However, both the American College of Pathologists and the American Association of Blood Banks (AABB) have mandated testing of all platelet products for bacteria.[21,22]

Alloimmunization

Allogeneic blood transfusions are in many ways similar to organ transplantation. Transfusing cells from one patient (the donor) to the recipient introduces multiple foreign cells, antigens, and other potential contaminants. An immunocompetent recipient often develops variable immune responses to the transfused agents that include graft versus host disease (to be considered later in this chapter). Multiple other antigens that are not routinely crossmatched for platelets and responsible for alloimmunization include HLAs, class I shared by platelets and leukocytes and class II present on some leukocytes; granulocyte-specific antigens; platelet-specific antigens (human platelet antigen); and RBC-specific antigens. Platelets are cross matched only to RBC specific antigens. The spectrum of additional antigenic components in platelets is why leukoreduction is part of an important management strategy.

Leukoreduction

Leukoreduced platelet and RBC products have many potential benefits. By reducing additional leukocyte exposure, sensitization and antibody formation to different white blood cell antigens (alloimmunization) is reduced.[21,22] CMV transmission is also reduced by reducing leukocyte burden, and as a result, there is also a reduction in febrile transfusion reactions.[21,22] Other potential benefits of leukoreduction include decreased exposure to white cells that potentially contribute to immunomodulatory effects of transfusion (transfusion-related immunomodulation or TRIM) that may present as increased risk for postoperative infections and tumor metastasis formation in cancer surgery. There is extensive controversy about the immunomodulatory effects of transfusions as patients often have multiple other risk factors that contribute to outcomes.[21,22] Several countries including Canada and many medical centers have instituted universal leukoreduction of the blood supply.

Graft versus Host Disease

In cancer patients and certain pediatric populations, platelets are irradiated to prevent transfusion-related graft versus host disease, a potentially fatal complication of transfusion. Graft versus host disease occurs more commonly after a bone marrow or stem cell transplant, or following platelet transfusions where viable white cells from the donor regard the recipient's body as foreign and create acute inflammatory responses and tissue and organ injury by attacking the recipient's body. For platelet transfusions, γ-irradiation is performed for patients receiving allogeneic stem cell transplants, for patients receiving blood products from related donors, and for patients who are severely immunocompromised, usually because of their disease or its treatment (e.g., patients with Hodgkin's disease or other lymphomas).[21,22]

Indications for Platelet Transfusions and Transfusion Triggers

In medical patients, a platelet transfusion trigger of approximately 10,000 platelets/μL in efforts to prevent bleeding is often described. However, data and prospective studies to evaluate the effects of platelet dose on hemostasis and rates of platelet use overall for perioperative management are often based on consensus guidelines rather than clinical studies. There are three important areas of controversy regarding the use of platelet transfusions without active bleeding[23]: first, the optimal prophylactic platelet dose to prevent thrombocytopenic bleeding even in medical patients is not well known. Second, the exact platelet count threshold that requires transfusion of platelets is not known. Finally, whether prophylactic platelet transfusions are superior to therapeutic platelet transfusions in surgical patients is not known.

A review of clinical trials[24] suggests that in hematologic malignancies, a target platelet count of more than 10,000 platelets/μL is acceptable in preventing spontaneous bleeding caused by thrombocytopenia alone,[25] although platelet dosing was not found to influence bleeding when administered prophylactically.[26] Guidelines for platelet transfusions exist in many countries.[27–32] Hematology patients receive about two-thirds of all platelet concentrates, depending on the medical center. Additional studies are needed to determine the optimal transfusion practice; however, the clinical use of platelet transfusions to obtain hemostasis is complicated because direct platelet function testing is rarely possible in the bleeding or coagulopathic patient. For instance, after cardiopulmonary bypass, platelet counts may be normal, but platelets are functioning poorly (qualitative platelet defect). Most recommendations are to maintain platelet counts of greater than 50,000/μL in surgical patients; however, this is also dependent on whether the circulating platelets are functional. While definitive data for the most effective platelet dosing strategy for maintaining perioperative hemostasis is not available, following platelet numbers is our only practical guide. However, clinicians must bear in mind that patients with abnormal platelet counts and/or hemostasis may not bleed at the same time that patients with normal platelets counts may bleed based on the platelet dysfunction that appears in many surgical settings.

In most surgical patients, there is little data to support prophylactic platelet transfusions; the exceptions are massive transfusion coagulopathy and certain closed procedures where bleeding may be highly problematic such as intracranial hemorrhage. Dilutional thrombocytopenia often occurs as an early manifestation of massive transfusion. However, studies also suggest thrombocytopenia may not always correlate with abnormal bleeding. In cardiac surgical patients, defective platelet function is part of the clinical problem, and the inability to have suitable platelet function testing for postoperative use complicates our ability to decide when to transfuse platelets.[21,22]

Studies in chronic thrombocytopenic patients suggested that significant spontaneous bleeding with an intact vascular system does not occur until the platelet count is 5,000 platelets/μL or less.[21,22] Previously, a platelet count of less than or equal to 20,000/μL was considered to be an indication for a prophylactic platelet transfusion. However, four randomized prospective transfusion trials comparing prophylactic platelet transfusion triggers of 10,000 platelets/μL versus 20,000 platelets/μL showed no differences in hemorrhagic risks.[33] Current recommendations are that a threshold of 10,000 platelets/μL for prophylactic platelet transfusion be used in hematology patients who are chronically thrombocytopenic.

Platelet Counts for Surgery and Invasive Procedures

For surgery or following trauma, expert recommendations suggest that a platelet count of greater than or equal to 50,000/μL be maintained. However, there is little data to support these recommendations. In neurosurgical patients or patients with intracerebral bleeding and for neurosurgical procedures, expert recommendations suggest that platelet counts should be maintained at greater than 100,000/μL. With platelet counts between 50,000 and 100,000/μL, clinical decisions to transfuse platelets should be based on the type of surgery, trauma, rates of bleeding, risk of bleeding, use of platelet inhibitors, and other potential coagulation abnormalities. An assessment of whether platelet function is normal should also weigh in to the decision about when to transfuse platelets.

Abnormal platelet function can arise from numerous causes, including multiple medications, sepsis, malignancy, tissue injury following trauma, obstetric issues including eclampsia, cardiopulmonary bypass, or hepatic or renal failure with azotemia/uremia. In the bleeding patient, laboratory testing can determine platelet counts but not platelet function, so bleeding due to tissue injury may occur at higher platelet counts. If platelet dysfunction is present in the face of trauma or surgery, platelet transfusions may be necessary, even in the presence of a normal platelet count. Unfortunately, there is little data to help clinicians manage these complex but common occurrences, and as a result, platelet transfusions must be guided by a logical approach that weighs each of these factors.

ABO Compatibility

Red cell antigens are expressed on platelets, and ABO-incompatible platelets have reduced posttransfusion platelet count recoveries but normal platelet survival.[21,22] ABO-compatible means the donor has no A or B antigens incompatible with the recipient's A or B antibodies.[21,22] Patients who receive ABO-incompatible platelets become refractory to additional platelet transfusions at a higher rate than the ABO-compatible recipients because sensitization produces anti-HLA and platelet-specific alloantibodies.[21,22] ABO-compatible platelets are important both to maximize posttransfusion platelet counts and to reduce the incidence of sensitization, which decreases platelet counts, shortens the half-life, and increases the potential for platelet dysfunction.[21,22]

Purified Protein Concentrates

Fibrinogen Concentrates

Fibrinogen is a critical clotting protein, with increasing data further reporting its importance for perioperative hemostasis.[34] Cryoprecipitate is routinely administered as the source of fibrinogen in many countries, while fibrinogen concentrates are also used in some countries. Although any biologic agent can potentially produce an adverse event, current reviews of published clinical data and pharmacovigilance reporting have not demonstrated significant thrombogenic concerns with fibrinogen concentrate to date.[35,36] However, fibrinogen concentrate administration in patients with hypofibrinogenemia and disseminated intravascular coagulation should be avoided and the focus placed on treatment of the underlying disease (i.e., sepsis).[37]

The advantage of factor concentrates is that the risk of viral infection is significantly reduced due to viral inactivation and removal that minimize the risk of transmitting viruses. Although fibrinogen concentrate is manufactured using human plasma from a large pool of donors, the production processes involved remove antibodies and antigens, largely mitigating the risk of immunologic and allergic reactions resulting from its administration, and provide a pure product without other cellular and protein contaminants.

Prothrombin Complex Concentrates

While warfarin reversal in the United States occurs with FFP,[38] most other countries use prothrombin complex concentrates (PCCs).[39] PCCs are recommended in guidelines as primary treatment for reversal in patients with life-threatening bleeding and an increased INR when urgent reversal is required. For reversal of warfarin and vitamin K antagonists, several therapies are used and include oral/intravenous vitamin K, human FFP, and PCCs. Although recombinant active factor VII (rFVIIa) has been used, better alternatives are currently available. Although vitamin K can be considered for nonemergency reversal, if rapid normalization of the INR is required, then PCCs should be used. Vitamin K is an active cofactor necessary to convert coagulation factor proteins to their active forms after they are synthesized in the liver. Because of the need for immediate reversal in the perioperative setting, FFP or PCCs should be considered.

Plasma/FFP is the agent most likely to be used in the United States, but for emergent reversal, clinicians should consider PCCs. Agents approved specifically for warfarin reversal include the 4 component PCC available in the US KCENTRA/Beriplex P/N (CSL Behring, King of Prussia, PA), Octaplex (Octapharma, Lachen,Switzerland) approved elsewhere, and there are also other 4 component PCCs available worldwide. Extensive clinical experience with the new purified PCCs available suggests the incidence of thrombotic complications is relatively low; however, they should be avoided in patients requiring surgery who were previously anticoagulated for a prothrombotic reason.

U.S. guidelines recommend PCCs as primary treatment for anticoagulation reversal in patients with life-threatening bleeding and elevated INR and are labeled as such. Clinical protocols for administering PCCS should be accompanied by discontinuing warfarin and its derivatives, and administering vitamin K. Many clinicians continue to use plasma/FFP to reverse an elevated INR even for urgent and emergency procedures, and use of plasma is one of the major causes of TRALI in the United States. The rapid onset of PCCs is important for emergency reversal of vitamin K antagonists including warfarin. Compared with FFP, PCCs provide quicker INR correction, have a lower infusion volume, and are more readily available without cross matching.[39,40] Although there are historical concerns about potential thrombotic risk with PCCs, present-day PCCs are much improved.[41]

Von Willebrand Factor

Human antihemophilic factor/von Willebrand factor complex is commercially available in the United States and is indicated for treatment and prevention of bleeding in adult patients with hemophilia A (classical hemophilia). This agent is also indicated in adult and pediatric patients with von Willebrand's disease (VWD) for (a) treatment of spontaneous and trauma-induced bleeding episodes and (b) prevention of excessive bleeding during and after surgery. This applies to patients with severe VWD and patients with mild and moderate VWD for whom use of desmopressin is known or suspected to be inadequate. This agent is not indicated for the prophylaxis of spontaneous bleeding episodes.

This product is the first plasma-derived von Willebrand factor/factor VIII (FVIII)–containing concentrate that was pasteurized to reduce the risk of virus infection and approved for use in Germany in 1981 and it is now available in many countries worldwide for on-demand treatment and long-term prophylaxis in patients with VWD or hemophilia A (factor VIII deficiency). This agent is used off label for bleeding with acquired VWD due to ventricular assist devices or aortic stenosis.

Hemophilia Management: Factors VIII and IX

Before the development of factor concentrates, FFP was the treatment for hemophilia A and hemophilia B. However, FFP contains minimal amounts of factor VIII and factor IX, thus large volumes are required to stop bleeding episodes, and this mandated hospitalization for treatment of joint bleeding. In the mid-1960s, the development of cryoprecipitate with concentrated factor VIII preparations allowed a concentrated form of factor VIII to be administered intravenously. By the late 1960s, methods for isolating both factor VIII and factor IX from pooled plasma allowed the development of lyophilized factor VIII or factor IX concentrates, which provided for more accurate dosing using true concentrates that could rapidly restore factor levels in hemophilia, and this also led to the ability to effectively treat patients at home. However, isolating factor concentrates requires combining plasma from multiple donors, and the associated risks of transmission of hepatitis viruses and HIV. Multiple steps were subsequently used to reduce viral contamination using heat, S/D treatment, and pasteurization, but not before many patients were infected. Better screening methods for blood donors improved the safety of donated plasma and included hepatitis B and HIV, and later hepatitis C virus. Recombinant human factor VIII (R factor VIII) was developed following cloning of the gene, and by 1992, two licensed factor VIII products for use in hemophilia A were available, and a factor IX product became available for people with hemophilia B in 1997. Other important developments for hemophilia patients include treatment for patients with inhibitors to factor VIII or factor IX and prophylaxis. Inhibitor antibodies develop in approximately 30% to 35% of people with hemophilia A and 1% to 3% with hemophilia B. A novel therapies for "bypassing" the inhibitor, recombinant activated factor VII (R factor VIIa), was first licensed for use in hemophilia in 1997.

Hereditary Angioedema and C1 Esterase Inhibitor Concentrates

Hereditary angioedema (HAE) is a life-threatening disease resulting from the absence or genetic mutation of a complement component inhibitor called ***C1 esterase inhibitor*** (C1 INH). Although there are several variants of HAE, they share a final common pathway following tissue injury, intubation, or other inciting events, leading to unopposed activation of multiple inflammatory pathways and mediators including kallikrein and bradykinin that increase vascular permeability.[42] Angioedema produces increased permeability of submucosal or subcutaneous capillaries and postcapillary venules leading to plasma extravasation and subsequent swelling of critical airway structures and other systemic effects. C1 INH concentrates have been used since 1974 in Europe and now are available in the United States for both preventing and terminating attacks. Two of these have now been licensed in the United States for use in HAE patients, one for prophylaxis (Cinryze [ViroPharma, Lexington, MA]) and the other for treating acute abdominal and facial HAE attacks (Berinert-P [CSL Behring, King of Prussia, PA]). The use of C1 INH concentrates is critical in the perioperative management of HAE patients.[42]

Adverse Effects of Transfusions

The risks of allogeneic transfusion extend beyond viral transmission and include allergy, alloimmunization, anaphylaxis, bacterial sepsis, graft versus host disease, TRALI, TACO, renal failure, volume overload, and immunosuppression.[43–45] Platelet transfusions also carry the added risk of bacterial contamination and they contain a high concentration of donor white blood cells. Transfusion of donor white blood cells has the potential to produce multiple adverse effects. Cytokines, such as interleukins 6 (IL-6), 8 (IL-8), tissue necrosis factor alpha (TNF-α), and other inflammatory mediators are especially concentrated in platelet products and could contribute to adverse outcomes.

Transfusion as an Inflammatory Response

Transfusions of allogeneic blood is reported to have multiple immunomodulatory effects including immunosuppression; they contain bioactive substances that cause febrile reactions, and they release inflammatory mediators.[46] Inflammatory responses to cardiac surgery are affected by giving packed RBCs during surgery as displayed by neutrophil activation.[47] Neutrophils in allogeneic cellular blood components are associated with adverse effects in the recipient.[48] In cardiac surgical patients who are already immunosuppressed by surgical trauma, added inhibition of immunomodulation may have harmful effects.

Because of increasing awareness and identification of TRALI and decreases in the incidence of infectious and hemolytic complications of transfusions, TRALI is now a primary cause of transfusion-associated mortality reported to the FDA and has become a frequent cause of transfusion-related morbidity and mortality.[49] TRALI can be confused with other transfusion and non–transfusion-related events such as anaphylaxis, hemolysis, circulatory overload and cardiac failure and present with acute shock, florid pulmonary edema and pulmonary hypertension.[48,50] Because TRALI is a major cause of mortality resulting from transfusion, strategies have evolved to reduce its incidence and will be considered in more detail later.

Transfusion-Associated Circulatory Overload

TACO is simply a volume overload state, where the rate of volume infusion of blood products is in excess of what the patient's cardiovascular status can handle. An example is the transfusion of 4 units of FFP to reverse warfarin in a patient with heart failure; in such a patient who can barely manage their own intravascular volume, they may well go on to develop orthopnea and paroxysmal nocturnal dyspnea following transfusion. TACO is characterized by the acute onset of dyspnea and is typically associated with hypertension, tachypnea, and tachycardia—an exacerbation of heart failure as shown in Table 28-4. Sometimes it can be difficult clinically to differentiate TRALI from TACO, but use of echocardiography, transthoracic or transesophageal, will reveal hypervolemia, ventricular dysfunction, and potentially reveal exacerbation of valvular dysfunction. In a TRALI patient, volume overload is not the cause of pulmonary edema, rather left ventricular size should be normal or low, and often the right ventricle is dilated. Alternately, attesting for brain-type natriuretic peptide (BNP) is another approach and this should be greatly elevated, usually several fold above a baseline of 100 to 200 in patients with TACO. TACO incidence ranges from approximately 1% to 8% of transfusions. TACO is increasingly report as a common cause of morbidity and mortality associated with transfusion, especially with the use of FFP.

Transfusion-Related Acute Lung Injury

The term ***transfusion-related acute lung injury*** was initially reported as the clinical presentation of hypoxia and bilateral noncardiogenic pulmonary edema within 6 hours of a transfusion.[51] Initially, this pathologic response was thought to be produced by donor IgG antibodies against recipient neutrophils, called ***leukoagglutinins***. From 2005 to 2009, half of the confirmed transfusion-related deaths in the United States reported to the FDA were secondary to TRALI. The most widely accepted current concept is that TRALI results from neutrophil and/or endothelial activation via multiple mechanisms in the lung, resulting in pulmonary vascular injury and pulmonary edema.[51] Multiple pathogenic transfused factors are associated with TRALI and predisposing events that may prime the response as will be covered in more detail later and as summarized in Figure 28-1.

Table 28-4

Presentation of Transfusion-Associated Circulatory Overload

Dyspnea
Elevated jugular venous pressure
Hypertension or hypotension
Tachycardia
Rales on lung auscultation
Pulmonary edema
Increased brain natriuretic peptide
Echocardiography: hypervolemia, mitral regurgitation due to volume overload

Clinical History of Transfusion-Related Acute Lung Injury

Initially, in the 1980s, this reaction was termed ***pulmonary hypersensitivity reaction*** and thought to be associated with leukocyte antibodies in the donor against the recipient, or in the recipient against the donor. In 1985, a series of 36 cases of TRALI were reported with acute respiratory failure characterized by hypoxemia and pulmonary edema occurring within 4 hours of transfusion. Granulocyte or lymphocytotoxic antibodies were detected in the donor of 89% of blood products. By 2006, more than 50% of transfusion-related fatalities reported to the FDA were due to TRALI. An NHLBI working group defined TRALI as new acute lung injury (ALI) occurring within 6 hours of the end of transfusion of one or more plasma-containing blood products in patients without other risk factors for ALI. Patients with preexisting ALI and ALI occurring more than 6 hours after transfusion are excluded.

Clinical presentation of TRALI, in its severe form, is indistinguishable from adult respiratory distress syndrome (ARDS) and is characterized by acute onset (within minutes to 6 hours after transfusion), bilateral pulmonary infiltrates and hypoxia without evidence of heart failure.[43,52,53] Because reports use different definitions of TRALI, the information on incidence, outcome, and blood product association are variable. In German hemovigilance data of 44 cases of TRALI, the fatal 18% of cases were antibody-mediated from female donor blood. However, from multiple reports and European countries, the rates vary from approximately 1:11,363 (Finland) to 1:250,000. Five of the blood products implicated in TRALI, 49% were FFP, 29% RBCs, 13% platelet concentrates, 2% whole blood, 0% S/D plasma, and 7% mixed products. The American Red Cross–estimated risk of fatal TRALI per distributed component was 1:202,673 for plasma, 1:320,572 for apheresis platelets, and 1:2,527,437 for RBC units.[51] TRALI mortality rates range from 5% to 35% in case series while leukocyte antibodies were identified in the implicated donor in 65% to 90% of TRALI cases.[51] Table 28-5 lists clinical presentation of TRALI.

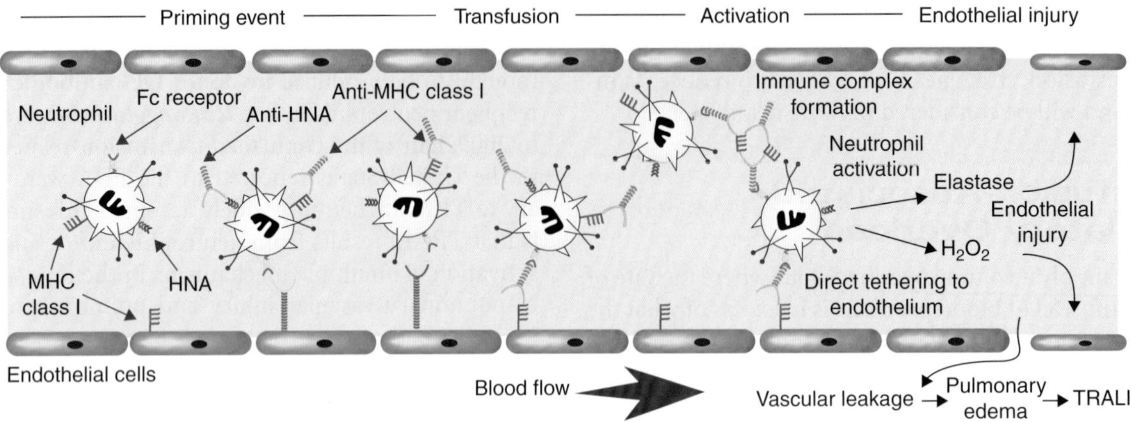

FIGURE 28-1 Transfusion-related acute lung injury (TRALI). Multiple priming events may or may not be required for TRALI but appear to be important factors in the inflammatory process that causes TRALI and may significantly potentiate the acute vasculitis that occurs. Transfusion of blood products from multiparous donors or other donors containing antibodies against white blood cell antigens that include human neutrophil antigen (HNA) and major histocompatibility complex (MHC) class I can result in direct binding and activation of intravascular polymorphonuclear leukocytes. These antibodies may also directly bind and tether neutrophils to the endothelium independent of the adhesion molecules, selectin and integrin. The antigen–antibody binding also produces immune complexes of multiple white blood cell antigens that may also be recognized by the Fc receptors (tail receptors of antibodies) resulting in neutrophil activation. The activated neutrophils bind to the pulmonary vascular endothelium, and aggregated clumps of neutrophils may lodge in the pulmonary microcirculation. Activated neutrophils release multiple proinflammatory substances including proteolytic enzymes, oxygen free radicals, thromboxane, and other inflammatory mediators both locally at the site of vascular injury and systemically. This complex series of events results in damage to endothelial cells, vascular leakage, and pulmonary edema.

Multiple Factors Influence Transfusion-Related Acute Lung Injury

Although multiple factors may produce TRALI, priming events that occur before actual blood product administration may also be needed in what is termed the ***two-hit model***.[51] First, an inciting inflammatory event may be required to activate and upregulate inflammatory cells and vascular endothelium (see "Role of Neutrophils and Other Inflammatory Cells" section), followed by a second, transfusion event that actually triggers an acute inflammatory response and injury. The initial priming event may be caused by lipids generated during prolonged storage of blood, recent infection including viral illnesses, and other events such as cardiopulmonary bypass that can trigger inflammatory responses and cytokine generation. Because neutrophils and endothelial cells are activated by multiple inflammatory events, there may be different thresholds for TRALI development in distinct settings from infection, lipid exposure, or extracorporeal circulation. Additional factors that likely contribute to the development of TRALI include complex factors such as antibody specificity and titer, antigen density, and the patient's underlying condition.[51]

Table 28-5

Transfusion-Related Acute Lung Injury

Onset within 6 hours, usually more acute, following transfusion
Bilateral infiltrates seen on frontal chest radiograph
Hypoxemia/ratio of Pao_2/Fio_2 300 mm Hg regardless of positive end-expiratory pressure level, or oxygen saturation of 90% on room air
Pulmonary artery occlusion ≤18 mm Hg when measured, or lack of clinical evidence of left atrial hypertension (volume overload)
Pathophysiologic mechanisms: human neutrophil antigen (HNA) and human leukocyte antigen (HLA) class I and II antibodies, CD40-ligand (CD40L), biologically active lipids

Acute Pulmonary Edema and Management

The multiple signaling mechanisms and inflammatory mediators in TRALI promote priming and activation of a patient's granulocytes leading to their pulmonary sequestration and release of proteases, oxidants, and leukotrienes, which cause alveolar epithelial and microvascular endothelial damage resulting in increased permeability and the eventual development of noncardiogenic pulmonary edema. The two-hit model of TRALI is similar to pathophysiology of acute respiratory failure/syndrome. With TRALI, several reactive lipid-like substances that accumulate in RBCs or platelets during storage, referred to as ***biologic response modifiers***, can act as the first pulmonary insult but are more likely the second. The first insult is generally a systemic inflammatory condition resulting from major surgery, sepsis, trauma, or pulmonary aspiration that causes activation of the pulmonary endothelium and priming of polymorphonuclear lymphocytes (PMNs) leading to their sequestration in the pulmonary vasculature. The second hit occurs when the primed PMNs are activated by the biologic response modifiers in the transfused component. Therapy for TRALI is supportive. Suspected cases of TRALI should be reported to the hospital transfusion service to assure a suitable investigation including testing of associated donors for antileukocyte and antiplatelet antibodies and typing recipients for HLA antigens (i.e., via leukocytes in a pretransfusion blood specimen or buccal swab technique). If donor leukocyte antibodies that react specifically to the patient's leukocytes are found, avoiding future transfusion of plasma-containing components from this donor is recommended. The patient, however, is not at an increased risk of future TRALI reactions with future transfusion.

A retrospective study of the incidence of acute pulmonary edema after transfusion in 8,902 ICU patients demonstrated 25 cases of TACO (incidence 1:356 units transfused), 7 cases of suspected TRALI (1:1,271 units transfused), and 14 cases of possible TRALI (1:534 units transfused).[54] Patients who developed suspected or possible TRALI received larger amounts of plasma, especially plasma from female donors. In addition, the mortality rate was 67% for suspected or possible TRALI, compared with 20% for TACO and 11% for matched controls.[54]

Decreasing the Incidence of Transfusion-Related Acute Lung Injury

Because antibodies are present in most TRALI cases, especially severe and fatal cases, most policy changes made to mitigate TRALI have targeted antibody-mediated TRALI. Decreasing TRALI through changes in blood product policies is supported through biovigilance data and includes use of plasma from men only, resuspending pooled buffy coat platelets in plasma from men only, and screening female donors (either all, or only those donors with a history of pregnancy, transfusion, or both) for leukocyte antibodies.[51] Recommendations for screening donors for leukocyte antibodies point to the need for screening patients at risk, including parous women and patients following transplantation and/or transfusion. Blood components with high plasma fractions that contain antibodies such as plasma, apheresis platelets, and whole blood should not be prepared from these donors.[51] AABB also recommends implementing measures to minimize the preparation of high plasma-volume components from donors known to be leukocyte-immunized or at increased risk of immunization.

Plasma from Male Donors

Because TRALI is usually secondary to donor HLA or human neutrophil antigen (HNA) antibodies, which are more common in females than males, the United Kingdom began using male donor plasma and resuspension of buffy coat–derived platelets in male-donated plasma. Since 2003, 80% to 90% of the United Kingdom FFP has been male-donated plasma. In 2004, the United Kingdom started using S/D plasma for plasma exchange procedures in thrombotic thrombocytopenic purpura patients. These changes resulted in a decrease in number of TRALI reports and deaths in the United Kingdom with a reduction from 1:65,000 to 1:317,000 ($P < .001$) for FFP, and 1:71,000 to 1:173,000 ($P = .068$) for platelets; the risks for RBCs (1:949,000) and cryoprecipitate (1:104,000) remained similar. Likewise, the American Red Cross reported a decrease in fatal and nonfatal TRALI cases after using only male-donated plasma in 2007 (from 26 cases in 2006 to 7 in 2008).[55]

Transfusion-Related Acute Inflammatory Responses and Immunomodulation

Although TRALI is an important example of the complex inflammatory responses associated with transfusions, multiple blood products have the potential for proinflammatory responses including acute hypersensitivity responses and anaphylaxis that may not affect the lung. Inflammatory mediators including cytokines, TNF-α, IL-6, and IL-8 are increased 100- to 1,000-fold over baseline in platelets and are also potentially elevated in other blood products.[56] Even though white cells are responsible for forming the high levels of inflammatory mediators including complement and cytokine factors, leukoreduction may be only partially effective in reducing the immunosuppressive effects of platelets.[57] In red cell transfusion, leukoreduction may affect T-cell activation and expression of key immune molecules on the surface of white cells.[58] Other mechanisms of immunosuppression not affected by leukoreduction may come into play.

Role of Neutrophils and Other Inflammatory Cells

Polymorphonuclear leukocytes are an important element of the innate immune response for host defense and are critical to controlling microbial pathogens after tissue injury following surgery or trauma. As part of all inflammatory responses, neutrophil-mediated events produce inflammatory responses that often become systemic producing widespread tissue damage and adverse sequelae. Neutrophils release multiple factors that kill both pathogens and surrounding tissue. Neutrophil activation is responsible for multiple inflammatory events, including reperfusion injury, a common issue following restoration of blood flow in occluded vessels. Following inflammatory insults, neutrophils and other inflammatory cells have important mechanisms of activation and recruitment, and interact with vascular endothelial cells for further activation, localization, and extravasation/transmigration to areas of tissue injury or actual microbial invasion. Important inflammatory mediators and interactions with endothelial cells orchestrate these events by upregulating adhesion molecules after hypoxic challenge and production of inflammatory cytokines or pathogen metabolites that facilitate margination of leukocytes. Cytokines liberated as part of the inflammatory response induce changes in integrins and increase adhesion to the vascular wall followed by transmigration across the vessel wall. Chemotactic factors released locally further attract neutrophils to areas of primary tissue damage to kill invading organisms and remove necrotic tissue.

Summary

Blood and blood products are used extensively in the perioperative setting in surgical and trauma patients. Blood products and transfusions should be considered in the same manner that we consider use of other drug therapies by carefully weighing their risks and benefits. The complex environment in which we transfuse patients, the wide range of reasons to transfuse, and the different indications for blood product administration all further emphasize the importance of considering risk and benefit for each unique patient. TRALI has emerged as a major cause of morbidity and mortality associated with transfusions, and many therapeutic approaches have been adopted to decrease the risk. Both purified and recombinant therapeutic proteins will have an important role to play in the perioperative management of patients; despite their cost, these products do not need crossmatching, and are likely to play an increasing role as alternatives to many blood products currently in use.

References

1. FDA Center for Biologics Evaluation and Research. Fatalities reported to the FDA following blood collection and transfusion: annual summary for fiscal year 2011,2012. http://transfusionnews.com/2012/07/20/fda-report-shows-decreasing-trend-of-transfusion-related-fatalities/ Accessed February 14, 2014.
2. Serious Hazards of Transfusion (SHOT) scheme. Annual SHOT Report 2011. ISBN 978-0-9558648-4-1. www.shotuk.org.
3. Goodnough LT, Despotis GJ, Hogue CW Jr, et al. On the need for improved transfusion indicators in cardiac surgery. *Ann Thorac Surg*. 1995;60(2):473–480.
4. Karkouti K, Cohen MM, McCluskey SA, et al. A multivariable model for predicting the need for blood transfusion in patients undergoing first-time elective coronary bypass graft surgery. *Transfusion*. 2001;41(10):1193–1203.
5. Practice guidelines for perioperative blood transfusion and adjuvant therapies: an updated report by the American Society of Anesthesiologists Task Force on Perioperative Blood Transfusion and Adjuvant Therapies. *Anesthesiology*. 2006;105:198–208.
6. Koch CG, Li L, Sessler DI, et al. Duration of red-cell storage and complications after cardiac surgery. *N Engl J Med*. 2008;358(12):1229–1239.
7. Koch CG, Li L, Van Wagoner DR, et al. Red cell transfusion is associated with an increased risk for postoperative atrial fibrillation. *Ann Thorac Surg*. 2006;82(5):1747–1756.
8. Koch CG, Khandwala F, Li L, et al. Persistent effect of red cell transfusion on health-related quality of life after cardiac surgery. *Ann Thorac Surg*. 2006;82(1):13–20.
9. Downes KA, Wilson E, Yomtovian R, et al. Serial measurement of clotting factors in thawed plasma stored for 5 days. *Transfusion*. 2001;41(4):570.
10. Stanworth SJ, Brunskill SJ, Hyde CJ, et al. Is fresh frozen plasma clinically effective? A systematic review of randomized controlled trials. *Br J Haematol*. 2004;126(1):139–152.
11. Yang L, Stanworth S, Hopewell S, et al. Is fresh-frozen plasma clinically effective? An update of a systematic review of randomized controlled trials. *Transfusion*. 2012;52(8):1673–1686.
12. Segal JB, Dzik WH. Paucity of studies to support that abnormal coagulation test results predict bleeding in the setting of invasive procedures: an evidence-based review. *Transfusion*. 2005;45(9):1413–1425.
13. Holland LL, Brooks JP. Toward rational fresh frozen plasma transfusion: The effect of plasma transfusion on coagulation test results. *Am J Clin Pathol*. 2006;126(1):133–139.
14. Stanworth SJ, Grant-Casey J, Lowe D, et al. The use of fresh-frozen plasma in England: high levels of inappropriate use in adults and children. *Transfusion*. 2011;51(1):62–70.
15. Li G, Rachmale S, Kojicic M, et al. Incidence and transfusion risk factors for transfusion-associated circulatory overload among medical intensive care unit patients. *Transfusion*. 2011;51(2):338–343.
16. Lin Y, Saw CL, Hannach B, et al. Transfusion-related acute lung injury prevention measures and their impact at Canadian Blood Services. *Transfusion*. 2012;52(3):567–574.
17. Chapman CE, Stainsby D, Jones H, et al. Ten years of hemovigilance reports of transfusion-related acute lung injury in the United Kingdom and the impact of preferential use of male donor plasma. *Transfusion*. 2009;49(3):440–452.
18. Pool JG, Gershgold EJ, Pappenhagen AR. High-potency antihaemophilic factor concentrate prepared from cryoglobulin precipitate. *Nature*. 1964;203:312.
19. Hershgold EJ, Pool JG, Pappenhagen AR, et al. A more potent human antihemophilic globulin concentrate: preparation and clinical trial. In: *10th Congress of the International Society of Blood Transfusion*. Stockholm, Sweden; 1964:1214–1218.
20. Leslie SD, Toy PT. Laboratory hemostatic abnormalities in massively transfused patients given red blood cells and crystalloid. *Am J Clin Pathol*. 1991;96(6):770–773.
21. Slichter SJ. Evidence-based platelet transfusion guidelines. *Hematology Am Soc Hematol Educ Program*. 2007:172–178.
22. Slichter SJ. Platelet transfusion therapy. *Hematol Oncol Clin North Am*. 2007;21(4):697–729; vii.
23. Estcourt LJ, Stanworth SJ, Murphy MF. Platelet transfusions for patients with haematological malignancies: who needs them? *Br J Haematol*. 2011;154(4):425–440.
24. Estcourt L, Stanworth S, Doree C, et al. Prophylactic platelet transfusion for prevention of bleeding in patients with haematological disorders after chemotherapy and stem cell transplantation. *Cochrane Database Syst Rev*. 2012;(5):CD004269.
25. Rebulla P, Finazzi G, Marangoni F, et al. The threshold for prophylactic platelet transfusions in adults with acute myeloid leukemia. Gruppo Italiano Malattie Ematologiche Maligne dell'Adulto. *N Engl J Med*. 1997;337(26):1870–1875.
26. Slichter SJ, Kaufman RM, Assmann SF, et al. Dose of prophylactic platelet transfusions and prevention of hemorrhage. *N Engl J Med*. 2010;362(7):600–613.
27. Murphy MF, Brozovic B, Murphy W, et al. Guidelines for platelet transfusions. British Committee for Standards in Haematology, Working Party of the Blood Transfusion Task Force. *Transfus Med*. 1992;2(4):311–318.
28. Practice parameter for the use of fresh-frozen plasma, cryoprecipitate, and platelets. Fresh-frozen plasma, cryoprecipitate, and platelets administration practice guidelines development task force of the college of american pathologists. *JAMA*. 1994;271(10):777–781.

29. Contreras M. Final statement from the consensus conference on platelet transfusion. *Transfusion*. 1998;38(8):796–797.
30. Schiffer CA, Anderson KC, Bennett CL, et al. Platelet transfusion for patients with cancer: clinical practice guidelines of the American Society of Clinical Oncology. *J Clin Oncol*. 2001;19(5):1519–1538.
31. British Committee for Standards in Haematology, Blood Transfusion Task Force. Guidelines for the use of platelet transfusions. *Br J Haematol*. 2003;122(1):10–23.
32. Liumbruno G, Bennardello F, Lattanzio A, et al. Recommendations for the transfusion of plasma and platelets. *Blood Transfus*. 2009;7(2):132–150.
33. Slichter SJ, Davis K, Enright H, et al. Factors affecting posttransfusion platelet increments, platelet refractoriness, and platelet transfusion intervals in thrombocytopenic patients. *Blood*. 2005; 105(10):4106–4114..
34. Levy JH, Welsby I, Goodnough LT. Fibrinogen as a therapeutic target for bleeding: a review of critical levels and replacement therapy. *Transfusion*. 2014;54(5):1389–1405.
35. Dickneite G, Pragst I, Joch C, et al. Animal model and clinical evidence indicating low thrombogenic potential of fibrinogen concentrate (Haemocomplettan P). *Blood Coagul Fibrinolysis*. 2009; 20(7):535–540.
36. Weinkove R, Rangarajan S. Fibrinogen concentrate for acquired hypofibrinogenaemic states. *Transfus Med*. 2008;18(3):151–157.
37. Fenger-Eriksen C, Ingerslev J, Sorensen B. Fibrinogen concentrate—a potential universal hemostatic agent. *Expert Opin Biol Ther*. 2009; 9(10):1325–1333.
38. Ozgonenel B, O'Malley B, Krishen P, et al. Warfarin reversal emerging as the major indication for fresh frozen plasma use at a tertiary care hospital. *Am J Hematol*. 2007;82(12):1091–1094.
39. Levy JH, Tanaka KA, Dietrich W. Perioperative hemostatic management of patients treated with vitamin K antagonists. *Anesthesiology*. 2008;109(5):918–926.
40. Dager WE, King JH, Regalia RC, et al. Reversal of elevated international normalized ratios and bleeding with low-dose recombinant activated factor VII in patients receiving warfarin. *Pharmacotherapy*. 2006;26(8):1091–1098.
41. Dickneite G. Prothrombin complex concentrate versus recombinant factor VIIa for reversal of coumarin anticoagulation. *Thromb Res*. 2007;119(5):643–651.
42. Levy JH, Freiberger DJ, Roback J. Hereditary angioedema: current and emerging treatment options. *Anesth Analg*. 2010;110(5): 1271–1280.
43. Sheppard CA, Logdberg LE, Zimring JC, et al. Transfusion-related acute lung injury. *Hematol Oncol Clin North Am*. 2007;21(1):163–176.
44. Spiess BD. Risks of transfusion: outcome focus. *Transfusion*. 2004;44(suppl 12):4S–14S.
45. Despotis GJ, Zhang L, Lublin DM. Transfusion risks and transfusion-related pro-inflammatory responses. *Hematol Oncol Clin North Am*. 2007;21(1):147–161.
46. Blajchman MA. Transfusion immunomodulation or TRIM: what does it mean clinically? *Hematology*. 2005;10(suppl 1):208–214.
47. Fransen E, Maessen J, Dentener M, et al. Impact of blood transfusions on inflammatory mediator release in patients undergoing cardiac surgery. *Chest*. 1999;116(5):1233–1239.
48. Silliman CC, Ambruso DR, Boshkov LK. Transfusion-related acute lung injury. *Blood*. 2005;105(6):2266–2273.
49. Mair DC, Hirschler N, Eastlund T. Blood donor and component management strategies to prevent transfusion-related acute lung injury (TRALI). *Crit Care Med*. 2006;34(suppl 5):S137–S143.
50. Levy JH, Adkinson NF Jr. Anaphylaxis during cardiac surgery: implications for clinicians. *Anesth Analg*. 2008;106(2):392–403.
51. Shaz BH, Stowell SR, Hillyer CD. Transfusion-related acute lung injury: from bedside to bench and back. *Blood*. 2011;117(5):1463–1471.
52. Moore SB. Transfusion-related acute lung injury (TRALI): clinical presentation, treatment, and prognosis. *Crit Care Med*. 2006;34 (suppl 5):S114–S117.
53. Kleinman S. A perspective on transfusion-related acute lung injury two years after the Canadian Consensus Conference. *Transfusion*. 2006;46(9):1465–1468.
54. Rana R, Afessa B, Keegan MT, et al. Evidence-based red cell transfusion in the critically ill: quality improvement using computerized physician order entry. *Crit Care Med*. 2006;34(7):1892–1897.
55. Eder AF, Herron RM Jr, Strupp A, et al. Effective reduction of transfusion-related acute lung injury risk with male-predominant plasma strategy in the American Red Cross (2006-2008). *Transfusion*. 2010;50(8):1732–1742.
56. Spiess BD, Royston D, Levy JH, et al. Platelet transfusions during coronary artery bypass graft surgery are associated with serious adverse outcomes. *Transfusion*. 2004;44(8):1143–1148.
57. Ferrer F, Rivera J, Corral J, et al. Evaluation of pooled platelet concentrates using prestorage versus poststorage WBC reduction: impact of filtration timing. *Transfusion*. 2000;40(7):781–788.
58. van de Watering L, Brand A. Independent association of massive blood loss with mortality in cardiac surgery. *Transfusion*. 2005; 45(7):1235–1236; author reply.

CHAPTER 29

Procoagulants

Jerrold H. Levy

Bleeding in a perioperative setting, following trauma or surgery, can arise from numerous causes that include activation of the coagulation, fibrinolytic, and inflammatory pathways; dilutional changes; hypothermia; and surgical factors.[1–3] Bleeding may be further exacerbated by the increasing use of multiple agents that affect coagulation, including oral and parenteral anticoagulants and platelet inhibitors. Hemostatic function and coagulation are complex and often altered in by multiple events that occur in the perioperative setting.[1–3] As a result, when patients bleed following surgery and trauma, multiple therapeutic approaches are often required in addition to blood transfusion, and procoagulants are now increasingly used to treat bleeding in the perioperative setting. This chapter will focus on the role of procoagulants used in a perioperative setting.

Antifibrinolytic Agents: Lysine Analogs

The two synthetic antifibrinolytic agents available are the lysine analogs epsilon aminocaproic acid (EACA) and tranexamic acid (TXA). These agents competitively inhibit activation of plasminogen to plasmin, an enzyme that degrades fibrin clots, fibrinogen, and other plasma proteins. TXA also inhibits plasmin at higher doses[4,5] and most of the efficacy data are reported with TXA. EACA does not consistently reduce transfusion requirements or surgical reexploration, especially in cardiac surgery, where these agents are best characterized.[6] Multiple meta-analyses examining the use of antifibrinolytic agents consistently report a decrease in bleeding with use of these agents as measured by chest tube drainage, but data are limited for any conclusions about safety. EACA has been removed from many European countries due to concerns about safety. Most studies reporting the use of antifibrinolytic agents are in cardiac surgical patients, but use in other patients, including orthopedic patients have also been reported. Aprotinin, a polypeptide protease inhibitor will be described later.

A review in cardiac surgical patients compared aprotinin, TXA, and EACA.[7] From 49 trials, 182 deaths among 7,439 participants were reported and the relative risk for mortality with aprotinin versus placebo was 0.93. In the 19 trials that included TXA versus placebo, there were 24 deaths in 1,802 patients, yielding a relative risk of mortality of 0.55. To calculate direct estimates of death for aprotinin versus TXA, 13 trials with 107 deaths among 3,537 patients were evaluated. The relative risk was 1.43. Among 1,840 patients, the calculated estimates of death for aprotinin compared directly to EACA yielded a relative risk of 1.49. There was no evidence of an increased risk of myocardial infarction with aprotinin compared with TXA or EACA in either direct or indirect analyses. Compared with placebo or no treatment, all three drugs were effective in reducing the need for red blood cell transfusion. The relative risk of transfusion with use of aprotinin was 0.66; the relative risk of transfusion was 0.70 for TXA and 0.75 for EACA. Aprotinin was also effective in reducing the need for reoperation because of bleeding (RR, 0.48; 95% CI, 0.34–0.67).[7]

One of the potential complications of TXA is seizures. The incidence of postoperative convulsive seizures at one institution was reported to increase from 1.3% to 3.8% following cardiac surgery, temporally coincident with high-dose TXA.[8] In 24 patients who developed perioperative seizures, all had received high doses of TXA intraoperatively ranging from 61 to 259 mg/kg, had a mean age of 69.9 years, and 21 of 24 had undergone open chamber cardiac procedures.[8] Additional reports have also noted seizures associated with TXA.[9] The ability of TXA to block γ-aminobutyric acid (GABA) receptors in the frontal cortex is the suspected mechanism. Despite the lack of safety data regarding these agents, they are widely used based on the available data on reduction in transfusion and mortality.

Antifibrinolytic agents also have been studied in other procedures, including orthopedic surgery, and all three agents reduce blood loss. Although most of the reported studies included small numbers of patients and lacked sufficient power, larger meta-analysis and more recent data suggest that these agents represent an important adjunct for reducing bleeding and the need for allogeneic transfusions. A recent meta-analysis examined the use of intravenous antifibrinolytics compared with placebo on red blood cell transfusion requirement in orthopedic surgery and the safety of these agents, including venous thromboembolic risk.[10] They evaluated 42 randomized trials in total hip and knee arthroplasty, spine fusion, musculoskeletal sepsis or tumor surgery performed up to 2004. There were 22 trials with 1,238 participants for aprotinin, 20 trials with 1,096 participants for TXA, and 3 trials with 141 participants for EACA. Aprotinin and TXA both significantly reduced allogeneic blood transfusions compared to placebo. There was a dose-effect relationship with TXA but EACA did not show any efficacy; antifibrinolytic use was not associated with an increased risk of venous thromboembolic events.

TXA has also been studied in trauma patients and is being used more commonly for this application. Much of this increase in use is based on the Clinical Randomization of an Antifibrinolytic in Significant Hemorrhage (CRASH-2) study, a study of the effects of early administration of TXA on death, vascular occlusive events, and blood transfusion in trauma patients conducted in 274 hospitals in 40 countries. A total of 20,211 adult trauma patients with (or at risk of) significant bleeding were randomly assigned within 8 hours of injury to receive either TXA (loading dose 1 g over 10 minutes then infusion of 1 g over 8 hours) or placebo. The primary outcome was in-hospital death within 4 weeks of injury and was described as bleeding, vascular occlusion (myocardial infarction, stroke, and pulmonary embolism), multiorgan failure, head injury, or other causes. A total of 10,096 patients were allocated to TXA and 10,115 to placebo, of whom 10,060 and 10,067, respectively, were analyzed. All-cause mortality was significantly reduced with TXA (1,463 [14.5%] TXA group vs. 1,613 [16.0%] placebo group; relative risk, 0.91; $P = .0035$). The risk of death due to bleeding was significantly reduced (489 [4.9%] vs. 574 [5.7%]; relative risk, 0.85; $P = .0077$).

In the United States, clinicians often use EACA instead of TXA; however, most of the efficacy and safety data with antifibrinolytic use is TXA and not EACA. Further, TXA is also approved in an oral form in the United States for the treatment of heavy menstrual bleeding. The recommended dose for women with normal renal function is two 650-mg tablets taken three times daily (3,900 mg per day) for a maximum of 5 days during monthly menstruation.

Antifibrinolytic Agents: Aprotinin

Aprotinin, a polypeptide serine protease inhibitor, inhibits plasmin and other serine proteases and has had a long history of use in different clinical applications. In cardiac surgery, multiple randomized, placebo-controlled trials reported aprotinin as effective in reducing bleeding and allogeneic transfusions.[11,12] However, more recent reports from observational databases[13–16] and one randomized study[17] have questioned the safety of aprotinin. Following publication of the *Blood Conservation Using Antifibrinolytics: A Randomized Trial in a Cardiac Surgery Population* (BART) study,[17] Bayer Pharmaceuticals removed the drug from the market, although it is still available for compassionate use.[18] The U.S. Food and Drug Administration (FDA)[18] noted "because . . . aprotinin . . . has been shown to decrease the need for RBC transfusions in patients undergoing CABG surgery, future supplies of [aprotinin] will continue to be available through the company as an investigational drug under a special treatment protocol." A recent retrospective, single-center cohort study reports on 15,365 cardiac surgical patients of which 1,017 received aprotinin and 14,358 received TXA. They noted aprotinin had a better risk-benefit profile than TXA in high-risk patients, but not in low- to moderate-risk patients and suggested its use in high-risk cases may be warranted.[19]

On September 21, 2011, Health Canada concluded that the benefits of aprotinin outweigh the risks when used as authorized by Health Canada. Aprotinin is authorized for patients undergoing coronary artery bypass graft (CABG) surgery. The evidence does not suggest any increased risk of death associated with use of this agent. As a result of this assessment, the manufacturer, Bayer Inc, can resume the marketing of aprotinin in Canada. (http://www.hc-sc.gc.ca/ahc-asc/media/advisories-avis/_2011/2011_124-eng.php). Health Canada's decision is based on a comprehensive review of the totality of evidence, which included an evaluation of BART study data, other clinical trial data, postmarket studies, and information from Bayer as well as an Expert Advisory Panel that was convened by Health Canada, and a summary of key findings include the following:

(a) Evidence from clinical trials and postmarket studies continues to support that aprotinin benefits outweigh the risks when it is used as authorized by Health Canada: for basic CABG surgery. (b) Clinical trial data involving aprotinin use as authorized does not show an increased risk of death. (c) Data suggesting an increased risk of death involved use of aprotinin in complex, higher risk surgeries for which it is not authorized, such as valve replacement/repair. The precise nature of this risk remains unclear and merits further study. (d) With respect to the BART study, Health Canada concluded that the study was not designed to reliably determine the risk of death (either within or outside of CABG surgery) relative to the two drugs it was being compared against, and that the increased number of deaths in aprotinin patients could have been due to chance. (e) Health Canada's review of the BART study revealed that aprotinin prolongs certain measures of blood clotting time differently than other drugs. This effect, if not recognized, can affect how blood clotting is managed during surgery in ways that can increase the risk of blood clots and death.

Protamine

Protamine is a polypeptide containing approximately 70% arginine residues and the only available agent to reverse unfractionated heparin. This basic protein inactivates the acidic heparin molecule via a simple acid–base interaction.[20] Protamine does not reverse low-molecular-weight heparin. Most patients receive too much protamine for anticoagulation reversal because plasma levels of heparin decrease over time, and most fixed dose regimens for reversal give protamine based on the initial or total heparin dose and do not account for elimination.

Excess protamine should be avoided when reversing heparin as it can contribute to coagulopathy as shown in Figure 29-1.[21] Protamine inhibits platelets and serine proteases involved in coagulation. Data suggests that maintaining heparin levels during cardiopulmonary bypass (CPB) and administering protamine based on the correct dose of circulating heparin reduces postoperative bleeding and the need for hemostatic factors.[22] Part of this efficacy may be related to the finding that excess protamine prolongs the activated clotting time (ACT) and causes additional platelet dysfunction. When protamine is dosed based on the exact amount needed to reverse circulating heparin levels, it produces the lowest ACT values.[21] Others have also reported lower protamine doses reduce bleeding and transfusion requirements.[23]

Heparin rebound can occur after initial reversal and is generally observed 2 to 3 hours after the first dose of protamine, when the patient is in the intensive care unit.[24] Heparin levels at this time may range from 0.1 to 0.3 IU/mL, equivalent to circulating levels of heparin, based on a 5 L blood volume, of 500 to 1,500 units. Protamine doses of 5 to 15 mg at this time may be effective at reversing heparin rebound rather than the dose of 50 mg commonly administered.[25] Studies have evaluated the ROTEM (Durham, NC) assay for determining the need for additional protamine administration and note that most patients do not need additional protamine administration within 30 minutes of initial administration. The ACT is not a sensitive indicator of low heparin concentrations because platelet counts and fibrinogen levels may also affect values.

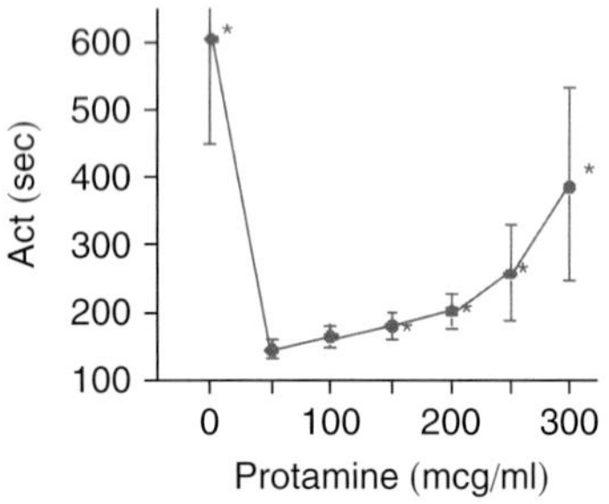

FIGURE 29-1 Excess protamine contribute to elevations in the activated clotting time (ACT), at excesses of the exact dose required to reverse systemic anticoagulation. Thus, overdosage of protamine should be strictly avoided.

Protamine can cause adverse reactions including anaphylaxis, acute pulmonary vasoconstriction and right ventricular failure, and hypotension.[20] Patients at an increased risk for adverse reactions are sensitized, often from exposure to neutral protamine Hagedorn (NPH), which contains insulin and protamine.[20] In a study of 1,551 cardiac surgery patients, the incidence of protamine reactions was 1/50 in insulin-dependent diabetics receiving NPH-insulin and 1/501 among other patients.[26] A subsequent prospective study found that reactions occurred in 0.6% (1/160) of patients with NPH-insulin–dependent diabetes.[27] Other individuals reported at risk for protamine reactions include patients with vasectomy, multiple drug allergies, and prior protamine exposure.[20] Despite the potential for anaphylaxis, there are no currently available alternatives to protamine.

Desmopressin

Desmopressin (DDAVP) is the V2 analog of arginine vasopressin that stimulates the release of ultra large von Willebrand factor (vWF) multimers from endothelial cells.[28] vWF mediates platelet adherence to vascular subendothelium by functioning as a protein bridge between glycoprotein Ib receptors on platelets and subendothelial vascular basement membrane proteins. DDAVP shortens the bleeding time of patients with mild forms of hemophilia A or von Willebrand's disease (VWD).[29] The specific surgical patients that might benefit from use of DDAVP are not clear. DDAVP is administered intravenously at a dose of 0.3 mg/kg and should be given over 15 to 30 minutes to avoid hypotension.[30] Most studies have not confirmed the early reported efficacy during complex cardiac surgery. There have been 18 trials of DDAVP in 1,295 patients undergoing cardiac surgery that show a small effect on perioperative blood loss (median decrease, 115 mL).[31,32] Because critically ill patients are often receiving vasopressin, which also has V2- and V1-mediated effects, there may not be a benefit to adding DDAVP to these patients.

DDAVP is also used to treat VWD; there are multiple types of this deficiency and therapy for each type varies. DDAVP is most useful in in type 3 (typically considered mild); in severe forms of types 1 and 2 VWD, DDAVP is not effective and vWF concentrates are available.[33] VWD is the most frequent inherited bleeding disorder and is due to quantitative (types 1 and 3) or qualitative (type 2) defects of vWF.[33] DDAVP is the treatment for type 1 VWD. In type 3 and in severe forms of types 1 and 2 VWD,

DDAVP is not effective and virally inactivated plasma vWF concentrates should be used in bleeding, surgery, and secondary long-term prophylaxis.[33]

DDAVP should be administered by slow intravenous infusion to avoid hypotension because it stimulates endothelial cells releasing vasoactive mediators in addition to vWF.[34,35] Prior reports that DDAVP reduced blood loss and transfusion needs approximately 30% during complex cardiac surgery[36–38] have not been confirmed.[30,35] There have been 18 trials of DDAVP in 1,295 patients undergoing cardiac surgery that show a small effect on perioperative blood loss (median decrease, 115 mL). Although DDAVP may stimulate release of vWF, its effect is likely minimal compared to multiple other factors involved in hemostasis. Also, DDAVP may be associated with other adverse effects as myocardial infarction was twofold higher compared to placebo with no improvement in clinical outcomes.[6] However, in another review evaluating 16 trials of DDAVP in cardiac surgery and in other high-risk operations, the rate of thrombosis did not differ significantly between patients who received DDAVP and patients who received placebo (3.4% vs. 2.7%).[39]

Fibrinogen

Fibrinogen is a 340-kDa plasma glycoprotein synthesized in the liver and a critical component of effective clot formation.[40] It is the substrate of three important enzymes involved in clot formation: thrombin, factor (F) XIIIa, and plasmin as previously reviewed. The half-life is ~3.7 days (range, 3.00 to 4.08 days). For clot formation, thrombin cleaves the fibrinogen molecule, producing a soluble fibrin monomer which polymerizes to form a loose network in trapping red blood cells and a clot begins to form. Cross-linking of the fibrin polymers, induced by FXIIIa, is fundamental to the coagulation process, increasing the elasticity of the clot and its resistance to fibrinolysis. Fibrinogen also acts as the binding site (ligand) for glycoprotein IIb/IIIa receptors, found on the platelet surface, which are responsible for platelet aggregation. These platelets then become enmeshed within the fibrin strands, stabilizing the growing clot, and create the ability to cross-link and expand the clot and seal the bleeding site. During major hemorrhage, hemodilution after blood loss and subsequent volume replacement leads to reduced fibrinogen levels impairing fibrin polymerization and reduces clot stability. Thus, fibrinogen supplementation to restore plasma fibrinogen is key to normalizing clotting function.

Fibrinogen is an underrecognized coagulation factor that is critical for producing effective clot in surgical patients, and data supports hypofibrinogenemia as a predictor of perioperative bleeding.[41–43] Normal fibrinogen levels are 200 to 400 mg/dL, although during the third trimester of pregnancy, fibrinogen levels are elevated to greater than 400 mg/dL. While the optimal fibrinogen level needed in a bleeding patient is not known, bleeding increases for each 100 mg/dL decrease in fibrinogen level in parturients.[44] Low fibrinogen levels can predict bleeding after prolonged CPB.[45,46] Treatment of fibrinogen deficiency is important for survival, and the amount of fibrinogen administered to trauma patients has been positively correlated with reductions in mortality.[40]

A major problem with managing bleeding is that many transfusion algorithms recommend therapy only when fibrinogen levels are less than 100 mg/dL. It is important to consider that such low levels of fibrinogen can increase laboratory measures of hemostasis including prothrombin time (PT) and partial thromboplastin time (PTT) that may not be corrected with transfusing fresh frozen plasma. In this situation, cryoprecipitate or fibrinogen concentrates are a better option to restore adequate plasma levels (~200 mg/dL) and need to be considered when treating life-threatening bleeding. Fibrinogen can be repleted by cryoprecipitate; 1 unit per 10 kg increases fibrinogen by 50 to 70 mg/dL. In Europe, fibrinogen concentrates are available and cryoprecipitate is not used. A fibrinogen concentrate (RiaSTAP [CSL Behring, King of Prussia, PA]) has just been granted licensing as an orphan drug for treating bleeding in patients with congenital afibrinogenemia or hypofibrinogenemia, but not for patients with dysfibrinogenemia.

Recombinant Coagulation Products

Recombinant proteins are becoming more readily available for managing bleeding, topical hemostasis and for other therapeutic interventions.[47,48] Recombinant proteins can also be modified to alter specific characteristics that may be important in therapeutic effects or provide quantities that can be administered supraphysiologically as a therapeutic agent.[47,48] Currently, they are used to manage bleeding in hemophilia, VWD, and in patients with acquired antibodies/inhibitors.[47]

Recombinant Activated Factor VIIa

Recombinant activated factor VIIa (rFVIIa; NovoSeven [Novo Nordisk, Princeton, NJ]) is most widely known and approved for hemophilia patients with inhibitors to treat bleeding but is increasingly used off-label as a prohemostatic agent for life-threatening hemorrhage.[49] Recombinant factor VIIa produces a prohemostatic effect by multiple mechanisms that include complexing with tissue factor (TF) expressed at the site of vascular injury to locally produce thrombin and amplify hemostatic activation.[50] Circulating FVIIa accounts for approximately 1% of

Table 29-1

Prohemostatic Agents

- Antifibrinolytic agents: aprotinin, epsilon aminocaproic acid, tranexamic acid
- DDAVP (desmopressin)
- Protamine
- Factor concentrates fibrinogen, factor XIII
- Prothrombin complex concentrates (PCCs): four components, three components, activated (FEIBA)
- Recombinant factor VIIa (rVIIa, NovoSeven [Novo Nordisk, Princeton, NJ])
- Topical thrombin/topical agents/fibrin glues

circulating FVII and has no effect until bound with TF.[50] An increasing number of publications report the off-label use of rFVIIa in cardiac surgical patients. The therapeutic dose of rFVIIa in nonhemophilia patients has not been established.[51] However, guidelines as reported by Goodnough et al.[51] and Despotis et al.[52] for off-label use in patients with life-threatening hemorrhage are listed in Table 29-1.

Controlled clinical trials report the incidence of thrombotic complications among patients who received rFVIIa was relatively low and similar to that among patients who received placebo (Table 29-2).[53] However, most case reports giving rFVIIa as rescue therapy include patients who have impaired coagulation, have received multiple transfusions, and are at a high risk for adverse events. The complex role that transfusion therapy has in producing adverse outcomes is emerging in the scientific literature.[54–56] A report using the FDA MedWatch database noted thromboembolic events in patients with diseases other than hemophilia in whom rFVIIa was used on an off-label basis and included 54% of the events as arterial thrombosis (e.g., stroke or acute myocardial infarction).[57] Venous thromboembolism (mostly, venous thrombosis or pulmonary embolism) occurred in 56% of patients. In 72% of the 50 reported deaths, thromboembolism was considered the probable cause. It is not clear to what extent the clinical conditions requiring the use of rFVIIa may have contributed to the risk of thrombosis.[31] Other major issues about rFVIIa include costs and dosing. This drug has also seen widespread use in treating battlefield injuries.

Table 29-2

Postoperative Rescue Therapy with Off-label Use of rVIIa in Cardiac Surgical Patients

- Severe (1 L/hr) or life-threatening bleeding without surgical source of bleeding
- Marginal response to routine hemostatic therapy (i.e., platelets, fresh frozen plasma, cryoprecipitate, desmopressin)
- Administration with appropriate hemostatic factors present
- Consider lower doses than used in hemophilia (30–40 μg/kg)
- Use in patients with multiple antibodies to platelets, crossmatch issues when factors or platelets not available
- Potential use for Jehovah's Witnesses

From Goodnough LT, Lublin DM, Zhang L, et al. Transfusion medicine service policies for recombinant factor VIIa administration. *Transfusion*. 2004;44(9):1325–1331; Despotis G, Avidan M, Lublin DM. Off-label use of recombinant factor VIIA concentrates after cardiac surgery. *Ann Thorac Surg*. 2005;80(1):3–5; Sniecinski RM, Chen EP, Levy JH, et al. Coagulopathy after cardiopulmonary bypass in Jehovah's Witness patients: management of two cases using fractionated components and factor VIIa. *Anesth Analg*. 2007;104(4):763–765; Sniecinski R, Levy JH. What is blood and what is not? Caring for the Jehovah's Witness patient undergoing cardiac surgery. *Anesth Analg*. 2007;104(4):753–754.

In the most recent cardiac surgical study,[58] patients bleeding postoperatively >200 mL per hour were randomized to placebo (n = 68), 40 μg/kg rFVIIa (n = 35), or 80 μg/kg rFVIIa (n = 69). The primary endpoints were the number of patients suffering critical serious adverse events. Secondary endpoints included rates of reoperation, blood loss, and transfusions. Although more adverse events occurred in the rFVIIa groups, they did not reach statistical significance (placebo, 7%; 40 μg/kg, 14%; $P = .25$; 80 μg/kg, 12%; $P = .43$). However, after randomization, significantly fewer patients in the rFVIIa group underwent a reoperation because of bleeding ($P = .03$) or needed allogeneic transfusions ($P = .01$).[58]

One of the difficulties in using rFVIIa is that it can normalize elevated international normalized ratio (INR)/PT values without actually correcting the coagulation defect, especially in patients receiving warfarin and other vitamin K antagonists.[59] The use of prothrombin complex concentrates (PCCs), including a new four-component PCC recently approved in the United States, offers an important and recommended approach for the urgent reversal of warfarin.

Factor XIII (FXIII)

Plasma FXIII is an important final step in clot formation that stabilizes the initial clot. Several investigators have demonstrated reductions in FXIII during CPB and an inverse relationship between postoperative blood loss and postoperative FXIII levels.[60,61] Addition of plasma-derived FXIII (Fibrogammin [CSL Behring, King of Prussia, PA]) at the end of CPB with concurrent antifibrinolytic therapy has reduced postoperative hemorrhage and transfusion requirement in two trials including 22 and 75 patients, respectively.[61,62] The addition of 2,500 units FXIII (Fibrogammin [CSL Behring, King of Prussia, PA]) quickly restored the plasma level of FXIII as measured by (Berichrom ≥70 [Dade Behring, Marburg, Germany]) and reduced transfusion requirements. A recombinant

FXIII has been recently reported in clinical studies and more studies are underway to evaluate this factor as a therapy to reduce bleeding.[60]

Prothrombin Complex Concentrates

PCCs are concentrates of coagulation factors that include factors II, VII, IX, and X in variable concentrations.[63] Two agents (e.g., KCENTRA/Beriplex P/N [CSL Behring, Marburg, Germany], Octaplex [Octapharma, Vienna, Austria]) are used worldwide for vitamin K antagonist–induced (i.e., warfarin) reversal. KCENTA was recently approved in 2013 in the United States. Other PCCs available in the United States include FEIBA VH (Baxter, Vienna, Austria), Profilnine SD (Grifols, Barcelona, Spain), and Bebulin VH (Baxter, Vienna, Austria). They are approved for use in hemophilia and contain mainly factor IX.[63]

The three-component and activated PCCs available in the United States are indicated for prevention/control of bleeding in patients with hemophilia B, although they are used extensively off-label for other indications. Only FEIBA contains FVII in an activated form, and Bebulin contains only low levels of FVII.[63] In general, it is considered preferable to give a PCC containing all four vitamin K–dependent coagulation factors and the natural anticoagulants antithrombin and activated protein C (APC) for anticoagulation reversal.

Although warfarin reversal in the United States is typically achieved with fresh frozen plasma (FFP),[64] most other countries use PCCs.[63] PCCs are recommended in guidelines as primary treatment for reversal in patients with life-threatening bleeding and an increased INR when urgent reversal is required. Recombinant factor VIIa can also be considered as an off-label alternative.[63,65] Compared with FFP, PCCs provide quicker INR correction, have a lower infusion volume, and are more readily available without crossmatching.[63,65] Although there are historical concerns about potential thrombotic risk with PCCs, present-day PCCs are much improved.[66]

Topical Hemostatic Agents

Topical hemostatic agents are used intraoperatively to promote hemostasis at the site of vascular injury and are classified based on their mechanism of action. They include physical and mechanical agents, caustic agents, biologic physical agents, and physiologic agents.[67] The agent to use depends on the type of bleeding, the agent's specific mechanism of action, its interaction with the environment, and the underlying coagulopathy.[67] Absorbable agents include gelatin sponges (Gelfoam [Pfizer, New York, NY]), derived from purified pork skin gelatin that increase contact activation to help create topical clot. Surgicel or Oxycel are oxidized regenerated cellulose that work like Gelfoam (Pfizer, New York, NY). Avitene (Bard Davol, Warwick, RI) is microfibrillar collagen derived from bovine skin. Collagen sponges are available in different commercial forms and are derived from bovine Achilles tendon or bovine skin. Gelatin foam should not be used near nerves or in confined spaces but can be administered topically with thrombin. CoSeal (Baxter, Deerfield, IL) is used where swelling and expansion are not a concern. BioGlue (CryoLife, Kennesaw, GA) has been used in cardiac surgery, but it contains a glutaraldehyde component that cross-links proteins to fix tissues it is applied to.[67]

Topically applied thrombin preparations are also used extensively. The first available thrombin was derived from bovine plasma (Thrombin JMI [Pfizer, New York, NY]). Bovine thrombin currently should be avoided due to its potential for antibovine thrombin antibody formation and immune-mediated coagulopathy.[68] Currently, there are two human thrombins available for clinical use including plasma-derived thrombin (Evithrom [Ethicon, Summerville, NJ]) and recombinant human thrombin RECOTHROM (The Medicines Company, Parsippany, NJ).

Fibrin sealants, also referred to as ***biologic glue*** or ***fibrin tissue adhesives***, are component products that combine thrombin (mostly human) and fibrinogen (usually plasma derived).[67] The first commercial fibrin sealant, Tisseel, (Baxter, Deerfield, IL) was approved in 1989. Additional fibrin sealants are currently in use and include Crosseal (Ethicon, Summerville, NJ), Evicel (Ethicon, Summerville, NJ) and FloSeal (Baxter, Deerfield, IL). They are packaged with a dual-syringe delivery system that combines the components to form a fibrin clot.[67] The thrombin concentration determines the onset and the tensile strength fibrin seal.[67] Crosseal (Ethicon, Summerville, NJ) contains human fibrinogen, human thrombin, and TXA. Evicel (Ethicon, Summerville, NJ) does not contain any fibrinolytic inhibitors. Several of these agents have been studied in cardiac surgical patients including FloSeal (Baxter, Deerfield, IL) [69] and is the subject of a recent review.[70]

Summary

The potential for bleeding in surgical patients represents an ongoing problem for clinicians. The increasing use of anticoagulation agents creates a need for multiple pharmacologic approaches as reviewed in the chapter on anticoagulation. Newer therapies, including purified protein concentrates such as the PCCs and potential recombinant therapies under development, will provide clinicians with the ability to administer key coagulation proteins to treat hemorrhage when standard therapies are ineffective, unavailable, or for other reasons that include no need for crossmatching. Therapy should be multimodal when managing perioperative hemostasis (Fig. 29-2).[71] Understanding the complex physiology of hemostatic function is an important part of therapy, and procoagulation agents are part of a multimodal approach.

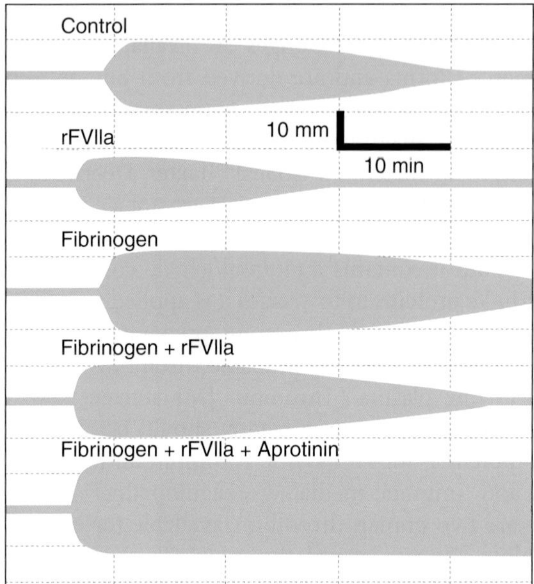

FIGURE 29-2 Thromboelastography recordings obtained with the ROTEM (Durham, NC) device after the addition of rF-VIIa and/or fibrinogen in the presence of tissue-type plasminogen activator in volunteer plasma. Tissue-type plasminogen activator was added to stimulate fibrinolysis. rFVIIa, rFVIIa in a final concentration 1.5 μg/mL; fibrinogen, fibrinogen in a final concentration 100 mg/dL. The maximum clot firmness (the width of clot tracing) was only improved after the addition of fibrinogen. The onset of clotting was shorter after the addition of rFVIIa, but the extent of lysis (i.e., decreased clot firmness) was increased in contrast to the samples with fibrinogen. Fibrinolysis was observed after the addition of rFVIIa and fibrinogen, and the clot structure was improved after the addition of an antifibrinolytic aprotinin.

References

1. Christensen MC, Krapf S, Kempel A, et al. Costs of excessive postoperative hemorrhage in cardiac surgery. *J Thorac Cardiovasc Surg.* 2009;138(3):687–693.
2. Karkouti K, Wijeysundera DN, Beattie WS, et al. Variability and predictability of large-volume red blood cell transfusion in cardiac surgery: a multicenter study. *Transfusion.* 2007;47(11):2081–2088.
3. Edmunds LH Jr. Managing fibrinolysis without aprotinin. *Ann Thorac Surg.* 2010;89(1):324–331.
4. Levy JH. Hemostatic agents. *Transfusion.* 2004;44(12)(suppl):58S–62S.
5. Levi MM, Vink R, de Jonge E. Management of bleeding disorders by prohemostatic therapy. *Int J Hematol.* 2002;76(suppl 2):139–144.
6. Levi M, Cromheecke ME, de Jonge E, et al. Pharmacological strategies to decrease excessive blood loss in cardiac surgery: a meta-analysis of clinically relevant endpoints. *Lancet.* 1999;354(9194):1940–1947.
7. Henry D, Carless P, Fergusson D, et al. The safety of aprotinin and lysine-derived antifibrinolytic drugs in cardiac surgery: a meta-analysis. *CMAJ.* 2009;180(2):183–193.
8. Martin K, Wiesner G, Breuer T, et al. The risks of aprotinin and tranexamic acid in cardiac surgery: a one-year follow-up of 1188 consecutive patients. *Anesth Analg.* 2008;107(6):1783–1790.
9. Murkin JM, Falter F, Granton J, et al. High-dose tranexamic acid is associated with nonischemic clinical seizures in cardiac surgical patients. *Anesth Analg.* 2009;110(2):350–353.
10. Zufferey P, Merquiol F, Laporte S, et al. Do antifibrinolytics reduce allogeneic blood transfusion in orthopedic surgery? *Anesthesiology.* 2006;105(5):1034–1046.
11. Royston D, Levy JH, Fitch J, et al. Full-dose aprotinin use in coronary artery bypass graft surgery: an analysis of perioperative pharmacotherapy and patient outcomes. *Anesth Analg.* 2006;103(5):1082–1088.
12. Sedrakyan A, Wu A, Sedrakyan G, et al. Aprotinin use in thoracic aortic surgery: safety and outcomes. *J Thorac Cardiovasc Surg.* 2006;132(4):909–917.
13. Mangano DT, Tudor IC, Dietzel C. The risk associated with aprotinin in cardiac surgery. *N Engl J Med.* 2006;354(4):353–365.
14. Mangano DT, Miao Y, Vuylsteke A, et al. Mortality associated with aprotinin during 5 years following coronary artery bypass graft surgery. *JAMA.* 2007;297(5):471–479.
15. Shaw AD, Stafford-Smith M, White WD, et al. The effect of aprotinin on outcome after coronary-artery bypass grafting. *N Engl J Med.* 2008;358(8):784–793.
16. Schneeweiss S, Seeger JD, Landon J, et al. Aprotinin during coronary-artery bypass grafting and risk of death. *N Engl J Med.* 2008;358(8):771–783.
17. Fergusson DA, Hebert PC, Mazer CD, et al. A comparison of aprotinin and lysine analogues in high-risk cardiac surgery. *N Engl J Med.* 2008;358(22):2319–2331.
18. McMullan V, Alston RP. III. Aprotinin and cardiac surgery: a sorry tale of evidence misused. *Br J Anaesth.* 2013;110(5):675–678.
19. Karkouti K, Wijeysundera DN, Yau TM, et al. The risk-benefit profile of aprotinin versus tranexamic acid in cardiac surgery. *Anesth Analg.* 2010;110(1):21–29.
20. Levy JH, Adkinson NF Jr. Anaphylaxis during cardiac surgery: implications for clinicians. *Anesth Analg.* 2008;106(2):392–403.
21. Mochizuki T, Olson PJ, Szlam F, et al. Protamine reversal of heparin affects platelet aggregation and activated clotting time after cardiopulmonary bypass. *Anesth Analg.* 1998;87(4):781–785.
22. Despotis GJ, Joist JH, Hogue CW Jr, et al. The impact of heparin concentration and activated clotting time monitoring on blood conservation. A prospective, randomized evaluation in patients undergoing cardiac operation. *J Thorac Cardiovasc Surg.* 1995;110(1):46–54.
23. DeLaria GA, Tyner JJ, Hayes CL, et al. Heparin-protamine mismatch. A controllable factor in bleeding after open heart surgery. *Arch Surg.* 1994;129(9):944–950; discussion 50–51.
24. Kuitunen AH, Salmenpera MT, Heinonen J, et al. Heparin rebound: a comparative study of protamine chloride and protamine sulfate in patients undergoing coronary artery bypass surgery. *J Cardiothorac Vasc Anesth.* 1991;5(3):221–226.
25. Teoh KH, Young E, Blackall MH, et al. Can extra protamine eliminate heparin rebound following cardiopulmonary bypass surgery? *J Thorac Cardiovasc Surg.* 2004;128(2):211–219.
26. Levy JH, Zaidan JR, Faraj B. Prospective evaluation of risk of protamine reactions in patients with NPH insulin-dependent diabetes. *Anesth Analg.* 1986;65(7):739–742.
27. Levy JH, Schwieger IM, Zaidan JR, et al. Evaluation of patients at risk for protamine reactions. *J Thorac Cardiovasc Surg.* 1989;98(2):200–204.
28. Mannucci PM. Desmopressin (DDAVP) in the treatment of bleeding disorders: the first 20 years. *Blood.* 1997;90(7):2515–2521.
29. Mannucci PM. Treatment of von Willebrand's disease. *N Engl J Med.* 2004;351(7):683–694.
30. de Prost D, Barbier-Boehm G, Hazebroucq J, et al. Desmopressin has no beneficial effect on excessive postoperative bleeding or blood product requirements associated with cardiopulmonary bypass. *Thromb Haemost.* 1992;68(2):106–110.
31. Mannucci PM, Levi M. Prevention and treatment of major blood loss. *N Engl J Med.* 2007;356(22):2301–2311.
32. Cattaneo M, Harris AS, Stromberg U, et al. The effect of desmopressin on reducing blood loss in cardiac surgery—a meta-analysis of double-blind, placebo-controlled trials. *Thromb Haemost.* 1995;74(4):1064–1070.
33. Federici AB, Mannucci PM. Management of inherited von Willebrand disease in 2007. *Ann Med.* 2007;39(5):346–358.

34. Frankville DD, Harper GB, Lake CL, et al. Hemodynamic consequences of desmopressin administration after cardiopulmonary bypass. *Anesthesiology*. 1991;74(6):988–996.
35. Rocha E, Llorens R, Paramo JA, et al. Does desmopressin acetate reduce blood loss after surgery in patients on cardiopulmonary bypass? *Circulation*. 1988;77(6):1319–1323.
36. Salzman EW, Weinstein MJ, Reilly D, et al. Adventures in hemostasis. Desmopressin in cardiac surgery. *Arch Surg*. 1993;128(2):212–217.
37. Salzman EW, Weinstein MJ, Weintraub RM, et al. Treatment with desmopressin acetate to reduce blood loss after cardiac surgery. A double-blind randomized trial. *N Engl J Med*. 1986;314(22):1402–1406.
38. Weinstein M, Ware JA, Troll J, et al. Changes in von Willebrand factor during cardiac surgery: effect of desmopressin acetate. *Blood*. 1988;71(6):1648–1655.
39. Mannucci PM, Carlsson S, Harris AS. Desmopressin, surgery and thrombosis. *Thromb Haemost*. 1994;71(1):154–155.
40. Levy JH, Welsby I, Goodnough LT. Fibrinogen as a therapeutic target for bleeding: a review of critical levels and replacement therapy. *Transfusion*. 2014;54(5):1389–1405.
41. Blome M, Isgro F, Kiessling AH, et al. Relationship between factor XIII activity, fibrinogen, haemostasis screening tests and postoperative bleeding in cardiopulmonary bypass surgery. *Thromb Haemost*. 2005;93(6):1101–1107.
42. Nielsen VG, Levy JH. Fibrinogen and bleeding: old molecule—new ideas. *Anesth Analg*. 2007;105(4):902–903.
43. Levy JH. Massive transfusion coagulopathy. *Semin Hematol*. 2006; 43(1)(suppl 1):S59–S63.
44. Charbit B, Mandelbrot L, Samain E, et al. The decrease of fibrinogen is an early predictor of the severity of postpartum hemorrhage. *J Thromb Haemost*. 2007;5(2):266–273.
45. Karlsson M, Ternstrom L, Hyllner M, et al. Prophylactic fibrinogen infusion reduces bleeding after coronary artery bypass surgery. A prospective randomised pilot study. *Thromb Haemost*. 2009; 102(1):137–144.
46. Karlsson M, Ternstrom L, Hyllner M, et al. Plasma fibrinogen level, bleeding, and transfusion after on-pump coronary artery bypass grafting surgery: a prospective observational study. *Transfusion*. 2008;48(10):2152–2158.
47. Pipe SW. Recombinant clotting factors. *Thromb Haemost*. 2008; 99(5):840–850.
48. Levy JH, Levi M. A modified recombinant factor VIIa: can we make it work harder, better, faster, stronger? *J Thromb Haemost*. 2009;7(9):1514–1516.
49. Steiner ME, Key NS, Levy JH. Activated recombinant factor VII in cardiac surgery. *Curr Opin Anaesthesiol*. 2005;18(1):89–92.
50. Hoffman M, Monroe DM III. A cell-based model of hemostasis. *Thromb Haemost*. 2001;85(6):958–965.
51. Goodnough LT, Lublin DM, Zhang L, et al. Transfusion medicine service policies for recombinant factor VIIa administration. *Transfusion*. 2004;44(9):1325–1331.
52. Despotis G, Avidan M, Lublin DM. Off-label use of recombinant factor VIIA concentrates after cardiac surgery. *Ann Thorac Surg*. 2005; 80(1):3–5.
53. Levy JH, Fingerhut A, Brott T, et al. Recombinant factor VIIa in patients with coagulopathy secondary to anticoagulant therapy, cirrhosis, or severe traumatic injury: review of safety profile. *Transfusion*. 2006;46(6):919–933.
54. Spiess BD, Royston D, Levy JH, et al. Platelet transfusions during coronary artery bypass graft surgery are associated with serious adverse outcomes. *Transfusion*. 2004;44(8):1143–1148.
55. Furnary AP, Wu Y, Hiratzka LF, et al. Aprotinin does not increase the risk of renal failure in cardiac surgery patients. *Circulation*. 2007;116(11)(suppl):I127–I133.
56. Koch CG, Li L, Sessler DI, et al. Duration of red-cell storage and complications after cardiac surgery. *N Engl J Med*. 2008;358(12): 1229–1239.
57. O'Connell KA, Wood JJ, Wise RP, et al. Thromboembolic adverse events after use of recombinant human coagulation factor VIIa. *JAMA*. 2006;295(3):293–298.
58. Gill R, Herbertson M, Vuylsteke A, et al. Safety and efficacy of recombinant activated factor VII: a randomized placebo-controlled trial in the setting of bleeding after cardiac surgery. *Circulation*. 2009;120(1):21–27.
59. Tanaka KA, Szlam F, Dickneite G, et al. Effects of prothrombin complex concentrate and recombinant activated factor VII on vitamin K antagonist induced anticoagulation. *Thromb Res*. 2008;122(1): 117–123.
60. Levy JH, Gill R, Nussmeier NA, et al. Repletion of factor XIII following cardiopulmonary bypass using a recombinant A-subunit homodimer. A preliminary report. *Thromb Haemost*. 2009;102(4): 765–771.
61. Godje O, Gallmeier U, Schelian M, et al. Coagulation factor XIII reduces postoperative bleeding after coronary surgery with extracorporeal circulation. *Thorac Cardiovasc Surg*. 2006;54(1):26–33.
62. Godje O, Haushofer M, Lamm P, et al. The effect of factor XIII on bleeding in coronary surgery. *Thorac Cardiovasc Surg*. 1998;46(5): 263–267.
63. Levy JH, Tanaka KA, Dietrich W. Perioperative hemostatic management of patients treated with vitamin K antagonists. *Anesthesiology*. 2008;109(5):918–926.
64. Ozgonenel B, O'Malley B, Krishen P, et al. Warfarin reversal emerging as the major indication for fresh frozen plasma use at a tertiary care hospital. *Am J Hematol*. 2007;82(12):1091–1094.
65. Dager WE, King JH, Regalia RC, et al. Reversal of elevated international normalized ratios and bleeding with low-dose recombinant activated factor VII in patients receiving warfarin. *Pharmacotherapy*. 2006;26(8):1091–1098.
66. Dickneite G. Prothrombin complex concentrate versus recombinant factor VIIa for reversal of coumarin anticoagulation. *Thromb Res*. 2007;119(5):643–651.
67. Achneck HE, Sileshi B, Jamiolkowski RM, et al. A comprehensive review of topical hemostatic agents: efficacy and recommendations for use. *Ann Surg*. 2010;251(2):217–228.
68. Lawson JH. The clinical use and immunologic impact of thrombin in surgery. *Semin Thromb Hemost*. 2006;32(suppl 1):98–110.
69. Nasso G, Piancone F, Bonifazi R, et al. Prospective, randomized clinical trial of the FloSeal matrix sealant in cardiac surgery. *Ann Thorac Surg*. 2009;88(5):1520–1526.
70. Barnard J, Millner R. A review of topical hemostatic agents for use in cardiac surgery. *Ann Thorac Surg*. 2009;88(4):1377–1383.
71. Tanaka KA, Taketomi T, Szlam F, et al. Improved clot formation by combined administration of activated factor VII (NovoSeven) and fibrinogen (Haemocomplettan P). *Anesth Analg*. 2008;106(3): 732–738, table of contents.

CHAPTER 30

Anticoagulants

Jerrold H. Levy

Anticoagulants are drugs that delay or prevent the clotting of blood. In a perioperative setting, patients receive anticoagulation for cardiovascular procedures, thromboprophylaxis, or for cardiovascular disease and/or atrial fibrillation. The therapeutic potential of anticoagulation must be considered against risks for increased bleeding. Many agents are also used in the perioperative setting that may not be routinely monitored, including drugs such as low-molecular-weight heparin, new oral anticoagulants that include direct thrombin inhibitors (dabigatran [Pradaxa] and factor Xa inhibitors rivaroxaban [Xarelto] and apixaban), or newer platelet inhibitors. This chapter will review the different anticoagulation agents, including antiplatelet agents, and considerations for their use in the perioperative use. The agents most commonly used will be considered in detail. Guidelines for management are published about every 4 years by the American College of Chest Physicians (ACCP) and should be referred to for more detail.[1–9]

Heparin

Unfractionated heparin (UFH) is an extract of porcine intestine or bovine lung, where heparin is stored in the mast cells. It is a mixture of highly sulfated glycosaminoglycans with molecular weights ranging from 3,000 to 30,000 daltons that produce their anticoagulant effects by binding to antithrombin (AT) (previously known as antithrombin III), a circulating serine protease. Heparin acts as an anticoagulant by binding to AT, enhancing the rate of thrombin–AT complex formation by 1,000 to 10,000 times. Other factors in the clotting cascade, including factor Xa but also XII, XI, and IX are also inhibited by AT.[10] Anticoagulation thus depends on the presence of adequate amounts of circulating AT as shown in the Figure 30-1.

Standardization of heparin potency is based on in vitro comparison with a known standard. A unit of heparin is defined as the volume of heparin-containing solution that will prevent 1 mL of citrated sheep blood from clotting for 1 hour after the addition of 0.2 mL of 1:100 calcium chloride. Heparin must contain at least 120 United States Pharmacopeia (USP) units per milliliter. Because the potency of different commercial preparations of heparin may vary greatly, the heparin dosing should always be prescribed in units, and most heparin is porcine in origin.

Pharmacokinetics

Heparin is a highly charged acidic molecule administered by intravenous (IV) or subcutaneous (SC) injection. The pharmacokinetics of heparin are based on measurements of its biologic activity using an anti-Xa assay. Over the range of heparin concentrations used clinically, the dose-response relationship is not linear for multiple reasons, including the need for AT to potentiate its effect, the effects of temperature, its highly charged nature that causes protein binding, and the variability of anticoagulation responses. The precise pathway of heparin elimination is uncertain, and the influence of renal and hepatic disease on its pharmacokinetics is less than with other anticoagulants. Heparin binds to many different proteins, which can affect its anticoagulant activity and contributes to heparin resistance.[11]

Laboratory Evaluation of Coagulation

The anticoagulant response to heparin varies widely especially in critically ill patients with alterations in AT and other plasma proteins. Different tests are used to monitor UFH and other anticoagulants as follows.[2]

Activated Partial Thromboplastin Time

Heparin treatment is usually monitored to maintain the ratio of the activated partial thromboplastin time (aPTT) within a defined range of approximately 1.5 to 2.5 times normal values, typically 30 to 35 seconds. An excessively prolonged aPTT (>120 seconds) is readily shortened by

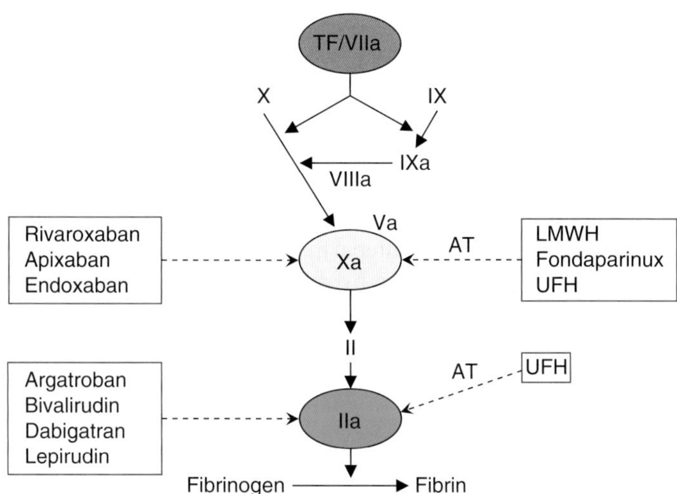

FIGURE 30-1 The major targets for anticoagulants in the coagulation pathway are directed against either factor Xa or thrombin (IIa). Unfractionated heparin (UFH) and low-molecular-weight heparin (LMWH) require circulating AT as a cofactor, and only UFH will inhibit thrombin. Fondaparinux is a synthetic pentasachharide and, like LMWH, indirectly inhibit factor Xa, requiring AT as a cofactor. The direct factor Xa inhibitors are AT-independent and include rivaroxaban, apixaban, and endoxaban. Both oral direct thrombin inhibitors (dabigatran) and IV agents directly inhibit thrombin. Vitamin K antagonists, such as warfarin, inhibit the activation of factors II, VII, IX, X, as factors are made but are not activated by the posttranslational carboxylation that is inhibited (mechanism not shown). (From Levy JH, Key NS, Azran MS. Novel oral anticoagulants: implications in the perioperative setting. *Anesthesiology.* 2010;113:726–745.)

omitting a dose because heparin has a brief elimination half-time. When low-dose heparin is used, laboratory tests may not be required to monitor treatment because the dosage and schedule are well known. However, some hospital laboratories have changed to anti-Xa assays instead of aPTT monitoring because of the variability of responses, with low-dose regimens targeting levels of 0.3 to 0.5 unit/mL and high-dose regimens targeting levels 0.5 to 0.8 unit/mL.

Activated Clotting Time

At higher heparin concentrations like those typically used during cardiopulmonary bypass, the activated clotting time is used to monitor anticoagulation. The activated clotting time (ACT) is performed by mixing whole blood with an activating substance that has a large surface area, such as celite (diatomaceous earth—silicon dioxide) or kaolin (clay—aluminum silicate). This is a contact activation through the classic intrinsic pathway where factor XII initiates activation of the clotting cascade. The activator speeds up the clotting time to normal values of approximately 100 to 150 seconds, depending on the device. Several commercially available timing systems used clinically to measure the ACT are based on detecting the onset of clot formation. Nevertheless, results between different commercial devices to measure the ACT may not be interchangeable, especially if the type of activator (celite or kaolin) is different.

Heparin effect and its antagonism by protamine are commonly monitored in patients undergoing cardiovascular procedures by measuring the ACT. Because the ACT is easy to use and reliable for high heparin concentrations (>1.0 unit/mL), it has become the mainstay of heparin anticoagulation monitoring in perioperative management and for cardiac catheterization. In addition to the presence of a heparin effect, the ACT may be influenced by hypothermia, thrombocytopenia, presence of contact activation inhibitors (aprotinin), and preexisting coagulation deficiencies (fibrinogen, factor XII, factor VII). With aprotinin therapy, the recommendation is to use kaolin-ACT rather than a celite-ACT determination as kaolin binds to aprotinin to minimize its effect.

For cardiac surgery, a baseline value for the ACT is determined (a) before the IV administration of heparin, (b) 3 to 5 minutes after administration, and (c) at 30-minute intervals, thereafter. The ACT response to heparin is not linear for multiple reasons, including the need for AT for its effectiveness and because of several other factors that affect ACT. During cardiopulmonary bypass, the target ACT value is still controversial but often considered adequate if the ACT is longer than 350 seconds, although most cardiac surgical centers target an ACT of longer than 400 seconds. The need to measure ACT repeatedly is emphasized by the fourfold variation in heparin sensitivity between patients and the threefold variation in the rate at which heparin is metabolized. Furthermore, ACT values can be misleading during cardiopulmonary bypass with respect to heparin-induced anticoagulation because of the effects of hypothermia and hemodilution on the measurement system.[12]

Clinical Uses

Heparin is used extensively for multiple purposes including the prevention and treatment of venous thrombosis and pulmonary embolism, for acute coronary syndromes, and for perioperative anticoagulation for extracorporeal circulation and hemodialysis. When administered intravenously, heparin has an immediate onset of action, whereas SC administration results in variable bioavailability with an onset of action in 1 to 2 hours.

Heparin-Induced Thrombocytopenia

Thrombocytopenia due to UFH is common and can begin within hours in patients exposed to heparin. However, a more severe and even life-threatening syndrome develops in 0.5% to 6.0% of patients, manifesting as severe thrombocytopenia (50% drop in platelet count or <100,000 cells/mm^3), that can be associated with thrombotic events (heparin-induced thrombocytopenia with thrombosis). This severe response typically develops after 4 to 5 days of heparin therapy and is caused by heparin-dependent antibodies to platelet factor IV that trigger platelet aggregation and result in thrombocytopenia (see the more detailed discussion in Physiology of Hemostasis, Chapter 27 Physiology of Hemostasis).[13]

Allergic Reactions

Heparin can cause allergic reactions, but these are rare and present in a manner typical of other hypersensitivity reactions. In patients that do experience immediate reactions, heparin-induced thrombocytopenia (HIT) should also be suspected due to the presence of preformed antibodies. Rapid IV infusion of large doses of heparin usually causes minimal hemodynamic changes.[13]

Reversal of Heparin-Induced Anticoagulation with Protamine

Protamine is one of the few agents available for reversing anticoagulation. Protamine is a strongly alkaline (nearly two-thirds of the amino acid composition is arginine), polycationic, low-molecular-weight protein found in salmon sperm. The positively charged alkaline protamine combines with the negatively charged acidic heparin to form a stable complex that is devoid of anticoagulant activity. These heparin–protamine complexes are removed by the reticuloendothelial system. Clearance of protamine by the reticuloendothelial system (within 20 minutes) is more rapid than heparin clearance and that may explain, in part, the phenomenon of heparin rebound. The dose of protamine required to antagonize heparin is typically 1 mg for every 100 units of circulating heparin activity. A more specific dose of protamine is calculated by heparin-protamine titration. Most clinicians give too much protamine because they reverse based on the total dose or heparin administered without accounting for heparin elimination prior to the administration of protamine. Heparin has a half life of approximately one hour, so determinations of protamine dosing should include considerations of the circulating heparin level for reversal. (See also "Protamine" in Chapter 29, Procoagulants.)

Low-Molecular-Weight Heparins

Enoxaparin and dalteparin are two commonly administered low-molecular-weight heparins (LMWHs) derived from standard commercial-grade UFH by chemical depolymerization to yield fragments with a mean molecular weight of 4,000 to 5,000 daltons. Depolymerization of heparin results in a change in its anticoagulant profile, pharmacokinetics, and effects on platelet function. Compared with heparin, which has an anti-Xa to anti-IIa activity of about 1:1, enoxaparin has a corresponding ratio that varies between 4:1 and 2:1.[14] The pharmacokinetics of enoxaparin and dalteparin between patients are more consistent than heparin because these drugs bind less avidly to proteins than heparin. This contributes to better bioavailability at low doses. Although protection against venous thromboembolism (VTE) in high-risk medical and surgical patients is often thought to be better with LMWH than with heparin, LMWH's effect is greatly prolonged with renal failure and anticoagulants such as UFH should be used in this population. Therefore, care should be taken to delay surgery for 12 hours after the last dose of LMWH in patients with normal renal function and longer with renal dysfunction. Protamine does not neutralize LMWH.[2,14]

Spinal and Epidural Hematomas

The risk of spontaneous hematoma formation may be increased in the presence of LMWH and indwelling epidural catheters for administration of postoperative analgesia and by concomitant use of other drugs that affect hemostasis (nonsteroidal antiinflammatory drugs, platelet inhibitors) and by traumatic or repeated attempts to accomplish entry into the epidural or subarachnoid space. This increased risk of hematoma formation is a consideration when selecting regional anesthesia in patients being treated with LMWH preparations. Recommendations for management of patients for regional anesthesia in the patient receiving antithrombotic or thrombolytic therapy are reported in American Society of Regional Anesthesia and Pain Medicine Evidence-Based Guidelines (Third Edition).[15]

Fondaparinux

Fondaparinux is a synthetic anticoagulant composed of the five saccharide units that make up the active site of heparin that binds AT, such as LMWH, to inhibit factor Xa but has no direct activity against thrombin. Administered subcutaneously, fondaparinux is rapidly absorbed and has an elimination half-time of 15 hours, allowing for once daily administration. Metabolism does not occur and the drug is eliminated by the kidneys and should not be used in patients with renal failure. Clinical uses of fondaparinux include prevention of deep vein thrombosis (DVT) and pulmonary embolism and as an alternate anticoagulant in patients with HIT. Because of its long duration of action, it is used primarily in patients with HIT or concerns about sensitization.[16]

Danaparoid

Danaparoid is a glycosaminoglycuronan that is derived from porcine intestinal mucosa and consists of a mixture mostly of dermatan sulfate, and chondroitin sulfate. This low-molecular-weight heparinoid compound attenuates fibrin formation principally by binding AT. Elimination of danaparoid is predominately through the kidneys. Danaparoid is effective in decreasing the incidence of DVT following total hip arthroplasty and was used for the treatment of HIT; this agent is no longer available in the United States (it was removed from the U.S. market in 2002 due to a shortage in drug substance) but is still in use in other countries.

Prophylaxis against Venous Thromboembolism

Surgical procedures have been associated with a 20-fold increase in risk for VTE, which is understandable considering that the majority of surgical patients have one or more risk factors for developing VTE.[17] The incidence of DVT is 10% to 40% among general surgery patients, and higher still in high-risk surgery patient populations (e.g., orthopedic, thoracic, cardiac, and vascular surgery).[2,3] Fortunately, thromboprophylaxis is known to effectively reduce VTE in a cost-effective manner.[2] However, despite their effectiveness, there are specific challenges regarding the use of currently recommended anticoagulants.[7]

To prevent VTE, patients are treated with anticoagulants. Although SC heparin and LMWH are commonly used, multiple novel agents are also approved for different indications including fondaparinux, rivaroxaban, and dabigatran with different indications depending on the country. Enoxaparin and dalteparin are commonly used LMWHs. Before the availability of LMWH, low-dose heparin, 5,000 units subcutaneously every 8 to 12 hours, was a common regimen. In those with renal failure or renal dysfunction, heparin and warfarin are the only drugs minimally affected because of nonrenal clearance.

Among surgical patients, those undergoing total hip replacement are at unique risk for developing DVT and many of the studies for approval of new anticoagulants have focused on this group and other orthopedic patients. The risk of DVT is more protracted after hip surgery than after general surgery, when it usually develops during the first few postoperative days. The surgical technique for hip surgery, which kinks the femoral vein, seems to stimulate proximal DVT in the operated leg, whereas calf vein thrombosis is more likely to develop in either leg. Another effect unique to hip surgery is impairment of venous hemodynamics, which may last several weeks in the operated leg. Indeed, there are significantly fewer venous thromboembolic complications in patients undergoing elective hip replacement when prophylaxis with LMWH is given for 1 month rather than only during the hospitalization. VTE is also a common, life-threatening complication of major trauma. Pulmonary embolism has been observed to occur in 2% to 22% of patients with major trauma, and fatal pulmonary embolism is the third most common cause of death in patients who survive the first 24 hours.[7,17]

Direct Thrombin Inhibitors: Parenteral Agents

An important class of anticoagulants that high-risk surgery patients at risk for HIT may receive are the direct thrombin inhibitors, including bivalirudin, argatroban, lepirudin, and desirudin (Table 30-1). Bivalirudin is also commonly used for cardiac interventional procedures. The direct thrombin inhibitors also vary in their binding affinities for thrombin. Desirudin, lepirudin, and bivalirudin bond in a bivalent manner to thrombin by interacting with both the catalytic site and fibrinogen-binding site. Bivalent direct thrombin inhibitors show higher affinity and specificity for thrombin compared with univalent direct thrombin inhibitors, which bind to the catalytic site only. Direct thrombin inhibitors vary substantially in their pharmacokinetic properties in terms of half life and metabolism. There are also differences in immunogenicity between the direct thrombin inhibitors and with 40% to 70% of patients developing antihirudin antibodies after 4 or more days of treatment.[18]

Bivalirudin

Bivalirudin, a synthetic analog of hirudin with a half-life of 25 minutes, has been widely studied in patients with and without acute coronary syndromes undergoing percutaneous coronary intervention (PCI). This agent is indicated for use in patients with unstable angina undergoing percutaneous transluminal coronary angioplasty (PTCA); in patients with or at risk for HIT or HIT with thrombosis syndrome (HITTS) undergoing PCI; and with provisional use of glycoprotein (GP) IIb/IIIa inhibitors in patients undergoing PCI. Although it is a polypeptide, bivalirudin is considered a safe anticoagulant in patients with HIT. In patients with HIT antibodies undergoing cardiopulmonary bypass, bivalirudin provided safe and effective anticoagulation, with a 94% success rate for the procedures.[19] Further, multiple studies have demonstrated its application as a heparin replacement in patients who are HIT positive and require on or off pump cardiac surgery, although this is an off-label use for the drug.[19–21]

Argatroban

Argatroban is an injectable, synthetic, univalent direct thrombin inhibitor indicated for prophylaxis or treatment

Table 30-1

Direct Thrombin Inhibitors Currently Available

Drug	Dose	Clinical Status	Indications Current (Future)	Recommended Monitoring	Time to Stop before Surgery
Bivalirudin	Intravenous	Available in United States, Europe, and Canada	• PCI in patients with HIT • PTCA • Cardiac surgery (Canada) • Acute coronary syndromes (Europe)	ACT	~4–6 h
Argatroban	Intravenous	Available in United States and Europe	• Prophylaxis and treatment of thrombosis in HIT • PCI in patients with HIT	aPTT ACT (PCI)	~4–6 h
Lepirudin	Intravenous	Available in United States and Europe	• HIT and prevention of further VTE	aPTT	~24 h: Lepirudin and desirudin are irreversible thrombin inhibitors.
Desirudin	Subcutaneous	Available in United States and Europe for hip arthroplasty	• Total hip arthroplasty • (HIT)	aPTT	~24 h
Ximelagatran	Oral	No longer in clinical development		None	
Dabigatran etexilate	Oral	Available in United States for stroke prevention for atrial fibrillation; approved in Europe and Canada for hip and knee arthroplasty.	• Total hip or knee arthroplasty • VTE • Atrial fibrillation	Thrombin times, aPTT	~48 hours with normal renal function; ~72–96 h or more if abnormal renal function. Drug effects can actually be measured as noted and potentially can be used to guide decision making.

ACT, activated clotting time; aPTT, activated partial thromboplastin time; HIT, heparin-induced thrombocytopenia; PCI, percutaneous coronary intervention; PTCA, percutaneous transluminal coronary angioplasty; VTE, venous thromboembolism.

of thrombosis in patients with or at risk of HIT undergoing PCI. It has a relatively short half-life of 40 to 50 minutes, and anticoagulation returns to baseline when stopping it after approximatrly 4 hours.[22] Patients with HIT are likely to have renal dysfunction and most of the agents used for HIT are all primarily renally eliminated. Argatroban is hepatically eliminated, thus no dose adjustments are required in patients with renal impairment. As lepirudin is renally eliminated and bivalirudin is partially (~20%) renally eliminated, their use may require dose adjustment in renally impaired patients to avoid accumulation. Antibodies to argatroban have not been detected after prolonged or repeated use due to its low molecular weight.[23]

Lepirudin and Desirudin

Lepirudin and desirudin are recombinant hirudins, synthetic analogs of hirudin, the direct thrombin inhibitor first isolated from leeches as *Hirudo medicinalis* is the name of the leech. These proteins are manufactured by recombinant methods. Lepirudin is approved for use in patients with HIT and associated thromboembolic disease to prevent further thromboembolic complications.

Lepirudin was initially reported for cardiac surgical patients; however, bleeding was a major problem due to its ability to irreversibly inhibit thrombin. HIT patients receiving lepirudin generate antibodies and require close monitoring (using aPTT) to avoid bleeding complications. In patients with renal dysfunction the drug may have a prolonged half-life.[16,23]

Desirudin (another recombinant hirudin) is approved for use in Europe and now in the United States for the prevention of VTE after total hip or knee replacement surgery and has been studied extensively in patients with stable angina or acute coronary syndromes undergoing PTCA. Antigenicity and anaphylaxis are also reported, although the risk of hypersensitivity to desirudin appears relatively low. Because desirudin is primarily eliminated by the kidneys, patients with renal impairment require monitoring and the aPTT can be used.[16]

Oral Anticoagulants

Vitamin K Antagonists—Warfarin

Oral anticoagulants are derivatives of 4-hydroxycoumarin (coumarin). Warfarin is the most frequently used anticoagulant because of its predictable onset and duration of action and its excellent bioavailability after oral administration (Table 30-2). Treatment usually begins with an oral warfarin dose of 5 to 10 mg, and the average maintenance dose is 5 mg; however, the dose varies widely among individuals due to pharmacogenetic differences. Warfarin has been the only oral agent available until the recent approval of new agents that are described in the sections that follow. Disadvantages of warfarin include delayed onset of action, the need for regular laboratory monitoring, and difficulty in reversal should a surgical procedure create concern about bleeding.[3]

Mechanism of Action

Warfarin inhibits vitamin K epoxide reductase that converts the vitamin K–dependent coagulation proteins (factors II [prothrombin], VII, IX, and X) to their active form, a posttranslational modification. The anticoagulant effect of oral or IV warfarin is delayed for 8 to 12 hours, reflecting the onset of inhibition of clotting factor synthesis and the elimination half-time of previously formed clotting factors that are not altered by the oral anticoagulant. Peak effects of warfarin do not occur for 36 to 72 hours.[3]

Pharmacokinetics

Warfarin is rapidly and completely absorbed, with peak concentrations occurring within 1 hour after ingestion. It is 97% bound to albumin, and this contributes to its negligible renal excretion and long elimination half-time of 24 to 36 hours after oral administration. Warfarin, however, does cross the placenta and produces exaggerated effects in the fetus, who has limited ability to synthesize clotting factors. Warfarin is metabolized to inactive metabolites that are conjugated with glucuronic acid and ultimately excreted in bile (enterohepatic circulation) and urine.

Laboratory Evaluation

Treatment with oral anticoagulants is best guided by measurement of the prothrombin time. The prothrombin time is particularly sensitive to three of the four vitamin K–dependent clotting factors (prothrombin and factors VII and X). Commercial prothrombin time reagents vary markedly in their responsiveness to warfarin-induced decreases in clotting factors. Therefore, prothrombin time results obtained with different reagents are not interchangeable between laboratories. This problem of variability in the responsiveness of prothrombin time reagents has been overcome by the introduction of a standardized system of reporting known as the international normalized ratio (INR). Each manufacturer assigns a specific value that indicates how a particular batch of tissue factor compares to an international reference tissue. The INR is the ratio of a patient's prothrombin time to a normal (control) sample, adjusted by the factor assigned by the manufacturer for the batch of factor being used in the assay. For most indications, a moderate anticoagulant effect with a targeted INR of 2.0 to 3.0 is appropriate, including prosthetic valve prophylaxis. An excessively prolonged prothrombin time is not readily shortened by omitting a dose because of the long elimination half-time of oral anticoagulants. Likewise, an inadequate therapeutic effect is not readily corrected by increasing the dose because of the delayed onset of therapeutic effect.

Unexpected fluctuations in the dose response to warfarin may reflect changes in diet, undisclosed drug use, poor patient compliance, surreptitious self-medication, or intermittent alcohol consumption. Concomitant medication with over-the-counter and prescription drugs can augment or inhibit the anticoagulant effect of coumarin drugs on hemostasis or interfere with platelet function. Patients receiving coumarin drugs are sensitive to fluctuating levels of dietary vitamin K, which is obtained predominantly from leafy green vegetables. The effect of coumarin can be potentiated in sick patients with poor vitamin K intake, particularly if they are treated with antibiotics and IV fluids without vitamin K supplementation. Preexisting liver disease and advanced age are associated with enhanced effects of oral anticoagulants.[3,24]

Clinical Uses

Vitamin K antagonists (VKAs) are effective in the prevention of VTE, the prevention of systemic embolization and resultant stroke in patients with prosthetic heart valves or atrial fibrillation, and for treatment of patients with thrombophilia who are hypercoagulable. Because of the extensive new range of oral anticoagulants for

Table 30-2

Current and Emerging Factor Xa Inhibitors and Vitamin K Antagonist

Drug	Administration	Clinical Status	Indications: Current (Future)	Monitoring	Time to Stop before Elective Surgery
Apixaban	Oral	Phase III	(Atrial fibrillation) (DVT) (Acute coronary syndrome) (Total knee arthroplasty)	None	Not yet approved; should be similar to rivaroxaban; half-life ~12 h
Danaparoid	Intravenous or subcutaneous	No longer available	Treatment of HIT; thromboprophylaxis in HIT patients	Calibrated plasma anti-Xa activity	No longer available
Low-molecular-weight heparin (LMWH)	Intravenous or subcutaneous	Available in Canada, Europe, and United States	Multiple: thromboprophylaxis, acute coronary syndromes	Plasma anti-Xa activity	At least 12 h before surgery; longer if renal dysfunction as elimination is prolonged, not reversible
Fondaparinux	Intravenous or subcutaneous	Available in Canada, Europe, and United States	Thromboprophylaxis and treatment of pulmonary embolism	Calibrated plasma anti-Xa activity	Long half-life of 17–21 h, should be stopped at least 2 d, longer if renal dysfunction
Rivaroxaban	Oral	Available in Canada, Europe, and United States	Total hip or knee arthroplasty (Treatment of DVT and PE) (Atrial fibrillation) (Acute coronary syndromes)	None current	At least 24 h based on prescribing information, but drug half-life may be prolonged with renal dysfunction and recommend holding ~48 h preoperatively with normal renal function and longer if abnormal.
Unfractionated heparin	Intravenous or subcutaneous			aPTT, heparin levels (plasma anti-Xa)	4–6 h before the procedure if possible but may need to continue for cardiovascular surgery; also reversible with protamine
Warfarin	Oral and intravenous		Anticoagulation for multiple reasons and treatment of thrombophilia	Prothrombin time/INR	~5 days before procedure to allow INR <1.5; patients may require bridging with heparin

aPTT, activated partial thromboplastin time; DVT, deep vein thrombosis; HIT, heparin-induced thrombocytopenia; INR, international normalized ratio; PE, pulmonary embolism.

perioperative VTE prophylaxis, these agents are used less and less for this indication.

Management before Elective Surgery

In patients receiving a VKA, the INR should be checked preoperatively. Although minor surgical procedures can be safely performed in patients receiving oral anticoagulants, for major surgery, discontinuation of oral anticoagulants 1 to 3 days preoperatively is recommended to permit the prothrombin time to return to within 20% of its normal range. This approach, followed by reinstitution of the oral anticoagulant regimen 1 to 7 days postoperatively, is not accompanied by an increased incidence of thromboembolic complications in vulnerable patients. However, patients at high risk, such as those with prosthetic heart valves, may require bridging with UFH.[3]

Bleeding is the main complication of any anticoagulant therapy, including the VKAs. The risk of bleeding is influenced by the intensity of the anticoagulant therapy, the patient's underlying disorder, and the concomitant use of aspirin. Bleeding that occurs when the INR is less than 3.0 are frequently associated with an obvious underlying cause (neoplasm, peptic ulcer). These drugs may increase the incidence of intracranial hemorrhage after a cerebrovascular accident. Compression neuropathy has been observed in treated patients after brachial artery puncture to obtain a sample for blood gas analysis. Treatment of bleeding depends on the severity and underlying patient and location. In emergency situations, oral or IV administration of vitamin K is used but will not immediately reverse the anticoagulant effect. If immediate reversal is needed, for performance of high-risk surgical procedures such as craniotomy, administration of prothrombin complex concentrates (PCCs) is needed if available or other reversal strategies as defined in Chapter 29 (Procoagulants).[3,25] Guidelines for perioperative management are available.[1]

New Oral Agents

For many years, warfarin has been the only oral anticoagulant available but has variabilities regarding dosing and effects and requires frequent monitoring and may take up to 5 days before therapeutic levels can be obtained. The newer therapeutic agents have a rapid onset with therapeutic anticoagulation within hours of administration and do not need routine monitoring. Dabigatran is an oral direct thrombin inhibitor, and rivaroxaban is a direct factor Xa inhibitor similar to LMWH.[16] Both of the newer agents require dose adjustments for renal failure and will be considered separately, along with agents still under investigation.[9,16] (Table 30-2)

Direct Factor Xa Inhibitors

Rivaroxaban (Xarelto)

Rivaroxaban is an oral, direct factor Xa inhibitor with >10,000-fold greater selectivity for factor Xa than for other related serine proteases. In contrast to LMWH and similar agents, rivaroxaban does not require AT as a cofactor. Direct factor Xa inhibitors, including rivaroxaban, can inhibit free factor Xa, clot-bound factor Xa, and factor Xa bound to the prothrombinase complex unlike indirect factor Xa inhibitors, such as fondaparinux, which are unable to inhibit factor Xa within the prothrombinase complex. Rivaroxaban is also a non-heparin-like molecule that may be suitable for the management of patients with HIT. Rivaroxaban has been approved for the reduction of risk of stroke and systemic embolism in nonvalvular atrial fibrillation, prophylaxis of deep vein thrombosis following hip or knee replacement surgery, treatment of DVTs, treatment of pulmonary embolism (PE), and reducing the risk of recurrence of DVTs and PE.[9,16]

When used with neuraxial anesthesia, an epidural catheter should not be removed earlier than 18 hours after the last administration of rivaroxaban, and the next rivaroxaban dose should be administered no earlier than 6 hours after the removal of the catheter and as noted in the manufacturer's package insert.

Apixaban

Apixaban is another oral, direct factor Xa inhibitor administered twice daily. Like rivaroxaban, apixiban is approved for the reduction of risk of stroke and systemic embolism in nonvalvular atrial fibrillation, prophylaxis of deep vein thrombosis following hip or knee replacement surgery, treatment of DVTs, treatment of pulmonary embolism (PE), and reducing the risk of recurrence of DVTs and PE.

Other Direct Factor Xa Inhibitors under Investigation

Several other direct factor Xa inhibitors are under investigation and are approved in certain countries. Edoxaban is being evaluated for atrial fibrillation and DVT prophylaxis.

Direct Thrombin Inhibitors

Ximelagatran

Ximelagatran is an oral, direct thrombin inhibitor that was approved in Europe for the VTE prophylaxis but later withdrawn from the market in 2006 due to concerns over potential liver toxicity. However, ximelagatran provided proof of principle that oral agents that act via direct inhibition of thrombin were an effective mode of action for new anticoagulants.[16]

Dabigatran Etexilate (Pradaxa)

Dabigatran etexilate is an oral, direct thrombin inhibitor approved to reduce the risk of stroke and systemic embolism in patients with non-valvular atrial fibrillation, for the treatment of DVT and PE in patients who have been treated with a parenteral anticoagulant for 5-10 days, and to reduce the risk of recurrence of DVT and PE in patients who have been previously treated. Dabigatran's effects can be measured best by thrombin times and also by aPTT values, although thrombin times are preferred.[9] Administration of the first dose should occur a minimum of 2 hours after the catheter is removed, and patients should be observed for neurologic signs and symptoms.[9,16] Dosing should also be adjusted for patients with renal dysfunction.

Perioperative Management of the New Oral Anticoagulants

The newer therapeutic agents have a rapid onset with therapeutic anticoagulation within hours of administration and do not need routine monitoring. Dabigatran is an oral direct thrombin inhibitor, and rivaroxaban is a direct factor Xa inhibitor similar to LMWH.[16] Both of the newer agents require dose adjustments for renal failure.[16] One of the new challenges with use of these agents is how to manage patients perioperatively. In the United States, warfarin is still a problem for clinicians because the PCCs effective for immediate INR reversal are not available.[25] Vitamin K takes days to work; use of 4 units of fresh frozen plasma (FFP) is often used, but associated with transfusion risk and volume overload, and FFP never restores the INR to baseline, but usually to approximately 1.4 to 1.6 which is the baseline INR for FFP.[25]

The French Study Group on thrombosis and hemostasis has proposed perioperative management strategies regarding the risk of bleeding and thrombosis for the new agents. The newer oral anticoagulants may increase surgical bleeding, they have no validated antagonists, they cannot be monitored by simple standardized laboratory assays, and their pharmacokinetics vary significantly between patients.[26] For procedures with low hemorrhagic risk, a therapeutic window of 48 hours (last administration 24 hours before surgery, restart 24 hours after) is proposed. For procedures with medium or high hemorrhagic risk, they suggest stopping therapy 5 days before surgery to ensure complete elimination in all patients. Treatment should be resumed only when the risk of bleeding subsides. In patients at high thrombotic risk (e.g., those in atrial fibrillation with a history of stroke), bridging with heparin (LMWH, or UFH, if the former is contraindicated) is proposed. In an emergency, the procedure should be postponed for as long as possible (minimum 1 to 2 half-lives) and nonspecific antihemorrhagic agents, such as recombinant human activated factor VIIa or PCCs should not be given for prophylactic reversal due to their uncertain benefit-risk.[26]

Although routine monitoring of the new anticoagulants is not standard, if needed they are best evaluated with specialized tests. For dabigatran, thrombin clotting time (TT), ecarin clotting time (ECT), and activated partial thromboplastin time (aPTT) can measure its effects.[27] Prothrombin time (INR) is not recommended. The aPTT, a standard test, can provide a useful qualitative assessment of anticoagulant activity but is less sensitive at supratherapeutic dabigatran levels and limited data exists for activated clotting time (ACT). Overall, the aPTT and TT are the most accessible qualitative methods for determining the presence or absence of anticoagulant effect. Although there is no specific antidote to antagonize the anticoagulant effect of dabigatran, because of its short duration of effect, drug discontinuation should be considered as previously noted. With overdose, dabigatran can also be dialyzed in patients with renal impairment. In instances of life-threatening bleeding, where conventional measures have failed or are unavailable, other prohemostatic agents such as recombinant activated factor VII and PCCs can be considered.[27] For rivaroxaban, prolongation of most standard hemostatic tests are too variable and specialized tests evaluating anti-Xa are required.[28] Recent data also suggests PCCs completely reverse the anticoagulant effect of rivaroxaban in healthy subjects but have minimal effects on dabigatran at the PCC doses of 50 IU/kg used in the study.[29]

In summary, for those who require urgent surgery, managing patients who receive dabigatran, rivaroxaban, and other novel oral anticoagulants is still not well defined. Risk versus benefit should be considered in logical decision making. It is important to note the therapies for reversal are off-label uses from the literature as referenced but provide important perspective for perioperative management for the clinician faced with managing patients receiving these agents.

Platelet Inhibitors

Aspirin

Antiplatelet agents are the mainstay therapy for patients with atherosclerotic vascular disease and coronary artery disease, therapy consistent with the role of platelets in atherosclerosis.[30] Treatment with aspirin reduces the incidence of occlusive arterial vascular events. Aspirin irreversibly acetylates cyclooxygenase and thereby prevents formation of thromboxane A_2. Despite rapid clearance from the body, the effects of aspirin on platelets are irreversible and last for the life of the platelet, 7 to 10 days. The ACCP's widely quoted guidelines suggest in patients who require temporary interruption of aspirin- or clopidogrel-containing drugs before surgery or a procedure, stopping this treatment 7 to 10 days before the procedure is recommended over stopping this treatment closer to surgery. In patients who have had temporary interruption of aspirin therapy because of surgery or a procedure, resuming aspirin approximately 24 hours (or the next morning) after surgery when there is adequate hemostasis is recommended instead of resuming aspirin closer to surgery.[1]

Thienopyridines: Clopidogrel, Prasugrel, and Ticagrelor

Currently approved thienopyridines include clopidogrel (Plavix), prasugrel (Effient), and ticagrelor. The first two agents are prodrugs requiring in vivo metabolism each to an active metabolite as shown in Table 30-3. Ticlopidine is

Table 30-3

Current Oral Antiplatelet Agents

	Clopidogrel	Prasugrel	Ticagrelor	Aspirin
Drug Class	Thienopyridine	Thienopyridine	Thienopyridine	Acetylsalicylate
Mechanism of Action	Selective, irreversible binding to and inhibition of $P2Y_{12}$ receptor on platelets	Selective, irreversible binding to and inhibition of $P2Y_{12}$ receptor on platelets	Selective, reversible binding to and inhibition of $P2Y_{12}$ receptor on platelets	Cyclooxygenase inhibition
Comments	Prodrug, metabolized to active form by two different metabolic steps, resistance due to metabolism	Prodrug, metabolized to active form one metabolic step, more potent and resistance rare	Direct-acting agent	Active drug but resistance can occur, likely due to absorption and other factors

now rarely used clinically and will not be considered. Thienopyridines irreversibly bind to $P2Y_{12}$ receptors thereby blocking adenosine diphosphate (ADP) binding. This $P2Y_{12}$ receptor antagonism inhibits ADP-mediated platelet activation and aggregation due to the critical role ADP plays in platelet function. When ADP is secreted from internal stores, it amplifies platelet responses induced by other platelet agonists to increase activation, an internal to external signaling mechanism.[31] The ADP-induced signal is again mediated by P2Y receptors, which are G-coupled 7-membrane-spanning proteins that are present in many different cells.[31] There are multiple other P2Y receptor subgroups, but the G_i-coupled $P2Y_{12}$ receptor mediates inhibition of adenylyl cyclase and amplifies the platelet aggregation response.[31]

Dual antiplatelet therapy—a thienopyridine (ADP $P2Y_{12}$ receptor antagonist) coadministered with aspirin—is commonly used for improving clinical outcomes in patients with acute coronary syndrome and undergoing percutaneous intervention. New agents include prasugrel and ticagrelor. Ticagrelor is a reversible, direct-acting $P2Y_{12}$ receptor antagonist. The $P2Y_{12}$ is a G_i-coupled platelet receptor for ADP that plays a central role in platelet function. Drugs that inhibit $P2Y_{12}$ are potent antithrombotic drugs. Clopidogrel is the most widely used agent, but resistance, as defined as its inability to inhibit adequately $P2Y_{12}$-dependent platelet function, occurs in 20% to 30% of patients. Prasugrel and ticagrelor appear to be more effective than clopidogrel in preventing thrombosis, although they increase the incidence of major bleeding, a problem with the efficacy of all anticoagulants.

Current recommendations are to discontinue thienopyridines 7 days before elective surgery and to avoid regional anesthesia until the effects of these drugs have dissipated. Guidelines for management of patients with coronary stents on antiplatelet agents have been proposed and are often elaborate (Table 30-4). The guidelines take in to consideration the type of coronary stent used and the interval since the stent was placed as well as the urgency of need for surgery in decision making.

Dipyridamole

Dipyridamole is an agent that increases cyclic adenosine monophosphate in platelets to inhibit their function. This agent was also used for cardiac stress testing because of its coronary vasodilatory effects (dipyridamole-thallium stress test). Currently, it is most frequently administered in combination with aspirin to prevent stroke in patients who cannot take a thienopyridine. It can increase bleeding and should be stopped preoperatively, but the aspirin component has a longer half life than dipyridamole.

Dextran

Dextran-70 (70,000 daltons) binds to platelets and inhibits their function. This agent was used clinically to reduce thrombosis after carotid surgery and a few other indications but is now rarely used for this indication.

Platelet Glycoprotein IIb/IIIa Antagonists

An important advance in managing ischemic cardiovascular disease was the development of platelet GP IIb/IIIa receptor inhibitors, although these agents are now often replaced with newer therapies. The IIb/IIIa receptor antagonists (abciximab, tirofiban, eptifibatide) either bind or competitively inhibit the corresponding fibrinogen receptor that is important for platelet aggregation. These drugs block fibrinogen binding to platelet GP IIb/IIIa receptors that are a common pathway of platelet aggregation. In multiple clinical trials, they have provided proof of concept on the critical role that platelet inhibition has in reducing ischemic events associated with acute coronary syndrome and PCIs. In recent years, thienopyridines and direct thrombin inhibitor (bivalirudin) in addition to PCIs including stenting have had a significant impact; nonetheless, inhibiting platelet function has been critical

Table 30-4

Antiplatelet Therapy following Stent Placement: A 2007 AHA/ACC Recommendations

1. Before implantation of a stent, the physician should discuss the need for dual-antiplatelet therapy. In patients not expected to comply with 12 months of thienopyridine therapy, whether for economic or other reasons, strong consideration should be given to avoiding a DES.
2. In patients who are undergoing preparation for PCI and who are likely to require invasive or surgical procedures within the next 12 months, consideration should be given to implantation of a bare-metal stent or performance of balloon angioplasty with provisional stent implantation instead of the routine use of a DES.
3. A greater effort by healthcare professionals must be made before patient discharge to ensure that patients are properly and thoroughly educated about the reasons they are prescribed thienopyridines and the significant risks associated with prematurely discontinuing such therapy.
4. Patients should be specifically instructed before hospital discharge to contact their treating cardiologist before stopping any antiplatelet therapy, even if instructed to stop such therapy by another healthcare provider.
5. Healthcare providers who perform invasive or surgical procedures and who are concerned about periprocedural and postprocedural bleeding must be made aware of the potentially catastrophic risks of premature discontinuation of thienopyridine therapy. Such professionals who perform these procedures should contact the patient's cardiologist if issues regarding the patient's antiplatelet therapy are unclear, to discuss optimal patient management strategy.
6. Elective procedures for which there is significant risk of perioperative or postoperative bleeding should be deferred until patients have completed an appropriate course of thienopyridine therapy (12 months after DES implantation if they are not at high risk of bleeding and a minimum of 1 month for bare-metal stent implantation).

   For patients treated with DES who are to undergo subsequent procedures that mandate discontinuation of thienopyridine therapy, aspirin should be continued if at all possible and the thienopyridine restarted as soon as possible after the procedure because of concerns about late stent thrombosis.

ACC, American College of Cardiology; AHA, American Heart Association; DES, drug-eluting stent; PCI, percutaneous coronary intervention.

From Fleisher LA, Beckman JA, Brown KA, et al. ACC/AHA 2007 Guidelines on perioperative cardiovascular evaluation and care for noncardiac surgery: executive summary: a report of the American College of Cardiology/American Heart Association Task Force on Practice Guidelines (Writing Committee to Revise the 2002 Guidelines on Perioperative Cardiovascular Evaluation for Noncardiac Surgery): developed in collaboration with the American Society of Echocardiography, American Society of Nuclear Cardiology, Heart Rhythm Society, Society of Cardiovascular Anesthesiologists, Society for Cardiovascular Angiography and Interventions, Society for Vascular Medicine and Biology, and Society for Vascular Surgery. *Circulation*. 2007;116: 1971–1996.

to prevent platelet responses to vascular injury and clot formation. These agents prevent thrombus formation initiated by platelets is in the pathogenesis of acute coronary syndrome (unstable angina, myocardial infarction), angioplasty failure, and stent thrombosis.[32,33] A summary of these agents is given in Table 30-5.

Various antagonists of GP IIb/IIIa are available. The first of these agents, the monoclonal antibody abciximab (ReoPro), was been approved for use in PCI. Tirofiban (Aggrastat), a nonpeptide, for treatment of acute coronary syndromes (unstable angina or non–Q-wave myocardial infarction) and eptifibatide (Integrelin), a peptide, for

Table 30-5

Properties of Glycoprotein IIb/IIIa Antagonists

Drug	Structure	Route of Administration	Elimination Half-Time (h)	Excretion	Clinical Uses	Stop before Surgery (h)	Prolong PT/PTT	Antidote
Abciximab	Monoclonal antibodies	Intravenous	12–24	Plasma proteases	ACS PCI	72	No/No	Dialysis
Eptifibatide	Peptide	Intravenous	2–4	Renal	ACS PCI	24	No/No	Dialysis
Tirofiban	Nonpeptide	Intravenous	2–4	Renal (30%–60%) Biliary (40%–70%)	ACS	24	No/No	Dialysis

ACS, acute coronary syndrome; PCI, percutaneous coronary intervention; PT, prothrombin time; PTT, partial thromboplastin time.

use both in PCI and acute coronary syndromes. New nonpeptide oral antagonists of GP IIb/IIIa intended for long-term use are in various stages of clinical development and may find application in a broad spectrum of atherothrombotic disease. Although GP IIb/IIIa antagonists are indicated for the acute coronary syndrome and in patients undergoing interventional cardiology procedures, thienopyridines have largely replaced these agents due to cost and increasing clinical data favoring the thienopyridines. Abciximab has the longest half-life of all these agents as a monoclonal antibody, whereas the other agents have shorter half-lives. All of three agents can cause thrombocytopenia.[33]

Perioperative Management of Patients on Platelet Inhibitors

Perioperative management of patients on various platelet inhibitors is complex and requires careful coordinated care with multiple specialties. The risks and benefits of discontinuing antiplatelet therapy must be carefully considered for each individual patient, especially prior to elective surgery. The most recent guidelines by Fleisher et al.[34] are listed in Table 30-4.

Thrombolytic Drugs

Pharmacologic thrombolysis is produced by drugs that act as plasminogen activators to convert the endogenous proenzyme plasminogen to the fibrinolytic enzyme plasmin that lysis clot and other proteins. The goal of thrombolytic therapy is to restore circulation through a previously occluded artery or vein, most often a coronary artery. Fibrinolytic therapy was used previously in the treatment of acute coronary syndrome but current American College of Cardiology and American Heart Association published evidence-based guidelines for the management of patients depend on whether a conservative (i.e., noninvasive) approach or an invasive strategy (i.e., PCI with possible angioplasty or coronary artery bypass graft [CABG] surgery) is possible, specifically whether cardiac catheterization is available.

Acute interventions with fibrinolytic agents can be lifesaving in patients with pulmonary emboli,[35] ischemic stroke (e.g., middle cerebral arterial occlusion),[6,36] and in patients suffering acute myocardial infraction without immediate access to PCIs.[37] Bleeding complications (5% to 30%) may occur whether fibrinolytics are injected systemically or directly into the affected arterial lesion.[38] Currently available fibrinolytics include streptokinase, urokinase, and tissue plasminogen activator (tPA). These agents activate plasminogen to plasmin, the major enzyme responsible for clot breakdown. Plasmin is a serine protease that degrades fibrin (ogen) and factors V and VIII. In clinical practice, tPA is most commonly used because of its localized catalytic effect on plasminogen activation in the presence of fibrin.[39] Blood flow to the thrombus is vital for the delivery of tPA, and thus localized activation of fibrinolysis via catheter-directed drug delivery is theoretically more favorable than systemic administration.

Thrombolytic agents have an associated risk of bleeding (particularly intracranial hemorrhage) and hemorrhagic complications occur more often in trauma, surgery, or following invasive diagnostic procedures. Intracranial hemorrhage occurs in 1.7% to 8.0% of treated patients.[40] Following lytic therapy, hemorrhagic transformation of ischemic infarcts can occur. The recommended treatment of intracranial or serious systemic bleeding after thrombolytic therapy is administration of cryoprecipitate and platelets, although evidence-based guidelines for such an approach are lacking.[40] Angioedema occurs in 1% to 5% of patients receiving IV rt-PA, and the use of angiotensin-converting enzyme inhibitors is strongly associated with this complication.[40]

References

1. Douketis JD, Spyropoulos AC, Spencer FA, et al; American College of Chest Physicians. Perioperative management of antithrombotic therapy: Antithrombotic Therapy and Prevention of Thrombosis, 9th ed: American College of Chest Physicians Evidence-Based Clinical Practice Guidelines. *Chest.* 2012;141(2)(suppl): e326S–e350S.
2. Gould MK, Garcia DA, Wren SM, et al; American College of Chest Physicians. Prevention of VTE in nonorthopedic surgical patients: Antithrombotic Therapy and Prevention of Thrombosis, 9th ed: American College of Chest Physicians Evidence-Based Clinical Practice Guidelines. *Chest.* 2012;141(2)(suppl):e227S–e277S.
3. Weitz JI, Eikelboom JW, Samama MM; American College of Chest Physicians. New antithrombotic drugs: Antithrombotic Therapy and Prevention of Thrombosis, 9th ed: American College of Chest Physicians Evidence-Based Clinical Practice Guidelines. *Chest.* 2012;141(2)(suppl):e120S–e151S.
4. Whitlock RP, Sun JC, Fremes SE, et al; American College of Chest Physicians. Antithrombotic and thrombolytic therapy for valvular disease: Antithrombotic Therapy and Prevention of Thrombosis, 9th ed: American College of Chest Physicians Evidence-Based Clinical Practice Guidelines. *Chest.* 2012;141(2)(suppl):e576S–e600S.
5. Linkins LA, Dans AL, Moores LK, et al; American College of Chest Physicians. Treatment and prevention of heparin-induced thrombocytopenia: Antithrombotic Therapy and Prevention of Thrombosis, 9th ed: American College of Chest Physicians Evidence-Based Clinical Practice Guidelines. *Chest.* 2012;141(2)(suppl):e495S–e530S.
6. Ageno W, Gallus AS, Wittkowsky A, et al; American College of Chest Physicians. Oral anticoagulant therapy: Antithrombotic Therapy and Prevention of Thrombosis, 9th ed: American College of Chest Physicians Evidence-Based Clinical Practice Guidelines. *Chest.* 2012;141(2)(suppl):e44S–e88S.
7. Kearon C, Akl EA, Comerota AJ, et al; American College of Chest Physicians. Antithrombotic therapy for VTE disease: Antithrombotic Therapy and Prevention of Thrombosis, 9th ed: American College of Chest Physicians Evidence-Based Clinical Practice Guidelines. *Chest.* 2012;141(2)(suppl):e419S–e494S.
8. Eikelboom JW, Hirsh J, Spencer FA, et al. Antiplatelet drugs: Antithrombotic Therapy and Prevention of Thrombosis, 9th ed: American College of Chest Physicians Evidence-Based Clinical Practice Guidelines. *Chest.* 2012;141(2)(suppl):e89S–e119S.
9. Garcia DA, Baglin TP, Weitz JI, et al; American College of Chest Physicians. Parenteral anticoagulants: Antithrombotic Therapy

and Prevention of Thrombosis, 9th ed: American College of Chest Physicians Evidence-Based Clinical Practice Guidelines. *Chest.* 2012;141(2)(suppl):e24S–e43S.

10. Levy JH. Novel intravenous antithrombins. *Am Heart J.* 2001;141: 1043–1047.
11. Hirsh J. Heparin. *N Engl J Med.* 1991;324:1565–1574.
12. Despotis GJ, Gravlee G, Filos K, et al. Anticoagulation monitoring during cardiac surgery: a review of current and emerging techniques. *Anesthesiology.* 1999;91:1122–1151.
13. Levy JH, Tanaka KA, Hursting MJ. Reducing thrombotic complications in the perioperative setting: an update on heparin-induced thrombocytopenia. *Anesth Analg.* 2007;105:570–582.
14. Weitz JI. Low-molecular-weight heparins. *N Engl J Med.* 1997;337: 688–698.
15. Horlocker TT, Wedel DJ, Rowlingson JC, et al. Executive summary: regional anesthesia in the patient receiving antithrombotic or thrombolytic therapy: American Society of Regional Anesthesia and Pain Medicine Evidence-Based Guidelines (Third Edition). *Reg Anesth Pain Med.* 2010;35:102–105.
16. Levy JH, Key NS, Azran MS. Novel oral anticoagulants: implications in the perioperative setting. *Anesthesiology.* 2010;113:726–745.
17. Geerts WH, Bergqvist D, Pineo GF, et al. Prevention of venous thromboembolism: American College of Chest Physicians Evidence-Based Clinical Practice Guidelines (8th Edition). *Chest.* 2008;133:381S–453S.
18. Di Nisio M, Middeldorp S, Buller HR. Direct thrombin inhibitors. *N Engl J Med.* 2005;353:1028–1040.
19. Koster A, Dyke CM, Aldea G, et al. Bivalirudin during cardiopulmonary bypass in patients with previous or acute heparin-induced thrombocytopenia and heparin antibodies: results of the CHOOSE-ON trial. *Ann Thorac Surg.* 2007;83:572–577.
20. Koster A, Spiess B, Jurmann M, et al. Bivalirudin provides rapid, effective, and reliable anticoagulation during off-pump coronary revascularization: results of the "EVOLUTION OFF" trial. *Anesth Analg.* 2006;103:540–544.
21. Merry AF, Raudkivi PJ, Middleton NG, et al. Bivalirudin versus heparin and protamine in off-pump coronary artery bypass surgery. *Ann Thorac Surg.* 2004;77:925–931; discussion 931.
22. McKeage K, Plosker GL. Argatroban. *Drugs.* 2001;61:515–522; discussion 523–524.
23. Levy JH, Hursting MJ. Heparin-induced thrombocytopenia, a prothrombotic disease. *Hematol Oncol Clin North Am.* 2007;21:65–88.
24. Vermeer C, Schurgers LJ. A comprehensive review of vitamin K and vitamin K antagonists. *Hematol Oncol Clin North Am.* 2000;14:339–353.
25. Levy JH, Tanaka KA, Dietrich W. Perioperative hemostatic management of patients treated with vitamin K antagonists. *Anesthesiology.* 2008;109:918–926.
26. Sie P, Samama CM, Godier A, et al. Surgery and invasive procedures in patients on long-term treatment with direct oral anticoagulants: thrombin or factor-Xa inhibitors. Recommendations of the Working Group on perioperative haemostasis and the French Study Group on thrombosis and haemostasis. *Arch Cardiovasc Dis.* 2011;104:669–676.
27. van Ryn J, Stangier J, Haertter S, et al. Dabigatran etexilate—a novel, reversible, oral direct thrombin inhibitor: interpretation of coagulation assays and reversal of anticoagulant activity. *Thromb Haemost.* 2010;103:1116–1127.
28. Samama MM, Contant G, Spiro TE, et al. Evaluation of the anti-factor Xa chromogenic assay for the measurement of rivaroxaban plasma concentrations using calibrators and controls. *Thromb Haemost.* 2011;107:379–387.
29. Eerenberg ES, Kamphuisen PW, Sijpkens MK, et al. Reversal of rivaroxaban and dabigatran by prothrombin complex concentrate: a randomized, placebo-controlled, crossover study in healthy subjects. *Circulation.* 2011;124:1573–1579.
30. Schneider DJ, Sobel BE. Conundrums in the combined use of anticoagulants and antiplatelet drugs. *Circulation.* 2007;116:305–315.
31. Cattaneo M. The platelet P2Y receptor for adenosine diphosphate: congenital and drug-induced defects. *Blood.* 2010;117:2102–2112.
32. Levy JH, Smith PK. Platelet inhibitors and cardiac surgery. *Ann Thoracic Surg.* 2000;70:S1–S2.
33. Atwater BD, Roe MT, Mahaffey KW. Platelet glycoprotein IIb/IIIa receptor antagonists in non-ST segment elevation acute coronary syndromes: a review and guide to patient selection. *Drugs.* 2005;65: 313–324.
34. Fleisher LA, Beckman JA, Brown KA, et al. ACC/AHA 2007 Guidelines on perioperative cardiovascular evaluation and care for noncardiac surgery: executive summary: a report of the American College of Cardiology/American Heart Association Task Force on Practice Guidelines (Writing Committee to Revise the 2002 Guidelines on Perioperative Cardiovascular Evaluation for Noncardiac Surgery): developed in collaboration with the American Society of Echocardiography, American Society of Nuclear Cardiology, Heart Rhythm Society, Society of Cardiovascular Anesthesiologists, Society for Cardiovascular Angiography and Interventions, Society for Vascular Medicine and Biology, and Society for Vascular Surgery. *Circulation.* 2007;116:1971–1996.
35. Hefer DVF, Munir A, Khouli H. Low-dose tenecteplase during cardiopulmonary resuscitation due to massive pulmonary embolism: a case report and review of previously reported cases. *Blood Coag Fibrin.* 2007;18:691–694.
36. Albers GW, Amarenco P, Easton JD, et al. Antithrombotic and thrombolytic therapy for ischemic stroke: the Seventh ACCP Conference on Antithrombotic and Thrombolytic Therapy. *Chest.* 2004;126:483S–512S.
37. Singh KP, Harrington RA. Primary percutaneous coronary intervention in acute myocardial infarction. *Med Clin North Am.* 2007;91:639–655; x–xi.
38. Alesh I, Kayali F, Stein PD. Catheter-directed thrombolysis (intrathrombus injection) in treatment of deep venous thrombosis: a systematic review. *Catheter Cardiovasc Interv.* 2007;70:143–148.
39. Hoylaerts M, Rijken DC, Lijnen HR, et al. Kinetics of the activation of plasminogen by human tissue plasminogen activator. Role of fibrin. *J Bio Chem.* 1982;257:2912–2919.
40. Wechsler LR. Intravenous thrombolytic therapy for acute ischemic stroke. *N Engl J Med.* 2011;364:2138–2146.

CHAPTER 31

Physiology and Management of Massive Transfusion

Jerrold H. Levy

Hemorrhage due to uncontrolled bleeding is a clinical problem commonly faced by clinicians managing traumatic injury, surgical patients, and obstetrical patients. There are many terms used to describe this life-threatening problem, including ***massive transfusion coagulopathy*** or ***trauma-induced coagulopathy***. The complex coagulopathy that occurs in these situations further compromises the efficacy of subsequent hemostatic treatments. Tissue injury due to trauma, surgical interventions, following delivery in obstetrical patients, or associated with extracorporeal circulation during cardiopulmonary bypass or extracorporeal membrane oxygenation may also contribute to the coagulopathic state.

Hemostasis is a physiologic response to vascular injury and disruption of the vascular endothelium and has been described in earlier chapters. Following surgery or trauma where there is extensive tissue injury, in addition to massive loss of blood, the endothelial integrity is compromised; the coagulopathy that follows tissue injury and blood loss produces a complex alteration in the vasculature often described as an ***endothelialopathy***. Loss of the critical aspects of vascular regulation can also manifest as disseminated intravascular coagulation (DIC), a perturbation of the balance between anticoagulant and procoagulant effects.

The management of hemostasis following traumatic injury and life-threatening hemorrhage has significantly changed over the years from initial resuscitation with crystalloid/colloids and red blood cells (RBCs) to routine administration of plasma/fresh frozen plasma (FFP) and platelets in addition to red cells. Experiences learned from the battlefield and civilian studies have been critical for developing multiple therapeutic approaches that have been combined in a rational massive transfusion protocol. Retrospective studies have reported improved survival with the initial use of plasma and platelets as part of these protocols. This chapter will review the physiology of massive transfusion and modern therapeutic approaches.

Pathophysiology of Hemostatic Abnormalities Associated with Trauma

Hemorrhage is a major cause of mortality following traumatic injury and responsible for approximately 50% of deaths within 24 hours of injury and approximately 80% of intraoperative trauma deaths.[1] The evolution of fluid resuscitation initially included crystalloid, followed by RBC transfusions, and the addition of FFP/plasma, platelets, and cryoprecipitate either empirically or as guided by additional laboratory testing. Therapy in the past was based on treating coagulopathy after the initial resuscitation and stabilization of the patient. More recent observations in trauma victims and on the battlefield found that early administration of plasma resulted in earlier improvement, whereas several studies reported that use of large crystalloid volumes were associated with increased bleeding and lower survival.[1–3]

Trauma and Endothelial Dysfunction

The effects of hemorrhagic shock on endothelial function have been described and the term ***endotheliopathy of trauma*** has been proposed to describe the systemic endothelial injury and dysfunction that contributes to coagulopathy, inflammation, vascular permeability, tissue edema, and multiorgan system dysfunction.[1,2] The endothelial dysfunction is secondary to vascular injury and other factors that result from shock, ischemic injury, and the release of inflammatory mediators. Plasma repletion is thought to have a restorative function on endothelial tight junctions to better modulate vascular integrity compared to crystalloid studying in vitro models. Plasma contains multiple serine protease inhibitors that may have antiinflammatory effects. The endothelium becomes permeable with hemorrhagic shock and extravascular fluid is mobilized intravascularly. Plasma contains proteins for osmotic maintenance but there are also multiple serine protease inhibitors that include antithrombin (also called ***antithrombin III***), C1 esterase inhibitor, tissue factor pathway inhibitor (TFPI), plasminogen activator inhibitor-1 (PAI-1), α_2-antiplasmin, and other inhibitors that may be critical for antiinflammatory responses. Crystalloids lack these factors and are thought to increase interstitial edema, increase lung injury, and promote multiorgan system dysfunction.[1,2]

Inflammatory activation following tissue injury contributes to the endothelial dysfunction as does the critical role of fibrinolysis. With tissue injury, the fibrinolytic system is activated converting plasminogen to plasmin, a critical enzyme that cleaves fibrin. Plasmin and its generation are inhibited by PAI-1, by thrombin-activatable fibrinolysis inhibitor (TAFI), and by α_2-antiplasmin. Thus, fibrinolysis is regulated by multiple circulating serine protease inhibitors under physiologic conditions that can be depleted with massive hemorrhage. As a result of this pathologic activation, antifibrinolytic therapy is a critical component of a multimodal approach, the success of which has been reported in multiple patient populations undergoing surgery. In addition to contributing to a bleeding diathesis, plasmin generation causes a multitude of other effects, including cell signalling, proinflammatory responses, and activation of the complement cascade.[4]

Massive Transfusion

Massive transfusion is defined as greater than 10 units of RBCs within 24 hours after initiating treatment and occurs in approximately 10% of military trauma and approximately 5% of civilian trauma patients.[1,2] Patients who acutely bleed and receive greater than 10 units of RBCs within 6 hours of a trauma have a higher mortality. However, the massive transfusion itself is likely a marker for more severe injury rather than a direct effect of the transfusions. The development of massive transfusion strategies and use of specific protocols improves survival and has been an important evolution in the management of trauma patients, wartime injuries, and even massive hospital bleeds that occur following postpartum hemorrhage or massive surgical bleeding.

Therapeutic Approaches for Massive Transfusion and Coagulopathy

Transfusion services, blood bankers, clinicians, and hospitals have developed and implemented protocols to rapidly provide blood products for patients suffering acute and massive hemorrhage. Observational studies and retrospective analyses of military and civilian trauma initially reported improved outcomes with the administration of whole blood or whole blood equivalents with massive transfusion that include transfusion ratios of 1:1:1 for RBCs, plasma, and platelets.[1,2] However, there is also conflicting data suggesting increased morbidity and mortality associated with plasma product transfusion. Recent studies evaluating the critical plasma ratios in trauma and will be considered in more detail later in this chapter.[5]

Adverse Effects of Transfusions

All transfusions have risk and certain concerns regarding plasma are important. Major life-threatening risks of plasma administration include transfusion-related acute lung injury, transfusion-associated circulatory overload, hemolytic transfusion reactions, and anaphylaxis (these phenomenons have been discussed in an earlier chapter, Chapter 28, Blood Products and Blood Components. Deciphering the causes of adverse outcomes following transfusions can be difficult because more critically injured patients who have worse outcomes will also require more transfusions, and the reason underlying the need for transfusion will invariably cloud any interpretation of the clinical outcomes.

Hemostatic Changes Associated with Massive Transfusion Coagulopathy

Hemostatic abnormalities following massive transfusions and/or trauma can develop as a result of multiple factors not necessarily directly related to blood administration. Along with coagulopathy, hypothermia and acidosis complete the triad that results in higher mortality in the management of acute trauma. These factors may play a role in the localized depletion or decreased function of hemostatic factors through blood loss, tissue injury, and/or consumption of factors. Volume resuscitation with crystalloids, colloids, and RBCs or the use of cell salvage systems following blood loss can lead to dilutional coagulopathy. The hemostatic balance between anticoagulant and procoagulant activity may be lost due to tissue injury following trauma (including head trauma), tissue hypoxia/acidosis, burns/sepsis, or other physical events especially in an intraoperative setting from suction and reinfusion of debris.

Hypothermia can be a critical factor that precipitates or worsens coagulopathy, as enzymatic cascades are impaired; this impairment may appear beginning at even small drops in core body temperatures, even as high as 35°C. Platelet function may also be impaired with hypothermia, and platelet dysfunction can also occur due to increased fibrinogen degradation products (FDP) and D-dimer levels. Other important considerations include anemia-related factors, that is, decreased RBC adenosine diphosphate and decreased platelet diffusivity; and the effects of acidemia, which may include hypocalcemia with massive transfusions.

Perioperative Hemostatic Changes

Trauma and surgical patients have varied degrees of vascular injury and exsanguination. Blood loss up to 30% of total blood volume is generally well tolerated with the fluid resuscitation alone. Coagulation factors are progressively diluted to 30% of normal after a loss of one blood volume, and down to 15% after a loss of two blood volumes.[6] With severe hemodilution, thrombin generation, a critical step in clot formation is impaired by reduction in procoagulant levels. Thrombin generation is also impaired by thrombocytopenia. Additionally, fibrinogen and factor XIII, critical substrates for clot formation also decrease without appropriate factor replacement during volume resuscitation. Although clot may form, low levels of fibrinogen and/or factor XIII will result in reduced clot strength, a finding that is often monitored with viscoelastic blood monitoring using thromboelastography or thromboelastometry. Low levels of clotting proteins affect the ability of fibrin to polymerize.[6]

Massive Transfusion Coagulopathy

Because standard laboratory tests often take too long to obtain, and with severe hemorrhage, several blood volumes may be replaced by the time the results are available, laboratory testing plays an uncertain role in decision making in many settings where massive transfusion is necessary. Thus, transfusion protocols have been developed where fixed doses of FFP and platelets are administered after a specific number of RBC units have been given, often in a 1:1:1 ratio.[6] Whether these fixed ratios prevent the development of coagulopathy or improve bleeding is not well established in cardiac surgery, but in trauma patients and in noncardiac surgical battlefield conditions, there is growing data that fixed ratios improve survival.[7,8]

With life-threatening hemorrhage, as seen in trauma patients, transfusion of fixed ratios of RBCs, FFP, and platelets should be administered.[6] Transfusion with fixed plasma/FFP:platelet:RBC ratios report a survival benefit. As a result, the Army Surgeon General established a clinical policy of 1:1:1 (plasma/FFP:platelets:RBCs) for combat casualties expected to receive massive transfusion. One large study of civilian massive transfusion patients demonstrated improved survival with increased use of platelets.[8] The current U.S. military resuscitation practice is to use a balanced approach, using 1:1:1 as the primary resuscitation fluid for the most seriously injured casualties (http://www.cs.amedd.army.mil/borden/book/ccc/UCLAchp4.pdf). Current studies are underway to determine what the optimal ratios should be in a variety of clinical settings.

Role of Red Blood Cells and Anemia

Anemia may also contribute to bleeding as reported in nonsurgical patients due to multiple mechanisms that include nitric oxide scavenging, margination of platelets, and contributions to the hemostatic processes, although the ideal hematocrit to minimize this risk is not clear. RBC transfusions are administered for multiple reasons and they are increasingly recognized for their critical role in hemostasis. RBCs can release adenosine diphosphate, an important activator of platelets. Platelets also contribute a surface for clot initiation by facilitating thrombin generation.[6] Studies suggest that the FXIII activation and fibrin cross-linking may play an important an important role in mediating RBC retention within clots.

Causes of Bleeding in the Setting of Massive Transfusion Coagulopathy

Risk factors for developing massive transfusion coagulopathy are often related to the surgical or traumatic injury that causes the hemorrhage. Patients should be evaluated for use of additional medications that can affect coagulation, including antiplatelet agents (clopidogrel, prasugrel, ticagrelor), anticoagulation agents (dabigatran, rivaroxaban, apixaban, warfarin), or parenteral agents such as low-molecular-weight heparin.[9] Monitoring these agents has been reviewed in other chapters. Many of the standard coagulation tests used for evaluating hemorrhage cannot adequately determine the effects of antiplatelet agents (e.g., aspirin, clopidogrel, prasugrel, or ticagrelor) as the complex platelet function tests used clinically are usually ineffective with significant bleeding.

Hypothermia, Acidosis, and Coagulopathy

Hypothermia has multiple effects because coagulation is an enzymatic process. As patient temperature decreases, the enzymatic processes that function maximally at normal body temperature are impaired. Hypothermia can produce multiple hemostatic defects that include reversible platelet dysfunction and increased fibrinolysis.[10] In addition, prothrombin time (PT) and activated partial thromboplastin time (aPTT) are prolonged at temperatures of 34°C or less when compared with measurements at 37°C.[10] When blood is sampled from a hypothermic patient, the test is actually conducted at 37°C, so the influence of hypothermia on coagulopathy and bleeding may not be readily appreciated by clinicians. Overall, hypothermia is an important contributing factor to the bleeding defect in coagulopathy in trauma patients and is part of the lethal triad defined as hypothermia, acidosis, and coagulopathy. Hypothermia and acidosis can also prevent thrombin generation, a critical component of clot formation. Hypothermia is thought to inhibit the initiation phase, whereas acidosis severely inhibits the propagation phase of thrombin generation.[11] Maintenance of normothermia is important as part of a multimodal therapeutic plan for minimizing blood loss with significant hemorrhage in trauma, surgery, or coagulopathy of any cause. In a perioperative setting, blood warmers and other warming devices should be used to prevent and treat hypothermia.

Dilutional Coagulopathy

Before the development of massive transfusion protocols, dilutional coagulopathy was a common cause of bleeding in the actively hemorrhaging patient. Bleeding and coagulopathy associated with massive transfusions in 21 acutely traumatized soldiers that occurred after transfusion of 20 to 25 units of stored whole blood was described.[12] In this report, dilutional thrombocytopenia was a primary cause of the bleeding and was thought to be due to decreased platelet levels in stored blood. Transfusion of approximately 15 to 20 units caused significant dilution of blood volumes, and critical decreases in platelet count to approximately 20,000 to 30,000/mm^3, far below the recommended platelet target goals in actively bleeding patients.[12]

Fibrinolysis

Fibrinolysis is a critical component of preventing excessive clot formation and balances for hemostasis but excessive fibrinolysis as occurs commonly in trauma patients can cause bleeding. Fibrinolysis is initiated by mechanisms that include stimulating tissue plasminogen activator (tPA) release in response to vascular endothelial damage, stress responses, and other mechanisms.[4] Plasmin degrades fibrinogen and von Willebrand's factor (vWF), cleaves receptors from platelets (glycoprotein Ib), and creates degradation products that bind glycoprotein IIb/IIIa receptors, thus interfering with platelet function. Contact activation associated with tissue injury and hemostatic activation also activates kallikrein that initiates plasmin generation but also is involved in other proinflammatory steps including neutrophil chemotaxis and chemokinesis.[4] Contact activation leads to the cleaving of glycoprotein Ib receptors from platelets, and generation of FDP resulted in the creation of multimers that bind with glycoprotein IIb/IIIa receptors to prevent platelet–fibrinogen cross-linking, similar to the effects of the glycoprotein IIb/IIIa receptor inhibitor, abciximab.[13] These alterations in fibrinolysis adversely affect platelet function.

Hypofibrinogenemia

Fibrinogen is a critical component in clot formation and an acute-phase reactant protein. Fibrinogen circulates in the highest concentration of all of the coagulation factors, and normal values for plasma levels are approximately 200 to 400 mg/dL but increase in pregnancy and as a nonspecific anabolic postoperative response following tissue injury.[14] In the late stages of pregnancy, the normal physiologic response is hypercoagulability to reduce the risk of bleeding complications during birth. Although benign dilutional thrombocytopenia often develops, with a platelet count of 80,000 to 150,000/mm^3, fibrinogen levels increase to approximately 400 to 600 mg/dL. During delivery, a systemic hemostatic state develops with consumption of platelets and coagulation factors (including fibrinogen) to allow clotting to occur; hemostasis then normalizes within 4 to 6 weeks postpartum.[14]

If fibrinogen levels fall to approximately 80 to 100 mg/dL, standard clot-based coagulation tests including PT and partial thromboplastin time (PTT) can be affected. These changes may not be corrected by transfusion of FFP/plasma; however, cryoprecipitate is used or fibrinogen concentrates in countries that do not have cryoprecipitate (see earlier chapters on blood and hemostasis). Older transfusion algorithms only recommend initiating treatment when fibrinogen levels are less than 100 mg/dL and it may be difficult to reverse the effects of such low levels of this vital component of hemostatic function. European guidelines have focused on the role of normal fibrinogen levels in the bleeding patient, and recent studies also support the potential blood-sparing effects of fibrinogen concentrates.[14]

Monitoring Hemostasis during Massive Transfusion

PT and aPTT are often used for monitoring coagulopathy during massive transfusion. The PT is considered proportional to coagulation factor loss and/or hemodilution but other factors may also be responsible. These standard coagulation tests have limitations for evaluating bleeding because of the multiple coagulation defects that occur. Standard plasma-based coagulation tests also do not provide information about platelet function or interactions with coagulation factors and can be prolonged even with normal clotting factor levels due to protein C deficiency. As a result, other coagulation tests are being used more and more for managing massive transfusions.

Whole blood viscoelastic measurements continue to expand for management of trauma, perioperative bleeding, and massive transfusion coagulopathy and include either thromboelastography (TEG; Hemonetics Corporation, Braintree, MA) or thromboelastometry (ROTEM; TEM International, Cary, NC). Some of the advantages of using these systems include the ability to rapidly have information for the diagnosis and management of coagulopathy and also provide methods for algorithm- and goal-directed management. Thromboelastometry provides information about clot formation and fibrin polymerization and its use has been reported for evaluating abnormal trauma-induced coagulopathy.[6] The clot strength as determined by maximal amplitude on TEG and maximal clot firmness on ROTEM is influenced by fibrinogen levels but also by platelet contributions to the clot. In addition, using the ROTEM FIBTEM assay, systemic fibrinogen levels can be rapidly determined. The role of these advanced tests during massive transfusion continues to evolve as therapeutic strategies for transfusion and treatment algorithms are developed. In European countries where cryoprecipitate may not be available, these assays are used as therapeutic guides for both fibrinogen concentrate and prothrombin complex concentrate administration.[6]

Treatment of Coagulopathy during Massive Transfusion

A flow chart and example for the activation and institution of a massive transfusion protocol are shown in Figures 31-1 and 31-2. Specific considerations for the management have been discussed and are also included in the following perspectives regarding individual component therapy.

Plasma/Fresh Frozen Plasma

Overall, developing massive transfusion protocols has been an important therapeutic tool for effectively managing life-threatening hemorrhage after trauma.[15] Plasma/FFP contains multiple factors for hemostasis and has increasingly been considered a critical component. Most of the analyses reporting beneficial effects of high plasma ratios are retrospective and include plasma/FFP transfusion:RBC ratios of 1:1 or more from trauma. The optimal ratio of plasma/FFP:RBCs is not known, but prospective studies including a current investigation from the North American Pragmatic, Randomized Optimal Platelets and Plasma Ratios study (ClinicalTrials.gov number, NCT01545232) will provide new information. This randomized trial from 12 different medical centers will evaluate outcomes from trauma patients who will require massive transfusions as defined by the administration of more than 10 units of RBCs within 24 hours and will assess overall mortality. There are major differences in the management of severe hemorrhage between the United States and Europe. Based on currently published European guidelines, clinicians are now using factor concentrates based on thromboelastometry (ROTEM) guidance, with prothrombin complex concentrates, fibrinogen, and factor XIII. Fibrinogen and other factor concentrates have been used for many years in Europe, as cryoprecipitate is not available in all countries. However, therapy is multimodal

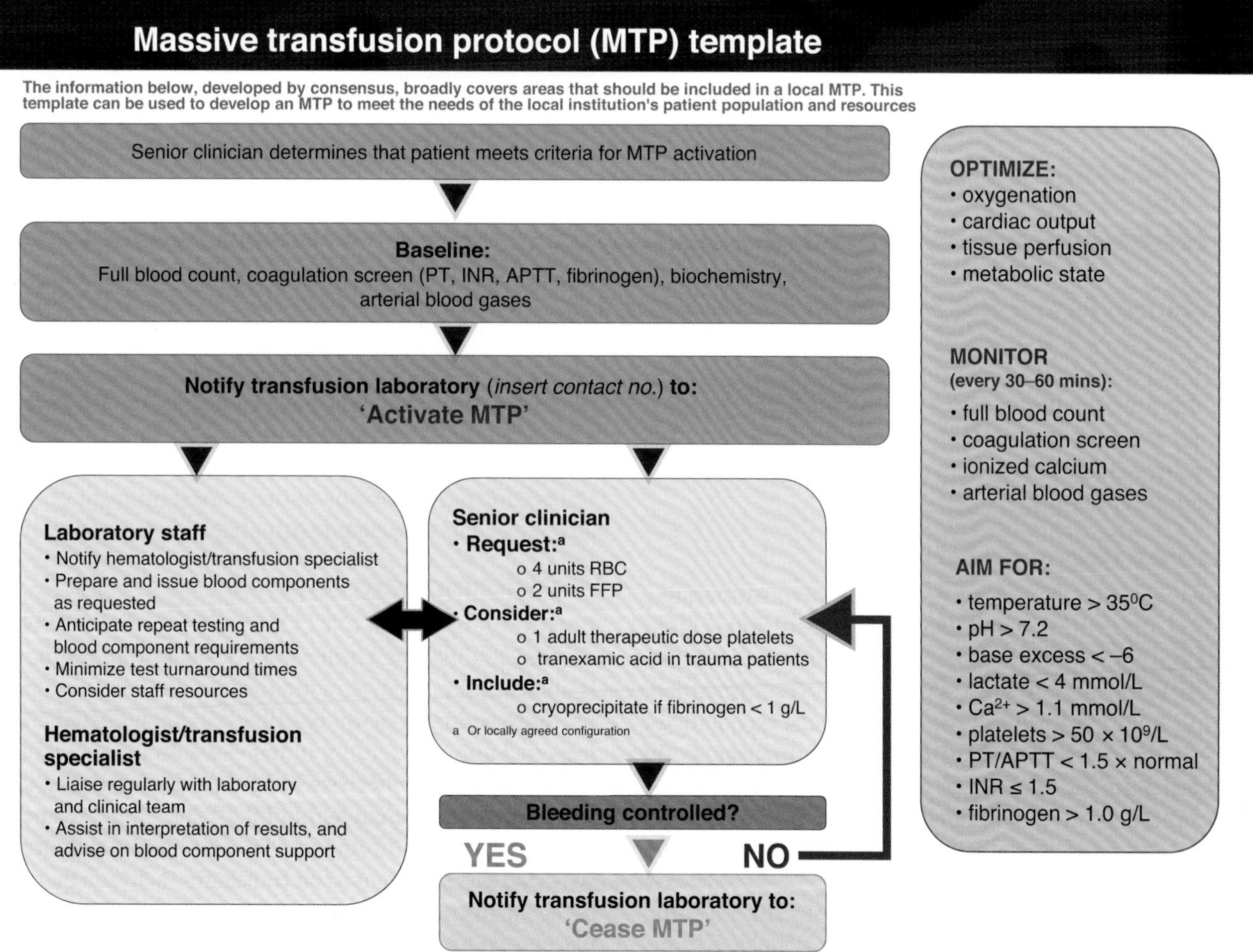

FIGURE 31-1 Massive transfusion protocol (MTP) template. (From http://www.blood.gov.au/pubs/pbm/module1/transfusion.html, with permission. Accessed September 12, 2014.

Suggested criteria for activation of MTP

- Actual or anticipated 4 units RBC in < 4 hrs, + hemodynamically unstable, +/– anticipated ongoing bleeding
- Severe thoracic, abdominal, pelvic or multiple long bone trauma
- Major obstetric, gastrointestinal or surgical bleeding

Initial management of bleeding

- Identify cause
- Initial measures:
  - compression
  - tourniquet
  - packing
- Surgical assessment:
  - early surgery or angiography to stop bleeding

Specific surgical considerations

- If significant physiological derangement, consider damage control surgery or angiography

Cell salvage

- Consider use of cell salvage where appropriate

Dosage

Platelet count < 50 x 10^9/L	1 adult therapeutic dose
INR > 1.5	FFP 15 mL/kg[a]
Fibrinogen < 1.0 g/L	cryoprecipitate 3–4 g[a]
Tranexamic acid	loading dose 1 g over 10 min, then infusion of 1 g over 8 hrs

a Local transfusion laboratory to advise on number of units needed to provide this dose

Resuscitation

- Avoid hypothermia, institute active warming
- Avoid excessive crystalloid
- Tolerate permissive hypotension (BP 80–100 mmHg systolic) until active bleeding controlled
- Do not use hemoglobin alone as a transfusion trigger

Special clinical situations

- Warfarin:
  - add vitamin K, prothrombin complex concentrates/FFP
- Obstetric hemorrhage:
  - early DIC often present; consider cryoprecipitate
- Head injury:
  - aim for platelet count > 100 x 10^9/L
  - permissive hypotension contraindicated

Considerations for use of rFVIIa[b]

The *routine* use of rFVIIa in trauma patients is not recommended due to its lack of effect on mortality (Grade B) and variable effect on morbidity (Grade C). Institutions may choose to develop a process for the use of rFVIIa where there is:

- uncontrolled hemorrhage in salvageable patient, and
- failed surgical or radiological measures to control bleeding, and
- adequate blood component replacement, and
- pH > 7.2, temperature > 34°C.

Discuss dose with hematologist/transfusion specialist

[b] rFVIIa is not licensed for use in this situation; all use must be part of practice review.

ABG	arterial blood gas	FFP	fresh frozen plasma	APTT	activated partial thromboplastin time
INR	international normalised ratio	BP	blood pressure	MTP	massive transfusion protocol
DIC	disseminated intravascular coagulation	PT	prothrombin time	FBC	full blood count
RBC	red blood cell	rFVIIa	activated recombinant factor VII		

FIGURE 31-2 Suggested criteria for activation of massive transfusion protocol (MTP) template. (From http://www.blood.gov.au/pubs/pbm/module1/transfusion.html, with permission. Accessed September 12, 2014.

and requires hemodynamic and hemostatic support as well as efforts to address the underlying bleeding source. An example of a massive transfusion protocol is shown in Figure 31-1.[6]

Platelet Administration

Following traumatic injury or significant postoperative bleeding, the critical platelet count for transfusion is often based on consensus therapy rather than true objective data. Although a count of 50,000 or more is recommended, the threshold for administration of platelets, especially in cases of dilutional coagulopathy, remains unclear as do the ideal ratio of platelets to other blood components. Most protocols attempt to develop a strategy that mimics whole blood replacement with RBC:plasma/FFP: platelets at a 1:1:1 ratio with massive bleeding.[13,14]

However, assessing platelet function in the bleeding patient is not possible; therefore, empiric platelet administration is often undertaken. If patients have received antiplatelet agents recently, then even the existing platelets and platelet counts may not be helpful. Therefore, if patients have received antiplatelet agents or are bleeding after separation from cardiopulmonary bypass, then platelet dysfunction should be suspected and platelet concentrates considered. However, there are significant potential adverse events associated with platelet administration.[6]

Antifibrinolytic Agents

Because of the critical role of fibrinolysis with severe bleeding and trauma, the antifibrinolytic agent tranexamic acid is increasingly used as a therapeutic strategy. Inhibiting fibrinolysis during acute bleeding has many beneficial effects including preserving initial clot formation at a bleeding site that may otherwise be broken down, similar to the clot destruction seen in hemophilia.[6] The Clinical Randomization of an Antifibrinolytic in Significant Hemorrhage (CRASH 2) study focused on tranexamic acid as a therapeutic agent in traumatic injury in a prospective randomized placebo-controlled trial of 1-g loading followed by 1 g over 8 hours in 20,211 trauma patients. Overall mortality was reduced from 14.5% to 16.0% (relative risk, 0.91; $P = 0.0035$), as were deaths due to bleeding (4.9% vs. 5.7%; relative risk,

0.85; $P = 0.0077$). Tranexamic acid is also approved in the United States for excessive menstrual bleeding at a dose of 1.3 g three times a day (~4 g total dose), without significant reported safety issues. Despite the efficacy and safety of tranexamic acid, clinicians often substitute epsilon-aminocaproic acid, another lysine analog, although this agent has not been studied as well as tranexamic acid and is not available in some European countries.

Procoagulants

Multiple other agents have been used or studied in trauma and massive transfusion coagulopathy, including recombinant activated factor VII and prothrombin complex concentrates. The off-label use of many of these agents to increase clot formation following major surgery and or traumatic injury is a reasonable but empiric approach for treating life-threatening bleeding and often used as a "last-ditch effort" in patients with ongoing bleeding and at risk for death or other adverse events. When clinicians are presented with a patient who continues to bleed despite standard therapeutic interventions, they have two choices. They can either continue to give their standard interventions (that have already failed to work) or administer a procoagulant such as recombinant activated factor VII and prothrombin complex concentrates. Clinicians are justified in choosing a procoagulant plan of action for several reasons.[16] First, it is clinically evident that patients with massive refractory bleeding will have adverse outcomes unless the blood loss is controlled in a timely manner. Second, persisting with standard interventions will likely not achieve this goal and will unnecessarily expose patients to the risks of excessive blood product administration. Third, the efficacy and safety data from most randomized trials are not applicable to these situations because patients with refractory bleeding were not studied. Fourth, even if the safety data from randomized trials do apply, which all suggest that procoagulants by virtue of their effects increase the risk of thromboembolic complications, this risk is relative to that of allowing bleeding and exsanguination to occur. Fifth, observational data from Europe and some randomized trial data in bleeding patients suggests that use of procoagulant therapy and concentrates is effective for refractory blood loss using factor concentrate driven algorithms. Finally, given the ethical implications and impracticality of such trials, it is unlikely that additional applicable data from placebo-controlled randomized trials to evaluate life-threatening hemorrhage will ever be performed.

Postpartum Hemorrhage

Postpartum hemorrhage is an important cause of life-threatening hemorrhage and continues to be a major cause of maternal mortality.[17] A recent published report from an international expert panel in obstetrics, gynecology, anesthesiology, hematology, and transfusion medicine performed a comprehensive literature review to identify patients at high risk of adverse outcomes.[17] They defined severe persistent postpartum hemorrhage as "active bleeding greater than 1,000 mL within the 24 hours following birth that continues despite the use of initial measures including first-line uterotonic agents and uterine massage." As in all life-threatening bleeding, a treatment algorithm that includes a massive transfusion protocol is important. The group suggested coagulation testing should be performed to guide therapy. If initial therapy fails to stop bleeding and uterine atony persists, second- and third-line interventions, including mechanical or surgical maneuvers, that is, intrauterine balloon tamponade or hemostatic brace sutures with hysterectomy are the final surgical option for uncontrollable bleeding.[17] Pharmacologic options include hemostatic agents, including tranexamic acid along with a massive transfusion protocol for blood product administration are also critical to minimize blood loss and optimize clinical outcomes in management of women with severe, persistent postpartum hemorrhage.[17]

Multimodal Resuscitation: Damage Control Resuscitation

Managing life-threatening and uncontrolled bleeding is a clinical problem that can occur following traumatic injury, during major surgical procedures, and following delivery. From information learned from combat and battlefield casualties, a multimodal and multispecialty approach has evolved that includes perspectives from surgeons, anesthesiologists, emergency medicine physicians, and transfusion medicine specialists for the optimal resuscitative approach to hemorrhagic shock.[1,10,18] Clinicians and investigators from multiple specialties have coined the term ***damage control resuscitation***, a multimodal strategy.[19] This concept calls for (a) early and increased use of plasma, platelets, and RBCs while minimizing crystalloid use; (b) hypotensive resuscitation strategies; (c) avoiding hypothermia and acidosis that may compound coagulopathy; (d) use of adjuncts such as calcium, THAM (tris-hydroxymethyl aminomethane, an alternate alkalizing agent to sodium bicarbonate), and tranexamic acid and off-label uses of procoagulation agents; and (d) early definitive hemorrhage control.[19]

Summary

Coagulopathy associated with massive transfusion is a complex, multifactorial clinical problem. When evaluating the causes of coagulopathy in this setting, preexisting pharmacotherapy including prior use of anticoagulants must be considered. The role of hypothermia, dilutional coagulopathy, platelet dysfunction and fibrinolysis should also be considered. Evaluating fibrinogen levels represents a critical aspect of all transfusion algorithms, especially for patients with massive transfusion and life-threatening hemorrhage. Transfusion algorithms are a critical and relatively new aspect of perioperative management; they attempt to provide adequate factor and hemostatic replacement, although the ideal ratio of various blood components and factor concentrates are still being determined. Significant changes in management have become important in resuscitation strategies and crystalloids are no longer a primary means of resuscitation; the primary strategy now is replacing acute blood loss with plasma and platelet-containing products instead of early and large amounts of crystalloids and RBCs.[1] Templates for a massive transfusion protocol and activation of a massive transfusion protocol are included in Figures 31-1 and 31-2. Several excellent reviews are available for additional reading on this subject.[1,2,6,18]

References

1. Holcomb JB, Pati S. Optimal trauma resuscitation with plasma as the primary resuscitative fluid: the surgeon's perspective. *Hematology Am Soc Hematol Educ Program*. 2013;2013:656–659.
2. Holcomb JB. Optimal use of blood products in severely injured trauma patients. *Hematology Am Soc Hematol Educ Program*. 2010; 2010:465–469.
3. Cotton BA, Au BK, Nunez TC, et al. Predefined massive transfusion protocols are associated with a reduction in organ failure and postinjury complications. *J Trauma*. 2009;66:41–48; discussion 8–9.
4. Levy JH. Antifibrinolytic therapy: new data and new concepts. *Lancet*. 2010;376:3–4.
5. Goodnough LT, Spain DA, Maggio P. Logistics of transfusion support for patients with massive hemorrhage. *Curr Opin Anesthesiol*. 2013;26(2):208–214.
6. Bolliger D, Gorlinger K, Tanaka KA. Pathophysiology and treatment of coagulopathy in massive hemorrhage and hemodilution. *Anesthesiology*. 2010;113:1205–1219.
7. Dente CJ, Shaz BH, Nicholas JM, et al. Improvements in early mortality and coagulopathy are sustained better in patients with blunt trauma after institution of a massive transfusion protocol in a civilian level I trauma center. *J Trauma*. 2009;66:1616–1624.
8. Holcomb JB, Wade CE, Michalek JE, et al. Increased plasma and platelet to red blood cell ratios improves outcome in 466 massively transfused civilian trauma patients. *Ann Surg*. 2008;248:447–458.
9. Levy JH, Faraoni D, Spring JL, et al. Managing new oral anticoagulants in the perioperative and intensive care unit setting. *Anesthesiology*. 2013;118:1466–1474.
10. Levy JH. Massive transfusion coagulopathy. *Semin Hematol*. 2006; 43:S59–S63.
11. Martini WZ. Coagulopathy by hypothermia and acidosis: mechanisms of thrombin generation and fibrinogen availability. *J Trauma*. 2009;67:202–208; discussion 8–9.
12. Miller RD, Robbins TO, Tong MJ, et al. Coagulation defects associated with massive blood transfusions. *Ann Surg*. 1971;174:794–801.
13. Rinder CS, Mathew JP, Rinder HM, et al. Modulation of platelet surface adhesion receptors during cardiopulmonary bypass. *Anesthesiology*. 1991;75:563–570.
14. Levy JH, Welsby I, Goodnough LT. Fibrinogen as a therapeutic target for bleeding: a review of critical levels and replacement therapy. *Transfusion*. 2014;54:1389–1405.
15. Roback JD, Caldwell S, Carson J, et al. Evidence-based practice guidelines for plasma transfusion. *Transfusion*. 2010;50:1227–1239.
16. Karkouti K, Levy JH. Recombinant activated factor vii: the controversial conundrum regarding its off-label use. *Anesth Analg*. 2011; 113:711–712.
17. Abdul-Kadir R, McLintock C, Ducloy AS, et al. Evaluation and management of postpartum hemorrhage: consensus from an international expert panel [published online ahead of print March 12, 2014]. *Transfusion*.
18. Levy JH, Dutton RP, Hemphill JC III, et al. Multidisciplinary approach to the challenge of hemostasis. *Anesth Analg*. 2010;110:354–364.
19. Holcomb JB, Jenkins D, Rhee P, et al. Damage control resuscitation: directly addressing the early coagulopathy of trauma. *J Trauma*. 2007;62:307–310.

CHAPTER 32

Gastrointestinal Physiology

Michael J. Murray

Liver

The liver lies in the right upper quadrant of the abdominal cavity and is attached to the diaphragm. It is the largest organ in the body, weighing approximately 1,500 g and representing 2% of body weight. In the neonate, the liver accounts for approximately 5% of body weight. Hepatocytes represent approximately 80% of the cytoplasmic mass within the liver. These cells perform diverse and complex functions (Table 32-1). The ability of hemopoietic stem cells to differentiate into hepatocytes introduces the possibility of treating inherited disorders of metabolism (reflecting absent to altered enzymes due to a single or multiple genetic defect) in the future.[1,2]

Anatomy

The liver is divided into four lobes consisting of 50,000 to 100,000 individual hepatic lobules (Fig. 32-1). Blood flows past hepatocytes via sinusoids from branches of the portal vein and hepatic artery to a central vein. There is usually only one layer of hepatocytes between sinusoids so the total area of contact with plasma is great. Central veins join to form hepatic veins, which drain into the inferior vena cava. Each hepatocyte is also located adjacent to bile canaliculi, which coalesce to form the common hepatic duct. This duct and the cystic duct from the gallbladder join to form the common bile duct, which enters the duodenum at a site surrounded by the sphincter of Oddi (Fig. 32-2).[3] The main pancreatic duct also unites with the common bile duct just before it enters the duodenum.

Hepatic lobules are lined by macrophages (derived from circulating monocytes) known as Kupffer cells, which phagocytize 99% or more of bacteria in the portal venous blood. This is crucial because the portal venous blood drains the gastrointestinal tract and usually contains colon bacteria.

Endothelial cells that line the hepatic lobules contain large pores, permitting easy diffusion of certain substances, including plasma proteins, into extravascular spaces of the liver that connect with terminal lymphatics. The extreme permeability of the lining of endothelial cells allows large quantities of lymph to form, which contain protein concentrations that are only slightly less than the protein concentration of plasma. Indeed, approximately one-third to one-half of all the lymph is formed in the liver.

Hepatic Blood Flow

The liver receives a dual afferent blood supply from the hepatic artery and portal veins (Fig. 32-3). Total hepatic blood flow is approximately 1,450 mL per minute or approximately 29% of the cardiac output. Of this amount, the portal vein provides 75% of the total flow but only 50% to 55% of the hepatic oxygen supply because this blood is partially deoxygenated in the preportal organs and tissues (gastrointestinal tract, spleen, pancreas). The hepatic artery provides only 25% of total hepatic blood flow but provides 45% to 50% of the hepatic oxygen requirements. Hepatic artery blood flow maintains nutrition of connective tissues and walls of bile ducts. For this reason, loss of hepatic artery blood flow can be fatal because of ensuing necrosis of vital liver structures. An increase in hepatic oxygen requirements is met by an increase in oxygen extraction rather than a further increase in the already high hepatic blood flow.

Control of Hepatic Blood Flow

Portal vein blood flow is controlled primarily by the arterioles in the preportal splanchnic organs. This flow,

Table 32-1

Functions of Hepatocytes

Functions of Hepatocytes
Absorb nutrients from portal venous blood
Store and release carbohydrates, proteins, and lipids
Excrete bile salts
Synthesize plasma proteins, glucose, cholesterol, and fatty acids
Metabolize exogenous and endogenous compounds

combined with the resistance to portal vein blood flow within the liver, determines portal venous pressure (normally 7 to 10 mm Hg) (see the section "Portal Venous Pressure"). Sympathetic nervous system innervation is from T3 to T11 and is mediated via α-adrenergic receptors. This innervation is principally responsible for resistance and compliance of hepatic venules. Changes in hepatic venous compliance play an essential role in overall regulation of cardiac output and the reservoir function of the liver (see the section "Reservoir Function").

Fibrotic constriction characteristic of hepatic cirrhosis (most often due to chronic alcohol abuse and hepatitis C) can increase resistance to portal vein blood flow, as evidenced by portal venous pressures of 20 to 30 mm Hg (portal hypertension). The resulting increased resistance to portal vein blood flow may result in development of shunts (varices) to allow blood flow to bypass the hepatocytes. Conversely, congestive heart failure and positive

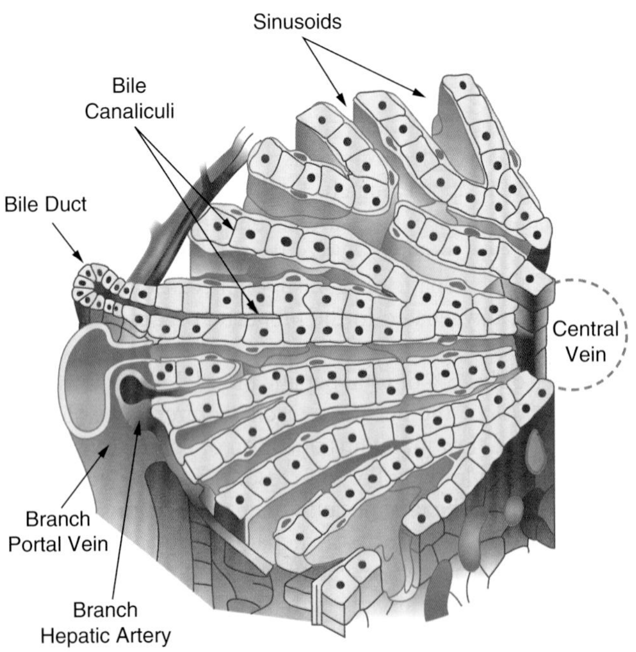

FIGURE 32-1 Schematic depiction of a hepatic lobule with a central vein and plates of hepatic cells extending radially. Blood from peripherally located branches of the hepatic artery and vein perfuses the sinusoids. Bile ducts drain the bile canaliculi that pass between the hepatocytes.

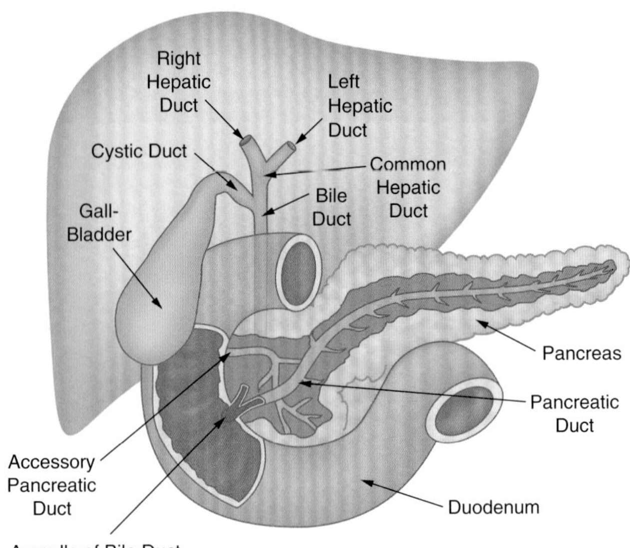

FIGURE 32-2 Connections of the ducts of the gallbladder, liver, and pancreas.

pressure ventilation of the lungs impair outflow of blood from the liver because of increased central venous pressure, which is transmitted to hepatic veins. Ascites results when increased portal venous pressures cause transudation of protein-rich fluid through the outer surface of the liver capsule and gastrointestinal tract into the abdominal cavity. Hepatic artery blood flow is influenced by arteriolar tone that reflects local and intrinsic mechanisms (autoregulation). For example, a decrease in portal vein blood flow is accompanied by an increase in hepatic artery blood flow by as much as 100%. Presumably, a vasodilating substance such as adenosine accumulates in the liver when portal vein blood flow decreases, leading to

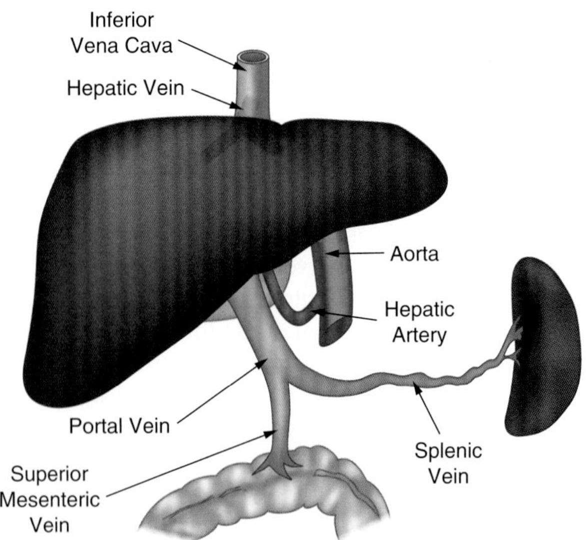

FIGURE 32-3 Schematic depiction of the dual afferent blood supply to the liver provided by the portal vein and hepatic artery.

subsequent hepatic arterial vasodilation and washout of the vasodilating material.

Halothane decreases hepatic oxygen supply more than isoflurane, enflurane, desflurane, or sevoflurane when administered in equal potent doses.[4] In contrast to the other volatile anesthetics, halothane preserves autoregulation of hepatic blood flow only to a limited extent and only when used in doses that do not decrease systemic blood pressure >20%. Surgical stimulation may further decrease hepatic blood flow, independent of the anesthetic drug administered. The greatest decreases in hepatic blood flow occur during intraabdominal operations, presumably due to mechanical interference of blood flow produced by retraction in the operative area, as well as the release of vasoconstricting substances such as catecholamines.

Reservoir Function

The liver normally contains approximately 500 mL of blood or approximately 10% of the total blood volume. An increase in central venous pressure causes back pressure, and the liver, being a distendible organ, may accommodate as much as 1 L of extra blood. As such, the liver acts as a storage site when blood volume is excessive, as in congestive heart failure, and is capable of supplying extra blood when hypovolemia occurs. Indeed, the large hepatic veins and sinuses are constricted by stimulation from the sympathetic nervous system, discharging up to 350 mL of blood into the circulation. Therefore, the liver is the single most important source of additional blood during strenuous exercise or acute hemorrhage.

Bile Secretion

Hepatocytes continually form bile (500 mL daily) and then secrete it into bile canaliculi, which empty into progressively larger ducts, ultimately reaching the common bile duct (see Fig. 32-2).[3] Between meals, the tone of the sphincter of Oddi, which guards the entrance of the common bile duct into the duodenum, is high. As a result, bile flow is diverted into the gallbladder, which has a capacity of 35 to 50 mL. The most potent stimulus for emptying the gallbladder is the presence of fat in the duodenum, which evokes the release of the hormone cholecystokinin by the duodenal mucosa. This hormone enters the circulation and passes to the gallbladder, where it causes selective contraction of the gallbladder smooth muscle. As a result, bile is forced from the gallbladder into the duodenum. When adequate amounts of fat are present, the gallbladder empties in approximately 1 hour.

The principal components of bile are bile salts, bilirubin, and cholesterol.

Bile Salts

Bile salts combine with lipids in the duodenum to form water-soluble complexes (micelles) that facilitate gastrointestinal absorption of fats (triglycerides) and fat-soluble vitamins. Once absorbed, bile salts return to the liver via the portal vein, where they enter hepatocytes (enterohepatic circulation). In the absence of bile secretion, steatorrhea and a deficiency of vitamin K develop in a few days. Vitamin K is necessary for activation of several of the clotting factors that contain glutamic acid residues.

Bilirubin

After approximately 120 days, the cell membranes of erythrocytes rupture, and the released hemoglobin is converted to bilirubin in reticuloendothelial cells (Fig. 32-4).[5] The resulting bilirubin is released into the circulation and transported in combination with albumin to the liver. In hepatocytes, bilirubin dissociates from albumin and conjugates principally with glucuronic acid. Unlike conjugated bilirubin, unconjugated bilirubin may be neurotoxic and may even cause a rapidly fatal encephalopathy. In the gastrointestinal tract, bilirubin is converted by bacterial action mainly into urobilinogen.

Jaundice

Jaundice is the yellowish tint of body tissues that accompanies accumulation of bilirubin in extracellular fluid. Skin color usually begins to change when the plasma concentration of bilirubin increases to approximately three times normal. The most common types of jaundice

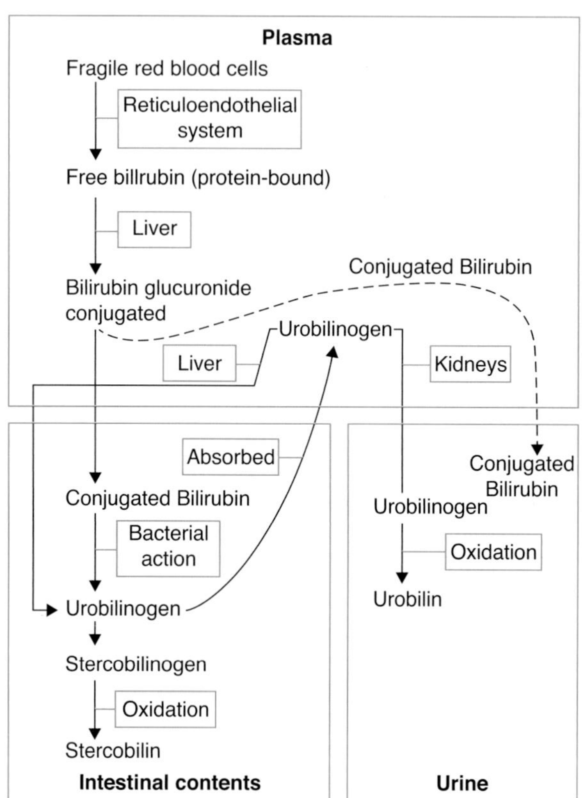

FIGURE 32-4 Schematic depiction of bilirubin formation and excretion. (From Guyton AC, Hall JE. *Textbook of Medical Physiology.* 10th ed. Philadelphia, PA: Saunders; 2000, with permission.)

are hemolytic jaundice, due to increased destruction of erythrocytes, and obstructive jaundice, due to obstruction of bile ducts.

Cholesterol

Cholesterol is an important component of cell walls (synthesized in tissues from acetate in a reaction catalyzed by β-hydroxy β-methylglutaryl coenzyme A) and is transported from the periphery to the liver as high-density lipoproteins (HDL). Once cholesterol has reached the liver, it can be excreted in the bile in association with bile acids. Cholesterol in the bile may precipitate as gallstones if there is excess absorption of water in the gallbladder or the diet contains too much cholesterol. Gallstones occur in 10% to 20% of individuals; 85% are cholesterol stones.

Metabolic Functions

Metabolism of carbohydrates, lipids, and proteins depends on normal hepatic function (see Chapter 33). Furthermore, the liver is an important storage site for vitamins and iron. Degradation of certain hormones (catecholamines and corticosteroids), as well as drugs, is an important function of the liver. Hepatocytes are the principal site for synthesis of all the coagulation factors, with the exception of von Willebrand factor and factor VIIIC. Because the half-life of clotting factors produced in the liver is short, coagulation is particularly sensitive to acute hepatocellular damage.

Carbohydrates

Regulation of blood glucose concentration is an important metabolic function of the liver. When hyperglycemia is present, glycogen is deposited in the liver, and when hypoglycemia occurs, glycogenolysis provides glucose. Amino acids can be converted to glucose by gluconeogenesis when the blood glucose concentration is decreased.

Lipids

The liver is responsible for β-oxidation of fatty acids and formation of acetoacetic acid. Triglycerides are formed from the esterification of glycerol with three molecules of fatty acid. Pancreatic lipases and esterases are important in facilitating the absorption of dietary fats. After absorption, fat may be stored as triglycerides (reserve energy) or metabolized to energy. Lipoproteins, cholesterol, and phospholipids, such as lecithin, are formed in the liver. Synthesis of fats from carbohydrates and proteins also occurs in the liver.

Proteins

The most important liver functions in protein metabolism are oxidative deamination of amino acids, formation of urea for removal of ammonia, formation of plasma proteins and coagulation factors, and interconversions (transfer of one amino group to another amino acid) among different amino acids. Albumin formed in the liver is critically important for maintaining plasma oncotic pressure as well as providing an essential transport role. The half-life for albumin is about 21 days; therefore, plasma albumin concentrations are unlikely to be significantly altered in acute hepatic failure. Deamination of amino acids is required before these substances can be used for energy or converted into carbohydrates or fats. Decreases in portal vein blood flow, as may occur with the surgical creation of a portocaval shunt to treat esophageal varices, can result in fatal hepatic coma because of accumulation of ammonia.

Gastrointestinal Tract

The primary function of the gastrointestinal tract is to provide the body with a continual supply of water, electrolytes, and nutrients. To achieve this goal, the contents of the gastrointestinal tract must move through the entire system at an appropriate rate for digestive and absorptive functions to occur. Each part of the gastrointestinal tract is adapted for specific functions such as (a) passage of food in the esophagus, (b) storage of food in the stomach or fecal matter in the colon, (c) digestion of food in the stomach and small intestine, and (d) absorption of the digestive end products and fluids in the small intestine and proximal parts of the colon. Overall, approximately 9 L of fluid and secretions enters the gastrointestinal tract daily, and all but approximately 100 mL is absorbed by the small intestine and colon (Fig. 32-5).[6] The pH of gastrointestinal secretions varies widely (Table 32-2).

Anatomy

The smooth muscle of the gastrointestinal tract is a syncytium such that electrical signals originating in one smooth muscle fiber are easily propagated from fiber to fiber. Mechanical activity of the gastrointestinal tract is enhanced by stretch and parasympathetic nervous system stimulation, whereas sympathetic nervous system stimulation decreases mechanical activity to almost zero.

Table 32-2

pH and Gastrointestinal Secretions

Secretions	pH
Saliva	6–7
Gastric fluid	1.0–3.5
Bile	7–8
Pancreatic fluid	8.0–8.3
Small intestine	6.5–7.5
Colon	7.5–8.0

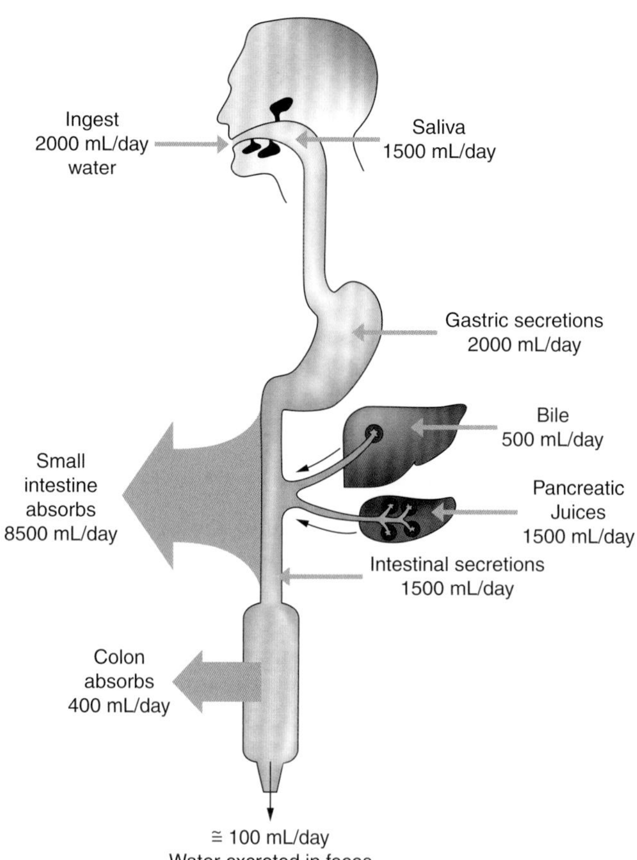

FIGURE 32-5 Overall fluid balance in the human gastrointestinal tract. Approximately 2 L of water are ingested each day and approximately 7 L of various secretions enter the gastrointestinal tract. Of this 9 L, about 8.5 L are absorbed from the small intestine. Approximately 0.5 L passes to the colon, which normally absorbs 80% to 90% of the water presented to it. (From Berne RM, Levy M, Koeppen BM, et al. *Physiology*. 5th ed. St Louis, MO: Mosby; 2004, with permission.)

Tonic contraction of gastrointestinal smooth muscle at the pylorus, ileocecal valve, and anal sphincter helps regulate the rate at which materials move through the gastrointestinal tract. In these parts of the gastrointestinal tract, rhythmic movements (peristalsis) occur 3 to 12 times per minute to facilitate mixing and movement of food.

Blood Flow

Most of the blood flow to the gastrointestinal tract is to the mucosa to supply energy needed for producing intestinal secretions and absorbing digested materials. Blood flow parallels digestive activity of the gastrointestinal tract. Approximately 80% of portal vein blood flow originates from the stomach and gastrointestinal tract, with the remainder coming from the spleen and pancreas.

Stimulation of the parasympathetic nervous system increases local blood flow at the same time it increases glandular secretions. Conversely, stimulation of the sympathetic nervous system causes vasoconstriction of the arterial supply to the gastrointestinal tract. The decrease in blood flow, however, is transient because local metabolic vasodilator mechanisms elicited by ischemia return blood flow toward normal. The importance of this transient sympathetic nervous system–induced vasoconstriction is that it permits shunting of blood from the gastrointestinal tract for brief periods during exercise, or when increased blood flow is needed by skeletal muscles or the heart.

Portal Venous Pressure

The liver offers modest resistance to blood flow from the portal venous system. As a result, the pressure in the portal vein averages 7 to 10 mm Hg, which is considerably higher than the almost zero pressure in the inferior vena cava. Cirrhosis of the liver, most frequently caused by alcoholism, is characterized by increased resistance to portal vein blood flow due to replacement of hepatic cells with fibrous tissue that contracts around the blood vessels. The gradual increase in resistance to portal vein blood flow produced by cirrhosis of the liver causes large collateral vessels to develop between the portal veins and the systemic veins. The most important of these collaterals are from the splenic veins to the esophageal veins. These collaterals may become so large that they protrude into the lumen of the esophagus, producing esophageal varicosities. The esophageal mucosa overlying these varicosities may become eroded, leading to life-threatening hemorrhage.

In the absence of the development of adequate collaterals, sustained increases in portal vein pressure may cause protein-containing fluid to escape from the surface of the mesentery, gastrointestinal tract, and liver into the peritoneal cavity. This fluid, known as ***ascites***, is similar to plasma, and its high protein content causes an increased colloid osmotic pressure in the abdominal fluid. This high colloid osmotic pressure draws additional fluid from the surfaces of the gastrointestinal tract and mesentery into the peritoneal cavity.

Splenic Circulation

The splenic capsule in humans, in contrast to that in many lower animals, is nonmuscular, which limits the ability of the spleen to release stored blood in response to sympathetic nervous system stimulation. A small amount (150 to 200 mL) of blood is stored in the splenic venous sinuses and can be released by sympathetic nervous system–induced vasoconstriction of the splenic vessels. Release of this amount of blood into the systemic circulation is sufficient to increase the hematocrit 1% to 2%.

The spleen functions to remove erythrocytes from the circulation. This occurs when erythrocytes reenter the venous sinuses from the splenic pulp by passing through pores that may be smaller than the erythrocyte. Fragile cells do not withstand this trauma, and the released hemoglobin that results from their rupture is ingested by the reticuloendothelial cells of the spleen. These same reticuloendothelial cells also function, much like lymph nodes, to remove bacteria and parasites from the circulation. Indeed, asplenic patients are more prone to developing bacterial infections.

During fetal life, the splenic pulp produces erythrocytes in the same manner as does the bone marrow in the adult. As the fetus reaches maturity, however, this function of the spleen is lost.

Innervation

The gastrointestinal tract receives innervation from both divisions of the autonomic nervous system as well as from an intrinsic nervous system consisting of the myenteric plexus, or Auerbach plexus, and the submucous plexus, or Meissner plexus. In the absence of sympathetic nervous system or parasympathetic nervous system innervation, the motor and secretory activities of the gastrointestinal tract continue, reflecting the function of the intrinsic nervous system. Signals from the autonomic nervous system influence the activity of the intrinsic nervous system. For example, impulses from the parasympathetic nervous system increase intrinsic activity, whereas signals from the sympathetic nervous system decrease intrinsic activity. A large number of neuromodulatory substances act in the gastrointestinal tract.

The cranial component of parasympathetic nervous system innervation to the gastrointestinal tract (esophagus, stomach, pancreas, small intestine, colon to the level of the transverse colon) is by way of the vagus nerves. The distal portion of the colon is richly supplied by the sacral parasympathetics via the pelvic nerves from the hypogastric plexus. Fibers of the sympathetic nervous system destined for the gastrointestinal tract pass through ganglia such as the celiac ganglia.

Motility

The two types of gastrointestinal motility are mixing contractions and propulsive movements characterized as ***peristalsis***. The usual stimulus for peristalsis is distension. Peristalsis occurs only weakly in portions of the gastrointestinal tract that have congenital absence of the myenteric plexus. Peristalsis is also decreased by increased parasympathetic nervous system activity and anticholinergic drugs.

Ileus

Trauma to the intestine or irritation of the peritoneum as follows abdominal operations causes adynamic (paralytic) ileus. Peristalsis returns to the small intestine in 6 to 8 hours, but colonic activity may take 2 to 3 days. Adynamic ileus can be relieved by a tube placed into the small intestine and aspiration of fluid and gas until the time when peristalsis returns.

Salivary Glands

The principal salivary glands (parotid and submaxillary) produce 0.5 to 1.0 mL per minute of saliva (pH 6 to 7), largely in response to parasympathetic nervous system stimulation. Saliva washes away pathogenic bacteria in the oral cavity as well as food particles that provide nutrition for bacteria. In the absence of saliva, oral tissues are likely to become ulcerated and infected. The bicarbonate ion concentration in saliva is two to four times that in plasma, and the high potassium content of saliva can result in hypokalemia and skeletal muscle weakness if excess salivation persists.

Esophagus

The esophagus serves as a conduit for passage of food from the pharynx to the stomach. The swallowing or deglutition center located in the medulla and lower pons inhibits the medullary ventilatory center, halting breathing at any point to allow swallowing to proceed. The upper and lower ends of the esophagus function as sphincters to prevent entry of air and acidic gastric contents, respectively, into the esophagus. The sphincters are known as the ***upper esophageal (pharyngoesophageal) sphincter*** and ***lower esophageal (gastroesophageal) sphincter***.

Lower Esophageal Sphincter

The lower esophageal sphincter regulates the flow of food between the esophagus and the stomach. The sphincter mechanism at the lower end of the esophagus consists of the intrinsic smooth muscle of the distal esophagus and the skeletal muscle of the crural diaphragm.[7] Under normal circumstances, the lower esophageal sphincter is approximately 4 cm long. The crural diaphragm, which forms the esophageal hiatus, encircles the proximal 2 cm of the sphincter. The intraluminal pressure of the esophagogastric junction is a measure of the strength of the antireflux barrier and is typically quantified with reference to the intragastric pressure (normal $<$7 mm Hg). Both the lower esophageal sphincter and the crural diaphragm contribute to the intragastric pressure. Muscle tone in the lower esophageal sphincter is the result of neurogenic and myogenic mechanisms. A substantial part of the neurogenic tone in humans is due to cholinergic innervation via the vagus nerves. The presynaptic neurotransmitter is acetylcholine, and the postsynaptic neurotransmitter is nitric oxide.

The normal lower esophageal sphincter pressure is 10 to 30 mm Hg at end-exhalation.[7] Transient relaxation of the lower esophageal sphincter is a neural reflex mediated through the brainstem. Gastric barrier pressure is calculated as lower esophageal sphincter pressure minus intragastric pressure. This barrier pressure is considered the major mechanism in preventing reflux of gastric contents into the esophagus. Gastric distension, meals high in fat, and pharyngeal stimulation are two possible mechanisms

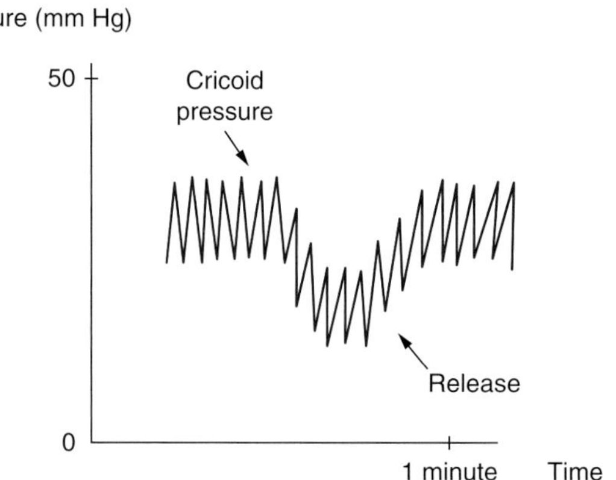

FIGURE 32-6 Application of cricoid pressure causes the lower esophageal sphincter pressure to decrease. (From Chassard D, Tournadre JP, Berrada KR, et al. Cricoid pressure decreases lower esophageal sphincter tone in anaesthetized pigs. *Can J Anaesth.* 1996;43:414–417, with permission.)

by which the afferent stimulus that initiates transient relaxation of the lower esophageal sphincter may originate.[8] Cricoid pressure decreases lower esophageal sphincter pressure, presumably reflecting stimulation of mechanoreceptors in the pharynx created by the external pressure on the cricoid cartilage (Fig. 32-6).[9–11] General anesthesia decreases lower esophageal sphincter pressure 7 to 14 mm Hg, depending on the degree of skeletal muscle relaxation.[12] Normally, upper esophageal sphincter pressure prevents regurgitation into the pharynx in the awake state. The administration of anesthetic drugs may decrease upper esophageal sphincter pressure even before the loss of consciousness.[12]

The influence, if any, of changes in lower esophageal sphincter tone and barrier pressure (lower esophageal sphincter tone minus gastric pressure) and subsequent inhalation of gastric fluid during anesthesia remains undocumented.[13] Despite decreases in lower esophageal sphincter pressure associated with anesthesia, the incidence of gastroesophageal reflux as reflected by decreases in esophageal fluid pH is rare in patients undergoing elective operations.[14,15]

Gastroesophageal Reflux Disease

Transient relaxation of the lower esophageal sphincter, rather than decreased lower esophageal sphincter pressure, is the major mechanism of gastroesophageal reflux disease (GERD). Transient relaxation of the lower esophageal sphincter is associated with simultaneous inhibition of the sphincter and crural diaphragm. Some patients with gastroesophageal reflux have a weak lower esophageal sphincter, some have a weak crural diaphragm, and some have both. In GERD, the reflux of gastric fluid into the esophagus or oropharynx causes symptoms (esophagitis characterized as "heartburn") and/or tissue injury (esophageal strictures). It is estimated that approximately 20% of adults in the United States experience symptoms of GERD at least weekly and many patients with severe GERD have a hiatal hernia.

Atropine and morphine decrease the frequency of transient relaxation of the lower esophageal sphincter in normal patients through an unknown mechanism.[7] Antisecretory drugs such as histamine (H_2) receptor antagonists or proton pump inhibitors may be useful in treating gastroesophageal reflux. Therapy with a prokinetic drug such as metoclopramide may be effective. Patients with severe gastroesophageal reflux may benefit from surgical fundoplication of the esophagus via a laparoscopic technique.

Hiatal Hernia

The majority of patients with moderate to severe gastroesophageal reflux have a hiatal hernia in which a portion of the stomach herniates into the chest.[7] Hiatal hernia may promote gastroesophageal reflux by trapping gastric acid in the hernia sac, which may then flow backward into the esophagus when the lower esophageal sphincter relaxes during swallowing. Hiatal hernia can also cause gastroesophageal reflux when contraction of the crural diaphragm during inspiration and other physical maneuvers lead to a compartmentalization of the stomach between the lower esophageal sphincter and the diaphragm. The presence of acid in the esophagus causes esophagitis, which decreases the lower esophageal sphincter pressure and impairs esophageal contractility.

Achalasia

Achalasia is the best characterized of all esophageal motility disorders reflecting degeneration of neurons in the wall of the esophagus, especially the nitric oxide–producing inhibitory neurons that affect the relaxation of esophageal smooth muscle necessary for opening the lower esophageal sphincter. The loss of inhibitory innervation in the lower esophageal sphincter causes basal sphincter pressure to increase and interferes with sphincter relaxation. In the body of the esophagus, the loss of intramural neurons manifests as aperistalsis. Dysphagia for both solid foods and liquids is the primary symptom of achalasia. A substantial number of patients complaining of heartburn and achalasia may be confused with GERD.

Achalasia can be confirmed with radiographic (barium swallow shows dilatation of the esophagus with a beaklike narrowing of esophagogastric junction), manometric, and endoscopic evaluation (often performed utilizing drugs to produce sedation). The diagnosis may be suggested by a routine radiograph of the chest that shows widening of the mediastinum from the dilated esophagus and the absence of the normal gastric air bubble, because lower esophageal sphincter contraction prevents swallowed air from entering the stomach.

Nitrates and calcium channel blockers relax the smooth muscle of the lower esophageal sphincter and may produce limited success in treating patients with achalasia. Pneumatic dilation therapy for achalasia (a large deflated balloon is passed through the mouth to the lower esophageal sphincter and then rapidly inflated) may be helpful. Esophageal perforation is a risk of this treatment. Surgical myotomy of the lower esophageal sphincter performed laparoscopically often results in excellent relief but may be followed by GERD. For this reason, the myotomy may be combined with an antireflux procedure (fundoplication). Endoscopic injection of botulinum toxin into the area of the lower esophageal sphincter blocks the excitatory (acetylcholine-releasing) neurons that contribute to lower esophageal sphincter tone. Unfortunately, the effect is usually short-lived (less than 6 to 12 months).

A patient with achalasia presenting for surgery unrelated to the underlying esophageal motility disorder represents a potential risk for pulmonary aspiration during the perioperative period.

Stomach

The stomach is a specialized organ of the digestive tract that stores and processes food for absorption (Fig. 32-7). The ability to secrete hydrogen ions in the form of hydrochloric acid is a hallmark of gastric function. The secretory unit of gastric mucosa is the oxyntic glandular mucosa. The stomach is richly innervated by the vagus nerves and celiac plexus.

Gastric Secretions

Total daily gastric secretion is approximately 2 L with a pH of 1.0 to 3.5. The stomach secretes only a few milliliters of gastric fluid each hour during the periods between digestion. Strong emotional stimulation, such as occurs preoperatively, can increase interdigestive secretion of highly acidic gastric fluid to >50 mL per hour. The major secretions are hydrochloric acid, pepsinogen, intrinsic factor, and mucus. Mucous secretion protects the gastric mucosa from mechanical and chemical destruction. Substances that disrupt the mucosal barrier and cause gastric irritation include ethanol and drugs that inhibit prostaglandin synthesis (aspirin, nonsteroidal antiinflammatory drugs).

Parietal Cells

Parietal cells secrete an hydrogen ion–containing solution with a pH of approximately 0.8. At this pH, the hydrogen ion concentration is approximately 3 million times that present in the arterial blood. Hydrochloric acid kills bacteria, aids protein digestion, provides the necessary pH for pepsin to start protein digestion, and stimulates the flow of bile and pancreatic juice.

Secretion of hydrochloric acid depends on stimulation of receptors in the membrane of parietal cells by histamine, acetylcholine (vagal stimulation), and gastrin.[16] All of these receptors increase the transport of hydrogen ions into the gastric lumen by the hydrogen-potassium adenosine triphosphatase (ATPase) enzyme system (Fig. 32-8).[17] Activation of one receptor type potentiates the response of the other receptors to stimulation. Blockade of receptors with specific antagonist drugs produces

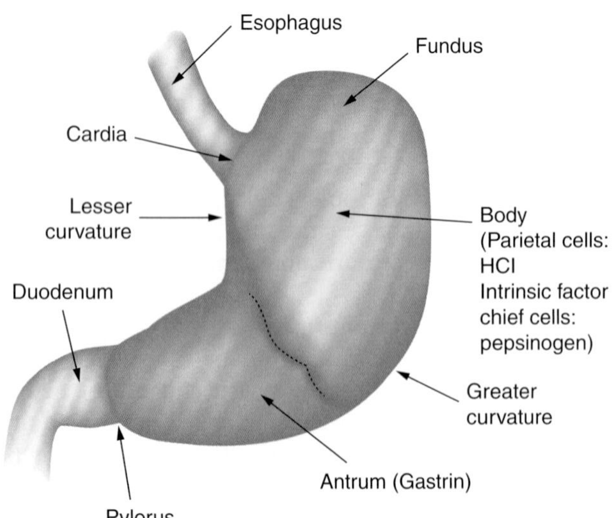

FIGURE 32-7 Anatomy of the stomach indicating the site of production of secretions. Mucus is secreted in all parts of the stomach.

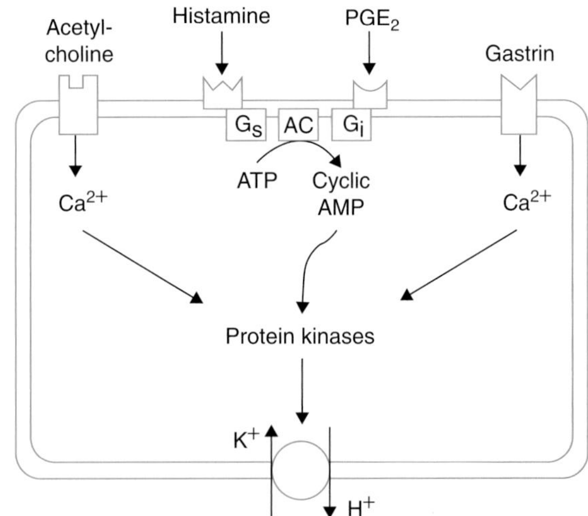

FIGURE 32-8 Gastric hydrogen ion secretion by parietal cells is increased by acetylcholine and gastrin acting on responsive receptors to increase intracellular calcium. Histamine activates receptors to activate stimulatory guanine proteins (G_s) to increase adenylate cyclase (AC) activity, whereas prostaglandins (PGE_2) activate inhibitory guanine proteins (G_i) to decrease AC activity. Cyclic adenosine monophosphate (cyclic AMP) and calcium act via protein kinases to increase transport of hydrogen ions into the gastric lumen. (Ganong WF. *Review of Medical Physiology*. 21st ed. New York, NY: Lange Medical Books/McGraw Hill; 2003, with permission.)

effective decreases in acid transport responses by removing the potentiating effect of stimulation of these receptors on the responses to other stimuli. Blockade of muscarinic receptors is produced by atropine or the more specific anticholinergic pirenzepine. Gastrin receptors can be inhibited by proglumide. Alternatively, the hydrogen-potassium-ATPase enzyme system can be inhibited by omeprazole. Pharmacologic manipulation of gastric fluid pH has special implications in the management of patients considered to be at risk for pulmonary aspiration during the perioperative period.

Intrinsic factor, which is essential for absorption of vitamin B_{12} from the ileum, is secreted by parietal cells. For this reason, destruction of parietal cells, as is associated with chronic gastritis, produces achlorhydria and often pernicious anemia.

Chief Cells

Pepsinogens secreted by chief cells undergo cleavage to pepsins in the presence of hydrochloric acid. Pepsins are proteolytic enzymes important for the digestion of proteins.

G Cells

Gastrin is secreted by gastric antral cells (G cells) into the circulation, which carries this hormone to responsive receptors in parietal cells to stimulate gastric hydrogen ion secretion. Gastrin also increases the tone of the lower esophageal sphincter and relaxes the pylorus.

Gastric Fluid Volume and Rate of Gastric Emptying

Neural and humoral mechanisms greatly influence gastric fluid volume and gastric-emptying time.[18–20] In general, parasympathetic nervous system stimulation enhances gastric fluid secretion and motility, whereas sympathetic nervous system stimulation has an opposite effect. The elimination of nonnutrient liquids is an exponential process (volume of liquid emptied per unit of time is directly proportional to the volume present in the stomach), whereas the emptying of solids is a linear process (Fig. 32-9).[19] In this regard, emptying of liquids from the stomach begins within 1 minute of ingestion, whereas emptying of solids typically begins after a lag time of 15 to 137 minutes (median 49 minutes).[18] Gastric emptying in healthy, term, nonobese parturients is not delayed after ingestion of 300 mL of water.[21] It is generally thought that the delay in gastric emptying of solids is caused by the time necessary for antral contractions to break solids down into small enough particles to exit through the pylorus. Clinical manifestations of delayed gastric emptying include anorexia, persistent fullness after meals, abdominal pain, and nausea and vomiting.

Several factors affect the rate of gastric emptying.[19] The primary determinant of the emptying of liquids from the stomach is volume. In addition to volume, another factor

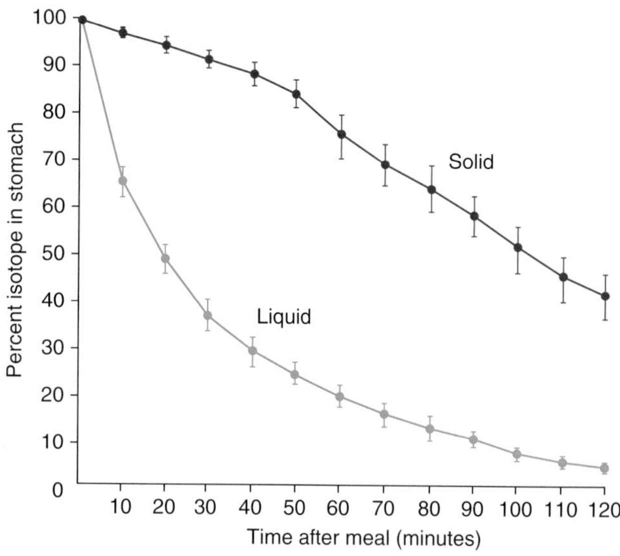

FIGURE 32-9 Gastric emptying of liquids is exponential, whereas emptying of solids is a linear process. (From Minami H, McCallum RW. The physiology of gastric emptying in humans. *Gastroenterology*. 1984;86:1592–1610, with permission.)

that influences the rate of gastric emptying is the composition of the liquids. Emptying of neutral, isoosmolar, and calorically inert solutions is rapid (250 mL of 500 mL of normal saline is emptied in 12 minutes). A small amount of water (up to 150 mL) to facilitate administration of oral medications shortly before the induction of anesthesia does not produce sustained increases in gastric fluid volume and could even contribute to gastric emptying.[22] Solutions that are hypertonic or contain acid, fat, or certain amino acids all retard gastric emptying. High lipid and/or caloric content (glucose) slows the emptying of solids from the stomach.[18,23]

The basic defect of diabetic gastroparesis appears to be one of impaired neural control. Delayed gastric emptying of solids is the most consistent abnormality in diabetics with gastroparesis and is the most predictably responsive to pharmacologic manipulation. Nevertheless, as diabetes progresses, it is possible that gastric retention of liquids will also occur.[19] Patients with GERD and documented slowing of gastric emptying of solids have been shown to have normal gastric emptying rates for liquids. Most patients with slowed gastric emptying of solids in association with GERD do not demonstrate symptoms such as nausea and vomiting, which are usually associated with gastric stasis. The existence of delayed gastric emptying in gastric ulcer disease is controversial. Some data suggest a slowing of gastric emptying of solids but not liquids in the presence of gastric ulcers. Although obesity and pregnancy are often assumed to slow gastric emptying, there are also data that fail to confirm this slowing, whereas other data suggest accelerated gastric emptying in obese individuals.[24–27] Contraction of the gastric fundus is responsible for facilitating the emptying of liquids, whereas antral contractions control the emptying of solids.[20] Gastrointestinal transit time has been shown to vary during the menstrual cycle, with prolongation occurring during the luteal phase when progesterone levels are increased. Acute viral gastroenteritis has been associated with delayed gastric emptying.

Certain drugs, including opioids, β-adrenergic agonists, and tricyclic antidepressants, may slow gastric emptying. Aluminum hydroxide antacid may slow gastric emptying. Alcohol, at least in concentrations present in wine, does not significantly affect gastric emptying of liquids or solids. Higher concentrations of alcohol, such as present in whiskey, do cause slowing of gastric emptying. The mechanism of this slowing is not clear but may be due to hyperosmolarity, changes in gastric acid secretion, or damage to gastric mucosa. Total parenteral nutrition may cause gastric stasis. Elemental diets, probably due to their high concentration of amino acids and hyperosmolarity, take longer to empty from the stomach than does blenderized food of comparable caloric composition. Cigarette smoking has been shown to delay emptying of solids although it may accelerate emptying of liquids. Gastric prokinetic drugs such as metoclopramide may speed the emptying of solids and liquids.

Gastric Emptying Prior to Elective Surgery

Clear liquids can be administered to adult patients scheduled for elective operations until 2 hours before induction of anesthesia without increasing gastric fluid volume. It takes 3 to 4 hours for the stomach to empty following a light breakfast (one slice of white bread with butter and jam, 150 mL of coffee without milk or sugar, 150 mL of pulp-free orange juice).[28] These data are consistent with the recommendation that a 6-hour fast should be enforced after a light breakfast.[29]

Opioid-Induced Slowing of Gastric Emptying

Opioid peptides and their receptors are found throughout the gastrointestinal system with particularly high concentrations in the gastric antrum and proximal duodenum. Central and peripheral μ opioid receptors can regulate gastric emptying, and opioid-induced delay in gastric emptying can be reversed with naloxone, which acts simultaneously at both central and peripheral sites. The demonstration that methylnaltrexone, a selective peripheral-acting opioid antagonist, attenuates morphine-induced changes in the rate of gastric emptying indicates that peripheral opioid receptors modulate this response in humans (see Chapter 7).[30]

Measurement of the Rate of Gastric Emptying

The rate of gastric emptying can be evaluated by a noninvasive electrical bioimpedance method (epigastric impedance method) and indirectly by the acetaminophen absorption technique.[31] Dye dilution techniques and scintigraphy also have been used to assess the rate of gastric emptying in humans.[32]

Electrical Bioimpedance Technique

The basis of the bioimpedance technique is that, after ingestion of fluids with a different conductivity from body tissues, the impedance to an electrical current through the upper abdomen changes. Electrodes are placed on the abdomen and back, and a constant current is applied. Impedance increases as the stomach fills and decreases as it empties. The slope of the plot of impedance versus time allows calculation of the emptying half-time of a meal.

The principal benefit of the bioimpedance method is that it is noninvasive and avoids gastric intubation or exposure to radioactivity. A limitation is that the subject must not move because alterations in body posture may alter baseline impedance readings and thus invalidate the recording. Another possible source of error is that gastric secretions might decrease the conductivity of gastric contents, thus reducing total surface impedance and producing inaccurate emptying rates. For this reason, deionized water may be used as the "test meal" because it does not appear to provoke sufficient gastric secretions to alter impedance.[30]

Acetaminophen Absorption Test

The appearance of acetaminophen in the systemic circulation is an indirect method of determining the rate of gastric emptying. The area under the plasma concentration curve of acetaminophen after oral administration is determined by the rate of gastric emptying, because acetaminophen is not absorbed from the stomach but is rapidly absorbed from the small intestine.

Absorption from the Stomach

The stomach is a poor absorptive area of the gastrointestinal tract because it lacks the villus structure characteristic of absorptive membranes. As a result, only highly lipid-soluble liquids such as ethanol and some drugs such as aspirin can be significantly absorbed from the stomach.

Vomiting

Vomiting is coordinated by the vomiting center in the medulla. This center receives input from multiple sites including the chemoreceptor trigger zone in the floor of the fourth ventricle, from the vestibular apparatus, from cortical centers and the gastrointestinal tract. The blood–brain barrier is poorly developed around the chemoreceptor trigger zone, and emetic substances present in the circulation are readily accessible to this site. Serotonin acting at 5-hydroxytryptamine receptors (5-HT_3) is an important emetic signal via neural pathways from the gastrointestinal tract ending at the chemoreceptor trigger zone. Likewise, dopamine and acetylcholine may provide emetic signals to the chemoreceptor trigger zone. Pharmacologic antagonism of these emetic signals results in antiemetic effects.

The role of specific opioid receptors in emetic responses is unresolved. Following stimulation of the vomiting center (directly or indirectly via neural pathways), vomiting is mediated by efferent pathways including the vagus and phrenic nerves, and innervation of the abdominal musculature. The initial manifestation of vomiting often involves nausea in which gastric peristalsis is reduced or absent and the tone of the upper small intestine is increased and gastric reflux occurs. Ultimately, the upper portion of the stomach relaxes while the pylorus constricts and the coordinated contraction of the diaphragm and abdominal muscles leads to expulsion of gastric contents. Risk factors for postoperative nausea and vomiting include female sex, young age (children), history of motion sickness, abstinence from tobacco, and obesity (perhaps reflecting emetic anesthetic drugs stored in adipose tissue).[33]

Small Intestine

The small intestine consists of the duodenum (from the pylorus to the ligament of Treitz), the jejunum, and the ileum (ending at the ileocecal valve). There is no distinct anatomic boundary between the jejunum and ileum, but the first 40% of small intestine after the ligament of Treitz is often considered the jejunum. The small intestine is presented with approximately 9 L of fluid daily (2 L from the diet and the rest representing gastrointestinal secretions), but only 1 to 2 L of chyme enters the colon. The small intestine is the site of most of the digestion and absorption of proteins, fats, and carbohydrates (Table 32-3).

Chyme moves through the 5 m of small intestine at an average rate of 1 cm per minute. As a result, it takes 3 to 5 hours for chyme to pass from the pylorus to the ileocecal valve. On reaching the ileocecal valve, chyme may remain in place for several hours until the person eats another meal. An inflamed appendix can increase the tone of the ileocecal valve to the extent that emptying of the ileum ceases. Conversely, gastrin causes relaxation of the ileocecal valve. When more than 50% of the small intestine is resected, the absorption of nutrients and vitamins is so compromised that development of malnutrition is likely.

Secretions of the Small Intestine

Mucus glands (Brunner glands) present in the first few centimeters of the duodenum secrete mucus to protect the duodenal wall from damage by acidic gastric fluid. Stimulation of the sympathetic nervous system inhibits the protective mucus-producing function of these glands, which may be one of the factors that causes this area of the gastrointestinal tract to be the most frequent site of peptic ulcer disease.

The crypts of Lieberkühn contain epithelial cells that produce up to 2 L daily of secretions that lack digestive enzymes and mimic extracellular fluid, having a pH of 6.5 to 7.5. This fluid provides a watery vehicle for absorption of substances from chyme as it passes through the small intestine. The most important mechanism for regulation of small intestine secretions is local neural reflexes, especially those initiated by distension produced by the presence of chyme.

The epithelial cells in the crypts of Lieberkühn continually undergo mitosis, with an average life cycle of approximately 5 days. This rapid growth of new cells allows prompt repair of any excoriation that occurs in the mucosa. This rapid turnover of cells also explains the vulnerability of the gastrointestinal epithelium to chemotherapeutic drugs (see Chapter 42).

The epithelial cells in the mucosa of the small intestine contain digestive enzymes that most likely are responsible for digestion of food substances because they are absorbed across the gastrointestinal epithelium. These enzymes include peptidases for splitting peptides into amino acids, enzymes for splitting disaccharides into monosaccharides, and intestinal lipases.

Table 32-3

Site of Absorption

	Duodenum	Jejunum	Ileum	Colon
Glucose	++	+++	++	0
Amino acids	++	+++	++	0
Fatty acids	+++	++	+	0
Bile salts	0	+	+++	0
Water-soluble vitamins	+++	++	0	0
Vitamin B_{12}	0	+	+++	0
Sodium	+++	++	+++	+++
Potassium	0	0	+	++
Hydrogen	0	+	++	++
Chloride	+++	++	+	0
Calcium	+++	++	+	?

Absorption from the Small Intestine

Mucosal folds (valvulae conniventes), microvilli (brush border), and epithelial cells provide an absorptive area of approximately 250 m^2 in the small intestine for nearly all the nutrients and electrolytes as well as approximately 95% of all the water. Daily absorption of sodium is 25 to 35 g, emphasizing the rapidity with which total body sodium depletion can occur if excessive intestinal secretions are lost as occurs with extreme diarrhea. Active transport of sodium ions in the small intestine is important for the absorption of glucose, which is the physiologic basis for treating diarrhea by oral administration of saline solutions containing glucose. Bacterial toxins as from cholera and staphylococci can stimulate the chloride-bicarbonate ion exchange mechanism, resulting in life-threatening diarrhea consisting of loss of sodium, bicarbonate, and an isosmotic equivalent of water.

Colon

The functions of the colon are absorption of water and electrolytes from the chyme and storage of feces. A test meal reaches the cecum in approximately 4 hours and then passes slowly through the colon during the next 6 to 12 hours, during which time 1 to 2 L of chyme are converted to 200 to 250 g of feces (Fig. 32-10). The circular muscle of the colon constricts and, at the same time, strips of longitudinal muscle (tinea coli) contract, causing the unstimulated portion of the colon to bulge outward into baglike sacs, or haustrations. Vagal stimulation causes segmental contractions of the proximal part of the colon and stimulation of the pelvic nerves causes explosive movements. Activation of the sympathetic nervous system inhibits colonic activity. Bacteria are predictably present in the colon.

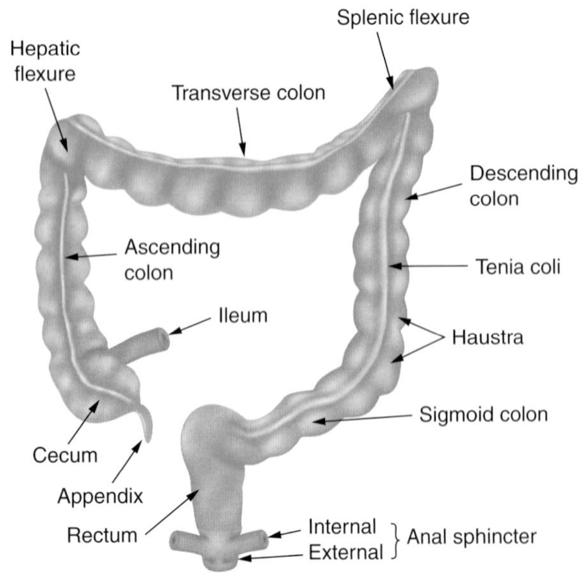

FIGURE 32-10 Anatomy of the colon.

Secretions of the Colon

Epithelial cells lining the colon secrete almost exclusively mucus, which protects the intestinal mucosa against trauma. The alkalinity of the mucus due to the presence of large amounts of bicarbonate ions provides a barrier to keep acids that are formed in the feces from attacking the intestinal wall. Irritation of a segment of colon as occurs with bacterial infection causes the mucosa to secrete large quantities of water and electrolytes in addition to mucus, diluting the irritating factors and causing rapid movement of feces toward the anus. The resulting diarrhea may result in dehydration and cardiovascular collapse.

Pancreas

The pancreas lies parallel to and beneath the stomach, serving as both an endocrine (insulin or glucagon) and exocrine gland. Exocrine secretions (approximately 1.5 L daily) are rich in bicarbonate ions to neutralize duodenal contents and digestive enzymes to initiate breakdown of carbohydrates, proteins, and fats.

Regulation of Pancreatic Secretions

Pancreatic secretions are regulated more by hormonal than neural mechanisms. For example, secretin is released by duodenal mucosa in response to hydrochloric acid. This hormone enters the circulation and causes the pancreas to produce large amounts of alkaline fluid necessary to neutralize the acidic pH of gastric fluid. In addition to the release of secretions, the presence of food in the duodenum causes the release of a second polypeptide hormone, cholecystokinin. Cholecystokinin also enters the circulation and causes the pancreas to secrete digestive enzymes (trypsins, amylase, lipases). Trypsins are activated in the gastrointestinal tract by the enzyme enterokinase, which is secreted by the gastrointestinal mucosa when chyme is exposed to the mucosa. Damage to the pancreas or blockade of a pancreatic duct may cause pooling of proteolytic enzymes, resulting in acute pancreatitis due to autodigestion by these enzymes. In general, pancreatic secretions are stimulated by the parasympathetic nervous system and inhibited by the sympathetic nervous system.

References

1. Alison MR, Poulsom R, Jeffery R, et al. Hepatocytes from non-hepatic adult stem cells. *Nature*. 2000;406:257–260.
2. Bloom W, Fawcell DW. *A Textbook of Histology*. 10th ed. Philadelphia, PA: Saunders; 1975.
3. Bell GH, Emslie-Smith D, Paterson CR. *Textbook of Physiology and Biochemistry*. 9th ed. New York, NY: Churchill Livingstone; 1976.
4. Gelman SI, Fowler KC, Smith LR. Liver circulation and function during isoflurane and halothane anesthesia. *Anesthesiology*. 1984; 61:726–730.
5. Guyton AC, Hall JE. *Textbook of Medical Physiology*. 10th ed. Philadelphia, PA: W.B. Saunders; 2000.
6. Berne RM, Levy M, Koeppen BM, et al. *Physiology*. 5th ed. St Louis, MO: Mosby; 2004.

7. Mittal RK, Balaban DH. The esophagogastric junction. *N Engl J Med.* 1997;336:924–932.
8. Mittal RK, Holloway RH, Penagini R, et al. Transient lower esophageal sphincter relaxation. *Gastroenterology.* 1995;109:601–610.
9. Brimacombe JR, Berry AM. Cricoid pressure. *Can J Anaesth.* 1997; 44:414–425.
10. Chassard D, Tournadre JP, Berrada KR, et al. Cricoid pressure decreases lower oesophageal sphincter tone in anaesthetized pigs. *Can J Anaesth.* 1996;43:414–417.
11. Tournadre JP, Chassard D, Berrada KR, et al. Cricoid cartilage pressure decreases lower esophageal sphincter tone. *Anesthesiology.* 1997;86:7–9.
12. Vanner RG, O'Dwyer JP, Pryle BJ, et al. Upper oesophageal sphincter pressure and the effect of cricoid pressure. *Anaesthesia.* 1992;47: 95–100.
13. Hardy JF. Large volume gastroesophageal reflux: a rationale for risk reduction in the perioperative period. *Can J Anaesth.* 1988;35:162–173.
14. Illing L, Ducan PG, Yip R. Gastroesophageal reflux during anaesthesia. *Can J Anaesth.* 1992;39:466–470.
15. Joshi GP, Morrison SG, Okonkwo NA, et al. Continuous hypopharyngeal pH measurements in spontaneously breathing anesthetized outpatients: laryngeal mask airway versus tracheal intubation. *Anesth Analg.* 1996;82:254–257.
16. Wolfe MM, Soll AH. The physiology of gastric acid secretion. *N Engl J Med.* 1988;319:1707–1715.
17. Ganong WF. *Review of Medical Physiology.* 21st ed. New York, NY: McGraw Hill; 2003.
18. Houghton LA, Read NW, Horowitz HM, et al. Relationship of the motor activity of the antrum, pylorus, and duodenum to gastric emptying of a solid–liquid mixed meal. *Gastroenterology.* 1988;94: 1285–1291.
19. Minami H, McCallum RW. The physiology and pathophysiology of gastric emptying in humans. *Gastroenterology.* 1984;86:1592–1610.
20. Read NW, Houghton LA. Physiology of gastric emptying and pathophysiology of gastroparesis. *Gastroenterol Clin North Am.* 1989; 18:359–373.
21. Wong CA, Loffredi M, Ganchiff JN, et al. Gastric emptying of water in term pregnancy. *Anesthesiology.* 2002;96:1395–1400.
22. Soreide E, Holst–Larsen K, Reite K, et al. Effects of giving water 20–450 mL with oral diazepam premedication 1–2 h before operation. *Br J Anaesth.* 1993;71:503–506.
23. Collins PJ, Horowitz M, Cook DJ, et al. Gastric emptying in normal subjects—a reproducible technique using a single scintillation camera and computer system. *Gut.* 1983;24:1117–1125.
24. Macfie AG, Magide AD, Richmond MN, et al. Gastric emptying in pregnancy. *Br J Anaesth.* 1991;67:54–57.
25. O'Sullivan GM, Sutton AJ, Thompson SA, et al. Noninvasive measurement of gastric emptying in obstetric patients. *Anesth Analg.* 1987;66:505–511.
26. Sandhar BK, Elliott RH, Windram I, et al. Peripartum changes in gastric emptying. *Anaesthesia.* 1992;47:196–198.
27. Wisen O, Johansson C. Gastrointestinal function in obesity: motility, secretion, and absorption following a liquid test meal. *Metabolism.* 1992;41:390–395.
28. Soreide E, Hausken T, Soreide A, et al. Gastric emptying of a light hospital breakfast. A study using real time ultrasonography. *Acta Anaesthesiol Scand.* 1996;40:549–553.
29. Warner MA, Caplan RA, Epstein BS, et al. Practice guidelines for preoperative fasting and the use of pharmacologic agents to reduce the risk of pulmonary aspiration: application to healthy patients undergoing elective procedures. *Anesthesiology.* 1999;90:896–905.
30. Murphy DB, Sutton JA, Prescott LF, et al. Opioid–induced delay in gastric emptying: a peripheral mechanism in humans. *Anesthesiology.* 1997;87:765–770.
31. McClelland GR, Sutton JA. Epigastric impedance: a noninvasive method for the assessment of gastric emptying and motility. *Gut.* 1985;26:607–614.
32. Sutton JA, Thompson S, Sobnack R. Measurement of gastric emptying rates by radioactive isotope scanning and epigastric impedance. *Lancet.* 1985;1:898–900.
33. Borgeat A, Ekatodramis G, Schenker CA. Postoperative nausea and vomiting in regional anesthesia. *Anesthesiology.* 2003;98:530–547.

CHAPTER 33

Metabolism

Michael J. Murray

One of the gastrointestinal tract's most important functions is for the ingestion of nutrients—carbohydrate, protein, lipid, minerals, vitamins, and water—that the organism uses for production of energy, creation of complex proteins and lipid moieties, and maintenance of electrolytes and total body water stores. The production of energy involves the oxidation of nutrients (carbohydrates, fats, and proteins) that results in creation of high-energy phosphate bonds in which energy is stored for life processes, with carbon dioxide and water produced as side products. The most important high-energy phosphate bond is adenosine triphosphate (ATP) (Fig. 33-1). This ubiquitous molecule is the energy storehouse for the body, providing the energy necessary for essentially all physiologic processes and chemical reactions. Probably the most important intracellular process that requires energy from hydrolysis of ATP is formation of peptide linkages between amino acids during protein synthesis. Likewise, skeletal muscle contraction cannot occur without energy derived from ATP hydrolysis. Metabolism of nutrients is necessary for creation of ATP that when hydrolyzed provides energy for transport of ions across cell membranes. Active transport is required to maintain the distribution of ions necessary for multiple cellular processes including the propagation of nerve impulses. In renal tubules, as much as 80% of ATP is used for membrane transport of ions. In addition to its function in energy transfer, ATP is also the precursor of cyclic adenosine monophosphate (cAMP), an important signaling molecule.

For adults, total energy expenditure averages 39 kcal/kg in males and 34 kcal/kg in females. Approximately 20 kcal/kg is expended as basal metabolism necessary to maintain integrity of the cell membrane and other energy-requiring tasks essential for life. In the resting state, the basal expenditure of calories is equivalent to approximately 1.1 kcal per minute, which requires approximately 200 to 250 mL per minute of oxygen in a 70-kg man for oxidation of nutrients. As the level of activities increase above the basal state, the caloric (and oxygen) requirements increase in proportion to the energy expenditure required (Table 33-1). The caloric values of carbohydrates, fats, and proteins are approximately 4.1 kcal/g, 9.3 kcal/g, and 4.1 kcal/g, respectively. Fat forms the major energy storage depot because of its greater mass and high caloric value (Fig. 33-2).[1] As a consequence, the primary form in which potential chemical energy is stored in the body is fat (triglyceride). The high caloric density and hydrophobic nature of triglycerides permit efficient energy storage without adverse osmotic consequences.

Carbohydrate Metabolism

Carbohydrates comprise a group of organic compounds that include sugars and starches and, in addition to carbon, contain hydrogen and oxygen in the same ratio as water (2:1). Three disaccharides are important in human biology—sucrose: glucose and fructose; lactose: glucose and galactose; and maltose: glucose and glucose. Starch, found in grains such as wheat, rice, and barley and other plants, including potatoes and corn, consists of many units of glucose joined by glycosidic bonds. Sugars are an important energy source for the body and the sole source of energy for the brain.

The liver is the site of carbohydrate metabolism where regulation, storage, and production of glucose takes place. The liver is the only organ that contains glucose kinase, an enzyme that has a high reaction rate (Km), capable of phosphorylating glucose, but only when its concentration is high. Adequate concentrations appear immediately after a meal when glucose concentration in the portal vein is increased. At least 99% of all the energy derived from carbohydrates is used by mitochondria to form ATP in the cells (Fig. 33-3). The final products of carbohydrate digestion in the gastrointestinal tract are glucose, fructose, and galactose. After absorption into the circulation, fructose and galactose are rapidly converted to glucose. As a result, glucose is the predominant molecule used to produce ATP. This glucose must be transported through cell membranes into cellular cytoplasm before it can be used by cells. This transport uses

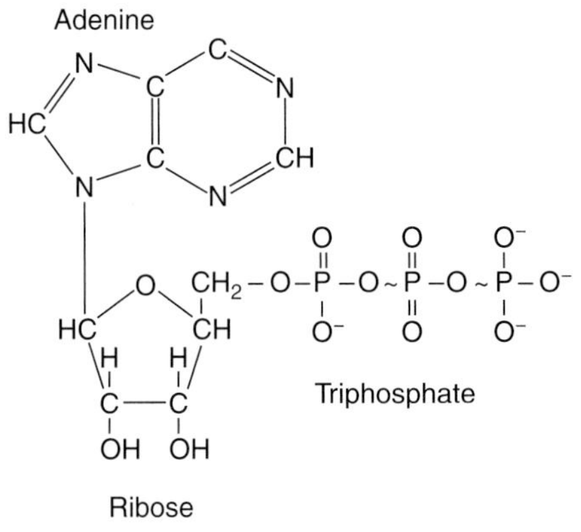

FIGURE 33-1 Metabolism of nutrients in cells is directed toward the ultimate synthesis of adenosine triphosphate (ATP). Energy necessary for physiologic processes and chemical reactions is derived from the high-energy phosphate bonds of ATP.

Table 33-1

Estimates of Energy Expenditure in Adults

Activity	Calorie Expenditure (kcal/minute)
Basal	1.1
Sitting	1.8
Walking (2.5 miles/hour)	4.3
Walking (4 miles/hour)	8.2
Climbing stairs	9.0
Swimming	10.9
Bicycling (13 miles/hour)	11.1

a protein carrier in ***carrier-mediated diffusion***, which is enhanced by insulin. Resistance to insulin, and thus transport of glucose into the cell in diabetes mellitus or sepsis,[2] results in hyperglycemia with associated adverse sequelae. Immediately upon entering cells, glucose is converted to glucose-6-phosphate under the influence of the enzyme hexose kinase. Phosphorylated glucose is ionized at pH 7 and, because plasma membranes are not permeable to the ions, the phosphorylated glucose cannot pass back through the membrane and is effectively trapped within the cell.

The fetus derives almost all its energy from glucose obtained from the maternal circulation. Immediately after birth, the infant stores of glycogen are sufficient to supply glucose for only a few hours. Furthermore, gluconeogenesis is limited in the neonate. As a result, the neonate is vulnerable to hypoglycemia if feeding is not initiated.

Glycogen

After entering cells, glucose can be used immediately for release of energy to cells or it can serve as a substrate for glycogen synthase. Dephosphorylation of the enzyme, glycogen synthase by protein phosphatase-1, which in turn is regulated by insulin and glucagon, activates the enzyme. Activated glycogen synthase combines molecules of glucose into a long polymer, similar to the way plants store carbohydrate as starch. Glycogen synthase is deactivated when it is phosphorylated—by glycogen synthase kinase-3, 5′-adenosine monophosphate–activated protein kinase, and protein kinase-A. The liver and skeletal muscles are particularly capable of storing large amounts of glycogen, but all cells can store at least some glucose as glycogen, and the glycogen in these cells is increasingly recognized as having important roles in both health and disease.[3] The liver stores glycogen for release of glucose during fasting, and muscle, which can store as much as 90% of the glucose contained in a meal, catabolizes glycogen during strenuous exercise.[4] The ability to form glycogen makes it possible to store substantial quantities of glucose without significantly altering the osmotic pressure of intracellular fluids. Glucose is cleaved from glycogen between meals, during fasting, and during exercise by glycogen phosphorylase and by a debranching enzyme.

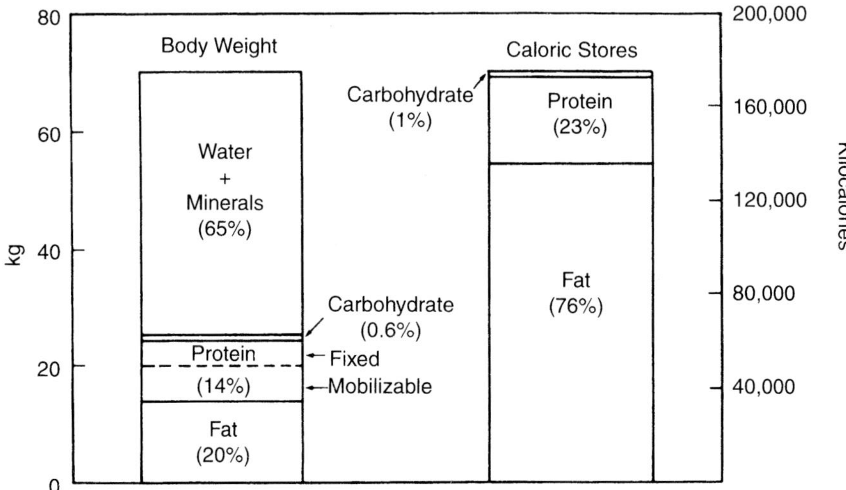

FIGURE 33-2 Comparison of the composition of body weight to caloric stores. (From Berne RM, Levy MN, Koeppen BM, et al. *Physiology*. 5th ed. St. Louis, MO: Mosby; 2004, with permission.)

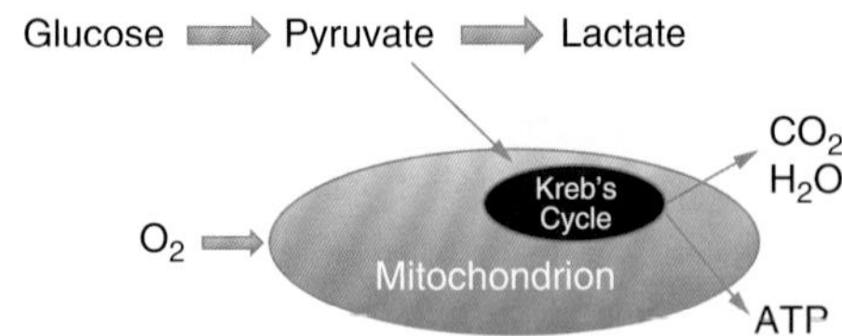

FIGURE 33-3 Formation of ATP from glucose.

Gluconeogenesis

Gluconeogenesis is the formation of glucose from amino acids and the glycerol portion of fat. Amino acids are first deaminated before entering the citric acid (Krebs) cycle (see Fig. 33-3). This process occurs when body stores of glycogen decrease below normal levels. An estimated 60% of the amino acids in the body's proteins can be converted easily to pyruvate and glucose, whereas the remaining 40% have chemical configurations that make this conversion difficult.

Gluconeogenesis is stimulated by hypoglycemia. Particularly in the liver, simultaneous release of cortisol mobilizes proteins, making them available for breakdown to amino acids used in gluconeogenesis. Thyroxine is also capable of increasing the rate of gluconeogenesis.

Energy Release from Glucose

Glucose is progressively broken down into two molecules of pyruvate, both of which can enter the citric acid cycle (Fig. 33-4), and the resulting energy is used to form ATP. For each mole of glucose that is completely degraded to carbon dioxide and water, a total of 38 moles of ATP is ultimately formed. The most important means by which energy is released from the glucose molecule is by glycolysis and the subsequent oxidation of the end products of glycolysis. Glycolysis is the splitting of the glucose molecule into two molecules of pyruvate, which enter the mitochondria where the pyruvate is converted to acetyl-coenzyme A (CoA), which enters the citric acid cycle and is converted to carbon dioxide and hydrogen ions with the formation of ATP (oxidative phosphorylation). Oxidative phosphorylation occurs only in the mitochondria and in the presence of adequate amounts of oxygen.

Anaerobic Glycolysis

In the absence of adequate amounts of oxygen, a small amount of energy can be released by anaerobic glycolysis, also known as fermentation in plants, fungi, and bacteria because conversion of glucose to pyruvate does not require oxygen. Indeed, glucose is the only nutrient that can serve as a substrate for the formation of ATP without oxygen. This release of glycolytic energy to cells can be lifesaving for a few minutes should oxygen become unavailable.

During anaerobic glycolysis, most pyruvic acid is converted to lactic acid, which diffuses rapidly out of cells into extracellular fluid. When oxygen is again available, this lactic acid can be reconverted to glucose. This reconversion occurs predominantly in the liver. Indeed, severe liver disease may interfere with the ability of the liver to convert lactic acid to glucose, leading to metabolic acidosis.

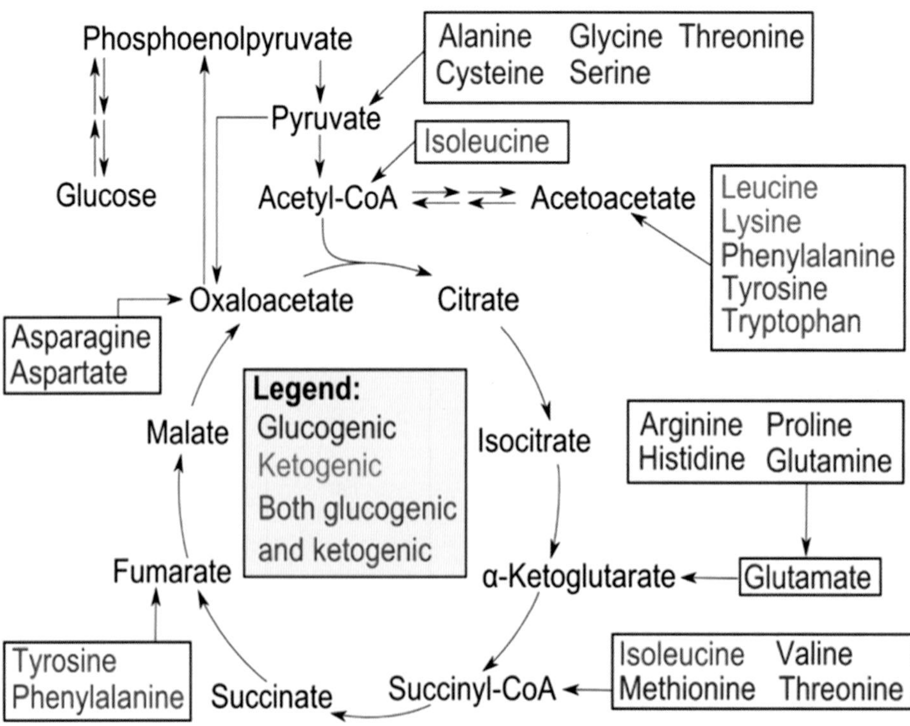

FIGURE 33-4 The citric acid cycle. (From Mikael Häggström, MD, Wikipedia Commons.)

Lipid Metabolism

Lipids are hydrophobic organic molecules that include waxes, sterols, fat-soluble vitamins, triglycerides (fats), phospholipids, and other substances. Lipids contain a high amount of potential energy, but are also important as structural components of cell membranes, in signaling pathways, and as precursors to a number of cytokines. Fatty acids and their derivatives as well as molecules that contain sterols such as cholesterol are also considered lipids. Although there are biosynthetic pathways to synt hesize and degrade lipids, some fatty acids are essential and must be ingested in the diet. Fatty acids are carboxylic acids consisting of a long hydrocarbon chain ending in a carboxyl group; the hydrocarbon chain can be saturated or unsaturated (Fig. 33-5). Humans can desaturate carbon atoms no closer than the 9th carbon from the tail of the aliphatic chain. However, humans require fatty acids (that are therefore essential) that are desaturated as close as the 6th and as close as the 3rd carbon to the terminus of the aliphatic chain—ω6 and ω3 fatty acids, respectively. Twenty carbon chain fatty acids are stored in the second position of phospholipids (see the following text), and when released, serve as substrates for a group of very important cytokines, the eicosanoids—prostaglandins, thromboxanes, and leukotrienes. Arachidonic acid (see Fig. 33-5), a 20 carbon chain ω6 fatty acid (C20:4ω6) is a precursor for prostaglandins and thromboxanes of the two series and leukotrienes of the four series, whereas eicosapentaenoic acid, C20:5ω3, is a precursor for prostaglandins and thromboxanes of the three series and leukotrienes of the five series.

A glycerol stem to which three fatty acid molecules are bound is known as a triglyceride (Fig. 33-6). A triglyceride molecule to which one of the terminal fatty acids is replaced with a phospate ion is known as a phospholipid (Fig. 33-7). Phospholipids are the building blocks of cell membranes (Fig. 33-8), form myelin, and, because of their unique structure and functions, are being used in other scientific applications.

Triglycerides, after absorption from the gastrointestinal tract, are transported in the lymph and then, by way of the thoracic duct, into the circulation in droplets known as ***chylomicrons***. Chylomicrons are rapidly removed from the circulation and stored as they pass through capillaries of adipose tissue and skeletal muscles. Triglycerides are used in the body mainly to provide energy for metabolic processes similar to those fueled by carbohydrates.

Cholesterol does not contain fatty acids, but it is a lipid, because it is composed of carbon and hydrogen, not

COOH

CH_3

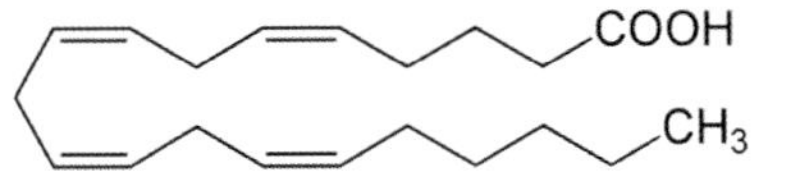

FIGURE 33-5 A long chain fatty acid, arachidonic acid. (From Yikrazuul via Wikimedia Commons.)

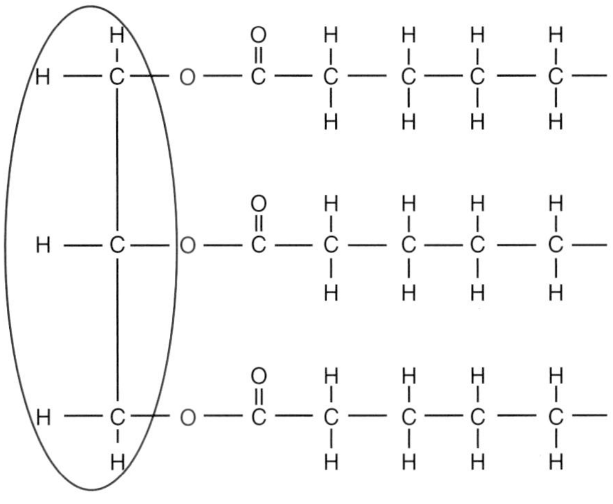

FIGURE 33-6 Triglyceride made up of a molecule of glycerol *(circled in red)* and three fatty acids.

as aliphatic chains of carbon but with four rings made up of carbon (Fig. 33-9). Seventy-five percent of cholesterol is produced in the liver in a synthetic process that involves 37 steps; the other 25% of cholesterol is ingested in the diet.

Molecules that are part lipid and part protein, lipoproteins, are also synthesized primarily in the liver (Table 33-2). The presumed function of lipoproteins is to provide a mechanism of transport for lipids throughout the body. Lipoproteins are classified according to their density, which is inversely proportional to their lipid content. All the cholesterol in plasma is found in lipoprotein complexes, with low-density lipoproteins (LDLs) representing the major cholesterol component in plasma. These LDLs provide cholesterol to tissues, where it is an essential component of cell membranes and is used in the synthesis of corticosteroids and sex hormones. In the liver, LDLs are taken up by receptor-mediated endocytosis. An intrinsic feedback control system increases the endogenous production of cholesterol when exogenous intake is decreased, explaining the relatively modest lowering

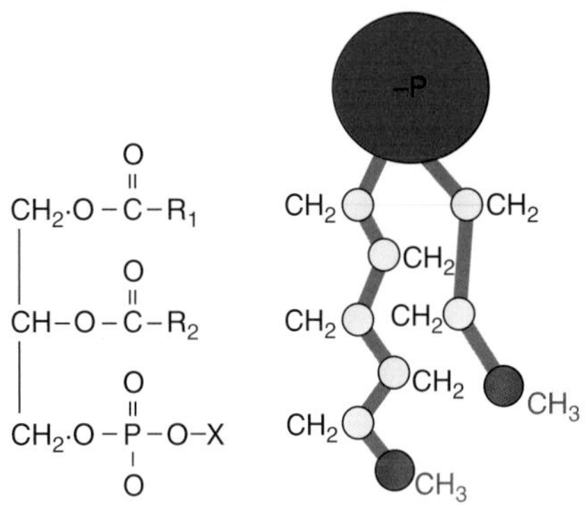

FIGURE 33-7 Substitution of one of the terminal fatty acids with a phosphate ion creates a phospholipid. Chemical structure on *left;* cartoon on *right* shows the hydrophilic phosphate group in *red,* with the hydrophobic hydrocarbon chains in *blue.* (From Wikipedia Commons.)

FIGURE 33-8 Cell membrane is a bilipid layer—made up of two opposing layers of phospholipids. The phosphate terminus is hydrophilic, whereas the two fatty acids, which are hydrophobic, orient to the interior of the membrane. (From Ties van Brusse, Wikipedia Commons.)

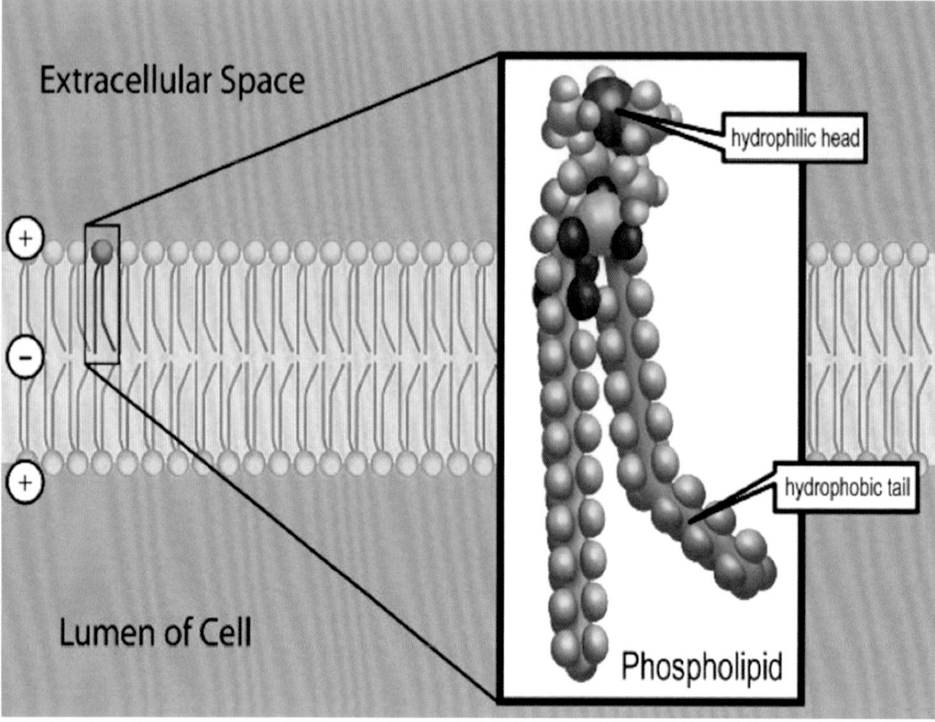

effect on plasma cholesterol concentrations produced by low-cholesterol diets. If this endogenous increase in cholesterol synthesis is blocked by drugs that inhibit hydroxymethylglutaryl coenzyme A (HMG-CoA) reductase, then there is an appreciable decrease in the plasma cholesterol concentration.

Drugs that selectively inhibit HMG-CoA are known as statins. Statins effectively lower plasma LDL cholesterol concentrations and seem to provide protection against acute cardiac events, perhaps reflecting antiinflammatory effects. In addition, statins lower plasma triglyceride concentrations and modestly increase high-density lipoprotein (HDL) cholesterol concentrations. Drugs that bind bile salts (cholestyramine, colestipol) prevent cholesterol from reentering the circulation as part of the enterohepatic circulation. A disadvantage of using drugs that bind bile salts to lower plasma cholesterol concentrations is an associated increase in plasma triglyceride concentrations.

The first step in the use of triglycerides for energy is hydrolysis into fatty acids and glycerol and subsequent transport of these products to tissues, where they are oxidized. Almost all cells, except for brain cells, can use fatty acids interchangeably with glucose for energy. Degradation and oxidation of fatty acids occur only in mitochondria, resulting in progressive release of two carbon fragments (β-oxidation) in the form of acetyl-CoA (Fig. 33-10). These acetyl-CoA molecules enter the citric acid cycle in the same manner as acetyl-CoA formed from pyruvate during the metabolism of glucose, ultimately leading to formation of ATP. In the liver, two molecules of acetyl-CoA formed from the degradation of fatty acids can combine to form acetoacetic acid (see Fig. 33-10). A substantial amount of acetoacetic acid is converted to

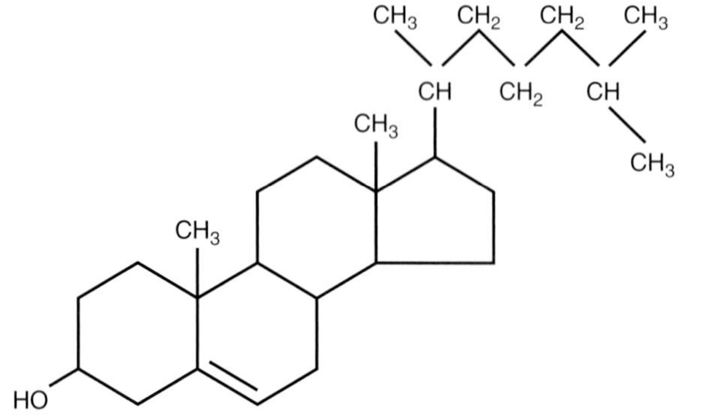

FIGURE 33-9 The chemical structure of a cholesterol molecule.

Table 33-2

Types of Proteins

Globular	Fibrous	Conjugated
Albumin	Collagen	Mucoprotein
Globulin	Elastin fibers	Structural components of cells
Fibrinogen	Keratin	
Hemoglobin	Actin	
Enzymes	Myosin	
Nucleoproteins		

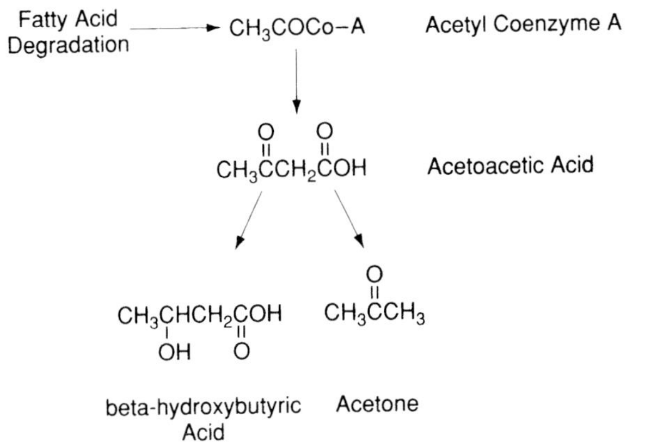

Fatty Acid Degradation → $CH_3COCo\text{-}A$ Acetyl Coenzyme A

$CH_3\overset{O}{\overset{\|}{C}}CH_2\overset{O}{\overset{\|}{C}}OH$ Acetoacetic Acid

$CH_3\underset{OH}{\underset{|}{C}}HCH_2\underset{O}{\underset{\|}{C}}OH$ beta-hydroxybutyric Acid

$CH_3\overset{O}{\overset{\|}{C}}CH_3$ Acetone

FIGURE 33-10 Fatty acid degradation in the liver leads to the formation of acetyl-CoA. Two molecules of acetyl-CoA combine to form acetoacetic acid, which, in large part, is converted to β-hydroxybutyric acid, and in lesser amounts, to acetone.

Table 33-4

Amino Acids

Essential	Nonessential
Arginine	Alanine
Histidine	Asparagine
Isoleucine	Aspartic acid
Leucine	Cysteine
Lysine	Glutamic acid
Methionine	Glutamine
Phenylalanine	Glycine
Threonine	Proline
Tryptophan	Serine
Valine	Tyrosine

β-hydroxybutyric acid and small amounts of acetone. In the absence of adequate carbohydrate metabolism (starvation or uncontrolled diabetes mellitus), large quantities of acetoacetic acid, β-hydroxybutyric acid, and acetone accumulate in the blood to produce ketosis because almost all the energy of the body must come from metabolism of lipids.

In contrast to glycogen, large amounts of lipids can be stored in adipose tissue and in the liver. A major function of adipose tissue is to store triglycerides until they are needed for energy. Epinephrine and norepinephrine activate triglyceride lipase in cells, leading to mobilization of fatty acids.

Protein Metabolism

Approximately 75% of the solid constituents of the body are proteins (Table 33-3). All proteins are composed of the same 20 amino acids, and several of these must be supplied in the diet because they cannot be formed endogenously (essential amino acids) (Table 33-4). Dietary proteins must be digested into amino acids and di- and tripeptides before they can be absorbed. The process begins in the stomach where pepsinogen is converted to pepsin in the acidic pH. The process continues in small intestine into which the pancreas secretes trypsin and chymotrypsin and carboxypeptidases. These gastric and pancreatic proteases hydrolyze proteins into medium and small chain peptides. Peptidases in the brush border of the small intestine hydrolyze these medium and small chain peptides into free amino acids and di- and tripeptides. These end products of digestion, formed on the surface of the enterocyte, are ready for absorption by sodium-dependent amino acid transporters.

Nonessential amino acids can be synthesized from the appropriate α-keto acid. For example, pyruvate formed during the glycolytic breakdown of glucose is the keto acid precursor of alanine. Each amino acid has an acidic carboxyl group (COOH) and an amino group (NH_3R), (Fig. 33-11). Proteins are formed by amino acids connected one to another by an amide bond, a covalent chemical bond between the carboxyl group of one amino acid with the amino group of another amino acid. The resulting C(O)NH bond is called a peptide bond, and the resulting molecule is an amide. The four-atom functional group -C(=O)NH- is

Table 33-3

Composition of Lipids in the Plasma

	Phospholipid (%)	Triglyceride (%)	Free Cholesterol (%)	Cholesterol Esters	Protein (%)	Density
Chylomicrons	3	90	2	3	2	0.94
LDL	21	6	7	46	20	1.019–1.063
HDL	25	5	4	16	50	1.063–1.21
IDL	20	40	5	25	10	1.006–1.019
VLDL	17	55	4	18	8	0.94–1.006

HDL, high-density lipoprotein; IDL, intermediate-density lipoprotein; LDL, low-density lipoprotein; VLDL, very-low-density lipoprotein.

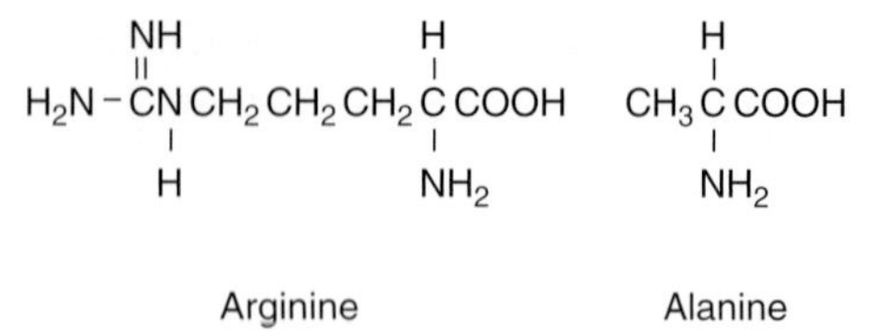

FIGURE 33-11 Examples of amino acids containing an acidic group (COOH) or an amino group (NH_2).

called a peptide link (Fig. 33-12). Even the smallest proteins characteristically contain more than 20 amino acids connected by peptide linkages, whereas complex proteins have as many as 100,000 amino acids. In addition, more than one amino acid chain in a protein may be bound to another amino acid chain by hydrogen bonds, hydrophobic bonds, or electrostatic forces.

Amino acids are relatively strong acids and exist in the blood principally in the ionized form. After a meal, the blood amino acid concentration increases only a few milligrams, reflecting rapid tissue uptake, especially by the liver. Passage of amino acids into cells requires active transport mechanisms because these substances are too large to pass by diffusion or through channels in cell membranes. In proximal renal tubules, amino acids that have entered the glomerular filtrate are actively transported back into the blood. These transport mechanisms have maximums above which amino acids appear in the urine. In the normal person, however, loss of amino acids in the urine each day is negligible. Failure to transport amino acids into the blood is indicative of renal disease.

Storage of Amino Acids

Immediately after entry into cells, amino acids are conjugated under the influence of intracellular enzymes into cellular proteins. As a result, concentrations of amino acids inside cells remain low. The concentration of amino acids within cells is low as the cell uses them as substrate to create proteins within the liver, kidneys, and gastrointestinal mucosa. Nevertheless, these proteins can be rapidly decomposed again into amino acids under the influence of intracellular liposomal digestive enzymes. The resulting amino acids can then be transported out of cells into blood to maintain optimal plasma amino acid concentrations. Tissues can synthesize new proteins from amino acids in blood. This response is especially apparent in relation to protein synthesis in cancer cells. Cancer cells are prolific users of amino acids, and, simultaneously, the proteins of other tissues become markedly depleted, contributing to cachexia.

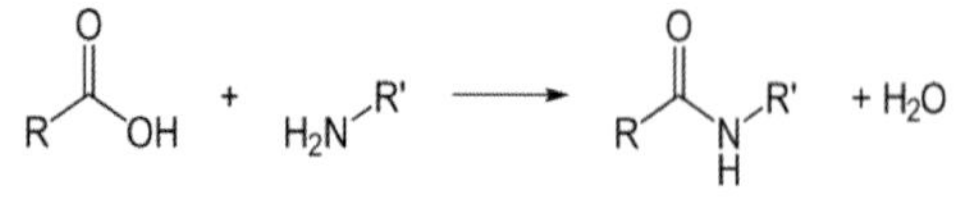

FIGURE 33-12 Formation of amides from carboxylic acid and primary amine.

Plasma Proteins

Plasma proteins are represented by (a) albumin, which provides colloid osmotic pressure; (b) globulins necessary for innate and acquired immunity; and (c) fibrinogen, which polymerizes into long fibrin threads during coagulation of blood. Essentially, all plasma albumin and fibrinogen and 60% to 80% of the globulins are formed in the liver. Additional globulins are formed in lymphoid tissues and other cells of the reticuloendothelial system. The rate of plasma protein formation by the liver can be greatly increased in situations, such as severe burns, where there is loss of large amounts of fluid and protein.

The hepatic synthetic rate of proteins depends on the blood concentration of amino acids. Even during starvation or severe debilitating diseases, the ratio of total tissue proteins to total plasma proteins in the body remains relatively constant at approximately 33:1. Because of the reversible equilibrium between plasma proteins and other proteins of the body, one of the most effective of all therapies for acute protein deficiency is the intravenous administration of plasma proteins. Within hours, amino acids of the administered protein become distributed throughout cells of the body to form proteins where they are needed.

Albumin

Albumin is the most abundant plasma protein and is principally responsible for maintaining plasma osmotic pressure. In addition, albumin is important as a transporter of plasma-bound substances often including exogenously administered drugs. Normal daily synthesis of albumin is about 10 g and the half-life for this protein may be as long as 22 days. Therefore, serum albumin concentrations may not be noticeably decreased in early states of acute hepatic failure. However, within hours of the onset of a critical illness or injury, albumin levels decrease by as much as 33% due to changes in the distribution between intravascular and extravascular compartments and rates of synthesis and degradation of protein. Despite the fact that low serum albumin is a poor prognostic factor in critical illness, supplementation has not been shown to improve prognosis.

Coagulation Factors

Hepatocytes synthesize all coagulation factors with the exception of von Willebrand factor and factor VIIIC. Coagulation may be rapidly impaired by acute liver failure, reflecting the short plasma half-life for many critical components (factor VII 100 to 300 minutes). Vitamin K (uptake dependent on bile salts) is necessary for modification of several of the clotting factors (prothrombin, antithrombin, protein S, and protein C) and may be deficient in malabsorptive states and malnutrition.

Use of Proteins for Energy

Once cells contain a maximum amount of amino acids, any additional amino acids are deaminated (oxidative deamination) to keto acids that can enter the citric acid cycle to become ATP or the keto acids are released into the bloodstream, taken up by adipocytes, and converted to and stored as fat. Ammonia resulting from deamination is converted to urea in the liver for excretion by the kidneys. Indeed, acute hepatic failure manifests by accumulation of toxic concentrations of ammonia. Certain deaminated amino acids are similar to the breakdown products that result from glucose and fatty acid metabolism. For example, deaminated alanine is pyruvic acid, which can be converted to glucose or glycogen, or it can become acetyl-CoA, which is polymerized to fatty acids. The conversion of amino acids to glucose or glycogen is ***gluconeogenesis***, and the conversion of amino acids into fatty acids is ***ketogenesis***. In the absence of protein intake, approximately 20 to 30 g of endogenous protein are degraded into amino acids daily. In severe starvation, cellular functions deteriorate because of protein depletion. Carbohydrates and lipids spare protein stores to a certain extent because they are used in preference but not exclusively to proteins for energy.

Growth hormone and insulin promote the synthetic rate of cellular proteins, possibly by facilitating the transfer of amino acids into cells. Glucocorticoids increase the breakdown rate of extrahepatic proteins, thereby making increased amino acids available to the liver. This allows the liver to synthesize increased amounts of cellular proteins and plasma proteins. Testosterone increases protein deposition in tissues, particularly the contractile proteins of skeletal muscles.

Effects of Stress on Metabolism

Carbohydrate, lipid, and protein metabolism are significantly altered by stress. In response to stress, the body increases secretion of cortisol, catecholamines, and glucagon, resulting in increased endogenous glucose production (hepatic gluconeogenesis) and hyperglycemia (to provide glucose to cells for ATP production in those cells involved in the fight or flight response. Stress-induced β-adrenergic stimulation increases the breakdown of fats (lipolysis). The products of lipolysis can be used for gluconeogenesis or directly by cells to produce ATP. Likewise, a predictable response to stress is catabolism of proteins in skeletal muscles, releasing keto acids that can be used for ATP production or for gluconeogenesis.

Exogenous glucose administered to injured or septic patients has a minimal effect on gluconeogenesis and lipolysis. Conversely, administration of glucose in the presence of starvation decreases gluconeogenesis and lipolysis.

Obesity

Given the importance of energy stores to individual survival and reproductive capacity, the ability to conserve energy in the form of adipose tissue would at one time have conferred a survival advantage.[5] For this reason, human genes that favor energy intake and storage are presumed to be present although not yet identified. Nevertheless, the combination of easy access to calorically dense foods and a sedentary lifestyle has made the metabolic consequences of these presumed genes maladaptive. In addition, certain medications are commonly associated with weight gain (Table 33-5).[6]

Obesity is the most common and costly nutritional problem in the United States. Based on body mass index (BMI) (weight in kilograms divided by the square of the height in meters), 67% of adult males and 62% of adult females are overweight (BMI ≥25) and 27.5% of adult males and 34% of adult females (BMI ≥30; class I obesity) are obese.[7] Individuals with a BMI >35 have class II obesity, and class III obesity if the BMI is >40. The prevalence of obesity peaks between 60 and 69 years of age but even 5-year-old children are increasingly found to be obese for their age.[8] A BMI of ≥28 is associated with a three to four times increase in the risk of ischemic heart disease, stroke, and diabetes mellitus compared with the general

Table 33-5

Drugs Commonly Associated with Weight Gain

Classification	Drug	Alternative Drug
Antidepressants	Tricyclic antidepressants Monoamine oxidase inhibitors	Selective serotonin reuptake inhibitors
Antidiabetics	Insulin Sulfonylureas Thiazolidinediones	Metformin Acarbose
Antiepileptics	Gabapentin Valproic acid	Lamotrigine Topiramate
Antipsychotics	Clozapine	Haloperidol
Steroids	Glucocorticoids	

Table 33-6

Criteria for Diagnosis of Metabolic Syndrome (Any Three of the following Characteristics)

Characteristic	Specific Finding
Waist circumference	Males >102 cm (40 inches) Females >88 cm (35 inches)
Blood glucose concentration (fasting)	>110 mg/dL
Increased systemic blood pressure	Systolic >130 mm Hg Diastolic >85 mm Hg
Serum triglyceride concentration	>150 mg/dL
High-density lipoprotein cholesterol concentration	Males <40 mg/dL Females <50 mg/dL

population. Increased waist circumference (>102 cm in adult males and >88 cm in adult females) is associated with an increased risk for ischemic heart disease, diabetes mellitus, and systemic hypertension. In this regard, an overweight person with a predominant abdominal fat distribution (common in elderly males with impaired glucose tolerance) may be at high risk for these diseases even if not considered obese by BMI criteria. The increased risk for morbidity and mortality extend beyond measurements of BMI and fat distribution, as reflected by the diagnosis of ***metabolic syndrome***, which is present if a patient has three of the following five risk factors: increased waist circumference (as described previously), low levels of HDL cholesterol, increased triglycerides, hypertension, and glucose intolerance (Table 33-6). The risk of anesthesia may be increased in classes II and III obese patients, reflecting mechanical difficulties (airway, positioning, and ventilation) and increased incidence of comorbid conditions (diabetes mellitus, systemic hypertension).

Treatment of obesity by decreasing caloric intake and increasing metabolic rate (exercise) directed toward a long-term decrease in body weight is largely ineffective, and 90% to 95% of persons who lose weight subsequently regain it.[9] Both proteins and carbohydrates can be metabolically converted to fat, and there is no evidence that changing the relative proportions of protein, carbohydrate, and fat in the diet without decreasing caloric intake will promote weight loss.[10] However, fat has a higher caloric density than protein and carbohydrate, and its contribution to the palatability of foods promotes its ingestion and increases the intake of calories.

Pharmacologic Treatment

Phentermine is an appetite suppressant that is utilized for short-term therapy intended to induce weight loss. In the past, this drug was frequently used in combination with fenfluramine (the latter induces the development of valvular heart disease, similar to that seen with carcinoid syndrome). It has been replaced by another combination drug, phentermine and topiramate, which is also somewhat effective; however, it may also be associated with heart problems. Orlistat inhibits lipases in the gastrointestinal lumen, thus antagonizing triglyceride hydrolysis and decreasing fat absorption by about 30%. Because orlistat is not absorbed, its ability to cause weight loss likely reflects the resulting low-fat diet and lower caloric intake. Weight loss with orlistat is modest, an average of 2.9 kg (6.4 lb) at 1 to 4 years.[11] Gastrointestinal side effects (abdominal discomfort, flatus, fecal urgency) reflecting the increased fat content in stool are dose limiting and occur in the majority of patients treated with orlistat. Concerns have also been raised about its negative effects on the kidneys.[12] It is recommended that orlistat not be prescribed for patients with known malabsorptive conditions, and daily multivitamin supplementation is useful. Lorcaserin is a third drug currently used in the United States, associated with a mean weight loss of 3.1 kg over 1 year compared to a placebo over a year.[13] Lorcaserin is a selective 5-HT_{2C} agonist, which activates proopiomelanocortin production and promotes weight loss through satiety.

References

1. Berne RM LM, Koeppen BM et al. *Physiology*. 5th ed. St. Louis, MO: Mosby; 2003.
2. Wakayama S, Haque A, Koide N, et al. Lipopolysaccharide impairs insulin sensitivity via activation of phosphoinositide 3-kinase in adipocytes. *Immunopharmacol Immunotoxicol*. 2014;36(2):145–149.
3. Greenberg CC, Jurczak MJ, Danos AM, et al. Glycogen branches out: new perspectives on the role of glycogen metabolism in the integration of metabolic pathways. *Am J Physiol Endocrinol Metab*. 2006;291(1):E1–E8.
4. Kollberg G, Tulinius M, Gilljam T, et al. Cardiomyopathy and exercise intolerance in muscle glycogen storage disease 0. *N Engl J Med*. 2007;357(15):1507–1514.
5. Rosenbaum M, Leibel RL, Hirsch J. Obesity. *N Engl J Med*. 1997;337(6):396–407.
6. Hockaday TD. Weight gain from common drugs. *QJM*. 2007;100(10):665; author reply 665–666.
7. Barnett R. Obesity. *Lancet*. 2005;365(9474):1843.

8. Cunningham SA, Kramer MR, Narayan KM. Incidence of childhood obesity in the United States. *N Engl J Med.* 2014;370(5):403–411.
9. Wadden TA. Treatment of obesity by moderate and severe caloric restriction. Results of clinical research trials. *Ann Intern Med.* 1993;119(7, pt 2):688–693.
10. Leibel RL, Hirsch J, Appel BE, et al. Energy intake required to maintain body weight is not affected by wide variation in diet composition. *Am J Clin Nutr.* 1992;55(2):350–355.
11. Rucker D, Padwal R, Li SK, et al. Long term pharmacotherapy for obesity and overweight: updated meta-analysis. *BMJ.* 2007;335(7631):1194–1199.
12. Weir MA, Beyea MM, Gomes T, et al. Orlistat and acute kidney injury: an analysis of 953 patients. *Arch Intern Med.* 2011;171(7):703–704.
13. Bays HE. Lorcaserin: drug profile and illustrative model of the regulatory challenges of weight-loss drug development. *Exp Rev Cardiovasc Ther.* 2011;9(3):265–277.

CHAPTER 34

Antiemetics

Michael J. Murray • David A. Grossblatt

Postoperative nausea and vomiting (PONV) is defined as nausea and/or vomiting occurring within 24 hours of surgery. Along with pain, PONV is the most important complaint patients report following surgery under anesthesia and is the leading cause of unanticipated hospital admission following outpatient surgery. Without prophylaxis, nausea occurs in up to 40% of patients who undergo general anesthesia but can be as high as 80% in high-risk patients.[1] There have been thousands of studies examining ways to prevent PONV and to effectively treat it when it does develop. Likewise, several anesthesia societies and organizations have developed guidelines on how to best address the problem. There have been a number of nonpharmacologic methods used to prevent and/or attenuate this disorder but this chapter will focus on the pharmacologic therapies used as prophylaxis and treatment of PONV.

Definition

PONV, recognized by the National Library of Medicine as a single medical subject heading term, actually refers to two distinct entities. Although nausea and emesis are intimately related, one can have one without the other or vice versa. Some drugs are more effective in treating one than the other. A patient who experiences nausea or has emesis within 24 hours of a surgical procedure that required anesthesia meets the criteria for the diagnosis of PONV. The classification is further divided into early PONV (within 6 hours of emergence from anesthesia) or late PONV (6 to 24 hours after the procedure).

Incidence

As mentioned previously, PONV occurs in 30% to 40% of all patients who undergo general anesthesia, but among patients with identified risk factors for developing PONV, it can occur in 70% to 80%. From a patient satisfaction point of view, PONV is a major issue. In a study of 195 surgical patients who were given a standardized questionnaire during the preoperative period, 130 questionnaires were returned prior to surgery. The patients rated emesis as the most important clinical anesthesia outcome to avoid, ahead of gagging on the tracheal tube (2), pain (3), nausea (4), and intraoperative recall (5). Independent of patient perception, PONV has been associated with morbidity including dehydration, electrolyte abnormalities, wound dehiscence, bleeding, esophageal rupture (Boerhaave's syndrome), and airway compromise.

Pathophysiology

Patients with nausea have a subjective feeling of the need to vomit; the sensation is very, very unpleasant. The nauseated patient does not necessarily vomit or retch, however. Emesis, which is the expulsion of stomach contents up the esophagus to the mouth, may or may not be preceded by nausea. The process often begins with antiperistalsis or muscular contractions within the ileum and jejunum, moving luminal contents back towards the stomach. The process of expelling these gastric contents involves closure of the glottis and contraction of the diaphragm, creating negative intrathoracic pressure at the same time that pharyngeal sphincters relax. Almost simultaneously, abdominal muscles contract creating increased intraabdominal pressure, which is transferred to the stomach; the stomach contents follow the path of least resistance and emesis occurs. If there are no stomach contents, the person may retch—the same events take place but no particulate or liquid material is expelled from the mouth. Emesis is different from regurgitation in which acidic gastric material passively reflexes into the esophagus because of an incompetent esophageal sphincter and elevated abdominal pressure.

The sequence of events that occur during emesis are controlled by the so-called vomiting "center," which lies in the medulla oblongata and consists of the nucleus of the tractus solitarius and parts of the reticular formation. A number of neurotransmitters modulate the activity of

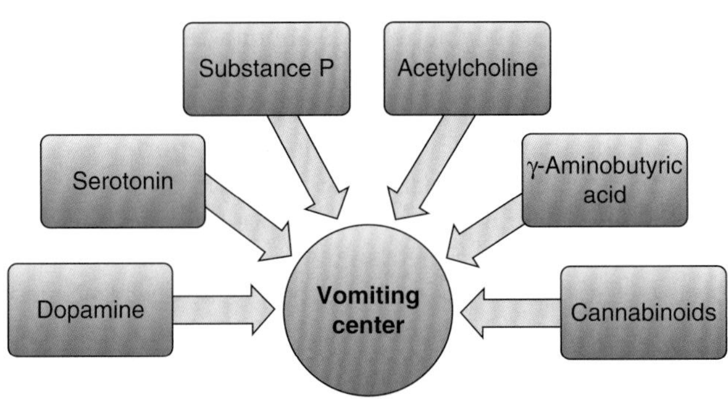

FIGURE 34-1 Pharmacological systems that interact with the vomiting center.

the vomiting center (Fig. 34-1); agonists and antagonists of these neurotransmitters are used to prevent nausea and vomiting. Slightly cephalad to the vomiting center is the chemoreceptor trigger zone (CRTZ), which detects noxious chemicals in the bloodstream, for example, ethanol at high concentration sends signals via neural networks, which activate the vomiting center. Other anatomic sites that can activate the vomiting center include the vestibular apparatus, the thalamus and cerebral cortex, and neurons within the gastrointestinal tract itself. The latter would occur for example if a small bowel obstruction triggered antiperistalsis, and as small intestinal contents were forced backwards filling the stomach, afferent signals would be transmitted to the vomiting center.

Upon activation, the vomiting center sends efferent signals via the cranial nerves V, VII, IX, X, and XII through the vagal parasympathetic fibers and sympathetic chain and to skeletal muscle through α motor neurons. Signals from the vomiting center via these nerves trigger the complex motor process resulting in emesis.

Prophylaxis

Preventing PONV is easier than treating it[2] but the side effects of the antiemetic drugs are such that the American Society of Anesthesiologists has recommended that antiemetic agents should be used for the prevention and treatment of nausea and vomiting when indicated but not routinely. In order to determine whether prophylaxis is indicated, it is important to assess a patient's propensity to develop PONV according to risk factors that increase or decrease a patient's chances of experiencing PONV. These risk factors are traditionally divided into patient, surgical, and anesthetic risk factors.

Patient Factors

Women, nonsmokers[3], and those with a history of motion sickness[4] or of previous episodes of PONV are at an increased risk of experiencing PONV if they undergo a surgical procedure under anesthesia. Women most likely are at increased risk for PONV because of the effects of progesterone and/or estrogen on the CRTZ or on the vomiting center itself as evidenced by the fact that the incidence of PONV varies within the menstrual cycle and is reduced after menopause.[5] Obese patients, because of exposure to greater amount of emetogenic lipophilic drugs such as the inhalational anesthetic agents stored in their adipose tissue, were once thought to have a higher incidence of PONV but a subsequent investigation did not show this to be true.[6]

Surgical Factors

The longer the surgical procedure, the greater is the risk for a patient to develop PONV, perhaps because of prolonged exposure to emetogenic lipophilic drugs.[7] Independent of duration, certain surgical procedures have been associated with an increased incidence of PONV, for example, laparotomies; gynecologic surgeries; laparoscopic procedures; as well as ear, nose, throat, breast, plastic, and orthopedic surgical procedures.[8] Age is only weakly associated with PONV; for pediatric patients having surgery under general anesthesia, the greatest association is with the surgical procedure itself. Herniorrhaphy, tonsillectomy, and adenoidectomy; strabismus procedures; and surgical procedures on male genitalia have the highest risk.[9] Among adults, risk is reduced with aging.

Anesthetic Factors

There have been a number of anesthetic-related factors that investigators have assessed for their relationship to the development of PONV. The inhalation anesthetic agents nitrous oxide, neostigmine, and opioids have all been implicated in the genesis of PONV. However, correlation is limited and most scoring systems used to identify patients at risk of PONV do not use anesthetic factors as risk factors.

Pharmacologic Interventions

A multimodal approach for prophylaxis in patients at high risk for developing PONV and as rescue therapy in patients who develop PONV in the postanesthetic care unit works well because of the complexity of systems involved in the pathogenesis of PONV. The drugs that modulate activity in the vomiting center and CRTZ are listed in Table 34-1 and will be discussed in the following sections.

Anticholinergics

Scopolamine

Prevention of Motion-Induced Nausea and of Postoperative Nausea and Vomiting

Transdermal absorption of scopolamine provides sustained therapeutic plasma concentrations, which protect against motion-induced nausea usually without

Table 34-1

Pharmacologic Therapies for Treatment of Nausea and Vomiting

Anticholinergics	Atropine
	Hyoscine
	Scopolamine
Benzamides	Metoclopramide
Benzodiazepines	Midazolam
Butyrophenones	Droperidol
	Haloperidol
Cannabinoids	Dronabinol
	Nabilone
Glucocorticoids	Dexamethasone
5-HT_3 antagonists	Dolasetron
	Granisetron
	Ondansetron
	Palonosetron
	Ramosetron
	Tropisetron
Neurokinin-1 antagonists	Aprepitant
	Fosaprepitant
Phenothiazines	Prochlorperazine
	Promethazine
	Chlorpromazine

introducing prohibitive side effects such as sedation, cycloplegia, or drying of secretions. For example, a postauricular application of scopolamine delivers the drug at about 5 μg per hour for 72 hours (total absorbed dose is <0.5 mg). Protection against motion-induced nausea is greatest if the transdermal application of scopolamine is initiated at least 4 hours before the noxious stimulus. Administration of transdermal scopolamine after the onset of symptoms is less effective than prophylactic administration. Similar protection against motion-induced nausea by oral or intravenous (IV) administration of scopolamine would require large doses, resulting in undesirable side effects and subsequent poor patient acceptance.

Transdermal application of a scopolamine patch has been shown to exert significant antiemetic effects in patients experiencing motion sickness and in those treated with patient-controlled analgesia or epidural morphine for the management of postoperative pain.[10] It is well known that motion sickness is caused by stimulation of the vestibular apparatus. It has also been shown that morphine and synthetic opioids increase vestibular sensitivity to motion. It is presumed that scopolamine blocks transmission to the medulla of impulses arising from overstimulation of the vestibular apparatus of the inner ear. Indeed, application of a transdermal scopolamine (TDS) patch before the induction of anesthesia protects against nausea and vomiting after middle ear surgery, which is likely due to altered function of the vestibular apparatus.[10] Furthermore, prophylactic TDS applied the evening before surgery decreases but does not abolish the occurrence of nausea and vomiting after outpatient laparoscopy using general anesthesia.[11] Conversely, not all reports describe an antiemetic effect in patients treated with TDS who are undergoing general anesthesia.[12] However, Apfel and colleagues[13] performed a meta-analysis of 25 studies of TDS used to treat PONV and found that TDS was associated with significant reductions in PONV with both early and late application during the first 24 hours after the start of anesthesia. TDS was associated with a higher prevalence of visual disturbances at 24 to 48 hours after surgery, but no other adverse events were noted.[13] Some of the visual disturbances may be due to anisocoria, which has been attributed to contamination of the eye after digital manipulation of the TDS patch.[14] More than 90% of unilateral dilated pupils occur on the same side as the patch. This diagnosis is confirmed by history and failure of the mydriasis to respond to topical installation of pilocarpine.

Central Anticholinergic Syndrome

Scopolamine and atropine can enter the central nervous system (CNS) and produce symptoms characterized as the central anticholinergic syndrome. Symptoms range from restlessness and hallucinations to somnolence and unconsciousness. Presumably, these responses reflect blockade of muscarinic cholinergic receptors and competitive inhibition of the effects of acetylcholine in the CNS. Glycopyrrolate does not easily cross the blood–brain barrier and thus is not likely to cause central anticholinergic syndrome. Nevertheless, central anticholinergic syndrome has been attributed to the IV administration of anticholinergic drugs before the induction of anesthesia.[15]

Physostigmine, a lipid-soluble tertiary amine anticholinesterase drug administered in doses of 15 to 60 μg/kg IV, is a specific treatment for the central anticholinergic syndrome. Treatment may need to be repeated every 1 to 2 hours. Edrophonium, neostigmine, and pyridostigmine are not effective antidotes because their quaternary ammonium structure prevents these drugs from easily entering the CNS. The central anticholinergic syndrome is often mistaken for delayed recovery from anesthesia. Ventilation may be depressed. Differentiation of this syndrome from other causes of perioperative confusion is possible with slow IV administration of physostigmine, 0.4 mg/kg.

Overdose

Deliberate or accidental overdose with an anticholinergic drug produces a rapid onset of symptoms characteristic of muscarinic cholinergic receptor blockade. The mouth becomes dry, swallowing and talking is difficult, vision is blurred, photophobia is present, and tachycardia is prominent. The skin is dry and flushed, and a rash may appear especially over the face, neck, and upper chest (blush area). Even therapeutic doses of anticholinergic drugs sometimes may selectively dilate cutaneous vessels in the blush area. Body temperature is likely to be increased by anticholinergic drugs, especially when the environmental temperature is also increased. This increase in body temperature largely reflects inhibition of sweating by anticholinergic drugs, emphasizing that innervation of sweat glands is by sympathetic nervous system nerves that release acetylcholine as the neurotransmitter. Small children are particularly vulnerable to drug-induced increases in body temperature, with "atropine fever" occurring occasionally in this age group after administration of even a therapeutic dose of anticholinergic drug. Minute ventilation may be slightly increased due to CNS stimulation and the impact of an increased physiologic dead space due to bronchodilation. Arterial blood gases are usually unchanged. Fatal events due to an overdose of an anticholinergic drug include seizures, coma, and medullary ventilatory center paralysis.

Small children and infants seem particularly vulnerable to developing life-threatening symptoms after an overdose with an anticholinergic drug. Physostigmine, administered in doses of 15 to 60 μg/kg IV, is the specific treatment for reversal of symptoms. Because physostigmine is metabolized rapidly, repeated doses of this anticholinesterase drug may be necessary to prevent the recurrence of symptoms.

Decreased Barrier Pressure

Barrier pressure is the difference between gastric pressure and lower esophageal sphincter pressure. Administration of atropine, 0.6 mg IV, or glycopyrrolate, 0.2 to 0.3 mg IV, decreases lower esophageal sphincter pressure and thus decreases barrier pressure and the inherent resistance to reflux of acidic fluid into the esophagus.[16] This effect may persist longer with glycopyrrolate (60 minutes) than after administration of atropine (40 minutes).

Benzamides

Metoclopramide

The benzamides stimulate the gastrointestinal tract via cholinergic mechanism, which results in (a) contraction of the lower esophageal sphincter and gastric fundus, (b) increased gastric and small intestinal motility, and (c) decreased muscle activity in the pylorus and duodenum when the stomach contracts. Metoclopramide and domperidone are the two benzamides currently in use, but domperidone is not available in the United States because the U.S. Food and Drug Administration (FDA) was concerned about its use in lactating women (increases milk production). This review will therefore focus on metoclopramide, which presumably has either a peripheral effect as just described or because it readily crosses the blood–brain barrier may have direct effects on the CRTZ and/or vomiting center because of its antidopaminergic effect.

A meta-analysis of 30 trials evaluating 10 mg of systemic metoclopramide on PONV outcomes concluded that compared to placebo metoclopramide, the incidence of 24-hour PONV was reduced with an odds ratio of .58 with a 95% confidence interval of 0.43 to 0.78. The number needed to treat was 7.8.[17]

Because of its antidopaminergic activity, metoclopramide should be used with caution if at all in patients with Parkinson's disease, restless leg syndrome, or who have movement disorders related to dopamine inhibition or depletion.[18] In patients with no known movement disorders, dystonic extrapyramidal reactions (oculogyric crises, opisthotonus, trismus, torticollis) occur in less than 1% of patients treated chronically with metoclopramide. Although usually a problem if large oral doses (40 to 80 mg daily) are administered chronically, there are reports of neurologic dysfunction related to the preoperative administration of metoclopramide.[19] These extrapyramidal reactions are identical to the Parkinson's syndrome evoked by antipsychotic drugs that antagonize the CNS actions of dopamine.[20] Akathisia, a feeling of unease and restlessness in the lower extremities, may follow the IV administration of metoclopramide, sometimes so severe that it can result in cancellation of surgery[21] or which may manifest in the postanesthesia care unit.[18,22]

Benzodiazepines

Midazolam

The activity of the benzodiazepines is relatively well known but with respect to a possible mechanism of action in PONV, benzodiazepines may decrease synthesis and release of dopamine within the CRTZ.[23,24] Because many, if not a majority of patients, receive benzodiazepines administered as part of general and regional anesthetics and for monitored anesthesia care, a lengthy discussion of their role in the prophylaxis and for rescue therapy of PONV is probably not warranted. However, in patients for whom the administration of benzodiazepine is not planned but who are at risk of PONV, if midazolam is used for its antiemetic effect, it should be administered IV toward the end of the surgical procedure[25] or by continuous infusion in intubated and ventilated patients in the intensive care unit.[26]

Butyrophenones

Droperidol and Haloperidol

After the FDA placed black box restrictions on droperidol due to its association with prolonged QT syndromes, many physicians stopped using droperidol. However, the FDA's restriction on droperidol was for a result of case reports with higher doses than are necessary for the treatment of PONV. Because of its efficacy at low dose, the use of droperidol has increased over the last several years for prophylaxis and as rescue therapy as an antiemetic.

Prophylactic doses of droperidol of 0.625 to 1.25 mg IV are effective for the prevention and treatment of PONV. Haloperidol also has antiemetic properties when used in low doses, 0.5 to 2 mg IV. At these doses, sedation does not occur. Extrapyramidal symptoms, however, are a risk of all medications that involve dopamine receptor blockade in the brain and therefore, these drugs should be used with caution if at all in patients with Parkinson's disease, restless leg syndrome, and other diseases related to dopaminergic activity. For patients in whom dopamine antagonism is not a concern, droperidol is as effective as dexamethasone or ondansetron in preventing and treating PONV.[27]

Corticosteroids

Dexamethasone

Dexamethasone has been shown to be useful in the management of PONV but the mechanism of antiemetic activity is unclear. Corticosteroids are proposed to centrally inhibit prostaglandin synthesis and control endorphin release. As discussed already, dexamethasone has efficacy similar to ondansetron and droperidol[27] and with a minimal side effect profile associated with one-time use. Obese and diabetic patients are at increased risk for perioperative hyperglycemia when they receive a single dose of dexamethasone.

5-HT_3 Receptor Antagonists

The 5-HT_3 receptors are excitatory ligand-gated nonselective cation. The ion channel is a pentamer consisting of five monomers that form a central pore, which can be readily permeated by small cations. The 5-HT_3 receptors are extensively distributed on enteric neurons in the gastrointestinal tract and brain. Serotonin is released from the enterochromaffin cells of the small intestine, stimulates the vagal afferents through 5-HT_3 receptors, and initiates the vomiting reflex. Antagonism of 5-HT_3 receptors results in an antiemetic effect. Clinically used 5-HT_3 receptor antagonists are selective for these receptors with almost no significant binding with other 5-HT receptor subtypes.

Clinical Uses

The 5-HT_3 receptor antagonists represent (ondansetron, tropisetron, granisetron, dolasetron) a significant advance in the prophylaxis and treatment of nausea and vomiting because they are highly specific and evoke minimal side effects. Drugs that act as competitive antagonists at 5-HT_3 receptors are useful antiemetics in the prophylaxis and treatment of chemotherapy- and radiation therapy–induced nausea and vomiting.[28] Furthermore, these 5-HT_3 receptor antagonists have proved to be highly effective in the prevention and treatment of PONV. Serotonin receptor antagonists are not effective in the treatment of motion-induced nausea and vomiting nor are they effective treatment for PONV caused by vestibular stimulation because the vestibular apparatus and the nucleus of the tractus solitarius are rich in muscarinic and histamine receptors that would not be blocked by a 5-HT_3 receptor antagonist.

The convenience of use, efficacy, and safety profile are some of the reasons for the popularity of 5-HT_3 receptor antagonists for management of PONV.

Comparison with Other Antiemetics

Ondansetron (4 mg), dexamethasone (4 mg), and droperidol (1.25 mg) administered IV as prophylactic therapy before induction of general anesthesia are equally effective in decreasing the incidence of PONV by about 26%.[27] However, a cost–benefit analysis did not support the use of 5-HT_3 receptor antagonists for routine antiemetic prophylaxis when studied in the early 2000s.[29] Now that some 5-HT_3 antagonists are available as lower cost generic preparations, the balance may have shifted.

Pharmacokinetics

The 5-HT_3 receptor antagonists are readily absorbed after oral administration and readily cross the blood–brain barrier. Following IV administration, the maximum brain concentration is achieved quickly. These antagonists are moderately bound to protein (60% to 75%). Metabolism is by different subtypes of cytochrome P450 enzymes and metabolites undergo principally renal excretion.

Ondansetron

Ondansetron is a carbazalone derivative that is structurally related to serotonin and possesses specific 5-HT_3 subtype receptor antagonist properties without altering dopamine, histamine, adrenergic, or cholinergic receptor activity.[30] As a result, ondansetron is free of neurologic side effects common to droperidol and metoclopramide.[31] Ondansetron is effective when administered orally or IV and has an oral bioavailability of about 60% with therapeutic blood concentrations appearing 30 to 60 minutes after administration. Metabolism to inactive metabolites occurs predominantly in the liver and the elimination half-time is 3 to 4 hours.

The most commonly reported side effects from treatment with ondansetron are headache and diarrhea. Transient increases in the plasma concentrations of liver transaminase enzymes have been observed only in patients receiving chemotherapy and may be due to these drugs rather than ondansetron. Cardiac arrhythmias and conduction disturbances (atrioventricular block) have been reported after the IV administration of ondansetron and metoclopramide.[28] Ondansetron and other 5-HT_3 receptor antagonists can cause slight prolongation of the QTc interval on the electrocardiogram of treated patients but this has not created the same level of concern as that ascribed to droperidol for unclear reasons.

It is estimated that for every 100 patients who receive ondansetron for the prevention of PONV, 20 patients will not vomit who would have vomited without treatment ("number needed to treat"), and three of those 100 patients will develop a headache who would have not had this adverse effect without the drug ("number needed to harm").[32] Ondansetron, 4 to 8 mg IV (administered over 2 to 5 minutes immediately before the induction of anesthesia), is highly effective in decreasing the incidence of PONV in a susceptible patient population (ambulatory gynecologic surgery, middle ear surgery). Oral (0.15 mg/kg) or IV (0.05 to 0.15 mg/kg) administration of ondansetron is effective in decreasing the incidence of postoperative vomiting in preadolescent children undergoing ambulatory surgery, including tonsillectomy and strabismus surgery.

Ondansetron, although highly effective in decreasing the incidence and intensity of PONV, does not totally eliminate this complication. The most significant feature of ondansetron prophylaxis and treatment is the relative freedom from side effects as compared with other described classes of antiemetic drugs. Use of propofol for induction and maintenance of anesthesia is almost as effective as ondansetron in preventing PONV (19% vs. 26%, respectively) and ondansetron continues to have antiemetic effects when used in propofol-based anesthetic.[27]

Tropisetron

Tropisetron is an indoleacetic acid ester of tropine that possesses highly selective 5-HT_3 receptor blocking effects. Compared with ondansetron, tropisetron has the benefit of a longer elimination half-time (7.3 hours vs. 3.5 hours). Overall, the beneficial effects and side effects of tropisetron resemble ondansetron.[33] This drug is also effective in the treatment of symptoms related to carcinoid syndrome and may also possess gastrokinetic properties. As an antiemetic, tropisetron is effective in prevention of chemotherapy- and radiotherapy-induced emesis and in the prevention of PONV when administered (2 to 5 mg IV) before the induction of general anesthesia.[34] Rescue treatment using a single dose of tropisetron is often effective in decreasing further nausea and vomiting.[35] Tropisetron did not prevent PONV associated with epidural morphine, whereas dexamethasone (5 mg IV) was effective.[36]

Granisetron

Granisetron is a more selective 5-HT_3 receptor antagonist than ondansetron. Like ondansetron, granisetron is effective orally and IV. Doses as low as 0.02 to 0.04 mg/kg IV have been described as effective in prevention of chemotherapy-induced emesis and prevention of PONV.[28] Concomitant administration of dexamethasone significantly improved the acute antiemetic efficacy of granisetron.[37,38] Metabolism to inactive metabolites occurs in the liver with only about 10% of the drug excreted unchanged by the kidneys. The elimination half-time of granisetron (9 hours) is 2.5 times longer than that of ondansetron and thus may require less frequent dosing. For example, a single dose of granisetron may be effective for 24 hours. Side effects are mild and include headache, sedation, and diarrhea.

Dolasetron

Dolasetron is a highly potent and selective 5-HT_3 receptor antagonist that is effective in the prevention of chemotherapy-induced nausea and vomiting and PONV following either oral or IV administration. After its administration, dolasetron is rapidly metabolized to hydrodolasetron, which is responsible for the antiemetic effect. Hydrodolasetron has an elimination half-time of approximately 8 hours and is approximately 100 times more potent as a serotonin antagonist than the parent compound.

A single IV dose of dolasetron, 1.8 mg, is equivalent to ondansetron, 32 mg IV, and granisetron, 3 mg IV, in preventing chemotherapy-induced nausea and vomiting. Established PONV is effectively blunted by treatment with dolasetron, 12.5 mg IV.[39] Oral dolasetron, 25 to 50 mg, is effective as prophylaxis for decreasing PONV. Although serotonergic pathways are involved in the development of postoperative shivering, dolasetron was not effective in preventing this complication.[40] Side effects include headache, dizziness, and increased appetite. It is unclear if an increased heart rate attributed to dolasetron is different from the incidence observed in placebo-treated patients.[28]

Histamine Receptor Antagonists

The effects of histamine are mediated via histamine receptors, and at least three histamine receptors subtypes have been identified and classified as H_1, H_2, and H_3. Histamine acting through H_1 receptors and inositol phospholipid hydrolysis evokes smooth muscle contraction in the gastrointestinal tract. Nonspecific antihistamines, likely acting on H_1 receptors including diphenhydramine, dimenhydrinate, cyclizine, and promethazine are used as antiemetics.

Dimenhydrinate (marketed as Dramamine) has been used to treat PONV as well as motion sickness. It is speculated that the efficacy of dimenhydrinate in motion sickness and inner ear diseases may be due to inhibition of the integrative functioning of the vestibular nuclei by decreasing vestibular and visual input. Manipulation of the extraocular muscles as in strabismus surgery may trigger an "oculoemetic" reflex similar to the well-described oculocardiac reflex. If the afferent arc of this reflex is also dependent on the integrity of the vestibular nuclei apparatus, then dimenhydrinate may attenuate or block this reflex and decrease the incidence of PONV. Administration of dimenhydrinate, 20 mg IV, in adults decreases vomiting after outpatient surgery.[41] In children, dimenhydrinate, 0.5 mg/kg IV, significantly decreases the incidence of vomiting after strabismus surgery.[42]

References

1. Apfel CC, Laara E, Koivuranta M, et al. A simplified risk score for predicting postoperative nausea and vomiting: conclusions from cross-validations between two centers. *Anesthesiology*. 1999; 91(3):693–700.
2. White PF, Watcha MF. Postoperative nausea and vomiting: prophylaxis versus treatment. *Anesth Analg*. 1999;89(6):1337–1339.
3. Sweeney BP. Why does smoking protect against PONV? *Br J Anaesth*. 2002;89(6):810–813.
4. Golding JF. Motion sickness susceptibility. *Autonomic Neurosci*. 2006;129(1–2):67–76.
5. Simurina T, Mraovic B, Skitarelic N, et al. Influence of the menstrual cycle on the incidence of nausea and vomiting after laparoscopic gynecological surgery: a pilot study. *J Clin Anesth*. 2012;24(3): 185–192.
6. Kranke P, Apefel CC, Papenfuss T, et al. An increased body mass index is no risk factor for postoperative nausea and vomiting. A systematic review and results of original data. *Acta Anaesthesiol Scand*. 2001;45(2):160–166.
7. Junger A, Hartmann B, Benson M, et al. The use of an anesthesia information management system for prediction of antiemetic rescue treatment at the postanesthesia care unit. *Anesth Analg*. 2001;92(5):1203–1209.
8. Apfel CC, Kranke P, Katz MH, et al. Volatile anaesthetics may be the main cause of early but not delayed postoperative vomiting: a randomized controlled trial of factorial design. *Br J Anaesth*. 2002;88(5):659–668.
9. Rose JB, Watcha MF. Postoperative nausea and vomiting in paediatric patients. *Br J Anaesth*. 1999;83(1):104–117.
10. Honkavaara P, Saarnivaara L, Klemola UM. Prevention of nausea and vomiting with transdermal hyoscine in adults after middle ear surgery during general anaesthesia. *Br J Anaesth*. 1994;73(6):763–766.
11. Bailey PL, Streisand JB, Pace NL, et al. Transdermal scopolamine reduces nausea and vomiting after outpatient laparoscopy. *Anesthesiology*. 1990;72(6):977–980.
12. Koski EM, Mattila MA, Knapik D, et al. Double blind comparison of transdermal hyoscine and placebo for the prevention of postoperative nausea. *Br J Anaesth*. 1990;64(1):16–20.
13. Apfel CC, Zhang K, George E, et al. Transdermal scopolamine for the prevention of postoperative nausea and vomiting: a systematic review and meta-analysis. *Clin Therapeut*. 2010;32(12):1987–2002.
14. Price BH. Anisocoria from scopolamine patches. *JAMA*. 1985; 253(11):1561.
15. Grum DF, Osborne LR. Central anticholinergic syndrome following glycopyrrolate. *Anesthesiology*. 1991;74(1):191–193.
16. Cotton BR, Smith G. Comparison of the effects of atropine and glycopyrrolate on lower oesophageal sphincter pressure. *Br J Anaesth*. 1981;53(8):875–879.
17. De Oliveira GS Jr, Castro-Alves LJ, Chang R, et al. Systemic metoclopramide to prevent postoperative nausea and vomiting: a meta-analysis without Fujii's studies. *Br J Anaesth*. 2012;109(5): 688–697.
18. Pasricha PJ, Pehlivanov N, Sugumar A, et al. Drug insight: from disturbed motility to disordered movement—a review of the clinical benefits and medicolegal risks of metoclopramide. *Nat Clin Pract*. 2006;3(3):138–148.
19. Scheller MS, Sears KL. Postoperative neurologic dysfunction associated with preoperative administration of metoclopramide. *Anesth Analg*. 1987;66(3):274–276.
20. Grimes JD, Hassan MN, Preston DN. Adverse neurologic effects of metoclopramide. *Canad Med Assoc J*. 1982;126(1):23–25.
21. LaGorio J, Thompson VA, Sternberg D, et al. Akathisia and anesthesia: refusal of surgery after the administration of metoclopramide. *Anesth Analg*. 1998;87(1):224–227.
22. Jo YY, Kim YB, Yang MR, et al. Extrapyramidal side effects after metoclopramide administration in a post-anesthesia care unit—a case report. *Kor J Anesthesiol*. 2012;63(3):274–276.
23. Di Florio T. Midazolam for PONV. What's new? *Anaesthesia*. 2002;57(9):941.
24. Di Florio T, Goucke R. Reduction of dopamine release and postoperative emesis by benzodiazepines. *Br J Anaesth*. 1993;71(2):325.
25. Safavi MR, Honarmand A. Low dose intravenous midazolam for prevention of PONV, in lower abdominal surgery—preoperative vs intraoperative administration. *Middle East J Anesthesiol*. 2009; 20(1):75–81.
26. Sanjay OP, Tauro DI. Midazolam: an effective antiemetic after cardiac surgery—a clinical trial. *Anesth Analg*. 2004;99(2):339–343, table of contents.
27. Apfel CC, Korttila K, Abdalla M, et al. A factorial trial of six interventions for the prevention of postoperative nausea and vomiting. *N Engl J Med*. 2004;350(24):2441–2451.
28. Wolf H. Preclinical and clinical pharmacology of the 5-HT3 receptor antagonists. *Scand J Rheumatol*. 2000;113:37–45.
29. White PF. Prevention of postoperative nausea and vomiting—a multimodal solution to a persistent problem. *N Engl J Med*. 2004; 350(24):2511–2512.
30. Bodner M, White PF. Antiemetic efficacy of ondansetron after outpatient laparoscopy. *Anesth Analg*. 1991;73(3):250–254.
31. Sprung J, Choudhry FM, Hall BA. Extrapyramidal reactions to ondansetron: cross-reactivity between ondansetron and prochlorperazine? *Anesth Analg*. 2003;96(5):1374–1376, table of contents.
32. Tramer MR, Reynolds DJ, Moore RA, et al. Efficacy, dose-response, and safety of ondansetron in prevention of postoperative nausea and vomiting: a quantitative systematic review of randomized placebo-controlled trials. *Anesthesiology*. 1997;87(6):1277–1289.
33. Scholz J, Hennes HJ, Steinfath M, et al. Tropisetron or ondansetron compared with placebo for prevention of postoperative nausea and vomiting. *Eur J Anaesthesiol*. 1998;15(6):676–685.
34. Alon E, Kocian R, Nett PC, et al. Tropisetron for the prevention of postoperative nausea and vomiting in women undergoing gynecologic surgery. *Anesth Analg*. 1996;82(2):338–341.
35. Alon E, Buchser E, Herrera E, et al. Tropisetron for treating established postoperative nausea and vomiting: a randomized, double-blind, placebo-controlled study. *Anesth Analg*. 1998;86(3): 617–623.
36. Wang JJ, Tzeng JI, Ho ST, et al. The prophylactic effect of tropisetron on epidural morphine-related nausea and vomiting: a comparison of dexamethasone with saline. *Anesth Analg*. 2002;94(3):749–753, table of contents.
37. Fujii Y, Saitoh Y, Tanaka H, et al. Granisetron/dexamethasone combination for the prevention of postoperative nausea and vomiting after laparoscopic cholecystectomy. *Eur J Anaesthesiol*. 2000; 17(1):64–68.
38. Fujii Y, Tanaka H, Kobayashi N. Granisetron/dexamethasone combination for the prevention of postoperative nausea and vomiting after thyroidectomy. *Anaesth Intens Care*. 2000;28(3): 266–269.
39. Diemunsch P, Leeser J, Feiss P, et al. Intravenous dolasetron mesilate ameliorates postoperative nausea and vomiting. *Can J Anaesth*. 1997;44(2):173–181.
40. Piper SN, Rohm KD, Maleck WH, et al. Dolasetron for preventing postanesthetic shivering. *Anesth Analg*. 2002;94(1):106–111, table of contents.
41. Bidwai AW, Meuleman T, Thatte WP. Prevention of postoperative nausea with dimenhydrinate (Dramamine) and droperidol (Inapsine). *Anesth Analg*. 1989;68:S25.
42. Vener D, Carr A, Sikich N, et al. Dimenhydrinate decreases vomiting in children after strabismus surgery. *Anesth Analg*. 1996;82: 728–731.

CHAPTER 35

Gastrointestinal Motility Drugs

Michael J. Murray • Jillian A. Maloney

Aspiration is the inhalation of gastric or oropharyngeal contents into the lungs. Aspiration during general anesthesia occurs in approximately 1 in 8,500 adults and 1 in 4,400 children younger than 16 years of age.[1] An earlier study of more than 56,000 patients younger than age 18 years identified an incidence of aspiration of approximately 1 in 2,600 anesthetics. The incidence was 1 in 4,500 patients undergoing elective procedures, but 1 in 400 undergoing emergency procedures. The authors commented that respiratory morbidity was rare and that there was no mortality associated with aspiration of gastric contents in this cohort.[2] Previous studies in adults have noted that, in addition to emergency procedures (many in patients with bowel obstruction), patients with an American Society of Anesthesiologists physical classification of 3 or greater had an increased risk of aspiration, associated pulmonary complications, and death. This study noted that approximately one-third of cases of aspiration occurred during laryngoscopy and intubation, one-third occurred during extubation, and the other one-third presumably during the procedure.[3]

Factors associated with pulmonary complications of aspiration include the volume and acidity of the aspirated gastric contents. Drugs then that increase the pH of gastric contents (antacids) and that decrease the volume of gastric contents (prokinetic drugs) have a role in decreasing the severity of the sequelae of aspirating gastric contents. Enforcement of the American Society of Anesthesiologists Task Force Fasting Recommendations can also reduce the risk of pulmonary aspiration.[4]

Oral Antacids

Antacids are drugs that neutralize (remove hydrogen ions) from gastric contents or decrease the secretion of hydrogen chloride into the stomach. Oral antacids have been used for centuries. In current practice, the oral antacids used most often are salts of aluminum, calcium, and magnesium; the hydrogen ions in stomach acid react with the base, forming a stable compound. As hydrogen ions are consumed, the pH of the stomach contents increases. The best known example would be sodium bicarbonate, $NaHCO_3$, which in the stomach would combine with HCl to produce NaCl, H_2O, and CO_2.

Increasing gastric pH relieves the symptoms of gastritis, but if the pH of the stomach is too high, digestion of food is inhibited as an acidic pH is necessary for the breakdown of many foods. In addition, increases in gastric fluid pH to >5 result in inactivation of pepsin and produce bile-chelating effects. Neutralization of gastric fluid pH increases gastric motility via the action of gastrin (aluminum hydroxide is an exception) and increases lower esophageal sphincter tone by a mechanism that is independent of gastrin.

$NaHCO_3$ results in a prompt and rapid antacid action, so much so that the pH is raised to the point that the stomach's pH is neutral, which can lead to **acid rebound**. Patients with hypertension or heart disease may not tolerate the increased sodium load associated with chronic use of this antacid.

Magnesium hydroxide (milk of magnesia) also produces prompt neutralization of gastric acid but is not associated with significant acid rebound. In contrast to aluminum hydroxide, a prominent laxative effect (osmotic diarrhea) is characteristic of magnesium hydroxide. Systemic absorption of magnesium may be sufficient to cause neurologic, neuromuscular, and cardiovascular impairment in patients with renal dysfunction. Renal dysfunction can also lead to the development of metabolic alkalosis in some patients.[5]

Calcium carbonate can also produce metabolic alkalosis with chronic therapy. The plasma concentration of calcium is increased transiently. Symptomatic hypercalcemia may occur in patients with renal disease. The administration of calcium carbonate–containing antacids may result in hypophosphatemia. Even small amounts of calcium carbonate–containing antacids evoke hypersecretion of hydrogen ions (acid rebound).[6] The chalky taste of calcium carbonate is an additional disadvantage. The release of CO_2 in the stomach may cause eructation and flatulence. Constipation is minimized by including magnesium oxide with calcium carbonate. Acute appendicitis has been reported due to impacted calcium carbonate fecaliths.

Aluminum hydroxide is actually a mixture of aluminum hydroxide, aluminum oxide, and some fixed CO_2 as carbonate. Systemic absorption of aluminum is minimal, but in patients with renal disease, the plasma and tissue concentrations of aluminum may become excessive.[7] Encephalopathy in patients undergoing hemodialysis has been attributed to intoxication with aluminum especially in patients who ingest solutions containing citrate.[8] Aluminum compounds, in contrast to other antacids, cause slowing of gastric emptying and marked constipation. These effects, in addition to an unpleasant taste, contribute to poor patient acceptance.

Occasional failure of particulate antacids to increase gastric fluid pH may reflect inadequate mixing with stomach contents or an unusually large volume of gastric fluid such that the standard dose of antacid is inadequate to neutralize gastric hydrogen ions. Layering is also common with particulate antacids.[9] Pneumonitis associated with functional and histologic changes in the lungs may reflect a foreign body reaction to inhaled particulate antacid particles.

Nonparticulate (clear) antacids such as sodium citrate are less likely to cause a foreign body reaction if aspirated, and their mixing with gastric fluid is more complete than is that of particulate antacids.[9,10] Furthermore, the onset of effect is more rapid with sodium citrate than with particulate antacids that require a longer time for adequate mixing with gastric fluid. Sodium citrate, 15 to 30 mL of a 0.3-mol per liter solution administered 15 to 30 minutes before the induction of anesthesia, is effective in reliably increasing gastric fluid pH in pregnant and nonpregnant patients.[11]

Complications of Antacid Therapy

The increase in urine and gastric volume pH resulting from antacid use has been associated with adverse events. Chronic alkalinization of gastric fluid has been associated with bacterial overgrowth in the duodenum and small intestine.[12] Alkalinization of the urine may predispose to urinary tract infections; if it is chronic, urolithiasis is possible. Increased urine pH may persist >24 hours after administration of an antacid, leading to changes in the renal elimination of drugs.

Acid rebound is a side effect that is unique to calcium-containing antacids. This response is characterized by a marked increase in gastric acid secretion that takes place several hours after neutralization of gastric acid. It is unclear if acid rebound persists with chronic calcium carbonate treatment.

The milk-alkali syndrome is characterized by hypercalcemia, increased blood urea nitrogen and plasma creatinine concentrations, and systemic alkalosis, as reflected by an above-normal plasma pH. The plasma calcium phosphate concentration is usually increased. There may be a marked decrease in renal function with calcification of the renal parenchyma. This syndrome is most commonly associated with ingestion of large amounts of calcium carbonate along with >1 L of milk every day.

Phosphorus depletion can occur in patients who ingest large doses of aluminum salts because they bind phosphate ions in the gastrointestinal tract, thus preventing their absorption. This effect may actually be beneficial in patients with renal disease because it can decrease the plasma phosphate concentration, but, unfortunately, patients with chronic renal failure are at risk of developing toxicity from the aluminum. Individuals with hypophosphatemia may experience anorexia, skeletal muscle weakness, and malaise. Osteomalacia, osteoporosis, and fractures may occur. If it is necessary to administer aluminum-containing antacids on a chronic basis to patients with osteomalacia or osteoporosis, phosphate supplements should be considered.

Drug Interactions

Gastric alkalinazation increases gastric emptying, resulting in a faster delivery of drugs into the small intestine. This may facilitate absorption of drugs that are poorly absorbed or it may shorten the time available for absorption, depending on where in the gastrointestinal tract absorbtion occurs. There are many drugs whose absorption is enhanced by antacids.[13] The rate of absorption of salicylates, indomethacin, and naproxen is increased when gastric fluid pH is increased. Aluminum hydroxide accelerates absorption and increases bioavailability of diazepam by an unknown mechanism. Conversely, bioavailability of certain drugs may be decreased because of their capacity to form complexes with antacids. For example, antacids decrease bioavailability of orally administered cimetidine by approximately 15%.[14] Antacids containing aluminum, and to a lesser extent, calcium or magnesium, interfere with the absorption of tetracyclines and possibly digoxin from the gastrointestinal tract. It is possible based on physicochemical properties to predict the effect of changes in pH on absorption.

Histamine-Receptor Antagonists

Histamine induces contraction of smooth muscles in the airways, increases the secretion of acid in the stomach, and stimulates the release of neurotransmitters in the central nervous system (CNS) through three receptor subtypes, H_1, H_2, H_3. Recently a fourth histamine receptor, designated as an H_4 receptor was cloned,[15] which has lead to the development of several drugs that inhibit its action.[16–18]

Depending on what responses to histamine are inhibited, drugs are classified as H_1-, H_2-, H_3-, and H_4-receptor antagonists. Histamine receptor antagonists bind to receptors on effector cell membranes, to the exclusion of agonist molecules, without themselves activating the receptor. For histamine-receptor antagonists, this is a competitive and reversible interaction. It is important to recognize that histamine-receptor antagonists do not inhibit release of histamine but, rather, attach to receptors and prevent responses mediated by histamine.

H_3- and H_4-receptor modulators do not currently play a role in anesthetic practice and as such are not described in detail. Activation of H_3 receptors inhibits the synthesis and release of histamine from neurons in the CNS; as such, they act as presynaptic autoreceptors. The H_4 receptor is expressed on mast cells, dendritic cells, basophils, and T lymphocytes. Activation of the H_4 receptor induces chemotaxis of immune cells.[17]

H_1-Receptor Antagonists

H_1-receptor antagonists are characterized as first-generation and second-generation receptor antagonists (Fig. 35-1).[19,20] First-generation drugs tend to produce sedation, whereas second-generation drugs are relatively nonsedating (Table 35-1). H_1-receptor antagonists are highly selective for H_1 receptors, having little effect on H_2, H_3, or H_4 receptors. First-generation H_1-receptor antagonists may also activate muscarinic, cholinergic, 5-hydroxytryptamine (serotonin), or α-adrenergic receptors, whereas few of the second-generation antagonists have any of these properties. The selectivity of the

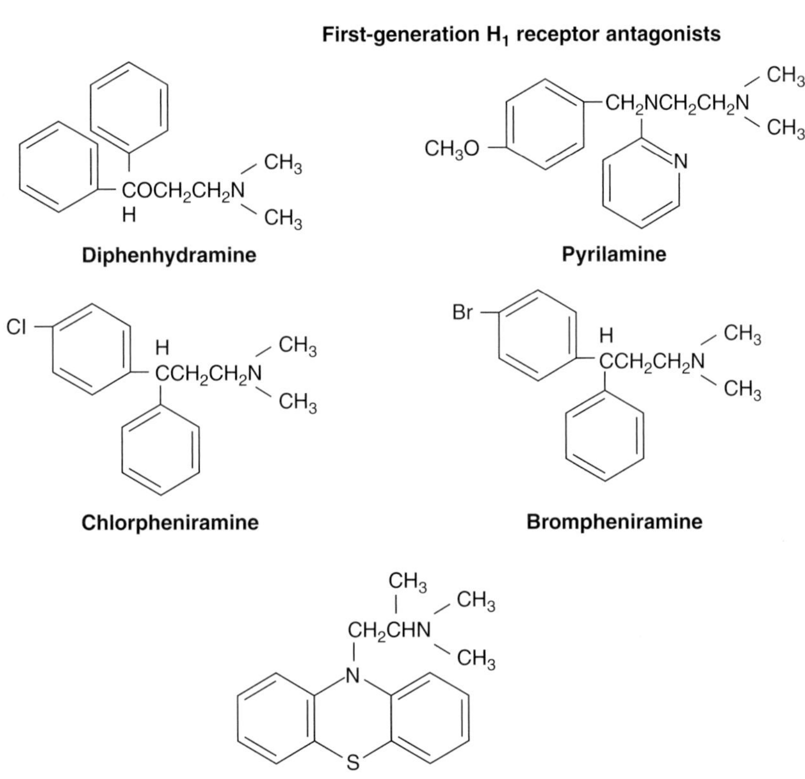

FIGURE 35-1 First-generation and second-generation H_1-receptor antagonists.

Table 35-1

Pharmacokinetics of H_1-Receptor Antagonists

	Time to Peak Plasma Level (h)	Elimination Half-Time (h)	Clearance Rate (mL/kg/min)
First-generation receptor antagonists			
Chlorpheniramine	2.8	27.9	1.8
Diphenhydramine	1.7	9.2	23.3
Hydroxyzine	2.1	20.0	98
Second-generation receptor antagonists			
Loratadine	1.0	11.0	202
Acrivastine	0.85–1.4	1.4–2.1	4.56
Azelastine	5.3	22	8.5

Data from Simons FE, Simons KJ. The pharmacology and use of H_1-receptor antagonist drugs. *N Engl J Med.* 1994;330:1663–1670.

second-generation antagonists for H_1 receptors decreases CNS toxicity. An increased understanding of the molecular pharmacologic features of these drugs has resulted in their reclassification as inverse agonists rather than as H_1-receptor antagonists.[19] H_1-receptor antagonists act as inverse agonists that combine with and stabilize the inactive form of the H_1 receptor, shifting the equilibrium toward the inactive state.

Pharmacokinetics

H_1-receptor antagonists are well absorbed after oral administration, often reaching peak plasma concentrations within 2 hours (see Table 35-1).[19,20] Many are highly protein bound, with ranges from 78% to 99%. Most of the new H_1-receptor antagonists do not accumulate in tissue to any extent. Interestingly, there is little tachyphyllaxis seen with their use.[21] Most H_1-receptor antagonists are metabolized by the hepatic microsomal mixed-function oxidase system. Plasma concentrations are relatively low after a single oral dose, which indicates first-pass hepatic extraction. Values for the elimination half-lives of these drugs are variable. For example, the elimination half-life of chlorpheniramine is >24 hours and that of acrivastine is about 2 hours (see Table 35-1).[19,20] Acrivastine is excreted mostly unchanged in urine, as is cetirizine, the active carboxylic metabolite of hydroxyzine.

Clinical Uses

H_1-receptor antagonists are among the most widely used of all medications.[19] H_1-receptor antagonists prevent and relieve the symptoms of allergic rhinoconjunctivitis (sneezing, nasal and ocular itching, rhinorrhea, tearing, and conjunctival erythema), but they are less effective for the nasal congestion characteristic of a delayed allergic reaction. In contrast to their role in the treatment of allergic rhinitis, H_1-receptor antagonists provide little benefit in the treatment of upper respiratory tract infections and are of no benefit in the management of otitis media. Depending on the H_1-receptor antagonist selected and its dose, pretreatment may provide some protection against bronchospasm induced by various stimuli (histamine, exercise, cold dry air). Earlier concerns about drying of secretions in patients with asthma have not been substantiated. In patients with chronic urticaria, H_1-receptor antagonists relieve pruritus and decrease the number, size, and duration of urticarial lesions. In some patients with refractory urticaria, concurrent treatment with an H_2-receptor antagonist (cimetidine, ranitidine) may enhance relief of pruritus. In addition to a direct effect on H_2 receptors, which account for 10% to 15% of all histamine receptors in the vasculature, this effect may be due in part to the ability of some H_2-receptor antagonists to inhibit the metabolism of H_1-receptor antagonists by the hepatic cytochrome P450 system, leading to an increased plasma and tissue concentration of H_1-receptor antagonists. The second-generation H_1-receptor antagonists (cetirizine, fexofenadine, loratadine, desloratadine, azelastine) are supplanting first-generation drugs (diphenhydramine, chlorpheniramine, cyproheptadine) in the treatment of allergic rhinoconjunctivitis and chronic urticarial. Their greater cost can be justified because of a more favorable risk-benefit ratio (e.g., they have fewer CNS side effects). For example, the first-generation H_1-receptor antagonists have sedating effects that result in delayed reaction times.

Diphenhydramine is prescribed as a sedative, an antipruritic, and as an antiemetic. When administered alone, it modestly stimulates ventilation by augmenting the interaction of hypoxic and hypercarbic ventilatory drives. When diphenhydramine is administered in combination with systemic or neuraxial opioids to control nausea and pruritus, there is the conceptual risk of depression of ventilation. However, diphenhydramine counteracts to some extent the opioid-induced decreases in the slope of the ventilatory response to CO_2 and does not exacerbate the opioid-induced depression of the hypoxic ventilatory response during moderate hypercarbia.[22]

The rich distribution of histamine receptors in the myocardium and coronary vasculature predisposes the heart to cardioregulatory changes during massive histamine release that characterizes type 1 immune-mediated hypersensitivity (anaphylactic) reactions. Use of antihistamines in the acute treatment of anaphylactic reactions is directed at blocking further histamine-mediated vasodilation and resulting homodynamic instability, as well as decreasing respiratory and other systemic complications. As such, the administration of H_1-receptor antagonists plus the administration of epinephrine is indicated in the treatment of acute anaphylaxis. H_1-receptor antagonists are also useful in the ancillary treatment of pruritus, urticaria, and angioedema. These drugs may also be administered prophylactically for anaphylactoid reactions to radiocontrast dyes. Second-generation H_1-receptor antagonists such as terfenadine, fexofenadine, and astemizole have low water solubility, and, unlike first-generation drugs, are not available for parenteral use. The addition of H_2-receptor antagonists to H_1-receptor antagonists in the treatment of anaphylaxis speeds the resolution of symptoms. Concerns of possible attenuation of H_2-mediated increases in inotropy and chronotropy, thereby limiting potential cardioexcitatory compensatory mechanisms, does not seem to be significant clinically.[23]

Dimenhydrinate is an H_1-receptor antagonist that is the theoclate salt of diphenhydramine. Dimenhydrinate has been used to treat motion sickness as well as postoperative nausea and vomiting. It is speculated that the efficacy of dimenhydrinate in motion sickness and inner ear diseases may be due to inhibition of the integrative functioning of the vestibular nuclei by decreasing vestibular and visual input. Manipulation of the extraocular muscles as in strabismus surgery may trigger an "oculoemetic" reflex similar to the well-described oculocardiac reflex. If the afferent arc of this reflex is also dependent on the integrity of the vestibular nuclei apparatus, then dimenhydrinate may attenuate or block this reflex and decrease the incidence of postoperative nausea and vomiting. Administration of dimenhydrinate, 20 mg intravenously (IV), to adults decreases vomiting after outpatient surgery.[24] In children, dimenhydrinate, 0.5 mg/kg IV, significantly decreases the incidence of vomiting after strabismus surgery and is not associated with prolonged sedation.[25] Compared with serotonin antagonists, dimenhydrinate is an inexpensive antiemetic.

Side Effects

First-generation H_1 antagonists often have adverse effects on the CNS, including somnolence, diminished alertness, slowed reaction time, and impairment of cognitive function. Because there is some cross-reactivity with muscarinic receptors, anticholinergic effects such as dry mouth, blurred vision, urinary retention, and impotence may be seen. Tachycardia is common, and prolongation of the QTc interval on the electrocardiogram (ECG), heart block, and cardiac arrhythmias have occurred. First-generation H_1-receptor antagonists are still prescribed because they are effective and inexpensive. Administration of these drugs at bedtime is sometimes recommended because drug-related somnolence is of no concern during the night. Indeed, H_1-receptor antagonists may be sold as nonprescription sleeping aids.

Second-generation H_1 antagonists are unlikely to produce CNS side effects such as somnolence unless the recommended doses are exceeded. Enhancement of the effects of diazepam or alcohol is unlikely by second-generation drugs. Fexofenadine, a metabolite of terfenadine, does not prolong the QTc interval on the ECG, even in large doses. Patients with hepatic dysfunction, cardiac disorders associated with prolongation of the QTc interval, or metabolic disorders such as hypokalemia or hypomagnesemia may be especially prone to adverse cardiovascular effects of H_1-receptor antagonists. Most second-generation H_1-receptor antagonists are not removed by hemodialysis.

Antihistamine intoxication is similar to anticholinergic poisoning and may be associated with seizures and cardiac conduction abnormalities resembling tricyclic antidepressant overdose. Older nonsedating antihistamine drugs (terfenadine, astemizole) were associated with prolongation of the QTc interval and atypical (torsades de pointes) ventricular tachycardia both after overdose and after coadministration with macrolide antibiotics, or other drugs that interfere with their elimination. These drugs were removed from the market in 1999.

H_2-Receptor Antagonists

Cimetidine, ranitidine, famotidine, and nizatidine are H_2-receptor antagonists that produce selective and reversible inhibition of H_2 receptor–mediated secretion of hydrogen ions by parietal cells in the stomach (Figs. 35-2 and 35-3).[26] The relationship between gastric hypersecretion of fluid containing high concentrations of hydrogen ions and peptic ulcer disease emphasizes the potential value of a drug that selectively blocks this response. Despite the presence of H_2 receptors throughout the body, inhibition of histamine binding to the receptors on gastric parietal cells is the major beneficial effect of H_2-receptor antagonists.

Mechanism of Action

The histamine receptors on the basolateral membranes of acid-secreting gastric parietal cells are of the H_2 type and thus are not blocked by conventional H_1 antagonists. The occupation of H_2 receptors by histamine released from mast cells and possibly other cells activates adenylate cyclase, increasing the intracellular concentrations of cyclic adenosine monophosphate (cAMP). The increased concentrations of cAMP activates the proton pump of gastric parietal cells (an enzyme designated as hydrogen-potassium-ATPase) to secrete hydrogen ions against a large concentration gradient in exchange for potassium ions.[26]

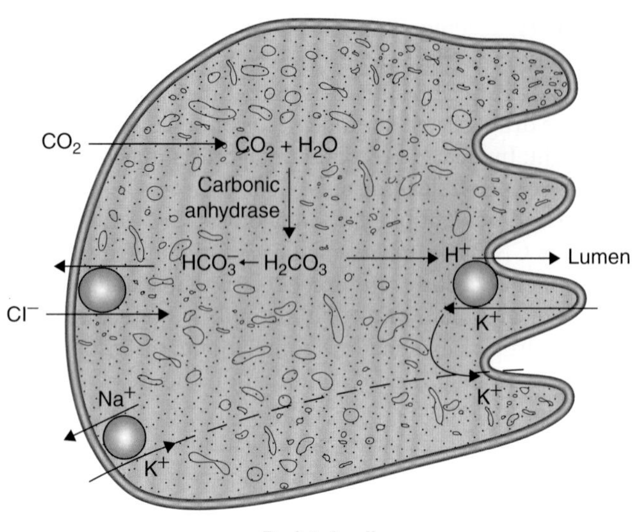

FIGURE 35-2 Ion flux through parietal cell.

Cimetidine: CH_3–(imidazole)–$CH_2SCH_2CH_2NHCNHCH_3$ (=NCN)

Ranitidine: $(CH_3)_2NCH_2$–(furan)–$CH_2SCH_2CH_2NHCNHCH_3$ (=$CHNO_2$)

Famotidine: $(H_2N)_2C{=}N$–(thiazole)–$CH_2SCH_2CH_2CNH_2$ (=NSO_2NH_2)

Nizatidine: $(CH_3)_2NCH_2$–(thiazole)–$CH_2SCH_2CH_2NHCNHCH_3$ (=$CHNO_2$)

FIGURE 35-3 H_2-receptor antagonists.

H_2-receptor antagonists competitively and selectively inhibit the binding of histamine to H_2 receptors, thereby decreasing the intracellular concentrations of cAMP and the subsequent secretion of hydrogen ions by the parietal cells.

The relative potencies of the four H_2-receptor antagonists for inhibition of secretion of gastric hydrogen ions varies from 20- to 50-fold, with cimetidine as the least potent and famotidine the most potent (Table 35-2).[26] The duration of inhibition ranges from approximately 6 hours for cimetidine to 10 hours for ranitidine, famotidine, and nizatidine. None of the four H_2-receptor antagonists have produced any consistent effects on lower esophageal sphincter function or the rate of gastric emptying.

Table 35-2

Pharmacokinetics of H_2-Receptor Antagonists

	Cimetidine	Ranitidine	Famotidine	Nizatidine
Potency	1	4–10	20–50	4–10
EC_{50} (μg/mL)[a]	250–500	60–165	10–13	154–180
Bioavailability (%)	60	50	43	98
Time to peak plasma concentration (hours)	1–2	1–3	1.0–3.5	1–3
Volume of distribution (L/kg)	0.8–1.2	1.2–1.9	1.1–1.4	1.2–1.6
Plasma protein binding (%)	13–26	15	16	26–35
Cerebrospinal fluid: plasma	0.18	0.06–0.17	0.05–0.09	Unknown
Clearance (mL/minute)	450–650	568–709	417–483	667–850
Hepatic clearance (%)				
Oral	60	73	50–80	22
Intravenous	25–40	30	25–30	25
Renal clearance (%)				
Oral	40	27	25–30	57–65
Intravenous	50–80	50	65–80	75
Elimination half-life (hours)	1.5–2.3	1.6–2.4	2.5–4	1.1–1.6
Decrease dose in presence of renal dysfunction	Yes	Yes	Yes	Yes
Hepatic dysfunction	No	No	No	No
Interfere with drug metabolism by cytochrome P450 enzymes	Yes	Minimal	No	No

[a] EC_{50} denotes the plasma concentration of the drug necessary to inhibit the pentagastrin-stimulated secretion of hydrogen ions by 50%.
Data from Feldman M, Burton ME. Histamine-$_2$-receptor antagonists. *N Engl J Med.* 1990;323:1672–1680.

Discontinuation of chronic H_2-receptor antagonist therapy is followed by rebound hypersecretion of gastric acid.

Pharmacokinetics

The absorption of cimetidine, ranitidine, and famotidine is rapid after oral administration. Because of extensive first-pass hepatic metabolism, however, the bioavailability of these drugs is approximately 50% (see Table 35-2).[26] Nizatidine does not undergo significant hepatic first-pass metabolism, and its bioavailability after oral administration approaches 100%. The average time to peak plasma concentrations of the four H_2-receptor antagonists ranges from 1 to 3 hours after oral administration. Because the volume of distribution for all four drugs exceeds the body's total body water content, some binding (13% to 35%) to proteins must occur (see Table 35-2).[26]

Cimetidine is widely distributed in most organs but not fat. Approximately 70% of the total body content of cimetidine is found in skeletal muscles. The volume of distribution is not altered by renal disease but is increased by severe hepatic disease and can be altered by changes in systemic blood pressure and cardiac output. All four drugs are present in breast milk and can cross the placenta and blood–brain barrier. The presence of cimetidine in cerebrospinal fluid is increased in patients with severe hepatic disease. The dose of cimetidine may need to be decreased to avoid mental confusion in patients with severe liver disease. The volume of distribution of cimetidine is also decreased about 40% in elderly patients, presumably reflecting the decrease in skeletal muscle mass associated with aging.

Although there is considerable variation in the clearance and elimination half-lives of H_2-receptor antagonists, their plasma elimination half-lives range from 1.5 to 4 hours (see Table 35-2).[26] The elimination of all four drugs occurs by a combination of hepatic metabolism, glomerular filtration, and renal tubular secretion. Hepatic metabolism is the principal mechanism for clearance from the plasma of oral doses of cimetidine, ranitidine, and famotidine, and renal excretion is the principal pathway for clearance from the plasma of an oral dose of nizatidine. The liver may metabolize 25% to 40% of an IV dose of nizatidine. Only nizatidine appears to have an active metabolite (*N*-2-monodesmethyl-nizatidine), possessing about 60% of the activity of the parent drug. Hepatic metabolism of cimetidine occurs primarily by conversion of its side-chain to a thioether or sulfoxide, and these inactive products appear in the urine as 5-hydroxymethyl and/or sulfoxide metabolites. The renal clearance of all four H_2-receptor antagonists is typically two to three times greater than creatinine clearance, reflecting extensive renal tubular secretion. Renal failure increases the elimination half-life of all four drugs, with the greatest effect on nizatidine and famotidine. Decreases in the doses of all four drugs are recommended for patients with renal dysfunction. Doses of H_2-receptor antagonists may also need to be decreased in patients with acute burns. Only 10% to 20% of total body cimetidine or ranitidine is cleared by hemodialysis.

Hepatic dysfunction does not seem to significantly alter the pharmacokinetics of H_2-receptor antagonists. Increasing age must be considered when determining the dose of H_2-receptor antagonists. For example, cimetidine clearance decreases 75% in patients between the ages of 20 years and 70 years.[26] There is also a 40% decrease in the volume of distribution of cimetidine in elderly patients. The elimination half-life of ranitidine and famotidine may be increased up to twofold in elderly patients.

Clinical Uses

H_2-receptor antagonists are most commonly administered for the treatment of duodenal ulcer disease associated with hypersecretion of gastric hydrogen ions. In the preoperative period, H_2-receptor antagonists have been administered as chemoprophylaxis to increase the pH of gastric fluid before induction of anesthesia. However, the American Society of Anesthesiologists' practice guidelines for preoperative fasting and the use of pharmacologic agents to reduce the risk of pulmonary aspiration state that the routine preoperative use of medications that block gastric acid secretion to decrease the risks of pulmonary aspiration in patients who have no apparent increased risk for pulmonary aspiration is not recommended.[4] When indicated though, H_2-receptor antagonists have been advocated as useful drugs in the preoperative period to decrease the risk of acid pneumonitis if inhalation of acidic gastric fluid were to occur in the perioperative period. One approach is to administer cimetidine, 300 mg orally (3 to 4 mg/kg), 1.5 to 2.0 hours before the induction of anesthesia, with or without a similar dose the preceding evening. Famotidine given the evening before and the morning of surgery or on the morning of surgery is equally effective in decreasing gastric fluid pH in outpatients and inpatients; there is no difference between famotidine doses of 20 mg or 40 mg.

The H_2-receptor antagonists also decrease gastric fluid volume.[27] Unfortunately, H_2-receptor antagonists, in contrast to antacids, have no influence on the pH of the gastric fluid that is already present in the stomach. Cimetidine crosses the placenta but does not adversely affect the fetus when administered before cesarean section. The other H_2-receptor antagonists have a profile to similar to that of cimetidine with respect to placental transfer.[28]

Preoperative preparation of patients with allergic histories or patients undergoing procedures associated with an increased likelihood of allergic reactions (radiographic contrast dye administration) may include prophylactic oral administration of an H_1-receptor antagonist (diphenhydramine, 0.5 to 1.0 mg/kg) and an H_2-receptor antagonist (cimetidine, 4 mg/kg) every 6 hours in the 12 to 24 hours preceding the possible triggering event. A corticosteroid administered at least 24 hours earlier is commonly added to this regimen. Dramatic reversals of life-threatening allergic reactions after the IV administration of cimetidine may reflect the cumulative effect of prior epinephrine administration in the presence of a prolonged circulation time.[29,30] In fact, such treatment could exacerbate bronchospasm due to sudden unmasking of unopposed histamine effects of H_1 receptors on bronchial smooth muscle. The risk of further hypotension is also a consideration with IV administration of cimetidine. Furthermore, H_2-receptor activity could have desirable effects during allergic reactions, including increased myocardial contractility and coronary artery vasodilation.

Drug-induced histamine release that may follow the rapid IV administration of certain drugs (morphine, atracurium, mivacurium, protamine) is not prevented by pretreatment with an H_1-receptor antagonist in combination with an H_2-receptor antagonist.[31] The magnitude of the systemic blood pressure decrease that occurs in response to drug-induced histamine release is less, confirming that prior occupation of histamine receptors with a specific antagonist drug attenuates the cardiovascular effects of subsequently released histamine.[32] Pretreatment with an H_1-receptor antagonist (diphenhydramine) or H_2-receptor antagonist (cimetidine) alone is not effective in preventing the cardiovascular effects of histamine that are released in response to drug administration, emphasizing the role of both H_1 and H_2 receptors in these responses. In fact, drug-induced histamine release may be exaggerated in patients pretreated with only H_2-receptor antagonists.

Side Effects

The frequency of severe side effects is low with all four H_2-receptor antagonists (Table 35-3). The risk for experiencing adverse side effects during treatment with an H_2-receptor antagonist is increased by the presence of multiple medical illnesses, hepatic or renal dysfunction, and advanced age. The most common adverse side effects are diarrhea, headache, fatigue, and skeletal muscle pain. Side effects that occur with a prevalence of <1% include mental confusion, dizziness, somnolence, gynecomastia, galactorrhea, thrombocytopenia, increased plasma levels of liver enzymes, drug fever, bradycardia, tachycardia, and cardiac arrhythmias. Cardiac reactions are most likely related to blockade of cardiac H_2 receptors. Mental confusion in patients being treated with cimetidine may be more likely in the presence of hepatic or renal dysfunction. Changes in mental status usually occur in the elderly and tend to be associated with high doses of cimetidine administered IV, often to patients in an intensive care unit. Most patients have an improvement in mental status 24 to 48 hours after discontinuing cimetidine. Ranitidine and famotidine also cross the blood–brain barrier and have been reported to produce mental confusion.[33] Mental confusion has rarely been observed in ambulatory patients being treated chronically with H_2-receptor antagonists.

Cimetidine and, to a lesser extent, ranitidine increase the plasma concentrations of prolactin, which may result in galactorrhea in females and gynecomastia in males. Famotidine and nizatidine do not appear to increase plasma prolactin levels. Cimetidine, but not the other H_2-receptor antagonists, inhibits the binding of dihydrotestosterone to androgen receptors. Indeed, impotence and loss of libido may occur in males receiving chronic high-dose treatment with cimetidine.

The adverse effects of H_2-receptor antagonists on hepatic function are typically reflected by reversible increases in the plasma level of aminotransaminase enzymes, mostly in patients receiving large IV doses of H_2-receptor antagonists. H_2-receptor antagonists probably do not markedly alter hepatic blood flow.

Cardiac arrhythmias (sinus bradycardia, sinus arrest, sinus arrest with idioventricular escape rhythm, complete atrioventricular heart block) have been described after either oral or IV administration of H_2-receptor antagonists.[34] Most of the described arrhythmias have occurred after chronic administration. Rare descriptions of prolonged QT interval and fatal cardiac arrest with famotidine have been reported.[35] Cardiac effects of H_2-receptor stimulation are similar to β_1 stimulation mediated by cAMP. This would explain why blockade of H_2-receptors might evoke bradycardia. Furthermore, blockade of H_2 receptors could increase H_1-receptor effects, including negative dromotropic effects. Bradycardia and hypotension are generally associated with rapid IV administration of these drugs, most often to critically ill or elderly patients.[36] The mechanism for hypotension appears to be peripheral vasodilation. A prudent approach is to administer these drugs over 15 to 30 minutes when IV administration is needed.

Prolonged H_2-receptor blockade and associated gastric achlorhydria may weaken the gastric barrier to bacteria and predispose to systemic infections.[37,38] Likewise, pulmonary infections from inhaled secretions may be more likely if the acid-killing effect on bacteria in the stomach is altered. Nevertheless, if acid suppression increases

Table 35-3

Side Effects of H_2-Receptor Antagonists

- Interaction with cerebral H_2 receptors (headache, somnolence, confusion)
- Interaction with cardiac H_2 receptors (bradycardia, hypotension, heart block)
- Hyperprolactinemia
- Acute pancreatitis
- Increased hepatic transaminase levels
- Alcohol dehydrogenase dehydration
- Thrombocytopenia
- Agranulocytosis
- Interstitial nephritis
- Interference with drug metabolism by cytochrome P450

the risk of pneumonia, that risk is small and usually amenable to therapy.[38] Sustained increases of gastric fluid pH may lead to an overgrowth of other organisms such as *Candida albicans*. This may account for the occasional case of *Candida* peritonitis observed after peptic ulcer perforation in patients treated with cimetidine. Prolonged increases of gastric fluid pH also result in the production of nitroso compounds because of an increase in nitrate-reducing bacteria.[39] Nitroso derivatives are potent mutagens in vitro, but there is no evidence that this occurs in vivo in association with chronic cimetidine therapy.

Cimetidine, but not ranitidine or famotidine, has been shown to augment cell-mediated immunity through its blockade of H_2 receptors on T lymphocytes.[26]

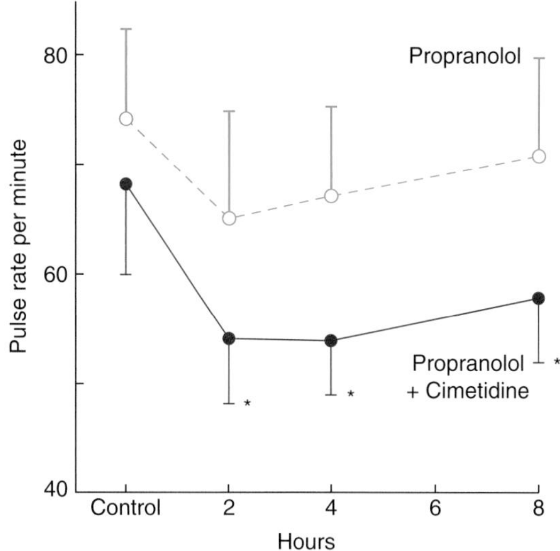

FIGURE 35-4 The effect of propranolol on resting heart rate is accentuated by the concomitant administration of cimetidine. (Mean ± SD; n = 5;*P <.05.) (From Feely J, Wilkinson GR, Wood AJJ. Reduction of liver blood flow and propranolol metabolism by cimetidine. *N Engl J Med.* 1981;304:692–696.)

Drug Interactions

Numerous drug interactions have been described between H_2-receptor antagonists, most commonly cimetidine, and other drugs (Table 35-4).[26] Drug interactions generally occur when a new drug is either started or discontinued. In this regard, measurement of plasma drug concentrations or laboratory measurements of an effect (prothrombin time) may be useful.

The principal type of drug interaction reported with cimetidine is impairment of the hepatic metabolism of another drug because of the binding of cimetidine to the heme portion of the cytochrome P450 oxidase system. Cimetidine retards metabolism of drugs such as propranolol and diazepam that normally undergo high hepatic extraction.[40,41] Slowed metabolism and prolonged elimination half-life with associated exaggerated pharmacologic effects of propranolol and diazepam have been documented with only 24 hours of treatment with cimetidine (Figs. 35-4 and 35-5).[41,42] In contrast, benzodiazepines, such as oxazepam and lorazepam that are eliminated almost entirely by glucuronidation are not altered by cimetidine-induced effects on P450 enzyme activity. Cimetidine may slow metabolism of lidocaine and thus increase the possibility of systemic toxicity.[43] In contrast, plasma

Table 35-4

Drug Interactions with Cimetidine

Drug	Effect of Cimetidine on Plasma Concentration	Clearance of Drug (% Decrease)	Mechanism
Ketoconazole	Decreased	No change	Decreased absorption due to increased gastric fluid pH that slows dissolution
Warfarin[a]	Increased	23–36	Decreased hydroxylation of dextrorotatory isomer
Theophylline[a]	Increased	12–34	Decreased methylation
Phenytoin[a]	Increased	21–24	Decreased hydroxylation (?)
Propranolol	Increased	20–27	Decreased hydroxylation
Nifedipine	Increased	38	Unknown
Lidocaine	Increased	14–30	Decreased *N*-dealkylation
Quinidine	Increased	25–37	Decreased 3-hydroxylation (?)
Imipramine	Increased	40	Decreased *N*-demethylation
Desipramine	Increased	36	Decreased hydroxylation in rapid metabolizers
Triazolam	Increased	27	Decreased hydroxylation
Meperidine	Increased	22	Decreased oxidation
Procainamide[a]	Increased	28	Competition for renal tubular secretion

[a] Lesser drug interactions also occur with ranitidine.

Data from Feldman M, Burton ME. Histamine-$_2$-receptor antagonists. *N Engl J Med.* 1990;323:1672–1680.

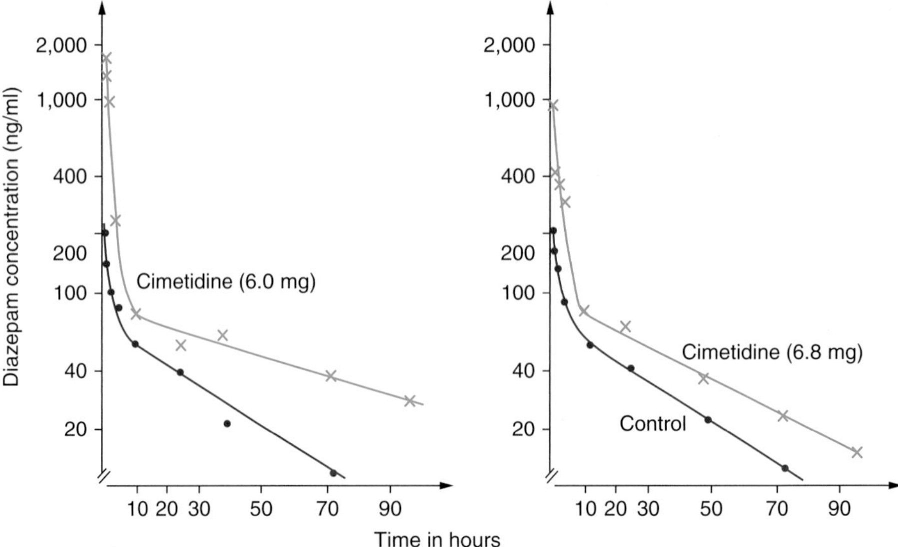

FIGURE 35-5 The rate of decline in the plasma concentration of diazepam, 0.1 mg/kg IV, is slowed by the prior administration of cimetidine, 6.0 to 6.8 mg/kg.

concentrations of bupivacaine after epidural anesthesia for cesarean section are not influenced by a single dose of cimetidine administered before induction of anesthesia (Fig. 35-6).[44,45] Indeed, plasma cholinesterase activity is not altered by cimetidine.[46] Ranitidine, although more potent than cimetidine, binds less avidly to the cytochrome P450 enzyme system and has less potential than cimetidine to alter the oxidative metabolism of other drugs. Famotidine and nizatidine do not bind notably to the cytochrome P450 enzyme system and thus have very limited potential for inhibiting the metabolism of other drugs.

H_2-receptor antagonists compete with cationic compounds for renal tubular secretion. Because of the competition of cimetidine and ranitidine with creatinine for renal tubular secretion, serum creatinine levels are increased about 15%. Cimetidine and ranitidine, but not famotidine, impair renal tubular secretion of procainamide and theophylline. Famotidine, however, has been reported to interfere with phosphate absorption, leading to the development of hypophosphatemia.[47] Impairment of renal theophylline clearance with cimetidine is probably negligible compared with impairment of the hepatic metabolism of theophylline.

All four H_2-receptor antagonists have the potential to alter the absorption of some drugs by increasing the gastric fluid pH. Cimetidine has been reported to enhance the absorption of ethanol from the stomach as a result of inhibition of gastric alcohol dehydrogenase.

In addition to drug interactions produced by H_2-receptor antagonists, several drugs alter the disposition

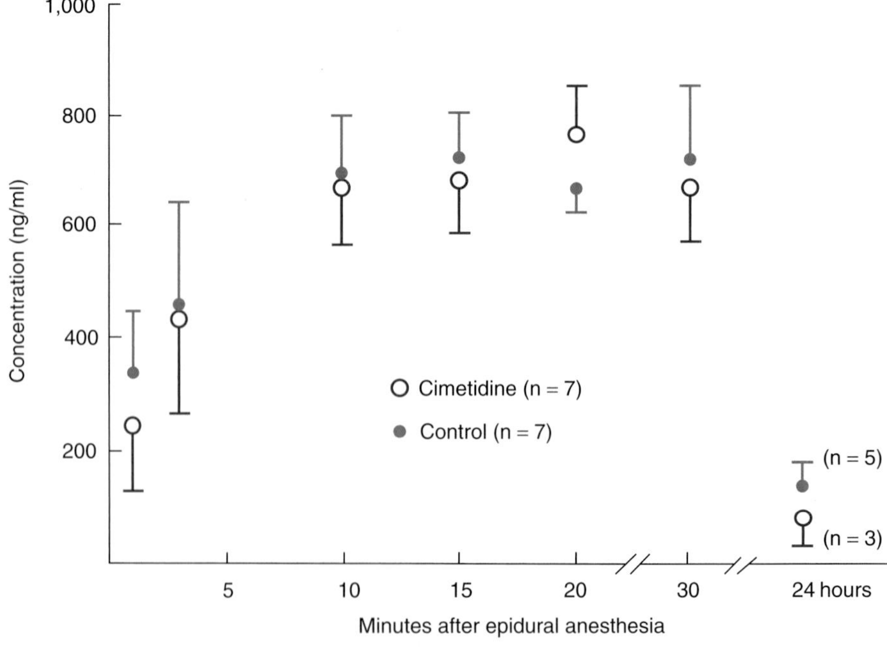

FIGURE 35-6 Maternal plasma levels of bupivacaine after epidural anesthesia. (From Kuhnert BR, Zuspan KJ, Kuhnert PM, et al. Lack of influence of cimetidine on bupivacaine levels during parturition. *Anesth Analg.* 1987; 66:986–990, with permission.)

of the antagonists. Magnesium and aluminum hydroxide antacids decrease by 30% to 40%, respectively, the bioavailability of cimetidine, ranitidine, and famotidine. Despite this impaired absorption, therapeutic blood levels of the H_2 antagonist can still be achieved, and rigorous separation of dosage schedules during combined drug therapy is probably unnecessary.[48] Hepatic metabolism of cimetidine may be enhanced if phenobarbital is administered concurrently.

Proton Pump Inhibitors

Proton pump inhibitors (PPIs) (omeprazole, esomeprazole, lansoprazole, pantoprazole, rabeprazole) are the most effective drugs available for controlling gastric acidity and volume (Table 35-5). The final step in gastric acid secretion is the membrane enzyme proton pump (hydrogen-potassium-ATPase) that moves hydrogen ions across the gastric parietal cell membranes in exchange for potassium ions. The secretion of hydrochloric acid by gastric parietal cells ultimately depends on the function of the proton (hydrogen ion) pump. PPIs are more effective than H_2-receptor antagonists for healing esophagitis and preventing relapse. PPIs also appear to be more effective than H_2-receptor antagonists for relieving heartburn, the cardinal feature of "gastroesophageal reflux disease."[49] However, for patients without esophagitis and infrequent symptoms H_2-receptor antagonists are probably more cost effective.

Omeprazole

Omeprazole is a substituted benzimidazole that acts as a prodrug that becomes a PPI.[50,51] (Fig. 35-7) As a weak base, omeprazole is concentrated in the secretory canaliculi of the gastric parietal cells. It is at this site that omeprazole is pronated to its active form, which inhibits the enzyme pump. The initial dose of omeprazole will only inhibit those proton pumps present and working on the luminal surface. As pumps are generated and inserted into the luminal surfaces, additional doses are required to inhibit these new pumps. Therefore, omeprazole takes several days to exert its maximal inhibitory effect on gastric acid secretion. Daily administration results in about 66% inhibition of gastric acid secretion by about 5 days. Likewise, discontinuation of omeprazole is not followed immediately by return of gastric acid secretion.[52]

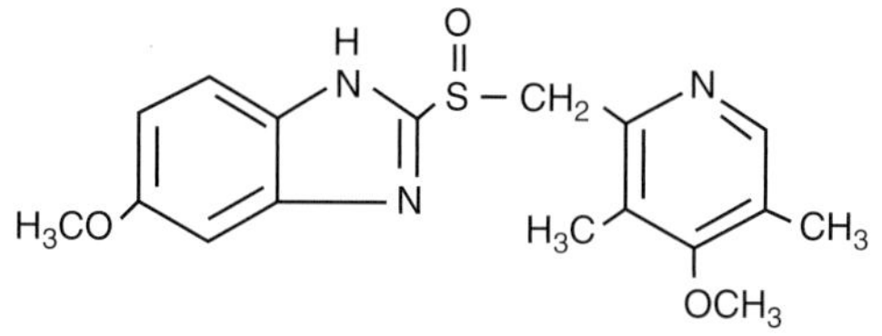

FIGURE 35-7 Omeprazole.

Omeprazole provides prolonged inhibition of gastric acid secretion, regardless of the stimulus, and it inhibits daytime and nocturnal acid secretion and meal-stimulated acid secretion to a significantly greater degree than do the H_2-receptor antagonists. This drug heals duodenal and possibly gastric ulcers more rapidly than do the H_2-receptor antagonists. In patients with bleeding peptic ulcers and signs of recent bleeding, treatment with omeprazole decreases the rate of bleeding and the need for surgery.[53] Omeprazole is superior to H_2-receptor antagonists for the treatment of reflux esophagitis[49] and is the best pharmacologic treatment of Zollinger-Ellison syndrome.[50]

Preoperative Medication

As preoperative medication, omeprazole effectively increases gastric fluid pH and decreases gastric fluid volume in children and adults.[54,55] In this regard, the onset of the gastric antisecretory effect of omeprazole after a single oral dose (20 mg) occurs within 2 to 6 hours. The duration of action is prolonged (>24 hours) because the drug is concentrated selectively in the acidic environment of gastric parietal cells. Omeprazole, 20 mg orally administered the night before surgery, increases gastric fluid pH, whereas administration on the day of surgery (up to 3 hours before induction of anesthesia) fails to improve the environment of the gastric fluid.[55] This suggests that

Table 35-5

Pharmacokinetics of Proton Pump Inhibitors

	Bioavailability	Time to Peak Plasma Concentration (h)	Protein Binding	Elimination Half-Life (h)	Hepatic Metabolism	Interference with Cytochrome P450
Omeprazole	60%	2–4	>90%	0.5–1.0	Yes	Minimal
Esomeprazole	60%	2–4	>90%	0.5–1.0	Yes	Minimal
Lansoprazole	85%	1.5–3.0	97%	1.5	Yes	Minimal
Pantoprazole	77%	2.5	98%	1.9	Yes	No
Rabeprazole	85%	2.9–3.8	96%	1	Yes	No

oral omeprazole should be administered >3 hours before anticipated induction of anesthesia to ensure adequate chemoprophylaxis.

Side Effects

Omeprazole crosses the blood–brain barrier and may cause headache, agitation, and confusion. Gastrointestinal side effects include abdominal pain, flatulence, nausea, and vomiting. Small bowel bacterial overgrowth may occur owing to acid suppression. The loss of the inhibitory effect of gastric acid results in increased plasma concentrations of gastrin. There is no need to decrease the dose of PPIs in the presence of renal or hepatic dysfunction.

Esomeprazole

Esomeprazole is the levorotatory isomer of omeprazole. This levoisomer is metabolized differently in the liver, resulting in greater plasma concentrations of the drug compared with the racemic drug, omeprazole.

Pantoprazole

Pantoprazole is a potent and fast-acting PPI. Memis et al.[56] studied two groups of 30 patients each and administered pantoprazole (40 mg) or ranitidine (50 mg) IV 1 hour before the induction of anesthesia and found that both were equally effective in decreasing gastric fluid volume and pH.

Gastrointestinal Prokinetics

Motility-modulating drugs exert their therapeutic effects by increasing lower esophageal sphincter tone, enhancing peristaltic contractions and accelerating the rate of gastric emptying.

Dopamine Blockers

Metoclopramide

Metoclopramide acts as a gastrointestinal prokinetic drug that increases lower esophageal sphincter tone and stimulates motility of the upper gastrointestinal tract in normal persons and parturients.[57] It is the only drug approved by the U.S. Food and Drug Administration (FDA) for the treatment of diabetic gastroparesis.[58] Gastric hydrogen ion secretion is not altered. The net effect is accelerated gastric clearance of liquids and solids (decreased gastric emptying time) and a shortened transit time through the small intestine.

Domperidone

Domperidone is a benzimidazole derivative that, like metoclopramide, acts as a specific dopamine antagonist that stimulates peristalsis in the gastrointestinal tract, speeds gastric emptying, and increases lower esophageal sphincter tone (Fig. 35-8).[59] Domperidone is currently not marketed in the Unites States.[60]

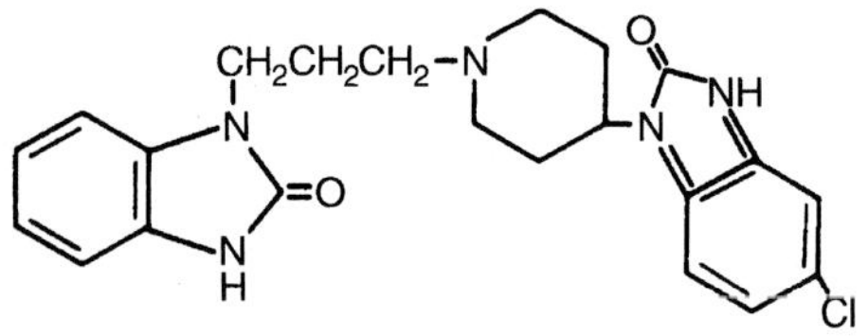

FIGURE 35-8 Domperidone.

Unlike metoclopramide, domperidone does not easily cross the blood–brain barrier and does not appear to have any anticholinergic activity. Its gastrokinetic actions have therefore been attributed to its peripheral dopaminergic activity. Because it lacks dopaminergic effects in the CNS, this drug is not associated with extrapyramidal symptoms. However, it does effect prolactin secretion by the pituitary. The FDA refused to give approval for domperidone's sale in the United States because of concerns about lactating women using dromperiodone to increase breast milk production because of the cardiac risks associated with domperidone use (e.g., cardiac arrhythmias, cardiac arrest, and sudden death). It is possible to obtain permission from the FDA for nonlactating adults with gastrointestinal motility disorders that are difficult to manage with available therapy, in whom domperidone's potential benefits outweigh its cardiac risks. The value of domperidone as prophylaxis against or treatment of postoperative nausea and vomiting is unclear.[61]

Mechanism of Action

Metoclopramide produces selective cholinergic stimulation of the gastrointestinal tract (gastrokinetic effect) consisting of (a) increased smooth muscle tension in the lower esophageal sphincter and gastric fundus, (b) increased gastric and small intestinal motility, and (c) relaxation of the pylorus and duodenum during contraction of the stomach.[62] The cholinergic stimulating effects of metoclopramide are largely restricted to smooth muscles of the proximal gastrointestinal tract and require some background cholinergic activity. There is evidence that metoclopramide sensitizes gastrointestinal smooth muscles to the effects of acetylcholine, which explains the observation that metoclopramide, unlike conventional cholinergic drugs, requires background cholinergic activity to be effective. Postsynaptic activity results from the ability of metoclopramide to cause the release of acetylcholine from cholinergic nerve endings. Indeed, atropine opposes metoclopramide-induced increases in lower esophageal sphincter tone and gastrointestinal hypermotility, indicating that metoclopramide acts on postganglionic cholinergic nerves intrinsic to the wall of the gastrointestinal tract.

Metoclopramide acts as a dopamine-receptor antagonist, but any effects on dopamine-induced inhibition of gastrointestinal motility are not considered to be clinically significant.[63] However, metoclopramide does cross the blood–brain barrier and, within the CNS, metoclopramide inhibiton of dopamine receptors can produce significant extrapyramidal side effects.[58] Metoclopramide's dopamine receptor antagomism also stimulates prolactin secretion but its risk-benefit ratio is considered safer than that of a domperidone. Metoclopramide-induced antagonism of dopamine-agonist effects on the chemoreceptor trigger zone (located outside the blood–brain barrier) contributes to an antiemetic effect.

Pharmacokinetics

Metoclopramide is rapidly absorbed after oral administration, reaching peak plasma concentrations in 40 to 120 minutes.[62] Extensive first-pass hepatic metabolism limits bioavailability to about 75%. Most patients achieve therapeutic plasma concentrations of 40 to 80 ng/mL after 10 mg of metoclopramide administered orally. The elimination half-life is 2 to 4 hours. Metoclopramide readily crosses the blood–brain barrier and the placenta. The concentration of metoclopramide in breast milk may exceed the plasma concentration. Approximately 85% of an oral dose of metoclopramide appears in the urine, equally divided between unchanged drug and sulfate and glucuronide conjugates. Impairment of renal function prolongs the elimination half-life and necessitates a decrease in metoclopramide dosage.

Clinical Uses

Clinical uses of metoclopramide include (a) preoperative decrease of gastric fluid volume, (b) production of an antiemetic effect, (c) treatment of gastroparesis, (d) symptomatic treatment of gastroesophageal reflux, and (e) intolerance to enteral feedings in patients who are critically ill.[64] Administration of metoclopramide, 10 to 20 mg IV, may be useful to speed gastric emptying before the induction of anesthesia, to facilitate small-bowel intubation, or to speed gastric emptying to improve radiographic examination of the small intestine. Metoclopramide has been used to improve the effectiveness of oral medication if other drugs or the patient's underlying condition slows gastric emptying.

Preoperative Decrease in Gastric Fluid Volume

Metoclopramide, 10 to 20 mg IV over 3 to 5 minutes administered 15[65] to 30[66] minutes before induction of anesthesia, results in increased lower esophageal sphincter tone and decreased gastric fluid volume. More rapid IV administration may produce abdominal cramping. This gastric-emptying effect of metoclopramide may be of potential benefit before the induction of anesthesia in (a) patients who have recently ingested solid food, (b) trauma patients, (c) obese patients, (d) patients with diabetes mellitus and symptoms of gastroparesis, and (e) parturients, especially those with a history of esophagitis ("heartburn"), suggesting lower esophageal sphincter dysfunction and gastric hypomotility. Nevertheless, beneficial effects of metoclopramide on gastric fluid volume may be difficult to document in otherwise normal patients with low gastric fluid volumes who are awaiting elective surgery (Table 35-6).[67]

Regardless of the effects of gastric fluid volume, the administration of metoclopramide does not reliably alter gastric fluid pH. Furthermore, it is important to recognize that opioid-induced inhibition of gastric motility may not be reversible with metoclopramide. Likewise, the beneficial cholinergic stimulant effects of metoclopramide on the gastrointestinal tract may be offset by concomitant administration of atropine in the preoperative medication. Metoclopramide and other prophylactic drugs (antacids or H_2 antagonists) do not replace the need for proper airway management, including placement of a cuffed tracheal tube.

Production of an Antiemetic Effect

The antiemetic effect of metoclopramide in preventing postoperative nausea and vomiting has been debated.[68] However, metoclopramide has been shown to decrease chemotherapy-induced nausea and vomiting and nausea and vomiting after cesarean section, although it is less efficacious than 5-HT_3 antagonsts.[69–71] The antiemetic property of metoclopramide probably results from antagonism

Table 35-6

Volume of Gastric Contents and pH in Study Groups (Mean ± SE)

	Metoclopramide (n = 30)	Placebo (n = 28)
Gastric volume (range)	24 ± 2 mL (3–600)	30 ± 5 mL (4–155)
Volume <25 mL	16[a] (53%)	15[a] (54%)
Gastric pH (range)	2.86 ± 0.27 (1–6)	2.55 ± 5 mL (1–5.5)
pH <2.5	12[a] (40%)	16[a] (57%)

[a]Number of patients.

Data from Cohen SE, Jasson J, Talafre ML, et al. Does metoclopramide decrease the volume of gastric contents in patients undergoing cesarean section? *Anesthesiology*. 1984;61:604–607, with permission.

of dopamine's effects in the chemoreceptor trigger zone. Additional antiemetic effects are provided by metoclopramide-induced increases in lower esophageal sphincter tone and facilitation of gastric emptying in the small intestine. These latter effects reverse the gastric immobility and cephalad peristalsis that accompany the vomiting reflex. Gastric stasis induced by morphine is reversed by metoclopramide, and opioid-induced nausea and vomiting, which can accompany preoperative medication or postoperative pain management, are blunted.

Side Effects

Metoclopramide should not be administered to patients with known Parkinson disease, restless leg syndrome, or who have movement disorders related to dopamine inhibition or depletion.[58] In patients with no known movement disorders, dystonic extrapyramidal reactions (oculogyric crises, opisthotonus, trismus, torticollis) occur in <1% of patients treated chronically with metoclopramide. Although extrapyramidal reactions may be a problem if large oral doses (40 to 80 mg daily) are administered chronically, there are reports of neurologic dysfunction related to the preoperative administration of metoclopramide.[72] These extrapyramidal reactions are identical to the parkinsonian syndrome evoked by antipsychotic drugs that antagonize the CNS actions of dopamine.[73] Akathisia, a feeling of unease and restlessness in the lower extremities, may follow the IV administration of metoclopramide, resulting in cancellation of scheduled surgery,[74] or may manifest in the postanesthesia care unit.[58,75]

Abdominal cramping may follow rapid IV administration (<3 minutes) of metoclopramide. IV administration of metoclopramide may also be associated with hypotension, tachycardia, bradycardia, and cardiac arrhythmias. Sedation, dysphoria, agitation, dry mouth, glossal or periorbital edema, hirsutism, and urticarial or maculopapular rash are rare side effects that have not been observed after single doses of metoclopramide. Breast enlargement, galactorrhea, or menstrual irregularities that occur rarely are presumed to reflect metoclopramide-induced increases in plasma prolactin concentrations. For this reason, patients with a history of breast cancer probably should not be treated chronically with metoclopramide.

Placental transfer of metoclopramide occurs rapidly, but adverse fetal effects with single doses have not been observed.[67] The usual dopamine-induced inhibition of aldosterone secretion is prevented by metoclopramide. As a result, the possibility of sodium retention and hypokalemia should be considered, especially in patients who develop peripheral edema during chronic therapy.

Metoclopramide may increase the sedative actions of CNS depressants and the incidence of extrapyramidal reactions caused by certain drugs. For this reason, metoclopramide should probably not be administered in combination with phenothiazine or butyrophenone drugs or to patients with preexisting extrapyramidal symptoms or signs, as mentioned previously, or with seizure disorders. Patients being treated with monoamine oxidase inhibitors or tricyclic antidepressants should likewise probably not receive metoclopramide. Metoclopramide decreases bioavailability of orally administered cimetidine by 25% to 50%.[14] It would seem prudent not to administer metoclopramide to a patient with a suspected or known mechanical obstruction to gastric emptying. Likewise, metoclopramide is not administered after gastrointestinal surgery such as pyloroplasty or intestinal anastomosis because it stimulates gastric motility and may delay healing.

Metoclopramide has an inhibitory effect on plasma cholinesterase activity when tested in vivo, which may explain occasional observations of prolonged responses to succinylcholine and mivacurium in patients receiving these drugs.[76,77] Parturients may be at increased risk for developing this response, considering the already decreased plasma cholinesterase activity associated with pregnancy. Likewise, the metabolism of ester local anesthetics could be slowed by metoclopramide-induced decreases in plasma cholinesterase activity.

Macrolides

The antibiotic erythromycin, as well as other macrolide antibiotics (i.e., azithromycin),[78] increases lower esophageal sphincter tone, enhances intraduodenal coordination, and promotes emptying of gastric liquids and solids in patients with diabetic gastroparesis,[79] in patients awaiting emergency surgery,[80] in normal patients,[81] and in patients in the intensive care unit with food intolerance[82] (Fig. 35-9). The macrolide antibiotics' prokinetic properties are attributed to their binding to motilin receptors in the stomach and duodenum,[78] although part of their prokinetic action may be secondary to cholinergic stimulatory properties.[83] Side effects of the macrolide compounds are the same as for any antibiotic, and therefore, because of concerns about tolerance, there are those that believe that erythromycin should be used if all other prokinetic agents have failed.[84]

5-HT_4–Receptor Agonists

Nonselective 5-HT_4–receptor agonists, such as cisapride and mosapride, decrease acid reflux, increase lower esophageal sphincter tone, improve gastric motility, and increase motility in the small and large intestine by enhancing the release of acetylcholine from nerve endings in the myenteric plexus of the gastrointestinal mucosa.[85] Opioid-induced gastric stasis, which is an important cause of postoperative nausea and vomiting, is reversed by cisapride.[86] Tegaserod, a partial 5-HT_4–receptor agonist improves small and large intestine transit and reduces constipation. Due to their relative nonselectivity, cisapride and mosapride are associated with prolongation of the QT interval.

Serotonin Agonists

Serotonin is involved in gastrointestinal motility and secretion, but studies of nonselective drugs that enhance serotonin action have not shown benefit.[87]

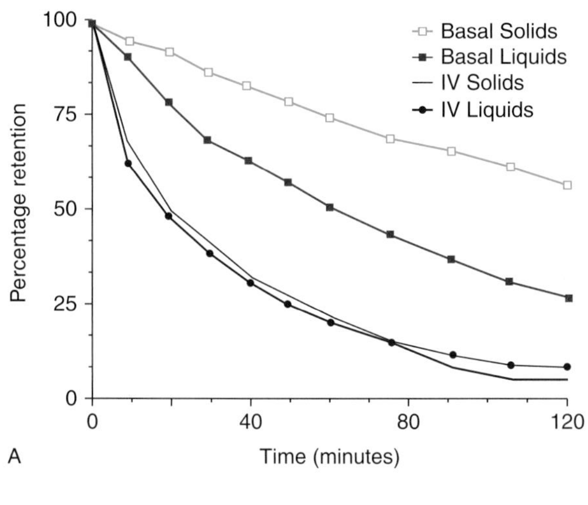

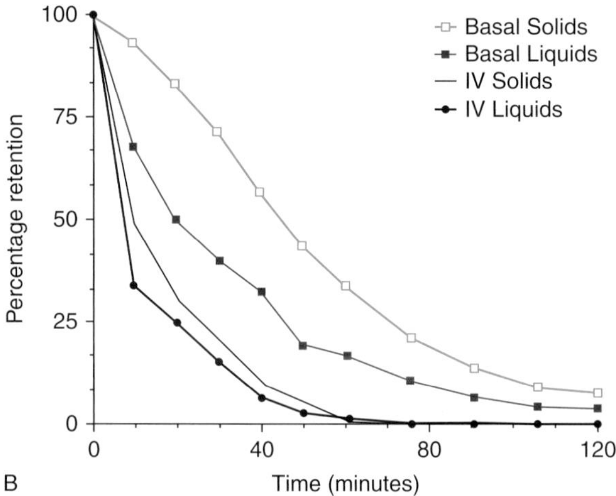

FIGURE 35-9 Erythromycin, 200 mg, administered intravenously over 15 minutes, followed by ingestion of a radioactive-labeled meal (scrambled egg, toast, and water) resulted in more rapid emptying of solids and liquids (IV solids and IV liquids) in patients with diabetic gastroparesis **(A)** and patients without diabetes **(B)** compared with gastric emptying times in the absence of erythromycin (basal solids and basal liquids). (From Urbain JLC, Vantrappen G, Janssens J, et al. Intravenous erythromycin dramatically accelerates gastric emptying in gastroparesis diabeticorum and normal and abolishes the emptying discrimination between solids and liquids. *J Nucl Med.* 1990;31:1490–1493, with permission.)

References

1. Neelakanta G, Chikyarappa A. A review of patients with pulmonary aspiration of gastric contents during anesthesia reported to the Departmental Quality Assurance Committee. *J Clin Anesth.* 2006;18(2):102–107.
2. Warner MA, Warner ME, Warner DO, et al. Perioperative pulmonary aspiration in infants and children. *Anesthesiology.* 1999;90(1):66–71.
3. Warner MA, Warner ME, Weber JG. Clinical significance of pulmonary aspiration during the perioperative period. *Anesthesiology.* 1993;78(1):56–62.
4. American Society of Anesthesiologists Committee. Practice guidelines for preoperative fasting and the use of pharmacologic agents to reduce the risk of pulmonary aspiration: application to healthy patients undergoing elective procedures: an updated report by the American Society of Anesthesiologists Committee on Standards and Practice Parameters. *Anesthesiology.* 2011;114(3):495–511.
5. Madias NE, Levey AS. Metabolic alkalosis due to absorption of "nonabsorbable" antacids. *Am J Med.* 1983;74(1):155–158.
6. Clayman CB. The carbonate affair: chalk one up. *JAMA.* 1980; 244(22):2554.
7. Berlyne GM, Ben-Ari J, Pest D, et al. Hyperaluminaemia from aluminum resins in renal failure. *Lancet.* 1970;2(7671):494–496.
8. Bakir AA, Hryhorczuk DO, Ahmed S, et al. Hyperaluminemia in renal failure: the influence of age and citrate intake. *Clin Nephrol.* 1989;31(1):40–44.
9. Holdsworth JD, Johnson K, Mascall G, et al. Mixing of antacids with stomach contents. Another approach to the prevention of the acid aspiration (Mendelson's) syndrome. *Anaesthesia.* 1980;35(7): 641–650.
10. Gibbs CP, Schwartz DJ, Wynne JW, et al. Antacid pulmonary aspiration in the dog. *Anesthesiology.* 1979;51(5):380–385.
11. Gibbs CP, Banner TC. Effectiveness of Bicitra as a preoperative antacid. *Anesthesiology.* 1984;61(1):97–99.
12. Theisen J, Nehra D, Citron D, et al. Suppression of gastric acid secretion in patients with gastroesophageal reflux disease results in gastric bacterial overgrowth and deconjugation of bile acids. *J Gastrointest Surg.* 2000;4(1):50–54.
13. Neuvonen PJ, Kivisto KT. Enhancement of drug absorption by antacids. An unrecognised drug interaction. *Clin Pharmacokinet.* 1994;27(2):120–128.
14. Gugler R, Brand M, Somogyi A. Impaired cimetidine absorption due to antacids and metoclopramide. *Eur J Clin Pharmacol.* 1981; 20(3):225–228.
15. Liu C, Ma X, Jiang X, et al. Cloning and pharmacological characterization of a fourth histamine receptor (H(4)) expressed in bone marrow. *Mol Pharmacol.* 2001;59(3):420–426.
16. Jablonowski JA, Grice CA, Chai W, et al. The first potent and selective non-imidazole human histamine H4 receptor antagonists. *J Med Chem.* 2003;46(19):3957–3960.
17. Marson CM. Targeting the histamine H4 receptor. *Chem Rev.* 2011;111(11):7121–7156.
18. Engelhardt H, Schultes S, de Graaf C, et al. Bispyrimidines as potent histamine H(4) receptor ligands: delineation of structure-activity relationships and detailed H(4) receptor binding mode. *J Med Chem.* 2013;56(11):4264–4276.
19. Simons FE. Advances in H1-antihistamines. *N Engl J Med.* 2004; 351(21):2203–2217.
20. Simons FE, Simons KJ. The pharmacology and use of H1-receptor-antagonist drugs. *N Engl J Med.* 1994;330(23):1663–1670.
21. Simons FE, Simons KJ. Clinical pharmacology of new histamine H1 receptor antagonists. *Clin Pharmacokinet.* 1999;36(5): 329–352.
22. Babenco HD, Blouin RT, Conard PF, et al. Diphenylhydramine increases ventilatory drive during alfentanil infusion. *Anesthesiology.* 1998;89(3):642–647.
23. Nault MA, Milne B, Parlow JL. Effects of the selective H1 and H2 histamine receptor antagonists loratadine and ranitidine on autonomic control of the heart. *Anesthesiology.* 2002;96(2):336–341.
24. Buckley DN. Best evidence in anesthetic practice: prevention: dimenhydrinate prevents postoperative nausea and vomiting. *Can J Anaesth.* 2003;50(1):11–12.
25. Vener DF, Carr AS, Sikich N, et al. Dimenhydrinate decreases vomiting after strabismus surgery in children. *Anesth Analg.* 1996; 82(4):728–731.
26. Feldman M, Burton ME. Histamine2-receptor antagonists. Standard therapy for acid-peptic diseases. 1. *N Engl J Med.* 1990;323(24): 1672–1680.
27. O'Connor TA, Basak J, Parker S. The effect of three different ranitidine dosage regimens on reducing gastric acidity and volume in ambulatory surgical patients. *Pharmacotherapy.* 1995;15(2): 170–175.
28. Dicke JM, Johnson RF, Henderson GI, et al. A comparative evaluation of the transport of H2-receptor antagonists by the human and baboon placenta. *Am J Med Sci.* 1988;295(3):198–206.

29. De Soto H, Turk P. Cimetidine in anaphylactic shock refractory to standard therapy. *Anesth Analg*. 1989;69(2):264–265.
30. Kelly JS, Prielipp RC. Is cimetidine indicated in the treatment of acute anaphylactic shock? *Anesth Analg*. 1990;71(1):104–105.
31. Moss J, Rosow CE, Savarese JJ, et al. Role of histamine in the hypotensive action of d-tubocurarine in humans. *Anesthesiology*. 1981; 55(1):19–25.
32. Philbin DM, Moss J, Akins CW, et al. The use of H1 and H2 histamine antagonists with morphine anesthesia: a double-blind study. *Anesthesiology*. 1981;55(3):292–296.
33. Boustani M, Hall KS, Lane KA, et al. The association between cognition and histamine-2 receptor antagonists in African Americans. *J Am Geriatr Soc*. 2007;55(8):1248–1253.
34. Shah RR. Symptomatic bradycardia in association with H2-receptor antagonists. *Lancet*. 1982;2(8307):1108.
35. Warning Famotidine2014.
36. Iberti TJ, Paluch TA, Helmer L, et al. The hemodynamic effects of intravenous cimetidine in intensive care unit patients: a double-blind, prospective study. *Anesthesiology*. 1986;64(1):87–89.
37. Cristiano P, Paradisi F. Can cimetidine facilitate infections by oral route. *Lancet*. 1982;2(8288):45.
38. Gregor JC. Acid suppression and pneumonia: a clinical indication for rational prescribing. *JAMA*. 2004;292(16):2012–2013.
39. Milton-Thompson GJ, Lightfoot NF, Ahmet Z, et al. Intragastric acidity, bacteria, nitrite, and N-nitroso compounds before, during, and after cimetidine treatment. *Lancet*. 1982;1(8281):1091–1095.
40. Donovan MA, Heagerty AM, Patel L, et al. Cimetidine and bioavailability of propranolol. *Lancet*. 1981;1(8212):164.
41. Klotz U, Reimann I. Delayed clearance of diazepam due to cimetidine. *N Engl J Med*. 1980;302(18):1012–1014.
42. Feely J, Wilkinson GR, Wood AJ. Reduction of liver blood flow and propranolol metabolism by cimetidine. *N Engl J Med*. 1981; 304(12):692–695.
43. Feely J, Wilkinson GR, McAllister CB, et al. Increased toxicity and reduced clearance of lidocaine by cimetidine. *Ann Int Med*. 1982; 96(5):592–594.
44. Flynn RJ, Moore J, Collier PS, et al. Does pretreatment with cimetidine and ranitidine affect the disposition of bupivacaine? *Br J Anaesth*. 1989;62(1):87–91.
45. Kuhnert BR, Zuspan KJ, Kuhnert PM, et al. Lack of influence of cimetidine on bupivacaine levels during parturition. *Anesth Analg*. 1987;66(10):986–990.
46. Kambam JR, Franks JJ. Cimetidine does not affect plasma cholinesterase activity. *Anesth Analg*. 1988;67(1):69–70.
47. Matsunaga C, Izumi S, Furukubo T, et al. Effect of famotidine and lansoprazole on serum phosphorus levels in hemodialysis patients on calcium carbonate therapy. *Clin Nephrol*. 2007;68(2):93–98.
48. Russell WL, Lopez LM, Normann SA, et al. Effect of antacids on predicted steady-state cimetidine concentrations. *Digest Dis Sci*. 1984;29(5):385–389.
49. Sigterman KE, van Pinxteren B, Bonis PA, et al. Short-term treatment with proton pump inhibitors, H2-receptor antagonists and prokinetics for gastro-oesophageal reflux disease-like symptoms and endoscopy negative reflux disease. *Cochrane Database Syst Rev*. 2013;(5):CD002095.
50. Maton PN. Omeprazole. *N Engl J Med*. 1991;324(14):965–975.
51. Storr M, Meining A. Pharmacologic management and treatment of gastroesophageal reflux disease. *Dis Esophagus*. 2004;17(3): 197–204.
52. Sachs G. Proton pump inhibitors and acid-related diseases. *Pharmacotherapy*. 1997;17(1):22–37.
53. Khuroo MS, Yattoo GN, Javid G, et al. A comparison of omeprazole and placebo for bleeding peptic ulcer. *N Engl J Med*. 1997; 336(15):1054–1058.
54. Nishina K, Mikawa K, Maekawa N, et al. A comparison of lansoprazole, omeprazole, and ranitidine for reducing preoperative gastric secretion in adult patients undergoing elective surgery. *Anesth Analg*. 1996;82(4):832–836.
55. Nishina K, Mikawa K, Maekawa N, et al. Omeprazole reduces preoperative gastric fluid acidity and volume in children. *Can J Anaesth*. 1994;41(10):925–929.
56. Memis D, Turan A, Karamanlioglu B, et al. The effect of intravenous pantoprazole and ranitidine for improving preoperative gastric fluid properties in adults undergoing elective surgery. *Anesth Analg*. 2003;97(5):1360–1363.
57. Brock-Utne JG, Dow TG, Welman S, et al. The effect of metoclopramide on the lower oesophageal sphincter in late pregnancy. *Anaesth Intens Care*. 1978;6(1):26–29.
58. Pasricha PJ, Pehlivanov N, Sugumar A, et al. Drug insight: from disturbed motility to disordered movement—a review of the clinical benefits and medicolegal risks of metoclopramide. *Nat Clin Pract Gastroenterol Hepatol*. 2006;3(3):138–148.
59. Brock-Utne JG, Downing JW, Dimopoulos GE, et al. Effect of domperidone on lower esophageal sphincter tone in late pregnancy. *Anesthesiology*. 1980;52(4):321–323.
60. U.S. Food and Drug Administration. Domperidone—how to obtain. http://www.fda.gov/Drugs/DevelopmentApprovalProcess/HowDrugsareDevelopedandApproved/ApprovalApplications/InvestigationalNewDrugINDApplication/ucm368736.htm. Accessed March 30, 2014.
61. Fragen RJ, Caldwell N. Antiemetic effectiveness of intramuscularly administered domperidone. *Anesthesiology*. 1979;51(5):460–461.
62. Schulze-Delrieu K. Drug therapy. Metoclopramide. *N Engl J Med*. 1981;305(1):28–33.
63. Klinkenberg-Knol EC, Festen HP, Meuwissen SG. Pharmacological management of gastro-oesophageal reflux disease. *Drugs*. 1995; 49(5):695–710.
64. Nguyen NQ, Mei SLCY. Current issues on safety of prokinetics in critically ill patients with feed intolerance. *Ther Adv Drug Saf*. 2011;2(5):197–204.
65. Hong JY. Effects of metoclopramide and ranitidine on preoperative gastric contents in day-case surgery. *Yonsei Med J*. 2006;47(3): 315–318.
66. Wyner J, Cohen SE. Gastric volume in early pregnancy: effect of metoclopramide. *Anesthesiology*. 1982;57(3):209–212.
67. Cohen SE, Jasson J, Talafre ML, et al. Does metoclopramide decrease the volume of gastric contents in patients undergoing cesarean section? *Anesthesiology*. 1984;61(5):604–607.
68. Henzi I, Walder B, Tramer MR. Metoclopramide in the prevention of postoperative nausea and vomiting: a quantitative systematic review of randomized, placebo-controlled studies. *Br J Anaesth*. 1999;83(5):761–771.
69. Griffiths JD, Gyte GM, Paranjothy S, et al. Interventions for preventing nausea and vomiting in women undergoing regional anaesthesia for caesarean section. *Cochrane Database Syst Rev*. 2012; (9):CD007579.
70. Navari RM. Comparison of intermittent versus continuous infusion metoclopramide in control of acute nausea induced by cisplatin chemotherapy. *J Clin Oncol*. 1989;7(7):943–946.
71. Navari RM, Province WS, Perrine GM, et al. Comparison of intermittent ondansetron versus continuous infusion metoclopramide used with standard combination antiemetics in control of acute nausea induced by cisplatin chemotherapy. *Cancer*. 1993;72(2):583–586.
72. Scheller MS, Sears KL. Postoperative neurologic dysfunction associated with preoperative administration of metoclopramide. *Anesth Analg*. 1987;66(3):274–276.
73. Grimes JD, Hassan MN, Preston DN. Adverse neurologic effects of metoclopramide. *Can Med Assoc J*. 1982;126(1):23–25.
74. LaGorio J, Thompson VA, Sternberg D, et al. Akathisia and anesthesia: refusal of surgery after the administration of metoclopramide. *Anesth Analg*. 1998;87(1):224–227.
75. Jo YY, Kim YB, Yang MR, et al. Extrapyramidal side effects after metoclopramide administration in a post-anesthesia care unit—a case report. *Kor J Anesthesiol*. 2012;63(3):274–276.
76. Kao YJ, Tellez J, Turner DR. Dose-dependent effect of metoclopramide on cholinesterases and suxamethonium metabolism. *Br J Anaesth*. 1990;65(2):220–224.

77. Skinner HJ, Girling KJ, Whitehurst A, et al. Influence of metoclopramide on plasma cholinesterase and duration of action of mivacurium. *Br J Anaesth.* 1999;82(4):542–545.
78. Broad J, Sanger GJ. The antibiotic azithromycin is a motilin receptor agonist in human stomach: comparison with erythromycin. *Br J Pharmacol.* 2013;168(8):1859–1867.
79. Janssens J, Peeters TL, Vantrappen G, et al. Improvement of gastric emptying in diabetic gastroparesis by erythromycin. Preliminary studies. *N Engl J Med.* 1990;322(15):1028–1031.
80. Kopp VJ, Mayer DC, Shaheen NJ. Intravenous erythromycin promotes gastric emptying prior to emergency anesthesia. *Anesthesiology.* 1997;87(3):703–705.
81. Urbain JL, Vantrappen G, Janssens J, et al. Intravenous erythromycin dramatically accelerates gastric emptying in gastroparesis diabeticorum and normals and abolishes the emptying discrimination between solids and liquids. *J Nucl Med.* 1990;31(9):1490–1493.
82. Chapman MJ, Fraser RJ, Kluger MT, et al. Erythromycin improves gastric emptying in critically ill patients intolerant of nasogastric feeding. *Crit Care Med.* 2000;28(7):2334–2337.
83. Chaussade S, Michopoulos S, Sogni P, et al. Motilin agonist erythromycin increases human lower esophageal sphincter pressure by stimulation of cholinergic nerves. *Digest Dis Sc.* 1994;39(2):381–384.
84. Hawkyard CV, Koerner RJ. The use of erythromycin as a gastrointestinal prokinetic agent in adult critical care: benefits versus risks. *J Antimicrob Chemother.* 2007;59(3):347–358.
85. Rowbotham DJ. Cisapride and anaesthesia. *Br J Anaesth.* 1989; 62(2):121–123.
86. Rowbotham DJ, Nimmo WS. Effect of cisapride on morphine-induced delay in gastric emptying. *Br J Anaesth.* 1987;59(5):536–539.
87. Parkman HP, Van Natta ML, Abell TL, et al. Effect of nortriptyline on symptoms of idiopathic gastroparesis: the NORIG randomized clinical trial. *JAMA.* 2013;310(24):2640–2649.

CHAPTER 36

Nutrition

Michael J. Murray

Enteral and Parenteral Nutrition

Enteral nutrition is defined as providing nourishment to a patient utilizing a diet that is delivered directly into the gastrointestinal tract (nasogastric tube, nasointestinal tube, gastrostomy tube, jejunostomy tube). Parenteral nutrition is defined as delivery of nutrients directly into the venous circulation (peripheral vein or central vein). The term ***total parenteral nutrition*** (TPN) is utilized when the only source of nutrient supply is via the parenteral route. Nutritional support is characterized as the use of enteral or parenteral nutrition rather than or in addition to an oral diet. Preexisting TPN should be continued during the perioperative period, whereas enteral nutrition should be discontinued about 6 hours before surgery (reflecting recommendations for food ingestion prior to elective surgery).

Nutritional Support

TPN is intended to supply all the essential inorganic and organic nutritional elements necessary to maintain optimal body composition. Alimentation by the gastrointestinal tract (enteral nutrition) is preferred to intravenous (IV) alimentation (parenteral nutrition) because it is more physiologic. Enteral nutrition provides nutrients that stimulate trophic factors (e.g., gastrin, cholecystokinin, bombesin) released from the lumen that maintains gut integrity (e.g., tight junctions between the intraepithelial cells and villous height) and the absorptive activity of the small intestine. These factors reduce the translocation of bacteria from the gastrointestinal tract and, at the same time, promote development of IgA-producing immunocytes, which reside in gut-associated lymphoid tissue (GALT).[1–3] Indeed, the route of feeding is more important than the amount of nutrition provided, and outcome correlates with the enteral protein intake in injured patients. Thus, even if the patient's caloric and nitrogen requirements cannot be met with luminal nutrition, the enteral route of feeding should be used unless it is contraindicated (bowel obstruction, inadequate bowel surface area, intractable diarrhea). If it is contraindicated and the patient is not malnourished or severely stressed, then parenteral nutrition is not necessary for the first week following surgery or intensive care unit (ICU) admission because it has not been shown to be of benefit.[4] The enteral and parenteral routes may be used simultaneously to meet nutritional requirements, although there is no evidence that the combination of the two to meet caloric needs improves outcome.[5] Furthermore, a recent large prospective study conducted in patients who were critically ill demonstrated that the administration of enteral glutamine supplemented with parenteral glutamine was correlated with an increase in hospital mortality, 28-day mortality, and 6-month mortality.[6] Preoperative nutritional support should be reserved for malnourished patients undergoing major elective surgery; this recommendation is not commonly followed for a variety of reasons, but if time permits, improvement in nutritional status is associated with an improvement in outcome.

Most patients do not need nutritional support, and clear-cut benefits of this expensive intervention have been established for only a select group of patients (Table 36-1).[7] Patients not expected to resume adequate oral feedings within 7 to 10 days of surgery should begin nutritional support within 2 to 4 days postoperatively, within 1 to 2 days if they are in an ICU. Although the benefits of parenteral nutrition in the perioperative period are controversial, postoperative enteral feeding has been shown to decrease complication rates in malnourished patients although mortality rates are unchanged.[8]

Severely injured patients, burn patients, and those with sepsis often are hypermetabolic, so directed nutritional support within 24 to 48 hours of admission may be beneficial. For example, energy requirements may double and protein requirements may triple in severely burned patients. Conversely, the increase in basal metabolic rate that occurs during and soon after major uncomplicated elective surgery is less than 10%, so that providing glucose

Table 36-1

Established Indications for Use of Nutritional Support

Major elective surgery in severely malnourished patients
Major trauma (blunt or penetrating injury, head injury)
Burns
Hepatic dysfunction
Renal dysfunction
Bone marrow transplant recipients undergoing intensive chemotherapy
Patients unable to eat or absorb nutrients for an indefinite period (neurologic impairment, pharyngeal dysfunction, or short bowel syndrome)
Well-nourished, minimally stressed patients unable to eat for 7 to 10 days

Adapted from Souba WW. Nutritional support. *N Engl J Med*. 1997;336: 41–48.

solutions (~500 kcal per day) in the postoperative period is sufficient, and further nutritional support does not improve outcome.

Minimally stressed patients require about 25 to 30 cal/kg and 1 g/kg of protein daily to remain in nitrogen and energy equilibrium. Moderately to severely stressed patients should be resuscitated first and then started on a hypocaloric regimen (20 cal/kg) until the stress response abates. Lipid calories from infusions of propofol may be significant and should be included when calculating caloric intake.[9]

Enteral Nutrition

Unless contraindicated (e.g., short gut syndrome, circulatory shock[10]), enteral nutrition is preferred over parenteral nutrition in almost every circumstance for the reasons mentioned earlier. Three decades ago, it was thought that the main goal of nutrition support in the hospitalized patient was to meet energy requirements and to make the patient anabolic. Current goals include meeting and attenuating the metabolic response to stress and, in addition, attenuating cellular injury and modulating the immune response to injury. Nutritional support of the moderately to severely injured patient includes enteral nutrition started sooner rather than later, pharmacotherapy (the provision of nutrients that modulate the body's response to injury) and glycemic control. Delivering early nutrition support, primarily using the enteral route, is seen as a proactive therapeutic strategy that may reduce disease severity, diminish complications, decrease length of stay in the ICU, and favorably impact patient outcome after severe injury. A variety of enteral solutions containing various amounts of protein (amino acids), carbohydrates (glucose), fat (medium- and long-chain triglycerides), micronutrients, macronutrients, and electrolytes are available. No single formulation has been found to be ideal for all patients. Carbohydrates can be the source of up to 90% of the calories, which increases the osmolarity of these solutions. Fat has a higher caloric density than carbohydrates, and because it does not increase the osmolarity of the formula as much as carbohydrates, iso-osmolar solutions can be constituted. Unless the patient has maldigestion or malabsorption of fat (and even then a formula containing medium-chain triglycerides can be tried), formulas with a normal range of fat content (~30%) are preferred. Selection of a formula that provides sufficient total nitrogen as protein (1 to 1.5 g protein per kilogram per day) or amino acids is essential for all patients. It was once thought that low-protein formulations were indicated for patients with severe renal dysfunction; however, we now recognize that these patients require the same amount of protein as do other patients, even if one has to resort to dialysis to maintain homeostasis.[11] Specialized formulas are available for nutritional deficiencies associated with renal disease, but they are rarely indicated.[12] The same can be said for patients with liver disease—standard enteral formulas work well. The only exception is the patient with hepatic encephalopathy for whom an enteral or parenteral formula containing branched-chain amino acids may improve the encephalopathy, but if not, one should change back to a standardized formula.[13] Increased amounts of protein are indicated when the nitrogen requirement is increased, as in patients with trauma, burns, or sepsis. The efficient use of protein for anabolism depends on adequate caloric intake. Enteral formulas containing glutamine, specifically when administered to patients with burns, reduce hospital and ICU length of stay, primarily through a reduction in infection.[14,15]

Enteral Tube Feeding

Enteral tube feeding may be necessary when patients are unable to consume nutritionally complete, liquefied food orally. Commercial formulations of natural foods can be so finely suspended that they pass through small-bore tubes. Defined-formula diets are necessary when luminal hydrolysis or absorption is impaired, as in malabsorption syndromes. An important consideration when utilizing enteral nutrition is placement and positioning of the small-bore (8 to 12 French) silastic delivery tube. Most often, patients receive continuous infusions of enteral nutrition through a nasoenteric tube positioned in the stomach, duodenum, or jejunum. Several groups of investigators have studied whether there is a clinical significance between gastric versus postpyloric feeding in various medical and surgical ICU settings. Two meta-analyses of these studies did not show a difference in the incidence of pneumonia whether the feeding tube was in the stomach or through the pylorus, nor was there a difference in mortality based on the position of the feeding tube; however, a contrary finding by Taylor was not included.[16–18]

Surgical placement of an esophagostomy or gastrostomy tube may be indicated for long-term feeding. For continuous enteral feeding, an automated infusion pump to control the rate of administration of the nutritional formula is useful. Indeed, absorption and tolerance are improved and the incidence of side effects is decreased by slow constant feeding over several hours. The rate of infusion is typically 100 to 120 mL per hour. This slow rate of infusion prevents the dumping syndrome, which may occur when hyperosmolar solutions are introduced rapidly into the small intestine.

Side Effects

Enteral feeding is frequently stopped because of patient's complaints of bloating or distention; emesis; high gastric residuals (usually 200 to 250 mL); diarrhea; distended abdomen on physical exam; reduced passage, or absence, of flatus; or abnormal findings on abdominal radiographs. With the exception of high gastric residuals and diarrhea, these are legimate criteria for interrupting enteral feedings. One should not interrupt enteral feedings for gastric residual volumes of less than 500 mL, in the absence of other symptoms or signs of intolerance.[19] The presence of diarrhea is always a concern, but one should consider alternative explanations before deciding that the diarrhea is caused by the osmolarity of the enteral product. Even if it is, osmotic diarrhea is relatively benign and short lasting.[20] Osmotic diarrhea in this situation is a diagnosis of exlusion, and one must try to identify other causes such as enteral medications containing sorbitol, *Clostridium difficile*, or other infection, by performing an abdominal exam, sending stool for an assessment for fecal leukocytes, stool culture, and toxin assay.[21] If clinically indicated, serum electrolyte levels should be measured to identify excessive loss or signs of dehydration.

Pulmonary aspiration is always a danger when enteral tube feeding is used. Patients should be maintained in a semi-sitting position (head of bed elevated 30 degrees) and, in patients at the highest risk of aspiration, the feeding tube should be placed through the pylorus. Preparations containing large amounts of electrolytes should be administered cautiously to patients with cardiovascular, renal, or hepatic disease. Many commercial formulas contain large amounts of sodium. Dry preparations mixed with water are excellent culture media unless they are kept sterile and refrigerated.

Parenteral Nutrition

Parenteral nutrition is indicated for patients who are unable to ingest or digest nutrients or to absorb them from the gastrointestinal tract. Parenteral nutrition using isotonic solutions delivered through a peripheral vein is acceptable when the patient requires less than 2,000 calories daily and the anticipated need for nutritional support is brief. Peripheral veins do not tolerate infusion of solutions with an osmolarity that exceeds 750 mOsm/L (equivalent to 12.5% glucose) thus limiting the number of calories that can be administered. When nutritional requirements are greater than 2,000 calories daily or prolonged nutritional support is required, a catheter is placed in the central venous system to permit infusion of a hypertonic (1,900 mOsm/L) nutrition solution.

Short-Term Parenteral Therapy

Short-term parenteral therapy (3 to 5 days in patients without nutritional deficits) after uncomplicated surgical procedures is most often provided by hypocaloric, non-nitrogen glucose-electrolyte solutions. For example, glucose solutions, 5% to 10%, with supplemental sodium, chloride, and other electrolytes are commonly administered for short-term therapy. These solutions provide total fluid and electrolyte needs and sufficient calories to decrease protein catabolism and prevent ketosis. For example, daily infusion of approximately 150 g of glucose maintains brain and erythrocyte metabolism and decreases protein catabolism from skeletal muscles and viscera.

Amino acids may have a greater protein-sparing effect than glucose, but amino acids without glucose do not completely prevent negative nitrogen balance after major surgery. The higher cost of amino acid solutions relative to potential benefit has prevented their popularity for use in place of glucose for short-term therapy.

Peripheral infusion of fat emulsions may be administered as a nonprotein source of calories to augment those supplied by glucose.

Long-Term TPN

TPN (IV hyperalimentation) is the technique of providing total nutrition needs by infusion of amino acids combined with glucose and varying amounts of lipids. Lean body mass is preserved, wound healing may be enhanced, and there may even be improvement of an impaired immune response mechanism.

TPN solutions contain a large proportion of calories from glucose and thus are hypertonic. For this reason, these solutions must be infused into a central vein with a high blood flow to provide rapid dilution. A catheter is often placed percutaneously into the subclavian vein and guided into the right atrium. The parenteral nutrition solution is usually infused continuously over 24 hours. Because the solutions in current use are not nearly as hypertonic and hypercaloric as they once were, there is little concern about the patient becoming hypoglycemic if the infusion is discontinued abruptly but should be considered.

Serum electrolytes, blood glucose concentrations, and blood urea nitrogen should be measured periodically during TPN. Tests of hepatic and renal function are also recommended but can be performed at less frequent intervals.

Side Effects

The side effects of TPN include infectious, mechanical, and metabolic complications. Amongst infectious complications, catheter-related sepsis is one of the most common and associated with significant morbidity. The mechanical complications such as pneumothorax and thrombosis if the catheter is left in place for extended periods, are complications related to the placement of a central line and with which anesthesiologists are familiar. There are a number of metabolic complications seen more often with parenteral nutrition than with enteral nutrition (Table 36-2).

Sepsis

TPN solutions infused through an IV catheter can support the growth of bacteria and fungi. A spiking temperature most likely reflects contamination via the delivery system or catheter. The catheter should be removed and the tip cultured to determine the appropriate antibiotic therapy. In view of the hazard of contamination, the use of a central venous hyperalimentation catheter for administration of medications, as during the perioperative period, or for sampling of blood is not recommended.

Fatty Acid Deficiency

Fatty acid deficiency may develop during prolonged TPN but only if no intralipid is administered as part of the 3-in-1 formulation (protein, glucose, lipid). Possible immunosuppressive effects of lipid emulsions and an increased incidence of infections has led to recommendations to limit fat calories to about 30% of total TPN calories.[22]

Hyperglycemia

Blood glucose concentrations should be monitored until glucose tolerance is demonstrated, which usually occurs after 2 to 3 days of therapy as endogenous insulin production increases. In addition, blood glucose concentrations should be periodically monitored during the perioperative period in patients maintained on TPN. The degree of hyperglycemia accompanying TPN is directly related to the rate of glucose infusion, and to the degree of stress. A 2001 study demonstrated improved outcomes in patients with hyperglycemia in whom blood glucose levels were kept below 110 mg/dL with intensive insulin therapy[23]; however, subsequent studies failed to confirm the original findings.[24] Current guidelines suggest a target of 140 to 200 mg/dL and avoidance of targets below 140 mg/dL.[25]

Table 36-2

Metabolic Complications of Parenteral Nutrition

Early Complications	Late Complications
Volume overload	Metabolic bone disease
Hyperglycemia	Hepatic steatosis
Hypophosphatemia (refeeding syndrome)	Hepatic cholestasis
Hypokalemia	Trace mineral deficiency
Hypomagnesemia	Vitamin deficiency
Hyperchloremic acidosis	

Hypoglycemia

Accidental sudden discontinuation of the infusion of TPN solutions containing large amounts of glucose (catheter kink or disconnection) may cause hypoglycemia. Indeed, TPN infusion should be discontinued gradually over 60 to 90 minutes. Hypoglycemia occurs because the pancreatic insulin response does not always cease in parallel with discontinuation of the parenteral nutrition solution. As a result, a high plasma concentration of insulin may persist in the absence of continued infusion of glucose. If administration of the TPN solution must be stopped abruptly, exogenous glucose should be infused for up to 90 minutes to prevent hypoglycemia. The incidence of hypoglycemia has decreased because clinicans have a lower daily caloric goal (e.g., 1,400 to 2,000 kcal per day) compared to prior therapies (3,000 to 4,000 kcal per day).[26]

Hepatobiliary Complications

Excessive caloric intake is associated with hepatic steatosis and steatohepatitis. An increased alkaline phosphatase or serum bilirubin concentrations warrant additional evaluation (e.g., cholehepatic ultrasound).

Metabolic Acidosis

Hyperchloremic metabolic acidosis may occur because most of the amino acids in TPN are administered as their chloride salts.

Hypercarbia

In a patient with inadequate respiratory reserve, respiratoy failure can develop with aggressive nutritional support that increases carbon dioxide production. Because glucose has a respiratory quotient of 1, excessive glucose was blamed on the respiratory failure associated with TPN, but we now know that excessive calories per se independent of their source increases carbon dioxide production and leads to respiratoy failure in susceptible patients.[27]

Monitoring during TPN

Acutely ill patients receiving TPN must be followed closely for the development of treatment-related complications. Access sites are observed for signs of infection. Substitution of sodium or potassium acetate (metabolized to bicarbonate) for sodium or potassium chloride may be helpful should signs of hyperchloric metabolic acidosis appear. Plasma triglyceride concentrations may increase in patients with diabetes mellitus, sepsis, and impaired hepatic or renal function. Vitamin K may need to be added to the TPN or administered intravenously based on measurement of prothrombin and plasma thromboplastin times. Monitoring of daily caloric intake, to ensure that caloric goals are being met, and fluid intake and output is needed as patients who are critically ill often experience significant fluid shifts.

Preparation of TPN Solutions

TPN solutions are prepared from commercially available solutions by mixing hypertonic glucose with an amino acid solution. Sodium, potassium, phosphorus, calcium, magnesium, and chloride are added to TPN solutions. Trace elements including zinc, copper, manganese, chromium, and selenium must also be added if the need for parenteral therapy is prolonged. Requirements for vitamins may be increased, emphasizing the need to add a multivitamin preparation to TPN solutions. Vitamin B_{12} and folic acid may be administered as components of a multivitamin preparation or separately. Vitamin D should be used sparingly because metabolic bone diseases may be associated with use of this vitamin in some patients on long-term parenteral nutrition. Vitamin K can be administered separately once every week. The U.S. Food and Drug Administration (FDA) disallowed routine addition of vitamin K to TPN because of concern about side effects, and its routine administration would complicate the use of anticoagulants such as warfarin in patients who require such therapy. The serum albumin concentration will usually increase over several days to weeks as the stress response abates and if patients receive adequate nutrition support. The administration of supplemental albumin is not necessary in the absence of symptoms or signs of hypoalbuminemia, which usually do not occur until the serum albumin concentration is less than 2.4 g/dL.

Fat emulsions (Intralipid) can be administered separately or together with the glucose and amino acids to create a 3-in-1 TPN solution, as mentioned previously. To decrease the possibility of bacterial contamination, TPN solutions are prepared aseptically under a laminar air-flow hood, refrigerated, and administered within 24 to 48 hours.

Immunonutrition

Cellular immunity decreases during acute stress, as may accompany multiple organ system failure, sepsis, and shock. Immunonutrition is an attempt to enhance immunity and cellular integrity by incorporating specific additives (omega-3 fatty acids, arginine to enhance lymphocyte cytotoxicity, purines as a precursor of RNA and DNA and antioxidants) into enteral diets. Currently, there are no well-controlled clinical studies that demonstrate improved outcomes with immunonutrition in patient populations that might benefit from their use, and there are no clinical guidelines that suggest their routine use in these patient populations.

Vitamins, Dietary Supplements, and Herbal Remedies

Vitamins

Vitamins are a group of structurally diverse organic substances (water soluble or fat soluble) that must be provided in small amounts in the diet for subsequent synthesis of cofactors that are essential for various metabolic reactions (Table 36-3). Food is the best source of vitamins, and healthy persons consuming an adequate balanced diet will not benefit from supplemental vitamins. Nevertheless, many persons do not consume adequate amounts of vitamin-rich foods, especially patients with alcoholism and malabsorbtion syndromes, the elderly, and the economically disadvantaged.

Antioxidant vitamins can retard atherogenesis, and antioxidants may lower the risk of carcinogenesis. There is a demonstrated relationship between low dietary intake of antioxidants or low plasma concentrations of antioxidants and an increased risk of atherosclerosis and cancer. Studies have linked low plasma concentrations of folic acid, vitamin B_6, and vitamin B_{12} with increased plasma concentrations of homocysteine and increased cardiovascular risks.[28] A vitamin supplement that combines antioxidants with zinc can slow progression of macular degneration. Individuals who consume multivitamins appear to have a decreased risk of cardiovascular disease and colon cancer, which may represent protection from folic acid and the B vitamins.[29]

It is clear that additional information and studies are necessary to clarify the need for vitamin supplements in the presence of an adequate diet. The present recommendation is for parturients, the elderly, and those individuals receiving a suboptimal nutritional diet to take a single multivitamin tablet daily. Strict vegetarians should take vitamin B_{12} supplements.

Use of megadose vitamin preparations is not encouraged. Brand name and so-called all-natural preparations are no more effective than generic vitamin preparations. Regardless, vitamin supplements should never be used as a substitute for a balanced healthful diet that provides abundant quantities of vitamin-rich foods.

Water-Soluble Vitamins

Water-soluble vitamins include members of the vitamin B complex (thiamine, riboflavin, nicotinic acid, pyridoxine, pantothenic acid, biotin, cyanocobalamin, folic acid) and ascorbic acid (vitamin C) (Fig. 36-1).

Thiamine

Thiamine (Vitamin B_1) is converted to a physiologically active coenzyme known as ***thiamine pyrophosphate***. This coenzyme is essential for the decarboxylation of α-keto acids such as pyruvate and in the use of pentose in the

Table 36-3

Vitamins

	Function	Deficiency	Toxic Effects	Sources
Thiamine (B_1)	Metabolism of carbohydrates, alcohol, amino acids	Beriberi Wernicke-Korsakoff syndrome	None	Grains Legumes Poultry Meat
Riboflavin (B_2)	Cellular oxidation-reduction reactions	Stomatitis Dermatitis Anemia	None	Grains Dairy products Meat Eggs Green vegetables
Nicotinic acid (niacin, B_3)	Oxidative metabolism Decreases LDL cholesterol Increases HDL cholesterol	Pellagra	Flushing Headaches Pruritus Hyperglycemia Hyperuricemia	Meat Poultry Fish Grains Peanuts Tryptophan in foods
Pyridoxine (B_6)	Amino acid metabolism Heme synthesis Neuronal excitability Decreases blood homocysteine levels	Anemia Cheilosis Dermatitis	Neurotoxicity	Liver Poultry Fish Grains Bananas
Pantothenic acid	Metabolic processes	Rare	None	Many foods
B_{12} (cobalamin, cyanocobalamin)	DNA synthesis Myelin synthesis Decreases blood homocysteine levels	Megaloblastic anemia Peripheral neuropathies	None	Liver Poultry Fish Dairy products
Folic acid	DNA synthesis Decreases blood homocysteine levels	Megaloblastic anemia Birth defects	None	Legumes Grains Fruit Poultry Meat
Ascorbic acid (vitamin C)	Collagen synthesis Possible protection against certain cancers	Scurvy	Nephrolithiasis Diarrhea	Fruits Green vegetables Potatoes Cereals
Vitamin A (retinol, retinoic acid)	Vision Epithelial integrity	Night blindness Susceptibility to infection	Teratogenicity Hepatotoxicity Cerebral edema	Liver Dairy products Green vegetables
Vitamin D (calciferol)	Intestinal calcium absorption	Osteomalacia Rickets	Hypercalcemia	Dairy products Fish Eggs Liver
Vitamin E (tocopherol)	Decreases peroxidation of fatty acids Possible protection against atherosclerosis	Rare	Antagonism of vitamin K Headaches	Vegetable oils Wheat germ Nuts
Vitamin K	Synthesis of clotting factors (VII, IX, X)	Hemorrhagic diathesis	None	Green vegetables Intestinal bacteria

LDL, low-density lipoprotein; HDL, high-density lipoprotein.

FIGURE 36-1 Chemical structure of water-soluble vitamins.

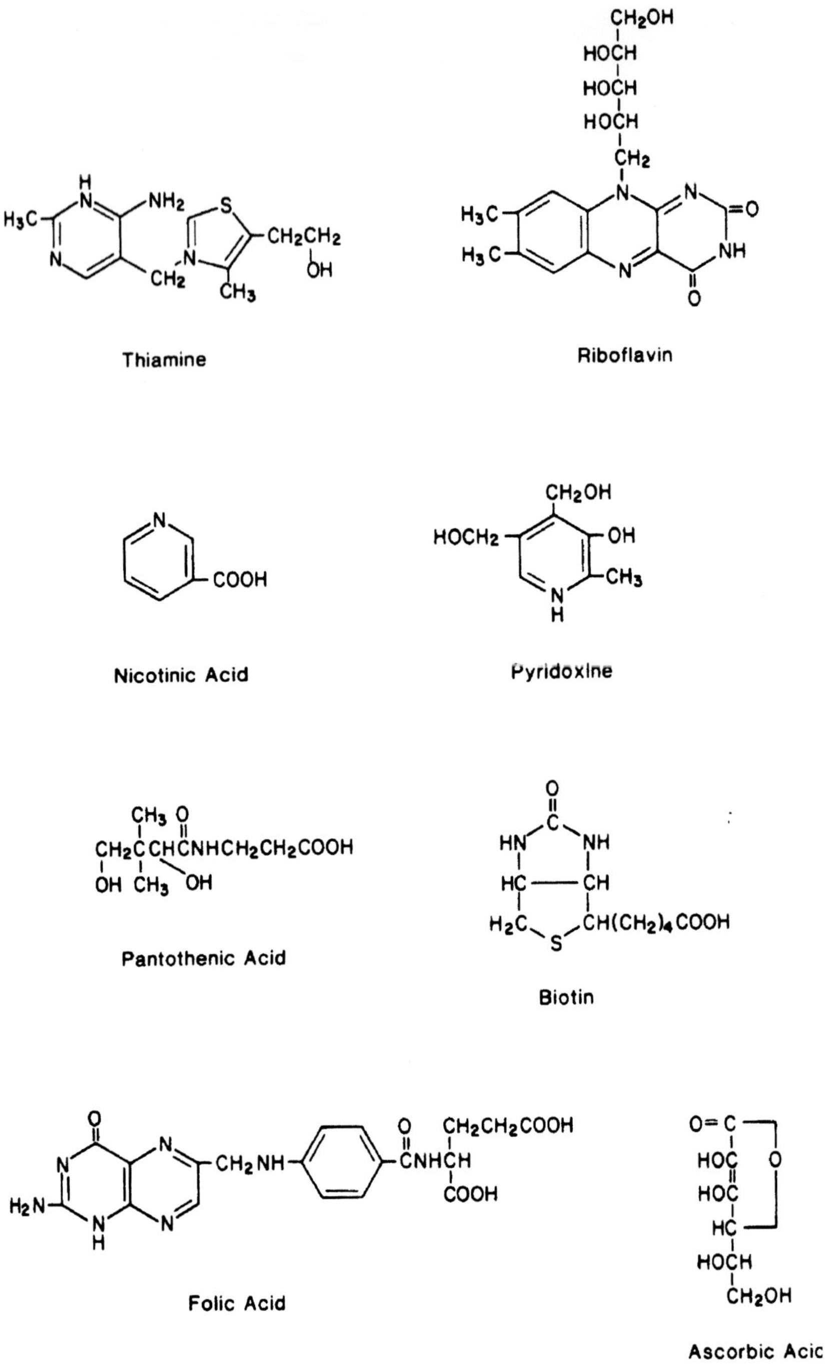

Thiamine

Riboflavin

Nicotinic Acid

Pyridoxine

Pantothenic Acid

Biotin

Folic Acid

Ascorbic Acid

hexose-monophosphate shunt pathway. Indeed, increased plasma concentrations of pyruvate are a diagnostic sign of thiamine deficiency.

Causes of Deficiency

The requirement for thiamine is related to the metabolic rate and is greatest when carbohydrate is the source of energy. This is important in patients maintained by hyperalimentation in which the majority of calories are provided in the form of glucose. Such patients should receive supplemental amounts of thiamine. Thiamine requirements are also increased during pregnancy and lactation[30] and in patients with chronic alcoholism.[31]

Symptoms of Deficiency

Symptoms of mild thiamine deficiency (beriberi) include loss of appetite, skeletal muscle weakness, a tendency to develop peripheral edema, decreased systemic blood pressure, and low body temperature. Severe thiamine deficiency (Korsakoff syndrome), which may occur in alcoholics, is associated with peripheral polyneuritis, including areas of hyperesthesia and anesthesia of the legs, impairment of memory, and encephalopathy. High-output cardiac failure with extensive peripheral edema reflecting hypoproteinemia is often prominent. There is flattening or inversion of the T-wave prolongation of the QTc interval on the electrocardiogram (ECG).

Treatment of Deficiency

Severe thiamine deficiency is treated with IV administration of the vitamin. Once severe thiamine deficiency has been corrected, oral supplementation is acceptable.

Riboflavin

Riboflavin (Vitamin B_2) is converted in the body to one of two physiologically active coenzymes: flavin mononucleotide (FMN) or flavin adenine dinucleotide (FAD). Because of their ability to "accept" two hydrogen atoms, these coenzymes primarily influence hydrogen ion transport in oxidative enzyme systems, including cytochrome C reductase, succinic dehydrogenase, and xanthine oxidase.

Symptoms of Deficiency

Pharyngitis and angular stomatitis are typically the first signs of riboflavin deficiency. Later, glossitis, red denuded lips, seborrheic dermatitis of the face, and dermatitis over the trunk and extremities occur. Riboflavin deficiency is classically associated with angular cheilitis, photophobia, and scrotal dermatitis—the oral-ocular-genital syndrome. Anemia and peripheral neuropathy may be prominent. Corneal vascularization and cataract formation occur in some subjects. Treatment is with oral vitamin supplements that contain riboflavin.

Nicotinic Acid

Nicotinic acid (Niacin, B_3) is converted to the physiologically active coenzyme nicotinamide adenine dinucleotide (NAD) and nicotinamide adenine dinucleotide phosphate (NADP); NAD is converted to NADP by phosphorylation. These coenzymes are necessary to catalyze oxidation-reduction reactions essential for tissue respiration.

Symptoms of Deficiency

Nicotinic acid is an essential dietary constituent, the lack of which leads to nausea, skin and mouth lesions, anemia, headaches, and tiredness. Chronic niacin deficiency is manifested by pellagra in which the skin characteristically becomes erythematous and rough in texture, especially in areas exposed to sun, friction, or pressure. The chief symptoms referable to the digestive tract are stomatitis, enteritis, and diarrhea. The tongue becomes very red and swollen. Salivary secretions are excessive, and nausea and vomiting are common. In addition to dementia, motor and sensory disturbances of the peripheral nerves also occur, mimicking changes that accompany a deficiency of thiamine.

The dietary requirement for niacin can be satisfied not only by nicotinic acid but also by nicotinamide and the amino acid tryptophan. The relationship between nicotinic acid requirements and the intake of tryptophan explains the association of pellagra with tryptophan-deficient corn diets. Carcinoid syndrome is associated with diversion of tryptophan from the synthesis of nicotinic acid to the production of serotonin (5-hydroxytryptamine), leading to symptoms of pellagra. Isoniazid inhibits incorporation of nicotinic acid into NAD and may produce pellagra.

Pellagra is uncommon in the United States, reflecting the supplementation of flour with nicotinic acid. Common causes of pellagra include chronic gastrointestinal disease and alcoholism, which are characteristically associated with multiple nutritional deficiencies. When pellagra is severe, IV administration of nicotinic acid is indicated. In less severe cases, oral administration of nicotinic acid is adequate. The response to nicotinic acid is dramatic, with symptoms waning within 24 hours after initiation of therapy.

Toxic effects of nicotinic acid include flushing, pruritus, hepatotoxicity, hyperuricemia, and activation of peptic ulcer disease. Nicotinic acid has also been prescribed to decrease the plasma concentrations of cholesterol and to increase the concentration of high-density lipoprotein (HDL).

Pyridoxine

Pyridoxine (Vitamin B_6) is converted to its physiologically active form, pyridoxal phosphate, by the enzyme pyridoxal kinase. Pyridoxal phosphate serves an important role in metabolism as a coenzyme for the conversion of tryptophan to serotonin and methionine to cysteine.

Symptoms of Deficiency

Pyridoxine deficiency is uncommon and, when present, is associated with deficiencies of other vitamins and, if seen, is more likely to be seen in the elderly, patients with alcoholism, and patients who are severly malnourished. Other patients who are at increased risk of manifesting deficiency are those with chronic renal failure on dialysis, those with hepatic failure, patients with rheumatoid arthritis, women with type 1 diabetes, and those patients infected with HIV. Certain drugs such as anticonvulsants and corticosteroids can interfere with pyridoxine metabolism, as can isoniazid, cycloserine, penicillamine, and hydrocortisone. Seizures accompanying deficiency of pyridoxine and peripheral neuritis such as carpal tunnel syndrome are common. The lowered seizure threshold may reflect decreased concentrations of the inhibitory neurotransmitter γ-aminobutyric acid, the synthesis of which requires a pyridoxal phosphate-requiring enzyme.

As described previously, a person with a deficiency of pyridoxine may also have a deficiency of the other B vitamins.

Drug Interactions

Isoniazid and hydralazine act as potent inhibitors of pyridoxal kinase, thus preventing synthesis of the active coenzyme form of the vitamin. Indeed, administration of pyridoxine decreases the incidence of neurologic side effects associated with the administration of these drugs.

Pyridoxine enhances the peripheral decarboxylation of levodopa and decreases its effectiveness for the treatment of Parkinson disease. There is a decrease in the plasma concentration of pyridoxal phosphate in patients taking oral contraceptives.

Pantothenic Acid

Pantothenic acid is converted to its physiologically active form, coenzyme A, which serves as a cofactor for enzyme-catalyzed reactions involving transfer of two carbon (acetyl) groups. Such reactions are important in the oxidative metabolism of carbohydrates, gluconeogenesis, and the synthesis and degradation of fatty acids.

Pantothenic acid deficiency in humans is rare, reflecting the ubiquitous presence of this vitamin in ordinary foods as well as its production by intestinal bacteria. No clearly defined uses of pantothenic acid exist, although it is commonly included in multivitamin preparations and in hyperalimentation solutions.

Biotin

Biotin is an organic acid that functions as a coenzyme for enzyme-catalyzed carboxylation reactions and fatty acid synthesis. In adults, a deficiency of biotin manifests as glossitis, anorexia, dermatitis, and mental depression. Seborrheic dermatitis of infancy is most likely a form of biotin deficiency. For this reason, it is recommended that formulas contain supplemental biotin.

Cyanocobalamin

Cyanocobalamin (Cobalamin, Vitamin B_{12}) and vitamin B_{12} are generic designations that are used interchangeably to describe several cobalt-containing compounds (cobalamins). Dietary vitamin B_{12} in the presence of hydrogen ions in the stomach is released from proteins and subsequently binds to a glycoprotein intrinsic factor. This vitamin-intrinsic factor complex travels to the ileum, where it interacts with a specific receptor and is then transported across the intestinal endothelium. After absorption, vitamin B_{12} binds to a β-globulin, transcobalamin II, for transport to tissues, especially the liver, which serves as its storage depot.

Causes of Deficiency

Although humans depend on exogenous sources of vitamin B_{12}, a deficient diet is rarely the cause of a deficiency state. Instead, gastric achlorhydria and decreased gastric secretion of intrinsic factor are more likely causes of vitamin B_{12} deficiency in adults. Antibodies to intrinsic factor may interfere with attachment of the complex to gastrin receptors in the ileum.[32] Bacterial overgrowth may also prevent an adequate amount of vitamin B_{12} from reaching the ileum. Surgical resection or disease of the ileum predictably interferes with the absorption of vitamin B_{12}. Nitrous oxide irreversibly oxidizes the cobalt atom of vitamin B_{12} such that the activity of two vitamin B_{12}–dependent enzymes, methionine synthetase and thymidylate synthetase, are decreased.

Diagnosis of Deficiency

The plasma concentration of vitamin B_{12} (cobalamin) is less than 200 pg/mL when there is a deficiency state. Measurements of gastric acidity may provide indirect evidence of a defect in gastric parietal cell function, whereas the Schilling test (radioactivity in the urine measured after oral administration of labeled vitamin B_{12}) can be used to quantitate ileal absorption of vitamin B_{12}. Observation of reticulocytosis after a therapeutic trial of vitamin B_{12} confirms the diagnosis.

Symptoms of Deficiency

Deficiency of vitamin B_{12} results in defective synthesis of DNA, especially in tissues with the greatest rate of cell turnover. In this regard, symptoms of vitamin B_{12} deficiency manifest most often in the hematopoietic and nervous systems. Changes in the hematopoietic system are most apparent in erythrocytes, but when vitamin B_{12} deficiency is severe, a pronounced cytopenia may occur. Clinically, the earliest sign of vitamin B_{12} deficiency is megaloblastic (pernicious) anemia. Anemia may be so severe that cardiac failure occurs, especially in elderly patients with limited cardiac reserves.

Encephalopathy is a well-recognized complication of vitamin B_{12} deficiency, manifesting as myelopathy, optic neuropathy, and peripheral neuropathy, either alone or in any combination. Neurologic complications do not parallel the presence of megaloblastic anemia. Damage to the myelin sheath is the most obvious symptom of nervous system dysfunction associated with vitamin B_{12} deficiency. Demyelination and cell death occur in the spinal cord and cerebral cortex, manifesting as paresthesias of the hands and feet and diminution of sensation of vibration and proprioception with resultant unsteadiness of gait. Deep tendon reflexes are decreased, and, in advanced states, loss of memory and mental confusion occur. Indeed, vitamin B_{12} deficiency should be considered in elderly patients with psychosis. Folic acid therapy corrects the hematopoietic, but not nervous system, effects produced by vitamin B_{12} deficiency.

Treatment of Deficiency

Vitamin B_{12} is available in a pure form for oral or parenteral use or in combination with other vitamins for oral administration. These preparations are of little value in the treatment of patients with deficiency of intrinsic factor or ileal disease. In the presence of clinically apparent vitamin B_{12} deficiency, oral absorption is not reliable; the preparation of choice is cyanocobalamin administered intramuscularly. For example, in the patient with neurologic changes, leukopenia, or thrombocytopenia, treatment must be aggressive. Initial treatment is with intramuscular administration of vitamin B_{12} and oral administration of folic acid. An increase in the hematocrit does not occur for 10 to 20 days. The plasma concentration of iron, however, usually declines within 48 hours, because iron is now used in the formation of hemoglobin. Platelet counts can be expected to reach normal levels within days of initiating treatment; the granulocyte count requires a longer period to normalize. Memory and sense of well-being may improve within 24 hours after initiation of therapy. Neurologic signs and symptoms that have been present for prolonged periods, however, often regress slowly and may never return to completely normal function. Indeed, neurologic damage after pernicious anemia develops that is not reversed after 12 to 18 months of therapy is likely to be permanent. Once initiated, vitamin B_{12} therapy must be continued indefinitely at monthly intervals. It is important to monitor plasma concentrations of vitamin B_{12} and examine the peripheral blood cells every 3 to 6 months to confirm the adequacy of treatment.

Hydroxocobalamin has hematopoietic activity similar to that of vitamin B_{12} but appears to offer no advantage despite its somewhat longer duration of action. Furthermore, some patients develop antibodies to the complex of hydroxocobalamin and transcobalamin II. Large doses of hydroxocobalamin have been approved for treatment of cyanide poisoning due to nitroprusside. Conceptually, cyanide reacts with the cobalt in cyanocobalamin, decreasing cyanide ion concentration.

Folic Acid

Folic acid is transported and stored as 5-methylhydrofolate after absorption from the small intestine, principally the jejunum. Conversion to the metabolically active form, tetrahydrofolate, is dependent on the activity of vitamin B_{12}. Tetrahydrofolate acts as an acceptor of 1-carbon units necessary for (a) conversion of homocysteine to methionine, (b) conversion of serine to glycine, (c) synthesis of DNA, and (d) synthesis of purines. Supplies of folic acid are maintained by ingestion of food and by enterohepatic circulation of the vitamin. Virtually all foods contain folic acid, but protracted cooking can destroy up to 90% of the vitamin.

Causes of Deficiency

Folic acid deficiency is a common complication of diseases of the small intestine, such as sprue, that interfere with absorption of the vitamin and its enterohepatic recirculation. Patients with alcoholism have reduced intake of folic acid because of their decreased intake of food, and enterohepatic recirculation may be impaired by the toxic effect of alcohol on hepatocytes. Indeed, alcoholism is the most common cause of folic acid deficiency, with decreases in the plasma concentrations of folic acid manifesting within 24 to 48 hours of continuous alcohol ingestion. Drugs that inhibit dihydrofolate reductase (methotrexate, trimethoprim) or interfere with absorption and storage of folic acid in tissues (phenytoin) may cause folic acid deficiency.

Symptoms of Deficiency

Megaloblastic anemia is the most common manifestation of folic acid deficiency. This anemia cannot be distinguished from that caused by a deficiency of vitamin B_{12}. Folic acid deficiency, however, is confirmed by the presence of a folic acid concentration in the plasma of less than 4 ng/mL. Furthermore, the rapid onset of megaloblastic anemia produced by folic acid deficiency (1 to 4 weeks) reflects the limited in vivo stores of this vitamin and contrasts with the slower onset (2 to 3 years) of symptoms and signs of vitamin B_{12} deficiency.

Treatment of Deficiency

Folic acid is available as an oral preparation alone or in combination with other vitamins and either an oral preparation or as a parenteral injection. The therapeutic uses of folic acid are limited to the prevention and treatment of deficiencies. For example, pregnancy increases folic acid requirements, and oral supplementation, usually in a multivitamin preparation, is indicated. In the presence of megaloblastic anemia because of folic acid deficiency, the administration of the vitamin is associated with a decrease in the plasma concentration of iron within 48 hours, reflecting new erythropoiesis. Likewise, the reticulocyte count begins to increase within 48 to 72 hours, and the hematocrit begins to increase during the second week of therapy.

Folate Therapy

Vitamin therapy to lower homocysteine levels has been recommended for the prevention of restenosis after coronary angioplasty. This is based on the belief that homocysteine is thrombogenic and is a risk factor for coronary artery disease. Folate supplementation is an effective treatment of homocystinemia. Nevertheless, folate therapy (combination of folic acid, vitamin B_6, and vitamin B_{12}) may actually increase the risk of in-stent restenosis and the need for revascularization.[33]

Leucovorin

Leucovorin (citrovorum factor) is a metabolically active, reduced form of folic acid. After treatment with folic acid antagonists, such as methotrexate, patients may receive leucovorin (rescue therapy), which serves as a source of tetrahydrofolate that cannot be formed due to drug-induced inhibition of dihydrofolate reductase.

Ascorbic Acid

Ascorbic acid (Vitamin C) is a six-carbon compound structurally related to glucose. This vitamin acts as a coenzyme and is important in a number of biochemical reactions, mostly involving oxidation. For example, ascorbic acid is necessary for the synthesis of collagen, carnitine, and corticosteroids. Ascorbic acid is readily absorbed from the gastrointestinal tract, and many foods, such as orange juice and lemon juice, have a high content of ascorbic acid. When gastrointestinal absorption is impaired, ascorbic acid can be administered intramuscularly or intravenously. Apart from its role in nutrition, ascorbic acid is commonly used as an antioxidant to protect the natural flavor and color of many foods.

Despite contrary claims, controlled studies do not support the efficacy of even large doses of ascorbic acid in treating viral respiratory tract infections.[34] A risk of large doses of ascorbic acid is the formation of kidney stones resulting from the excessive secretion of oxalate. Excessive ascorbic acid doses can also enhance the absorption of iron and interfere with anticoagulant therapy.

Symptoms of Deficiency

A deficiency of ascorbic acid is known as scurvy. Humans, in contrast to many other mammals, are unable to synthesize ascorbic acid, emphasizing the need for dietary sources of the vitamin to prevent scurvy. Specifically, humans lack the hepatic enzyme necessary to produce ascorbic acid from gluconate. Manifestations of scurvy include gingivitis, rupture of the capillaries with formation of numerous petechiae, and failure of wounds to heal. An associated anemia may reflect a specific function of ascorbic acid on hemoglobin synthesis. Scurvy is evident when the plasma concentration of ascorbic acid is less than 0.15 mg/dL.

Scurvy is encountered among the elderly, alcoholics, and drug addicts. Ascorbic acid requirements are increased during pregnancy, lactation, and stresses such as infection or after surgery. Infants receiving formula diets with inadequate concentrations of ascorbic acid can develop scurvy. Patients receiving TPN should receive supplemental ascorbic acid. Urinary loss of infused ascorbic acid is large, necessitating daily doses of 200 mg to maintain normal concentrations in plasma of 1 mg/dL. Increased urinary excretion of ascorbic acid is caused by salicylates, tetracyclines, and barbiturates.

Fat-Soluble Vitamins

The fat-soluble vitamins are vitamins A, D, E, and K (Fig. 36-2). They are absorbed from the gastrointestinal tract by a complex process that parallels absorption of fat. Thus, any condition that causes malabsorption of fat, such as obstructive jaundice, may result in deficiency of one or all these vitamins. Fat-soluble vitamins are stored principally in the liver and excreted in the feces. Because these vitamins are metabolized very slowly, overdose may produce toxic effects.

Vitamin A (Retinol, Retinoic Acid)

Vitamin A exists in a variety of forms, including retinal and 3-dehydroretinal. This vitamin is important in the function of the retina, integrity of mucosal and epithelial surfaces, bone development and growth, reproduction, and embryonic development. It also has a stabilizing effect on various membranes and regulates membrane permeability. Vitamin A may exert transcriptional control of the production of specific proteins, a process that has important implications with respect to regulation of cellular differentiation and development of malignancies. Limitations in the therapeutic use of vitamin A for antineoplastic uses are the associated hepatotoxicity and its failure to distribute to specific organs.

Major dietary sources of vitamin A are liver, butter, cheese, milk, certain fish, and various yellow or green fruits and vegetables. Fish liver oils contain large amounts of vitamin A. Sufficient vitamin A is stored in the liver of well-nourished persons to satisfy requirements for several months. Plasma concentrations of vitamin A are maintained at the expense of hepatic reserves and thus do

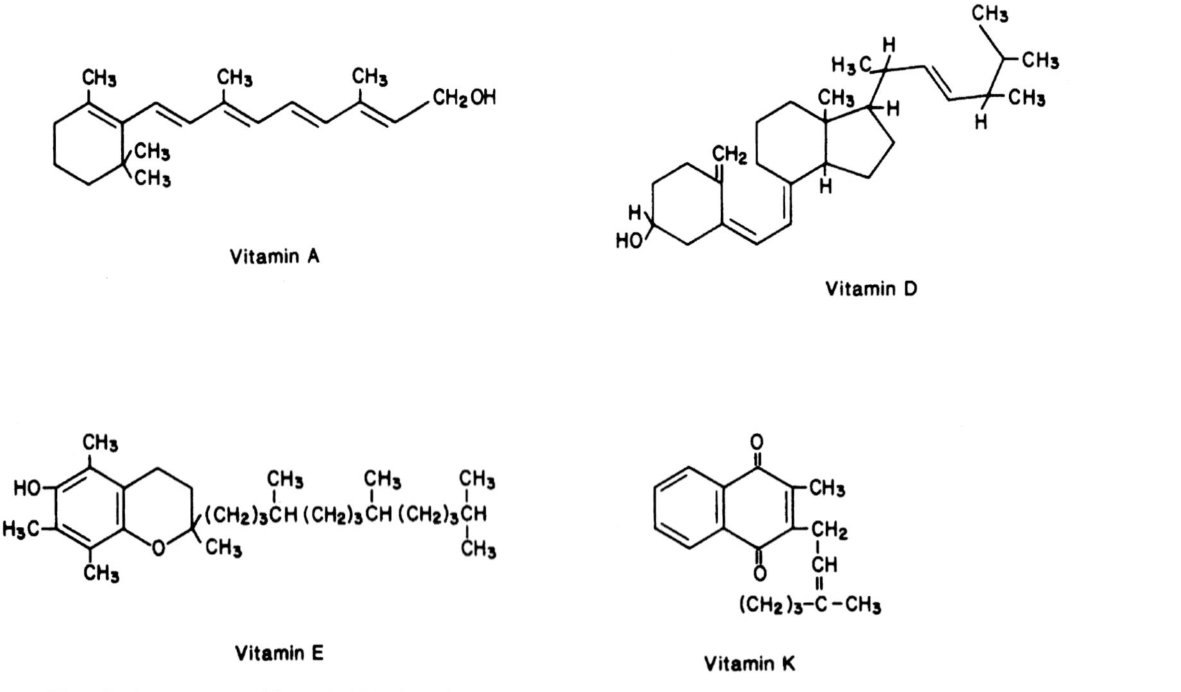

Vitamin A

Vitamin D

Vitamin E

Vitamin K

FIGURE 36-2 Chemical structure of fat-soluble vitamins.

not always reflect a person's vitamin A status. Vitamin A may interact with cellular proteins, which function analogously to receptors for estrogens and other steroids.

Symptoms of Deficiency

Plasma concentrations of vitamin A of less than 20 μg/dL indicate the risk of deficiency. Most deficiencies occur in infants or children. Signs and symptoms of mild vitamin A deficiency are easily overlooked. Skin lesions such as follicular hyperkeratosis and infections are often the earliest signs of deficiency. Nevertheless, the most recognizable manifestation of vitamin A deficiency is night blindness (nyctalopia), which occurs only when the depletion is severe. Pulmonary infections are increased as mucous secretion from bronchial epithelium is decreased because the epithelial cells undergoe keratinization. Keratinization and drying of the epidermis occurs. Urinary calculi are frequently associated with vitamin A deficiency, which may reflect epithelial changes that provide a nidus around which a calculus is formed. Abnormalities of reproduction include impairment of spermatogenesis and spontaneous abortion. Impairment of taste and smell is common in patients with vitamin A deficiency, presumably reflecting a keratinizing effect. Decreased erythropoiesis may be masked by abnormal losses of fluids.

Hypervitaminosis A

Hypervitaminosis A is the toxic syndrome that results from excessive ingestion of vitamin A, particularly in children. Typically, high vitamin A intake has resulted from overzealous prophylactic vitamin A therapy. Plasma concentrations of vitamin A of greater than 300 μg/dL are diagnostic of hypervitaminosis A. Treatment consists of withdrawal of the vitamin source, which is usually followed within 7 days by disappearance of the manifestations of excess vitamin A activity.

Early signs and symptoms of vitamin A intoxication include irritability, vomiting, and dermatitis. Fatigue, myalgia, loss of body hair, diplopia, nystagmus, gingivitis, stomatitis, and lymphadenopathy have been observed. Hepatosplenomegaly is accompanied by cirrhosis of the liver, portal vein hypertension, and ascites. Intracranial pressure may be increased, and neurologic symptoms, including papilledema, may mimic those of a brain tumor (pseudotumor cerebri). The diagnosis is confirmed by radiologic demonstration of hyperostoses underlying tender swellings on the extremities and the occipital region of the head. Plasma alkaline phosphatase concentrations are increased, reflecting osteoblastic activity. Hypercalcemia may occur because of bone destruction. Bones continue to grow in length but not in thickness, with increased susceptibility to fractures. Congenital abnormalities may occur in infants whose mothers have consumed excessive amounts of vitamin A during pregnancy. Psychiatric disturbances may mimic mental depression or schizophrenia.

Vitamin D

Vitamin D (Calciferol) has two forms, D2 (ergocalciferol) and D3 (cholecalciferol) with identical chemical structure except that D2 has an additional methyl group on Carbon 24. D2 comes from the diet, whereas D3 is synthesized in the skin by ultraviolet light's action on 7-dehydrocholesterol. D2 and D3 are metabolically inert and require two chemical reactions to acquire activity. In hepatic cells 25-hydroxylase adds a hydroxyl group to the molecule to form 25-hydroxyvitamin D or 25-(OH)D, and the second reaction takes place in the kidney where 1α-hydroxylase converts 25-(OH)D to the biologically active $1,25(OH)_2$ vitamin D (calcitriol), which regulates calcium and phosphate concentrations in the blood. 25-(OH)D is transported in the blood by vitamin D–binding protein (DBP). Following its production in the kidney, calcitriol binds to DBP for transport to sites of action. 25-(OH)D bound to DBP circulates in the blood, and, when calcium levels decrease, 25-(OH)D is absorbed by the kidney and hydroxylated to the biologically active calcitriol, and then released back into the bloodstream. The process is quite regulated and, unless there is a need, calcitriol is not produced in the kidney. Traditionally, calcitriol has been thought to be the biologically active molecule and 25-(OH)D is a prohormone, but more recent studies in knockout mice deficient in 1α-hydroxylase have demonstrated that sufficient calcium in diet can normalize serum calcium levels,[35] presumably because of the action of 25-(OH)D.

Calcitriol exerts its effects by binding and activating vitamin D receptors (VDRs) in the nuclei of many different cell types.

Calcitriol's primary function is to maintain calcium and phosphorous homeostasis.[36] Calcium levels are maintained through three mechanisms: absorption of calcium in the duodenum and jejunum, release of calcium from bone,[37] and increased uptake of calcium in the distal tubule of the kidney.[38]

When phosphate levels are low, calcitriol inceases its absorption in the small intestine, or conversely, when phosphate levels are elevated, calcitriol acts on osteocytes to release fibroblast growth factor 23, which in turn increases the loss of phosphorous in the renal distal tubule.[39]

VDRs are identified in the nuclei of a wide variety of cells that do not play a role in calcium or phosphorus homeostasis, and it is not suprising then that vitamin D has a role in the regulation of many different genes.[36]

Retrospective studies have shown a 21% reduction in mortality from cardiovascular disease and conversely a reduction by as much as 28% in mortality in those with vitamin D levels twice that of controls. However, supplementation with vitamin D to decrease the incidence of cardiovascular disease has not been shown,[40] but there are advocates of such an approach to decrease the morbidity associated with cardiovascular disease.[41]

Other studies have demonstrated a correlation between vitamin D concentrations and outcome in cancer patients. Calcitriol has a role in malignant disease,[42] attenuating the proliferation of malignant cells through several mechanisms.[43,44] Calcitriol may regulate the progression of malignant cell growth by suppressing the protooncogene myc, the cyclin-dependent kinases, and retinoblastoma protein phosphorylation and via interference of growth factor receptor–mediated signaling pathways.[45–48] Calcitriol's impact on apoptosis may also have a role in its modulation of malignant cancerous cells.[45,46]

Calcitriol may also influence immune function,[49] through similar metabolic pathways. In monocytes, calcitriol stimulates cathelicidin, a peptide with bactericidal and mycobactericidal properties. Calcitriol also inhibits the number and activity of T helper cells. These effects may be clinically important with the former benefiting patients who are septic, and the latter, patients with myeloproliferative diseases.

Calcitriol might have a role in both type I and type II diabetes through its binding to the VDRs of pancreatic cells or through its effects on calcium metabolism.[50] In addition to calcitriol's theoretical role in cardiovascular disease, cancer, immune function, and diabetes, it may also have an effect on morbidity and mortality patients who are critically ill.[51]

Symptoms of Deficiency

A deficiency of vitamin D results in decreased plasma concentrations of calcium and phosphate ions, with the subsequent stimulation of parathyroid hormone secretion. Parathyroid hormone acts to restore plasma calcium concentrations at the expense of bone calcium. In infants and children, this results in failure to mineralize newly formed osteoid tissue and cartilage, causing formation of soft bone, which, with weight bearing, results in deformities known as rickets. In adults, vitamin D deficiency results in osteomalacia. Anticonvulsant therapy with phenytoin increases target organ resistance to vitamin D, resulting in an increased incidence of rickets and osteomalacia. There is evidence that vitamin D supplementation reduces the risk of falling among elderly individuals.[52]

Hypervitaminosis D

Administration of excessive amounts of vitamin D results in hypervitaminosis, manifesting as hypercalcemia, skeletal muscle weakness, fatigue, headache, and vomiting. Early impairment of renal function from hypercalcemia manifests as polyuria, polydipsia, proteinuria, and decreased urine-concentrating ability. In addition to withdrawal of the vitamin, treatment includes increased fluid intake, diuresis, and administration of corticosteroids.

Vitamin E

Vitamin E (α-Tocopherol) is not a single molecule but, rather, a group of fat-soluble substances occurring in plants. There is little persuasive evidence that vitamin E is nutritionally significant in humans.[53] α-Tocopherol is the most abundant and important of the eight naturally occurring tocopherols that constitute vitamin E. An important chemical feature of the tocopherols is that they are antioxidants. In acting as an antioxidant, vitamin E presumably prevents oxidation of essential cellular constituents or prevents the formation of toxic oxidation products. There seems to be a relationship between vitamins A and E in which vitamin E facilitates the absorption, hepatic storage, and use of vitamin A. In addition, vitamin E seems to protect against the development of hypervitaminosis A by enhancing the use of the vitamin. Vitamin E is stored in adipose tissue and is thought to stabilize the lipid portions of cell membranes. Other functions attributed to vitamin E are inhibition of prostaglandin production and stimulation of an essential cofactor in corticosteroid metabolism.

Vitamin E requirements may be increased in individuals exposed to high oxygen environments or in those receiving therapeutic doses of iron or large doses of thyroid hormone replacement. Vitamin E may be important in hematopoiesis, with occasional forms of anemia responding favorably to the administration of α-tocopherol.

Despite absence of conclusive supportive evidence, vitamin E has been administered to women with a history of recurrent spontaneous abortions and for sterility in both sexes. In animals, vitamin E deficiency leads to the development of muscular dystrophy, but there is no evidence that a similar sequence occurs in humans. Changes similar to those observed in skeletal muscles have occurred in cardiac muscle of animals. A necrotizing myopathy with proximal skeletal muscle weakness and increased plasma concentrations of creatine kinase may occur in patients self-medicated with large doses of vitamin E. There are data that support an association between low plasma levels of vitamin E and the risk of developing lung cancer.[54]

Epidemiologic studies have provided evidence of an inverse relationship between coronary artery disease and antioxidant intake, and vitamin E supplementation in particular.[55] This association has been attributed to the finding that antioxidants prevent oxidation of lipids in low-density lipoproteins. It is proposed that oxidation of lipids in low-density lipoproteins (lipid peroxidation) initiates the process of atherogenesis.

Vitamin K

Vitamin K is a lipid-soluble dietary compound that is essential for the biosynthesis of several factors required for normal blood clotting. Phytonadione (vitamin K_1) is present in a variety of foods and is the only natural form of vitamin K available for therapeutic use. Vitamin K_2 represents a series of compounds that are synthesized by gram-positive bacteria in the gastrointestinal tract. Synthesis of vitamin K provides approximately 50% of the estimated daily requirement of vitamin K; the rest is supplied by the diet. Vitamin K is absorbed from the gastrointestinal tract only in the presence of adequate quantities of bile salts. Vitamin K accumulates in the liver, spleen, and lungs, but, despite its lipid solubility, significant amounts are not stored in the body for prolonged periods.

Mechanism of Action

Vitamin K functions as an essential cofactor for the hepatic microsomal enzyme that converts glutamic acid residues to γ-carboxyglutamic acid residues in factors II (prothrombin), VII, IX, and X. The γ-carboxyglutamic acid residues make it possible for these coagulation factors to bind calcium ions and attach to phospholipid surfaces, leading to clot formation. If vitamin K deficiency occurs, the plasma concentrations of these coagulation factors decrease and a hemorrhagic disorder develops. Vitamin K deficiency is characterized by ecchymoses, epistaxis, hematuria, and gastrointestinal bleeding. Vitamin K activity is assessed by monitoring the prothrombin time.

Clinical Uses

Vitamin K is administered to treat its deficiency and attendant decrease in plasma concentrations of prothrombin and related clotting factors. Deficiency of vitamin K may be due to (a) inadequate dietary intake, (b) decreased bacterial synthesis due to antibiotic therapy, (c) impaired gastrointestinal absorption resulting from obstructive biliary tract disease and absence of bile salts, or (d) hepatocellular disease. Neonates have hypoprothrombinemia due to vitamin K deficiency until adequate dietary intake of the vitamin occurs and normal intestinal bacterial floras are established. Indeed, at birth, the normal infant has only 20% to 40% of the adult plasma concentrations of clotting factors II, VII, IX, and X. These plasma concentrations decrease even further during the first 2 to 3 days after birth and then begin to increase toward adult values after approximately 6 days. In premature infants, plasma concentrations of clotting factors are even lower. Human breast milk has low concentrations of vitamin K. Administration of vitamin K, 0.5 to 1.0 mg intramuscularly at birth, to the normal neonate prevents the decrease in concentration of vitamin K–dependent clotting factors in the first days after birth but does not increase these concentrations to adult levels.

Vitamin K replacement therapy is not effective when severe hepatocellular disease is responsible for the decreased production of clotting factors. In the absence of severe hepatocellular disease and the presence of adequate bile salts, the administration of oral vitamin K preparations is effective in reversing hypoprothrombinemia. Phytonadione and menadione are the vitamin K preparations most often used to treat hypoprothrombinemia.

Phytonadione

Phytonadione (vitamin K_1) is the preferred drug to treat hypoprothrombinemia, particularly if large doses or prolonged therapy is necessary. Hypoprothrombinemia of the neonate is treated with phytonadione, 0.5 to 1.0 mg intramuscularly, within 24 hours of birth. A frequent indication for phytonadione is to reverse the effects of oral anticoagulants. For example, phytonadione, 10 to 20 mg orally or administered intravenously at a rate of 1 mg per minute, is usually adequate to reverse the effects of oral anticoagulants. The oral and intramuscular routes of administration are less likely than the IV injections of phytonadione to cause side effects and are thus preferred for nonemergency reversal of oral anticoagulants. Even large doses of phytonadione are ineffective against heparin-induced anticoagulation. Vitamin K supplementation is also indicated for patients receiving prolonged TPN, especially if antibiotics are concomitantly administered.

IV injection of phytonadione may cause life-threatening allergic reactions characterized by hypotension and bronchospasm. Intramuscular administration may produce local hemorrhage at the injection site in hypoprothrombinemic patients. In neonates, doses of phytonadione of greater than 1 mg may cause hemolytic anemia and increase the plasma concentrations of unbound bilirubin, thus increasing the risk of kernicterus. The occurrence of hemolytic anemia reflects a deficiency of glycolytic enzymes in some neonates.

Menadione

Menadione has the same actions and uses as phytonadione (Fig. 36-3). Water-soluble salts of menadione do not require the presence of bile salts for their systemic absorption after oral administration. This characteristic becomes important when malabsorption of vitamin K is due to biliary obstruction.

Menadione hemolyzes erythrocytes in patients genetically deficient in glucose-6-phosphate dehydrogenase, as well as in neonates, particularly premature infants. This hemolysis and occasionally hepatic toxicity reflect a combination of menadione with sulfhydryl groups in tissues. Kernicterus has occurred after menadione administration to neonates. For this reason, menadione is not recommended for treatment of hemorrhagic disease of the neonate. Administration of large doses of menadione or phytonadione may depress liver function, particularly in the presence of preexisting liver disease.

Dietary Supplements

Dietary supplements (vitamins, minerals, herbs, amino acids, enzymes) are products ingested orally and intended to supplement the diet with nutrients thought to improve health. Herbs include flowering plants, shrubs, seaweed, and algae. It is estimated that 25% of patients use alternative therapies characterized as dietary supplements or herbal remedies (more than 3 billion doses). These

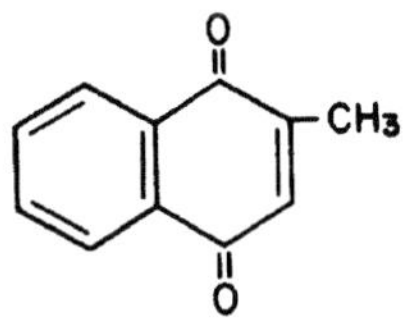

FIGURE 36-3 Chemical structure of menadione.

products are not subject to FDA approval because they are considered nutrients (do not undergo scientific testing to prove efficacy and plants and parts of plants are not patent eligible) although they cannot be promoted specifically for treatment, prevention, or cure of disease. Nevertheless, these products can be labeled with statements describing their alleged effects. The FDA has no control over the herbal industry in terms of safety guidelines that would regulate purity and consistency of therapeutic medications.

Adverse Effects and Drug Interactions

Individuals who take dietary supplements and/or herbal remedies in combination with prescription drugs may be at risk for experiencing adverse interactions (Tables 36-4 and 36-5).[56] The most serious side effects associated with

Table 36-4

Suggested Uses, Potential Toxicities, and Drug Interactions of Dietary Supplements and Herbal Remedies

	Suggested Uses	Potential Toxicity	Drug Interactions
Black cohosh	Menopausal symptoms	Gastrointestinal discomfort	
Chaste tree berries	Premenstrual symptoms	Pruritus	Dopamine-receptor antagonists
Cranberry	Urinary tract infections	Nephrolithiasis	
Dong quai	Menopausal symptoms	Rash	Warfarin
Echinacea	Upper respiratory infections	Hypersensitivity reactions Hepatic inflammation	
Evening primrose	Eczema Irritable bowel syndrome Premenstrual symptoms Rheumatoid arthritis	Nausea Vomiting Diarrhea Flatulence	Antiepileptic drugs
Feverfew	Prevent migraine Arthritis Allergies	Hypersensitivity reactions Inhibits platelet activity	Warfarin
Garlic	Hypertension Hypertriglyceridemia Hypercholesterolemia	Gastrointestinal discomfort Hemorrhage	Warfarin
Ginger	Motion sickness Vertigo		Warfarin
Ginkgo biloba	Dementia Claudication Tinnitus	Gastrointestinal discomfort Headache Dizziness Bleeding Seizures	Warfarin
Ginseng	Fatigue Diabetes	Tachycardia Hypertension	Warfarin
Goldenseal	Laxative	Hypertension Edema	
Kava-kava	Anxiety	Rash Sedation Liver toxicity	Benzodiazepines Alcohol Anesthetic drugs
Kola nut	Fatigue	Irritability Insomnia	Stimulants
Licorice	Gastric ulcers	Hypertension	
Saw palmetto	Prostatic hyperplasia	Gastrointestinal discomfort	
St. John's wort	Depression Anxiety	Headache Insomnia Dizziness Gastrointestinal discomfort	Digoxin Oral contraceptives Serotonin antagonists Anesthetic drugs
Valerian	Insomnia	Headaches	Benzodiazepines Anesthetic drugs Antiepileptic drugs

Table 36-5

Suggested Uses, Potential Toxicities, and Drug Interactions of Nonherbal Dietary Supplements

	Suggested Uses	Potential Toxicity	Drug Interactions
Coenzyme Q10	Congestive heart failure Hypertension	Dyspepsia Nausea Diarrhea	Warfarin
Glucosamine	Osteoarthritis	Gastrointestinal discomfort	Warfarin
Melatonin	Insomnia Jet lag	Fatigue Sedation	
S-adenosylmethionine	Osteoarthritis Depression	Nausea Gastrointestinal discomfort	Tricyclic antidepressants

these substances include cardiovascular instability, bleeding tendency particularly in conjunction with other anticoagulants such as warfarin, and delayed awakening from anesthesia.

Ephedra (ma huang) is a common ingredient in herbal weight-loss products, stimulants, decongestants, and bronchodilators. The active moiety in ephedra is ephedrine, a sympathomimetic amine structurally related to amphetamines. Serious adverse reactions, including hypertension, cardiac arrhythmias, prolonged QTc interval on the ECG, myocardial infarction, stroke, and death, have been described in patients taking ephedra.[57] The chances of experiencing an adverse reaction when taking ephedra are estimated to be 100-fold greater than with any other dietary supplement or herbal remedy. Although tachycardia and vasoconstriction can occur in healthy patients, those with heart disease or systemic hypertension, or those who engage in strenuous physical exercise, seem to be at greatest risk for ephedra-related side effects. Based on the risk of adverse reactions, the FDA concluded that dietary supplements containing ephedra present an unreasonable risk of illness or injury. The FDA banned sales of dietary supplements containing ephedra in April 2004.

Ginseng may cause tachycardia or systemic hypertension, particularly in combinations with other cardiac stimulant drugs. In addition, ginseng may decrease the anticoagulant effects of warfarin. Fever may enhance bleeding by inhibition of platelet activity. Warfarin may also be potentiated by concomitant use of garlic, ginkgo biloba, and ginger. Ginkgo biloba has been suggested to possess antiplatelet effects, and spontaneous hemorrhage has been reported.[58] St. John's wort, which is alleged to be a natural antidepressant, has been shown to inhibit serotonin, dopamine, and norepinephrine reuptake and thus presents the possibility of interactions with monoamine oxidase inhibitors and other serotoninergic drugs.[59] Valerian, kava-kava, and possibly St. John's wort may delay awakening from anesthesia by prolonging sedative effects of anesthetic drugs.

References

1. Braunschweig CL, Levy P, Sheean PM, et al. Enteral compared with parenteral nutrition: a meta-analysis. *Am J Clin Nutr*. 2001;74(4): 534–542.
2. Jabbar A, Chang WK, Dryden GW, et al. Gut immunology and the differential response to feeding and starvation. *Nutr Clin Pract*. 2003;18(6):461–482.
3. Kang W, Kudsk KA. Is there evidence that the gut contributes to mucosal immunity in humans? *JPEN J Parenter Enteral Nutr*. 2007;31(3):246–258.
4. Doig GS, Simpson F, Sweetman EA, et al. Early parenteral nutrition in critically ill patients with short-term relative contraindications to early enteral nutrition: a randomized controlled trial. *JAMA*. 2013;309(20):2130–2138.
5. Clemens MG, Radermacher P, Thiemermann C. Nutritional support in critically ill patients: enteral, parenteral, or not at all? *Shock*. 2014;41(1):87–88.
6. Heyland D, Muscedere J, Wischmeyer PE, et al. A randomized trial of glutamine and antioxidants in critically ill patients. *N Engl J Med*. 2013;368(16):1489–1497.
7. Souba WW. How should we evaluate the efficacy of nutrition support? *J Trauma*. 1997;42(2):343–344.
8. Andersen HK, Lewis SJ, Thomas S. Early enteral nutrition within 24h of colorectal surgery versus later commencement of feeding for postoperative complications. *Cochrane Database Syst Rev*. 2006; (4):CD004080.
9. Lowrey TS, Dunlap AW, Brown RO, et al. Pharmacologic influence on nutrition support therapy: use of propofol in a patient receiving combined enteral and parenteral nutrition support. *Nutr Clin Pract*. 1996;11(4):147–149.
10. McClave SA, Chang WK. Feeding the hypotensive patient: does enteral feeding precipitate or protect against ischemic bowel? *Nutr Clin Pract*. 2003;18(4):279–284.
11. Cano N, Fiaccadori E, Tesinsky P, et al. ESPEN guidelines on enteral nutrition: adult renal failure. *Clin Nutr*. 2006;25(2):295–310.
12. Fiaccadori E, Maggiore U, Giacosa R, et al. Enteral nutrition in patients with acute renal failure. *Kidney Int*. 2004;65(3): 999–1008.
13. Plauth M, Cabre E, Riggio O, et al. ESPEN guidelines on enteral nutrition: liver disease. *Clin Nutr*. 2006;25(2):285–294.
14. Hall JC, Dobb G, Hall J, et al. A prospective randomized trial of enteral glutamine in critical illness. *Intensive Care Med*. 2003; 29(10):1710–1716.
15. Garrel D, Patenaude J, Nedelec B, et al. Decreased mortality and infectious morbidity in adult burn patients given enteral glutamine supplements: a prospective, controlled, randomized clinical trial. *Crit Care Med*. 2003;31(10):2444–2449.

16. Marik PE, Zaloga GP. Gastric versus post-pyloric feeding: a systematic review. *Crit Care.* 2003;7(3):R46–R51.
17. Ho KM, Dobb GJ, Webb SA. A comparison of early gastric and post-pyloric feeding in critically ill patients: a meta-analysis. *Intensive Care Med.* 2006;32(5):639–649.
18. White H, Sosnowski K, Tran K, et al. A randomised controlled comparison of early post-pyloric versus early gastric feeding to meet nutritional targets in ventilated intensive care patients. *Crit Care.* 2009;13(6):R187.
19. McClave SA, DeMeo MT, DeLegge MH, et al. North American Summit on Aspiration in the Critically Ill Patient: consensus statement. *JPEN J Parenter Enteral Nutr.* 2002;26(6)(suppl):S80–S85.
20. Kenneally C, Rosini JM, Skrupky LP, et al. Analysis of 30-day mortality for clostridium difficile-associated disease in the ICU setting. *Chest.* 2007;132(2):418–424.
21. Maroo S, Lamont JT. Recurrent clostridium difficile. *Gastroenterology.* 2006;130(4):1311–1316.
22. Chan S, McCowen KC, Blackburn GL. Nutrition management in the ICU. *Chest.* 1999;115(5)(suppl):145S–148S.
23. van den Berghe G, Wouters P, Weekers F, et al. Intensive insulin therapy in critically ill patients. *N Engl J Med.* 2001;345(19): 1359–1367.
24. Wiener RS, Wiener DC, Larson RJ. Benefits and risks of tight glucose control in critically ill adults: a meta-analysis. *JAMA.* 2008; 300(8):933–944.
25. Qaseem A, Chou R, Humphrey LL, et al; Clinical Guidelines Committee of the American College of Physicians. Inpatient glycemic control: best practice advice from the Clinical Guidelines Committee of the American College of Physicians. *Am J Med Qual.* 2014; 29(2):95–98.
26. Nirula R, Yamada K, Waxman K. The effect of abrupt cessation of total parenteral nutrition on serum glucose: a randomized trial. *Am Surg.* 2000;66(9):866–869.
27. Talpers SS, Romberger DJ, Bunce SB, et al. Nutritionally associated increased carbon dioxide production. Excess total calories vs high proportion of carbohydrate calories. *Chest.* 1992;102(2):551–555.
28. Debreceni B, Debreceni L. The role of homocysteine-lowering B-vitamins in the primary prevention of cardiovascular disease. *Cardiovasc Ther.* 2014;32(3):130–138.
29. Cui R, Iso H, Date C, et al; Japan Collaborative Cohort Study Group. Dietary folate and vitamin b6 and B12 intake in relation to mortality from cardiovascular diseases: Japan collaborative cohort study. *Stroke.* 2010;41(6):1285–1289.
30. Bowman BA, Pfeiffer CM, Barfield WD. Thiamine deficiency, beriberi, and maternal and child health: why pharmacokinetics matter. *Am J Clin Nutr.* 2013;98(3):635–636.
31. Pitel AL, Zahr NM, Jackson K, et al. Signs of preclinical Wernicke's encephalopathy and thiamine levels as predictors of neuropsychological deficits in alcoholism without Korsakoff's syndrome. *Neuropsychopharmacology.* 2011;36(3):580–588.
32. de Aizpurua HJ, Ungar B, Toh BH. Autoantibody to the gastrin receptor in pernicious anemia. *N Engl J Med.* 1985;313(8):479–483.
33. Lange H, Suryapranata H, De Luca G, et al. Folate therapy and in-stent restenosis after coronary stenting. *N Engl J Med.* 2004; 350(26):2673–2681.
34. Moertel CG, Fleming TR, Creagan ET, et al. High-dose vitamin C versus placebo in the treatment of patients with advanced cancer who have had no prior chemotherapy. A randomized double-blind comparison. *N Engl J Med.* 1985;312(3):137–141.
35. Hoenderop JG, Chon H, Gkika D, et al. Regulation of gene expression by dietary Ca2+ in kidneys of 25-hydroxyvitamin D3-1 alpha-hydroxylase knockout mice. *Kidney Int.* 2004;65(2):531–539.
36. Jurutka PW, Whitfield GK, Hsieh JC, et al. Molecular nature of the vitamin D receptor and its role in regulation of gene expression. *Rev Endocr Metab Disord.* 2001;2(2):203–216.
37. Lips P. Vitamin D physiology. *Prog Biophys Mol Biol.* 2006;92(1):4–8.
38. Yamamoto M, Kawanobe Y, Takahashi H, et al. Vitamin D deficiency and renal calcium transport in the rat. *J Clin Invest.* 1984;74(2): 507–513.
39. Liu S, Gupta A, Quarles LD. Emerging role of fibroblast growth factor 23 in a bone-kidney axis regulating systemic phosphate homeostasis and extracellular matrix mineralization. *Curr Opin Nephrol Hypertens.* 2007;16(4):329–335.
40. Kassi E, Adamopoulos C, Basdra EK, et al. Role of vitamin D in atherosclerosis. *Circulation.* 2013;128(23):2517–2531.
41. Grant WB. An estimate of the global reduction in mortality rates through doubling vitamin D levels. *Eur J Clin Nutr.* 2011;65(9): 1016–1026.
42. Masuda S, Jones G. Promise of vitamin D analogues in the treatment of hyperproliferative conditions. *Mol Cancer Ther.* 2006;5(4): 797–808.
43. Lopes N, Sousa B, Martins D, et al. Alterations in vitamin D signalling and metabolic pathways in breast cancer progression: a study of VDR, CYP27B1 and CYP24A1 expression in benign and malignant breast lesions. *BMC Cancer.* 2010;10:483.
44. Kovalenko PL, Zhang Z, Cui M, et al. 1,25 dihydroxyvitamin D-mediated orchestration of anticancer, transcript-level effects in the immortalized, non-transformed prostate epithelial cell line, RWPE1. *BMC Genomics.* 2010;11:26.
45. Yanagisawa J, Yanagi Y, Masuhiro Y, et al. Convergence of transforming growth factor-beta and vitamin D signaling pathways on SMAD transcriptional coactivators. *Science.* 1999;283(5406):1317–1321.
46. Sundaram S, Chaudhry M, Reardon D, et al. The vitamin D3 analog EB 1089 enhances the antiproliferative and apoptotic effects of adriamycin in MCF-7 breast tumor cells. *Breast Cancer Res Treat.* 2000;63(1):1–10.
47. Li P, Li C, Zhao X, et al. p27(Kip1) stabilization and G(1) arrest by 1,25-dihydroxyvitamin D(3) in ovarian cancer cells mediated through down-regulation of cyclin E/cyclin-dependent kinase 2 and Skp1-Cullin-F-box protein/Skp2 ubiquitin ligase. *J Biol Chem.* 2004;279(24):25260–25267.
48. Gaschott T, Stein J. Short-chain fatty acids and colon cancer cells: the vitamin D receptor—butyrate connection. *Recent Results Cancer Res.* 2003;164:247–257.
49. Adams JS, Hewison M. Unexpected actions of vitamin D: new perspectives on the regulation of innate and adaptive immunity. *Nat Clin Pract Endocrinol Metab.* 2008;4(2):80–90.
50. Pittas AG, Dawson-Hughes B. Vitamin D and diabetes. *J Steroid Biochem Mol Biol.* 2010;121(1-2):425–429.
51. Murray MJ. Vitamin d-do our patients need not just a room with a view, but one with sunshine? *Crit Care Med.* 2014;42(6):1540–1542.
52. Murad MH, Elamin KB, Abu Elnour NO, et al. Clinical review: the effect of vitamin D on falls: a systematic review and meta-analysis. *J Clin Endocrinol Metab.* 2011;96(10):2997–3006.
53. Roberts HJ. Perspective on vitamin E as therapy. *JAMA.* 1981; 246(2):129–131.
54. Basu TK, Hill GB, Ng D, et al. Serum vitamins A and E, beta-carotene, and selenium in patients with breast cancer. *J Am Coll Nutr.* 1989;8(6):524–529.
55. Diaz MN, Frei B, Vita JA, et al. Antioxidants and atherosclerotic heart disease. *N Engl J Med.* 1997;337(6):408–416.
56. Cupp MJ. Herbal remedies: adverse effects and drug interactions. *Am Fam Physician.* 1999;59(5):1239–1245.
57. McBride BF, Karapanos AK, Krudysz A, et al. Electrocardiographic and hemodynamic effects of a multicomponent dietary supplement containing ephedra and caffeine: a randomized controlled trial. *JAMA.* 2004;291(2):216–221.
58. Matthews MK Jr. Association of Ginkgo biloba with intracerebral hemorrhage. *Neurology.* 1998;50(6):1933–1934.
59. Haller CA, Benowitz NL. Adverse cardiovascular and central nervous system events associated with dietary supplements containing ephedra alkaloids. *N Engl J Med.* 2000;343(25):1833–1838.

CHAPTER 37

Normal Endocrine Function

Vivek K. Moitra

Anesthesiologists face several preoperative challenges when patients with endocrine disorders need surgery. Patients may present with an endocrinopathy requiring surgery or more commonly have an endocrine abnormality, which complicates surgical and anesthetic management. Physiologic perturbations from the stress response of surgery may precipitate an endocrine crisis perioperatively.

Endocrine glands secrete hormones into the blood, which can act at distant sites (endocrine), adjacent to the site of origin (paracrine), at the site of origin (autocrine), and even within the site of origin (intracrine) to provoke a physiologic response. The endocrine system is evaluated by measuring hormone levels. In most cases, hormone output is regulated by a negative feedback system in which increased circulating plasma concentrations of the hormone decrease its subsequent release from the parent gland. The nervous system (via hypothalamic-releasing factors and peptides produced by the brain) and the immune system (via cortisol, cytokines, and interleukins) also modulate the endocrine system to regulate hormone levels. Defects in the pathway such as genetic receptor mutations or excessive circulating serum factors can cause endocrinologic dysfunction (hormone excess, hormone deficiency, and hormone resistance). Management of endocrinopathies includes hormone replacement and medical or surgical reduction of hormone levels produced by tumors.

Mechanism of Hormone Action

Hormones bind to membrane and nuclear receptors to trigger selective and diverse cellular responses. Membrane receptor binding (peptides and catecholamines) initiates signal transduction through enzymes such as adenylate cyclase, tyrosine kinase, and serine kinase. Receptor binding in the nucleus (steroids and vitamin D) regulates gene expression in the cytoplasm and nucleus to produce specific intracellular proteins and enzymes.

Hypothalamus and Pituitary Gland

The hypothalamus is located at the base of the brain and above the pituitary gland. Environmental factors such as light and temperature, adrenergic and dopaminergic receptors, pain signals, emotions, and olfactory sensations stimulate the hypothalamus to secrete hypothalamic-releasing and hypothalamic inhibitory hormones. The hypothalamus is a collecting and coordinating center for information and links the central nervous system and endocrine system to the environment.

Hormones designated as hypothalamic-releasing or hypothalamic inhibitory hormones originate in the hypothalamus and control secretions from the anterior pituitary (Table 37-1). The hormones travel via hypothalamic-hypophyseal portal vessels (undiluted by peripheral blood) to interact with cell membrane receptors in the anterior pituitary, which increase the intracellular concentrations of calcium ions and cyclic adenosine monophosphate (cAMP). Hypothalamic and pituitary secretion is pulsatile rather than tonic, and the pulses are superimposed on broader biologic rhythms such as the circadian release of adrenocorticotrophic hormone (ACTH), the sleep-entrained release of human growth hormone (HGH), and the monthly cycle of gonadotropins in females.

The pituitary gland lies in the sella turcica at the base of the brain and is connected to the hypothalamus by the

Table 37-1

Hypothalamic Hormones

Hormone	Target Anterior Pituitary Hormone
Human growth hormone–releasing hormone	HGH
Human growth hormone–inhibiting hormone (somatostatin)	HGH, prolactin, TSH
Prolactin-releasing factor	Prolactin
Prolactin-inhibiting factor	Prolactin
Luteinizing hormone–releasing hormone	LH, FSH
Corticotropin-releasing hormone	ACTH, β-lipotropins, endorphins
Thyrotropin-releasing hormone	TSH

ACTH, adrenocorticotrophic hormone; FSH, follicle-stimulating hormone; HGH, human growth hormone; LH, luteinizing hormone; TSH, thyroid-stimulating hormone.

pituitary stalk. Physiologically, the gland is outside the blood–brain barrier and is divided into the anterior pituitary (adenohypophysis) and posterior pituitary (neurohypophysis). The anterior pituitary synthesizes, stores, and secretes six tropic hormones. ACTH, prolactin, and HGH are polypeptides; thyroid-stimulating hormone (TSH), luteinizing hormone (LH), and follicle-stimulating hormone (FSH) are glycoproteins. The anterior pituitary also secretes β-lipotropin, which contains the amino acid sequences of several endorphins that bind to opioid receptors. The posterior pituitary stores and secretes two hormones—arginine vasopressin (AVP), formerly designated antidiuretic hormone (ADH) and oxytocin. Both are initially synthesized in the hypothalamus and subsequently transported (via axons) to the posterior pituitary (Table 37-2). During the perioperative period, secretion of pituitary hormones increases with activation of the sympathetic nervous system.[1]

The response to pituitary stalk destruction differs in the anterior and posterior pituitary gland. Stalk destruction causes axonal atrophy and subsequent loss of posterior pituitary function. After stalk destruction, the anterior pituitary can still respond to hypothalamic hormones in the peripheral blood via the inferior hypophyseal artery.

Anterior Pituitary

Anterior pituitary cells have been traditionally classified on the basis of their staining characteristics as agranular chromophobes or granular chromophils. Chromophils are subdivided into acidophils and basophils depending on the staining response to acidic or basic dyes. With more modern techniques, including electron microscopy and immunochemistry, it is possible to identify at least five types of cells, some of which secrete more than one tropic hormone (see Table 37-2).

Growth Hormone (Somatotropin)

Growth hormone (GH) is the most abundant anterior pituitary hormone. GH stimulates growth of all tissues in

Table 37-2

Pituitary Hormones

Hormone	Cell Type	Principal Action
Anterior pituitary		
Human growth hormone (HGH, somatotropin)	Somatotropes	Accelerates body growth; insulin antagonism
Prolactin	Lactotropes	Stimulates secretion of milk and maternal behavior, inhibits ovulation
Luteinizing hormone (LH)	Gonadotropes	Stimulates ovulation in females and testosterone secretion in males
Follicle-stimulating hormone (FSH)	Gonadotropes	Stimulates ovarian follicle growth in females and spermatogenesis in males
Adrenocorticotrophic hormone (ACTH)	Corticotropes	Stimulates adrenal cortex secretion and growth; steroid production
Thyroid-stimulating hormone (TSH)	Thyrotropes	Stimulates thyroid secretion and growth
β-Lipotropin	Corticotropes	Precursor of endorphins
Posterior pituitary		
Arginine vasopressin	Supraoptic nuclei	Promotes water retention and regulates plasma osmolarity
Oxytocin	Paraventricular nuclei	Causes ejection of milk and uterine contraction

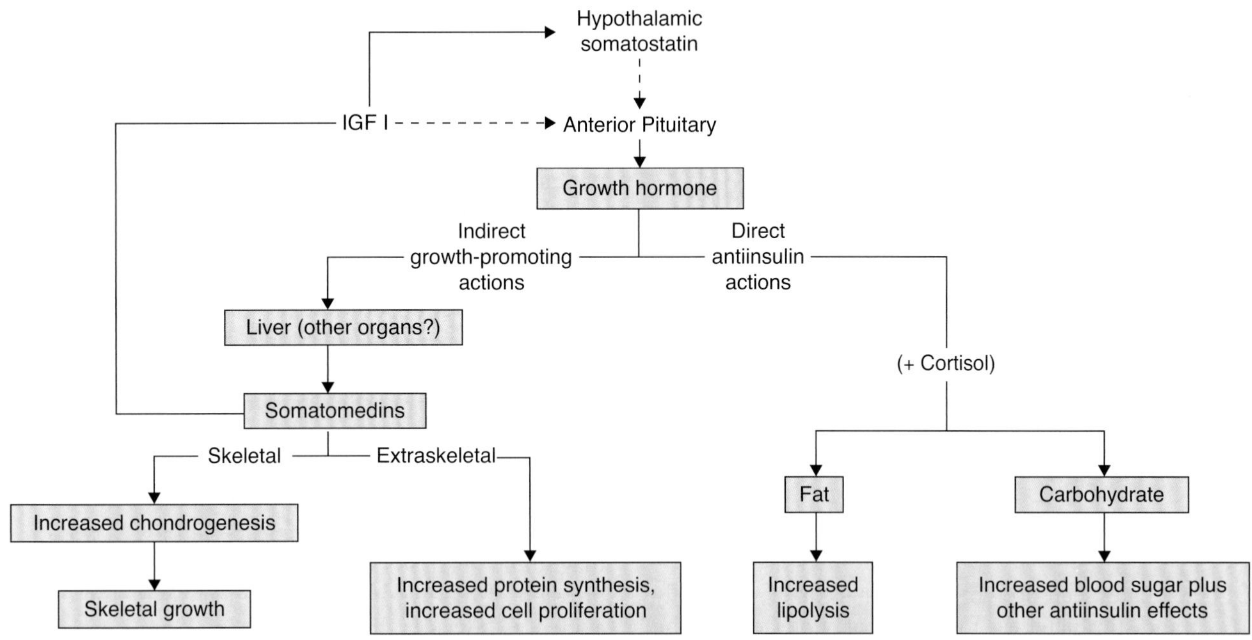

FIGURE 37-1 Effects of human growth hormone manifesting as direct effects or via production of somatomedins in the liver. (From Ganong WF. *Review of Medical Physiology*. 21st ed. New York, NY: Lange Medical Books/McGraw Hill; 2003, with permission.)

the body and evokes intense metabolic effects (Fig. 37-1).[2] The most striking and specific effect is stimulation of linear bone growth that results from GH action on the epiphyseal cartilage plates of long bones. Excess secretion of GH before epiphyseal closure occurs causes gigantism. When excess GH secretion is excessive after epiphyseal closure and long bones can no longer increase in length but only in thickness, acromegaly results. The metabolic effects of GH include increased rates of protein synthesis (anabolic effect), increased mobilization of free fatty acids (ketogenic effect), antagonism of insulin action (diabetogenic effect) and sodium and water retention. Many of the activities of GH require the generation of a family of peptides known as ***somatomedins***.

Releasing (growth hormone–releasing hormone) and inhibitory (somatostatin) hormones, physiologic events, and medications regulate GH secretion (Table 37-3). For example, perioperative anxiety and stress may evoke the release of GH.[1] Plasma concentrations of GH characteristically increase during physiologic sleep. Drugs may influence the secretion of GH, presumably via effects on the hypothalamus. In this regard, large doses of corticosteroids suppress secretion of GH, which may be responsible for the inhibitory effects on growth observed in children receiving high doses of corticosteroids for prolonged periods of time. Conversely, dopaminergic agonists acutely increase the secretion of GH.

Prolactin

Prolactin has little metabolic activity but it prompts the growth and development of the breast in preparation for breast-feeding. Pregnancy stimulates the release of prolactin; dopamine inhibits its release (Table 37-4). Preoperative anxiety also increases plasma concentrations of prolactin.[1] Prolactin secretion in response to suckling inhibits ovarian function, explaining the usual lack of ovulation and resulting infertility during breast-feeding.

Gonadotropins

LH and FSH are gonadotropins responsible for pubertal maturation and secretion of steroid sex hormones by the gonads of either sex. These hormones bind to cell membrane receptors in the ovaries or testes to stimulate the synthesis of cAMP.

Table 37-3

Regulation of Growth Hormone Secretion

Stimulation	Inhibition
GH-releasing hormone	GH-inhibiting hormone (somatostatin)
Stress	Insulin-like growth factor 1 (IGF-1)
Physiologic sleep	Pregnancy
Hypoglycemia	Hyperglycemia
Free fatty acid decrease	Free fatty acid increase
Amino acid increase	Cortisol
Fasting	Obesity
Estrogens	
Dopamine	
α-Adrenergic agonists	

GH, growth hormone.

Table 37-4

Regulation of Prolactin Secretion

Stimulation	Inhibition
Prolactin-releasing factor	Prolactin-inhibiting factor
Pregnancy	Prolactin
Suckling	Dopamine
Stress	L-dopa
Physiologic sleep	
Metoclopramide	
Cimetidine	
Opioids	
α-Methyldopa	

Adrenocorticotrophic Hormone

ACTH regulates secretions of the adrenal cortex, especially cortisol, and stimulates the formation of cholesterol in the adrenal cortex. Cholesterol is the initial building block for the synthesis of corticosteroids. Secretion of ACTH responds dramatically to stress under the control of corticotropin-releasing hormone from the hypothalamus, as well as a negative feedback mechanism from the circulating plasma concentration of cortisol (Table 37-5).[3] Secretory rates of corticotropin-releasing hormone and ACTH are high in the morning and low in the evening. This diurnal variation results in high plasma cortisol concentrations in the morning (~20 μg/dL) and low levels (~5 μg/dL) around midnight. For this reason, plasma concentrations of cortisol are interpreted in terms of the time of day of the measurement. Surgical incision, reversal of anesthesia, and postoperative pain stimulate ACTH release.[1,4,5]

In the absence of ACTH, the adrenal cortex undergoes atrophy, but the zona glomerulosa, which secretes aldosterone, is least affected. Indeed, hypophysectomy has minimal effects on electrolyte balance because of the continued release of aldosterone from the adrenal cortex. Pigmentary changes that may accompany certain endocrine diseases most likely reflect changes in plasma concentrations of ACTH, revealing the melanocyte-stimulating effects of this hormone. For example, pallor is a hallmark of hypopituitarism. Conversely, hyperpigmentation in patients with adrenal insufficiency from primary adrenal gland disease reflects high concentrations of ACTH circulating in plasma as the anterior pituitary attempts to stimulate corticosteroid secretion.

Table 37-5

Regulation of Adrenocorticotrophic Hormone Secretion

Stimulation	Inhibition
Corticotropin-releasing hormone	ACTH
Cortisol decrease	Cortisol increase
Stress	Opioids
Sleep-wake transition	Etomidate
Hypoglycemia	Suppression of the hypothalamic-pituitary axis
Trauma	
α-Adrenergic agonists	
β-Adrenergic antagonists	

ACTH, adrenocorticotrophic hormone.

Chronic administration of corticosteroids suppresses corticotropin-releasing hormone and leads to atrophy the hypothalamic-pituitary axis. Several months may be required for recovery of this axis after removal of the suppressive influence. In such patients, stressful events during the perioperative period might evoke life-threatening hypotension. For this reason, it is a common practice to administer supplemental exogenous corticosteroids (based on the magnitude of stress) to patients considered at risk for suppression of the hypothalamic-pituitary axis. There is little evidence, however, that supplemental corticosteroids in excess of normal daily physiologic secretion are necessary or beneficial intra- or postoperatively.[6] See Chapter 40 for dosing of corticosteroids during the perioperative period.

Thyroid-Stimulating Hormone

TSH accelerates all the steps in the formation of thyroid hormones, including initial uptake of iodide into the thyroid gland. TSH causes proteolysis of thyroglobulin in the follicles of thyroid cells to release thyroid hormones into the circulation. Secretion of TSH from the anterior pituitary is under the control of thyrotropin-releasing hormone from the hypothalamus as well as a negative feedback mechanism, depending on the concentrations of thyroid hormones circulating in plasma. Sympathetic nervous system stimulation and corticosteroids also suppress the secretion of TSH and thus diminish activity of the thyroid gland. Thyrotropin-releasing hormone is widely distributed in the central nervous system and is a potent analeptic. TRH stimulates respiratory rate, induces tremor, and reduces sleep time.

A long-acting thyroid stimulator is an immunoglobulin A antibody that binds to receptor sites on thyroid cells. Binding can mimic the effects of TSH and account for hyperthyroidism, and patients with hyperthyroidism often have detectable circulating concentrations of these proteins. Hypothyroidism with increased plasma concentrations of TSH indicates a primary defect at the thyroid gland (primary hypothyroidism) and an attempt by the anterior pituitary to stimulate hormonal output by releasing TSH. A defect at the hypothalamus or anterior pituitary is indicated by low concentrations of both TSH and thyroid hormones circulating in plasma (secondary hypothyroidism).

Posterior Pituitary

The cells in the posterior pituitary act as supports for the terminal nerve endings of fibers from the supraoptic and paraventricular nuclei of the hypothalamus. AVP is synthesized in the supraoptic nuclei and oxytocin in the paraventricular nuclei. These hormones are transported in secretory granules along axons from corresponding nuclei in the hypothalamus to the posterior pituitary for subsequent release in response to appropriate stimuli.

Arginine Vasopressin

The physiologic functions of AVP include vasoconstriction, water retention, and corticotropin secretion. Decreases in blood volume, increased plasma osmolality, and decreased arterial pressure stimulate AVP release[7] (Table 37-6). With hydration and establishment of an adequate blood volume before induction of anesthesia, urine output is maintained by blunting the release of AVP associated with painful stimulation or fluid deprivation before surgery. Concentrations of AVP in the plasma in response to acute decreases in the volume of extracellular fluid may exert direct vasopressor effects on arterioles and thus contribute to maintenance of systemic blood pressure. Administration of morphine, or other opioids, in the absence of painful stimulation does not evoke the release of AVP. Ethanol inhibits the secretion of AVP. Decreases in urine output and fluid retention previously attributed to release of AVP during positive pressure ventilation of the lungs are more likely the result of changes in cardiac filling pressures that impair the release of atrial natriuretic hormone.

There are three subtypes of AVP receptors, V1, V2, and V3. Stimulation of V1 receptors (found on vascular smooth muscle) causes vasoconstriction. AVP is used as a vasopressor during intraoperative hypotension, sepsis, and cardiopulmonary resuscitation. Activation of the V2 receptors, which are located on collecting duct cells in the kidney, increases reabsorption of water. AVP is transported in the blood to the kidneys, where it attaches to receptors on the capillary side of epithelial cells lining the distal convoluted renal tubules and collecting ducts of the renal medulla. The receptor-hormone interaction results in the formation of large amounts of cAMP, which causes insertion of aquaporin-2 into the collecting duct walls for exit of water to minimize osmolality. Hypokalemia, hypercalcemia, cortisol, and lithium also interfere with renal responsiveness to AVP. AVP binds to V3 receptors in the adenohypophysis to release corticotropin, which suggests that this hormone affects the stress response.[7]

Destruction of neurons in or near the supraoptic and paraventricular nuclei of the hypothalamus from pituitary surgery, trauma, cerebral ischemia, or malignancy may decrease vasopressin release to cause central diabetes insipidus.[7] If the posterior pituitary alone is damaged, however, the transected fibers of the pituitary stalk can still continue to secrete AVP. Diabetes insipidus from lack of vasopressin release during pituitary surgery is usually transient. (See Chapter 40 for hormonal treatment of central diabetes insipidus.)

Unnecessary or excessive secretion of AVP with subsequent retention of water and dilutional hyponatremia may result from head injuries, intracranial tumors, meningitis, or pulmonary infections. Aberrant production of AVP is observed most commonly in patients with cancer, especially oat cell carcinoma, in which the tumor itself produces AVP. In cancer patients, the antibiotic demeclocycline promotes diuresis by antagonizing the effects of AVP on renal tubules.

Table 37-6

Regulation of Arginine Vasopressin Secretion

Stimulation	Inhibition
Increased plasma osmolarity	Decreased plasma osmolarity
Hypovolemia	Ethanol
Pain	α-Adrenergic agonists
Hypotension	Cortisol
Hyperthermia	Hypothermia
Stress	
Nausea and vomiting	
Opioids (?)	

Oxytocin

Breast suckling and cervical and vaginal dilation stimulate oxytocin secretion. Oxytocin ejects milk from the lactating mammary gland via contraction of the myoepithelial cells that surround the alveoli of the mammary glands. Oxytocin binds to G proteins on the surface of uterine myocytes to trigger the release of calcium from the sarcoplasmic reticulum, exerting a contracting effect on the pregnant uterus.[8] Oxytocin also augments the action potential of the uterine smooth muscle.[9] Large amounts of oxytocin cause sustained uterine contraction as necessary for postpartum hemostasis. Oxytocin has only 0.5% to 1.0% the antidiuretic activity of AVP and can be released abruptly and independently of AVP.

Thyroid Gland

The thyroid gland maintains optimal metabolism for normal tissue function.[10] The principal hormonal secretions of the thyroid gland are thyroxine (T_4) and triiodothyronine (T_3) (Fig. 37-2). T_4, a prohormone synthesized from tyrosine, represents 80% of the body's thyroid hormone production. T_3, five times more active than T_4, is produced directly from tyrosine metabolism or from conversion of T_4 in peripheral tissues. Two distinct deiodases (located in the liver, kidneys, and central nervous system) metabolize T_4 and T_3 to inactive compounds. The half-lives of endogenously or exogenously administered T_3 and T_4 are 1.5 and 7 days, respectively. T_3 and T_4 are both highly protein bound to albumin, thyroid-binding prealbumin, and thyroid-binding globulin with only 0.2% of T_3 and 0.3% of T_4

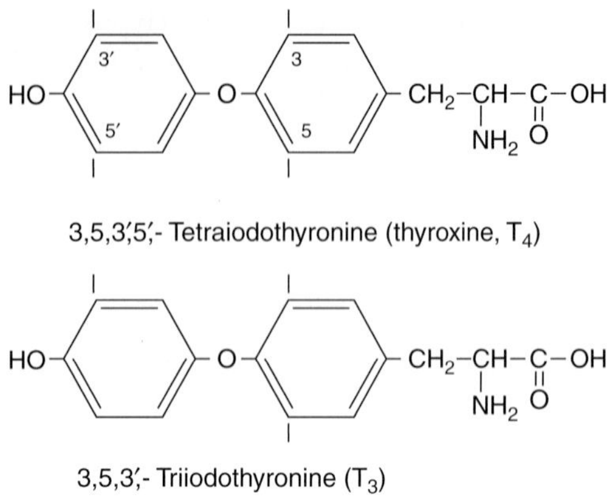

3,5,3′,5′- Tetraiodothyronine (thyroxine, T_4)

3,5,3′- Triiodothyronine (T_3)

FIGURE 37-2 Chemical structure of thyroid hormones.

freely circulating unbound and pharmacologically active.[10] It is of interest that iodine present in thyroid hormones is not necessary for biologic activity (see Fig. 37-2). In addition to thyroid hormones, the thyroid gland secretes calcitonin, which is important for calcium ion use.

The thyroid hormones increase oxygen consumption in nearly all tissues, except for the brain. Failure of thyroid hormones to greatly alter the oxygen consumption of the brain is consistent with the minimal changes in anesthetic requirements (MAC) that accompany hyperthyroidism or hypothyroidism.[11] Cardiovascular changes are often the earliest clinical manifestations of abnormal thyroid hormone levels. Absence of thyroid gland hormones decreases minute oxygen consumption to approximately 40% less than normal; excesses of thyroid hormones can expand oxygen consumption as much as 100% more than normal. Thyroid hormones stimulate carbohydrate metabolism and facilitate the mobilization of free fatty acids. Despite the latter effect, plasma concentrations of cholesterol usually decrease, reflecting stimulation of low-density lipoprotein receptor synthesis by thyroid hormones.

Anatomically, the thyroid gland consists of two lobes connected by a bridge of tissues known as the ***thyroid isthmus*** (Fig. 37-3). The gland is highly vascularized and receives innervation from the autonomic nervous system. Structurally, the gland consists of multiple follicles (acini) that are filled with colloid, which consists principally of thyroglobulin. Thyroid hormones are stored in combination with thyroglobulin. Stimulation of proteases by TSH results in cleavage of hormones from thyroglobulin and their release into the systemic circulation.

Mechanism of Action

When thyroid hormones enter cells, T_3 binds to nuclear receptors. T_4 also binds to these receptors but not as avidly. Indeed, T_4 serves principally as a prohormone for T_3, so that the biologic effects of T_4 are largely a result of its intracellular conversion to T_3.

Thyroid hormones exert most, if not all, of their effects through control of protein synthesis. Thyroid hormones

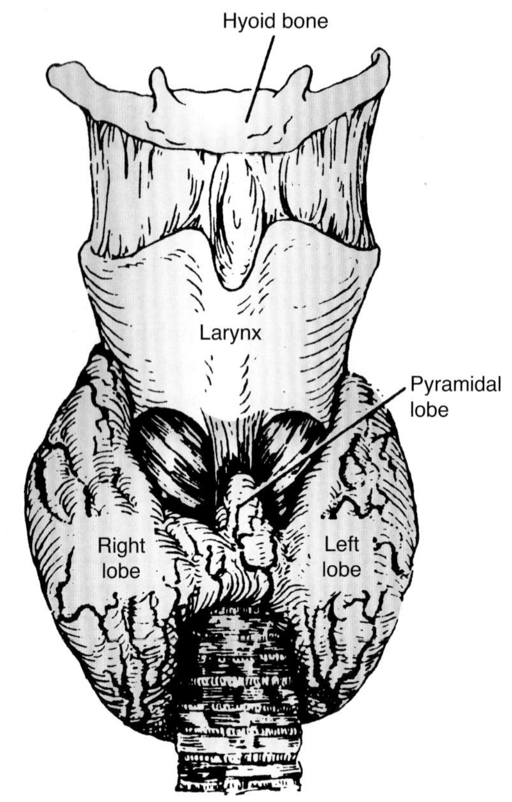

FIGURE 37-3 The two lobes of the thyroid and their relationship to the larynx and trachea.

activate the DNA transcription process in the cell nucleus to form new cell proteins and enzymes. Sympathomimetic effects that accompany thyroid hormone stimulation most likely reflect a greater number and sensitivity of β-adrenergic receptors to release of T_4 and T_3. It has been proposed that thyroid hormones modulate conversion of α-adrenergic to β-adrenergic receptors. Cardiac cholinergic receptor numbers are decreased by thyroid hormones, which is consistent with an increase in heart rate that is out of proportion to the increase in cardiac output.

When thyroid hormones accelerate metabolism, tissues vasodilate and blood flow delivers necessary oxygen and carries away metabolites and heat. As a result, cardiac output often increases but systemic blood pressure is unchanged because peripheral vasodilation offsets the impact of more blood flow. Excess protein catabolism associated with greater secretion of thyroid hormones is the mechanism behind skeletal muscle weakness characteristic of hyperthyroidism. The fine muscle tremor that accompanies hyperthyroidism stems from the sensitivity of neuronal synapses in the area of the spinal cord that controls skeletal muscle tone. Diarrhea reflects additional motility in the gastrointestinal tract with excessive activity of the thyroid gland.

Calcitonin

Calcitonin, a polypeptide hormone secreted by the thyroid gland, decreases the concentration of calcium ions in plasma by weakening the activity of osteoclasts and strengthening the activity of osteoblasts. Calcitonin works in the early moments after ingestion of high-calcium meals. A total thyroidectomy and subsequent absence of calcitonin, however, does not measurably influence the plasma concentration of calcium, because of the predominance of parathyroid hormone.

Parathyroid Glands

The four parathyroid glands secrete parathyroid hormone (PTH), an amino and acid polypeptide that regulates plasma concentration of calcium ions. Secretion of PTH is inversely related to plasma ionized calcium concentration. Small declines in the plasma concentration of calcium ions stimulate the release of PTH. PTH promotes mobilization of bone calcium (osteoclastic activity); enhances conversion of vitamin D to its active form, 1,25-dihydroxycholecalciferol, to increase gastrointestinal absorption of calcium; increases renal tubular absorption of calcium; and inhibits renal reabsorption of phosphate to increase calcium and to decrease phosphate concentrations in plasma.

Parathyroid hormone exerts its effect on target cells in bones, renal tubules, and the gastrointestinal tract by stimulating the formation of cAMP. Because a portion of cAMP synthesized in the kidneys escapes into the urine, its assay serves as a measure of parathyroid gland activity.

Adrenal Cortex

The adrenal cortex secretes three major classes of corticosteroids: mineralocorticoids, glucocorticoids, and androgens. The precursor of all corticosteroids is cholesterol. More than 30 different corticosteroids have been isolated from the adrenal cortex, but only two are important: aldosterone, a mineralocorticoid, and cortisol, the principal glucocorticoid (Table 37-7). The corticosteroids are not stored in the adrenal cortex; the rate of synthesis determines the subsequent plasma concentration. Anatomically, the adrenal cortex is divided into three zones designated the (a) ***zona glomerulosa*** that secretes mineralocorticoids, (b) ***zona fasciculata*** that secretes glucocorticoids, and (c) ***zona reticularis*** that secretes androgens and estrogens.

Mineralocorticoids: Aldosterone

Aldosterone accounts for approximately 95% of the mineralocorticoid activity of the corticosteroids. Desoxycorticosterone, the other naturally occurring mineralocorticoid, has only 3% of the sodium ion–retaining potency of aldosterone. Cortisol induces retention of sodium ions and secretion of potassium ions but much less effectively than aldosterone.

Physiologic Effects

Aldosterone sustains extracellular fluid volume by conserving sodium and by maintaining a normal plasma concentration of potassium. Sodium ions are absorbed at the same time potassium ions are secreted by the lining of epithelial cells of the distal renal tubules and collecting ducts. As a result, sodium is conserved in the extracellular fluid, and potassium is excreted in the urine. Water follows sodium such that extracellular fluid volume changes in proportion to the rate of aldosterone secretion. If aldosterone secretion is excessive, extracellular fluid volume, cardiac output, and systemic blood pressure increase. If plasma concentration of potassium decreases approximately 50% after excess secretion of aldosterone, skeletal muscle weakens or paralysis occurs because nerve and muscle membranes are hyperpolarized and the transmission of action potentials is prevented.

Aldosterone affects sweat glands and salivary glands. It increases the reabsorption of sodium and secretion of potassium by sweat glands. This effect conserves sodium in hot environments or during excess salivation. Aldosterone also enhances sodium ion reabsorption by the gastrointestinal tract.

Mechanism of Action

Aldosterone diffuses to the interior of renal tubular epithelial cells, where it induces DNA to form messenger RNA (mRNA) necessary for the transport of sodium and potassium ions. It is speculated that this mRNA is a specific

Table 37-7

Physiologic Effects of Endogenous Corticosteroids (mg)

	Daily Secretion	Sodium Retention[a]	Glucocorticoid Effect[a]	Antiinflammatory Effect[a]
Aldosterone	0.125	3,000	0.3	Insignificant
Desoxycorticosterone	—	100	0	0
Cortisol	20	1	1	1
Corticosterone	Minimal	15	0.35	0.3
Cortisone	Minimal	0.8	0.8	0.8

[a]Relative to cortisol.

adenosine triphosphatase (ATPase) that catalyzes energy from cytoplasmic adenosine triphosphate (ATP) to the sodium ion transport mechanism of cell membranes. It takes as long as 30 minutes before the new mRNA appears and approximately 45 minutes before the rate of sodium ion transport begins to increase.

Regulation of Secretion

The most important stimulus for aldosterone secretion is an accumulation of potassium in the plasma. A powerful negative feedback system maintains the plasma concentration of potassium ions in a normal range. The renin-angiotensin system also affects aldosterone secretion (see Chapter 16). The elimination half time of aldosterone is approximately 20 minutes, and nearly 90% is cleared by the liver in a single passage. Mineralocorticoid secretion is not under the primary control of ACTH. For this reason, hypoaldosteronism does not accompany loss of ACTH secretion from the anterior pituitary.

Glucocorticoids: Cortisol

At least 95% of the glucocorticoid activity results from the secretion of cortisol. A small amount of glucocorticoid activity is provided by corticosterone and an even smaller amount by cortisone. Cortisol is one of the few hormones essential for life.

Physiologic Effects

Cortisol (a) increases gluconeogenesis, (b) breaks down protein, (c) mobilizes fatty acid, and (d) has antiinflammatory effects. Cortisol may improve cardiac function by increasing the number or responsiveness of β-adrenergic receptors. In addition to sustaining cardiac function and maintaining systemic blood pressure, cortisol promotes the normal responsiveness of arterioles to the constrictive action of catecholamines. Cortisol inhibits bone formation.

Developmental Changes

Plasma concentrations of cortisol increase progressively during the last trimester of pregnancy to reach a peak plasma concentration at term, so that systems critical for survival are mature for the onset of extrauterine life. These systems include production of pulmonary surfactant, maturation of various enzyme systems in the liver, and the expression of phenylethanolamine *N*-methyltransferase, the enzyme necessary for the synthesis of epinephrine from norepinephrine.

Gluconeogenesis

Cortisol stimulates gluconeogenesis by the liver as much as 10-fold. Amino acids are mobilized from extrahepatic sites and transferred to the liver for conversion to glucose. An accelerated rate of gluconeogenesis with a moderate decline in glucose use caused by cortisol results in larger concentrations of blood glucose known as ***adrenal diabetes***. Adrenal diabetes is responsive to the administration of insulin.

Protein Catabolism

Cortisol breaks down protein stores in nearly all cells except hepatocytes, to mobilize amino acids for gluconeogenesis. When excesses of cortisol are sustained, skeletal muscle weakness may become pronounced.

Fatty Acid Mobilization

Cortisol promotes mobilization of fatty acids from adipose tissue and enhances oxidation of fatty acids in cells. Despite these effects, with excess amounts of cortisol, fat is deposited in the neck and chest regions, giving rise to a "buffalo-like" torso. Fat deposits at these sites at a rate that exceeds its mobilization.

Antiinflammatory Effects

In large amounts, cortisol has antiinflammatory effects when it stabilizes lysosomal membranes and stops migration of leukocytes into the inflamed area. When lysosomal membranes are stable, the release of inflammation-causing lysosomes is attenuated. Cortisol lessens capillary permeability to prevent loss of plasma into tissues. Even after inflammation has been well established, the administration of cortisol weakens its manifestations. This effect of cortisol is useful for disease states with inflammation such as rheumatoid arthritis and acute glomerulonephritis.

Cortisol minimizes the number of eosinophils and leukocytes in the blood within a few minutes after its administration. Atrophy of lymphoid tissue throughout the body reduces the production of antibodies. As a result, the level of immunity against bacterial or viral infection is diminished, and infection can fulminate. Conversely, suppressing immunity is useful to prevent immunologic rejection of transplanted tissues.

In the treatment of allergic reactions, cortisol prevents the life-threatening inflammatory responses of allergic reactions such as laryngeal edema. Cortisol may also interfere with activation of the complement pathway and formation of chemical mediators derived from arachidonic acid, such as leukotrienes. Cortisol does not, however, alter the antigen–antibody interaction or histamine release associated with allergic reactions.

Mechanism of Action

Steroids are intracrine hormones that interact with intracellular (often nuclear) receptors. Cortisol stimulates DNA-dependent synthesis of mRNA in the nuclei of responsive cells, leading to the synthesis of necessary enzymes.

Regulation of Secretion

The most important stimulus for the secretion of cortisol (13 to 20 mg daily) is the release of ACTH from the anterior pituitary (see Table 37-5). The secretion of ACTH in the anterior pituitary is determined by two hypothalamic neurohormones, diurnal release of corticotropin-releasing hormone and arginine vasopressin (AVP) that act synergistically. Circulating cortisol has a direct negative feedback effect on the hypothalamus and anterior pituitary to decrease the discharge of corticotropin-releasing hormone and ACTH from these respective sites. Immediately following migration from the adrenal gland, cortisol is bound to the α-globulin, transcortin (cortisol-binding globulin). Plasma concentrations of cortisol are higher in females than males with additional concentrations accompanying the menstrual cycle just before ovulation. If stress from the perioperative period overrides the normal negative feedback control mechanisms, plasma concentrations of cortisol increase. The beneficial effect of a greater plasma concentration of cortisol and other hormones in response to stressful stimuli may be the acute mobilization of cellular proteins and fat stores for energy and synthesis of other compounds, including glucose.

Cortisol is secreted and released by the adrenal cortex at a basal rate of approximately 20 to 30 mg daily. In response to maximal stressful stimuli (sepsis, burns), the output of cortisol is increased to approximately 150 mg daily.[12] This amount should be a sufficient replacement for patients who lack adrenal function and who are acutely ill or undergoing major surgery. The peak plasma cortisol concentration of 8 to 25 μg/dL occurs in the morning shortly after awakening. Stress-induced changes in the plasma concentration of cortisol are superimposed on the circadian tone and vary in onset, magnitude, and duration, depending on the intensity of the stress. In the systemic circulation, 80% to 90% of cortisol is bound to a specific globulin known as ***transcortin***. It is the relatively small amount of unbound cortisol that exerts a biologic effect. The elimination half-time of cortisol is approximately 70 minutes. Cortisol is degraded mainly in the liver with the formation of inactive 17-hydroxycorticosteroids that appear in the urine. Cortisol is also filtered at the glomerulus and may be excreted unchanged in urine.

Effect of Anesthesia and Surgery

Perioperative stress stimulates hormonal secretion of ACTH and cortisol.[1] This response may be diminished by less invasive surgeries such as laparoscopy and blunted by choice of anesthetic technique. During the perioperative period, ACTH stimulation, tissue damage, and proinflammatory mediators can release cortisol. As with other types of stress, the episodic release of cortisol remains intact but the amplitude of episodic releases is greater. Large concentrations of cortisol in plasma in the perioperative period may be prompted by baroreceptor and spinal reflexes that signal tissue injury to the hypothalamus.[13]

Plasma cortisol concentrations typically return to normal levels within 24 hours postoperatively but may remain elevated for as long as 72 hours, depending on the severity of the surgical trauma. In addition, disturbances in the circadian rhythm may be associated with postoperative fatigue and debility. Return of plasma cortisol concentrations to normal following surgery is characterized by increased plasma concentrations of ACTH and cortisol (consistent with sustained, stress-induced stimulation of the hypothalamus) followed by a second phase in which plasma ACTH concentrations are low and larger cortisol concentrations in plasma are independent of the hypothalamic-pituitary system. Cytokines released from traumatized tissue may stimulate synthesis of cortisol directly despite low plasma concentrations of ACTH. Alternatively, prior increases in ACTH concentrations in plasma may stimulate production of ACTH receptors in the adrenal glands resulting in greater cortisol production.

Plasma cortisol concentrations in the perioperative period are designed to provide protection during and after surgery. In adrenalectomized animals who received subphysiologic doses of cortisol, hemodynamic instability and mortality followed surgery. Animals treated with physiologic or supraphysiologic doses of cortisol were indistinguishable from control animals.[14] A key feature of hypothalamic-pituitary-adrenal (HPA) physiology is negative feedback that suppresses release of ACTH by the pituitary by high levels of endogenous or exogenous glucocorticoids. Suppression of the hypothalamic-pituitary axis by regular administration of corticosteroids prevents the release of cortisol in response to stressful stimuli.

The acute phase response to surgery is also mediated by the release of proinflammatory cytokines such as interleukin-1, tumor necrosis factor-α, and interleukin-6 from damaged tissue and activation of the sympathetic nervous system. Cytokines may stimulate ACTH and cortisol production and are subject to a negative feedback system. Cytokine levels peak 24 hours after surgery and can remain elevated for several days. Hepatic production of acute phase proteins (C-reactive protein, fibrinogen, and α_2-macroglobulin) is generated in response to trauma and surgery.[1]

In addition to surgical trauma, the choice of anesthetic drugs and techniques may influence the HPA response. Large doses of opioids may attenuate the cortisol response to surgical stimulation.[15,16] Volatile anesthetics do not suppress the stress-induced endocrine response as much. Etomidate, unique among drugs administered to induce anesthesia, inhibits cortisol synthesis even in the absence of surgical stimulation (see Chapter 5). Although studies of regional anesthetics show a potential to decrease perioperative complications, a reduction in surgical stress-induced release of cortisol has not been proven in abdominal or thoracic surgeries.

Reproductive Glands

In both sexes, the reproductive glands (testes and ovaries) produce germ cells and steroid sex hormones.

Testes

The testes secrete male sex hormones, which are collectively designated ***androgens***. All androgens are steroid compounds that can be synthesized from cholesterol.

Testosterone, the most potent and abundant of the androgens, develops and maintains male sex characteristics. Skeletal muscle growth is an anabolic effect of testosterone in the male. Testosterone is produced in the testes only with stimulation from LH, and FSH is necessary for spermatogenesis. Puberty is characterized by the production of testosterone rapidly in response to hypothalamic-releasing hormones that evoke the release of LH and FSH. Hypertrophy of the laryngeal mucosa accompanies secretion of testosterone, leading to changes in voice at puberty. Testosterone increases secretion of sebaceous glands, leading to acne. Beard growth is the last manifestation of puberty. Testosterone production continues throughout life, although the amount produced lessens gradually after 40 years. At age 80 years, it is approximately one-fifth the peak value.

At most sites of action, testosterone is not the active form of the hormone. It is converted in target tissues to the more active dihydrotestosterone by a reductase enzyme. Dihydrotestosterone binds to a cytoplasmic protein receptor for synthesis of specific mRNA protein. In the absence of sufficient reductase enzyme, external genitalia fail to develop (pseudohermaphroditism) despite secretion of adequate amounts of testosterone. Not all target tissues, however, require the conversion of testosterone to dihydrotestosterone for activity. For example, effects of testosterone on skeletal muscles and bone marrow are mediated by the hormone or a metabolite other than dihydrotestosterone.

The adrenal cortex also secretes androgens, but the effects of these hormones are usually inconsequential unless a hormone-secreting tumor develops. For example, in males, approximately 10% of androgens are produced in the adrenal cortex, an insufficient amount to maintain spermatogenesis or secondary sexual features in an adult male. In abnormal conditions, such as the adrenogenital syndrome, the adrenal cortex can secrete large quantities of steroids and androgenic precursors.

Ovaries

The two ovarian hormones, estrogen and progesterone, are secreted in response to LH and FSH, which are released from the anterior pituitary in response to hypothalamic-releasing hormones. In postpubertal females, an orderly secretion of LH and FSH is necessary for menstruation, pregnancy, and lactation. The Stein-Leventhal syndrome is characterized by virilization when ovarian secretion of androgens is excessive.

Estrogens

Estrogens give the female sexual characteristics. In the nonpregnant female, most of the estrogen comes from the ovaries; small amounts are also secreted by the adrenal cortex. The three most important estrogens are β-estradiol, estrone, and estriol. These estrogens are conjugated in the liver to inactive metabolites that appear in urine.

Progesterone

Progesterone prepares the uterus for pregnancy and the breasts for lactation. Almost all of the progesterone in the nonpregnant female is secreted by the corpus luteum during the lateral phase of the menstrual cycle. The adrenal cortex forms small amounts of progesterone. Progesterone is metabolized to pregnanediol, which appears in the urine and is a valuable index of the secretion and metabolism of this hormone.

Menstruation

The overall duration of a normal menstrual cycle is 21 to 35 days and consists of three phases designated as follicular, ovulatory, and luteal. The follicular phase begins with the onset of menstrual bleeding after the plasma concentration of progesterone decreases. After a variable length of time, the follicular phase is followed by the ovulatory phase lasting 1 to 3 days and culminating in ovulation. The increase in body temperature (~0.5°C) that accompanies ovulation most likely reflects a thermogenic effect of progesterone. The luteal phase follows ovulation and is characterized by the development of a corpus luteum that secretes progesterone and estrogen. The corpus luteum degenerates after a fairly constant period of 13 to 14 days and the menstrual cycle repeats.

Pregnancy

During pregnancy, the placenta forms large amounts of estrogens, progesterone, chorionic gonadotropin, and chorionic somatomammotropin. Chorionic gonadotropin prevents the usual involution of the corpus luteum or the onset of menstrual bleeding. The first key hormone of pregnancy, chorionic gonadotropin, which can be detected in the maternal plasma within 9 days after conception, is the basis for pregnancy tests. After approximately 12 weeks, the placenta secretes sufficient amounts of progesterone and estrogens to maintain pregnancy and the corpus luteum involutes. Chorionic somatomammotropin attenuates insulin activity, making more glucose available to the fetus.

Circulating concentrations of estrogen enlarge the breasts and uterus; progesterone is necessary to develop decidual cells in the uterine endometrium and to suppress uterine contractions that could result in spontaneous abortion. Greater concentrations of progesterone in plasma and associated sedative effects during pregnancy may explain why requirements for volatile anesthetics lessen in gravid animals. In animals, anesthetic requirements return to nonpregnant values within 5 days postpartum, whereas the plasma concentration of progesterone remains increased, suggesting that the decrease in MAC cannot be attributed entirely to progesterone.[17] Progesterone concentrations are the stimulus for increased alveolar ventilation that accompanies pregnancy. Near term, the ovaries secrete the hormone relaxin, which relaxes pelvic ligaments so the sacroiliac joints become limber and the symphysis pubis becomes elastic.

The parturient with asthma may experience unpredictable changes in airway reactivity. Exacerbation of asthma from bronchoconstriction is evoked by prostaglandins of the F series, which are present in all trimesters of pregnancy but especially during labor. Conversely, prostaglandins of the E series are bronchodilators and predominate during the third trimester. That corticosteroids alter airway responsiveness is questionable, because the plasma concentrations of cortisol associated with pregnancy are offset by the carrier protein transcortin, with the net effect being an unchanged level of available cortisol.

Menopause

Between the ages of 45 and 55 years, a woman's ovaries gradually become unresponsive to the stimulatory effects of LH and FSH, and the sexual cycles disappear. Because the negative feedback control of estrogen and progesterone on the anterior pituitary is decreased, output of LH and FSH accumulates in circulating plasma concentrations. Sensations of warmth spreading from the trunk to the face (hot flashes) coincide with surges of LH secretion and are prevented by exogenous administration of estrogens.

Pancreas

The exocrine pancreas secretes digestive substances into the duodenum. The islets of Langerhans are organized endocrine cells that secrete four hormones (insulin, glucagon, somatostatin, and pancreatic polypeptide) into the systemic circulation. The pancreas contains 1 to 2 million islets, which, based on staining characteristics and morphology, are classified as α, β, δ, and pancreatic polypeptide cells.[18] β cells account for about 60% of the islet cells and are the site of insulin production. The α cells account for 25% of islet cells and produce glucagon. Each islet receives a generous blood supply, which unlike any other endocrine organ, drains into the portal vein.

Insulin

Insulin is a 51-amino acid peptide hormone synthesized in the β cells of the islets of Langerhans as a single polypeptide proinsulin, which is the precursor molecule to insulin (Fig. 37-4).[19,20] The peptide that connects the amino terminus of the A chain to the carboxyl terminus of the B chain is designated the connecting (C) peptide. Proinsulin is converted to insulin and C-peptide, and these two molecules are stored together in secretory granules. When pancreatic β cells are stimulated, equimolar amounts of insulin C-peptide are released. Thus, plasma concentrations of insulin C-peptide reflect functional activity of

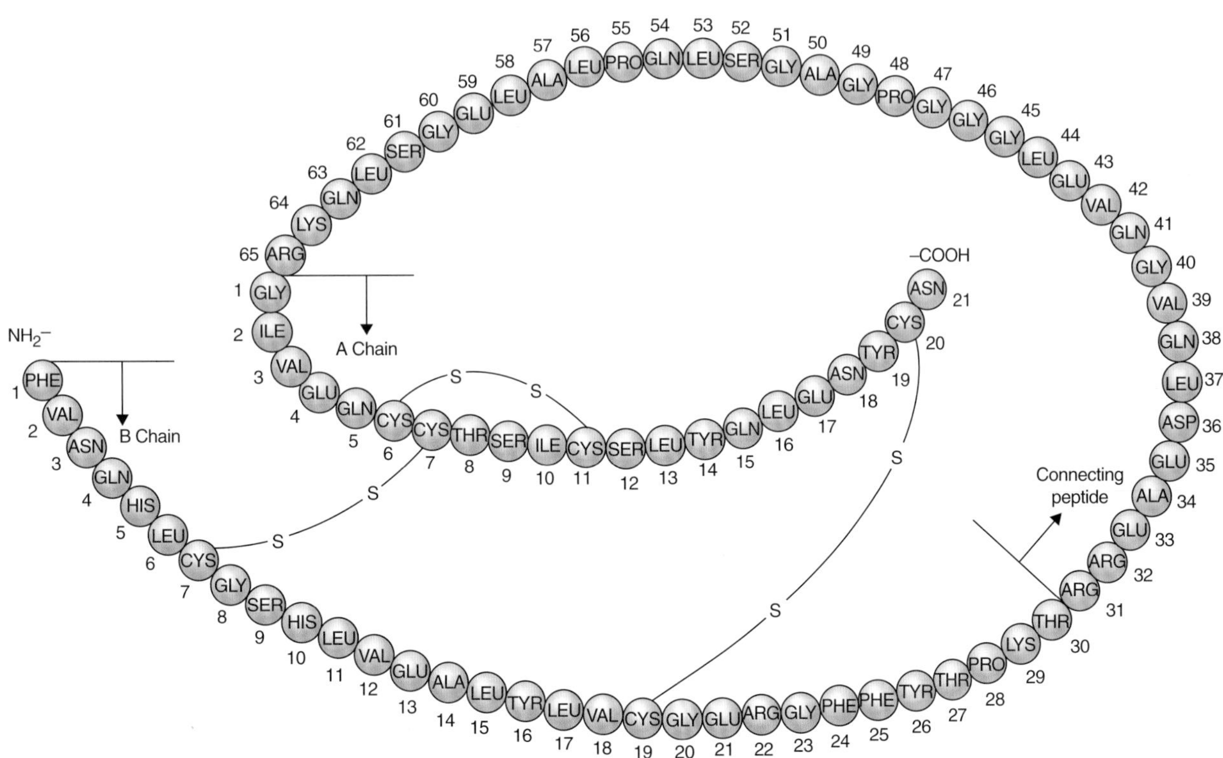

FIGURE 37-4 Proinsulin, which is converted to insulin by proteolytic cleavage of amino acids 31, 32, 64, 65, and the connecting peptide. (From Larner J. Insulin and oral hypoglycemic drugs: glucagon. In: Gilman AG, Goodman LS, Rall TW, et al, eds. *The Pharmacological Basis of Therapeutics*. 7th ed. New York, NY: Macmillan; 1985, with permission.)

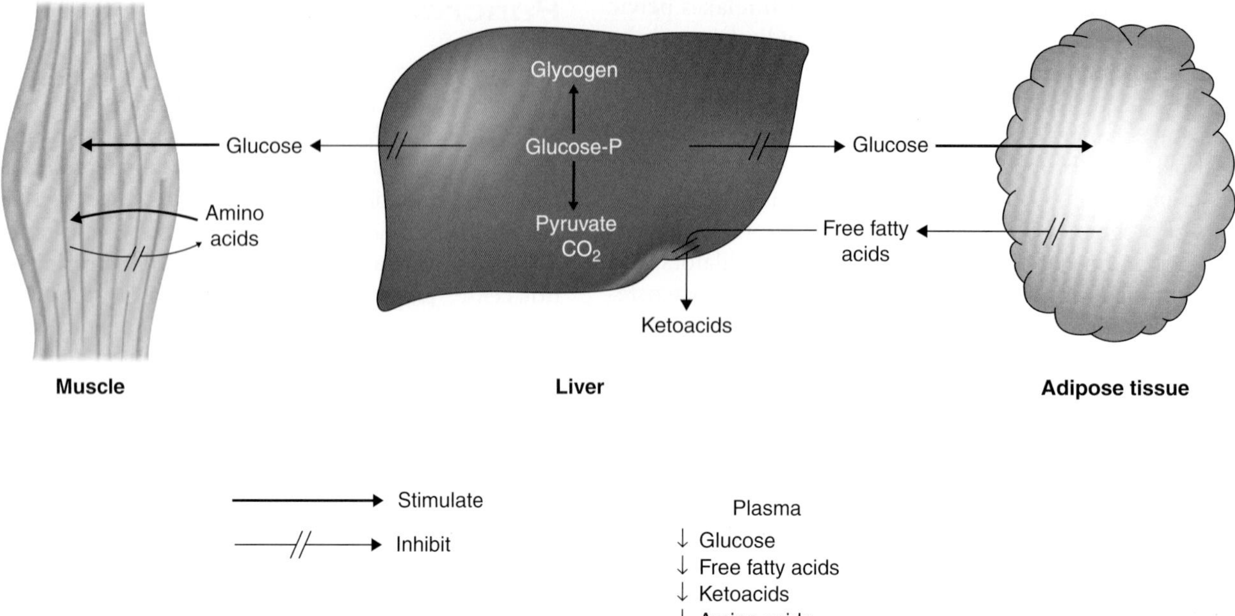

FIGURE 37-5 Insulin stimulates tissue uptake of glucose and amino acids, whereas release of fatty acids is inhibited. As a result, the plasma concentrations of glucose, free fatty acids, amino acids, and ketoacids decrease. (From Berne RM, Levy MN, Koeppen BM, et al. *Physiology*. 5th ed. St. Louis, MO: Mosby; 2004, with permission.)

pancreatic β cells. Insulin is an anabolic hormone promoting the storage of glucose, fatty acids, and amino acids (Fig. 37-5).[21] The amount of insulin secreted daily is equivalent to approximately 40 units. In the systemic circulation, insulin has an elimination half-time of approximately 5 minutes, with greater than 80% degraded in the liver and kidneys.

Insulin binds to a transmembrane, glycoprotein receptor with two distinct insulin-binding domains (an extracellular domain of α subunits and an intracellular domain of β subunits) to regulate metabolic function. When insulin binds to the extracellular domain, a conformational change of the α subunits facilitates ATP binding to the β subunits. As a result, tyrosine molecules in the intracelluar portions of the transmembrane receptors are autophosphorylated. The phosphorylated receptor phosphorylates other protein substrates such as insulin receptor substrates (IRS) that mediates enzyme activation (mitogen-activated protein), inactivation, and metabolic signaling. (Fig. 37-6).[2] The insulin cascade stimulates translocation of glucose (GLUT-4) transporters from the cytosol to plasma membranes to (a) facilitate glucose diffusion into cells; (b) shift intracellular glucose metabolism toward glycogen storage via glycogen synthetase activation; (c) stimulate cellular uptake of amino acids, phosphate, potassium, and magnesium; (d) stimulate protein synthesis and inhibit proteolysis; and (e) regulate gene expression via insulin regulatory elements in target DNA molecules. Activation of sodium-potassium ATPase in cell membranes by insulin moves potassium ions into cells and decreases concentration of potassium in plasma.

Regulation of Secretion

The principal control of insulin secretion is via a negative feedback effect of the blood glucose concentration in the pancreas (Table 37-8). Virtually no insulin is secreted by the pancreas when the blood glucose concentrations are less than 50 mg/dL, and maximum stimulation for release of insulin is at concentrations greater than 300 mg/dL. Thus, blood glucose concentrations are maintained

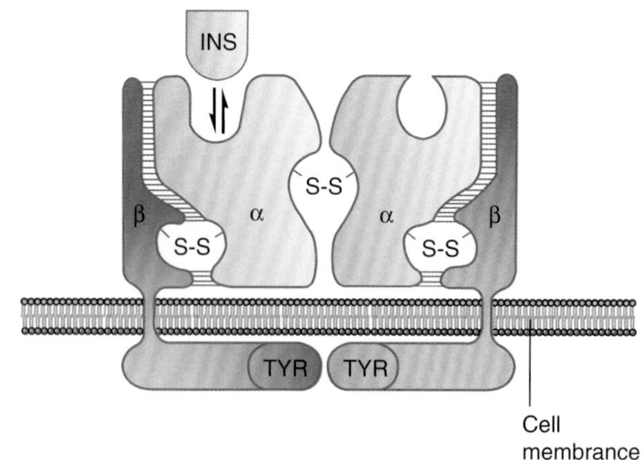

FIGURE 37-6 Schematic depiction of the insulin receptor consisting of two α and two β subunits joined by disulfide bonds (-S-S-). Insulin (INS) attaches to the α subunits, which triggers autophosphorylation of the tyrosine kinase (TYR) portions of the β subunits inside the cell and the resultant effects of insulin. (From Ganong WF. *Review of Medical Physiology*. 21st ed. New York, NY: Lange Medical Books/McGraw Hill; 2003, with permission.)

Table 37-8

Regulation of Insulin Secretion

Stimulation	Inhibition
Hyperglycemia	Hypoglycemia
β-Adrenergic agonists	β-Adrenergic antagonists
Acetylcholine	α-Adrenergic agonists
Glucagon	Somatostatin
	Diazoxide
	Thiazide diuretics
	Volatile anesthetics
	Insulin

within a narrow range. The pancreas is richly innervated by the autonomic nervous system, so that insulin is released in response to β-adrenergic stimulation or to acetylcholine. Conversely, α-adrenergic stimulation or β-adrenergic blockade inhibits insulin release. Oral glucose is more effective than glucose administered intravenously in evoking the release of insulin, suggesting the presence of an anticipatory signal from the gastrointestinal tract to the pancreas. Glycosuria is more likely after intravenous rather than oral glucose administration. Glucagon, HGH, and corticosteroids potentiate glucose-induced stimulation of insulin secretion. Prolonged secretion of these hormones or their exogenous administration can exhaust pancreatic β cells and lead to diabetes mellitus. Indeed, diabetes mellitus is found in patients who develop acromegaly or in individuals with a diabetic tendency who are treated with corticosteroids.

Physiologic Effects

Insulin receptor expression is highest in tissues, which regulate glucose, lipid, and protein metabolism (adipose, skeletal muscle, and liver) via insulin. Insulin promotes the use of carbohydrates for energy while depressing the use of fats and amino acids. For example, insulin facilitates storage of fat in adipose cells by inhibiting lipase enzyme, which normally hydrolyzes triglycerides in fat cells. In the liver, insulin inhibits enzymes necessary for gluconeogenesis, thus conserving amino acid stores.

Insulin facilitates glucose uptake and storage in the liver through effects on specific enzymes. When insulin induces the activity of glucokinase, uptake of glucose into liver cells is enhanced. Glucokinase is the enzyme that causes initial phosphorylation of glucose after it diffuses into hepatocytes. Once phosphorylated, glucose is trapped and unable to diffuse back through cell membranes. Storage is further enhanced by insulin-induced inhibition of phosphorylase enzyme, which normally causes liver glycogen to split into glucose. The net effects of these actions of insulin on enzymes is to increase hepatic stores of glycogen up to a maximum of approximately 100 g. Ordinarily, approximately 60% of the glucose in a meal is stored in the liver as glycogen.

Resting skeletal muscles are almost impermeable to glucose except in the presence of insulin. Glucose that enters resting skeletal muscles under the influence of insulin is stored as glycogen for subsequent use as energy. The amount of glycogen that can be stored in skeletal muscles, however, is much less than the amount that can be stored in the liver. Furthermore, glycogen in skeletal muscles, unlike that stored in the liver, cannot be reconverted to glucose and released into the systemic circulation because skeletal muscles lack glucose phosphatase enzyme, which is necessary for splitting glycogen. Exercise increases the permeability of skeletal muscle membranes to glucose, perhaps because insulin is released from within the skeletal muscle itself or its vasculature.

Brain cells are unique in that the permeability of their membranes to glucose does not depend on the presence of insulin. This characteristic is crucial because brain cells use only glucose for energy, thus the importance of maintaining blood glucose concentrations above a critical level of approximately 50 mg/dL. Indeed, lack of insulin causes the use mainly of fat for energy to the exclusion of glucose, except by brain cells.

Deficiencies in insulin signaling are associated with insulin resistance. When an impaired intracellular signal decreases recruitment of proteins that transport glucose to the plasma membrane for glucose uptake, an individual is said to have insulin resistance. Compensatory hyperinsulinemia overcomes peripheral tissue resistance to insulin. A feedback loop exists between insulin responsiveness in target tissues and insulin secretion by pancreatic β cells.

Glucagon

Glucagon is a catabolic hormone acting to mobilize glucose, fatty acids, and amino acids into the systemic circulation (Fig. 37-7).[21] These responses are the reciprocal of the insulin effects, emphasizing that these two hormones are also reciprocally secreted (Table 37-9). Indeed, the principal stimulus for secretion of glucagon is hypoglycemia. Glucagon abruptly increases the blood glucose concentration by stimulating glycogenolysis in the liver. Glucagon activates adenylate cyclase for the subsequent formation of cAMP. The metabolic effects of glucagon at the liver mimic those produced by epinephrine. Indeed, the study of the mechanism by which glucagon and epinephrine act as hyperglycemics led to the discovery of cAMP.[22] Glucagon also causes hyperglycemia by stimulating gluconeogenesis in hepatocytes. Enhanced myocardial contractility and more secretion of bile are effects when exogenous administration increases plasma concentrations of glucagon far above normal levels Amino acids help the release of glucagon and thus prevent hypoglycemia from ingestion of a pure protein meal, which stimulates insulin secretion. Glucagon undergoes

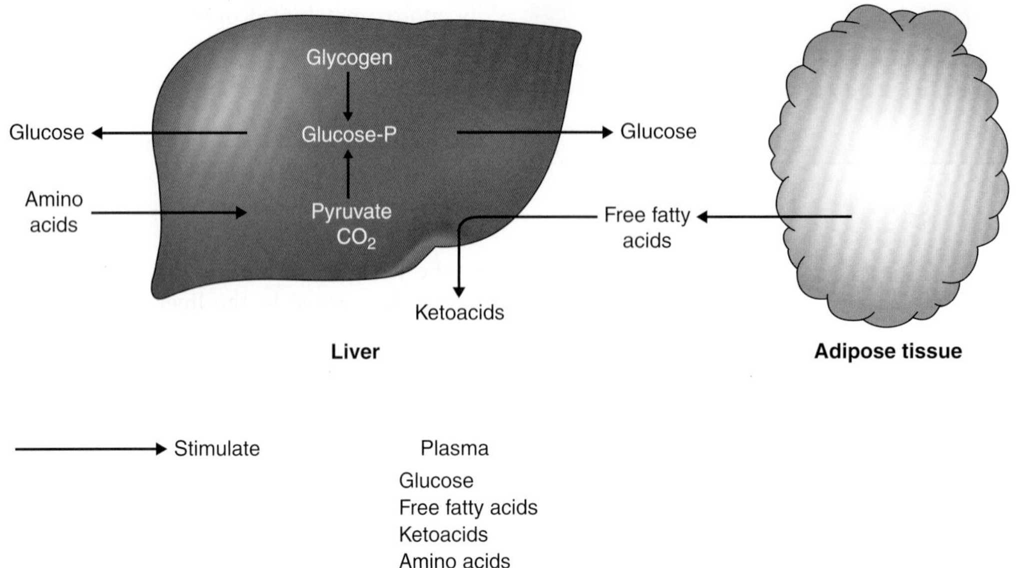

FIGURE 37-7 Glucagon stimulates tissue release of glucose, free fatty acids, and ketoacids and hepatic uptake of amino acids. (From Berne RM, Levy MN, Koeppen BM, et al. *Physiology*. 5th ed. St. Louis, MO: Mosby; 2004, with permission.)

enzymatic degradation to inactive metabolites in the liver and kidneys and at receptor sites in cell membranes. The elimination half-time of glucagon is brief—only 3 to 6 minutes.

Somatostatin

Somatostatin regulates islet cell secretion, inhibits both insulin and glucagon release, and inhibits several gastrointestinal processes including gallbladder contraction, gastric motility, and splanchnic blood flow.[23] This peptide is the same as growth hormone–releasing inhibitory hormone that is secreted by the hypothalamus.

Pancreatic Polypeptide

Pancreatic polypeptide inhibits pancreatic exocrine secretion, gallbladder contraction, vagally stimulated gastric acid secretion, and gut motility.[24–26]

Table 37-9

Regulation of Glucagon Secretion

Stimulation	Inhibition
Hypoglycemia	Hyperglycemia
Stress	Somatostatin
Sepsis	Insulin
Trauma	Free fatty acids
β-Adrenergic agonists	α-Adrenergic agonists
Acetylcholine	
Cortisol	

References

1. Desborough JP. The stress response to trauma and surgery. *Br J Anaesth*. 2000;85:109–117.
2. Ganong WF. *Review of Medical Physiology*. 21st ed. New York, NY: Lange Medical Books/McGraw Hill; 2003.
3. Taylor AL, Fishman LM. Corticotropin-releasing hormone. *N Engl J Med*. 1988;319:213–221.
4. Udelsman R, Norton JA, Jelenich SE, et al. Responses of the hypothalamic-pituitary-adrenal and angiotensin axes and the sympathetic system during controlled surgical and anesthetic stress. *J Clin Endocrinol Metab*. 1987;64:986–994.
5. Raff H, Norton JA, Flemma RJ, et al. Inhibition of the adrenocorticotropin response to surgery in humans: interaction between dexamethasone and fentanyl. *J Clin Endocrinol Metab*. 1987;65:295–298.
6. Stoelting RK. Perioperative management of the patient receiving glucocorticoids. *Curr Opin Anaesth*. 1997;10:227–228.
7. Treschan T, Jurgen P. The vasopressin system: physiology and clinical strategies. *Anesthesiology*. 2006;105:599–612.
8. Gimpl G, Fahrenholz F. The oxytocin receptor system: structure, function, and regulation. *Physiol Rev*. 2001;81:629–683.
9. Nakao K, Inoue Y, Okabe K, et al. Oxytocin enhances action potentials in pregnant human myometrium: a study with microelectrodes. *Am J Obstet Gynecol*. 1997;177:222–228.
10. Bennett-Guerrero E, Kramer DC, Schwinn DA. Effect of chronic and acute thyroid hormone reduction on perioperative outcome. *Anesth Analg*. 1997;85:30–36.
11. Babad AA, Eger EI II. The effects of hyperthyroidism and hypothyroidism on halothane and oxygen requirements in dogs. *Anesthesiology*. 1968;29:1087–1093.
12. Hume DM, Bell CC, Bartter FC. Direct measurement of adrenal secretion during operative trauma and convalescence. *Surgery*. 1962;52:174–187.
13. Udelsmann R, Holbrook NJ. Endocrine and molecular responses to surgical stress. *Curr Prob Surg*. 1994;31:653–658.
14. Udelsman R, Goldstein DS, Loariaus DL, et al. Catecholamine-glucocorticoid interactions during surgical stress. *J Surg Res*. 1987;43:539–545.
15. Bovill JG, Sebel PS, Fiolet JW, et al. The influence of sufentanil on endocrine and metabolic responses to cardiac surgery. *Anesth Analg*. 1983;62:391–397.

16. Sebel PS, Bovill JG, Schellekens APM, et al. Hormonal responses to high-dose fentanyl anesthesia. *Br J Anaesth.* 1981;53:941–948.
17. Strout CD, Nahrwold ML. Halothane requirement during pregnancy and lactation in rats. *Anesthesiology.* 1981;55:322–323.
18. Collombat P, Hecksher-Sorensen J, Serup P, et al. Specifying pancreatic endocrine cell fates. *Mech Dev.* 2006;123:501–512.
19. Genuth S. Diabetes mellitus. *Sci Am Med.* 2001;9:VI:1–34.
20. Larner J. Insulin and oral hypoglycemic drugs: glucagon. In: Gilman AG, Goodman LS, Rall TW, et al, eds. *The Pharmacological Basis of Therapeutics.* 7th ed. New York, NY: MacMillan; 1985: 1490–1516.
21. Berne RM, Levy MN, Koeppen BM, et al. *Physiology.* 5th ed. St. Louis, MO: Mosby; 2004.
22. Rall TW, Sutherland EW. Formation of a cyclic adenine ribonucleotide by tissue particles. *J Biol Chem.* 1958;232:1065–1076.
23. Lamberts SWJ, van der Lely A, de Herder WW, et al. Octreotide. *N Engl J Med.* 1996;334:246–254.
24. Lin TM, Evans, DC, Chance RE, et al. Bovine pancreatic peptide: action on gastric and pancreatic secretion in dogs. *Am J Physiol.* 1977;232:E311–E315.
25. Hazelwood RL. The pancreatic polypeptide (PP-fold) family: gastrointestinal, vascular, and feeding behavioral implications. *Proc Soc Exp Biol Med.* 1993;202:44–63.
26. Adrian TE, Mitchenere P, Sagor G, et al. Effect of pancreatic polypeptide on gallbladder pressure and hepatic bile secretion. *Am J Physiol.* 1982;243:G204–G207.

CHAPTER 38

Drugs that Alter Glucose Regulation

Vivek K. Moitra

Diabetes Mellitus

According to recent recommendations by the American Diabetes Association and the World Health Organization, diabetes mellitus is classified by the underlying disease etiology (i.e., type 1 vs. type 2) rather than by age-of-onset (i.e., juvenile-onset vs. adult-onset diabetes) or treatment modality (i.e., insulin-dependent vs. non–insulin-dependent diabetes).[1] The insulin deficiency in type 1 diabetes is the result of autoimmune-mediated destruction of pancreatic β cells. Patients depend on exogenous insulin to regulate metabolism. Onset of type 1 diabetes is at a younger age than onset of type 2 diabetes, and sensitivity to insulin is normal. Lack of insulin may precipitate diabetic ketoacidosis, a complex and potentially life-threatening metabolic derangement. In contrast, the peripheral insulin resistance of type 2 diabetes is often coupled with a failure to secrete insulin because of pancreatic β cell dysfunction. Oral hypoglycemic drugs are alternatives to exogenous administration of insulin to patients with type 2 diabetes. The vast majority of cases of diabetes are either type 1 or type 2 in an approximate ratio of 1:9. Gestation, exocrine pancreas disease, medications, endocrinopathies, genetic defects in insulin action and β cell function, infections, and uncommon immune-mediated disorders also cause diabetes[2] (Table 38-1).

Without sufficient insulin, transport of glucose across certain cell membranes slows markedly to cause hyperglycemia. The formation of glucose from protein accounts for the discovery that glucose in urine may exceed oral intake. Much of the protein used for glucose formation comes from skeletal muscles; glucose loss may manifest in extreme cases as skeletal muscle wasting. Elevations in blood glucose levels and hypoinsulinemia cause diabetic myopathy via muscle proteolysis. Increased free fatty acid concentrations in the plasma of diabetic patients show inhibition of the lipase enzyme system so that mobilization of fatty acids proceeds unopposed. The insulin-deficient liver is likely to use fatty acids to produce ketones, which can serve as an energy source for skeletal muscles and cardiac muscle. Production of ketones can lead to ketoacidosis; urinary excretion of ketones contributes to the depletion of electrolytes, especially potassium. Hypokalemia, however, may not be apparent, because intracellular potassium ions are exchanged for extracellular ions to compensate for the acidosis.

Low plasma concentrations of insulin, although inadequate to prevent hyperglycemia, may block lipolysis. This differential effect of insulin explains why hyperglycemia can exist without the presence of ketone bodies. Ketosis can be reliably prevented by continuously providing all diabetic patients with glucose and insulin.[3] Prevention is uniquely important in the perioperative period when nutritional intake is altered.

Hyperglycemia impairs vasodilation and induces a chronic proinflammatory, prothrombotic, and proatherogenic state leading to vascular complications.[4] Although all tissues are affected, of greatest relevance for anesthesia are atherosclerotic vascular, renal, and nervous system effects with peripheral vascular disease, renal insufficiency, and cerebrovascular disease.

The goals of therapy for patients with diabetes mellitus include preventing the adverse consequences of hypoglycemia and hyperglycemia, avoiding weight gain, and reducing microvascular and macrovascular complications. Symptoms often resolve when blood glucose levels are less than 200 mg/dL. Long-term metabolic control of diabetes is best monitored by measurement of glycosylated hemoglobin (HbA_{1c}), which reflects glucose control over the previous 2 to 3 months. In general, HbA_{1c} values less than 6.0% to 7.0% are associated with fewer microvascular complications. Therapy choices consider compliance, age, comorbidities, and impact on organ function (heart, kidney, liver).[5]

Insulin

Because patients with type 1 diabetes mellitus do not produce insulin, they require insulin therapy to survive. Insulin is prescribed for patients with type 2 diabetes mellitus

Table 38-1

Etiologic Classification of Diabetes Mellitus

Type 1 diabetes mellitus (absolute insulin deficiency from pancreatic β cell destruction)
Type 2 diabetes mellitus (insulin resistance vs. insulin deficiency)
Gestational diabetes mellitus
Exocrine pancreas disease (pancreatitis, pancreatectomy, cystic fibrosis, hemochromatosis)
Drug-induced (glucocorticoids, thiazides, thyroid hormone, β-adrenergic agonists)
Endocrinopathies (acromegaly, Cushing syndrome, glucagonoma)
Genetic defects in pancreatic β cell function
Genetic defects in insulin action (resistance)
Infections (congenital rubella, cytomegalovirus)
Uncommon immune-mediated diabetes ("stiff man" syndrome, anti-insulin receptor antibodies)

if treatment with oral glucose regulators fails. In these patients, pancreatic β cells have been destroyed or autoantibodies have developed (see Chapter 37 for insulin's mechanism of action). Insulin therapy mirrors the normal pattern of insulin secretion (pulsatile secretion that occurs under basal conditions and in response to meals) with basal supplementation and by short-acting insulin taken before food absorption. Insulin receptors become fully saturated with low concentrations of insulin. For example, continuous infusion of insulin, 1 to 2 units per hour, has the same or even greater pharmacologic effect than a single larger intravenous (IV) dose that is cleared rapidly from the circulation. Large doses of insulin, however, will last longer and exert a greater net effect than small doses. The number of insulin receptors seems to be inversely related to the plasma concentration of insulin, which reflect the ability of insulin to regulate the population of its receptors. Obesity and type 1 diabetes mellitus appear to be associated with fewer insulin receptors.

Pharmacokinetics

The elimination half-time of IV insulin is 5 to 10 minutes in both healthy and diabetic patients. Insulin is metabolized in the kidneys and liver by a proteolytic enzyme. Approximately 50% of the insulin that reaches the liver through its portal vein is metabolized in a single passage. Nevertheless, renal dysfunction alters the disappearance rate of circulating insulin to a greater extent than does hepatic disease. Indeed, unexpected prolonged effects of insulin are found in patients with renal disease, reflecting impairment of both its metabolism and excretion by the kidneys. Peripheral tissues such as skeletal muscles and fat can bind and inactivate insulin, but this effect is of minor quantitative significance. Despite rapid clearance from plasma after IV injection of insulin, the pharmacologic effect lasts for 30 to 60 minutes because insulin is tightly bound to tissue receptors. Insulin administered subcutaneously releases slowly into the circulation to produce a sustained biologic effect.

Insulin is secreted into the portal venous system in the basal state at a rate of approximately 1 unit per hour. After food intake, the rate of insulin secretion increases to 5- to 10-fold. The total daily secretion of insulin is approximately 40 units. The sympathetic and parasympathetic nervous systems innervate the insulin-producing islet cells to influence the basal rate of hormone secretion as well as the response to stress. For example, α-adrenergic stimulation decreases and β-adrenergic or parasympathetic nervous system stimulation increases the basal secretion of insulin. The insulin response to glucose is greater after oral ingestion than after IV infusion because glucose-dependent insulinotropic polypeptide is released after oral ingestion of glucose and the pancreatic β cell response is augmented. To gain adequate glycemic control in type 1 diabetes, at least two daily subcutaneous injections of intermediate- or long-acting insulin combined with rapid-acting insulin are nearly always required.

Insulin Preparations and Delivery

Human insulin manufactured using recombinant DNA technology has replaced insulin extracted from beef and pork pancreas. Allergy or immunoresistance to animal insulins is no longer a serious problem. In rare instances of local allergy to human insulin, pure porcine insulin or lispro insulin is substituted. The basic principle of replacement is to provide a slow, long-acting, continuous supply of insulin (neutral protamine Hagedorn [NPH] insulin, insulin glargine, insulin detemir, or insulin degludec) that mimics the nocturnal and interprandial basal secretion of normal pancreatic β cells.[6] A rapid and relatively short-acting form of insulin (insulin aspart, lispro, or glulisine) delivered before meals mimics the normal meal-stimulated (prandial) release of insulin.

A number of insulin preparations for subcutaneous administration are available (Table 38-2).[7] The pharmacokinetics of these insulins vary from individual to individual and even within the same individual from day to day. Rates of insulin absorption from subcutaneous sites differ with the injection site (absorption from abdominal sites is least variable), depth and angle of injection, ambient temperature, and exercise of an injected extremity.

Commercially prepared insulin is bioassayed, and its physiologic activity (potency), based on the ability to decrease blood glucose concentration, is expressed in units. The potency of insulin is 22 to 26 U/mg. Insulin U-100 (100 U/mL) is the most commonly used commercial preparation. The total daily exogenous dose of insulin

Table 38-2

Classification of Insulin Preparations

Insulin Preparation	Hours after Subcutaneous Administration		
	Onset	Peak	Duration (h)
Very rapid-acting			
Lispro	5–15 min	45–75 min	2–4
Insulin aspart	5–15 min	45–75 min	2–4
Glulisine	5–15 min	45–75 min	2–4
Rapid-acting			
Regular	30 min	2–4 h	6–8
Intermediate-acting			
NPH	2 h	4–12 h	18–28
Long-acting			
Detemir	2 h	3–9 h	6–24
Glargine	1.5 h	None	20–>24
Ultra long-acting			
Degludec	2 h	None	>40

NPH, neutral protamine Hagedorn.

for treatment of type 1 diabetes mellitus is usually in the range of 0.5 to 1 U/kg/day. This insulin requirement, however, may be increased dramatically by stress associated with sepsis or trauma.

Continuous subcutaneous insulin infusion (CSII) through an external pump delivers basal insulin (0.01 to 0.015 U/kg/hour) and bolus doses before meals. With this system, nocturnal versus daytime basal requirements can be accommodated, infusions can be altered during exercise, and doses can be calculated via algorithms of previous glucose values and insulin delivery. Short-acting insulin (regular) and ultra rapid–acting insulins (lispro, aspart, and glulisine) are the only preparations used for CSII delivery pumps.

Lispro

Lispro is a short-acting insulin analogue that more closely parallels physiologic insulin secretion and needs. A feature of natural or synthetic human insulin is that six molecules associate with a zinc molecule to form hexamers. Insulin hexamers must dissociate to monomers before absorption from subcutaneous injection sites. This feature is the reason that crystalline zinc insulin (regular insulin) has a peak action 2 to 4 hours after its subcutaneous injection. It must be administered 30 to 60 minutes before eating to effectively limit postprandial hyperglycemia. By exchanging lysine and proline at positions 28 and 29 of the insulin B chain, hexamer formation is prevented and the monomer is rapidly absorbed from the injection site. Therefore, lispro insulin injected subcutaneously begins to act within 15 minutes, the peak effect is reached in 45 to 75 minutes, and the duration of action is only 2 to 4 hours. Lispro injected just before eating provides a postprandial plasma insulin concentration profile similar to that of normal insulin secretion. An important benefit of lispro is a decrease in postprandial hyperglycemia and less risk of hypoglycemia, which may follow injection of regular insulin. Loss of the late action of regular insulin, however, may result in recurrent hyperglycemia before the next meal. In patients treated with lispro, HbA_{1c} may not decrease unless the doses of basal insulin (NPH, detemir, or glargine) are increased.

Insulin Aspart and Glulisine

Insulin aspart and glulisine are synthetic rapid-acting analogues with a profile of action and therapeutic benefits similar to those of lispro.

Regular Insulin (Crystalline Zinc Insulin)

Regular insulin is a fast-acting preparation and is the only form of insulin that can be administered IV as well as subcutaneously. This form can be mixed in the same syringe with other insulin preparations if the pH of the solutions is similar.

Administration of regular insulin is preferred for treating the abrupt onset of hyperglycemia or the appearance of ketoacidosis. In the perioperative period, regular insulin is administered as a single IV injection (1 to 5 units) or as a continuous infusion (0.5 to 2.0 units per hour) to treat metabolic derangements associated with diabetes mellitus.

Neutral Protamine Hagedorn

NPH is an intermediate-acting preparation whose absorption from its subcutaneous injection site is delayed because the insulin is conjugated with protamine. The acronym NPH designates a neutral solution (N), protamine (P), and origin in Hagedorn's (H) laboratory.[8] This insulin preparation contains 0.005 mg protamine/U of insulin.

Glargine, Detemir, Degludec

Glargine, detemir, and degludec are long-acting insulin analogues for basal insulin replacement. Compared to NPH insulin, these long-acting insulins have a later onset of action and less pronounced peaks. Glargine or detemir can be administered as a single bedtime injection to provide basal insulin for 24 hours with less nocturnal hypoglycemia.[9] Unlike glargine and detemir, degludec can be mixed with rapid-acting insulins. Degludec is not approved for use in the United States.

Side Effects

Side effects of treatment with insulin may manifest as (a) hypoglycemia, (b) allergic reactions, (c) lipodystrophy, (d) insulin resistance, or (e) drug interactions.

Hypoglycemia

The most serious side effect of insulin therapy is hypoglycemia. Patients are vulnerable to hypoglycemia if they receive exogenous insulin in the absence of carbohydrate intake, as during a perioperative period, especially before surgery. The first symptoms of hypoglycemia are the compensatory effects of increased epinephrine secretion: diaphoresis, tachycardia, and hypertension. Rebound hyperglycemia caused by sympathetic nervous system activity in response to hypoglycemia (Somogyi effect) may mask the correct diagnosis. Symptoms of hypoglycemia involving the central nervous system (CNS) include mental confusion progressing to seizures and coma. The CNS effects are intense because the brain depends on glucose as a selective substrate for oxidative metabolism. A prolonged period of hypoglycemia may result in irreversible brain damage.

The diagnosis of hypoglycemia during general anesthesia is difficult because anesthetic drugs mask the classic signs of sympathetic nervous system stimulation. The signs of sympathetic nervous system stimulation are likely to be confused with responses evoked by painful surgical stimulation in an anesthetized patient. The anesthesiologist may then decide to increase the dose of anesthetic drugs. Changes in heart rate and systemic blood pressure may be caused by hypoglycemia.[10] Nonselective β-adrenergic antagonists also may mask the symptoms of hypoglycemia.

Severe hypoglycemia is treated with 50 to 100 mL of 50% glucose solution administered IV. Alternatively, glucagon, 0.5 to 1.0 mg IV or administered subcutaneously, is given. Nausea and vomiting are frequent side effects of glucagon treatment. In the absence of CNS depression, carbohydrates may be administered orally.

Allergic Reactions

Use of human insulin preparations has eliminated the problem of systemic allergic reactions that could result from administration of animal-derived insulins. Local allergic reactions to insulin are approximately 10 times more frequent than systemic allergic reactions. Local allergic reactions are characterized by an erythematous indurated area that develops at the site of insulin injection. The cause of local allergic reactions is likely to be noninsulin materials in the insulin preparation. Chronic exposure to low doses of protamine in NPH insulin may stimulate the production of antibodies against protamine. Patients remain asymptomatic until a large dose of protamine is administered IV to antagonize the anticoagulant effects of heparin. Indeed, patients with diabetes who are treated with NPH insulin have had allergic reactions to protamine.[11] Yet allergic reactions to protamine are not found more in patients treated with NPH insulin than in nondiabetics.[12]

Lipodystrophy

Lipodystrophy results when fat atrophies at the site of subcutaneous injection of insulin. This side effect is minimized by frequently changing the site used for injection of insulin.

Insulin Resistance

Patients requiring greater than 100 units of exogenous insulin daily are in a state of insulin resistance. Even this value is high, because insulin requirements for pancreatectomized adults are often as low as 30 units. The use of human insulins has eliminated the problem of immunoresistance that could accompany administration of animal insulins. Acute insulin resistance is associated with trauma from infection or surgery.

Drug Interactions

There are hormones administered as drugs that counter the hypoglycemic effect of insulin: adrenocorticotrophic hormone, estrogens, and glucagon. Epinephrine inhibits the secretion of insulin and stimulates glycogenolysis. Certain antibiotics (tetracycline or chloramphenicol), salicylates, and phenylbutazone increase the duration of action of insulin and may have a direct hypoglycemic effect. The hypoglycemic effect of insulin may be potentiated by monoamine oxidase inhibitors.

Oral Glucose Regulators

Oral drugs with different mechanisms of action are available for controlling plasma glucose concentrations in patients with type 2 diabetes mellitus (Table 38-3). None of these drugs will adequately control hyperglycemia indefinitely. Therefore, use of combinations of oral drugs from the onset of treatment may be indicated.[13] Insulin itself

Table 38-3

Oral Drugs for Treatment of Type 2 Diabetes Mellitus

Sulfonylureas (stimulate insulin secretion; hypoglycemia a risk)
Glyburide
Glipizide
Glimepiride
Gliclazide
Tolbutamide
Tolazamide
Chlorpropamide
Acetohexamide
Meglitinides (stimulate insulin secretion; hypoglycemia a risk)
Repaglinide
Nateglinide
Biguanides (inhibit glucose production by the liver; hypoglycemia not a risk)
Metformin
Thiazolidinediones (increase sensitivity to insulin for glucose uptake by skeletal muscles and adipose tissues; hypoglycemia not a risk)
Rosiglitazone
Pioglitazone
α-**Glucosidase inhibitors** (slow digestion and absorption of carbohydrates from the diet; hypoglycemia not a risk)
Acarbose
Miglitol

may be administered with sulfonylureas and meglitinides. The effect on HbA_{1c} is similar for these drugs.

Metformin

Metformin is an oral biguanide that is often prescribed as the initial agent to prevent hyperglycemia in patients with type 2 diabetes (Fig. 38-1). Metformin decreases blood glucose concentrations in both the fasting and postprandial state and rarely causes hypoglycemia. It can be used in combination with other medications such as insulin and sulfonylureas. Metformin should not be prescribed for patients with lactic acidosis, acute kidney injury, gastrointestinal intolerance, or acute hepatic disease. Metformin has pleiotropic effects. It improves lipid profiles and fibrinolysis and promotes mild to moderate weight loss.[14]

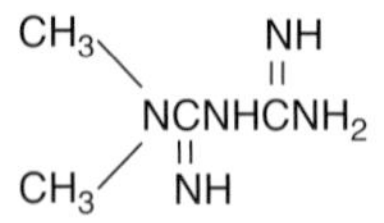

$$(CH_3)_2N\text{-}C(=NH)\text{-}NH\text{-}C(=NH)\text{-}NH_2$$

FIGURE 38-1 Metformin.

Metformin also has been used in patients with polycystic ovarian disease, nonalcoholic fatty liver disease, and premature puberty.

Pharmacokinetics

In contrast to sulfonylureas, metformin is not bound to plasma proteins and does not undergo metabolism. It is eliminated by the kidneys, with 90% of an oral dose excreted in approximately 12 hours. Peak plasma concentrations of metformin occur approximately 2 hours after oral administration. The drug has an elimination half-time of 2 to 4 hours, which means that it is taken up to three times a day (500 to 1,000 mg with meals). In view of its dependence on renal clearance, metformin is prescribed with caution, if at all, to patients with renal dysfunction.

Mechanism of Action

The blood glucose–lowering effect of metformin is not mediated through stimulation of endogenous insulin secretion.[15] Metformin activates adenosine monophosphate–activated protein kinase to suppress hepatic glucose production by decreasing gluconeogenesis and glycogenolysis and to enhance postprandial insulin suppression of hepatic glucose production. Metformin also regulates glucose levels by decreasing gastrointestinal glucose absorption, increasing insulin sensitivity in peripheral tissues, and enhancing synthesis of glucagon-like peptide-1 (GLP-1) in the ileum.[14]

Side Effects

The most common side effects of metformin are anorexia, nausea, and diarrhea, which are dose related. Up to 15% of patients experience side effects sufficient to warrant withdrawal of the drug.[5] In contrast to sulfonylureas, metformin does not cause hypoglycemia. Metformin is associated with vitamin B_{12} deficiency.[5] The most serious, although rare, side effect of metformin therapy is lactic acidosis.

Lactic Acidosis

Lactic acidosis is a possible side effect associated with metformin that has been described during the intraoperative period.[15–17] For this reason, some have recommended discontinuing metformin 48 hours or longer before elective operations.[16] If metformin cannot be discontinued before surgery, the patient is monitored for the development of lactic acidosis (arterial blood gases and pH, serum lactate concentrations, renal function) in the perioperative period.

Metformin binds to mitochondrial membranes to decrease intracellular adenosine triphosphate and increase adenosine monophosphate concentrations. Glucose is metabolized anaerobically. The resulting pyruvate is reduced to lactate, which is usually metabolized quickly in the liver. For this reason, metformin should be administered with caution, if at all, to patients with a history of hepatic dysfunction, renal insufficiency (creatinine level

>1.5 mg/dL), IV administration of radiographic iodinated contrast media, acute myocardial infarction, congestive heart failure, arterial hypoxemia, or sepsis. Hemodialysis along with bicarbonate administration can be effective therapy for metformin-induced lactic acidosis. Management of biguanide-induced lactic acidosis is supportive because the underlying pathologic change (blockade of the mitochondrial respiratory chain) cannot be treated.

Sulfonylureas

Sulfonylurea compounds are drugs capable of lowering blood glucose concentrations even to hypoglycemic levels (Fig. 38-2).[15,18] The drug-induced improvement in blood glucose control is associated with decreased hepatic production of very-low-density lipoproteins as well as amelioration of hypertriglyceridemia. Yet as many as 20% of patients with type 2 diabetes mellitus who begin sulfonylurea therapy do not have an adequate hypoglycemic response to maximal doses (*primary failures*), and each year, an additional 10% to 15% of patients who responded initially fail to respond to sulfonylurea therapy (*secondary failure*). Successful management of glucose control with sulfonylureas requires some β cell function. The sulfonylureas have no effect on and no role in the treatment of patients with type 1 diabetes mellitus. Although sulfonylureas are derivatives of sulfonamides, they have no antibacterial actions. These drugs should not be administered to patients with known allergy to sulfa drugs.

Mechanism of Action

Sulfonylurea receptors are found on pancreatic and cardiac cells. These drugs inhibit adenosine triphosphate–sensitive potassium ion channels (now known as the ***sulfonylurea receptor-1***) on pancreatic β cells.[5] As a result, there is an influx of calcium and stimulation of exocytosis (release) of insulin storage granules. Although sulfonylureas decrease insulin resistance, this effect is minor, if at all, in decreasing blood glucose concentrations.

Pharmacokinetics

Oral hypoglycemics are readily absorbed from the gastrointestinal tract, with the most important distinguishing features being differences in duration of action and elimination half-time (Table 38-4).[18] The biological effects of sulfonylureas such as glyburide may be longer than plasma half-lives because of the formation of active metabolites.[19] Weakly acidic, sulfonylureas circulate bound to protein (90% to 98%), principally to albumin. Metabolism in the liver is extensive, and the active and inactive metabolites are eliminated by renal tubular secretion. Approximately 50% of glyburide is excreted in feces.

Side Effects

Sulfonylureas are generally well tolerated; the most common severe complication of these drugs is hypoglycemia. The greatest risk of hypoglycemia occurs with drugs with the longest elimination half-times, glyburide and chlorpropamide; sulfonylureas may act for up to 7 days.

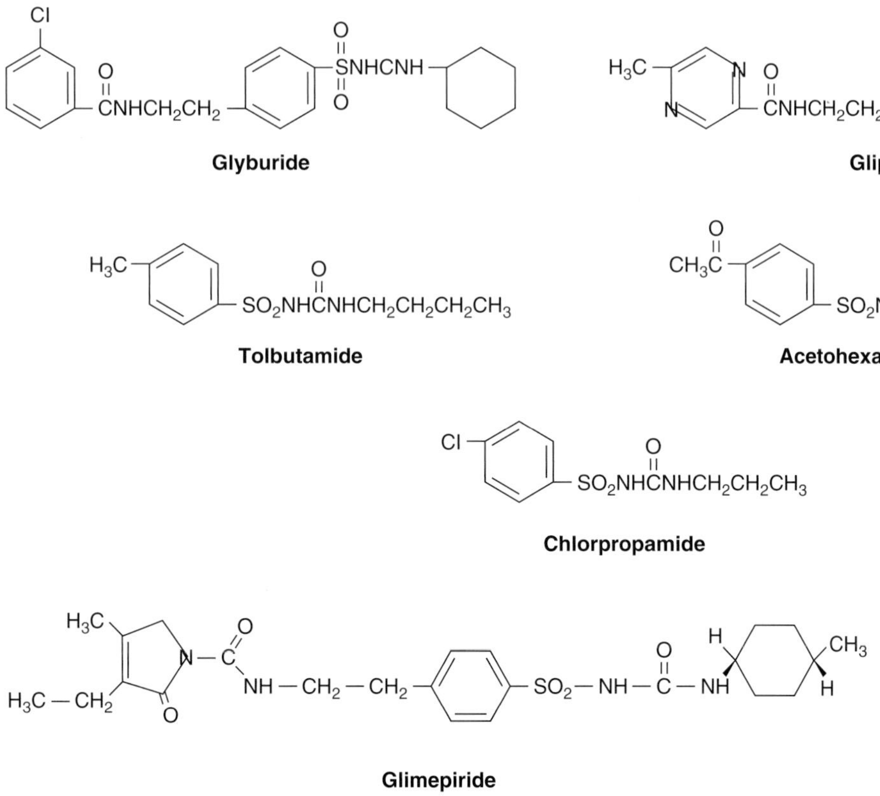

Glyburide

Glipizide

Tolbutamide

Acetohexamide

Chlorpropamide

Glimepiride

FIGURE 38-2 Oral hypoglycemics derived from sulfonylurea.

Table 38-4

Classification and Pharmacokinetics of Sulfonylurea Oral Hypoglycemics

	Equivalent Daily Dose (mg)	Daily Dose Range (mg)	Doses/Day	Duration of Action (h)	Elimination Half-Time (h)[a]
Glyburide	2.5–5	2.5–20	1–2	18–24	4.6–12
Glipizide	5–10	5–40	1–2	12–24	4–7
Glimepiride	2	2–4	1	24+	5–8
Tolbutamide	1,000	500–1,000	2–3	6–12	4–8
Tolazamide	250	200–1,000	1–2	16–24	7
Acetohexamide	500	250–1,500	2	12–18	1.3–6
Chlorpropamide	100–250	100–750	1	36	30–36

[a]Approximate.

Although hypoglycemia from sulfonylureas may be infrequent, it is often more prolonged and more dangerous than hypoglycemia from insulin (Table 38-5).

Hypoglycemia caused by sulfonylureas is treated with prolonged infusion of glucose-containing solutions. Risk factors for sulfonylurea-induced hypoglycemia include (a) impaired nutrition, as in the perioperative period; (b) age older than 60 years; (c) impaired renal function; and (d) concomitant drug therapy that potentiates sulfonylureas (phenylbutazone, sulfonamide antibiotics, warfarin) or itself produces hypoglycemia (alcohol or salicylates). Renal disease decreases elimination of sulfonylureas and their active metabolites, thus increasing the likelihood of hypoglycemia. In this regard, only small amounts of tolbutamide and glipizide are excreted unchanged in urine, making these drugs preferable for patients with renal disease. Sulfonylureas cross the placenta and may produce fetal hypoglycemia.

Sulfonylureas close K_{ATP} channels and inhibit ischemic preconditioning, a cardioprotective mechanism.[20] Cardiovascular mortality has been associated with some sulfonylureas, especially in patients who have had a prior myocardial infarction.[21,22] Gliclazide, a newer sulfonylurea selective for pancreatic β cells may not be associated with the same cardiac morbidity.[23,24] For this reason, sulfonylureas may be discontinued 24 to 48 hours before elective surgery in high-risk patients. Approximately 1% to 3% of patients treated with oral hypoglycemics experience gastrointestinal disturbances including nausea, vomiting, abnormal liver function tests, and cholestasis. Sulfonylureas are not recommended for patients with hepatic dysfunction as liver disease prolongs their elimination half-time and enhances their hypoglycemic action, with the exception of acetohexamide. Disulfiram-like reactions and inappropriate secretion of arginine vasopressin hormone that results in hyponatremia are unique side effects of chlorpropamide.

Table 38-5

Comparison of Sulfonylurea Therapy with Insulin Therapy

Sulfonylurea	Insulin
Failed initial response in 10% to 15% of patients	No maximum dose
Secondary failure rate each year among treated patients is about 10%	
Hypoglycemia may be more severe	Hypoglycemia may be more frequent
Associated cardiac complications	Lipid levels lowered
Patients may prefer oral medication	Patients may resist injections

Glyburide

Glyburide stimulates insulin secretion over a 24-hour period after a morning oral dose.[25] Peak plasma levels occur approximately 3 hours after an oral dose. Glyburide increases sensitivity to insulin and inhibits the production of glucose by the liver. Metabolism is in the liver, with metabolites excreted equally in urine and feces. One of the hepatic metabolites of glyburide has approximately 15% of the activity of the parent compound. A mild diuretic effect accompanies use of this drug. When administration is discontinued, the drug is cleared from plasma in about 36 hours.

Glipizide

Glipizide stimulates insulin secretion over a 12-hour period after a morning oral dose. Peak plasma levels occur approximately 1 hour after oral administration. Glipizide increases glucose uptake and suppresses glucose output by the liver.[26] These effects persist for prolonged periods (at least 3 years) without evidence of tolerance. Unlike glyburide, metabolism of glipizide in the liver produces inactive substances that are excreted in urine. A mild diuretic effect accompanies use of this drug. Relatively rapid clearance from the plasma minimizes the potential for long-lasting hypoglycemia.

Glimepiride

Glimepiride decreases blood glucose concentrations by stimulating release of insulin from the pancreas and may decrease hepatic glucose production. It is combined with insulin therapy when oral sulfonylureas are not effective.

Tolbutamide

Tolbutamide is the shortest acting and least potent sulfonylurea (see Table 38-4).[18] It is extensively metabolized in the liver to much less potent compounds before excretion in urine. Of all the sulfonylureas, tolbutamide probably causes the fewest side effects, although it can produce hypoglycemia and hyponatremia.

Acetohexamide

Acetohexamide differs from other sulfonylureas in that most of its hypoglycemic action comes from its principal metabolite hydroxyhexamide, which is 2.5 times as potent as the parent compound. After oral ingestion, peak plasma concentrations of acetohexamide and its active metabolite occur after 1.5 hours and 3.5 hours, respectively. This drug is not recommended for patients with renal disease because the kidneys excrete the active metabolite. Acetohexamide is the only sulfonylurea with uricosuric properties (urocosuric drugs increase the excretion of uric acid in the urine), making it an appropriate drug for the diabetic patient with gout.

Chlorpropamide

Chlorpropamide is the longest acting sulfonylurea, with a duration of action that may approach 72 hours (see Table 38-4).[18] The maximal effect of chlorpropamide may not be apparent for 7 to 14 days, and several weeks are needed for complete elimination of the drug. Because 20% of a dose is excreted unchanged, impaired renal function can lead to accumulation and an enhanced hypoglycemic effect. Chlorpropamide is associated with reactions similar to those produced by disulfiram (facial flushing after ingestion of alcohol) and can cause severe hyponatremia. Approximately 5% of patients treated with chlorpropamide have serum sodium concentrations of less than 129 mEq/L, but they are usually asymptomatic. Risk factors for the development of hyponatremia include age older than 60 years, female gender, and the concomitant administration of thiazide diuretics. If all these risk factors are present, the frequency of hyponatremia increases threefold.

Meglitinides

Repaglinide and the phenylalanine derivative, nateglinide, differ in structure and timing of action from sulfonylurea drugs. Although these drugs exert effects on β cells similar to those of sulfonylurea drugs, their peak effect is about 1 hour and duration of action is about 4 hours. β cell stimulants lower HbA_{1c} about 1%. Repaglinide and nateglinide must be administered 15 to 30 minutes before a meal and should never be ingested while fasting. The short duration of action and activity only in the presence of glucose should decrease the risk of prolonged hypoglycemic episodes.[27] Nateglinide is metabolized by the liver, and its metabolites are excreted by the kidney. The accumulation of active metabolites may cause hypoglycemia. Excretion of repaglinide by the kidneys is minimal so adjustment is not necessary for patients with renal insufficiency.

α-Glucosidase Inhibitors

Acarbose and miglitol are α-glucosidase inhibitors (AGI) that decrease carbohydrate digestion and absorption of disaccharides by interfering with intestinal glucosidase activity.[18] As a result, both release of glucose from food and absorption from the gastrointestinal tract are slow. HbA_{1c} generally decreases 0.5% to 0.8%. These drugs are useful only as monotherapy when postprandial hyperglycemia is the main problem. Flatulence, abdominal cramping, and diarrhea are side effects that frequently result from undigested carbohydrates that reach bacteria in the lower colon. With the exception of occasional increases in liver transaminases, these drugs are considered nontoxic.[15] Although hypoglycemia does not occur with monotherapy, it can occur when AGI are added to sulfonylureas or insulin.

Thiazolidinediones

Thiazolidinediones (TZDs), such as rosiglitazone and pioglitazone, act principally at skeletal muscle, liver, and adipose tissue via peroxisome proliferator activator receptor-γ (PPAR-γ) to decrease insulin resistance and hepatic glucose production and to increase use of glucose by the liver.[5] Like metformin, TZDs act in the presence of insulin and are especially effective in obese patients. As monotherapy, these drugs decrease HbA_{1c} 1% to 1.5%. The clinical effect takes 4 to 12 weeks. TZDs can cause weight gain, which is partly extracellular fluid. The accumulation of extracellular fluid as edema is undesirable in patients with congestive heart failure. These drugs also are contraindicated in patients with liver failure. The possibility of drug-induced liver dysfunction is the reason that plasma concentrations of hepatic transaminases must be measured periodically. TZDs tend to decrease plasma concentrations of triglycerides and increase high-density lipoprotein and low-density lipoprotein cholesterol levels. Although rosiglitazone has been associated with cardiovascular risk, particularly heart failure, this risk may be similar to the cardiovascular risks observed with other standard diabetes medications.[28]

Glucagon-Like Peptide-1 Receptor Agonists

GLP-1 receptor agonists such as exenatide and liraglutide are injectable agents that bind to receptors in the pancreas, gastrointestinal tract, and brain to increase insulin secretion from β cells (glucose dependent), decrease glucagon production from α cells, and reduce gastric emptying. Nausea and vomiting is associated with GLP-1 receptor agonists. The risk of hypoglycemia increases when GLP-1 receptor agonists are combined with sulfonylureas. Exenatide formulations include a short-acting formulation and a long-acting formulation that is injected once weekly. Liraglutide has a half-life of 8 to 14 hours and is injected once daily.[5]

Dipeptidyl-Peptidase-4 Inhibitors

Dipeptidyl-peptidase-4 (DDP-4) inhibitors (saxagliptin, sitagliptin, linagliptin, alogliptin, vildagliptin) enhance the incretin effect via inhibition of native GLP-1 degradation. Similar to GLP-1 receptor agonists, DPP-4 inhibitors increase insulin secretion from α cells (glucose dependent) and reduce pancreatic α cell secretion of glucagon.[5] This class of drugs has a duration of action of 12 to 24 hours, and doses are reduced for patients with renal insufficiency.

Amylin Agonists

Pancreatic β cells secrete insulin and amylin. Although amylin agonists (pramlintide) do not alter insulin levels, they suppress gastric emptying, inhibit glucagon release, and reduce HbA_{1c} levels. Side effects of pramlintide include nausea and vomiting.

Other Medications

Colesevelam (bile acid sequestrant) and bromocriptine mesylate (dopamine receptor agonist) lower glucose levels and decrease HbA_{1c} values, but the mechanisms are unclear. Neither of these medications is associated with hypoglycemia and both may cause gastrointestinal intolerance.[5]

Combination Therapy

Combination therapies target two or more different causes of hyperglycemia simultaneously. For example, insulin resistance in the liver is decreased with metformin while insulin secretion is increased with sulfonylureas or meglitinide. AGI complement the different actions of these two classes of drugs. Exogenous insulin also may be part of combination therapy. The primary aim of combination therapy is to decrease HbA_{1c}; reductions in the daily insulin dose are a secondary benefit.

References

1. Expert Committee on the Diagnosis and Classification of Diabetes Mellitus. Report of the expert committee on the diagnosis and classification of diabetes mellitus. *Diabetes Care*. 2003;26(suppl 1): S5–S20.
2. American Diabetes Association. Diagnosis and classification of diabetes mellitus. *Diabetes Care*. 2010;33(suppl 1):S62–S69.
3. Hirsch IB, McGill JB, Cryer PE, et al. Perioperative management of surgical patients with diabetes mellitus. *Anesthesiology*. 1991;74: 346–359.
4. Beckman JA, Creager MA, Libby P. Diabetes and atherosclerosis. *JAMA*. 2002;287:2570–2581.
5. Garber AJ, Abrahamson MJ, Barzilay JI, et al. American Association of Clinical Endocrinologists' Comprehensive diabetes management algorithm 2013 consensus statement. *Endocr Pract*. 2013;19(S2): 1–48.
6. Hirsch IB. Type 1 diabetes mellitus and the use of flexible insulin regimens. *Am Fam Physician*. 1999;60:2343–2349.
7. Genuth S. Diabetes mellitus. *Sci Am Med*. 2001;9:VI:1–34.
8. Hagedorn HC, Jensen BN, Krarup NB, et al. Protamine insulinate. *JAMA*. 1936;106:179–180.
9. Ratner RE, Hirsch IB, Neifing JL, et al. Less hypoglycemia with insulin glargine in intensive insulin therapy for type 1 diabetes. *Diabetes Care*. 2000;23:639–645.
10. Burgos LG, Ebert TJ, Asiddao C, et al. Increased intraoperative cardiovascular morbidity in diabetics with autonomic neuropathy. *Anesthesiology*. 1989;70:591–597.
11. Steward WJ, McSweeney SM, Kellett MA, et al. Increased risk of severe protamine reactions in NPH insulin–dependent diabetics undergoing cardiac catheterization. *Circulation*. 1984;70:788–792.
12. Levy JH, Schwieger IM, Zaidan JR, et al. Evaluation of patients at risk for protamine reactions. *J Thorac Cardiovasc Surg*. 1989;98: 200–204.
13. Riddle M. The 2 defects of type 2 diabetes: combining drugs to treat both insulin deficiency and insulin resistance. *Am J Med*. 2000;108: S1–S6.
14. Rodbard HW, Jellinger PS, Davidson JA, et al. Statement by an American Association of Clinical Endocrinologists/American College of Endocrinology consensus panel on type 2 diabetes mellitus: an algorithm for glycemic control. *Endocr Pract*. 2009;15: 540–559.
15. Mooradian AD. Drug therapy of non–insulin-dependent diabetes mellitus in the elderly. *Drugs*. 1996;51:931–941.
16. Mercker SK, Maier C, Doz P, et al. Lactic acidosis as a serious perioperative complication of antidiabetic biguanide medication with metformin. *Anesthesiology*. 1997;87:1003–1005.
17. Stumvoll M, Nurjhan N, Perriello G, et al. Metabolic effects of metformin in non–insulin-dependent diabetes mellitus. *N Engl J Med*. 1995;333:550–554.
18. Gerich JE. Oral hypoglycemic agents. *N Engl J Med*. 1989;321: 1231–1243.
19. Rydberg T, Jonsson A, Roder M, et al. Hypoglycemic activity of glyburide (gibenclamide) metabolites in humans. *Diabetes Care*. 1994;17:1026–1030.
20. Brady PA, Terzic A. The sulfonylurea controversy: more questions from the heart. *J Am Coll Cardiol*. 1998;31:950–956.
21. Garratt KN, Brady PA, Hassinger NL, et al. Sulfonylurea drugs increase early mortality in patients with diabetes mellitus after direct angioplasty for acute myocardial infarction. *J Am Coll Cardiol*. 1999;33:119–124.
22. Simpson SH, Majumdar SR, Tsuyuki RT, et al. Dose-response relation between sulfonylurea drugs and mortality in type 2 diabetes mellitus: a population-based cohort study. *CMAJ*. 2006;174: 169–174.
23. Zeller M, Danchin N, Simon D, et al. Impact of type of preadmission sulfonylureas on mortality and cardiovascular outcomes in

diabetic patients with acute myocardial infarction. *J Clin Endocrinol Metab*. 2010;95:4993–5002.

24. Schramm TK, Gislason GH, Vaag A, et al. Mortality and cardiovascular risk associated with different insulin secretagogues compared with metformin in type 2 diabetes, with or without a previous myocardial infarction: a nationwide study. *Eur Heart J*. 2011;32: 1900–1908.
25. Feldman JM. Glyburide: second-generation sulfonylurea hypoglycemic agent; history, chemistry, metabolism, pharmacokinetics, clinical use and adverse effects. *Pharmacotherapy*. 1985;5: 43–62.
26. Lebovitz HE. Glipzide: second-generation sulfonylurea hypoglycemic agent. Pharmacology, pharmacokinetics, and clinical use. *Pharmacotherapy*. 1985;5:63–77.
27. Lebovitz HE. Insulin secretagogues: old and new. *Diabetes Rev*. 1999;7:139–146.
28. Mitka M. FDA eases restrictions on the glucose-lowering drug rosiglitazone. *JAMA*. 2013;10:2604.

CHAPTER 39

Drugs for the Treatment of Hypothyroidism and Hyperthyroidism

Vivek K. Moitra

Hypothyroidism

The primary treatment of hypothyroidism is hormone replacement therapy. In primary hypothyroidism, thyroid-stimulating hormone (TSH) concentrations can be used to monitor this treatment. Free T_4 is an insensitive indicator and may be within the normal range when TSH is inhibited. However, measurement of free T_4 is warranted in secondary hypothyroidism when TSH release is impaired. The goals of therapy include correction of hypothyroidism to a euthyroid state (reduction of symptoms and normalization of TSH secretion), reduction in goiter size, and/or prevention of thyroid cancer recurrence.

Synthetic Thyroxine (T_4: Levothyroxine)

Synthetic thyroxine (T_4) is the treatment of choice for primary hypothyroidism. In the peripheral tissues, T_4 is deiodinated to form triiodothyronine (T_3; the active form of thyroid hormone) (Fig. 39-1). In young healthy patients, initial doses range from 50 to 200 μg per day. Although formulations of T_4 (Synthroid, Levoxyl, generic preparations) may have minor differences in bioavailability, one study suggests that bioequivalence among formulations may be equivalent.[1,2] Doses may be decreased in older patients and increased during pregnancy.[3,4] Because T_4 has a half-life of 7 to 10 days, hypothyroid patients can miss several days of T_4 without adverse consequences. If the patient is unable to eat for more than a week, parenteral T_4 (80% of the patient's oral dose) can be administered.

T_3 Formulations (Liothyronine)

Liothyronine is the levorotatory isomer of T_3 and is 2.5 to 3.0 times as potent as levothyroxine. Its rapid onset and short duration of action preclude the use of liothyronine for long-term thyroid replacement. T_4-T_3 combination therapy may improve symptoms in a small subgroup of patients with a polymorphism in type 2 deiodinase, which converts T_4 to T_3.[5]

Hyperthyroidism

The treatments for hyperthyroidism are antithyroid drugs, radioiodine, and/or surgery. TSH levels are useful for the diagnosis of hyperthyroidism, but not for determining its degree of severity. Therefore, measuring free T_3 and T_4 is necessary to assess the efficacy of treatment. Once steady state is achieved, TSH can be used to assess the efficacy of therapy.

A large number of substances interfere with the synthesis of thyroid hormones or reduce the amount of thyroid tissue. These compounds include (a) thionamides, (b) inhibitors of the iodide transport mechanism, (c) iodide, and (d) radioactive iodine.

Thionamides (Methimazole, Propylthiouracil, Carbimazole)

Thionamides are antithyroid drugs that inhibit the formation of thyroid hormone by inhibiting thyroid peroxidase to prevent incorporation of iodine into tyrosine residues of thyroglobulin (Fig. 39-2). Thionamides exert immunosuppressive effects via a reduction in concentrations of antithyrotropin-receptor antibodies. In addition to blocking hormone synthesis, propylthiouracil also inhibits the peripheral deiodination of T_4 and T_3.[6] Antithyroid drugs are useful in the treatment of hyperthyroidism before elective thyroidectomy.

Serum levels of thionamides peak 1 to 2 hours after ingestion.[6] Thionamides are not available as parenteral preparations. The half-life of methimazole (4 to 6 hours, dosed once daily) is longer than the half-life of propylthiouracil (75 minutes, dosed several times per day). Drug-induced decreases in excessive thyroid activity usually require several days, because preformed hormone

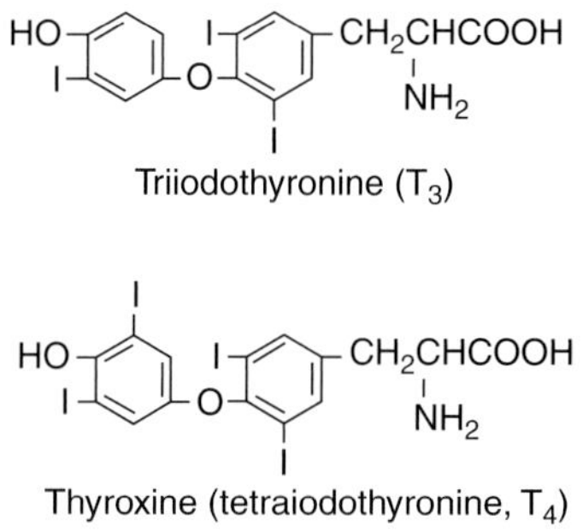

Triiodothyronine (T_3)

Thyroxine (tetraiodothyronine, T_4)

FIGURE 39-1 Thyroid gland hormones.

must be depleted before symptoms begin to wane. In a few patients, especially those with severe hyperthyroidism, definite improvement is evident in 1 to 2 days.

Side Effects

Minor side effects of thionamide therapy are observed in approximately 5% of patients and include urticarial or macular skin rash, arthralgias, and gastrointestinal discomfort.[6] Granulocytopenia and agranulocytosis are serious but rare side effects that are most likely to occur in the first 3 months of therapy with an antithyroid drug.[6] Periodic white blood cell counts, although helpful for detecting gradual decreases in the leukocyte count, should not be relied on to detect agranulocytosis because of the rapidity with which this complication can develop. Fever or pharyngitis may be the earliest manifestation of the development of agranulocytosis. Recovery is likely if the antithyroid drug is discontinued at the first sign of this side effect. Hepatic toxicity has been reported with thionamide use, particularly propylthiouracil.[7,8] Methimazole crosses the placenta and appears in breast milk. Placental passage, however, is limited for propylthiouracil, making it the preferred drug for use in the parturient.[6]

Iodine (Saturated Potassium Iodide Solutions, Potassium Iodide-Iodine [Lugol's Solution])

Iodide is the oldest available therapy for hyperthyroidism, providing a paradoxical treatment that is effective for reasons that are not fully understood. The response of the patient with hyperthyroidism to iodide is acute and often discernible within 24 hours, emphasizing that release of hormone into the circulation is quickly interrupted. Indeed, the most important clinical effect of high doses of iodide is inhibition of the release of thyroid hormone. This may reflect the ability of iodide to antagonize the ability of TSH and cyclic adenosine monophosphate to stimulate hormone release.

Iodide is particularly useful in the treatment of hyperthyroidism before elective thyroidectomy. Indeed, the combination of oral potassium iodide and propranolol is a recommended approach.[9] The vascularity of the thyroid gland is also decreased by iodide therapy.[10] Chronic treatment with iodide, however, is often associated with a recurrence of previously suppressed excessive thyroid gland activity.[11]

Allergic reactions may accompany treatment with iodide or administration of organic preparations that contain iodide. Angioedema and laryngeal edema may become life-threatening.

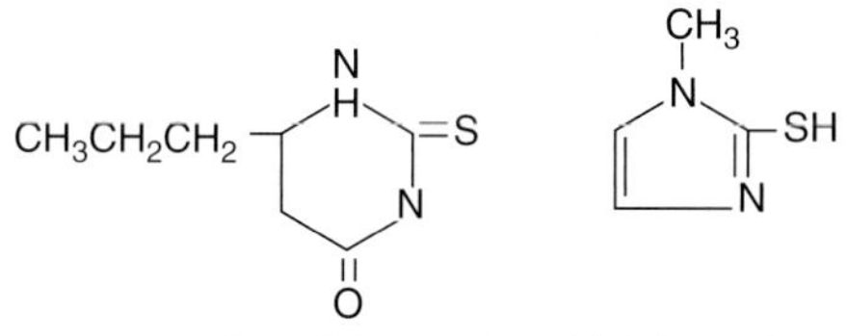

Propylthiouracil Methimazole

FIGURE 39-2 Antithyroid drugs.

Radioactive Iodine

Radioiodine is commonly administered as the therapy of choice for Graves' hyperthyroidism.[12] Many practitioners administer radioactive iodine therapy to patients after euthyroidism is achieved via thionamides. Among the radioactive isotopes of iodine, ^{131}I is the most frequently administered. This isotope is rapidly and efficiently trapped by thyroid gland cells, and the subsequent emission of destructive β rays acts almost exclusively on these cells, with little or no damage to surrounding tissue. It is possible to completely destroy the thyroid gland with ^{131}I within 6 to 18 weeks.[13] Indeed, hypothyroidism occurs in about 10% of treated patients in the first year after ^{131}I administration and increases about 2% to 3% each year thereafter. For this reason, iatrogenic hypothyroidism must be considered preoperatively in any patient who has previously been treated with ^{131}I.

Hyperthyroidism is treated with orally administered ^{131}I, with symptoms of excessive thyroid gland activity gradually abating over a period of 2 to 3 months. One-half to two-thirds of patients are cured by a single dose of isotope, and the remainder require an additional one to two doses. The use of ^{131}I is contraindicated during pregnancy because the fetal thyroid gland would concentrate the isotope. Most thyroid cancers except for follicular cancer accumulate little radioactive iodine. As a result, the therapeutic effectiveness of ^{131}I for treatment of thyroid cancer is limited.

References

1. Dong BJ, Hauck WW, Gambertoglio JG, et al. Bioequivalence of generic and brand-name levothyroxine products in the treatment of hypothyroidism. *JAMA*. 1997;277:1205–1213.
2. American Thyroid Association, Endocrine Society, American Association of Clinical Endocrinologists. Joint statement on the U.S. Food and Drug Administration's decision regarding bioequivalence of levothyroxine sodium. *Thyroid*. 2004;14:486.

3. Sawin CT, Herman T, Molitch ME, et al. Aging and the thyroid. Decreased requirement for thyroid hormone in older hypothyroid patients. *Am J Med.* 1983;75:206–209.
4. Abalovich M, Guiterrez S, Alcaraz G, et al. Overt and subclinical hypothyroidism complicating pregnancy. *Thyroid.* 2002;12:63–68.
5. Panicker V, Saravanan P, Vaidya B, et al. Common variation in the DIO2 gene predicts baseline psychological well-being and response to combination thyroxine plus triiodothyronine therapy in hypothyroid patients. *J Clin Endocrinol Metab.* 2009;94:1623–1629.
6. Cooper DS. Antithyroid drugs. *N Engl J Med.* 2005;352:905–917.
7. Cooper DS. The side effects of antithyroid drugs. *Endocrinologist.* 1999;9:457–476.
8. Williams KV, Nayak S, Becker D, et al. Fifty years of experience with propylthiouracil-associated hepatotoxicity: what have we learned? *J Clin Endocrinol Metab.* 1997;82:1727–1733.
9. Feek CM, Stewart J, Sawers A, et al. Combination of potassium iodide and propranolol in preparation of patients with Grave's disease for thyroid surgery. *N Engl J Med.* 1980;302:883–885.
10. Erbil Y, Ozluk Y, Giris M, et al. Effect of lugol solution on thyroid gland blood flow and microvessel density in the patients with Graves' disease. *J Clin Endocrinol Metab.* 2007;92:2182–2189.
11. Philippou G, Koutras DA, Piperingos G, et al. The effect of iodide on serum thyroid hormone levels in normal persons, in hyperthyroid patients, and in hypothyroid patients on thyroxine replacement. *Clin Endocrinol.* 2002;36:573–578.
12. Burch HB, Burman KD, Cooper DS. A 2011 survey of clinical practice patterns in the management of Graves' disease. *J Clin Endocrinol Metab.* 2012;97:4549–4558.
13. Franklyn JA. The management of hyperthyroidism. *N Engl J Med.* 1994;330:1731–1738.

CHAPTER 40

Other Endocrine Drugs

Vivek K. Moitra

Preparations that contain synthetic hormones identical to those secreted endogenously by endocrine glands may be administered as drugs. These synthetic hormones resemble the endogenous substances in structure and activity. Typically, the clinical application of these drugs is for hormone replacement to provide a physiologic effect. In certain patients, however, large doses of synthetic hormones are used to exert a pharmacologic effect. Recombinant DNA technology permits the incorporation of synthetic genes that code for the synthesis of specific human hormones by bacteria, thus permitting production of pure hormones devoid of allergic properties.

Corticosteroids

The actions of corticosteroids are classified according to the potencies of these compounds to (a) evoke distal renal tubular reabsorption of sodium in exchange for potassium ions (mineralocorticoid effect) or (b) produce an antiinflammatory response (glucocorticoid effect). Naturally occurring corticosteroids are cortisol (hydrocortisone), cortisone, corticosterone, desoxycorticosterone, and aldosterone (Fig. 40-1). Several synthetic corticosteroids are available, principally for use to produce antiinflammatory effects. Although it is possible to separate mineralocorticoid and glucocorticoid effects using synthetic drugs, it has not been possible to separate the various components of glucocorticoid effects. Consequently, all synthetic corticosteroids, when used in pharmacologic doses for their antiinflammatory effects, also produce less desirable effects, such as suppression of the hypothalamic-pituitary-adrenal (HPA) axis, weight gain, and skeletal muscle wasting.

Structure–Activity Relationships

All corticosteroids are constructed on the same primary molecular framework, designated as the steroid nucleus (see Fig. 40-1). Changes in molecular structure may result in altered biologic responses due to changes in absorption, protein binding, rate of metabolism, and intrinsic effectiveness of the drug at receptors. Modifications of structure, such as introduction of a double bond in prednisolone and prednisone, have resulted in synthetic corticosteroids with more potent glucocorticoid effects than the two closely related natural hormones, cortisol and cortisone, respectively (Table 40-1). At the same time, mineralocorticoid effects and the rate of hepatic metabolism of these synthetic drugs are less than those of the natural hormones. Despite increased antiinflammatory effects, it has not been possible to separate this response from alterations in carbohydrate and protein metabolism. This suggests that the multiple manifestations of drug-induced glucocorticoid effects are mediated by the same receptor.

Mechanism of Action

Glucocorticoids attach to cytoplasmic receptors to enhance or suppress changes in the transcription of DNA and thus the synthesis of proteins. Glucocorticoids also inhibit the secretion of cytokines via posttranslational effects.[1] Two distinct types of corticosteroid receptors have been identified (mineralocorticoid and glucocorticoid). Mineralocorticoid receptors are present in distal renal tubules, colon, salivary glands, and the hippocampus. In contrast, glucocorticoids receptors are more widely distributed and do not bind aldosterone, making these receptors glucocorticoid-selective. Local mechanisms that result in release of steroids from their carrier proteins serve to facilitate steroid entry into cells. Target cells also contain an enzyme, 11-β hydroxysteroid dehydrogenase that controls the interconversion of cortisol (active) and cortisone (inert). The concentration of glucocorticoids receptors may fluctuate and thus influence responsiveness to glucocorticoids.

Maintenance of Homeostasis

Permissive and protective effects of glucocorticoids are critical for the maintenance of homeostasis during severe

Cortisol

Cortisone

Corticosterone

Desoxycorticosterone

Aldosterone

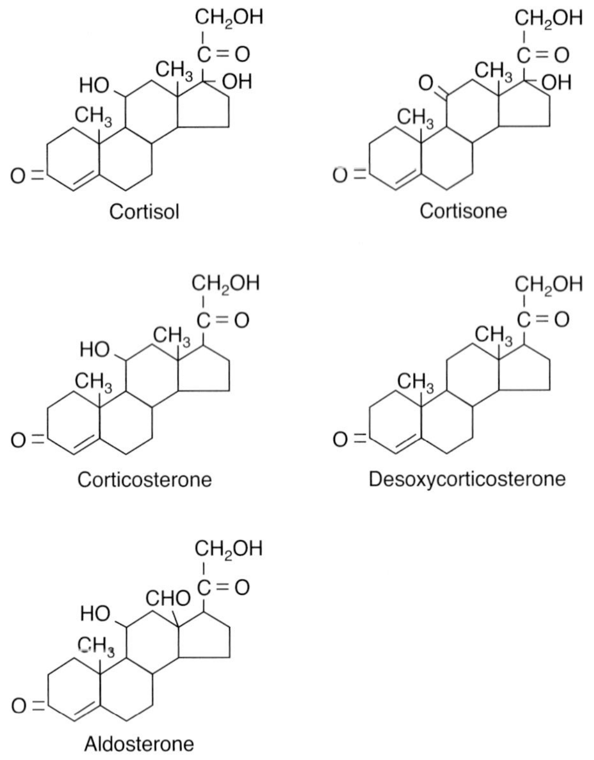

FIGURE 40-1 Endogenous corticosteroids.

stress. The permissive and protective actions of glucocorticoids are complementary and permit the individual to affect an appropriate stress response and to maintain homeostasis.

Permissive Actions

Permissive actions of glucocorticoids occur at low physiologic steroid concentrations and serve to prepare the individual for responding to stress. These permissive actions of glucocorticoids maintain basal activity of the HPA by providing negative feedback and by setting the threshold for a response to stress.

Protective Actions

The protective mode of glucocorticoids occurs when high plasma concentrations of steroids exert antiinflammatory and immunosuppressive effects. This protective response prevents the host-defense mechanisms that are activated during stress from overshooting and damaging the organism. Other important protective actions of glucocorticoids include redirection of metabolism to meet energy needs during stress.

Pharmacokinetics

Synthetic cortisol and its derivatives are effective orally (see Table 40-1). Antacids, but not food, interfere with the oral absorption of corticosteroids. Water-soluble cor-

Table 40-1

Comparative Pharmacology of Endogenous and Synthetic Corticosteroids

	Antiinflammatory Potency	Sodium Retaining Potency	Equivalent Dose (mg)	Elimination Half-Time (h)	Duration of Action (h)	Route of Administration
Cortisol	1	1	20	1.5–3.0	8–12	Oral, topical, IV, IM, IA
Cortisone	0.8	0.8	25	0.5	8–36	Oral, topical, IV, IM, IA
Prednisolone	4	0.8	5	2–4	12–36	Oral, topical, IV, IM, IA
Prednisone	4	0.8	5	2–4	12–36	Oral
Methylprednisolone	5	0.5	4	2–4	12–36	Oral, topical, IV, IM, IA, epidural
Betamethasone	25	0	0.75	5	36–54	Oral, topical, IV, IM, IA
Dexamethasone	25	0	0.75	3.5–5.0	36–54	Oral, topical, IV, IM, IA
Triamcinolone	5	0	4	3.5	12–36	Oral, topical, IV, IM, epidural
Fludrocortisone	10	250	2	—	24	Oral, topical, IV, IM
Aldosterone	0	3,000				

IV, intravenous; IM, intramuscular; IA, intraarticular.

tisol succinate can be administered intravenously (IV) to achieve prompt increases in plasma concentrations. More prolonged effects are possible with intramuscular (IM) injection. Cortisone acetate may be given orally or intramuscularly but cannot be administered IV. The acetate preparation is a slow-release preparation lasting 8 to 12 hours. After release, cortisone is converted to cortisol in the liver. Corticosteroids are also promptly absorbed after topical application or aerosol administration.

Cortisol is highly bound (90% or more) in the plasma to corticosteroid-binding globulin. Cortisol also binds albumin and erythrocytes.[2] Nevertheless, cortisol and related compounds readily cross the placenta. Small amounts of cortisol appear unchanged in the urine, but at least 70% is conjugated in the liver to inactive or poorly active metabolites. These water-soluble conjugated metabolites appear in the urine and bile. The elimination half-time of cortisol is 1.5 to 3.0 hours but its biologic effects persist for several hours. The half-lives of synthetic glucocorticoids range from 1 hour (prednisolone) to more than 4 hours (dexamethasone) and clearance may be prolonged in older individuals.[3] Individuals who clear glucocorticoids slowly may be subject to an increased incidence of side effects.[4]

Cortisol is released from the adrenal glands in an episodic manner and the frequency of pulses follows a circadian rhythm that is linked to the sleep-wake cycle. Maximal plasma concentrations of cortisol occur just before awakening and the lowest levels occur 8 to 10 hours later. Stress-induced changes in the plasma concentrations of cortisol are superimposed on the background baseline release of cortisol. Synthesis of cortisol is governed by adrenocorticotrophic hormone (ACTH) that is controlled by the hypothalamic hormones, corticotropin-releasing hormone and arginine vasopressin.

Synthetic Corticosteroids

Synthetic corticosteroids administered for their glucocorticoid effects include prednisolone, prednisone, methylprednisolone, betamethasone, dexamethasone, and triamcinolone (see Table 40-1, Fig. 40-2). Fludrocortisone is a synthetic halogenated derivative of cortisol that is administered for its mineralocorticoid effect (see Table 40-1 and Fig. 40-2). Naturally occurring corticosteroids, such as cortisol and cortisone, are also available as synthetic drugs (see Table 40-1 and Fig. 40-1).

Prednisolone

Prednisolone is an analogue of cortisol that is available as an oral or parenteral preparation. The antiinflammatory effect of 5 mg of prednisolone is equivalent to that of 20 mg of cortisol. This drug and prednisone are suitable for sole replacement therapy in adrenocortical insufficiency because of the presence of glucocorticoid and mineralocorticoid effects.

Prednisolone

Prednisone

Methylprednisolone

Betamethasone

Triamcinolone

Fludrocortisone

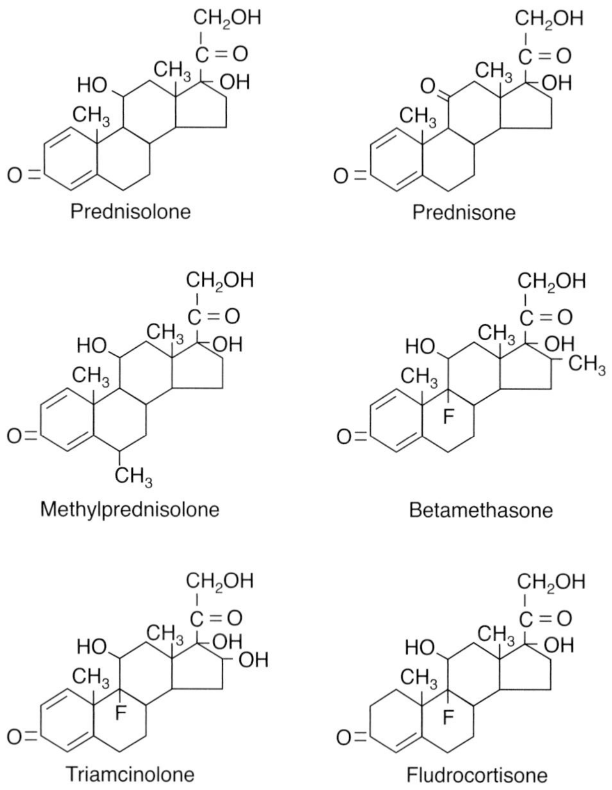

FIGURE 40-2 Synthetic corticosteroids.

Prednisone

Prednisone is an analogue of cortisone that is available as an oral or parenteral preparation. It is rapidly converted to prednisolone after its absorption from the gastrointestinal tract. Its antiinflammatory effect and clinical uses are similar to those of prednisolone.

Methylprednisolone

Methylprednisolone is the methyl derivative of prednisolone. The antiinflammatory effect of 4 mg of methylprednisolone is equivalent to that of 20 mg of cortisol. The acetate preparation administered intraarticularly has a prolonged effect. Methylprednisolone succinate is highly soluble in water and is used IV to produce an intense glucocorticoid effect.

Betamethasone

Betamethasone is a fluorinated derivative of prednisolone. The antiinflammatory effect of 0.75 mg is equivalent to that of 20 mg of cortisol. Betamethasone lacks the mineralocorticoid properties of cortisol and thus is not acceptable for sole replacement therapy in adrenocortical insufficiency. Oral or parenteral administration is acceptable.

Dexamethasone

Dexamethasone is a fluorinated derivative of prednisolone and an isomer of betamethasone. The antiinflammatory effect of 0.75 mg is equivalent to that of 20 mg of cortisol. Oral and parenteral preparations are available. The acetate preparation is used as a long-acting repository suspension. Dexamethasone sodium phosphate is water soluble, rendering it appropriate for parenteral use. This corticosteroid is commonly chosen to treat certain types of cerebral edema.

Triamcinolone

Triamcinolone is a fluorinated derivative of prednisolone. The antiinflammatory effect of 4 mg is equivalent to that of 20 mg of cortisol. Triamcinolone has less mineralocorticoid effect than does prednisolone. Oral and parenteral preparations are available. The hexacetonide preparation injected intraarticularly may provide therapeutic effects for 3 months or longer. This drug is often used for epidural injections in the treatment of lumbar disc disease.

During the first days of treatment with triamcinolone, mild diuresis with sodium loss may occur. Conversely, edema may occur in patients with decreased glomerular filtration rates. Triamcinolone does not increase urinary potassium loss except when administered in large doses.

An unusual adverse side effect of triamcinolone is an increased incidence of skeletal muscle weakness. Likewise, anorexia rather than appetite stimulation, and sedation rather than euphoria may accompany administration of triamcinolone.

Clinical Uses

The only universally accepted clinical use of corticosteroids and their synthetic derivatives is as replacement therapy for deficiency states. With this exception, the use of corticosteroids in disease states is empirical and not curative, although antiinflammatory responses exert an intense palliative effect. The safety of corticosteroids is such that it is acceptable to administer a single large dose in a life-threatening situation on the presumption that unrecognized adrenal or pituitary insufficiency may be present.

Prednisolone or prednisone is recommended when an antiinflammatory effect is desired. The low mineralocorticoid potency of these drugs limits sodium and water retention when large doses are administered to produce the desired glucocorticoid effect. It must be recognized, however, that the antiinflammatory effect of corticosteroids is palliative because the underlying cause of the response remains. Nevertheless, suppression of the inflammatory response may be lifesaving in some situations. Conversely, masking of the symptoms of inflammation may delay diagnosis of life-threatening illness, such as peritonitis due to perforation of a peptic ulcer.

Deficiency States

Acute adrenal insufficiency requires electrolyte and fluid replacement as well as supplemental corticosteroids. Cortisol is administered at a rate of 100 mg IV every 8 hours after an initial injection of 100 mg. Management of chronic adrenal insufficiency in adults is with the daily oral administration of cortisone, 25.0 to 37.5 mg. A typical regimen is 25.0 mg in the morning and 12.5 mg in the late afternoon. This schedule mimics the normal diurnal cycle of adrenal secretion. An orally effective mineralocorticoid such as fludrocortisone, 0.1 to 0.3 mg daily, is required by most patients.

Allergic Therapy

Topical corticosteroids are capable of potent antiinflammatory effects and are the mainstay of allergic therapy. These medications interfere with the inflammatory response, induce cutaneous vasoconstriction, and have antimitotic activity.[5] Corticosteroids work by inhibiting the production of inflammatory cytokines and chemokines, thus decreasing inflammation, cellular edema, and cellular recruitment to sites of disease. Oral administration of steroids is effective but the risk of unacceptable side effects with chronic treatment limits use by this route. Side effects, although possible with topical administration of corticosteroids, are usually not significant. Unlike antihistamines that provide pharmacologic effects within 1 to 2 hours, topical corticosteroids may require 3 to 5 days of treatment to produce a therapeutic effect.

Manifestations of allergic diseases that are of limited duration, such as hay fever, contact dermatitis, drug reactions, angioneurotic edema, and anaphylaxis, can be suppressed by adequate doses of corticosteroids. Life-threatening allergic reactions, however, must be treated with epinephrine, because the onset of the antiinflammatory effect produced by corticosteroids is delayed. Indeed, any beneficial effect of corticosteroids in the management of severe allergic reactions is probably related to suppression of the antiinflammatory response rather than to inhibition of production of immunoglobulins.

Asthma

Asthma is an inflammatory disease of the lungs and inhaled glucocorticoids (beclomethasone, budesonide, fluticasone, ciclesonide, and triamcinolone) are often recommended as first-line therapy for controlling the symptoms of asthma, improving quality of life and lung function, and in preventing exacerbations.[6] Inhaled glucocorticoids are highly lipophilic and rapidly enter airway cells, where they have direct inhibitory effects on many of the cells involved in airway inflammation. One possible antiinflammatory mechanism is the modulation of the release of cytokines from inflammatory cells. It is estimated that 80% to 90% of the dose inhaled from the metered-dose inhaler is deposited in the oropharynx and swallowed. Inhaled glucocorticoids have oropharyngeal side effects that include dysphonia and candidiasis. Dysphonia occurs in approximately one-third of treated patients and may reflect myopathy of the laryngeal muscles that is reversible when treatment is stopped. Inhaled glucocorticoids, in doses of 1,500 μg per day or less in adults and 400 μg per day or less in children, have little, if any, effect on pituitary adrenal function.

Parenteral corticosteroids are important in the emergent preoperative preparation of patients with active reactive airway disease and in the treatment of intraoperative bronchospasm. Doses equivalent to 1 to 2 mg/kg of cortisol (or the equivalent dose of prednisolone) are commonly recommended. Preoperative corticosteroid administration 1 to 2 hours before induction of anesthesia is important because the beneficial effects of corticosteroids may not be fully manifest for several hours. Corticosteroids also enhance and prolong the responses to β-adrenergic agonists. Some enhancement of β-agonist effect may be present within 1 hour, but 4 to 6 hours are required for an antiinflammatory effect. In noncompliant or newly diagnosed patients with bronchial hyperactivity, preoperative treatment with combined corticosteroids (40 mg orally for 5 days) and salbutamol (0.2 mg puffs for 5 days) but not salbutamol alone minimizes intubation-evoked bronchoconstriction.[7]

Antiemetic Effect

Dexamethasone prevents postoperative nausea and vomiting only when administered near the beginning of surgery, probably by reducing surgery-induced inflammation due to inhibition of prostaglandin synthesis.[8] In addition, dexamethasone may exert antiemetic effects by increasing the release of endorphins resulting in mood elevation and appetite stimulation. Prophylactic administration of dexamethasone 4 mg, ondansetron 4 mg, or droperidol 1.25 mg produced similar decreases (about 26%) in the incidence of postoperative nausea and vomiting.[9] Because antiemetic interventions are similarly effective and act independently, it is recommended that the safest and least expensive antiemetic should be selected for prophylaxis. Prophylaxis is rarely warranted in low-risk patients, moderate-risk patients may benefit from a single intervention, and multiple interventions should be reserved for high-risk patients.[9] Rescue treatments are ineffective when the same drug has already been administered for prophylaxis. A suggested treatment strategy is to administer dexamethasone in conjunction with total intravenous anesthesia as first-line and second-line methods of prophylaxis against postoperative nausea and vomiting and to reserve serotonin antagonists as a rescue treatment.[9] Administration of higher doses (8 to 10 mg) of dexamethasone has a similar clinical effect to lower doses (4 to 5 mg).[10] Dexamethasone is also effective in suppressing chemotherapy-induced nausea and vomiting. The elimination half-time of dexamethasone is about 3 hours, but antiemetic effects, unlike other classes of antiemetics, often persist as long as 24 hours.

Postoperative Analgesia

Glucocorticoids peripherally inhibit phospholipase enzyme that is necessary for the inflammatory chain reaction along both the cyclooxygenase and lipoxygenase pathways.[11] As a result, glucocorticoids may be effective in decreasing postoperative pain but with a different side effect profile than nonsteroidal antiinflammatory drugs. For example, administration of betamethasone 12 mg intramuscularly 30 minutes before induction of anesthesia for outpatient foot or hemorrhoid surgery, resulted in reductions in postoperative pain and the incidence of postoperative nausea and vomiting.[12] A meta-analysis of perioperative intravenous dexamethasone suggests that dexamethasone at doses more than 0.1 mg/kg decreases acute postoperative pain and reduces opioid use, especially when administered preoperatively.[13]

Cerebral Edema

Corticosteroids in large doses are of value in the reduction or prevention of vasogenic cerebral edema and the resulting increases in intracranial pressure that may accompany intracranial tumors and metastatic lesions and bacterial meningitis.[14] Dexamethasone, with minimal mineralocorticoid activity, is frequently selected to decrease cerebral edema and associated increases in intracranial pressure. Conversely, the administration of glucocorticoids to patients with severe head injury, cerebral infarction, and intracranial hemorrhage is not useful and can be associated with worse outcomes.[15,16]

Aspiration Pneumonitis

The use of corticosteroids in the treatment of aspiration pneumonitis is controversial. There is evidence in animals that corticosteroids administered immediately after the inhalation of acidic gastric fluid may be effective in decreasing pulmonary damage.[17] Conversely, other data show no beneficial effect or suggest that the use of corticosteroids may enhance the likelihood of gram-negative pneumonia.[18,19] Despite the absence of confirming evidence that corticosteroids are beneficial, it is not uncommon for the treatment of aspiration pneumonitis to include the empiric use of pharmacologic doses of these drugs.

Lumbar Disc Disease

An alternative to surgical treatment of lumbar disc disease is the epidural placement of corticosteroids.[20] Corticosteroids may decrease inflammation and edema of the nerve root that has resulted from compression. A common regimen is epidural injection of 25 to 50 mg of triamcinolone, or 40 to 80 mg of methylprednisolone, in a solution containing lidocaine at or near the interspace corresponding to the distribution of pain. In animals, the epidural injection of triamcinolone, 2 mg/kg, interferes with the ability of the adrenal cortex to release cortisol in response to hypoglycemia for 4 weeks. Injection of triamcinolone, 80 mg, into the lumbar epidural space of patients with lumbar disc disease results in acute suppression of plasma concentrations of ACTH and cortisol between 15 minutes (midazolam sedation) and 45 minutes (midazolam not administered) of corticosteroid injection.[21] Median suppression of the HPA axis was less than 1 month and all patients had recovered by 3 months. Exogenous corticosteroid coverage during this potentially vulnerable period should be considered in patients undergoing major stress, especially if the adrenocortical response to ACTH is subnormal. Although epidural injections of methylprednisolone may result in short-term improvement of symptoms (pain, sensory loss) due to sciatic nerve compression from a herniated nucleus pulposus, this treatment offers no significant functional benefit nor does it decrease the need for surgery.[22]

Immunosuppression

In organ transplantation, high doses of corticosteroids are often administered at the time of surgery to produce immunosuppression and decrease the risk of rejection of the newly transplanted organ. Smaller maintenance doses of corticosteroids are continued indefinitely, and the dosage is increased if rejection of the transplanted organ is threatened.

Arthritis

The criterion for initiating corticosteroid therapy in patients with rheumatoid arthritis is rapid control of symptomatic flares and progressive disability despite maximal medical therapy. Corticosteroids are administered in the smallest dose possible that provides significant but not complete symptomatic relief. The usual initial dose is prednisolone, 10 mg or its equivalent, in divided doses. Intraarticular injection of corticosteroids is recommended for treatment of episodic manifestations of acute joint inflammation associated with osteoarthritis. However, painless destruction of the joint is a risk of this treatment.

Collagen Diseases

Manifestations of collagen diseases, such as polymyositis, polyarteritis nodosa, and Wegener granulomatosis, but not scleroderma, are decreased and longevity is improved by corticosteroid therapy. Fulminating systemic lupus erythematosus is a life-threatening illness that is aggressively treated initially with large doses of prednisone, 1 mg/kg, or its equivalent. Large doses of corticosteroids are effective for inducing a remission of sarcoidosis. In temporal arteritis, corticosteroid therapy is necessary to prevent blindness, which occurs in about 20% of untreated patients. Some forms of nephrotic syndrome respond favorably to corticosteroids. Rheumatic carditis may be suppressed by large doses of corticosteroids.

Ocular Inflammation

Corticosteroids are used to suppress ocular inflammation (uveitis and iritis) and thus preserve sight. Instillation of corticosteroids into the conjunctival sac results in therapeutic concentrations in the aqueous humor. Topical and intraocular corticosteroid therapy often increases intraocular pressure and is associated with cataractogenesis. For this reason, it is recommended that intraocular pressure be monitored when topical corticosteroids are used for more than 2 weeks. Corticosteroids are not recommended in herpes simplex infections (dendritic keratitis) of the eye. Topical corticosteroids should not be used for treatment of ocular abrasions because delayed healing and infections may occur.

Cutaneous Disorders

Topical administration of corticosteroids is frequently effective in the treatment of skin diseases. Effectiveness is increased by application of the corticosteroid as an ointment under an occlusive dressing. Systemic absorption is also occasionally enhanced to the degree that suppression of the HPA axis occurs or manifestations of Cushing syndrome appear. Corticosteroids may also be administered systemically for treatment of severe episodes of acute skin disorders and exacerbations of chronic disorders.

Postintubation Laryngeal Edema

Treatment of postintubation laryngeal edema may include administration of corticosteroids, such as dexamethasone, 0.1 to 0.2 mg/kg IV. Nevertheless, the efficacy of corticosteroids for treatment of this condition has not been confirmed. Dexamethasone, 0.6 mg/kg orally is an effective treatment for children with mild croup.[23]

Ulcerative Colitis

Corticosteroid therapy is indicated in selected patients with chronic ulcerative colitis. A disadvantage of this therapy is that signs and symptoms of intestinal perforation and peritonitis may be masked.

Myasthenia Gravis

Corticosteroids are usually reserved for patients with myasthenia gravis who are unresponsive to medical or surgical therapy. These drugs seem to be most effective after thymectomy. The mechanism of beneficial effects produced by corticosteroids is not known but may reflect drug-induced suppression of the production of an immunoglobulin that normally binds to the neuromuscular junction.

Respiratory Distress Syndrome

Administration of corticosteroids at least 24 hours before delivery decreases the incidence and severity of respiratory distress syndrome in neonates born between 24 and 36 weeks' gestation. Dexamethasone administered for prolonged periods (42 days) improves pulmonary and neurodevelopmental outcome of low-birth-weight infants at risk for bronchopulmonary dysplasia.[24] Glucocorticoid administration in the setting of acute respiratory distress syndrome is controversial and the effect may vary according to timing. Early administration ($\leq$72 hours) of methylprednisolone in one small study has been associated with improved outcomes.[25] Later administration ($>$14 days) of glucocorticoids is associated with increased mortality, ventilator-free days, oxygenation, and compliance.[26]

Leukemia

The antilymphocytic effects of glucocorticoids are used to advantage in combination chemotherapy of acute lymphocytic leukemia and lymphomas, including Hodgkin disease and multiple myeloma. For example, prednisone and vincristine produce remissions in about 90% of children with lymphoblastic leukemia.

Cardiac Arrest

Cardiac arrest is associated with lower cortisol levels (relative adrenal insufficiency), vasoplegia, and myocardial dysfunction. Recent studies preliminarily suggest that the administration of glucocorticoids (along with vasopressin and epinephrine) during a cardiac arrest may improve survival and is associated with better neurologic outcomes.[27] Potential explanations include attenuation of the systemic inflammatory response syndrome and enhancement of myocardial and vascular function.[28]

Side Effects

The side effects of chronic corticosteroid therapy include (a) suppression of the HPA axis, (b) electrolyte and metabolic changes, (c) osteoporosis, (d) peptic ulcer disease, (e) skeletal muscle myopathy, (f) central nervous system dysfunction, (g) peripheral blood changes, and (h) inhibition of normal growth. Increased susceptibility to bacterial or fungal infection accompanies treatment with corticosteroids. Corticosteroid administration is associated with greater clearance of salicylates and decreased effectiveness of anticoagulants. Systemic corticosteroids used for short periods of time (<7 days) even at high doses are unlikely to cause adverse side effects. Inhaled corticosteroids are unlikely to evoke adverse systemic effects.

Corticosteroid Supplementation in the Perioperative Period

Corticosteroid supplementation should be increased whenever the patient being treated for chronic hypoadrenocorticism undergoes a surgical procedure. This recommendation is based on the concern that these patients are susceptible to cardiovascular collapse because they cannot release additional endogenous cortisol in response to the stress of surgery. More controversial is the management of patients who may manifest suppression of the HPA axis because of current or previous administration of corticosteroids for treatment of a disease unrelated to pituitary or adrenal function. Recommendations that prescribe supraphysiologic doses have been advocated despite the absence of supporting scientific data.[29] In adrenalectomized primates undergoing general anesthesia and surgery, the animals receiving physiologic replacement doses of cortisol were indistinguishable from those receiving supraphysiologic doses (10 times the normal production rate) of cortisol.[30] Subphysiologically treated animals (one-tenth the normal production rate) were hemodynamically unstable during surgery and had a significantly higher mortality rate. Based on these animal data, it was concluded that there is no advantage in supraphysiologic glucocorticoid prophylaxis during surgical stress, and replacement doses of cortisol equivalent to the daily unstressed cortisol production rate are sufficient to allow homeostatic mechanisms to function during surgery.[30]

Patients taking greater than 20 mg per day of prednisone or its equivalent for more than 3 weeks have a suppressed HPA axis. Patients taking less than 5 mg per day of prednisone or its equivalent can be considered not to have suppression of their HPA axis. However, patients taking 5 to 20 mg per day of prednisone or its equivalent for more than 3 weeks may or may not have suppression of the HPA axis.

A rational regimen for corticosteroid supplementation in the perioperative period is to avoid steroid supplementation in patients who do not have a suppressed HPA axis (patients taking any dose of glucocorticoids for less than 3 weeks or a daily dose of prednisone <5 mg).

Patients taking 5 to 20 mg per day of prednisone or its equivalent for more than 3 weeks may or may not have suppression of the HPA axis. These patients may benefit from further assessment of their HPA axis. Glucocorticoid supplementation considers preoperative doses and the stress of surgery.

For patients with a suppressed HPA axis (patients taking >20 mg prednisone per day for more than 3 weeks), glucocorticoid supplementation should consider the stress of surgery. For minor surgical stress (inguinal hernia repair), the daily cortisol secretion rate and static plasma cortisol measurements suggest that a glucocorticoid replacement dose of 25 mg of hydrocortisone or 5 mg of methylprednisolone is sufficient. If the postoperative course is uncomplicated, the patient can be returned the next day to the prior glucocorticoid maintenance dose. For moderate surgical stress (nonlaparoscopic cholecystectomy, colon resection, total hip replacement), cortisol production rates suggest the glucocorticoid requirement is about 50 to 75 mg daily of hydrocortisone for 1 to 2 days. For major surgical stress (pancreatoduodenectomy, esophagectomy, cardiopulmonary bypass), the glucocorticoid dose should be 100 to 150 mg of hydrocortisone daily for 2 to 3 days. Even with this coverage, vascular collapse has been described in a patient experiencing massive hemorrhage during surgery.[31] This approach maintains the plasma concentration of cortisol above normal during major surgery in patients receiving chronic treatment with corticosteroids and manifesting a subnormal response to the preoperative infusion of ACTH (Fig. 40-3).[32] In those instances in which events such as burns or sepsis could exaggerate the need for exogenous corticosteroid supplementation, the continuous infusion of cortisol, 100 mg every

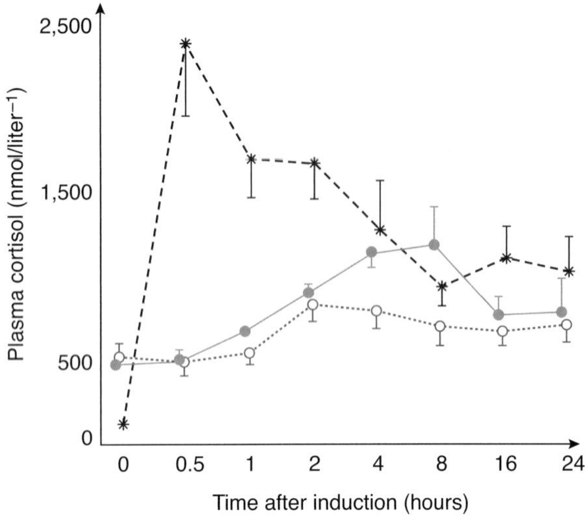

FIGURE 40-3 Administration of cortisol, 25 mg IV, plus a continuous infusion of 100 mg over 24 hours, maintains the plasma cortisol concentration above normal in patients (*) receiving chronic treatment with corticosteroids and manifesting a subnormal response to the preoperative infusion of adrenocorticotropic hormone. (From Symreng T, Karlberg BE, Kagedal B, et al. Physiological cortisol substitution of long-term steroid-treated patients undergoing major surgery. *Br J Anesth.* 1981;53:949–953; with permission.)

12 hours, should be sufficient. Indeed, endogenous cortisol production during stress introduced by major surgery or extensive burns is not greater than 150 mg daily.[33,34] It is likely that patients undergoing minor operations will need minimal to no additional corticosteroid coverage during the perioperative period.

In addition to intravenous supplementation with cortisol, patients receiving daily maintenance doses of a corticosteroid should also receive this dose with the preoperative medication on the day of surgery. There is no objective evidence to support increasing the maintenance dose of corticosteroid preoperatively.

Electrolyte and Metabolic Changes and Weight Gain

Hypokalemic metabolic alkalosis reflects mineralocorticoid effects of corticosteroids on distal renal tubules, leading to enhanced absorption of sodium and loss of potassium. Edema and weight gain accompany this corticosteroid effect. Corticosteroids inhibit the use of glucose in peripheral tissues and promote hepatic gluconeogenesis. The resulting corticosteroid-induced hyperglycemia can usually be managed with diet, insulin, or both. The dose requirement for oral hypoglycemics may be increased by corticosteroids. There is a redistribution of body fat characterized by deposition of fat in the back of the neck (buffalo hump), supraclavicular area, and face (moon facies) and loss of fat from the extremities. The mechanism by which corticosteroids elicit this redistribution of fat is not known. Peripherally, corticosteroids mobilize amino acids from tissues. This catabolic effect manifests as decreased skeletal muscle mass, osteoporosis, thinning of the skin, and a negative nitrogen balance.

Osteoporosis

Osteoporosis, vertebral compression fractures, and rib fractures are common and serious complications of corticosteroid therapy that can be found in patients of all ages. Corticosteroids appear to inhibit the activities of osteoblasts and stimulate osteoclasts by inhibition of calcium absorption from the gastrointestinal tract, which causes an increased secretion of parathyroid hormone. Osteoporosis is an indication for withdrawal of corticosteroid therapy. Evidence of osteoporosis should be sought on radiographs of the spines of patients being treated chronically with corticosteroids. The presence of osteoporosis could predispose patients to fractures during positioning in the operating room. Bisphosphonates are effective in decreasing vertebral fractures in patients taking corticosteroids.[35]

Peptic Ulcer Disease

Although a cause-and-effect relationship has not been proved, the incidence of peptic ulcer disease seems to be increased by chronic corticosteroid therapy. Indeed, corticosteroids may decrease the normal protective barrier provided by gastric mucus.

Skeletal Muscle Myopathy

Skeletal muscle myopathy characterized by weakness of the proximal musculature is occasionally observed in patients taking large doses of corticosteroids. In some patients, this skeletal muscle weakness is so severe that ambulation is not possible and corticosteroid therapy must be discontinued.

Central Nervous System Dysfunction

Corticosteroid therapy is associated with an increased incidence of neuroses and psychoses. Behavioral changes include manic depression and suicidal tendencies. Cataracts develop in almost all patients who receive prednisone, 20 mg daily, or its equivalent for 4 years.

Peripheral Blood Changes

Corticosteroids tend to increase the hematocrit and number of circulating leukocytes. Conversely, a single dose of cortisol decreases by almost 70%—the number of circulating lymphocytes, and by more than 90%—the number of circulating monocytes in 4 to 6 hours. This acute lymphocytopenia most likely reflects sequestration from the blood rather than destruction of cells.

Inhibition of Normal Growth

Inhibition or arrest of growth can result from the administration of relatively small doses of glucocorticoids to children. The mechanism of this effect is presumed to be the generalized inhibitory effect of glucocorticoids on DNA synthesis and cell division.

Inhibitors of Corticosteroid Synthesis

Metyrapone

Metyrapone decreases cortisol synthesis by inhibition of the 11-β-hydroxylation reaction, resulting in accumulation of 11-deoxycortisol. Metyrapone may induce acute adrenal insufficiency in patients with decreased adrenocortical function. A deficiency of mineralocorticoids does not occur, because metyrapone-induced inhibition of 11-β-hydroxylation results in increased production of the mineralocorticoid 11-desoxycorticosterone.

Metyrapone has been used in the diagnosis of adrenal insufficiency and treatment of excessive adrenocortical function that results from adrenal neoplasms that function autonomously or as a result of ectopic production of ACTH by tumors.

Aminoglutethimide

Aminoglutethimide inhibits the conversion of cholesterol to 20-α-hydroxycholesterol, which interrupts production of both cortisol and aldosterone. Thus, this drug is effective in decreasing the excessive secretion of cortisol in autonomously functioning adrenal tumors and in hypersecretion resulting from ectopic production of ACTH.

Drugs that Regulate Calcium

Calcium is ingested and absorbed in the gastrointestinal tract; resorbed by bone; and filtered and reabsorbed by the kidney. The effects of parathyroid hormone, calcitonin, and vitamin D metabolites regulate calcium homeostasis (see Chapter 37). Parathyroid hormone (PTH) regulates extracellular calcium concentration through action on the bone, kidney, and intestine. PTH secretion is activated by hypocalcemia and elevated phosphorous levels. The net effect of PTH is to increase extracellular calcium. An excess or deficiency of calcium can disrupt coagulation, neurotransmitter and hormone secretion, neuromuscular excitability, muscle contraction, hormone action, and enzyme function.

Hypercalcemia

Hypercalcemia can be categorized as either parathyroid dependent or non–parathyroid dependent. Disorders of the parathyroid gland that result in hypercalcemia include primary and tertiary hyperparathyroidism, familial hypocalciuric hypercalcemia, and lithium-induced hypercalcemia. Hypercalcemia of malignancy is usually associated with destructive bone lesions or secretion of a PTH-like tumor peptide (PTH-RP). Hypercalcemia from parathyroid disease is associated with bone loss and osteoporosis. Management of hypercalcemia includes intravenous fluids, bisphosphonates, calcitonin (see Chapter 37), glucocorticoids and other less commonly used medications such as cinacalcet and denosumab.

Bisphosphonates

Bisphosphonates (pamidronate, zoledronate, alendronate, etc) are pyrophosphate analogues that lower calcium levels by inhibiting osteoclastic-mediated bone reabsorption. Hypercalcemia from malignancy, primary hyperparathyroidism, vitamin A intoxication, granulomatous disease, and Paget's disease has been successfully managed with bisphosphonate therapy. Renal injury and jaw osteonecrosis has been reported in patients who take bisphosphonates. These medications should be prescribed early in the course of hypercalcemia because clinically significant reductions in calcium levels may not be observed for 2 days.

Glucocorticoids

In the setting of hypercalcemia from solid tumors and primary hyperparathyroidism, glucocorticoids are minimally effective agents. Glucocorticoids decrease synthesis of 1,25-dihydroxyvitamin D to decrease intestinal absorption of calcium and increase renal excretion of calcium.

Hypocalcemia

Preoperative patients with rhabdomyolysis, pancreatitis, sepsis, burns, fat embolism syndrome, recent massive transfusion, hypoalbuminemia, hypomagnesemia, or renal insufficiency are at risk for hypocalcemia. Chronic hypocalcemia may have few clinical signs or symptoms, whereas rapidly developing hypocalcemia may have impressive clinical effects. The most common setting for symptomatic hypocalcemia is within 12 to 24 hours after surgery, particularly after total or subtotal thyroidectomy or four-gland parathyroid exploration or removal.

Long-standing hypocalcemia with hyperphosphatemia and PTH deficiency is associated with calcification of the basal ganglia with extrapyramidal signs. Hypocalcemia can cause neuromuscular irritability, arrhythmias, congestive heart failure (decreased myocardial contractility), and hypotension. Acute, severe hypocalcemia (total serum calcium levels $<$7.5 mg/dL, normal albumin) is a medical emergency associated with death from laryngeal spasm or grand mal seizures. Intravenous calcium is indicated for acute symptomatic hypocalcemia. Ten percent calcium gluconate contains less elemental calcium than calcium chloride but is less likely to cause tissue necrosis during an extravasation.

Drugs for Pituitary Function

Anterior Pituitary Hormones

Anterior pituitary hormones include (a) growth hormone; (b) prolactin; (c) gonadotropins, including luteinizing hormone and follicle-stimulating hormone; (d) ACTH; and (e) thyroid-stimulating hormone (TSH). Growth hormone, gonadotropins, and ACTH can be administered in the form of synthetic drugs.

Perioperative replacement of anterior pituitary hormones may be necessary for patients receiving exogenous hormones because of a prior hypophysectomy. For example, cortisol must be provided continuously. Conversely, thyroid hormones have such a long elimination half-time that they can be omitted for several days without adverse effects. Likewise, the loss of other anterior pituitary hormones has no immediate physiologic implications.

Growth Hormone

Recombinant growth hormone is administered subcutaneously and daily to treat growth hormone deficiency. Growth hormone is also used to manage growth failure from chronic kidney disease and short stature from Turner syndrome, Prader-Willi syndrome, Noonan's syndrome, and mutations in the Short Stature Homeobox gene. Radioimmunoassays for growth hormone are used to measure plasma concentrations of the hormone. Treatment is maintained and titrated for months to years in response to growth velocity and insulin-like growth factor 1 (IGF-1) levels (which are associated with growth velocity) and is often discontinued when linear growth decreases to less than 1 in per year.[36,37]

Octreotide

Octreotide is a somatostatin analogue that inhibits the release of growth hormone, making it an effective treatment for patients with acromegaly.[38] Long-term treatment with octreotide (>1 month) is associated with an increased incidence of cholesterol gallstones (occurring in 20% to 30% of treated patients). Because somatostatin analogues inhibit the secretion of insulin, decreased glucose tolerance and even overt hyperglycemia might be expected during treatment with octreotide. Octreotide may be a lifesaving treatment in patients experiencing an acute carcinoid crisis although bolus injection of this somatostatin analog may be accompanied by bradycardia and second- and third-degree heart block.[39]

Gonadotropins

Gonadotropins are used most often for the treatment of infertility and cryptorchism. Induction of ovulation can be stimulated in females who are infertile because of pituitary insufficiency. Excessive ovarian enlargement and maturation of many follicles, leading to multiple births, is a possibility. Gonadotropins are effective only by parenteral injection. Radioimmunoassays are useful in measuring plasma and urine concentrations of gonadotropins.

Adrenocorticotrophic Hormone

The physiologic and pharmacologic effects of ACTH result from this hormone's stimulation of secretion of corticosteroids from the adrenal cortex, principally cortisol. An important clinical use of ACTH is as a diagnostic aid in patients with suspected adrenal insufficiency. For example, a normal increase in the plasma concentration of cortisol in response to the administration of ACTH rules out primary adrenocortical insufficiency. Furthermore, ACTH may be administered therapeutically to evoke the release of cortisol. Treatment of disease states with ACTH is not physiologically equivalent to administration of a specific hormone because ACTH exposes the tissues to a mixture of glucocorticoids, mineralocorticoids, and androgens. Indeed, there may be associated retention of sodium, development of hypokalemic metabolic alkalosis, and appearance of acne, which are unlikely to accompany selective-acting corticosteroids.

Absorption of ACTH after IM injection is prompt. After intravenous injection, ACTH disappears rapidly from the plasma, with an elimination half-time of about 15 minutes. Allergic reactions ranging from mild fever to life-threatening anaphylaxis may be associated with administration of ACTH.

Melatonin

Melatonin (*N*-acetyl-5-methoxytryptamine) is the principal substance secreted by the pineal gland (Fig. 40-4).[40] The mammalian pineal gland is a neuroendocrine transducer. Photic information from the retina is transmitted to the pineal gland through the suprachiasmatic nucleus of the hypothalamus and the sympathetic nervous system. The neural input to the gland is norepinephrine and the output is melatonin. The synthesis and release of melatonin are stimulated by darkness and inhibited by light. As the synthesis of melatonin increases, the hormone enters the bloodstream through passive diffusion. Melatonin is rapidly metabolized, chiefly in the liver, by hydroxylation to 6-hydroxymelatonin, and, after conjugation with sulfuric or glucuronic acid, is excreted in the urine. Intravenous melatonin is rapidly distributed, and the elimination half-time is 0.5 to 5.6 minutes. The bioavailability of orally administered melatonin varies widely.

Dose-dependent physiologic effects of melatonin include biologic regulation of circadian rhythms, sleep, mood, and perhaps reproduction, tumor growth, and aging.[40] In humans, the circadian rhythm for the release of melatonin from the pineal gland is closely synchronized with the habitual hours of sleep. Alterations in synchronization due to phase shifts (acute change in time zones or working hours) are correlated with sleep disturbances. Ingestion of melatonin affects the speed of falling asleep as well as the duration and quality of sleep and has hypnotic effects. The circadian cycle of body temperature is linked to the 24-hour cycle of subjective sleepiness and inversely related to serum melatonin concentrations. Nevertheless, sleep-promoting doses

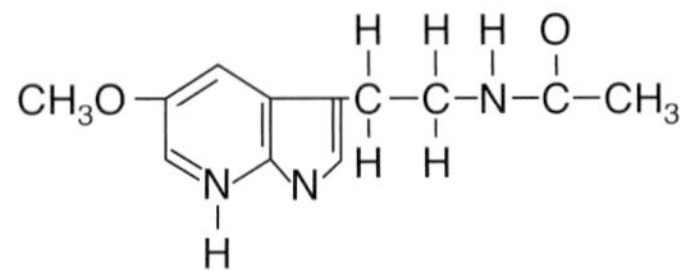

FIGURE 40-4 Melatonin.

of melatonin do not have any effect on body temperature. It is unclear whether the beneficial effect of exogenous melatonin on symptoms of jet lag is due to a hypnotic effect or resynchronization of the circadian rhythm.

Posterior Pituitary Hormones

Arginine vasopressin (AVP) (also known as ***antidiuretic hormone*** [ADH]) and oxytocin are the two principal hormones secreted by the posterior pituitary. AVP targets the renal collecting ducts to increase permeability of cell membranes to water and promote passive water reabsorption from renal collecting ducts into extracellular fluid. AVP also elicits intense arterial vasoconstriction via activation of vascular V1a receptors.[41] Oxytocin elicits contractions of the uterus, which are indistinguishable from those that occur in spontaneous labor.

Arginine Vasopressin

Vasopressin is the exogenous preparation of AVP used for (a) treatment of AVP-sensitive diabetes insipidus, (b) management of refractory hypotension during anesthesia, (c) management of uncontrolled hemorrhage from esophageal varices, (d) hemodynamic stabilization in the presence of hemorrhagic and septic shock, and (e) management of refractory cardiac arrest. This drug is not effective in the management of patients with nephrogenic diabetes insipidus.

Diabetes Insipidus

Inadequate secretion of vasopressin by the posterior pituitary causes diabetes insipidus. Excessive water loss and hypernatremia via polyuria follow. Neurotrauma and surgery of the pituitary and hypothalamus, cerebral ischemia, or cerebral malignancy can cause diabetes insipidus.[41] Nephrogenic diabetes insipidus resulting from an inability of the renal tubules to respond to adequate amounts of centrally produced AVP does not respond to exogenous administration of the hormone or its congeners.

Vasopressin administered IV is used for the initial evaluation of patients with suspected diabetes insipidus, which may follow head trauma or hypophysectomy. Under these circumstances, polyuria may be transient, and a longer antidiuretic effect (1 to 3 days) as produced by IM vasopressin tannate in oil could produce water intoxication. Oral administration of vasopressin is followed by rapid inactivation by trypsin, which cleaves a peptide linkage. Likewise, intravenous administration of vasopressin results in a brief effect because of rapid enzymatic breakdown of peptides in the tissues, especially the kidneys.

Administration of the synthetic selective V2 receptor agonist, desmopressin (DDAVP), treats central diabetes insipidus. DDAVP has an intense antidiuretic (V_2) effect and decreased pressor (V_1) effect. Through its V_2 effects, DDAVP also causes endothelial cells to release von Willebrand factor, tissue-type plasminogen activator, and prostaglandins. The elimination half-time of DDAVP is 2.5 to 4.4 hours.[42] There are fewer side effects produced by DDAVP than are associated with vasopressin, although nausea and increases in systemic blood pressure can occur. DDAVP, which is not inactivated by trypsin can be administered orally (0.3 to 0.6 mg per day), IV (1 to 4 μg per day), or nasally (5 to 40 μg per day).[41]

Administered intranasally twice daily, using a calibrated catheter (Rhinyle), DDAVP is the drug of choice in the treatment of diabetes insipidus due to inadequate production of AVP by the posterior pituitary. DDAVP, like all the AVP analogues, is not effective in the treatment of nephrogenic diabetes insipidus. Increased release of von Willebrand factor accounts for the hemostatic activity of DDAVP in patients with uremia, chronic liver disease, and certain types of hemophilia by promoting platelet adhesiveness to the vascular endothelium. DDAVP has also been reported to minimize intraoperative blood loss in patients undergoing cardiac surgery with cardiopulmonary bypass, whereas other reports find no effect on blood loss in patients undergoing cardiac surgery or spinal fusion surgery.[43–45] DDAVP does not decrease bleeding following cardiopulmonary bypass in patients who were maintained on aspirin therapy until the day before surgery.[46] DDAVP administered IV may decrease systemic vascular resistance leading to hypotension.[43]

Lypressin is a synthetic analogue of AVP that produces antidiuresis for about 4 hours after intranasal administration. Its short duration of action limits its usefulness in the treatment of diabetes insipidus.

Hypotension During Anesthesia

Perioperative administration of angiotensin-converting enzyme inhibitors (ACE-I) or angiotensin II receptor blockers (ARB) inhibits the renin-angiotensin system and can cause refractory hypotension after administration of anesthesia.[47] In these cases, catecholamine administration may be unsuccessful.[48] The synthetic vasopressin analog, terlipressin (1 mg), has been used to manage refractory hypotension in patients who have taken ACE- I or ARB.[49,50] Vasopressin may be effective to treat hypotension from anaphylaxis and from severe catecholamine deficiency after resection of a pheochromocytoma.[51,52]

Septic Shock

Excess generation of nitric oxide, activation of the renin-angiotensin system, and low plasma concentrations of vasopressin contribute to progressive loss of vascular tone during sepsis.[53] Vasopressin levels are initially elevated with the onset of sepsis but decrease to normal levels after 24 hours producing a relative vasopressin deficiency.[54] Vasopressin infusion (0.01 to 0.04 unit per minute) can reverse systemic hypotension and decrease norepinephrine dosages in catecholamine-resistant septic shock.[55]

Refractory Cardiac Arrest

Vasopressin is an alternative to epinephrine for vasopressor therapy during cardiopulmonary resuscitation. Vasopressin, 40 units IV, was similar to epinephrine 1 mg IV for management of ventricular fibrillation and pulseless electrical activity. Vasopressin was more effective than epinephrine for management of asystole and the treatment of refractory cardiac arrest.[56] The American Heart Association recommends that vasopressin, at a one-time only dose of 40 units IV be considered instead of epinephrine 1 mg IV every 3 to 5 minutes for patients who are being treated for cardiac arrest. Vasopressin functions as a vasoconstrictor when it is administered in supraphysiologic doses which serve to displace peripheral blood volume to the central circulation without some of the adverse effects produced by epinephrine. This drug needs to only be administered once during cardiopulmonary resuscitation because of its 10- to 20-minute elimination half-time. Vasopressin administered during cardiac arrest and hemorrhagic shock may improve vital organ blood flow during cardiopulmonary resuscitation and stabilize cardiocirculatory function after successful resuscitation.[57]

Esophageal Varices

Vasopressin may serve as an adjunct in the control of bleeding esophageal varices and during abdominal surgery in patients with cirrhosis and portal hypertension. Infusion of 20 units over 5 minutes results in marked decreases in hepatic blood flow lasting about 30 minutes. Only a moderate increase in systemic blood pressure occurs. This effect on the portal circulation is attributable to marked splanchnic vasoconstriction. An alternative to systemic administration is the infusion of vasopressin directly into the superior mesenteric artery. It has not been established whether selective arterial administration is safer than systemic administration with respect to cardiac and vascular side effects.

Side Effects

Vasoconstriction and increased systemic blood pressure occur only with doses of vasopressin that are much larger than those administered for the treatment of diabetes insipidus. This response is because of a direct and generalized effect on vascular smooth muscles that is not antagonized by denervation or adrenergic-blocking drugs. Facial pallor due to cutaneous vasoconstriction may also accompany large doses of vasopressin. The magnitude of increase in systemic blood pressure caused by vasopressin depends, to some extent, on the reactivity of the baroreceptor reflexes. For example, when baroreceptor reflexes are depressed by anesthesia, smaller amounts of vasopressin are capable of evoking a pressor response. Pulmonary artery pressures are also increased by vasopressin. Higher doses of vasopressin may cause splanchnic, digit, and coronary ischemia.[58]

Vasopressin, even in small doses, may produce selective vasoconstriction of the coronary arteries, with decreases in coronary blood flow manifesting as angina pectoris, electrocardiographic evidence of myocardial ischemia, and, in some instances, myocardial infarction. Ventricular cardiac dysrhythmias may accompany these cardiac effects.

Large doses of vasopressin stimulate gastrointestinal smooth muscle, and the resulting increased peristalsis may manifest as abdominal pain, nausea, and vomiting. Smooth muscle of the uterus is also stimulated by large doses of vasopressin.

A decrease in platelet count has been attributed to AVP-mediated platelet aggregation via V_1 receptors.[55] AVP infusion in advanced vasodilatory shock does not increase plasma concentrations of factor VIII, von Willebrand factor antigen, and ristocetin cofactor. Allergic reactions ranging from urticaria to anaphylaxis may occasionally follow the administration of vasopressin. Prolonged use of vasopressin may result in antibody formation and a shortened duration of action of the drug.

Oxytocin

Oxytocin stimulates uterine muscle and is administered to induce labor at term, reduce and prevent uterine atony, and decrease hemorrhage in the postpartum or postabortion period.[59] By stimulating smooth muscle uterine contraction, blood loss at the site of placental attachment is reduced. All preparations of oxytocin used clinically are synthetic, and their potency is described in units. These synthetic preparations are identical to the hormone normally released from the posterior pituitary but devoid of contamination by other polypeptide hormones and proteins found in natural proteins.

For induction of labor, a continuous infusion is preferred, because the low dose of oxytocin needed can be precisely controlled. Indeed, the sensitivity of the uterus to oxytocin increases as pregnancy progresses. To induce labor, a dilute solution (10 mU/mL) is administered by a constant infusion pump beginning at 1 to 2 mU per minute. This infusion rate is increased 1 to 2 mU per minute every 15 to 30 minutes until an optimal response (uterine contraction every 2 to 3 minutes) is obtained. The average dose of oxytocin to induce labor is 8 to 10 mU per minute. Infusion rates up to 40 mU per minute of oxytocin may be necessary to treat uterine atony initially after delivery. IM injections of oxytocin are commonly used to provide sustained uterine contractions in the postpartum period.

To prevent uterine atony, slow administration (to reduce adverse side effects) of 1 to 3 International Unit of oxytocin over 30 seconds is recommended. Coadministration with phenylephrine may be required if higher doses are used. To manage uterine atony and postpartum hemorrhage, 3 to 5 International Unit of intravenous oxytocin over 30 seconds is recommended.[60] Prior oxytocin exposure promotes oxytocin receptor downregulation and desensitization and may be a risk factor for postpartum hemorrhage from uterine atony.[61,62]

Side Effects

High and bolus doses of oxytocin are more likely to decrease systolic and diastolic blood pressure via a direct relaxant effect on vascular smooth muscles.[63] Reflex tachycardia and increased cardiac output accompany the transient decrease in systemic blood pressure.[64] The amounts of oxytocin administered for most obstetric purposes are inadequate to produce marked alterations in systemic blood pressure. A marked decrease in blood pressure, however, may occur if oxytocin is administered to patients with blunted compensatory reflex responses, as may be produced by anesthesia. Likewise, hypovolemic patients may be particularly susceptible to oxytocin-induced hypotension. The hemodynamic effects of a second dose of oxytocin are diminished compared to the initial dose.[65]

In the past, oxytocin preparations were often contaminated with ergot alkaloids, resulting in exaggerated systemic blood pressure increases when administered to patients previously treated with a sympathomimetic. Modern synthetic commercial preparations are pure oxytocin and do not introduce the risk of exaggerated vasoconstriction when administered in the presence of a sympathomimetic drug.

Oxytocin exhibits a slight AVP-like activity when administered in high doses, introducing the possibility of water intoxication, hyponatremia, and neurologic dysfunction if an excessive volume of fluid is administered.[66] The risk of this complication can be minimized by infusion of oxytocin in an electrolyte-containing solution rather than glucose in water.

Drugs for Reproductive Regulation

Ovarian Hormones

An understanding of the synthesis and action of ovarian hormones, including estrogens and progesterone, permits therapeutic interventions in certain disease states. Equally important is the therapeutic use of drugs that can mimic effects of these hormones and act as contraceptives.

Estrogens

Estrogens are effective in treating unpleasant side effects of menopause (Fig. 40-5). Hormone replacement therapy may reduce the depressive symptoms during menopause.[67] Senile or atrophic vaginitis responds to topical estrogen. There is no evidence that administration of estrogens delays the progression of atherosclerosis in postmenopausal women. There is abundant evidence that administration of estrogen to postmenopausal women prevents bone loss (protects against osteoporosis) and also prevents vertebral and femoral bone fractures.[68] Estrogens are administered to decrease milk production in the postpartum period. The presence of receptors for estrogen increases the likelihood of a palliative response to estrogen therapy in women with metastatic breast cancer. An important use of estrogens is in combination with progestins as oral contraceptives.

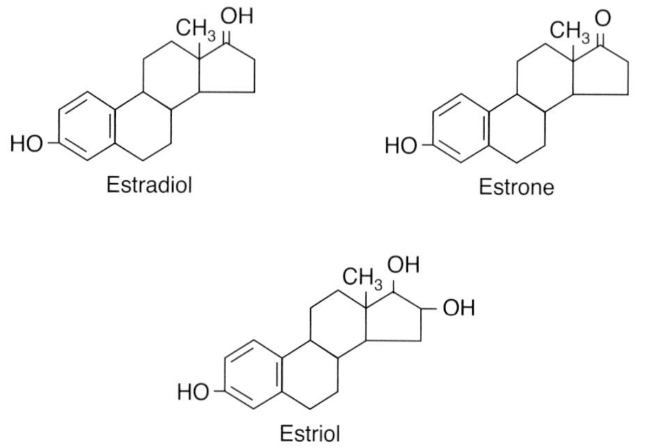

CH3 OH
HO
Estradiol
CH3 O
HO
Estrone
CH3 OH
OH
HO
Estriol

FIGURE 40-5 Estrogens.

Route of Administration

The absorption of most estrogens and their derivatives from the gastrointestinal tract is prompt and nearly complete. Metabolism in the liver, however, limits the effectiveness of orally administered estrogens. Topical and IM administration of estrogens is also effective. Radioimmunoassay methods are highly specific and sensitive for measuring the plasma concentrations of estrogens.

Side Effects

The most frequent unpleasant symptom associated with the use of estrogens is nausea. Large doses of estrogens may cause retention of sodium and water, which is particularly undesirable in patients with cardiac or renal disease. There is an increased incidence of vaginal and cervical adenocarcinoma in daughters of mothers treated with diethylstilbestrol or other synthetic estrogens during the first trimester of pregnancy. Most of the affected women have been 20 to 25 years old when diagnosed. Use of estrogen by postmenopausal women increases the risk of developing endometrial cancer.

Antiestrogens

Clomiphene and tamoxifen act as antiestrogens by binding to estrogen receptors (Fig. 40-6). Tamoxifen is administered for a period of 5 years to postmenopausal women with breast cancer that was characterized by estrogen-responsive receptors. It is of interest that tamoxifen has estrogenic activity in some tissues, including bone. The loss of normal feedback inhibition of estrogen synthesis causes an increased secretion of gonadotropins. The most prominent effect on increased plasma concentrations of gonadotropins is the enlargement of the ovaries and enhancement of fertility in otherwise infertile women. Endometrial stimulation and an increased incidence of

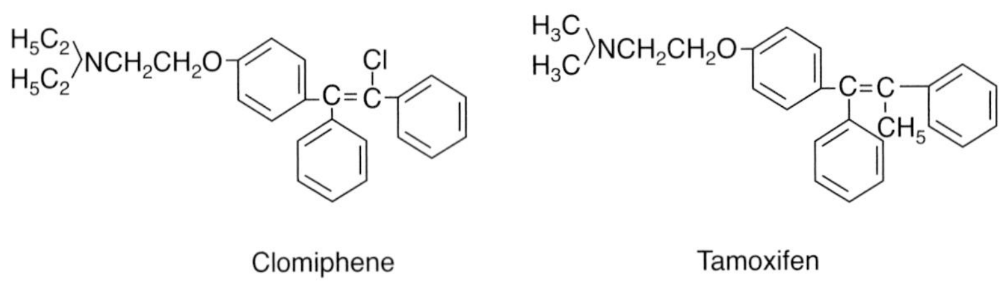

FIGURE 40-6 Antiestrogens.

Clomiphene

Tamoxifen

temperature disturbances ("hot flashes") may accompany treatment with tamoxifen.

Tissue-Specific Estrogens

Raloxifene is a nonsteroidal benzothiophene that acts as a selective estrogen-receptor modulator.[69] In this regard, raloxifene preserves the beneficial effects of estrogens (prevention of bone loss and lowering of plasma cholesterol concentrations) without any associated effects on reproductive organs. For example, endometrial stimulation does not accompany treatment with raloxifene. Tissue-specific estrogen agonist or antagonist actions of raloxifene may be related to estrogen receptor-mediated gene activation.

Progesterone

Orally active derivatives of progesterone are designated ***progestins*** (Fig. 40-7). Progestins are often combined with estrogens as oral contraceptives. Dysfunctional uterine bleeding can be treated with small doses of a progestin for a few days, with the goal being induction of progesterone-withdrawal bleeding. Progestins, like estrogens, are effective in suppressing lactation in the immediate postpartum period. Palliative treatment of metastatic endometrial carcinoma is achieved with progestins. Absorption of progestins from the gastrointestinal tract is rapid, but hepatic first-pass metabolism is extensive.

Antiprogestins

Antiprogestins inhibit the hormonal effects of progesterone and are the most effective and safest means of medical abortion.[70] In this regard, mifepristone (RU 486) can be administered in a single oral dose to produce termination of pregnancy (Fig. 40-8). The combination of mifepristone with a prostaglandin administered 48 hours later by IM injection (sulprostone), by vaginal suppository (gemeprost), or orally (misoprostol) has resulted in a rate of complete abortion approaching 100%. Mifepristone has been used as a postcoital contraceptive within 72 hours of unprotected intercourse. In addition to its antiprogesterone properties, mifepristone has antiglucocorticoid activity and is useful in the treatment of patients with hypercortisolism. Side effects of mifepristone include vaginal bleeding, nausea, vomiting, abdominal pain, and fatigue.

Oral Contraceptives

Oral contraceptives are most often a combination of an estrogen and a progestin. This combination inhibits ovulation, presumably by preventing release of follicle-stimulating hormone by estrogen and luteinizing hormone by progesterone.

Side Effects

Estrogens in combined preparations are believed to be responsible for most, if not all of the side effects of oral

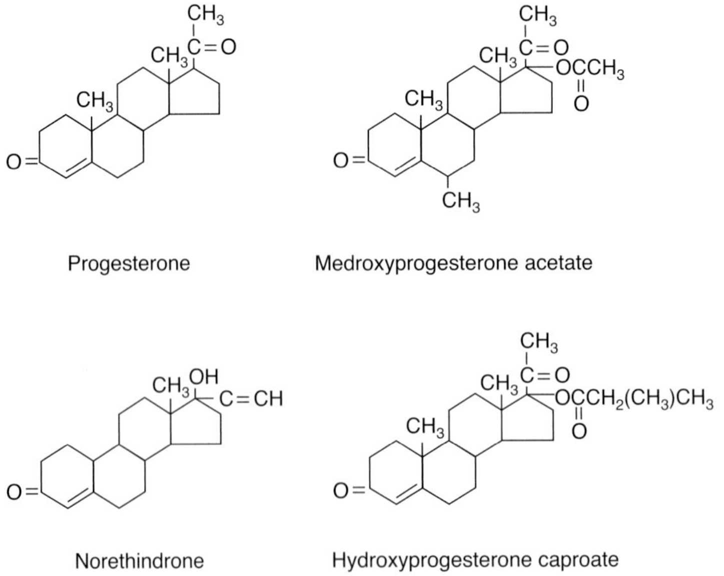

FIGURE 40-7 Progestins.

Progesterone

Medroxyprogesterone acetate

Norethindrone

Hydroxyprogesterone caproate

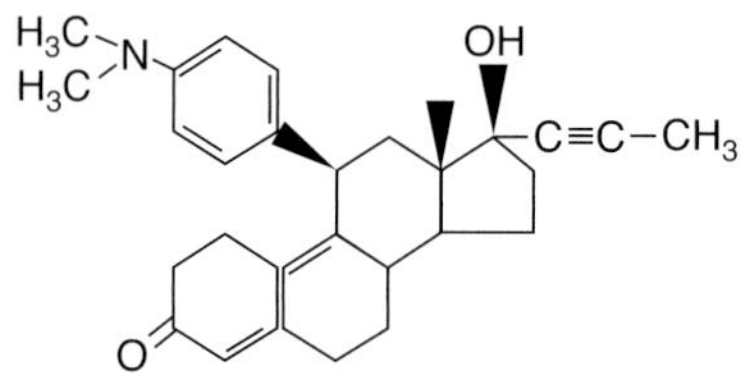

FIGURE 40-8 Mifepristone (RU 486).

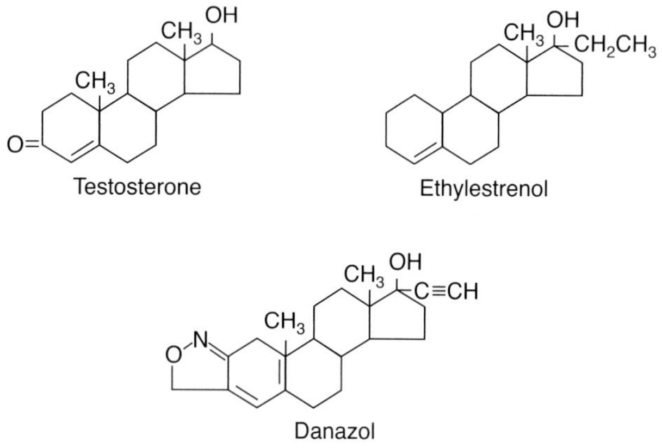

Testosterone

Ethylestrenol

Danazol

FIGURE 40-9 Androgens.

contraceptives. For example, estrogens seem to be responsible for the increased incidence of thromboembolism. Indeed, patients taking estrogens manifest increased blood concentrations of some clotting factors as well as increased platelet aggregation. Nausea, vomiting, weight gain, and breast discomfort resembling early pregnancy are attributed to the estrogen component of oral contraceptives. The incidence of myocardial infarction and stroke is increased in patients who chronically take oral contraceptives.[71] Hypertension occurs in about 5% of women taking oral contraceptives chronically.[72] This response probably reflects estrogen-induced increases in circulating plasma concentrations of renin and angiotensin, with associated retention of sodium and water.

Oral contraceptives containing high doses of estrogen may produce alterations in the glucose tolerance curves of patients with preclinical diabetes mellitus. These drugs increase the concentration of cholesterol in bile, which is consistent with an increased incidence of cholelithiasis. Benign hepatomas have been associated with the use of oral contraceptives. An increased incidence of breast cancer in patients taking oral contraceptives has not been documented. Depression of mood and fatigue have been attributed to the progestin component of oral contraceptives.

Androgens

Androgens are administered to males to stimulate the development and maintenance of secondary sexual characteristics (Fig. 40-9). Testosterone is also prescribed to hypogonadal men who have evidence of androgen deficiency and a low serum testosterone concentration. The most common indication of androgen therapy in females is palliative management of metastatic breast cancer. Androgens enhance erythropoiesis by stimulation of renal production of erythropoietin as well as by direct dose-related stimulation of erythropoietin-sensitive elements in bone marrow. In addition, there is a drug-induced increase in 2,3-diphosphoglycerate levels, which decreases hemoglobin affinity for oxygen, thus enhancing the availability of oxygen to tissues. For these reasons, androgen therapy is often instituted in patients with aplastic anemia or hemolytic anemia. Androgen-anabolic steroids have been used in the treatment of chronic debilitating diseases. These drugs promote a feeling of well-being and may improve appetite when administered to patients with terminal illnesses. The efficacy of anabolic steroids to improve athletic performance is not documented and is condemned on ethical grounds. Certain androgens may be useful in the treatment of hereditary angioedema.

Route of Administration

About 99% of testosterone circulating in the plasma is bound to sex hormone–binding globulin. As a result, this globulin determines the concentration of free testosterone in the plasma and thus its elimination half-time, which is 10 to 20 minutes. Testosterone administered orally is readily absorbed but is metabolized so extensively by the liver that therapeutic effects do not occur. Alkylation of androgens at the 17 position retards their hepatic metabolism and permits such derivatives to be effective (see Fig. 40-9). Alkylated testosterones are rarely prescribed because of their association with hepatic dysfunction. Intramuscular injection of esters of testosterone (i.e., testosterone enanthate and testosterone cypionate), which are more lipophilic than testosterone alone, prolongs the duration of time that testosterone is present in the blood. Testosterone can also be delivered via patch and gels.

Side Effects

Dose-related cholestatic hepatitis and jaundice are particularly likely to accompany androgen therapy for palliation in neoplastic disease. Increases in the plasma alkaline phosphatase, hematocrit, and transaminase enzymes are also likely. Prolonged therapy (>1 year) with androgens, as for management of anemia, is associated with an increased incidence of hepatic cancer. Retention of sodium and water is also likely to accompany palliative treatment of cancer with high doses of androgens. Androgens increase the potency of coumarin anticoagulants and the likelihood of spontaneous hemorrhage. Androgens can decrease the concentration of thyroid-binding globulin in plasma and thus influence thyroid function tests.

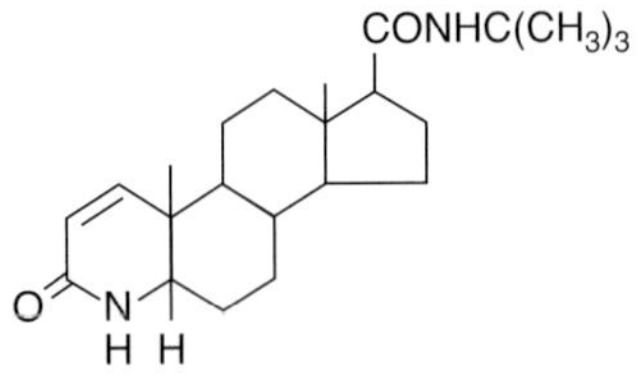

$CONHC(CH_3)_3$

FIGURE 40-10 Finasteride.

Danazol

The low androgenic activity of danazol makes it the preferred androgen for treatment of hereditary angioedema (see Fig. 40-9). In treated patients, there is a remission of symptoms as well as increased production of previously deficient plasma protein factors. As with other androgens, danazol therapy has been associated with abnormal liver function tests and jaundice. Danazol also decreases breast pain and nodularity in many women with fibrocystic breast disease. Symptoms of endometriosis are decreased, and fertility may be restored in danazol-treated women. In patients with hemophilia A, danazol increases factor VIII activity and decreases the incidence of hemorrhage.[73]

Finasteride

Finasteride is a competitive 5-α-reductase inhibitor that does not bind to the androgen receptor (Fig. 40-10).[74] As a result of this drug-induced enzyme inhibition, dihydrotestosterone production from testosterone does not occur. In the absence of dihydrotestosterone, the androgen effects on the prostate and skin do not occur. Finasteride is administered orally (5 mg once daily) for the treatment of benign prostatic hyperplasia. Treatment of male pattern baldness, hirsutism, and acne may represent other potentially useful applications for finasteride. There is no evidence that finasteride is beneficial in men with established prostate cancer. The elimination half-time after oral administration is 6 to 8 hours. The only important side effects of finasteride are related to decreased sexual function. Finasteride has no effect on serum lipids or bone density. Prostate-specific antigen concentrations are decreased by treatment with finasteride, introducing the concern that detection of prostate cancer could be masked in patients treated with this drug.

References

1. Tobler A, Meier R, Seitz M, et al. Glucocorticoids downregulate gene expression of GM-CSF, NAP-1/IL-8, and IL-6, but not of M-CSF in human fibroblasts. *Blood.* 1992;79:45–51.
2. Migeon CJ, Lawrence B, Bertrand J, et al. In vivo distribution of some 17-hydroxycorticoids between the plasma and red blood cells of man. *J Clin Endocrinol Metab.* 1959;19:1411–1419.
3. Tornatore KM, Logue G, Venuto RC, e t al. Cortisol pharmacodynamics after methylprednisolone administration in young and elderly males. *J Clin Pharmacol.* 1997;37:304–311.
4. Kozower M, Veatch L, Kaplan MM. Decreased clearance of prednisolone, a factor in the development of corticosteroid side effects. *J Clin Endocrinol Metab.* 1974;38:407–412.
5. Cornell RC, Stoughton RB. Correlation of the vasoconstriction assay and clinical activity in psoriasis. *Arch Dermatol.* 1985;121:63–67.
6. Bel EH. Mild asthma. *New Engl J Med.* 2013;369:549–557.
7. Silvanus M-T, Groeben H, Peters J. Corticosteroids and inhaled salbutamol in patients with reversible airway obstruction markedly decrease the incidence of bronchoconstriction after tracheal intubation. *Anesthesiology.* 2004;100:1052–1057.
8. Wang JJ, Ho ST, Tzeng JI, et al. The effect of timing of dexamethasone administration on its efficacy as a prophylactic antiemetic for postoperative nausea and vomiting. *Anesth Analg.* 2000;91:136–139.
9. Apfel CC, Korttila K, Abdalla M, et al. A factorial trial of six interventions for the prevention of postoperative nausea and vomiting. *N Engl J Med.* 2004;350:2441–2451.
10. De Oliveira GS, Santana Castro-Alves LJ, Ahmad S, et al. Dexamethasone to prevent postoperative nausea and vomiting: an updated meta-analysis of randomized controlled trials. *Anesth Analg.* 2013;116:58–74.
11. Sapolsky RM, Romero LM, Munck AU. How do glucocorticoids influence stress responses? Integrating permissive, suppressive, stimulatory, and preparative pain. *Anesth Analg.* 2005;21:55–89.
12. Aasboe V, Raeder JC. Groegaard B. Betamethasone reduces postoperative pain and nausea after ambulatory surgery. *Anesth Analg.* 1998;87:319–323.
13. De Oliveira GS, Almeida M, Benzon H, et al. Perioperative single dose systemic dexamethasone for postoperative pain: a meta-analysis of randomized controlled trials. *Anesthesiology.* 2011;115:575–588.
14. De Gans J, van de Beek D; European Dexamethasone in Adulthood Bacterial Meningitis Study Investigators. Dexamethasone in adults with bacterial meningitis. *N Engl J Med.* 2002;347:1549–1556.
15. Roberts I, Yates D, Sandercock P, et al. Effect of intravenous corticosteroids on death within 14 days in 10008 adults with clinically significant head injury (MRC CRASH trial): a randomised placebo-controlled trial. *Lancet.* 2004;364:1321–1328.
16. Edwards P, Arango M, Balica L, et al. Final results of MRC CRASH, a randomized placebo-controlled trial of intravenous corticosteroid in adults with head-injury-outcomes at 6 months. *Lancet.* 2005;365:1957–1959.
17. Dudley WR, Marshall BE. Steroid treatment for acid-aspiration pneumonia. *Anesthesiology.* 1974;40:136–141.
18. Downs JB, Chapman RL, Modell JH, et al. An evaluation of steroid therapy in aspiration pneumonitis. *Anesthesiology.* 1974;40:129–135.
19. Wynne JW, DeMarco FJ, Hood CI. Physiological effects of corticosteroids in foodstuff aspiration. *Arch Surg.* 1981;116:46–49.
20. Haddox JD. Lumbar and cervical epidural steroid therapy. *Anesth Clin North Am.* 1992;10:179–203.
21. Kay J, Findling JW, Raff H. Epidural triamcinolone suppresses the pituitary-adrenal axis in human subjects. *Anesth Analg.* 1994;79: 501–505.
22. Carette S, Leclaire R, Marcoux S, et al. Epidural corticosteroid injections for sciatica due to herniated nucleus pulposus. *N Engl J Med.* 1997;336:1634–1640.
23. Bjornson CL, Klassen TP, Williamson J, et al. A randomized trial of a single dose of oral dexamethasone for mild croup. *N Engl J Med.* 2004;351:1306–1313.
24. Cummings JJ, D'Eugenio DB, Gross SJ. A controlled trial of dexamethasone in preterm infants at high risk for bronchopulmonary dysplasia. *N Engl J Med.* 1989;320:1505–1510.
25. Meduri GU, Golden E, Freire AX et al. Methyprednisolone infusion in early severe ARDS: results of a randomized controlled trial. *Chest.* 2007;131:954–963.
26. Steinberg JP, Hudson LD, Goodman RB, et al. Efficacy and safety of corticosteroids for persistent acute respiratory distress syndrome. *N Engl J Med.* 2006;354:1671–1684.
27. Mentzelopoulos SD, Malachias S, Chamos C, et al. Vasopressin, steroids, and epinephrine and neurologically favorable survival after in-hospital cardiac arrest. *JAMA.* 2013;310:270–279.

28. Mentzelopoulos SD, Zakynthinos SG, Tzoufi M, et al. Vasopressin, epinephrine, and corticosteroids for in-hospital cardiac arrest. *Arch Intern Med.* 2009;169:15–24.
29. Salem M, Tainsh RE Jr, Bromberg J, et al. Perioperative glucocorticoid coverage. A reassessment 42 years after emergence of a problem. *Ann Surg.* 1994;219:416–425.
30. Udelsman R, Ramp J, Gallucci WT, et al. Adaptation during surgical stress: a reevaluation of the role of glucocorticoids. *J Clin Invest.* 1986;77:1377–1381.
31. Ratner EF, Allen R, Mihm F, et al. Failure of steroid supplementation to prevent operative hypotension in a patient receiving chronic steroid therapy. *Anesth Analg.* 1996;82:1294–1296.
32. Symreng T, Karlberg BE, Kagedal B, et al. Physiological cortisol substitution of long-term steroid-treated patients undergoing major surgery. *Br J Anaesth.* 1981;53:949–953.
33. Hardy JD, Turner MD. Hydrocortisone secretion in man: studies of adrenal vein blood. *Surgery.* 1957;42:194–201.
34. Hume DM, Bell C, Bartter FC. Direct measurement of adrenal secretion during operative trauma and convalescence. *Surgery.* 1962;52: 174–187.
35. O'Dell JR. Therapeutic strategies for rheumatoid arthritis. *N Engl J Med.* 2004;350:2591–2602.
36. Silvers JB, Marinova D, Mercer MB, et al. A national study of physician recommendations to initiate and discontinue growth hormone for short stature. *Pediatrics.* 2010;126:468–476.
37. Cohen P, Germak J, Rogol AD, et al. Variable degree of growth hormone (GH) and insulin-like growth factor (IGF) sensitivity in children with idiopathic short stature compared with GH-deficient patients: evidence from an IGF-based dosing study of short children. *J Clin Endocrinol Metab.* 2010;95:2089–2098.
38. Lamberts SWJ, van der Lely AJ, de Herder WW, et al. Octreotide. *N Engl J Med.* 1996;334:246–254.
39. Dilger JA, Rho EH, Que FG, et al. Octreotide-induced bradycardia and heart block during surgical resection of a carcinoid tumor. *Anesth Analg.* 2004;98:318–320.
40. Brzezinski A. Melatonin in humans. *N Engl J Med.* 1997;336:186–195.
41. Treschan T, Jurgen P. The vasopressin system: physiology and clinical strategies. *Anesthesiology.* 2006;105:599–612.
42. Horrow JC. Desmopressin and antifibrinolytics. *Int Anesthesiol Clin.* 1990;28:230–236.
43. Frankville DD, Harper GB, Lake CL, et al. Hemodynamic consequences of desmopressin administration after cardiopulmonary bypass. *Anesthesiology.* 1991;74:988–996.
44. Guay J, Reinberg C, Poitras B, et al. A trial of desmopressin to reduce blood loss in patients undergoing spinal fusion for idiopathic scoliosis. *Anesth Analg.* 1992;75:405–410.
45. Mongan PD, Hosking MP. The role of desmopressin acetate in patients undergoing coronary artery bypass surgery: a controlled clinical trial with thromboelastographic risk stratification. *Anesthesiology.* 1992;77:38–46.
46. Pleym H, Stenseth R, Waqhba A, et al. Prophylactic treatment with desmopressin does not reduce postoperative bleeding after coronary surgery in patients treated with aspirin before surgery. *Anesth Analg* 2004;98:578–584.
47. Bertrand M, Godet G, Meersschaert K, et al. Should the angiotensin II antagonists be discontinued before surgery. *Anesth Analg.* 2001;92:26–30.
48. Brabant SM, Eyraud D, Bertrand M, et al. Refractory hypotension after induction of anesthesia in a patient chronically treated with angiotensin receptor antagonists. *Anesth Analg.* 1999;89:887–888.
49. Boccara G, Outtara A, Godet G, et al. Terlipressin versus norepinephrine to correct refractory arterial hypotension after general anesthesia in patients chronically treated with renin-angiotensin system inhibitors. *Anesthesiology.* 2003;98:1338–1344.
50. Eyraud D, Brabant S, Nathalie D, et al. Treatment of intraoperative refractory hypotension with terlipressin in patients chronically treated with an antagonist of the renin-angiotensin system. *Anesth Analg.* 1999;88:980–984.
51. Augoustides JG, Abrams M, Berkowitz D, et al. Vasopressin for hemodynamic rescue in catecholamine-resistant vasoplegic shock after resection of massive pheochromocytoma. *Anesthesiology.* 2004;101:1022–1024.
52. Schummer C, Wirsing M, Schummer W. The pivotal role of vasopressin in refractory anaphylactic shock. *Anesth Analg.* 2008;107:620–624.
53. Landry DW, Levin HR, Gallant EM, et al. Vasopressin deficiency contributes to the vasodilation of septic shock. *Circulation.* 1997; 95:1122–1125.
54. Sharshar T, Blanchard A, Paillard M, et al. Circulating vasopressin levels in septic shock. *Crit Care Med.* 2003;31:1752–1758
55. Dünser MW, Mayr AJ, Ulmer H, et al. Arginine vasopressin in advanced vasodilatory shock: a prospective, randomized, controlled study. *Circulation.* 2003;107:2313–2319.
56. Wenzel V, Krismer AC, Arntz HR, et al. A comparison of vasopressin and epinephrine for out-of-hospital cardiopulmonary resuscitation. *N Engl J Med.* 2004;350:105–113.
57. Voelckel WG, Lurie KG, Lindner KH, et al. Vasopressin improves survival after cardiac arrest in hypovolemic shock. *Anesth Analg.* 2000;91:627–634.
58. Dünser MW, Mayr AJ, Tür A, et al. Ischemic skin lesions as a complication of continuous vasopressin infusion in catecholamine-resistant vasodilatory shock: incidence and risk factors. *Crit Care Med.* 2003;31:1394–1398.
59. Winkioff B, Dabash R, Durocher J, et al. Treatment of postpartum haemorrhage with sublingual misoprostol versus oxytocin in women not exposed to oxytocin during labour: a double-blind, randomized, non-inferiority trial. *Lancet.* 2010;375:210–216.
60. Dyer RA, Butwick AJ, Carvalho B. Oxytocin for labour and caesarean delivery: implications for the anaesthesiologist. *Curr Opin Anesthesiol.* 2011;24:255–261.
61. Phaeneuf S, Rodriguez Linares B, TambyRaja RL, et al. Loss of myometrial oxytocin receptors during oxytocin-induced and oxytocin-augmented labour. *J Reprod Fertil.* 2000;120:91–97.
62. Grotegut CA, Paglia MJ, Johnson LN, et al. Oxytocin exposure during labor among women with postpartum hemorrhage secondary to uterine atony. *Am J Obstet Gynecol.* 2011;204:56.e1–56.e6.
63. Thomas JS, Koh SH, Cooper GM. Haemodynamic effects of oxytocin given as i.v. bolus or infusion on women undergoing Caesarean section. *Br J Anaesth.* 2007;98:116–119.
64. Dyer R, Reed A, van Dyk D, et al. Hemodynamic effects of ephedrine, phenylephrine, and the coadministration of phenylephrine with oxytocin during spinal anesthesia for elective cesarean delivery. *Anesthesiology.* 2009;111:753–765.
65. Langesaeter E, Rosseland LA, Stubhaug A. Haemodynamic effects of repeated doses of oxytocin during Caesarean delivery in healthy parturients. *Br J Anaesth.* 2009;103:260–262.
66. Bergum D, Lonne H, Hakli TF. Oxytocin infusion: acute hyponatremia, seizures, and coma. *Acta Anaesthesiol Scand.* 2009;53:826–827.
67. Zweifel JE, O'Brien WH. A meta-analysis of the effect of hormone replacement therapy upon depressed mood. *Psychoneuroendrocrinology.* 1997;22:189–212.
68. Belchetz PE. Hormonal treatment of postmenopausal women. *N Engl J Med.* 1994;330:1062–1072.
69. Delmas PD, Bjarnason NH, Mitlak BH, et al. Effects of raloxifene on bone mineral density, serum cholesterol concentrations, and uterine endometrium in postmenopausal women. *N Engl J Med.* 1997;337:1641–1647.
70. Spitz IM, Bardin CW. Mifepristone (RU 486)—a modulator of progestin and glucocorticoid action. *N Engl J Med.* 1993;329:404–412.
71. Kaplan NM. Cardiovascular complications of oral contraceptives. *Ann Rev Med.* 1978;29:31–40.
72. Laragh JH. Oral contraceptive-induced hypertension: nine years later. *Am J Obstet Gynecol.* 1976;126:141–147.
73. Gralnick HR, Maisonneuve P, Sultan Y, et al. Benefits of danazol treatment in patients with hemophilia A (classic hemophilia). *JAMA.* 1985;253:1151–1153.
74. Rittmaster RS. Finasteride. *N Engl J Med.* 1994;330:120–126.

CHAPTER 41

Antimicrobials, Antiseptics, Disinfectants, and Management of Perioperative Infection

Pamela Flood

The excessive use of antimicrobials (antibiotics) for the treatment of conditions for which these drugs provide little or no benefit (upper respiratory tract infections, bronchitis) has contributed to the emergence of bacterial resistance. It is estimated that 21% of all prescriptions written for antimicrobials are for ambulatory patients seen in physicians' offices with the diagnosis of upper respiratory tract infections or bronchitis.[1]

Misuse of antibiotics in the general population is in contrast to the proven benefit of antibiotic prophylaxis for selected surgical procedures, which has been part of a national initiative to enhance compliance, the Surgical Care Improvement Project (SCIP). SCIP, based originally on the Surgical Infection Project (SIP), was designed to combat a perceived national crisis of preventable surgical site infections, identified in the 1990s, which were associated with doubled risk of mortality, 60% higher likelihood of spending time in an intensive care unit, and fivefold risk of readmission.[2] The SIP was expanded to the SCIP to include additional perioperative quality measures related to infection control (Table 41-1).[3] Each of these measures has been independently associated with a reduction in surgical site infection in clinical trials. The original SCIP goal was a 25% reduction in surgical site infection by 2010. This goal was not met. However, a new goal of 25% reduction was set for 2013 and the latest data analysis suggests that the goal may have been met with 20% reduction achieved in 2012.[4]

The baseline risk for perioperative infection is highly dependent on factors that require risk adjustment in clinical trials and consideration in clinical care. Patient-related risk factors for surgical site infection include extremes of age (younger than 5 and older than 65 years), poor nutritional status, obesity, diabetes mellitus and perioperative glycemic control, peripheral vascular disease, tobacco use, coexistent infections, altered immune response, corticosteroid therapy, preoperative skin preparation (surgical scrub and hair removal), and length of preoperative hospitalization. Institutional variables include surgical experience and technique (i.e., open vs. laparoscopic), duration of procedure, hospital environments including sterilization of instruments, and maintenance of perioperative normothermia.[5,6]

Of the aforementioned variables, few are modifiable at the time of surgery. Good perioperative glucose control can reduce infection risk. Perioperative glucose control has been studied predominantly in the cardiothoracic surgery population where it is associated with about a 50% decrease in deep sternal infection.[7] Continuous insulin infusion was associated with an additional reduction in surgical site infection compared to intermittent subcutaneous injection.[8] These trials are the basis of SCIP measure 4. These findings have been generalized to bowel surgery where patients whose glucose was maintained below 200 mg/dL for 48 hours after surgery compared with those having concentrations greater than 200 mg/dL had significantly fewer surgical site infections (29.7% vs. 14.3%).[9] However, intensive insulin regimens designed to keep blood sugar ultralow have shown higher hypoglycemia and mortality compared to conventional treatment.[10]

Although more difficult to achieve, smoking cessation is a perioperative goal. Perioperative education on smoking cessation by surgeons and anesthesiologists in preoperative evaluation is important. The preoperative period has been called a "teachable moment" and even brief smoking cessation can reduce infection risk. A meta-analysis of four studies that have assessed the effect of 4 to 8 weeks of preoperative smoking cessation demonstrates a risk reduction of approximately 50%.[11]

Table 41-1

SCIP Measures Related to Prevention of Surgical Site Infection

SCIP-Inf 1:	Prophylactic antibiotic received within 1 h prior to surgical incision
SCIP-Inf 2:	Prophylactic antibiotic selection for surgical patients
SCIP-Inf 3:	Prophylactic antibiotics discontinued within 24 h after surgery end time (48 h for cardiac patients)
SCIP-Inf 4:	Cardiac surgery patients with controlled 6 am postoperative serum glucose (≤200 mg/dL)
SCIP-Inf 5:	Postoperative wound infection diagnosed during index hospitalization
SCIP-Inf 6:	Surgical patients with appropriate hair removal
SCIP-Inf 7:	Colorectal surgical patients with immediate postoperative normothermia

SCIP, Surgical Care Improvement Project.
From Rosenberger LH, Politano AD, Sawyer RG. The surgical care improvement project and prevention of post-operative infection, including surgical site infection. *Surg Infect (Larchmt)*. 2011;12(3):163–168.

The anesthesiologist should contribute to the maintenance of perioperative normothermia. It is logical that hypothermia will result in peripheral vasoconstriction, decreased wound oxygen tension and recruitment of leukocytes, favoring infection and impaired healing. In a meta-analysis of trials comparing intraoperative warming to control, warming was associated with a 64% decrease in surgical site infections.[12] Prewarming patients before surgery reduces the peripheral to core temperature gradient and has the added advantage of making placement of intravenous lines easier because of peripheral vasodilation. Active prewarming of volunteers for 2 hours resulted in maintenance of core temperatures above 36°C for 60 minutes of general anesthesia at ambient temperature, whereas core temperatures in unwarmed subjects dropped an average of 1.9°C to below 35°C.

Immunosuppression on the basis of long-term use of corticosteroids has been considered a risk factor for surgical site infection. However, there are surprisingly few studies to support this supposition. In a study of infection after mastectomy, steroid use was not found to be associated with surgical site infection. In contrast, long-term steroid treatment was associated with anastomotic leaks in bowel surgery.[13] There is clear evidence that a single dose of corticosteroid given to prevent nausea and vomiting and reduce pain does not promote infection. For example, in a study of open abdominal surgery for gynecologic cancer, there were no excess wound infections in patients treated with a single dose of dexamethasone for nausea and vomiting prophylaxis.[14]

Antimicrobial Prophylaxis for Surgical Procedures

The use of antimicrobial prophylaxis in surgery involves a risk-to-benefit evaluation, which varies depending on the nature of the operative procedure. SCIP measure 1 recommends that prophylactic antimicrobials should be administered intravenously (IV) within 1 hour of surgical incision. The general concept is that tissue concentration of the antibiotic should exceed the minimum inhibitory concentration (MIC) associated with the procedure and or patient characteristics from the time of incision to the completion of surgery. For short-acting antibiotics, this may require redosing (Table 41-2). Antibiotic treatment is not recommended for no longer than 24 hours. This recommendation is based on findings of no benefit to prolonged dosing but rather an increased incidence of drug-resistant organisms.

The antibiotic chosen should be appropriate for the most likely microorganism related to the procedure and patient characteristics (SCIP measure 2). For clean elective surgical procedures such as mastectomy and thyroidectomy in which no tissue (other than the skin) carrying an indigenous flora is penetrated, the risks of routine antimicrobial prophylaxis outweigh the possible benefits. The predominant organisms causing surgical site infections after clean procedures are skin flora (*Staphylococcus aureus* and *Staphylococcus epidermidis*). In clean-contaminated procedures, including abdominal procedures and solid organ transplantation, the most common organisms include gram-negative rods and enterococci in addition to skin flora.[15] Antibiotic recommendations for specific procedure prophylaxis can be found in Table 41-3.[16]

Because of their wide therapeutic index and low incidence of side effects, cephalosporins (most often a cost-effective first-generation cephalosporin such as cefazolin) are the antimicrobials of choice for surgical procedures in which skin flora and normal flora of the gastrointestinal and genitourinary tracts are the most likely pathogens. Patients with documented immunoglobulin E (IgE) reaction to cephalosporins are rare and often mistaken for more common intolerances such as nausea or yeast infection. IgE-mediated anaphylactic reactions to antimicrobials usually occur 30 to 60 minutes after dosing and often include urticaria, bronchospasm, and hemodynamic collapse. This reaction is a life-threatening emergency that precludes subsequent use of the drug. Cephalosporins can safely be used in patients with an allergic reaction to penicillins that is not an IgE-mediated reaction (e.g., anaphylaxis, urticaria, bronchospasm) or exfoliative dermatitis (Stevens-Johnson syndrome, toxic epidermal necrolysis).[17] Although early reports of cross-reactivity were high due to contaminated drug lots, the actual rate of cross-reactivity is only 1%.[17] However, the consequences of true anaphylaxis are severe. Patients should be carefully questioned about the nature of any drug allergy.

Table 41-2

Recommended Doses and Redosing Intervals for Commonly Used Antimicrobials for Surgical Prophylaxis

Antimicrobial	Recommended Dose: Adults[a]	Recommended Dose: Pediatrics[b]	Half-life in Adults with Normal Renal Function, h	Recommended Redosing Interval (From Initiation of Preoperative Dose), h[c]
Ampicillin–sulbactam	3 g (ampicillin 2 g/ sulbactam 1 g)	50 mg/kg of the ampicillin component	0.8–1.3	2
Ampicillin	2 g	50 mg/kg	1–1.9	2
Aztreonam	2 g	30 mg/kg	1.3–2.4	4
Cefazolin	2 g, 3 g for pts weighing ≥120 kg	30 mg/kg	1.2–2.2	4
Cefuroxime	1.5 g	50 mg/kg	1–2	4
Cefotaxime	1 g[d]	50 mg/kg	0.9–1.7	3
Cefoxitin	2 g	40 mg/kg	0.7–1.1	2
Cefotetan	2 g	40 mg/kg	2.8–4.6	6
Ceftriaxone	2 g[e]	50–75 mg/kg	5.4–10.9	NA
Ciprofloxacin[f]	400 mg	10 mg/kg	3–7	NA
Clindamycin	900 mg	10 mg/kg	2–4	6
Ertapenem	1 g	15 mg/kg	3–5	NA
Fluconazole	400 mg	6 mg/kg	30	NA
Gentamicin[g]	5 mg/kg based on dosing weight (single dose)	2.5 mg/kg based on dosing weight	2–3	NA
Levofloxacin[f]	500 mg	10 mg/kg	6–8	NA
Metronidazole	500 mg	15 mg/kg Neonates weighing <1,200 g should receive a single 7.5-mg/kg dose	6–8	NA
Moxifloxacin[f]	400 mg	10 mg/kg	8–15	NA
Piperacillin–tazobactam	3.375 g	Infants 2–9 mo: 80 mg/kg of the piperacillin component Children >9 mo and ≤40 kg: 100 mg/kg of the piperacillin component	0.7–1.2	2
Vancomycin	15 mg/kg	15 mg/kg	4–8	NA
Oral antibiotics for colorectal surgery prophylaxis (used in conjunction with a mechanical bowel preparation)				
Erythromycin base	1 g	20 mg/kg	0.8–3	NA
Metronidazole	1 g	15 mg/kg	6–10	NA
Neomycin	1 g	15 mg/kg	2–3 (3% absorbed under normal gastrointestinal conditions)	NA

[a]Adult doses are obtained from the studies cited in each section. When doses differed between studies, expert opinion used the most-often recommended dose.

[b]The maximum pediatric dose should not exceed the usual adult dose.

[c]For antimicrobials with a short half-life (e.g., cefazolin, cefoxitin) used before long procedures, redosing in the operating room is recommended at an interval of approximately two times the half-life of the agent in patients with normal renal function. Recommended redosing intervals marked as "not applicable" (NA) are based on typical case length; for unusually long procedures, redosing may be needed.

[d]Although FDA-approved package insert labeling indicates 1 g, 14 experts recommend 2 g for obese patients.

[e]When used as a single dose in combination with metronidazole for colorectal procedures.

[f]While fluoroquinolones have been associated with an increased risk of tendinitis/tendon rupture in all ages, use of these agents for single-dose prophylaxis is generally safe.

[g]In general, gentamicin for surgical antibiotic prophylaxis should be limited to a single dose given preoperatively. Dosing is based on the patient's actual body weight. If the patient's actual weight is more than 20% above ideal body weight (IBW), the dosing weight (DW) can be determined as follows: DW = IBW + 0.4 (actual weight − IBW).

From Bratzler DW, Dellinger, EP, Olsen KM, et al; American Society of Health-System Pharmacists; Infectious Diseases Society of America; Surgical Infection Society; Society for Healthcare Epidemiology of America. Clinical practice guidelines for antimicrobial prophylaxis in surgery. *Am J Health Syst Pharm.* 2013;70(3):195–283. http://www.ashp.org/surgical-guidelines. Accessed February 24, 2014.

Table 41-3

Common Antimicrobials Used for Prophylaxis in Various Surgical Settings

Type of Procedure	Recommended Agents[a,b]	Alternative Agents in Patients with β-Lactam Allergy	Strength of Evidence[c]
Cardiac			
Coronary artery bypass	Cefazolin, cefuroxime	Clindamycin,[d] vancomycin[d]	A
Cardiac device insertion procedures (e.g., pacemaker implantation)	Cefazolin, cefuroxime	Clindamycin, vancomycin	A
Ventricular assist devices	Cefazolin, cefuroxime	Clindamycin, vancomycin	C
Thoracic			
Noncardiac procedures, including lobectomy, pneumonectomy, lung resection, and thoracotomy	Cefazolin, ampicillin–sulbactam	Clindamycin,[d] vancomycin[d]	A
Video-assisted thoracoscopic surgery	Cefazolin, ampicillin–sulbactam	Clindamycin,[d] vancomycin[d]	C
Gastroduodenale			
Procedures involving entry into lumen of gastrointestinal tract (bariatric, pancreaticoduodenectomy[f])	Cefazolin	Clindamycin or vancomycin + aminoglycoside[g] or aztreonam or fluoroquinolone[h–j]	A
Procedures without entry into gastrointestinal tract (antireflux, highly selective vagotomy) for high-risk patients	Cefazolin	Clindamycin or vancomycin + aminoglycoside[g] or aztreonam or fluoroquinolone[h–j]	A
Biliary tract			
Open procedure	Cefazolin, cefoxitin, cefotetan, ceftriaxone,[k] ampicillin–sulbactam[h]	Clindamycin or vancomycin + aminoglycoside[g] or aztreonam or fluoroquinolone[h–j] Metronidazole + aminoglycoside[g] or fluoroquinolone[h–j]	A
Laparoscopic procedure			
Elective, low-risk[l]	None	None	A
Elective, high-risk[l]	Cefazolin, cefoxitin, cefotetan, ceftriaxone,[k] ampicillin–sulbactam[h]	Clindamycin or vancomycin + aminoglycoside[g] or aztreonam or fluoroquinolone[h–j] Metronidazole + aminoglycoside[g] or fluoroquinolone[h–j]	A
Appendectomy for uncomplicated appendicitis	Cefoxitin, cefotetan, cefazolin + metronidazole	Clindamycin + aminoglycoside[g] or aztreonam or fluoroquinolone[h–j] Metronidazole + aminoglycoside[g] or fluoroquinolone[h–j]	A

Table 41-3

Common Antimicrobials Used for Prophylaxis in Various Surgical Settings *(continued)*

Type of Procedure	Recommended Agents[a,b]	Alternative Agents in Patients with β-Lactam Allergy	Strength of Evidence[c]
Small intestine			
Nonobstructed	Cefazolin	Clindamycin + aminoglycoside[g] or aztreonam or fluoroquinolone[h–j]	C
Obstructed	Cefazolin + metronidazole, cefoxitin, cefotetan	Metronidazole + aminoglycoside[g] or fluoroquinolone[h–j]	C
Hernia repair (hernioplasty and herniorrhaphy)	Cefazolin	Clindamycin, vancomycin	A
Colorectal[m]	Cefazolin + metronidazole, cefoxitin, cefotetan, ampicillin–sulbactam,[h] ceftriaxone + metronidazole,[n] ertapenem	Clindamycin + aminoglycoside[g] or aztreonam or fluoroquinolone[h–j] metronidazole + aminoglycoside[g] or fluoroquinolone[h–j]	A
Head and neck			
Clean	None	None	B
Clean with placement of prosthesis (excludes tympanostomy tubes)	Cefazolin, cefuroxime	Clindamycin[d]	C
Clean-contaminated cancer surgery	Cefazolin + metronidazole, cefuroxime + metronidazole, ampicillin–sulbactam	Clindamycin[d]	A
Other clean-contaminated procedures with the exception of tonsillectomy and functional endoscopic sinus procedures	Cefazolin + metronidazole, cefuroxime + metronidazole, ampicillin–sulbactam	Clindamycin[d]	B
Neurosurgery			
Elective craniotomy and cerebrospinal fluid-shunting procedures	Cefazolin	Clindamycin,[d] vancomycin[d]	A
Implantation of intrathecal pumps	Cefazolin	Clindamycin,[d] vancomycin[d]	C
Cesarean delivery	Cefazolin	Clindamycin + aminoglycoside[g]	A
Hysterectomy (vaginal or abdominal)	Cefazolin, cefotetan, cefoxitin, ampicillin–sulbactam[h]	Clindamycin or vancomycin + aminoglycoside[g] or aztreonam or fluoroquinolone[h–j] Metronidazole + aminoglycoside[g] or fluoroquinolone[h–j]	A

(continued)

Table 41-3

Common Antimicrobials Used for Prophylaxis in Various Surgical Settings (continued)

Type of Procedure	Recommended Agents[a,b]	Alternative Agents in Patients with β-Lactam Allergy	Strength of Evidence[c]
Ophthalmic	Topical neomycin–polymyxin B–gramicidin or fourth-generation topical fluoroquinolones (gatifloxacin or moxifloxacin) given as 1 drop every 5–15 min for 5 doses[o] Addition of cefazolin 100 mg by subconjunctival injection or intracameral cefazolin 1–2.5 mg or cefuroxime 1 mg at the end of procedure is optional	None	B
Orthopedic			
Clean operations involving hand, knee, or foot and not involving implantation of foreign materials	None	None	C
Spinal procedures with and without instrumentation	Cefazolin	Clindamycin,[d] vancomycin[d]	A
Hip fracture repair	Cefazolin	Clindamycin,[d] vancomycin[d]	A
Implantation of internal fixation devices (e.g., nails, screws, plates, wires)	Cefazolin	Clindamycin,[d] vancomycin[d]	C
Total joint replacement	Cefazolin	Clindamycin,[d] vancomycin[d]	A
Urologic			
Lower tract instrumentation with risk factors for infection (includes transrectal prostate biopsy)	Fluoroquinolone,[h–j] trimethoprim–sulfamethoxazole, cefazolin	Aminoglycoside[g] with or without clindamycin	A
Clean without entry into urinary tract	Cefazolin (the addition of a single dose of an aminoglycoside may be recommended for placement of prosthetic material [e.g., penile prosthesis])	Clindamycin,[d] vancomycin[d]	A
Involving implanted prosthesis	Cefazolin ± aminoglycoside, cefazolin ± aztreonam, ampicillin–sulbactam	Clindamycin ± aminoglycoside or aztreonam, vancomycin ± aminoglycoside or aztreonam	A

Table 41-3

Common Antimicrobials Used for Prophylaxis in Various Surgical Settings *(continued)*

Type of Procedure	Recommended Agents[a,b]	Alternative Agents in Patients with β-Lactam Allergy	Strength of Evidence[c]
Clean with entry into urinary tract	Cefazolin (the addition of a single dose of an aminoglycoside may be recommended for placement of prosthetic material [e.g., penile prosthesis])	Fluoroquinolone,[h–j] aminoglycosidee[g] with or without clindamycin	A
Clean-contaminated	Cefazolin + metronidazole, cefoxitin	Fluoroquinolone,[h–j] aminoglycoside[g] + metronidazole or clindamycin	A
Vascular[p]	Cefazolin	Clindamycin,[d] vancomycin[d]	A
Heart, lung, heart–lung transplantation[q]			
Heart transplantation[r]	Cefazolin	Clindamycin,[d] vancomycin[d]	A (based on cardiac procedures)
Lung and heart–lung transplantation[r,s]	Cefazolin	Clindamycin,[d] vancomycin[d]	A (based on cardiac procedures)
Liver transplantation[q,t]	Piperacillin–tazobactam, cefotaxime + ampicillin	Clindamycin or vancomycin + aminoglycoside[g] or aztreonam or fluoroquinolone[h–j]	B
Pancreas and pancreas–kidney transplantation[r]	Cefazolin, fluconazole (for patients at high risk of fungal infection [e.g., those with enteric drainage of the pancreas])	Clindamycin or vancomycin + aminoglycoside[g] or aztreonam or fluoroquinolone[h–j]	A

(continued)

Table 41-3

Common Antimicrobials Used for Prophylaxis in Various Surgical Settings *(continued)*

Type of Procedure	Recommended Agents[a,b]	Alternative Agents in Patients with β-Lactam Allergy	Strength of Evidence[c]
Plastic surgery	Cefazolin	Clindamycin or vancomycin + aminoglycoside[g] or aztreonam or fluoroquinolone[h–j]	A
Clean with risk factors or clean-contaminated	Cefazolin, ampicillin–sulbactam	Clindamycin,[d] vancomycin[d]	C

[a]The antimicrobial agent should be started within 60 minutes before surgical incision (120 minutes for vancomycin or fluoroquinolones). While single-dose prophylaxis is usually sufficient, the duration of prophylaxis for all procedures should be less than 24 hours. If an agent with a short half-life is used (e.g., cefazolin, cefoxitin), it should be readministered if the procedure duration exceeds the recommended redosing interval (from the time of initiation of the preoperative dose [see Table 41-2]). Readministration may also be warranted if prolonged or excessive bleeding occurs or if there are other factors that may shorten the half-life of the prophylactic agent (e.g., extensive burns). Readministration may not be warranted in patients in whom the half-life of the agent may be prolonged (e.g., patients with renal insufficiency or failure).

[b]For patients known to be colonized with methicillin-resistant *Staphylococcus aureus*, it is reasonable to add a single preoperative dose of vancomycin to the recommended agent(s).

[c]Strength of evidence that supports the use or nonuse of prophylaxis is classified as A (levels I–III), B (levels IV–VI), or C (level VII). Level I evidence is from large, well-conducted, randomized controlled clinical trials. Level II evidence is from small, well-conducted, randomized controlled clinical trials. Level III evidence is from well-conducted cohort studies. Level IV evidence is from well-conducted case–control studies. Level V evidence is from uncontrolled studies that were not well conducted. Level VI evidence is conflicting evidence that tends to favor the recommendation. Level VII evidence is expert opinion.

[d]For procedures in which pathogens other than staphylococci and streptococci are likely, an additional agent with activity against those pathogens could be considered. For example, if there are surveillance data showing that gram-negative organisms are a cause of surgical-site infections (SSIs) for the procedure, practitioners may consider combining clindamycin or vancomycin with another agent (cefazolin if the patient is not β-lactam allergic; aztreonam, gentamicin, or single-dose fluoroquinolone if the patient is β-lactam allergic).

[e]Prophylaxis should be considered for patients at highest risk for postoperative gastroduodenal infections, such as those with increased gastric pH (e.g., those receiving histamine H_2-receptor antagonists or proton-pump inhibitors), gastroduodenal perforation, decreased gastric motility, gastric outlet obstruction, gastric bleeding, morbid obesity, or cancer. Antimicrobial prophylaxis may not be needed when the lumen of the intestinal tract is not entered.

[f]Consider additional antimicrobial coverage with infected biliary tract. See the biliary tract procedures section of this article.

[g]Gentamicin or tobramycin.

[h]Due to increasing resistance of *Escherichia coli* to fluoroquinolones and ampicillin–sulbactam, local population susceptibility profiles should be reviewed prior to use.

[i]Ciprofloxacin or levofloxacin.

[j]Fluoroquinolones are associated with an increased risk of tendonitis and tendon rupture in all ages. However, this risk would be expected to be quite small with single-dose antibiotic prophylaxis. Although the use of fluoroquinolones may be necessary for surgical antibiotic prophylaxis in some children, they are not drugs of first choice in the pediatric population due to an increased incidence of adverse events as compared with controls in some clinical trials.

[k]Ceftriaxone use should be limited to patients requiring antimicrobial treatment for acute cholecystitis or acute biliary tract infections which may not be determined prior to incision, not patients undergoing cholecystectomy for noninfected biliary conditions, including biliary colic or dyskinesia without infection.

[l]Factors that indicate a high risk of infectious complications in laparoscopic cholecystectomy include emergency procedures, diabetes, long procedure duration, intraoperative gallbladder rupture, age of >70 years, conversion from laparoscopic to open cholecystectomy, American Society of Anesthesiologists classification of 3 or greater, episode of colic within 30 days before the procedure, reintervention in less than 1 month for noninfectious complication, acute cholecystitis, bile spillage, jaundice, pregnancy, nonfunctioning gallbladder, immunosuppression, and insertion of prosthetic device. Because a number of these risk factors are not possible to determine before surgical intervention, it may be reasonable to give a single dose of antimicrobial prophylaxis to all patients undergoing laparoscopic cholecystectomy.

[m]For most patients, a mechanical bowel preparation combined with oral neomycin sulfate plus oral erythromycin base or with oral neomycin sulfate plus oral metronidazole should be given in addition to i.v. prophylaxis.

[n]Where there is increasing resistance to first- and second-generation cephalosporins among gram-negative isolates from SSIs, a single dose of ceftriaxone plus metronidazole may be preferred over the routine use of carbapenems.

[o]The necessity of continuing topical antimicrobials postoperatively has not been established.

[p]Prophylaxis is not routinely indicated for brachiocephalic procedures. Although there are no data in support, patients undergoing brachiocephalic procedures involving vascular prostheses or patch implantation (e.g., carotid endarterectomy) may benefit from prophylaxis.

[q]These guidelines reflect recommendations for perioperative antibiotic prophylaxis to prevent SSIs and do not provide recommendations for prevention of opportunistic infections in immunosuppressed transplantation patients (e.g., for antifungal or antiviral medications).

[r]Patients who have left-ventricular assist devices as a bridge and who are chronically infected might also benefit from coverage of the infecting microorganism.

[s]The prophylactic regimen may need to be modified to provide coverage against any potential pathogens, including gram-negative (e.g., *Pseudomonas aeruginosa*) or fungal organisms, isolated from the donor lung or the recipient before transplantation. Patients undergoing lung transplantation with negative pretransplantation cultures should receive antimicrobial prophylaxis as appropriate for other types of cardiothoracic surgeries. Patients undergoing lung transplantation for cystic fibrosis should receive 7–14 days of treatment with antimicrobials selected according to pretransplantation culture and susceptibility results. This treatment may include additional antibacterial or antifungal agents.

[t]The prophylactic regimen may need to be modified to provide coverage against any potential pathogens, including vancomycin-resistant enterococci, isolated from the recipient before transplantation.

Bratzler DW, Dellinger, EP, Olsen KM, et al; American Society of Health-System Pharmacists; Infectious Diseases Society of America; Surgical Infection Society; Society for Healthcare Epidemiology of America. Clinical practice guidelines for antimicrobial prophylaxis in surgery. *Am J Health Syst Pharm.* 2013;70(3):195–283. http://www.ashp.org/surgical-guidelines. Accessed February 24, 2014.

In patients with documented IgE-mediated anaphylactic reactions, β-lactam antibiotics can usually be substituted with clindamycin or vancomycin.[16] Vancomycin may also be considered when methicillin-resistant *S. aureus* (MRSA) is considered likely, for example in children or elderly patients known to be colonized with MRSA. Nasal application of mupirocin has been considered as an alternative and has been found to be effective in eliminating MRSA colonization in adults and children. It is U.S. Food and Drug Administration approved for eradication of colonization in adults and health care workers. Treatment with mupirocin is effective in reducing *S. aureus* infection in documented carriers. Preoperative screening is recommended to identify high-risk patients who would benefit from decolonization and to guide appropriate preoperative antibiotic selection for those with resistant organisms. Routine prophylaxis with vancomycin is not recommended for any patient population in the absence of documented or highly suspected colonization or infection with MRSA (recent hospitalization of nursing home stay and hemodialysis patients) or known IgE-mediated response to β-lactam antibiotics.[18] The recommendation against routine prophylaxis with vancomycin is due to concerns about selection of resistant organisms, its risk of inducing hemodynamic instability due to histamine release (red man syndrome; Fig. 41-1) if given rapidly, and evidence that vancomycin is less effective than cephazolin in methicillin-susceptible *S. aureus*.[19,20]

Clean-contaminated procedures such as colorectal and abdominal surgeries require additional coverage for gram-negative rods and anaerobes in addition to skin flora. Metronidazole can be added to cefazolin or cefoxitin, cefotetan, ampicillin-sulbactam, ertapenem, or ceftriaxone.

Bowel preparation with oral antimicrobials has been studied as a potentially less costly alternative. Mechanical bowel preparation alone does not reduce infection, but selective decontamination of the digestive tract with oral topical polymyxin, tobramycin, and amphotericin eradicates the colonization gram-negative microorganisms, *S. aureus*, and yeasts from oral cavity to rectum. Vancomycin would be active against MRSA but is not recommended because gram-positive flora plays an important role in the resistance to colonization.[21] In a meta-analysis of eight studies, the combination of oral treatment and perioperative venous prophylaxis was found to be superior to IV prophylaxis alone in preventing surgical site infection and anastomotic leak. However, older studies found that oral antibiotics alone are not a solution. A randomized controlled study was stopped because of higher rate of infection in the oral neomycin and erythromycin group (41%) compared with the single-dose IV metronidazole and ceftriaxone group.[22] Another trial of oral metronidazole and kanamycin compared with the same medications given IV found an increased rate of postoperative sepsis and pseudomembranous colitis in the oral group.[23] Pseudomembranous colitis is the most frequent complication of prophylactic antimicrobials, including the IV cephalosporins. Additional toxicities are covered in Table 41-4.

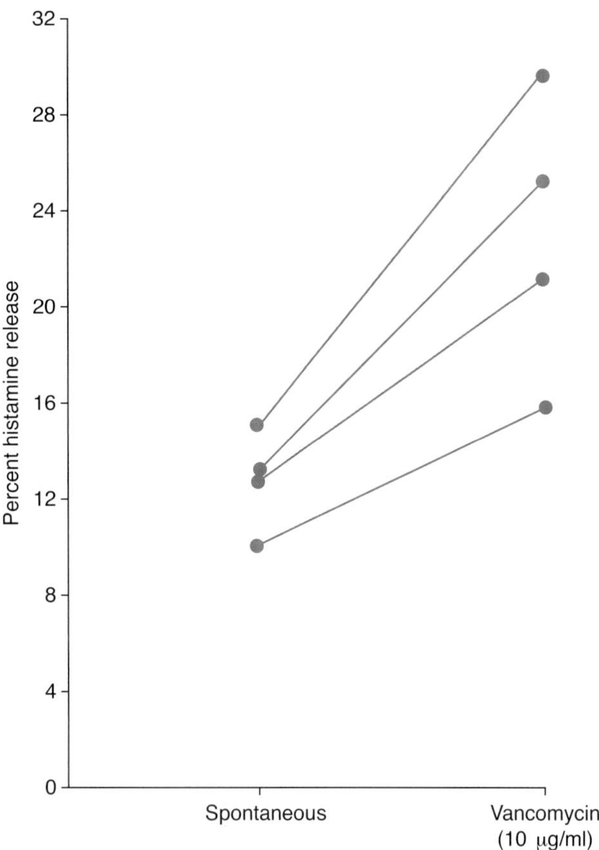

FIGURE 41-1 Histamine release (%) from dispersed human cutaneous mast cells after the administration of vancomycin. (From Levy JH, Kettlekamp N, Goertz P, et al. Histamine release by vancomycin. A mechanism for hypotension in man. *Anesthesiology*. 1987;67:122–125, with permission.)

Antimicrobial Selection

Prompt identification of the causative organism is essential for the selection of appropriate antimicrobial drugs to treat ongoing infection. The efficacy of antimicrobial therapy depends on drug delivery to the site of infection. Transport across the blood–brain barrier varies greatly among antimicrobials. Antimicrobial therapy is more likely to be effective if the infected material (foreign body, prosthesis) is removed. Infections behind obstructing lesions such as pneumonia behind a blocked bronchus will not respond to antimicrobials until the obstruction is relieved.

Nosocomial Infections

Nearly 80% of nosocomial infections occur in three sites (urinary tract, respiratory system, and bloodstream). The incidence of nosocomial infections is highly associated

Table 41-4

Direct Drug Toxicity Associated with Administration of Antimicrobials

Toxicity	Antimicrobial
Allergic reactions	All antimicrobials but most often with β-lactam derivatives
Nephrotoxicity	Aminoglycosides
	Polymyxins
	Amphotericin B
Neutropenia	Penicillins
	Cephalosporins
	Vancomycin
Inhibition of platelet aggregation	Penicillins (high doses)
Prolonged prothrombin time	Cephalosporins
Bone marrow suppression (aplastic anemia, pancytopenia)	Chloramphenicol
	Flucytosine
	Linezolid (reversible)
Hemolytic anemia	Chloramphenicol
	Sulfonamides
	Nitrofurantoin
	Primaquine
Agranulocytosis	Macrolides
	Trimethoprim-sulfamethoxazole
Leukopenia and thrombocytopenia (folate deficiency)	Trimethoprim
Normocytic normochromic anemia	Amphotericin B
Ototoxicity	Aminoglycosides
	Vancomycin (auditory neurotoxicity)
	Minocycline (vestibular toxicity)
Seizures	Penicillins and other β-lactams (high doses, azotemic patients, history of epilepsy)
	Metronidazole
Neuromuscular blockade	Aminoglycosides
Peripheral neuropathy	Nitrofurantoin (renal failure)
	Isoniazid (prevent with pyridoxine)
	Metronidazole
Benign intracranial hypertension	Tetracyclines
Optic neuritis	Ethambutol
Hepatotoxicity	Isoniazid
	Rifampin
	Tetracyclines (high doses)
	β-Lactam antimicrobials (high doses)
	Nitrofurantoin
	Erythromycin
	Sulfonamides
Increased plasma bilirubin concentrations	Quinupristin-dalfopristin
	Erythromycin
Gastrointestinal irritation	Tetracyclines
Prolongation of QTc interval	Erythromycin
	Fluoroquinolones
Exaggerated sympathomimetic effects in patients receiving monoamine oxidase inhibitors	Linezolid
Hyperkalemia	Trimethoprim-sulfamethoxazole

Table 41-4

Direct Drug Toxicity Associated with Administration of Antimicrobials *(continued)*

Toxicity	Antimicrobial
Tendinitis	Fluoroquinolones
Arthralgias and myalgias	Quinupristin-dalfopristin
Photosensitivity	Sulfonamides Tetracyclines Fluoroquinolones
Teratogenicity	Tetracyclines Metronidazole Rifampin Trimethoprim Fluoroquinolones

with the use of devices such as ventilators, vascular access catheters, and urinary catheters. Intravascular access catheters are the most common causes of bacteremia or fungemia in hospitalized patients.[24] The organism infecting access catheters most commonly comes from the colonized hub or lumen and reflect skin flora (*S. aureus* and *S. epidermidis*). Initial therapy of suspected intravascular catheter infection usually includes vancomycin because of the high incidence of MRSA and methicillin-resistant *S. epidermidis* in the nosocomial environment.

Special Patient Groups

Parturients

Administration of antimicrobials during pregnancy introduces the question of safety for the mother and fetus (Table 41-5). Most antimicrobials cross the placenta and enter maternal milk. The immature fetal liver may lack enzymes necessary to metabolize certain drugs such that pharmacokinetics and toxicities in the fetus are often different from those in older children and adults. Teratogenicity is a concern when any drug is administered during early pregnancy. Increases in maternal blood volume, glomerular filtration rate, and hepatic metabolic activity may decrease plasma antimicrobial concentrations (10% to 50%), especially late in pregnancy and in the early postpartum period. In some parturients, delayed gastric emptying may decrease absorption of orally administered antimicrobials.

Elderly Patients

Physiologic changes that occur with increasing age can alter oral absorption (decreased gastric acidity, reduced gastrointestinal motility), distribution (increased total body fat, decreased plasma albumin concentrations), metabolism (decreased hepatic blood flow), and excretion (decreased glomerular filtration rate) of antimicrobials. Penicillins and cephalosporins, because of their large therapeutic index, obviate the need for significant changes in dosage schedules in elderly patients who have normal serum creatinine concentrations. Conversely, administration of aminoglycosides and vancomycin to elderly patients may require adjustments in dosing regimens. Measurement of plasma concentrations of antimicrobials and monitoring of renal function may be indicated when administering certain antimicrobials to elderly patients.

HIV-Infected Patients

There has been concern about increased risk of postoperative infection in HIV-infected patients based on their increased risk for opportunistic infection in the setting of reduced T4 cell counts. Several recent studies have addressed this issue and produced conflicting results.[25–27] Favorable results appear to be related to good preoperative control on an antiretroviral regimen with preserved T4 cell counts.[28]

Antibacterial Drugs Commonly Used in the Perioperative Period

Penicillins

The basic structure of penicillins is a dicyclic nucleus (aminopenicillanic acid) that consists of a thiazolidine ring connected to a β-lactam ring. The penicillins may be classified into subgroups because of their structure, β-lactamase susceptibility, and spectrum of activity. The bactericidal action of penicillins reflects the ability of

Table 41-5

Antimicrobials in Pregnancy

Drug	Maternal Toxicity	Fetal Toxicity	Excreted in Colostrum
Considered safe			
Penicillins	Allergic reactions	None known	Trace
Cephalosporins	Allergic reactions	None known	Trace
Erythromycin base	Allergic reactions Gastrointestinal irritation	None known	Yes
Use cautiously			
Aminoglycosides	Ototoxicity Nephrotoxicity	Ototoxicity	Yes
Clindamycin	Allergic reactions Colitis	None known	Trace
Ethambutol	Optic neuritis	None known	Unknown
Isoniazid	Allergic reactions Hepatotoxicity	Neuropathy Seizures	Yes
Rifampin	Allergic reactions Hepatotoxicity	None known	Yes
Sulfonamides	Allergic reactions	Kernicterus (at term) Hemolysis (G6PD deficiency)	Yes
Avoid			
Metronidazole	Allergic reactions Alcohol intolerance Peripheral neuropathy	None known (teratogenic in animals)	Yes
Contraindicated			
Chloramphenicol	Bone marrow depression	Gray syndrome	Yes
Erythromycin estolate	Hepatotoxicity	None known	Yes
Nalidixic acid	Gastrointestinal irritation	Increased intracranial pressure	Unknown
Fluoroquinolones	Gastrointestinal irritation	Arthropathies (animals)	Unknown
Nitrofurantoin	Allergic reactions Peripheral neuropathy Gastrointestinal irritation	Hemolysis (G6PD deficiency)	Trace
Tetracyclines	Hepatotoxicity Nephrotoxicity	Tooth discoloration and dysplasia Impaired bone growth	Yes
Trimethoprim	Allergic reactions	Teratogenicity	Yes

these antimicrobials to interfere with the synthesis of peptidoglycan, which is an essential component of cell walls of susceptible bacteria. Penicillins also decrease the availability of an inhibitor of murein hydrolase such that the uninhibited enzyme can then destroy (lyse) the structural integrity of bacterial cell walls. Cell membranes of resistant gram-negative bacteria are in general resistant to penicillins because they prevent access to sites where synthesis of peptidoglycan is taking place.

Clinical Indications

Penicillin is the drug of choice for treatment of pneumococcal, streptococcal, and meningococcal infections. Gonococci have gradually become more resistant to penicillin, requiring higher doses for adequate treatment. Treatment of syphilis with penicillin is highly effective. Penicillin is the drug of choice for treating all forms of actinomycosis and clostridial infections causing gas gangrene.

Prophylactic administration of penicillin is highly effective against streptococcal infections, accounting for its value in patients with rheumatic fever. Transient bacteremia occurs in the majority of patients undergoing dental extractions, emphasizing the importance of prophylactic penicillin in patients with congenital or acquired heart disease or tissue implants undergoing dental procedures. Transient bacteremia may also accompany surgical procedures, such as tonsillectomy and operations on the genitourinary and gastrointestinal tracts, and vaginal delivery.

Administration of high doses of penicillin G IV to patients with renal dysfunction may result in neurotoxicity and hyperkalemia (10 million U of penicillin G contains 16 mEq of potassium). If this amount of potassium introduces a risk to the patient, a sodium salt of penicillin G or a sodium salt of a similar penicillin, such as ampicillin or carbenicillin, can be substituted for the aqueous penicillin G.

Other drugs should not be mixed with penicillin as the combination may inactivate the antimicrobial. Intrathecal administration of penicillins is not recommended because these drugs are potent convulsants when administered by this route. Furthermore, arachnoiditis and encephalopathy may follow intrathecal penicillin administration.

Excretion

Renal excretion of penicillin is rapid (60% to 90% of an intramuscular [IM] dose is excreted in the first hour), such that the plasma concentration decreases to 50% of its peak value within 1 hour after injection. Approximately 10% is eliminated by glomerular filtration, and 90% is eliminated by renal tubular secretion. Anuria increases the elimination half-time of penicillin G approximately 10-fold.

Duration of Action

Methods to prolong the duration of action of penicillin include the simultaneous administration of probenecid, which blocks the renal tubular secretion of penicillin. Alternatively, the IM injection of poorly soluble salts of penicillin, such as procaine or benzathine, delays absorption and thus prolongs the duration of action. Procaine penicillin contains 120 mg of the local anesthetic for every 300,000 U of the antimicrobial. Possible hypersensitivity to procaine must be considered when selecting this form of the antimicrobial for administration.

Penicillinase-Resistant Penicillins

The major mechanism of resistance to the penicillins is bacterial production of β-lactamase enzymes that hydrolyze the β-lactam ring, rendering the antimicrobial molecule inactive. Methicillin (dimethoxybenzylpenicillin), oxacillin, nafcillin, cloxacillin, and dicloxacillin are not susceptible to hydrolysis by staphylococcal penicillinases that would otherwise hydrolyze the cyclic amide bond of the β-lactam ring and render the antimicrobial inactive. Specific indications for these drugs are infections caused by staphylococci known to produce this enzyme. Penetration of nafcillin into the central nervous system (CNS) is sufficient to treat staphylococcal meningitis. Parenteral methicillin has largely been superseded by oxacillin and nafcillin. Hemorrhagic cystitis and an allergic interstitial nephritis (hematuria, proteinuria) may accompany administration of methicillin. Hepatitis has been associated with high-dose oxacillin therapy. Renal excretion of methicillin, oxacillin, and cloxacillin is extensive. More than 80% of an IV dose of nafcillin is excreted in the bile, which may be an advantage when high-dose therapy is necessary in a patient with impaired renal function.

Oxacillin and nafcillin, unlike methicillin, are relatively stable in an acidic medium, resulting in adequate systemic absorption after oral administration. Nevertheless, variable absorption from the gastrointestinal tract often dictates a parenteral route of administration for treatment of serious infections caused by penicillinase-producing staphylococci. Cloxacillin and dicloxacillin are available only as oral preparations and may be preferable because they produce higher blood levels than do oxacillin and nafcillin.

Penicillinase-Susceptible Broad-Spectrum Penicillins (Second-Generation Penicillins)

Broad-spectrum penicillins, such as ampicillin, amoxicillin, and carbenicillin, have a wider range of activity than other penicillins, being bactericidal against gram-positive and gram-negative bacteria. They are, nevertheless, all inactivated by penicillinase produced by certain gram-negative and gram-positive bacteria. Therefore, these drugs are not effective against most staphylococcal infections.

Ampicillin

Ampicillin (α-aminobenzylpenicillin) has a broader range of activity than penicillin G. Its spectrum encompasses not only pneumococci, meningococci, gonococci, and various streptococci but also a number of gram-negative bacilli, such as *Haemophilus influenzae* and *Escherichia coli*. Ampicillin is stable in acid and thus is well absorbed after oral administration, although peak plasma concentrations are lower than those achieved after administration of penicillin V. Approximately 50% of an oral dose of ampicillin is excreted unchanged by the kidneys in the first 6 hours, emphasizing that renal function greatly influences the duration of action of this antimicrobial. Ampicillin also appears in the bile and undergoes enterohepatic circulation. Among the penicillins, ampicillin is associated with the highest incidence of skin rash (9%), which typically appears 7 to 10 days after initiation of therapy. Many of these rashes are due to protein impurities in the commercial preparation of the drug and do not represent true allergic reactions.

Amoxicillin

Amoxicillin is chemically identical to ampicillin except for an −OH substituent instead of an −H on the side chain. Its spectrum of activity is identical to that of ampicillin, but it is more efficiently absorbed from the gastrointestinal tract than ampicillin, and effective concentrations are present in the circulation for twice as long.

Extended-Spectrum Carboxypenicillins (Third-Generation Penicillins)

Carbenicillin

Carbenicillin (α-carboxybenzylpenicillin) results from the change from an amino to carboxy substituent on the side chain of ampicillin. The principal advantage of carbenicillin is its effectiveness in the treatment of infections caused by *Pseudomonas aeruginosa* and certain *Proteus* strains that are resistant to ampicillin. This antimicrobial is penicillinase susceptible and therefore ineffective against most strains of *S. aureus*. Carbenicillin is not absorbed from the gastrointestinal tract; therefore, it must be administered parenterally. The elimination half-time is approximately 1 hour and is prolonged to approximately 2 hours when there is hepatic or renal dysfunction. Approximately 85% of the unchanged drug is recovered in urine over 9 hours. Probenecid, by delaying renal excretion of the drug, increases the plasma concentration of carbenicillin by approximately 50%.

The sodium load administered with a large dose of carbenicillin (30 to 40 g) is considerable because greater than 10% of carbenicillin is sodium (about 5 mEq/g). Congestive heart failure may develop in susceptible patients in response to this acute drug-produced sodium load. Hypokalemia and metabolic alkalosis may occur because of obligatory excretion of potassium with the large amount of nonreabsorbable carbenicillin. Carbenicillin interferes with normal platelet aggregation such that bleeding time is prolonged but platelet count remains normal.

Extended-Spectrum Acylaminopenicillins (Fourth-Generation Penicillins)

The acylaminopenicillins (mezlocillin, piperacillin, azlocillin) have the broadest spectrum of activity of all the penicillins. Like the carboxypenicillins, the acylaminopenicillins are derivatives of ampicillin. These drugs are ineffective against penicillinase-producing strains of *S. aureus*. The acylaminopenicillins have lower sodium content than the carboxypenicillins but otherwise the side effects are similar. Clinical studies have not demonstrated that these antimicrobials are superior to the carboxypenicillins.

Penicillin β-Lactamase Inhibitor Combinations

Clavulanic acid, sulbactam, and tazobactam are β-lactam compounds that have little intrinsic antimicrobial activity. However, these compounds bind irreversibly to the β-lactamase enzymes, which are produced by many bacteria, thus inactivating these enzymes and rendering the organisms sensitive to β-lactamase–susceptible penicillins. Clavulanic acid is available with oral amoxicillin and parenteral ampicillin preparations have been combined with sulbactam.

Cephalosporins

Cephalosporins, like the penicillins, are bactericidal antimicrobials that inhibit bacterial cell wall synthesis and have a low intrinsic toxicity. These antimicrobials are derived from 7-aminocephalosporanic acid. Resistance to the cephalosporins, as to the penicillins, may be due to an inability of the antimicrobial to penetrate to its site of action. Bacteria can also produce cephalosporinases (β-lactamases), which disrupt the β-lactam structure of cephalosporins and thus inhibit their antimicrobial activity. Like the newer penicillins, the new cephalosporins have an extraordinarily broad spectrum of antimicrobial action but are expensive.

Individual cephalosporins differ significantly with respect to the extent of absorption after oral ingestion, severity of pain produced by IM injection, and protein binding. IV administration of any of the cephalosporins can cause thrombophlebitis. Diacetyl metabolites of cephalosporins can occur and are associated with decreased antimicrobial activity.

A positive Coombs' reaction frequently occurs in patients who receive large doses of cephalosporins. Hemolysis, however, is rarely associated with this response. Nephrotoxicity owing to cephalosporins, with the exception of cephaloridine, is less frequent than after administration of aminoglycosides or polymyxins.

The incidence of allergic reactions in patients being treated with cephalosporins ranges from 1% to 10%. The majority of the allergic reactions consist of cutaneous manifestations, which occur 24 hours after drug exposure. Life-threatening anaphylaxis is estimated to occur in 0.02% of treated patients.[29] Because the cephalosporins share immunologic cross-reactivity, patients who are allergic to one cephalosporin are likely to be allergic to others. The possibility of cross-reactivity between cephalosporins and penicillins seems to be very infrequent, and cephalosporins are often selected as alternative antimicrobials in patients with a history of penicillin allergy.[29]

Cephalosporins and Allergy to Penicillins

Hypersensitivity is the most common adverse reaction to β-lactam antimicrobials. Allergic reactions are noted in 1% to 10% of patients treated with penicillins, making these antimicrobials the most allergenic of all drugs.[30] Most often, the allergic response is a delayed reaction characterized by a maculopapular rash and/or fever. Less often but more serious is immediate hypersensitivity that is mediated by IgE antibodies. Manifestations of immediate hypersensitivity may include laryngeal edema, bronchospasm, and cardiovascular collapse. Allergic reactions may occur in the absence of previous known exposure to any of the penicillins. This may reflect prior unrecognized exposure to penicillin, presumably in ingested foods. Allergic reactions can occur with any dose or route of administration, although severe anaphylactic reactions are more often associated with parenteral than with oral administration. Some patients who experience cutaneous reactions may continue to receive the offending penicillin or receive the same penicillin in the future without experiencing a similar response.

The penicillin molecule itself is probably unable to form a complete antigen, but instead the ring structure of penicillin is opened to form a hapten metabolite, penicilloyl. Approximately 95% of patients allergic to penicillin form this penicilloyl-protein conjugate (the major antigenic determinant); the remaining allergic patients form 6-aminopenicillic acid and benzylpenamaldic acid (minor antigenic determinants). Skin testing with a polyvalent skin test antigen, penicilloyl-polylysine, makes it possible to detect most patients who would develop a life-threatening allergic reaction if treated with a penicillin antimicrobial. Nevertheless, minor antigenic determinants that would not be detected by skin testing may produce severe allergic reactions.

Cross-Reactivity

The presence of a common nucleus (β-lactam ring) in the structure of all penicillins means that allergy to one penicillin increases the likelihood of an allergic reaction to another penicillin. Furthermore, there would seem to be the potential for cross-reactivity between penicillins and cephalosporins as they both share a common β-lactam ring. However, actual cross-reactivity is rare.[17,29]

Classification

Cephalosporins are classified as first-, second-, and third-generation because of their antimicrobial spectrum. In general, activity against gram-positive cocci decreases, and activity against gram-negative cocci increases from the first- to third-generation cephalosporins. First-generation cephalosporins are inexpensive, exhibit low toxicity, and are as active as second- and third-generation cephalosporins against staphylococci and nonenterococcal streptococci. For these reasons, first-generation cephalosporins have been commonly selected for antimicrobial prophylaxis in patients undergoing cardiovascular, orthopedic, biliary, pelvic, and intraabdominal surgery (see the section "Antimicrobial Prophylaxis for Surgical Procedures"). All cephalosporins can penetrate into joints and can readily cross the placenta.

First-Generation Cephalosporins

Cephalothin is the prototype of first-generation cephalosporins. Like most other cephalosporins, cephalothin is excreted largely unaltered by the kidneys, emphasizing the need to decrease the dose in the presence of renal dysfunction. Oral absorption is poor and IM injection is painful, accounting for its common administration by the IV route. Although cephalothin is present in many tissues and fluids, it does not enter the cerebrospinal fluid in significant amounts and is not recommended for treatment of meningitis. Cefazolin has essentially the same antimicrobial spectrum as cephalothin but has the advantage of achieving higher blood levels, presumably due to slower renal elimination. In this regard, cefazolin is viewed as the drug of choice for antimicrobial prophylaxis for many surgeries. This drug is well tolerated after IM or IV injection.

Second-Generation Cephalosporins

Cefoxitin and cefamandole are examples of second-generation cephalosporins with extended activity against gram-negative bacteria. Cefoxitin is resistant to cephalosporinases produced by gram-negative bacteria. Cefamandole is pharmacologically similar to cefoxitin, but its methylthiotetrazole side chain poses a risk of bleeding and disulfiram-like reactions with concurrent use of alcohol. Both drugs are excreted predominantly unchanged by the kidneys. Cefuroxime is more effective than cefamandole against *H. influenzae* and is the only second-generation cephalosporin effective in the treatment of meningitis.

Third-Generation Cephalosporins

Third-generation cephalosporins have an enhanced ability to resist hydrolysis by the β-lactamases of many gram-negative bacilli including *E. coli*, *Klebsiella*, *Proteus*, and *H. influenzae*. Unlike older cephalosporins, the third-generation cephalosporins achieve therapeutic levels in the cerebrospinal fluid and can be used to treat meningitis. The third-generation cephalosporins seem to have the same relatively low toxicities as the older cephalosporins.

Cefotaxime was the first third-generation cephalosporin and has been effective in a broad range of infections, including meningitis caused by gram-negative bacilli other than *Pseudomonas*. The elimination half-time of this antimicrobial is approximately 1 hour, with clearance via the kidneys and hepatic metabolism. An adjustment in dosage or dosing interval is indicated in patients with renal dysfunction who are being treated with this drug. Approximately 30% of cefotaxime is excreted as a desacetyl derivative that has antibacterial activity and is synergistic with the parent compound. Ceftriaxone has the longest elimination half-time of any third-generation cephalosporin and is highly effective against gram-negative bacilli, especially *Neisseria* and *Haemophilus*. Cefixime is an orally effective third-generation cephalosporin that is as active as other cephalosporins against pneumococci, group A streptococci, and *H. influenzae* but less active against *S. aureus* and not active against anaerobes such as *Pseudomonas*. The spectrum of activity of cefixime and a single daily dose make it attractive for upper respiratory tract infections, but less expensive alternatives are available.

Other β-Lactam Antimicrobials

Aztreonam

Aztreonam is a monobactam antimicrobial that lacks the thiazolidine ring present in penicillins and the dihydrothiazine ring found in cephalosporins. The antimicrobial activity of this drug is limited to gram-negative bacteria. Aztreonam is not absorbed from the gastrointestinal tract, but therapeutic blood levels are achieved after IM or IV administration in most body tissues and fluids, including cerebrospinal fluid. The elimination half-time is about 1.5 hours, and clearance is principally by glomerular filtration. Neither nephrotoxicity nor bleeding disorders have been reported. A unique advantage is the absence of any cross-reactivity between aztreonam and circulating antibodies of penicillin- or cephalosporin-allergic patients.[31] Because aztreonam combines the activity of the aminoglycosides with the low toxicity of the β-lactam antimicrobials, it can replace aminoglycosides in the treatment of many gram-negative infections. A potential disadvantage of aztreonam is the development of enterococcal superinfections. This antimicrobial is significantly more expensive than aminoglycosides.

Aminoglycoside Antimicrobials

Aminoglycosides are poorly lipid-soluble antimicrobials that are rapidly bactericidal for aerobic gram-negative bacteria. As would be predicted with the poor lipid solubility of these drugs, less than 1% of an orally administered aminoglycoside is absorbed into the systemic circulation. Aminoglycosides have a volume of distribution similar to the extracellular fluid volume and undergo extensive renal excretion due almost exclusively to glomerular filtration. There is a linear relationship between the plasma creatinine concentration and the elimination half-time of aminoglycosides. In the presence of normal renal function, the elimination half-time of aminoglycosides is 2 to 3 hours and is prolonged 20- to 40-fold in the presence of renal failure. Determination of the plasma concentration of aminoglycosides is an essential guide to the safe administration of these antimicrobials in the setting of renal dysfunction. The role of aminoglycosides is influenced by their toxicity (see the section "Side Effects") and cost-effectiveness relative to other antibiotics with broad gram-negative coverage.

Streptomycin was the first parenterally administered antimicrobial that was active against many gram-negative bacilli and *Mycobacterium tuberculosis*. Current use of this drug is limited because of the rapid emergence of resistant organisms, the frequent occurrence of vestibular damage during prolonged treatment, and the availability of less toxic antimicrobials.

Gentamicin is active against *P. aeruginosa* as well as the gram-negative bacilli. Gentamicin penetrates pleural, ascitic, and synovial fluids in the presence of inflammation. Monitoring plasma concentrations of gentamicin is the best approach for recognizing potentially toxic levels (>9 μg/mL). If plasma concentrations of gentamicin cannot be monitored, the dose can be adjusted based on the plasma creatinine concentration.

Amikacin is a semisynthetic derivative of kanamycin that has the advantage of not being associated with the development of resistance. The principal use of amikacin is in the treatment of infections caused by gentamicin- or tobramycin-resistant gram-negative bacilli. Unlike other aminoglycosides, this drug should not be administered in combination with penicillin, which may result in antagonism of the bactericidal actions of penicillin against some strains of *Enterococcus faecalis*. The incidence of nephrotoxicity and ototoxicity is similar to that produced by gentamicin.

Neomycin is commonly used for topical application to treat infections of the skin (as after burn injury), cornea, and mucous membranes. Allergic reactions occur in 6% to 8% of patients treated with topical neomycin. Oral neomycin does not undergo systemic absorption and is thus administered to decrease bacterial flora in the intestine before gastrointestinal surgery and as an adjunct to the therapy of hepatic coma (decreases blood ammonia concentrations).

Side Effects

The side effects of aminoglycosides that limit their clinical usefulness include ototoxicity, nephrotoxicity, skeletal muscle weakness, and potentiation of nondepolarizing neuromuscular blocking drugs. These side effects parallel the plasma concentration of the aminoglycoside, emphasizing the need to decrease the dose of these drugs in patients with renal dysfunction.

Ototoxicity

Ototoxicity manifests as vestibular dysfunction, auditory dysfunction, or both and parallels the accumulation of aminoglycosides in the perilymph of the inner ear. There is drug-induced destruction of vestibular or cochlear sensory hairs that is dose-dependent and most likely occurs with chronic therapy, especially in elderly patients, in whom renal dysfunction is more likely. Furosemide, mannitol, and probably other diuretics seem to accentuate the ototoxic effects of aminoglycosides. Vestibular toxicity manifests as nystagmus, vertigo, nausea, and the acute onset of Ménière's syndrome. Auditory dysfunction manifests as tinnitus or a sensation of pressure or fullness in the ears. Deafness may develop suddenly.

Nephrotoxicity

Aminoglycosides accumulate in the renal cortex and can produce acute tubular necrosis that initially manifests as an inability to concentrate urine and the appearance of proteinuria and red blood cell casts. These changes are usually reversible if the drug is discontinued. Neomycin is the most nephrotoxic of the aminoglycosides and therefore is not administered by the parenteral route.

Skeletal Muscle Weakness

Skeletal muscle weakness can occur with the intrapleural or intraperitoneal institution of large doses of aminoglycosides. This effect is most likely because of the ability of aminoglycosides to inhibit the prejunctional release of acetylcholine while also decreasing postsynaptic sensitivity to the neurotransmitter. IV administration of calcium overcomes the effect of aminoglycosides at the neuromuscular junction. Patients with myasthenia gravis are uniquely susceptible to skeletal muscle weakness if treated with an aminoglycoside. Administration of a single dose of an aminoglycoside is unlikely to produce skeletal muscle weakness in an otherwise healthy patient.

Macrolides

Macrolides are stable in the presence of acidic gastric fluid, and as a result, these antimicrobials are well absorbed from the gastrointestinal tract. Structurally, these antimicrobials are characterized by 14 to 16 carbon atoms joined together in a complex, central molecule that is linked to various side chains.

Erythromycin

Erythromycin has a spectrum of activity, which includes most gram-positive bacteria, *Streptococcus pneumoniae*, *S. aureus*, *Moraxella catarrhalis*, *H. influenzae*, *Mycoplasma*, *Chlamydia pneumoniae*, and *Corynebacterium diphtheriae*. In patients who cannot tolerate penicillins or cephalosporins, erythromycin or clindamycin are an effective alternative for the treatment of streptococcal pharyngitis, bronchitis, and pneumonia. Gastrointestinal intolerance is the most common side effect which severely limits its use. IV preparations are available for treatment of severe infections, but prolonged use by this route of administration is limited by the common occurrence of thrombophlebitis at the injection site and development of tinnitus or hearing loss in many patients. Severe nausea and vomiting may accompany infusion of erythromycin. Erythromycin is excreted largely in bile and only to a minor degree in urine. The dosage need not be altered in the presence of renal failure.

Effects on QTc

Oral erythromycin prolongs cardiac repolarization and is associated with reports of torsades de pointes.[32] Because erythromycin is extensively metabolized by cytochrome P-450 3A (CYP3A) isozymes, commonly used medications that inhibit the effects of CYP3A may increase plasma erythromycin concentrations thus increasing the risk of ventricular dysrhythmias and sudden death. The concurrent use of erythromycin and strong inhibitors of CYP3A such as ketoconazole is not recommended.

Azithromycin

Azithromycin resembles erythromycin in its antimicrobial spectrum, but an extraordinarily prolonged elimination half-time (68 hours) permits once-a-day dosing for 5 days (500 mg on day 1 and 250 mg on days 2 to 5). Tissue levels of azithromycin can be expected to remain at therapeutic levels for 4 to 7 days after a 5-day treatment course. Unlike clarithromycin, bioavailability of azithromycin is decreased by food such that the drug should be administered 1 hour before or 2 hours after meals.

Clindamycin

Clindamycin resembles erythromycin in antimicrobial activity, but it is more active against many anaerobes. Because severe pseudomembranous colitis can be a complication of clindamycin therapy, this drug should be used only to treat infections that cannot be adequately treated by less toxic antimicrobials. Significant diarrhea in patients treated with clindamycin is an indication to discontinue this drug and initiate evaluation for pseudomembranous colitis. However, clindamycin is indicated in the treatment of or prophylaxis for serious infections caused by susceptible anaerobes, particularly those originating in the gastrointestinal tract and female genital tract.

Only about 10% of administered clindamycin is excreted in an active form in urine; the remainder is changed into inactive metabolites. In patients with renal dysfunction, the elimination half-time of clindamycin is only slightly prolonged, and little change in dosage is required. In patients with severe liver disease, the dose of clindamycin may need to be decreased.

Side Effects

Clindamycin produces prejunctional and postjunctional effects at the neuromuscular junction, and these effects cannot be readily antagonized with calcium or anticholinesterase drugs. Large doses of clindamycin can induce profound and long-lasting neuromuscular blockade in the absence of nondepolarizing muscle relaxants and after full recovery from the effects of succinylcholine has occurred.[33] Skin rashes occur in about 10% of patients treated with clindamycin.

Vancomycin

Vancomycin is a bactericidal glycopeptide antimicrobial that impairs cell wall synthesis of gram-positive bacteria. The oral route of administration is used only for the treatment of staphylococcal enterocolitis and antimicrobial-associated pseudomembranous enterocolitis, taking advantage of the fact that vancomycin is poorly absorbed from the gastrointestinal tract. Vancomycin is administered IV for the treatment of severe staphylococcal infections or streptococcal or enterococcal endocarditis in patients who are allergic to penicillins or cephalosporins. Concomitant administration of an aminoglycoside is often necessary when vancomycin is used in the treatment of enterococcal endocarditis. Vancomycin is the drug of choice in the treatment of infections caused by MRSA.

Vancomycin can be useful in the therapy of prosthetic heart valve endocarditis caused by *S. epidermidis*. In this setting, vancomycin is often administered in combination with gentamicin or rifampin. Vancomycin is also used for prophylaxis against endocarditis in penicillin- and cephalosporin-allergic patients who have valvular heart disease and are undergoing dental procedures.

When vancomycin is administered IV, the recommendation is to infuse the calculated dose (10 to 15 mg/kg) over 60 minutes to minimize the occurrence of drug-induced histamine release and hypotension. As such it can be begun 2 hours prior to surgery for prophylaxis. Infusion over 60 minutes produces sustained plasma concentrations for up to 12 hours. Vancomycin is principally excreted by the kidneys, with 90% of a dose being recovered unchanged in urine. The elimination half-time is approximately 6 hours and may be greatly prolonged (as long as 9 days) in the presence of renal failure. Determination of plasma vancomycin levels is an important guide to dosage (20 to 30 μg/mL is considered ideal) when this antimicrobial must be administered in the presence of renal dysfunction.

Side Effects

Rapid infusion (<30 minutes) of vancomycin has been associated with profound hypotension and even cardiac arrest.[34–37] Hypotension is often accompanied by signs of histamine release characterized by intense facial and truncal erythema ("red man syndrome"). The red man syndrome may occur even with slow infusion of vancomycin and is not always associated with hypotension.[38] Cardiovascular side effects most likely reflect nonimmunologic histamine release induced by vancomycin.[39] Although drug-induced histamine release initially causes increases in myocardial contractility, this effect is promptly followed by venodilation, a sudden decrease in left ventricular filling, and decreased contractility. Histamine produces hypotension in humans by directly dilating peripheral blood vessels. Direct myocardial depression produced by vancomycin does not seem to be important in causing hypotension in humans.[39] Vancomycin may also produce allergic reactions characterized as anaphylactoid with associated hypotension, erythema, and occasionally bronchospasm.[37] Plasma tryptase concentrations are not increased following vancomycin-induced anaphylactoid reactions thus permitting a method to distinguish anaphylactic from anaphylactoid reactions.[40] Arterial hypoxemia manifesting as an unexpected decrease in the Spo_2 may occur in association with vancomycin administration, perhaps reflecting drug-induced vasodilation in the lungs leading to an increase in ventilation to perfusion mismatching.[41] Oral H_1 (diphenhydramine 1 mg/kg) and H_2 (cimetidine 4 mg/kg) receptor antagonists administered 1 hour before induction of anesthesia decreased histamine-related side effects of rapid vancomycin infusion (1 g over 10 minutes).[42] In ambulatory anesthesia settings, as for orthopedic procedures, the time available for vancomycin administration before surgical incision or tourniquet inflation is often limited and may result in inadequate levels of antibiotic in blood and tissues if vancomycin cannot be administered more rapidly than 10 to 15 mg/kg over 60 minutes.

Ototoxicity is likely when persistent high plasma concentrations (>30 μg/mL) are present. The incidence of nephrotoxicity in association with vancomycin treatment is low. Particular attention to ototoxicity and nephrotoxicity is required when vancomycin is administered with an aminoglycoside. The administration of vancomycin to a patient recovering from succinylcholine-induced neuromuscular blockade has resulted in a return of neuromuscular blockade.[43]

Bacitracins

Bacitracins are a group of polypeptide antibiotics effective against a variety of gram-positive bacteria. Use of these antimicrobials is limited to topical application in ophthalmologic and dermatologic ointments. Despite a perception that topical application of bacitracin rarely results in allergic reactions, there are reports of anaphylactic reactions following bacitracin nasal packing and mediastinal irrigation.[44,45] Established topical uses of bacitracin include treatment of furunculosis, carbuncle, impetigo, suppurative conjunctivitis, and infected corneal ulcer.

Metronidazole

Metronidazole is bactericidal against most anaerobic gram-negative bacilli and *Clostridium* species. If administered orally, the drug is well absorbed and widely distributed in body tissues, including the CNS. As such, this antimicrobial has been useful in treating a variety of CNS, bone and joint infections, abdominal and pelvic sepsis, and endocarditis. Administered orally, metronidazole is useful for treating pseudomembranous colitis. Metronidazole is a useful part of preoperative prophylactic regimens for elective colorectal surgery. For serious anaerobic infections, the drug is administered IV.

Side effects of metronidazole include dry mouth (metallic taste) and nausea. Concurrent ingestion of alcohol may cause a reaction similar to that produced when alcohol is ingested by patients taking disulfiram. Neuropathy and pancreatitis are infrequent.

Fluoroquinolones

The fluoroquinolones are broad-spectrum antimicrobials that are bactericidal against most enteric gram-negative bacilli.[46] They are rapidly absorbed from the gastrointestinal tract, and penetration into body fluids and tissues is excellent. Their elimination half-time is prolonged (3 to 8 hours), and the principal route of excretion is via the kidneys, including glomerular filtration and renal tubular secretion. The dose of the fluoroquinolones should be decreased in the presence of renal dysfunction. Side effects are minimal, with mild gastrointestinal disturbances (nausea, vomiting) and CNS disturbances (dizziness, insomnia) occurring in less than 10% of treated patients. Fluoroquinolones have been useful clinically in the treatment of genitourinary and gastrointestinal infections, but soft tissue and bone infections have not responded to these drugs. Fluoroquinolones are bactericidal against most mycobacteria and are useful as part of multidrug regimens.[47] Fluoroquinolones are associated with an increased risk of tendinitis and tendon rupture that is enhanced in patients older than 60 years of age, taking corticosteroid drugs, and in patients with kidney, heart, or lung transplants. In addition, fluoroquinolones may exacerbate muscle weakness in patients with myasthenia gravis.

Ciprofloxacin

Ciprofloxacin is highly effective in the treatment of urinary and genital tract infections, including prostatitis, and gastrointestinal infections. The major advantage of ciprofloxacin is its greatly enhanced serum concentration and its availability as an IV preparation. Because of high blood levels and good tissue penetration, ciprofloxacin has been useful in the treatment of a variety of systemic infections, including upper and lower respiratory tract infections, skin and soft tissue infections, and bone and joint infections. Most strains of *M. tuberculosis* are susceptible to ciprofloxacin.

Moxifloxacin

Moxifloxacin is long acting for the treatment of acute bacterial sinusitis, acute bacterial exacerbation of chronic bronchitis, community-acquired pneumonia, skin infections, and complicated intraabdominal infections. Because of serious adverse effects including peripheral neuropathy, syndrome of inappropriate secretion of antidiuretic hormone, tendonitis, acute liver failure, QTc prolongation, toxic epidermal necrolysis, psychotic reactions, and Stevens-Johnson syndrome, use is recommended only when less toxic options are not available.

Antiseptic and Disinfectant Prophylaxis for Surgical Procedures

Contamination of the surgical site is a requirement for surgical site infection. Decontamination of the skin with antiseptic preparations reduces the burden of skin flora but the effect on the incidence of surgical site infection is not clear.[48] Centers for Disease Control and Prevention guidelines recommend showering or bathing with an antiseptic solution before surgery and the clinical practice guidelines from the National Institute for Health and Care Excellence recommend bathing or showering with soap, use of an iodine-impregnated drape, and immediate preparation with an antiseptic solution. Neither set of guidelines puts forth a preference of type of antiseptic solution. The main types of disinfectants are alcohols, chlorhexidine, and iodine-containing preparations which can be used alone or in combination.

Topical Antiseptics

Alcohols

Alcohols are applied topically to decrease local cutaneous bacterial flora (quick drying and antisepsis) before penetration of the skin with needles. Their antiseptic action can be enhanced by prior mechanical cleansing of the skin with water and a detergent and gentle rubbing with sterile gauze during application.

Ethyl alcohol is an antiseptic of low potency but moderate efficacy, being bactericidal to many bacteria. On the skin, 70% ethyl alcohol kills nearly 90% of the cutaneous bacteria within 2 minutes, provided the area is kept moist. Greater than a 75% decrease in cutaneous bacterial count is unlikely with a single wipe of an ethyl alcohol–soaked sponge followed by evaporation of the residual solution. Isopropyl alcohol has a slightly greater bactericidal activity than ethyl alcohol. Alcohols reduce bacterial contamination and are not fungicidal or virucidal.

Fire Risks

It is important to recognize that alcohol-based preparations are flammable until all the liquid has evaporated.[49,50] Alcohol-based surgical solutions can create a fire hazard (flash fire) especially if the solution is allowed to pool (for example in the umbilicus) or the patient is draped before the solution is completely dry resulting in trapped alcohol vapors being channeled to the surgical site where a heat source may be used. Sterile towels may be used to absorb excess alcohol-based solutions.

Chlorhexidine

Chlorhexidine is a colorless chlorophenol biguanide solution that disrupts cell membranes of the bacterial cells and is effective against both gram-positive and gram-negative bacteria. It persists on the skin to provide continued antibacterial protection. As a hand wash or surgical scrub, 2% chlorhexidine causes a greater initial decrease in the number of normal cutaneous bacteria than does povidone-iodine or hexachlorophene, and it has a persistent effect equal to or greater than that of hexachlorophene. Chlorhexidine is mainly used for the preoperative reduction of cutaneous flora for the surgeon and patient. It is also used to treat superficial infections caused by gram-positive bacteria and to disinfect wounds. As an antiseptic, chlorhexidine is rapid acting, has considerable residual adherence to the skin, has a low potential for producing contact sensitivity and photosensitivity, and is poorly absorbed even after many daily hand washings. Chlorhexidine solutions in an alcohol base are not appropriate for instillation into the eye (corneal injury) or middle ear (deafness).

Iodine

Iodine is a rapid-acting antiseptic that, in the absence of organic material, kills bacteria, viruses, and spores. For example, on the skin, 1% tincture of iodine will kill 90% of the bacteria in 90 seconds, whereas a 5% solution achieves this response in 60 seconds. In the presence of organic matter, some iodine is bound covalently, diminishing the immediate but not eventual effect. Nevertheless, commercial preparations contain iodine in such excess that minimal organic matter does not adversely influence immediate efficacy. The local toxicity of iodine is low, with cutaneous burns occurring only with concentrations of greater than 7%. In rare instances, an individual may be allergic to iodine and react to topical application. An allergic reaction usually manifests as fever and generalized skin eruption.

The most important use of iodine is disinfection of the skin. For this use, it is best used in the form of a tincture of iodine because the alcohol vehicle facilitates spreading and skin penetration. Iodine may also be used in the treatment of wounds and abrasions. Applied to abraded tissue, 0.5% to 1.0% iodine aqueous solutions are less irritating than the tinctures.

Iodophors

An iodophor is a loose complex of elemental iodine with an organic carrier that not only increases the solubility of iodine but also provides a reservoir for sustained release. The most widely used iodophor is povidone-iodine, in which the carrier molecule is polyvinylpyrrolidone. A 10% solution contains 1% available iodine, but the free iodine concentration is less than 1 ppm. This is sufficiently low that little, if any, staining of the skin occurs. Because of the low concentrations, the immediate bactericidal action is only moderate compared with that of iodine solutions.

Clinical Uses

The iodophors have a broad antimicrobial spectrum and are widely used as hand washes, including surgical scrubs; preparation of the skin before surgery or needle puncture; and treatment of minor cuts, abrasions, and burns. A standard surgical scrub with 10% povidone-iodine solutions (Betadine) will decrease the usual cutaneous bacterial population by greater than 90%, with a return to normal in about 6 to 8 hours. Compared with povidone-iodine, a disinfectant that contains an iodophor in isopropyl alcohol (DuraPrep) is more effective than povidone-iodine in decreasing the number of positive skin cultures immediately after disinfection as well as in bacterial regrowth and colonization of epidural catheters.[51] As vaginal disinfectants, iodophors may be absorbed, introducing the risk of fetal hypothyroidism if used in a parturient.[52]

Corneal Toxicity

Chemical burns to the cornea may follow exposure (accidental splashes) to a variety of disinfectant solutions (chlorhexidine, hexachlorophene, iodine, alcohol, detergents containing iodine-based solutions). Povidone-iodine solution without detergent appears to be least toxic to the cornea.[53]

Preference for Chlorhexidine or Iodine for Skin Disinfection

Central vascular catheters are a common site of hospital-acquired infection. The superiority of chlorhexidine compared to iodine-based solutions has been examined in several studies. A meta-analysis of eight studies concluded that the incidence of bloodstream infections was significantly less when central vascular lines were inserted after skin preparation with chlorhexidine gluconate compared to povidone-iodine.[54] In contrast, no difference was detected in catheter colonization when skin was prepared with iodine or chlorhexidine before epidural catheter insertion.[55] An iodophor in isopropyl alcohol solution was found to be superior to povidone-iodine, decreasing the number of positive skin cultures immediately after disinfection as well as in bacterial regrowth and colonization of epidural catheters[51] and chlorhexidine-impregnated split dressing may reduce colonization of epidural catheters.[56] However, concerns have been raised about potential neurotoxicity of chlorhexidine, which is inadvertently introduced into the neuraxial space.[57]

Quaternary Ammonium Compounds

Quaternary ammonium compounds are bactericidal in vitro to a wide variety of gram-positive and gram-negative bacteria. Many fungi and viruses are also susceptible. *M. tuberculosis*, however, is relatively resistant. Alcohol enhances the germicidal activity of quaternary ammonium compounds so that tinctures are more effective than aqueous solutions. The major site of action of quaternary ammonium compounds appears to be the cell membrane, where these solutions cause a change in permeability.

Benzalkonium and cetylpyridinium (mouthwash) are examples of quaternary ammonium compounds. These compounds may be used preoperatively to decrease the number of microorganisms on intact skin. There is a rapid onset of action, but the availability of more efficacious solutions has decreased their frequency of use. Quaternary ammonium compounds have been widely used for the sterilization of instruments. Endoscopes and other instruments made of polyethylene or polypropylene, however, absorb quaternary ammonium compounds, which may decrease the concentration of the active ingredient to below a bactericidal concentration.

Hexachlorophene

Hexachlorophene (pHisoHex) is a polychlorinated bisphenol that exhibits bacteriostatic activity against gram-positive but not gram-negative organisms. Immediately after a hand scrub with hexachlorophene, the cutaneous bacterial population may be decreased by only 30% to

50% compared with greater than 90% following use of an iodophor. Nevertheless, 60 minutes later, the bacterial population surviving a hexachlorophene scrub will have decreased further to about 4%, whereas with the iodophor scrub, the bacterial population will have recovered to about 16% of normal.

Because most of the potentially pathogenic bacteria on the skin are gram-positive, 3% hexachlorophene is commonly used by physicians and nurses to decrease the spread of contaminants from caregivers' hands. This antiseptic is also used to cleanse the skin of patients scheduled for certain surgical procedures. Hexachlorophene may be absorbed through intact skin in sufficient amounts to produce neurotoxic effects, including cerebral irritability.

Methods for Sterilization of Instruments

Formaldehyde

Formaldehyde is a volatile, wide-spectrum disinfectant that kills bacteria, fungi, and viruses by precipitating proteins. A 0.5% concentration requires 6 to 12 hours to kill bacteria and 2 to 4 days to kill spores. A 2% to 8% concentration is used to disinfect inanimate objects such as surgical instruments. Formaldehyde can be toxic, allergenic, and was named a known carcinogen by the U.S. National Toxicology Program in 2011. Most exposure is through volatilization and use under with fume hoods is recommended.

Glutaraldehyde

Glutaraldehyde is superior to formaldehyde as a disinfectant because it is rapidly effective against all microorganisms, including viruses and spores. This disinfectant also possesses tuberculocidal activity. Glutaraldehyde is less volatile than formaldehyde and hence causes minimal odor and irritant fumes. A period of 10 hours is necessary to sterilize dried spores, whereas an acid-stabilized solution kills dried spores in 20 minutes. Neither alkaline nor acidic solutions are damaging to most surgical instruments and endoscopes. As a sterilizing solution for endoscopes, glutaraldehyde is superior to iodophors and hexachlorophene.

Pasteurization

Pasteurization (hot water disinfection) is a process that destroys microorganisms in a liquid medium by application of heat. Pasteurizing water temperatures in the range of 55°C to 75°C will destroy all vegetative bacteria of significance in human disease, as well as many fungi and viruses. Pasteurization kills bacteria by coagulating cell proteins, and water acts as a very effective medium for transferring the heat required to destroy organisms. This is the rationale for maximizing direct water contact with surfaces to be disinfected. Water temperatures of greater than 75°C may cause some plastic parts to deform. Equipment (respiratory therapy breathing circuits, anesthesia breathing circuits) should be submerged in water at 68°C for a minimum of 30 minutes. With respect to breathing circuits, pasteurization is effective against gram-negative rods, *M. tuberculosis*, and most fungi and viruses. Pasteurization may be a cost-effective alternative to potentially toxic disinfecting solutions such as glutaraldehyde and formaldehyde.

Cresol

Cresol is bactericidal against common pathogenic organisms including *M. tuberculosis*. It is widely used for disinfecting inanimate objects. Cresol should not be used to disinfect materials that can absorb this solution because burns could result from subsequent tissue contact.

Silver Nitrate

Silver nitrate is used as a caustic, antiseptic, and astringent. A solid form is used for cauterizing wounds and removing granulation tissue. It is conveniently dispensed in pencils that should be moistened before use. Solutions of silver nitrate are strongly bactericidal, especially for gonococci, accounting for its frequent use as prophylaxis for ophthalmia neonatorum.

Silver sulfadiazine or nitrate is used in the treatment of burns. With this use, hypochloremia may occur, reflecting the combination of silver ions with chloride. Hyponatremia also may result because the sodium ions are attracted by chloride ions into the exudate. Furthermore, absorbed nitrate can cause methemoglobinemia.

Ethylene Oxide

Ethylene oxide is a readily diffusible gas that is noncorrosive and antimicrobial to all organisms at room temperature. This gaseous alkylating material is widely used as an alternative to heat sterilization. It reacts with chloride and water to produce two additional active germicides, ethylene chlorohydrin and ethylene glycol. Special sterilizing chambers are required because the gas must remain in contact with the objects for several hours. Adequate airing of sterilized materials, such as tracheal tubes, is essential to ensure removal of residual ethylene oxide and thus minimize tissue irritation. Ethylene oxide sensitization has been described in children with spina bifida experiencing preoperative anaphylactic reactions, always in association with latex sensitization.[58]

References

1. Gonzales R, Steiner JF, Sande MA. Antibiotic prescribing for adults with colds, upper respiratory tract infections, and bronchitis by ambulatory care physicians. *JAMA*. 1997;278:901–904.
2. Kirkland KB, Briggs JP, Trivette SL, et al. The impact of surgical-site infections in the 1990s: attributable mortality, excess length of hospitalization, and extra costs. *Infect Contr Hosp Epidemiol*. 1999;20:725–730.

3. Rosenberger LH, Politano AD, Sawyer RD. The surgical care improvement project and prevention of post-operative infection, including surgical site infection. *Surg Infect.* 2011;12:163–168.
4. U.S. Department of Health and Human Services. National action plan to prevent health care-associated infections: road map to elimination. Health.gov Web site. http://www.health.gov/hai/prevent_hai.asp#table1. Accessed February 2, 2014.
5. Anderson DJ, Kaye KS, Classen D, et al. Strategies to prevent surgical site infections in acute care hospitals. *Infect Control Hosp Epidemiol.* 2008;29(suppl 1):S51–S61.
6. Mangram AJ, Horan TC, Pearson ML, et al. Guideline for prevention of surgical site infection. *Infect Control Hosp Epidemiol.* 1999;20:250–278.
7. Zerr KJ, Furnary AP, Grunkemeier GL, et al. Glucose control lowers the risk of wound infection in diabetics after open heart operations. *Ann Thorac Surg.* 1997;63:356–361.
8. Furnary AP, Zerr KJ, Grunkemeier GL, et al. Continuous intravenous insulin infusion reduces the incidence of deep sternal wound infection in diabetic patients after cardiac surgical procedures. *Ann Thorac Surg.* 1999;67:352–360.
9. McConnell YJ, Johnson PM, Porter GA. Surgical site infections following colorectal surgery in patients with diabetes: association with postoperative hyperglycemia. *J Gastrointest Surg.* 2009;13:508–515.
10. NICE-SUGAR Study Investigators; Finfer S, Chittock DR, Su SY, et al. Intensive versus conventional glucose control in critically ill patients. *N Engl J Med.* 2009;360(13):1283–1297.
11. Sorensen LT. Wound healing and infection in surgery. The clinical impact of smoking and smoking cessation: a systematic review and meta-analysis. *Arch Surg.* 2012;147(4):373–383.
12. Mahoney CB, Odom J. Maintaining intraoperative normothermia: a meta-analysis of outcomes with costs. *AANA J.* 1999;67(2): 155–163.
13. Suding P, Jensen E, Abramson MA, et al. Definitive risk factors for anastomotic leaks in elective open colorectal resection. *Arch Surg.* 2008;143:907–912.
14. Bolac CS, Wallace AH, Broadwater G, et al. The impact of postoperative nausea and vomiting prophylaxis with dexamethasone on postoperative wound complications in patients undergoing laparotomy for endometrial cancer. *Anesth Analg.* 2013;116(5):1041–1047.
15. Hidron AI, Edwards JR, Patel J, et al; National Healthcare Safety Network Team and participating National Healthcare Safety Network facilities. Antimicrobial-resistant pathogens associated with healthcare-associated infections: annual summary of data reported to the National Healthcare Safety Network at the Centers for Disease Control and Prevention, 2006–2007. *Infect Control Hosp Epidemiol.* 2008;29:996–1011.
16. Bratzler DW, Dellinger, EP, Olsen KM, et al; American Society of Health-System Pharmacists; Infectious Diseases Society of America; Surgical Infection Society; Society for Healthcare Epidemiology of America. Clinical practice guidelines for antimicrobial prophylaxis in surgery. *Am J Health Syst Pharm.* 2013;70(3):195–283. http://www.ashp.org/surgical-guidelines. Accessed February 24, 2014.
17. Frumin J, Gallagher JC. Allergic cross-sensitivity between penicillin, carbapenem, and monobactam antibiotics: what are the chances? *Ann Pharmacother.* 2009;43:304–315.
18. Gould FK, Brindle R, Chadwick PR, et al. Guidelines (2008) for the prophylaxis and treatment of methicillin-resistant Staphylococcus aureus (MRSA) infections in the United Kingdom. *J Antimicrob Chemother.* 2009;63:849–861.
19. Bull AL, Worth LJ, Richards MJ. Impact of vancomycin surgical prophylaxis on the development of methicillin-sensitive Staphylococcus aureus surgical site infections: report from Australian surveillance data (VICNISS). *Ann Surg.* 2012;256(6):1089–1092.
20. Finkelstein R, Rabino G, Mashiah T, et al. Vancomycin versus cefazolin prophylaxis for cardiac surgery in the setting of a high prevalence of methicillin-resistant staphylococcal infections. *Thorac Cardiovasc Surg.* 2002;123:326–332.
21. van der Waaij D, Manson WL, Arends JP, et al. Clinical use of selective decontamination: the concept. *Intens Care Med.* 1990;16(suppl 3): S212–S216.
22. Weaver M, Burdon DW, Youngs DJ, et al. Oral neomycin and erythromycin compared with single-dose systemic metronidazole and ceftriaxone prophylaxis in elective colorectal surgery. *Am J Surg.* 1986;151:437–442.
23. Keighley MR, Arabi Y, Alexander-Williams J, et al. Comparison between systemic and oral antimicrobial prophylaxis in colorectal surgery. *Lancet.* 1979;1:894–897.
24. Wenzel RP, Edmond MB. The evolving technology of venous access. *N Engl J Med.* 1999;340:48–50.
25. Harbell J, Fung J, Nissen N, et al; HIV-TR Investigators. Surgical complications in 275 HIV-infected liver and/or kidney transplantation recipients. *Surgery.* 2012;152(3):376–381.
26. Muchuweti D, Jönsson KU. Abdominal surgical site infections: a prospective study of determinant factors in Harare, Zimbabwe [published online ahead of print September 19, 2013]. *Int Wound J.*
27. Coleman J, Green I, Scheib S, et al. Surgical site infections after hysterectomy among HIV-infected women in the HAART era: a single institution's experience from 1999–2012. *Am J Obstet Gynecol.* 2014;210(2):117.e1–117.e7.
28. Kigera JW, Straetemans M, Vuhaka SK, et al. Is there an increased risk of post-operative surgical site infection after orthopaedic surgery in HIV patients? A systematic review and meta-analysis. *PLoS One.* 2012;7(8):e42254.
29. Annè S, Reisman RE. Risk of administering cephalosporin antibiotics to patients with histories of penicillin allergy. *Ann Allergy Asthma Immunol.* 1995;74(2):167–170.
30. Pallasch TJ. Principles of pharmacotherapy: III. Drug allergy. *Anesth Prog.* 1988;35:178–189.
31. Adkinson NF. Immunogenicity and cross-allergenicity of aztreonam. *Am J Med.* 1990;88:12S–15S.
32. Ray WA, Murray KT, Meredith S, et al. Oral erythromycin and the risk of sudden death from cardiac causes. *N Engl J Med.* 2004;351(11):1089–1096.
33. Ahdal OA, Bevan DR. Clindamycin-induced neuromuscular blockade. *Can J Anaesth.* 1995;42:614–617.
34. Lyon GD, Bruce DL. Diphenhydramine reversal of vancomycin-induced hypotension. *Anesth Analg.* 1988;67:1109–1110.
35. Mayhew JF, Deutsch S. Cardiac arrest following administration of vancomycin. *Can Anaesth Soc J.* 1985;32:65–66.
36. Southorn PA, Plevak DJ, Wilson WR. Adverse effects of vancomycin administered in the perioperative period. *Mayo Clin Proc.* 1986;61:721–724.
37. Symons NLP, Hobbes AFT, Leaver HK. Anaphylactoid reactions to vancomycin. *Can Anaesth Soc J.* 1985;32:65–66.
38. Davis RL, Smith AL, Koup JR. The "red-man's syndrome" and slow infusion of vancomycin. *N Engl J Med.* 1985;313:756–757.
39. Levy JH, Kettlekamp N, Goertz P, et al. Histamine release by vancomycin. A mechanism for hypotension in man. *Anesthesiology.* 1987;67:122–125.
40. Renz CL, Thurn JD, Finn HA, et al. Oral antihistamines reduce the side effects from rapid vancomycin infusion. *Anesth Analg.* 1998;87:681–685.
41. Gopalan K, Dhandha SK. Hypoxia following perioperative administration of vancomycin. *Anesth Analg.* 1993;76:200–201.
42. Renz CL, Laroche D, Thurn JD, et al. Tryptase levels are not increased during vancomycin-induced anaphylactoid reactions. *Anesthesiology.* 1998;89:620–625.
43. Albrecht RF, Lanier WL. Potentiation of succinylcholine-induced phase II block by vancomycin. *Anesth Analg.* 1993;77:1300–1302.
44. Blas M, Briesacher K, Lobato E. Bacitracin irrigation: a cause of anaphylaxis in the operating room. *Anesth Analg.* 2000;91:1027–1028.
45. Gail R, Blakley B, Warrington R, et al. Intraoperative anaphylactic shock from bacitracin nasal packing after septorhinoplasty. *Anesthesiology.* 1999;91:1545–1547.

46. Hooper DC, Wolfson JS. Fluoroquinolone antimicrobial agents. *N Engl J Med.* 1991;324:384–394.
47. Alangaden GJ, Lerner SA. The clinical use of fluoroquinolones for the treatment of mycobacterial diseases. *Clin Infect Dis.* 1997;25:1213–1218.
48. Kamel C, McGahan L, Polisena J, et al. Preoperative skin antiseptic preparations for preventing surgical site infections: a systematic review. *Infect Control Hosp Epidemiol.* 2012;33:608–617.
49. Barker SJ, Polson JS. Fire in the operating room: a case report and laboratory study. *Anesth Analg.* 2001;93:960–965.
50. Improper use of alcohol-based skin preps can cause surgical fires. *Health Devices.* 2003;32:441–443.
51. Birnbach DJ, Meadows W, Stein DJ, et al. Comparison of povidone iodine and DuraPrep, an iodophor-in-isopropyl alcohol solution, for skin disinfection prior to epidural catheter insertion in parturients. *Anesthesiology.* 2003;98:164–169.
52. Vorherr H, Vorherr UF, Mehta P, et al. Vaginal absorption of povidone-iodine. *JAMA.* 1980;244:2628–2629.
53. Rae SCC, Brown B, Edelhauser HF. The corneal toxicity of presurgical skin antiseptics. *Am J Ophthalmol.* 1984;97:221–232.
54. Chaiyakunapruk N, Veenstra DL, Lipsky BA, et al. Chlorhexidine compared with povidone-iodine solution for vascular catheter–site care: a meta-analysis. *Ann Intern Med.* 2002;136:792–801.
55. Kasuda H, Fukuda H, Togashi H, et al. Skin disinfection before epidural catheterization: comparative study of povidone-iodine versus chlorhexidine ethanol. *Dermatology.* 2002;204(suppl 1): 42–46.
56. Kinirons B, Mimoz O, Lafendi L, et al. Chlorhexidine versus povidone iodine in preventing colonization of continuous epidural catheters in children. *Anesthesiology.* 2001;94:239–244.
57. Milstone AM, Bamford P, Aucott SW, et al. Chlorhexidine inhibits L1 cell adhesion molecule-mediated neurite outgrowth in vitro. *Pediatr Res.* 2014;75:8–13.
58. Porri F, Pradal M, Lemiere C, et al. Association between latex sensitization and repeated latex exposure in children. *Anesthesiology.* 1997;86:599–602.

CHAPTER 42

Chemotherapeutic Drugs

Updated by: James P. Rathmell • Mihir M. Kamdar

Chemotherapy is a term that was coined to refer to a broad range of chemicals (drugs) aimed at treating cancer by eradicating malignant cells anywhere in the body.[1] Conventional wisdom is that the effectiveness of chemotherapy requires that there be complete destruction (total cell kill) of all cancer cells because a single surviving cell with the ability to divide can give rise to sufficient progeny to ultimately kill the host. The role of the immune system in identifying and eliminating foreign tumor cells has gained increasing recognition, and harnessing our intrinsic immune surveillance system has become more and more a part of contemporary investigations of cancer and its treatment.[2] The use of several chemotherapeutic drugs (also called ***antineoplastic drugs***) concurrently or in a planned sequence is commonly done in efforts to eradicate even small residual tumor cell populations that have survived treatment with a single or previous agent. In practice, combination chemotherapy regimens typically use the largest tolerated doses of each chemotherapeutic drug; drugs that work via different mechanisms and that do not share similar toxic effects are combined. Using a combination of agents that have different mechanisms also decreases the chances that drug-resistant tumor cell populations will emerge. Chemotherapeutic drugs used in combination are usually administered over short periods at specific treatment intervals rather than as continuous therapy. This approach is based on the empiric observation that normal cells usually recover more rapidly from a pulse of maximal chemotherapy than do malignant cells. Furthermore, immunosuppression is less profound with intermittent administration of chemotherapy. With rare exceptions, the optimal dose of chemotherapeutic drugs requires repetitive dosing because even if all cells in a tumor are sensitive to a drug, a single dose of the drug is not usually sufficient to kill the typically hundreds of millions of cells that are present in patients with cancer.

Malignant cells are often characterized by rapid division and synthesis of DNA. Most conventional chemotherapeutic drugs exert their antineoplastic effects on cells that are actively undergoing division (mitosis) or DNA synthesis. Many chemotherapeutic drugs act only at specific phases of the cell cycle (Fig. 42-1).[1] The biology of the cancer under treatment and the cell cycle specificity of agents effect how drugs are scheduled and combined for maximal effect. Slow-growing malignant cells with a slow rate of division, like carcinoma of the lung and colon, are often unresponsive or at best partially responsive to conventional chemotherapy. Conversely, rapidly dividing normal cells, like the cells found in the bone marrow, gastrointestinal mucosa, skin, and hair follicles, are more vulnerable to the toxic effects of chemotherapeutic drugs. Thus, it is predictable that clinical manifestations of toxicity caused by chemotherapeutic drugs often include myelosuppression (leukopenia, thrombocytopenia, or anemia), nausea, vomiting, diarrhea, mucosal ulceration, dermatitis, and alopecia as these represent activity at normal rapidly dividing cells. Myelosuppression is the dose-limiting factor for many chemotherapeutic drugs and is the most common toxicity that leads to temporary or permanent withdrawal of therapy. Drug-induced myelosuppression is usually reversible with discontinuation of the chemotherapeutic agent.

Drug Resistance

Resistance to chemotherapeutic drugs often occurs and has many causes.[3] Some chemotherapy agents lead to induction of drug-metabolizing enzymes in the liver, other tissues, or tumor cells, accelerating drug conversion to nontoxic metabolites. Many solid tumors grow so rapidly that portions of the tumor are poorly vascularized, preventing therapeutic concentrations from reaching many target cells. In poorly perfused areas of some tumors, cells remain resistant to chemotherapeutic drugs because of relative hypoxia. Indeed, hypoxia causes resistance to both radiation and most chemotherapeutic drugs (with the exception of malignancies susceptible to treatment with the mitomycins).

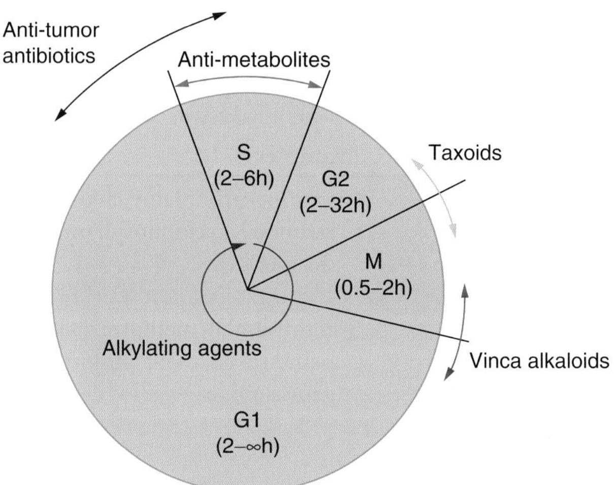

FIGURE 42-1 Cell cycle specificity of chemotherapy agents. The cell cycle is divided into a number of phases: G1 (gap 1, cells increase in size and prepare for DNA synthesis), S (synthesis, DNA replication occurs), G2 (gap 2, cells continue to grow and prepare for mitosis), and M (mitosis, cellular growth stops and preparation for cell division takes place), each of which can vary in length according to the type of cell and the growth rate of the cell. The activity of different classes of certain chemotherapy agents (antibiotics, antimetabolites, taxoids, vinca alkaloids) is optimal in different phases of the cell cycle, whereas alkylating agents are relatively non–phase-specific. (From Caley A, Jones R. The principles of cancer treatment by chemotherapy. *Surgery (Oxford)*. 2012;30:186–190, with permission.)

As in the treatment of infections, multiple drug resistance describes the clinical circumstance in which a tumor is no longer susceptible to several chemotherapeutic drugs. For a number of agents, P-glycoprotein spans the plasma membrane and acts to pump chemotherapeutic drugs (anthracyclines, vinca alkaloids, and taxanes but not alkylating drugs, platinating drugs, and antimetabolites) to the extracellular space such that an effective toxic intracellular concentration is not reached. In addition to P-glycoprotein, there is an additional family of multidrug resistance proteins (MRPs) that are located on plasma membranes and endoplasmic reticulum of some tumor cell types, which confer drug resistance via an adenosine triphosphate (ATP)–dependent decrease in cellular drug accumulation (with the exception of malignancies susceptible to treatment with the taxanes). Collectively, P-glycoprotein and the MRPs are members of the ATP-binding cassette (ABC) class of transporter proteins that protect normal tissues from a variety of toxicants and are overexpressed in some tumor cells. The breast cancer resistance protein (also known as the ***ATP-binding cassette subfamily G member 2*** or ***ABCG$_2$ protein or the mitoxantrone resistance–associated protein***) is a specific example of an ABC protein that confers tumor resistance to certain chemotherapeutic agents via active transport of the offending agent out of cells expressing this transporter.

Topoisomerases, enzymes that regulate the overwinding or underwinding of DNA during replication, are the targets for many chemotherapeutic drugs. Resistance to chemotherapeutic drugs can also occur through mutations in the drug-binding domain of the target enzyme. Resistance to the drug methotrexate may reflect mutations in the drug target, the enzyme dihydrofolate reductase; dihydrofolate reductase converts dihydrofolate into tetrahydrofolate and is required for the de novo synthesis of purines and thymidylic acid, which are important for cell growth and proliferation. Resistance to alkylating drugs occurs through overexpression of drug-neutralizing substances and metabolizing proteins.

Classification

Chemotherapeutic drugs are classified according to their mechanism of action (Table 42-1)[1]; adverse effects associated with these drugs are generally similar among drugs with similar mechanisms of action (Table 42-2).[4–6] Knowledge of drug-induced adverse effects and evaluation of appropriate laboratory tests (hemoglobin, platelet count, white blood cell count, coagulation profile, arterial blood gases, blood glucose, plasma electrolytes, liver and renal function tests, electrocardiogram [ECG], and radiograph of the chest) are useful in the preoperative evaluation of patients being treated with specific chemotherapeutic drugs. Immunosuppression makes these patients susceptible to iatrogenic infections, thus asepsis and the use of appropriate prophylactic antibiotics is critical. A history of severe vomiting or diarrhea may be associated with electrolyte disturbances and decreased intravascular fluid volume. The existence of mucositis makes placement of pharyngeal airways, laryngeal mask airways, and esophageal catheters questionable. The response to inhaled and injected anesthetic drugs may be altered by drug-induced cardiac, hepatic, or renal dysfunction and induction of hepatic enzymes. The response to older nondepolarizing neuromuscular blocking drugs may be altered by impaired renal function. Theoretically, the effects of succinylcholine may be prolonged if plasma cholinesterase activity is decreased by chemotherapeutic drugs.

Toxicities

Chemotherapeutic drugs typically target proteins or nucleic acids, which are common to malignant and nonmalignant cells and thus possess a narrow therapeutic index. Indeed, using the standard definition of therapeutic index (the dose that causes toxicity divided by the minimum effective dose) is not useful, as these agents all produce significant, even life-threatening toxicities at doses which may not reach levels that are high enough

Table 42-1

Biochemical Classification of Chemotherapy Drugs

Drug Class	Mechanism of Action	Examples
Alkylating agents	Impair cell function by forming covalent bonds on important molecules in proteins, DNA, and RNA. Classified by their chemical structure and mechanism of covalent bonding.	Cisplatin, carboplatin, chlorambucil, cyclophosphamide, ifosfamide
Antimetabolites	Structural analogues of naturally occurring metabolites involved in DNA and RNA synthesis. They either substitute for a metabolite that is normally incorporated into DNA or RNA or compete for the catalytic site of a key enzyme.	5-Fluorouracil, methotrexate, pemetrexed, mercaptopurine, gemcitabine
Antitumor antibiotics	Intercalate DNA at specific sequences, creating free radicals, which cause strand breakage. Anthracyclines are products of the fungus having *Streptomyces*, also mechanism of action of topoisomerase I and II, required for the uncoiling of DNA during replication.	Bleomycin, anthracyclines (doxorubicin, epirubicin)
Topoisomerase inhibitors	Topoisomerases are enzymes that control the 3-D structure of DNA. Topoisomerase I and topoisomerase II are enzymes responsible for the uncoiling of DNA during replication.	Topoisomerase I—irinotecan, topotecan Topoisomerase II—etoposide
Tubulin-binding drugs	Vinca alkaloids bind to tubulin and prevent the formation of the microtubule, which is important during mitosis, but also for cell shape, intracellular transport, and axonal function. Taxoids prevent the disassembly of the microtubules, thereby inhibiting normal function.	Vinca alkaloids—vincristine, vinorelbine Taxoids—docetaxel, paclitaxel
Signal transduction modifiers	Hormonal treatment of cancer results in a disruption of the normal growth factor receptor interactions which lead to cell proliferation and is effective in cancer cells where mutations have resulted in uncontrolled cell proliferation utilizing activated signaling pathways. Monoclonal antibodies bind to specific antigens on tumor cells and thereby modify cell proliferation. Aromatase inhibitors work by inhibiting the action of the enzyme aromatase, which converts androgens into estrogens.	Antiestrogens—tamoxifen, toremifene, raloxifene Antiandrogens—flutamide, bicalutamide, nilutamide Monoclonal antibodies—rituximab, trastuzumab Aromatase inhibitors—aminoglutethimide, anastrazole, letrozole Gonadotropin-releasing drugs—leuprolide, buserelin Progestins—megestrol acetate

Modified from Caley A, Jones R. The principles of cancer treatment by chemotherapy. *Surgery (Oxford)*. 2012;30:186–190, with permission.

to eradicate cancer (therapeutic index <1). Furthermore, chemotherapeutic drugs are usually administered at maximum tolerated doses. Although toxicities may be unique for specific drugs, many toxicities are shared (nausea and vomiting, myelosuppression, mucositis, alopecia) (see Table 42-2).[4] Nausea and vomiting result from local gastrointestinal effects as well as activation of the chemoreceptor trigger zone in the central nervous system. Patients who have a history of chemotherapy-induced nausea and vomiting are not necessarily prone to postoperative nausea and vomiting, as there is only weak positive association between the two; however, patients who have a history of tolerating emetogenic chemotherapy regimens are unlikely to develop postoperative nausea and vomiting.[7] Development of serotonin antagonists as effective antiemetics in addition to combination antiemetic regimens has facilitated the tolerance of emetogenic chemotherapeutic drugs. Mucositis and diarrhea are common gastrointestinal toxicities that reflect the high proliferative rate of gastrointestinal tissues, which makes these tissues more susceptible to the cytotoxic effects of certain chemotherapeutic drugs. Myelosuppression and alopecia reflect similar chemotherapeutic drug effects on highly proliferative tissues. Chemotherapeutic drugs that damage DNA (alkylating drugs, topoisomerases) are associated with secondary malignancies.

Table 42-2

Chemotherapeutic Drugs, Therapeutic Uses, and Associated Side Effects

Group and Class	Therapeutic Uses	Side Effects (Other than Nausea and Vomiting)
Alkylating agents		
Nitrogen mustards		
Mechlorethamine	Hodgkin disease Non-Hodgkin lymphoma	Myelosuppression Mucositis Alopecia
Cyclophosphamide	Acute lymphocytic leukemia Chronic lymphocytic leukemia Lymphomas Myeloma Neuroblastoma Breast, ovarian, cervical, and testicular cancer Lung cancer Wilms tumor Sarcoma	Myelosuppression Mucositis Alopecia Hemorrhagic cystitis Skin pigmentation Seizures Renal failure Cardiac failure Inappropriate secretion of vasopressin (ADH)
Melphalan	Myeloma Breast cancer	Myelosuppression
Chlorambucil	Hodgkin disease Non-Hodgkin lymphoma Macroglobulinemia	Myelosuppression Secondary leukemias
Ethyleneimine		
Hexamethylmelamine	Ovarian cancer	Myelosuppression
Thiotepa	Bladder, breast, and ovarian cancer	
Alkyl sulfonates		
Busulfan	Acute myelogenous leukemia Chronic myelogenous leukemia	Myelosuppression Thrombocytopenia
Nitrosoureas		
Carmustine (BCNU)	Hodgkin disease Non-Hodgkin lymphoma Astrocytoma Myeloma Melanoma	Myelosuppression Hepatitis Interstitial pulmonary fibrosis Renal failure Flushing
Lomustine (CCNU)	Hodgkin disease Non-Hodgkin lymphoma Astrocytoma Small cell lung cancer	Myelosuppression
Semustine (methyl-CCNU)	Colon cancer	Myelosuppression
Streptozotocin	Insulinoma Carcinoid tumor	Myelosuppression Hepatitis Renal failure
Triazenes		
Dacarbazine (DTIC)	Hodgkin disease Melanoma Sarcomas	Myelosuppression Flulike syndrome
Temozolomide	Astrocytoma Melanoma	Hepatic toxicity Hyperglycemia Anemia Thrombocytopenia Lymphocytopenia

(continued)

Table 42-2

Chemotherapeutic Drugs, Therapeutic Uses, and Associated Side Effects *(continued)*

Group and Class	Therapeutic Uses	Side Effects (Other than Nausea and Vomiting)
Bioreductive alkylating drugs		
Mitomycin-C	Head and neck, breast, lung, gastric, colon, rectal, and cervical cancer	Myelosuppression Mucositis Cardiac failure Interstitial fibrosis Hemolytic uremic syndrome
Platinum compounds		
Cisplatin	Head and neck, thyroid, lung, ovarian, endometrial, cervical, and testicular cancer Neuroblastoma Osteogenic sarcoma	Myelosuppression Peripheral neuropathy Allergic reactions Renal toxicity Electrolyte abnormalities (hypocalcemia, hypomagnesemia, hypophosphatemia)
Carboplatin	As for cisplatin	Myelosuppression
Oxaliplatin	Colon cancer	Myelosuppression Peripheral neuropathy
Antimetabolites		
Folate analogues		
Methotrexate	Head and neck, breast, and lung cancer Acute lymphocytic leukemia Non-Hodgkin lymphoma Osteogenic sarcoma	Myelosuppression Mucositis Pneumonitis Hepatic fibrosis
Pyrimidine analogues		
Fluorouracil (5-FU)	Head and neck, breast, gastric, pancreatic, bladder, ovarian, cervical, and prostate cancer Hepatoma	Myelosuppression Mucositis Alopecia Pigmentation Chest pain
Cytarabine	Acute lymphocytic leukemia Acute myeloid leukemia Non-Hodgkin lymphoma	Myelosuppression Mucositis Hepatitis
Gemcitabine	Breast, lung, pancreatic, and bladder cancer	Myelosuppression Flulike syndrome
Purine analogues		
Mercaptopurine	Acute lymphocytic leukemia Acute myeloid leukemia Chronic myeloid leukemia	Myelosuppression Anorexia Jaundice
Thioguanine	As for mercaptopurine	Myelosuppression Anorexia
Fludarabine	Chronic lymphocytic leukemia Non-Hodgkin lymphoma	Myelosuppression Optic neuritis Peripheral neuropathy Seizures Coma Depletion of CD4 cells
Pentostatin	Chronic lymphocytic leukemia Cutaneous T-cell lymphoma Hairy cell leukemia	Myelosuppression Depletion of T cells Hepatitis

Table 42-2

Chemotherapeutic Drugs, Therapeutic Uses, and Associated Side Effects *(continued)*

Group and Class	Therapeutic Uses	Side Effects (Other than Nausea and Vomiting)
Cladribine	Chronic lymphocytic leukemia Cutaneous T-cell lymphoma Hairy cell leukemia Waldenström macroglobulinemia	Myelosuppression Tumor lysis syndrome Asthenia
Hydroxyurea	Chronic myeloid leukemia Polycythemia vera Thrombocytopenia Melanoma	Myelosuppression Dermatologic changes
Topoisomerase inhibitors		
Anthracyclines		
Doxorubicin	Hodgkin disease Non-Hodgkin lymphoma Acute lymphocytic leukemia Neuroblastoma Thyroid, breast, lung, and gastric cancer	Myelosuppression Cardiomyopathy Mucositis
Daunomycin	Acute myeloid leukemia Acute lymphocytic leukemia	
Idarubicin	As for daunomycin	
Epirubicin	Hodgkin disease Non-Hodgkin lymphoma Acute lymphocytic leukemia Breast, lung, gastric, and bladder cancer	Myelosuppression Cardiomyopathy Alopecia Phlebitis
Anthracenediones		
Mitoxantrone	Acute myeloid leukemia Breast cancer	Myelosuppression Mucositis
Epipodophyllotoxins		
Etoposide	Hodgkin disease Non-Hodgkin lymphoma Acute myeloid leukemia Kaposi sarcoma Breast, lung, and testicular cancer	Myelosuppression Systemic hypotension Hepatitis Mucositis
Teniposide	Acute lymphocytic leukemia (children) Acute myeloid leukemia (children)	Myelosuppression Systemic hypotension
Dactinomycin	Wilms tumor Rhabdomyosarcoma Choriocarcinoma Kaposi sarcoma Ewing sarcoma Testicular cancer	Myelosuppression Mucositis Cheilitis Glossitis Alopecia Cutaneous erythema
Camptothecins		
Irinotecan	Colon cancer Ovarian cancer	Myelosuppression Alopecia
Topotecan	Lung cancer Ovarian cancer	As for irinotecan
Antitumor antibiotics		
Antibiotic		
Bleomycin	Hodgkin disease Non-Hodgkin lymphoma Head and neck cancer Testicular cancer	Interstitial pulmonary fibrosis Allergic reactions Skin pigmentation

(continued)

Table 42-2

Chemotherapeutic Drugs, Therapeutic Uses, and Associated Side Effects *(continued)*

Group and Class	Therapeutic Uses	Side Effects (Other than Nausea and Vomiting)
Tubulin-binding drugs		
Vinca alkaloids		
Vinblastine	Hodgkin disease Non-Hodgkin lymphoma Breast cancer Testicular cancer	Myelosuppression Peripheral neuropathy
Vincristine	Hodgkin disease Non-Hodgkin lymphoma Small cell lung cancer Neuroblastoma Wilms tumor Rhabdomyosarcoma Acute lymphocytic leukemia	Myelosuppression Peripheral neuropathy
Vinorelbine	Breast cancer Lung cancer	Myelosuppression Peripheral neuropathy
Taxanes		
Paclitaxel	Breast, lung, bladder, and ovarian cancer	Myelosuppression Peripheral neuropathy Allergic reactions Alopecia totalis
Docetaxel	Breast, lung, bladder, and ovarian cancer	Myelosuppression Peripheral neuropathy Allergic reactions Alopecia totalis Cardiac dysrhythmias Capillary leakage
Signal transduction modulators		
Antiestrogens		
Tamoxifen	Breast cancer	Venous thrombosis Weight gain Amenorrhea Hypercalcemia Endometrial cancer Hot flashes
Toremifene	Breast cancer	Venous thrombosis Hot flashes
Raloxifene	Breast cancer	Venous thrombosis Hot flashes
Antiandrogens		
Flutamide	Prostate cancer	Gynecomastia Hot flashes
Bicalutamide	Prostate cancer	Gynecomastia Hot flashes
Nilutamide	Prostate cancer	Gynecomastia Hot flashes Delayed visual adaptation to dark

Table 42-2

Chemotherapeutic Drugs, Therapeutic Uses, and Associated Side Effects *(continued)*

Group and Class	Therapeutic Uses	Side Effects (Other than Nausea and Vomiting)
Monoclonal antibodies		
Rituximab	Chronic lymphocytic leukemia Non-Hodgkin lymphoma	Infusion-related chills, rash, and fever Non–infusion-related myalgias, angioedema, bronchospasm, cardiac dysrhythmias Myelosuppression
Trastuzumab	Breast cancer	Fever and chills
Aromatase inhibitors		
Aminoglutethimide	Breast cancer	Orthostatic hypotension Glucocorticoid deficiency Cutaneous rash
Anastrazole	Breast cancer	Asthenia Headache Hot flashes
Letrozole	Breast cancer	Headache Heartburn
Gonadotropin-releasing drugs		
Leuprolide	Breast cancer Prostate cancer	Impotence Hot flashes Pain at sites of bony metastases (tumor flare)
Buserelin	Breast cancer	As for leuprolide
Progestin		
Megestrol acetate	Breast cancer Prostate cancer Endometrial cancer	Weight gain

ADH, antidiuretic hormone; BCNU, bischloroethylnitrosourea; CCNU, 1-(2-chloroethyl)-3-cyclohexyl-1-nitrosourea; DTIC, dimethyl triazeno imidazole carboxamide.

Adapted from Rubin EH, Hait WN. Principles of cancer treatment. *Sci Am Med.* 2003;12(IV):1–17.

Alkylating Agents

Alkylating drugs include nitrogen mustards, alkyl sulfonates, nitrosoureas, and triazenes. These chemotherapeutic drugs form covalent alkyl bonds with nucleic acid bases, resulting in intrastrand or interstrand DNA cross-links which are toxic to cells undergoing division. By altering the structure of DNA, these drugs inhibit DNA replication and transcription. DNA damage produced by alkylating chemotherapeutic drugs is more likely to kill malignant cells than nonmalignant cells because rates of proliferation are greater for the cancer cells. Acquired resistance to alkylating drugs is a common occurrence and may reflect decreased cell membrane permeability to the drugs and increased production of nucleophilic substances that can compete with target DNA for alkylation.

Side Effects

Bone marrow suppression is the most important dose-limiting factor in the clinical use of alkylating drugs, especially busulfan. Cessation of mitosis is evident within 6 to 8 hours. Lymphocytopenia is usually present within 24 hours. Variable degrees of depression of platelet and erythrocyte counts may occur. Hemolytic anemia is predictably present.

Treatment with alkylating drugs is often associated with gonadal dysfunction, including oligospermia and amenorrhea. Hemorrhagic cystitis can result from irritation by the acrolein metabolite of cyclophosphamide or ifosfamide. Gastrointestinal mucosa is sensitive to the effects of alkylating drugs, manifesting as mitotic arrest, cellular hypertrophy, and desquamation of the epithelium. Damage to hair follicles, often leading to alopecia, is a common side effect. Increased skin pigmentation is frequent. All alkylating drugs are powerful central nervous system (CNS) stimulants, manifesting most often as nausea and vomiting. Skeletal muscle weakness and seizures may be present. Pneumonitis and pulmonary fibrosis are potential adverse effects of alkylating drugs. Symptomatic patients may demonstrate a decreased pulmonary diffusing capacity. Inhibition of plasma cholinesterase activity may be present for as long as 2 to 3 weeks after administration of chemotherapy regimens that include an alkylating agent and can lead to prolonged skeletal muscle paralysis after administration of succinylcholine.[8,9]

Rapid drug-induced destruction of malignant cells can produce increased purine and pyrimidine breakdown, leading to uric acid–induced nephropathy. To minimize the likelihood of this complication, it is recommended that adequate fluid intake, alkalinization of the urine, and administration of allopurinol be established before drug treatment.

Nitrogen Mustards

The most commonly used nitrogen mustards are mechlorethamine, cyclophosphamide, melphalan, and chlorambucil.

Mechlorethamine

Mechlorethamine is a rapidly acting nitrogen mustard administered intravenously (IV) to minimize local tissue irritation. This drug must be freshly prepared before each administration. Mechlorethamine and other nitrogen mustards are intensely powerful vesicants, requiring that gloves be worn by personnel handling the drug. A course of therapy with mechlorethamine consists of the injection of a total dose of 0.4 mg/kg. The drug undergoes rapid chemical transformation in tissues such that active drug is no longer present after a few minutes. For this reason, it is possible to prevent tissue toxicity from the drug by isolating the blood supply to that tissue. Alternatively, it is theoretically possible to localize the action of mechlorethamine in a specific tissue by injecting the drug into the arterial blood supply to the tissue.

Clinical Uses

Mechlorethamine produces beneficial effects in the treatment of Hodgkin disease and, less predictably, in other lymphomas. The drug is most often used in combination with vincristine, procarbazine, and prednisone (MOPP regimen) for the treatment of Hodgkin disease.

Side Effects

The major side effects of mechlorethamine include nausea, vomiting, and myelosuppression. Leukopenia and thrombocytopenia constitute the principal limitation on the amount of drug that can be given. Herpes zoster is a type of skin lesion frequently associated with nitrogen mustard therapy. Latent viral infections may be unmasked by treatment with mechlorethamine. Thrombophlebitis is a potential complication, and extravasation of the drug results in severe local tissue reactions, with brawny and tender induration that may persist for prolonged periods.

Cyclophosphamide

Cyclophosphamide is well absorbed after oral administration and is subsequently activated in the liver to aldophosphamide for transport to target tissues. Parenteral administration is also effective. Target cells are able to convert aldophosphamide to highly cytotoxic metabolites, phosphoramide, and acrolein that then alkylate DNA. Maximal plasma concentrations of cyclophosphamide are achieved about 1 hour after oral administration, and the elimination half-time is 6 to 7 hours. Urinary elimination accounts for approximately 14% of this drug in an unchanged form.

Clinical Uses

Cyclophosphamide is one of the most frequently used chemotherapeutic drugs, as it is effective in the treatment of a wide range of cancers and inflammatory diseases. Its versatility is improved because of its effectiveness after oral as well as parenteral administration. Given in combination with other drugs, favorable responses have been shown in patients with Hodgkin disease, lymphosarcoma, Burkitt lymphoma, and acute lymphoblastic leukemia of childhood. Cyclophosphamide is frequently used in combination with methotrexate and fluorouracil as adjuvant therapy after surgery for breast cancer when there is involvement of the axillary nodes. Cyclophosphamide has potent immunosuppressive properties, leading to its use in nonneoplastic disorders associated with altered immune reactivity, including Wegener granulomatosis and rheumatoid arthritis.

Side Effects

Hypersensitivity reactions and fibrosing pneumonitis have been noted in patients treated with cyclophosphamide; the incidence is less than 1% and symptoms may develop months to years after initiation of the drug. Large doses of cyclophosphamide are associated with a high incidence of pericarditis and pericardial effusion, which in some cases has progressed to cardiac tamponade.[10] Smaller numbers of treated patients develop hemorrhagic myocarditis with symptoms of congestive heart failure, which may not occur for as long as 2 weeks after the last dose of drug.

Cyclophosphamide differs from other nitrogen mustards in that significant degrees of thrombocytopenia are less common but alopecia is more frequent. Nausea and vomiting occur with equal frequency regardless of the route of administration. Mucosal ulcerations, increased skin pigmentation, and hepatotoxicity are possible side effects. Sterile hemorrhagic cystitis occurs in 5% to 10% of patients, presumably reflecting chemical irritation produced by reactive metabolites of cyclophosphamide. Dysuria and hematuria are indications to discontinue the drug. Inappropriate secretion of arginine vasopressin hormone has been observed in patients receiving cyclophosphamide, usually with doses of greater than 50 mg/kg. It is important to consider the possibility of water intoxication because these patients are usually being hydrated to minimize the likelihood that hemorrhagic cystitis will develop. Extravasation of the drug does not produce local reactions, and thrombophlebitis does not complicate IV administration.

Melphalan

Melphalan is a phenylalanine derivative of nitrogen mustard with a range of activity similar to other alkylating drugs. It is not a vesicant. Oral absorption is excellent, resulting in drug concentrations similar to those achieved by the IV route of administration. The elimination half-time is approximately 1.5 hours, and up to 15% of the drug is eliminated unchanged in urine.

Side Effects

The side effects of melphalan are primarily hematologic and are similar to those of other alkylating drugs. It is usually necessary to maintain a significant degree of bone marrow depression (leukocyte count 3,000 to 5,000 cells/mm^3) to achieve optimal therapeutic effects. Pulmonary fibrosis is possible. Nausea and vomiting are not common side effects of melphalan. Alopecia does not occur, and changes in renal or hepatic function have not been reported.

Chlorambucil

Chlorambucil is the aromatic derivative of mechlorethamine. Oral absorption is adequate. The drug has an elimination half-time of approximately 1.5 hours and is almost completely metabolized. Chlorambucil is the slowest acting nitrogen mustard in clinical use. It is the treatment of choice in chronic lymphocytic leukemia and in primary (Waldenström) macroglobulinemia. A marked increase in the incidence of leukemia and other tumors has been noted with the use of this drug for the treatment of polycythemia vera.

Side Effects

Cytotoxic effects of chlorambucil on the bone marrow, lymphoid organs, and epithelial tissues are similar to those observed with other alkylating drugs. Its myelosuppressive action is usually moderate, gradual, and rapidly reversible. Pulmonary fibrosis is possible. Nausea and vomiting are frequent. CNS stimulation can occur but has been observed only with large doses. Hepatotoxicity may rarely occur.

Alkyl Sulfonates

Busulfan is a cell cycle nonspecific alkylating antineoplastic agent in the class of alkyl sulfonates. Busulfan is well absorbed after oral administration. IV administration is also effective. Almost the entire drug is eliminated by the kidneys as methane sulfonic acid. Busulfan produces remissions in up to 90% of patients with chronic myelogenous leukemia. The drug is of no value in the treatment of acute leukemia.

Side Effects

Busulfan can produce progressive pulmonary fibrosis in up to 4% of patients. The prognosis after appearance of clinical symptoms is poor, with a median survival of 5 months.[11] Enhanced toxicity with administration of supplemental oxygen has not been noted. Myelosuppression and thrombocytopenia are important side effects of busulfan. Nausea, vomiting, and diarrhea occur. Hyperuricemia resulting from extensive purine catabolism accompanying the rapid cellular destruction and renal damage from precipitation of urates have been noted. Allopurinol is recommended to minimize renal complications.

Nitrosoureas

The nitrosoureas are mustard gas–related compounds used as an alkylating agent in chemotherapy. Nitrosoureas, represented by carmustine, lomustine, semustine, and streptozocin, possess a wide spectrum of activity for human malignancies including intracranial tumors, melanomas, and gastrointestinal and hematologic malignancies. Indeed, the high lipid solubility results in passage across the blood–brain barrier and efficacy in the treatment of meningeal leukemias and brain tumors. These drugs appear to act by carboxylation and alkylation of nucleic acids. With the exception of streptozocin, the clinical use of nitrosoureas is limited by profound drug-induced myelosuppression.

Carmustine

Carmustine is the nitrosourea in widest clinical use. It is capable of inhibiting synthesis of both RNA and DNA. Although oral absorption is rapid, the drug is injected IV because tissue uptake and metabolism occur quickly. Local burning may accompany infusion. Carmustine disappears from plasma in 5 to 15 minutes. Because of its ability to rapidly cross the blood–brain barrier, carmustine is used to treat meningeal leukemia and primary as well as metastatic brain tumors.

Side Effects

Carmustine has been associated with interstitial pneumonitis and fibrosis much like bleomycin.[12] The incidence of pulmonary toxicity is in the range of 20% to 30%, with a mortality in those affected of 24% to 90%. The cumulative dose is the major risk factor, with 50% of patients exhibiting toxicity at doses above the range of 1,200 to 1,500 mg/m^2. A unique side effect of carmustine is a delayed onset (after approximately 6 weeks of treatment) of leukopenia and thrombocytopenia. Active metabolites may be responsible for this toxicity. CNS toxicity, nausea and vomiting, flushing of the skin and conjunctiva, nephrotoxicity, and hepatotoxicity have been reported.

Lomustine and Semustine

Lomustine and its methylated analogue semustine possess similar clinical toxicity to carmustine, including delayed bone marrow depression manifesting as leukopenia and thrombocytopenia. Lomustine appears to be more effective than carmustine in the treatment of Hodgkin disease.

Streptozocin

Streptozocin has a methylnitrosourea moiety attached to the number 2 carbon atom of glucose. It has a unique affinity for β cells of the islets of Langerhans and has proved useful in the treatment of human pancreatic islet cell carcinoma and malignant carcinoid. In animals, the drug is used to produce experimental diabetes mellitus.

Side Effects

Approximately 70% of patients receiving this drug develop hepatic or renal toxicity. Renal toxicity may manifest as tubular damage and progress to renal failure and death. Hyperglycemia can occur as a result of selective destruction of pancreatic β cells and resultant hypoinsulinism.[6] Myelosuppression is not produced by this drug.

Mitomycin

Mitomycin is the prototypical alkylating agent and is of value in the palliative treatment of gastric adenocarcinoma in combination with fluorouracil and doxorubicin. The drug is administered IV and is widely distributed in tissues but does not readily enter the CNS. Metabolism is in the liver, with less than 10% of mitomycin excreted unchanged in bile or urine.

Side Effects

Myelosuppression is a prominent side effect of mitomycin and is characterized by severe leukopenia and thrombocytopenia, which may be delayed in appearance. Mitomycin is capable of inducing pulmonary fibrosis, with an incidence ranging between 3% and 12%.[13] Like bleomycin, mitomycin appears to act synergistically to induce pulmonary fibrosis with thoracic radiation and oxygen therapy, suggesting the need to limit exposure of treated patients to hyperoxia. Nausea, vomiting, gastrointestinal mucositis, and alopecia are recognized toxic effects. Glomerular damage resulting in renal failure is a rare but well-recognized complication.

Platinating Drugs

Cisplatin

Although cisplatin is frequently designated as an alkylating agent, it has no alkyl group and so cannot carry out alkylating reactions. It is correctly classified as alkylating-like. Cisplatin contains a platinum atom, two amines, and two chlorides, which result in chemotherapeutic effects resembling DNA alkylating drugs by cross-linking adjacent or opposing guanine bases to disrupt DNA. The drug must be administered IV because oral ingestion is ineffective. High concentrations of cisplatin are found in the kidneys, liver, intestines, and testes, but there is poor penetration into the CNS. Cisplatin and its analogue carboplatin are components of the treatment of many nonhematologic malignancies, including lung, bladder, testicular, and ovarian cancer.

Side Effects

Renal toxicity is prominent and becomes the dose-limiting toxic effect of cisplatin. Decreased glomerular filtration rate and renal tubular dysfunction produced by cisplatin may begin as early as 3 to 5 days after initiating treatment with this drug. Along with increasing blood urea nitrogen and plasma creatinine concentrations, proteinuria, and hyperuricemia, there is a magnesium-wasting defect in as many as 50% of patients manifesting as some degree of cisplatin-induced renal dysfunction. Acute tubular necrosis may progress to acute renal failure, necessitating hemodialysis. Hydration and diuresis induced with mannitol and furosemide may protect against the development of renal toxicity by dilution of the tubular urinary concentration of cisplatin. The hypomagnesemia that is associated with cisplatin's renal tubular injury may predispose to cardiac dysrhythmias and decrease the dose requirements for neuromuscular blocking drugs.

Ototoxicity caused by cisplatin is manifested by tinnitus and hearing loss in the high-frequency range. Cisplatin is considered highly emetogenic, with marked nausea and vomiting occurring in almost all patients who do not receive antiemetics, although prophylactic antinausea regimens can be highly effective. Mild to moderate myelosuppression may develop, with transient leukopenia and thrombocytopenia. Peripheral sensory neuropathies, paresthesias, and loss of vibratory and position sense are common findings. Most neuropathies are reversible, although symptoms may persist for months. Hyperuricemia, seizures, and cardiac dysrhythmias have been observed. Allergic reactions characterized by facial edema, bronchoconstriction, tachycardia, and hypotension may occur minutes after injection of the drug.

Antimetabolites

Nucleic acid synthesis inhibitors (antimetabolites) include folate analogues, pyrimidine analogues, and purine analogues. These drugs are particularly effective in destroying cells during the S phase of the cell cycle, which is when DNA is synthesized. Selective effects on cancer cells may relate to greater rates of DNA replication in cancer cells than normal cells. Nevertheless, side effects (myelosuppression and mucositis) reflect effects on proliferating but nonmalignant cells.

Folate Analogues

Methotrexate

Methotrexate is a poorly lipid-soluble folate analogue that is effective in the treatment of different hematologic and nonhematologic cancers and is classified as an antimetabolite (folic acid antagonist). This drug inhibits dihydrofolate reductase, which is the enzyme that uses reduced folate as a methyl donor in the synthesis of pyrimidine and purine nucleosides. Inhibition of dihydrofolate reductase by methotrexate prevents the formation of tetrahydrofolic acid and causes disruption of cellular metabolism by producing an acute intracellular deficiency of folate enzymes. As a result, 1-carbon transfer reactions necessary for the eventual synthesis of DNA and RNA cease.

Methotrexate is readily absorbed after oral administration. Significant metabolism of methotrexate does not seem to occur, with more than 50% of the drug appearing unchanged in urine. Renal excretion reflects glomerular filtration and tubular secretion. Toxic concentrations of methotrexate may occur in patients with renal insufficiency. Methotrexate remains in tissues for weeks, suggesting binding of the drug to dihydrofolate reductase.

Clinical Uses

Methotrexate is widely used in the treatment of malignant and some nonmalignant disorders. It is a useful drug in the treatment of acute lymphoblastic leukemia in children but not adults. Choriocarcinoma is effectively treated with this drug. Improvement in the clinical manifestations of psoriasis in patients reflects the effect of methotrexate on rapidly dividing epidermal cells characteristic of this disease. This drug may also be useful in the treatment of rheumatoid arthritis.

Methotrexate is poorly transported across the blood–brain barrier, and neoplastic cells that have entered the CNS probably are not affected by the usual plasma concentrations of the drug. Intrathecal injection is used to treat cerebral involvement with either leukemia or choriocarcinoma.

Acquired resistance to methotrexate develops as a result of (a) impaired transport of methotrexate into cells, (b) production of altered forms of dihydrofolate reductase that have decreased affinity for the drug, and (c) increased concentrations of intracellular dihydrofolate reductase.

Side Effects

The most important side effects of methotrexate occur in the gastrointestinal tract and bone marrow. Leukopenia and thrombocytopenia reflect bone marrow depression. Ulcerative stomatitis and diarrhea are frequent side effects and require interruption of treatment. Hemorrhagic enteritis and death from intestinal perforation may occur. Pulmonary toxicity may take the form of fulminant noncardiogenic pulmonary edema, or a more progressive inflammation, with interstitial infiltrates and pleural effusions.[14] The incidence of pulmonary toxicity attributed to methotrexate is in the range of 8%, but its frequent use in combination with other chemotherapeutic drugs makes this number uncertain.[15] Methotrexate is associated with renal toxicity, with an incidence approaching 10% in higher doses.[16] Renal insufficiency may be prevented by hydration and urinary alkalinization. Short-term or intermittent therapy with methotrexate results in increases in liver transaminase enzymes. Hepatic dysfunction is usually reversible but may sometimes lead to cirrhosis. It may be useful to measure liver function tests preoperatively in patients who have recently received methotrexate. Encephalopathic syndromes may accompany intrathecal or IV administration of methotrexate and may be transient or permanent.[17] Alopecia and dermatitis may accompany administration of methotrexate. Folic acid antagonists also interfere with embryogenesis, emphasizing the risk in administering these drugs to pregnant patients. Normal cells can be protected from lethal damage by folate antagonists with sequential administration of folinic acid (leucovorin), thymidine, or both. This approach has been termed the ***rescue technique***.

Pyrimidine Analogues

Pyrimidine analogues have in common the ability to prevent the biosynthesis of pyrimidine nucleotides or to mimic these natural metabolites to such an extent that they interfere with vital cellular activities such as the synthesis and functioning of nucleic acids. Examples of antimetabolite chemotherapeutic drugs that function as pyrimidine analogues are fluorouracil and cytarabine.

Fluorouracil

Fluorouracil blocks production of thymine nucleotides by inhibiting thymidylate synthase. This chemotherapeutic drug lacks significant inhibitory activity on cells and must be converted enzymatically to a 5′-monophosphate nucleotide. Administration of fluorouracil is usually by IV injection because absorption after oral ingestion is unpredictable and incomplete. Metabolic degradation occurs primarily in the liver, with an important metabolite being urea. Only approximately 10% of fluorouracil appears unchanged in urine. Fluorouracil readily enters the cerebrospinal fluid, with therapeutic concentrations being present within 30 minutes after IV administration.

Clinical Uses

Fluorouracil may be of palliative value in certain types of carcinoma, particularly of the breast and gastrointestinal tract. The drug is often used for the topical treatment of premalignant keratoses of the skin and superficial basal cell carcinomas.

Side Effects

Side effects caused by fluorouracil are difficult to anticipate because of their delayed appearance. Fluorouracil-induced myocardial ischemia is a rare cardiac toxicity that may lead to myocardial infarction up to 1 week after treatment.[18] The incidence of this side effect is low in patients without underlying heart disease but may increase to 4.5% of treated patients with preexisting coronary artery disease. Stomatitis manifesting as a white patchy membrane that ulcerates and becomes necrotic is an early sign of toxicity and warns of the possibility that similar lesions may be developing in the esophagus and gastrointestinal tract. Myelosuppression, most frequently manifesting as leukopenia between 9 and 14 days of therapy, is a serious side effect. Thrombocytopenia and anemia may complicate treatment with fluorouracil. Loss of hair progressing to total alopecia, nail changes, dermatitis, and increased pigmentation and atrophy of the skin may occur. Hand-foot syndrome has also been associated with fluorouracil. Neurologic manifestations, including an acute cerebellar syndrome (ataxia), have been reported.

Capecitabine

Capecitabine is an orally administered drug that is metabolized to fluorouracil by thymidine phosphorylase after absorption from the gastrointestinal tract. Because there is more activity of thymidine phosphorylase in cancer cells (especially breast cancer) than in normal cells, capecitabine has the potential to be more selective than fluorouracil.

Pemetrexed

Pemetrexed is a folate antagonist that is effective in the treatment of mesothelioma and lung cancer. This drug inhibits multiple enzymes involved in the folate pathway, including thymidylate synthase and dihydrofolate reductase.

Cytarabine

Cytarabine (cytosine arabinoside), like other pyrimidine antimetabolites, must be activated by conversion to the 5′-monophosphate nucleotide before inhibition of DNA synthesis can occur. Both natural and acquired resistance to cytarabine develops, reflecting the activity of cytidine deaminase, an enzyme capable of converting cytarabine to the inactive metabolite arabinosyl uracil.

Clinical Uses

In addition to its chemotherapeutic activity, particularly in acute leukemia in children and adults, cytarabine has potent immunosuppressive properties. The drug is particularly useful in chemotherapy of acute granulocytic leukemia in adults. IV administration of cytarabine is recommended because oral absorption is poor and unpredictable.

Side Effects

Cytarabine is a potent myelosuppressive drug capable of producing severe leukopenia, thrombocytopenia, and anemia. Cerebellar toxicity and ataxia can occur at high doses. Other side effects include gastrointestinal disturbances, stomatitis, and hepatic dysfunction. Thrombophlebitis at the site of infusion is common. Alternatively, the drug may be given subcutaneously.

Gemcitabine

Gemcitabine resembles cytarabine structurally yet gemcitabine is active in several nonhematologic cancers, whereas cytarabine is not effective. Gemcitabine is also used in solid organ carcinomas, such as of the pancreas, breast, and lung. This most likely reflects unique effects of this chemotherapeutic drug on DNA and RNA metabolism. Common side effects associated with use of gemcitabine include bone marrow suppression, flulike symptoms, fever, fatigue, mild nausea/vomiting, and diarrhea.

Purine Analogues

Antimetabolite chemotherapeutic drugs that function as purine analogues include mercaptopurine, azathioprine, thioguanine, pentostatin (2′-deoxycoformycin), and cladribine (2-chlorodeoxyadenosine). Mercaptopurine and thioguanine are analogues of the natural purines hypoxanthine and guanine, respectively.

Mercaptopurine

Mercaptopurine is incorporated into DNA or RNA strands and either blocks further strand synthesis or causes structural alterations that damage DNA. This drug is useful in the treatment of acute leukemia in children. Oral absorption is prompt, and gastrointestinal epithelium is not damaged. The elimination half-time is brief (about 90 minutes) due to rapid tissue uptake, renal excretion, and hepatic metabolism. One pathway of metabolism is methylation and subsequent oxidation of the methylated derivatives. A second pathway involves the enzyme xanthine oxidase, which oxidizes mercaptopurine to 6-thiouric acid. Allopurinol, as an inhibitor of xanthine oxidase, prevents conversion of mercaptopurine to 6-thiouric acid and thus increases the exposure of cells to mercaptopurine. The dose of mercaptopurine is decreased by about one-third when the drug is combined with allopurinol.

Side Effects

The principal side effect of mercaptopurine is a gradual development of bone marrow depression manifesting as thrombocytopenia, granulocytopenia, or anemia several weeks after initiation of therapy. Anorexia, nausea, and vomiting are common side effects; stomatitis and diarrhea rarely occur. Jaundice occurs in approximately one-third of patients and is associated with bile stasis and occasional hepatic necrosis. Hyperuricemia and hyperuricosuria may occur during treatment with mercaptopurine, presumably reflecting destruction of cells. This effect may require the use of allopurinol.

Thioguanine

Thioguanine is of particular value in the treatment of acute myelogenous leukemia, especially if given with cytarabine. After oral administration, thioguanine appears in the urine as a methylated metabolite and inorganic sulfate. Minimal amounts of 6-thiouric acid are formed, suggesting that deamination is not important in the metabolic inactivation of thioguanine. For this reason, thioguanine may be administered concurrently with allopurinol without a decrease in dosage, unlike mercaptopurine. Toxic manifestations of thioguanine treatment include bone marrow depression and, occasionally, gastrointestinal effects.

Pentostatin and Cladribine

Pentostatin and cladribine are purine analogues that have clinical activity against a variety of indolent lymphoid tumors, with the most dramatic effects occurring in patients with hairy-cell leukemia.[19] These drugs act by irreversibly binding to adenosine deaminase (pentostatin) or by chemical modification of enzyme substrate, rendering it resistant to the action of adenosine deaminase (cladribine). Patients with acute leukemia and cells with high levels of adenosine deaminase activity are most likely to respond to these drugs. Fever, which is likely due to cytokines, is a side effect of treatment with cladribine. Both drugs are capable of producing immunosuppression. The recovery from immunosuppression seems to be more rapid after treatment with cladribine than after treatment with pentostatin, perhaps because of the shorter duration of administration of the former. Indeed, cladribine is emerging as the treatment of choice for hairy cell leukemia because of its minimal toxicity and its ability to induce a complete and sustained response with a single course of therapy.

Hydroxyurea

Hydroxyurea acts on the enzyme ribonucleoside diphosphate reductase to interfere with the synthesis of DNA. Oral absorption is excellent, and approximately 80% of the drug appears in the urine within 12 hours after oral or IV administration. The primary use of hydroxyurea is in the treatment of chronic myelogenous leukemia. Temporary remissions in patients with metastatic malignant melanoma have been reported.

Side Effects

Myelosuppression manifesting as leukopenia, megaloblastic anemia, and occasionally thrombocytopenia is the major side effect produced by hydroxyurea. Nausea and vomiting may accompany administration of this drug. Hyperpigmentation of the skin, stomatitis, and alopecia occur infrequently.

Topoisomerase Inhibitors

Topoisomerases are enzymes that correct alterations in DNA which occur during replication and transcription. Certain chemotherapeutic drugs inhibit either topoisomerase I or topoisomerase II. Because cancer cells possess more topoisomerase activity than normal cells, there is more drug-induced DNA damage and resultant cell death. Toxicity reflects effects of inhibition of topoisomerase enzymes on normal proliferating tissues (myelosuppression, mucositis). Topoisomerase II inhibitors that include doxorubicin, daunorubicin, etoposide, and teniposide are part of most combination chemotherapy treatment regimens. Topoisomerase I inhibitors include topotecan and irinotecan. These drugs exhibit a broad spectrum of chemotherapeutic activity being useful in the treatment of leukemia and lung, colon, and ovarian cancer.

Doxorubicin and Daunorubicin

Doxorubicin and daunorubicin are anthracycline antibiotics that are natural products of certain soil fungi. Structurally, they contain a tetracycline ring attached to the sugar daunosamine by a glycosidic linkage. These drugs most likely act by binding to DNA, resulting in changes in the DNA helix that interfere with the ability of nucleic acids to serve as a template during replication. These drugs are also a likely cause of disruptive effects on cellular membranes. Drug-induced free radicals may overwhelm the heart's antioxidant defenses, leading to the oxidation of critical cardiac proteins and membrane components (unsaturated free fatty acids), leading to cardiotoxicity.[20] Laboratory studies demonstrate that each subsequent dose of doxorubicin appears to diminish the heart's ability to withstand subsequent oxidant stress. Evidence that free radicals have a role is the protective effect of free radical scavengers.

Daunorubicin and doxorubicin are administered IV, with care taken to prevent extravasation because local vesicant action may result. There is rapid clearance from the plasma into the heart, kidneys, lungs, and liver. These drugs do not cross the blood–brain barrier to any significant extent. The urine may become red for 1 to 2 days after administration of these drugs.

Daunorubicin is metabolized primarily to daunorubiconol, whereas doxorubicin is excreted unchanged and as metabolites, including adriamycinol in the urine. Ultimately, approximately 40% of daunorubicin and doxorubicin are metabolized. Indeed, clinical toxicity may result in patients with hepatic dysfunction.

Clinical Uses

Daunorubicin is used primarily in the treatment of acute lymphocytic and myelocytic leukemia. Doxorubicin, which differs from daunorubicin only by a single hydroxyl group on the number 14 carbon atom, is also effective against a wide range of solid tumors. For example, doxorubicin is one of the most active single drugs for treating metastatic adenocarcinoma of the breast, carcinoma of the bladder, bronchogenic carcinoma, metastatic thyroid carcinoma, oat cell carcinoma, and osteogenic carcinoma.

Resistance is observed to the anthracycline antibiotics, as with other chemotherapeutic drugs. Furthermore, cross-tolerance occurs between daunorubicin and doxorubicin. Cross-resistance also occurs between these antibiotics and the vinca alkaloids, suggesting that an alteration of cellular permeability may be involved.

Side Effects

Cardiomyopathy and myelosuppression are side effects of the chemotherapeutic antibiotics. Leukopenia typically manifests during the second week of therapy. Thrombocytopenia and anemia occur but are usually less pronounced. Stomatitis, gastrointestinal disturbances, and alopecia are common side effects.

Cardiomyopathy

Cardiomyopathy is a unique dose-related and often irreversible side effect of the anthracycline antibiotics. Increased plasma concentrations of troponin T reflect drug-induced injury to myocardial cells. Congestive heart failure develops in less than 3% of patients with a cumulative dose of doxorubicin of less than 400 mg/m^2, rising to 18% at 700 mg/m^2 (Fig. 42-2).[21] Prior mediastinal radiation or previous treatment with cyclophosphamide increases the subsequent risk of cardiomyopathy in response to administration of an anthracycline antibiotic. Marked impairment of left ventricular function for as long as 3 years after discontinuing doxorubicin has been observed. Previous treatment with anthracycline antibiotics may enhance myocardial depressant effects of anesthetic drugs even in patients with normal resting cardiac function.[22] Acute left ventricular failure 2 months after cessation of treatment with doxorubicin has been described during general anesthesia.[23]

Two types of cardiomyopathies may occur.[6,20] An acute form of cardiomyopathy occurs in approximately 10% of patients and is characterized by relatively benign changes on the ECG that include nonspecific ST-T changes and decreased QRS voltage. Other cardiac changes include premature ventricular contractions, supraventricular tachydysrhythmias, cardiac conduction abnormalities, and left axis deviation. These abnormalities occur during therapy at all dose levels and, except for decreased QRS voltage on the ECG, resolve 1 to 2 months after discontinuation of therapy. There is an associated acute reversible decrease in the ejection fraction within 24 hours after a single dose.

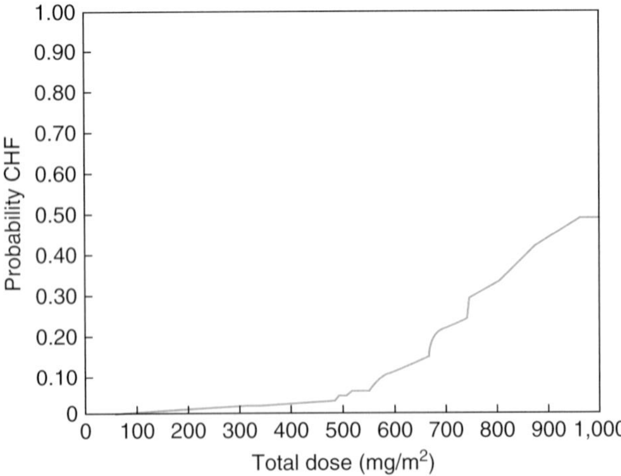

FIGURE 42-2 The probability of developing doxorubicin-induced congestive heart failure (CHF) versus the total cumulative dose of doxorubicin. (From Von Hoff DD, Layard MW, Basa P, et al. Risk factors for doxorubicin-induced congestive heart failure. *Ann Intern Med.* 1979;91:710–707, with permission.)

The second form of cardiomyopathy is characterized by the insidious onset of symptoms such as dry nonproductive cough, suggesting bronchitis, followed by rapidly progressive heart failure that is unresponsive to inotropic drugs and mechanical ventricular assistance.[6] This severe form of cardiomyopathy occurs in almost 2% of treated patients and is fatal approximately 3 weeks after the onset of symptoms in nearly 60% of affected patients. Predictive tests to permit early recognition of impending cardiomyopathy are not available, although diminution in QRS voltage on the ECG is consistent with the diffuse character of the myocardial damage. Increased plasma concentrations of cardiac enzymes occur late in the course of cardiac failure and are of limited value in achieving an early diagnosis. Systolic time intervals and echocardiograms have been used to detect cardiotoxicity before the occurrence of clinically significant damage. Dexrazoxane is a free radical scavenger that protects the heart from doxorubicin-associated damage.[24]

Dactinomycin

Dactinomycin (actinomycin D) is an antibiotic with chemotherapeutic activity resulting from its ability to bind to DNA, especially in rapidly proliferating cells. As a result of this binding, the function of RNA polymerase and thus the transcription of the DNA molecule are blocked. After IV injection, dactinomycin rapidly leaves the circulation. In animals, approximately 50% of an injected dose is excreted unchanged in bile and 10% in urine. There is no evidence that the drug undergoes metabolism. Dactinomycin does not cross the blood–brain barrier in amounts sufficient to produce a pharmacologic effect.

Clinical Uses

The most important clinical use of dactinomycin is the treatment of Wilms tumor in children and of rhabdomyosarcoma. It may be effective in some women with methotrexate-resistant choriocarcinoma. Occasionally, this drug is used to inhibit immunologic responses associated with organ transplantation.

Side Effects

The toxic effects of dactinomycin include the early onset of nausea and vomiting, often followed by myelosuppression manifesting as pancytopenia 1 to 7 days after completion of therapy. Pancytopenia may be preceded by thrombocytopenia as the first manifestation of bone marrow suppression. Glossitis, ulcerations of the oral mucosa, diarrhea, alopecia, and cutaneous erythema are commonly associated with dactinomycin therapy. Extravasation of the drug results in tissue necrosis.

Bleomycin

Bleomycins are water-soluble glycopeptides that differ from one another (there are more than 200 congeners) in their terminal amine moiety. The terminal amine is coupled through an amide linkage to a carboxylic acid. Bleomycin possesses a tripeptide component that binds DNA and a metal-binding region. In the presence of oxygen and either iron or copper, bleomycin produces free radicals which create DNA breaks.

Bleomycin is administered IV, and high concentrations occur in the skin and lungs. The drug accumulates in tumors, suggesting the presence of a lower level of inactivating enzyme. Bleomycin is eliminated primarily by renal excretion, with approximately 50% of the dose cleared within 4 hours and 70% by 24 hours.[25] Indeed, excessive concentrations of drug occur if usual doses are administered to patients with impaired renal function.

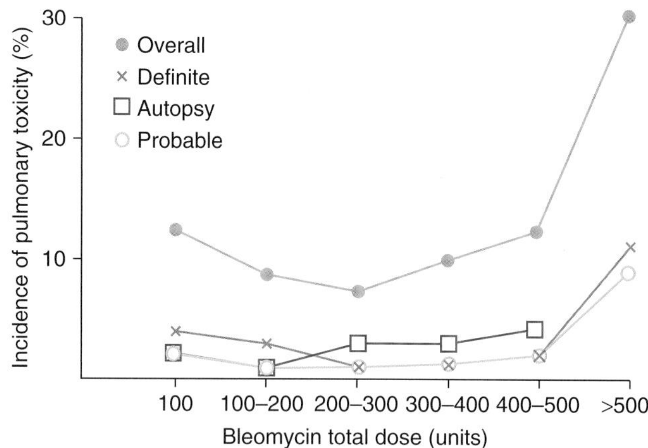

FIGURE 42-3 The relationship between the total dose of bleomycin and the incidence of pulmonary toxicity. (From Ginsberg SJ, Comis RL. The pulmonary toxicity of antineoplastic agents. *Semin Oncol.* 1982;9:34–51, with permission.)

Clinical Uses

Bleomycin is effective in the treatment of testicular carcinoma, particularly if administered in combination with vinblastine. It is also useful in the palliative treatment of squamous cell carcinomas of the head, neck, esophagus, skin, and genitourinary tract.

Side Effects

The most common side effects of bleomycin are mucocutaneous reactions, including stomatitis, alopecia, pruritus, erythema, and hyperpigmentation, which occur in approximately 45% of patients. In contrast to other chemotherapeutic drugs, bleomycin causes minimal myelosuppression. Unexplained exacerbations of rheumatoid arthritis have occurred.

Patients with lymphomas who are receiving bleomycin may develop an acute reaction characterized by hyperthermia, hypotension, and hypoventilation. The likely mechanism is the release of an endogenous pyrogen, presumably from destroyed tumor cells. An initial small test dose of bleomycin is recommended to minimize the occurrence of this syndrome.

Pulmonary Toxicity

The most serious side effect of bleomycin is dose-related pulmonary toxicity (Fig. 42-3).[11] Indeed, bleomycin is concentrated preferentially in the lungs and is inactivated by a hydrolase enzyme, which is relatively deficient in lung tissue. Initially, bleomycin produces pulmonary capillary endothelial damage, progressing to alveolar epithelial injury with necrosis of type 1 and proliferation of type 2 alveolar cells. Interstitial fibrosis develops and may progress to involve the entire lung. It is estimated that some form of pulmonary toxicity (most often pulmonary fibrosis) occurs in 4% of patients treated with bleomycin. Fatal pulmonary toxicity has occurred with bleomycin doses as low as 100 mg but more often in the presence of other risk factors (Table 42-3).

The first signs of pulmonary toxicity are cough, dyspnea, and basilar rales, which progress in one of two directions. A mild form of pulmonary toxicity is characterized by exertional dyspnea and a normal resting $Pa{O_2}$. A more severe form of arterial hypoxemia at rest is associated with radiographic findings of interstitial pneumonitis and fibrosis. Lesions are found more frequently in lower lobes and subpleural areas, and radiographs of the chest often reveal basilar and perihilar infiltrates. The alveolar–arterial gradient for oxygen is increased, and pulmonary diffusion capacity may be decreased. Pulmonary function studies have been of no greater value than clinical signs in detecting the onset of pulmonary toxicity.

Early reports of postoperative respiratory failure in bleomycin-treated patients suggested that either arterial hyperoxia or excessive crystalloid administration played a role in the exacerbation of pulmonary fibrosis.[26–28] One speculation is that acutely increased inhaled concentrations of oxygen facilitate production of superoxide and other free radicals in the presence of bleomycin. For this

Table 42-3

Risk Factors for Development of Chemotherapy-Induced Pulmonary Toxicity

Total drug dose
Age
Concurrent or prior chest radiation
Oxygen therapy
Combination chemotherapy
Preexisting pulmonary disease
Genetic predisposition
Cigarette smoking (?)

reason, it has been recommended that inhaled oxygen concentrations be maintained below 30% in bleomycin-treated patients. Animal model literature confirms that the continuous administration of inspired oxygen concentrations of greater than 30% immediately after exposure to bleomycin increases pulmonary damage.[29] Nevertheless, it is unlikely that patients will present to the operating room immediately after treatment with bleomycin. A more practical question is whether hyperoxia for short periods of time several days after treatment is a risk factor for bleomycin-induced pulmonary damage.[30] In this regard, animal studies have confirmed that delayed exposure to supplemental oxygen after bleomycin treatment is not harmful.[31] Nevertheless, there are case reports of respiratory failure with inspired oxygen concentrations greater than 30% in patients last exposed to bleomycin up to 6 to 12 months before hyperoxia. Patients with prior exposure to bleomycin but with no risk factors appear to be at a minimum risk from hyperoxia. In contrast, those patients with one or more major risk factors (preexisting pulmonary damage from bleomycin, which is more likely if the total dose is greater than 450 mg; renal dysfunction, which slows clearance of the drug from the lungs; and/or prior exposure to bleomycin within a 1- to 2-month period) may be at higher risk for the development of bleomycin-induced hyperoxic pulmonary injury in the operating room. It may be prudent to maintain these patients on the minimum inspired oxygen concentration that can be used safely intraoperatively to provide oxygen saturations of greater than 90% by pulse oximetry.[30] The value of corticosteroids as pretreatment in patients with risk factors and in whom greater than 30% oxygen may be needed, for example, operations requiring cardiopulmonary bypass, has not been confirmed by controlled studies. The role of excessive crystalloid administration has not received the same scrutiny as increased delivered oxygen concentrations. A consideration in this regard is replacement of fluids with colloids rather than crystalloids to decrease or prevent pulmonary interstitial edema in bleomycin-treated patients undergoing surgery. Accumulation of interstitial fluid may reflect impaired lymphatic function caused by bleomycin-induced fibrotic changes in the lungs. In the future, bleomycin may be replaced with phleomycin, an analogue of bleomycin that has lower pulmonary toxicity and a broader effectiveness against multiple types of tumors.[32]

Tubulin-Binding Drugs

Microtubules are subcellular structures that are essential for normal function of cells. They form the architecture to maintain cell shape, organize the location of organelles, and mediate intracellular transport and secretion, neurotransmission, axonemal flow, and cell motility.[33] Vinca alkaloids and taxanes are examples of antimitotic chemotherapeutic drugs that disrupt the normal function of microtubules. Vinca alkaloids bind to depolymerized microtubules and inhibit microtubule formation. Taxanes bind to polymerized microtubules and inhibit their breakdown. The result of these interactions is the failure of the cell to undergo normal mitosis leading to cell death.

Vinca Alkaloids

Vinca alkaloids represent the active medicinal ingredients from the pink periwinkle plant and include vincristine, vinblastine, vinorelbine, and vindesine. Vincristine is highly effective against Hodgkin disease, non-Hodgkin lymphoma, and pediatric solid tumors, yet it has little activity against adult solid tumors. Vinorelbine, in contrast, is active against breast and lung cancer. Vinblastine is most often used in the treatment of testicular cancer and non-Hodgkin lymphoma.

Side Effects

Myelosuppression manifesting as leukopenia, thrombocytopenia, and anemia are the most prominent side effects of vinca alkaloids, appearing 7 to 10 days after initiation of treatment. Vincristine is less likely than vinblastine and vinorelbine to cause bone marrow depression.

Symmetric peripheral sensory–motor neuropathy often occurs during administration of therapeutic doses of vincristine and may become the dose-limiting side effect.[34,35] Clinical manifestations may include several aspects of peripheral nerve function with areflexia (loss of Achilles tendon reflex) being the earliest finding. Paresthesias in the hands and feet, weakness and atrophy of the extremities, and skeletal muscle pain make use of the hands and feet difficult (ataxia). Tremors frequently develop, neuropathic pain and foot drop are common. Autonomic neuropathy with orthostatic hypotension, bowel motility dysfunction, and cranial nerve involvement (laryngeal nerve paralysis with hoarseness, weakness of the extraocular muscles) are present in about 10% of treated patients.[36] CNS effects (confusion, insomnia, seizures, hallucinations) due to vincristine are rare, presumably because of poor penetration of the blood–brain barrier by the drug. The peripheral neuropathy is mainly axonal, but demyelination may also occur as demonstrated by measurement of somatosensory evoked potentials.[35] Vincristine-induced peripheral neuropathy is said to be reversible after discontinuing the drug, although this may require months, and in some patients, the resolution may be incomplete.[34] There is limited evidence that suggests that neuraxial anesthesia and peripheral nerve blocks can be safely and effectively used in patients with preexisting peripheral neuropathy without significant risk of worsening of the neuropathy. The concentration of local anesthetic should be reduced, epinephrine should be avoided, and a nerve localization technique that minimizes the likelihood of intraneuronal injection should be used in efforts to minimize the risk of worsening the neuropathy.[37] Neuropathies do worsen during the perioperative period in a small number of patients whether general or regional anesthesia is used, thus a careful risk-benefit assessment and informed decision making along with each individual patient is essential.

The syndrome of hyponatremia associated with high urinary sodium and inappropriate secretion of arginine vasopressin hormone has occasionally been observed during vincristine therapy. An effect on the autonomic nervous system may be responsible for paralytic ileus and abdominal pain, which commonly develops during vinblastine therapy. Urinary retention, tenderness of the parotid glands, dryness of the mouth, and sinus tachycardia are other occasionally experienced manifestations of altered autonomic nervous system activity. Transient mental depression is most likely to occur on the second or third day of treatment with vinblastine. Alopecia appears to occur more frequently with vincristine than with vinblastine. Vinorelbine may cause chest pain, bronchospasm, dyspnea, and pulmonary infiltrations.

Taxanes

Paclitaxel (active extract from the Pacific yew tree) and docetaxel (more water-soluble semisynthetic derivative) share a broad spectrum of similar chemotherapeutic activity against breast, lung, ovarian, and bladder cancer.[38] Both drugs are also active against lymphoid malignancies. Taxanes block the function of the mitotic apparatus by impeding the normal function of microtubules. Unlike vinca alkaloids, which affect the rates of tubulin polymerization, the taxanes inhibit microtubule depolymerization in a dose-dependent manner. The microtubules formed in the presence of taxanes are extraordinarily stable and dysfunctional, thereby causing the death of the cell by disrupting the normal microtubule dynamics required for cell division.

Taxanes are rapidly cleared from the plasma despite extensive binding to proteins. The volume of distribution is large, suggesting binding to cellular proteins, possibly tubulin. Renal clearance accounts for a small proportion (<10%) of total clearance. Hepatic metabolism, biliary excretion, fecal elimination, or extensive tissue binding appears to be responsible for most of the plasma clearance.

Side Effects

Taxanes are associated with myelosuppression, peripheral neuropathy, and alopecia. Severe neurotoxicity precludes the administration of high doses of taxanes. The peripheral neuropathy is characterized by sensory symptoms such as numbness and paresthesia in a glove-and-stocking distribution. Patients may also experience transient taxane-associated arthralgias and myalgias for several days following treatment. Cardiac effects, including dysrhythmias, myocardial ischemia, and transient asymptomatic bradycardia may be more common with paclitaxel than docetaxel. Docetaxel seems to have unique vascular permeability properties which may result in peripheral edema, pleural effusion, and ascites. Fluid retention produced by docetaxel is dose-dependent and may be decreased by pretreatment with dexamethasone. Docetaxel also produces skin toxicities including an erythematous maculopapular rash on the forearms and hands. Hypersensitivity reactions (flushing, bronchospasm, dyspnea, systemic hypotension) caused by direct release of histamine or other chemical mediators may occur in 25% to 30% of patients treated with taxanes.[38]

Estramustine

Estramustine exerts its chemotherapeutic effects by inhibition of microtubule assembly and depolymerization. This drug also binds to an estramustine-binding protein in prostate tissue explaining the possible usefulness of this drug as part of combination therapy of hormone-refractory prostate cancer.

Signal Transduction Modulators

Signal transduction modulators (hormones) that may be useful in the treatment of neoplastic disease include antiestrogens, antiandrogens, aromatase inhibitors, gonadotropin-releasing drugs, and progestin. Normal cell division results from the interaction of growth factors with specific receptors. This interaction initiates a series of enzyme reactions (signal transduction), culminating in activation of nuclear transcription factors that produce cell proliferation molecules. Mutations in cancer cells result in uncontrolled cell proliferation using activated signaling pathways. Hormonal treatment of cancer disrupts growth factor receptor interactions.

Progestins

Progestational drugs are useful in the management of patients with endometrial carcinoma. Progestins act by reducing the production of hormones that stimulate the neoplastic endometrium.

Estrogens and Androgens

Malignant changes in the breast and prostate often depend on hormones for their continued growth. For example, prostatic cancer is stimulated by androgens, whereas orchiectomy or estrogens (diethylstilbestrol) slow the growth of the tumor cells. Eventually, prostatic tumors become insensitive to the lack of androgen or the presence of estrogens, presumably because of the survival of progressively undifferentiated cells that favor the emergence of cell types that no longer depend on androgens for their growth.

Malignant tissues that are responsive to estrogens contain receptors for the hormone, whereas malignant tissues lacking these receptors are unlikely to respond to hormonal manipulation. The onset of action of hormone therapy is slow, requiring 8 to 12 weeks.

Hypercalcemia may be associated with androgen or estrogen therapy, requiring adequate hydration in an attempt to facilitate renal excretion of calcium. Plasma calcium concentrations should be determined in patients receiving treatment with these hormones.

Antiestrogens

Antiestrogens, such as tamoxifen, are useful in the treatment of breast cancer that expresses estrogen or progesterone receptors. The estrogen receptor resides in the cytosol and, upon occupation by estradiol, is transported to the nucleus, where it activates genes (including those genes that encode proliferation molecules) containing estrogen-response elements. Tamoxifen binds to estrogen receptors and disrupts receptor interactions with estrogen in some but not all estrogen-responsive tissues. For example, tamoxifen is antiestrogenic in breast and ovarian tissue but is estrogenic in the uterus, liver, and bone. As a result, tamoxifen is effective in the prevention and treatment of breast cancer but produces undesired estrogen side effects including deep vein thrombosis (<1% of patients), endometrial cancer (about 0.3% of patients), and early menopausal symptoms (hot flashes). In addition, tamoxifen lowers plasma cholesterol concentrations and increases bone density.

The response to tamoxifen is proportional to the degree of expression of estrogen receptors in the breast cancer. Tamoxifen is of little benefit in women with breast cancer that does not express hormone receptors. After surgical removal of the primary breast cancer, adjuvant treatment of women with tumors that are hormone-positive decreases the odds of recurrence by more than 30%. Other antiestrogens that may have greater selectivity for breast estrogen receptors include raloxifene, toremifene, and fulvestrant.

Antiandrogens

Antiandrogens such as flutamide, bicalutamide, and nilutamide are competitive antagonists of the interactions between androstenedione and androgen receptors. Flutamide is a nonsteroidal antiandrogenic that possesses pure antiandrogenic activity when metabolized to its hydroxylated derivative. Administered with other drugs that decrease androgen production, flutamide is an effective treatment for hormone-dependent prostate cancer. Androgenic blockade results in feminizing side effects in men, including gynecomastia, hot flashes, and loss of facial hair. Skeletal muscle weakness and development of osteoporosis reflect a male menopause–like state. Flutamide can induce methemoglobinemia.[39] Pulse oximetry readings in the presence of methemoglobinemia can overestimate the hemoglobin saturation levels. At levels of methemoglobinemia of greater than 35%, the pulse oximetry readings tend to approach a minimal level of 85%.[40]

Monoclonal Antibodies

Antibody-based therapies for treatment of cancer include the monoclonal antibodies trastuzumab, alemtuzumab, rituximab, and imatinib, which target specific antigen sites on cancer cells.[41] The mechanisms of action of these agents are specific and varied depending on the target. Rituximab is used to treat leukemias and lymphomas. Rituximab binds to a specific protein (CD20) that is expressed on the cell surface of B cells; the rituximab–CD20 complex appears to improve the effectiveness of natural killer cells in killing these diseased cells. Imatinib is a monoclonal antibody that binds to the extracellular domain of a specific tyrosine kinase (BCR-ABL) and inhibits this enzyme, which is responsible for cell proliferation in Philadelphia chromosome–positive chronic myelocytic leukemia. Vaccines are also being developed that may include genetic manipulation of cancer cells to make them more antigenic and thus susceptible to immune responses. Two types of vaccines aimed at preventing infection related to subsequent development of cancer have been approved by the U.S. Food and Drug Administration (FDA): vaccines against the hepatitis B virus, which can cause liver cancer, and vaccines against specific human papillomaviruses, which are responsible for the majority of cases of cervical cancer. The FDA has approved one cancer treatment vaccine for certain men with metastatic prostate cancer.

Aromatase Inhibitors

Aromatase is an enzyme complex consisting of two proteins, aromatase cytochrome P450 (CYP19) and nicotinamide adenine dinucleotide phosphate cytochrome P450 reductase. Inhibition of aromatase blocks the conversion of androgens to estrone in peripheral tissues including breast tissue. The high affinity of the aromatase inhibitors anastrozole and letrozole for CYP19 results in intense inhibition of estrogen effects on responsive receptors. Inhibition of aromatase is an effective treatment for postmenopausal women with breast cancer, in which the greatest source of estrone comes from conversion of androstenedione to estrone in liver, skeletal muscles, and fat. Exemestane is a steroidal aromatase inhibitor that binds to the enzyme complex and promotes enzyme degradation.

A partial medical hypophysectomy is produced by luteinizing hormone–releasing hormone agonists, such as leuprolide, buserelin, and goserelin, which inhibit secretion of follicle-stimulating hormone and luteinizing hormone by downregulating receptors that respond to these hormones. The result is insignificant plasma concentrations of sex hormones and palliation of breast and prostate cancer.

References

1. Caley A, Jones R. The principles of cancer treatment by chemotherapy. *Surgery (Oxford)*. 2012;30:186–190.
2. Finn OJ. Immuno-oncology: understanding the function and dysfunction of the immune system in cancer. *Ann Oncol*. 2012; 23(suppl 8):viii6–viii9.
3. Damia G, Garattini S. The pharmacological point of view of resistance to therapy in tumors. *Cancer Treat Rev*. 2014:40(8):909–916.
4. Rubin EH, Hait WN. Principles of cancer treatment. *Sci Am Med*. 2003;12(IV):1–17.
5. Chung F. Cancer, chemotherapy, and anesthesia. *Can Anaesth Soc J*. 1982;29:364–371.
6. Selvin BF. Cancer chemotherapy: implications for the anesthesiologist. *Anesth Analg*. 1981;60:425–434.
7. Oddby-Muhrbeck E, Öbrink E, Eksborg S, et al. Is there an association between PONV and chemotherapy-induced nausea and vomiting? *Acta Anaesthesiol Scand*. 2013;57:749–753.
8. Norris JC. Prolonged succinylcholine apnoea resulting from acquired deficiency of plasma cholinesterase. *Anaesthesia*. 2003;58:1137.
9. Zsigmond EK, Robins G. The effect of a series of anticancer drugs on plasma cholinesterase activity. *Can Anaesth Soc J*. 1972;19:75–82.
10. Gottdiener JS, Appelbaum FR, Ferrans VJ, et al. Cardiotoxicity associated with high-dose cyclophosphamide therapy. *Arch Intern Med*. 1981;141:758–762.
11. Ginsberg SJ, Comis RL. The pulmonary toxicity of antineoplastic agents. *Semin Oncol*. 1982;9:34–51.
12. Weiss RB, Poster DS, Penta JS. The nitrosoureas and pulmonary toxicity. *Cancer Treat Rev*. 1981;8:111–125.
13. Gunstream SR, Seidenfeld JJ, Cobonya RE, et al. Mitomycin-associated lung disease. *Cancer Treat Rev*. 1983;67:301–304.
14. White DA, Orenstein M, Godwin TA, et al. Chemotherapy-associated pulmonary toxic reactions during treatment for breast cancer. *Arch Intern Med*. 1984;144:953–956.
15. Cooper JA Jr, White DA, Matthay RA. Drug-induced pulmonary disease. Part 1: cytotoxic drugs. *Am Rev Respir Dis*. 1986;133:321–340.
16. Perazella MA, Moeckel GW. Nephrotoxicity from chemotherapeutic agents: clinical manifestations, pathobiology, and prevention/therapy. *Semin Nephrol*. 2010;30:570–581.
17. Kaplan RS, Wienik PH. Neurotoxicity of antineoplastic drugs. *Semin Oncol*. 1982;9:103–110.
18. Labianca R, Beretta G, Clerici M. Cardiac toxicity of 5-fluorouracil: a study of 10,083 patients. *Tumor*. 1982;68:505–509.
19. Saven A, Piro L. Newer purine analogues for the treatment of hairy-cell leukemia. *N Engl J Med*. 1994;330:691–697.
20. Doroshow JH. Doxorubicin-induced cardiac toxicity. *N Engl J Med*. 1991;324:843–845.
21. Von Hoff DD, Layard MW, Basa P, et al. Risk factors for doxorubicin-induced congestive heart failure. *Ann Intern Med*. 1979;91:710–717.
22. Huettemann E, Junker T, Chatzinikolaou KP, et al. The influence of anthracycline therapy on cardiac function during anesthesia. *Anesth Analg*. 2004;98:941–947.
23. Borgeat A, Chiolero R, Baylon P, et al. Perioperative cardiovascular collapse in a patient previously treated with doxorubicin. *Anesth Analg*. 1988;67:1189–1191.
24. Lipshultz SE, Rifai N, Dalton VM, et al. The effect of dexrazoxane on myocardial injury in doxorubicin-treated children with acute lymphoblastic leukemia. *N Engl J Med*. 2004;351:145–153.
25. Dorr RT. Bleomycin pharmacology: mechanism of action and resistance, and clinical pharmacokinetics. *Semin Oncol*. 1992;19:3–8.
26. Allen SC, Riddell GS, Butchart EG. Bleomycin therapy and anaesthesia: the possible hazards of oxygen administration to patients after treatment with bleomycin. *Anaesthesia*. 1981;60:121–124.
27. Eigen H, Wyszomierski D. Bleomycin lung injury in children. Pathophysiology and guidelines for management. *Am J Pediatr Hematol Oncol*. 1985;7:71–78.
28. Hulbert JC, Grossman JE, Cummings KB. Risk factors of anesthesia and surgery in bleomycin-treated patients. *J Urol*. 1983;130:163–164.
29. Hay JG, Haslam PL, Dewar A, et al. Development of acute lung injury after the combination of intravenous bleomycin and exposure to hyperoxia in rats. *Thorax*. 1987;42:374–382.
30. Mathes DD. Bleomycin and hyperoxia exposure in the operating room. *Anesth Analg*. 1995;81:624–629.
31. Blom-Muilwijk MC, Vriesendorp R, Veninga TS, et al. Pulmonary toxicity after treatment with bleomycin along or in combination with hyperoxia. Studies in the rat. *Br J Anaesth*. 1988;60:91–97.
32. Comis RL. Bleomycin pulmonary toxicity: current status and future directions. *Semin Oncol*. 1992;19:64–70.
33. Wilson L, Jordan MA. Microtubule dynamics: taking aim at a moving target. *Chem Biol*. 1995;2:569–575.
34. Postma TJ, Benard BA, Huijgens PC, et al. Long term effects of vincristine on the peripheral nervous system. *J Neurooncol*. 1993;15:23–27.
35. Vainionpaa L, Kovala T, Tolonen U, et al. Vincristine therapy for children with acute lymphoblastic leukemia impairs conduction in the entire peripheral nerve. *Pediatr Neurol*. 1995;13:314–318.
36. Delaney P. Vincristine-induced laryngeal nerve paralysis. *Neurology*. 1982;32:1285–1288.
37. Lirk P, Birmingham B, Hogan Q. Regional anesthesia in patients with preexisting neuropathy. *Int Anesthesiol Clin*. 2011;49:144–165.
38. Rowinsky EK, Donehower RC. Paclitaxel (Taxol). *N Engl J Med*. 1995;332:1004–1014.
39. Jackson SH, Barker SJ. Methemoglobinemia in a patient receiving flutamide. *Anesthesiology*. 1995;82:1065–1067.
40. Barker SJ, Tremper KK, Hyatt J. Effects of methemoglobinemia on pulse oximetry and mixed venous oximetry. *Anesthesiology*. 1989;70: 112–117.
41. Dillman RO. Radiolabled anti-CD20 monoclonal antibodies for the treatment of B-cell lymphoma. *J Clin Oncol*. 2002;20:3345–3351.

CHAPTER 43

Drugs Used for Psychopharmacologic Therapy

Joseph Kwok • Pamela Flood

Drugs used for psychopharmacologic therapy include antidepressants, anxiolytics, lithium, antipsychotics, and anticonvulsants. The development of relatively safe and effective psychotherapeutic drugs has made it possible to effectively treat as ambulatory patients many individuals with depression and anxiety disorders. Antidepressants and anxiolytics are the drugs most likely to be prescribed by primary care physicians for the treatment of depression in adults. Lithium, anticonvulsants, and antipsychotic drugs are useful for treatment of bipolar disorders and psychotic disorders including schizophrenia. It is estimated that up to 10% of the population is treated for a depressive illness at some time in life, and mood disorders requiring antidepressant therapy are an increasingly frequent occurrence in the elderly population in whom side effects may be less well tolerated due to coexisting disease.

It is well accepted that anesthesia can be safely administered to patients being treated with drugs used to treat mental illness.[1,2] There appears to be growing acceptance that the problem of drug interactions between psychopharmacologic drugs and drugs administered in the perioperative period is less than previously perceived and that past recommendations for discontinuation of antidepressant therapy are not justified. Nevertheless, it remains important to remain alert for potential drug interactions.[3] This is particularly true in elderly patients who are at particular risk for toxicity.

Antidepressants

Considering the wide range of disorders for which antidepressant drugs are effective, the term ***antidepressant*** has become a misnomer (Table 43-1). The broad spectrum of effectiveness of antidepressants does not imply a common pathophysiology but rather reflects the diverse roles of monoamine neurotransmitters in the human nervous system.

Antidepressants are logically classified based on their chemical structures and their acute neuropharmacologic effects (Table 43-2). The precise mechanism by which antidepressants work is unknown, but they appear to act by altering noradrenergic neurotransmission and/or serotoninergic neurotransmission (see Table 43-2). This suggests that antidepressants work by increasing the amount of norepinephrine and serotonin in synapses. Nevertheless, the most important observation not explained by this hypothesis is the time course of clinical improvement. Neurobiologically, reuptake blockade or monoamine oxidase (MAO) inhibition (necessary for breakdown of free norepinephrine and serotonin) occurs promptly after initiation of antidepressant therapy, but clinical improvement typically does not occur for 2 to 4 weeks. Perhaps adaptive changes including downregulation of neurotransmitter receptors are necessary before evidence of clinical improvement appears.

Selective Serotonin Reuptake Inhibitors

The selective serotonin reuptake inhibitors (SSRIs) are the most broadly prescribed class of antidepressants and are the drugs of choice for the treatment of mild to moderate depression.[4] SSRIs are the first-line pharmacotherapy for panic disorder and obsessive-compulsive syndrome. These drugs are also effective in treatment of social phobia and posttraumatic stress disorder. SSRIs that share the ability to block the reuptake of serotonin (and thus enhance serotonergic activity) include fluoxetine, paroxetine, sertraline, fluvoxamine, citalopram, and escitalopram. Other newer SSRIs are believed to act on serotonin and norepinephrine pathways in the brain by a variety of mechanisms, including dual serotonin and norepinephrine reuptake blockade (venlafaxine) and α_2-receptor blockade (mirtazapine).[5] Different SSRIs have different side effect profiles, and patients who do not respond to one drug or who fail to tolerate the drug may do well on a different SSRI. Standard practice dictates trying several SSRIs before moving to another class of medication.

Table 43-1

Clinical Uses of Antidepressant Drugs

Unipolar and bipolar depression
Panic disorder
Social phobia
Posttraumatic stress syndrome
Neuropathic pain
Migraine prophylaxis
Obsessive-compulsive disorder
Bulimia
Childhood attention deficit hyperactivity disorder

There is abundant evidence that serotonin receptors are involved in the etiology of anxiety. Potent inhibition of serotonin reuptake appears to be necessary for effectiveness in the treatment of obsessive-compulsive disorders. Compared with tricyclic antidepressants, SSRIs lack anticholinergic properties, do not cause postural hypotension or delayed conduction of cardiac impulses, and do not appear to have a major effect on the seizure threshold. Perhaps the most important advantage of SSRIs compared with tricyclic antidepressants is the relative safety of SSRIs when taken in overdose.[6] The exception may be venlafaxine that may be similar to tricyclic antidepressants with respect to elevated

Table 43-2

Comparative Pharmacology of Antidepressant Drugs

	Sedative Potency	Anticholinergic Potency	Orthostatic Hypotension
Selective serotonin reuptake inhibitors			
Fluoxetine	+	+	+
Sertraline	+	+	+
Paroxetine	+	+	+
Fluvoxamine	+	+	+
Citalopram	+	+	+
Escitalopram	+	+	+
Bupropion	+	+	+
Venlafaxine	+	+	May cause hypertension in some individuals
Trazodone	+ + +	+	+ + + Associated with cardiac dysrhythmias
Nefazodone	+ + +	+	+ +
Tricyclic and related cyclic compounds[a]			
Amitriptyline	+ + +	+ + + +	+ + +
Amoxapine	+	+	+ +
Clomipramine	+ + +	+ + +	+ + +
Desipramine	+	+	+ +
Doxepin	+ + +	+ +	+ +
Imipramine	++	+ +	+ + +
Nortriptyline	+	+	0
Protriptyline	+	+ + +	+
Trimipramine	+ + +	+ +	+ +
Mirtazapine			
Monoamine oxidase inhibitors			
Phenelzine	+	+	+ + +
Tranylcypromine	+	+	+ + +
Isocarboxazid	+	+	+ + +

[a]All tricyclic and related cyclic compounds may produce cardiac dysrhythmias.
0, none; +, mild; + +, moderate; + + +, marked; + + + +, greatest.

overdose-associated risk associated with proconvulsant and cardiac side effects.[7] Common side effects of SSRIs include insomnia, agitation, headache, nausea, and diarrhea. A prominent cause of noncompliance with SSRI therapy is drug-induced sexual dysfunction in both men and women (delayed ejaculation, anorgasmia, decreased libido).[8]

Abrupt discontinuation of SSRIs with short elimination half-times (paroxetine, venlafaxine) may be associated with dizziness, paresthesias, myalgias, irritability, insomnia, and visual disturbances. Tapering all SSRIs before discontinuance is recommended especially for drugs with short elimination half-times.[9]

In September 2004, the U.S. Food and Drug Administration recommended a "black box" warning for newer antidepressant drugs, primarily SSRIs.[10] This warning is based on evidence that suicidal tendencies in children and adolescents may be increased in those age groups when they are treated with SSRIs. Nevertheless, the risk is small and many patients benefit from treatment with SSRIs emphasizing the need to individualize therapy.

Fluoxetine

Fluoxetine was the first SSRI introduced in the United States in 1988.[11] The drug is commonly administered once daily in the morning to decrease the risk of insomnia. Because fluoxetine has a prolonged elimination half-time (1 to 3 days for acute administration and 4 to 6 days for chronic administration), the drug can be taken every other day. An active metabolite, norfluoxetine, has an elimination half-time of 4 to 16 days. A therapeutic effect produced by fluoxetine is usually evident in 2 to 4 weeks. Because of this drug's prolonged elimination half-time, increases in dosage are often limited to no more often than once every 4 weeks.

Side Effects

The most common side effects of fluoxetine are nausea, anorexia, insomnia, sexual dysfunction, agitation, and neuromuscular restlessness, which may mimic akathisia. Appetite suppression associated with fluoxetine therapy may help patients achieve weight loss.[12] Like tricyclic antidepressants, fluoxetine may be an effective analgesic for treatment of chronic pain as may be associated with rheumatoid arthritis.[13] Fluoxetine does not cause hypotension, and changes in conduction of cardiac impulses seem infrequent. Bradycardia causing syncope has been reported in occasional elderly patients.[14] Because of its long elimination half-time, fluoxetine should be discontinued for about 5 weeks before initiating treatment with an MAO inhibitor. The long elimination half-time of fluoxetine appears to prevent withdrawal symptoms induced by abrupt discontinuance of the drug. An overdose with fluoxetine alone is not associated with the risk of cardiovascular and central nervous system (CNS) toxicity.

Drug Interactions

Among the SSRIs, fluoxetine is the most potent inhibitor of certain hepatic cytochrome P-450 enzymes. As a result, this drug may increase the plasma concentrations of drugs that depend on hepatic metabolism for clearance. For example, the addition of fluoxetine to treatment with a tricyclic antidepressant drug may result in a two- to fivefold increase in the plasma concentration of the tricyclic drug. Neuroleptic drugs may inhibit the metabolism of fluoxetine or vice versa. Several cardiac antidysrhythmic drugs as well as some β-adrenergic antagonists may be metabolized by the same enzyme system that is inhibited by fluoxetine, resulting in potentiation of these drug effects. MAO inhibitors combined with fluoxetine may cause the development of a serotonin syndrome characterized by anxiety, restlessness, chills, ataxia, and insomnia.[14] The combination of fluoxetine and lithium or carbamazepine may also provoke this potentially fatal syndrome.

Sertraline

Sertraline was the second SSRI introduced in the United States and has a spectrum of efficacy similar to fluoxetine. This drug has a shorter elimination half-time (25 hours) than fluoxetine and is a less potent inhibitor of hepatic microsomal enzymes. A potentially active metabolite has an elimination half-time of 60 to 70 hours.

Compared with fluoxetine, sertraline may cause more gastrointestinal symptoms (nausea, diarrhea) but may be less likely to cause insomnia and agitation. The recommended washout period before starting an MAO inhibitor is 14 days.

Paroxetine

Paroxetine was the third SSRI introduced in the United States and has an efficacy similar to that of fluoxetine. This drug has a relatively short elimination half-time (24 hours), and there are no active metabolites. Side effects resemble those of other SSRIs with the exception of a possibly increased incidence of sedation. The levels of paroxetine in breast milk are greater than levels in patients receiving fluoxetine or sertraline. Paroxetine produces less inhibition of hepatic cytoplasmic P-450 enzymes than is fluoxetine. Enhancement of the anticoagulant effect of warfarin reflects competition for common protein-binding sites. The recommended washout period before starting an MAO inhibitor is 14 days.

Citalopram/Escitalopram

Citalopram was the fourth SSRI introduced in the United States. Escitalopram is simply the S isomer of citalopram, which is the more pharmacologically active stereoisomer. Citalopram causes dose-dependent QT interval prolongation, which can place patients at risk for torsades de pointes.[15,16] Escitalopram may also prolong the QT interval but possibly to a lesser degree. Citalopram should be used with caution in patients at risk for prolonged QT intervals.

Fluvoxamine

Fluvoxamine is effective in the management of obsessive-compulsive disorders. In addition, this drug probably has a spectrum of therapeutic efficacy similar to that of other SSRIs. The most common side effects associated with this drug are nausea, vomiting (possibly a greater frequency than with other SSRIs), headache, sedation, insomnia, and sexual dysfunction. Although it produces less inhibition of hepatic cytoplasmic P-450 enzymes than the other SSRIs, fluvoxamine may still cause clinically significant drug interactions.

Bupropion

Bupropion, which is structurally related to amphetamine, is effective in the treatment of major depression, producing improvement in 2 to 4 weeks. In addition, bupropion is effective for smoking cessation. The mechanism of action of bupropion is obscure but may include inhibition of dopamine and norepinephrine reuptake. This drug does not inhibit MAO. Bupropion is associated with a greater incidence of seizures (about 0.4%) than other antidepressants.[17] Some patients experience stimulant-like effects early in therapy. Like the SSRIs, bupropion has no anticholinergic effects, does not cause postural hypotension, and lacks significant effects on conduction of cardiac impulses. Unlike the SSRIs, bupropion is not associated with significant drug interactions and is not commonly associated with sexual dysfunction. Ataxia and myoclonus have occurred rarely. Bupropion should not be administered in combination with an MAO inhibitor; elevated blood pressure and serotonin syndrome have been reported.[18]

Venlafaxine

Venlafaxine is perceived to have a profile of efficacy similar to that of the tricyclic antidepressants but has a more favorable side effect profile. Like the tricyclic antidepressants, this drug inhibits the reuptake of norepinephrine and serotonin and may potentiate the action of dopamine in the CNS. Unlike tricyclic antidepressants, venlafaxine does not produce anticholinergic effects or postural hypotension. Side effects include insomnia, sedation, and nausea. At high doses, a modest but persistent increase in diastolic blood pressure occurs in 5% to 7% of patients. Some studies have suggested that venlafaxine may be beneficial in patients with neuropathic pain. Venlafaxine is metabolized by cytochrome P-450 enzymes and also acts as a weak inhibitor of these enzymes. The elimination half-time is 5 hours and that of its active metabolite is 11 hours. Venlafaxine should not be used in combination with an MAO inhibitor, and the recommended washout period is 14 days.

Duloxetine

Duloxetine is a serotonin and noradrenaline reuptake inhibitor, similar to venlafaxine. Indications for its use include major depression, fibromyalgia, and diabetic neuropathy.[19,20] Its side effect profile includes nausea, dry mouth, insomnia, and sexual dysfunction. It does not cause significant changes in blood pressure and is a moderate inhibitor of CYP2D6.[21] Duloxetine should be avoided in patients with severe renal dysfunction and chronic liver disease. Like venlafaxine, duloxetine should not be used in combination with an MAO inhibitor. The potential for the development of serotonin syndrome is present when this drug is used in conjunction with another serotonergic drug.

Trazodone

Trazodone inhibits serotonin reuptake and may also act as a serotonin agonist via an active metabolite. Although effective in the management of depression, its greatest efficacy may be treatment of insomnia induced by SSRIs or bupropion. Common side effects of trazodone include sedation, orthostatic hypotension, nausea, and vomiting. Priapism may occur in males. This drug lacks effects on conduction of cardiac impulses but on rare occasions has been associated with cardiac dysrhythmias. The elimination half-time of this drug is brief (3 to 9 hours), and toxicity associated with an overdose is less than what accompanies an overdose of tricyclic antidepressants and MAO inhibitors. Combination therapy with an MAO inhibitor is not recommended.

Nefazodone

Nefazodone is chemically related to trazodone but with fewer α_1-adrenergic blocking properties. Like trazodone, this drug inhibits reuptake of serotonin and norepinephrine. The risk of sedation and priapism may be less than in patients treated with trazodone. The principal side effects are nausea, dry mouth, and sedation. Orthostatic hypotension may occur. Nefazodone-induced inhibition of cytochrome P-450 results in elevated plasma concentrations of benzodiazepines, antihistamines, and of protease inhibitors used in the treatment of HIV infection. Combination therapy with an MAO inhibitor is not recommended.

Management of Anesthesia

Several studies have suggested that SSRIs may have antiplatelet activity and increase the risk of bleeding particularly in the setting of antiplatelet medication use.[22–24] The risks of discontinuing an SSRI may take 2 to 3 weeks for full washout and reinitiation may require 2 to 4 weeks for reestablishment of clinical antidepressant effect. Furthermore, discontinuation of a patient's SSRI may expose them to the risks of a major depressive episode. Anesthesia providers may consider holding antiplatelet medication in the perioperative setting if their patients are taking SSRIs, as there may be increased risk of bleeding in the setting of SSRI and antiplatelet medication use.

Tricyclic and Related Antidepressants

Before the availability of SSRIs, tricyclic antidepressants and related cyclic antidepressants were the most commonly used drugs to treat depression (see Table 43-2). Although tricyclic antidepressants are highly effective, they have been supplanted as first-line drugs in many clinical situations because of their unfavorable side effect profile (largely resulting from their anticholinergic, antiadrenergic, and antihistaminic properties). Tricyclic antidepressants also have a narrow therapeutic index and are potentially lethal in overdose (resulting in part from inhibition of sodium ion channels) reflecting a slowing of conduction of cardiac impulses and appearance of life-threatening cardiac dysrhythmias.

Measurement of plasma drug levels for the tricyclics imipramine, desipramine, and nortriptyline can be useful in guiding therapeutic decisions. Generally, plasma levels should not exceed 225 ng/mL when imipramine is administered. Plasma levels should not exceed 125 ng/mL when desipramine is administered, and the therapeutic range for nortriptyline is 50 to 150 ng/mL. It is preferable to taper tricyclic and tetracyclic antidepressants during a 4-week period to avoid the risk of withdrawal symptoms (chills, coryza, muscle aches). These symptoms have been attributed to supersensitivity of the cholinergic nervous system.

Chronic Pain Syndromes

The tricyclic antidepressants (especially amitriptyline and imipramine), in doses lower than those used to treat depression, may be useful in the treatment of chronic neuropathic pain and other chronic pain syndromes including fibromyalgia. Although there is no consensus on the mechanism of pain relief, current hypotheses include serotonin activity and reuptake inhibition, potentiation of CNS endogenous opioids, and antiinflammatory effects.[25] Because of their structural similarities to local anesthetics and known sodium channel blockade, it is possible that tricyclic antidepressants produce antiinflammatory effects similar to local anesthetics. Because many chronic pain syndromes include an inflammatory component, it is possible that the clinical efficacy of tricyclic antidepressants in chronic pain patients is due to inhibition of an overactive inflammatory system.[26] The efficacy of tricyclic antidepressants on chronic pain syndromes may be limited by a narrow therapeutic index and intolerability of side effects.

Structure–Activity Relationships

The structure of tricyclic antidepressants resembles that of local anesthetics and phenothiazines. Similar to local anesthetics, tricyclic antidepressants include a hydrophobic portion linked to an amide via a linear intermediate moiety. Tricyclic denotes the three-ring chemical structure of the central portion of the molecule. Imipramine, which is the prototype of the tricyclic antidepressants, differs from phenothiazine only in the replacement of the sulfur atom with an ethylene linkage to produce a seven-membered central ring. Desipramine is the principal metabolite of imipramine, and nortriptyline is the demethylated metabolite of amitriptyline. Maprotiline is a tetracyclic antidepressant with a clinical profile that resembles imipramine. Mirtazapine is a tetracyclic antidepressant that may enhance central norepinephrine and serotonin activity in the CNS. Maprotiline and mirtazapine should not be administered to patients being treated with MAO inhibitors.

Mechanism of Action

Tricyclic antidepressants act at several transporters and receptors, but their antidepressant effect is likely produced by blocking the reuptake (uptake) of serotonin and/or norepinephrine at presynaptic terminals, thereby increasing the availability of these neurotransmitters. These drugs can be categorized into tertiary amines, which inhibit reuptake of both serotonin and norepinephrine (amitriptyline, imipramine, clomipramine) and secondary amines, which are primarily norepinephrine reuptake inhibitors (desipramine, nortriptyline). Despite the prompt onset of this effect, the development of a therapeutic antidepressant effect is inexplicably delayed for 2 to 3 weeks. For this reason, there is doubt that antidepressant effects are totally due to an accumulation of biogenic amines in the brain. Furthermore, some drugs without effects on uptake of biogenic amines are effective antidepressants. It seems likely that potentiation of monoaminergic neurotransmission in the brain is only an early event in a complex cascade of events that eventually results in an antidepressant effect. Indeed, chronic administration of these drugs is associated with (a) decreased sensitivity of postsynaptic β_1 and serotonin$_2$ receptors and of presynaptic α_2 receptors, and (b) increased sensitivity of postsynaptic α_1 receptors.

Pharmacokinetics

Tricyclic antidepressants are efficiently absorbed from the gastrointestinal tract after oral administration, reflecting high lipid solubility. Peak plasma concentrations occur within 2 to 8 hours after oral administration. Therapeutic plasma concentrations (parent drug plus the pharmacologically active demethylated metabolites) are 100 to 300 ng/ mL, whereas toxicity is likely at levels greater than 500 ng/mL. Tricyclic antidepressants are strongly bound to plasma and tissue proteins, which, in combination with high lipid solubility, results in a large volume of distribution (up to 50 L/kg) for these drugs. The long elimination half-time (17 to 30 hours) and wide range of therapeutic plasma concentrations make once-daily dosing intervals effective.

Metabolism

Tricyclic antidepressants are oxidized by microsomal enzymes in the liver with subsequent conjugation with glucuronic acid. The individual variation in rate of metabolism between patients is 10- to 30-fold. Metabolism is likely to be slowed in elderly patients. The elimination of tricyclic antidepressants occurs over several days, with 1 week or longer required for excretion.

Imipramine is metabolized to the active compound desipramine. Both these active compounds are inactivated by oxidation of hydroxy metabolites and by conjugation with glucuronic acid. Nortriptyline, which is the pharmacologically active demethylated metabolite of imipramine and amitriptyline, can accumulate to levels that exceed the precursors. Doxepin also appears to be converted to an active metabolite, nordoxepin, by demethylation.

Side Effects

The side effects of tricyclic antidepressants occur frequently, most commonly manifesting as (a) anticholinergic effects, (b) cardiovascular effects, and (c) CNS effects (see Table 43-2). Individual variation in the incidence and type of side effects may be related to the plasma concentrations of the tricyclic antidepressant and its active metabolites.

Anticholinergic Effects

The anticholinergic effects of tricyclic antidepressants are prominent, especially at high doses. Amitriptyline causes the highest incidence of anticholinergic effects (dry mouth, blurred vision, tachycardia, urinary retention, slowed gastric emptying, ileus), whereas desipramine produces the fewest such effects (see Table 43-2). Anticholinergic delirium may occur in elderly patients even at therapeutic doses of these drugs. Serious anticholinergic toxicity may reflect the results of polypharmacy with more than one anticholinergic drug (over-the-counter preparations to treat diarrhea or insomnia). Elderly patients have greater sensitivity to anticholinergic and other receptor effects compared with younger patients being treated with tricyclic antidepressants.

Cardiovascular Effects

Orthostatic hypotension and modest increases in heart rate are the most common cardiovascular side effects of tricyclic antidepressants, presumably reflecting drug-induced inhibition of norepinephrine reuptake into presynaptic nerve terminals. Orthostatic hypotension may be particularly hazardous in elderly patients, who are at increased risk of fractures when they fall. The risk of hypotension during general anesthesia in patients treated with tricyclic antidepressants is low but has been reported.[27] Previous suggestions that tricyclic antidepressants increase the risks of cardiac dysrhythmias and sudden death have not been substantiated in the absence of drug overdose.[28] Furthermore, in the absence of severe preexisting cardiac dysfunction, tricyclic antidepressants lack adverse effects on left ventricular function and may even possess cardiac antidysrhythmic properties.[29]

Tricyclic antidepressants produce depression of conduction of cardiac impulses through the atria and ventricles, manifesting on the electrocardiogram (ECG) as prolongation of the P-R interval, widening of the QRS complex, and flattening or inversion of the T wave. Nevertheless, these changes on the ECG are probably benign and gradually disappear with continued therapy.[28] Atropine is a useful treatment when tricyclic antidepressants dangerously slow atrioventricular or intraventricular conduction of cardiac impulses.

Direct cardiac depressant effects may reflect quinidine-like actions of tricyclic antidepressants on the heart. Conceivably, there could also be enhancement of depressant cardiac effects of anesthetics by tricyclic antidepressants. Quinidine-like properties of tricyclic antidepressants are thought to reflect slowing of sodium ion flux into cells, resulting in altered repolarization and conduction of cardiac impulses.

Central Nervous System Effects

Sedation associated with tricyclic antidepressant therapy may be desirable for management of depressed patients with insomnia. Amitriptyline and doxepin produce the greatest degree of sedation (see Table 43-2). Tricyclic antidepressants, especially maprotiline and clomipramine, lower the seizure threshold, raising the question of the advisability of administering these drugs to patients with seizure disorders or to those receiving drugs that may produce seizures. Children seem to be especially vulnerable to the seizure-inducing effects of tricyclic antidepressants. Treatment with tricyclic antidepressants may enhance the CNS-stimulating effects of enflurane. Weakness and fatigue are attributable to CNS effects and may resemble those seen in patients treated with phenothiazines. Extrapyramidal reactions are rare, although a fine tremor develops in about 10% of patients, especially the elderly. Because of their cardiac toxicity, tendency to cause seizures, and depressant properties on the CNS, the tricyclic antidepressants may be fatal if taken in an overdose. The combination of a tricyclic antidepressant and an MAO inhibitor may result in CNS toxicity manifesting as hyperthermia, seizures, and coma.

Drug Interactions

The anticholinergic effects and catecholamine uptake blocking properties of tricyclic antidepressants are most likely to be responsible for drug interactions. Drug interactions may be prominent with (a) sympathomimetics, (b) inhaled anesthetics, (c) anticholinergics, (d) antihypertensives, and (e) opioids. Binding of tricyclic antidepressants to plasma albumin can be decreased by competition from other drugs, including phenytoin, aspirin, and scopolamine.

Sympathomimetics

The systemic blood pressure response to the administration of sympathomimetics to patients treated with tricyclic antidepressants is complex and unpredictable. It has been suggested that indirect-acting sympathomimetics may produce exaggerated pressor responses due to an increased amount of norepinephrine available to stimulate postsynaptic adrenergic receptors. Although acute administration of tricyclic antidepressants increases sympathetic nervous system synaptic activity due to norepinephrine reuptake blockade, chronic administration of these drugs may result in decreased sympathetic nervous system transmission due to downregulation of β-adrenergic receptors.[30,31] It would appear that for patients recently started on tricyclic antidepressants, exaggerated pressor responses should be anticipated whether or not direct-acting or indirect-acting sympathomimetics are administered, although pressor responses may be more pronounced with an indirect-acting drug such as ephedrine. Smaller than usual doses of direct-acting sympathomimetics that are titrated to a specific hemodynamic response are recommended. For individuals chronically treated with tricyclic antidepressants (>6 weeks), administration of either a direct-acting or indirect-acting sympathomimetic is acceptable, although a prudent approach may be to decrease the initial dose of drug to about one-third the usual dose. Conversely, conventional sympathomimetics may not be effective in restoring systemic blood pressure in patients chronically treated with tricyclic antidepressants because adrenergic receptors are either desensitized or catecholamine stores are depleted. In these patients, a potent direct-acting sympathomimetic such as norepinephrine may be the only effective management for hypotension.[32]

Induction of anesthesia may be associated with an increased incidence of cardiac dysrhythmias in patients treated with tricyclic antidepressants. Likewise, the dose of exogenous epinephrine necessary to produce cardiac dysrhythmias during anesthesia with a volatile anesthetic is decreased by tricyclic antidepressants.[33] Theoretically, increased availability of norepinephrine in the CNS could result in increased anesthetic requirements for inhaled anesthetics.

Anticholinergics

Because the anticholinergic side effects of drugs may be additive, the use of centrally active anticholinergic drugs for preoperative medication of patients treated with tricyclic antidepressants could increase the likelihood of postoperative delirium and confusion (central anticholinergic syndrome). Glycopyrrolate would theoretically be less likely to evoke this type of drug interaction in patients being treated with tricyclic antidepressants.

Antihypertensives

Rebound hypertension after abrupt discontinuation of clonidine may be accentuated and prolonged by concomitant tricyclic antidepressant therapy.[34] Conceivably, increased plasma concentrations of catecholamines can persist for longer periods in the presence of tricyclic antidepressants that prevent uptake of norepinephrine back into sympathetic nerve endings.

Opioids

In animals, tricyclic antidepressants augment the analgesic and ventilatory depressant effects of opioids. If these responses also occur in patients, doses of these drugs should be carefully titrated to avoid exaggerated or prolonged depressant effects.

Tolerance

Tolerance to anticholinergic effects (dry mouth, blurred vision, tachycardia) and orthostatic hypotension develops during chronic therapy with tricyclic antidepressants. Conversely, tolerance to desirable effects often fails to develop. Abrupt discontinuation of high doses of tricyclic antidepressants may be associated with a mild withdrawal syndrome characterized by malaise, chills, coryza, and skeletal muscle aching.

Overdose

Tricyclic antidepressant overdose is life-threatening, as the progression from an alert state to unresponsiveness may be rapid.[35] Intractable myocardial depression or ventricular cardiac dysrhythmias are the most frequent terminal events.

Presenting features of tricyclic antidepressant overdose include agitation and seizures followed by coma, depression of ventilation, hypotension, hypothermia, and striking evidence of anticholinergic effects including mydriasis, flushed dry skin, urinary retention, and tachycardia. The QRS complex on the ECG may be prolonged to greater than 100 milliseconds. Indeed, the likelihood of seizures and ventricular dysrhythmias is increased when the duration of the QRS complex is greater than 100 milliseconds.[36] Conversely, plasma concentrations of tricyclic antidepressants do not allow prediction of the likely occurrence of seizures or cardiac dysrhythmias.[36]

The comatose phase of tricyclic antidepressant overdose lasts 24 to 72 hours. Even after this phase passes, the risk of life-threatening cardiac dysrhythmias persists for up to 10 days, necessitating continued monitoring of the ECG in these patients.

Treatment of a life-threatening overdose of a tricyclic antidepressant is directed toward management of CNS and cardiac toxicity (Table 43-3).[35] Coma usually resolves in 24 hours but is frequently severe enough to require invasive airway support. Extrapyramidal effects and organic brain syndrome usually require supportive care only, although judicious use of physostigmine, 0.5 to 2 mg given intravenously (IV), for treatment of anticholinergic psychosis may be indicated.

Seizures may precede cardiac arrest and should be treated aggressively with a benzodiazepine. After initial suppression of seizure activity with diazepam, it may be necessary to provide sustained effects with a longer acting drug such as phenytoin. Acidosis associated with seizure activity may abruptly increase the unbound fraction of tricyclic antidepressants in the circulation and predispose

Table 43-3

Pharmacologic Treatment of Tricyclic Antidepressant Overdose

Symptom	Treatment
Seizures	Diazepam Sodium bicarbonate Phenytoin
Ventricular cardiac dysrhythmias	Sodium bicarbonate Lidocaine Phenytoin
Heart block	Isoproterenol
Hypotension	Crystalloid or colloid solutions Sodium bicarbonate Sympathomimetics Inotropics

Data from Frommer DA, Kulig KW, Marx JA, et al. Tricyclic antidepressant overdose. *JAMA*. 1987;257:521–526, with permission.

Table 43-4

Dietary Restrictions in Patients Treated with Monoamine Oxidase Inhibitors

Prohibited foods
Cheese
Liver
Fava beans
Avocados
Chianti wine
Prohibited drugs
Cyclic antidepressants
Fluoxetine
Cold or allergy medications
Nasal decongestants
Sympathomimetic drugs
Opioids (especially meperidine)

to cardiac dysrhythmias. In this regard, alkalization of the plasma (pH >7.45) either by IV administration of sodium bicarbonate or deliberate hyperventilation of the patient's lungs can temporarily reverse drug-induced cardiotoxicity. Lidocaine and phenytoin may be used subsequently to provide sustained suppression of cardiac ventricular dysrhythmias.

Hypotension may be the result of direct tricyclic antidepressant–induced vasodilation, α-adrenergic blockade, or myocardial depression. Patients remaining hypotensive despite intravascular fluid replacement and alkalinization of the plasma may require systemic blood pressure support with sympathomimetics, inotropes, or both.

Gastric lavage may be useful in the early treatment, but this is most safely performed with a cuffed tracheal tube already in place. Activated charcoal significantly absorbs drugs throughout the gastrointestinal tract ("intestinal dialysis"). Conversely, avid protein binding of tricyclic antidepressants negates any therapeutic value of hemodialysis or drug-induced diuresis.

Monoamine Oxidase Inhibitors

MAO inhibitors constitute a heterogenous group of drugs, which block the enzyme that metabolizes biogenic amines, increasing the availability of these neurotransmitters in the CNS and peripheral autonomic nervous system. MAO inhibitors are used less commonly because their administration is complicated by side effects (hypotension), lethality in overdose, and lack of simplicity in dosing. Patients treated with MAO inhibitors must follow a specific tyramine-free diet because of the potential for pharmacodynamic interactions with tyramine that can result in systemic hypertension (Table 43-4). However, many patients with major depression who do not respond to cyclic antidepressants improve with MAO inhibitors. MAO inhibitors are also effective in the treatment of panic disorder. The dosage of MAO inhibitors is the same in the elderly as in younger adults because elderly persons often have higher levels of MAO and because the metabolism of these drugs does not seem to be affected by age.

The only MAO inhibitors approved in the United States for the treatment of depression or panic disorder are phenelzine, tranylcypromine, and isocarboxazid. Selegiline, which is a MAO-B selective inhibitor (formerly termed *deprenyl*), has been shown to be effective in the treatment of early Parkinson's disease. These drugs are administered orally, being readily absorbed from the gastrointestinal tract.

Monoamine Oxidase Enzyme System

MAO is a flavin-containing enzyme found principally on outer mitochondrial membranes. The enzyme functions via oxidative deamination to inactivate several monoamines including dopamine, serotonin (5-hydroxytryptamine), norepinephrine, and epinephrine. MAO is divided into two subtypes (MAO-A and MAO-B) based on different substrate specificities (Fig. 43-1).[2,3] MAO-A preferentially deaminates serotonin, norepinephrine, and epinephrine, whereas MAO-B preferentially deaminates phenylethylamine. Platelets contain exclusively MAO-A and the placenta exclusively MAO-B. About 60% of human brain MAO activity is of the A subtype.

Mechanism of Action

MAO inhibitors act by forming a stable, irreversible complex with MAO enzyme, especially with cerebral neuronal MAO.[37] As a result, the amount of neurotransmitter (norepinephrine) available for release from CNS neurons increases. These effects, however, are not limited to the brain, and the concentration of norepinephrine also increases in the sympathetic nervous system. Because MAO inhibitors

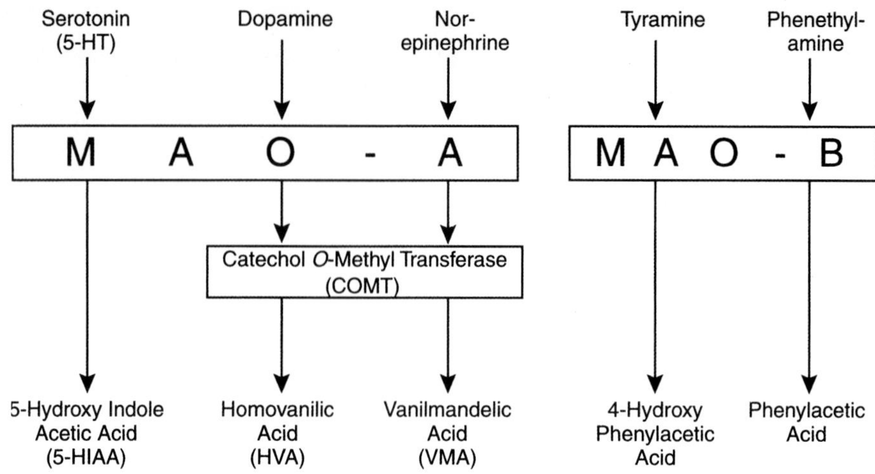

FIGURE 43-1 The two forms of monoamine oxidase enzyme (MAO-A and MAO-B) exhibit substrate selectivity. (From Michaels I, Serrins M, Shier NQ, et al. Anesthesia for cardiac surgery in patients receiving monoamine oxidase inhibitors. *Anesth Analg.* 1984;63:1041–1044, with permission.)

cause irreversible enzyme inhibition, their effects are prolonged, as the synthesis of new enzyme is a slow process.

Due to its location in the outer mitochondrial membrane, MAO in neurons is only capable of deaminating substrates that are free within the cytoplasm and are unable to gain access to substrates once they are bound in the storage vesicles. As a result, cytoplasmic concentrations of monoamines are maintained at a low level.

Side Effects

The most common serious side effect of MAO inhibitors is orthostatic hypotension, which may be especially prominent in elderly patients. Orthostatic hypotension may reflect accumulation of the false neurotransmitter octopamine in the cytoplasm of postganglionic sympathetic nerve endings. Release of this less potent vasoconstrictor in response to neural impulses is the most likely explanation for orthostatic hypotension as well as the antihypertensive effect that has been associated with chronic MAO inhibitor therapy.

Phenelzine has anticholinergic-like side effects and may produce sedation in some patients. Tranylcypromine has no anticholinergic side effects but has mild stimulant effects, which may cause insomnia. Impotence and anorgasmy are side effects of MAO inhibitors. Some patients complain of paresthesias, which may respond to pyridoxine therapy. Weight gain is a common side effect of treatment with MAO inhibitors. Hepatitis is a rare complication of MAO inhibitor therapy. Effects of MAO inhibitors on the electroencephalogram (EEG) are minimal and not seizure-like, which contrasts with tricyclic antidepressants. Also in contrast with tricyclic antidepressants is the failure of MAO inhibitors to produce cardiac dysrhythmias.[33]

Dietary Restrictions

MAO enzyme present in the liver, gastrointestinal tract, kidneys, and lungs seems to perform a protective function in deactivating circulating monoamines. In particular, this enzyme appears to form the initial defense against monoamines absorbed from foods, such as tyramine and β-phenylethanolamine, which would otherwise produce an indirect sympathomimetic response and precipitous hypertension. MAO-A is found in the gastrointestinal tract and liver, where it acts to metabolize bioactive amines such as tyramine. The MAO inhibitors used in the United States as antidepressants inhibit MAO-A and MAO-B nonselectively. Selegiline, when used to treat Parkinson's disease, selectively inhibits MAO-B and patients do not need to follow a tyramine-free diet. At high doses (30 mg per day), however, even selegiline becomes a nonselective MAO inhibitor, making dietary precautions necessary (see Table 43-4).

Because patients treated with MAO inhibitors cannot metabolize dietary tyramine and other monoamines, these compounds can enter the systemic circulation and be taken up by sympathetic nervous system nerve endings. This uptake can elicit massive release of endogenous catecholamines and result in a hyperadrenergic crisis characterized by hypertension, hyperpyrexia, and cerebral vascular accident. Therefore, patients taking MAO inhibitors should be instructed to report promptly the onset of serious headache, nausea, vomiting, or chest pain. The precipitous hypertension resembles that which occurs with the release of catecholamines from a pheochromocytoma. Treatment of hypertension is with a peripheral vasodilator such as nitroprusside. Cardiac dysrhythmias that persist after control of systemic blood pressure are treated with lidocaine or a β-adrenergic antagonist.

Drug Interactions

In addition to interacting with foods, MAO inhibitors can interact adversely with opioids, sympathomimetic drugs, tricyclic antidepressants, and SSRIs. These interactions can result in hypertension, CNS excitation, delirium, seizures, and death. In animals, anesthetic requirements for volatile anesthetics are increased, presumably reflecting accumulation of norepinephrine in the CNS.

Opioids and Monoamine Oxidase Inhibitors

Administration of meperidine to a patient treated with MAO inhibitors may result in an excitatory (type I) response (agitation, headache, skeletal muscle rigidity, hyperpyrexia) or a depressive (type II) response characterized by hypotension, depression of ventilation, and coma.[38] Enhanced serotonin activity in the brain is presumed to be responsible for excitatory reactions evoked by meperidine. Meperidine is capable of inhibiting neuronal serotonin uptake. Slowed breakdown of meperidine due to *N*-demethylase inhibition by MAO inhibitors is the presumed explanation for hypotension and depression of ventilation. About 20% of MAO inhibitor–treated patients have experienced excitatory reactions in response to meperidine. There is evidence that meperidine toxicity is increased only when both MAO-A and MAO-B are inhibited.[3] Derivatives of meperidine (fentanyl, sufentanil, alfentanil) have been associated with adverse reactions in patients treated with MAO inhibitors, although the incidence seems to be less than with meperidine.[39] Morphine does not inhibit uptake of serotonin, but its opioid effects may be potentiated in the presence of MAO inhibitors.

Sympathomimetics and Monoamine Oxidase Inhibitors

There is no experimental evidence to support the recommendation that all sympathomimetic drugs be avoided in patients treated with MAO inhibitors. The most consistent observation has been an occasional patient who experienced an exaggerated systemic blood pressure response after the administration of an indirect-acting vasopressor such as ephedrine. The hypertensive response is presumed to reflect an exaggerated release of norepinephrine from neuronal nerve endings. If needed, the use of a direct-acting sympathomimetic (phenylephrine) is preferable to an indirect-acting drug, keeping in mind that receptor hypersensitivity may enhance the systemic blood pressure response to these drugs as well. Regardless of the drug selected, the recommendation is to decrease the dose to about one-third of normal, with additional titration of doses based on cardiovascular responses.[3]

Overdose

Overdose with an MAO inhibitor is reflected by signs of excessive sympathetic nervous system activity (tachycardia, hyperthermia, mydriasis), seizures, and coma. Treatment is supportive in addition to gastric lavage. Dantrolene has been suggested as a treatment for skeletal muscle rigidity and associated symptoms of hypermetabolism after an overdose with MAO inhibitors.[40]

Management of Anesthesia

In the past, it was a common recommendation to discontinue MAO inhibitors 2 to 3 weeks before elective surgery based on the concern that life-threatening cardiovascular and CNS instability could occur during anesthesia and surgery when these drugs were present. This policy of drug withdrawal seems to be based more on anecdotes and isolated responses than on controlled scientific studies. Furthermore, discontinuation of effective therapy potentially places patients at risk from their psychiatric disturbances. There is growing appreciation that anesthesia can be safely administered in most patients being chronically treated with MAO inhibitors.[3] When anesthesia is administered to patients treated with MAO inhibitors, it remains prudent to consider certain drug interactions and to avoid certain drugs, if possible.[3,37]

Selection of Drugs Used during Anesthesia

The anesthetic technique selected should minimize the possibility of sympathetic nervous system stimulation or drug-induced hypotension. Regional anesthesia as in parturients is acceptable, recognizing the disadvantage of these techniques should hypotension require administration of a sympathomimetic.[38] If regional anesthesia is performed, a cautious approach is not to add epinephrine to the local anesthetic solution, although problems have not been reported with a 1:200,000 dilution. An advantage of regional anesthesia is postoperative analgesia such that the need for opioids is negated or minimized. Etomidate and thiopental have been administered to MAO inhibitor–treated patients undergoing electroconvulsive therapy without adverse effects. Responses to nondepolarizing neuromuscular blocking drugs are not altered by MAO inhibitors.

Serotonin Syndrome

Serotonin syndrome occurs when there is an excess of serotonin agonism in the central and peripheral nervous systems. The clinical findings can vary widely from mild tremor to altered mental status, clonus, and hyperthermia.[41] SSRIs, tricyclic antidepressants, and MAO inhibitors, particularly in combination, have all been associated with serotonin syndrome. The differential diagnosis includes malignant hyperthermia, neuroleptic malignant syndrome, and anticholinergic poisoning (Table 43-5). Management of serotonin syndrome includes hemodynamic and respiratory supportive care, discontinuation of offending serotonergic agents, control of agitation with sedatives, control of hyperthermia, and administration of 5-HT2A antagonists.

Anxiolytics

Benzodiazepines

Benzodiazepines (see Chapter 5) are used clinically as anxiolytics, sedatives, anticonvulsants, and muscle relaxants. They appear to produce all these effects by facilitating the actions of γ-aminobutyric acid (GABA), the major inhibitory neurotransmitter in the nervous system.

Table 43-5

Serotonin Syndrome and Commonly Mistaken Diagnoses

Diagnosis	Inciting Agent	Time Course	Fever	Physical Examination
Serotonin syndrome	Serotonergic agonists	<12 h	>41°	Mydriasis, drooling, sweating, hyperactive reflexes, agitation, coma
Anticholinergic syndrome	Muscarinic antagonists	<12 h	<39°	Mydriasis, dry mouth and skin, normal reflexes, delirium
Neuroleptic malignant syndrome	Dopamine antagonists	1–3 d after dosing	>41°	Normal pupils, drooling, pallor, lead-pipe rigidity, hyporeflexia, alert mutism, coma
Malignant hyperthermia	Volatile anesthetic and/or succinylcholine	Onset immediate to 24 h after administration	To 46°	Normal pupils, mottled sweaty skin, total body rigidity, hyporeflexia, agitation

Adapted from Boyer EW, Shannon M. The serotonin syndrome. *NEJM*. 2005;352:11.

The effectiveness of benzodiazepines, combined with the high frequency of anxiety and insomnia in the adult population, has led to these drugs being widely prescribed. Few patients who receive benzodiazepines for valid indications abuse them or become addicted. Benzodiazepines have less of a tendency to produce tolerance, less potential for abuse, and a large margin of safety if taken as an overdose in isolation. A history of alcohol abuse or substance abuse is a relative contraindication to use of benzodiazepines for treatment of anxiety.

When benzodiazepines are used to treat situational anxiety or generalized anxiety disorder, low doses (diazepam, 2 to 5 mg three times daily) are typically selected to minimize sedation. Sedation associated with administration of benzodiazepines to treat anxiety usually subsides within 2 weeks. For short-term treatment of situational anxiety or long-term treatment of generalized anxiety disorders, a total daily dose of greater than 30 mg of diazepam or its equivalent is almost never needed. For the treatment of panic disorder, the high-potency, short-acting benzodiazepine alprazolam has the longest record of efficacy, although the long-acting benzodiazepine clonazepam is gaining increasing acceptance. Use of benzodiazepines for anxiety and panic disorders is frequently being replaced with SSRIs. Problems with benzodiazepine rebound and withdrawal symptoms can be minimized if low-potency, long-acting drugs are used for the treatment of generalized anxiety disorders. Elderly patients manifest greater sedation and greater impairment of psychomotor performance than younger persons receiving the same dose.

Buspirone

Buspirone is a nonbenzodiazepine that is effective in the treatment of generalized anxiety disorders (onset of anxiolytic effects over several days) but not panic disorder. This drug is a partial agonist at serotonin receptors, resulting in decreased serotonin turnover and anxiolytic effects. Buspirone has no direct effects on GABA receptors and thus no pharmacologic cross-reactivity with benzodiazepines, barbiturates, or alcohol. Buspirone lacks sedative, anticonvulsant, and skeletal muscle–relaxing effects characteristic of benzodiazepines. Absorption from the gastrointestinal tract is 100%, but extensive hepatic first-pass metabolism decreases bioavailability to 4%. The elimination half-time is 2 to 11 hours. Buspirone does not produce dependence and does not appear to be highly toxic if taken in overdose. The principal disadvantage seems to be a slow onset of effect (1 to 2 weeks), which may be interpreted as ineffectiveness by patients experiencing acute anxiety.

Lithium

Lithium, anticonvulsants, and antipsychotics are considered drugs of choice for the treatment of bipolar disorders. Because of the multiple drug interactions with lithium and severe toxicity, alternative drugs are being used frequently in its place in the treatment of bipolar disorder. Lithium has many neurobiologic effects, but it is not known which components are necessary for its efficacy in the treatment of bipolar disorders.[42] One possible mechanism is the ability of lithium to inhibit a second messenger system that transduces signals from many neurotransmitter receptors, which ultimately lead to release of calcium ions from intracellular storage sites. With repeated firing, a neuron that has been exposed to lithium would become relatively depleted of second messengers and signal transmission would be dampened, especially in hyperactive neurons. Full therapeutic effects of lithium may take several weeks. The goal for treatment of acute mania is to maintain plasma lithium concentrations between 1.0 and 1.2 mEq/L. Plasma lithium concentrations should be measured 10 to 12 hours after the last oral dose, and levels should not be drawn sooner than 4 to 5 days after the latest change in dosage.

Pharmacokinetics

Lithium is distributed throughout the total body water and is excreted almost entirely by the kidneys. Lithium, like sodium, is filtered by the glomerulus and reabsorbed by the proximal, but not distal, renal tubules. Thus, its renal excretion is not enhanced by thiazide diuretics, which act selectively on the distal renal tubules. In fact, because proximal reabsorption of lithium and sodium is competitive, depletion of sodium as produced by dehydration, decreased sodium intake, and thiazide and loop diuretics may increase reabsorption of lithium by proximal renal tubules, resulting in as much as a 50% increase in the plasma concentration of lithium. Potassium-sparing diuretics (triamterene, spironolactone) do not facilitate reabsorption of lithium and, in fact, may increase excretion. Nonsteroidal antiinflammatory drugs, by altering renal blood flow, may produce marked increases in the plasma concentration of lithium and should be used with care.

Safe and effective use of lithium can be monitored only by measuring plasma concentrations. The therapeutic range for acute mania is 1.0 to 1.2 mEq/L, with oral doses averaging 900 to 1,800 mg per day. Plasma lithium concentrations should be measured about 12 hours after the last oral dose. Because the elimination half-time is about 24 hours and the time to reach steady state is four or five elimination half-times, plasma concentrations should be measured no sooner than 5 days after a change in dosage, unless toxicity is suspected. In elderly patients and in patients with renal disease, the elimination half-time for lithium is prolonged; the time to equilibration can be delayed to 7 days or longer. If toxicity is suspected, lithium should be withheld and the plasma concentration determined immediately, taking into account the time that has elapsed since the last dose.

Side Effects

The most common serious side effects of lithium occur at the kidneys, manifesting as polydipsia and polyuria. An estimated 20% of treated patients excrete greater than 3 L of urine daily, reflecting an impaired renal concentrating ability due to the inhibitory effect of lithium on intracellular adenosine monophosphate formation in the renal tubules. The potassium-sparing diuretic amiloride is effective in decreasing urine volume without affecting the plasma concentrations of either lithium or potassium. It is recommended that renal function be evaluated by measuring blood urea nitrogen or plasma creatinine every 6 months.

Changes on the ECG characterized by T wave flattening or inversion occur in some patients being treated with lithium, but there seem to be no related clinical effects. These changes are reversible within 2 weeks when lithium is discontinued. Clinically significant lithium-induced cardiac conduction disturbances are rare, although sinoatrial node dysfunction and sinoatrial node block have been described. Patients with preexisting sinoatrial node dysfunction (sick sinus syndrome) should probably be treated with lithium only if they have an artificial cardiac pacemaker in place.

Hypothyroidism develops in about 5% of patients treated with lithium and is more common in women than men. For this reason, it is recommended that thyroid-stimulating hormone levels be measured every 6 months. If necessary, levothyroxine therapy may be initiated without discontinuing lithium.

Clinically important dermatologic toxicities of lithium include acne and exacerbations of psoriasis or a new onset of psoriasis. Patients may complain of memory disturbance and cognitive slowing. Hand tremor occurs in 25% to 50% of treated patients and diminishes with time and in response to a decrease in the dose of lithium or treatment with a β-adrenergic antagonist. Rarely, lithium may cause extrapyramidal effects.

The association of sedation with lithium therapy suggests that anesthetic requirements for injected and inhaled drugs could be decreased. High plasma concentrations of lithium may delay recovery from the CNS depressant effects of barbiturates.[43] Responses to depolarizing and nondepolarizing neuromuscular blocking drugs may be prolonged in the presence of lithium.[44]

Drug Interactions (Table 43-6)

Toxicity

Diuretic therapy, sodium restriction, and sodium wasting increase reabsorption of lithium and thus increase plasma lithium concentrations. Patients being treated with lithium should avoid nonsteroidal antiinflammatory drugs and diuretics.

Many symptoms and signs of toxicity are closely correlated with the plasma lithium concentration (Table 43-7).[42] Mild lithium toxicity is reflected by sedation, nausea, skeletal muscle weakness, and changes on the ECG characterized by widening of the QRS complex. Atrioventricular heart block, hypotension, cardiac dysrhythmias, and seizures may occur when plasma concentrations of lithium are greater than 2 mEq/L. It is not uncommon for elderly patients who excrete lithium slowly to become confused, even in the presence of therapeutic plasma concentrations of this ion. Significant lithium toxicity is a medical emergency that may require aggressive treatment, including hemodialysis. If renal function is adequate, excretion of lithium ions can be modestly accelerated by osmotic diuresis and IV administration of sodium bicarbonate.

Table 43-6

Drug Interactions with Lithium

Drug	Interaction
Thiazide diuretics	Increased plasma lithium concentration as a result of decreased renal clearance
Furosemide	Usually no change in the plasma lithium concentration
Nonsteroidal antiinflammatory drugs	Increased plasma lithium concentration as a result of decreased renal clearance (exceptions are aspirin and sulindac)
Aminophylline	Decreased plasma lithium concentration as result of increased renal clearance
Angiotensin-converting enzyme inhibitors	May increase plasma lithium concentration
Neuroleptic drugs	Lithium may exacerbate extrapyramidal symptoms or increase the risk of the neuroleptic malignant syndrome
Anticonvulsant drugs (carbamazepine)	Concurrent use with lithium may result in additive neurotoxicity
β-Adrenergic antagonists	Decrease lithium-induced tremor
Neuromuscular blocking drugs	Lithium may prolong the duration of action

Adapted from Price LH, Heninger GR. Lithium in the treatment of mood disorders. *N Engl J Med.* 1994;331:591–598.

Anticonvulsants in Treatment of Bipolar Disorder

The anticonvulsants carbamazepine and valproic acid are used commonly in the treatment of bipolar disorder and valproic acid is used for migraine off label. Side effects of valproic acid that occur between 1% and 10% include headache, somnolence, dizziness, insomnia, nervousness, pain, alopecia, nausea, vomiting, diarrhea, abdominal pain, dyspepsia, anorexia, thrombocytopenia (dose related), tremor, weakness, diplopia, amblyopia/blurred vision, infection, and flulike syndrome. Despite this wide array of common side effects, valproic acid is often better tolerated than lithium, which has life-threatening side effects. Side

Table 43-7

Signs and Symptoms of Lithium Toxicity

Toxic Effects	Plasma Lithium Concentration (mEq/L)	Signs and Symptoms
Mild	1.0–1.5	Lethargy Irritability Skeletal muscle weakness Tremor Slurred speech Nausea
Moderate	1.6–2.5	Confusion Drowsiness Restlessness Unsteady gait Coarse tremor Dysarthria Skeletal muscle fasciculations Vomiting
Severe	>2.5	Impaired consciousness (coma) Delirium Ataxia Extrapyramidal symptoms Seizures Impaired renal function

Adapted from Price LH, Heninger GR. Lithium in the treatment of mood disorders. *N Engl J Med.* 1994;331:591–598.

effects of carbamazepine, although rare, include leukopenia, aplastic anemia, and hepatitis. It is recommended that liver function tests and complete blood counts be followed in patients being treated with carbamazepine.

Antipsychotic (Neuroleptic) Drugs

The antipsychotic drugs are a chemically diverse group of compounds (phenothiazines, thioxanthenes, butyrophenones) that are useful in the treatment of schizophrenia, mania, depression with psychotic features, and certain organic psychoses (Table 43-8). Schizophrenic patients who have not responded to standard antipsychotics may respond to clozapine. In addition, antipsychotic drugs are used to treat Tourette's syndrome and certain movement disorders. Some of these drugs may also be used as antiemetics at low doses.

Phenothiazines and thioxanthenes have a high therapeutic index and relatively flat dose-response curve, accounting for the remarkable safety of these drugs over a wide dose range. Even large overdoses are unlikely to cause life-threatening depression of ventilation. These drugs do not produce physical dependence, although abrupt discontinuation may be accompanied by skeletal muscle discomfort.

Structure–Activity Relationships

Phenothiazines have a three-ring structure in which two benzene rings are linked by a sulfur and a nitrogen atom. If the nitrogen atom at position 10 is replaced by a carbon atom with a double bond to the side chain, the compound becomes a thioxanthene. Phenothiazines and thioxanthenes used to treat psychiatric disease have three carbon atoms interposed between position 10 of the central ring and the first amino nitrogen atom of the side chain at this position. In addition, the amine is always tertiary. This structure contrasts with that of phenothiazines with significant antihistamine activity (promethazine) or phenothiazines with significant anticholinergic activity (ethopropazine, diethazine), which have only two carbon atoms separating the amino group from position 10 of the central ring. Loss of a methyl group or other substituents on the tertiary amino group, as can occur during metabolism, results in a loss of pharmacologic activity.

Mechanism of Action

The mechanism of action of antipsychotic drugs is thought to be due to blockade of dopamine receptors (especially dopamine$_2$ receptors) in the basal ganglia and limbic portions of the forebrain.[45,46] All antipsychotic drugs achieve maximum clinical efficacy over a period of weeks, emphasizing the importance of distinguishing the acute receptor

Table 43-8

Comparative Pharmacology of Antipsychotic (Neuroleptic) Drugs

Category and Drug	Sedative Potency	Anticholinergic Potency	Orthostatic Hypotension Potency	Extrapyramidal Potency
Phenothiazines				
Chlorpromazine	+ + +	+ +	+ + +	+
Triflupromazine	+ + +	+ +	+ + +	+ +
Thioridazine	+ + +	+ + +	+ + +	+
Fluphenazine	+ +	+	+	+ + +
Perphenazine	+	+	+	+ + +
Trifluoperazine	+ +	+	+	+ + +
Thioxanthenes				
Chlorprothixene	+ + +	+ + +	+ + +	+
Thiothixene	+	+	+	+ + +
Dibenzodiazepines				
Clozapine	+ + +	+ + +	+ + +	0
Loxapine	+ +	+ +	+ +	+ + +
Butyrophenones				
Haloperidol	+	+	+	+ + +
Droperidol	+	+	+	+ + +
Diphenylbutylpiperidines				
Pimozide	+	+	+	+ + +
Benzisoxazole				
Risperidone	+	+	+ +	+

0, none; +, mild; + +, moderate; + + +, marked.

antagonist effects of antipsychotic drugs from their chronic effects. Interference with the neurotransmitter functions of dopamine by these drugs is suggested by extrapyramidal side effects. Blockade of dopamine receptors in the chemoreceptor trigger zone of the medulla is responsible for the antiemetic effect of these drugs.

Pharmacokinetics

Phenothiazines and thioxanthenes often display erratic and unpredictable patterns of absorption after oral administration. These drugs are highly lipid soluble and accumulate in well-perfused tissues such as the brain. Passage across the placenta and accumulation of drug in the fetus is possible. Avid binding to protein in plasma and tissues limits the effectiveness of hemodialysis in removing these drugs.

Metabolism

Metabolism of phenothiazines and thioxanthenes is principally by oxidation in the liver followed by conjugation. Most oxidative metabolites are pharmacologically inactive, with a notable exception being 7-hydroxychlorpromazine. Metabolites appear primarily in urine and to a lesser extent in bile. Typical elimination half-times of these drugs are 10 to 20 hours, permitting once-daily dosing intervals. The elimination half-time may be prolonged in the fetus and in the elderly, who have decreased capacity to metabolize these drugs.

Side Effects

With the exception of clozapine, the chronic use of phenothiazines and thioxanthenes may be complicated by serious side effects, most likely reflecting drug-induced blockade of dopamine receptors, especially in the forebrain.[45] Despite the common occurrence of side effects, these drugs have a large margin of safety and overdoses are rarely fatal.

Extrapyramidal Effects

Tardive dyskinesia may occur in 20% of patients who receive antipsychotic drugs for greater than 1 year. Only clozapine has not been implicated as a cause of this potentially permanent side effect. Elderly patients and women of all ages seem to be more susceptible to the development of tardive dyskinesia. Manifestations of tardive dyskinesia include abnormal involuntary movements, which may affect the tongue, facial and neck muscles, upper and lower extremities, truncal musculature, and, occasionally, skeletal muscle groups involved in breathing and swallowing. Tardive dyskinesia only rarely remits, and there is no treatment. Compensatory increases in the function of dopamine activity in the basal ganglia may be responsible for the development of tardive dyskinesia.

Acute dystonic reactions occur in approximately 2% of treated patients and are most likely to occur within the first 72 hours of therapy. Dystonic reactions are most common in young men and in patients taking high-potency antipsychotics. Acute skeletal muscle rigidity and cramping may develop, usually in the musculature of the neck, tongue, face, and back. Opisthotonos and oculogyric crises may occur. The sudden onset of respiratory distress in a patient on neuroleptics may reflect laryngeal dyskinesia (laryngospasm).[47] Acute dystonia responds dramatically to diphenhydramine, 25 to 50 mg IV. Extrapyramidal side effects including tremor, masked facies, and skeletal muscle rigidity may occur, especially in elderly patients. Patients with antipsychotic-induced akathisia often appear restless (inability to tolerate inactivity), which may be confused with the underlying psychotic disorder.

Cardiovascular Effects

IV administration of chlorpromazine causes a decrease in systemic blood pressure resulting from (a) depression of vasomotor reflexes mediated by the hypothalamus or brainstem, (b) peripheral α-adrenergic blockade, (c) direct relaxant effects on vascular smooth muscle, and (d) direct cardiac depression. Risperidone is an antipsychotic drug that has been associated with exaggerated systemic hypotension during a spinal anesthetic, perhaps reflecting risperidone-induced α blockade.[48] α-Adrenergic blockade produced by chlorpromazine is sufficient to blunt or prevent the pressor effects of epinephrine. Miosis that occurs predictably may also be due to α-adrenergic blockade. A cardiac antidysrhythmic effect of chlorpromazine may reflect the potent local anesthetic activity of this drug. These drugs usually do not cause cardiac dysrhythmias. Rarely, antipsychotic drugs prolong the QTc interval on the ECG and therefore predispose to the development of ventricular tachycardia.[49] Thioridazine and pimozide are potent calcium channel blockers, which may contribute to their cardiac toxicity, including prolongation of the QTc interval on the ECG.

Oral administration of these drugs is associated with less pronounced systemic blood pressure–lowering effects. Indeed, tolerance to the hypotensive effect develops so that after several weeks of therapy, the blood pressure returns toward normal. Nevertheless, some element of orthostatic hypotension may persist for the duration of therapy.

Neuroleptic Malignant Syndrome

Neuroleptic malignant syndrome occurs in 0.5% to 1.0% of all patients treated with antipsychotic drugs. Risk factors for the development of this syndrome may include dehydration and intercurrent illness. The syndrome typically develops over 24 to 72 hours in young men and is characterized by (a) hyperthermia; (b) generalized hypertonicity of skeletal muscles; (c) instability of the autonomic nervous system manifesting as alterations in systemic blood pressure, tachycardia, and cardiac dysrhythmias; and (d) fluctuating levels of consciousness.[50] Autonomic nervous system dysfunction may precede the onset of other symptoms. Increased skeletal muscle tone may so decrease chest wall expansion that it becomes necessary to provide mechanical support of ventilation. Skeletal muscle rigidity may be severe enough to cause myonecrosis leading to increased creatine phosphokinase levels, myoglobinuria, and renal failure. Liver transaminase enzymes are likely to be increased. Mortality is 20% to 30%, with common causes of death being ventilatory failure, cardiac failure and/or dysrhythmias, renal failure, and thromboembolism.

The cause of neuroleptic malignant syndrome is not known and, as a result, treatment is empirical and includes supportive measures and the administration of the direct-acting muscle relaxant dantrolene and the dopamine agonists bromocriptine or amantadine.[51] The reported efficacy of dopamine agonists in the treatment of skeletal muscle rigidity as well as the prevention of the onset of the syndrome with abrupt withdrawal of levodopa therapy suggests a role of dopamine receptor blockade in the development of this syndrome.[52]

Malignant hyperthermia associated with anesthesia as well as the central anticholinergic syndrome may mimic the neuroleptic malignant syndrome.[50] A distinguishing feature is the ability of nondepolarizing muscle relaxants to produce flaccid paralysis in patients experiencing the neuroleptic malignant syndrome but not in those experiencing malignant hyperthermia (see Table 43-2).[53]

Endocrine Effects

Prolactin levels are increased as a result of blockade of dopamine receptors and loss of the normal inhibition of prolactin secretion. Galactorrhea and gynecomastia may accompany excess prolactin secretion. Amenorrhea is a possible but rare complication of therapy. Decreased secretion of corticosteroids may be due to diminished corticotropin release from the anterior pituitary. Chlorpromazine may impair glucose tolerance and the release of insulin in some patients. Hypothalamic effects may manifest as weight gain and occasionally abnormalities of thermoregulation.

Sedation

Sedation produced by antipsychotic drugs appears to be due to antagonism of α_1-adrenergic, muscarinic, and histamine (H_1) receptors. With chronic therapy, tolerance develops to the sedative effects produced by these drugs.

Antiemetic Effects

The antiemetic effects of antipsychotic drugs reflect their interaction with dopaminergic receptors in the chemoreceptor trigger zone of the medulla. These drugs seem most effective in preventing opioid-induced nausea and vomiting. Perphenazine, 5 mg IV, has been shown to be as effective as ondansetron, 4 mg IV, and droperidol, 1.25 mg IV, for prevention of postoperative vomiting after gynecologic surgery.[54] Unlike these other antiemetics, perphenazine was not associated with side effects such as sedation or hypotension, making this phenothiazine derivative useful as an inexpensive prophylactic antiemetic. Perphenazine, 70 μg/kg IV, decreases the incidence of vomiting in children during the first 24 hours after tonsillectomy.[55] The CNS dopaminergic activity of phenothiazines, which results in their antiemetic effects, may also produce extrapyramidal symptoms. These symptoms, which are easily treated with benztropine, appear to be rare.

Obstructive Jaundice

Obstructive jaundice that is considered to be an allergic reaction occurs rarely 2 to 4 weeks after administration of phenothiazines or thioxanthenes. Indeed, there is prompt recurrence of jaundice if the offending drug, usually chlorpromazine, is again administered. If jaundice is not observed in the first month of therapy, it is unlikely to occur at a later date.

Hypothermia

An effect of chlorpromazine on the hypothalamus is most likely responsible for the poikilothermic effect of this drug. In the past, this effect was used to facilitate the production of surgical hypothermia.

Seizure Threshold

Many antipsychotic drugs decrease the seizure threshold and produce a pattern on the EEG similar to that associated with seizure disorders. Chlorpromazine causes slowing of the EEG pattern, with some increase in burst activity and spiking. Sensory evoked potentials are often decreased in amplitude, and there is an increase in latency.

Skeletal Muscle Relaxation

Chlorpromazine causes skeletal muscle relaxation in some types of spastic conditions, presumably by actions on the CNS because the drug is devoid of actions at the neuromuscular junction.

Drug Interactions

The ventilatory depressant effects of opioids are likely to be exaggerated by antipsychotic drugs. Likewise, the miotic and sedative effects of opioids are increased, and the analgesic actions are likely to be potentiated. These drugs may interfere with the actions of exogenously administered dopamine, and the effects of alcohol are enhanced.

Clozapine

Clozapine is the only antipsychotic that does not seem to cause tardive dyskinesia or extrapyramidal side effects.[45] Among the most common side effects are sedation, nausea and vomiting, and orthostatic hypotension. Excessive salivation, especially during sleep, is a common but paradoxical and poorly explained effect of this strongly anticholinergic drug. Another presumed manifestation of a parasympatholytic effect is sustained mild sinus tachycardia. Caution is advised in the use of such an anticholinergic drug in patients at risk for glaucoma, ileus, or urinary retention. Low-grade fever sometimes occurs early in the use of clozapine. Clozapine has been combined safely with lithium and antidepressant drugs, but there may be a risk of excessive sedation if this drug is combined with a benzodiazepine.

Agranulocytosis is a particularly serious side effect of clozapine, occurring in less than 1% of patients.[45] For this reason, weekly monitoring of the white blood cell count is recommended in treated patients.

The incidence of seizures is 2% to 4% in those treated with high doses of clozapine. Some clinicians prescribe an anticonvulsant when high doses of clozapine (>500 mg per day) are administered or in patients with a history of epilepsy. Valproic acid may be selected as the anticonvulsant, as this drug does not alter the metabolism of clozapine.

Butyrophenones

Butyrophenones, such as droperidol and haloperidol, structurally resemble and evoke pharmacologic effects similar to those of phenothiazines and thioxanthenes. Butyrophenones can decrease anxiety that accompanies psychoses. Conversely, butyrophenones are less effective against anxiety such as that present in the preoperative period.

Droperidol is the butyrophenone most often administered in the preoperative period. Haloperidol has a longer duration of action than droperidol and lacks significant α-adrenergic antagonist effects such that decreases in systemic blood pressure are unlikely. The principal use of haloperidol is as a long-acting antipsychotic drug and for treatment of agitation and delirium in the intensive care unit.

Ziprasidone is an atypical antipsychotic drug that may be a useful alternative to haloperidol for the treatment of delirium.[56] Like haloperidol, ziprasidone is associated with antidopaminergic side effects (extrapyramidal effects, tardive dyskinesia) and can cause prolongation of the QTc interval on the ECG (not recommended in patients with QTc >500 milliseconds, recent myocardial infarction, uncompensated congestive heart failure).

Pharmacokinetics

In patients anesthetized with nitrous oxide-fentanyl, the elimination half-time of droperidol is 104 minutes, clearance is 14.1 mL/kg per minute, and the volume of distribution is 2.04 L/kg.[57] The total body clearance of droperidol is similar to hepatic blood flow (perfusion dependent), emphasizing the importance of hepatic metabolism rather than hepatic enzyme activity (capacity dependent) in elimination of this drug. In this regard, potential accumulation of droperidol is more likely to occur when the hepatic blood flow is decreased rather than with an alteration in hepatic enzyme activity. The short elimination half-time is not consistent with the prolonged CNS effects of droperidol, which may reflect slow dissociation of the drug from receptors or retention of droperidol in the brain. Droperidol is metabolized in the liver, with maximal excretion of metabolites occurring during the first 24 hours.

Side Effects

The side effects of butyrophenones resemble those described for phenothiazines and thioxanthenes.

Central Nervous System

The outwardly calming effect of droperidol may mask an overwhelming fear of surgery. This dysphoric response detracts from the use of droperidol in the preoperative period, especially as preoperative medication.[58] Akathisia (most often a feeling of restlessness in the legs) may accompany administration of droperidol as preoperative medication.[59] As a dopamine antagonist, droperidol evokes extrapyramidal reactions in about 1% of patients.[60,61] For this reason, droperidol should not be administered to patients who are concurrently being treated for Parkinson's disease. Acute laryngeal dystonia (laryngospasm) is a rare extrapyramidal reaction to the butyrophenones.[47] Diphenhydramine administered IV is an effective treatment for droperidol-induced extrapyramidal reactions.

Droperidol is a cerebral vasoconstrictor that causes a decrease in cerebral blood flow, but cerebral metabolic rate for oxygen is not greatly altered. Failure to decrease the metabolic rate despite decreased cerebral blood flow could be undesirable in patients with cerebral vascular disease. The reticular activating system is not depressed, and α rhythm persists on the EEG. Droperidol does not produce amnesia nor does it have an anticonvulsant action.

Cardiovascular Effects

Droperidol can decrease systemic blood pressure as a result of actions in the CNS and by peripheral α-adrenergic blockade.[62] The decrease in blood pressure is usually minimal, although occasionally a patient may experience marked hypotension. Systemic and pulmonary vascular resistance is only modestly and transiently decreased. Myocardial contractility is not altered by droperidol.

Hypertension has been reported after administration of droperidol to patients with pheochromocytoma.[63,64] This systemic blood pressure response reflects droperidol-induced release of catecholamines from the adrenal medulla as well as inhibition of catecholamine uptake into chromaffin granules (Fig. 43-2).[65]

Droperidol is a cardiac antidysrhythmic and protects against epinephrine-induced dysrhythmias.[63] The mechanism for the cardiac antidysrhythmic effect has not been established but may reflect blockade of α-adrenergic receptors in the myocardium, stabilization of excitable membranes of cardiac cells by local anesthetic effects of

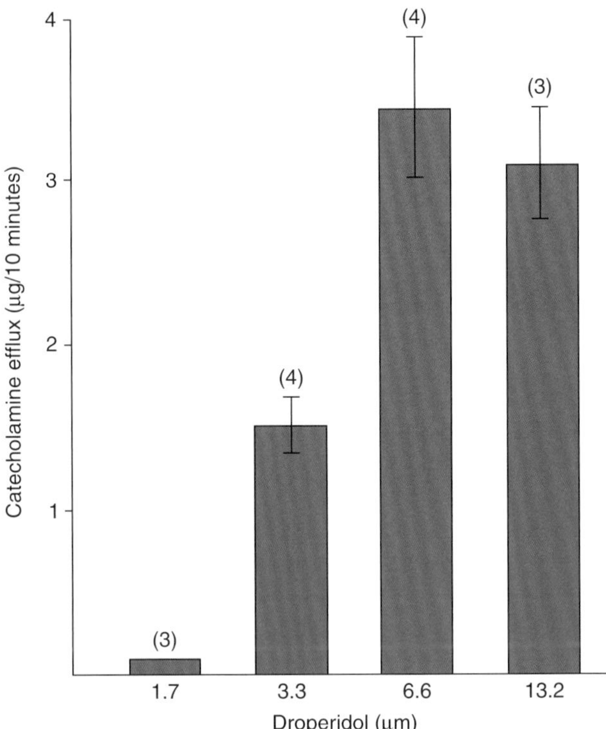

FIGURE 43-2 Catecholamine efflux (mean ± SE) from the perfused dog adrenal medulla is increased by droperidol. The number of experiments is indicated by the figure in parentheses. (From Sumikawa K, Hirano H, Amakata Y, et al. Mechanism of the effect of droperidol to induce catecholamine efflux from the adrenal medulla. *Anesthesiology.* 1985;62:17–22, with permission.)

droperidol, and decreases in systemic blood pressure, which decrease the likelihood of pressure-dependent cardiac dysrhythmias. Large doses of droperidol, 0.2 to 0.6 mg/kg IV, decrease conduction of cardiac impulses along accessory pathways responsible for tachydysrhythmias that occur in patients with Wolff-Parkinson-White syndrome (Fig. 43-3).[66]

Prolonged QTc Interval

Prolonged QTc syndrome is a malfunction of cardiac ion channels resulting in impaired ventricular repolarization that can lead to a characteristic polymorphic ventricular tachycardia known as torsades de pointes.[67] The single most common cause of the withdrawal or restriction of the use of drugs that are already in clinical use is the prolongation of the QTc interval on the ECG associated with torsades de pointes (polymorphic ventricular tachycardia).[68,69] This prolongation most often results from delayed ventricular repolarization, a process that is mediated by the efflux of intracellular potassium. The channels responsible for the current are susceptible to blockade by many drugs, producing a suitable environment for the development of torsades de pointes, which may lead to sudden death. Nondrug factors associated with prolongation of the QTc interval include female gender, advanced age, electrolyte disturbances (hypokalemia, hypomagnesemia), congestive heart failure, bradycardia, myocardial ischemia, and congenital long Q-T syndromes.

Several classes of noncardiac drugs (droperidol, thiopental, propofol, isoflurane, sevoflurane, succinylcholine, neostigmine, atropine, glycopyrrolate, metoclopramide, macrolide and quinolone antibiotics, SSRIs, $5HT_3$ receptor antagonists) produce dose-dependent prolongation of the QTc interval on the ECG in some patients.[68] Although these drugs can provoke torsades de pointes in susceptible patients, the risk of this response in patients with no other risk factors is minimal. Nevertheless, even in low-risk patients, drug interactions can lead to life-threatening torsades de pointes. These drug interactions are characterized by (a) additive or synergistic effects when two drugs capable of prolonging the QTc are administered (haloperidol and amitriptyline) or (b) the simultaneous administration of a drug that interferes with the metabolism of a second drug capable of prolonging the QTc interval (resulting increased plasma concentration of the second drug increases the risk of torsades de pointes). Drugs capable of inhibiting P-450 enzyme and thus delaying the metabolism of second drugs capable of prolonging the QTc interval include calcium channel blockers, antifungal drugs, SSRIs, macrolide and quinolone antibiotics, antiretroviral drugs, and amiodarone.

Droperidol is capable of prolonging the QTc interval on the ECG.[70–73] Although the QTc prolongation effect peaks 2 to 3 minutes following IV administration of droperidol, the effects may persist for several hours.

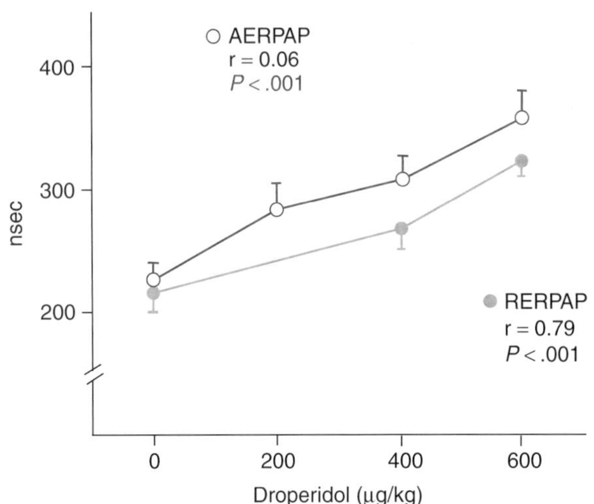

FIGURE 43-3 Droperidol produces dose-dependent prolongation of the antegrade and retrograde effective refractory period of accessory pathways. AERPAP, antegrade effective refractory period of accessory pathways; RERPAP, retrograde effective refractory period of accessory pathways. (From Gomez-Arnau J, Marquez-Montes J, Avello F. Fentanyl and droperidol effects on the refractoriness of the accessory pathway in the Wolff-Parkinson-White syndrome. *Anesthesiology.* 1983;58:307–313, with permission.)

Cases of QTc prolongation and/or torsades de pointes have occurred in patients receiving droperidol at (1.25 to 2.5 mg) as well as doses (0.625 to 1.25 mg) below those approved by the U.S. Food and Drug Administration.[71] Some of these responses occurred in patients without known risk factors and some have been fatal. Nevertheless, there were many confounding factors in these cases that make it impossible to establish the precise cause of the adverse cardiac events.[71] Of note, since droperidol was approved in 1970, there has not been a single case report where droperidol in doses used for the management of postoperative nausea and vomiting has been associated with cardiac dysrhythmias or cardiac arrest.[74,75] Although even small doses of droperidol (<1.25 mg IV) may cause prolongation of the QTc interval, this prolongation is considered clinically insignificant.[76,77]

Based on these reports, a "black box warning" has been added to the package insert for droperidol. This warning includes the requirement that all patients should undergo a 12-lead ECG prior to the administration of droperidol to determine if a prolonged QTc interval is present (>440 milliseconds for males and >450 milliseconds for females). When treatment with droperidol is selected, ECG monitoring should be performed before administration of droperidol and continued for 2 to 3 hours. Furthermore, droperidol should be administered with caution to patients who may be at risk for development of prolonged QTc syndrome (congestive heart failure, bradycardia, hypokalemia, elderly, concomitant administration of other drugs known to prolong the QTc interval). Sudden death during treatment with haloperidol has been attributed to drug-induced prolongation of the QTc interval on the ECG.[49]

When considering the effects of drugs on the QTc interval, it is important to recognize that it is difficult to measure this interval with precision.[75] There is inherent imprecision in identifying the end of the T wave and variation in the onset of the QRS complex on some ECG leads providing different QT values, depending on the leads selected for the measurement. Even paper speed and sensitivity can influence QT measurements. Automatic QTc measurement techniques have been found to be less accurate in cardiac patients than in healthy controls. Indeed, calculation of the QTc interval is ambiguous, as there are numerous different formulae and each produces different results.

Ventilation

Resting ventilation and the ventilatory response to carbon dioxide are not altered by droperidol.[78] Furthermore, droperidol administered IV augments the ventilatory response evoked by arterial hypoxemia, presumably by blocking the action of the inhibitory neurotransmitter dopamine at the carotid body (Fig. 43-4).[59] For this reason, droperidol may be an acceptable preoperative medication in patients with chronic obstructive airway disease who depend on carotid body drive to prevent hypoventilation.

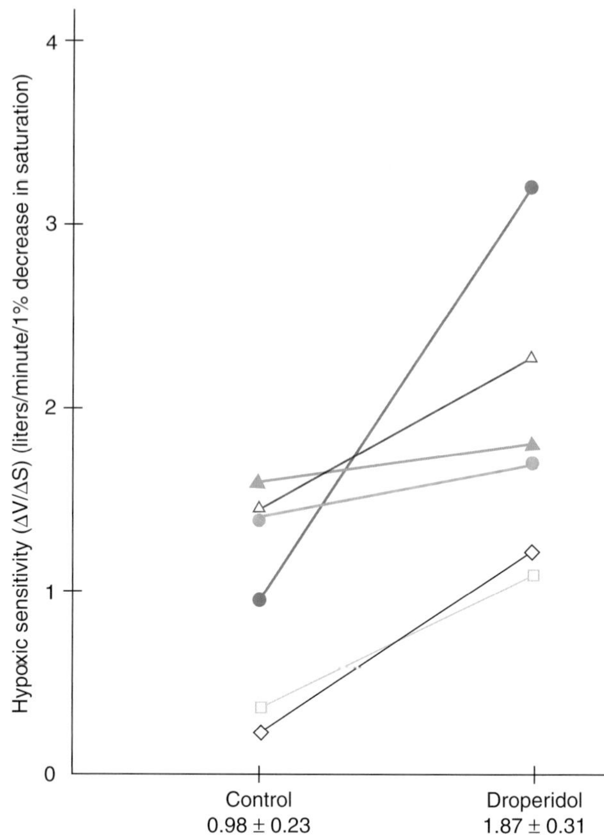

FIGURE 43-4 The ventilatory response to arterial hypoxemia (hypoxic sensitivity) is enhanced by droperidol. Solid symbols represent repeated experiments on the same subjects as those represented by the open symbols. (From Ward DS. Stimulation of hypoxic ventilatory drive by droperidol. *Anesth Analg.* 1984;63:106–110, with permission.)

Clinical Uses

Clinical uses of droperidol are limited to its use as an antiemetic.

Neuroleptanalgesia

Droperidol combined with fentanyl is administered for the production of neuroleptanalgesia. A commercially available 50:1 combination of droperidol with fentanyl was known as *Innovar.* This fixed combination of drugs is not associated with enhanced depression of ventilation as compared with either drug alone.[79] Droperidol does not enhance analgesia produced by fentanyl but rather prolongs its duration of action. Orthostatic hypotension and dysphoria are more likely to occur after the administration of Innovar compared with fentanyl alone.

Neuroleptanalgesia is characterized by trance-like (cataleptic) immobility in an outwardly tranquil patient who is dissociated and indifferent to the external surroundings. Analgesia is intense, allowing performance of a variety of diagnostic and minor surgical procedures such as bronchoscopy and cystoscopy. The disadvantages of neuroleptanalgesia are prolonged CNS depression and failure to depress sympathetic nervous system responses predictably to painful stimulation.

The mechanism by which droperidol produces anesthesia is not known but likely involves inhibition of synaptic transmission by ligand-gated ion channels. GABA and neuronal nicotinic acetylcholine receptors (nAChRs) are important in the mechanism of action of injected and inhaled anesthetics. There is evidence that droperidol inhibits activation of GABA and nAChRs receptors within a concentration range, which might result in anxiety, dysphoria, and restlessness that limit the clinical usefulness of high-dose droperidol anesthesia.[80]

Antiemetic

Droperidol is a powerful antiemetic agent as a result of inhibition of dopamine$_2$ receptors in the chemoreceptor trigger zone of the medulla. Despite the black box warning, there is a question whether small antiemetic doses ($\leq$1.25 mg) introduce the risk of prolonged QTc interval on the ECG.[71] Over nearly three decades, droperidol, 0.625 to 1.25 mg IV, has become widely accepted as a safe, cost-effective first-line therapy for the management of postoperative nausea and vomiting.[81,82] The use of droperidol, 1.25 mg IV is associated with greater effectiveness, lower cost, and similar patient satisfaction compared with 0.625 mg droperidol IV or ondansetron 4 mg IV.[83] Droperidol (1.25 mg) was as effective as dexamethasone (4 mg) and ondansetron (4 mg) in decreasing the incidence of postoperative nausea and vomiting by about 26% when administered as preoperative prophylaxis.[84] Labyrinthine-induced vomiting (motion sickness) is not influenced by droperidol.

Cannabis

Cannabis is an alkaloid mixture of more than 400 compounds derived from the *Cannabis sativa* plant. Cannabis has been used for thousands of years and is presently the most commonly used illicit drug in the world. The most abundant cannabinoids are δ-9-tetrahydrocannabinol (D9THC), cannabidiol, and cannabinol.[85] D9THC is the main psychotropically active cannabinoid. Two principal endogenous cannabis receptors (CB1 and CB2) have been identified. CB1 receptors are present in the CNS (especially spinal cord) and CB2 receptors are located peripherally and linked with cells in the immune system. Both receptors are members of the G protein family and like opioid receptors exert their actions by modulating second messenger activity (adenylate cyclase activity) and calcium ion function. Endogenous cannabinoid agonists (anandamide, 2-arachidonylglycerol) have been identified and produce effects similar to D9THC.

Pharmacokinetics

Cannabinoids undergo substantial hepatic first-pass metabolism following oral administration such that only 10% to 20% of the ingested dose reaches the systemic circulation. This metabolism produces large amounts of active metabolite, 11-hydroxy-δ-9-tetrahydrocannabinol, which is as active as the parent compound (D9THC) and has a prolonged half-time. The peak clinical effect after oral administration occurs after 1 to 2 hours and duration of action is 4 to 6 hours. In contrast, inhalation administration results in onset of action within seconds.

Toxicity

Euphoria and feeling of relaxation occurs at plasma cannabinoid concentrations of about 3 ng/mL and this can be produced by 2 to 3 mg of D9THC. Acute intoxication may cause perceptual alterations, distortion of time, intensification of normal sensory experiences, decreased reaction times, poor motor skills, increased appetite, impairment of skilled activities, tachycardia, and hypotension. The greatest concern is the creation of long-term toxicity, development of physical dependence associated with withdrawal symptom during a period of abstinence after frequent use.[86] Cannabis is often mixed with tobacco to make it burn more efficiently. Materials that are present in cannabis smoke are carcinogenic. Chronic inhalation of cannabis smoke is associated with an increased incidence of chronic obstructive lung disease and carcinoma of the lung and larynx. Persistent use of cannabis may be associated with decreased reproductive potential and reduced production of testosterone.

Clinical Uses

D9THC is increasingly used for the long-term treatment of nausea, vomiting, cachexia, and management of chronic pain including migraine.[87] The role of the endogenous cannabinoid system is not fully understood but evidence suggests it is involved with analgesia, cognition, appetite, vomiting, bronchodilation, inflammation, and immune control.[85] Cannabinoids are highly lipid soluble and the presence of CB1 receptors in the spinal cord suggests potential analgesic efficacy if placed in the epidural or intrathecal space. Although use of cannabis for analgesia introduces the potential for psychic and physical dependence, there is considerably less risk of life-threatening side effects compared to those associated with opioids. Pure D9THC may be effective in the treatment of chemotherapy-induced nausea and vomiting and is a recognized appetite stimulant in patients with terminal disease. Relief of skeletal muscle spasms in patients with multiple sclerosis has been described. The use of D9THC may be associated with an increased risk of myocardial infarction and thromboangiitis obliterans, perhaps reflecting D9THC-induced platelet activation.[87]

Two receptors for endogenous and exogenous cannabinoids have been described, CB1 and CB2. CB1 receptors are principally expressed on neurons and their activation has been associated with antinociception. CB2 receptors are principally expressed on glia and immune cells and their activation is associated with antiinflammatory activity and reduction in chronic and neuropathic pain. Subtype-specific agonists are under investigation for pain therapy in order to overcome the problem of a narrow therapeutic window seen with nonsubtype selective cannabinoid drugs between pain relief and psychogenic effects.[88]

PSYCHOSTIMULANTS

Methylphenidate is a psychostimulant used for the treatment of attention deficit hyperactivity disorder and narcolepsy. Similar to amphetamines, it blocks the reuptake of norepinephrine and dopamine. The data is limited as to the effect these psychostimulants may have on the anesthetized patient when used at clinical doses, but it is commonly thought that the risk of intraoperative hemodynamic instability and arrhythmias may be increased. A small case study showed that patients who take chronic prescription amphetamines are hemodynamically stable during anesthesia.[89] It is unclear what the effects anesthesia may have when methylphenidate is being abused, but anesthesia providers should be aware of its abuse potential.

References

1. El-Ganzouri AR, Ivankovich AD, Braverman B, et al. Monoamine oxidase inhibitors: should they be discontinued preoperatively? *Anesth Analg*. 1985;64:592–596.
2. Michaels I, Serrins M, Shier NQ, et al. Anesthesia for cardiac surgery in patients receiving monoamine oxidase inhibitors. *Anesth Analg*. 1984;63:1041–1044.
3. Wells DG, Bjorksten AR. Monoamine oxidase inhibitors revisited. *Can J Anaesth*. 1989;36:64–74.
4. Richelson E. Where are all the novel antidepressants? *Curr Opin Investig Drugs*. 2001;2(2):256–258.
5. Harvey AT, Rudolph RL, Preskorn SH. Evidence of the dual mechanism of action of venlafaxine. *Arch Gen Psychiatry*. 2000;57:503–508.
6. Buckley NA, McManus PR. Fatal toxicity of serotonergic and other antidepressant drugs: analysis of United Kingdom mortality data. *Br Med J*. 2002;325:1332–1336.
7. Whyte IM, Dawson AH, Buckley NA. Relative toxicity of venlafaxine and selective serotonin reuptake inhibitors in overdose compared to tricyclic antidepressants. *QJM*. 2003;96(5):369–374.
8. Hirschfeld RM. Efficacy of SSRIs and newer antidepressants in severe depression: comparison with TCAs. *J Clin Psychiatry*. 1999; 60(5):326–335.
9. Coupland NJ, Bell CJ, Potokar JP. Serotonin reuptake inhibitor withdrawal. *J Clin Psychopharmacol*. 1996;16:356–360.
10. Newman TB. A black-box warning for antidepressants in children? *N Engl J Med*. 2004;351:1595–1597.
11. Kennedy SH, Rizvi S. Sexual dysfunction, depression, and the impact of antidepressants. *J Clin Psychopharmacol*. 2009;29(2): 157–164.
12. Goldstein DJ, Rampey AH, Enas GG, et al. Fluoxetine: a randomized clinical trial in the treatment of obesity. *Int J Obes Relat Metab Disord*. 1994;18:129–135.
13. Rani PU, Naidu MUR, Prasad VB, et al. An evaluation of antidepressants in rheumatic pain conditions. *Anesth Analg*. 1996;83:371–375.
14. Gram LF. Fluoxetine. *N Engl J Med*. 1994;331:1354–1361.
15. Castro VM, Clements CC, Murphy SN, et al. QT interval and antidepressant use: a cross sectional study of electronic health records. *BMJ*. 2013;346:f288.
16. Girardin F, Gex-Fabry M, Berney P, et al. Drug-induced long QT in adult psychiatric inpatients: the 5-year cross-sectional ECG screening outcome in psychiatry study. *Am J Psychiatry*. 2013;170:1468–1476.
17. Johnston AJ, Lineberry CG, Ascher JAA. 102-Center prospective study of seizure in association with bupropion. *J Clin Psychiatry*. 1991;52:450–456.
18. Morrison EK, Rowe AS. Probable drug-drug interaction leading to serotonin syndrome in a patient treated with concomitant buspirone and linezolid in the setting of therapeutic hypothermia. *J Clin Pharm Ther*. 2012;37(5):610–613.
19. Häuser W, Wolfe F, Tölle T, et al. The role of antidepressants in the management of fibromyalgia syndrome: a systematic review and meta-analysis. *CNS Drugs*. 2012;26(4):297–307.
20. Lunn MP, Hughes RA, Wiffen PJ. Duloxetine for treating painful neuropathy or chronic pain. *Cochrane Database Syst Rev*. 2009;4: CD007115.
21. Spina E, Trifirò G, Caraci F, et al. Clinically significant drug interactions with newer antidepressants. *CNS Drugs*. 2012;26(1):39–67.
22. Yuan Y, Choi K, Hunt RH, et al. Selective serotonin reuptake inhibitors and risk of upper GI bleeding: confusion or confounding? *Am J Med*. 2006,119(9).719.
23. Ziegelstin RC, Meuchel J, Kim TJ, et al. Selective serotonin reuptake inhibitor use by patients with acute coronary syndromes. *Am J Med*. 2007;120(6):525–530.
24. Labos C, Dasgupta K, Nedjar H, et al. Risk of bleeding associated with combined use of selective serotonin reuptake inhibitors and antiplatelet therapy following acute myocardial infarction. *CMAJ*. 2011;183(16):1835.
25. Godfrey RG. A guide to the understanding and use of tricyclic antidepressants in the overall management of fibromyalgia and other chronic pain syndromes. *Arch Intern Med*. 1996;156(10):1047.
26. Strumper D, Durieux ME, Hollmann MW, et al. Effects of antidepressants on function and viability of human neutrophils. *Anesthesiology*. 2003;98:1356–1362.
27. Malan TP, Nolan PE, Lichtenthal PR, et al. Severe, refractory hypotension during anesthesia in a patient on chronic clomipramine therapy. *Anesthesiology*. 2001;95:264–266.
28. Thompson TL, Moran MG, Nies AS. Psychotropic drug use in the elderly. *N Engl J Med*. 1983;308:194–198.
29. Veith RC, Raskind MA, Caldwell JH, et al. Cardiovascular effects of tricyclic antidepressants in depressed patients with chronic heart disease. *N Engl J Med* 1982;306:954–959.
30. Spiss CK, Smith CM, Maze M. Halothane-epinephrine arrhythmias and adrenergic responsiveness after chronic imipramine administration in dogs. *Anesth Analg*. 1984;63:825–828.
31. Braverman B, McCarthy RJ, Ivankovich AD. Vasopressor challenges during chronic MAOI or TCA treatment in anesthetized dogs. *Life Sci* 1987;40:2587–2595.
32. Sprung J, Schoenwald PK, Levy P, et al. Treating intraoperative hypotension in a patient on long-term tricyclic antidepressants: a case of aborted aortic surgery. *Anesthesiology*. 1997;86:990–992.
33. Wong KC, Puerto AX, Puerto BA, et al. Influence of imipramine and pargyline on the arrhythmogenicity of epinephrine during halothane, enflurane, or methoxyflurane anesthesia in dogs. *Anesthesiology*. 1980;53:S25.
34. Stiff JL, Harris DB. Clonidine withdrawal complicated by amitriptyline therapy. *Anesthesiology*. 1983;59:73–74.
35. Frommer DA, Kulig KW, Marx JA, et al. Tricyclic antidepressant overdose. *JAMA*. 1987;257:521–526.
36. Boehnert MT, Lovejoy FH. Value of the QRS duration versus the serum drug level in predicting seizures and ventricular arrhythmias after an acute overdose of tricyclic antidepressants. *N Engl J Med*. 1985;313:474–479.

37. Stack CG, Rogers P, Linter PSK. Monoamine oxidase inhibitors and anaesthesia. *Br J Anaesth.* 1988;60:222–227.
38. Pavy TJG, Kliffer AP, Douglas MJ. Anaesthetic management of labour and delivery in a woman taking long-term MAOI. *Can J Anaesth.* 1995;42:618–620.
39. Insler SR, Kraenzler EJ, Licina MR, et al. Cardiac surgery in a patient taking monoamine oxidase inhibitors: an adverse fentanyl reaction. *Anesth Analg.* 1994;78:593–597.
40. Kaplan RF, Feinglass NG, Webster W, et al. Phenelzine overdose treated with dantrolene sodium. *JAMA.* 1986;255:642–644.
41. Boyer EW, Shannon M. The serotonin syndrome. *N Engl J Med.* 2005;352;1112–1120.
42. Price LH, Heninger GR. Lithium in the treatment of mood disorders. *N Engl J Med.* 1994;331:591–598.
43. Mannisto PT, Saarnivaara L. Effect of lithium and rubidium on the sleeping time caused by various anaesthetics in the mouse. *Br J Anaesth.* 1976;48:185–189.
44. Hill GE, Wong KC, Hodges MR. Lithium carbonate and neuromuscular blocking agents. *Anesthesiology.* 1977;46:122–126.
45. Baldessarini RJ, Frankenburg FR. Clozapine: a novel antipsychotic agent. *N Engl J Med.* 1991;324:746–754.
46. Richter JJ. Current theories about the mechanisms of benzodiazepines and neuroleptic drugs. *Anesthesiology.* 1981;54:66–72.
47. Koek RJ, Pi EH. Acute laryngeal dystonic reactions to neuroleptics. *Psychosomatics.* 1989;30:359–364.
48. Williams JH, Hepner DL. Risperidone and exaggerated hypotension during a spinal anesthetic. *Anesth Analg.* 2004;98:240–241.
49. Kriwisky M, Perry GY, Tarchitsky D, et al. Haloperidol-induced torsades de pointes. *Chest.* 1990;98;482–484.
50. Guze BH, Baxter LR. Neuroleptic malignant syndrome. *New Engl J Med.* 1985;313:163–166.
51. Rosenberg MR, Green M. Neuroleptic malignant syndrome: review of response to therapy. *Arch Intern Med.* 1989;149:1927–1931.
52. Granato JE, Stern BJ, Ringel A, et al. Neuroleptic malignant syndrome: successful treatment with dantrolene and bromocriptine. *Ann Neurol.* 1983;14:89–90.
53. Sangal R, Dimitrijevic R. Neuroleptic malignant syndrome: successful treatment with pancuronium. *JAMA.* 1985;254:2795–2796.
54. Desilva PHDP, Darvish AH, McDonald SM, et al. The efficacy of prophylactic ondansetron, droperidol, perphenazine, and metoclopramide in the prevention of nausea and vomiting after major gynecologic surgery. *Anesth Analg.* 1995;81:139–143.
55. Splinter WM, Roberts DJ. Perphenazine decreases vomiting by children after tonsillectomy. *Can J Anaesth.* 1997;44:1308–1310.
56. Young CC, Lujan E. Intravenous ziprasidone for treatment of delirium in the intensive care unit. *Anesthesiology.* 2004;101:794–795.
57. Fischler M, Bonnet F, Trang H, et al. The pharmacokinetics of droperidol in anesthetized patients. *Anesthesiology.* 1986;64:486–489.
58. Lee CM, Yeakel AE. Patient refusal of surgery following Innovar premedication. *Anesth Analg.* 1975;54:224–226.
59. Ward DS. Stimulation of hypoxic ventilatory drive by droperidol. *Anesth Analg.* 1984;63:106–110.
60. Rivera VM, Keichian AH, Oliver RE. Persistent parkinsonism following neuroleptanalgesia. *Anesthesiology.* 1975;42:635–637.
61. Wiklund RA, Ngai SH. Rigidity and pulmonary edema after Innovar in a patient on levodopa therapy: report of a case. *Anesthesiology.* 1971;35:545–547.
62. Whitwam JG, Russell WJ. The acute cardiovascular changes and adrenergic blockade by droperidol in man. *Br J Anaesth.* 1971;43:581–591.
63. Bittar DA. Innovar-induced hypertensive crisis in patients with pheochromocytoma. *Anesthesiology* 1979;50:366–369.
64. Sumikawa K, Amakata Y. The pressor effect of droperidol on a patient with pheochromocytoma. *Anesthesiology.* 1977;46:359–361.
65. Sumikawa K, Hirano H, Amakata Y, et al. Mechanism of the effect of droperidol to induce catecholamine efflux from the adrenal medulla. *Anesthesiology.* 1985;62:17–22.
66. Gomez-Arnau J, Marquez-Montes J, Avello F. Fentanyl and droperidol effects on the refractoriness of the accessory pathway in the Wolff-Parkinson-White syndrome. *Anesthesiology.* 1983;58:307–313.
67. Kies SJ, Pabelick CM, Hurley HA, et al. Anesthesia for patients with congenital long QT syndrome. *Anesthesiology.* 2005;102:204–210.
68. Liu BA, Juurlink DN. Drugs and the QT interval—caveat doctor. *N Engl J Med.* 2004;351:1053–1056.
69. Roden DM. Drug-induced prolongation of the QT interval. *N Engl J Med.* 2004;350:1013–1022.
70. Drolet B, Zhang S, Deschenes D et al. Droperidol lengthens cardiac repolarization due to block of the rapid component of the delayed rectifier potassium current. *J Cardiovasc Electrophysiol.* 1999;10:1597–1604.
71. Habib AS, Gan TJ. Food and Drug Administration black box warning on the perioperative use of droperidol: a review of the cases. *Anesth Analg.* 2003;96:1377–1379.
72. Reilly JG, Ayis SA, Ferrier IN, et al. QTc-interval abnormalities and psychotropic drug therapy in psychiatric patients. *Lancet.* 2000;355:1048–1052.
73. Scuderi PE. Droperidol: many questions, few answers. *Anesthesiology.* 2003;98:289–290.
74. Gan TJ, White PF, Scuderi PE, et al. FDA "black box" warning regarding use of droperidol for postoperative nausea and vomiting: is it justified? *Anesthesiology.* 2002;97:287–290.
75. Gan TJ. "Black box" warning on droperidol: a report of the FDA convened expert panel. *Anesth Analg.* 2004;98:1809.
76. Zhang Y, Luo Z, White PF. A model for evaluating droperidol's effect on the median QTc interval. *Anesth Analg.* 2004;98:1330–1335.
77. White PF. Prevention of postoperative nausea and vomiting—a multimodal solution to a persistent problem. *N Engl J Med.* 2004;350:2511–2512.
78. Soroker D, Barjilay E, Konichezky S. Respiratory function following premedication with droperidol or diazepam. *Anesth Analg.* 1978;57:695–699.
79. Harper MH, Hickey RF, Cromwell TH, et al. The magnitude and duration of respiratory depression produced by fentanyl plus droperidol in man. *J Pharmacol Exp Ther.* 1976;199:464–468.
80. Flood P, Coates KM. Droperidol inhibits $GABA_A$ and neuronal nicotinic receptor activation. *Anesthesiology.* 2002;96:987–993.
81. Henzi I, Sondergegger J, Tarmer MR. Systematic review. Efficacy, dose-response, and adverse effects of droperidol for prevention of postoperative nausea and vomiting. *Can J Anesth.* 2000;47:537–551.
82. White PF. Droperidol: a cost-effective antiemetic for over thirty years. *Anesth Analg.* 2002;95:789–790.
83. Hill RP, Lubarsky DA, Phillips-Bute B, et al. Cost-effectiveness of prophylactic antiemetic therapy with ondansetron, droperidol, or placebo. *Anesthesiology.* 2000;92:958–967.
84. Apfel CC, Korttila K, Abdalla M, et al. A factorial trial of six interventions for the prevention of postoperative nausea and vomiting. *N Engl J Med.* 2004;350:2441–2451.
85. Smith G. Cannabis: time for scientific evaluation of this ancient remedy? *Anesth Analg.* 2000;90:237–240.
86. Lee D, Schroeder JR, Karschner EL, et al. Cannabis withdrawal in chronic, frequent cannabis smokers during sustained abstinence within a closed residential environment. *Am J Addict.* 2014;23(3):234–242.
87. Deusch E, Kress HG, Kraft B, et al. The procoagulatory effects of delta-9-tetrahydrocannabinol in human platelets. *Anesth Analg.* 2004;99:1127–1130.
88. Karst M, Wippermann S, Ahrens J. Role of cannabinoids in the treatment of pain and (painful) spasticity. *Drugs.* 2010;70(18):2409–2438.
89. Fischer SP, Schmiesing CA, Guta CG, et al. General anesthesia and chronic amphetamine use: should the drug be stopped preoperatively? *Anesth Analg.* 2006;103(1):203.

CHAPTER 44

Physiology of the Newborn

Pamela Flood

In the absence of inborn metabolic dysfunction or birth trauma, the neonate is able to meet their physiologic needs when not under stress. However, neonatal physiology is characterized by decreased functional reserve. Increased physiologic demands may place a significant burden on organ systems that have not yet developed normal adult functional reserve.

Neonatal Physiology

Neonatal oxygen consumption is approximately 6 mL/kg per minute compared to 3 mL/kg per minute in the adult. The high metabolic rate of the neonate is the crucial determinant of cardiopulmonary function. Even under normal physiologic circumstances, the immature cardiac and respiratory systems operate near the edge of their functional reserve to support this metabolic demand. Immaturity of multiple neonatal organ systems creates important developmental differences in drug handling and response when compared to the older child and adults.[1]

Neonatal Cardiovascular Physiology

The newborn infant is in a state of transition from the fetal, intrauterine to the newborn, extrauterine circulatory pattern. As described in Chapter 45, the fetal circulation is characterized by high pulmonary vascular resistance, low systemic vascular resistance (including the placenta), and right-to-left cardiac shunting via the foramen ovale and ductus arteriosus. Expansion of the lungs at birth increases Po_2 and causes a rapid decline in pulmonary vascular resistance and an increase in pulmonary blood flow. The decrease in pulmonary vascular resistance at birth is mediated by the endogenous production of nitric oxide. Increasing blood return to the heart via the pulmonary veins raises the pressure of the left atrium above that of the right, causing a functional closure of the foramen ovale. Anatomic closure of the foramen ovale usually occurs between 3 months and 1 year of age, but the foramen remains anatomically patent in 10% to 30% of people throughout life.[2] These individuals are described as having a "probe patent" foramen ovale, meaning that a probe or other surgical instrument can be passed through the foramen ovale. In most of these individuals, the foramen is functionally closed by the lack of any significant pressure gradient between the left and right atria; however, in conditions where the pulmonary vascular resistance rises, significant right-to-left shunting can occur. Individuals with a probe patent foramen ovale are also at risk for systemic air embolism and resultant stroke when air emboli pass from the pulmonary to the systemic circulation. The functional closure of the ductus arteriosus is, in part, mediated by an increase in arterial oxygen partial pressure and is normally complete within the first 10 to 15 hours of life in the term neonate. However, anatomic closure does not occur until 2 months of age.

Because the foramen ovale and ductus arteriosus are only functionally closed in the neonatal period, the neonatal circulation is able to readily revert to the fetal pattern, particularly in response to physiologic stresses occasionally encountered in the perinatal period. The neonatal pulmonary circulation is very reactive. Hypoxemia, hypercarbia, or acidosis cause both pulmonary vasoconstriction and dilation of the ductus arteriosus. Increases in pulmonary vascular resistance result in right-to-left shunting across the foramen ovale and ductus arteriosus. Right-to-left shunting, by causing arterial hypoxemia, causes a further increase in pulmonary vascular resistance, thus creating a vicious cycle. Persistent pulmonary hypertension may be seen in premature neonates and those with diaphragmatic hernia, meconium aspiration, infection, congenital heart disease, and polycythemia.

The neonatal myocardium contains immature contractile elements and is less compliant than the adult myocardium. The Frank-Starling relationship is functional only within a very narrow range of left ventricular end diastolic pressure (Fig. 44-1).[3] Thus, there is a limited increase in cardiac output to be gained from aggressive volume loading in the normovolemic newborn. However, if preload is reduced by hypovolemia or dehydration, normalization of volume status will generally restore cardiac output. However, because stroke volume cannot be significantly augmented by volume loading, and because contractile reserve is limited, neonatal cardiac output is exquisitely dependent on heart rate.

Although adrenergic receptors are thought to be mature at birth, sympathetic innervation is incomplete. After birth, neurotransmitter concentrations increase progressively, reflecting the maturation of sympathetic innervation. When compared to the adult, neonatal myocardium is more sensitive to norepinephrine.[4] This phenomenon is a reflection of the relatively denervated status of neonatal myocardium. Dopamine is an indirectly acting inotrope that depends, in part, upon endogenous norepinephrine release for its action. Neonatal myocardium, being deficient in sympathetic innervation, is therefore less responsive to dopamine.

To meet the elevated metabolic demand, neonatal cardiac output, relative to body weight, is twice that of the adult. This is achieved with a relatively rapid heart rate (140 beats per minute) because as described earlier,

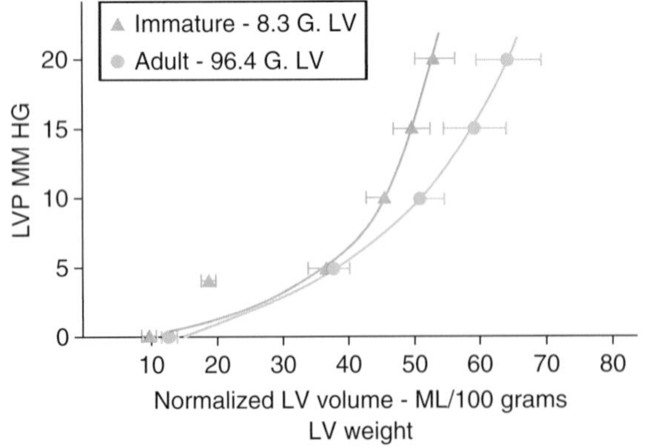

FIGURE 44-1 Pressure volume curve for neonatal and adult heart. Pressure volume curves for adult and neonatal canine heart. The immature heart is less compliant than the adult heart. As a result, the pressure volume curves diverge above a left ventricular pressure (LVP) of about 5 mm Hg.

stroke volume cannot be significantly increased. The neonatal circulation is characterized by centralization (increased peripheral vascular resistance and distribution of cardiac output primarily to vital organs), a situation comparable to an adult in compensated shock. Because neonatal baroreflex activity is impaired, the response to hemorrhage produces little increase in heart rate or change in total peripheral resistance. Thus, even a modest (10%) reduction in blood volume will cause a 15% to 30% decrease in mean blood pressure in the newborn infant. The structural and functional immaturity of the neonatal cardiovascular system severely limits the reserve that is available in the face of common perinatal and perioperative events such as hypovolemia, anesthetic-induced depression of contractility, relative bradycardia and positive pressure ventilation–induced decreases venous return. The marginal cardiovascular reserve of the neonate and leftward shift of the fetal hemoglobin dissociation curve are the rationale underlying the recommendation that the hematocrit be maintained at 30% or higher to prevent tissue ischemia in the newborn.

Respiratory Physiology of the Newborn

The respiratory system of a term neonate at birth is immature and postnatal development continues through early childhood. Although the conducting airways are fully developed by 16 weeks of gestation, the number of alveoli is reduced at birth. A premature infant born at 24 to 28 weeks of gestation is just beginning to develop alveoli from the distal saccules of the lung.[5] Complete alveolar maturation does not occur until 8 to 10 years of age. Thus, the ratio of alveolar surface area to body surface area is one-third that of the adult. At birth, the infant possesses approximately one-tenth of the adult population of alveoli. To satisfy increased oxygen demand, neonatal alveolar minute ventilation is twice that of the adult. Increasing respiratory rate rather than tidal volume is the most efficient means to increase alveolar ventilation in the newborn. The diaphragm is the primary muscle of respiration in the neonate but has fewer high-oxidative muscle fibers and is thus less fatigue-resistant than in the adult. Ventilation-perfusion imbalance occurs as a result of distal airway closure during normal tidal breathing in the neonate. This phenomenon is responsible for an increase in the alveolar-arterial oxygen tension gradient compared to adults.

Adequate gas exchange depends on adequate alveolar recruitment and thus surfactant function. Production of surfactant begins by 23 to 24 weeks of gestation and reaches maturity at approximately 35 weeks of gestation. Surfactant-deficient preterm infants have decreased lung compliance and are at risk for the development of respiratory distress syndrome (RDS).[5] Administration of corticosteroids to mothers in preterm labor may accelerate lung maturation in the fetus. Furthermore, the instillation of intratracheal exogenous surfactant in preterm babies has considerably improved the prognosis for premature infants. Infants born to mothers with intrauterine infection have a paradoxical increase in pulmonary maturation. The enhancement in lung maturation can be mimicked with lipopolysaccharide, suggesting that the effect is due to local inflammatory mediators rather than a downstream effect of corticosteroids.[6] In humans, the effect of inflammation on lung maturation is not enhanced by corticosteroid administration.[7]

The neonatal chest wall is more compliant and has less outward recoil than that of the adult. Thus, the neonatal lung has a greater tendency to collapse and the infant is obliged to utilize active mechanisms to maintain normal lung volumes (Table 44-1). First, by breathing at a relatively rapid rate, the duration of expiration is limited. In this way, inspiration is initiated before the lung has completed recoiling to its end-expiratory volume. Second, the neonate utilizes intercostal muscle activity during expiration to stabilize the chest wall, thus retarding the decline in lung volume during expiration. Last, the neonate exhales through a partially closed glottis, also retarding expiratory flow and maintaining end-expiratory lung volume. The awake neonate has a functional residual capacity (FRC) that is similar, when normalized to body weight, to that of an adult. However, because neonatal alveolar ventilation is twice that of an adult, the ratio of alveolar ventilation to FRC in the neonate is twice that of the adult. The high ratio of minute ventilation to FRC causes a much more rapid wash-out or wash-in of oxygen and anesthetic drugs in response to changes in inspired concentrations.

The active mechanisms utilized by the newborn to protect lung volume are exquisitely sensitive to the effects of general anesthesia. Therefore, the neonatal FRC may decrease significantly during anesthesia, particularly during periodic breathing and apnea. The combination of increased oxygen consumption and a reduced ratio of alveolar ventilation to FRC in the newborn explains why apnea and hypoventilation are associated with marked and rapid arterial oxygen desaturation.

Table 44-1

Active Mechanisms Used by Neonates to Maintain Lung Volume[a]

Rapid respiratory rate—early termination of expiration
Intercostal muscle activity in expiration—stabilizes compliant chest wall
Expiration against partially closed glottis—retards expiratory flow

[a]Significantly attenuated by general anesthesia.

Although the peripheral chemoreceptors are active from 28 weeks of gestation, their function is immature until several days after birth. Therefore, the neonate and preterm infant exhibit an altered response to hypoxia and hypercarbia. When challenged with hypoxic inspired gas mixtures, both the term and preterm infant have an initial 1- or 2-minute period of hyperventilation followed by sustained hypoventilation. As postnatal age increases, the hyperventilatory response becomes sustained. However, this protective response develops more slowly in the preterm infant and the ventilatory response to hypercarbia is impaired. The impaired neonatal ventilatory responses to hypoxia and hypercarbia are contributing factors to the development of life-threatening apnea and hypoventilation in the postoperative period.[8]

Although airway resistance is relatively low in infants, in absolute terms, the airways are very narrow. Relatively minor quantities of secretions or trivial inflammatory disease can produce serious respiratory embarrassment in small infants.

Neonatal Thermoregulation

The neonate tends to become hypothermic during general anesthesia much more rapidly than the adult. Accelerated heat loss in the neonate is related to its relatively large surface area compared to body mass, thinner layer of insulating subcutaneous fat, and a limited capability for thermogenesis. The neonate primarily relies on nonshivering or chemical thermogenesis in brown adipose tissue for heat production. Thermogenesis in brown fat is mediated by the sympathetic nervous system and is stimulated by norepinephrine, resulting in triglyceride hydrolysis. The thermoregulatory range is the ambient temperature range within which an unclothed subject can maintain normal body temperature. The lower limit of the thermoregulatory range (ambient temperature at which core temperature can be maintained) is 1¼°C for an adult, but is as high as 23°C and 28°C for the full-term infant and premature infant, respectively. Therefore, the thermoregulatory range of the neonate is much narrower than that of the adult. During anesthesia and surgery, heat loss in the pediatric patient is further enhanced by decrease in the thermoregulatory threshold due to anesthesia, low ambient temperatures of the operating suite (20°C to 22°C), preparation of skin with cold solutions, infusion of cold solutions, anesthesia-induced vasodilatation, and use of dry anesthetic gases in high flow, nonrebreathing systems. Intraoperative hypothermia will markedly delay emergence. Furthermore, with the return of the thermostatic reflexes, oxygen consumption increases by three- to fourfold as the metabolic rate is increased in an attempt to generate heat. This additional demand on an immature cardiorespiratory system that is already compromised due to the residual effects of anesthesia and surgery may precipitate cardiorespiratory failure. However, the loss of heat during anesthesia and surgery can be prevented by a number of simple measures, such as raising operating room temperature to 28°C to 30°C, radiant heat lamps, wrapping the extremities with insulating material, using nonvolatile warmed solutions for skin preparation, and administration of warmed intravenous fluids and blood products. Inhaled gases should be heated and humidified. Forced air warming devices are also effective in maintaining perioperative normothermia in neonates.

Neonatal Fluid, Electrolyte, and Renal Physiology

The neonate is characterized by an increased total body water, increased extracellular fluid volume, increased water turnover rate, and reduced glomerular filtration rate. The neonatal renal tubules have a decreased ability to absorb sodium, bicarbonate, glucose, amino acids, and phosphates. Neonates are obligate sodium wasters and require sodium supplementation. All of these factors contribute to the potential for overhydration, dehydration, metabolic acidosis, and hyponatremia, necessitating meticulous attention to intraoperative fluid therapy. Although third-space translocation of fluids is relatively similar in neonates and adults, neonatal insensible losses vary greatly. Fever, radiant warmers, phototherapy, increased ambient temperature, and decreased humidity all increase insensible loss.

Neonates have decreased glycogen stores and are prone to hypoglycemia after relatively brief periods of starvation. The preterm infant is at even greater risk for hypoglycemia. Glucose is therefore an essential element of the intraoperative fluid plan. The term neonate requires 3 to 5 mg/kg per minute and preterm neonates 5 to 6 mg/kg per minute of glucose to maintain serum glucose between 35 and 125 mg/dL.

Neonatal Neurophysiology

EEG rhythms that are mediated by subcortical integration of cortical and subcortical processes are present from 20 weeks' gestation.[9] Somatosensory evoked potentials can be recorded from the fetal cerebral cortex at 29 weeks' gestation.[10] As such, the functional circuitry required for sensation of pain is likely to be present between 20 and 30 weeks' gestation. Although myelination is incomplete, and nerve conduction velocity may be diminished, the shorter conduction distances found in the neonate facilitate rapid transmission of nociceptive impulses to the brain.[11] As in adults, most nociceptive impulses are transmitted by unmyelinated C fibers and by poorly myelinated Aδ fibers. Painful stimuli produce withdrawal, autonomic stimulation, and neuroendocrine stress responses. The concept of plasticity of the nervous system has important implications for the management of pain in newborns. The failure to provide analgesia for neonates leads to changes in nociceptive pathways in the dorsal horn of the spinal cord and in the brain. As a result, future painful insults result in exaggerated pain perception. Indeed, in human newborns, the failure to provide adequate anesthesia or analgesia for circumcision is associated with long-term changes, including an increased response to immunization later in childhood.[12] The adequate treatment of pain in the neonatal period is challenging because of the fear of respiratory depression associated with opioid administration. Fortunately, several nonpharmacologic behavioral interventions have analgesic effects in infants.[13] Analgesia may be induced by the administration of sucrose and by suckling. These effects are mediated via descending endogenous opioid and nonopioid mechanisms originating in the brainstem and may be partially reversed by the administration of naloxone.[14]

The germinal matrix has a rich blood supply, thin vessel walls, and scant vascular supporting tissue, causing the vessels of this region to be susceptible to rupture. With increasing gestational age, the germinal matrix involutes and is absent in the full-term infant. Intraventricular hemorrhage in the premature infant and in the fetus originates predominantly in the germinal matrix and occasionally in the choroid plexus. Periventricular-intraventricular hemorrhage occurs in 40% to 50% of premature infants and is a major cause of neonatal morbidity and mortality. The factors in the pathogenesis of intraventricular hemorrhage include abrupt changes in cerebral hemodynamics, changes in intracranial pressure, disturbances in osmotic equilibrium, and coagulopathy. Preterm infants are also at risk for retinopathy of prematurity (ROP) in which abnormal growth of retinal vessels can lead to scarring and blindness. Although gestational age is the primary etiologic factor in the development of ROP, hyperoxia, hypocarbia, vitamin E deficiency, and acidemia have also been implicated as contributing factors. The neonatal brain is comparatively large at birth compared to the adult. Myelination is incomplete at birth and is typically accomplished before the third year of age.

References

1. Hillier SC, Krishna G, Brasoveanu E. Neonatal anesthesia. *Semin Ped Surg.* 2004;13:142–151.
2. Fisher DC, Fisher EA, Budd JH, et al. The incidence of patent foramen ovale in 1,000 consecutive patients. A contrast transesophageal echocardiography study. *Chest.* 1995;107(6):1504–1509.
3. Spotnitz WD, Spotnitz HM, Truccone NJ, et al. Relation of ultrastructure and function. Sarcomere dimensions, pressure-volume curves, and geometry of the intact left ventricle of the immature canine heart. *Circ Res.* 1979;44(5):679–691.
4. Tanaka H, Manita S, Matsuda T, et al. Sustained negative inotropism mediated by alpha-adrenoceptors in adult mouse myocardia: developmental conversion from positive response in the neonate. *Br J Pharmacol.* 1995;114(3):673–677.
5. Moss TJ. Respiratory consequences of preterm birth. *Clin Exp Pharmacol Physiol.* 2006;33(3):280–284.
6. Jobe AH, Newnham JP, Willet KE, et al. Endotoxin-induced lung maturation in preterm lambs is not mediated by cortisol. *Am J Respir Crit Care Med.* 2000;162:1656–1661.

7. Foix-L'helias L, Baud O, Lenclen R, et al. Benefit of antenatal glucocorticoids according to the cause of very premature birth. *Arch Dis Child Fetal Neonatal Ed.* 2005;90:F46–F48.
8. Abu-Shaweesh JM. Maturation of respiratory reflex responses in the fetus and neonate. *Semin Neonatol.* 2004;9(3):169–180.
9. Brusseau R. Developmental perspectives: is the fetus conscious? *Int Anesthesiol Clin.* 2008;46(3):11–23.
10. Salihagic Kadic A, Predojevic M. Fetal neurophysiology according to gestational age. *Semin Fetal Neonatal Med.* 2012;17(5):256–260.
11. Benatar D, Benatar M. A pain in the fetus: toward ending confusion about fetal pain. *Bioethics.* 2001;15:57–76.
12. Marcus DA. A review of perinatal acute pain: treating perinatal pain to reduce adult chronic pain. *J Headache Pain.* 2006;7(1):3–8.
13. Kaufman GE, Cimo S, Miller LW, et al. An evaluation of the effects of sucrose on neonatal pain with 2 commonly used circumcision methods. *Am J Obstet Gynecol.* 2002;186:564–568.
14. Stevens B, Yamada J, Lee GY, et al. Sucrose for analgesia in newborn infants undergoing painful procedures. *Cochrane Database Syst Rev.* 2013;(1):CD001069.

CHAPTER 45

Maternal and Fetal Physiology and Pharmacology

Pamela Flood

As many as 1 out of every 50 pregnant women will undergo some type of surgery during their pregnancy. This rate is likely to increase in the face of improving outcomes from fetal surgery. Pregnancy causes significant physiologic changes that allow for the metabolic demands of the growing fetus. The pharmacokinetics and pharmacodynamics of many drugs are altered during pregnancy. When possible, surgery is performed during the second trimester of pregnancy to avoid affecting major organogenesis during the first trimester and to reduce the risk of preterm delivery which is increased in the third trimester. The effects of anesthesia are normally well tolerated by the fetus. The fetus does not depend on alveolar ventilation for oxygenation or carbon dioxide removal and has the maternal organs to help manage drug metabolism and excretion. However, the fetal cardiac output is sensitive to depression by anesthetic drugs. Drugs used in anesthesia cross the placenta to a variable extent (Table 45-1).[1–82] As a general rule, drugs that do not cross the blood–brain barrier do not cross the placenta to any appreciable degree. Knowledge of the fetal/maternal ratio of drugs used during pregnancy is important because in some cases it is preferred that the fetus not be exposed and in other cases drugs are given to the mother with the purpose of treating the fetus. During cesarean section, it is preferable to limit cardiac and respiratory depressant drugs that will cross the placenta and potentially depress the neonate at birth. In contrast, during fetal surgery, anesthetics that cross the placenta are used when possible to provide fetal anesthesia and analgesia.

Maternal Physiology

Physiologic Changes during Pregnancy and Delivery

During pregnancy and the peripartum period, substantial changes in maternal anatomy and physiology occur secondary to changes in hormone activity, increased maternal metabolic demands, and biochemical alterations from the fetus and the mechanical effects of an enlarging uterus.

Cardiovascular Changes

Pregnancy-induced changes in the maternal cardiovascular system include increased blood volume and cardiac output, decreased vascular resistance, and supine hypotension.

Intravascular Volumes and Hematology

Maternal intravascular fluid volume begins to increase in the first trimester of pregnancy as the result of increased production of rennin, angiotensin, and aldosterone, which together promote sodium absorption and water retention. These changes are likely induced by progesterone.[83] With increases in plasma volume, there is an associated reduction in maternal plasma protein concentration. By term gestation, the plasma volume increases approximately 50%, and the red cell volume increases about 25%. The greater increase in plasma volume is the cause of the "physiologic anemia of pregnancy" (Fig. 45-1).[84] Because the increase in red cell mass lags behind the increase in plasma volume, hematocrit typically reaches a nadir in the second trimester and increases by term. Maternal hemoglobin normally remains at 11 g/dL or greater even at term, and lower values at any time during pregnancy represent anemia. The physiologic anemia of pregnancy does not cause a reduction in oxygen delivery because of a coincident increase in cardiac output. The additional intravascular fluid volume (1,000 to 1,500 mL at term) compensates for an average 300 to 500 mL blood loss with vaginal delivery and 800 to 1,000 mL estimated blood loss with cesarean section. Following delivery, uterine contraction creates an autotransfusion of blood often in excess of 500 mL that also compensates for the acute blood loss from delivery. Mild thrombocytopenia is a normal finding.[85] However, 8% of otherwise healthy women have thrombocytopenia

Table 45-1

Maternal and Fetal Drug Distribution

Drug	F/M Ratio	Reference(s)
Induction Agents		
Thiopental	0.43–1.1	1–4
Propofol	0.74–1.13	5–7
Ketamine	1.26	8–10
Etomidate	0.5	4, 11, 12
Neuromuscular Blocking Agents		
Succinylcholine	undetected[a]	13–15
Rocuronium	0.16	16, 17
Atracurium	0.12	18, 19
Pancuronium	0.19	20–22
Vecuronium	0.056–0.11	20, 23
Inhalation Agents		
Desflurane	NR	
Sevoflurane	0.15	24
Nitrous oxide	0.785–0.812	25–27
Isoflurane	0.71	28
Halothane	0.71–0.87	28, 29
Enflurane	0.6	30
Opioids		
Fentanyl	0.37	31
Sufentanil	0.4	32
Remifentanil	0.88	33
Alfentanil	0.28–0.31	34–36
Meperidine	0.35–1.5	37, 38
Morphine	0.61	39
Nalbuphine	0.69–0.75	40, 41
Local Anesthetics		
Lidocaine	0.76–0.9	42, 43
Bupivacaine	0.3–0.56	44–47
Ropivacaine	0.25	48–50
Mepivacaine	0.53	51
Chloroprocaine	NR	
Anticholinergic Agents		
Atropine	1.0	52
Glycopyrrolate	0.13	52
Scopolamine	1.0	53
Anticholinesterase Agents		
Neostigmine	NR	
Edrophonium	NR	
Vasoactive Agents		
Ephedrine	0.71	54, 55
Phenylephrine	0.17	55
Terbutaline	0.55	56
Benzodiazepines		
Diazepam	2.0	57, 58
Midazolam	0.15–0.28	2, 59
Lorazepam	1.0	60
Cardioactive Agents		
Propranolol	1.0	61
Propranolol (single dose)	0.26	62
Sotalol	1.1	63
Phenoxybenzamine	1.6	64
Labetalol	0.38	65
Hydralazine	0.72	66
Metoprolol	1.0	62
Atenolol	0.94	67
Esmolol	0.2	68
Methyldopa	1.17	69
Clonidine	1.04	70
Dexmedetomidine	0.88	70
Nitroglycerine	0.18	71
Nitroprusside	1.0	72, 73
Antiemetics		
Ondansetron	0.41	74
Metoclopramide	0.57	75
Dexamethasone	0.2	76
Oral Hypoglycemics		
Glyburide	<0.3	77–81
Metformin	0.3	82

F/M Ratio is the concentration of a drug in the fetal circulation as a ratio of the drug concentration in the maternal circulation. Values of less than 1 represent incomplete transfer and values greater than 1 represent accumulation of drug.

Notations in blue represent adaptations.

Adapted from Campbell D, San Vicente M. Placental transfer of drugs and perinatal pharmacology. In: Suresh M, Segal BS, Preston R, et al, eds. *Shnider and Levinson's Anesthesia for Obstetrics*. 5th ed. Philadelphia, PA: Lippincott Williams & Wilkins; 2013.

with a platelet count less than 150,000/mm^3. In the absence of other hematologic abnormalities, the cause for gestational thrombocytopenia is a diagnosis of exclusion. Platelet count does not usually drop below 70,000/mm^3 and is not associated with abnormal bleeding. Gestational thrombocytopenia is thought to result from a combination of hemodilution and accelerated platelet turnover.

Mild leukocytosis unrelated to infection is common during pregnancy.[86] In particular, the neutrophil count increases at term and is further increased during labor. These changes revert to normal during the week after delivery.

In spite of mild thrombocytopenia, pregnancy is a hypercoagulable state with important increases in fibrinogen

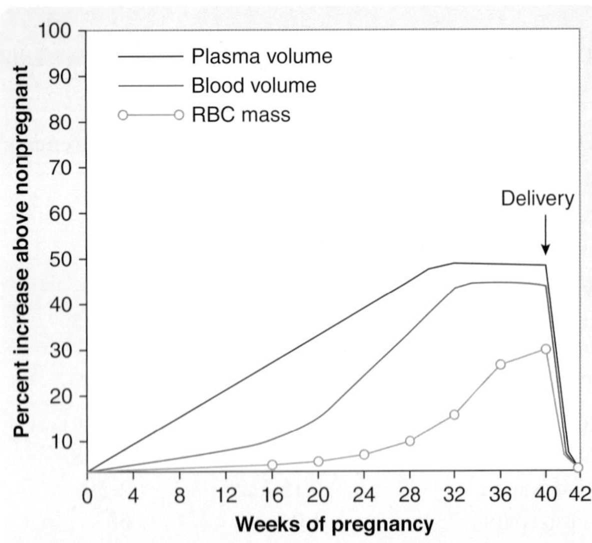

FIGURE 45-1 Blood volume changes during pregnancy. Plasma volume increases during pregnancy more rapidly than red cell mass leading to a physiologic anemia of pregnancy. (Modified from Scott D. Anemia during pregnancy. *Obstet Gynecol Ann.* 1972;1:219.)

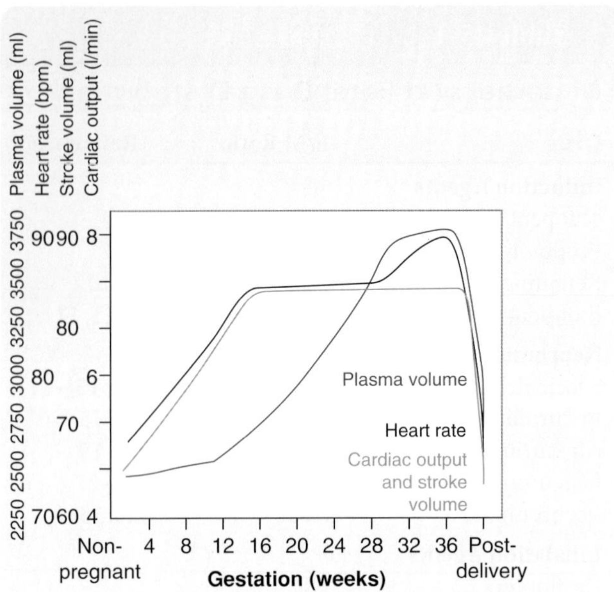

FIGURE 45-2 Maternal hemodynamic changes of pregnancy. Maternal heart rate and cardiac output increase early in the first trimester and plateau in the second trimester. There is an additional increase in heart rate during the third trimester. Plasma volume increases throughout the first and second trimester and reaches a plateau during the third trimester. All values drop rapidly in the days after delivery. (From Thorn SA. Pregnancy in heart disease. *Heart.* 2004;90:450–456.)

and factor VII.[85] Factor XI and XIII and antithrombin III are decreased and factors II and V typically remain unchanged. These changes result in an approximately 20% decrease in prothrombin time (PT) and partial thromboplastin time (PTT) during a normal pregnancy. One specific type of antithrombin III deficiency (homozygous type II antithrombin deficiency) is a relatively common, genetically determined form of this disorder that is exacerbated during pregnancy and may result in fetal loss, thrombosis, and pulmonary emboli.

Cardiac Output

By the end of the first trimester, maternal cardiac output increases, on average, by 35% above prepregnancy values and continues to increase to 50% above nonpregnant values by the end of the second trimester, remaining at similar, elevated levels throughout the third trimester. This increased cardiac output is the result of both increases in stroke volume and heart rate (Fig. 45-2).[87] Labor is associated with further increases in cardiac output, which increases with each uterine contraction. Increases above prelabor values of 10% to 25% are noted during the first stage of labor and a 40% increase occurs during the second stage. The largest increase in cardiac output occurs immediately after delivery, when cardiac output can be increased by 80% to 100% above prelabor values. This large increase is secondary to the autotransfusion from the final uterine contraction, reduced vascular capacitance from loss of the placenta, and decreased lower extremity venous pressure from release of the aortocaval compression. This massive increase in cardiac output represents a moment of unique risk for patients with cardiopulmonary disease, particularly those with valvular stenosis and pulmonary hypertension. Cardiac output returns toward pre-labor values by about 24 hours postpartum and returns to nonpregnant levels within 12 weeks after delivery. It is critical to monitor patients with cardiac disease closely in the postpartum period.

Systemic Vascular Resistance

In spite of increases in cardiac output and plasma volume, systemic blood pressure normally decreases secondary to a 20% reduction in systemic vascular resistance by term. Blood pressure decreases approximately 20% by 20 weeks gestational age and then increases toward nonpregnant values as the pregnancy reaches term. Central venous pressure and pulmonary capillary wedge pressure are unchanged during normal pregnancy despite the increase in plasma volume because of the concurrent increase in venous capacitance.

Aortocaval Compression

In the supine position, blood pressure commonly decreases as the result of aortocaval compression by the gravid uterus. Supine hypotension is manifest by symptoms of diaphoresis, nausea, vomiting, and dizziness. At term, there is almost complete occlusion of the inferior vena cava in the supine position, with return of blood from the lower extremities through the epidural, azygos, and vertebral veins. Vena caval compression may exacerbate lower extremity venous stasis and thereby result in ankle edema, varices, and the risk of venous thromboembolism.

Compensatory adaptations mitigate supine hypotension due to aortocaval compression. One example is a reflexive increase in peripheral sympathetic nervous system activity. This enhanced sympathetic activity increases systemic vascular resistance and maintains systemic blood pressure in spite of reduced cardiac output. Reduced sympathetic tone resulting from neuraxial or general anesthesia will impair this compensatory response and worsen the hypotensive response to supine positioning. A lateral tilt is used to avoid the hypotension that can be associated with supine positioning with neuraxial techniques for labor analgesia and operative deliveries.

The earlier described cardiovascular changes of a pregnancy produce significant changes in the normal cardiac exam. Auscultation reveals an accentuated first heart sound (S1) with an increased splitting of the first heart sound caused by dissociated closure of the tricuspid and mitral valves. A third heart sound (S3) is often heard in the final trimester and a fourth heart sound (S4) can also be heard in a minority of pregnant patients as a result of increased volume and turbulent flow. A mild systolic ejection (grade 2/6) murmur is commonly noted over the left sternal border and is secondary to mild regurgitation at the tricuspid valve from increased cardiac volume.

Pulmonary Changes

Pregnancy results in significant alterations in the upper airway, lung volumes, minute ventilation, oxygen consumption, and metabolic rate.

Airway

During pregnancy, there is vascular engorgement with friability and edema of the mucosal lining of the oro- and nasopharynx. As a result, there is danger of bleeding with instrumentation of the airway and increased risk of difficult ventilation and intubation. Attempts at laryngoscopy should be minimized and a smaller size cuffed endotracheal tube (6.0- to 6.5-mm internal diameter) should be considered to avoid airway edema and bleeding. Airway edema can be particularly problematic in the setting of preeclampsia, upper respiratory tract infections, and after prolonged pushing due to the associated increases in venous pressure. In addition, pregnancy-associated weight gain, particularly in women of short stature or with preexisting obesity, can exacerbate difficult laryngoscopy because of a shorter neck and heavy breast tissue. The patient's position should be optimized and all necessary equipment for airway management should be available before attempts are made at intubation.

Minute Ventilation and Oxygenation

In order to accommodate the increased oxygen demand and carbon dioxide production of the growing placenta and fetus, minute ventilation is increased 45% to 50% above nonpregnant values during the first trimester and remains at this increased level for the remainder of the pregnancy. This greater minute ventilation is attained primarily as a result of a greater tidal volume with a small increase in the respiratory rate (Fig. 45-3).[88] Maternal $Paco_2$ is commonly reduced from 40 mm Hg to approximately

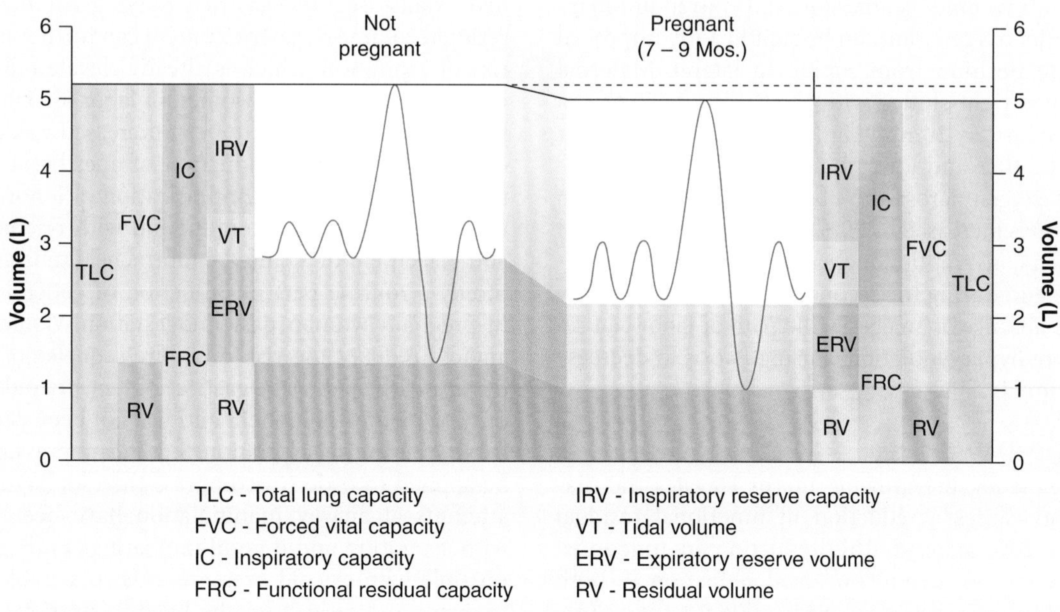

FIGURE 45-3 Changes in maternal pulmonary function. Functional residual capacity (FRV) is reduced by virtue of reductions in expiratory reserve volume (ERV) and residual volume (RV) during pregnancy. Inspiratory capacity (IC) is increased resulting from an increase in tidal volume (VT). (From Hegewald MJ, Crapo RO. Respiratory physiology in pregnancy. *Clin Chest Med.* 2011;32[1]:1–13.)

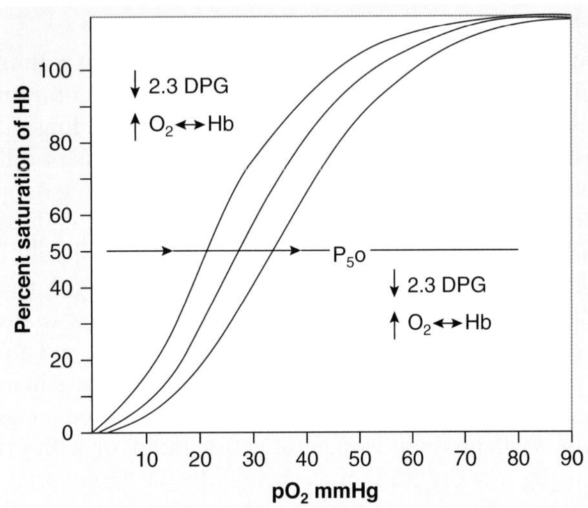

FIGURE 45-4 Right shift of maternal hemoglobin oxygen dissociation curve. Increased interaction with 2,3-DPG results in hemoglobin with lower oxygen affinity and a right shift in the hemoglobin oxygen saturation curve. As a result, oxygen is more easily off-loaded to fetal hemoglobin, which has a left-shifted hemoglobin oxygen dissociation curve. (From Jepson JH. Factors influencing oxygenation in mother and fetus. *Obstet Gynecol.* 1974;44[6]:906–914.)

30 mm Hg during the first trimester. Arterial pH, however, is only slightly increased (pH 7.42 to 7.44) because of metabolic compensation from increased renal excretion of bicarbonate (HCO_3^- is typically 20 or 21 mEq/L at term). During the first trimester, maternal Pao_2 may be above 100 mm Hg due to hyperventilation and decreased alveolar CO_2. Later, Pao_2 becomes normal or even slightly decreased, most likely reflecting small airway closure with normal tidal volume ventilation and intrapulmonary shunt. Arterial oxygenation can be significantly improved by changing position from supine to lateral. Maternal hemoglobin is right-shifted with the P_{50} increasing from 27 to approximately 30 mm Hg (Fig. 45-4).[89] The higher P_{50} in the mother and lower P_{50} in the fetus favors off-loading of oxygen across the placenta. At term, oxygen consumption is increased by 20%. During the first stage of labor, oxygen consumption increases above pre-labor values by 40% and during the second stage it is increased by 75%. In the absence of analgesia, the pain of labor can result in severe hyperventilation causing $Paco_2$ to decrease below 20 mm Hg.

Lung Volumes

During pregnancy, the growing uterus elevates the diaphragm and causes a reduction in functional residual capacity by 20% at term. This reduction in functional residual capacity is a result of equal reduction in both the expiratory reserve volume and residual volume (see Fig. 45-3). The closing capacity remains unchanged. The reduced ratio of functional residual capacity to closing capacity favors small airway closure with reduced lung volumes and in the supine position causing atelectasis. Vital capacity is not significantly changed with pregnancy.

The combination of increased minute ventilation and decreased functional residual capacity results in a greater rate at which changes in the alveolar concentration of inhaled anesthetics can be achieved with spontaneous ventilation in the case of mask induction.

During induction of general anesthesia in a pregnant patient, desaturation occurs more rapidly than in a nonpregnant patient because of decreased functional residual capacity and increased metabolic rate. Administration of 100% oxygen prior to the induction of general anesthesia is critical to allow as much time as possible for safe airway management. Inhalation of 100% oxygen for 3 minutes or, in an emergency, 4 maximal breaths over the 30 seconds will significantly prolong the period between apnea and arterial oxygen desaturation.

Gastrointestinal Changes

After midgestation, pregnant women are thought to be at increased risk of aspiration pneumonia with administration of general anesthesia. This increased risk is caused by several factors. There is upward movement of the esophageal sphincter by the gravid uterus. Increased progesterone and estrogen concentrations during pregnancy also contribute to reduced esophageal sphincter tone. Gastrin is secreted by the placenta which increases gastric acid secretion. Together, these changes result in an increased incidence of gastroesophageal reflux during pregnancy. Gastric emptying is not changed during pregnancy before the onset of labor in women who are of normal weight or obese.[90,91] However, during labor, pain, anxiety, and the administration of opioids (including those administered neuraxially) decrease gastric emptying. An increase in the residual volume of gastric content can further increase the risk of aspiration, which is already elevated during pregnancy.[92] As a result, all women in labor are considered to have full stomachs and to be at increased risk for pulmonary aspiration with induction of anesthesia. To reduce the risk of aspiration, administration of a nonparticulate antacid, rapid sequence induction with cricoid pressure, and placement of a cuffed endotracheal tube are all commonly a routine part of induction of general anesthesia in pregnant woman past midgestation. While use of an antacid reduces the risk of severe sequelae of aspiration by raising the pH of the gastric content, cricoid pressure is only of theoretical benefit and has not been proven effective in preventing aspiration. Significant pressure needs to be applied in order to compress the esophagus. Multiple attempts at airway manipulation have been associated with aspiration and if good intubating conditions are not possible with cricoid pressure, it is reasonable to release pressure and reposition the head to improve intubating conditions prior to additional attempts at intubation.

While blood flow to the liver does not change during pregnancy, markers of liver function including aspartate aminotransferase (AST), alanine aminotransferase (ALT), and bilirubin all increase to the upper limits of normal.

Alkaline phosphatase levels more than double secondary to placental production of this enzyme. Hemodilution during pregnancy is responsible for lower plasma protein concentrations. Lower serum albumin concentrations can result in elevated free blood levels of highly protein-bound drugs. Plasma cholinesterase (pseudocholinesterase) activity is decreased about 30% from the 10th week of gestation up to 6 weeks postpartum, but this decreased cholinesterase activity is not associated with clinically relevant prolongation of neuromuscular blockade from succinylcholine or mivacurium in patients with normal baseline levels of the enzyme. Gallbladder disease is common during pregnancy due to incomplete gallbladder emptying and changes in bile composition.

Renal Changes

Renal blood flow and the glomerular filtration rate are increased 50% by the second trimester and remain elevated until 3 months postpartum. As a result, clearance of creatinine, urea, and uric acid are increased during pregnancy. Increased urine protein and glucose result from decreased renal tubular resorption capacity. The upper limit of the normal 24-hour urine elimination during pregnancy is 300 mg of protein and 10 g glucose.

Neurologic Changes

Pregnant patients are more sensitive to both inhaled and local anesthetic agents. MAC is reduced by 30% by the first trimester of pregnancy. MAC or immobility in response to volatile anesthetics occurs at the level of the spinal cord. A recent electroencephalographic study suggests that anesthetic effects of sevoflurane on the brain are similar in the pregnant and nonpregnant state.[93] Fortunately, anesthetic concentrations required for hypnosis and amnesia are approximately half of MAC or the concentration required to prevent activation of spinal reflexes. Unanticipated awareness is more common during cesarean section. The reasons are likely multifactorial. There is often a desire to prevent anesthetic exposure to an already depressed fetus and the requirement for rapid surgery to allow for neonatal resuscitation may not allow the anesthetic to come to steady state before surgery begins.

Pregnant women are more sensitive to the local anesthetics and a lower dose is able to obtain the same level of either spinal or epidural neuraxial blockade compared to nonpregnant women. At term, distention of epidural veins decreases the size of the epidural space, and volume of cerebrospinal fluid (CSF) in the subarachnoid space. CSF pressure is not increased during the course of pregnancy until labor, when it is increased both during uterine contractions and expulsion of the fetus. Although the decreased volume of these spaces may facilitate spread of local anesthetics, the decreased local anesthetic required during pregnancy occurs as early as the first trimester, before mechanical or pressure related changes occur. As such, hormonal changes likely play a role in causing increased nerve sensitivity to local anesthetics.

Uteroplacental Physiology

The placenta is composed of both maternal and fetal tissues and is the interface of maternal and fetal circulation systems. It provides a substrate for physiologic exchange between mother and fetus without immunologic rejection. Maternal blood is delivered to the placenta by the uterine arteries and enters the intervillous space via the spiral arteries. The deoxygenated fetal blood arrives at the placenta via two umbilical arteries that form umbilical capillaries that cross the chorionic villi. Following placental exchange, oxygenated, nutrient-rich and waste-free blood is returned from the placenta to the fetus through a single umbilical vein (Fig. 45-5).

Uterine Blood Flow

An understanding of uteroplacental blood flow is important for the anesthesiologist caring for a pregnant patient. Uterine blood flow increases progressively during pregnancy from about 100 mL per minute in the nonpregnant state to 700 mL per minute (about 10% of cardiac output) at term gestation. Uterine blood flow has minimal autoregulation and the vasculature remains essentially fully dilated during normal pregnancy. Uterine and placental blood flows are dependent on maternal cardiac output and are directly related to uterine perfusion pressure. Decreased perfusion pressure can result from maternal hypotension secondary to hypovolemia, aortocaval compression, or decreased systemic resistance from either general or neuraxial anesthesia. Increased uterine venous pressure can also decrease uterine perfusion. This can occur from supine positioning with vena caval compression, frequent or prolonged uterine contractions, or significant prolonged abdominal musculature contraction (Valsalva) during pushing. Additionally, extreme hypocapnia ($Paco_2$ <20 mm Hg) associated with hyperventilation secondary to labor pain can reduce uterine blood flow with resultant fetal hypoxemia and acidosis. Neuraxial blockade does not alter uterine blood flow as long as maternal hypotension does not occur.

Endogenous maternal catecholamines and exogenous vasopressors may cause an increase in uterine arterial resistance and a decrease in uterine blood flow, depending on the type and dose given. In early studies in pregnant ewes, ephedrine was found to have no effect on uterine blood flow despite drug-induced increases in maternal arterial blood pressure, whereas other vasopressors including phenylephrine resulted in vasoconstriction and fetal acidosis.[94,95] From this animal data, ephedrine was long considered the vasopressor of choice for the treatment of hypotension caused by the administration of neuraxial anesthesia to pregnant women. In complete contrast, however, clinical trials demonstrate the use of phenylephrine is not only effective in preventing hypotension but is associated

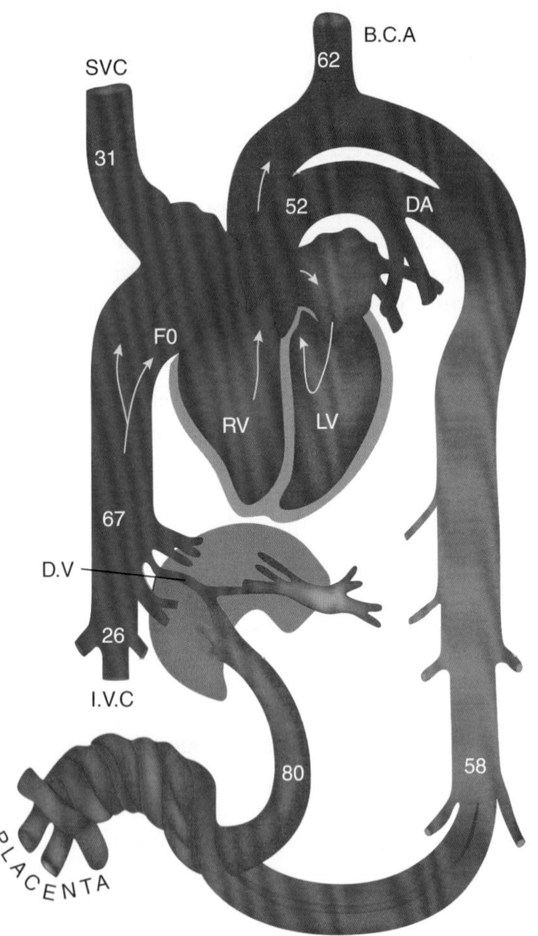

FIGURE 45-5 Diagram of the fetal circulation. Oxygenated blood flows in through the umbilical vein. It passes through the ductus venosus (DV) where it is diluted by deoxygenated blood returning from the inferior vena cava (IVC). Oxygenated blood passes to the right atrium, where little passes through the fetal lungs because of high pulmonary vascular resistance. Part of the circulation passes through the foramen ovale (FO) directly to the left atrium to enter the fetal systemic circulation. Another portion bypasses the lungs by passing from the pulmonary artery through the ductus arteriosus (DA) where it proceeds directly to the aorta. The numbers represent oxygen saturation at various points in the fetal circulation. BCA, brachial cephalic artery; SVC, superior vena cava. (Modified from Meschia G. Fetal oxygenation and maternal ventilation. *Clin Chest Med.* 2011;32[1]:15–19.)

with less fetal acidosis and base deficit than the use of ephedrine.[96,97] Thus, many clinicians have now switched from ephedrine to phenylephrine as the vasopressor of first choice for treating hypotension during labor and delivery.

Oxygen Transfer

The delivery of oxygen from the mother to the fetus is dependent on a variety of factors including placental blood flow, the oxygen partial pressure gradient between the two circulations, the diffusion capacity of the placenta, the respective maternal and fetal hemoglobin concentrations and oxygen affinities, and the acid–base status of the fetal and maternal blood (Bohr effect). The fetal oxyhemoglobin dissociation curve is left-shifted (P_{50} = 19 mm Hg, greater oxygen affinity), whereas the maternal oxyhemoglobin dissociation curve is right-shifted (P_{50} = 27 mm Hg, less oxygen affinity). This occurs because fetal hemoglobin does not interact with 2,3-disphosphoglycerate (2,3-DPG), facilitating oxygen transfer to the fetus (see Fig. 45-4). Fetal Pao_2 is normally 40 mm Hg and does not exceed 60 mm Hg even if the mother is breathing 100% oxygen. This is because significant oxygen has been extracted by the mother's tissues prior to arrival at the feto-placental unit. Carbon dioxide easily crosses the placenta and is limited by blood flow and not diffusion.

Fetal Heart Rate Monitoring

After 18 weeks, fetal heart rate monitoring is practical, and after 25 weeks, variability in fetal heart rate is a reliable sign of well-being. The American College of Obstetrics and Gynecology states, "although there are no data to support specific recommendations regarding non-obstetric surgery and anesthesia in pregnancy, it is important for non-obstetric physicians to obtain obstetric consultation before performing non-obstetric surgery. The decision to use fetal monitoring should be individualized and each case warrants a team approach for optimal safety of the woman and her baby."[98] Under general anesthesia and with the use of opioids and maternal cooling, the loss of fetal heart rate variability may not be indicative of fetal acidemia but may be a result of anesthetic alteration of autonomic tone. Fetal bradycardia is more concerning but can also be affected by hypothermia, maternal acidosis, or the maternal administration of drugs such as β blockers that cross the placenta and reduce fetal heart rate.

Pain Management

When nonobstetric surgery is conducted under regional anesthesia, effective analgesia can be provided by administering a long-acting narcotic neuraxially or by continuation of an epidural infusion postoperatively. Systemic opioids including those used in patient-controlled intravenous analgesia cross the placenta and may reduce fetal heart rate variability. However, there is no evidence that this is detrimental to the fetus. If the fetus is born prematurely shortly after exposure to maternal systemic opioids, reversal with naloxone and/or respiratory support may be necessary. Maternal pain control after nonobstetric surgery is of paramount importance to maternal and fetal well-being. Nonsteroidal antiinflammatory drugs, although useful adjuvant analgesics outside of pregnancy, should be used with caution in pregnancy. They are associated with an increased risk of miscarriage and fetal malformation when used in early pregnancy and premature closure of the ductus arteriosus and oligohydramnios when used after 30 weeks' gestation. Acetaminophen is generally accepted as safe in pregnancy.

Following surgery, both the fetal heart rate and uterine activity should be evaluated. Preterm labor can be managed with appropriate tocolytic drugs. Postoperative pain medications may make it difficult for the patient to note early contractions and patient perception should not be considered a substitute for standard monitoring. In addition, venous thrombosis prophylaxis should be instituted unless surgically contraindicated.

Fetal Physiology

Characteristics of the Fetal Circulation

Approximately two-thirds of the fetal-placental blood volume is contained within the placenta. The fetal blood volume increases throughout gestation. During the second and third trimester, the fetal blood volume has been estimated to be approximately 120 to 160 mL/kg of fetal body weight.

The fetal blood passes from the placenta through the umbilical vein (see Fig. 45-5).[99] Approximately one-third of the blood volume passes through the ductus venosus to the inferior vena cava. The rest of the blood volume passes to the fetal liver, joins the portal vein, and passes to the right atrium. As a result, drugs and toxic substances are detoxified by the fetal liver prior to exposure to the fetal brain and heart. The fetal circulation is characterized by high pulmonary vascular resistance, low systemic vascular resistance (including the placenta), and right-to-left cardiac shunting via the foramen ovale and ductus arteriosus. As such, the majority of the blood bypasses the fetal lungs. The blood is pumped from the fetal left ventricle through the body to the internal iliac arteries where it passes through the umbilical arteries back to the placenta to be detoxified and reoxygenated.

Drug Transfer

Maternal-fetal exchange of most drugs and other substances with molecular weights of less than 1,000 Daltons occurs primarily by diffusion. The rate of diffusion and peak levels in the fetus depend on maternal-to-fetal concentration gradients, maternal protein binding, molecular weight of the substance, lipid solubility, and the degree of ionization of that substance. The maternal blood concentration of a drug is normally the primary determinant of how much drug will ultimately reach the fetus. The high molecular weight and poor lipid solubility of nondepolarizing neuromuscular blocking drugs result in minimal transfer of these drugs across the placenta.[16–23] Succinylcholine has a low molecular weight but is highly ionized and therefore does not readily cross the placenta unless given in very large doses.[13–15] Thus, during administration of a general anesthetic for cesarean delivery, the fetus/neonate is not paralyzed. If paralysis is desired, for example, during fetal surgery, muscle relaxants must be injected directly into the umbilical vein. Both heparin and glycopyrrolate have minimal placental transfer because they are highly charged.[52] Placental transfer of volatile agents,[24–30] benzodiazapines,[2,57–60] local anesthetics,[42–51] and opioids[31–41] is facilitated by the relatively low molecular weights, neutral charge and relative lipophilicity of these drugs.

Fetal blood is more acidic than maternal and the lower pH creates an environment where weakly basic drugs such as local anesthetics can cross the placenta as a nonionized molecule and become ionized in the fetal circulation. Because the newly ionized molecule has more resistance to diffusion back across the placenta, the drug can accumulate in the fetal circulation and reach levels higher than the maternal blood. This process is named "ion trapping." During fetal distress (lower pH in the fetal circulation), higher concentrations of weakly basic drugs, such as local anesthetics, can be trapped. High concentrations of local anesthetics in the fetal circulation decrease neonatal neuromuscular tone. Extremely high levels such as those associated with unintended maternal intravascular local anesthetic injection result in a variety of fetal effects that include bradycardia, ventricular arrhythmias, acidosis, and severe cardiac depression.

Fetal Liver Function and Drug Metabolism

Although fetal liver function is not yet mature, coagulation factors are synthesized independent of the maternal circulation. These factors do not cross the placenta and their serum concentrations increase with gestational age. However, fetal clot formation in response to tissue injury is less robust in comparison to adults. The anatomy of the fetal circulation helps to decrease fetal exposure to potentially high concentrations of drugs in umbilical venous blood. Approximately 75% of umbilical venous blood initially passes through the fetal liver, which may result in significant drug metabolism by the fetal liver before the drug reaches the fetal heart and brain (first-pass metabolism). Fetal/neonatal enzyme activities are less developed than those of adults, but most drugs that cross the placenta can be metabolized. In addition, drugs entering the fetal inferior vena cava via the ductus venosus are initially diluted by drug-free blood returning from the fetal lower extremities and pelvic viscera of the fetus. These anatomic characteristics of the fetal circulation markedly decrease fetal plasma drug concentrations compared to maternal concentrations.

Anesthetic Toxicity in the Fetus

All general anesthetic drugs cross the placenta. While there is no clear evidence for toxicity of specific anesthetic drugs in humans, there is concerning animal data in rodents and primates that suggest that prolonged exposure to general anesthetic drugs including inhaled anesthetics,[100] propofol,[101] and ketamine[102] may induce inappropriate neuronal apoptosis that is associated with long lasting behavioral abnormalities. Although these preclinical results are concerning, it is not clear whether or when these drugs might cause toxicity in humans. The critical period of rapid synaptic development is extended in humans from the prenatal period through 2 years of postnatal life. Analyses of existing human data have yielded conflicting results. In population-based cohorts evaluating the effect of general anesthesia before birth, there was a suggestion that multiple exposures increase the risk for learning disability.[103] The results of these types of studies are difficult to interpret because the reason for the anesthesia cannot be separated for the impact of the anesthesia itself. Also, the timing, type, and duration of anesthesia were not considered. Changes in practice have not been recommended in the absence of any anesthetic regimen that has been proven to provide more safety than others.

Studies have found an excess of birth defects in women who underwent general anesthesia during pregnancy but most have found a small increase in the risk of preterm delivery or miscarriage during the first trimester. In general, the second trimester is preferred for surgical intervention as this is a period after much organogenesis has taken place and yet minimizes the risk of preterm labor associated with the third trimester. Monitoring for contractions is recommended and in some situations suppression with magnesium is recommended after surgery. As the long-term impact of general anesthesia on the fetus is unknown, regional anesthesia is favored when possible for the surgical procedure but should not be undertaken unless both the anesthesiologist and surgeon are experienced in using the technique for a given procedure.

Fetal Neurophysiology

Fetal Pain

The gestational age at which the fetus can feel pain is highly controversial. The experience of pain requires two conditions: (a) nociception and (b) perception with emotional response. Afferent sensory fibers required for nociception are in place and a functional spinal reflex is present by 20 weeks' gestation (Fig. 45-6).[104] The second

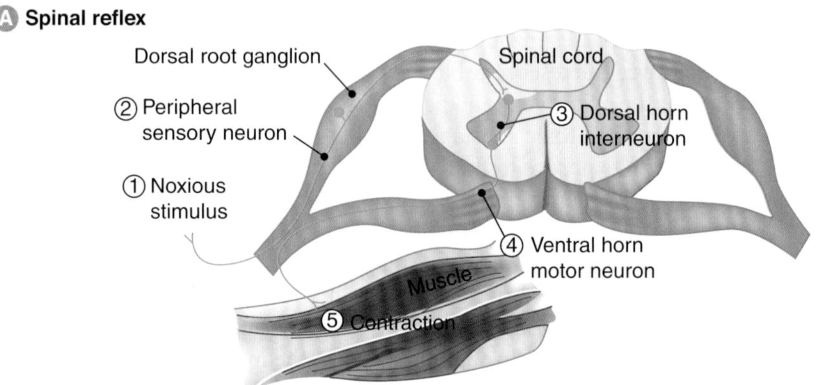

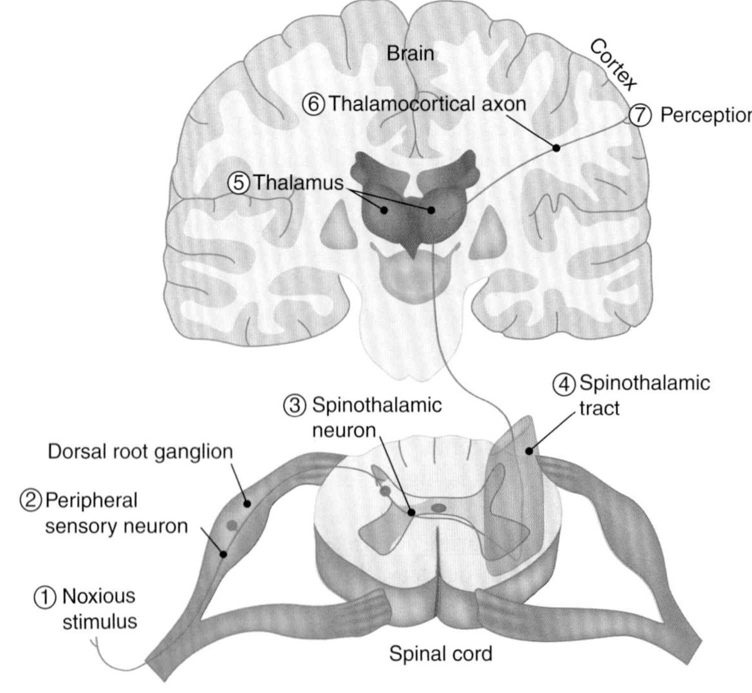

FIGURE 45-6 Spinal reflex and pain perception pathways. **A.** Spinal reflex responses to noxious stimuli occur early in fetal development before cortical connections are functional. **B.** Later in fetal development, a noxious stimulus will activate a peripheral sensory neuron that projects to neurons that form the spinothalamic tract. These neurons in turn project to neurons in the thalamus. Thalamic neurons project to neurons in the subplate zone and the somatosensory cortex. This sequence is the anatomic basis for nociception, the sequence of neuronal events that lead to the conscious perception of pain. The functional circuitry required for apprehension of pain is likely to be present between 20 and 30 weeks' gestation. (Modified from Lowery CL, Hardman MP, Manning N, et al. Neurodevelopmental changes in fetal pain. *Semin Perinatol.* 2007;31:275–282.)

requirement for the experience of pain, perception with emotional response, is much more difficult to establish. In the verbal patient, pain is established by self-report. In the nonverbal, it is measured with observation of complex behaviors thought to be representative of emotional response such as grimace. Neither measurement is practical or necessarily representative in the fetus because of coincident development of motor and intermediary circuitry.

In humans, after about 2 to 3 months of age, pain can be both apprehended and comprehended. Comprehension requires a relationship with the object. The fetus can likely not comprehend, but only apprehend. Consciousness requires certain anatomic structures to be in place and functional. The neural circuitry that is required for apprehension includes thalamocortical pathways (see Fig. 45-6). The subplate zone contains the earliest cortical cells and is partially a transient compartment that is required for normal cortical maturation. There is thalamic fiber penetration of an outer layer of brain cells which stimulate development of the subplate zone by 11 weeks' gestation. Most nociceptive pathways connect from the thalamus to the subplate zone by gestational week 17.[105] Maturation of the primary somatosensory cortex continues into neonatal life. Evidence for the functionality required for consciousness, thought to be represented by certain EEG rhythms that are mediated by subcortical integration of cortical and subcortical processes are present from 20 weeks' gestation.[106] Somatosensory evoked potentials can be recorded from the fetal cerebral cortex at 29 weeks' gestation.[107] As such, the functional circuitry required for apprehension of pain is likely to be present between 20 and 30 weeks' gestation. These details are of concern to the anesthesiologist to inform decisions about anesthesia for fetal surgery and whether and at what point a live fetus requires anesthesia and analgesia prior to abortion.

References

1. Finster M, Perel JM, Papper EM. Uptake of thiopental by fetal tissue and the placenta. *Fed Proc.* 1968;27:706.
2. Bach V, Carl P, Ravlo O, et al. A randomized comparison between midazolam and thiopental for elective cesarean section anesthesia: III placental transfer and elimination in neonates. *Anesth Analg.* 1989;68:238–242.
3. Gaspari F, Marraro G, Penna GF, et al. Elimination kinetics of thiopentone in mothers and their newborn infants. *Eur J Clin Pharmacol.* 1985;28:321–325.
4. Downing JW, Buley RJR, Brock-Utne JG, et al. Etomidate for induction of anaesthesia at caesarean section: comparison with thiopentone. *Br J Anaesth.* 1979;51:135–140.
5. He Y, Tsujimoto S, Tanimoto M, et al. Effects of protein binding on the placental transfer of propofol in the human dually-perfused cotyledon. *Br J Anaesth.* 2000;85:281–286.
6. He Y, Seno H, Tsujimoto S, et al. The effects of uterine and umbilical blood flows on the transfer of propofol across the human placenta during in vitro perfusion. *Anesth Analg.* 2001;93:151–156.
7. Sanchez-Alcaraz A, Quintana MB, Laguarda M, et al. Placental transfer and neonatal effects of propofol in caesarean section. *J Clin Pharm Ther.* 1998;23:19–23.
8. Ellingson A, Haram K, Sagen N, et al. Transplacental passage of ketamine after intravenous administration. *Acta Anaesth Scand.* 1977;21:41–44.
9. Maduska AL, Hajghassemali M. Arterial blood gases in mother and infants during ketamine anesthesia for vaginal delivery. *Anesth Analg.* 1978;57:121–123.
10. Houlton PC, Downing JW, Buley RJ, et al. Anaestheic induction of caesarean section with thiopentone, methohexitone and ketamine. *S Afr Med J.* 1978;54(20):818–820.
11. Gregory MA, Davidson DG. Plasma etomidate levels in mother and fetus. *Anaesthesia.* 1991;46:716–718.
12. Fresno L, Andaluz A, Moll X, et al. Placental transfer of etomidate in pregnant ewes after an intravenous bolus dose and continuous infusion. *Vet J.* 2008;175:395–402.
13. Moya F, Kvisselgaard N. The placental transmission of succinylcholine. *Anesthesiology.* 1961;22:1–6.
14. Kvisselgaard N, Moya F. Investigation of placental thresholds to succinylcholine. *Anesthesiology.* 1961;22:7–10.
15. Drabkova C, Van Der Kleijn E. Placental transfer of C14 labeled succinylcholine in near term macaca mulatta monkeys. *Br J Anesth.* 1973;45:1087–1096.
16. Abouleish E, Abboud T, Lechevalier T, et al. Rocuronium for caesarean section. *Br J Anaesth.* 1994;73:336–341.
17. Baraka AS, Sayyid SS, Assaf BA. Thiopental-rocuronium versus ketamine–rocuronium for rapid-sequence intubation in parturients undergoing cesarean section. *Anesth Analg.* 1997;84:1104–1107.
18. Flynn P, Frank M, Hughes R. Use of atracurium in cesarean section. *Br J Anaesth.* 1984;56:599–605.
19. Shearer ES, Fahy LT, O'Sullivan EP, et al. Transplacental distribution of atracurium, laudanosine and monoquaternary alcohol during elective caesarean section. *Br J Anaesth.* 1991;66:551–556.
20. Dailey P, Fisher D, Shnider S, et al. Pharmacokinetics, placental transfer, and neonatal effects of vecuronium and pancuronium administered during cesarean section. *Anesthesiology.* 1984;60:569–574.
21. Duvaldestin P, Demetriou M, Henzel D, et al. The placental transfer of pan-curonium and its pharmacokinetics during caesarean section. *Acta Anaesthesiol Scand.* 1978;22:327–333.
22. Abouleish E, Wingard LB Jr, de la Vega S, et al. Pancuronium in caesarean section and its placental transfer. *Br J Anaesth.* 1980;52: 531–536.
23. Iwama H, Kaneko T, Tobishima S, et al. Time dependency of the ratio of umbilical vein/maternal artery concentrations of vecuronium in caesarean section. *Acta Anaesthesiol Scand.* 1999:43:9–12.
24. Ueki R, Tatara T, Kariya N, et al. Effect of decreased fetal perfusion on placental clearance of volatile anesthetics in a dual perfused human placental cotyledon model [ahead of print January 3, 2014]. *J Anesth.*
25. Marx GF, Joshi CW, Orkin LR. Placental transmission of nitrous oxide. *Anesthesiology.* 1970;32:429–432.
26. Polvi HJ, Pirhonen JP, Erkkola RU. Nitrous oxide inhalation: Effects on maternal and fetal circulations at term. *Obstet Gynecol.* 1996;87:1045–1048.
27. Mankowitz E, Brock-Utne JG, Downing JW. Nitrous oxide elimination by the newborn. *Anaesthesia.* 1981;36:1014–1016.
28. Dwyer R, Fee JPH, Moore J. Uptake of halothane and isoflurane by mother and baby during caesarean section. *Br J Anaesth.* 1995;74:379–383.
29. Kangas L, Erkkola R, Kanto J, et al. Halothane anaesthesia in caesarean section. *Acta Anaesthesiol Scand.* 1976;20:189–194.
30. Dick W, Knoche E, Traub E. Clinical investigations concerning the use of Ethrane for cesarean section. *J Perinat Med.* 1979;7: 125–133.
31. Loftus JR, Hill H, Cohen SE. Placental transfer and neonatal effects of epidural sufentanil and fentanyl administered with bupivacaine during labor. *Anesthesiology.* 1995;83:300–308.
32. Johnson RF, Herman N, Arney T, et al. The placental transfer of sufentanil: effects of fetal pH, protein binding, and sufentanil concentration. *Anesth Analg.* 1997;84:1262–1268.

33. Kan R, Hughes S, Rosen M, et al. Intravenous remifentanil: placental transfer, maternal and neonatal effects. *Anesthesiology*. 1998;88:467–474.
34. Gepts E, Heytens L, Camu F. Pharmacokinetics and placental transfer of intravenous and epidural alfentanil in parturient women. *Anesth Analg*. 1986;65:1155–1160.
35. Zakowski MI, Ham AA, Grant GJ. Transfer and uptake of alfentanil in the human placenta during in vitro perfusion. *Anesth Analg*. 1994;79:1089–1093.
36. Cartwright DP, Dann WL, Hutchinson A. Placental transfer of alfentanil at caesarean section. *Eur J Anaesthesiol*. 1989;6:103–109.
37. Wilson CM, McClean E, Moore J, et al. A double-blind comparison of intramuscular pethidine and nalbuphine in labour. *Anaesthesia*. 1986;41(12):1207–1213.
38. Tomson G, Garle R, Thalme B, et al. Maternal kinetics and transplacental passage of pethidine during labour. *Br J Clin Pharmac*. 1982;13:653–659.
39. Kopecky E, Ryan ML, Barrett J, et al. Fetal response to maternally administered morphine. *Am J Obstet Gynecol*. 2000;183:424–430.
40. Nicolle E, Devillier P, Delanoy B, et al. Therapeutic monitoring of nalbuphine: transplacental transfer and estimated pharmacokinetics in the neonate. *Eur J Clin Pharmacol*. 1996;49:485–489.
41. Wilson SJ, Errick JK, Balkon J. Pharmacokinetics of nalbuphine during parturition. *Am J Obstet Gynecol*. 1986;155:340–345.
42. Biehl D, Shnider S, Levinson G, et al. Placental transfer of lidocaine: effects of fetal acidosis. *Anesthesiology*. 1978;48:409–412.
43. Morishima H, Santos A, Pedersen H, et al. Effect of lidocaine on the asphyxial responses in the mature fetal lamb. *Anesthesiology*. 1987;66:502–507.
44. Reynolds F. Placental transfer of drugs. *Curr Anaesth Crit Care*. 1991;2:108–116.
45. Johnson R, Herman N, Arney T, et al. Bupivacaine transfer across the human term placenta. *Anesthesiology*. 1995;82:459–468.
46. Reynolds F, Laishley R, Morgan B, et al. The effect of time and adrenaline on the transplacental distribution of bupivacaine. *Br J Anaesth*. 1989;62:509–514.
47. Laishley R, Carson R, Reynolds F. Effect of adrenaline on placental transfer of bupivacaine in the perfused in situ rabbit placenta. *Br J Anaesth*. 1989;63:439–443.
48. Ueki R, Tatara T, Kariya N, et al. Comparison of placental transfer of local anesthetics in perfusates with different pH values in a human cotyledon model. *J Anesth*. 2009;23:526–529.
49. Reiz S, Haggmark G, Johansson G, et al. Cardiotoxicity of ropivacaine—a new amide local anaesthetic agent. *Acta Anaesthesiol Scand*. 1989;33:93–98.
50. Porter JM, Kelleher N, Flynn R, et al. Epidural ropivacaine hydrochloride during labour: protein binding, placental transfer and neonatal outcome. *Anaesthesia*. 2001;56:418–423.
51. Bremerich DH, Schlosser RL, L'Allemand N, et al. Mepivacaine for spinal anesthesia in parturients undergoing elective cesarean and neonatal plasma concentrations and neonatal outcome. *Zentralbl Gynakol*. 2003;125:518–521.
52. Murad S, Conklin K, Tabsh K, et al. Atropine and glycopyrrolate. Hemodynamic effects and placental transfer in the pregnant ewe. *Anesth Analg*. 1981;60:710–714.
53. Kanto J, Kentala E, Kaila T, et al. Pharmacokinetics of scopolamine during caesarean section: relationship between serum concentration and effect. *Acta Anaesthesiol Scand*. 1989;33:482–486.
54. Hughes S, Ward M, Levinson G, et al. Placental transfer of ephedrine does not affect neonatal outcome. *Anesthesiology*. 1985;63:217–219.
55. Ngan Kee WD, Khaw KS, Tan PE, et al. Placental transfer and fetal metabolic effects of phenylephrine and ephedrine during spinal anesthesia for cesarean delivery. *Anesthesiology*. 2009;111:506–512.
56. Ingemarsson I, Westgren M, Lindberg C, et al. Single injection of terbutaline in term labor: placental transfer and effects on maternal and fetal carbohydrate metabolism. *Am J Obstet Gynecol*. 1981;139:697–701.
57. Erkkola R, Kangas L, Pekkarinen A. The transfer of diazepam across the placenta during labour. *Acta Obstet Gynecol Scand*. 1973;52:167–170.
58. Bakke OM, Haram K. Time-course of transplacental passage of diazepam: influence of injection-delivery interval on neonatal drug concentration. *Clin Pharm*. 1982;7:353–362.
59. Vree TB, Reekers-Kettling JJ, Fragen RJ, et al. Placental transfer of midazolam and its metabolite 1-hydroxymethylmidazolam in the pregnant ewe. *Anesth Analg*. 1984;63:31–34.
60. McBride RJ, Dundee JW, Moore J, et al. A study of the plasma concentrations of lorazepam in mother and neonate. *Br J Anaesth*. 1979;51:971–978.
61. Cottrill C, McAllister R, Gettes L, et al. Propranolol therapy during pregnancy, labor, and delivery: evidence for transplacental drug transfer and impaired neonatal drug disposition. *J Pediatr*. 1977;91:812–814.
62. Lindeberg S, Sandström B, Lundborg P, et al. Disposition of the adrenergic blocker metoprolol in the late-pregnant woman, the amniotic fluid, the cord blood and the neonate. *Acta Obstet Gynaecol*. 1984;118:61–64.
63. Oudijk M, Ruskamp J, Ververs T, et al. Treatment of fetal tachycardia with sotalol: transplacental pharmacokinetics and pharmacodynamics. *J Am Coll Cardiol*. 2003;42(4):765–770.
64. Santeiro ML, Stromquist C, Wyble L. Phenoxybenzamine placental transfer during the third trimester. *Ann Pharmacother*. 1996;30:1249–1251.
65. Macpherson M, Broughton-Pipkin F, Rutter N. The effect of maternal labetalol on the newborn infant. *Br J Obstet Gynaecol*. 1986;93:539–542.
66. Magee K, Bawdon R. Ex vivo human placental transfer and the vasoactive properties of hydralazine. *Am J Obstet Gynecol*. 2000;182:167–169.
67. Gregory YH, Beevers M, Churchill D, et al. Effect of atenolol on birth weight. *Am J Cardiol*. 1997;79:1436–1438.
68. Östman PL, Chestnut DH, Robillard JE, et al. Transplacental passage and hemodynamic effects of esmolol in gravid ewe. *Anesthesiology*. 1988;69:738–741.
69. Jones HMR, Cummings AJ, Setchell KD, et al. A study of the disposition of alpha-methyldopa in newborn infants following its administration to the mother for treatment of hypertension during pregnancy. *Br J Clin Pharmacol*. 1979;8:433–440.
70. Ala-Kokko TI, Pienimaki P, Lampela E, et al. Transfer of clonidine and dexmedetomidine across the isolated perfused human placenta. *Acta Anaesthesiol Scand*. 1997;41:313–319.
71. De Rosayro M, Nahrwold ML, Hill AB, et al. Plasma levels and cardiovascular effects of nitroglycerin in pregnant sheep. *Can J Anesth*. 1980;27:560–564.
72. Naulty J, Cefalo RC, Lewis PE. Fetal toxicity of nitroprusside in the pregnant ewe. *Am J Obstet Gynecol*. 1981;139(6):708–711.
73. Donchin Y, Amirav B, Sahar A, et al. Sodium nitroprusside for aneurysm surgery in pregnancy. *Br J Anaesth*. 1978;50:849–851.
74. Siu S, Chan M, Lau T. Placental transfer of ondansetron during early human pregnancy. *Clin Pharmacokinet*. 2006;45:419–423.
75. Riggs KW, Rurak DW, Taylor SM, et al. Fetal and maternal placental and nonplacental clearances of metoclopramide in chronically instrumented pregnant sheep. *J Pharm Sci*. 1990;79(12):1056–1061.
76. Samtani MN, Schwab M, Nathanielsz PW, et al. Area/moment and compartmental modeling of pharmacokinetics during pregnancy: applications to maternal/fetal exposures to corticosteroids in sheep and rats. *Pharm Res*. 2004;21(12):2279–2292.
77. Kraemer J, Klein J, Lubetsky A, et al. Perfusion studies of glyburide transfer across the human placenta: implications for fetal safety. *Am J Obstet Gynecol*. 2006;195:270–274.
78. Nanovskaya TN, Nekhayeva I, Hankins GDV, et al. Effect of human serum albumin on transplacental transfer of glyburide. *Biochem Pharmacol*. 2006;72:632–639.

79. Jain S, Zharikova OL, Ravindran S, et al. Glyburide metabolism by placentas of healthy and gestational diabetics. *Am J Perinatol.* 2008;25(3):169–174.
80. Gedeon C, Behravan J, Koren G, et al. Transport of glyburide by placental ABC transporters: implication in fetal drug exposure. *Placenta.* 2006;27:1096–1102.
81. Pollex EK, Feig DS, Koren G. Oral hypoglycemic therapy: understanding the mechanisms of transplacental transfer. *J Matern Fetal Neonatal Med.* 2010;23(3):224–228.
82. Nanovskaya TN, Nekhayeva IA, Patrikeeva SL, et al. Transfer of metformin across the dually perfused human placental lobule. *Am J Obstet Gynecol.* 2006;195:1081–1085.
83. Tamai T, Matsuura S, Tatsumi N, et al. Role of sex steroid hormones in relative refractoriness to angiotensin II during pregnancy. *Am J Obstet Gynecol.* 1984;149(2):177–183.
84. Scott D. Anemia during pregnancy. *Obstet Gynecol Ann.* 1972; 1:219.
85. Battinelli EM, Marshall A, Connors JM. The role of thrombophilia in pregnancy. *Thrombosis.* 2013;2013:516420.
86. Branch DW. Physiologic adaptations of pregnancy. *Am J Reprod Immunol.* 1992;28(3–4):120–122.
87. Thorn SA. Pregnancy in heart disease. *Heart.* 2004;90:450–456.
88. Hegewald MJ, Crapo RO. Respiratory physiology in pregnancy. *Clin Chest Med.* 2011;32(1):1–13.
89. Jepson JH. Factors influencing oxygenation in mother and fetus. *Obstet Gynecol.* 1974;44(6):906–914.
90. Wong CA, Loffredi M, Ganchiff JN, et al. Gastric emptying of water in term pregnancy. *Anesthesiology.* 2002;96(6):1395–1400.
91. Wong CA, McCarthy RJ, Fitzgerald PC, et al. Gastric emptying of water in obese pregnant women at term. *Anesth Analg.* 2007; 105(3):751–755.
92. Kelly MC, Carabine UA, Hill DA, et al. A comparison of the effect of intrathecal and extradural fentanyl on gastric emptying in laboring women. *Anesth Analg.* 1997;85(4):834–838.
93. Ueyama H, Hagihira S, Takashina M, et al. Pregnancy does not enhance volatile anesthetic sensitivity on the brain: an electroencephalographic analysis study. *Anesthesiology.* 2010;113(3):577–584.
94. Ralston DH, Shnider SM, DeLorimier AA. Effects of equipotent ephedrine, metaraminol, mephentermine, and methoxamine on uterine blood flow in the pregnant ewe. *Anesthesiology.* 1974; 40(4):354–370.
95. Danielson L, McMillen IC, Dyer JL, et al. Restriction of placental growth results in greater hypotensive response to alpha-adrenergic blockade in fetal sheep during late gestation. *J Physiol.* 2005; 563(pt 2):611–620.
96. Allen TK, George RB, White WD, et al. A double-blind, placebo-controlled trial of four fixed rate infusion regimens of phenylephrine for hemodynamic support during spinal anesthesia for cesarean delivery. *Anesth Analg.* 2010;111(5):1221–1229.
97. Lee A, Ngan Kee WD, Gin T. A quantitative, systematic review of randomized controlled trials of ephedrine versus phenylephrine for the management of hypotension during spinal anesthesia for cesarean delivery. *Anesth Analg.* 2002;94(4):920–926.
98. Goodman S. Anesthesia for nonobstetric surgery in the pregnant patient. *Semin Perinatol.* 2002;26(2):136–145.
99. Meschia G. Fetal oxygenation and maternal ventilation. *Clin Chest Med.* 2011;32(1):15–19.
100. Wise-Faberowski L, Aono M, Pearlstein RD, et al. Apoptosis is not enhanced in primary mixed neuronal/glial cultures protected by isoflurane against N-methyl-D-aspartate excitotoxicity. *Anesth Analg.* 2004;99(6):1708–1714.
101. Creeley C, Dikranian K, Dissen G, et al. Propofol-induced apoptosis of neurones and oligodendrocytes in fetal and neonatal rhesus macaque brain. *Br J Anaesth.* 2013;110(suppl 1):i29–i38.
102. Bosnjak ZJ, Yan Y, Canfield S, et al. Ketamine induces toxicity in human neurons differentiated from embryonic stem cells via mitochondrial apoptosis pathway. *Curr Drug Saf.* 2012;7(2):106–119.
103. Hays SR, Deshpande JK. Newly postulated neurodevelopmental risks of pediatric anesthesia. *Curr Neurol Neurosci Rep.* 2011; 11(2):205–210.
104. Lowery CL, Hardman MP, Manning N, et al. Neurodevelopmental changes of fetal pain. *Semin Perinatol.* 2007;31(5):275–282.
105. Derbyshire SW. Foetal pain? *Best Pract Res Clin Obstet Gynaecol.* 2010;24(5):647–655.
106. Brusseau R. Developmental perspectives: is the fetus conscious? *Int Anesthesiol Clin.* 2008;46(3):11–23.
107. Salihagic Kadic A, Predojevic M. Fetal neurophysiology according to gestational age. *Semin Fetal Neonatal Med.* 2012;17(5):256–260.

CHAPTER 46

Physiology and Pharmacology of the Elderly

Pamela Flood

There are a lot of old people. In the 2010 United States census, patients older than the age of age 65 years comprised 13% of the U.S. population or 40,300,000 people.[1] It is important that anesthesiologists understand the differences in pharmacology and physiology in elderly patients in order to be able to properly use anesthetic and analgesic drugs and compensate for aging-related functional decline in major organ systems. Some fortunate individuals remain physically vigorous until very late in life, whereas others deteriorate physically at a younger age. The cumulative effects of smoking, alcohol, and environmental toxins can accelerate the deterioration of aging in exposed individuals. Thus, it is not surprising that variability in physiology increases throughout life.[2] Increased physiologic variability results in increased pharmacokinetic and pharmacodynamic variability in elderly subjects.[3] The clinical result of this increased variability is an increased incidence of adverse drug reactions in elderly patients.[4] Thus, elderly patients require more careful attention to drug titration. The elderly have in common with the newborn limited physiologic reserve.

Aging and the Cardiovascular System

Increasing age is associated with increasing cardiac morbidity. Aging is associated with an increasing prevalence of cardiovascular disease and decreasing cardiovascular functional reserve.[5] Heart failure is the most frequent cause of hospitalization in patients older than 65 years of age. However, it is important to separate the cardiovascular effects of aging from those of common diseases with increased prevalence in the elderly, such as atherosclerosis, hypertension, and diabetes mellitus. The decline in cardiac function that occurs with aging in the healthy individual appears to be related, in part, to decreasing functional demand. Indeed, when exercise and low-calorie diet are maintained into the later decades, the decline in cardiovascular function is markedly attenuated.[6] It has been suggested that cardiovascular function is directly related to skeletal muscle mass. Aging also has discrete effects on the heart, large vessels, endothelial function, cardiac conduction system, and the cardiovascular autonomic response (Fig. 46-1).[6]

Heart

The heart increases in size during aging as a result of concentric ventricular hypertrophy. This occurs in response to the increase in left ventricular afterload. This increase in afterload occurs as the result of fibrosis and endothelial damage, which increase arterial stiffness and reduce the capacity for nitric oxide–induced vasodilation. Hypertrophy of cardiac myocytes occurs and accounts for a 30% increase in left ventricular wall thickness. Meanwhile, the number of cardiac myocytes is decreased due to necrosis and apoptosis. Despite these changes, resting systolic function tends to be well preserved in healthy individuals. However, the heart rate response to severe exercise is diminished. As a result, increases in cardiac output in response to severe exertion are attenuated by approximately 20% to 30%.

Cardiac dysfunction in aging is largely related to impaired diastolic left ventricle function with increased prevalence of diastolic heart failure.[7] There is an age-related increase in cardiac connective tissue that, when combined with ventricular hypertrophy, increases wall stiffness and reduces diastolic compliance. Ventricular filling in the elderly is especially dependent on active diastolic relaxation. In this process, calcium is removed from troponin C binding sites, triggering the dissociation of actin and myosin, thus facilitating isometric relaxation. Active diastolic relaxation uses approximately 15% of the energy consumed during the cardiac cycle. This process is significantly impaired in the elderly and exacerbates the adverse effects of ventricular hypertrophy on diastolic filling. As such, the elderly heart is markedly dependent on the atrial "kick" for adequate ventricular preload. It is estimated that atrial contraction contributes approximately 30% of ventricular filling in the elderly versus 10% in younger individuals. Because of the importance of atrial contraction,

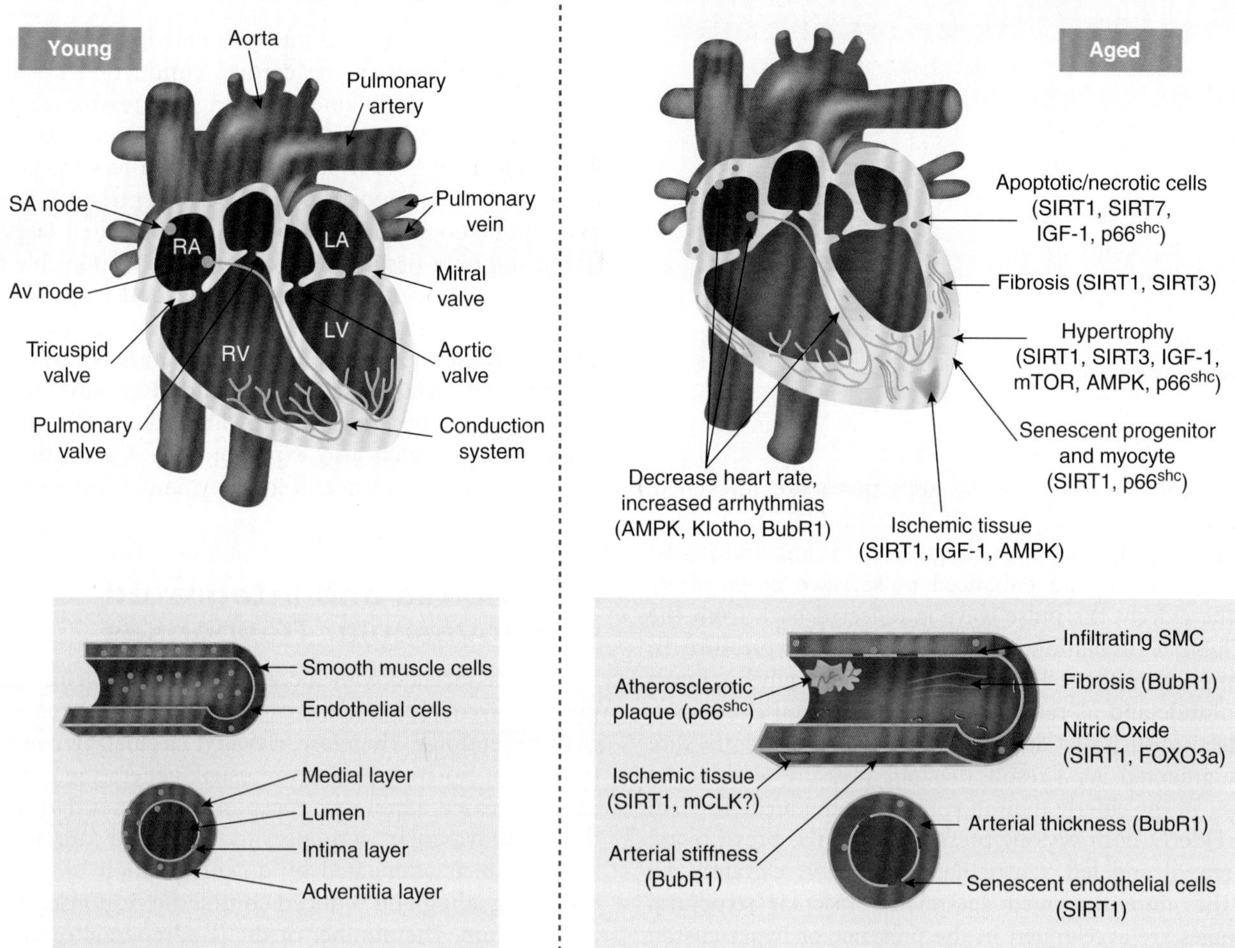

FIGURE 46-1 Age-dependent changes to cardiovascular tissues. Both the heart and vasculature undergo numerous alterations during aging as a result of deregulation of molecular longevity pathways, leading to compromised function. Important functional changes include arterial hypertrophy resulting in increased afterload, ventricular hypertrophy resulting in elevated systolic blood pressure, loss of cells in the electrical conduction system predisposing to arrhythmia, and loss of sensitivity to catecholamines resulting in reduced maximal heart rate and heart rate variability. (Adapted from North BJ, Sinclair DA. The intersection between aging and cardiovascular disease. *Circ Res.* 2012;110(8):1097–1108. Illustration credit: Cosmocyte/Ben Smith.)

and because filling is delayed by reduced ventricular compliance, ventricular filling is typically not complete until very late in diastole. Tachycardia and shortened diastolic intervals are associated with marked decreases in ventricular preload in the elderly. Atrial fibrillation is a common rhythm in the elderly. Loss of the atrial kick is particularly poorly tolerated by elderly patients because of decreased capacitance of the left ventricle from the previously noted changes. Perioperative events that reduce venous return, such as hypovolemia, positive pressure ventilation, and increased venous capacitance, may be accompanied by significant decreases in cardiac output. Conversely, excessive perioperative increases in blood volume or decreases in contractility can precipitate congestive cardiac failure. Diastolic dysfunction is now recognized as a major contributor to cardiovascular disease in the elderly population and is exacerbated by several coexisting diseases[8,9] (Table 46-1).

It is difficult to distinguish systolic dysfunction from diastolic dysfunction during routine clinical evaluation. Furthermore, routine preoperative echocardiographic indices of function such as left ventricular ejection fraction will fail to identify diastolic dysfunction. However, diastolic filling can be evaluated by comparing Doppler echocardiographic measurements of mitral valve inflow velocities during the early and late (atrial contraction) phases of diastole. Dyspnea in the elderly may indicate congestive cardiac failure and/or pulmonary disease.

Large Vessels

Structural changes in the large vessels are an important element of the aging process and contribute significantly to the age-related changes in the heart described earlier.[10] The large vessels become elongated, tortuous, and dilated

Table 46-1

Diseases Commonly Encountered in the Elderly that are Associated with Diastolic Dysfunction

Systemic hypertension
Coronary artery disease
Cardiomyopathy
Aortic stenosis
Atrial fibrillation
Diabetes
Chronic renal disease

in the elderly. Their intima and media are thickened, causing these vessels to be less distensible. The normal cushioning function of the large vessels is impaired; causing accelerated and enhanced pulse wave propagation. In the elderly, the pulse wave is reflected back from the peripheral circulation and augments systolic pressure. In young adults, the reflected pulse wave generally has lower amplitude and its return from the peripheral circulation is delayed such that diastolic rather than systolic pressure is augmented. As a result, diastolic pressure tends to be lower in the elderly than in younger individuals. Thus, in the elderly, both systolic pressure and pulse pressure are increased and left ventricular afterload is elevated. All of the aforementioned age-related vascular structural changes are accelerated in the presence of hypertension or atherosclerosis.

Endothelial Function

The vascular endothelium is an important regulator of vasomotor response, coagulation, fibrinolysis, immunomodulation, and vascular growth and proliferation. Endothelial dysfunction is an important element in the early pathogenesis of atherosclerosis, diabetes mellitus, and systemic hypertension.[11] Aging is associated with altered endothelial structure and function, even in the absence of disease. Reactive oxygen species, such as superoxide anions, have been implicated in age-related endothelial dysfunction. Endothelial dysfunction is accelerated by smoking, diabetes, hypertension, and hyperlipidemia. In the elderly, endothelial nitric oxide release is decreased in all vascular beds, including the coronary circulation.[12] Furthermore, the vasodilator response to nitric oxide of the adjacent vascular smooth muscle is also reduced. Vasodilator responses to β_2 agonists and vasoconstrictor responses to α-adrenergic stimulation are similarly attenuated in the elderly. Thus, age-related endothelial dysfunction can be characterized as a decrease in the ability of the endothelium to dilate or contract blood vessels in response to physiologic and pharmacologic stimuli.

Conduction System

There are several important age-related structural and functional changes in the cardiac conduction system.[5] The sinoatrial node undergoes a progressive change over time such that the proportion of pacemaker cells decreases from 50% in late childhood to less than 10% at 75 years. The sinoatrial node, atrioventricular node, and conduction bundles also become infiltrated with fibrous and fatty tissue. These changes are responsible for the increased incidence of first- and second-degree heart block, sick sinus syndrome, and atrial fibrillation in the elderly. The development of atrial fibrillation is also facilitated by left atrial enlargement, which typically accompanies aging in otherwise healthy individuals. Otherwise, healthy elderly men also experience an age-related increase in the prevalence, frequency, and complexity of ventricular ectopy.

Autonomic and Integrated Cardiovascular Responses

Aging is associated with increased norepinephrine entry into the circulation and deficient catecholamine reuptake at nerve endings. Therefore, elevated circulating concentrations of norepinephrine are usual, generating chronically increased adrenergic receptor occupancy. However, the cardiovascular response to increased adrenergic stimulation is attenuated by downregulation of postreceptor signaling and reduced contractile response of the myocardium. The number of the β-adrenergic receptors is reduced in the elderly myocardium.[7] The decreased chronotropic and inotropic response of elderly patients to β-adrenergic drugs also has a contribution from downstream changes in the mechanism by which binding at the receptor is coupled to cyclic adenosine monophosphate. The response to exogenously administered β agonists, such as isoproterenol, is similarly attenuated. Receptor downregulation is responsible for the age-related decline in maximum heart rate during exercise. Indeed, receptor downregulation in the elderly makes their cardiovascular function similar to that of a younger individual who has received β-adrenergic antagonists.

Orthostatic hypotension is common in the elderly and is associated with syncope, falls, and cognitive decline. Impaired baroreceptor reflexes and attenuated peripheral vasoconstriction are partially responsible. Hypovolemia and salt depletion also contribute and are the result of iatrogenic diuretic administration or increased atrial natriuretic peptide release. Orthostatic hypotension is more common in patients who are hypertensive at baseline. It is difficult to separate the effects of aging per se from those of age-related chronic increases in systolic pressure. Straining against a closed glottis (Valsalva maneuver) typically produces a decrease in venous return and cardiac output. The normal baroreceptor response to this maneuver includes an increase in heart rate and peripheral vascular tone and restoration of blood pressure. However, this response is markedly attenuated in the elderly. Age-related impairment of baroreceptor responses makes hypotension more likely after the initiation of positive pressure ventilation, particularly in the presence of hypovolemia. Similarly, neuraxial local anesthetic–induced sympathetic blockade is more likely to be accompanied by hypotension in the presence of an impaired baroreceptor response. In the Irish Longitudinal Aging Study, antidepressants and β blockers were associated with orthostatic hypotension, and hypnotics and sedatives worsened preexisting orthostatic intolerance.[13] Antihypertensive drugs that did not act through β-adrenergic blockade were not associated with orthostatic hypotension. These findings should be considered in the mobilization of elderly patients who may have received these drugs in the perioperative period.

Anesthetic and Ischemic Preconditioning in the Aging Heart

It is now recognized that, under certain circumstances, exposure to volatile anesthetics (anesthetic preconditioning) or several brief periods of ischemia (ischemic preconditioning) may enhance tolerance to subsequent ischemia, enhance cardiac function, and reduce infarction size.[14] Because the incidence of atherosclerosis and coronary artery disease is age-related, the elderly would seem be most likely to benefit from a preconditioning strategy. However, both anesthetic and ischemic preconditioning may be markedly attenuated in the elderly, potentially explaining the difficulty of translating promising preclinical results to treatment.[15,16] Furthermore, potent volatile drugs may induce significant cardiovascular depression in this age group. Therefore, the use of preconditioning strategies in this age group is uncertain.

Aging and the Respiratory System

The respiratory system undergoes a multifactorial decline in functional reserve with aging (Tables 46-2 and 46-3).[17] Under normal circumstances, this decrease in respiratory function is not associated with significant limitation of daily activity. However, decreased respiratory reserve may be unmasked by illness, surgery, anesthesia, and other perioperative events. Common respiratory diseases and the effects of smoking and environmental pollution frequently exacerbate the decline in respiratory function with aging. The anticipation and amelioration of their effects is critically important to anesthetic management in the elderly, as postoperative respiratory complications result in 40% of perioperative deaths in patient older than 65 years.[18]

Table 46-2

Intrinsic and Extrinsic Events that Influence the Respiratory System during Aging

Intrinsic to the Aging Process	Environmental, Behavioral, and Disease Related
Decreased bronchiolar caliber	Industrial and environmental pollution
Decreased alveolar surface area	Smoking
Increased lung collagen content	General deconditioning
Decreased lung elastin content	Coexisting disease
Kyphoscoliosis	
Increased thoracic cage rigidity	
Decreased diaphragmatic strength	

Respiratory System Mechanics and Architecture

The chest wall becomes less compliant with aging, presumably related to changes in the thoracic skeleton and a decline in costovertebral joint mobility. These changes produce a restrictive functional impairment. The noncompliant thoracic cage makes intercostal muscle activity less efficient. Therefore, the diaphragm and abdominal muscles assume a greater role in tidal breathing. However, diaphragmatic function declines with age, predisposing the elderly to respiratory fatigue when required to significantly increase minute ventilation. Although the diaphragm does not appear to undergo significant atrophy or change in muscle fiber type with aging, it does occupy a flatter position and therefore has a less favorable mechanical advantage. These changes predispose the elderly to respiratory insufficiency in the setting of high regional anesthesia.

Table 46-3

Functional Consequences of the Intrinsic and Extrinsic Events that Influence the Respiratory System during Aging

Decrease in lung elastic recoil
Increase in lung compliance
Decrease in oxygen diffusing capacity
Premature airway closure causing V/Q mismatch and increased alveolar-to-arterial oxygen gradient
Small airway closure and gas trapping
Decreased expiratory flow rates

V/Q, ventilation to perfusion.

Aging is associated with a loss of lung elasticity that is responsible for a decrease in lung recoil, thus making the lung more distensible. Changes in surfactant function may also contribute to age-related changes in lung compliance. The net result of these changes in the elastic properties of the lung and chest wall is an increase in intrapleural pressure that significantly impacts on respiratory function. Intrapleural pressure is a critical determinant of small airway caliber. Increased intrapleural pressures increase the tendency for small airway collapse to occur, thus causing gas trapping and/or expiratory airflow limitation.

Lung Volumes and Capacities

Vital Capacity

Vital capacity (VC) is the volume generated when a maximal inspiration is followed by a maximal expiration. There is a progressive loss of VC with aging that results from increased chest wall stiffness, decreased lung elastic recoil, and decreased respiratory muscle strength.

Residual Volume

The residual volume is the volume remaining in the lungs after a maximal expiration. In young individuals, the residual volume is determined primarily by ability of the expiratory muscles to overcome the elastic recoil properties of the lung and chest wall. However, in the elderly, dynamic airway closure also limits expiration. Therefore, aging is associated with a progressive increase in residual volume of up to 10% per decade (Fig. 46-2).[19]

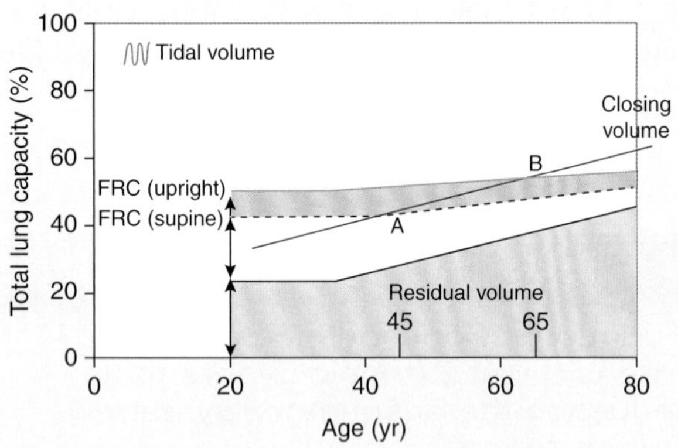

FIGURE 46-2 Effect of aging on lung volumes. Functional residual capacity (FRC) increases with age as a result of increasing residual volume. Closing volume also increases with age and exceeds FRC in the upright position around age 65 years and in the supine position at age 45 years. These changes lead to ventilation perfusion mismatch and shunt, resulting in reduced resting PO_2 with age. (From Sprung J, Gajic O, Warner DO. Review article: age related alterations in respiratory function—anesthetic considerations. *Can J Anaesth.* 2006;53[12]:1244–1257).

Total Lung Capacity

Total lung capacity is the sum of the residual volume and the VC. Thus, the combined effect of the decline in VC and increase in residual volume is that the total lung capacity remains relatively constant with aging.

Functional Residual Capacity

The functional residual capacity (FRC) is the volume remaining in the lungs at the end of a normal expiration. The FRC is the volume at which the elastic recoil forces of the lung and chest wall are at equilibrium. The opposing recoil forces of the lung and chest wall generate the subatmospheric intrapleural pressure. Aging is associated with a progressive increase in FRC that occurs as a result of the decreased elastic recoil force of the lungs. However, the increase in FRC is less than would be predicted from the change in lung elastic recoil alone. This is because the increased stiffness of the chest wall counteracts the increase in lung volume.

Closing Capacity

Airway closure may occur in small airways (<1 mm) whose caliber is determined by their transmural pressure. Airway closure typically occurs in dependent areas of the lung where the surrounding intrapleural pressure is likely to be greater. In young adults, airway closure occurs only at low lung volumes (approximately 10% of VC). Thus, airway closure is unlikely during normal tidal breathing. However, as intrapleural pressure increases with age, airway closure occurs at progressively greater lung volumes. Indeed, in the elderly, airway closure occurs at approximately 40% of the VC reflecting lung volumes that exceed FRC. Although the FRC increases by up to 3% per decade, closing capacity increases at a greater rate. Thus, gas exchange impairment due to shunting in regions of airway closure is typical in the elderly during normal tidal breathing. The supine position is associated with a decrease in FRC when compared to the standing position. In this regard, the supine position makes airway closure during normal tidal breathing more likely. Indeed, airway closure may occur during tidal breathing as early as the mid-40s in the supine position.

Expiratory Flow

There is a progressive decline in forced exhaled volume in 1 second (FEV_1) and forced vital capacity (FVC) with age that is independent of smoking or environmental exposure. Age-related loss of lung elastic recoil predisposes to dynamic airway collapse during forced expiratory maneuvers. Expiratory muscle strength also declines with age.

Diffusing Capacity and Alveolar-to-Arterial Oxygen Gradient

Gas exchange efficiency declines with aging as a result of increasing intrapulmonary shunting and decreasing lung diffusing capacity. The result is a linear decline in resting

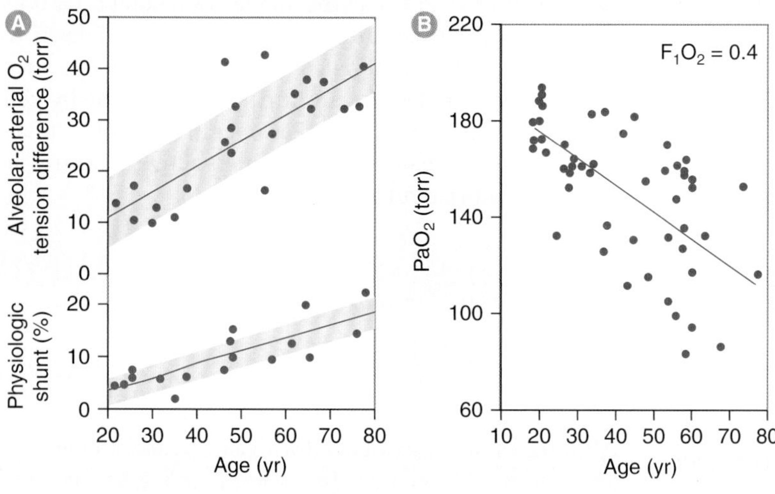

FIGURE 46-3 Effect of aging on gas exchange. **A:** The change in alveolar/arterial oxygen tension with age (shunt fraction or percent shunt). **B:** Relationship of PO_2 with age during spontaneous breathing of 40% oxygen and 60% nitrous oxide under general anesthesia with enflurane. (From Wahba WM. Influence of aging on lung function—clinical significance of changes from age 20 years. *Anesth Analg.* 1983;62:764–776).

supine PaO_2 between early adulthood and 65 years of age (Fig. 46-3).[20] Small airway closure causes ventilation to perfusion (V/Q) mismatch and shunting. Cardiac output is often decreased in the elderly to the extent that mixed venous oxygen tension is decreased. Thus, even modest amounts of shunting may produce a significant decrease in PaO_2 because of the contribution of desaturated venous blood. The diameter of the alveolar ducts is increased and their respective alveoli are wider and shallower. These architectural changes significantly reduce alveolar surface area. As a result, diffusing capacity for carbon monoxide may decline by up to 50% between early adulthood and 80 years of age.

Upper Airway Protective Reflexes

Cough effectiveness is reduced in the elderly because of diminished reflex sensitivity and impaired muscle function. Cough reflex attenuation is associated with an increased incidence of aspiration pneumonia. The mechanisms of cough reflex impairment include desensitization of airway epithelial irritant receptors and impaired swallowing.[21] Smoking causes airway sensory nerve neuropeptide depletion and nicotine inhibits C fiber transmission in the lower respiratory tract.[22] Coexisting medical conditions that are associated with cough reflex suppression include stroke, laryngectomy, and Parkinson disease. General anesthetics inhibit the cough reflex through inhibition of central respiratory neurons.[23] Care is needed during intubation and extubation of patients with risk factors for impaired airway protection.

Control of Breathing, Chemoreceptors, and Integrated Responses

The cardiorespiratory responses to hypoxia and hypercarbia are mediated via central and peripheral chemoreceptors. The increases in heart rate and minute ventilation in response to elevations in $PaCO_2$ or decreases in PaO_2 are markedly attenuated in the elderly. The attenuated ventilatory response is multifactorial and reflects decreased peripheral chemoreceptor sensitivity, reduced respiratory muscle activity, decreased respiratory mechanical efficiency, and general respiratory deconditioning. These important protective reflexes are further attenuated by the administration of opioids and sedative/hypnotic drugs. Thus, the elderly are at particular risk from life-threatening respiratory depression in the perioperative period. In a recent report, investigators found that the risk of opioid-induced ventilatory depression increased with increasing age, with patients 61 to 70 years of age having 2.8 times the risk of ventilatory depression compared with patients 16 to 45 years old.[24] Although the risk of respiratory depression from opioids is greater in the elderly, the same is not true for all opioid side effects. Opioids are a major cause of postoperative nausea and vomiting in young and middle-aged patients, increasing the risk nearly four-fold[25]; age was not a risk factor for nausea and vomiting in other reports.[24] In fact, age may actually decrease the risk of nausea and vomiting; one group of investigators reported a 13% decrease in the risk of postoperative nausea and vomiting with each additional decade of life.[26]

Sleep Disordered Breathing

The incidence of sleep disordered breathing increases with age, especially in men. It is estimated that approximately 20% of elderly people have clinically significant obstructive sleep apnea.[27] The prevalence of snoring is highest in the seventh decade and is associated with an increased risk of stroke and heart disease. Morbidity associated with sleep apnea includes systemic and pulmonary hypertension, dysrhythmias, myocardial infarction, stroke, sudden death, and automobile accidents. In addition, obstructive sleep apnea doubles the risk for postoperative delirium in the elderly.[28]

Thermoregulation in the Elderly

There is ample evidence that hyperthermia and hypothermia in the elderly are poorly tolerated and that extreme cold and heat stress are associated with increased mortality compared to younger individuals.[29] However, it is not clear whether the greater susceptibility to thermal stress is related to aging per se or to underlying socioeconomic conditions, general fitness, activity levels, and the effects of coexisting disease in the elderly.

Resting Core Temperature

Aging is associated with a greater variability in core temperature. Indeed, it is estimated that up to 10% of people greater than 65 years of age have early morning core temperatures of less than 35.5°C (Table 46-4). However, when the effects of coexisting disease, socioeconomic circumstances, and medication are eliminated, there is no evidence of declining body temperature with advancing age in healthy individuals under thermoneutral conditions. Circadian temperature variations are not significantly different in the healthy elderly compared to younger individuals.

Response to Cold Stress

The elderly do not have a normal response to cold stress. The usual physiologic response to cold stress is to decrease heat loss by peripheral vasoconstriction and to increase heat production via shivering and nonshivering thermogenesis. Aging is associated with attenuated vasoconstrictor responses to cold. The inability to efficiently conserve heat in the elderly is exacerbated by the age-related decrease in skeletal muscle mass. Loss of skeletal muscle mass is responsible for the age-related decline in basal heat production. It is estimated that resting heat production declines by 20% between the ages of 30 and 70 years. There is a significant gender-related difference in cold stress response in the elderly. Mortality during cold weather is higher in men compared to age-matched women. It is likely that the higher percentage of body fat and lower surface area-to-mass ratio in females is responsible for this difference. The attenuated cold stress responses of the elderly are further diminished by general and regional anesthesia. Perioperative hypothermia is very likely in the elderly patient unless active measures are taken to maintain normothermia.

Table 46-4

Factors Associated with Reduced Resting Core Temperatures in the Elderly

- Neurologic disease
- Diabetes
- Low body weight
- Lack of self-sufficiency
- Consumption of less than two meals per day
- Smoking
- Alcohol consumption

Gastrointestinal Function in the Elderly

Liver

Although aging is associated with a decrease in liver mass and hepatic blood flow, hepatocellular metabolic function appears to be relatively well preserved throughout life. Protein synthetic function may be diminished in some elderly individuals, particularly those with poor nutritional intake. Reduced serum albumin concentrations will affect drug binding. On the other hand, the concentration of another important drug-binding protein, α-1-acid glycoprotein, is typically increased in the elderly. Hepatic synthesis of plasma cholinesterase may be diminished, particularly in men. There is evidence of an increase in the duration of mivacurium activity but not succinylcholine with age.[30]

Although hepatic enzyme function may be qualitatively normal in the elderly, the reduction in hepatic mass and blood flow is responsible for a significant decrease in first-pass metabolism of several drugs that are important in the aging population.[31] Because first-pass metabolism is reduced, the oral bioavailability of propranolol and labetalol are increased in the elderly. Conversely, prodrugs, such as the angiotensin-converting enzyme (ACE) inhibitor enalapril, require activation by the liver before they exert their pharmacologic effect. Therefore, the bioavailability of these drugs may be decreased in the elderly.

Gastroesophageal Physiology

Gastric emptying of solid material appears to be relatively normal in the healthy elderly population. However, gastric emptying of liquids may be delayed compared to younger individuals.[32] Emptying of both liquids and solids is commonly delayed in the presence of certain coexisting diseases that are common with aging such as gastroesophageal reflux disease (GERD) (Table 46-5). However, the typical symptoms of GERD seen in the younger population (heartburn and regurgitation) are less frequent in the elderly, making diagnosis more difficult. Dysphagia, vomiting, respiratory symptoms, weight loss, and anemia are more common presenting symptoms in the elderly. Several medications that are commonly prescribed in the elderly population predispose to GERD by decreasing lower esophageal sphincter tone (Table 46-6).

Table 46-5

Factors that Predispose to the Increased Incidence of Gastroesophageal Reflux Disease in the Elderly

Increased prevalence of sliding hiatal hernia
Shortened intraabdominal segment of the lower esophageal sphincter
Impaired clearance of refluxed acid
Use of medications that reduce lower esophageal sphincter pressure
Decreased esophageal peristalsis pressure

Renal Function in the Elderly

Aging is accompanied by a decrease in the cortical nephron population and a reduction in renal mass. Renal blood flow and glomerular filtration rate (GFR) both decline with age.[31] The average male GFR is 125 mL per minute. This value decreases by approximately 1 mL/min/yr after the age of 40 years as a result of the decline in nephron population and hyalinization of cortical afferent arterioles. The medullary nephron population is relatively preserved, and age-related vascular changes in the medulla are minimal. Despite the significant decline in GFR with aging, the serum creatinine concentration increases minimally because there is also an age-related decrease in skeletal muscle mass. Although renal function is diminished in the elderly, it is sufficient to maintain homeostasis under normal physiologic conditions. However, the renal response to common perioperative stresses may be insufficient to maintain homeostasis.[31] Although the elderly individual is able to maintain acid–base balance under every day physiologic conditions, the response to increased acid loads such as during ischemia and sepsis is attenuated due to impaired renal tubular ammonium secretion.

The elderly are at risk for both dehydration and free water overload because of impaired renal responses. Urine concentrating ability is critically dependent upon the presence of a hypertonic renal medulla. However, medullary perfusion is relatively increased in the elderly, resulting in a washout of solute and a reduction in osmolality in that region. Thus, the collecting tubules are not exposed to the usual concentration gradient necessary to produce concentrated urine.[33] Reduced numbers of cortical nephrons also contribute to impaired salt conservation. This suboptimal renal response to dehydration is compounded by age-related deficiencies in thirst mechanisms. Water deprivation is associated with a reduced thirst response in elderly subjects despite significant increases in plasma osmolality.[34] As a result of these factors, the elderly are at enhanced risk of dehydration.

The response to free water excess is similarly attenuated in the elderly. This is particularly relevant because the perioperative neuroendocrine stress response is associated with arginine vasopressin (antidiuretic hormone) release and water retention. When combined with iatrogenic hypotonic fluid administration, these factors make the elderly patient particularly susceptible to perioperative free water overload and hyponatremia.

Table 46-6

Medications that Are Commonly Administered in the Elderly that Reduce Lower Esophageal Sphincter Tone and Predispose to Gastroesophageal Reflux

Anticholinergics
Antidepressants
Nitrates
Calcium channel blockers
Theophylline

Skeletal Muscle Mass and Aging

Aging is associated with a significant decline in neuromuscular performance. Loss of neuromuscular function causes functional disability and loss of independence.[35] By the seventh and eighth decades, maximal voluntary contractile strength is reduced by 20% to 40%. Neuromuscular decline results predominantly from loss of skeletal muscle mass, which declines by approximately 40% between the ages of 20 and 60 years (sarcopenia). However, strength losses with aging may be attenuated by continued physical activity, particularly resistance training. The decline in muscle function is multifactorial (Table 46-7). Diminished skeletal muscle mass has significant implications for the elderly patient in the perioperative period (Table 46-8).

Table 46-7

Factors that Are Thought to Be Responsible for the Significant Decrease in Lean Muscle Mass that Occurs with Aging

Decreased motor neuron innervation
Decreased physical activity
Endocrine shift toward catabolism (reduced insulin-like growth factor 1 secretion)
Decreased androgen (testosterone and estrogen) secretion
Decreased total caloric intake
Decreased protein consumption and protein synthesis
Inflammatory mediators and cytokines (interleukins 1 and 6, tumor necrosis factor)

Table 46-8

Perioperative Functional Consequences of the Loss of Skeletal Muscle Mass that Typically Accompanies Aging

Impaired postoperative mobilization and ambulation
Reduced cough effectiveness
Reduced shivering thermogenesis
Altered drug disposition
Reduced neuromuscular functional reserve
Prolonged recovery and hospitalization

Neurophysiology of Aging

The elderly demonstrate increased sensitivity to benzodiazepines, opioids, and volatile anesthetic drugs. The minimum alveolar concentration (MAC) of potent volatile anesthetic drugs is decreased by approximately 25% at 80 years of age when compared to MAC values obtained at 40 years of age.[36] The addition of nitrous oxide is more effective in reducing the requirements for potent inhaled anesthetic drugs in the elderly.

Perhaps as a function of limited neurologic reserve, the elderly are at risk for postoperative delirium (POD) and postoperative cognitive dysfunction (POCD) that are strong risks factor for mortality.[37] POD is a syndrome of fluctuating consciousness, inattention, memory impairment, and perceptual abnormalities that typically occurs after a lucid interval of 1 to 3 days after emergence from general anesthesia. In comparison to the validated criteria for POD, the definition of POCD is much looser. One of the largest studies, International Study of Postoperative Cognitive Dysfunction 1 described POCD in 26% of elderly patients 1 week after anesthesia and 10% after 3 months using a variety of well-recognized tests.[38]

Although POCD and POD are distinct syndromes, there are a large number of risk factors for POCD and POD that overlap, which suggests a shared pathogenesis. POD is equally common after both regional and general anesthesia, whereas POCD may be more common after general anesthesia.[39] The pathophysiology of acute POD in the elderly is undetermined. However, a neuroinflammatory response exacerbated by a faulty blood–brain barrier is thought to be mechanistically important. Surgical trauma induces an inflammatory response, which leads to an inflammatory cascade mediated by cytokines and macrophages in the central nervous system resulting in POCD.[40]

Although POCD is a risk factor for early mortality, in an 11-year follow-up of the ISPOCD cohort, it was not found to be a risk factor for dementia. As the population ages and requires more surgical intervention, the pathogenesis of this syndrome and its best management are important areas for investigation.

Pain and Aging

Pain is a part of daily life for many elderly patients, with about 50% of patients older than the age of 70 years reporting chronic pain.[41] Elderly patients are particularly more prone to chronic pain than younger people.[42] There are some interesting differences between young and older subjects in their response to experimental pain. There is some evidence that older patients are more sensitive to experimental pain, which may be explained, at least in part, by a reduction in the endogenous analgesic response to pain, possibly mediated by reduced production of β-endorphin in response to noxious stimulation.[43,44] Older patients experience a more prolonged hyperalgesia following capsaicin injection compared with younger subjects. However, older patients appear to also require a higher intensity of noxious stimulation before first reporting pain.[45] Some of the differences between studies may also depend on exactly which pain pathways are activated during the assessment. Chakour and colleagues[46] demonstrated that pain transmission via C fibers was unchanged in young versus elderly subjects. However, there was a substantial reduction in pain transmission via Aδ fibers. Thus, the relative perceptions of pain in elderly subjects versus younger subjects were influenced by the extent of pain transmission via Aδ fibers.

As a general rule, elderly patients are more sensitive to opioids. Electroencephalographic studies of subjects treated with fentanyl, alfentanil, sufentanil, and remifentanil support a 50% dose reduction for elderly patients.[47–50] Aging results in less important pharmacokinetic effects of these drugs with variable reports of small reductions in clearance.

In contrast, morphine and meperidine have active metabolites, which accumulate in the elderly.

Morphine is metabolized by glucuronidation into two metabolites, morphine-3-glucuronide, which is mostly inactive, and morphine-6-glucuronide, which is itself a potent analgesic. Although the potency of intrathecal morphine-6-glucuronide is 650-fold higher than that of morphine, morphine-6-glucuronide crosses the blood–brain barrier very slowly, so slowly that it is unlikely that it contributes to the acute analgesia provided by morphine. However, with chronic administration, the levels of morphine-6-glucuronide will rise to pharmacologically active concentrations.[51] Morphine-6-glucuronide is eliminated by the kidneys. Creatinine clearance is reduced with advancing age. Thus, morphine-6-glucuronide will accumulate more in elderly patients, necessitating a reduction in dose of chronically administered morphine. Of course, if the patient has renal insufficiency, it might be better to select an opioid without an active metabolite.

Elderly patients have reduced meperidine clearance, resulting in a longer half-life for meperidine. Meperidine will accumulate in elderly subjects with repeated administration.[52] A worrisome aspect of meperidine is the toxic metabolite, normeperidine. Renal excretion of normeperidine was particularly reduced in elderly patients. The result is that normeperidine will likely accumulate with repeated doses in elderly patients.[53] Because normeperidine is highly epileptogenic, meperidine is probably a poor choice for patient-controlled analgesia or other forms of continuous opioid delivery in elderly patients.

The alterations in physiology and pharmacology discussed earlier make the anesthetic management of elderly patients more challenging. The increasing elderly population requiring surgery makes knowledge of these factors critical. With careful drug titration and pre- and postoperative management, even the extreme elderly can safely undergo surgery in order to improve the quality of their lives.

References

1. Werner CA. *Census 2010 Brief C2010BR-09: The Older Population: 2010*. Suitland, MD: U.S. Census Bureau; 2011.
2. Bafitis H, Sargent F II. Human physiological adaptability through the life sequence. *J Gerontol*. 1977;32:402–410.
3. Klein U, Klein M, Sturm H, et al. The frequency of adverse drug reactions as dependent upon age, sex and duration of hospitalization. *Int J Clin Pharmacol Biopharm*. 1976;13:187–195.
4. Crooks J. Aging and drug disposition pharmacodynamics. *J Chronic Dis*. 1983;36:85–90.
5. Lakatta EG, Levy D. Arterial and cardiac aging: major shareholders in cardiovascular disease enterprises. Part II: the aging heart in health: links to disease. *Circulation*. 2003;107:346–354.
6. North BJ, Sinclair DA. The intersection between aging and cardiovascular disease. *Circ Res*. 2012;110:1097–1108.
7. Ferrara N, Komici K, Corbi G, et al. β-Adrenergic receptor responsiveness in aging heart and clinical implications. *Front Physiol*. 2014;4:396.
8. Phillip BK, Pastor D, Bellows W, et al. The prevalence of preoperative diastolic filling abnormalities in geriatric surgical patients. *Anesth Analg*. 2003;97:1214–1221.
9. Aurigemma GP, Gaasch WH. Diastolic heart failure. *N Engl J Med*. 2004;351:1097–1105.
10. Ferrari AU, Radaelli A, Centola M. Aging and the cardiovascular system. *J Appl Physiol*. 2003;95:2591–2597.
11. Matz RL, Andriantsitohaina R. Age-related endothelial dysfunction. *Drugs Aging*. 2003;20:527–550.
12. Toro L, Marijic J, Nishimaru K, et al. Aging, ion channel expression, and vascular function. *Vascul Pharmacol*. 2002;38(1):73–80.
13. Romero-Ortuno R, O'Connell MD, Finucane C, et al. Insights into the clinical management of the syndrome of supine hypertension—orthostatic hypotension (SH-OH): the Irish Longitudinal Study on Ageing (TILDA). *BMC Geriatr*. 2013;13:73.
14. Zaugg M, Schaub MC, Foex P. Myocardial injury and its prevention in the perioperative setting. *Br J Anaesth*. 2004;93:21–33.
15. Mio Y, Bienengraeber MW, Marinovic J, et al. Age-related attenuation of isoflurane preconditioning in human atrial cardiomyocytes: roles for mitochondrial respiration and sarcolemmal adenosine triphosphate-sensitive potassium channel activity. *Anesthesiology*. 2008;108(4):612–620.
16. van den Munckhof I, Riksen N, Seeger JP, et al. Aging attenuates the protective effect of ischemic preconditioning against endothelial ischemia-reperfusion injury in humans. *Am J Physiol Heart Circ Physiol*. 2013;304(12):H1727–H1732.
17. Chan ED, Welsch CH. Geriatric respiratory medicine. *Chest*. 1998;114:1704–1733.
18. Zaugg M, Lucchinetti E. Respiratory function in the elderly. *Anesthesiol Clin N Am*. 2000;18:47–58.
19. Sprung J, Gajic O, Warner DO. Review article: age related alterations in respiratory function—anesthetic considerations. *Can J Anaesth*. 2006;53(12):1244–1257.
20. Wahba WM. Influence of aging on lung function—clinical significance of changes from age twenty. *Anesth Analg*. 1983;62:764–776.
21. Kikawada M, Iwamoto T, Takasaki M. Aspiration and infection in the elderly: epidemiology, diagnosis and management. *Drugs Aging*. 2005;22(2):115–130.
22. Watando A, Ebihara S, Ebihara T, et al. Daily oral care and cough reflex sensitivity in elderly nursing home patients. *Chest*. 2004;126:1066–1070.
23. Kondo T, Hayama N. Cough reflex is additively potentiated by inputs from the laryngeal and tracheobronchial [corrected] receptors and enhanced by stimulation of the central respiratory neurons. *J Physiol Sci*. 2009;59(5):347–353.
24. Cepeda MS, Farrar JT, Baumgarten M, et al. Side effects of opioids during short-term administration: effect of age, gender, and race. *Clin Pharmacol Ther*. 2003;74(2):102–112.
25. Junger A, Hartmann B, Benson M, et al. The use of an anesthesia information management system for prediction of antiemetic rescue treatment at the postanesthesia care unit. *Anesth Analg*. 2001;92(5):1203–1209.
26. Sinclair DR, Chung F, Mezei G. Can postoperative nausea and vomiting be predicted? *Anesthesiology*. 1999;91(1):109–118.
27. Nishihata Y, Takata Y, Usui Y, et al. Continuous positive airway pressure treatment improves cardiovascular outcomes in elderly patients with cardiovascular disease and obstructive sleep apnea [published online ahead of print December 8, 2013]. *Heart Vessels*.
28. Flink BJ, Rivelli SK, Cox EA, et al. Obstructive sleep apnea and incidence of postoperative delirium after elective knee replacement in the nondemented elderly. *Anesthesiology*. 2012;116(4):788–796.
29. Kenney WL, Munce TA. Invited review: aging and human temperature regulation. *J Appl Physiol (1985)*. 2003;95(6):2598–2603.
30. Cope TM, Hunter JM. Selecting neuromuscular-blocking drugs for elderly patients. *Drugs Aging*. 2003;20(2):125–140.
31. Mangoni AA, Jackson SHD. Age-related changes in pharmacokinetics and pharmacodynamics: basic principles and applications. *Br J Clin Pharm*. 2004;57:6–14.
32. Thompson ABR. Gastro-esophageal reflux in the elderly. Role of drug therapy in management. *Drugs Aging*. 2001;18:409–414.
33. Guyton AC, Hall JE. *Textbook of Medical Physiology*. 10th ed. Philadelphia, PA: Saunders; 2000.
34. Phillips PA, Rolls BJ, Ledingham JG, et al. Reduced thirst after water deprivation in healthy elderly men. *N Engl J Med*. 1984;311:753–759.
35. Doherty TJ. Invited review: aging and sarcopenia. *J Appl Physiol*. 2003;95:1717–1727.
36. Gold MI, Abello D, Herrington C. Minimum alveolar concentration of desflurane in patients older than 65yr. *Anesthesiology*. 1993;79:710–714.
37. Steinmetz J, Christensen KB, Lund T, et al; ISPOCD Group. Long-term consequences of postoperative cognitive dysfunction. *Anesthesiology*. 2009;110(3):548–555.
38. Moller JT, Cluitmans P, Rasmussen LS, et al. Long-term postoperative cognitive dysfunction in the elderly ISPOCD1 study. *Lancet*. 1998;351(9106):857–861.
39. Mason SE, Noel-Storr A, Ritchie CW. The impact of general and regional anesthesia on the incidence of post-operative cognitive dysfunction and post-operative delirium: a systematic review with meta-analysis. *J Alzheimers Dis*. 2010;22(suppl 3):67–79.
40. Riedel B, Browne K, Silbert B. Cerebral protection: inflammation, endothelial dysfunction, and postoperative cognitive dysfunction. *Curr Opin Anaesthesiol*. 2014;27(1):89–97.
41. Helme RD, Gibson SJ. The epidemiology of pain in elderly people. *Clin Geriatr Med*. 2001;17:417–431.

42. Verhaak PF, Kerssens JJ, Dekker J, et al. Prevalence of chronic benign pain disorder among adults: a review of the literature. *Pain*. 1998;77:231–239.
43. Edwards RR, Fillingim RB. Age-associated differences in responses to noxious stimuli. *J Gerontol A Biol Sci Med Sci*. 2001;56(3): M180–M185.
44. Edwards RR, Fillingim RB, Ness TJ. Age-related differences in endogenous pain modulation: a comparison of diffuse noxious inhibitory controls in healthy older and younger adults. *Pain*. 2003;101(1–2):155–165.
45. Zheng Z, Gibson SJ, Khalil Z, et al. Age-related differences in the time course of capsaicin-induced hyperalgesia. *Pain*. 2000;85: 51–58.
46. Chakour MC, Gibson SJ, Bradbeer M, et al. The effect of age on A delta- and C-fibre thermal pain perception. *Pain*. 1996;64: 143–152.
47. Scott JC, Ponganis KV, Stanski DR. EEG quantitation of narcotic effect: the comparative pharmacodynamics of fentanyl and alfentanil. *Anesthesiology*. 1985;62:234–241.
48. Scott JC, Stanski DR. Decreased fentanyl/alfentanil dose requirement with increasing age: a pharmacodynamic basis. *J Pharmacol Exp Ther*. 1987;240:159–166.
49. Matteo RS, Schwartz AE, Ornstein E, et al. Pharmacokinetics of sufentanil in the elderly surgical patient. *Can J Anaesth*. 1990;37: 852–856.
50. Minto CF, Schnider TW, Shafer SL. The influence of age and gender on the pharmacokinetics and pharmacodynamics of remifentanil. II. Model application. *Anesthesiology*. 1997;86:24–33.
51. Portenoy RK, Foley KM, Stulman J, et al. Plasma morphine and morphine-6-glucuronide during chronic morphine therapy for cancer pain: plasma profiles, steady-state concentrations and the consequences of renal failure. *Pain*. 1991;47:13–19.
52. Holmberg L, Odar-Cederlof I, Boreus LO, et al. Comparative disposition of pethidine and norpethidine in old and young patients. *Eur J Clin Pharmacol*. 1982;22:175–179.
53. Odar-Cederlöf I, Boréus LO, Bondesson U, et al. Comparison of renal excretion of pethidine (meperidine) and its metabolites in old and young patients. *Eur J Clin Pharmacol*. 1985;28(2):171–175.

CHAPTER 47

Physiology and Pharmacology of Resuscitation

Michael J. Murray

The term ***resuscitation*** for many people means resuscitation from cardiac arrest, so much so that the term ***cardiopulmonary resuscitation*** and its acronym "CPR" is widely used not only by health care professionals but by laypeople as well. This is understandable as cardiovascular disease is the number one cause of death in the United States, and in 2010, it is estimated that 746,000 Americans died of cardiovascular disease.[1] Unfortunately, the first manifestation of cardiovascular disease is often sudden death due to ventricular tachycardia, ventricular fibrillation, or asystole. In order to improve outcome from cardiac arrest, the American College of Cardiology, American Heart Association, and many other organizations have joined together to educate health care professionals and laypeople on how to resuscitate patients who have had a cardiac arrest by promoting the American Heart Association's Basic Life Support and Advanced Cardiac Life Support courses.

However, resuscitation is also applied to resuscitation from other near-death events. Death from traumatic injury is the third leading cause of death overall in the United States and the primary cause of death in individuals younger than the age of 45 years.[2] These individuals most often die because of hemorrhage. As such, the American College of Surgeons Committee on Trauma has developed the Advanced Trauma Life Support course to standardize proven treatment and improve the outcome of patients who have sustained traumatic injury.

For the neonatologist, resuscitation might bring to mind the resuscitation of neonates whose cardiorespiratory function is depressed at birth.[3] Primary and secondary apnea is the most common etiology of the need for resuscitation of the neonate and the most common antecedent of cardiac arrest (see Chapter 44, Physiology of the Newborn). In adults, respiratory arrest can precede cardiac arrest and vice versa. If either is not recognized in a timely manner and treated effectively, one will but quickly precipitate the other.

Common to all these scenarios and the actual mechanism by which patients die is inadequate oxygen delivery to tissues. Oxygen delivery is defined as:

$$\dot{D}o_2 = CO \times Cao_2$$

where $\dot{D}o_2$ is equal to oxygen delivery, CO represents cardiac output, and Cao_2 is the O_2 content of arterial blood.

In a 70-kg person, oxygen delivery is assumed to be 1 L per minute, derived by multiplying cardiac output (5 L per minute) times arterial oxygen content (200 mL O_2/L). Arterial oxygen content can be calculated by multiplying 15 g hemoglobin/dL (or 150g/L) times 1.39 (the amount of oxygen each gram of hemoglobin can hold when fully saturated) times the arterial oxygen saturation. For this calculation, we are assuming a hemoglobin oxygen saturation of 100%.

From these equations, one can gain insight into the three mechanisms from which death might occur from cardiac and brain ischemia if the patient is not resuscitated in a timely and effective fashion. (a) During ventricular tachycardia, ventricular fibrillation, or during asystole, cardiac output decreases to zero as will oxygen delivery to the tissues. (b) During hemorrhagic shock, as hemoglobin levels decrease, the arterial oxygen content decreases and cardiac output falls because of decreased intravascular volume resulting in decreased left ventricular end diastolic volume. (c) During apnea from whatever cause, as whatever oxygen is contained in the functional residual capacity of the lung decreases, the amount of oxygen available to bind with hemoglobin decreases, which also results in a steadily decreasing oxygen delivery and eventually, cell death.

For the purposes of this chapter then, the focus will be on resuscitation from cardiac events, traumatic injury, and decreased fractional inspired concentration of oxygen (F_IO_2).

Pathophysiology

The basic physiology of death due to decreased oxygen delivery is in some ways straightforward but at the same time, quite complex. As oxygenated hemoglobin is delivered to peripheral tissues, O_2 dissociates from hemoglobin because of the concentration gradient between the oxygenated hemoglobin in red blood cells and the capillary blood perfusing the tissue. The dissociation of O_2 from hemoglobin is facilitated by the respiratory acidosis created by CO_2 released through cellular respiration. Oxygen diffuses out of red blood cells through the plasma, across cell membranes, and into the cytoplasm where it is taken up by mitochondria. In oxidative metabolism, O_2 breaks down pyruvate, derived from glucose, amino acids, and fatty acids in the Krebs cycle. Water and CO_2 are the byproducts and the energy produced is used by the coenzymes nicotinamide, adenine, dinucleotide, and flavin adenine dinucleotide to add a phosphate molecule to adenosine diphosphate to create adenosine triphosphate (ATP). The third phosphate bond is readily broken and the energy that is released is used by cells for protein synthesis, for endocytosis and exocytosis, to provide energy for other transporter processes, for maintenance of the electrical potential across the membrane, and to maintain the integrity of the cell membrane itself. Oxygen is the molecule that serves as the electron acceptor by which nicotinamide adenine dinucleotide and flavin adenine dinucleotide produce more ATP than can be created by anaerobic metabolism. Based strictly on the byproducts of the chemical reactions involved, anaerobic metabolism of pyruvate leads to the production of 4 molecules of ATP, whereas the metabolism of pyruvate in the presence of O_2 can potentially produce 38 molecules of ATP. Anaerobic metabolism is insufficient in the long term to produce enough ATP molecules to maintain cell integrity. In the absence of oxygen, cells die (Fig. 47-1) at a variable rate depending on their metabolic rate. Typically, neurons are the most sensitive to lack of O_2 and will develop irreversible damage within 3 to 5 minutes; myocytes and hepatocytes on the other hand can survive 1 to 2 hours in the absence of O_2; muscle cells may survive for several hours. By decreasing metabolic rate, hypothermia can prolong the "safe" ischemic time. Neurons for example decrease their metabolic rate by approximately 7% for every 1°C decrease in temperature.[4] There is a limit, however, to how much hypothermia can delay a cell's demise. For example, during circulatory arrest while a patient is on cardiopulmonary bypass, at 15°C to 20°C, neurons do not display

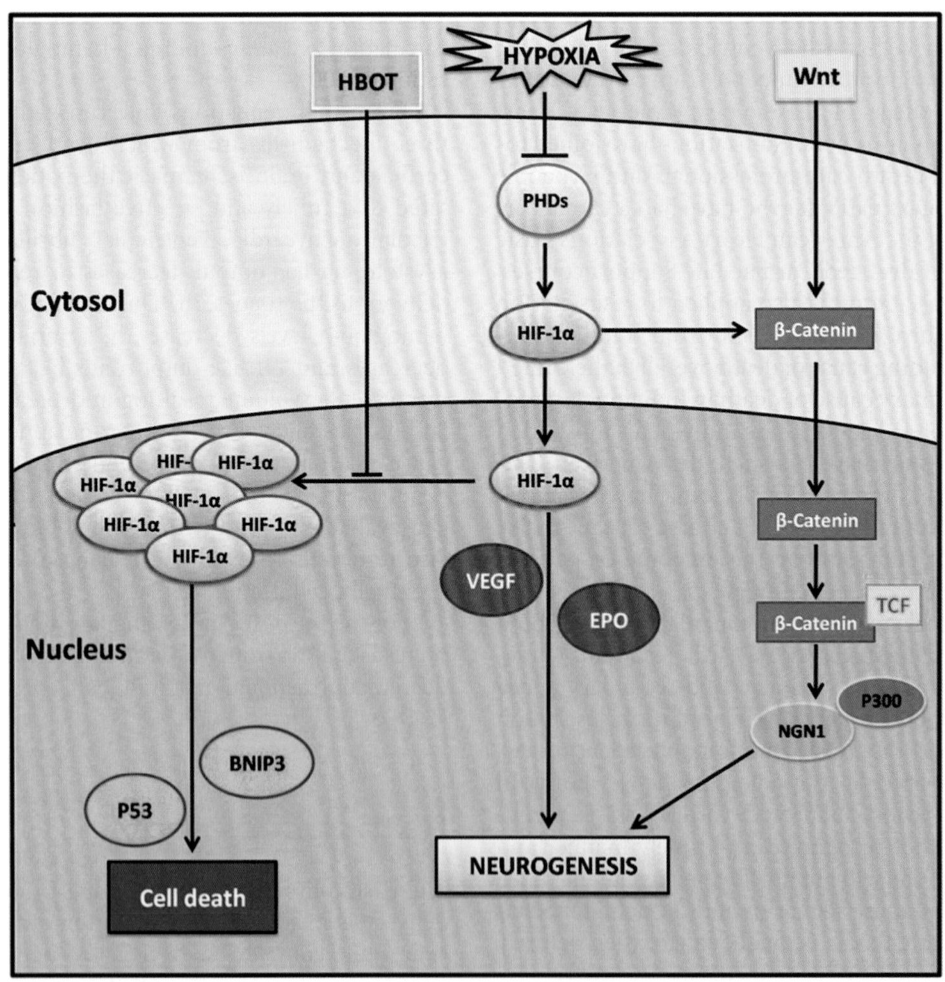

FIGURE 47-1 Physiological pathways underlining hypoxic cellular responses in the brain.

irreversible cell damage for as long as 30 to 60 minutes, but after 60 minutes, the risk for potential irreversible neuronal damage increases markedly. Hypothermia has the same effect on other cells such as myocytes and hepatocytes, as well as cells in other organs. This factor allows transplant surgeons to prolong the amount of time between when an organ is harvested and when it is transplanted, thus improving the matching potential for transplantable organs.

Although temperature has an impact on survivability of ischemic cells, time is the factor that most directly and importantly impacts the reversibility of ischemia—the safe ischemic time. Independent of all other factors, the number of minutes that cardiac function is arrested, the amount of time that the hemoglobin concentration is below 6 to 7 g/dL, or the duration of apnea or asphyxia all directly correlate with morbidity and mortality. For cardiac arrest, evidence from assessment of the effect of duration of the arrest on survivability suggests that mortality increases by 8% to 10% for each minute for which there is no cardiac output.[5] From a physiologic perspective, the most vital factor then in determining outcome is the timely restoration of normal cardiac, pulmonary, and hemostatic function. Drugs play a limited, but very important, role in the return of the aforementioned functions in certain circumstances as will be described later.

Cardiac Arrest

The National Library of Medicine in its MeSH (Medical Subject Headings) terms defines "heart arrest" as the cessation of effective cardiac function, which if not recognized and treated within minutes will lead to "sudden cardiac death." Sudden cardiac death in turn is the unexpected rapid natural death due to cardiovascular collapse within 1 hour of the onset of symptoms usually caused by the worsening of existing heart disease.

Ventricular tachyarrhythmias account for many cardiac arrests; 6% to 14% of the time, no known structural lesions of the heart can be identified.[6] If no structural cause can be identified, individuals who have a prolonged QT interval are at increased risk of developing polymorphic ventricular tachycardia, that is, *torsades de pointes* especially if they receive certain drugs that are also known to prolong the QT. Mutations in genes that code for ion channels that generate the cardiac action potential have been identified in patients with the long QT syndrome.[7,8] There are more than 150 drugs that have been reported to prolong the QT interval; list the drugs that are most relevant to anesthesiologists. Drugs that prolong the QT interval are thought to do so by modifying the activity of the same ion channels responsible for the long QT syndrome. The effects of the different drugs range from mild to severe with the latter having the greatest probability of precipitating *torsades de pointes*.[9] The ability of a drug to precipitate a malignant tachyarrhythmia is related not just to the drug itself but also to the dose, to drug interactions, to genetic factors, to the gender of the patient, and to the type and severity of preexisting cardiac disease.

Ventricular fibrillation is the cause for most of the other instances of sudden cardiac arrest with a relatively small proportion of people developing asystole as the initial manifestation of sudden cardiac arrest. The true incidence of the precipitating arrhythmia is not known because most sudden cardiac arrests occur out of hospital and typically, several minutes pass before the rhythm can be assessed. The cardiac diseases that lead to the genesis of ventricular fibrillation resulting in cardiac collapse are varied, and the association with sudden death in some cases is not well understood. Similar to patients who have cardiovascular collapse from ventricular tachyarrhythmias, there are patients who develop ventricular fibrillation who do not have identifiable structural heart disease. There is a correlation between what is normally considered to be benign, early repolarization (defined as an elevation of the QRS–ST segment of at least 0.1 mV in the inferior or lateral leads on the electrocardiogram) and the development of ventricular fibrillation.[10,11] As such, early repolarization may be a sign of electrochemical imbalance within the myocardium.

Independent of the etiology of the cardiac collapse, for resuscitation to be successful, CPR must be initiated as soon as possible. Weisfeldt and Becker[12] have proposed a three-phase model of resuscitation: the electrical phase, the circulatory phase, and the metabolic phase. The electrical phase begins with the cardiac collapse and lasts for approximately 4 minutes; the circulatory phase represents an approximation of 6 minutes window from 4 to 10 minutes; and the metabolic window which commences at approximately 10 minutes. The best outcomes are achieved if the heart is defibrillated within the first 4 minutes after the cardiac arrest, during the electrical phase. This observation has been borne out by studies of patients who have an implantable cardioverter defibrillator. One meta-analysis of three large such studies that compared the administration of amiodarone to implantation of an implantable cardioverter defibrillator demonstrated decreased arrhythmias and improved survivability in patients who had an internal defibrillator.[13] In a canine model, Yakaitis and colleagues[14] demonstrated that for defibrillation *per se* to be successful, the electroshock had to be delivered within 3 minutes of the onset of ventricular fibrillation. Once the circulatory phase has begun, the most important intervention to achieve the return of spontaneous circulation (ROSC) is to commence chest compressions that will deliver some oxygenated blood to tissues. Another animal study showed that once the circulatory phase has begun, a threefold improvement in results is obtained if chest compressions are performed first, along with the administration of epinephrine and then defibrillation attempted compared to performing the defibrillation first and then performing chest compressions.[15]

Once the patient transitions into the metabolic phase, the chances of ROSC and more importantly, the chances of a full neurologic recovery are quite low—neither immediate countershock nor chest compressions followed by countershock are associated with good outcomes. Investigators have speculated that even with ROSC, 10 minutes or more of global ischemia induces cells to release cytotoxins,[16] and bacteria are more able to translocate across the intestinal endothelial barrier.[17] Cytotoxins and endotoxin may further injure an already damaged heart, and worse, may disrupt mechanisms maintaining cellular integrity.[18] As circulation returns, the hyperoxia that is often present will exacerbate the reperfusion syndrome and has been associated with increased mortality.[19]

In those patients with ROSC, the enthusiasm clinicians had for the ability of hypothermia to attenuate the neurologic injury that many of these patients developed has been tempered by a more recent well-performed study that did not demonstrate an improvement in neurologic outcome with hypothermia (33°C vs. 36°C).[20]

Once patients enter the metabolic phase after 10 minutes of untreated cardiac arrest, the chances of meaningful recovery are slim. Improvement in outcome in patients who do have ROSC will require development of therapies to attenuate the ischemia-reperfusion syndrome.

Hemorrhagic Shock

In patients who sustain traumatic injury, hemorrhage accounts for 30% to 40% of the deaths. Of these, a majority occur before the patients arrive at a hospital. Among traumatized patients who arrive at the hospital, mortality in the first several hours correlates with inadequate resuscitation and the presence of coagulopathy.[21] During the recent combat experiences in Iraq and Afghanistan, particularly during the later years of the combat in Afghanistan when dismounted complex blast injury was recognized, there was a strong correlation between the degree of hemorrhage, the severity of the injury, and the overall mortality.[22] However, service members who were alive upon arrival at a level III medical facility had a greater than 95% chance of survival. These results were obtained because of the military's emphasis on controlling hemorrhage at the point of injury, recognition and treatment of acute traumatic coagulopathy (ATC), and the use of damage control surgery. In both civilians and wounded warriors, it is impossible to quantify the amount of blood that is lost from the intravascular circulation, but an estimate can be made from the amount of blood transfused, the degree of lactic acidosis, and the alterations and vital signs. In an observational study of patients who refused blood transfusions because of religious beliefs, there was no 30-day mortality among patients whose hemoglobin was greater than 7.1 g/dL. However, as the hemoglobin level decreased below 6 g/dL, mortality increased significantly.[23]

Although the volume of blood lost cannot be accurately measured, the number of units of blood given and changes in coagulation factors are readily recorded and analyzed. Improvements in early hemorrhage control and resuscitation and the prevention and aggressive treatment of coagulopathy appear to have the greatest potential to improve outcomes in severely injured trauma patients. A cascade of life-threatening medical problems can begin with severe hemorrhage, and many of these occur simultaneously: (a) hemorrhage, (b) impaired resuscitation, (c) shock, (d) inflammation, and (e) coagulopathy. The severity of each problem is commonly associated with the extent of overall blood loss. Low blood pressure due to blood loss indicates immediate complications, including the incidence of multiple organ failure and life-threatening infections.

Respiratory Arrest

Respiratory and cardiac arrest are distinct, but if untreated, one inevitably leads to the other. There are a multitude of etiologies of respiratory arrest, and respiratory arrest per se implies any process that inhibits the delivery of sufficient oxygen to the mitochondria to maintain aerobic metabolism. The respiratory centers in the brainstem can be injured by penetrating injury and by increased intracranial pressure due to infection or intraventricular hemorrhage. Even blunt trauma to the head of sufficient force can produce a similar result. Atkinson et al.,[24] using a mechanical blow to the head, demonstrated in a rodent model that as the force of the blow incrementally increased, there came a point that the animal became completely apneic. There are a number of drugs that can depress the respiratory centers, most notably opioids, sedatives, and hypnotics. These drugs can suppress ventilation or induce complete apnea even at low doses in patients with central sleep apnea,[25] in patients with chronic obstructive pulmonary disease (COPD) and hypercarbia, and in geriatric patients with comorbid conditions. Although it is true that opioids suppress ventilation, some have used this relationship to justify withholding opioids from patients with severe COPD at the end of their lives.[26] One study of over 2,000 patients with severe COPD found that there was a correlation between the dose of opioids and mortality at high doses, but at lower doses, the effect was not seen, and yet at lower doses, the patients' dyspnea was atenuated.[27]

Whatever the cause, be it through a central nervous system mechanism, or a peripheral mechanism such as glottic edema from anaphylactic shock, or airway disruption from trauma or a foreign body, death does not occur immediately. The hemoglobin in the circulating blood carries enough O_2 for maintenance of aerobic metabolism for 1 to 3 minutes. In addition, there is O_2 that has already entered the lungs. During normal breathing at end expiration, there is O_2 in the functional residual capacity (FRC) that can be calculated as the F_IO_2 times the volume of air in the FRC which in turn is equal to the person's weight in kilograms times 15 mL/kg. For a 70-kg person, breathing room air the FRC would contain approximately 220 mL of O_2 ([70 kg × 15mL/kg] × .21), enough to meet metabolic demand. At 3 to 4 minutes of complete apnea, evidence of tissue ischemia would become apparent and at longer than 5 minutes, irreversible damage would occur, especially in the brain. Cardiac arrest would soon follow unless oxygenation and ventilation were immediately rapidly restored.

Other causes of hypoxemic death are related to the neuromuscular system. A spinal cord transection above C4 would result in apnea because the phrenic nerves arise from C1 through C4. Likewise, patients with amyotrophic lateral sclerosis in which upper and lower motor neurons in the motor cortex, in the brainstem, and in the spinal cord die over time are unable to maintain respiratory effort. The cause is not understood but genetic factors play a role.[28] Neuromuscular blocking agents produce the same effect albeit more quickly. Any process that decreases the alveolar to arterial O_2 gradient can likewise interfere with the delivery of O_2 to tissues, for example, drowning or acute respiratory distress syndrome. Cyanide poisoning is the most well-known cause of inhibition of O_2 use within mitochondria by inhibiting cytochrome C oxidase. Adequate oxygen is supplied but cannot be used for aerobic metabolism.

All the causes of hypoxemic death discussed so far come about from inhibition or destruction of the body's normal physiologic mechanisms. There are also environmental factors that play a role as well, the most important of which would be any factor that decreases the F_IO_2 would interrupt aerobic metabolism. The best example for anesthesiologists would be a helium quench from a magnetic resonance imaging scanner. If the required safety valves in the room were not working correctly, the helium could displace all the O_2 in the room.

Pharmacology

Cardiopulmonary Resuscitation

The primary goal when resuscitating a patient from cardiac arrest is the ROSC, which is best achieved with effective chest compressions delivered immediately by a bystander, and if the patient has ventricular fibrillation, the delivery of electroshock therapy to defibrillate the heart. However, if these maneuvers are unsuccessful in restoring cardiac function and an advanced practitioner is present, drug therapy has been shown to increase the rate of ROSC. Recommendations for advanced cardiac life support (ACLS) are continually updated and provided by the American Heart Association. Although the drugs currently recommended for ACLS improve the likelihood of ROSC, none has improved long-term outcome.[29]

Epinephrine

Epinephrine is a catecholamine (vasoactive compound with a catechol—benzene ring with two hydroxyl groups

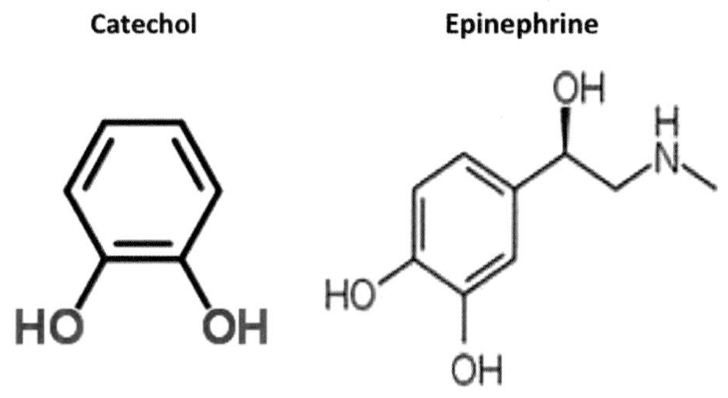

FIGURE 47-2 Molecular structure for the common catechol ring and for epinephrine.

[Fig. 47-2] in its structure). Dopamine is its precursor, and in turn, epinephrine is the precursor for norepinephrine. Chromaffin cells in the adrenal medulla and the terminal boutons of certain nerves produce and release epinephrine, which gains its biologic activity by binding to α- and β-adrenergic receptors. Among its many effects, epinephrine activation of α receptors produces vasoconstriction in the peripheral vasculature, whereas activation of β receptors within the heart increases chronotropy, inotropy, dromotropy, and lusitropy. The majority of epinephrine produced is metabolized within the same cells; it was synthesized simply because there is so much leakage of the catecholamine from the vesicles where it is stored into the cytoplasm. There is a very dynamic equilibrium between vesicular and cytoplasmic epinephrine.[30]

When administered intravenously during a cardiac arrest, epinephrine is thought to increase the ROSC primarily by binding to and activating α-adrenergic receptors.[31] Activation of these receptors on the venules[32] in the periphery increases venous return to the heart, allowing chest compressions to better increase cardiac output. On the arterial side, the vasoconstriction caused by α receptor activation constricts the peripheral arterial system further centralizing the circulation to perfuse vital organs with the highest oxygen requirement. The increase in cardiac output with an increased systemic vascular resistance is hypothesized to improve coronary artery and carotid artery blood flow.[33] By activating β receptors within the heart, epinephrine augments cardiac output even further, with additional benefit to the patient. However, some believe that epinephrine's effect on β receptors is more detrimental than beneficial because of increased metabolic demand.

Epinephrine has been repeatedly demonstrated to improve ROSC when administered to patients in cardiac arrest but without an improvement in overall outcome. Ditchey and Lindenfeld[34] observed that even with an improvement in coronary perfusion pressure in a canine model of cardiac arrest 10 minutes after the administration of epinephrine during chest compression, myocytes had decreased ATP compared to controls and an accompanying lactic acidosis. In a clinical study, Olasveengen and colleagues observed that patients arriving at the hospital following a cardiac arrest who had received epinephrine as part of their CPR regimen had no improvement in tissue perfusion nor was there any difference in long-term survival compared to case-matched controls.[35] Other studies, one in rodents[36] and one in patients,[37] demonstrated decreased survival in subjects who had received epinephrine following cardiac arrest that was treated with CPR. The difficulty with interpreting clinical studies is that patients who receive epinephrine are more likely to have had a longer period without cardiac activity and therefore greater duration of CPR—and therefore less likely to have a good outcome no matter the intervention.

If the effects of epinephrine are attributed to its effect on α-adrenergic receptors, then drugs with even more α receptor specificity might be indicated. However, studies of epinephrine compared to either norepinephrine[38] or phenylephrine[39] during cardiac arrest with CPR showed no benefit to the more α receptor–specific drugs. If it is vasoconstriction that explains the better ROSC of epinephrine but its β receptor properties that offset the benefit, then perhaps the administration of a drug such as vasopressin that works through a different mechanism than does epinephrine might result in better outcomes. However, a study comparing vasopressin to epinephrine for out-of-hospital CPR following cardiac arrest found no difference in outcomes between the two drugs.[40]

The most recent guidelines of the American Heart Association recommend 1 mg of epinephrine administered intravenously or by the intraosseous injection every 3 to 5 minutes with recognition of the fact that although there may be ROSC, there are no prospective randomized controlled trials that demonstrate an improvement in outcome.

Vasopressin

Vasopressin (antidiuretic hormone) is an oligopeptide composed of nine amino acids and is a nonapeptide synthesized in the hypothalamus. The axons of the neuronal cells that produce vasopressin extend into the posterior pituitary where it is released.[41] Because there is no blood brain barrier in the capillaries in the posterior pituitary, the vasopressin can be readily released into blood.[42] Vasopressin is released in response to a decrease in mean arterial pressure, a decrease in end diastolic left ventricular pressure, or an increase in plasma osmolality.[43] In the periphery, vasopressin can bind to one of three subtypes of vasopressin receptors, V1, V2, or V3, all of which are transmembrane proteins, but the G proteins to which these receptors are coupled are unique to each receptor.[44] Activation of these receptors results in a number of actions, but most importantly in the kidney, activation of these receptors results in an antidiuretic effect.

When administered intravenously, vasopressin distributes from the plasma into the extracellular fluid rapidly, exerting its effects within just a few minutes. The plasma $t_{1/2}$ is between 4 and 20 minutes. Vasopressin is metabolized in the liver and kidneys, with a small amount excreted unchanged in the urine.[45]

The use of vasopressin to treat sudden cardiac arrest came about from the results of several reports. In one study of patients who had a sudden cardiac arrest in whom vasopressin levels were measured before the initiation of CPR, it was found that the levels were quite high compared to control. Of most interest to investigators was the observation that patients who had ROSC had higher levels of vasopressin in their blood than those patients who were not successfully resuscitated.[46,47] These results served as a stimulus for additional studies. Vasopressin administered during CPR to patients who had had a sudden cardiac arrest improved coronary perfusion pressure, even in some patients whose coronary artery perfusion pressure was unresponsive to epinephrine.[47] In three prospective studies of patients in whom CPR was initiated to treat cardiac arrest, either vasopressin or epinephrine were administered intravenously as the initial pharmacologic intervention. In one study of 40 patients who had had out-of-hospital cardiac arrest and who had continuing ventricular fibrillation despite electric defibrillation, either epinephrine (1 mg) or vasopressin (40 units) were administered intravenously. Significantly more patients who received vasopressin had ROSC and significantly more patients were alive at 24 hours.[48] In a second larger study of 200 hospitalized patients who were administered either epinephrine (1 mg) or vasopressin (40 units) intravenously during CPR for cardiac arrest, there were no differences in the ROSC.[49] In a third even larger study, vasopressin compared to epinephrine for the treatment of out-of-hospital cardiac arrest in over 1,000 patients, there was no significant difference between vasopressin and epinephrine in ROSC or survival in patients with ventricular tachycardia or pulseless electrical activity but significantly more patients with asystole who received vasopressin had ROSC.[40]

Independent of these findings, the current guidelines of the American Heart Association for ACLS state that vasopressin (40 units) can be administered intravenously or by the intraosseous route to instead or either the first or second dose of epinephrine.

Amiodarone

Electric defibrillation is first-line treatment for ventricular fibrillation. Amiodarone is the second pharmacologic treatment (after either epinephrine or vasopressin) in patients who have ventricular fibrillation refractory to electric defibrillation. Administered intravenously at a dose of 300 mg[50] or 5 mg/kg,[51] amiodarone compared to lidocaine has been shown to be superior for ROSC in patients with ventricular fibrillation refractory to electric defibrillation. However, no study has yet demonstrated that long-term outcome in terms of morbidity or mortality is improved. The American Heart Association has recommended amiodarone to treat refractory ventricular fibrillation or pulseless ventricular tachycardia.[52]

Following intravenous administration, amiodarone enters the central compartment and from there it undergoes extensive tissue redistribution. The distribution half-life of amiodarone from the central compartment (t1/2α) may be as short as 4 hours. The terminal half-life (t1/2β) is lengthy and also variable (9 to 77 days) because of prolonged release of amiodarone out of adipocytes due to the lipophilicity of the drug.[53,54]

Hemodynamic effects of orally administered amiodarone are usually negligible. When administered as an intravenous bolus, there have been reports of hypotension that was thought due to the vasoactive solvents (polysorbate and benzyl alcohol) in which it was compounded. When administered with a different diluent, rapid administration of amiodarone intravenously is not associated with hypotension.[55]

Effects on the thyroid gland and the liver are of more significance.[56,57] The similarity between the chemical structures of amiodarone and thyroid hormone explain the former, and the latter is most likely due to direct injury to lipid bilayers of the hepatocyte cell membrane and inhibition of lysosomal function.[58] However, these adverse effects are only seen in patients taking the drug in high dose for extended periods of time, not in patients who are administered one or two doses of the drug during sudden cardiac arrest.

Hemorrhage

The most critical intervention in hemorrhage is to stop the bleeding—either by applying a tourniquet in the field to an extremity or if there is massive internal bleeding from a crush injury or ruptured aortic aneurysm—by transporting the patient as quickly as possible to a level I trauma hospital and from the emergency department directly to the operating room. The importance of surgical intervention as quickly as possible was underscored by Maddox and colleagues in a study of patients who were transported by emergency medical personnel randomized to the (at the time) conventional therapy of placing an intravenous cannula and initiating the infusion of crystalloid during transport to the hospital or to essentially no therapy, the "scoop and run" approach. Emergency personnel evaluated the patient, treated the ABCs (airway, breathing, and circulation), and then placed the patient in the ambulance with immediate transport back to the hospital. The latter group not only received less crystalloid but had better survival than the conventionally treated group.[59]

Other components of damage control resuscitation include maintaining normothermia, limiting intravenous crystalloid, using a hemoglobin target of 7 to 8 g/dL, and identifying patients at risk of developing ATC. As with resuscitation from cardiac arrest, there is a limited role for drugs in improving outcome in patients who sustained traumatic injury with possibly one exception. In the CRASH-2 trial, such patients were randomized to a tranexamic acid group or control. The group that received tranexamic acid within an hour of admission had a small reduction in mortality (1.6% in all comers—a recent subgroup analysis suggested 2.5%). Beyond 3 hours, there appeared to be an increase in mortality.[60]

Tranexamic Acid

Tranexamic acid, a synthetic analog of the amino acid lysine, is an antifibrinolytic that has found widespread use following the removal of aprotinin from the market. By binding to specific sites on plasminogen and plasmin, it inhibits the transformation of plasminogen to plasmin. Circulating plasmin degrades fibrin, an integral part of blood clots. The role of tranexamic acid in managing patients with traumatic injury has not yet been determined, but there are a number of level I trauma centers in the United States who administer it routinely to their patients. It is also commonly used in massive hemorrhage during cancer surgery, removal of invasive placenta, and major orthopedic surgery.

Oxygenation/Ventilation

In patients with pulmonary failure or respiratory arrest, immediate assisted ventilation and oxygenation is the intervention most likely to increase the chances of survival. There are no drugs that have been demonstrated in large prospective randomized trials to improve the chances of successful resuscitation in this setting. Respiratory arrest due to specific drug overdose is an exception. Respiratory arrest secondary to an opioid is reversed with naloxone. Less commonly, for respiratory arrest secondary to or contributed to by benzodiazepine overdose, flumazenil antagonizes the drug effects. Likewise, for patients with cyanide toxicity and respiratory arrest at the cellular level, sodium thiosulfate is indicated.

As stated at the onset, resuscitation is simple in some ways. In patients with cardiac arrest, defibrillation in the first 3 minutes and CPR/defibrillation during the next 5 to 7 minutes achieves the best results. In patients with profound hemorrhage, immediate control of bleeding and infusion of red blood cells has the biggest impact on outcome. In patients with pulmonary or respiratory arrest, immediate assisted ventilation and oxygenation is the most likely intervention to increase the chances of survival. The difficulty is in the absence of therapies that can preserve tissue integrity until an energy source can be reestablished.

References

1. Go AS, Mozaffarian D, Roger VL, et al. Heart disease and stroke statistics—2013 update: a report from the American Heart Association. *Circulation.* 2013;127(1):e6–e245.
2. Murphy SL, Kochanek KD. *Deaths: Final Data for 2010.* Vol 61. Hyattsville, MD: National Center for Health Statistics; 2013.

3. Finer NN, Rich W, Wang C, et al. Airway obstruction during mask ventilation of very low birth weight infants during neonatal resuscitation. *Pediatrics*. 2009;123(3):865–869.
4. Mrozek S, Vardon F, Geeraerts T. Brain temperature: physiology and pathophysiology after brain injury. *Anesthesiol Res Pract*. 2012;2012:989487.
5. Valenzuela TD, Roe DJ, Cretin S, et al. Estimating effectiveness of cardiac arrest interventions: a logistic regression survival model. *Circulation*. 1997;96(10):3308–3313.
6. Cobb LA, Fahrenbruch CE, Olsufka M, et al. Changing incidence of out-of-hospital ventricular fibrillation, 1980–2000. *JAMA*. 2002; 288(23):3008–3013.
7. Newton-Cheh C, Guo CY, Larson MG, et al. Common genetic variation in KCNH2 is associated with QT interval duration: the Framingham Heart Study. *Circulation*. 2007;116(10):1128–1136.
8. Splawski I, Timothy KW, Tateyama M, et al. Variant of SCN5A sodium channel implicated in risk of cardiac arrhythmia. *Science*. 2002;297(5585):1333–1336.
9. Heist EK, Ruskin JN. Drug-induced arrhythmia. *Circulation*. 2010; 122(14):1426–1435.
10. Haissaguerre M, Derval N, Sacher F, et al. Sudden cardiac arrest associated with early repolarization. *N Engl J Med*. 2008;358(19): 2016–2023.
11. Kim SH, Kim do Y, Kim HJ, et al. Early repolarization with horizontal ST segment may be associated with aborted sudden cardiac arrest: a retrospective case control study. *BMC Cardiovasc Disord*. 2012;12:122.
12. Weisfeldt ML, Becker LB. Resuscitation after cardiac arrest: a 3-phase time-sensitive model. *JAMA*. 2002;288(23):3035–3038.
13. Connolly SJ, Hallstrom AP, Cappato R, et al. Meta-analysis of the implantable cardioverter defibrillator secondary prevention trials. *Eur Heart J*. 2000;21(24):2071–2078.
14. Yakaitis RW, Ewy GA, Otto CW, et al. Influence of time and therapy on ventricular defibrillation in dogs. *Crit Care Med*. 1980;8(3): 157–163.
15. Niemann JT, Cairns CB, Sharma J, et al. Treatment of prolonged ventricular fibrillation. Immediate countershock versus high-dose epinephrine and CPR preceding countershock. *Circulation*. 1992; 85(1):281–287.
16. White BC, Grossman LI, Krause GS. Brain injury by global ischemia and reperfusion: a theoretical perspective on membrane damage and repair. *Neurology*. 1993;43(9):1656–1665.
17. Cerchiari EL, Safar P, Klein E, et al. Visceral, hematologic and bacteriologic changes and neurologic outcome after cardiac arrest in dogs. The visceral post-resuscitation syndrome. *Resuscitation*. 1993;25(2):119–136.
18. Adrie C, Laurent I, Monchi M, et al. Postresuscitation disease after cardiac arrest: a sepsis-like syndrome? *Curr Opin Crit Care*. 2004;10(3):208–212.
19. Kilgannon JH, Jones AE, Shapiro NI, et al. Association between arterial hyperoxia following resuscitation from cardiac arrest and in-hospital mortality. *JAMA*. 2010;303(21):2165–2171.
20. Nielsen N, Wetterslev J, Cronberg T, et al. Targeted temperature management at 33°C versus 36°C after cardiac arrest. *N Engl J Med*. 2013;369(23):2197–2206.
21. Kauvar DS, Lefering R, Wade CE. Impact of hemorrhage on trauma outcome: an overview of epidemiology, clinical presentations, and therapeutic considerations. J *Trauma*. 2006;60(6)(suppl):S3–S11.
22. Andersen RC, Fleming M, Forsberg JA, et al. Dismounted complex blast injury. *J Surg Orthop Adv*. 2012;21(1):2–7.
23. Carson JL, Noveck H, Berlin JA, et al. Mortality and morbidity in patients with very low postoperative Hb levels who decline blood transfusion. *Transfusion*. 2002;42(7):812–818.
24. Atkinson JL, Anderson RE, Murray MJ. The early critical phase of severe head injury: importance of apnea and dysfunctional respiration. *J Trauma*. 1998;45(5):941–945.
25. Mogri M, Khan MI, Grant BJ, et al. Central sleep apnea induced by acute ingestion of opioids. *Chest*. 2008;133(6):1484–1488.
26. Goodridge D, Lawson J, Rocker G, et al. Factors associated with opioid dispensation for patients with COPD and lung cancer in the last year of life: a retrospective analysis. *Int J Chron Obstruct Pulmon Dis*. 2010;5:99–105.
27. Ekstrom MP, Bornefalk-Hermansson A, Abernethy AP, et al. Safety of benzodiazepines and opioids in very severe respiratory disease: national prospective study. *BMJ*. 2014;348:g445.
28. Deng HX, Chen W, Hong ST, et al. Mutations in UBQLN2 cause dominant X-linked juvenile and adult-onset ALS and ALS/dementia. *Nature*. 2011;477(7363):211–215.
29. Papastylianou A, Mentzelopoulos S. Current pharmacological advances in the treatment of cardiac arrest. *Emerg Med Int*. 2012; 2012:815857.
30. Eisenhofer G, Kopin IJ, Goldstein DS. Catecholamine metabolism: a contemporary view with implications for physiology and medicine. *Pharmacol Rev*. 2004;56(3):331–349.
31. Yakaitis RW, Otto CW, Blitt CD. Relative importance of alpha and beta adrenergic receptors during resuscitation. *Crit Care Med*. 1979;7(7):293–296.
32. Greenway CV, Lawson AE. The effects of adrenaline and noradrenaline on venous return and regional blood flows in the anaesthetized cat with special reference to intestinal blood flow. *J Physiol*. 1966; 186(3):579–595.
33. Michael JR, Guerci AD, Koehler RC, et al. Mechanisms by which epinephrine augments cerebral and myocardial perfusion during cardiopulmonary resuscitation in dogs. *Circulation*. 1984;69(4): 822–835.
34. Ditchey RV, Lindenfeld J. Failure of epinephrine to improve the balance between myocardial oxygen supply and demand during closed-chest resuscitation in dogs. *Circulation*. 1988;78(2):382–389.
35. Olasveengen TM, Wik L, Sunde K, et al. Outcome when adrenaline (epinephrine) was actually given vs. not given—post hoc analysis of a randomized clinical trial. *Resuscitation*. 2012;83(3):327–332.
36. McCaul CL, McNamara PJ, Engelberts D, et al. Epinephrine increases mortality after brief asphyxial cardiac arrest in an in vivo rat model. *Anesth Analg*. 2006;102(2):542–548.
37. Holmberg M, Holmberg S, Herlitz J. Low chance of survival among patients requiring adrenaline (epinephrine) or intubation after out-of-hospital cardiac arrest in Sweden. *Resuscitation*. 2002;54(1): 37–45.
38. Callaham M, Madsen CD, Barton CW, et al. A randomized clinical trial of high-dose epinephrine and norepinephrine vs standard-dose epinephrine in prehospital cardiac arrest. *JAMA*. 1992;268(19): 2667–2672.
39. Silfvast T, Saarnivaara L, Kinnunen A, et al. Comparison of adrenaline and phenylephrine in out-of-hospital cardiopulmonary resuscitation. A double-blind study. *Acta Anaesthesiol Scand*. 1985;29(6):610–613.
40. Wenzel V, Krismer AC, Arntz HR, et al. A comparison of vasopressin and epinephrine for out-of-hospital cardiopulmonary resuscitation. *N Engl J Med*. 2004;350(2):105–113.
41. Treschan TA, Peters J. The vasopressin system: physiology and clinical strategies. *Anesthesiology*. 2006;105(3):599–612; quiz 639–540.
42. Leng G, Brown CH, Russell JA. Physiological pathways regulating the activity of magnocellular neurosecretory cells. *Prog Neurobiol*. 1999;57(6):625–655.
43. Goldsmith SR. Baroreceptor-mediated suppression of osmotically stimulated vasopressin in normal humans. *J Appl Physiol*. 1988;65(3): 1226–1230.
44. Thibonnier M, Berti-Mattera LN, Dulin N, et al. Signal transduction pathways of the human V1-vascular, V2-renal, V3-pituitary vasopressin and oxytocin receptors. *Prog Brain Res*. 1998;119:147–161.
45. Baumann G, Dingman JF. Distribution, blood transport, and degradation of antidiuretic hormone in man. *J Clin Invest*. 1976;57(5): 1109–1116.
46. Lindner KH, Haak T, Keller A, et al. Release of endogenous vasopressors during and after cardiopulmonary resuscitation. *Heart*. 1996;75(2):145–150.

47. Morris DC, Dereczyk BE, Grzybowski M, et al. Vasopressin can increase coronary perfusion pressure during human cardiopulmonary resuscitation. *Acad Emerg Med.* 1997;4(9):878–883.
48. Lindner KH, Dirks B, Strohmenger HU, et al. Randomised comparison of epinephrine and vasopressin in patients with out-of-hospital ventricular fibrillation. *Lancet.* 1997;349(9051): 535–537.
49. Stiell IG, Hebert PC, Wells GA, et al. Vasopressin versus epinephrine for inhospital cardiac arrest: a randomised controlled trial. *Lancet.* 2001;358(9276):105–109.
50. Kudenchuk PJ, Cobb LA, Copass MK, et al. Amiodarone for resuscitation after out-of-hospital cardiac arrest due to ventricular fibrillation. *N Engl J Med.* 1999;341(12):871–878.
51. Dorian P, Cass D, Schwartz B, et al. Amiodarone as compared with lidocaine for shock-resistant ventricular fibrillation. *N Engl J Med.* 2002;346(12):884–890.
52. Neumar RW, Otto CW, Link MS, et al. Part 8: adult advanced cardiovascular life support: 2010 American Heart Association guidelines for cardiopulmonary resuscitation and emergency cardiovascular care. *Circulation.* 2010;122(18)(suppl 3):S729–767.
53. Freedman MD, Somberg JC. Pharmacology and pharmacokinetics of amiodarone. *J Clin Pharmacol.* 1991;31(11):1061–1069.
54. Chow MS. Intravenous amiodarone: pharmacology, pharmacokinetics, and clinical use. *Ann Pharmacother.* 1996;30(6):637–643.
55. Somberg JC, Timar S, Bailin SJ, et al. Lack of a hypotensive effect with rapid administration of a new aqueous formulation of intravenous amiodarone. *Am J Cardiol.* 2004;93(5):576–581.
56. Narayana SK, Woods DR, Boos CJ. Management of amiodarone-related thyroid problems. *Ther Adv Endocrinol Metab.* 2011;2(3):115–126.
57. Varma RR, Troup PJ, Komorowski RA, et al. Clinical and morphologic effects of amiodarone on the liver. *Gastroenterology.* 1985;88(4):1091–1093.
58. Poucell S, Ireton J, Valencia-Mayoral P, et al. Amiodarone-associated phospholipidosis and fibrosis of the liver. Light, immunohistochemical, and electron microscopic studies. *Gastroenterology.*1984;86(5)(pt 1):926–936.
59. Bickell WH, Wall MJ Jr, Pepe PE, et al. Immediate versus delayed fluid resuscitation for hypotensive patients with penetrating torso injuries. *N Engl J Med.* 1994;331(17):1105–1109.
60. Shakur H, Roberts I, Bautista R, et al; CRASH-2 Trial Collaborators. Effects of tranexamic acid on death, vascular occlusive events, and blood transfusion in trauma patients with significant haemorrhage (CRASH-2): a randomised, placebo-controlled trial. *Lancet.* 2010;376(9734):23–32.

DRUG INDEX

Note: Page numbers followed by *f* indicate figures; page numbers followed by *t* indicate tables.

SUBJECT INDEX

Note: Page numbers followed by *f* indicate figures; page numbers followed by *t* indicate tables.

C

D

E

F

CCS0119